TEXTBOOK OF
DIAGNOSTIC
MICROBIOLOGY

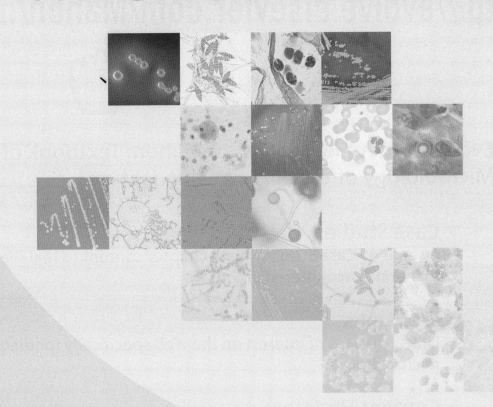

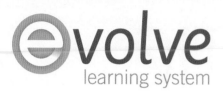
learning system

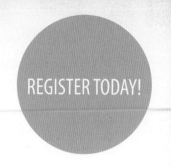
REGISTER TODAY!

To access your Student Resources, visit:

http://evolve.elsevier.com/Mahon/microbiology/

Evolve Student Resources for Mahon: Textbook of Diagnostic Microbiology offers the following features

- ### Case Studies
  A set of 41 Case Studies relate chapter content to real-life scenarios encountered in the lab.

- ### WebLinks
  Links to places of interest on the Web specifically for diagnostic microbiology.

- ### Content Updates
  Find out the latest information on relevant issues in the field of microbiology.

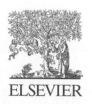
ELSEVIER

TEXTBOOK OF
DIAGNOSTIC
MICROBIOLOGY

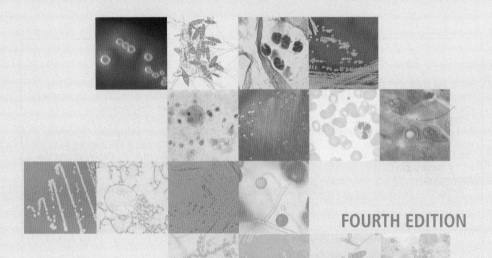

FOURTH EDITION

Connie R. Mahon, MS

Director, Staff College
Center for Veterinary Medicine
Food and Drug Administration
Rockville, Maryland
Adjunct Faculty
Department of Clinical Laboratory Sciences
School of Medicine and Health Sciences
The George Washington University
Washington, D.C.

Donald C. Lehman, EdD, MT(ASCP), SM(NRM)

Associate Professor
Department of Medical Technology
University of Delaware
Newark, Delaware

George Manuselis, MA, MT(ASCP)

Emeritus
Medical Technology Division
The Ohio State University
Columbus, Ohio
Adjunct Faculty
Department of Natural Sciences and Forensic Science
Central Ohio Technical College
Newark, Ohio

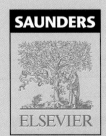

SAUNDERS

ELSEVIER

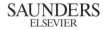

3251 Riverport Lane
Maryland Heights, Missouri 63043

TEXTBOOK OF DIAGNOSTIC MICROBIOLOGY   ISBN: 978-1-4160-6165-6
FOURTH EDITION
Copyright © 2011 by W.B. Saunders Company

Notice

Previous editions copyrighted 2007, 2000, 1995

Library of Congress Cataloging-in-Publication Data

Textbook of diagnostic microbiology / [edited by] Connie R. Mahon, Donald C. Lehman, George Manuselis.—4th ed.
    p. ; cm.
  Includes bibliographical references and index.
  ISBN 978-1-4160-6165-6 (pbk. : alk. paper) 1. Diagnostic microbiology. I. Mahon, Connie R. II. Lehman, Donald C. III. Manuselis, George.
  [DNLM: 1. Microbiological Techniques. 2. Communicable Diseases—diagnosis. 3. Laboratory Techniques and Procedures. QW 25 T355 2011]
  QR67.T49 2011
  616.9′041—dc22

          2009036108

Publishing Director: Andrew Allen
Managing Editor: Ellen Wurm-Cutter
Publishing Services Manager: Patricia Tannian
Senior Project Manager: Sharon Corell
Designer: Teresa McBryan

Working together to grow
libraries in developing countries

www.elsevier.com | www.bookaid.org | www.sabre.org

ELSEVIER   BOOK AID International   Sabre Foundation

Printed in China

Last digit is the print number: 9 8 7 6 5 4 3 2

To my husband, Dan, for his love and continued support
and understanding; my son, Sean, who inspires me; and my daughter,
Kathleen, for showing me courage.

CRM

To my wife, Terri, who has given me constant support and
encouragement and whose love makes anything I do possible;
my parents, Gerald and Sherrie, who have always been proud of me;
even though they have passed away, I know they still look over me.

DCL

To my daughters, Kristina and Shellie; my sisters, Libby and Helen;
my brother Demetrious; and in memory of my parents,
Katherine and George, for their love and encouragement.

GM

Reviewers

Kim Boyd, AAS, BAAS, MS, MLT(ASCP), MT(AMT)
Assistant Professor
Amarillo College
Amarillo, Texas

Russell F. Cheadle, MS, MT(ASCP)
Associate Professor
Program Director of Clinical Laboratory Science
Western Carolina University
Cullowhee, North Carolina

Donna M. Duberg, MA, MS, MT(ASCP)SM, CLS(NCA)
Assistant Professor
Clinical Laboratory Science Department
Saint Louis University
St. Louis, Missouri

Rosemary Duda, MS, MT(ASCP), SM(ASCP)
Director, Medical Technology Program
St. Margaret Hospital
Hammond, Indiana

Rita M. Heuertz, PhD, MT(ASCP)
Associate Professor
Clinical Laboratory Science Department
Internal Medicine Department
Molecular Microbiology and Immunology Department
Saint Louis University
St. Louis, Missouri

Paula C. Mister, MS, MT (ASCP), SM(ASCP)
Educational Coordinator and Clinical Microbiology
    Laboratory Instructor
Microbiology Department
Johns Hopkins Hospital
Instructor, The Community College of Baltimore Country,
    Essex Campus
Baltimore, Maryland
Pathogenic Microbiology Laboratory Instructor
Stevenson University, Stevenson, Maryland

Hamida Nusrat, PhD
Lecturer, Clinical Laboratory Science Internship Program
College of Health and Human Services
San Francisco State University
San Francisco, California

Eric Landon Parnell, M(ASCP)
Regional Medical Laboratories
Battle Creek Health Systems
Adjunct Professor
Kellogg Community College
Medical Laboratory Technology Program
Battle Creek, Michigan

Alisa J. Petree, MHSM, MT(ASCP)
Instructor/Clinical Coordinator
Medical Laboratory Technician Program
McLennan Community College
Waco, Texas

Tania Puro, EdD, CA CLS, MT(ASCP)
Instructor and Laboratory Coordinator
Medical Laboratory Technician and Phlebotomy Program
Hartnell College
Salinas, California
Education Coordinator
Clinical Laboratory Science School
Clinical Laboratory Scientist
Marian Medical Center
Santa Maria, California
Consultant
Clinical Laboratory Science Program
San Francisco State University
San Francisco, California

Anne T. Rodgers, PhD, MT(ASCP)
Professor of Medical Technology (Retired)
Armstrong Atlantic State University
Savannah, Georgia

Perry M. Scanlan, PhD, MT(ASCP)
Assistant Professor
Department of Allied Health Sciences
Austin Peay State University
Clarksville, Tennessee

Jeremy Spinney, MT(ASCP)
Technical Manager
Regional Medical Laboratories, Inc.
Adjunct Faculty
Clinical Microbiology
Kellogg Community College
Battle Creek, Michigan

Maria Lorraine Torres, EdD, MT(ASCP)
Clinical Laboratory Science Program Director
College of Health Sciences
University of Texas at El Paso
El Paso, Texas

K. Nisi Zell, EdD, MT(ASCP), SH, CLS(NCA)
Professor (Retired)
Division of Health Sciences
College of Coastal Georgia
Brunswick, Georgia

Contributors

Wade K. Aldous, PhD
Lieutenant Colonel, Medical Service Corps, United States Army
Chief, Microbiology
Department of Pathology and Area Laboratory Services
Brooke Army Medical Center
Fort Sam Houston, Texas

Leona W. Ayers, MD
Professor
Department of Pathology
School of Allied Medical Sciences
College of Medicine
The Ohio State University
Columbus, Ohio

Carl Brinkley, PhD
Chief, Microbiology
U.S. Army Medical Department Center and School
Fort Sam Houston, Texas

Maximo O. Brito, MD, FACP
Assistant Professor of Medicine
Director
Infectious Diseases Fellowship Training Program
Section of Infectious Diseases
Immunology and International Medicine
University of Illinois at Chicago
Chicago, Illinois

Nina M. Clark, MD
Associate Professor
University of Illinois at Chicago
Director of Transplant Infectious Diseases
University of Illinois Medical Center
Chicago, Illinois

James L. Cook, MD
Chief, Section of Infectious Diseases
Immunology and International Medicine
Professor of Medicine, Microbiology, and Immunology
University of Illinois at Chicago
Chief, Infectious Diseases
University of Illinois Hospital
Jesse Brown Veterans Administration Hospital
Chicago, Illinois

Robert C. Fader, PhD, D(ABMM)
Section Chief, Microbiology/Virology Laboratory
Scott and White Memorial Hospital
Assistant Professor
Department of Pathology
Texas A&M University College of Medicine
Temple, Texas

Maribeth Laude Flaws, PhD, SM(ASCP)SI
Associate Professor
Rush University
Chicago, Illinois

Annette W. Fothergill, MA, MBA, MT(ASCP), CLS(NCA)
Assistant Professor
Department of Pathology
Technical Director, Fungus Testing Lab
University of Texas Health Science Center at San Antonio
San Antonio, Texas

Olarae Giger, PhD
Lecturer, BioScience Technologies Department
Jefferson College of Health Professions
Thomas Jefferson University
Main Line Health Laboratories
Lankenau Hospital
Philadelphia, Pennsylvania

Gerri S. Hall, PhD, D(ABMM), F(AAM)
Section Head, Clinical Microbiology
Medical Director, Bacteriology and Mycobacteriology
Department of Clinical Pathology
Director, PBL Facilitator Recruitment and Development
Cleveland Clinic Lerner College of Medicine
Case Western Reserve University School of Medicine
The Cleveland Clinic
Cleveland, Ohio

Amanda T. Harrington, PhD, D(ABMM)
Assistant Director, Microbiology and Molecular Diagnostics
Department of Pathology and Laboratory Medicine
VA Puget Sound Health Care System
Seattle, Washington

Amy J. Horneman, PhD, SM(ASCP)
Associate Professor
Department of Medical and Research Technology
University of Maryland School of Medicine
Baltimore, Maryland

Michelle M. Jackson, PhD
Microbiologist
U.S. Food and Drug Administration
Center for Drug Evaluation and Research
Silver Spring, Maryland

Deborah Ann Josko, PhD
Associate Professor
University of Medicine and Dentistry of New Jersey
Newark, New Jersey

Preeti Kaur, MD, MPH
Transplant Infectious Disease Fellow
Massachusetts General Hospital
Boston, Massachusetts

Edward F. Keen III, PhD, M(ASCP)
Assistant Chief, Microbiology
Captain, Medical Service Corps, United States Army
Department of Pathology and Area Laboratory Services
Brooke Army Medical Center
Fort Sam Houston, Texas

Jennifer E. Layden, MD, PhD
Section of Infectious Diseases
University of Illinois at Chicago
Chicago, Illinois

Donald C. Lehman, EdD, MT(ASCP), SM(NRM)
Associate Professor
Department of Medical Technology
University of Delaware
Newark, Delaware

Karen S. Long, MS, CLS(NCA), MT(ASCP)
Associate Professor
Medical Technology Program
West Virginia University
Morgantown, West Virginia

Steven D. Mahlen, PhD, D(ABMM)
Medical Director
Microbiology & Immunology Department of Pathology
Madigan Army Medical Center
Tacoma, Washington

Connie R. Mahon, MS, MT(ASCP), CLS
Microbiologist and Senior Education Program Specialist
Staff College
Center for Veterinary Medicine
Food and Drug Administration
Rockville, Maryland
Adjunct Faculty
Department of Clinical Laboratory Sciences
School of Medicine and Health Sciences
The George Washington University
Washington, D.C.

George Manuselis, MA, MT(ASCP)
Emeritus
Medical Technology Division
The Ohio State University
Columbus, Ohio
Adjunct Faculty
Department of Natural Sciences and Forensic Science
Central Ohio Technical College
Newark, Ohio

Patrick McDermott, PhD
Director, Division of Animal & Food Microbiology
Director, National Antimicrobial Resistance Monitoring
   System (NARMS)
U.S. Food & Drug Administration
Center for Veterinary Medicine
Office of Research
Laurel, Maryland

Frederic J. Marsik, PhD, ABMM
Team Leader, Clinical Microbiology
Division of Antiinfective and Ophthalmology Products
Center for Drug Evaluation and Research
U.S. Food and Drug Administration
White Oak Campus
Silver Spring, Maryland

Darlene Miller, DHSc, MPH, SM (ASCP, NRM), CIC
Research Assistant Professor
Department of Ophthalmology
Scientific Director
Abrams Ocular Microbiology Laboratory
Bascom Palmer Eye Institute
Anne Bates Leach Eye Hospital
Miller School of Medicine
University of Miami
Miami, Florida

Sarojini R. Misra, MS, SM(ASCP), SM(AAM)
University of Delaware
Manager, Microbiology, Immunology, Virology
Christiana Care Health Services
Newark, Delaware

Linda S. Monson, MS, MT(ASCP)
Supervisory Microbiologist
Brooke Army Medical Center
Fort Sam Houston, Texas

Sumathi Nambiar, MD, MPH
Division of Antiinfective and Ophthalmology Products
Center for Drug Evaluation and Research
U.S. Food and Drug Administration
Silver Spring, Maryland

William F. Nauschuetz, PhD
Clinical Coordinator for Biopreparedness
U.S. Army Coordinator for the Lab Response Network for
    Bioterrorism
U.S. Army Medical Command
Fort Sam Houston, Texas

Sarah L.L. Pierson, MS
Captain, United States Army
Chief, Endemic Disease Section
1st Area Medical Laboratory
Aberdeen Proving Ground, Maryland

Gail E. Reid, MD
Assistant Professor of Medicine
Division of Infectious Diseases
University of Illinois, Chicago, School of Medicine
Chicago, Illinois

Brian Robinson, CPT, MS, USA
Chief, Immunology
Brooke Army Medical Center
Fort Sam Houston, Texas

Lauren Roberts, MS, MT(ASCP)
Associate Clinical Professor
Clinical Laboratory Science Program
School of Life Sciences
Arizona State University
Tempe, Arizona

Barbara L. Russell, EdD, MT, SH
Associate Professor and Program Director
Program of Clinical Laboratory Science
Department of Biomedical and Radiological Technologies
Medical College of Georgia
Augusta, Georgia

Vanessa Sarda, MD
Fellow
Section of Infectious Disease
University of Illinois at Chicago
Chicago, Illinois

Linda A. Smith, PhD, CLS
Professor and Chair
Graduate Program Director
Department of Clinical Laboratory Sciences
The University of Texas Health Science Center
San Antonio, Texas

Becky B. Stone, MEd, MT(ASCP)
Department of Biomedical and Radiological Technologies
Medical College of Georgia
Augusta, Georgia

Kalavati Suvarna, PhD
Microbiologist
Division of Manufacturing and Product Quality
Office of Compliance
Center for Drug Evaluation and Research
Food and Drug Administration
Rockville, Maryland

David L. Taylor, PhD, ABMM
Infection Control Practitioner
Department of Epidemiology
The Ohio State University Medical Center
Columbus, Ohio

Suzanne Templer, DO
Fellow
University of Illinois at Chicago
Chicago, Illinois

Kimberly E. Walker, PhD, MT(ASCP)
Assistant Professor
Graduate Program Director
Department of Medical and Research Technology
University of Maryland School of Medicine
Baltimore, Maryland

A. Christian Whelen, PhD, (D)ABMM
Chief, State Laboratories Division
Hawaii Department of Health
Honolulu, Hawaii

David G. White, MS, PhD
Director
Office of Research
Center for Veterinary Medicine
U.S. Food and Drug Administration
Laurel, Maryland

Preface

The fourth edition of the *Textbook of Diagnostic Microbiology* has enhanced all the features that have made this textbook user-friendly. We have maintained a tradition of providing a well-designed and -organized textbook.

This edition has been revised and updated and continues to facilitate and enhance learning as well as provide opportunities for critical thinking and problem solving. This edition has been responsive to users' needs and has kept its building-block approach, a characteristic that clinical laboratory science and clinical laboratory technician students, entry-level clinical laboratory practitioners, microbiologists, and educators have found effective. Students and other readers are provided with valuable learning tools to help them sort through the vast amount of information—background theoretical concepts, disease mechanisms, identification schemas, diagnostic characteristics, biochemical reactions, and isolation techniques—to produce clinically relevant results. Because the goal of the *Textbook of Diagnostic Microbiology* is to provide a strong foundation for clinical laboratory science students, entry-level practitioners, and other health care professionals, discussions of organisms are limited to those that are medically important and commonly encountered, as well as new and emerging pathogens.

NEW TO THIS EDITION

Despite significant strides in improving diagnosis and treatment, infectious diseases still have a dramatic effect on human life. Developing global events and new threats that have besieged our lives are reflected in the fourth edition of the *Textbook of Diagnostic Microbiology*: the continuing spread of antimicrobial resistant bacteria, such as community-associated methicillin-resistant *Staphylococcus aureus*, and the perplexing sudden appearance of swine influenza viruses in North America. This edition discusses these emerging public health issues and others.

Whereas the recovery of etiologic agents in cultures has remained the gold standard in microbiology in determining the probable cause of an infectious disease, molecular diagnostic techniques are becoming more important in clinical laboratories. Chapter 11 has been updated to reflect these changes. In addition, a discussion on immunochromatographic assays was added to Chapter 10. New for this edition is a single chapter covering *Chlamydia*, *Rickettsia*, and *Rickettsia*-like bacteria, whereas the *Mycoplasma* and *Ureaplasma* are in a separate chapter. This edition has a new appendix with procedures for commonly performed clinical microbiology tests.

ORGANIZATION

Part I has remained the backbone of the textbook, whereas Part II emphasizes the laboratory identification of etiologic agents. Part I presents basic principles and concepts of diagnostic microbiology, including quality assurance, which provide students with a firm theoretical foundation. Chapters 7 (Microscopic Examination of Infected Materials) and 8 (Use of Colonial Morphology for the Presumptive Identification of Microorganisms) still play vital roles in the textbook. These two chapters help students and practitioners who may have difficulty recognizing bacterial morphology on direct smear preparations, as well as colony morphology on primary culture plates, develop these skills through the use of color photomicrographs of stained direct smears and cultures from clinical samples. These two chapters also illustrate how microscopic and colony morphology of organisms can aid in the initial identification of the bacterial isolate. A summary of the principles of the various biochemical identification methods for gram-negative bacteria is described in Chapter 9. This chapter contains several color photographs to help students understand the principles and interpretations of these important tests.

Part II highlights methods for the identification of clinically significant isolates. Bacterial isolates are presented based on a taxonomic approach. Although diseases caused by the organisms are discussed, the emphasis is on the characteristics and methods used to recover and identify each group of organisms. Numerous tables summarize the major features of organisms, and schematic networks are used to show relationships and differences between similar or closely related species. Chapters devoted to anaerobic bacterial species, medically important fungi, parasites, and viruses affirm the significance of these agents. Chapter 29 describes viral pathogens, including severe acute respiratory syndrome and the highly pathogenic avian influenza virus. Chapter 31 describes an increasingly complex entity—biofilms. Recently it has become evident that microbial biofilms are involved in the pathogenesis of several human diseases.

Part III focuses on the clinical and laboratory diagnoses of infectious diseases at various body sites—the organ system approach. The organ system approach has been the foundation of the *Textbook of Diagnostic Microbiology* and provides an opportunity for students and other readers to "pull things together." In Part III, each chapter begins with the anatomic considerations of the organ system to be discussed and the role of the usual microbiota found at the particular site in the pathogenesis of disease. Before students can recognize the significance of the opportunistic infectious agents they are most likely to encounter, it is important for them to know the usual inhabitants at a body site. The case studies included in the chapters in Part III enhance problem solving and critical thinking skills, and help students apply knowledge acquired in Parts I and II. The case studies describe the clinical and laboratory findings associated with the patients, allowing students opportunities to correlate these observations with possible etiologic agents. In most cases the cause of the illness is not disclosed in the case study; rather it is revealed elsewhere in the chapter to give students time to think the case through.

PEDAGOGICAL FEATURES

This edition of the *Textbook of Diagnostic Microbiology*, as was the case in the previous editions, incorporates the expertise of the contributors along with elements such as full-color photographs and photomicrographs, an engaging and easy-to-follow design, learning assessment questions and answers, opening case scenarios, hands-on procedures, and lists of key terms to strengthen the learning strategy. Each chapter is introduced by a Case in Point. These introductory case studies represent an important pathogen, infectious disease, concept, or principle that is discussed in the chapter text. The Case in Point is used to introduce the learner to the main context discussed in the chapter and is followed by Issues to Consider. These are points that the learners should be thinking about as they read the chapter. Issues to Consider lists the main points of the chapter text in bulleted format.

To reinforce learning, identification tables, flow charts, and featured illustrations have been updated, and new ones have been added. Learning objectives and a list of key terms are also found at the beginning of each chapter. The key terms include abbreviations used in the text; this places abbreviations where students can easily find them. At the end of each chapter, readers will find Points to Remember and Learning Assessment Questions to reinforce comprehension and understanding of important concepts. Points to Remember includes a bulleted list of important concepts that the reader should have learned from reading the chapter.

ANCILLARIES FOR INSTRUCTORS AND STUDENTS

For this edition, we continue offering a variety of instructor ancillaries specifically geared for this book. For instructors, the Evolve website includes a test bank in ExamView containing more than 1200 questions. It also includes an electronic image collection in addition to a laboratory manual in PDF format that can be customized to meet the needs of particular programs. For students, the Evolve website includes case studies to test their knowledge with real-life scenarios, WebLinks, and content updates.

Connie R. Mahon
Donald C. Lehman
George Manuselis

Acknowledgments

We are grateful to all contributing authors, students, and instructors, and to many other individuals who have made significant suggestions and invaluable comments on ways to improve this edition.

Connie R. Mahon
Donald C. Lehman
George Manuselis

Contents

TEXTBOOK OF
DIAGNOSTIC
MICROBIOLOGY

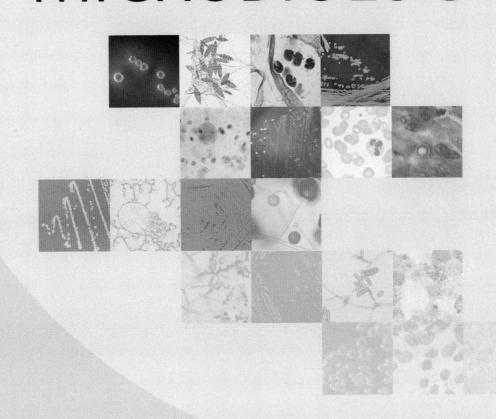

PART I

Introduction to Clinical Microbiology

Bacterial Cell Structure, Physiology, Metabolism, and Genetics

George Manuselis, Connie R. Mahon*

- **SIGNIFICANCE**
- **OVERVIEW OF THE MICROBIAL WORLD**
  Bacteria
  Parasites
  Fungi
  Viruses
- **CLASSIFICATION/TAXONOMY**
  Nomenclature
  Classification by Phenotypic and Genotypic
    Characteristics
  Classification by Cellular Type: Prokaryotes,
    Eukaryotes, and Archaeobacteria
- **COMPARISON OF PROKARYOTIC AND EUKARYOTIC CELL STRUCTURE**
  Prokaryotic Cell Structure
  Eukaryotic Cell Structure
- **BACTERIAL MORPHOLOGY**
  Microscopic Shapes
  Common Stains Used for Microscopic Visualization

- **MICROBIAL GROWTH AND NUTRITION**
  Nutritional Requirements for Growth
  Environmental Factors Influencing Growth
  Bacterial Growth
- **BACTERIAL BIOCHEMISTRY AND METABOLISM**
  Metabolism
  Fermentation and Respiration
  Biochemical Pathways from Glucose to Pyruvic
    Acid
  Anaerobic Utilization of Pyruvic Acid (Fermentation)
  Aerobic Utilization of Pyruvate (Oxidation)
  Carbohydrate Utilization and Lactose Fermentation
- **BACTERIAL GENETICS**
  Anatomy of a DNA and RNA Molecule
  Terminology
  Genetic Elements and Alterations
  Mechanisms of Gene Transfer

OBJECTIVES

After reading and studying this chapter, you should be able to:

1. Describe microbial classification (taxonomy) and accurately apply the rules of scientific nomenclature for bacterial names.

2. List and define five methods used by epidemiologists to subdivide bacterial species.

3. Differentiate between prokaryotic (bacterial and archaeobacteria) and eukaryotic cell types.

4. Compare and contrast prokaryotic and eukaryotic cytoplasmic and cell envelope structures and functions.

5. Describe the cell walls of gram-positive and gram-negative bacteria. Explain the Gram stain reaction of each cell wall type. Describe two other bacterial cell wall types, and give microbial examples of each.

6. Explain the use of the following stains in the diagnostic microbiology laboratory: Gram stain, acid-fast stains (Ziehl-Neelsen, Kinyoun, auramine-rhodamine), acridine orange, methylene blue, calcofluor white, lactophenol cotton blue, and India ink).

7. List the nutritional and environmental requirements for bacterial growth and define the categories of media used for culturing bacteria in the laboratory.

8. Define the atmospheric requirements of obligate aerobes, microaerophiles, facultative anaerobes, obligate anaerobes, and capnophilic bacteria.

9. Describe the stages in the growth of bacterial cells.

10. Describe the importance of microbial metabolism in clinical microbiology.

11. Differentiate between fermentation and oxidation (respiration).

---

*This chapter was prepared by C.R. Mahon in her private capacity. No official support or endorsement by the FDA is intended or implied.

12. Name and compare three biochemical pathways that bacteria use to convert glucose to pyruvate.

13. Identify and compare the two types of fermentation that explain positive results with the methyl red or Voges-Proskauer test.

14. Define the following genetic terms: *genotype, phenotype, constitutive, inducible, replication, transcription, translation, genome, chromosome, plasmids, IS element, transposon, point mutations, frame-shift mutations,* and *recombination.*

15. Discuss the development and transfer of antibiotic resistance in bacteria.

16. Differentiate among the mechanisms of transformation, transduction, and conjugation in the transfer of genetic material from one bacterium to another.

17. Define the terms *bacteriophage, lytic phage, lysogeny,* and *temperate phage.*

18. Define *restriction endonuclease enzyme* and explain the use of such enzymes in the clinical microbiology laboratory.

Case in Point

A 4-year-old girl had the presenting symptoms of redness, burning, and light sensitivity in both eyes. She also complained of her eyelids sticking together because of exudative discharge. A Gram stain of the conjunctival exudates (product of acute inflammation with white blood cells and fluid) showed gram-positive intracellular and extracellular, faint-staining, coccobacillary organisms. The organisms appeared to have small, clear, nonstaining "halos" surrounding each one. This clear area was noted to be between the stained organism and the amorphous (no definite form; shapeless) background material. The Gram stain of the stock staphylococci (gram-positive) *Escherichia coli* (gram negative) showed gram-positive reactions for both organisms on review of the stained quality control organisms.

Issues to Consider

After reading the case study, consider:
- The role of microscopic morphology in identification
- Significance of the clear halo surrounding the organism
- Importance of quality control procedures in the identification process
- Unique characteristics; for example, metabolic and physiologic pathways, and cell structure, which produce infection and disease in hosts

Key Terms

Acid-fast	Differential media
Aerotolerant anaerobes	Dimorphic
Anticodon	Eukarya
Archaea	Eukaryotes
Archaeobacteria	Facultative anaerobes
Autotrophs	Family
Bacteria	Fermentation
Bacteriophage	Fimbriae
Capnophilic	Flagella
Capsule	Fusiform
Codon	Genotype
Competent	Genus
Conjugation	Gram-negative

Gram-positive	Prokaryotes
Heterotrophs	Protein expression
Hyphae	Psychrophiles
Lysogeny	Respiration
Mesophiles	Restriction enzymes
Microaerophilic	Selective media
Minimal medium	Species
Mycelia	Spores
Nutrient media	Strains
Obligate aerobes	Taxa
Obligate anaerobes	Taxonomy
Pathogenic bacteria	Temperate
Phenotype	Thermophiles
Phyla	Transduction
Pili	Transformation
Plasmids	Transport medium
Pleomorphic	

In this chapter the basic concepts of prokaryotic and eukaryotic cells, viral and bacterial cell structure physiology, metabolism, and genetics are reviewed. Common stains used to visualize microorganisms microscopically also are presented. The reader is made aware of the practical importance of each topic to diagnostic microbiologists in their efforts to culture, identify, and characterize the microbes that cause disease in humans. As presented in the opening Case in Point, proper characterization of the bacterial cells in human samples is critical in the correct identification of the infecting organism.

SIGNIFICANCE

Microbial inhabitants have evolved to survive in a variety of ecologic niches (way in which an organism uses its resources) and habitats (organism's location and where its resources may be found). Some grow rapidly, some slowly. Some can replicate with a minimal number of nutrients present, whereas others require enriched nutrients to survive. Variation exists in atmospheric growth conditions, temperature requirements, and cell structure. This diversity is also found in the microorganisms that inhabit the human body as normal biota (normal flora), as opportunistic pathogens, or as true pathogens. Each microbe has its own unique physiology and metabolic pathways that allow it to survive in its particular habitat. One of the main roles of a diagnostic or clinical microbiologist is to isolate, identify, and analyze the bacteria that cause disease in humans. Knowledge of microbial structure and physiology is extremely important to clinical microbiologists in three areas:

- Culture of organisms from patient specimens
- Classification and identification of organisms after they have been isolated
- Prediction and interpretation of antimicrobial susceptibility patterns

Understanding the growth requirements of a particular bacterium enables the microbiologist to select the correct medium for primary culture and optimize the chance of isolating the pathogen. Determination of staining characteristics, based on differences in cell wall structure, is the first step in bacterial classification. Metabolic biochemical differences between organisms form the basis for most bacterial identification systems in use today. The cell structure and biochemical pathways of an organism determine its susceptibility to various antibiotics.

The ability of microorganisms to change rapidly, acquire new genes, and undergo mutations presents continual challenges to diagnostic microbiologists as they isolate and characterize the microorganisms associated with humans.

OVERVIEW OF THE MICROBIAL WORLD

The study of microorganisms by the Dutch biologist/lens maker Anton van Leeuwenhoek has evolved immensely from its early historical beginnings. Because of Leeuwenhoek's discovery of what he affectionately called *beasties* in a water droplet in his homemade microscope, the scientific community acknowledged him as the "father of protozoology and bacteriology."

Today we know that there are enormous numbers of microbes in, on, and around us in our environment. Many of these microbes do not cause disease. The focus of this chapter and this textbook is on microbes that are associated with disease.

Bacteria

Bacteria are unicellular organisms that lack a nuclear membrane and true nucleus. They are classified as **prokaryotes** (Gr: before kernel [nucleus]), having no mitochondria, endoplasmic reticulum (ER), or Golgi bodies. The absence of the preceding bacterial cell structures differentiates them from **eukaryotes.** Table 1-1 compares prokaryotic and eukaryotic cell organization; Figure 1-1 shows both types of cells.

Parasites

Eukaryotic parasites exist as unicellular organisms of microscopic size, whereas others are multicellular organisms. Protozoa are unicellular organisms within the kingdom Protista, which obtain their nutrition through ingestion. Some are capable of locomotion (motile), whereas others are nonmo-

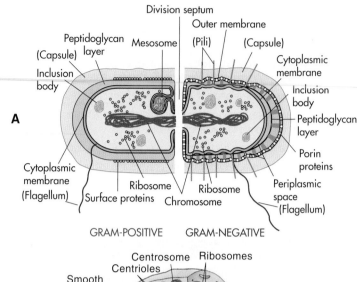

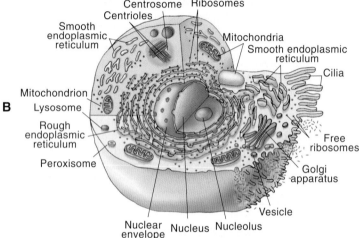

FIGURE 1-1 Comparison of prokaryotic and eukaryotic cell organization and structures. **A,** Prokaryotic gram-positive and gram-negative bacteria. (From Murray PR, Rosenthal KS, Pfaller MA: *Medical microbiology,* ed 6, Philadelphia, 2009 Mosby.) **B,** Structure of the generalized eukaryotic cell. (From Thibodeau GA, Patton KT: *Anatomy and physiology,* ed 6, St Louis, 2007, Mosby.)

tile. They are categorized by their locomotive structures: flagella (Latin: whiplike), pseudopodia (Gr: false feet), or cilia (Latin: eyelash). Many multicellular parasites (e.g., tapeworms) may be as long as 7 to 10 meters (see Chapter 28).

Fungi

Fungi are heterotrophic eukaryotes that obtain nutrients through absorption. Yeasts are a group of unicellular fungi that reproduce asexually. "True" yeasts do not form **hyphae** or **mycelia.** Most fungi are multicellular and many can reproduce sexually and asexually. The bodies of multicellular fungi are composed of filaments called *hyphae,* which interweave to form mats called *mycelia.* Moulds are filamentous forms that can reproduce asexually and sexually. Certain fungi can assume both morphologies (yeast and hyphae/mycelial forms), growing as yeast at incubator or human temperature, and the filamentous form at room temperature. These fungi are called **dimorphic.** Many of the dimorphic fungi produce systemic diseases in human hosts (see Chapter 27).

TABLE 1-1 Comparison of Prokaryotic and Eukaryotic Cell Organization

Characteristic	Prokaryote	Eukaryote
Typical size	0.4-2 μm in diameter 0.5-5 μm in length	10-100 μm in diameter >10 μm in length
Nucleus	No nuclear membrane; nucleoid region of the cytosol	Classic membrane-bound nucleus
Genome		
Location	In the nucleoid, at the mesosome	In the nucleus
Chromosomal DNA	Circular; complexed with RNA	Linear; complexed with basic histones and other proteins
Genome: extrachromosomal circular DNA	Plasmids, small circular molecule of DNA containing accessory information; most commonly found in gram-negative bacteria; each carries genes for its own replication; can confer resistance to antibiotics	In mitochondria and chloroplasts
Reproduction	Asexual (binary fission)	Sexual and asexual
Membrane-bound organelles	Absent	All
Golgi bodies	Absent in all	Present in some
Lysosomes	Absent in all	Present in some; contain hydrolytic enzymes
Endoplasmic reticulum	Absent in all	Present in all; lipid synthesis, transport
Mitochondria	Absent in all	Present in most
Nucleus	Absent in all	Present in all
Chloroplasts for photosynthesis	Absent in all	Present in algae and plants
Ribosomes: site of protein synthesis (nonmembranous)	Present in all	Present in all
Size	70S in size, consisting of 50S and 30S subunits	80S in size, consisting of 60S and 40S subunits
Electron transport for energy	In the cell membrane if present; no mitochondria present	In the inner membrane of mitochondria and chloroplasts
Sterols in cytoplasmic membrane	Absent, except in *Mycoplasma* spp.	Present
Plasma membrane	Lacks carbohydrates	Also contains glycolipids and glycoproteins
Cell wall, if present	Peptidoglycan in most bacteria	Cellulose, phenolic polymers, lignin (plants), chitin (fungi), other glycans (algae)
Glycocalyx	Present in most as an organized capsule or unorganized slime layer	Present; some animal cells
Cilia	Absent	Present; see description of flagella
Flagella, if present	Simple flagella; composed of polymers of flagellin; movement by rotary action at the base; spirochetes have MTs	Complex cilia of flagella composed of MTs, polymers of tubulin with dynein connecting the MTs; movement by sliding filaments by one another
Pili and fimbriae	Present	Absent

MT, Microtubule.

Viruses

Viruses are the smallest infectious particles (virions); they cannot be seen under an ordinary light microscope. They are neither prokaryotic nor eukaryotic. Many times we can see their effects on cell lines, such as inclusions, rounding up of cells, and syncytium (cell fusion of host cells into multinucleated infected forms), where these characteristics become diagnostic for many viral diseases. They are distinguished from living cells by the following characteristics:

- Viruses consist of DNA or RNA, but not both. Their genome may be double-stranded DNA (dsDNA), single-stranded DNA (ssDNA), double-stranded RNA (dsRNA), or single-stranded RNA (ssRNA).
- They are acellular (not composed of cells), lack cytoplasmic membranes, and are surrounded by a protein coat.
- They are obligate intracellular parasites that require host cells for replication (increase in number does not involve mitosis, meiosis, or binary fission) and metabolism. Because they lack enzymes, ribosomes, and other metabolites, they "take over" host cell function to produce virus. Growth (increase in size) does not occur in viruses.
- Viruses are mostly host and/or host cell specific. For example, human immunodeficiency virus (HIV) infects T helper lymphocytes, not muscle cells, in humans; others such as the rabies virus can infect dogs, skunks, bats, and humans. A virus that infects and possibly destroys bacterial cells is known as a bacteriophage (Gr *phage*: to eat).

Viruses are becoming better known by their DNA or RNA makeup, host disease signs and symptoms, chemical makeup, geographic distribution, resistance to lipid solvents and detergents, resistance to changes in pH and temperature, and antigenicity (serologic methods). Currently, the organization and type (either DNA or RNA), of the virus's genome, how the virus replicates, and the virus's virion (a virus outside of a cell) structure are used to differentiate virus order, family, and genera. More than 2000 descriptions of viruses can be found in The Universal Virus Database of the International Committee on Taxonomy of Viruses (www.ncbi.nlm.nih.gov/ICTVdb/). See Chapter 29 for a further discussion of viruses.

CLASSIFICATION/TAXONOMY

Taxonomy (Gr *taxes*: arrangement; Gr *nomos*: law) is the orderly classification and grouping of organisms into **taxa** (categories). Taxonomy involves three structured, interrelated categories: classification/taxonomy, nomenclature, and identification. It is based on similarities and differences in **genotype** (genetic makeup of an organism, or combinations of forms of one or a few genes under scrutiny in an organism's genome) and **phenotype** (readily observable physical and functional features of an organism expressed by its genotype). Examples of genotypic characteristics include base sequencing of DNA or RNA and DNA base composition ratio to measure the degree of relatedness of two organisms (see later in this chapter and Chapter 11). Examples of phenotypic characteristics include macroscopic (colony morphology on media) and microscopic (size, shape, arrangement into groups or chains of organisms) morphology, staining characteristics (gram-positive or gram-negative), nutritional requirements, physiologic and biochemical characteristics, and susceptibility or resistance to antibiotics or chemicals. See Chapters 5, 8, and 9 for more detailed information.

Taxa (plural of *taxon*), for example the levels of classification, are the categories or subsets in taxonomy. The formal levels of bacterial classification in successively smaller taxa or subsets are as follows: domain, kingdom, division (or phylum in kingdom Animalia), class, order, family, tribe, genus, species, and subspecies. Below the subspecies level, designations, such as serotype or biotype, may be given to organisms that share specific minor characteristics. Protists (protozoans) of clinical importance are named like animals; instead of divisions, one uses **phyla** (plural of *phylum*), but the names of the others remain the same. Bacteria are placed in domains Bacteria and Archaea, separate from the animals; plants and protists are placed in domain Eukarya. The domains Bacteria and Archaea include unicellular prokaryotic organisms.

Diagnostic microbiologists traditionally emphasize placement and naming of bacterial species into three (occasionally four or five) categories: the **family** (similar to a human "clan"), a genus (equivalent to a human last name), and a species (equivalent to a human first name). The plural of **genus** is *genera*, and there are many genera in the family Enterobacteriaceae. The proper word for the name of a **species** is an *epithet*. Although order and tribe may be useful for the classification of plants and animals, these taxa are not always used for the classification of bacteria. For example, *Staphylococcus* (genus) *aureus* (species epithet) belongs to the family Micrococcaceae. In addition, there are usually different **strains** within a given species of the same genus. For example, there are many different strains of *S. aureus*. If the *S. aureus*

isolated from one patient is resistant to penicillin and another *S. aureus* from another patient is susceptible to penicillin, then the two isolates are considered to be different strains of the same species. For an additional example, see *Corynebacterium diphtheriae* in the Transduction section later in this chapter.

Nomenclature

Nomenclature provides naming assignments for each organism in this textbook. The following standard rules for denoting bacterial names are used. The family name is capitalized and has an *-aceae* ending (e.g., Micrococcaceae). The genus name is capitalized and followed by the species epithet, which begins with a lowercase letter; both the genus and species should be italicized in print but underlined when written in script (e.g., *Staphylococcus aureus* or Staphylococcus aureus). Often the genus name is abbreviated by using the first letter (capitalized) of the genus followed by a period and the species epithet (e.g., *S. aureus*). To eliminate confusion, the first two letters or the first syllable are used when two or more genera names begin with the same first letter (e.g., *Staph.* and *Strept.* for when *Staphylococcus* and *Streptococcus* are discussed). The reason for combining the two allows the species epithet to be used for a different species in another genus. For example, *Escherichia coli* (*E. coli* or *Esch. coli*) is a bacterium, but *Entamoeba coli* (*Ent. coli*) is an intestinal parasite. The genus name followed by the word *species* (e.g., *Staphylococcus* species) may be used to refer to the genus as a whole. Species are abbreviated "sp." (singular) or "spp." (plural) when the species is not specified. When bacteria are referred to as a group, their names are neither capitalized nor underlined (e.g., staphylococci).

Classification by Phenotypic and Genotypic Characteristics

The traditional method of placing an organism into a particular genus and species is based on the similarity of all members in a number of phenotypic characteristics. In the diagnostic microbiology laboratory, this is accomplished by testing each bacterial culture for a variety of metabolic characteristics and comparing the results with those listed in established charts. In many rapid identification systems, a numeric taxonomy is used, in which phenotypic characteristics are assigned a numeric value and the derived number indicates the genus and species of the bacterium.

Epidemiologists constantly seek means of further subdividing bacterial species to follow the spread of bacterial infections. Species may be subdivided into subspecies, based on phenotypic differences (abbreviated "subsp."); serovarieties, based on serologic differences (abbreviated "serovar"); or biovarieties, based on biochemical test result differences (abbreviated "biovar"). Phage typing (based on susceptibility to specific bacterial phages) has also been used for this purpose. Current technology has allowed the analysis of genetic relatedness (DNA and RNA structure and homology) for taxonomic purposes. The analysis of ribosomal RNA (rRNA) has proved particularly useful for this purpose. The information obtained from these studies has resulted in the reclassification of some bacteria.

Classification by Cellular Type: Prokaryotes, Eukaryotes, and Archaeobacteria

Another method of classifying organisms is by cell organization. It is now recognized that organisms fall into three distinct groups based on type of cell organization and function: the prokaryotes, the eukaryotes, and the **archaeobacteria.** However, recently taxonomists have placed all organisms into three domains that have replaced some kingdoms: **Bacteria, Archaea,** and **Eukarya.** These three domains are the largest and most inclusive taxa. Each of these domains is divided into kingdoms based on the similarities of RNA, DNA, and protein sequences. Prokaryotes ("before nucleus") includes the domains Archaea and Bacteria (Eubacteria), whereas fungi, algae, protozoa, animals, and plants are eukaryotic in nature.

The domain Archaea (archaeobacteria) cell type appears to be more closely related to eukaryotic cells than to prokaryotic cells and is found in microorganisms that grow under extreme environmental conditions. Archaeal cell walls lack peptidoglycan, a major reason they are placed in a domain separate from bacteria. These microbes share some common characteristics with bacteria; they too can stain gram-positive and gram-negative. Gram-positive archaea have a thick wall and stain purple. Gram-negative archaeal cells, unlike the typical gram-negative bacterial lipid membrane, have a layer of protein covering the cell wall and stain pink. See the Gram stain discussion later in this chapter.

The structure of the cell envelope and enzymes of *archaea* (Gr: ancient, origin from the earliest cells) allows them to survive under stressful or extreme (*extremophiles*; lovers of the extreme) conditions. Examples include halophiles (salt-loving cells) in Utah's Great Salt Lake or thermophiles (heat-loving cells) in hot springs and deep ocean vents, and the anaerobic methanogens that give off swamp gas and inhabit the intestinal tracts of animals. Because *archaea* are not encountered in clinical microbiology, they are not discussed further in this chapter.

In general, the interior organization of eukaryotic cells is more complex than that of prokaryotic cells (see Figure 1-1). The eukaryotic cell is usually larger and contains membrane-encased organelles ("little organs") or compartments that serve specific functions; the prokaryotic cell is noncompartmentalized. Differences also exist in the processes of DNA synthesis, protein synthesis, and cell envelope synthesis and structure. Table 1-1 compares the major characteristics of eukaryotic and prokaryotic cells.

Pathogenic (disease-causing) **bacteria** are prokaryotic cells that infect eukaryotic hosts. Targeting antibiotic action against unique prokaryotic structures and functions inhibits bacterial growth without harming eukaryotic host cells. This is one reason that pharmaceutical companies have been so successful in developing effective antibiotics against bacterial pathogens but have been less successful in finding drugs effective against parasites, medically important fungi, and viruses, which are eukaryotic like their human hosts.

COMPARISON OF PROKARYOTIC AND EUKARYOTIC CELL STRUCTURE

Prokaryotic Cell Structure

The bacterial cell is smaller and less compartmentalized than the eukaryotic cell. A variety of structures are, however, unique to prokaryotic cells (see Figure 1-1).

Cytoplasmic Structures

Bacteria do not contain a membrane-bound nucleus. Their genome consists of a single circular chromosome. This appears as a diffuse nucleoid or chromatin body (nuclear body), which is attached to a mesosome, a saclike structure in the cell membrane.

Bacterial ribosomes, consisting of RNA and protein, are found free in the cytoplasm and attached to the cytoplasmic membrane. They are the site of protein biosynthesis. They are 70S in size and dissociate into two subunits, 50S and 30S in size (see Table 1-1). The *S* stands for *Svedberg* units that refer to sedimentation rates (unit of time) during high-speed centrifugation. It is named for Theodor Svedberg, Nobel prize winner, and inventor of the ultracentrifuge. Larger particles have higher S values. It is important to remember that the S value is *not additive.* When the two subunits 50S and 30S above bind together, there is a loss of surface area, and therefore the two subunits will add up to only 70S in size. The same occurs in the eukaryotic cell where the two subunits, 60S and 40S, add up to 80S.

Stained bacteria sometimes reveal the presence of granules in the cytoplasm (cytoplasmic granules). These granules are storage deposits and may consist of polysaccharides such as glycogen, lipids such as poly-β-hydroxybutyrate, or polyphosphates.

Certain genera, such as *Bacillus* and *Clostridium*, produce endospores in response to harsh environmental conditions. Endospores are small, dormant (inactive), asexual spores that develop inside the bacterial cell (active vegetative cell) as a means of survival, although they do become vegetative when the harsh conditions are removed. Their thick protein coat makes them highly resistant to chemical agents, temperature change, starvation, dehydration, ultraviolet and gamma radiation, and desiccation. It is important to remember that endospores are not a means of reproduction. Each vegetative cell (active, capable of growing and dividing), under harsh conditions, produces internally one endospore (inactive), which germinates under favorable environmental conditions into one vegetative cell (active). Endospores should not confused with the reproductive spores of fungi (see Chapter 27).

Spores appear as highly refractile bodies in the cell. Spores are visualized microscopically as unstained areas in a cell with the use of traditional bacterial stains (Gram) or by using specific spore stains. *Schaeffer-Fulton* is the most commonly used endospore stain. The size, shape, and interior location of the spore, for example at one end (terminal), subterminal, or central, can be used as identifying characteristics. For example, the terminal spore of *Clostridium tetani*, the etiologic (causative) agent of tetanus, gives the organism a characteristic "racquet (tennis) or lollipop" shaped appearance.

Cell Envelope Structures

The cell envelope consists of the membrane and structures surrounding the cytoplasm. In bacteria, these are the cell membrane and the cell wall. Some species also produce capsules and slime layers.

Plasma Membrane (Cell Membrane). The plasma membrane is a phospholipid bilayer with embedded proteins that envelop the cytoplasm. The prokaryotic plasma membrane is made of phospholipids and proteins but does not contain sterols, unlike eukaryotic plasma membranes (except for *Mycoplasma*). The plasma membrane acts as an osmotic barrier (prokaryotes have a high osmotic pressure inside the cell) and is the location of the electron transport chain, where energy is generated. The general functions of the prokaryotic plasma membrane are identical to those in eukaryotes (see Figure 1-2).

Cell Wall. The cell wall of prokaryotes is a rigid structure that maintains the shape of the cell and prevents bursting of the cell from the high osmotic pressure inside it. There are several different types of cell wall structures in bacteria, which have traditionally been categorized according to their staining characteristics. The two major types of cell walls are the **gram-positive** and the **gram-negative** types. In addition, mycobacteria have a modified gram-positive cell wall called an **acid-fast** cell wall, although they do stain gram-positive, and mycoplasmas have no cell wall.

Gram-Positive Cell Wall. The gram-positive cell wall is composed of a very thick protective peptidoglycan (murein) layer. Because the peptidoglycan layer is the principal component of the gram-positive cell wall, many antibiotics effective against gram-positive organisms (e.g., penicillin) act by preventing synthesis of peptidoglycan. Gram-negative bacteria, which have a thinner layer of peptidoglycan and a different cell wall structure, are less affected by these antibiotics.

The peptidoglycan or murein layer consists of glycan (polysaccharide) chains of alternating *N*-acetyl-d-glucosamine (NAG) and *N*-acetyl-d-muramic acid (NAM) (Figure 1-3). Short peptides, each consisting of four amino acid residues, are attached to a carboxyl group on each NAM residue. The chains are then cross-linked to form a thick network via a peptide bridge (varying in number of peptides) connected to the tetrapeptides on the NAM.

Other components of the gram-positive cell wall that penetrate to the exterior of the cell are teichoic acid (anchored to the peptidoglycan) and lipoteichoic acid (anchored to the plasma membrane). These two components are unique to the gram-positive cell wall. Other antigenic polysaccharides may be present on the surface of the peptidoglycan layer.

Gram-Negative Cell Wall. The cell wall of gram-negative microorganisms is composed of two layers. The inner peptidoglycan layer is much thinner than in gram-positive cell walls. Outside the peptidoglycan layer is an additional outer membrane unique to the gram-negative cell wall. The outer membrane contains proteins, phospholipids, and lipopolysaccharide (LPS). LPS contains three regions: an antigenic O–specific polysaccharide, a core polysaccharide, and an inner lipid A (also called *endotoxin*). The lipid A moiety is responsible for producing fever and shock conditions in patients infected with gram-negative bacteria. The outer membrane functions in the following ways:

- It acts as a barrier to hydrophobic compounds and harmful substances.
- It acts as a sieve, allowing water-soluble molecules to enter through protein-lined channels called *porins*.
- It provides attachment sites that enhance attachment to host cells.

Between the outer membrane and the inner membrane, and encompassing the thin peptidoglycan layer, is an area referred to as the *periplasmic space*. Within the periplasmic

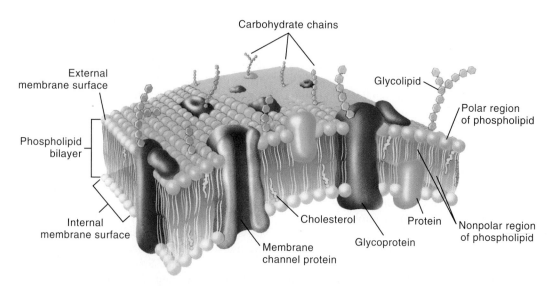

FIGURE 1-2 Structure of the plasma membrane. (From Thibodeau GA, Patton KT: *Anatomy & physiology*, ed 6, St Louis, 2007, Mosby.)

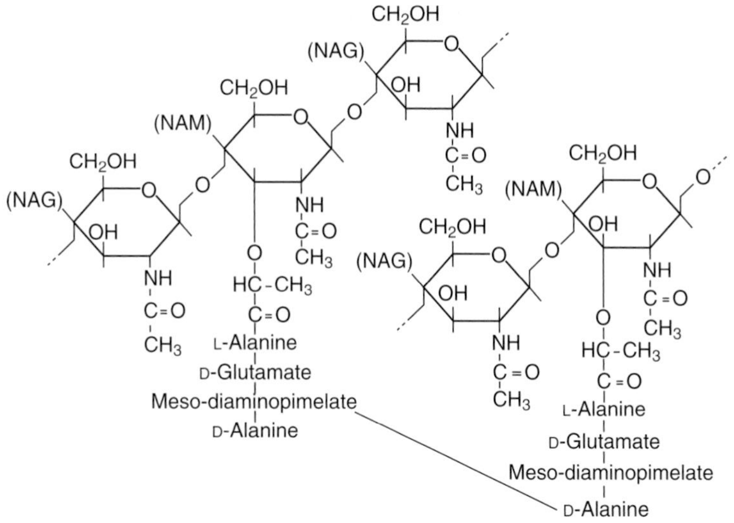

CH₂OH

(NAG)

CH₂OH

(NAM)

CH₂OH

(NAG)

CH₂OH

(NAG)

CH₂OH

(NAM)

NH

C=O

CH₃

NH

C=O

CH₃

HC-CH₃

C=O

L-Alanine

D-Glutamate

Meso-diaminopimelate

D-Alanine

NH

C=O

CH₃

HC-CH₃

C=O

L-Alanine

D-Glutamate

Meso-diaminopimelate

D-Alanine

FIGURE 1-3 A diagram that demonstrates the structure of the peptidoglycan layer in the cell wall of *Escherichia coli*. The amino acids in the cross-linking tetrapeptides may vary among species. NAG, *N*-acetyl-d-glucosamine; NAM, *N*-acetyl-d-muramic acid. (From Neidhardt FC, Ingraham M, Schaechter M: *Physiology of bacterial cell: a molecular approach*, Sunderland, Mass, 1990, Sinauer Associates.)

space is a gel-like matrix containing nutrient-binding proteins and degradative and detoxifying enzymes. The periplasmic space is absent in gram-positive bacteria.

Acid-Fast Cell Wall. Certain genera (*Mycobacterium* and *Nocardia*) have a gram-positive cell wall structure but, in addition, contain a waxy layer of glycolipids and fatty acids (mycolic acid) bound to the exterior of the cell wall. More than 60% of the cell wall is lipid, and the major lipid component is mycolic acid. This is a strong "hydrophobic" molecule that forms a lipid shell around the organism and affects its permeability. This makes *Mycobacterium* spp. difficult to stain with the Gram stain. Because of their gram-positive nature, they stain a faint blue (gram-positive) color. The mycobacteria and nocardiae are best stained with an acid-fast stain, in which the bacteria are stained with carbolfuchsin, followed by acid-alcohol as a decolorizer. Other bacteria are decolorized by acid-alcohol, whereas mycobacteria and nocardiae retain the stain. They have therefore been designated *acid-fast bacteria*.

Absence of Cell Wall. Prokaryotes that belong to the *Mycoplasma* and *Ureaplasma* genera are unique in that they lack a cell wall and contain sterols in their cell membranes. Because they lack the rigidity of the cell wall, they are seen in a variety of shapes microscopically. Gram-positive and gram-negative cells can lose their cell walls and grow as L-forms in media supplemented with serum or sugar to prevent osmotic rupture of the cell membrane.

Surface Polymers

A variety of pathogenic bacteria produce a discrete organized covering termed a **capsule**. Capsules are usually made of polysaccharide polymers, although they may also be made of polypeptides. Capsules act as virulence factors in helping the pathogen evade phagocytosis. During identification of certain bacteria by serologic typing, capsules sometimes must be

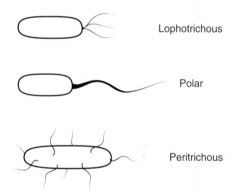

Lophotrichous

Polar

Peritrichous

FIGURE 1-4 Diagram of three flagellar arrangements that occur in bacteria. Other variations do occur.

removed in order to detect the somatic (cell wall) antigens present underneath them. Capsule removal is accomplished by boiling a suspension of the microorganism. *Salmonella typhi* must have its capsular (Vi) antigen removed in order for the technologist to observe agglutination with *Salmonella* somatic (O) antisera. The capsule does not ordinarily stain with use of common laboratory stains, such as Gram or India ink. Instead, it appears as a clear area ("halolike") between or surrounding the stained organism and the stained amorphous background material in a direct smear from a clinical specimen.

Slime layers are similar to capsules but are more diffuse layers surrounding the cell. They also are made of polysaccharides and serve either to inhibit phagocytosis or, in some cases, to aid in adherence to host tissue or synthetic implants.

Cell Appendages. The flagellum is the organ of locomotion. **Flagella** are exterior protein filaments that rotate and cause bacteria to be motile. Bacterial species vary in their possession of flagella from none (nonmotile) to many (Figure 1-4). Flagella that extend from one end of the bacterium are polar. Polar flagella may occur singly at one or both ends or multiply in tufts at one end termed *lophotrichous.* Flagella that occur on all sides of the bacterium are peritrichous. The number and arrangement of flagella are sometimes used for identification purposes. Flagella can be visualized microscopically with special flagellum stains.

Pili (plural of *pilus*), also known as *conjugation pili*, are nonmotile, long, hollow protein tubes that connect two bacterial cells and mediate DNA exchange. **Fimbriae** (plural of *fimbria*) are nonflagellar, sticky, proteinaceous, hairlike appendages that adhere some bacterial cells to one another and to environmental surfaces.

Eukaryotic Cell Structure

The following structures are associated with eukaryotic cells (see Table 1-1 and Figure 1-1). In the diagnostic microbiology laboratory, the eukaryotic cell type occurs in medically important fungi and in parasites.

Cytoplasmic Structures

The nucleus of the eukaryotic cell contains the DNA of the cell in the form of discrete chromosomes (structures in the nucleus that carry genetic information; the genes). They are covered with basic proteins called *histones*. The number of chromosomes in the nucleus varies according to the particular organism.

A rounded, refractile body called a *nucleolus* is also located within the nucleus. The nucleolus is the site of ribosomal RNA synthesis. The nucleus is bounded by a bilayered lipoprotein nuclear membrane.

The ER is a system of membranes that occur throughout the cytoplasm. It is found in two forms. The "rough" ER is covered with ribosomes, the site of protein synthesis. It is the ribosomes that give the ER the rough appearance. The smooth ER does not have ribosomes on the outer surface of its membrane, hence the smooth appearance. Smooth ER does not synthesize proteins, but it does synthesize phospholipids (like rough ER). The major function of the Golgi apparatus or complex is to modify and package proteins sent to it by the rough ER depending on the protein's final destination.

Eukaryotic ribosomes, where protein synthesis occurs, are 80S in size and dissociate into two subunits: 60S and 40S. They are attached to the rough ER. Eukaryotic cells contain several membrane-enclosed organelles. Mitochondria are the main sites of energy production. They contain their own DNA and the electron transport system that produces energy for cell functions. Lysosomes contain hydrolytic enzymes for degradation of macromolecules and microorganisms within the cell. Peroxisomes contain protective enzymes that break down hydrogen peroxide and other peroxides generated within the cell. Chloroplasts, found in plant cells, are the sites of photosynthesis. Chloroplasts are the sites of energy production. Photosynthesis produces glucose from carbon dioxide and water. Fungi are not plants and therefore have no chloroplasts.

Cell Envelope Structures

Plasma Membrane. The plasma membrane (PM) (see Figure 1-2) is a phospholipid bilayer with embedded proteins that envelops the cytoplasm and regulates transport of macromolecules into and out of the cell. A substantial amount of cholesterol is found. Cholesterol has a stabilizing effect and helps keep the membrane fluid. The polar heads of the phospholipids are hydrophilic (water loving) and lie on both the intracellular and extracellular fluids; their nonpolar tails are hydrophobic (water hating) and avoid water by lining up in the center of the PM "tail to tail." It is this type of hydrophobic makeup of the interior of the PM that makes it potentially impermeable to water-soluble molecules. Proteins perform several important functions of the membrane. They may act as enzymes, hormone receptors, pore channels, and carriers. The presence of sterols is also a trait of eukaryotic cell membranes.

Cell Wall. The function of a cell wall is to provide rigidity and strength to the exterior of the cell. Most eukaryotic cells do not have cell walls. Fungi, however, have cell walls principally made of polysaccharides such as chitin, mannan, and glucan. Chitin is a distinct component of fungal cell walls.

Motility Organelles. Cilia are short projections (3 to 10 μm), usually numerous, that extend from the cell surface and are used for locomotion. They are found in certain protozoa and in ciliated epithelial cells of the respiratory tract. Flagella are longer projections (greater than 150 μm) used for locomotion by cells such as spermatozoa. The basal body, or kinetosome, is a small structure located at the base of cilia or flagella, where microtubule proteins involved in movement originate.

BACTERIAL MORPHOLOGY

Microscopic Shapes

Bacteria vary in size from 0.4 to 2 μm. They occur in three basic shapes (Figure 1-5):
- Cocci (spherical)
- Bacilli (rod-shaped)
- Spirochetes (spiral)

Individual bacteria may form characteristic groupings. Cocci (plural of *coccus*) may occur singly, in pairs (diplococci), in chains (streptococci), or in clusters (staphylococci). Bacilli (plural of *bacillus*) may vary greatly in size and length from very short coccobacilli to long filamentous rods. The ends may be square or rounded. Bacilli with tapered, pointed ends are termed **fusiform.** Some bacilli are curved. When a species varies in size and shape within a pure culture, the bacterium is **pleomorphic.** Bacilli may occur as single rods or in chains or may align themselves side by side (palisading). Spirochetes vary in length and in the number of helical turns (not all helical bacteria are called *spirochetes*).

Common Stains Used for Microscopic Visualization

Stains that impart color or fluorescence are needed to visualize bacteria under the microscope. The microscopic staining characteristics, shapes, and groupings are used in the classification of microorganisms (Figure 1-6).

Microscopic Morphology of Bacteria

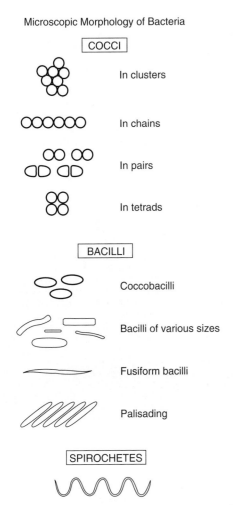

FIGURE 1-5 Diagram of the microscopic shapes and arrangements of bacteria.

Gram Stain. The Gram stain is the most commonly used stain in the clinical microbiology laboratory. It places bacteria into one of the two main groups: gram-positive (blue to purple) or gram-negative (pink) (see Figure 1-6, *A* and *B*). Some organisms are gram variable or do not stain at all. As mentioned previously, the cell wall structure determines the Gram-staining characteristics of a species. The Gram stain consists of gentle heat fixing (methyl alcohol may also be used to fix) of the smear and the addition of four sequential components: crystal violet (the primary stain, 1 minute), iodine (the mordant or fixative, 1 minute), alcohol or an alcohol acetone solution (the decolorizer, quick on and rinse), and safranin (the counterstain, 30 seconds). The time frames listed are not exact and vary with the organism; rinsing with water between each step is important. The bacteria are initially stained purple by the crystal violet, which is bound to the cell wall with the aid of iodine. When decolorizer is applied to bacteria with a gram-negative type of cell wall structure, the crystal violet washes out of the cells, which then take up the pink counterstain, safranin. Gram-negative bacteria therefore appear pink under the light microscope. Bacteria with a gram-positive cell wall retain the primary crystal violet stain during the decolorizing treatment and therefore remain purple. Cells in a direct smear from a patient specimen, such as epithelial cells, white blood cells, red blood cells, and amorphous background material, should appear pink (gram-negative) if the Gram stain was performed correctly. As presented in the case in point at the beginning of the chapter, review of quality control slides is important in the detection of errors in the performance of the Gram stain procedure and in interpretation.

Acid-Fast Stains. Acid-fast stains are used to stain bacteria that have a high lipid and wax content in their cell walls and do not stain well with traditional bacterial stains. Carbolfuchsin (a red dye) is used as the primary stain (see Figure 1-6, *C*). The cell wall is treated to allow penetration of the dye either by heat (Ziehl-Neelsen method) or by a detergent (Kinyoun method). Acidified alcohol is used as a decolorizer, and methylene blue is the counterstain. Acid-fast bacteria retain the primary stain and are red. Bacteria that are not acid-fast are blue.

Two other gram-positive genera, *Nocardia* and *Rhodococcus*, may stain acid-fast by a modified method. Acid-fast staining is used to identify a yeast, *Saccharomyces*, and coccidian parasites, such as *Isospora belli*, *Cryptosporidium*, and other coccidia-like bodies. A fluorochrome (i.e., fluorescent) stain, auramine-rhodamine, has also been used to screen for acid-fast bacteria (see Figure 1-6, *D*). This stain is selective for the cell wall of acid-fast bacteria. Acid-fast bacteria appear yellow or orange under a fluorescent microscope, making them easier to find.

Acridine Orange. Acridine orange is a fluorochrome dye that stains both gram-positive and gram-negative bacteria, living or dead. It binds to the nucleic acid of the cell and fluoresces as a bright orange when a fluorescent microscope is used. Acridine orange is used to locate bacteria in blood cultures and other specimens where discerning bacteria might otherwise be difficult (see Figure 1-6, *E*).

Calcofluor White. Calcofluor white is a fluorochrome that binds to chitin in fungal cell walls. It fluoresces as a bright apple-green or blue-white, allowing visualization of fungal structures with a fluorescent microscope. This was the original "blueing" used in high-volume laundries to whiten yellow-appearing white cotton and other fabrics.

Methylene Blue. Methylene blue has been traditionally used to stain *Corynebacterium diphtheriae* for observation of metachromatic granules (see Figure 1-6, *F*). It is also used as a counterstain in the acid-fast staining procedures.

Lactophenol Cotton Blue. Lactophenol cotton blue is used to stain the cell walls of medically important fungi grown in slide culture (see Figure 1-6, *G*).

India Ink. India ink is a negative stain used to visualize capsules surrounding certain yeasts, such as *Cryptococcus* spp. (see Figure 1-6, *H*). The fine ink particles are excluded from the capsule, leaving a dark background and a clear capsule surrounding the yeast.

Endospore Stain. To a heat-fixed smear, the primary stain, malachite green, is applied (flooded) and heated to steaming for about 5 minutes. Then the preparation is washed for about 30 seconds to remove the primary stain. Next, the counterstain safranin is applied to the smear. The endospores appear green, within pink- or red-appearing bacterial cells.

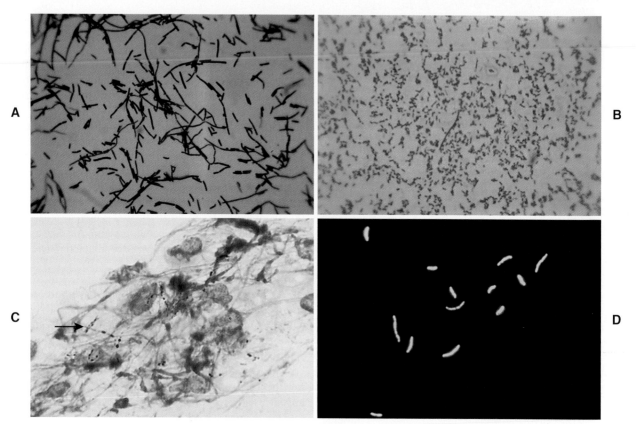

FIGURE 1-6   A, Gram stain of *Lactobacillus* species illustrating gram-positive bacilli, singly and in chains. A few gram-negative–staining bacilli are also present. (Courtesy Dr. Andrew G. Smith, Baltimore.) **B,** Gram stain of *Escherichia coli* illustrating short gram-negative bacilli. (Courtesy Dr. Andrew G. Smith, Baltimore.) **C,** Acid-fast stain, carbolfuchsin based. A sputum smear demonstrating the presence of acid-fast *Mycobacterium* species stained by the Kinyoun or Ziehl-Neelsen carbolfuchsin method. **D,** Acid-fast stain, fluorochrome based. *Mycobacterium* species stained with the acid-fast fluorescent auramine-rhodamine stain. This stain is useful for screening for the presence of acid-fast bacteria in clinical specimens. (Courtesy Clinical Microbiology Audiovisual Study Units, Health and Education Resources, Inc., Bethesda, Md.)

MICROBIAL GROWTH AND NUTRITION

All bacteria have three major nutritional needs for growth:

- A source of carbon (for making cellular constituents). Carbon represents 50% of the dry weight of a bacterium.
- A source of nitrogen (for making proteins). Nitrogen makes up 14% of the dry weight.
- A source of energy (ATP, for performing cellular functions).

Smaller amounts of molecules, such as phosphate for nucleic acids and phospholipids of cell membranes, and sulfur for protein synthesis make up an additional 4% of the weight. A variety of metals and ions for enzymatic activity must also be present. Important mineral ions, such as Na^+, K^+, Cl^-, and Ca^{2+}, are also required. Although the basic building blocks required for growth are the same for all cells, bacteria vary widely in their ability to use different sources of these molecules.

Nutritional Requirements for Growth

Bacteria are classified into two basic groups according to how they meet their nutritional needs. Members of the first group, the **autotrophs** (lithotrophs), are able to grow simply, using carbon dioxide as the sole source of carbon, with only water and inorganic salts required in addition. Autotrophs obtain energy either photosynthetically (phototrophs) or by oxidation of inorganic compounds (chemolithotrophs). Autotrophs occur in environmental milieus.

The second group of bacteria, the **heterotrophs,** require more complex substances for growth. They require an organic source of carbon, such as glucose, and obtain energy by oxidizing or fermenting organic substances. Often, the same substance (e.g., glucose) is used as both the carbon source and the energy source.

All bacteria that inhabit the human body fall into the heterotrophic group. Within this group, however, nutritional needs vary greatly. Bacteria such as *E. coli* and *Pseudomonas aeruginosa* can use a wide variety or organic compounds as carbon sources and therefore grow on most simple laboratory media. Other pathogenic bacteria, such as *Haemophilus influenzae* and the anaerobes, are fastidious, requiring additional metabolites such as vitamins, purines, pyrimidines, and hemoglobin supplied in the growth medium. Some pathogenic bacteria, such as *Chlamydia* spp., cannot be cultured on laboratory

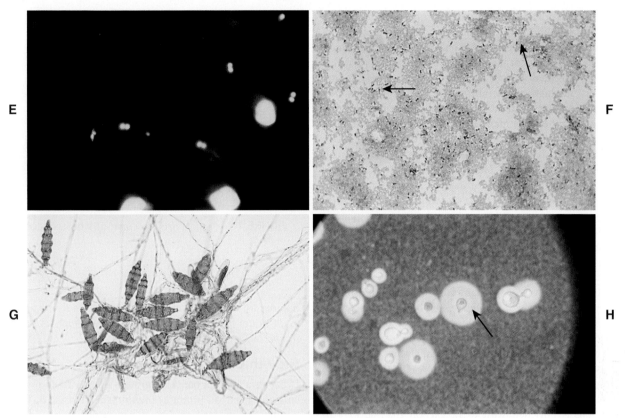

FIGURE 1-6, cont'd   **E,** Acridine orange stain. A fluorescent stain demonstrating the presence of staphylococci in a blood culture broth. This stain is useful for detecting bacteria in situations where debris may mask the bacteria. (Courtesy Dr. John E. Peters Baltimore.) **F,** Methylene blue stain. A methylene blue stain demonstrating the typical morphology of *Corynebacterium diphtheriae (arrows)*. **G,** Lactophenol cotton blue stain. Lactophenol cotton blue-stained slide of macroconidia and hyphae of the fungal dermatophyte *Microsporum gypseum*. **H,** India ink. An India ink wet mount of *Cryptococcus neoformans* demonstrating the presence of a capsule *(arrow)*. (Courtesy Dr. Andrew G. Smith, Baltimore.)

media at all and must be grown in tissue culture or detected by other means.

Types of Growth Media

A laboratory growth medium whose contents are simple and completely defined is termed **minimal medium.** This type of medium is not usually used in the diagnostic microbiology laboratory. Media that are more complex and made of extracts of meat or soybeans are termed **nutrient media** (e.g., nutrient broth, trypticase soy broth). A growth medium that contains added growth factors, such as blood, vitamins, and yeast extract, is referred to as *enriched* (e.g., blood agar, chocolate agar). Media containing additives that inhibit the growth of some bacteria but allow others to grow are called **selective media** (e.g., MacConkey agar [MAC] selective for gram-negatives while inhibiting gram positives and colistin-nalidixic acid [CNA] selective for gram-positives while inhibiting gram negatives). Ingredients in media that allow visualization of metabolic differences between groups or species of bacteria are called **differential media.** Therefore MacConkey agar can also be a differential medium because it distinguishes between lactose fermenters (pink) and nonlactose fermenters (clear).

A blood agar plate can also be, in a nonstrict sense, differential, because it distinguishes between hemolytic and nonhemolytic organisms. When a delay between collection of the specimen and culturing the specimen is necessary, a **transport medium** is used. A transport medium is a holding medium designed to preserve the viability of microorganisms in the specimen but not allow multiplication. Stuart broth and Amies and Cary-Blair transport media are common examples.

Environmental Factors Influencing Growth

Three environmental factors influence the growth rate of bacteria and must be considered when bacteria are cultured in the laboratory:

- pH
- Temperature
- Gaseous composition of the atmosphere

Most pathogenic bacteria grow best at a neutral pH. Diagnostic laboratory media for bacteria are usually adjusted to a final pH between 7.0 and 7.5. Temperature influences the rate of growth of a bacterial culture. Microorganisms have been categorized according to their optimal temperature for growth. Bacteria that grow best at cold temperatures are called **psychrophiles** (optimal growth at 10° to 20° C). Bacteria that grow optimally at moderate temperatures are called **mesophiles** (optimal growth at 20° to 40° C). Bacteria that grow best at high temperatures are called **thermophiles** (optimal growth at 50° to 60° C). Psychrophiles and thermophiles are found environmentally in places such as the arctic seas and hot springs, respectively. Most bacteria that have adapted to humans are mesophiles that grow best near human body temperature (37° C). Diagnostic laboratories routinely incubate cultures for bacterial growth at 35° C. Some pathogenic species, however, prefer a lower temperature for growth; when these organisms are suspected, the specimen plate is incubated at a lower temperature. Fungal cultures are incubated at 30° C. The ability to grow at room temperature (25° C) or at an elevated temperature (42° C) is used as diagnostic characteristics for some bacteria.

Bacteria that grow on humans vary in their atmospheric requirements for growth. **Obligate aerobes** require oxygen for growth. **Aerotolerant anaerobes,** previously referred to as *facultative aerobes*, can survive in the presence of oxygen but do not use oxygen in metabolism (e.g., certain *Clostridium* spp.). **Obligate anaerobes** cannot grow in the presence of oxygen. **Facultative anaerobes** can grow either with or without oxygen. **Capnophilic** organisms grow best when the atmosphere is enriched with extra carbon dioxide (5% to 10%).

Air contains approximately 21% oxygen and 1% carbon dioxide. When the carbon dioxide content of an aerobic incubator is increased to 10%, the oxygen content of the incubator is lowered to approximately 18%. Obligate aerobes must have oxygen to grow; incubation in air or an aerobic incubator with 10% carbon dioxide present satisfies their oxygen requirement. **Microaerophilic** bacteria require a reduced level of oxygen to grow. An example of a pathogenic microaerophile is *Campylobacter* spp., which requires 5% to 6% oxygen. This type of atmosphere can be generated in culture jars or pouches using a commercially available microaerophilic atmosphere-generating system. Obligate anaerobes must be grown in an atmosphere either devoid of oxygen or with a significantly reduced oxygen content. Facultative anaerobes (aerobes that can grow anaerobically) are routinely cultured in an aerobic atmosphere because aerobic culture is easier and less expensive than anaerobic culture; an example is *E. coli.* Capnophilic bacteria require extra carbon dioxide (5% to 10%) for growth; an example is *H. influenzae.* Because many bacteria grow better in the presence of increased carbon dioxide, diagnostic microbiology laboratories often maintain their aerobic incubators at a 5% to 10% carbon dioxide level.

Bacterial Growth

Generation Time

Bacteria replicate by binary fission, with one cell dividing into two cells. The time required for one cell to divide into two cells is called the *generation time* or *doubling time.* The generation time of a bacterium in culture can be as little as 20

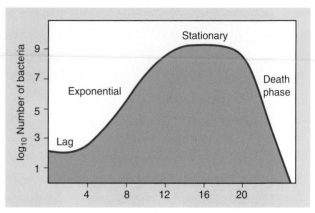

FIGURE 1-7 Typical growth curve of a bacterial culture.

minutes for a fast-growing bacterium such as *E. coli* or as long as 24 hours for a slow-growing bacterium such as *Mycobacterium tuberculosis.*

Growth Curve

If bacteria are in a balanced growth state, with enough nutrients and no toxic products present, the increase in bacterial numbers is proportional to the increase in other bacterial properties, such as mass, protein content, and nucleic acid content. Thus measurement of any of these properties can be used as an indication of bacterial growth. When the growth of a bacterial culture is plotted during balanced growth, the resulting curve shows four phases of growth: (1) a lag phase, during which bacteria are preparing to divide, (2) a log phase, during which bacteria numbers increase logarithmically, (3) a stationary phase, in which nutrients are becoming limited and the numbers of bacteria remain constant (although viability may decrease), and (4) a death phase, when the number of nonviable bacterial cells exceeds the number of viable cells. An example of such a growth curve is shown in Figure 1-7.

Determination of Cell Numbers

In the diagnostic laboratory the number of bacterial cells present is determined in one of three ways:
- *Direct counting under the microscope:* This method can be used to estimate the number of bacteria present in a specimen. It does not distinguish between live and dead cells.
- *Direct plate count:* By growing dilutions of broth cultures on agar plates, one can determine the number of colony-forming units per milliliter (CFU/mL). This provides a count of viable cells only. This method is used in determining the bacterial cell count in urine cultures.
- *Density measurement:* The density (referred to as *cloudiness* or *turbidity*) of a bacterial broth culture in log phase can be correlated to CFU/mL of the culture. This method is used to prepare a standard inoculum for antimicrobial susceptibility testing.

BACTERIAL BIOCHEMISTRY AND METABOLISM

Metabolism

Microbial metabolism consists of the biochemical reactions bacteria use to break down organic compounds as well as those they use to synthesize new bacterial parts from the resulting carbon skeletons. Energy for the new constructions is generated during the metabolic breakdown of the substrate.

The occurrence of all biochemical reactions in the cell depends on the presence and activity of specific enzymes. Thus metabolism can be regulated in the cell either by regulating the production of an enzyme itself (a genetic type of regulation, in which production of the enzyme can be induced or suppressed by molecules present in the cell) or by regulating the activity of the enzyme (via feedback inhibition, in which the products of the enzymatic reaction or a succeeding enzymatic reaction inhibit the activity of the enzyme).

Bacteria vary widely in their ability to use various compounds as substrates and in the end products generated. A variety of biochemical pathways exist for substrate breakdown in the microbial world, and the particular pathway used determines the end product and final pH of the medium (Figure 1-8). Microbiologists use these metabolic differences as phenotypic markers in the identification of bacteria. Diagnostic schemes analyze each unknown microorganism for (1) utilization of a variety of substrates as a carbon source, (2) production of specific end products from various substrates, and (3) production of an acid or alkaline pH in the test medium. Thus knowledge of the biochemistry and metabolism of bacteria is important in the clinical laboratory.

Fermentation and Respiration

Bacteria use biochemical pathways to catabolize (break down) carbohydrates and produce energy by two mechanisms—**fermentation** and **respiration** (commonly referred to as *oxida-*

tion). Fermentation is an anaerobic process carried out by both obligate and facultative anaerobes. In fermentation, the electron acceptor is an organic compound. Fermentation is less efficient in energy generation than respiration (oxidation) because the beginning substrate is not completely reduced; therefore all the energy in the substrate is not released. When fermentation occurs, a mixture of end products (e.g., lactate, butyrate, ethanol, and acetoin) accumulates in the medium. Analysis of these end products is particularly useful for the identification of anaerobic bacteria. End-product determination is also used in the Voges-Proskauer (VP) and methyl red tests, two important diagnostic tests used in the identification of the Enterobacteriaceae. (The term *fermentation* is often used loosely in the diagnostic microbiology laboratory to indicate any type of utilization—fermentative or oxidative—of a carbohydrate—sugar—with the resulting production of an acid pH.)

Respiration (not an act of breathing) is an efficient energy-generating process in which molecular oxygen is the final electron acceptor. Obligate aerobes and facultative anaerobes carry out aerobic respiration, in which oxygen is the final electron acceptor. Certain anaerobes can carry out anaerobic respiration, in which inorganic forms of oxygen, such as nitrate and sulfate, act as the final electron acceptors.

Biochemical Pathways from Glucose to Pyruvic Acid

The starting carbohydrate for bacterial fermentations or oxidations is glucose. When bacteria use other sugars as a carbon source, they first convert the sugar to glucose, which is then processed by one of three pathways. These pathways are designed to generate pyruvic acid, a key three-carbon intermediate. The three major biochemical pathways bacteria use to break down glucose to pyruvic acid are (1) the Embden-Meyerhof-Parnas (EMP) glycolytic pathway (Figure 1-9), (2) the pentose phosphate pathway (Figure 1-10), and (3) the Entner-Doudoroff pathway (see Figure 1-10). Pyruvate can then be further processed either fermentatively or oxidatively.

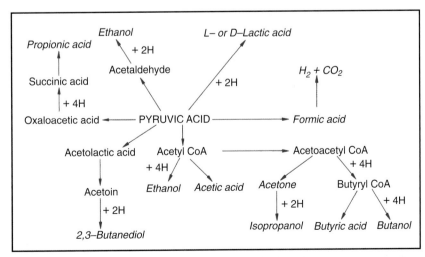

FIGURE 1-8   The fate of pyruvate in major fermentation pathways by microorganisms. (From Joklik WK et al: *Zinsser microbiology*, ed 20, Norwalk, Conn, 1992, Appleton & Lange.)

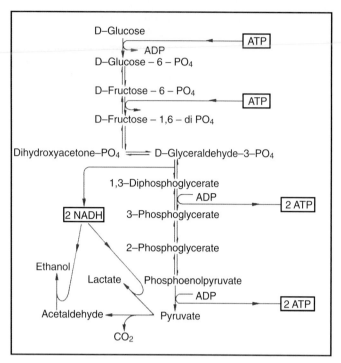

FIGURE 1-9 The Embden-Meyerhof-Parnas glycolytic pathway. (From Joklik WK et al: *Zinsser microbiology*, ed 20, Norwalk, Conn, 1992, Appleton & Lange.)

The three major metabolic pathways and their key characteristics are described in Box 1-1.

Anaerobic Utilization of Pyruvic Acid (Fermentation)

Pyruvic acid is a key metabolic intermediate. Bacteria process pyruvic acid further using a variety of fermentation pathways. Each pathway yields different end products, which can be analyzed and used as phenotypic markers (see Figure 1-8). Some of the fermentation pathways used by the microbes that inhabit the human body are as follows:

- *Alcoholic fermentation:* The major end product is ethanol. This is the pathway used by yeasts when they ferment glucose to produce ethanol.
- *Homolactic fermentation:* The end product is almost exclusively lactic acid. All members of the *Streptococcus* genus and many members of the *Lactobacillus* genus ferment pyruvate using this pathway.
- *Heterolactic fermentation:* Some lactobacilli use this mixed fermentation pathway, of which, in addition to lactic acid, the end products include carbon dioxide, alcohols, formic acid, and acetic acid.
- *Propionic acid fermentation:* Propionic acid is the major end product of fermentations carried out by *Propionibacterium acnes* and some anaerobic non–spore-forming gram-positive bacilli.

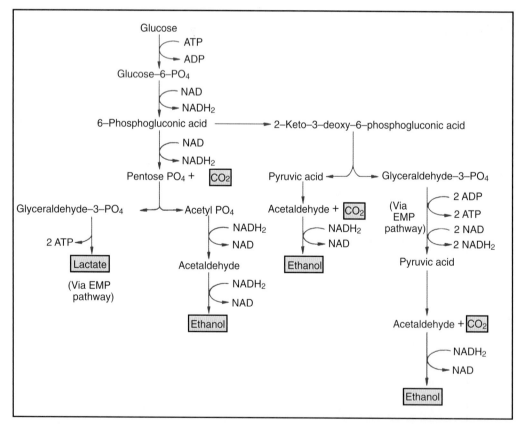

FIGURE 1-10 Alternative microbial pathways to the Embden-Meyerhof-Parnas pathway for glucose fermentation. The pentose phosphate pathway is on the left, and the Entner-Doudoroff pathway is on the right. (From Joklik WK et al: *Zinsser microbiology*, ed 20, Norwalk, Conn, 1992, Appleton & Lange.)

BOX 1-1 The Three Major Metabolic Pathways

EMP Glycolytic Pathway
- The major pathway in conversion of glucose to pyruvate
- Generates reducing power in the form of $NADH_2$
- Generates energy in the form of ATP
- Anaerobic; does not require oxygen
- Used by many bacteria, including all members of Enterobacteriaceae

Pentose Phosphate (Phosphogluconate) Pathway
- An alternative to EMP pathway for carbohydrate metabolism
- Conversion of glucose to ribulose-5-phosphate, which is then rearranged into other 3-, 4-, 5-, 6-, and 7-carbon sugars
- Provides pentoses for nucleotide synthesis
- Produces glyceraldehyde-3-phosphate, which can be converted to pyruvate
- Generates NADPH, which provides reducing power for biosynthetic reactions
- May be used to generate ATP (yield is less than with the EMP pathway)
- Used by heterolactic fermenting bacteria, such as lactobacilli, and by *Brucella abortus,* which lacks some of the enzymes required in the EMP pathway

Entner-Doudoroff Pathway
- Converts glucose-6-phosphate (rather than glucose) to pyruvate and glyceraldehyde phosphate, which can then be funneled into other pathways
- Generates one NADPH per molecule of glucose but uses one ATP
- Aerobic process used by *Pseudomonas, Alcaligenes, Enterococcus faecalis,* and other bacteria lacking certain glycolytic enzymes

ATP, Adenosine triphosphate; *EMP,* Embden-Meyerhof-Parnas; *NADH₂,* nicotinamide adenine dinucleotide dehydrogenase; *NADPH,* nicotinamide adenine dinucleotide phosphate.

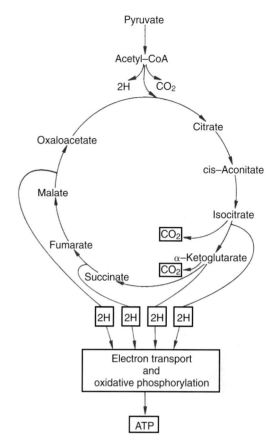

FIGURE 1-11 The Krebs tricarboxylic acid cycle allowing the complete oxidation of a substrate. (From Joklik WK et al: *Zinsser microbiology,* ed 20, Norwalk, Conn, 1992, Appleton & Lange.)

- *Mixed acid fermentation:* Members of the genera *Escherichia, Salmonella,* and *Shigella* within the Enterobacteriaceae use this pathway for sugar fermentation and produce a number of acids as end products—lactic, acetic, succinic, and formic acids. The strong acid produced is the basis for the positive reaction on the methyl red test exhibited by these organisms.
- *Butanediol fermentation:* Members of the genera *Klebsiella, Enterobacter,* and *Serratia* within the Enterobacteriaceae use this pathway for sugar fermentation. The end products are acetoin (acetyl methyl carbinol) and 2,3-butanediol. Detection of acetoin is the basis for the positive VP reaction characteristic of these microorganisms. Little acid is produced by this pathway. Thus organisms that have a positive VP reaction usually have a negative reaction on the methyl red test, and vice versa.
- *Butyric acid fermentation:* Certain obligate anaerobes, including many *Clostridium* species, *Fusobacterium,* and *Eubacterium,* produce butyric acid as their primary end product along with acetic acid, carbon dioxide, and hydrogen.

Aerobic Utilization of Pyruvate (Oxidation)

The most important pathway for the complete oxidation of a substrate under aerobic conditions is the Krebs or TCA (tri-carboxylic acid) cycle. In this cycle, pyruvate is oxidized, carbon skeletons for biosynthetic reactions are created, and the electrons donated by pyruvate are passed through an electron transport chain and used to generate energy in the form of ATP. This cycle results in the production of acid and the evolution of carbon dioxide (Figure 1-11).

Carbohydrate Utilization and Lactose Fermentation

The ability of microorganisms to use various sugars (carbohydrates) for growth is an integral part of most diagnostic identification schemes. The fermentation of the sugar is usually detected by acid production and a concomitant change of color resulting from a pH indicator present in the culture medium. In general, bacteria ferment glucose preferentially over other sugars, and therefore glucose must not be present if the ability to ferment another sugar is being tested.

One of the important steps in classifying members of the Enterobacteriaceae family is the determination of the microorganism's ability to ferment lactose. These bacteria are classified as either lactose fermenters or lactose nonfermenters. Lactose is a disaccharide consisting of one molecule of glucose and one molecule of galactose linked together by a galactoside bond. Two steps are involved in the utilization of lactose by a bacterium. The first step requires an enzyme, β-galactoside permease, for the transport of lactose across the cell wall into the bacterial cytoplasm. The second step occurs inside the cell and requires the enzyme β-galactosidase to break the galactoside bond, releasing glucose, which can then be fermented. Thus all organisms that can ferment lactose can also ferment glucose.

BACTERIAL GENETICS

No discussion of bacterial genetics is complete without first describing deoxyribonucleic acid (DNA) and ribonucleic acid (RNA). Historically, DNA was first discovered by Frederick Miescher in 1869. In the 1920s, Phoebus A.T. Levine discovered that DNA contained phosphates, five-carbon sugars (cyclic pentose), and nitrogen-containing bases. Later, Rosalind Franklin discovered the helical structure by x-ray crystallography. Most everyone is familiar with James Watson and Francis Crick, who both described the three-dimensional structure of the DNA molecule in the 1950s.

Anatomy of a DNA and RNA Molecule

DNA is a double helical chain of nucleotides. The helix is a double strand twisted together, which many scientists refer to as a "spiral staircase" (resembling the handrail, sides, and steps of a spiral staircase). Others refer to it as a "zipper with teeth."

A nucleotide is a complex combination of the following:
- A phosphate group (PO_4).
- A cyclic five-carbon pentose (the carbons in the pentose are numbered 1′ through 5′) sugar (deoxyribose), which makes up the "handrails and sides."
- A nitrogen-containing base, or the "steps," either a purine or a pyrimidine. A purine consists of a fused ring of nine carbon atoms and nitrogen. There are two purines in the molecule: adenine *(A)* and guanine *(G)*. A pyrimidine consists of a single ring of six atoms of carbon and nitrogen. There are two pyrimidines in the molecule: thymine *(T)* and cytosine *(C)*. A nucleotide is formed when the 5′ carbon of the sugar and one of the nitrogenous bases attaches to the 1′ carbon of the pentose sugar. These are the basic building blocks of DNA (Figure 1-12).

In the chain of nucleotides, bonds form between the phosphate group of one nucleotide and the 3′ sugar of the next nucleotide. The base extends out of the sugar. Adenine of one chain always pairs with thymine of the other chain, and cytosine of one chain pairs with guanine of the other chain. The bases are held together by hydrogen bonds. The information contained in DNA is determined primarily by the sequence of letters along the "staircase" or "zipper." The sequence *ACGCT* represents different information than the sequence *AGTCC*. This would be like taking the word "stops" and using the same letters to form the word "spots" or "posts," which have different meanings but all the same letters. The two complementary sugar phosphate strands run in opposite directions (antiparallel), 3′ to 5′ and 5′ to 3′, like one train with its engine going one way alongside a caboose of a train going the opposite direction (Figure 1-13). The direction is based on what is found at the ends of the strands; for example, phosphate attaches to the 5′ carbon of the sugar and OH group is attached to the 3′ carbon of the sugar.

DNA is also involved in the production of RNA. In RNA, the nitrogenous base thymine is replaced by uracil, another pyrimidine. Unlike DNA, RNA is single stranded and short, not double stranded and long, and contains the sugar ribose, not deoxyribose.

An interesting aspect is introduced. Human beings are 99.9% identical. In a human genome of 3 billion "letters," even one tenth of 1% translates into 3 million separate lettering differences, an important characteristic useful in forensic science, but with related importance in diagnostic microbiology using the bacterial genome. Bacterial genetics is increasingly important in the diagnostic microbiology laboratory. New diagnostic tests have been developed that are based on identifying unique RNA or DNA sequences present in each bacterial species. The polymerase chain reaction (PCR) technique is a means of amplifying specific DNA sequences and thus detecting very small numbers of bacteria present in a specimen. Genetic tests circumvent the need to culture bacteria, providing a more rapid method of identifying pathogens.

An understanding of bacterial genetics is also necessary to understand the development and transfer of antimicrobial resistance by bacteria. The occurrence of mutations can result

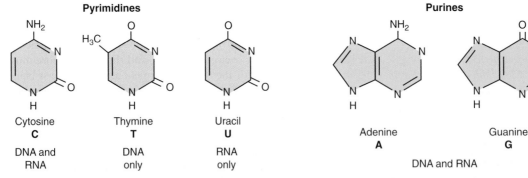

FIGURE 1-12 Molecular structure of nucleic acid bases. Pyrimidines: cytosine, thymine, and uracil. Purines: adenine and guanine.

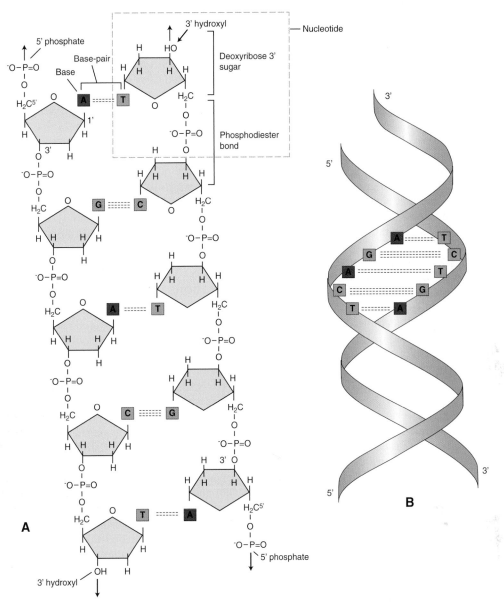

FIGURE 1-13   A, Molecular structure of DNA showing nucleotide structure, phosphodiester bond connecting nucleotides, and complementary pairing of bases (*A,* adenine; *T,* thymine; *G,* guanine; *C,* cytosine) between antiparallel nucleic acid strands. **B,** 5′ and 3′ antiparallel polarity and "twisted ladder" configuration of DNA.

in a change in the expected phenotypic characteristics of an organism and provides an explanation for atypical results sometimes encountered on diagnostic biochemical tests. This section briefly reviews some of the basic terminology and concepts of bacterial genetics. For a detailed discussion of DNA and molecular diagnostics, see Chapter 11.

Terminology

The genotype of a cell is the genetic potential of the DNA of an organism. It includes all the characteristics that are coded for in the DNA of a bacterium and that have the potential to be expressed. Some genes are silent genes, expressed only under certain conditions. Genes that are always expressed are constitutive. Genes that are expressed only under certain conditions are inducible. The phenotype of a cell consists of the genetic characteristics of a cell that actually are expressed and can be observed. The ultimate aim of a cell is to produce the proteins that are responsible for cellular structure and function and to transmit the information for accomplishing this to the next generation of cells. Information for protein synthesis is encoded in the bacterial DNA and transmitted in the chromosome to each generation. The general flow of information in a bacterial cell is from DNA (which contains the genetic information) to messenger RNA (mRNA) (which acts as a blueprint for protein construction) to the actual protein itself. Replication is the duplication of chromosomal DNA for insertion into a daughter cell. Transcription is the synthesis of single-stranded RNA (with the aid of the enzyme RNA polymerase) using one strand of the DNA as a template. Translation is the actual synthesis of a specific protein from the mRNA code. The term **protein expression** also refers to the synthesis (i.e., translation) of a protein. Proteins are polypeptides composed of amino acids. The number and sequence of amino acids in a polypeptide, and thus the character of that particular protein, are determined by sequence of codons in the mRNA molecule. A **codon** is a group of three nucleotides in an mRNA molecule that signifies a specific amino acid. During translation, ribosomes containing ribosomal RNA (rRNA) sequentially add amino acids to the growing polypeptide chain. These amino acids are brought to the ribosome by transfer RNA (tRNA) molecules that "translate" the codons. Transfer RNA molecules temporarily attach to the mRNA using their complementary anticodon regions. An **anticodon** is the triplet of bases on the tRNA that bind the triplet of bases on the mRNA. It identifies which amino acid will be in a specific location in the protein.

Genetic Elements and Alterations

Bacterial Genome

The bacterial chromosome (also called the *genome*) consists of a single, closed, circular piece of double-stranded DNA that is supercoiled in order to fit inside the cell. It contains all the information needed for cell growth and replication. Genes are specific DNA sequences that code for the amino acid sequence in one protein (e.g., one gene equals one polypeptide), but this may be sliced up and/or combined with other polypeptides to form more than one protein. In front of each gene on the DNA strand is an untranscribed area containing a promoter region, which the RNA polymerase recognizes for transcription initiation. This area may also contain regulatory regions to which molecules may attach and cause either a decrease or an increase in transcription.

Extrachromosomal Elements

In addition to the genetic information encoded in the bacterial chromosome, many bacteria contain extra information on small circular pieces of *extrachromosomal,* double-stranded DNA called **plasmids.** They are *not* essential for bacterial growth, so they can be gained or lost. Genes that code for antibiotic resistance (and sometimes toxins or other virulence factors) are often located on plasmids. Antibiotic therapy selects for bacterial strains containing plasmids encoding antibiotic resistance genes; this is one reason antibiotics should not be overprescribed. The number of plasmids present in a bacterial cell may vary from one (low copy number) to hundreds (high copy number). Plasmids are located in the cytoplasm of the cell and are self-replicating and passed to daughter cells, just like chromosomal DNA. They may also sometimes be passed (nonsexually) from one bacterial species to another through **conjugation** (horizontal transfer of genetic material by cell-to-cell contact). This is one way resistance to antibiotics is acquired.

Mobile Genetic Elements

Certain pieces of DNA are mobile and may jump from one place in the chromosome to another place. These are sometimes referred to as *jumping genes*. The simplest mobile piece of DNA is an insertion sequence (IS) element. It is approximately 1000 base pairs long with inverted repeats on each end. Each IS element codes for only one gene, a transposase enzyme that allows the IS element to pop into and out of DNA. Bacterial genomes contain many IS elements. The main effect of IS elements in bacteria is that when an IS element inserts itself into the middle of a gene, it disrupts and inactivates the gene. This can result in loss of an observable characteristic, such as the ability to ferment a particular sugar. Transposons are related mobile elements that contain additional genes. Transposons often carry antibiotic-resistance genes and are usually located in plasmids.

Mutations

A gene sequence must be read in the right "frame" for the correct protein to be produced. This is because every set of three bases (known as a *codon*) specifies a particular amino acid, and when the reading frame is askew, the codons are interpreted incorrectly. Mutations are changes that occur in the DNA code and often (not always; "silent mutations" do not make a change in the protein) results in a change in the coded protein or in the prevention of its synthesis. A mutation may be the result of a change in one nucleotide base (a point mutation) that leads to a change in a single amino acid within a protein or may be the result of insertions or deletions in the genome that lead to disruption of the gene and/or a frameshift mutation. Incomplete, inactive proteins are often the result. Spontaneous mutations occur in bacteria at a rate of about one in 10^9 cells. Mutations also occur as the result of error during DNA replication at a rate of about one in 10^7 cells. Exposure to certain chemical and physical agents can greatly increase the mutation rate.

Genetic Recombination

Genetic recombination is a method by which genes are transferred or exchanged between homologous (similar) regions on two DNA molecules. This method provides a way for organisms to obtain new combinations of biochemical pathways and copy with changes in their environment.

Mechanisms of Gene Transfer

Genetic material may be transferred from one bacterium to another in three basic ways:
- Transformation
- Transduction
- Conjugation

Transformation

Transformation is the uptake and incorporation of naked DNA into a bacterial cell (Figure 1-14, *A*). Once the DNA has been taken up, it can be incorporated into the bacterial genome by recombination. If the DNA is a circular plasmid and the recipient cell is compatible, the plasmid can replicate in the cytoplasm and be transferred to daughter cells. Cells

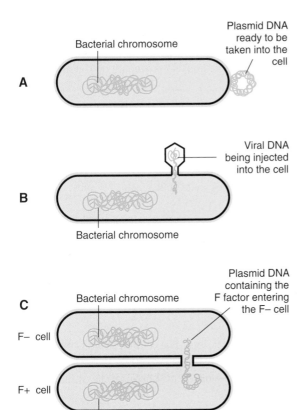

FIGURE 1-14 Diagram of methods of gene transfer into bacterial cells. **A,** Bacterial transformation. Free or "naked" DNA is taken up by a competent bacterial cell. After uptake, the DNA may take one of three courses: (1) it is integrated into existing bacterial genetic material, (2) it is degraded, or (3) if it is a compatible plasmid, it may replicate in the cytoplasm. **B,** Bacterial transduction. A phage injects DNA into the bacterial cell. The phage tail combines with a receptor of the bacterial cell wall and injects the DNA into the bacterium. One of two courses may then be taken. In the lytic cycle, replication of the bacterial chromosome is disrupted; phage components are formed and assembled into phage particles. The bacterial cell is lysed, releasing mature phage. In the lysogenic cycle, the phage DNA is incorporated into the bacterial genetic material, and genes encoded on the phage DNA may be expressed from this site. At a later time the phage may be "induced," and a lytic cycle will then ensue. **C,** Bacterial conjugation. An F– cell connects with an F– cell via sex pili. DNA is then transferred from one cell to the other.

that can take up naked DNA are referred to as being **competent.** Only a few bacterial species, such as *Streptococcus pneumoniae, Neisseria gonorrhoeae,* and *H. influenzae,* do this naturally. Bacteria can be made competent in the laboratory, and transformation is the main method used to introduce genetically manipulated plasmids into bacteria, such as *E. coli,* during cloning procedures.

Transduction

Transduction is the transfer of bacterial genes by a **bacteriophage** (virus-infected bacteria) from one cell to another (see

Figure 1-14, *B*). A bacteriophage consists of a chromosome (DNA or RNA) surrounded by a protein coat. When a phage infects a bacterial cell, it injects its genome into the bacterial cell, leaving the protein coat outside. The phage may then take a lytic pathway, in which the bacteriophage DNA directs the bacterial cell to synthesize phage DNA and phage protein and package it into new phage particles. The bacterial cell then lyses (lytic phase), releasing new phage, which can infect other bacterial cells. In some instances, the phage DNA instead becomes incorporated into the bacterial genome, where it is replicated along with the bacterial chromosomal DNA; this state is known as **lysogeny,** and the phage is referred to as being **temperate.** During lysogeny, genes present in the phage DNA may be expressed by the bacterial cell. An example of this in the clinical laboratory is *Corynebacterium diphtheriae.* Strains of *C. diphtheriae* that are lysogenized with a temperate phage carrying the gene for diphtheria toxin cause disease. Strains lacking the phage do not produce the toxin and do not cause disease. Under certain conditions a temperate phage can be induced, the phage DNA is excised from the bacterial genome, and a lytic state occurs. During this process, adjacent bacterial genes may be excised with the phage DNA and packaged into the new phage. The bacterial genes may then be transferred when the phage infects a new bacterium. In the field of biotechnology, phages are often used to insert cloned genes into bacteria for analysis.

Conjugation

Conjugation is the transfer of genetic material from a donor bacterial strain to a recipient strain (see Figure 1-14, *C*). It requires close contact between the two cells. In the *E. coli* system, the donor strain (F+) possesses a fertility factor (F factor) on a plasmid that carries the genes for conjugative transfer. The donor strain produces a hollow surface appendage called a *sex pilus,* which binds to the recipient F–cell and brings the two cells in close contact. Transfer of DNA then occurs. Both plasmids and chromosomal genes can be transferred by this method. When the F factor is integrated into the bacterial chromosome rather than a plasmid, there is a higher frequency of transfer of adjacent bacterial chromosomal genes. These strains are known as *high-frequency* (Hfr) *strains.*

Restriction Enzymes

Bacteria have evolved a system to restrict the incorporation of foreign DNA into their genomes. Specific **restriction enzymes** are produced that cut incoming, foreign DNA at specific DNA sequences. The bacteria methylate their own DNA at these same sequences so that the restriction enzymes do not cut the DNA in their own cell. Many restriction enzymes with a variety of recognition sequences have now been isolated from various microorganisms. The first three letters in the restriction endonuclease name indicate the bacterial source of the enzyme. For instance, the enzyme *Eco*RI was isolated from *E. coli,* and the enzyme *Hind*III was isolated from *H. influenzae* type d. These enzymes are used in the field of biotechnology to create sites for insertion of new genes. In clinical microbiology, epidemiologists use restriction enzyme fragment analysis to determine whether strains of bacteria have identical restriction sites in their genomic DNA.

BIBLIOGRAPHY

Baumann RW: *Microbiology*, San Francisco, 2004, Pearson Benjamin Cummings.

Campbell NA, Reece JB: *Essential biology*, San Francisco, 2001, Pearson Benjamin Cummings.

Forbes BA et al: *Bailey and Scott's diagnostic microbiology*, ed 12, St Louis, 2007, Mosby.

Holt JG et al: *Bergey's manual of determinative bacteriology*, ed 9, Baltimore, 1993, Williams & Wilkins.

Howard BJ: *Clinical and pathogenic microbiology*, ed 2, St Louis, 1994, Mosby.

Marieb EN: *Essentials of human anatomy and physiology*, ed 8, San Francisco, 2006, Pearson Benjamin Cummings.

Murray PR et al: *Medical microbiology*, ed 5, St Louis, 2005, Mosby.

Murray PR et al: *Manual of clinical microbiology*, ed 8, vol 1, Washington, DC, 2003, ASM.

Tortora GJ et al: *Microbiology: an introduction*, ed 7, San Francisco, 2002, Benjamin Cummings.

Points to Remember

- There are many organisms that inhabit our environment. The majority of these microorganisms are nonpathogenic.
- Prokaryotes, including bacteria, do not have membrane-enclosed nuclei and organelles.
- Eukaryotes differ from prokaryotes in that they have membrane-enclosed nuclei and organelles.
- Viruses cannot be seen under an ordinary light microscope, although their cytopathic effects on cell lines are visible. They are obligate parasites, and antibiotics are ineffective for their treatment. Viruses have DNA or RNA, but never both, in contrast to the prokaryotes and eukaryotes.
- Bacteria utilize two biochemical pathways, fermentation and respiration (oxidation) to catabolize carbohydrates to produce energy.
- The major way bacteria are classified in the diagnostic microbiology laboratory is by the Gram stain reaction. Whether an organism is gram-positive (blue or purple) or gram-negative (pink or red) is an important first step in identifying bacteria and in determining appropriate antimicrobial therapy.
- Bacterial spores are formed due to harsh environments. They are a means of survival, not reproduction.

Learning Assessment Questions

1. Explain the reason why the technologist should repeat the Gram stain procedure on the exudate.

2. What may have occurred to make the results invalid?

3. Differentiate the role of the pili from that of the flagella.

4. What is the role of the capsule in the pathogenesis of infectious diseases?

5. If the technologist forgets to add the Gram's iodine to the staining procedure, what will most likely occur?

6. Why is lipopolysaccharide (LPS) a significant outer-membrane structure in gram-negative bacteria?

7. Fimbriae present on the outer surface of bacteria are used for:
   a. Sexual reproduction
   b. Bacterial motility
   c. Adherence to surfaces
   d. Antibiotic resistance

8. Why are older bacterial cells more easily decolorized than younger colonies?

9. All of the following are characteristic of fermentation **except:**
   a. It follows glycolysis and produces NAD.
   b. It produces acids, alcohols, and gases.
   c. It occurs in the presence of oxygen.
   d. It begins with the breakdown of pyruvic acid.

10. Why are spore-forming organisms more resistant than non–spore-forming species?

11. Explain the three ways in which genetic material may be transferred from one bacterium to another.

12. For the following DNA, write the complementary sequence. Include labeling the 3' and 5' end.

    TTACGGACAAC

    _____

13. In RNA, thymine is replaced by_____.

Host-Parasite Interaction

Connie R. Mahon*, Maribeth L. Flaws

A. Role of the Usual Microbial Flora

- **ORIGIN OF MICROBIAL FLORA**
  Characteristics of Indigenous Microbial Flora
  Factors That Determine the Composition of the Usual
     Microbial Flora
- **COMPOSITION OF THE MICROBIAL FLORA AT DIFFERENT BODY SITES**
  Usual Flora of the Skin
  Usual Flora of the Mouth

Usual Flora of the Respiratory Tract
Usual Flora of the Gastrointestinal Tract
Usual Flora of the Genitourinary Tract
- **ROLE OF THE MICROBIAL FLORA IN THE PATHOGENESIS OF INFECTIOUS DISEASE**
- **ROLE OF THE MICROBIAL FLORA IN THE HOST DEFENSE AGAINST INFECTIOUS DISEASE**

OBJECTIVES

After reading and studying this chapter, you should be able to:

1. Define the following terms: *parasitism, indigenous flora, commensal, symbiont, opportunist, resident flora, transient flora,* and *carrier.*

2. Explain how the following factors determine the composition of the microbial flora at various body sites:
   - Amounts and types of nutrients available in the environment
   - pH
   - Oxidation-reduction potential
   - Resistance to antibacterial substances

3. List the predominant flora of various body sites in a healthy individual.

4. Describe the role of the usual microbial flora in the pathogenesis of infectious disease.

5. Describe the role of the indigenous flora in host defense against infectious diseases.

Case in Point

A 48-year-old woman had a complete hysterectomy. After 3 days of uneventful hospitalization, the patient was discharged from the hospital with a 10-day regimen of prophylactic antimicrobial. On the fifth day after her discharge, she noticed the presence of creamy-white, cheesy material on her tongue and buccal cavity. Wet mount preparations of the material showed budding yeast cells and hyphal elements.

Issues to Consider

After reading the patient's case history, consider:
- Factors that predisposed this patient to her current condition
- Clues that indicate the source of the infection
- Significance of the microbial flora in protecting the host against pathogenic organisms

Key Terms

Carrier
Carrier state
Commensalism
Indigenous flora
Opportunists
Parasite

Parasitism
Pathogen
Resident microbial flora
Symbiosis
Transient flora

*This chapter was prepared by C.R. Mahon in her private capacity. No official support or endorsement by the FDA is intended or implied.

The outcome from the interactions between host and **pathogen** is influenced by numerous factors. The status of the host's immune system and ability of the host to defend itself from microbial invasion, combined with microbial factors inherent to the invading organism, often determine whether disease will occur. To appreciate and understand the concepts involved in the pathogenesis of infectious diseases, knowledge and understanding of the host-pathogen relationship is important.

This chapter describes the interactions between the host and infectious agent in the pathogenesis of disease. The first section of the chapter describes the origin of the indigenous microbial flora and the composition at different body sites. It presents the role of the microbial flora at each body site in the host immune defense and as a source of opportunistic infections. Factors that determine the composition of the flora at different body sites are described. The second section of the chapter discusses the virulence factors that contribute to the invasiveness of organisms, protective mechanisms the host employs, and how microbes are able to evade the host's defenses. Lastly, this chapter describes factors that may make the host more susceptible to microbial infections and how microbes are transmitted and acquired.

ORIGIN OF MICROBIAL FLORA

The fetus is in a sterile environment until birth. During the first few days of life, the newborn is introduced to the many and varied microorganisms present in the environment. Each organism has the opportunity to find an area on or in the infant into which it is to adapt. Those that find their niche colonize various anatomic sites and become the predominant organisms. Others are transient or fail to establish themselves at all. As the infant grows, the microbial flora eventually becomes similar to that seen in older individuals.

Once established onto or into a particular body site of the host, microorganisms develop a particular relationship with that host. The host-microbe relationship, depending on the circumstance, may be one of **symbiosis, commensalism,** or **parasitism.** Symbiosis is defined as the association of two organisms living together. The organisms are called *symbionts*. Symbiosis as a biological relationship between two or more organisms where both (host and organism) benefit from one another may be described as *mutualism*. Lactobacilli in the urogenital tract of women offer a mutual association, providing the host protection by preventing colonization of pathogenic species at that site while the lactobacilli derive nutrients from the host. In the relationship where the organism benefits, but there is no beneficial or harmful effect to the host, the association between organisms is called *commensalism. Proteus mirabilis* is a commensal species in the gastrointestinal tract of humans. In parasitism, one species (microbe) benefits at the expense of the other (host). The parasite *Entamoeba histolytica* is a pathogenic intestinal amoeba that derives nutrients from the host at the expense of the host, causing intestinal ulcers and amebic dysentery.

Characteristics of Indigenous Microbial Flora

Microorganisms that are commonly found on or in body sites of healthy persons are called *normal, usual,* or **indigenous flora.** The different body sites may have the same or different flora, depending on local conditions. Local conditions select for those organisms that are suited for growth in a particular area. For example, the environment found on the dry skin surface is different from that found on the moist surfaces of the mouth and so the flora is different at the two sites.

Microorganisms that colonize an area for months or years are called **resident microbial flora,** whereas **transient flora** are those that are present at a site temporarily. Transient flora comes to "visit" but does not usually live or stay. They are eliminated by either the host inherent immune defenses or by competition with the resident flora. Some pathogenic organisms may establish themselves in a host without manifesting symptoms. However, these hosts, called **carriers,** are capable of transmitting the infection. These hosts' condition is called the **carrier state.** The carrier state may be acute (short-lived or transient) or chronic (lasting for months, years, or permanently). An example of a chronic carrier state is found in post-*Salmonella typhi* infection. This organism may establish itself in the bile duct and be excreted in the stool over years. In contrast, *Neisseria meningitidis* may be found in the nasopharynx of asymptomatic individuals during an outbreak of meningitis. After a few days or weeks at most, these individuals may no longer harbor the organism, in which case the carrier state would be termed *acute*. The most transient of carrier states is the inoculation of a person's hands or fingers with an organism (e.g., with *Staphylococcus aureus* that has colonized the person's anterior nares) that is carried only until the hands are washed.

The organisms colonizing different body sites play a significant role in providing host resistance to infections. The efficiency of the microbial flora in providing protection to the human host is indicated by the relatively small number of infections caused by these organisms in immune-competent individuals. Nevertheless, these organisms may cause significant, often serious, infections or may exacerbate existing infections in individuals lacking a fully responsive immune system.

Factors That Determine the Composition of the Usual Microbial Flora

Which organisms are present at a particular body site is influenced by the nutritional and environmental factors such as the amount and types of nutrients available at the site. For example, more organisms inhabit moist areas than dry areas; these areas are dominated by diphtheroids. Although lipids and fatty acids are bactericidal to most bacteria, *Propionibacterium* spp. colonize the ducts of hair follicles because these bacteria are able to break down the skin lipids to fatty acids. *Propionibacterium acnes* cannot be removed by washing or scrubbing. The affinity of microorganisms for a specific site depends on the ability of those organisms to resist the antibacterial effects of substances such as bile, lysozyme, or fatty acids. The composition of the microbial flora is also affected by pH. For example, the female genital tract flora depends on the pH of that environment, which in women of child-bearing age is approximately 4.0 to 5.0. Most bacteria do not survive at these extreme pH ranges. Another example is that of the fecal flora found in babies who are breast-fed, which differs from those in babies fed with cow's milk. Human milk has a high lactose concentration and maintains a pH of 5.0 to 5.5, an environment supportive of *Bifidobacterium* spp. Cow's milk, on the other hand, has a greater buffering capacity and is therefore less acidic. Infants fed with cow's milk do not have the high colonization by *Bifidobacterium* spp. found in breast-fed babies, but have instead colon flora similar to that seen in older children and adults (see Box 2-5). In areas of the body that have a low oxidation-reduction potential, the environment will support only organisms capable of fermentation, such as is seen in the gingival crevices colonized with *Bacteroides* and *Fusobacterium*.

The environmental conditions described here certainly may change with age, nutritional status, disease states, and drug or antibiotic effects. These changes may predispose an individual to infection by the indigenous flora, a type of infection referred to as an *opportunistic infection*. For example, two groups at increased risk for gram-negative rod pneumonia are diabetics and alcoholics. As described in the introductory case study, antibiotics may reduce a particular population of bacteria, allowing the proliferation of other organisms such as *Candida albicans*. An increase in age brings with it a decrease in the effectiveness of the immune response. As a result, the incidence of infection caused by opportunistic organisms increases.

COMPOSITION OF THE MICROBIAL FLORA AT DIFFERENT BODY SITES

The human host is colonized by approximately 100 different species of microorganisms and has a total organism load of about 100 trillion. The effectiveness of the various host defenses is evidenced by the relatively low incidence of infection in immune-competent individuals by members of the usual or indigenous flora. However, infections caused by members of the microbial flora are frequently encountered among immune-compromised patients. Because of this, the clinical microbiologist must be able to recognize and identify the types of microorganisms found at the various body sites.

Usual Flora of the Skin

Normal skin has a number of mechanisms to prevent infection and protect the underlying tissue from invasion by potential pathogens. These include the mechanical separation of microorganisms from the tissues, presence of fatty acids that inhibit many microorganisms, excretion of lysozyme by sweat glands, and the desquamation of the epithelium. The skin contains a wide variety of microorganisms, most of which are found on the most superficial layers of cells and the upper parts of hair follicles. The number of bacteria present on the skin can be reduced by about 90% by scrubbing and washing,

but they are not completely eliminated and their numbers return to normal within a few hours.

The composition of the flora on the skin depends on the activity of the sebaceous or sweat glands. Organisms concentrate the most in areas that are moist such as the armpit, groin, and perineum. The apocrine sweat glands in these areas secrete substances metabolized by the skin bacteria, releasing odorous amines. Aerobic diphtheroids are usually found in moist areas such as the axillae and between toes. *Staphylococcus epidermidis* and *Propionibacterium* spp. reside in hair follicles and colonize the sebaceous glands because they are resistant to skin lipids and fatty acids as well as to superficial antiseptic agents commonly used to cleanse the skin. The presence of skin bacteria inhibits the growth of more pathogenic bacterial species, thus providing benefits to the host.

Microorganisms such as *P. acnes* colonize the deep sebaceous glands. Superficial antisepsis of the skin does not eliminate this organism, which may be found as a contaminant in those culture specimens obtained by invasive procedures (e.g., blood, cerebrospinal fluid), as a result of contamination of the needle.

Box 2-1 lists the microorganisms most commonly found on the skin. Other organisms have been isolated from the skin but are found only occasionally or rarely and are therefore not listed.

Usual Flora of the Mouth

The mouth contains large numbers of bacteria, with *Streptococcus* being the predominant genus. Many organisms bind to the buccal mucosa and tooth surfaces. Bacterial plaques that develop on teeth may contain as many as 10^{11} streptococci per gram. Plaque also results in a low oxidation-reduction potential at the tooth surface; this supports the growth of strict anaerobes, particularly in crevices and in the areas between the teeth. Box 2-2 gives a partial list of microorganisms found in the mouth.

Usual Flora of the Respiratory Tract

The respiratory tract, commonly divided into upper and lower tracts, is responsible for the exchange of oxygen and carbon dioxide as well as for the delivery of air from the outside of the body to the pulmonary tissues responsible for that exchange. The upper respiratory tract is composed of the mouth, nasopharynx, oropharynx, and larynx; the lower respiratory tract is composed of the trachea, bronchi, and pulmonary parenchyma. The trachea, bronchi, and lungs are protected by the action of ciliary epithelial cells and by the

---

BOX 2-1 Microorganisms Found on the Skin

Common	Less Common
Candida spp.	*Streptococcus* spp.
Micrococcus spp.	*Acinetobacter* spp.
Staphylococcus spp.	*Bacteroides* spp.
Clostridium spp.	Gram-negative rods (fermenters
Propionibacterium spp.	and nonfermenters)
Diphtheroids	*Moraxella* spp.

BOX 2-2 Microorganisms Found in the Mouth

Common

Staphylococcus epidermidis
Streptococcus mitis
Streptococcus sanguis
Streptococcus salivarius
Streptococcus mutans
Peptostreptococcus spp.
Veillonella spp.
Lactobacillus spp.
Actinomyces israelii
Bacteroides spp.

Prevotella/Porphyromonas
Bacteroides oralis
Treponema denticola
Treponema refringens

Less Common

Staphylococcus aureus
Enterococcus spp.
Eikenella corrodens
Fusobacterium nucleatum
Candida albicans

BOX 2-3 Microorganisms Found in the Nose and Nasopharynx

Common

Staphylococcus aureus
Staphylococcus epidermidis
Diphtheroids
Haemophilus parainfluenzae
Streptococcus spp.

Less Common

Streptococcus pneumoniae
Moraxella catarrhalis
Haemophilus influenzae
Neisseria meningitidis
Moraxella spp.

BOX 2-4 Microorganisms Found in the Oropharynx

Common

α-Hemolytic and nonhemolytic
  streptococci
Diphtheroids
Staphylococcus aureus
Staphylococcus epidermidis
Streptococcus pneumoniae
Streptococcus mutans
Streptococcus milleri
Streptococcus mitis
Streptococcus sanguis
Streptococcus salivarius
Moraxella catarrhalis

Haemophilus parainfluenzae
Anaerobic streptococci
Bacteroides spp.
Prevotella/Porphyromonas
Bacteroides oralis
Fusobacterium necrophorum

Less Common

Streptococcus pyogenes
Neisseria meningitidis
Haemophilus influenzae
Gram-negative rods

---

movement of mucus. The tissues of these structures are normally sterile as a result of this protective action.

The mouth, nasopharynx, and oropharynx are colonized predominantly with viridans streptococci such as *Streptococcus mitis, Streptococcus mutans, Streptococcus milleri, Streptococcus sanguis*, and *Moraxella catarrhalis, Neisseria* spp., and diphtheroids. Obligate anaerobes reside in the gingival crevices where the anaerobic environment supports these organisms. The organisms found in the mouth, nasopharynx, oropharynx, and nose, although similar show some differences. Box 2-3 lists common microorganisms encountered in the nose and nasopharynx. Opportunistic pathogens such as *S. aureus*, found in approximately 30% of healthy individuals, colonize the anterior nares. The population of the nasopharynx mirrors that of the nose, even if the environment is different enough from that of the nose to select for several additional organisms. *Haemophilus influenzae, Streptococcus pneumoniae*, and *N. meningitidis*, all potential pathogens, are also found in the nasopharynx of healthy individuals. Individuals who are hospitalized for several days may become colonized in the upper respiratory tract by gram-negative bacteria, particularly members of the Enterobacteriaceae.

The oropharynx contains a mixture of streptococci. A number of species of the viridans group can be isolated, including *S. mitis, S. mutans, S. milleri, S. sanguis*, and *S. salivarius*. In addition, diphtheroids and *M. catarrhalis* can be readily isolated. Hospitalized patients often show colonization with gram-negative rods. The usual flora of the oropharynx is listed in Box 2-4.

Usual Flora of the Gastrointestinal Tract

The gastrointestinal tract comprises the esophagus, stomach, small intestine, and colon. The gastrointestinal tract is equipped with numerous defenses and effective antimicrobial factors. Because intestinal pathogens are usually acquired by ingesting organisms contained in contaminated food or drink, host defenses against infections are present throughout the intestinal tract.

Microorganisms usually do not multiply in the esophagus and stomach, but are present in ingested food and as transient flora. The stomach is usually sterile, especially after ingestion of a meal, when gastric juices, acids, and enzymes, which help to protect the stomach from microbial attack, are produced. Most microorganisms are susceptible to the acid pH of the stomach and are destroyed, with the exception of spore-forming bacterial species in their spore phase, the cysts of **parasites,** and *Helicobacter pylori*. Organisms that are pH-susceptible and survive are generally protected by being enmeshed in food, and they move to the small intestine. The stomach acidity greatly reduces the number of organisms that reach the small intestine.

The small intestine contains few microorganisms; organisms that are present are usually from the colon. Microorganisms prevalent in the colon may produce a count between 10^8 and 10^{11} bacteria per gram of solid material. Although we usually think of the facultative anaerobes as being the predominant organisms, anaerobes far outnumber the facultative gram-negative rods, making up more than 90% of the microbial flora of the large intestine. Gram-positive cocci, yeasts, and *Pseudomonas aeruginosa* are also usually present in the large intestine.

The gastrointestinal tract population may be altered by antibiotics. In some cases, certain populations or organisms are eradicated or suppressed and other members of the indigenous flora are able to proliferate. This can be the cause of a severe necrotizing enterocolitis *(Clostridium difficile)*, diarrhea *(C. albicans, S. aureus)*, or other superinfection. The bacteria constituting the usual intestinal flora also carry out a variety of metabolic degradations and syntheses that appear to play a role in the health of the host. A summary of the organisms found in the gastrointestinal tract is shown in Box 2-5.

Usual Flora of the Genitourinary Tract

The kidneys, bladder, and fallopian tubes are normally free of microorganisms, although there are a few organisms origi-

---

BOX 2-5 Common Microorganisms Found in the Gastrointestinal Tract

Bacteroides spp.	*Peptostreptococcus* spp.
Clostridium spp.	*Peptococcus* spp.
Enterobacteriaceae	*Staphylococcus aureus*
Eubacterium spp.	*Enterococcus* spp.
Fusobacterium spp.	

BOX 2-6 Microorganisms Found in the Genitourinary Tract

Common	Less Common
Lactobacillus spp.	Group B streptococci
Bacteroides spp.	Enterobacteriaceae
Clostridium spp.	*Acinetobacter* spp.
Peptostreptococcus spp.	*Candida albicans*
Staphylococcus aureus	
Staphylococcus epidermidis	
Enterococcus spp.	
Diphtheroids	

---

nating from the perineum that may be found in the distal centimeter of the urethra, particularly in women. The urethra is colonized in its outermost segment by those organisms found on the skin. The composition of the vaginal flora is consistent with hormonal changes and age. Before puberty and in postmenopausal women, vaginal flora primarily consists of yeasts, gram-negative bacilli, and gram-positive cocci. During child-bearing years, high estrogen levels promote the deposition of glycogen in vaginal epithelial cells. Lactobacilli metabolize glycogen in vaginal epithelial cells to maintain a low pH, creating an environment that is inhibitory to many organisms. The low pH, however, encourages colonization of the vagina with lactobacilli, anaerobic gram-negative bacilli, and gram-positive cocci. Microorganisms expected to be isolated from the genitourinary tract are listed in Box 2-6.

ROLE OF THE MICROBIAL FLORA IN THE PATHOGENESIS OF INFECTIOUS DISEASE

Some organisms that comprise the usual microbial flora are actually parasites that live off the host's nutrients, but in most cases provide some benefit to the host, creating a symbiotic relationship with the host, as mentioned earlier. However, certain members of the usual flora are **opportunists**; they cause disease when their habitat is damaged, disturbed, or changed, or when the host's immune system is weakened or compromised. In the case of trauma, either accidental or surgical, enough of the usual microbial flora found in the traumatized area may reach other areas in the body where these organisms are not part of the usual microbial flora. For example, patients who undergo surgery become susceptible to infections caused by organisms that colonize the particular surgical site (e.g., abdominal cavity); leakage following perforation of the colon spills the contents of the colon into the

peritoneal cavity, leading to an overwhelming infection by the colon flora.

The host's immune response may be reduced or altered due to suppression by immunosuppressive drugs, chemotherapy, or radiation. Individuals with lymphoma, leukemia, or other blood disorders in which there is a functional defect in phagocytic activity or a decrease in the number of functioning cells, or in which chemotactic activity is impaired, also may have a reduced immune response. Members of the usual microbial flora also may initiate an infection or make an infection more serious in patients with chronic illnesses such as diabetes or severe hepatic disease such as cirrhosis.

ROLE OF THE MICROBIAL FLORA IN THE HOST DEFENSE AGAINST INFECTIOUS DISEASE

The microbial flora provides beneficial effects. The development of immunologic competence depends on this flora. The immune system is constantly primed by contact with the microorganisms. Animals born and raised in a germ-free environment have a poorly functioning immune system. Exposure to otherwise innocuous organisms can be fatal to such animals. Likewise, consider how a sterile environment might affect a newborn. Antibody production would not be stimulated and the reticuloendothelial system would remain undeveloped. Serum IgG and other antibodies effective against microorganisms would be suppressed that would make the individual more susceptible to pathogenic species. Without activation by microorganisms and the supporting action of antigen-presenting cells and cytokines, cell-mediated immunity would not develop normally.

The microbial flora produces conditions at the microenvironmental level that block colonization by extraneous pathogens. When the composition of the indigenous flora is altered (e.g., by antibiotic therapy with broad-spectrum antibiotics), other organisms capable of causing disease may fill the void. For example, gastroenteritis due to *Salmonella* is generally not treated with antibiotics and is better eliminated by natural exclusion by the colon flora. If the microbial flora is eliminated, such as in patients receiving antimicrobial therapy or some types of chemotherapy, resistant or more pathogenic species may be able to establish infection. *C. albicans* may multiply and cause diarrhea or possibly infections in the mouth or vagina as illustrated in the Case in Point presented at the beginning of this chapter.

The microbial flora plays an important role in both health and disease. Eradication of the usual flora may have profound negative effects, yet many common infections are caused by members of the usual flora. Knowledge of the role of these organisms in the pathogenesis of an infectious disease is helpful in assessing their significance when isolated from clinical samples.

BIBLIOGRAPHY

Hentschel U, Steinert M, Hacker J: Common molecular mechanisms of symbiosis and pathogenesis, *Trends Microbiol* 8:226, 2000.

Kumar V, Fausto N, Abbas A, editors: *Robbins & Cotran pathologic basis of disease*, ed 7, Philadelphia, 2004, Saunders.

Mandell G, Bennett J, Dolin R: *Mandell, Douglas and Bennett's principles and practice of infectious diseases*, ed 6, New York, 2005, Churchill Livingstone.

McKenzie SB: *Clinical laboratory hematology*, Upper Saddle River, NJ, 2009, Pearson Prentice Hall.

Mims C, Nash A, Stephen J: *Mim's pathogenesis of infectious disease*, ed 5, San Diego, 2001, Academic Press.

Moran NA, Baumann P: Bacterial endosymbionts in animals, *Curr Opin Microbiol* 3:270, 2000.

Nelson KE, Masters Williams CF: *Infectious disease epidemiology: theory and practice*, ed 2, 2006, Jones & Bartlett.

Sheldon GF: *Boyd's introduction to the study of disease*, ed 11, Philadelphia, 1992, Lea & Febiger.

Sharp S: Commensal and pathogenic microorganisms of humans. In Murray PR et al, editors: *Manual of clinical microbiology*, ed 9, Washington DC, 2007, ASM Press.

Winn W et al, editors: *Koneman's color atlas and textbook of diagnostic microbiology*, ed 6, Philadelphia, 2005, Lippincott Williams & Wilkins.

Points to Remember

- Humans do not exist in a sterile environment. Colonization of the body by microorganisms begins at birth.
- The usual microbial flora present at each site in the body is dictated by nutritional and environmental factors.
- Some species of the usual microbial flora may be opportunists, capable of causing disease in an immunocompromised host.
- The usual microbial flora benefits the normal host by priming the immune system, out-competing potential pathogens for nutrients, and creating a hostile environment for other microbes.

Learning Assessment Questions

1. How did the patient in the case study develop the yeast infection in her mouth?
2. What is the difference between resident and transient flora?
3. What is a carrier?
4. What is the significance of the carrier in the pathogenesis of disease?
5. What determines the composition of the indigenous flora at the different body sites?
6. A long-term resident species of bacteria in the gastrointestinal tract produces vitamin K, which is required for blood clotting in mammals. Of what type of host-parasite relationship is this an example?
7. What are the functions of the microbial flora as a host protective mechanism?

B. Pathogenesis of Infection

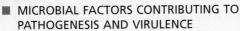

- ■ MICROBIAL FACTORS CONTRIBUTING TO PATHOGENESIS AND VIRULENCE
  - Pathogenesis
  - Virulence
  - Ability to Resist Phagocytosis
  - Surface Structures That Promote Adhesion to Host Cells and Tissues
  - Ability to Survive Intracellularly and Proliferate
  - Ability to Produce Extracellular Toxins and Enzymes
- ■ HOST RESISTANCE FACTORS
  - Physical Barriers
  - Cleansing Mechanisms
  - Antimicrobial Substances
  - Indigenous Microbial Flora

  - Phagocytosis
  - Inflammation
  - Immune Responses
- ■ MECHANISMS BY WHICH MICROBES MAY OVERCOME THE HOST DEFENSES
- ■ ROUTES OF TRANSMISSION
  - Airborne Transmission
  - Transmission by Food and Water
  - Close Contact
  - Cuts and Bites
  - Arthropods
  - Zoonoses

OBJECTIVES

After reading and studying this chapter, you should be able to:

1. Define the following terms: *true pathogen, opportunistic pathogen,* and *virulence.*

2. Differentiate the mechanisms of infections caused by true pathogens from those caused by opportunistic pathogens.

3. Discuss the conditions that must be present or events that must occur for a microorganism to cause disease.

4. Name the characteristics of infectious agents that enable them to cause disease in the host.

5. Describe the factors and mechanisms by which the human host is protected from microbial invasion.

6. Discuss the sequence of events in the phagocytosis and killing of an infectious agent.

7. Name the routes of transmission that microorganisms use to initiate infection in a host and give examples of each.

Case in Point

A 52-year-old man was taken to the emergency department in a disoriented and unresponsive state, experiencing shortness of breath. The patient had a history of poorly controlled diabetes, chronic obstructive pulmonary disease, and Kaposi's sarcoma of the right leg. He had a history of homosexual activities and for several years had received steroid therapy. The patient had a diagnosis of acquired immunodeficiency syndrome.

On admission, physical examination showed that the patient was slightly febrile and in respiratory failure. A few days later he became progressively anemic, his mental status deteriorated, and a diagnosis of meningitis was made. Microbiologic studies performed on the cerebrospinal fluid identified *Cryptococcus neoformans.*

Issues to Consider

After reading the case history, consider:

- Factors that predisposed this patient to his current condition
- Role of the host innate and acquired immunity in protecting the host from infection

- Significance of microbial virulence factors in promoting infection

Key Terms

Adaptive immunity	Fimbriae
Adhesin	Glycolysis
Anamnestic immune response	Humoral immune response
Antibody	Iatrogenic infection
Antigen	Immune response
Bacteriocidal effect	Immune system
Bacteriocin	Immunoglobulin A (IgA)
Chemotactic agent	Immunoglobulin E (IgE)
Chemotaxis	Immunoglobulin G (IgG)
Complement	Immunoglobulin M (IgM)
Diapedesis	Immunoglobulins
Dissemination	Innate immunity
Endotoxin	Interferon
Exotoxin	Lactoferrin

Leukocidin

Lymphocyte

Lymphokine

Lysozyme

Opsonin

Opsonization

Panton-Valentine

Pathogenicity

Phagocyte

Phagocytosis

Pili

Respiratory burst

True pathogen

Virulence

Zoonoses

TABLE 2-1 Abbreviated List of Opportunistic Microorganisms

Conditions Compromising Host Defenses	Organism(s)
Foreign bodies (catheters, shunts, prosthetic heart valves)	*Staphylococcus epidermidis* *Propionibacterium acnes* *Aspergillus* spp. *Candida albicans* Viridans streptococci *Serratia marcescens* *Pseudomonas aeruginosa*
Alcoholism	*Streptococcus pneumoniae* *Klebsiella pneumoniae*
Burns	*Pseudomonas aeruginosa*
Hematoproliferative disorders	*Cryptococcus neoformans* Varicella-zoster virus
Cystic fibrosis	*Pseudomonas aeruginosa* *Burkholderia cepacia*
Immunosuppression (drugs, congenital disease)	*Candida albicans* *Pneumocystis jiroveci* (*carinii*) Herpes simplex virus *Aspergillus* spp. Diphtheroids Cytomegalovirus *Staphylococcus* spp. *Pseudomonas* spp.

The relationship that exists between the human host and the microbial world is exceedingly complex. Each component of this relationship is in constant interaction with the other. The relationship is an equilibrium that is in constant motion and subject to change. Nutrition, stress, genetic background, and the presence of other diseases are additional influences that have an effect on the outcome of the meeting of human and microbe. This part of Chapter 2 discusses the role of each of the factors in host-pathogen interaction and how the host interacts with the microbe to prevent the onset of a disease process.

MICROBIAL FACTORS CONTRIBUTING TO PATHOGENESIS AND VIRULENCE

Pathogenesis

Pathogenicity is the ability of a microbe to produce disease in a susceptible individual. An organism may be described as a frank or true pathogen or as an opportunistic pathogen. **True pathogens** are organisms recognized to cause disease in healthy immune-competent individuals. Bacterial species such as *Yersinia pestis* and *Bacillus anthracis* are pathogenic in nearly all situations; when recovered in clinical samples taken from a body site, the clinical significance of these species is well established.

Over the last several years, patient populations have changed. Patients are living longer with their disease and are more likely to undergo highly invasive medical procedures, organ transplantation, and insertion of prosthetic devices, making them more susceptible to infections. As a result, organisms that are found as normal biota (normal flora) are being seen with increasing frequency in clinical infections among immunosuppressed and immunocompromised individuals. *Haemophilus influenzae* colonizes the upper respiratory tract of healthy individuals without causing disease, but given the opportunity, it may rapidly produce a life-threatening infection. Organisms such as *Staphylococcus epidermidis* under usual conditions do not cause disease, but can induce an infectious process in patients with prosthetic devices. *Haemophilus influenzae* and *S. epidermidis* are called *opportunistic pathogens* and the infections they cause are called *opportunistic infections*. Table 2-1 lists some of the common opportunistic microorganisms and the conditions with which they are most commonly associated.

Because of these situations, our definition of a pathogen must be expanded to apply to virtually any microorganism when conditions for infection are met. In deciding whether the isolation of a particular organism is a pathogen or not, we also must consider the human host from whom the organism was isolated and whether that host has underlying disease that may affect susceptibility to infection. For example, the potential pathogen list for a healthy 20-year-old college student is much shorter than for a healthy 90-year-old person, a transplant recipient, or a 20-year-old college student with AIDS. Because almost any organism in the right place can cause an infection, this needs to be considered when performing invasive procedures, because an inadvertent result of intervention can be the transfer of an organism from where it is present as part of the indigenous flora to a place where it can replicate and cause infection.

An **iatrogenic infection** is an infection that occurs as the result of medical treatment or procedures. For example, many patients who have indwelling urinary catheters develop a urinary tract infection. Although the catheter was a necessary procedure in the medical treatment of the individual, its use may result in an infection. Patients who are given immunosuppressive drugs because they have received a transplant are more susceptible to infection. Because any infection in such a patient would probably be the result of the physician-ordered drug therapy, it would be an iatrogenic infection.

Virulence

Virulence is the relative ability of a microorganism to cause disease or the degree of pathogenicity. It is usually measured by the numbers of microorganisms necessary to cause infection in the host. Those organisms that can establish infection with a relatively low infective dose are considered more virulent than those that require high numbers for infection. For example, because *Shigella* spp. causes disease with a relatively low infective dose, as few as 100 organisms, it is considered more virulent than *Salmonella* spp., wherein 10^5 colony-forming units (CFU) per milliliter of organisms are necessary to cause symptoms. This generalization is somewhat misleading because the severity of disease caused by different organisms varies from one to another. If a microorganism requires a relatively high infective dose but the disease it causes is often fatal, we tend to think of the microorganism as highly virulent. On the other hand, a different organism may require a low infective dose but produces a relatively mild disease.

Microbial Virulence Factors

Infectious organisms have a wide variety of mechanisms or virulence factors that allow them to persist in a host and cause disease. Some virulence factors, such as capsules and toxins, are used by many organisms. Other virulence factors tend to be specialized and specific to one particular organism, such as the tissue tropism of the gonococcus. Virulence factors allow the pathogen to evade or overcome host defenses and cause disease and encompass functions such as inhibiting phagocytosis, facilitating adhesion to host cells or tissues, enhancing intracellular survival after phagocytosis, and damaging tissue through the production of toxins and extracellular enzymes. Many virulence factors are well defined, such as the diphtheria and cholera toxins, the capsule of *Streptococcus pneumoniae*, and the fimbriae of *Neisseria gonorrhoeae*. Certain microorganisms produce extracellular factors that appear to aid in infection, but the exact role of these factors is unknown.

Ability to Resist Phagocytosis

Phagocytic cells such as macrophages and polymorphonuclear cells play a major role in defending the host from microbial invasion. In fact, the lack of phagocytic cells leaves the host susceptible to overwhelming infection. Therefore an extremely important event in the life of an invading pathogen that wants to survive in the host is avoiding phagocytosis. There are many ways by which microbial species evade phagocytosis. Table 2-2 lists some of the ways microorganisms interfere with phagocytic activities.

The most common mechanism for evading phagocytosis that is used by many different microorganisms is that of having a polysaccharide capsule on the surface. Many of those possessing a capsule are highly virulent (as in the Case in Point) until its removal, at which point their virulence becomes extremely low. Encapsulated strains of *S. pneumoniae* and *H. influenzae* are associated with highly invasive infections and are known to be more virulent than nonencapsulated strains. The capsule is composed usually of polysaccharides, but can also be made of proteins or a combination of protein and carbohydrate. The capsule inhibits phagocytosis primarily by masking the cell surface structures that are recognized by receptors on the surface of the phagocytic cell and in the same manner, inhibits the activation of complement by masking structures to which complement proteins bind.

TABLE 2-2 Microbial Interference with Phagocytic Activities

Microorganisms*	Type of Interference†	Mechanism (or Responsible Factor)
Streptococci	Kill phagocyte	Streptolysin induces lysosomal discharge into cell cytoplasm
	Inhibit chemotaxis	Streptolysin
	Resist phagocytosis	M substance
	Resist digestion	
Staphylococci	Kill phagocyte	Leucocidin induces lysosomal discharge into cell cytoplasm
	Inhibit opsonization	Protein A blocks Fc portion of Ab
	Resist killing	Cell wall mucopeptide
Bacillus anthracis	Kill phagocyte	Toxic complex
	Resist killing	Capsular polyglutamic acid
Haemophilus influenzae *Streptococcus pneumoniae*	Resist phagocytosis (unless Ab present)	Polysaccharide capsule
Klebsiella pneumoniae	Resist digestion	
Pseudomonas aeruginosa	Resist phagocytosis (unless Ab present) Resist digestion	"Surface slime" (polysaccharide)
Escherichia coli	Resist phagocytosis (unless Ab present)	O antigen (smooth strains) K antigen (acid polysaccharide)
	Resist killing	K antigen
Salmonella typhi	Resist phagocytosis (unless Ab present) Resist killing	Vi antigen
Cryptococcus neoformans	Resist phagocytosis	Polysaccharide capsule
Treponema pallidum	Resist phagocytosis	Cell wall
Yersinia pestis	Resist killing	Protein-carbohydrate cell wall
Mycobacteria	Resist killing and digestion	Cell wall structure
	Inhibit lysosomal fusion	?
Brucella abortus	Resist killing	Cell wall substance
Toxoplasma gondii	Inhibit attachment to PMN	?
	Inhibit lysosomal fusion	?

Adapted from Mims CA: *The pathogenesis of infectious disease,* ed 5, New York, 2001, Academic Press.
PMN, Polymorphonuclear neutrophil.
*Often only the virulent strains show the type of interference listed.
†Sometimes the type of interference listed has been described only in a particular type of phagocyte (polymorph or macrophage) from a particular host, but it generally bears a relationship to pathogenicity in that host.

Another bacterial structure that protects organisms from phagocytosis is Protein A. Protein A in the cell wall of *Staphylococcus aureus* helps the organism avoid phagocytosis by interfering with the binding of the host's antibodies to the surface of the organism. Antibodies bind to antigens via their

Fab or antigen-binding portion. Protein A binds to the Fc portion of IgG (at the opposite end of the Fab), preventing opsonization and phagocytosis by turning the antibody around on the surface.

Some organisms evade phagocytic cell killing by releasing potent materials in tissues that kill **phagocytes.** Streptococci produce hemolysins that lyse red blood cells but also induce toxic effects on white blood cells and macrophages. Pathogenic staphylococci release **leukocidins** that cause lysosomal discharge into cell cytoplasm. Staphylococcal leukocidin, called **Panton-Valentine,** is lethal to leukocytes and contributes to the invasiveness of the organism. Others inhibit chemotaxis, and thus the host is less able to direct polymorphonuclear neutrophils (PMNs) and macrophages into the site of infection.

Surface Structures That Promote Adhesion to Host Cells and Tissues

Most infectious agents must attach to host cells before infection occurs. In some diseases caused by exotoxins (e.g., botulism, staphylococcal food poisoning), adherence is not important. In virtually all other cases, however, the bacterium, virus, or fungus requires adherence to the host cell before infection and disease can progress. The cell surface structures that mediate attachment are called **adhesins.** The host cells must possess the necessary receptors for the adhesins. If the host or the infectious agent undergoes a mutation that changes the structure of the adhesin or the host receptor, adherence likely will not take place, and the virulence of the infectious agent is affected. Figure 2-1 illustrates surface bacterial structures that are involved in the pathogenesis of disease.

Virus infections depend on the cell being able to maintain an appropriate receptor for the virus particle. Infection of the cell occurs only if attachment is the initial event. The main adhesins in bacteria are the **fimbriae (pili)** and surface polysaccharides. Fimbriae enable bacteria to adhere to host cell surfaces, offering resistance by attachment to target cells, thereby increasing the organism's colonizing ability. Once attached, phagocytosis is less likely to occur. For example, the strains of *Escherichia coli* that cause traveler's diarrhea use their fimbriae to adhere to cells of the small intestine, where they secrete a toxin that causes the disease symptoms. Similarly, fimbriae are essential for gonococci to infect the epithelial cells of the genitourinary tract. Antibodies to the fimbriae of *N. gonorrhoeae* are protective by preventing the organism from attaching to the epithelial cells.

Ability to Survive Intracellularly and Proliferate

Some pathogens are able to survive within the phagocytic cell after they have been engulfed. These organisms have developed methods to prevent being killed intracellularly. Some prevent fusion of phagosomes and lysosomes, others have a resistance to the effects of the lysosomal contents, and still others escape from the phagosome into the cytoplasm.

To establish itself and cause disease, a pathogen must be able to replicate after attachment to host cells. Numerous host factors work to prevent proliferation. Secretory antibody, **lactoferrin,** and **lysozyme** are all produced by the host as a way to protect against infection. To be successful in establishing infection, infectious agents must be able to avoid or overcome these local factors. For example, lactoferrin competes with bacteria for free iron; meningococci can use lactoferrin as a source of iron. They are not inhibited by the presence of lactoferrin and, in fact, are able to use it for growth. On the other hand, the nonpathogenic *Neisseria* spp. are usually unable to use the iron in lactoferrin and thereby are inhibited by its presence.

Several pathogens (*H. influenzae, N. gonorrhoeae,* and *N. meningitidis*) produce an IgA protease that degrades the IgA found at mucosal surfaces. Other pathogens (influenza virus, *Borrelia* spp.) circumvent host antibodies by shifting key cell surface antigens. The host produces antibodies against the "old" antigens, which are no longer effective because the organism now has "new" antigens that do not bind to antibodies made against the old antigens.

In most situations when an organism is engulfed by macrophages, lysosomal contents are released into the phagocytic vacuoles and the organism is killed. If the engulfed organism is not exposed to intracellular killing and digestive processes, however, it is able to survive and multiply inside the macro-

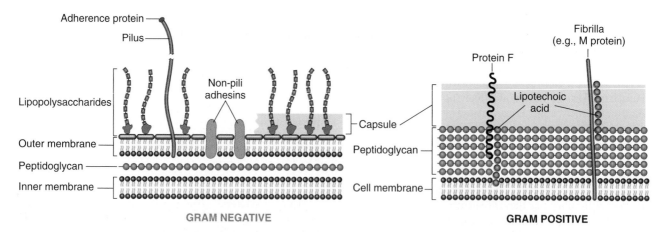

FIGURE 2-1 Surface bacterial structures that are involved in the pathogenesis of disease. (From Kumar V, Abbas AK, Fausto M: *Robbins and Cotran pathologic basis of disease,* ed 7, Philadelphia, 2005, Saunders.)

phage. Bacterial species such as *Chlamydia, Mycobacterium, Brucella,* and *Listeria* species are easily engulfed by macrophages and phagocytes; however, these species are not only able to survive inside the macrophages—protected from the host's other immune defenses—but are also able to multiply intracellularly.

Pathogens exhibit an ability to penetrate and grow in tissues. This process is called *invasion*. With some organisms, the invasion is localized and involves only a few layers of cells. With others, it involves deep tissues; for example, the gonococcus organism is invasive and may infect the fallopian tubes. With some organisms, such as *Salmonella* spp., the disease or organisms spread to distant sites (organs and tissues). This is called **dissemination.** Other organisms such as *Corynebacterium diphtheriae* do not spread beyond their initial site of infection, yet the disease they produce is serious and often fatal. Certain organisms that survive phagocytosis may be disseminated rapidly to many body sites, but the organisms themselves are not invasive. The phagocyte simply carries the organism, but the bacterium itself is incapable of penetrating tissues. *Clostridium perfringens* is an example of a highly invasive organism that may not necessarily disseminate.

Ability to Produce Extracellular Toxins and Enzymes

Generally, disease from infection is noticeable only if tissue damage occurs. This damage may be from toxins, either **exotoxins** or **endotoxins,** or from inflammatory substances that cause host-driven, immunologically mediated damage. The ability of organisms to produce exotoxins and extracellular enzymes is another major factor that contributes to the virulence and invasiveness of organisms. Toxins are poisonous substances produced by organisms that interact with host cells, disrupting normal metabolism and causing harm. Exotoxins are produced by both gram-negative and gram-positive bacteria and are secreted by the organism into the extracellular environment, or they are released upon lysis of the organism. Exotoxins can mediate direct spread of the microorganisms through the matrix of connective tissues and can cause cell and tissue damage. Some organisms produce soluble substances, such as proteases and hyaluronidases that liquefy the hyaluronic acid of the connective tissue matrix, helping to spread bacteria in tissues, thereby promoting the dissemination of infection. Endotoxins, on the other hand, are a constituent, the lipopolysaccharide (LPS), of the outer cell membrane of gram-negative bacteria exclusively. Endotoxins, in contrast to exotoxins, do not have enzyme activity, are secreted in only very small amounts, do not have specificity in their activity on host cells, are not very potent, and are not destroyed by heating.

Exotoxins

Many of the bacterial exotoxins are highly characterized. Most are composed of two subunits: the first is nontoxic and binds the toxin to the host cells; the second is toxic. The toxin gene is commonly encoded by phages, plasmids, or transposons. Therefore only those organisms that carry the extrachromosomal DNA coding for the toxin gene produce toxin.

Isolates of *Clostridium difficile,* for example, have to be tested for toxin production. Other pathogenic bacteria show similarities. Diphtheria toxin inhibits protein synthesis and affects the heart, nerve tissue, and liver. Botulinum toxin is a neurotoxin that blocks nerve impulse transmission, causing flaccid paralysis, especially in infants. *Streptococcus pyogenes* and *S. aureus* both produce exfoliatin, which causes rash and massive skin peeling or exfoliation. Table 2-3 lists many of the bacterial exotoxins that are important in disease production as examples.

Endotoxins

Endotoxins are composed of the LPS portion of the outer membrane on the cell wall of gram-negative bacteria. The cell wall of gram-negative microorganisms is composed of two layers, the inner peptidoglycan layer and an outer membrane. The LPS is contained in the outer membrane along with proteins and phospholipids (see Figure 2-1). LPS contains three regions: an antigenic O–specific polysaccharide, a core polysaccharide, and an inner lipid A (also called *endotoxin*). The toxic activity of endotoxin is found in the lipid A portion of the LPS. The effects of endotoxin consist of dramatic changes in blood pressure, clotting, body temperature, circulating blood cells, metabolism, humoral immunity, cellular immunity, and resistance to infection. Endotoxin stimulates the fever centers in the hypothalamus. An increase in body temperature occurs within an hour after exposure. Exposure to endotoxin also causes hypotension. Severe hypotension occurs within 30 minutes after exposure. Septic or endotoxic shock is a serious and potentially life-threatening problem. Unlike shock caused by fluid loss, such as that seen in severe bleeding, septic shock is unaffected by fluid administration. The endotoxin also initiates coagulation, which can result in intravascular coagulation. This process depletes clotting factors and activates fibrinolysis so that fibrin-split products accumulate in the blood. These fragments are anticoagulants and can cause serious bleeding. Another feature of patients with endotoxic shock is severe neutropenia, which can occur within minutes after exposure. It results from sequestration of neutrophils in capillaries of the lung and other organs. Leukocytosis follows neutropenia because neutrophils are released from the bone marrow.

Endotoxin also produces a wide variety of effects on the immune system. It stimulates proliferation of B lymphocytes in some animal species, activates macrophages, activates complement, and has an adjuvant effect with protein antigens. It also stimulates interferon production and causes changes in carbohydrates, lipids, iron, and sensitivity to epinephrine. A severe infection with gram-negative bacteria therefore can lead to serious and often life-threatening situations. A comparison of bacterial exotoxins and endotoxins is given in Table 2-4.

HOST RESISTANCE FACTORS

Physical Barriers

Humans have evolved a complex system of defense mechanisms to prevent infectious agents from gaining access to and

TABLE 2-3 Examples of Exotoxins of Pathogenic Bacteria

Bacterium	Disease Caused in Humans	Toxins
Bacillus anthracis	Anthrax	Complex, lethal, edema-producing toxin
Bordetella pertussis	Whooping cough	Lethal, dermonecrotizing toxin
Clostridium botulinum	Botulism	6 type-specific lethal neurotoxins*
Clostridium oedematiens	Gas gangrene	Alpha, lethal, dermonecrotizing
		Beta, lethal, dermonecrotizing, hemolytic
		Gamma, lethal, dermonecrotizing, hemolytic
		Delta, hemolytic
		Epsilon, lethal, hemolytic
		Zeta, hemolytic
Clostridium perfringens	Gas gangrene and enteritis necroticans	Alpha, lethal, dermonecrotizing, hemolytic*
		Beta, lethal
		Gamma, lethal
		Delta, lethal
		Epsilon, lethal, dermonecrotizing
		Eta, lethal (?)
		Iota, lethal, dermonecrotizing
		Theta, lethal, cardiotoxic, hemolytic
		Kappa, lethal, proteolytic
		Enterotoxin*
Clostridium septicum	Gas gangrene	Alpha, letal, hemolytic
Clostridium sordellii	Gas gangrene	Edema-producing toxin
		Hemorrhagic toxin
Clostridium tetani	Tetanus	Tetanospasmin, lethal, neurotoxic*
		Neurotoxin, nonspasmogenic
		Tetanolysin, lethal, cardiotoxic, hemolytic
Corynebacterium diphtheriae	Diphtheria	Diphtheria toxin, lethal, dermonecrotizing*
Escherichia coli	Diarrhea	Heat-labile enterotoxin*
		Heat-stable enterotoxin
		Shiga toxin
Pseudomonas aeruginosa	Pyogenic infections	Exotoxin A
Staphylococcus aureus	Pyogenic infections, enterotoxemia	Alpha, lethal, dermonecrotizing, hemolytic
		Beta, lethal, hemolytic
		Gamma, lethal, hemolytic
		Delta, hemolytic
		Exfoliating toxin*
		Enterotoxin*
Streptococcus pyogenes	Pyogenic infections, scarlet fever, rheumatic fever	Dick toxin, erythrogenic, nonlethal
		Streptolysin O, lethal, hemolytic, cardiotoxic
		Streptolysin S, lethal, hemolytic
Vibrio cholerae	Cholera	Cholera toxin, lethal, enterotoxic*
Salmonella typhimurium	Enteritis	Enterotoxin?*
Shigella sp.	Dysentery	Enterotoxin*
Yersinia pestis	Plague	Murine toxin

From Braude AI, Davis CE, Fierer J, editors: *Infectious diseases and medical microbiology*, Philadelphia, 1986, Saunders.
*Indicates toxins that produce harmful effects of infectious disease.

replicing in the body. Healthy skin is an effective barrier against infection. The stratified and cornified epithelium presents a mechanical barrier to penetration by most microorganisms. Organisms that can cause infection by penetrating the mucous membrane epithelium usually cannot penetrate unbroken skin. Only a few microorganisms are capable of entering the body by way of intact skin. Some of these microorganisms, and others that normally enter when the skin barrier is compromised, are listed in Table 2-5. Most of the organisms listed in Table 2-5 require help in breaking the skin barrier (e.g., animal or arthropod bite). Those capable of penetrating normal, healthy skin are few and include *Lepto-spira* spp., *Francisella tularensis*, *Treponema* spp., and some fungi. Even these organisms probably require microscopic breaks in the skin surface. Healthy, intact skin is clearly the primary mechanical barrier to infection. The skin also has substantial numbers of microbial flora that are usually not pathogens, organisms that contribute to a low pH, compete for nutrients, and produce bactericidal substances. In addition, the low pH resulting from long-chain fatty acids secreted by sebaceous glands ensures that relatively few organisms can survive and prosper in the acid environment of the skin. These conditions prevent colonization by transient, possibly pathogenic organisms.

TABLE 2-4 Differences Between Bacterial Exotoxins and Endotoxins

Characteristic	Exotoxins	Endotoxins
Organism type	Gram-positive and gram-negative	Gram-negative
Part of or secreted from organism	Part of and secreted from organism	Part of organism
Chemical nature	Simple protein	Protein-lipid-polysaccharide
Stability to heating (100° C)	Labile	Stable
Detoxification by formaldehyde	Detoxified	Not detoxified
Neutralization by homologous antibody	Complete	Partial
Biologic activity	Individual to toxin	Same for all toxins
Toxicity compared with strychnine as 1	100 to 1,000,000	0.1

Modified from Braude AI, Davis CE, Fierer J, editors: *Infectious diseases and medical microbiology*, Philadelphia, 1986, Saunders.

TABLE 2-5 Microorganisms That Infect Skin or Enter the Body via the Skin

Microorganisms	Disease	Comments
Arthropod-borne viruses	Various fevers, encephalitides	150 distinct viruses, transmitted by infected arthropod bites
Rabies virus	Rabies	Bites from infected animals
Vaccinia virus	Skin lesion	Vaccination against smallpox
Rickettsieae	Typhus, spotted fevers	Infestation with infected arthropods
Leptospira	Leptospirosis	Contact with water containing infected animal urine
Staphylococci	Boils, impetigo	Most common skin invaders
Streptococci	Impetigo, erysipelas	
Bacillus anthracis	Cutaneous anthrax	Systemic disease following local lesion at inoculation site
Treponema pallidum and *pertenue*	Syphilis, yaws	Warm, moist skin is more susceptible
Yersinia pestis	Plague	Bite from infected rat flea
Plasmodium spp.	Malaria	Bite from infected mosquito
Dermatophytes	Ringworm, athlete's foot	Infection restricted to skin, nails, and hair

From Mims CA: *The pathogenesis of infectious disease*, ed 5, San Diego, 2001, Academic Press.

Cleansing Mechanisms

Normally the term *cleansing* brings to mind a liquid. One of the most effective cleansing mechanisms humans have, however, is the desquamation of the skin surface. The keratinized squamous epithelium or outer layer of skin is being shed continuously. Many of the microorganisms colonizing the skin are disposed of with the sloughing of the epithelium.

More obvious is the cleansing action of the fluids of the eye and the respiratory, digestive, urinary, and genital tracts. The eye is continually exposed to microorganisms, which means this organ has some highly developed antimicrobial mechanisms. Tears bathe the cornea and sclera. This not only lubricates the eye but also washes foreign matter and infectious agents away from the surface. Additionally, tears contain IgA and lysozyme.

The respiratory tract is also continuously exposed to microorganisms and is protected by nasal hairs, ciliary epithelium, and mucous membranes. A continuous flow of mucus emanates from the membranes lining the nasopharynx, which traps particles and microbes and sweeps them to the oropharynx, where they are either expectorated or swallowed. The trachea is lined with ciliary epithelium. These cells have hairlike extensions (cilia) that sweep particles and organisms upward toward the oropharynx. This material is then expectorated or swallowed. Heavy smokers have a significant reduction in ciliated epithelial cells and therefore are more susceptible to respiratory infections. The purpose of these mechanisms is to prevent infectious agents and other particles from reaching the bronchioles and lungs. Under normal conditions, they are very effective, and the air moving into and out of the lungs is sterile.

Bacteria are swallowed into the gastrointestinal tract either as part of the mouth flora and upper respiratory tract or in liquids and food. Most bacteria are easily destroyed by the low pH found in the stomach. Some bacteria, however, are able to survive and pass into the small intestine. The number of bacteria in the intestine increases as the distance from the stomach increases. The distal portion of the colon contains the highest number of organisms. The gastrointestinal tract is protected by mucous secretions and peristalsis that prevent the organisms from attaching to the intestinal epithelium. Additionally, secretory antibody and phagocytic cells lining the mucosa defend the gastrointestinal tract against infection.

The genitourinary tract is cleansed by voiding urine. Consequently, only the outermost portions of the urethra have a microbial population. The vagina contains a large population of organisms as part of the indigenous flora. The acidity of the vagina, resulting from the breakdown of glycogen by the resident flora, tends to inhibit transient organisms from colonizing.

Antimicrobial Substances

A variety of substances produced in the human host have antimicrobial activity. Some are produced as part of the phagocytic defense and are discussed later. Others, such as fatty acids, hydrogen chloride (HCl) in the stomach, and secretory IgA have already been mentioned. A substance that plays a major role in resistance to infection is lysozyme, a low–molecular-weight (approximately 20,000 daltons) enzyme that hydrolyzes the peptidoglycan layer of bacterial cell walls. In some bacteria, the peptidoglycan layer is directly accessible to lysozyme. These bacteria are killed by the enzyme alone. In other bacteria, the peptidoglycan layer is exposed after other agents have damaged the cell wall (e.g., antibody and complement, hydrogen peroxide). In these cases, lysozyme acts with the other agents to cause death of the infecting bacteria. Lysozyme is found in serum, tissue fluids, tears, breast milk, saliva, and sweat.

Antibodies, especially secretory IgA, are found in mucous secretions of the respiratory, genital, and digestive tracts. They may serve as opsonins, thereby enhancing phagocytosis, or they may fix complement and neutralize the infecting organism.

Serum also contains low–molecular-weight cationic proteins, termed *β-lysins*. These proteins are lethal against gram-positive bacteria and are released from platelets during coagulation. The site of action is the cytoplasmic membrane.

These antimicrobial substances and systems work best together. A combination of antibody, complement, lysozyme, and β-lysin is significantly more effective in killing bacteria than each alone or than any combination in which one or more are missing.

Proliferation of viruses is inhibited by **interferon.** The interferons are a group of cellular proteins induced in eukaryotic cells in response to virus infection or other inducers. Uninfected cells that have been exposed to interferon are refractory to virus infection. A number of bacteria, viruses, and their products induce interferon production. The interferon produced binds to the surface receptors on noninfected cells. This binding stimulates the cell to synthesize enzymes that inhibit viral replication over several days. The antiviral effect of interferon is only one action it exhibits.

One type of interferon, interferon-gamma, plays an especially important role in the immune response. It inhibits cell proliferation and tumor growth, and enhances phagocytosis by macrophages, the activity of natural killer cells, and the generation of cytotoxic T cells.

Indigenous Microbial Flora

Nonpathogenic microorganisms compete with pathogens for nutrients and space. This competition lessens the chance that the pathogen will colonize the host. Some normal flora species produce **bacteriocins,** substances that inhibit the growth of closely related bacteria. These proteins are produced by a variety of gram-positive and gram-negative bacteria and appear to give the secreting bacterium an advantage, because they can eliminate other bacteria that would compete for nutrients and space. Some species of bacteria produce metabolic by-products that result in a microenvironment hostile to potential pathogens. Vitamins and other essential nutrients are synthesized by certain bacteria in the intestine and appear to contribute to the overall health of the host.

Phagocytosis

Phagocytosis is an essential component in the resistance of the host to infectious agents. It is the primary mechanism in the host defense against extracellular bacteria and a number of viruses and fungi. The PMNs and macrophages (monocytes in the peripheral blood) are the body's first line of defense.

The stem cells for neutrophils arise in the bone marrow, where they differentiate to form mature neutrophils. During this maturation, the cells synthesize myeloperoxidase, proteases, cathepsin, lactoferrin, lysozyme, and elastase. These products are incorporated into membrane-bound vesicles called *lysosomes.* The lysosomes contain the enzymes and other substances necessary for the killing and digestion of the engulfed particles. They show up as azurophilic granules on a Wright's stain. The PMN also has receptors on the cell membrane for some complement components that stimulate cell motion, the metabolic burst, and secretion of the lysosome contents into a phagosome. The PMN is an end-stage cell and has a circulating half-life of 2 to 7 hours. It may migrate to the tissues, where its half-life is less than 1 week.

Macrophages also originate in the bone marrow. They circulate as monocytes for 1 to 2 days and then migrate through the blood vessel walls into the tissues and reside in specific tissues as part of the reticuloendothelial system. These cells are widely distributed in the body and play a central role in specific immunity and nonspecific phagocytosis (Table 2-6).

Four activities must occur for phagocytosis to take place and be effective in host defense: (1) migration of the phagocyte to the area of infection (chemotaxis), (2) attachment of the particle to the phagocyte, (3) ingestion, and (4) killing.

Chemotaxis

The PMNs circulate through the body, followed by movement into the tissues by an action called **diapedesis,** which is movement of the neutrophils between the endothelial cells of the blood vessels into the tissues. The body is under constant surveillance by these and other phagocytic cells. When an infection occurs, massive numbers of PMNs accumulate at the site. This accumulation is not a random event; rather it is a directed migration of PMNs into the area needing their services. This migration is called **chemotaxis** (a chemical "taxi" or chemically caused movement). Several substances serve as **chemotactic agents.** These are certain components of complement, a number of bacterial products, products from damaged tissue cells, and products from responding immune cells. The initial contact of the PMN with an invading organism may be random. As the organism causes the body's defense mechanisms to respond via inflammation, directed

TABLE 2-6 Tissue Distribution of Monocytes/ Macrophages

Cell Name	Tissue Distribution
Monocyte	Blood
Kupffer cell	Liver
Alveolar macrophage	Lung
Histiocyte	Connective tissue
Peritoneal macrophage	Peritoneum
Microglial cell	Central nervous system
Mesanglial cell	Kidney
Macrophage	Spleen, lymph nodes

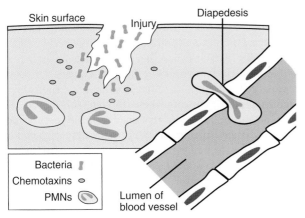

FIGURE 2-2   Phagocytosis: chemotaxis migration of phagocytes.

migration of phagocytes occurs (chemotaxis; Figure 2-2). The speed and magnitude of this response are easily visualized by recalling how quickly a splinter or similar injury becomes infected and how much pus is produced.

Attachment

One of the most effective defenses bacteria have against phagocytosis is the capsule. This structure prevents attachment of the organism to the neutrophil's membrane, which must occur before ingestion can take place. Attachment is facilitated by the binding of specific antibodies to the microorganism. The neutrophil membrane has a variety of receptors, including receptors for the Fc portion of IgG1, IgG3, and the C3b component of complement. These three factors can and do bind to the invading microorganism resulting in the invading microorganisms being coated with one or more of these factors. The receptor on the PMN for the particular factor coating the bacterium binds to the factor and forms a bridge that brings the bacterium into close physical contact with the leukocyte membrane. The coating of the bacterium with antibody or complement components results in enhanced phagocytosis by the PMN. This process or phenomenon is called **opsonization.**

The antibody and complement components are termed **opsonins.** Opsonization can be accomplished by three different types of responses: (1) IgG1 or IgG3 binding to the organism, (2) the antibody response is insufficient for opsonization, but complement is fixed on the surface of the organism, or (3) the alternative complement pathway is activated by the endotoxin or polysaccharides of the organism.

Ingestion

The next step of phagocytosis is ingestion. This process occurs rapidly following attachment. The cell membrane of the phagocytic cell invaginates and surrounds the attached particle. The particle is taken into the cytoplasm and enclosed within a vacuole called a *phagosome* (Figure 2-3). The phagosome fuses with lysosomes, which are vacuoles containing hydrolytic enzymes. The lysosomes release their contents into the phagosome, a process called *degranulation.* The list of enzymes found within the lysosomes is long—more than 20

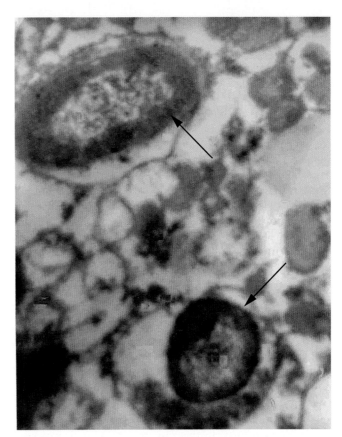

FIGURE 2-3   Engulfed bacterial cells inside phagosomes.

enzymes, including proteases, lipases, RNase, DNase, peroxidase, and acid phosphatase. Several of these are important in the killing and digestion of the engulfed bacterial cell.

Killing

The phagocytosis of a particle triggers a significant increase in the metabolic activity of the neutrophil or macrophage. This increase is termed a *metabolic* or **respiratory burst.** The cell demonstrates increases in **glycolysis,** the hexose monophosphate shunt pathway, oxygen use, and production of lactic acid and hydrogen peroxide. The hydrogen peroxide produced at this time diffuses from the cytoplasm into the phagosome. It acts in conjunction with other compounds to exert a **bactericidal effect.** In addition, other enzymes from the lysosome have antimicrobial action. They include lactoferrin, which chelates iron and prevents bacterial growth, lysozyme, and several basic proteins. The usual result is that a phagocytosed organism is quickly engulfed, killed, and digested.

Organisms that are "intracellular" (e.g., *Mycobacterium tuberculosis, Listeria monocytogenes, Brucella* spp.) are able to survive phagocytosis and, in fact, may actually multiply within the phagocyte. Obviously, other defense mechanisms must play a major role in immunity to these intracellular organisms.

The importance of phagocytosis is seen in patients with defects in the numbers or function of phagocytic cells. Such patients have frequent infections despite possessing high levels of serum antibody.

Many of the organisms listed in Table 2-2 are common isolates, which is not surprising, because they have developed a means to interfere with phagocytosis, thereby increasing their pathogenicity.

Inflammation

Inflammation is the body's response to injury or foreign body. Figure 2-4 illustrates the components involved in acute and chronic inflammatory responses. A hallmark of inflammation is the accumulation of large numbers of phagocytic cells. These leukocytes release mediators or cause other cell types to release mediators. The mediators cause erythema as a result of greater blood flow, edema from an increase in vascular permeability, and continued phagocyte accumulation, resulting in pus. The enzymes released by the phagocytes digest the foreign particles, injured cells, and cell debris. After the removal of the invading object, the injured tissue is repaired.

Immune Responses

This chapter gives a brief discussion on the immune system response to infection to provide the reader with an appreciation of its role and complexity. The balance between health and infectious disease is complex and mediated by humoral and cellular factors. As illustrated in the Case in Point at the beginning of this section, the relative importance of each factor depends on the microbe, route of infection, condition and genetic makeup of the host, and other factors yet to be clearly characterized. In this case, this AIDS patient would become susceptible to opportunistic organisms as his immune system continues to deteriorate.

Table 2-7 summarizes the defenses used by the human host against infection. Classically, the term *immunity* has been defined as a complex mechanism whereby the body is able to protect itself from invasion by disease-causing organisms. This mechanism, known as the **immune system,** consists of numerous cells and protein molecules that are responsible for recognizing and removing these foreign substances. This general definition has been broadened over the years to mean a reaction to any foreign substance, including proteins and polysaccharides, as well as invading microorganisms. Research advances over the years have dramatically increased our understanding of the basic **immune response** and given us an appreciation of the cellular interrelationships. The immune response can be divided into two broad categories. The first is known as *innate* or *natural immunity* with little or no specificity, and the second, called *adaptive* or *specific,* is highly specialized.

Innate, or Natural, Immunity

Innate immunity, also referred to as *natural* or *nonspecific immunity*, consists of several components. These include (1) physical and chemical barriers such as the skin and mucous membranes, (2) blood proteins that act as mediators of infection, and (3) a cellular mechanism capable of phagocytosis such as neutrophils and macrophages and other leukocytes such as natural killer cells. Figure 2-5 shows examples of the innate immune defenses located at different body sites. This first line of defense has a limited capacity to distinguish one organism from another; however, previous exposure to a particular foreign substance is not required. Physical barriers,

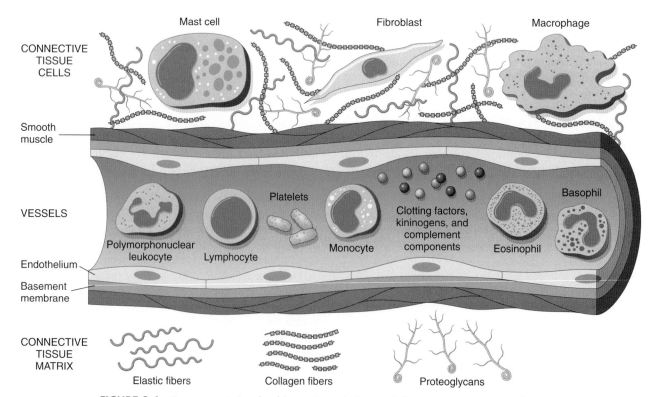

FIGURE 2-4   Components involved in acute and chronic inflammatory responses. (From Kumar V, Abbas AK, Fausto M: *Robbins and Cotran pathologic basis of disease*, ed 7, Philadelphia, 2005, Saunders.)

TABLE 2-7 Summary of Defenses of the Human or Animal Host to Infection and Evasion Mechanisms Attributed to Various Microorganisms

Host Defense	Mechanism of Evasion	Example
Hydrodynamic flow	Attachment	Fimbriae, surface proteins, lipoteichoic acid pseudomembrane of diphtheria
Mucus barrier	Attachment Penetration	Mannose-sensitive fimbriae
Deprivation of essential nutrients	Systems of high-affinity uptake	Iron metabolism
Lysozyme in secretions	Resistance to lysis	Substitution of peptidoglycan
Surface immunoglobulins	Absent or low immunogenicity Antigenic heterogeneity Masking of antigens Destruction	Hyaluronic acid, capsules Fimbriae, capsules, LPS, M protein, etc. Capsules, IgA-binding proteins IgA protease
Unbroken surface (epithelial cell surface)	Penetration	*Neisseria gonorrhoeae, Shigella* spp.
Unknown defenses in lymphatics (intercellular space)		*N. gonorrhoeae, Shigella* spp.
Serum defenses		
Recognition by antibody	Antigenic heterogeneity Masking of antigen Destruction of antibody Antigenic variation	Fimbriae, capsules, LPS, M protein Capsules, Ig-binding proteins *Borrelia*
Complement system	Failure to activate alternative pathway Inactivation of complement components Resistance to bacteriolysis Formation of abscess	Sialic acid capsules Cleavage of C3b in empyema fluids ColV plasmid *Bacteroides fragilis* capsule
Localization		
Fibrin tapping	Fibrinolysis	*Streptococcus* spp.
Abscess formation	Collagenase, elastase	*Pseudomonas, Clostridium*
Secondary immune response	Nonspecific B-cell activation Inhibition of delayed hypersensitivity Rapidly fatal (toxin)	LPS, lipoprotein Anergy of miliary tuberculosis Anthrax, plague, *Clostridium*
Phagocytosis	Inhibition of chemotaxis Inhibition of attachment and ingestion Inhibition of metabolic burst Inhibition of degranulation Resistance to permeability inducing cationic protein Resistance to oxidative attack Escape from phagosome Destruction of phagocyte	*Brucella, Salmonella, Neisseria, Staphylococcus, Pseudomonas* Capsules, M protein, Ig-binding proteins, gonococcal pili *Salmonella typhi* Mycobacteria Gram-positive cell wall, smooth LPS, polyanionic capsules Catalase, superoxide dismutase, carotenoid pigments *Mycobacterium bovis, Legionella pneumophila* *Streptococcus pneumoniae, Streptococcus pyogenes, Staphylococcus aureus, Pseudomonas aeruginosa*

Adapted from Gotschlich EC: Thoughts on the evolution of strategies used by bacteria for evasion of host defenses, *Rev Infect Dis* 5:S779, 1983.
LPS, Lipopolysaccharide.

mentioned earlier, may be as simple as the keratinized outer layer of the skin. Also, the secretions of the mucous membranes and the ciliated epithelial cells of the respiratory tract promote trapping and removal of microorganisms. In addition, many secretions provide a chemical barrier, such as the acidic pH of the stomach and vagina. Saliva and tears contain enzymes such as lysozyme, and the sebaceous glands of the skin contain oils capable of inhibiting invasion by pathogenic organisms. The normal biota of all of these sites adds another dimension to the host's ability to resist invading pathogens.

Once the physical and chemical barriers to infection have been penetrated, nonspecific mechanisms of innate immunity become operational. Phagocytic cells ingest and kill microorganisms, whereas activated complement components contribute to a wide variety of immunologic events, including promotion of attachment and engulfment of bacteria by neutrophils (opsonization) and attraction of neutrophils to sites of infection (chemotaxis). Collectively, these immunologic defense mechanisms, along with host tissue damage caused by the invading organisms, combine to produce an acute inflammatory response in the host. The importance of natural immune mechanisms rests in their rapid response to invading organisms. However, these mechanisms are effective primarily against extracellular bacterial pathogens, playing only a minor role by themselves in immunity to intracellular bacterial pathogens, viruses, and fungi.

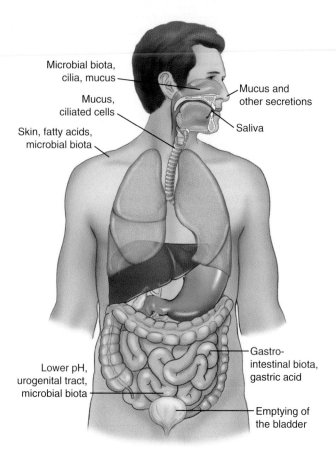

Microbial biota, cilia, mucus

Mucus, ciliated cells

Skin, fatty acids, microbial biota

Mucus and other secretions

Saliva

Lower pH, urogenital tract, microbial biota

Gastro-intestinal biota, gastric acid

Emptying of the bladder

FIGURE 2-5   Innate immune defenses located at different body sites.

Adaptive, or Specific, Immunity

Adaptive immunity is much more highly evolved and complex than innate immunity and enhances the protective capability of the innate defense. This arm of the immune response is capable of being specific for distinct molecules, responding in particular ways to different types of foreign substances, and developing memory, which allows for a more vigorous response to repeated exposures to the same foreign invader. Lymphocytes and their products, known as **antibodies,** are the major constituents of the adaptive or specific immune response. Antibodies are produced in response to antigens, substances that are capable of inducing the immune response.

An interrelationship exists between the mechanisms of the innate and the adaptive. For instance, inflammation, a non-specific response of the innate system, provides a signal that triggers an adaptive type of immune response. The adaptive immune system is able to enhance the protective mechanisms of the innate system, as previously mentioned. For instance, the activation of **complement** (a component of innate immunity) by invading bacteria is enhanced by the presence of specific antibodies (components of adaptive immunity). This activation leads to phagocytic clearance and elimination of the bacteria. The adaptive immune response adds a high degree of specialization to the passive mechanisms of the innate response. The nature of the adaptive immune response varies according to the type of organism and is designed to eliminate it efficiently. For example, antibodies are produced by B lymphocytes in response to blood-borne organisms and aid in their elimination. However, the response to phagocytosed antigens is primarily by T lymphocytes that produce chemicals that enhance the activities of the phagocytic cells. The nature and origin of these cells are described in the following paragraph. Most importantly, the specific response is able to remember each time it encounters a particular foreign antigen, called *immunologic memory*. Subsequent exposure to that antigen stimulates an increasingly effective and specific defense. Ultimately, the adaptive or specific immune response is the second line of defense and is able to significantly improve upon the first.

Lymphocytes originate in the bone marrow from stem and progenitor cells. Lymphocytes mature and take up residence in various body tissues and organs, including the thymus, lymph nodes, and spleen. They are a diverse group of cells that can be classified into two major types—T (thymus-derived) cells and B (bone marrow–derived) cells—on the basis of cell surface markers. The uniqueness of these cells lies in the presence of specific cell surface receptor molecules that recognize and bind a unique antigen, activating the cell to divide, differentiate, and secrete a number of effector substances. The millions of lymphocytes found in the body have been preengineered during embryogenesis to recognize a vast array of substances as foreign while learning which substances constitute self. Thus the result of encounter with the antigen is an expanded clone or clones of activated lymphocytes.

Nature of the Immune Response to Infectious Agents

Although both humoral immunity and cell-mediated immunity are important in protecting the human from a wide variety of infectious agents, each contributes differently, in terms of overall importance, according to the type of pathogen and virulence mechanisms. Whereas B lymphocytes play the predominant role in the **humoral immune response,** T lymphocytes mediate cellular immunity. Each B lymphocyte has surface receptors that recognize only one type of antigen. After antigen binding, the B lymphocyte undergoes multiple divisions, and the resulting cells, known as *plasma cells,* actively secrete proteins known as **immunoglobulins** or antibodies. All of the antibody molecules derived from a single clone of B cells are of a single specificity (recognize a unique antigen), identical to the receptor molecule on the original activated B cell. These antibody molecules circulate in the bloodstream and lymphatics, bathe body tissues, and bind to infectious agents or substances to aid the host in eliminating them from the body. The detection and quantification of these antibody molecules, obtained from a patient's serum, constitute the primary goal of diagnosing infectious diseases through serologic methods.

Classification and Characteristics of Antibodies

Antibody molecules, found in serum and other body fluids and secretions, may be classified into one of five distinct

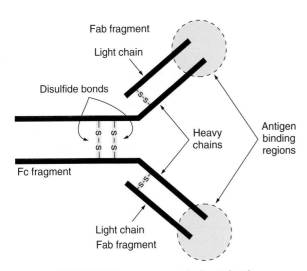

FIGURE 2-6   Immunoglobulin G (IgG).

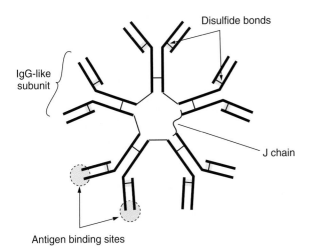

FIGURE 2-7   Immunoglobulin M (IgM).

TABLE 2-8 IgG versus IgM

Property	Immunoglobulin Class	
	IgG	IgM
Molecular weight (daltons)	150,000	900,000
Number of 4-polypeptide subunits	1	5
Number of antigen-binding sites	2	10
Serum concentration (mg/dL)	800-1600	50-200
Percentage of total immunoglobulin	75	10
Ability to cross placenta	+	−
Half-life (days)	23-25	5-8

developing fetus in the second or third trimester, as well as a newborn, may respond to an infectious agent with an IgM antibody response of its own. The IgM antibody molecules are large; the whole molecule has a molecular weight of about 900,000 daltons and consists of five basic subunits—each composed of two heavy chains and two light chains (similar to an IgG molecule) and linked to another polypeptide chain (J chain) by disulfide bonds (Figure 2-7). Thus the IgM molecule has up to 10 antigen-binding sites available. Both IgG and IgM antibodies are commonly assayed in a variety of serologic tests. The differences in size and configuration of IgG and IgM molecules result in differences in functional activity of the molecules in serologic tests (Table 2-8).

Immunoglobulin A (IgA) antibodies represent 15% to 20% of the total serum immunoglobulin pool. Immunoglobulin A constitutes the predominant immunoglobulin class in certain body secretions, such as saliva, tears, and intestinal secretions. Because of this association of IgA with mucosal surfaces, it provides protection against microorganisms invading at those sites. Serum IgA occurs primarily as two subunits (each similar to an IgG molecule) linked together by a J chain. When found in secretions, however, the molecule also contains a secretory component that stabilizes the molecule. Although significant increases in serum IgA may occur in association with certain infections, the function of serum IgA is unclear, and few serologic tests for the diagnosis of infectious disease are designed to specifically detect IgA antibody.

The remaining two immunoglobulin classes, IgD and IgE, are found in very low concentrations in serum (less than 1%). **Immunoglobulin E (IgE)** antibody levels rise during infection by a number of parasites and may play a role in eliminating these infectious agents from the host. Total serum IgE levels may rise during parasitic infection, and IgE-specific serologic tests for the diagnosis of a few parasitic agents have been developed. The role of serum IgD antibodies during infection is not known.

Primary and Secondary Antibody Responses

After exposure to an infectious agent, the host's acquired humoral immunity may respond through the production of various classes of antibody directed to one or more antigens associated with the agent. If the host has not been previously

immunoglobulin groups or classes. The classes differ from one another in several ways, including chemical structure, serum concentration, half-life, and functional activity.

Immunoglobulin G (IgG) class antibodies constitute about 70% to 75% of the total serum immunoglobulin pool. Their half-life in serum is about 3 to 4 weeks, and IgG can cross the maternal placenta to the fetus, possibly conferring some protection in both the prenatal and postnatal periods. Structurally, IgG is a protein with a molecular weight of about 150,000 daltons consisting of four polypeptides (two identical light chains and two identical heavy chains) bridged by several disulfide bonds (Figure 2-6). Although the amino acid sequence of some regions of the polypeptides is nearly identical among all IgG molecules (conserved regions), one of the ends of each polypeptide is highly variable. These variable regions create two active sites for antigen binding on each IgG molecule (see Figure 2-6). Thus IgG antibodies are said to be bivalent—capable of binding two antigen molecules.

Antibodies of the **immunoglobulin M (IgM)** class account for 10% to 15% of serum immunoglobulins. Their half-life in serum is about 5 days, and IgM cannot cross the placenta. A

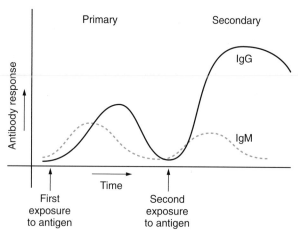

FIGURE 2-8 Primary versus secondary response.

exposed to the antigen, a primary immune response, characterized by the relatively rapid appearance of IgM antibodies, occurs. IM antibody levels usually peak in 1 to 2 weeks followed by a gradual decline to undetectable levels over the next few months. At the time when IgM levels have nearly peaked, IgG (and in some cases IgA) antibodies become detectable and continue to increase for about 1 month, surpassing peak IgM levels. IgG levels remain elevated for months and then decline slowly, often persisting at low but detectable levels for years (Figure 2-8).

A subsequent exposure to the same antigen elicits a secondary or **anamnestic immune response,** characterized by a rapid increase in IgG antibody associated with higher levels, a prolonged elevation, and a more gradual decline (see Figure 2-8). IgM antibody synthesis plays a minor role in a secondary immune response. Serologic tests that are designed to separately detect IgG and IgM antibodies take advantage of the differences in IgM production between a primary and a secondary immune response. Thus a positive test result for IgM antibody is considered indicative of a primary current or very recent infection, whereas the presence of IgG antibody alone suggests a previous infection or exposure. Similarly, the presence of significant levels of IgM antibody (with or without IgG) in a newborn suggests in utero infection (IgM can be synthesized by the fetus and cannot cross the placenta), whereas IgG antibody only in the newborn is indicative of passive maternal transfer of IgG across the placenta, not in utero infection.

Cell-Mediated Immune Response

In contrast to humoral immunity, the primary effector cell in cell-mediated immunity is the T lymphocyte. The T cell does not secrete antibody molecules; however, the result of antigen binding, activation, cell division, and differentiation of the T cell is the production of a number of low–molecular-weight proteins known as **lymphokines.** Lymphocytes affect their immunologic function through direct cell-to-cell contact or through the activity of the lymphokines on other cells, such as macrophages. The measurement and diagnostic significance of cell-mediated immunity are beyond the scope of this book, and cellular immune function tests generally are not performed in microbiology or microbial serology laboratories.

In essence, the wide variety and complexity of infectious agents necessitate flexibility in the immune mechanisms of the host. Immunity to extracellular bacterial pathogens, such as *S. aureus* and *S. pyogenes*, is mediated primarily by antibody functioning either alone (neutralization of toxins and extracellular bacterial enzymes) or with complement and neutrophils (chemotaxis and phagocytosis of bacterial cells). Immunity to intracellular bacterial pathogens, such as *M. tuberculosis*, is primarily cell mediated, through the activities of T lymphocytes, lymphokines, and macrophages. If antibody is produced, it plays little role in eliminating this pathogen, because the pathogen is sequestered (hidden) intracellularly where antibody cannot reach.

Meanwhile, viral infections often elicit both humoral and cell-mediated immune responses. Antibody may bind directly to and neutralize viral particles (render the virus noninfectious—unable to infect other cells) when they are found free in the bloodstream or other body fluids. For example, central nervous system infection by arboviruses (which cause encephalitis) or by certain enteroviruses (which cause meningitis) may be prevented if neutralizing antibody against these organisms is present when the virus reaches the bloodstream, and before it enters the central nervous system. Some viruses, however, cause infections that spread by cell-to-cell transmission (e.g., herpes simplex virus, which causes cold sores); they would not be subject to the neutralizing effect of antibodies. In these cases, cell-mediated immunity plays a predominant role in eliminating the agent. Immunity to both fungal and parasitic infections is also primarily cell mediated; antibody plays little or no role in prevention of or recovery from infection resulting from these agents. Although antibodies may not have protective value for certain infectious agents, they may nonetheless have diagnostic and prognostic value in serologic tests. Methods for detecting the presence and significance of antibodies for diagnostic purposes are discussed in Chapter 10.

MECHANISMS BY WHICH MICROBES MAY OVERCOME THE HOST DEFENSES

Because organisms can use a variety of antihost mechanisms, infectious agents are able to establish disease despite the host's defenses. The strategies that microbes employ to counter the host's defenses consist of bringing about tolerance, immune suppression, change in the appropriate target for the immune response, and antigenic variation.

Sometimes the host immune system fails to respond to specific antigens of the infecting microorganisms. This failure to respond is not necessarily due to immune suppression. The inability to induce an immune response to a microbial antigen, referred to as *tolerance*, may be due to a "feeble antigen"; that is, an antigen or antigenic component of an organism that is incapable of stimulating an immune response from the host. The host therefore fails to initiate a response or is sometimes slow in responding. This lack of response suggests tolerance to this antigen. Tolerance to an organism may also develop when the infection occurs during fetal life or in a neonate. For example, it is believed that although the fetus, when infected by the rubella virus, responds and makes its own antibodies, the antibodies are often weak and unable to contain the infection. Because the T-cell response is also poor, the virus is able to persist in the fetus and during the neonatal period. Hence microorganisms can persist if they are able to survive in the host during prenatal infections without producing an overt form of the disease.

Certain microorganisms do cause immune suppression in the infected individual. The decreased immune response is often more far reaching than simply to the antigen of the involved microorganism. Viruses, certain bacteria, and protozoans are examples of microorganisms likely to cause immune suppression in the infected host. These infectious agents multiply in macrophages or in lymphoid tissues. The exact mechanisms of immunosuppression used by the infecting organism have not been defined for all organisms. However, individuals infected with viruses such as Epstein-Barr virus and cytomegalovirus show depressed T-cell or antibody responses to other unassociated antigens. Reduced immune reactivity caused by an infectious agent is exemplified by that caused by the human immunodeficiency virus (HIV), which targets CD4+ T cells. Because the virus destroys the major cells that defend the host against viral, fungal, and protozoan infections, the infected person becomes susceptible to opportunistic infections caused by these organisms.

Certain organisms have the ability to systematically change their surface antigens during the course of a single infection, even while inside the host, thereby evading the host immune defenses. This occurs in relapsing or recurring fever infections with *Borrelia recurrentis*. After an initial incubation period of 2 to 15 days following transmission of the spirochetes from a tick or louse, high numbers of the organism are found in the blood. The infected individual experiences high fever, rigors, severe headache, muscle pains, and weakness. The febrile period lasts for about 3 to 7 days but ends quickly with the induction of an immune response. However, a similar but less severe course of symptoms recurs several days to weeks later. The relapses are caused by antigen variation by the borreliae. Spirochetemia worsens during febrile periods and diminishes between recurrences.

Certain organisms such as *Brucella* spp., *Listeria* spp., and mycobacteria avoid the host's immune response by surviving inside infected cells. This is another evasion strategy used by microorganisms, making themselves unavailable as targets to the host's immune system. Macrophages that engulfed these microbial species protect them from antibacterial substances and support their growth inside the macrophage. For example, during the exoerythrogenic cycle in liver cells, the parasite *Plasmodium* spp. avoids being a target for the immune response. Malarial parasites can therefore infect red blood cells and cause disease while being protected from the host's defense mechanisms.

Hosts also produce antibodies against specific antigenic stimuli as an immune defense. However, if the antibodies produced against an infecting organism are of low avidity or have a weak antimicrobial effect on the infecting organisms, the ability of the infected host to control the infection is decreased. Therefore in certain microbial infections, antibodies, although produced, provide little or no protection to the host.

Similarly, interferons play a significant role in the host defense against foreign invaders. The main function of these cytokines is to stimulate the expression of major histocompatibility complex (MHC) proteins by T cells. Interferons (IFNs) are also antiviral; IFN-alpha and IFN-beta work against double-stranded RNA viruses, whereas IFN-gamma is produced following the activation of T cells. There are instances when viruses escape the effects of interferons, either because they are resistant to the antiviral effects or because the induction of interferon in the host does not take place. For example, vaccinia virus is able to resist the effects of interferons by inactivating IFN-gamma. Other viruses may produce persistent infections because these viruses do not induce interferon production.

ROUTES OF TRANSMISSION

The last portion of this chapter is devoted to the routes by which a pathogen may be transmitted to a susceptible host—an important factor in the establishment of infection, which is often explained by the characteristics of the pathogen. Although some organisms may be naturally transmitted by more than one route, most have a limited number of routes. These routes can be characterized as in the air (inhalation), via food and water (ingestion), through close contact (includes sexual transmission), through cuts and bites, and via arthropods; animal diseases that can infect humans are transmitted through animal contact (**zoonoses**). A summary of the routes of transmission is given in Table 2-9. Figure 2-9 shows the routes of entry to and exit of microbes from the body.

Airborne Transmission

Respiratory spread of infectious disease is common. Often, the respiratory secretions are aerosolized by coughing, sneezing, and talking. Very small particles, referred to as *droplet nuclei*, are the residue from the evaporation of fluid from larger droplets and are light enough to remain airborne for long periods. Pathogens that are spread through the air generally must be resistant to drying and inactivation by ultraviolet light. Some infectious agents may be transmitted by dust particles that have become airborne. As discussed earlier in this chapter, the body has a number of defenses against airborne infectious agents. The nasal turbinates, oropharynx, and larynx provide a twisting, mucus-lined passageway that makes direct access to the lower respiratory tract mechanically difficult. In addition, the lower portions of the respiratory tract contain ciliary epithelium that sweeps organisms upward. For a microorganism to cause disease, it must circumvent these defenses, penetrate the mucous layer, and attach to the epithelium. The host also produces secretory IgA, lysozyme, alveolar macrophages, and other factors that act on the pathogen that manages to get beyond the physical defenses.

Respiratory tract infections are the most common reason that patients of all ages seek medical attention. Although most upper respiratory tract infections are self-limiting and can be treated with over-the-counter medications, some are

TABLE 2-9 Common Routes of Transmission*

Route of Exit	Route of Transmission	Example
Respiratory	Aerosol droplet inhalation	Influenza virus; tuberculosis
	Nose or mouth → hand or object → nose	Common cold (rhinovirus)
Salivary	Direct salivary transfer (e.g., kissing)	Oral-labial herpes; infectious mononucleosis
	Animal bite	Rabies
Gastrointestinal	Stool → hand → mouth and/or stool → object → mouth	Enterovirus; hepatitis A
	Stool → water or food → mouth	Salmonellosis; shigellosis
Skin	Skin discharge → air → respiratory tract	Varicella; poxvirus infection
	Skin to skin	Human papillomavirus (warts); syphilis
Blood	Transfusion or needle prick	Hepatitis B; cytomegalovirus infection; malaria; human immunodeficiency virus
	Insect bite	Malaria; relapsing fever; West Nile Virus
Genital secretions	Urethral or cervical secretions	Gonorrhea; herpes simplex; *Chlamydia* infection
	Semen	Cytomegalovirus infection
Urine	Urine → hand → catheter	Hospital-acquired urinary tract infection
	Urine → aerosol (rare)	Tuberculosis
Eye	Conjunctival	Adenovirus
Zoonotic	Animal bite	Rabies
	Contact with carcasses	Tularemia
	Arthropod	Plague; Rocky Mountain spotted fever; Lyme disease

From Sherris JC, editor: *Medical microbiology: an introduction to infection diseases,* ed 4, New York, 2003, McGraw-Hill.
*The examples cited are incomplete, and in some cases more than one route of transmission exists.

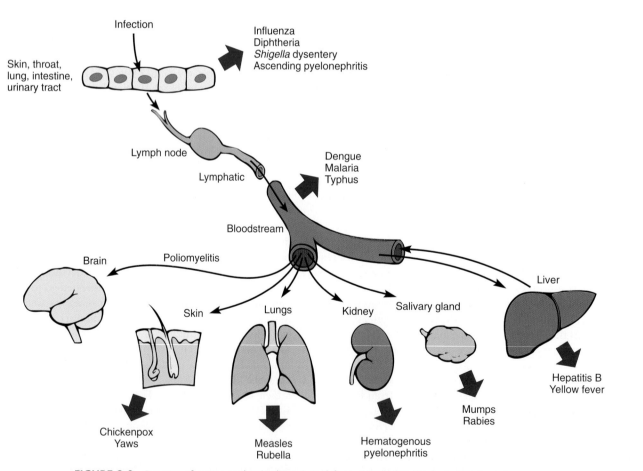

FIGURE 2-9 Routes of entry and exit. (Reprinted from Mims CA, Nash A, Stephen J: *Mims pathogenesis of infectious disease,* ed 5, San Diego, 2001, Elsevier Ltd, permission from Elsevier.)

more serious. Streptococcal sore throat, sinusitis, otitis media, acute epiglottitis, and diphtheria can be serious and even life threatening. Viral diseases causing the common cold and infectious mononucleosis are usually not life threatening but can result in much discomfort and absenteeism from work or school.

Although all the diseases mentioned can be spread via aerosols, some may also be transmitted via the fingers and hands; this is especially true of the common cold–causing rhinovirus. The fingers and hands are contaminated with infectious nasal secretions because of hand-to-nose contact. The infectious viral particles are passed from the infected individual to a susceptible recipient via hand-to-hand or hand-to-face contact. The recipient transmits the virus picked up from the hands of the infected individual by touching the face and nose. In this case, the disease is transmitted via the respiratory route, but not in the normal, classic manner of respiratory transmission.

Transmission may also result from contact with inanimate objects contaminated with the infectious agent. For example, a doorknob is contaminated by the hand and fingers of an infected individual, and the virus is transmitted to a susceptible person's hand and fingers when that person opens the door. Control of such transmission is often as simple as frequent handwashing.

Infections of the lower respiratory tract are less common but more serious than those of the upper respiratory tract. The organisms causing these infections have managed to bypass host defenses, or the host defenses have been compromised (e.g., by alcoholism, heavy smoking), allowing the pathogen access to the deeper portions of the respiratory tract.

The most common microorganism causing lower respiratory tract infection of individuals older than 30 years of age is *S. pneumoniae*. Although the pneumococcus is the most common community-acquired pneumonia, it is also often seen in aspiration pneumonia, a common type of hospital-acquired pneumonia. Pneumococcal pneumonia begins suddenly and is a serious, life-threatening disease, particularly in older patients. Among younger people, the common causes of pneumonia are *Mycoplasma* organisms and viruses. The onset of these pneumonias is more gradual than with pneumococcal pneumonia and the outcome is far more favorable.

In chronic lower respiratory tract infections, the survival of the infecting agent within phagocytes plays a role in the pathogenic mechanism. As the agent of tuberculosis, a chronic debilitating infection, *M. tuberculosis* is the classic example of an intracellular pathogen. This organism is highly virulent, is invasive, survives well, and multiplies within phagocytes.

Transmission by Food and Water

Transmission of gastrointestinal infections is usually a result of ingestion of contaminated food or water. In some situations, infection occurs via the fecal-oral route.

The digestive tract is colonized with vast numbers of different microorganisms. Under usual conditions, the gut flora maintains a harmless relationship with the host. Gastric enzymes and juices in the stomach prevent survival of most organisms, but many survive and colonize the small intestine and colon.

Gastrointestinal infections result from organisms that survive the harsh conditions of the stomach and competition with the microbial flora, and then produce damage to the tissues of the gastrointestinal tract. This damage is a result of either a preformed toxin or disruption of the normal functioning of the intestinal cells by invasion of the pathogen or production of a toxin within the intestine.

Organisms that can cause disease by means of a preformed toxin include *Clostridium botulinum*, *Bacillus cereus*, and *S. aureus*. The severity of disease ranges from a mild diarrhea to a rapidly fatal intoxication. Food poisoning by *B. cereus* and *S. aureus* is relatively common and is self-limiting. Botulism, caused by *C. botulinum*, although rare, can be life threatening.

Other bacteria produce a toxin after infection of the intestinal tract. Generally, to be effective as a disease producer, an organism must survive, adhere to, and colonize the intestinal mucosa and either produce a toxin or invade deeper tissues. A commonly seen cause of diarrhea and intestinal infection is *E. coli*. This organism is a member of the intestinal flora; however, some strains of *E. coli* produce cytotoxins that cause alterations in the biochemical activity of the intestinal epithelial cells, resulting in problems with fluid and electrolyte control by the intestinal cells. These strains of *E. coli*, referred to as *enterotoxigenic*, are a common cause of traveler's diarrhea and other intestinal problems.

Probably the classic intestinal pathogen is *Vibrio cholerae*, the cause of cholera. This organism produces an enterotoxin that causes the outpouring of fluid from the cells into the lumen of the intestine. Massive amounts (up to 20 L per day) of fluid can be lost. Other intestinal pathogens are *C. difficile*, *Shigella* spp., *Aeromonas hydrophila*, *Campylobacter jejuni*, and *Salmonella* spp. The infective dose, severity, and incidence of disease vary with the agent.

A number of viruses also cause diarrheal disease. They multiply within the cells of the intestinal mucosa and affect the normal functioning of the cells. Viral agents in this category include hepatitis A and E, rotavirus, adenovirus, coxsackievirus, and *Norovirus* spp. The incidence of diarrhea caused by these agents is high, especially when people are in close contact (e.g., in daycare centers, nursing homes, military camps). Numerous parasites, such as *Fasciolopsis buski*, *Giardia lamblia*, *Entamoeba histolytica*, and *Balantidium coli*, also infect the gastrointestinal tract.

Close Contact

All of the routes of transmission of infectious diseases require close contact. For a respiratory pathogen to be transmitted via aerosols, the susceptible host must be relatively close. For this discussion, however, *close contact* refers to passage of organisms by salivary, skin, and genital contact. Two prominent infections passed by direct transfer of saliva (e.g., kissing) are herpes simplex virus and Epstein-Barr virus. Skin-to-skin transfer of infectious disease is not as common as for some of the other routes, but diseases such as warts (human papillomavirus), syphilis, and impetigo result when material from infectious lesions inoculates a susceptible host's skin. The list

TABLE 2-10 Zoonoses

Disease	Organism
Anthrax	*Bacillus anthracis*
Brucellosis	*Brucella* spp.
Erysipeloid	*Erysipelothrix rhusiopathiae*
Leptospirosis	*Leptospira interrogans*
Tularemia	*Francisella tularensis*
Ringworm	*Trichophyton* spp.
	Microsporum spp.
Lyme disease	*Borrelia burgdorferi*
Plague	*Yersinia pestis*
Rocky Mountain spotted fever	*Rickettsia rickettsii*
Yellow fever	Flavivirus
Encephalitis	Alphavirus
Colorado tick fever	Orbivirus
Leishmaniasis	*Leishmania* spp.
Rabies	Rhabdovirus
Blastomycosis	*Blastomyces dermatitidis*
Tuberculosis	*Mycobacterium bovis*
Q fever	*Coxiella burnetii*
Ornithosis	*Chlamydia psittaci*
Gastroenteritis	*Campylobacter* spp.
	Salmonella spp.
Listeriosis	*Listeria monocytogenes*
Giardiasis	*Giardia lamblia*
Toxoplasmosis	*Toxoplasma gondii*
Tapeworms	*Taenia saginata*
	Taenia solium
	Diphyllobothrium latum
	Echinococcus spp.
Trichinosis	*Trichinella spiralis*

of sexually transmitted diseases is a long one. In North America, the most commonly transmitted venereal diseases or agents are gonorrhea, herpes simplex virus, hepatitis B and C, *Chlamydia* spp., syphilis, *Trichomonas* spp., and HIV.

Cuts and Bites

The classic example of a bite-wound infection is rabies. Human rabies though is relatively rare. Of more concern with animal bites, and especially human bites, is infection by the mouth flora. Dog-bite and cat-bite infections often yield *Pasteurella multocida*, but the possibilities are extensive. Human bites are extremely dangerous because they are difficult to treat and because the human oral flora comprises many different organisms in extremely high numbers.

Arthropods

Infection as a result of a tick, flea, or mite bite is a common occurrence in many parts of the world. The diseases spread by arthropods include malaria, relapsing fever, plague, Rocky Mountain spotted fever, Lyme disease, typhus, and untold numbers of regional hemorrhagic fevers. In most cases, the infectious agent multiplies in the arthropod, which then feeds off a human host and transmits the microorganism.

Zoonoses

The route of transmission known as *zoonosis* depends on contact with animals or animal products. Certain organisms causing disease in animals may also infect humans who have contact with them. These diseases may be passed by animal bites (rabies), arthropod vectors (plague), contact with secretions (brucellosis), and contact with animal carcasses and products (tularemia, listeriosis). The diseases are transmitted by routes already discussed. The common factor is that, regardless of the route, the disease is a disease of animals that is transmitted to humans. A partial list of zoonotic diseases and infecting organisms is given in Table 2-10.

BIBLIOGRAPHY

Ceciliani F, Giordano A, Spagnolo V: The systemic reaction during inflammation: the acute-phase proteins, *Protein Pept Lett* 9:211, 2002.

Chapel H et al: *Essentials of clinical immunology*, ed 5, Malden, Mass, 2006, Wiley Blackwell.

Fu YX, Chaplin DD: Development and maturation of secondary lymphoid tissues, *Annu Rev Immunol* 17:399, 1999.

Gabay C, Kushner I: Acute-phase proteins and other systemic responses to inflammation, *N Engl J Med* 340:448, 1999.

Grewal IS, Flavell RA: CD40 and CD154 in cell-mediated immunity, *Annu Rev Immunol* 16:111, 1998.

Hiemstra PS, Bals R: Series introduction: innate host defense of the respiratory epithelium, *J Leukoc Biol* 75:3-4, 2004.

Johnson HL, Chiou CC, Cho CT: Applications of acute phase reactant in infectious diseases, *J Microbiol Immunol Infect* 32:73, 1999.

Kamradt T, Mitchison NA: Tolerance and autoimmunity, *N Engl J Med* 344:655, 2001.

Kumar V, Abbas A, Aster J, editors: *Robbins and Cotran pathologic basis of disease*, ed 8, Philadelphia, 2010, Saunders.

Lanzavecchia A, Sallusto F: Dynamics of T lymphocyte responses: intermediates, effectors, and memory cells, *Science* 290:92, 2000.

Mandell G, Bennett J, Dolin R: *Mandell, Douglas, and Bennett's principles and practice of infectious diseases*, ed 7, New York, 2010, Churchill Livingstone.

McKenzie SB: *Clinical laboratory hematology*, ed 2, Upper Saddle River, NJ, 2010, Prentice Hall.

Medzhitov R, Janeway C Jr: Innate immunity, *N Engl J Med* 343:338, 2000.

Mims C, Nash A, Stephen J: *Mim's pathogenesis of infectious disease*, ed 5, San Diego, 2001, Academic Press.

Nemazee D: Receptor selection in B and T lymphocytes, *Annu Rev Immunol* 18:19, 2000.

Sheldon H: *Boyd's introduction to the study of disease*, ed 11, Philadelphia, 1992, Lea & Febiger.

Sompayac LM: *How the immune system works*, ed 3, Malden, Mass, 2008, Wiley-Blackwell.

Wilson JW, et al: Mechanism of bacterial pathogenicity, *Postgrad Med J* 78:216, 2002.

Winn W et al, editors: *Koneman's color atlas and textbook of diagnostic microbiology*, ed 6, Philadelphia, 2006, Lippincott Williams & Wilkins.

Points to Remember

- Some species of the usual microbial flora may be opportunists, capable of causing disease in an immunocompromised host.
- True pathogens cause disease in all individuals.

- The host defense system against microorganisms includes physical, mechanical, and chemical barriers; components of the innate immune system such as phagocytes, complement, cytokines, and the products of inflammation; and the components of the adaptive immune response.
- Microbes have mechanisms to evade the host's defenses, including the ability to evade phagocytosis, production of enzymes and exotoxins, the ability to induce tolerance in the adaptive immune system or to suppress the adaptive immune system, and the ability to avoid recognition by the adaptive immune system by varying the antigens present on the surface of the microorganism.

Learning Assessment Questions

1. What host resistance factor is compromised in the patient described in the Case in Point?
2. What microbial factor contributes to the virulence of the infecting organism?
3. What is the difference between true pathogens and opportunistic pathogens?
4. How does inflammation play a role as a host immune defense?
5. What is the difference between exotoxins and endotoxins?
6. What cells and soluble mediators are involved in the innate immune response versus the adaptive immune response? Humoral versus cellular?
7. How can microorganisms evade the immune response?
8. How are organisms transmitted?
9. Name the major immune response that is responsible for eliminating extracellular and intracellular bacteria and viruses.
10. What are the steps involved in phagocytosis, and how can microorganisms evade each step?
11. What are the differences between and functions of IgG and IgM?
12. What are zoonoses, and what organisms are considered zoonotic agents?

Laboratory Role in Infection Control

David L. Taylor

- ■ **GENERAL CONCEPTS IN INFECTION CONTROL PRACTICE**
  Infection Control in Health Care Settings
  Infection Control Surveillance
  Frequently Identified Microbes
- ■ **OUTBREAK INVESTIGATION**
  Local
  Widespread
  Steps of Outbreak Investigation
  Investigation Support from the Laboratory

Environmental Culturing
  Reporting
- ■ **EDUCATION**
  Technologists and ICPs
  Safety
- ■ **EMERGING AND REEMERGING PATHOGENS**
  Emerging Pathogens
  Reemerging Pathogens
  Response Plans

OBJECTIVES

After reading and studying this chapter, you should be able to:

1. Delineate the various roles the laboratory and the laboratory technologist may play in an infection control program.
2. List the facilities/settings in which an infection control program is important.
3. Define *surveillance* and the ways in which surveillance is conducted.
4. Describe outbreak investigation and the steps followed in an outbreak investigation.
5. List the ways in which a microbiology laboratory may support an outbreak investigation.
6. Define when and how environmental culturing is appropriate in an infection control program.
7. Describe agencies/entities to which an infection control program would provide reports.
8. Discuss educational activities that encompass an infection control program.
9. Correlate the activities of the laboratory with the safety and prevention activities of an infection control program.
10. Describe the roles of the microbiology laboratory and the epidemiology program in preparing for potential bioterrorism activities.

Case in Point

An 82-year-old man was admitted to an intensive care unit (ICU) from an **extended care facility (ECF);** he was confused and short-of-breath. His chest radiograph revealed consolidation in the left lower lobe. A bronchoalveolar lavage was performed and the specimen was sent to the laboratory for culture and antibiotic susceptibilities. An **endotracheal** tube was placed and the patient was attached to a ventilator for respiratory support. The cultures grew a multidrug-resistant strain of *Acinetobacter baumannii*. Within 3 days, two more patients in the ICU had respiratory cultures positive for *A. baumannii*. Over the next 4 days, three additional ventilated patients had tracheal aspirate cultures that grew the same microbe.

Infection control was notified by the microbiology technologist of the unusual occurrence of several isolates of the resistant *Acinetobacter*. The infection control practitioner, the microbiology technologist, the ICU nurse manager, and the physician in

charge of the ICU met to review the situation. The patients were placed into Contact Precautions, education was initiated that highlighted hand hygiene practices, and environmental cultures were taken. Data were collected and analyzed. The occurrence of the multidrug-resistant strain of *Acinetobacter* decreased and eventually no new cases were observed.

Issues to Consider

After reading the patient's case history, consider:
- The role of the laboratory worker and the microbiology laboratory in an infection control program
- The surveillance of health care–associated infections and the required laboratory support
- The information needed in an outbreak investigation
- The role of the laboratorian as an educator in infection control
- Bioterrorism and emerging pathogens

Key Terms

Antibiograms

Antibiotic pressures

Baseline data

Case definition

Central line–associated bloodstream infections (CLA-BSIs)

Communal living

Community-acquired infections

Data mining

Emergency response plans

Emerging pathogens

Endotracheal

Environmental cultures

Epidemiologic curve

Extended care facility (ECF)

Hand hygiene

Health care–associated infections

Iatrogenic

Index case

Infection control practitioner (ICP)

Infection control risk assessment

Infection rate

Interventions

Intravascular device

Outbreaks

Outbreak investigation

Prevalence

Public health

Pulsed-field gel electrophoresis

Reemerging pathogens

Standard Precautions

Surgical site infections (SSIs)

Surveillance

Targeted surveillance

Total surveillance

Urinary tract infections (UTIs)

Ventilator-associated pneumonias (VAPs)

TABLE 3-1 Health Care Settings Involving Infection Control

Setting	Description
Public health	Community settings (e.g., daycare centers, schools)
Acute care	Hospitals
Ambulatory care	Outpatient surgery, chronic dialysis and infusion centers, physicians' offices, emergency care facilities
Extended care	Skilled nursing facilities, nursing homes, assisted living centers
Home care	Skilled nursing provided in the home
Communal living	Prisons and jails, behavioral health facilities

Every year, more than 2 million health care–associated infections occur that cost the health care system countless dollars and impact millions of lives. An effective infection control program must be established in a health care setting to recognize and prevent these health care–associated infections. This chapter covers the settings, the activities, and the analytic practices involved in implementing an effective infection control program, specifically from the laboratory technologist's perspective.

GENERAL CONCEPTS IN INFECTION CONTROL PRACTICE

The clinical laboratory and the laboratory technologists play a vital role in the functioning of an effective infection control program. In some settings, the technologists provide supportive data; in other settings, the technologist may function as a part-time **infection control practitioner (ICP)** as well as a part-time laboratorian. Not infrequently, the technologist may leave the laboratory bench and become the ICP or work as a member of an infection control department.

As the term implies, *infection control* involves activities aimed at preventing infections in persons in broad and varied settings. The activities sweep the gamut from surveillance activities to outbreak investigation to education. They require an inquisitive and analytic mind, both of which are characteristics seen in clinical laboratory scientists and technologists.

Infection Control in Health Care Settings

Infection control practices are important in many health care settings. Table 3-1 lists different health care environments wherein infection control practices play a vital role. In all of the settings, the goal is to prevent the spread of infectious agents. In **public health** or community-at-large settings, the transmission of microorganisms occurs through many events in daily living. Microbes are spread at home, in daycare centers, in schools, in crowds (malls), and by individuals. There are sexually transmitted diseases, diseases spread by respiratory routes, diseases spread by contact, food-borne diseases, and waterborne diseases, all of which occur in the public arena. In acute care hospitals, infections occur as **surgical site infections (SSIs), central line–associated bloodstream infections (CLA-BSIs), urinary tract infections (UTIs),** and **ventilator-associated pneumonias (VAPs).** They are found in adults, teenagers, children, and neonates, as well as in healthy individuals, and immunocompromised patients. These infections occur as **community-acquired infections**, health care–associated infections, and **iatrogenic** infections. They occur because of instrumentation, increased use of antimicrobial agents, breaks in aseptic techniques, and lack of **hand hygiene.** Ambulatory care settings include outpatient surgical, chronic dialysis, and infusion centers as well as physician offices and emergency care facilities. Patients are seen, treated, and released. Infection control must be practiced in these settings even though the patients may not be seen again. In extended care facilities (ECFs), patients are frequently immunosuppressed by disease, age, or therapy. Extended care settings include skilled nursing facilities, nursing homes, assisted living centers, rehabilitation centers, and hospice care settings. Because of their suppressed defenses, these patients are prime candidates to acquire infections. Patients who are at home and receive home care from family or from professional home care providers sometimes acquire infections. Most often, home care involves intravascular-related or some other device-related care. As in extended care settings, the immune defenses of these patients are often suppressed by their disease or by their therapy.

Communal living programs can also be settings in which infections occur. These community living programs might include prisons and behavioral health facilities. In these facilities, infections might be found that are spread by contact (illicit tattooing) or by intimate contact with blood and body fluids.

The microbiology laboratory may receive specimens from any of these settings, all of which represent opportunities for infections to spread and opportunities for infection control to be practiced. Microbiology technologists must know who their customers are and be poised to insert themselves into infection control activities for the varied customer base.

Infection Control Surveillance

Infection control programs include many activities aimed at preventing the spread of infections. To determine where to most efficiently direct these preventive activities, an effective infection control program must collect statistics on existing infections. By comparing baseline figures with periodic numbers, the ICP can recognize **outbreaks,** upward trends, and positive effects of **interventions.** Ongoing, systematic collection of these data and the analysis and interpretation of the details surrounding a disease or event is termed **surveillance.** The laboratory contributes on a daily basis to these records.

Surveillance Definitions

Surveillance data can best be done and the data compared internally, locally, and nationally if standard definitions are used. Table 3-2 lists the common terms used in surveillance and their definitions. The Centers for Disease Control and Prevention (CDC) have recommended definitions that are generally used in the infection control profession. Most infection control programs are concerned about infections that are acquired within the setting. These infections occur after the patient arrives (generally not within the first 48 hours) and were not incubating in the community before the patient arrived. These acquired infections are generally called **health care–associated infections**. These health care–associated infections can be followed within a setting to determine when infection numbers increase above baseline, thereby requiring some investigation and intervention.

Infections are generally defined by site, risk factors, and procedures as shown in Table 3-2; primary infections are those infections that occur at one site, for example, a primary bacteremia. A primary bacteremia would not have another site that might be the source of the infection, as would be seen in urosepsis, in which the primary site would most likely be the urinary tract. Using primary bacteremia as an example, the laboratorian recognizes a bloodstream infection by the recovery of clinically significant organisms from blood cultures, whereas the ICP determines whether the infection was health care associated and primary. If the infection control program was monitoring CLA-BSIs, then the ICP would determine whether the bloodstream infection was related to an **intravascular device.** For this reason, the site of the blood culture draw (e.g., peripheral internal jugular catheter, femoral catheter) is important to include with the specimen description on the microbiology laboratory report.

The incidence of SSIs is frequently reviewed by the ICP. To the laboratorian, the isolation of pathogens from the surgical site is indicative of postsurgical wound infection; the ICP determines whether the infection was superficial, deep, or an organ-space infection. Therefore the site of the wound culture is an important component of the specimen description on the laboratory report. The ICP relates the infection to other risk factors, such as the length of surgery, the degree of contamination of the surgical site (gunshot wound to the abdomen versus a hernia repair), and whether any breaks in surgical technique occurred.

Because UTIs are determined by microbial growth from a urine specimen, the method of urine specimen collection should be described and differentiated between a voided clean-catch urine specimen and a specimen collected by catheterization. The definition of a health care–associated UTI includes the presence or absence of a urinary catheter. Health care–associated pneumonias are difficult to assess from the perspectives of both the laboratory and the ICP. From the ICP perspective, the criteria to define a hospital-acquired pneumonia include the presence of an endotracheal tube or some other respiratory device, and whether the pneumonia was incubating or present when the patient arrived. In the laboratory, the microbiologist should include in the specimen description on the laboratory report the type and source of the respiratory specimens (bronchoalveolar lavage, tracheal aspirate, expectorated sputum). With sputum specimens, the quality of the specimen as evaluated by the presence of white blood cells and single bacterial morphotypes, and the absence of squamous epithelial cells, is an important adjunct. The use of these definitions is important in guiding the ICP and in allowing the comparison of data.

General or Targeted Surveillance. Infection control programs may have all the health care–associated infections within the setting under surveillance or, because of budget or personnel restraints, they may be observant for only specific infections. In **total surveillance** programs, all infections are

TABLE 3-2 Surveillance Definitions

Term	Definition
Primary infection	An infection related to a single, specific site, not from multiple sites.
Bloodstream infection	An infection found in the bloodstream.
Central line–associated bloodstream infection	A bloodstream infection related to the presence of an intravascular device such as a central venous catheter.
Surgical site infection	An infection at a site where a surgical procedure was performed. Usually risk is stratified by length of surgery, site of infection, and degree of anticipated contamination.
Urinary tract infection	Infection of the urinary tract, frequently associated with a urinary catheter.
Ventilator-associated pneumonia	A pneumonia in a patient associated with a ventilator device such as an endotracheal tube or a tracheotomy.

recorded and analyzed to determine whether the infections are health care associated. Risk assessments determine whether the situation is a high or low risk and whether the infections are occurring in an unanticipated number. The **infection rate** is determined and analyzed to establish whether the number of infections has increased or decreased. These rates can be compared with previous rates in the setting or with rates in similar local or national health care facilities. There are several ways of calculating infection rates. For example, the SSI rate is defined as the number of infections per number of procedures expressed as percentages. Infection rates of CLA-BSIs and VAPs are calculated as number of infections per 1000 device-days. If an unexpected change in rates is seen, the ICP may conduct further investigations to determine, if possible, the cause of the change and to propose the course of action to reverse the situation. Based on the results of the investigation, the ICP would recommend the appropriate intervention such as a change in procedure, education, or increased emphasis on hand hygiene. The ICP would continue to monitor the infection to determine whether the rate of infection decreases.

Unlike in total surveillance, **targeted surveillance** involves a close watch of only specific, high-risk, high-volume procedures. For example, the program may follow CLA-BSIs in the ICU only and SSI in gynecologic surgical procedures, whereas another program may conduct surveillance on VAP in the neonatal intensive care unit and in the adult intensive care unit. Which infections to target would largely be based on review of previously ascertained data on infection rates **(baseline data),** recognition of high-volume and high-risk procedures within the setting, and sometimes on requests by others (e.g., insurance companies, physicians). This process is often termed a *risk assessment.* The targeted surveillance may change from year to year depending on recognized outbreaks or changes in the number of procedures performed. All of the surveillance data must be carefully collected, must use high-quality laboratory data, and should be protected from legal discovery as determined by the risk management team for the setting.

Baseline Data. To recognize when infections constitute an outbreak or when an upward trend is occurring, the infection control program must have established baseline data; that is, the historical occurrence of infections over time. Data at the national level that can be derived from the National Healthcare Safety Network (NHSN) may also serve as the baseline data. However, baseline data from within the specific health care setting more accurately reflects happenings within that setting. The baseline data are collected and analyzed by numbers, by percentages, or by rates per 1000 device-days. Baseline data are an important component of the decision-making process regarding which types of infections to target.

Data Gathering

Culture Review. Many infection control programs rely heavily on review of culture results, which is initiated informally by the laboratory technologist who may then inform the ICP of what appears to be an increased number of specific isolates. For example, the technologist may notice the isolation of an increased number of *Serratia marcescens* or *Sal-monella* spp. isolates, which may be infrequently seen in this particular health care facility. Or, the technologist may think that there is an unusual number of isolated methicillin-resistant *Staphylococcus aureus* (MRSA) from skin sites in a prison setting. The appearance of an increase in the number of surgical site specimens with various microorganisms may trigger a call to the ICP. These are informal data gathering activities that are significant to the infection control program. To report data, laboratorians use their experience and sense of what is usual regarding types of specimens and microbes encountered.

A more formal data review involves the daily review of actual culture results done either by the technologist or by the ICP. Such a review requires laboratory-generated results, generally from a laboratory information system (LIS). For example, the ICP or microbiologist reviews positive cultures and categorizes them into groups based on sites, units, organisms, or procedures. From this categorization, the ICP may recognize a trend, such as an upward trend in the number of *Pseudomonas aeruginosa* isolates from a skilled nursing facility or an increased number of positive cultures in laminectomy patients. Even more important is when the ICP determines that there are more *S. aureus* isolates than usual in the home health care setting. In this instance, an initiation of detailed investigations may be indicated. These fact-gathering activities are more formal and specific than the informal monitoring done by the technologist based on experience.

Recent advances in statistical correlation interface the LIS with a more sophisticated data review system for the purpose of **data mining.** In this type of data presentation, a multitude of events are analyzed and reported to the ICP. Data mining removes much of the day-to-day detail of the culture result review. It also adds other health care parameters to the analysis that are frequently not available to the ICP without detailed examination. This type of analysis may require the LIS and other hospital information systems to interface with the data mining system.

No matter how the culture results are screened and analyzed, a timely review is an integral component of an infection control program. Not only are the patients and their health care providers dependent on high-quality microbiology results, but the effectiveness of an infection control program is also dependent on such results.

Cases. The laboratory must be attuned to what is happening in the community and in the various settings within the community in regard to infection control issues. Infection control in the public health arena impacts the local microbiology laboratory. For instance, there may be an increase in the number of cases of whooping cough in surrounding counties. Even though the laboratory in the immediate county may not have seen any *Bordetella pertussis* isolates, they need to be aware of these other cases. Similarly, the anticipated appearance of influenza cases is a seasonal occurrence that influences the activities of a microbiology laboratory as well. The laboratory can be proactive in educating health care providers on specimen collection and transportation if those are unique to a specific public health concern. Awareness of infection control activities within the public health setting allows the laboratory to acquire the necessary media or reagents to meet emerging needs. Potential infection control issues that might become apparent within a setting may drive activities within the microbiology laboratory. For example, a product used in the health care setting is recalled because of suspected bacterial contamination. Effective communication between the infection control program and the microbiology laboratory is needed to establish screening techniques in anticipation of cases involving contaminated products that might arise in the health care setting. The technologists need to increase their knowledge of the specific product, the types of specimens to anticipate, and the expected isolates that may be unique or previously unrecognized by the laboratory. Collaboration among the microbiology laboratory, the infection control program, and the health care customer becomes paramount. Reporting of cases, both to the laboratory and from the laboratory to the infection control community, is an important tool in surveillance activities.

Laboratory Support and Data Gathering. In addition to providing culture results, the microbiology laboratory also provides the ICP with other details. These may include specimen contamination rates, the numbers of isolates per site, or the number of isolates per unit within the health care facility. Knowledge of specimen contamination rates helps the ICP with the interpretation of culture results and provides guidance in developing educational activities to improve collection of quality specimens. For example, if respiratory specimens are frequently contaminated with upper respiratory flora, interpretation of the results for the health care provider as well as for the ICP becomes more difficult. Contaminated specimens also prove costly for the patient and the payer because they do not provide useful or appropriate information. Attempts to determine VAP become futile if the specimens are contaminated with upper respiratory flora. A similar situation is encountered in blood culture contamination, which lessens the likelihood of high-level interpretive abilities. Blood culture contamination rates greater than 3% are generally considered high and may indicate educational opportunities for the microbiology laboratory and the infection control program.

The types of pathogens isolated from given specimens represent important information that can be generated by the laboratory to support the infection control program. By knowing what organisms would most likely be recovered from a given body site, the ICP can guide the health care provider in considering the appropriate empirical therapy. For example, if *S. aureus* is frequently isolated from skin infections in a jail setting, then the health care provider can anticipate the success of anti-staphylococcal antimicrobials in routinely treating those infections. If MRSA, however, is more frequently isolated, the health care provider would change the empirical therapy.

The **prevalence** of a particular pathogen is another piece of information that the microbiology laboratory can provide to the ICP. Prevalence is the number of cases of disease that occur in a given moment in time or specific time period in a given population. Therefore not only knowing what pathogens are isolated from a given body site but also being familiar with what pathogens are frequently isolated from a given location within a health care facility is important to the ICP. For

instance, a skilled nursing facility may be reassured that the lack of negative airflow rooms is acceptable if *Mycobacterium tuberculosis* has not been isolated from any of their patients over the past 7 years.

Being able to recognize what pathogens are isolated from patients in a medical intensive care unit may provide the opportunity for the ICP to inform health care providers the effects of **antibiotic pressures**. For example, if extended-spectrum β-lactamase (ESBL)–producing *Klebsiella pneumoniae* isolates were seen in that medical intensive care unit, then the physicians may be advised to limit the use of antimicrobial agents that tend to induce the formation of ESBLs. The microbiology laboratory then serves as an important adjunct to an infection control program by providing a multiplicity of types of data. The technologist must be aware of the customer needs and, in some cases, anticipate the customer needs in regard to these types of information.

Frequently Identified Microbes

Although the types of microorganisms seen in health care–associated infections vary from setting to setting, there are common pathogens that are frequently encountered. This discussion of the role of the laboratory in infection control addresses some of these common microbes to focus the attention of the laboratory technologist to the health care setting, the specimens, and the likely isolates. Table 3-3 delineates some of the most common organisms identified.

Public Health and Community Setting

The laboratory serving a public health or community setting is likely to identify infectious diseases of infection control importance that are less frequently seen in other health care situations. Some of the microbes frequently associated in water- or food-borne community outbreaks include *Giardia lamblia, Salmonella, Shigella, Campylobacter,* and *Cryptosporidium* species. Sexually transmitted diseases (STDs) such as syphilis, gonorrhea, and chlamydial infections are

---

TABLE 3-3   Health Care Settings and Common Microbes of Infection Control Significance

Health Care Setting	Microorganisms/Infectious Disease
Public health	*Salmonella* spp., *Shigella* spp., *Campylobacter* spp., *Giardia* spp., *Cryptosporidium* spp., syphilis, gonorrhea, *Chlamydia* spp., HIV, *Neisseria meningitidis,* encephalitis viruses, hepatitis B, hepatitis C
Acute care	*Staphylococcus aureus,* MRSA, VRE, *Escherichia coli, Pseudomonas aeruginosa, Clostridium difficile*
Ambulatory care	Hepatitis B, hepatitis C, HIV, *S. aureus,* MRSA, *P. aeruginosa,* VRE
Extended care facilities, home care	Opportunistic pathogens, *P. aeruginosa, Candida albicans, S. aureus,* MRSA, *Acinetobacter, C. difficile,* VRE
Communal living	*S. aureus,* MRSA, hepatitis C, lice

HIV, Human immunodeficiency virus; *MRSA,* methicillin-resistant *S. aureus; VRE,* vancomycin-resistant enterococci.

community-acquired infectious diseases that are identified in public health laboratories as well as laboratories serving acute care facilities. Some organisms that are important in public health settings may be more likely to be recovered in an acute care hospital but reported to a public health jurisdiction for the latter to follow up as a potential outbreak. Organisms such as *Neisseria meningitidis,* encephalitis viruses, coronaviruses (severe acute respiratory syndrome [SARS]), and West Nile virus are examples.

Acute Care Setting

Although a great variety of infectious agents can cause concern as health care–associated infections in acute care settings, some are more frequently seen than others. These are listed in Table 3-3. *S. aureus,* especially MRSA, is an important health care–associated pathogen, causing BSIs, SSIs, VAPs, and other infections. Although community-acquired MRSA is becoming more prevalent, health care–associated MRSA is worrisome because of its resistance to multiple antimicrobial agents. Similarly, enterococci are pathogens of concern in health care–associated infections because of their possible resistance to vancomycin and their potential ability to pass that resistance on to other microbes. *Escherichia coli* is a common fecal organism and is seen in a variety of health care–associated infections in a variety of sites including BSIs, SSIs, VAPs, and UTIs. In patients who are immunosuppressed by disease or by therapy, *P. aeruginosa* is seen as a cause of health care–associated infections. *Clostridium difficile* is an organism whose toxic products cause diarrhea associated with health care infections. Recovery of the organism is not the significant finding, but rather demonstration of the toxin. Although many other microbes are implicated in health care–associated infections, these are the top six in most acute care facilities.

Ambulatory Care Setting

Ambulatory care settings include a variety of different locations. However, the commonly encountered microorganisms of infection control importance do not vary. Most often, the patients have chronic illnesses, are immunosuppressed, and have infectious diseases caused by opportunistic pathogens. Other patients are likely to acquire community-acquired infections such as hepatitis B, hepatitis C, and human immunodeficiency virus (HIV). Other bacterial isolates include pathogens seen in other settings such as *S. aureus,* MRSA, vancomycin-resistant enterococci (VRE), and *P. aeruginosa.*

Extended Care Facility and Home Care Settings

Patients in both ECF and home care settings are frequently immunosuppressed by disease or therapy and often need intravascular or other device-related care. The microbes identified in these patients are often opportunistic pathogens. Infectious etiologic agents of infection control significance identified in these patients include *P. aeruginosa, Candida, S. aureus,* MRSA, VRE, *Acinetobacter* spp., and *C. difficile.*

Communal Living

People who are housed together in some form of communal living, such as prisons or behavioral health facilities, have infection control–related pathogens similar to those in the other settings previously described. The infectious diseases are more likely related to the activities of the persons within the facility. For example, *S. aureus* and MRSA are recovered from prisoners who practice illicit tattooing with nonsterile, shared equipment, whereas lice and hepatitis C are more frequently seen in behavioral health settings because of the community source of the clients and their intimate contact with blood and body fluids.

OUTBREAK INVESTIGATION

When numbers of isolates or infection rates increase above the baseline, or when an isolate of a rare or potential bioterrorism agent is recovered, an outbreak may have occurred. The microbiology laboratory may be the first to recognize the event and will likely participate in the **outbreak investigation.**

Local

In a given setting, an outbreak may be suspected when an unanticipated increase in infections occurs. Figure 3-1 shows infection rates that might trigger an outbreak investigation. In that figure, the baseline infection rate is seen for January through August as 3.3. In addition, the NHSN benchmark of 5.0 is also plotted. In September, the infection rate rose above the baseline and the NHSN benchmark. This might indicate that an outbreak has taken place, or the change in the rate of infections may have been due to other reasons. A more detailed investigation would reveal more.

As represented by the Case in Point at the beginning of this chapter, an outbreak may also involve the unexpected isolation of a microorganism. During the investigation and introduction of infection control interventions, an epidemiology curve is created. Figure 3-2 shows the **epidemiologic curve**

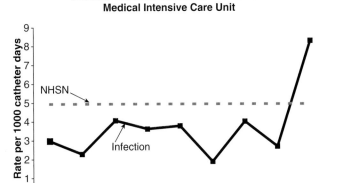

FIGURE 3-1 Plot of the rate of central line–associated bloodstream infections in a medical intensive care unit. The figure shows the National Healthcare Safety Network (NHSN) benchmark and the calculated monthly infection rate. The increase in the rate above the baseline and above the NHSN benchmark in September would trigger an investigation of a possible outbreak.

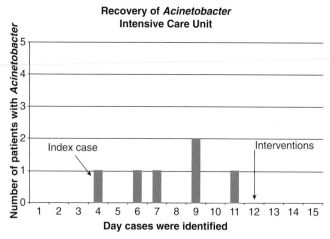

FIGURE 3-2 An epidemiologic curve of the occurrence of *Acinetobacter* spp. in respiratory specimens in an intensive care unit. Data were gathered as the result of a suspected outbreak. The graph plots the number of patients with *Acinetobacter* spp. infection by the day on which the cases were identified. Both the index case and the point when infection control interventions were implemented are indicated on the graph.

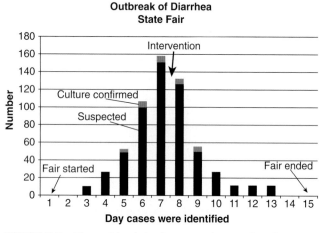

FIGURE 3-3 The epidemiologic curve of an outbreak investigation of diarrhea over a 15-day period at a state fair. The number of cases includes both suspected cases *(black bars)* and culture-proven cases *(colored bars)*. Infection control interventions were implemented on day 8 of the outbreak, and the number of cases decreased.

and the recovery of the *Acinetobacter* sp. The case first described on the fourth of the month is termed the **index case,** and it was to be determined whether the other infections that followed were related to that case. The investigation used the laboratory results provided by microbiologists.

Widespread

Widespread outbreaks occur outside the confines of a given health care setting. These outbreaks might be found in a statewide outbreak or a worldwide outbreak. An example of a statewide outbreak is the occurrence of diarrheal disease in persons attending a state fair. Figure 3-3 depicts an epide-

miologic curve from such an outbreak. The outbreak involved reported cases in 565 fair attendees. A total of 47 cultures were obtained, and 26 of those cultures were positive for *Salmonella* spp. Contaminated well water at the fairgrounds was suspected as the source, and increased hand hygiene and use of bottled water were instituted 5 days after the first case was reported. After the interventions, the numbers of suspected cases decreased. Cases involved individuals from seven states and Canada. Some of the cases were in food handlers at the fair as well as fair attendees. Many suspected cases (more than 500) were reported but not cultured. The *Salmonella* spp. isolates recovered were all the same serogroup. Well water, food, and food preparation sites were cultured.

Another example involves the investigation of a potential measles outbreak involving an international flight from Russia to the United States. The patient involved in the suspected index case flew from Russia to London, where she changed planes for a flight to New York. She then changed planes in New York for a flight to Chicago, where she lived. The patient was a college student who visited her parents in Russia for the summer. While in Russia, she had contact with several young children who had measles. On her return flight to the United States, she complained of a fever but did not develop a rash until she had been home in Chicago for a day.

Imagine the complexity of an investigation of this potential outbreak. This scenario was recognized as a potential outbreak and not an actual outbreak when the investigation was undertaken. The recognition of measles by the microbiology laboratory set the investigation into motion, not the occurrence of any additional cases. Several issues must be examined. Did the student have measles? Most, but not all, people in the United States are immune. The people on the flight from Russia to London were the first exposed persons, followed by the people on the flight from New York to Chicago. Were they immune? Where did they go after their flight landed? How does the health department follow up with them? The incubation period for measles is approximately 10 days (8 to 13 days to the fever, 14 days to the rash). People are contagious before the development of the fever and the rash. Persons who are not immune are susceptible.

All three of these examples (*Acinetobacter* spp., *Salmonella* spp., measles) represent scenarios of potential infectious disease outbreaks. The investigation of these outbreaks depends heavily on the support of the microbiology laboratory to assist in ruling in or ruling out the infections and in identifying cases and sources. Laboratory support is described in detail later.

Steps of Outbreak Investigation

When an outbreak is suspected, steps are taken to investigate the event. The laboratory is integral in several of the steps. Table 3-4 lists the steps that are followed in an outbreak investigation. The first step is to establish a **case definition**. This step ensures that all of the remaining investigation is based on a single definition. This may involve the microbiology laboratory in the search for a specific pathogen or the recovery of several pathogens.

TABLE 3-4 Steps of an Outbreak Investigation

Steps	Description
1. Verify diagnosis of suspected cases	Establish a case definition.
2. Confirm that an outbreak exists	Be certain that all suspected cases meet the definition.
3. Find additional cases	Investigate to determine whether additional cases exist.
4. Characterize cases	Collect as much information as possible about the cases, including people, place, and time elements. Develop an epidemiologic curve.
5. Form hypothesis	Establish a "best guess" hypothesis about the outbreak.
6. Test hypothesis	Test the hypothesis with control groups and data collected.
7. Institute control measures	Implement intervention activities to control the outbreak.
8. Evaluate effectiveness of control measures	Determine whether the implemented activities have an impact on the outbreak. Does the number of cases diminish or disappear?
9. Communicate the findings	Document the investigation and communicate with all involved parties.

The second step is to confirm that an outbreak exists. One needs to be certain that all of the suspected cases match the definition and that there is more than an expected number of cases. At this point, the investigator seeks as much consultative assistance as possible. The laboratory is frequently asked for additional input. The third step is to find additional cases that may be added to the initial number of cases. Additional suspected cases may be discovered by more detailed investigation or by the new occurrence of cases. The laboratory may be asked to review microbiology data over a previous period of time to determine whether unrecognized cases have occurred.

The fourth step is to gather as much information as possible about the cases with respect to person, place, and time. An epidemiologic curve may be drawn to assist in the visualization of the outbreak numbers over time.

The fifth and sixth steps are to form a hypothesis about the event and then to test that hypothesis. In the fifth step, a tentative hypothesis is established as a "best guess" of what are the likely reservoir, source, and means of transmission. In testing that hypothesis, a control group is established; then the event is compared in both the incident and the control groups. Again, the microbiology laboratory may provide insight into the hypothesis and the relationship to the control group.

The seventh step in the investigation may actually occur at any point along the investigation time line. The establishment of interventions to stop the outbreak probably results from the initial recognition and the heightened awareness of a problem. The formal steps of the intervention process may not be developed until after the hypothesis is developed and

tested. Undoubtedly, interventions of some type (e.g., increased hand hygiene) are introduced early in the investigation. The eighth step, which comes after the development of interventional strategies, is to evaluate the effectiveness of the interventions. Did the outbreak cease or at least decrease in its intensity? Step nine, the final step and one of extreme and often overlooked importance, is to communicate the findings of the investigation. This communication step must include a written report that is kept on file and provided to all responsible individuals.

It is not unusual for an outbreak to end before all data are collected and analyzed. This is probably due to early intervention. An early end to the outbreak does not ameliorate the need for communication and a written report.

Investigation Support from the Laboratory

The microbiology laboratory plays a crucial role in providing investigative support both in an outbreak investigation and in the creation of routine surveillance information. The availability of culture reviews, which may result in the initiation of an outbreak investigation, was discussed earlier. Other types of laboratory support are often important as well.

Cultures and Serology

In an outbreak investigation and in the collection of routine surveillance data, the collection, processing, reporting, and reviewing of pertinent cultures becomes critical. In the *Salmonella* spp. outbreak at the state fair, consider the number of fecal specimens that the health department laboratory processed, although cultures from patients are only one component of the investigative activity. Cultures from other sites may provide additional significant information. Well water and food may have been cultured in addition to specimens from the patients with diarrhea and the food handlers. In the outbreak of infections owing to *Acinetobacter* spp., the laboratory may have cultured respiratory therapy equipment and water samples.

One of the major difficulties in a large outbreak (e.g., the state fair outbreak) is the reduced ability to collect and transport specimens from persons from out of state. Individuals may have cultures processed in their home state, but those results may be difficult to retrieve. In the state fair example, only a few of the affected individuals had cultures processed and results included in the investigation. In the example of 565 suspected cases, only 47 cultures were processed. Reasons for this low number of cultures include the following: (1) the diarrhea lasts 24 to 48 hours and people may not seek medical help, (2) people not from the immediate area may not know of the potential outbreak and the need to provide culture material, (3) people do not want to be bothered with the expense and the time spent to collect cultures, and (4) the specimens may be collected too late in the infection or not transported properly, so no organisms are recovered.

In addition to the actual culture results, the laboratory may be asked to determine the serologic relationship of the isolates. Were all the *Salmonella* spp. of the same serogroup?

What was the epidemiologic profile of the serogroup? Both the isolate identification and the serologic relatedness may be important determinants in the outbreak investigation.

Antibiograms

Antibiograms can often be used in the investigation of an outbreak. As discussed in Chapter 13, there are times when antibiograms must be viewed with suspicion. Although these laboratory figures are not always as precise as other results, they may give guidance to the microbial relatedness of the isolates. Table 3-5 demonstrates comparisons of two antibiograms of isolates with the antibiogram of the index case. If the isolates all had identical antibiograms (such as isolate #1) or if some of the isolates were quite different in their susceptibility patterns (isolate #2), the inclusion or exclusion from the case definitions might have been affected. For example, relatively susceptible *S. aureus* can be distinguished from MRSA in an outbreak of skin infections in prisoners.

Pulsed-Field Gel Electrophoresis

Pulsed-field gel electrophoresis is a strain typing technique that can be an important adjunct to epidemiologic investigations. In this methodology, electrophoretic separation of enzyme-digested chromosomal fragments of bacteria is accomplished. The patterns of the fragments are compared among strains of microbes recovered in a possible outbreak. Strains with dissimilar patterns would be determined to be unrelated. However, if the patterns are similar, the strains can be identified as possibly related. This potential relatedness is an additional epidemiologic tool that can be incorporated into the investigation of an outbreak.

Environmental Culturing

As part of an effective infection control program, the microbiology laboratory may be called upon to perform cultures of various environmental sites. Recommendations surrounding environmental infection control have been extensively discussed in a CDC document, *Guidelines for Environmental Control in Health Care Facilities*. The environment is rarely implicated in disease transmission except with immunosuppressed patients. Although **environmental cultures** are generally to be avoided, there are times when they become an important and often required element of an infection control program that impacts the microbiology laboratory.

Air

Most often, infections traced to air quality occur during construction activities in a health care setting. Because microbes in the air can be incriminated in health care–associated infections, cultures of the air can be a component of air quality investigations. Initially, an **infection control risk assessment** should be conducted to determine whether the air is a likely source of infectious particles. Such an assessment is necessary in construction activities and must be done before any decision to culture the air can be made. The CDC makes no recommendation regarding "routine microbiologic air sampling" before, during, or after construction. If a fungal infection, such as aspergillosis, occurs during or immediately after construction, an outbreak investigation may be initiated and control measures implemented. Such an investigation may involve collecting environmental samples (e.g., searching for sources of airborne fungi). High-volume air samplers are the preferred method for collection, although settle plates may also be used. The results of these microbiologic cultures must be reported to the infection control team and evaluated.

Water

Water is incriminated in outbreaks in many of the settings for which microbiology laboratories provide service. Outbreaks may occur in various environmental situations such as those associated with contaminated drinking water (e.g., hospitals, extended care facilities, prisons) or recreation water (e.g., swimming pools, whirlpools, lakes, streams). They may take place in homes, aboard a plane or ship, in a city or state, or in a foreign country. In the United States alone, 15 to 20 outbreaks owing to waterborne pathogens cause diarrheal illness and affect several thousand people annually. Other waterborne diseases include respiratory illnesses (e.g., legionellosis), hepatitis (hepatitis A or hepatitis E), skin infections (from *Pseudomonas* spp. or mycobacteria), and central nervous system infections (*Naegleria* spp.). Because of these infection control implications, the laboratory must be prepared to offer diagnostic services or recommend laboratories that do offer those services for waterborne pathogens.

TABLE 3-5 Comparison of Antibiograms from Microbial Isolates

Antimicrobial Agent	Index Case	Isolate #1	Isolate #2
Ampicillin-sulbactam	R	R	S
Piperacillin	R	R	S
Cefepime	R	R	S
Imipenem	S	S	S
Ciprofloxacin	R	R	S
Gentamicin	R	R	S
Tobramycin	R	R	R
Amikacin	R	R	I

R, Resistant; *S,* sensitive; *I,* intermediate.

TABLE 3-6 Pathogens Related to Waterborne Infections

Viruses	Bacteria	Parasites
Noroviruses	*Salmonella* spp.	*Entamoeba histolytica*
Rotavirus	*Campylobacter* spp.	*Giardia enterolitica*
Hepatitis A	*Yersinia lamblia*	*Cryptosporidium* spp.
Hepatitis E	*Escherichia coli* (O157:H7)	Amoeba (*Naegleria* spp.)
	Legionella spp.	
	Pseudomonas spp.	
	Mycobacterium spp.	
	Aeromonas spp.	

Table 3-6 lists examples of waterborne pathogens. Some of the waterborne agents can be recovered by routine microbiology procedures such as cultures, but others may require specialized techniques. When asked to do environmental cultures of water, the microbiology laboratory must determine what specific pathogens are sought, if that information is known. If legionellosis is suspected, for example, the laboratory needs to have standard procedures for recovering this microbe. If the outbreak involves diarrheal diseases due to unknown etiology or etiologies, the recovery techniques must be broader and may require the use of a specialized laboratory. Consultation with the ICPs involved in the outbreak investigation must be obtained before routine culturing of environmental water is undertaken.

In some settings, routine water cultures must be performed because of specific guidelines. For example, for chronic dialysis centers, the CDC recommendations include performing bacteriologic assays of water and dialysis fluids at least once a month using standard methods. The infection control program or the managers of the specific area of concern must be familiar with regulations and guidelines addressing water cultures. The laboratory must be aware of the standard methods to ensure that proper procedures and proper media are used. The laboratory technologist, the ICP, and the manager should maintain a close working relationship to ensure compliance with culturing requirements.

Surfaces

The culturing of environmental surfaces should be performed only under the combined direction of the laboratory and the infection control program. In an outbreak investigation, surface culturing would be needed; however, such cultures should not be routinely obtained. The laboratory must be consulted before environmental surface cultures are undertaken to ensure that proper procedures and media are used. The laboratory technologist should be instrumental in the interpretation of the results.

Reporting

The role of the microbiology laboratory does not stop with providing culture results. Depending on statutory requirements, the laboratory may also be responsible for the reporting of certain infectious diseases to public health jurisdictions. Other groups may expect reports as well, such as committees, persons managing specific programs, and the news media.

Reporting to Public Health

There is the requirement to report the identification or suspicion of certain infectious diseases to the local, state, or federal public health entities. As shown in Table 3-7, diseases designated as Class A1 are considered public health concerns and are to be reported as soon as they are suspected or identified. Some of these requirements are federally mandated by the CDC, whereas some may be designated by the state. It is imperative that the laboratory technologist knows what infectious diseases are reportable, to what agency they are to be reported, and in what time frame they are to be reported.

Reporting to Committees and Programs

Depending on the setting in which the microbiology laboratory serves, there may be expectations of reports of infectious diseases to committees within that setting. For example, in an acute care hospital, infection control committees may desire reports of various microbiologic information. Periodic antibiograms, lists of reportable diseases, pathogens recovered in certain hospital units, isolates recovered from certain sites, and blood culture contamination rates are examples of reports that might be requested.

In other settings, physicians may expect periodic updates including antibiograms and pathogen prevalence. They may expect these to be delineated by office practice, by physician, by site, or by patient type. The settings making these requests may be home health care, extended care, or communal living.

Schools and businesses may request updated reports especially related to outbreaks that affect their operation. These reports must be tempered by public health needs and individual confidentiality restrictions. Recently, insurance companies and community advocacy groups have expressed interest in knowing about infection control rates. Some states require periodic reporting of these rates. The microbiology laboratory may be involved in providing data for these reports.

TABLE 3-7 Examples of Reportable Diseases*

Class	Description	Examples
Class A1	Diseases of major public health concern—reported immediately on recognition of a case, a suspected case, or positive laboratory results	Anthrax, botulism (food-borne), diphtheria, plague, rabies, smallpox
Class A2	Diseases of public health concern needing timely response reported by the end of the next business day after the recognition of a case, a suspected case, or positive laboratory results	Encephalitis (viral), food-borne disease outbreaks, hepatitis A, Legionnaires' disease, pertussis, syphilis, tuberculosis, typhoid fever
Class A3	Diseases of significant public health concern—reported by the end of the work week	Brucellosis, giardiasis, hepatitis B, hepatitis C, Lyme disease, Rocky Mountain spotted fever, trichinosis
Class B	Diseases reported only by number of cases—reported by the end of the work week	Chickenpox, influenza
Class C	Report of outbreak, unusual incidence, or epidemic—reported by the end of next working day	Blastomycosis, histoplasmosis, scabies, staphylococcal skin infections, toxoplasmosis

*These are reporting regulations from the Ohio Administrative Code and may vary from state to state.

Reporting to the Media

Among the activities of a microbiology laboratory, discussing microbiology and infection control activities with the media (e.g., television, radio, newspapers) may become necessary. Media relations for the laboratory technologist should be discussed with the risk management area associated with the laboratory. Media relations represent an educational opportunity that might be investigated before the laboratory technologist speaks to media personnel. One must balance the public's need for knowledge as perceived by the news media with privacy restraints for the patient, the laboratory, and the setting.

EDUCATION

Technologists and ICPs

The role of the microbiology laboratory in education is a further extension of its activities related to infection control. The laboratory technologists must not only keep themselves educated in their contribution to the infection control team, but also keep the infection control personnel educated regarding the laboratory's contribution to the team. Seminars, scientific articles and books, computer-based learning, and discussion with the infection control personnel are ways in which technologists can maintain their knowledge of infection control and laboratory techniques that can aid the infection control program. The technologist should continuously educate the ICP regarding the abilities of the laboratory in contributing meaningful information to the infection control program. As new techniques become available or old techniques are replaced, the technologist needs to relay that information to the ICP.

Similar knowledge needs to be provided for other people associated with the health care setting and the infection control program. Ancillary personnel, such as housekeeping and maintenance personnel, benefit from knowing the laboratory perspective of an infection control program. What cleaning and disinfecting agents work against viruses? How long does the environment need to be in contact with the agent to kill the virus? When do the maintenance personnel need to worry about fungi? What does mold growing on wet drywall look like? These and other questions arise among ancillary health care personnel to which the laboratory technologist needs to be prepared to respond.

Consultation with the laboratory technologist often is sought when construction is anticipated. Sometimes that education needs to be provided even when it is not sought. What microbes may be harbored in standing water? When should high-efficiency particulate air (HEPA) filters be used? What might spread through a facility if proper barriers are not used to control demolition dust and debris? These are samples of questions that might be addressed by the microbiology laboratory technologist while acting as a consultant to the infection control program.

Safety

The infection control program impacts the microbiology laboratory by emphasizing the need for laboratory safety. As discussed in Chapter 4, Section C, Microbiology Safety, safety within the microbiology laboratory embraces the infection control program. Hand hygiene is a critical part of laboratory safety. Hand hygiene involves handwashing when hands are soiled or the use of alcohol hand rubs when hands are not soiled. The practice of **Standard Precautions** further extends infection control to the microbiology laboratory. Gloves are always to be worn when handling blood or body fluids. Proper disposal of microbiologic waste, according to state or local regulations and national guidelines, is another critical component of the infection control program in the microbiology laboratory. Receiving available vaccines (for hepatitis B, chickenpox, influenza) is one step to protect susceptible laboratory personnel. All of these functions connect the microbiology laboratory safety program and the infection control program.

EMERGING AND REEMERGING PATHOGENS

With the advent of terroristic activities in the world, the microbiology laboratory has become an integral part of that area of the infection control program. Whether dealing with emerging diseases, such as SARS, or reemerging diseases, such as smallpox and anthrax, the laboratory must stay closely aligned with the infection control activities in the setting that the laboratory serves. Box 3-1 lists examples of **emerging pathogens** and **reemerging pathogens**.

Emerging Pathogens

Sometimes infectious agents that have not been previously recognized appear. Agents such as the West Nile virus, the coronavirus associated with SARS, and the avian influenza virus are three examples of emerging diseases. The laboratory must not only quickly learn how to identify these agents in human infections but also collaborate with the infection control program in dealing with the agents in the human population. How are these microbes spread? What reservoirs may harbor them? What is their incubation period? What antimicrobial agents can successfully treat them? How can the environment be disinfected? These are questions that the

---

BOX 3-1 Examples of Emerging and Reemerging Pathogens

Emerging Pathogens
- Avian influenza virus
- Coronavirus (SARS)
- Viral hemorrhagic fever viruses
- West Nile virus

Reemerging Pathogens
- Anthrax (Bacillus anthracis)
- Botulism (Clostridium botulinum)
- Plague (Yersinia pestis)
- Smallpox virus
- Tularemia (Francisella tularensis)

infection control program must ask. The laboratory technologist, the ICP, and the infectious disease physicians all must combine their knowledge to address these issues. The educational role of the laboratory technologist once again becomes evident in teaching specimen collection, specimen transport, disinfection, and safety methods.

Reemerging Pathogens

The reemergence or potential reemergence of pathogens once thought to be eliminated demands collaboration with the infection control program. Smallpox, anthrax, and plague are examples of agents that have been learned about but have not been identified by the average microbiology laboratory in many years. The laboratory technologist must relearn information once thought to be out of date. Media selection, identification techniques, and safety precautions must all be reexamined and implemented. Interaction with the infection control program strengthens the establishment of prevention and control strategies.

Response Plans

With the potential use of biologic agents in terrorism, the development of **emergency response plans** is paramount. The microbiology laboratory is an integral part of that infection control activity. Safety, specimen collection, agent identification, and agent control are components of the response plan to which the laboratory can contribute its input.

Whether in everyday activities or in activities in response to an outbreak or emerging diseases, the microbiology laboratory and the laboratory technologist constitute a critical component of an efficient and successful infection control program. The lessons of the chapter must be carefully learned and implemented.

BIBLIOGRAPHY

Arias KM: *Quick reference to outbreak investigation and control in health care facilities*, Gaithersburg, Md, 2000, Aspen Publishers.

Association for the Advancement of Medical Instrumentation: *Water treatment equipment for hemodialysis applications*, ANSI/AAMI RD62-2001, Arlington, Va, 2001, American National Standards Institute.

Carrico R et al: *APIC text of infection control and epidemiology*, ed 2, Washington, DC, 2005, Association for Professionals in Infection Control and Epidemiology.

Emori TG, Gaynes RP: An overview of nosocomial infections, including the role of the microbiology laboratory, *Clin Microbiol Rev* 6:428, 1993.

Garner JS et al: CDC definitions for nosocomial infections, *Am J Infect Cont* 16:28, 1988.

Guidelines for environmental infection control in health-care facilities, recommendations of CDC and the Healthcare Infection Control Practices Advisory Committee (HICPAC), *MMWR Morbid Mortal Wkly Rep* 52(RR-10), 2000.

Guidelines for hand hygiene in health-care settings, recommendations of the Healthcare Infection Control Practices Advisory Committee and the HICPAC/SHEA/APIC/IDSA Hand Hygiene task force, *MMWR Morbid Mortal Wkly Rep* 51(RR-16), 2002.

Guideline for isolation precautions: preventing transmission of infectious agents in healthcare settings, June 2007. Available at: www.cdc.gov/ncidod/dhgp/pdf/isolation 2007.pdf.

National Healthcare Safety Network (NHSN) Report, data summary for 2006, issued June 2007, *Am J Infect Cont* 35:290-301, 2007.

Schiffman RB et al: Blood culture contamination: a College of American Pathologists Q-Probe study involving 640 institutions and 497,134 specimens from adults, *Arch Pathol Lab Med* 122:216, 1998.

Points to Remember

- The microbiology laboratory interacts with the infection control program in many different health care settings.
- Surveillance is important to establish baseline data and to recognize the need to investigate potential outbreaks.
- The microbiology laboratory supports outbreak investigations by providing consultative services including epidemiologic correlation of isolates.
- Although infrequently performed, environmental cultures may play a role in outbreak investigation.

- Microbiology technologists must recognize their role in providing reports to health departments, to committees, to the infection control program, and, on occasion, to the public.
- The microbiology laboratory must maintain competencies in new techniques.
- In anticipation of potential bioterrorism events, the microbiology laboratory must be equipped to participate in emergency preparedness programs.

Learning Assessment Questions

1. Surveillance is defined as:
   a. The systematic collection and analysis of data
   b. The review of health care–associated infections in laboratory personnel
   c. The recognition of emerging pathogens
   d. The development of an infection control risk assessment

2. Microbes commonly encountered in health care–associated infections in hospitals are:
   a. *Salmonella* spp., *Shigella* spp., hepatitis C, *Neisseria meningitides*
   b. *Staphylococcus aureus, Pseudomonas aeruginosa,* MRSA, *Escherichia coli*
   c. *Pseudomonas aeruginosa,* hepatitis C, lice, *Giardia* spp.
   d. All of the above

3. Pulsed-field gel electrophoresis might be performed to:
   a. Identify staphylococcal species
   b. Assist in an outbreak investigation
   c. Develop a new isolation precaution
   d. All of the above

4. The occurrence of surgical site infections (SSIs) is generally calculated as:
   a. A rate of infections in 1000 device-related events
   b. A percent of infections in 100 device-related events
   c. A percent of infections in surgical sites or procedures
   d. All of the above

5. Health departments frequently require the reporting by the laboratory of:
   a. Diseases of major health concerns (e.g., smallpox)
   b. Diseases needing timely response (e.g., food-borne outbreaks)
   c. Outbreaks of public health concern (e.g., scabies)
   d. All of the above

6. Microbial pathogens of potential bioterrorism activity include:
   a. *Bacillus anthracis, Staphylococcus aureus,* West Nile virus
   b. *Yersinia pestis, Staphylococcus aureus,* hepatitis C
   c. *Bacillus anthracis, Yersinia pestis, Francisella tularensis*
   d. *Bacillus anthracis, Escherichia coli,* coronaviruses, *Giardia* spp.

7. Environmental cultures are usually to be avoided except in:
   a. An outbreak investigation
   b. The occurrence of infections following construction
   c. Compliance with specific regulatory requirements
   d. All of the above

8. The formal steps in an outbreak investigation include:
   a. Establishing a case definition and culturing air and water
   b. Establishing a case definition, forming and testing a hypothesis, and communicating findings
   c. Forming and testing a hypothesis, performing PFGE, and calculating an infection rate
   d. Confirming an outbreak exists, calculating an infection rate, and performing serology and culture tests

9. Infection control programs rely on microbiology laboratory support in:
   a. Public health settings
   b. Acute care facilities
   c. Home care settings
   d. All of the above

10. The microbiology laboratory interacts with the infection control program by providing:
    a. Culture results
    b. Antibiograms and pathogen prevalence reports
    c. Environmental cultures when appropriate
    d. All of the above

Control of Microorganisms

A. Disinfection and Sterilization

Michelle M. Jackson*

- ■ **STERILIZATION VERSUS DISINFECTION**
- ■ **FACTORS THAT INFLUENCE THE DEGREE OF KILLING**
  Types of Organisms
  Number of Organisms
  Concentration of Disinfecting Agent
  Presence of Organic Material
  Nature of Surface to Be Disinfected
  Contact Time
  Temperature
  pH
  Biofilms
  Compatibility of Disinfectants
- ■ **METHODS OF DISINFECTION AND STERILIZATION**
  Physical Methods
  Chemical Methods

- ■ **DISINFECTANTS VERSUS ANTISEPTICS**
  Alcohols
  Aldehydes
  Halogens
  Chlorine and Chlorine Compounds
  Detergents: Quaternary Ammonium Compounds
  Phenolics
  Heavy Metals
  Gases
- ■ **EPA REGULATIONS ON CHEMICAL SURFACE DISINFECTANTS**
- ■ **FDA REGULATIONS ON CHEMICAL SKIN ANTISEPTICS**
  Hygienic Handwashing and Waterless Handrubs
  Surgical Hand Scrub and Waterless Surgical Handrubs
  Presurgical Skin Disinfection

OBJECTIVES

After reading and studying this chapter, you should be able to:

1. Define the following terms: *sterilization, disinfection,* and *antiseptic.*

2. Differentiate the functions and purposes of a disinfectant and an antiseptic.

3. Describe the general modes of antimicrobial action.

4. Describe the way each physical agent controls the growth of microorganisms.

5. Give the mechanism of action for each type of chemical agent commonly used in antiseptics and disinfectants.

6. Describe the different heat methods and their respective applications.

7. Describe EPA regulations on chemical surface disinfectants and FDA regulations on chemical skin antiseptics.

8. Describe the following hospital-use skin antiseptics: health care personnel handwash, surgical hand scrub, and patient preoperative skin preparation.

Case in Point

A 35-year-old infectious disease specialist complained of experiencing fever, chills, myalgia, and severe headache for the past several days. The patient had otherwise been healthy until 2

weeks ago, when he began to experience fatigue and felt the slightly swollen lymph nodes. The patient then recalled that he had demonstrated to his medical students and residents a culture of *Brucella melitensis* isolated from a patient's blood sample. He remembered that, while handling the Petri dish without gloves, he picked up the telephone to answer a page. While talking on the telephone, he touched his mustache as he habitually does when he speaks.

---

*This section was prepared by the author in her private capacity. No official support or endorsement by the FDA is intended or implied.

Issues to Consider

After reading the patient's case history, consider:
- Potential risks to which laboratory workers are exposed while working in the microbiology laboratory
- Exposure control plan to minimize the risks
- Laboratory safety guidelines to protect the laboratory personnel

Case in Point

Dr. Adams is a pediatrician at a busy metropolitan medical clinic. This morning, she arrived late to work because she had to take her sick son to her mother's house and dropped off her dog to the vet. When Dr. Adams arrived at the clinic, many children were waiting for her, so she immediately began seeing her patients. At one point, she thought about washing her hands, but she felt guilty about coming to work late and did not want to keep her patients waiting any longer. Besides, her hands did not look soiled or dirty.

Issues to Consider

After reading the Case in Point, consider:
- Potential risks that the doctor is taking in spreading germs to her patients
- Importance of handwashing and use of an appropriate antiseptic
- Quality control plan to minimize the risks to her patients

Key Terms

Antisepsis	Lister
Antiseptic	Microbial load
Antiseptic drug	Moist heat
Biofilms	Monograph
Destruction	New drug application (NDA)
Disinfectants	Over-the-counter (OTC)
Disinfection	drug
Environmental Protection	Pasteurization
Agency (EPA)	Patient preoperative skin
Fast-acting antiseptic	preparation
Filtration	Persistent
Food and Drug Administra-	Prions
tion (FDA)	Recognized as safe and
Generally recognized as safe	effective (RASE)
and effective (GRASE)	Resident flora
Germ theory	Semmelweis
Health care antiseptic drug	Sporicidal
products	Sterilization
Health care personnel	Surgical hand scrub
handwash	Transient flora

Safety in the laboratory cannot be overemphasized. Quantization of the risk of working with an infectious agent is difficult. Risk to an individual increases with the frequency and type of organism, and level of contact with the agent, as demonstrated by the Cases in Point. Therefore each laboratory must develop and institute a plan that will effectively minimize exposure to infectious agents. This chapter provides information on standard disinfection and sterilization techniques and laboratory safety guidelines for the clinical laboratory.

This section provides a practical overview of the following topics:
- Sterilization and disinfection
- Chemical and physical methods of disinfection and sterilization
- Principles and application of each method
- Common disinfectants and antiseptics used in health care settings
- Principles and applications of disinfectants and antiseptics
- Regulatory process of disinfectants and antiseptics

STERILIZATION VERSUS DISINFECTION

The scientific use of **disinfection** and **sterilization** methods originated more than 100 years ago when Joseph **Lister** introduced the concept of aseptic surgery. Since then, the implementation of effective sterilization and disinfection methods remains crucial in the control of infections in the laboratory and health care facilities (nosocomial infections).

To fully understand the principles of disinfection and sterilization, we need to have accurate definitions of certain terms. *Sterilization* refers to the **destruction** of all forms of life, including bacterial spores. By definition, there are no degrees of sterilization—it is an all-or-nothing process. Chemical or physical methods may be used to accomplish this form of microbial destruction. The word *sterile* is a term that is relevant to the method used. For example, a solution that has been filtered through a certain pore-size filter (less than 0.22 μm) is often referred to as *sterile*. Even though the filtered solution may be free of large microorganisms such as bacteria and fungi and their spores, in actuality, any microorganisms (e.g., viruses) that are smaller than the pore size of the filter were not removed and therefore the filtered solution is not truly sterilized or sterile. *Disinfection* refers to a process that eliminates a defined scope of microorganisms, including some spores. Physical or chemical methods may be used, but most **disinfectants** are chemical agents applied to inanimate objects. A substance applied to the skin for the purpose of eliminating or reducing the number of bacteria present is referred to as an **antiseptic**. Antiseptics do not kill spores and cannot be used as disinfectants.

FACTORS THAT INFLUENCE THE DEGREE OF KILLING

Before discussing methods used to kill microorganisms, a review of the factors that influence the degree of killing of organisms is important. The following factors play a significant role in the selection and implementation of the appropriate method of disinfection:
- Types of organisms
- Number of organisms

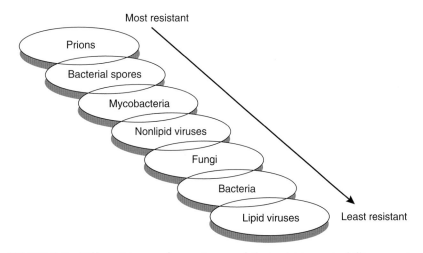

FIGURE 4-1 Different types of organisms and their resistance to killing agents.

- Concentration of disinfecting agent
- Presence of organic material (e.g., serum, blood)
- Nature of surface to be disinfected
- Contact time
- Temperature
- pH
- Biofilms
- Compatibility of disinfectants and sterilants

Types of Organisms

Organisms vary greatly in their ability to withstand chemical and physical treatment (Figure 4-1). This is due to the biochemical composition of microorganisms and various mechanisms that they can use to protect themselves. For example, spores have coats rich in proteins, lipids, and carbohydrates as well as cores rich in dipicolinic acid and calcium, all of which protect the spores. Cell walls of mycobacteria are rich in lipids, which may account for their resistance to chemical and environmental stresses, particularly desiccation. In contrast, viruses containing lipid-rich envelopes are more susceptible to the effects of detergents and wetting agents. Microorganisms living together in communities, referred to as **biofilms,** also provide protection to the microorganisms against chemical and physical means of destruction.

The organisms known today to be the most resistant to the actions of heat, chemicals, and radiation are **prions.** Prions are naked pieces of protein, similar to a virus, but without the nucleic acid. Prions are thought to be the agents that cause a number of degenerative diseases of the nervous system (transmissible spongiform encephalopathy—mad cow disease, Creutzfeldt-Jakob disease). These agents are transmitted to humans through contaminated medicinal products, therapeutic devices, body fluids, and food products. These infectious agents are extremely resistant to chemical and physical methods of destruction. Prions can withstand temperatures exceeding 121° C for several hours while immersed in acid or basic solutions. It is best to handle all body secretions as potentially being contaminated with this agent. When an object or material is thought to be contaminated with a prion, special methods need to be taken to

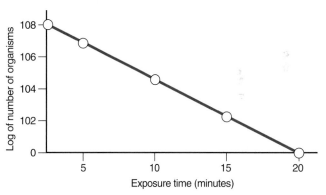

FIGURE 4-2 The effect of exposure time versus number of organisms.

destroy the agent. Simple disinfection or sterilization may not be sufficient.

Number of Organisms

Another factor to consider is the total number of organisms present, referred to as the **microbial load** (bioburden). If the number of organisms is plotted against the time they are exposed to the killing agent (exposure time) logarithmically, the result is a straight line (Figure 4-2). The death curve is logarithmic. Because the microbial load is most likely composed of organisms with varying degrees of susceptibility to killing agents, not all the organisms die at the same time. The microbial load determines the exposure time that is necessary for 99.9% elimination of the microorganisms. In general, higher numbers of organisms require longer exposure times.

Concentration of Disinfecting Agent

The concentration of a disinfecting agent is also important. The amount of disinfectant needed to destroy microorganisms varies with the different agents. Therefore manufacturers' instructions on preparation, dilution, and use must be followed very carefully. Concentrated disinfectants, such as povidone-iodine, may actually allow microorganisms to survive because there is not enough free iodine to kill microorganisms. Proper concentrations of disinfecting agents ensure the inactivation of target organisms and promote safe and cost-effective practices.

Presence of Organic Material

Organic material, such as blood, mucus, and pus, affects killing activity by actually inactivating the disinfecting agent. In addition, by coating the surface to be treated, organic material prevents full contact between object and agent (see Glutaraldehyde). Bleach (sodium hypochlorite) is easily inactivated by organic material. For optimal killing activity, instruments and surfaces should be cleansed of excess organic material before disinfection.

Nature of Surface to Be Disinfected

Certain medical instruments are manufactured of biomaterials that exclude the use of certain disinfection or sterilization methods because of possible damage to the instruments. For example, endoscopic instruments are readily damaged by the heat generated in an autoclave. Alternative methods must be used for this class of instruments.

Contact Time

The amount of time a disinfectant or sterilant is in contact with the object is critical. Too little contact time will not allow the agent to work properly. The contact time is a function not only of the agent itself, but also of the bioburden on the object, the type of microorganism that is to be killed, and the presence of organic material and temperature at which the agent is being used. When disinfecting or sterilizing a contaminated object, it is critical to know what organisms may be present and the contact time to use based on the microorganism that is most resistant. The amount of time that an agent is in contact with an object can also determine whether it is disinfecting or sterilizing the object. For example, glutaraldehyde can be used as a disinfectant or a sterilant, with the difference being the amount of time the glutaraldehyde is in contact with the contaminated object. When glutaraldehyde is used as a sterilant, the contact time is much longer than when it is used as a disinfectant. Alcohol and iodine preparations such as Betadine must be in contact with an object for at least 1 to 2 minutes in order for them to kill microorganisms. The spores of both bacteria and fungi must be in the presence of disinfectants or sterilants for a much longer time than their vegetative counterpart before they are killed.

Temperature

Disinfectants are generally used at room temperature (20° to 22° C). Generally their activity is increased to some degree by an increase in temperature and decreased by a drop in temperature. Therefore a disinfectant that is used on the workbench will generally work faster than if that disinfectant is used on a cold surface such as the walls of a refrigerator. Disinfection of blood spills in a refrigerator can take longer than disinfection of blood spills on a room temperature countertop. Disinfectants as well as sterilants can be rendered inactive by too high or too low a temperature.

pH

The pH of the material to be disinfected or sterilized can have an effect on the activity of the disinfecting or sterilizing agent. It is critical to make sure at what pH the agent is active and what the pH of the material to be exposed to the agent is at the time the process will be done.

Biofilms

Biofilms can be considered as a community of bacteria or other microorganisms. These communities are generally layers of microorganisms that often have a protective material over them that protects them from outside environmental factors. These communities of microorganisms can be on the surface of either inanimate or animate objects. A critical place where biofilms are seen in the hospital is on catheters. Other places may be inside of pipes that carry water and on deionizing columns used to make processed water. When dealing with the disinfection of objects that may have a biofilm, it is critical to realize that the presence of the biofilm will make disinfection more difficult. To disinfect materials that may have a biofilm present, the concentration of the disinfectant may need to be increased, the contact time may need to be increased, or both.

Compatibility of Disinfectants

A common mistake is to believe that two disinfectants are better than one. This is not necessarily incorrect, but when more than one disinfectant is used, then the compatibility of the disinfectants must be taken into consideration. Some disinfectants may actually inactivate other disinfectants. For example, the use of bleach and a quaternary ammonium compound together may negate the activity of both disinfectants.

METHODS OF DISINFECTION AND STERILIZATION

Having discussed the way factors that affect the survival of microorganisms influence disinfection and sterilization, the following looks at the ways in which methods are selected. E.H. Spaulding categorized medical materials into three device classifications:

1. Critical materials
2. Semicritical materials
3. Noncritical materials

Critical materials are those that invade sterile tissues or enter the vascular system. These materials are most likely to produce infection if contaminated and therefore require sterilization. Before semicritical materials come into contact with mucous membranes, they require high-level disinfection agents. Noncritical materials require intermediate-level to low-level disinfection before contact with intact skin. High-level disinfectants have activity against bacterial endospores, whereas intermediate-level disinfectants have tuberculocidal activity but not **sporicidal** activity. Finally, low-level disinfectants have a wide range of activity against microorganisms but do not demonstrate sporicidal or tuberculocidal activity. Table 4-1 presents a summary of these principles.

TABLE 4-1 Device Classification and Methods of Effective Disinfection

Device Classification	Disinfection Method	Killing Action Against				
		Spores	Mycobacteria	Nonlipid Viruses	Fungi	Bacteria
Critical	**Sterilization**					
	Steam	+	+	+	+	+
	Dry heat	+	+	+	+	+
	Gas	+	+	+	+	+
	Chemical	+	+	+	+	+
	Ionizing radiation	+	+	+	+	+
Semicritical	**High-level disinfection**					
	2% glutaraldehyde	±	+	+	+	+
	Chlorine dioxide	±	+	+	+	+
	Wet pasteurization	−	+	+	+	+
	Low-level disinfection					
	Sodium hypochlorite	−	+	+	+	+
	Quaternary ammonium compounds	−	−	±	+	+
	Ethyl, isopropyl alcohol (70% to 90%)	−	−	+	+	+
	Phenolics	−	±	+	+	+
	Iodophors	−	−	+	+	+

+, Positive kill; −, no kill; ±, variable.

Physical Methods

As mentioned earlier, sterilization and disinfection can be performed by both physical and chemical methods. Although several physical methods are available, this discussion is restricted to those methods most commonly used in a laboratory or hospital setting.

Heat

Because of its reliable effects, ease of use, and economy, heat is the most common method used for the elimination of microorganisms. Heat can be used in several ways. **Moist heat,** or *heat under steam pressure*, is the agent used in autoclaves. Putting steam under 1 atm of pressure, or 15 psi, achieves a temperature of 121° C. At this temperature, all microorganisms (an exception being prions) and their endospores are destroyed within approximately 15 minutes of exposure. The time varies somewhat according to the density of the material; the important factor is that the moisturized heat comes in contact with the material, and the contact time is sufficient. An added advantage of moist heat is the shorter time required for sterilization than for dry heat sterilization. (Heat in water is transferred more readily to a cool body than heat in air.) Moist heat is the sterilization method of choice for heat-stable objects.

Dry heat may also be used as a sterilizing agent, although it requires much longer exposure times and higher temperatures than moist heat. This method may be used for heat-stable substances that are not penetrated by moist heat, such as oils. Dry heat is commonly used to sterilize glassware.

Boiling and **pasteurization** are both methods that achieve disinfection but not sterilization; neither method eliminates spores. Boiling (100° C) kills most microorganisms in approximately 10 minutes. Pasteurization, used mostly in the food industry, eliminates food-borne pathogens as well as organisms responsible for food spoilage. It is performed at 63° C

TABLE 4-2 Control of Microorganisms Using Health Methods

Method	Temperature (° C)	Time Required	Applications
Boiling water (steam)	100	15 minutes	Kills microbial vegetative forms; endospores survive
Autoclave (steam under pressure)	121.6	15 minutes at 15 psi	Sterilizes and kills endospores
Pasteurization			
Batch method	63	30 minutes	Disinfects and kills milk-borne pathogens and vegetable forms; endospores survive
Flash method	72	15 seconds	Same, but shorter time at higher temperature
Over (dry heat)	160-180	1.5-3 hours	Sterilizes; keeps materials dry

Adapted from VanDemark PJ, Batzing BL: *The microbes: an introduction to their nature and importance*, Redwood City, Calif, 1987, Benjamin-Cummings.

for 30 minutes. The main advantage of pasteurization is that treatment at this temperature reduces spoilage of food without affecting its taste. Table 4-2 summarizes the applications of heat.

Filtration

Filtration methods may be used with both liquid and air. **Filtration** of liquids is accomplished through the use of thin membrane filters composed of plastic polymers or cellulose

TABLE 4-3 Chemical Agents Commonly Used as Disinfectants and Antiseptics

Type	Agent(s)	Action(s)	Applications and Precautions
Alcohols (50%-70%)	Ethanol, isopropanol, benzyl alcohol	Denature proteins; make lipids soluble	Skin antiseptics
Aldehydes (in solution)	Formaldehyde (8%), glutaraldehyde (2%)	React with NH_2, $-SH$, and $-COOH$ groups	Disinfectants; kills endospores; toxic to humans
Halogens	Tincture of iodine (2% in 70% alcohol)	Inactivates proteins	Skin disinfectants
	Chlorine and chlorine compounds	Reacts with water to form hypochlorous acid (HClO); oxidizing agent	Used to disinfect drinking water; surface disinfectants
Heavy metals	Silver nitrate ($AgNO_3$)	Precipitates proteins	Eye drop (1% solution)
	Mercuric chloride ($HgCl_2$)	Reacts with $-SH$ groups; lyses cell membrane	Disinfectant: toxic at high concentrations
Detergents	Quaternary ammonium compounds	Disrupt cell membranes	Skin antiseptics; disinfectants
Phenolics	Phenol, carbolic acid, Lysol, hexachlorophene	Denature proteins; disrupt cell membranes	Disinfectants at high concentrations; used in soaps at low concentrations
Gases	Ethylene oxide	Alkylating agent	Sterilization of heat-sensitive objects

Adapted from VanDemark PJ, Batzing BL: *The microbes: an introduction to their nature and importance,* Redwood City, Calif, 1987, Benjamin-Cummings.

esters containing pores of a certain size. The liquid is pulled (vacuum) or pushed (pressure) through the filter matrix. Organisms larger than the size of the pores are retained. Filters with various pore sizes are available. Most bacteria, yeasts, and moulds are retained by pore sizes of 0.45 and 0.80 μm; however, this pore size may allow passage of *Pseudomonas*-like organisms, and therefore a 0.22-μm size is available for critical sterilizing (e.g., parenteral solutions). Membranes with pore sizes as small as 0.01 μm are capable of retaining small viruses. The most common application of filtration is in the sterilization of heat-sensitive solutions, such as parenteral solutions, vaccines, and antibiotic solutions. Filtration of air is accomplished with the use of high-efficiency particulate air (HEPA) filters. These filters are able to remove microorganisms larger than 0.3 μm and are used in laboratory hoods and in rooms of immune-compromised patients.

Radiation

Radiation may be used in two forms, ionizing and nonionizing. Ionizing radiation, in the form of gamma rays or electron beams, is of short wavelength and high energy. This method of sterilization is used by the medical industry for the sterilization of disposable supplies, such as syringes, catheters, and gloves. Nonionizing radiation in the form of ultraviolet rays is of long wavelength and low energy. Because of its poor penetrability, the usefulness of nonionizing radiation is limited; it can be used to disinfect surfaces, although the parameters (distance to surface, potential microorganisms to be destroyed) under which it is to be used need to be determined.

Chemical Methods

Just as physical methods are used mainly to achieve sterilization, chemical agents are used mainly as disinfectants. Some chemical agents, however, may be used to sterilize. These are known as *chemosterilizers*. All disinfectants are regulated by the U.S. Environmental Protection Agency (EPA). Agents that are classified as *sterilants* are regulated by the Food and Drug Administration (FDA) when they are to be used to sterilize

devices that will come in contact with patients. Chemical agents exert their killing effect by the following mechanisms:
- Reaction with components of the cytoplasmic membrane
- Denaturation of cellular proteins
- Reaction with the thiol (–SH) groups of enzymes
- Damage of RNA and DNA

The fact that agents can exert one or a combination of actions on microorganisms is important to remember. Damage to the integrity of the cytoplasmic membrane causes the cytoplasm and its contents to leak out, resulting in cell death. Denaturation of proteins effectively disrupts the metabolism of the cells. Some agents specifically react with the thiol (–SH) groups of enzymes, thereby inactivating them. Thiol groups occur usually as the amino acid cysteine. Finally, damage to RNA and DNA inhibits the replication of the organism. For ease of discussion, the chemical agents are grouped on the basis of chemical composition. Table 4-3 summarizes the applications of chemicals commonly used as disinfectants and antiseptics.

DISINFECTANTS AND ANTISEPTICS

The **germ theory** of disease was one of the most important contributions by the scientific community of microbiologists to the general welfare of the worldwide population. The medical community gradually grew aware of the problem of nosocomial (hospital-acquired) infections and the need to practice asepsis to prevent the contamination of wounds, dressings, and surgical instruments. The germ theory of disease also contributed to the development of antimicrobial chemotherapeutics.

Ignatz **Semmelweis** (1816-1865) and Joseph Lister (1827-1912) are considered to be important pioneers for the promotion of asepsis. More than 100 years ago, Semmelweis demonstrated that routine handwashing can prevent the spread of disease. Semmelweis worked in a hospital in Vienna where maternity patients were dying an alarming rate. Most of those dying maternity patients had been treated by medical students who worked on cadavers during an anatomy class before beginning their rounds in the maternity ward. Because the students did not wash their hands between touching the dead and the living (handwashing was an unrecognized hygienic practice at the time), pathogenic bacteria from the cadavers were transmitted by the hands of the students to the mothers. The result was a death rate five times higher for mothers who delivered in the hospital in contrast to the mothers who delivered at home. As many as 25% of women who delivered their babies in hospitals died of childbed fever (puerperal sepsis), later found to be caused by infection with *Streptococcus pyogenes*. In an experiment considered quaint at best by his colleagues, Semmelweis insisted that his students wash their hands before treating the mothers, and deaths on the maternity ward were reduced fivefold. Despite these remarkable results, Semmelweis' colleagues greeted his findings with hostility. Because of this hostility, he eventually resigned his position. Later in another maternity clinic, he had similar dramatic results when handwashing was implemented. Ironically, Semmelweis died in 1865 of an *S. pyogenes* infection, with his views still largely ridiculed.

After the death of Semmelweis, Joseph Lister, an academic surgeon, benefited by reading Pasteur's works about bacteria as causes of infection before he ventured into the studies of **antisepsis**. In 1867, Lister introduced British surgery to handwashing and the use of phenol as an antimicrobial agent for surgical wound dressings. His principles were gradually, although reluctantly, adopted in Britain, and the mortality rate for amputation decreased from 45% to 15%. The Listerian technique was approved in the United States at the first official meeting of the American Surgical Association in 1883, 20 years after Semmelweis' initial publications. This was the beginning of infection control.

Health care workers' hands are frequently contaminated by direct contact while caring for a patient or by indirect contact while touching a contaminated surface or device. Several factors should be included in the evaluation of a disinfectant and an antiseptic. A prerequisite for a disinfectant or antiseptic is its effectiveness against the expected spectrum of pathogens. The implementation of effective disinfection and antiseptic chemicals remains crucial in the control of nosocomial infections.

Alcohols

The two most effective alcohols used in hospitals for disinfection purposes are ethyl alcohol and isopropyl alcohol. Alcohols have excellent in vitro bactericidal activity against most gram-positive and gram-negative bacteria. They also kill *Mycobacterium tuberculosis,* various fungi, and certain enveloped viruses; however, they are not sporicidal and have poor activity against certain nonenveloped viruses. Because alcohols are not sporicidal solutions, alcohol may actually be contaminated with spores. Any solution of an alcohol that is used as an antiseptic or disinfectant should be filtered through a 0.22-µm filter to remove any spores that may be present. In addition, because alcohols are not sporicidal, any time that alcohol is used to saturate cotton balls to be used to prepare the skin for blood collection or inoculation, the cotton balls

that are saturated with the alcohol should be sterile, and the alcohol that is used should be filtered to remove the presence of any spores. There have been many reports of false-positive blood cultures that have been traced back to the use of alcohol-soaked cotton balls contaminated with spores that were used to prepare the skin for blood collection. Alcohols are inactivated by the presence of organic material. Because their action is greatly reduced in concentrations less than 50%, alcohols should be used in concentrations between 60% and 90%. For alcohols to be effective, they must be allowed to evaporate from the surface to which they were applied. Alcohols inactivate microorganisms by denaturing proteins. Alcohols are used principally as antiseptics and disinfectants. Commonly, alcohols are used to disinfect laboratory surfaces and gloved hands. The 1994 Tentative Final Monograph (TFM) for **health care antiseptic drug products** establishes ethanol (60% to 95%) as Category I, safe and effective for health care personnel handwash, surgical hand scrub, and patient preoperative skin preparation (for preparation of the skin before injection). Their use as an antiseptic is generally for preparing skin sites from which blood is to be collected or where an inoculation is to be placed. Alcohols are flammable, so they should not be used in the presence of ignition sources such as open flames or incinerators. They may be used as a housekeeping disinfectant for damp-dusting furniture and lights or wiping electrical cords without leaving a residue on treated surfaces. They are nonstaining and can disinfect semicritical instruments.

Aldehydes

Formaldehyde

Formaldehyde is an aldehyde generally used as formalin, a 37% aqueous solution or formaldehyde gas. Formaldehyde gas is often used to disinfectant biosafety hoods. This type of procedure should be left to professionals. Although formalin can be used as a chemosterilizer in high concentrations, its usefulness is limited by its irritability factor and its potential carcinogenicity. Formaldehyde has been found to be a carcinogen, and the U.S. Occupational Safety and Health Administration (OSHA) has set worker exposure limits. It is not recommended that formaldehyde in any form be used as a disinfectant or sterilant on a routine basis. *Mycobacterium tuberculosis* has been known to survive for many years in tissue fixed in formaldehyde.

Glutaraldehyde

Glutaraldehyde is also an aldehyde—more precisely, a saturated five-carbon dialdehyde that has broad-spectrum activity and rapid killing action and remains active in the presence of organic matter. Glutaraldehyde is extremely susceptible to pH changes because it is active only in an alkaline environment. When used as a 2% solution, it is germicidal in approximately 10 minutes and sporicidal in 3 to 10 hours. Its killing activity is due to inactivation of DNA and RNA through alkylation of sulfhydryl and amino groups. Even though glutaraldehyde is not inactivated by organic material, it does not penetrate organic material well. Therefore objects coated with organic material should be cleaned before glutaraldehyde is used. Glutaraldehyde solutions may be reused; however, a decrease in the activity of the glutaraldehyde may be seen due to accumulation of organic material, dilution, and change in the pH of the solution. Because it does not corrode lenses, metal, or rubber, it is the sterilizer of choice for medical equipment that is not heat-stable and therefore cannot be autoclaved as well as for material that cannot be sterilized with gas. It is a safe, high-level disinfectant for most plastic and rubber items, such as those used for administering anesthetic agents or respiratory therapy.

Glutaraldehyde is bactericidal, pseudomonacidal, fungicidal, and virucidal (against human immunodeficiency virus [HIV] and hepatitis B virus [HBV]) in a minimum of 10 minutes' exposure at a temperature between 20° and 30° C. It is tuberculocidal. Variations in formulations of products available affect the exposure time and temperature of the solution, especially after reuse. A 2% solution at 25° to 30° C may be 100% tuberculocidal. Users should follow the label instructions of the manufacturer. Most of the products labeled as *cold sterilants* are sporicidal in a minimum of 10 hours' exposure at room temperature. It remains active in the presence of organic matter and does not coagulate protein material.

Halogens

Iodophors

Iodine can be used as a disinfectant in one of two forms: tincture or iodophor. Tinctures are alcohol and iodine solutions, used mainly as antiseptics. An iodophor is a combination of iodine and a neutral polymer carrier that increases the solubility of the agent. This combination allows the slow release of iodine. Iodophors must be diluted properly them to be effective. Improperly diluted iodophors may not kill microorganisms because of the lack of free iodine in solution. Iodophors have the added advantage of being less irritating, nonstaining, and more stable than iodine in its pure form. Iodophors may be used as antiseptics or disinfectants, depending on the concentration of free iodine. The best known iodophor is povidone-iodine, which is mainly used as an antiseptic. Povidone-iodine provides slow and continuous release of free iodine. Free iodine degrades microbial cell walls and cytoplasm, denatures enzymes, and coagulates chromosomal material. Iodophors are commonly used as skin preparations from sites where blood is to be drawn. When iodophors are used for this purpose, it is critical that there is the proper amount of contact time, which is generally more than 30 seconds. All iodine tinctures and iodophors must be completely removed from the skin in order to avoid irritancy. Iodophors are used only as disinfectants because they are not sporicidal. Their bactericidal action is due to the oxidative effects of molecular iodine (I_2) and hypoiodic acid (HOI), both of which are found in solution. The FDA classifies povidone-iodine 5% to 10% as Category I for use as a topical antiseptic in health care personnel handwash, surgical hand scrub, and patient preoperative skin preparation.

Chlorine and Chlorine Compounds

Chlorine and chlorine compounds are some of the oldest and most commonly used disinfectants. They are usually used in the form of hypochlorite, such as the liquid sodium hypochlorite (household bleach) and solid calcium hypochlorite. Their killing activity is based on the oxidative effects of hypochlorous acid, formed when chloride ions are dissolved in water. Hypochlorites are inexpensive and have a broad spectrum of activity; however, they are not used as sterilants because of the long exposure time required for sporicidal action and their inactivation by organic matter. Hypochlorites are corrosive; therefore concentrated bleach solutions should not be used for disinfection. The activity of hypochlorite solutions is greatly influenced by the pH of the surrounding medium. These solutions are commonly used as surface disinfectants (e.g., for tabletops). A solution containing 0.5% to 1% sodium hypochlorite is generally used for disinfecting. Such solutions are generally stable for no longer than 30 days with as much as 50% of the original concentration of chlorine dissipating by 30 days. As with the use of any disinfectant, proper contact time is critical for bleach solutions. Solutions should be allowed a contact time of a least 3 minutes and longer if there is the presence of organic material. A 1 : 10 dilution of a 5.25% concentration of sodium hypochlorite is recommended by the Centers for Disease Control and Prevention (CDC) for cleaning up blood spills. The most common use of chlorine is disinfection of water.

Detergents: Quaternary Ammonium Compounds

Quaternary ammonium compounds (quacs) are derived by substitution of the four-valence ammonium ion with alkyl halides. They are cationic, surface-active agents, or surfactants, that work by reducing the surface tension of molecules in a liquid. Their effectiveness is reduced by hard water and soap, and they are inactivated by excess organic matter. Their action is mediated through disruption of the cellular membrane, resulting in leakage of cell contents. Certain bacteria, particularly gram-negative bacteria such as *Pseudomonas aeruginosa*, are intrinsically resistant to quaternary ammonium compounds. *Pseudomonas* spp. growing in ammonium acetate containing quacs and disease outbreaks associated with contaminated quacs have been reported. Because they are not sporicidal or tuberculocidal, the use of quaternary ammonium compounds is limited to disinfection of noncritical surfaces such as bench tops and floors.

Phenolics

Phenolics are molecules of phenol (carbolic acid) that have been chemically substituted, typically by halogens, alkyl, phenyl, or benzyl groups. These groups reduce the toxicity of phenol and increase its effectiveness. The most common phenolics are ortho-phenylphenol and ortho-benzyl-para-chlorophenol. Phenolics have a fairly broad spectrum of activity but are not sporicidal. The addition of detergents to the phenol formulation makes products that clean and disinfect in one step. They are stable, biodegradable, and relatively active in the presence of organic material. Their mechanism of inactivation is disruption of cell walls, resulting in precipitation of proteins. At lower concentrations, phenolics are able to disrupt enzyme systems. Their main use is in the disinfection of hospital, institutional, and household environments. They are also commonly found in germicidal soaps.

Chlorhexidine Gluconate

Chlorhexidine gluconate (CHG) has been used for more than 30 years in the hospital setting. In 1976, the FDA granted approval of CHG for use as a topical antiseptic based on its high level of antimicrobial activity, low toxicity, and strong affinity for binding to the skin and mucous membranes. CHG was not an OTC drug monograph active ingredient at that time. CHG disrupts the microbial cell membrane and precipitates the cell contents. CHG (0.5% to 4%) is more effective against gram-positive than gram-negative bacteria and has less activity against fungi and tubercle bacilli. CHG is inactive against bacteria spores, except at elevated temperatures. Lipid-enveloped viruses (e.g., herpes virus, HIV, respiratory viruses, influenza virus, cytomegalovirus) are rapidly inactivated. Nonenveloped viruses (e.g., rotavirus, adenovirus, enteroviruses) are not inactivated by exposure to CHG. Numerous studies indicate that CHG is safe and nontoxic. It is not absorbed through the skin and has a low skin-irritancy potential. However, severe skin reactions may occur in infants younger than 2 months of age. The potential for allergic contact sensitization and photosensitization is reported to be minimal. However, CHG should not come into contact with eyes, the middle ear, or meninges. Although not as rapidly effective as the alcohols, a major attribute of CHG is its persistence, in that it binds to the skin and remains active for at least 6 hours. Although it is not significantly affected by organic matter such as blood, it is pH-dependent; hence the formulation significantly affects activity. The optimum range of 5.5 to 7.0 corresponds to the pH of body surfaces and tissues.

Chlorhexidine gluconate is used extensively for disinfection of surgical personnel's hands and provides whole-body disinfection of patients undergoing surgery. Low concentration (0.5% to 1%) CHG is added to alcohol-based preparations to provide greater residual activity than alcohol alone. The immediate bactericidal action of CHG surpasses antiseptic preparations containing povidone-iodine, triclosan, hexachlorophene, or chloroxylenol. Its persistence, which prevents regrowth of microorganisms on the skin, is comparable to that of hexachlorophene or triclosan. CHG has a broader spectrum of activity than the others, especially against gram-negative bacteria.

Hexachlorophene

Hexachlorophene is primarily effective against gram-positive bacteria. It is a chlorinated bisphenol that interrupts bacterial electron transport, inhibits membrane-bound enzymes at low concentrations, and ruptures bacterial membranes at high concentrations. Three percent hexachlorophene kills gram-positive bacteria within 15 to 30 seconds, but a longer time is needed for gram-negative bacteria. Hexachlorophene has residual activity for several hours after application and has a cumulative effect after multiple uses. Hexachlorophene has been associated with severe toxic effects, including deaths. It can be absorbed through damaged skin of adults and the skin of premature infants. The FDA classified 3% hexachloro-

phene to be available only by prescription and designated it as unsafe for OTC distribution. Hexachlorophene is indicated to control outbreaks of gram-positive infections when other infection control procedures have been unsuccessful. Hexachlorophene should be used only as long as necessary for infection control.

Chloroxylenol

Chloroxylenol (PCMX) is a halogen-substituted phenolic compound that has been used in the United States since the 1940s. PCMX at concentrations of 0.5% to 4% acts by microbial cell wall disruption and enzyme inactivation. PCMX has good activity against gram-positive bacteria, but it is less active against gram-negative bacteria, *M. tuberculosis*, fungi, and viruses. The antimicrobial activity of PCMX is unaffected by organic materials such as blood or sputum, but it is neutralized by nonionic surfactants and polyethylene glycol. It is considered intermediate to slow acting and has minimal **persistent** effect of over a few hours. PCMX has low antimicrobial efficacy compared to iodines, iodophors, and CHG in reducing skin flora. The FDA classified PCMX (0.24% to 3.75%) as Category I for safety and Category III for effectiveness for short-term use such as patient preoperative skin preparation. PCMX is classified as Category III for safety and effectiveness for long-term uses; that is, health care personnel handwash and surgical hand scrub. The FDA is currently evaluating the safety and efficacy of PCMX for use as a health care antiseptic under the OTC drug review.

Triclosan

Triclosan is a diphenyl ether that disrupts the cell wall. The reaction time is intermediate while the persistence is excellent. It has good activity against gram-positive bacteria, gram-negative bacteria, and viruses. It has fair activity against *M. tuberculosis* and poor activity against fungi. Triclosan is not significantly affected by organic matter such as blood, but is affected by pH and the presence of surfactants and emollients, and hence formulation significantly affects activity. Triclosan can be absorbed through intact skin but appears to be nonallergenic and nonmutagenic with short-term use. The FDA classified triclosan as Category I for safety and Category III for effectiveness for short-term use such as patient preoperative skin preparation. It is classified as Category III for safety and effectiveness for long-term repeat uses for health care personnel handwash and surgical hand scrub.

Safety and efficacy evaluation of triclosan for use as a health care antiseptic is currently underway at the FDA. Triclosan has been incorporated into a variety of personal care products, including toothpaste, deodorant soap, underarm deodorant, shower gel, and health care personnel handwash.

Heavy Metals

Disinfectants containing heavy metals are rarely used in clinical applications; they have been replaced by safer and more effective compounds. Slowly bactericidal, the action of heavy metal disinfectants is primarily bacteriostatic. Because of the toxic effects of mercuric chloride and other mercury compounds, their use as disinfectants has declined, and they are used mainly as preservatives for paint. Silver nitrate (1%

eyedrop solution) has been used as a prophylactic treatment to prevent gonococcal *(Neisseria gonorrhoeae)* conjunctivitis in newborns.

Gases

Ethylene Oxide

Ethylene oxide is the gas most commonly used for sterilization. Because it is explosive in its pure form, it is mixed with nitrogen or carbon dioxide before use. Factors such as temperature, time, and relative humidity are extremely important in determining the effectiveness of gas sterilization. The recommended concentration is 450 to 700 mg of ethylene oxide per liter of chamber space at 55° to 60° C for 2 hours. A relative humidity of 30% is optimal for the destruction of spores. The killing mechanism of ethylene oxide is the alkylation of nucleic acids in the spore and vegetative cell. Gas sterilization is widely used in hospitals for materials that cannot withstand steam sterilization. This method is also used extensively by the manufacturing industry for the sterilization of low-cost thermoplastic products.

Hydrogen Peroxide

Vaporized hydrogen peroxide (H_2O_2) is primarily used as a sterilant in the pharmaceutical and medical device manufacturing industries. It is active against all vegetative microorganisms as well as bacterial and fungal spores.

Periacetic Acid

Periacetic acid is used in a gaseous form as a sterilant primarily in the pharmaceutical and medical device manufacturing industries. It is active against all vegetative microorganisms as well as bacterial and fungal spores.

Hydrogen Peroxide and Periacetic Acid

The combination of H_2O_2 and periacetic acid vapors is used in the pharmaceutical and medical device manufacturing industries. Just like each of its individual components, the combination of H_2O_2 and periacetic acid is active against all vegetative forms of microorganisms as well as bacterial and fungal spores. The major advantage to the use of the combination of H_2O_2 and periacetic acid over each of its individual components is a shorter contact time. The activity of the combination of H_2O_2 and periacetic acid, as well as each of the individual components against prions, is not fully known.

EPA REGULATIONS ON CHEMICAL SURFACE DISINFECTANTS

The Antimicrobial Division of the **Environmental Protection Agency (EPA)** regulates the registration on the use, sale, and distribution of antimicrobial pesticide products for certain inanimate, hard nonporous surfaces, or incorporation of antimicrobial pesticide products into substances under the pesticide law—the Federal Insecticide, Fungicide and Rodenticide Act (FIFRA). An EPA registration number is granted only when the requirement of laboratory test data, toxicity data, product formula, and label copy are approved. The disinfectant label should indicate several highlighted points impor-

---

BOX 4-1 Type of Information to Review on a Disinfectant Label

Front Panel
- Product name, brand, or trademark
- Ingredient statement (concentration or strength)
- "Keep Out of Reach of Children"
- EPA registration number and establishment number

Back Panel
- Precautionary statements
  - Hazards to humans and domestic animals
  - First aid
  - Environmental hazard
  - Physical or chemical hazard
- Directions for use
  - How to use the product
  - Application sites and rates
  - Worker protection issues
- Aftercare
  - Equipment
  - Treated surfaces
  - Cleaning supplies
  - Storage and disposal

EPA, Environmental Protection Agency.

---

tant in selecting the appropriate agents for the designated use (Box 4-1).

FDA REGULATIONS ON CHEMICAL SKIN ANTISEPTICS

When developing an **antiseptic drug** product, there are two options a manufacturer can pursue: the **new drug application (NDA)** process or the **over-the-counter (OTC) drug** review known as the **monograph** system. NDAs are defined by law as being **recognized as safe and effective (RASE).** A new chemical entity never before marketed in the United States would be classified as a new drug and, in most cases, initially approved for prescription use only. The approved NDA is manufacturer-specific and allows only that particular sponsor to market the product. Other manufacturers wanting to market a similar product would also need to seek **Food and Drug Administration (FDA)** approval through an NDA. The FDA considers a drug safe enough to approve when the benefits outweigh the risks. This risk-to-benefit assessment is critical in the drug approval process.

Over-the-counter drugs are defined as **generally recognized as safe and effective (GRASE)** for their intended use as long as they are neither misbranded nor marketed using false or misleading statements. The FDA classifies OTC drug products into three categories: (1) Category I: GRASE for the claimed therapeutic indication; (2) Category II: not GRASE or having unacceptable indications; and (3) Category III: insufficient data available to permit final classification.

A manufacturer desiring to market a monographed (therapeutic classes of ingredients that are GRASE) drug need not seek clearance from the FDA before marketing. In this case, marketing is not exclusive and all data and information sup-

TABLE 4-4 FDA Product Categories of Topical Antiseptics

Category	Definition
Antiseptic drug	The representative of a drug, in its labeling, as an antiseptic shall be considered to be representation that it is a germicide, except in the case of a drug purporting to be, or represented as, an antiseptic for inhibitory use as a wet dressing, ointment, dusting powder, or such other use as involves prolonged contact with the body.
Broad spectrum activity	A properly formulated drug product, containing an ingredient included in the monograph, that possesses in vitro activity against the microorganisms listed in §333.470(a)(1)(ii), as demonstrated by in vitro minimum inhibitory concentration determinations conducted according to methodology established in §333.470(a)(1)(ii).
Health care antiseptic drug product	An antiseptic-containing drug product applied topically to the skin to help prevent infection or help prevent cross contamination.
Antiseptic handwash or health care personnel handwash drug product	An antiseptic-containing preparation designed for frequent use; it reduces the number of transient microorganisms on intact skin to an initial baseline level after adequate washing, rinsing, and drying; it is broad-spectrum, fast-acting and, if possible, persistent.
Surgical hand scrub drug product	An antiseptic-containing preparation that significantly reduces the number of microorganisms on intact skin; it is broad-spectrum, fast-acting, and persistent.
Patient preoperative skin preparation drug product	A fast-acting, broad-spectrum, and persistent antiseptic-containing preparation that significantly reduces the number of microorganisms on intact skin.

porting GRASE status are publicly available. Monographs mainly address active ingredients in the product, and in most cases, final formulations are not subject to monograph specifications. Manufacturers are free to include any inactive ingredients that serve a pharmaceutical purpose, as long as those ingredients are considered safe and do not interfere with product effectiveness or required final product testing. In some instances, even though the product may contain GRASE ingredients, the final formulation may need to meet a monograph testing procedure. An example would be the antiseptic drug products that are for **health care personnel handwash, surgical hand scrub,** and **patient preoperative skin preparation.** Table 4-4 lists terms and definitions frequently used for topical antiseptics in health care settings. These are required to meet in vivo and in vitro efficacy testing requirements to ensure that their formulated products are effective as an antiseptic. Inactive ingredients and emollients, when included in the products, may inhibit the antiseptic action; therefore testing must be performed to show effectiveness.

Hygienic Handwashing and Waterless Handrubs

The main goal of handwashing is to eliminate the **transient flora.** Transient flora is contracted from the environment or from other people. In most cases, these organisms are not part of the established normal biota (normal flora). For example, the health care worker in the second Case in Point may acquire microbes including methicillin-resistant *Staphylococcus aureus* (MRSA) during direct contact with animals, patients, or contaminated surfaces. Hands should always be washed immediately after arriving at work. Even though the health care worker's hands appeared to be clean, after having contact with her sick child and her dog, her hands harbored many bacteria and infectious microorganisms. She should have stopped seeing patients and washed her hands as soon as she remembered, and she should wash her hands before and after contact with each patient. Although transient organisms are easily removed from the upper layer of the skin along with dirt particles and oil, they may become part of the resident

established flora of individuals. Interventions against the bacterial load of the hands should balance two goals: protecting the skin with its **resident flora** and killing the transient flora. Intact skin on health care workers' hands helps to protect both patients and health care workers from getting or transmitting nosocomial infections.

Routine handwashing procedure in health care settings is performed in the following situations:

- Removing physical dirt (including blood, excretions, secretions or discharge from lesions)
- Before and after routine patient contact
- After contact with infected or colonized patients or their immediate surroundings
- In high-risk units such as intensive care and burn units
- On entering protective isolation units and leaving source isolation units
- Before antiseptic procedures (e.g., dressing techniques, minor invasive procedures)

The FDA requires that all antiseptic handwashing products used in the hospital setting reduce the number of sampled test bacteria by 2 $\log_{10}$ on each hand within 5 minutes after the first wash application and demonstrate a 3 $\log_{10}$ reduction within 5 minutes after the tenth wash application. The technique involves treating the hands with the antiseptic product according to the manufacturer's instructions for the specified time period. The lower third of the forearm is also washed. After completion of the wash, hands and forearms are rinsed under tap water ($40 \pm 2°$ C) and dried thoroughly with disposable or sterilized towels.

Waterless handrubs (alcohol handrubs)—either liquid or gel—are used for hygienic hand antiseptics. They can also be used as an alternative to routine handwashing when there is no visible soiling and for patient contacts. They are often more convenient than handwashing and can be particularly useful if sinks are not readily available. Dispensers for alcohol handrubs can be fitted next to sinks and placed beside each bed or carried around by each health care worker. The technique involves rubbing small portions (3 to 5 mL) of a **fast-acting antiseptic,** usually an alcoholic preparation, into the hands and rubbing until dry or for a preset duration recommended by the manufacturer. All areas of the hands must be covered completely with the antiseptic, including the subungual spaces of the fingers.

Surgical Hand Scrub and Waterless Surgical Handrubs

The objective of the surgical hand scrub and waterless surgical handrubs is to eliminate the transient flora and most of the resident flora. Resident flora can be persistently isolated from the hands of most people. These organisms include coagulase-negative staphylococci, *Corynebacterium* spp. (diphtheroids or coryneforms), *Propionibacterium* spp., and *Acinetobacter* spp.

The rationale is to limit bacterial exposure of the surgeon's hands in case the surgical glove is punctured or torn. Tiny holes are observed in 30% or more of surgeons' gloves after operation, even when high-quality gloves are used. A surgical hand scrub drug product is defined as an antiseptic containing a preparation that significantly reduces the number of microorganisms on intact skin; it is broad spectrum, fast acting, and persistent. The FDA requires that the product (1) reduce on the first day the number of bacteria by 1 log_{10} on each hand within 1 minute after application and that the count on each hand does not subsequently exceed baseline within 6 hours; (2) produce a 2 log_{10} reduction within 1 minute after use by the end of the second day; and (3) produce a 3 log_{10} reduction within 1 minute by the end of the fifth day. Surgical hand scrub procedures are performed according to the manufacturer's instruction but for no longer than 5 minutes. They offer the advantage of cleaning and disinfecting the hands at the same time.

Surgical handrubs, alcohol solutions (60% to 70% ethanol or isopropanol) with an emollient and with or without an added antiseptic as recommended for hygienic waterless handrubs, are used, but larger volumes and longer exposure times are needed than for hygienic waterless handrubs. Surgical handrub application technique is accomplished by pouring a specified amount of antiseptic into the cupped dry hands and rubbing vigorously all over the hands and forearms, which must be kept wet with the handrub solution for the scheduled period of 3 to 5 minutes by adding additional portions as necessary and continuing to rub. Before the application of an alcohol, the hands must be dry, and before donning gloves, the alcohol must have completely evaporated.

Presurgical Skin Disinfection

In order to be effective, preoperative skin preparation formulations must degerm an intended surgical site rapidly as well as provide a high level of bacterial inactivation and persistent antimicrobial activity, up to 6 hours after preparing the skin. A patient preoperative skin preparation drug product is defined as a fast-acting, broad-spectrum, and persistent antiseptic-containing preparation that significantly reduces the number of microorganisms on intact skin. Like the surgeon's hands, the patient's operation site requires surgical disinfection, directed against resident as well as transient flora, and it often requires maximum disinfection in a single treatment, without the benefit from progressive effects of repeated application. The FDA requires that the product reduce the number of bacteria 2 log_{10} per square centimeter on an abdomen test site and 3 log_{10} per square centimeter on a groin test site within 10 minutes after product use and that the bacterial count for each test site does not exceed baseline 6 hours after product use. For preinjection sites, the product must reduce the number of bacteria 1 log_{10} per square centimeter square on a dry skin test site within 30 seconds of product use. It has long been debated whether or not a preoperative skin preparation is adequate in degerming the skin before making a surgical incision. Many surgeons recognize this problem, and to promote greater degerming of the surgical site area, patients are requested to wash the area daily or more often, before surgery. The intent is to reduce the microbial population at the presurgical site area so that the region is prepared before surgery; the organisms then being few in number, they would be virtually totally removed from the skin.

BIBLIOGRAPHY

Ali Y et al: Alcohols. In Block SS, editor: *Disinfection, sterilization, and preservation*, ed 5, Philadelphia, 2001, Lippincott Williams & Wilkins.

Block SS, editor: *Disinfection, sterilization, and preservation*, ed 5, Philadelphia, 2001, Lippincott Williams & Wilkins.

Clinical and Laboratory Standards Institute (CLSI): *Clinical laboratory waste management GP5-A2*, Wayne, Pa, 2002, CLSI.

Denny V, Marsik F: Disinfection practices in parenteral manufacturing. In *Microbial contamination control in parenteral manufacturing*, New York, 2004, Marcel Dekker.

Denton GW: Chlorhexidine. In Block SS, editor: *Disinfection, sterilization, and preservation*, ed 5, Philadelphia, 2001, Lippincott Williams & Wilkins.

Fleming D, Hunt DL: *Biological safety: principles and practices*, ed 3, Washington, DC, 2000, American Society for Microbiology.

Food and Drug Administration: OTC topical antimicrobial products. Tentative final monograph for healthcare antiseptic drug products, *Fed Reg* 59:31402, 1994.

Food and Drug Administration: Statements of general policy or interpretation. Hexachlorophene as a component in drug and cosmetic products for human use: final rule, *Fed Reg* 37:20160, 1972.

Goddard PA, McCue KA: Phenolic compounds. In Block SS, editor: *Disinfection, sterilization, and preservation*, ed 5, Philadelphia, 2001, Lippincott Williams & Wilkins.

Gottardi W: Iodine and iodine compounds. In Block SS, editor: *Disinfection, sterilization, and preservation*, ed 5, Philadelphia, 2001, Lippincott Williams & Wilkins.

Hoffman P, Bradley C, Ayliffe G, editors: *Disinfection in healthcare*, ed 3, Malden, Mass, 2004, Blackwell.

Jackson MM: Topical antiseptics in healthcare, *Clin Lab Science J* 18:160-169, 2005.

Manivannan G, editor: *Disinfection and decontamination: principles, applications and related issues*, Boca Raton, Fla, 2007, CRC Press.

Marsik FJ, Denys GE: Sterilization, decontamination, and disinfection procedures for the microbiology laboratory. In *Manual of clinical microbiology*, ed 6, Washington, DC, 1995, American Society for Microbiology.

McDonnell GE, editor: *Antisepsis, disinfection, and sterilization*, Washington, DC, 2007, American Society for Microbiology.

Moore SL, Payne DN: Types of antimicrobial agents. In Fraise AP, Lambert PA, Maillard JY, editors: *Russell, Hugo and Ayliffe's principles and practice of disinfection, preservation and sterilization*, Malden, Mass, 2004, Blackwell.

Newman JL, Seitz JC: Intermittent use of an antimicrobial hand gel for reducing soap-induced irritation of health care personnel, *Am J Infect Control* 18:194, 1990.

Occupational Safety and Health Administration: *Bloodborne pathogens standards*, CFR, Washington, DC, 1991, OSHA.

Paulson DS: Nosocomial infection. In Paulson DS, editor: *Handbook of topical antimicrobials*, New York, 2003, Marcel Dekker.

Phillips NF, editor: *Berry & Kohn's operating room technique*, ed 11, St Louis, 2007, Mosby.

Ranganathan NS: Chlorhexidine. In Ascenzi JM, editor: *Handbook of disinfectants and antiseptic*, New York, 1996, Marcel Dekker.

Rotter ML: Special problems in hospital antisepsis. In Fraise AP, Lambert PA, Maillard JY, editors: *Russell, Hugo and Ayliffe's principles and practice of disinfection, preservation and sterilization*, Malden, Mass, 2004, Blackwell.

Rutala WA, Weber DJ: *Draft guideline for disinfection and sterilization in healthcare facilities*, HIPAC 2b, Atlanta, 2002, Centers for Disease Control and Prevention and DHHS.

Sheldon AT: Food and Drug Administration perspective on topical antiseptic drug product development. In Paulson DS, editor: *Handbook of topical antimicrobials*, New York, 2003, Marcel Dekker.

Tooher R, Maddern GJ, Simpson J: Surgical fires and alcohol-based skin preparations, *Aust N Z J Surg* 74:382, 2004.

Voss A, Nulens E: Prevention and control of laboratory acquired infections. In *Manual of clinical microbiology*, ed 8, Washington, DC, 2003, American Society for Microbiology.

World Health Organization: *Infection control guidelines for transmissible spongiform encephalopathies*. Report of a WHO Consultation, Geneva, March 23-24, 1999, WHO/CDS/CSR/APH/20003.

Points to Remember

- Physical and chemical methods may be used in the process of sterilization in order to remove all forms of life.
- Disinfection involves removal of pathogenic organisms but may not include removal of bacterial or other spores, and most disinfectants are chemical agents.
- Factors that influence the degree of killing include the types of organisms, number of organisms present, concentration of disinfecting agent, amount of soil present, and the nature of the surface to be disinfected.
- Antiseptics are designed to reduce the bacterial load of living tissues.
- Disinfectants are designed to be used on inanimate objects to kill or destroy disease-producing microorganisms.
- There are two options a manufacturer can pursue in seeking approval for a disinfectant product: submission of a new drug application (NDA) or over-the-counter (OTC) drug review known as the *monograph system*.
- Antimicrobial agents for health care personnel use must meet certain standards that demonstrate the product's safety and efficacy.

Learning Assessment Questions

1. What is the difference between sterilization and disinfection?
2. When is an antiseptic used?
3. Describe the difference between physical and chemical methods of disinfection and sterilization.
4. What method is required to effectively kill endospores?
5. List and describe factors that influence the degree of killing during disinfection and sterilization.
6. What is the difference between disinfectant and antiseptic?
7. Transient flora of the skin is defined as:
   a. Organisms that are contracted from the environment
   b. Organisms that are contracted from other persons
   c. Not part of the established normal biota
   d. All of the above
8. Give the mechanism of action for each type of chemical agent commonly used in antiseptics and disinfectants.
9. Alcohol drug products have excellent in vitro bacteriocidal activity against most vegetative gram-positive and gram-negative bacteria; however, they are:
   a. Not fast acting
   b. Not sporicidal
   c. Not bacteriocidal
   d. None of the above
10. Describe EPA regulations on chemical surface disinfectants and FDA regulations on chemical skin antiseptics.
11. Describe the following hospital-use skin antiseptics: health care personnel handwash, surgical hand scrub, and patient preoperative skin preparation.
12. Which of the following characteristics should be considered when selecting an antimicrobial agent?
    a. Spectrum of activity
    b. Rate of action
    c. Mechanism of action
    d. All of the above

B. Microbiology Safety

Barbara L. Russell, Rebecca B. Stone

- **GENERAL LABORATORY SAFETY**
  Safety Program for the Clinical Laboratory
  Safety from Infectious Agents in the Microbiology
    Laboratory
  Hazardous Waste
  Chemical Safety
  Fire Safety
  Storage of Compressed Gases

  Electrical Safety
  Miscellaneous Safety Considerations
  Safety Training
- **BIOTERRORISM AND THE CLINICAL MICROBIOLOGY LABORATORY**
  Laboratory Response Network
  Safety During a Possible Bioterrorism Event
  Packaging and Shipping of Infectious Substances

OBJECTIVES

After reading and studying this chapter, you should be able to:

1. Describe the hazards that can be encountered in a microbiology laboratory.
2. List the elements included in an exposure control plan.
3. Discuss the practice of Standard Precautions.
4. Define and give examples of engineering controls, work practice controls, and personal protective equipment.
5. Discuss the WHO classification of infectious microorganisms by risk group.
6. Differentiate the three types of biosafety cabinets.
7. Describe the four categories of biosafety levels.
8. Explain the information that must be included in the MSDS sheets.
9. Describe the components of basic fire safety and electrical safety within the microbiology laboratory.
10. Understand the special safety considerations that must be addressed in the clinical microbiology laboratory during a possible bioterrorism event.

Case in Point

In 1979 a microbiologist at the bench was examining a stool culture from a patient in a pediatric hospital with a suspected case of a food-borne enteric disease. She spilled the selenite F (a liquid enrichment media for the growth of *Salmonella* and *Shigella* spp.) on her work area. She cleaned the area with alcohol and proceeded to work on additional cultures. Within 48 hours, she started having watery diarrhea progressing to abdominal cramps and bloody stools. Because of her signs and symptoms, a stool culture was performed. *Shigella sonnei* was isolated from both the patient's and the technologist's stool culture. An inquiry by the laboratory supervisor was performed. Her co-workers said that she had eaten her lunch that day at the bench and was seen chewing her pen. In addition, she was not wearing gloves.

Issues to Consider

After reading the patient's and technologist's case history, consider:

- The identity of the organism causing the infections
- Risk factors for the acquisition of the organism
- Importance of laboratory safety procedures

Key Terms

Biosafety cabinet
Biosafety level
Blood-borne pathogens
Employee right-to-know
Engineering controls
Exposure control plan
Hazard-rating diamond
Laboratory Response Network
Material Safety Data Sheets
  (MSDSs)

National Fire Protection
  Association (NFPA)
Personal protective
  equipment (PPE)
Risk groups
Sentinel laboratories
Standard Precautions
Work practice controls

The concept of laboratory safety has changed drastically in the past decade. Before 1980, safety practices in most microbiology laboratories were lax. Mouth pipetting was a widely used technique, and eating, drinking, and smoking in the laboratory, although discouraged, were common. Beginning in the early 1980s, this relaxed attitude toward safety among personnel changed dramatically. The impetus behind the change was the arrival in the United States of a previously unheard-of disease with an apparent 100% mortality rate. This disease became known as the acquired immunedeficiency syndrome (AIDS). In addition to being a global calamity, AIDS initiated a major rethinking of employee risk for laboratory-acquired infections in hospitals around the country. Beginning with an emphasis on reducing the risks of biologic hazards (biohazards), safety became a priority for laboratory personnel. The attitude "What you don't know can't hurt you," common among laboratory employees, rapidly went out of date. With the passage of time, the concept of laboratory safety expanded to include chemical, radioactive, electrical, and fire hazard protection.

GENERAL LABORATORY SAFETY

Safety in the clinical laboratory is the responsibility of the institution, laboratory directors, and laboratory managers, as well as the laboratory employees. Laboratory employees must be provided a safe work environment. Laboratory directors, managers, and employees must know the current safety regulations, safety procedure manuals must be provided, and training in safe laboratory practices must occur on an annual basis through in-service education and should be the duties of an assigned safety officer. Although the provision of a safe work environment is ultimately the employer's responsibility, it cannot be achieved without the commitment of all persons in that environment to practice safe techniques for their own and their co-workers' protection.

Safety Program for the Clinical Laboratory

The comprehensive safety program for the clinical laboratory needs to fulfill the following:
- Address biologic hazards by performing Biologic Risk Assessments and the development of safety procedures for working with these hazards.
- Describe the safe handling, storage, and disposal of chemicals and radioactive substances.
- Clearly outline the laboratory or hospital policies for correct procedures in the event of fire, natural disasters, and even bomb threats.
- Perform initial safety training for all employees in all aspects of laboratory safety and update annually.
- Teach correct techniques for lifting and moving heavy objects and patients.

This safety program needs to be ongoing and consistent with current federal and state regulations. Most important, it must be presented in a way that encourages employees to incorporate the safety practices into their daily routines and take responsibility for keeping the work environment safe.

Occupational Safety and Health Administration

Laboratorians must always remember that they work in a hazardous environment. Hazards can be classified as biologic, chemical, radiologic, or physical. Training programs are instituted in all of these areas for employees who are exposed to any of these hazards. It is imperative for the individual to

follow the rules that are set forth in the safety procedure manuals.

The mission of the Occupational Safety and Health Administration (OSHA) is to protect workers within the United States. The clinical laboratory falls under these regulations. In 1991 the *Bloodborne Pathogen Final Standard,* which is one of the OSHA standards created to protect health care workers, was released. This standard was revised in 2001 in conformance with Public Law 106-430, the Needlestick Safety and Prevention Act.

Exposure Control Plan

The OSHA Bloodborne Pathogen Standard clearly states the safety requirements that the employer must have in place to protect the employee from **blood-borne pathogens.** Employers are required to have an **exposure control plan,** which must be annually reviewed and updated. This plan must be available to all employees and should include the following:
- A determination of tasks and procedures that may result in an occupational hazard
- A plan to investigate all exposure incidents and a plan to prevent these from reoccurring
- Methods of compliance for standard precautions (universal precautions)
- Engineering and work practice controls
- Personal protective equipment (PPE)
- Guidelines for ensuring that the work site is maintained in a clean and sanitary manner
- Guidelines for the handling and disposal of regulated waste
- A training program for all employees

Universal/Standard Precautions

In 1985 the CDC instituted safety guidelines for the handling of blood and body fluids. These guidelines, called *universal precautions,* were intended to protect hospital personnel from blood-borne infections. In 1996, these guidelines were updated and renamed. This new set of guidelines, **Standard Precautions,** is still in effect. These guidelines require that blood and body fluids from *all* patients be considered infectious and capable of transmitting disease. Blood and all body fluids, including secretions and excretions, except sweat, regardless of whether visible blood is present, is considered infectious. Standard Precautions also include nonintact skin and mucous membranes.

To ensure that the guidelines required in standard precautions are followed within the laboratory, engineering controls and work practice controls are instituted, and employers must provide PPE. Standard Precautions address the following:
- *Handwashing* must be done after touching blood, body fluids, secretions, excretions, and any items considered contaminated. Hands must be washed after removing gloves and between patients.
- *Gloves* should be worn when handling blood, body fluids, secretions, excretions, and any items considered contaminated. Clean gloves must be put on before touching mucous membranes and nonintact skin. Hands must be washed after removal of gloves.

- *Mask, eye protection, and a face shield* must be worn anytime there is a potential for splashes or sprays of blood, body fluids, secretions, and excretions.
- *Lab coats* must be worn to protect skin and clothing when contact with blood, body fluids, secretions, and excretions could occur.
- *Appropriate sharps disposal* must be implemented with care to prevent injuries with sharps, needles, and scalpels. These devices must be placed in appropriate puncture-resistant containers after use.
- *Environmental control* must be adequate such that it provide procedures for routine care, cleaning, and disinfection of environmental surfaces.

Engineering Controls

Engineering controls are defined by OSHA as controls that isolate or remove the hazard from the workplace. Some examples of engineering controls are the use of closed tube sampling by laboratory equipment, the use of safety needles and single-use holders, eyewash stations, emergency showers, and plastic shield barriers. Ideally laboratories should have negative air pressure, access to the laboratory should be limited, and there should be a plan to prevent insect infestation.

Work Practice Controls

Altering the manner in which a task is performed in order to reduce the likelihood of exposure to infectious agents is defined by OSHA as **work practice controls.** Examples of work practice controls are:
- No mouth pipetting
- No eating, drinking, smoking, or applying cosmetics in the laboratory
- Disinfecting workstations at the end of each shift and after any spill of infectious material
- No recapping or breaking of contaminated needles
- Disposal of needles in an appropriate puncture resistant container
- Procedures performed in a manner that minimizes splashing and the generation of air droplets
- Specimens transported by way of well-constructed containers with secure lids to prevent leakage of infectious materials
- Frequent handwashing

Personal Protective Equipment

Specialized clothing or equipment that is worn by an employee for protection B is defined by OSHA as **personal protective equipment (PPE),** which must be provided and maintained by the employer. Gloves, lab coats, masks, respirators, face shields, and safety glasses are all examples of PPE. For PPE to be protective and considered appropriate, blood and body fluids must not be able to penetrate the PPE material. The equipment must be accessible to the employee and must be worn whenever there is the potential for exposure to infectious material; it must be removed before leaving the work area and must be placed in an area designated for PPE. Gloves should be removed whenever they become contaminated, and disposable gloves should *never* be washed and reused. Again, hands must be washed after the removal of gloves.

Personal protective equipment must fit properly to be the most effective. Respirators that are used for protection against airborne transmission of infectious agents must be fit-tested to ensure the protection of the worker. Figure 4-3 illustrates goggles, masks, and laboratory garments appropriate for use in laboratory workstations.

Safety from Infectious Agents in the Microbiology Laboratory

For an infection to occur, including a laboratory-acquired infection (LAI), there must be a susceptible host, the infectious agent must have a route of transmission to the susceptible host, and the concentration of the agent must be high enough to cause disease. The biologic hazards in the microbiology laboratory come from two major sources: (1) processing of the patient specimens and (2) handling of the actively growing cultures of microorganisms. Either activity puts the employee at risk of potential contact with infectious agents through direct skin, eye or mucous membrane exposure (e.g., rubbing the nose or eyes with contaminated hands), inhalation of aerosols of microorganisms, accidental ingestion (e.g., putting pens or fingers into the mouth), or needlesticks. Families of microbiology personnel and persons who work in adjacent laboratories may also be at risk.

Many infectious agents pose a high risk to laboratory employees. *Mycobacterium tuberculosis* has long been known to cause tuberculosis in laboratory workers exposed to aerosols created in processing sputum samples. A laboratory accident involving a spill of active *M. tuberculosis*, which could easily aerosolize through the ventilation system, is every microbiologist's nightmare. *Brucella* spp. and *Francisella tularensis* are other infectious agents that can be transmitted through inhalation of an aerosol created during the processing or handling of specimens (e.g., blood, which may harbor these organisms) or cultures of the organism. *Coccidioides immitis*, the most infectious of all the fungi, can infect several people in a room if culture plates on which the organism is growing are not sealed with tape or are open in the absence of a biosafety hood. In the 1970s, *Bacillus anthracis* was responsible for the deaths of a laboratory worker's wife and infant who were infected through handling his contaminated laboratory coat. Emerging pathogens, such as severe acute respiratory syndrome–coronavirus (SARS-CoV), pose a major risk due to the fact that there is often a lack of knowledge and experience when working with these emerging infectious agents.

Blood-borne pathogens pose a high risk also. Hepatitis B virus can be transmitted to laboratory workers through needlestick injuries or cuts from other sharp instruments that have been contaminated with an infected patient's blood or body fluids or through contact with mucous membranes. The Centers for Disease Control and Prevention (CDC) stated that before the institution of the HBV vaccine in 1982, more than 10,000 health care workers were accidentally infected with this blood-borne pathogen annually. However, in 2001 the number dropped to fewer than 400. Human immunodeficiency virus (HIV) and hepatitis C virus are other blood-borne pathogens that may be transmitted to laboratory personnel from contaminated specimens through a needle-

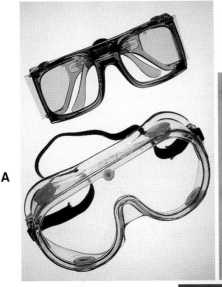

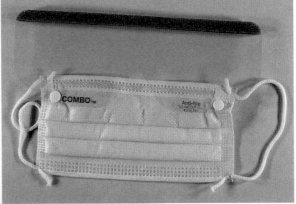

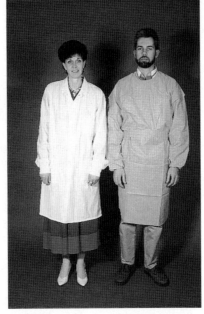

FIGURE 4-3 **A,** Eye protection used when chemical splashing could occur. **B,** Integrated eye protection and mask. **C,** Laboratory coats. The material of the white laboratory coat slows the penetration of liquids that splash or soak it. The coat on the right is disposable.

stick injury or another percutaneous route. All these infectious agents must be handled with extreme care.

Because microbiology laboratory personnel frequently deal with a variety of infectious agents—viral, fungal, bacterial, parasitic, and mycobacterial—LAIs are an obvious hazard and should be a concern for all laboratorians. Therefore all laboratorians must understand that they are at risk for an LAI, because of the environment in which they work, and it should be the goal of laboratory management and laboratory workers to minimize this risk and follow all of the safety procedures employed by the laboratory for their protection.

The Case in Point illustrates a laboratory-acquired infection that could have been prevented with the use of proper precautions. There are, however, many unseen hazards that also need to be addressed to provide a comprehensive and thorough safety program.

Biologic Risk Assessment

Biologic risk assessment is an important part of every microbiology laboratory safety program. Biologic risk assessment is a process used to recognize the hazardous characteristics of infectious agents that may be encountered in the clinical microbiology laboratory. Also included in the risk assessment process are the laboratory practices that could result in an infectious exposure, the likelihood that the LAI will occur, and the consequences of that infection. It is through this

---

BOX 4-2 Classification of Infective Microorganisms by Risk Group

Risk Group 1 (no or low individual and community risk)
A microorganism that is unlikely to cause human or animal disease.

Risk Group 2 (moderate individual risk, low community risk)
A pathogen that can cause human or animal disease but is unlikely to be a serious hazard to laboratory workers, the community, livestock, or the environment. Laboratory exposures may cause serious infection, but effective treatment and preventive measures are available and the risk of spread of infection is limited.

Risk Group 3 (high individual risk, low community risk)
A pathogen that usually causes serious human or animal disease but does not ordinarily spread from one infected individual to another. Effective treatment and preventive measures are available.

Risk Group 4 (high individual and community risk)
A pathogen that usually causes serious human or animal disease and that can be readily transmitted from one individual to another, directly or indirectly. Effective treatment and preventive measures are not usually available.

From World Health Organization: *Laboratory biosafety manual*, ed 3, 2004.

---

process that appropriate safety practices can be identified to protect laboratorians.

The hazardous risk characteristics of an agent are determined by the agent's ability to infect and cause disease in humans or animals, its virulence, the availability of treatment for the disease, and whether there are any preventive measures, such as a vaccine, that can be used to prevent disease by the microorganism. The World Health Organization (WHO) defined four **risk groups** for infectious agents based on the hazardous characteristics listed previously. The four risk groups, defined in the WHO Classification of Infectious Microorganisms by Risk Group, correlates with the biosafety levels discussed later in this chapter, but are not always equal. Other factors that must be considered when determining the correct biosafety level needed are the mode of transmission, the microbiological procedures that will be performed, and the experience of the staff members (Box 4-2).

Processing of Patient Specimens

Labeling only those specimens from patients with known hepatitis or AIDS and requiring "extra precautions" for dealing with these specimens does not provide adequate protection for laboratory workers. Many patients come into emergency departments or are admitted to the hospital with no apparent diagnosis. These patients may be in the early stages of either disease and may be asymptomatic but still contagious. Because the incidence of both hepatitis and AIDS is increasing steadily, the likelihood of exposure to one or both of these blood-borne pathogens is also increasing. For this reason, Standard Precautions should be used when handling all patient samples.

As stated earlier, when samples are received in the microbiology laboratory, there is often not enough information to assess the risk involved with processing the sample. Microbiologists do not know what infectious agents are present in the sample and will not know until the agent or agents have been identified. For this reason, it must be assumed that the specimen contains agents that correlate with at least a biosafety level (BSL) 2 unless there is additional information suggesting that there may be an agent present from a higher risk group. A common practice is to perform all specimen processing in a **biosafety cabinet** because of the uncertainty regarding the infectious agents that might be present in the sample.

Working with Actively Growing Cultures

Many of the guidelines in place for the protection of microbiology personnel against exposure to blood-borne pathogens also apply to working with cultures of microorganisms at the bench. Hands must be washed frequently and kept away from the nose, mouth, and eyes. Adhesive bandages or small finger cots should be worn directly over cuts or hangnails. Plates should not be waved in front of the face in order to determine the odor of the organism. Any plates growing a fungus should immediately be sealed, and the culture should then be worked on in a biosafety cabinet. Any cultures suspected of growing other potentially aerosolized infectious agents, such as *M. tuberculosis* or *Brucella* spp., should also be worked on only in a biosafety cabinet. In an effort to educate those at risk for laboratory-acquired infection, the CDC publishes a manual entitled *Biosafety in Microbiological and Biomedical Laboratories* every few years, which contains important information on the degree of risk of biologic agents for laboratory workers and the safety procedures that should be used when working with infections agents.

Biologic Safety Cabinet

Biologic safety cabinets (BSCs) are a form of engineering control that is used throughout the microbiology laboratory. These hoods are a type of containment barrier that protects the worker from the aerosolized transmission of organisms. Any procedure that has the ability to create aerosols should be performed in a BSC. Specimen handling of microbiology samples should also be handled within a BSC. There are three types of BSC: Class I, Class II, and Class III (Figure 4-4).

A BSC must be used properly, and it is imperative that the laboratory worker understand the functions and limitations of the unit. The most common type of BSC used in a microbiology laboratory is the Class II. Box 4-3 gives a few guidelines to follow to ensure the proper use of a BSC.

Biosafety Levels

Laboratory-acquired infections may occur through error, accident, or carelessness. However, in many laboratory-acquired infections the mode of transmission is unknown. For this reason, strict guidelines have been instituted to protect the worker during all laboratory tasks. Earlier in this chapter, the classification of infectious microorganisms into risk groups was discussed. When considering which **biosafety**

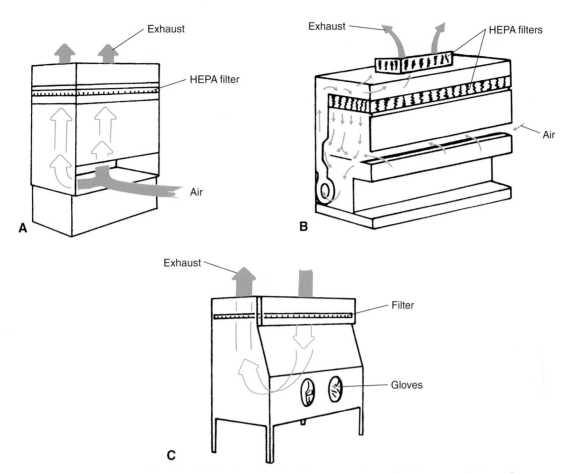

FIGURE 4-4 **A,** The Class I biologic safety hood uses an exhaust fan to move air inward through the open front. The air is circulated within the safety hood, passing through a high-efficiency particulate air (HEPA) filter before reaching the environment outside the hood. **B,** The Class II biologic safety hood is the most common in microbiology laboratories. Air is pulled inward and downward by a blower and passed up through the airflow plenum where it passes through an HEPA filter before reaching the work surface. A percentage of the remaining air is HEPA filtered before reaching the environment. **C,** The Class III biologic safety hood is a self-contained ventilated system for highly infectious microorganisms or materials and provides the highest level of personal protection. The closed front contains attached gloves for manipulation on the work surface. NOTE: Chemical fume hoods cannot be used as biologic safety cabinets, and biologic safety cabinets cannot be used as chemical fume hoods.

level to use, the laboratorian should know the risk group for the agents being handled, the mode of transmission for the agent or agents, and the procedures that will be performed (e.g., whether will aerosols be created). The CDC's *Biosafety in Microbiological and Biomedical Laboratories* has recommended the biosafety levels that should be used when working with particular agents and performing certain procedures. Four biosafety levels (BSLs) with guidelines were established for each level for protection.

Biosafety Level-1. The infectious agents that would be classified as requiring a BSL-1 level of containment are those that are well classified and are not known to consistently cause disease in healthy adult humans. These agents pose a minimal threat to laboratory personnel and the environment. Some of the safety guidelines for handling these agents are described as follows:

1. Access to the laboratory is limited or restricted, and there must be a biohazard sign posted at the entrance of the laboratory.
2. Employees must wash their hands after they have removed their gloves, after they have handled live organisms, and before they leave the laboratory.
3. Employees must follow basic work practice controls.
4. Employees must follow OSHA guidelines for handling needles and sharps.
5. Work surfaces must be decontaminated after completion of work and anytime there has been a spill of potentially infectious material.
6. Lab coats and gloves should be worn and other PPE, such as face shields and eye protection, may be needed when there is a potential for splashes or sprays of infectious or other hazardous materials.

BOX 4-3 Proper Use of a Biologic Safety Cabinet

1. Be aware of the functioning and limitations of the unit. You and your specimen are being protected solely by an air curtain barrier, and anything that disrupts this curtain threatens your safety. Ensure that the cabinet has been inspected within the last year and that the air pressure readings across the HEPA filter are within specifications.
2. Plan your work, anticipating the order of events.
3. Turn on the incandescent lights and the blower fan. Be sure the UV light is off. Wait 15 to 30 minutes to ensure satisfactory establishment of the air curtain.
4. Wash your hands, then gown and glove. Wear mask or other personal protective equipment as appropriate.
5. Decontaminate the interior work surfaces by cleansing thoroughly with 70% ethanol.
6. Organize all necessary work materials and place in cabinet. Do not place any extra items in the cabinet. Ensure that both the front intake grill and the rear-wall or floor exhaust grills are unobstructed.
7. Segregate clean and contaminated items and place them to minimize subsequent movement with the BSC. The discard bucket/pan should be near the rear of the cabinet but not obstructing the exhaust grill.
8. Do not use open flames in the unit. Instead, use disposable supplies or a microburner/incinerator.
9. All arm movements into and within the cabinet should be slow and deliberate so as to minimize disruption of the air curtain. Allow adequate time at the conclusion of movement for the air curtain to reestablish itself.
10. When work is completed, remove all nonpermanent items from the BSC and allow the cabinet fans to continue running for at least 30 minutes to ensure thorough filtering of the inside air (assuming the fans are not left on permanently). Turn on the UV lights to disinfect the interior of the cabinet.

Data from Kruse RH, Puckett WH, Richardson JH: Biological safety cabinetry, *Clin Microbiol Rev* 2:207, 1991.

BSC, Biologic safety cabinet; *HEPA*, high-efficiency particulate air; *UV*, ultraviolet.

---

7. Cultures and stock material must be decontaminated before disposal.
8. An insect and rodent control plan must be in effect.
9. The laboratory facility should be designed so that it can be easily cleaned. Carpets and rugs should not be used. The laboratory must be equipped with handwashing sinks, eyewashes, and adequate illumination.

Laboratory work can be conducted on open bench tops in a BSL-1 laboratory. Employees should be trained in laboratory procedures and supervised by a scientist with training in microbiology or a related science. Standard microbiology practices should be followed at all times. Examples of BSL-1 organisms are *Bacillus subtilis* and *Naegleria gruberi*.

Biosafety Level-2. Infectious agents that require BSL-2 containment and practices are those that can cause a moderate potential hazard for the employees and the environment. The guidelines are the same as for BSL-1 with added precautions for BSL-2 agents such as:

1. Employees in the laboratory must have specific training in the handling of pathogenic agents and should receive annual updates or additional training as needed.

2. Access to the laboratory is limited when work is being conducted. The laboratory director is ultimately responsible for determining who may enter or work in the laboratory.
3. Laboratorians should receive immunizations or tests for agents handled or for those agents that could potentially be in the laboratory environment; for example, hepatitis B vaccination and the tuberculosis skin test.
4. A biosafety manual must be developed and updated.
5. A BSC must be used whenever there is a potential for creating infectious aerosols or splashes or when high concentrations of infectious agents are used. The recommended BSC is the Class 2.
6. All PPE must be worn. Gloves must be worn to protect hands from exposure to hazardous materials.
7. Extreme precautions are taken with contaminated sharp items. The use of needles and syringes is restricted within the laboratory to only those times when there is no alternative equipment that can be used.

Examples of BSL-2 organisms are hepatitis B virus, HIV, *Salmonella* spp., and *Toxoplasma* spp.

Biosafety Level-3. Biosafety level-3 containment and practices are required for infectious agents that are either indigenous or exotic. These agents have the potential for aerosol transmission, and diseases with these agents may have serious lethal consequences. The guidelines for BSL-2 laboratories must be followed along with the more stringent guidelines needed to safely handle BSL-3 agents. Laboratory personnel must have specific training in handling of these pathogenic and potentially lethal organisms. A few of the special BSL-3 guidelines are:

1. The handling of infectious materials, samples, and cultures must occur within a BSC or other physical containment device.
2. Personnel must wear appropriate PPE. Gloves must be worn to protect hands from exposure to hazardous materials.
3. The BSL-3 laboratory should be separated from the other parts of the building by an anteroom or by access through a BSL-2 laboratory.
4. The BSL-3 laboratory requires a ducted air ventilation system that must provide for sustained directional air flow. This directional air flow pulls air from "clean" areas toward "potentially contaminated" areas.
5. The ceilings and floors must be solid, and any seams must be sealed.
6. All parts of the laboratory must be constructed for easy cleaning and decontamination.

Examples of BSL-3 organisms are *M. tuberculosis*, St. Louis encephalitis virus, and *Coxiella burnetii*.

Biosafety Level-4. Biosafety level-4 containment and practices are required when working with agents that are dangerous and exotic. These agents have a high risk of causing life-threatening infections, can be transmitted by aerosols, or have an unknown risk of transmission. As in all microbiology practices, specific training is required. Laboratory personnel must receive thorough training in the handling of these dangerous agents, and they must be trained in how to use the containment barriers that are in place for protection. The

BSL-4 facility is either a separate building or it is in a isolated zone within a building. This facility is isolated from all other areas, and access is strictly controlled. The guidelines listed for BSL-3 must be followed along with additional guidelines for handling BSL-4 agents. There are two types of BSL-4 laboratories, Cabinet and Suit. In the Cabinet laboratory, all work is performed within a Class III BS. In a Suit laboratory, personnel wear a positive protective suit to perform all work. Some of the additional guidelines are:

1. Access is strictly controlled and the supervisor has the ultimate responsibility for who has access. A logbook is maintained to document all personnel who enter and exit the laboratory.
2. As required by all levels, a biohazard sign must be posted outside the door with the potential hazards, the laboratory director's name, and any special requirements, such as immunizations, for entering the area.
3. All personnel must demonstrate high proficiency in standard and special microbiologic practices.
4. Policies and procedure are established on the collection and storage of serum samples from at-risk personnel.
5. Personnel enter and exit the laboratory through the clothing change room. When personnel leave the laboratory, they must completely change clothes and shower. The clothes are then decontaminated before being laundered.
6. The BSL-4 laboratory has a dedicated nonrecirculating ventilation system, which is filtered through a high-efficiency particulate air (HEPA) filter before being exhausted.
7. All material is decontaminated before leaving the BSL-4 laboratory.

Examples of BSL-4 agents are Marburg and Congo-Crimean hemorrhagic fever.

Hazardous Waste

The clinical laboratory is responsible for the proper handling and disposal of all of the waste it generates. The scope of hazardous waste comprises more than just infectious waste. The Clinical Laboratory Standards Institute, *Clinical Laboratory Waste Management Approved Guideline*, 2nd edition, provides information for laboratory managers on the regulations governing hazardous wastes and addresses the following types of waste: chemical, infectious, radioactive, sharps, multihazardous, and nonhazardous. The guideline also emphasizes methods to reduce waste generation and methods to reduce the volume of and toxicity of unavoidable wastes. The definition of hazardous waste for the clinical laboratory is:

> Those substances which singly, or in combination, pose a significant present or potential threat or hazard to human health or to the environment and which singly or in combination require special handling, processing, or disposal because they are flammable, oxidizers, explosive, reactive, corrosive, toxic, infectious, carcinogenic, bioconcentrative-persistent in nature, potentially lethal, an irritant or a strong sensitizer.

Disposal of Infectious Waste

In addition to laboratory employees who work with potentially infectious material, the general public must be protected from exposure to these same materials after the laboratory or hospital has disposed of them. The surfacing of contaminated needles and other sharps along lake and ocean beaches has led to a public outcry to make hospitals accountable for their infectious waste disposal. In an effort to deal with this increasing problem, the U.S. Congress passed the Medical Wastes Tracking Act in 1988 to regulate the states of New York, New Jersey, Connecticut, and Rhode Island as well as Puerto Rico. These regulations went into effect on June 24, 1989, and expired on June 21, 1999. This act allowed the EPA to gather information and focus attention on the problem of medical waste and provided a basis for other states and federal agencies to develop policies on the disposal of medical waste.

The microbiology laboratory's safety program must follow state and local regulations for the safe disposal of its infectious wastes, usually by either autoclaving or incineration. Warning signs containing the warning symbol for biohazardous materials must be placed on all biohazard wastes and material disposal containers. Figures 4-5 and 4-6 show disposal containers appropriate for contaminated and biohazardous materials.

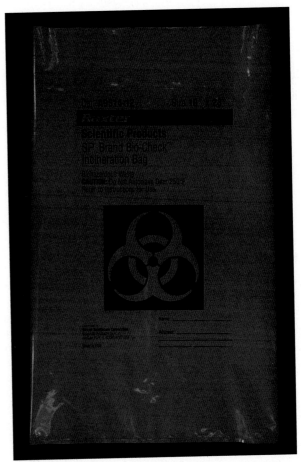

FIGURE 4-5 Biohazard bag used to dispose of culture plates and other nonsharp contaminated materials. The bag is sealed and incinerated. In the center of the bag is the biohazard symbol.

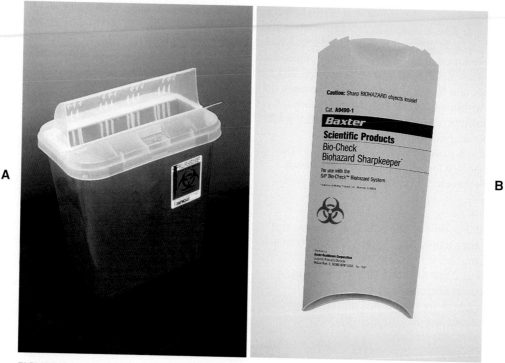

FIGURE 4-6 Examples of biohazard containers for disposable needles, glass slides, and other sharp materials.

Hazardous Waste Reduction

The EPA has also made recommendations for hazardous waste reduction through the following methods:

1. Substitute less hazardous chemicals when possible.
2. Develop procedures that use less of a hazardous chemical.
3. Recycle chemicals when possible.
4. Segregate infectious wastes from uncontaminated trash.
5. Substitute micromethodology in antibiotic susceptibility testing and identification of organisms to reduce volume of chemical reagents as well as infectious waste.

Chemical Safety

Chemicals used in the clinical laboratory can be hazardous to the laboratorian. The toxic risks of a chemical are related to the extent of exposure and to the inherent toxicity of the chemical. The possible routes of exposure for chemicals are through the skin, eyes, mucosa, gastrointestinal tract, and/or respiratory tract. OSHA addresses employee safety with hazardous chemicals in 29 CFR 1910.1200, Hazard Communication Standard (HCS). This provides for a laboratory chemical hygiene plan and a hazard communication, which states that all clinical laboratory personnel should have a thorough working knowledge of the hazards of the chemicals with which they come into contact, or **employee right-to-know,** and must receive chemical safety training annually. The National Research Council's publication *Prudent Practices in the Laboratory: Handling and Disposal of Chemical* can be used by laboratory managers when developing a laboratory's chemical

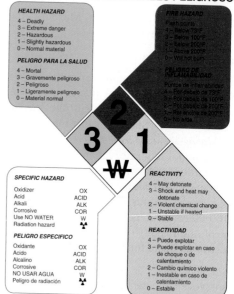

FIGURE 4-7 Hazardous material classification symbol. (Courtesy Lab Safety Supply, Inc., Janesville, Wis.)

hygiene plan. All hazardous chemicals in the workplace must be identified and clearly labeled with the **National Fire Protection Association (NFPA)** 704 **hazard-rating diamond,** stating risk for flammability, reactivity, and health (Figure 4-7).

3. International Agency for Cancer Research Monographs

> **BOX 4-4** Hazardous Chemicals Commonly Used in the Microbiology Laboratory
>
> **Flammables**
> - Methanol
> - Acetone
> - Ethanol
>
> **Potential or Proven Carcinogens**
> - Formaldehyde
> - Aniline (crystal violet) stain
> - Auramine-rhodamine (Truant) stain
>
> **Irritants and Corrosives**
> - Hydrogen peroxide
> - Acids: HCl, H_2SO_4, acetic acid
> - NaOH

Material Safety Data Sheets

Material Safety Data Sheets (MSDSs) are provided by the manufacturer or distributor for hazardous chemicals. Although there is no accepted format to what is contained in an MSDS, some of the information that should be provided is:

- The name, address and telephone number of the manufacturer
- The chemical and synonym names, and a list of the hazardous ingredients
- Physical and chemical characteristics of the hazardous chemical (e.g., vapor pressure, flash point) and the physical characteristics (potential for fire, explosion, and reactivity)
- The health hazards of the hazardous chemical (signs and symptoms of exposure, and any medical conditions that can be caused by exposure)
- The primary route(s) of entry and the target organs
- Precautions for safe handling and use, including appropriate hygienic practices
- Any generally applicable control measures, such as appropriate engineering controls, work practices, or personal protective equipment
- Emergency and first aid procedures
- Spill cleanup procedure
- Disposal recommendations

An example of an MSDS is shown in Figure 4-8. These documents should be kept on file and made available to every employee. Some of the more common hazardous chemicals that can be found in the microbiology laboratory are listed in Box 4-4.

Hazardous Chemicals Inventory

The laboratory must maintain a current inventory of hazardous chemicals, which must be updated annually, and the MSDSs for those particular chemicals. The following four sources should be consulted in preparing an inventory:

1. 29 CFR Part 1910, Subpart Z, Toxic and Hazardous Substances, OSHA
2. National Toxicology Program Annual Report on Carcinogens
3. International Agency for Cancer Research Monographs
4. Manufacturers' MSDSs

Laboratory Safety for Hazardous Chemicals

Laboratory fume hoods are one of the most important pieces of equipment for protecting workers from exposure to hazardous chemicals. Fume hoods must be provided to prevent inhalation of fumes and should be evaluated at least annually for adequate face velocity (average velocity of the air drawn through the face of the hood) and proper operation. Fume hoods should be vented. Personal protective equipment, such as appropriate gloves, aprons, and eyewear, must be used in the case of a small spill to protect the workers from exposure. A dust mask or respirator may be appropriate depending on the material spilled. Acid spill kits and flammable spill kits should be kept in areas where such substances are used. Warning signs and symbols, as shown in Figure 4-9, must be placed in appropriate locations. Employees must be able to recognize each of these symbols and must be knowledgeable about the danger each indicates and the proper precautions that must be observed. In the event of a large spill, call your Environmental Health & Safety Department for assistance.

Fire Safety

Bunsen burners and other open-flame burners, in most cases, have been replaced with other methods or techniques, such as fixing slides with methanol or using disposable loops. However, Bunsen burners and open-flame burners, if used, are among the biggest sources of fire hazards in the clinical microbiology laboratory. Employees must strive not to be careless or negligent in the use of this equipment. Flammable materials should never be opened near a Bunsen burner in use. Do not leave open flames unattended, and always make sure to turn off the gas when finished. Another hazard associated with Bunsen burners and other open-flame burners is the fuel. Bunsen burners use a gas. A leaking gas line may be a source of explosion or may cause illness in employees who work near the leak. Always inspect the gas hose for cracks, holes, pinched points or other defects, and replace the hose if any defects are found. If a leak is suspected or the appliance is newly connected, leaks can be checked for by lightly spraying the tubing with soapy water. If bubbles appear when the gas is on, there is a leak at that point. Other burners use a flammable liquid as the fuel, which is in itself a hazard. Other sources of ignition are heating elements, hot plates, and spark gaps in motors and light switches.

OSHA requires employers to have an emergency action plan, which includes what to do in the event of a fire. The emergency action plan must be written, and it must be kept in the workplace and available to all employees. All personnel must be thoroughly trained in the procedure for responding to a fire emergency. Most institutions use the acronym *RACE*:

*R*escue: Remove anyone who is in danger. The safety of handicapped personnel (deaf or physically disabled) should be a priority.

*A*larm: Know where the nearest fire pull box or alarm station is located and the number to call to report the fire.

Text continued on page 88

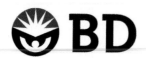

Material Safety Data Sheet
acc. to ISO/DIS 11014

Page 1/5

Date Prepared: 02/16/2009

Reviewed On: 12/21/2007

1 Identification of substance:

· **Product name:** <u>Streptococus pneumoniae Antibody-Coated Latex</u>
<u>(Pneumoslide Test Kit)</u>
· **Catalog number:** *240840*

· **Manufacturer/Supplier:**
BD Diagnostic Systems
7 Loveton Circle
Sparks, MD 21152
Telephone: (410) 771 - 0100 or (800) 638 - 8663
· **Information department:** *Technical Services*
· **Emergency information:**
In case of a chemical emergency, spill, fire, exposure, or accident contact BD Diagnostic Systems (410) 771-0100 or (800)-638-8663, or ChemTrec at (800) 424-9300.

2 Composition/Data on components:

· **Chemical characterization**
· **Description:** *Mixture consisting of the following components.*

· **Dangerous components:** *Void*

3 Hazards identification

· **Hazard description:**
This product contains no hazardous constituents, or the concentration of all chemical constituents are below the regulatory threshold limits described by Occupational Safety Health Administration Hazard Communication Standard 29 CFR 1910.1200, the Canada's Workplace Hazardous Materials Information System (WHMIS) and the European Directive 91/155/EEC, and 93/112/EC.
· **NFPA ratings (scale 0-4)**

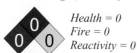

Health = 0
Fire = 0
Reactivity = 0

· **HMIS ratings (scale 0-4)**

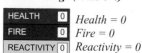

Health = 0
Fire = 0
Reactivity = 0

4 First aid measures

· **General information** *No special measures required.*
· **After inhalation** *Seek medical treatment in case of complaints.*
· **After skin contact** *Immediately wash with water and soap and rinse thoroughly.*
· **After eye contact**
Rinse opened eye for several minutes under running water. If symptoms persist, consult a doctor.
· **After swallowing** *If symptoms persist consult doctor.*
· **Information for doctor** *Show this product label or this MSDS.*

— USA —

(Contd. on page 2)

FIGURE 4-8   Material safety data sheet. (Courtesy and © Becton, Dickinson and Company, Franklin Lakes, N.J.)

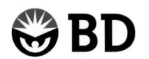

Material Safety Data Sheet
acc. to ISO/DIS 11014

Date Prepared: 02/16/2009

Reviewed On: 12/21/2007

> **Product name: Streptococus pneumoniae Antibody-Coated Latex**
> **(Pneumoslide Test Kit)**

(Contd. of page 1)

5 Fire fighting measures

· **Suitable extinguishing agents**
CO_2, ABC multipurpose dry chemical or water spray. Fight larger fires with water spray or alcohol resistant foam.
· **Protective equipment:** *No special measures required.*

6 Accidental release measures

· **Person-related safety precautions:** *Not required.*
· **Measures for environmental protection:** *Wipe up with damp sponge or mop.*
· **Measures for cleaning/collecting:** *No special measures required.*
· **Additional information:** *No dangerous substances are released.*

7 Handling and storage

· **Handling**
· **Information for safe handling:** *No special measures required.*
· **Information about protection against explosions and fires:** *No special measures required.*

· **Storage**
· **Requirements to be met by storerooms and receptacles:** *2 - 8 C*
· **Information about storage in one common storage facility:** *Store away from oxidizing agents.*
· **Further information about storage conditions:** *Store in cool, dry conditions in well sealed containers.*

8 Exposure controls and personal protection

· **Additional information about design of technical systems:** *No further data; see item 7.*

· **Components with limit values that require monitoring at the workplace:**
The product does not contain any relevant quantities of materials with critical values that have to be monitored at the workplace.
· **Additional information:** *The lists that were valid during the creation were used as basis.*

· **Personal Protective Equipment**
· **General protective and hygienic measures**
The usual precautionary measures for handling chemicals should be followed.
· **Breathing equipment:**
In case of brief exposure, use a chemical fume hood or a NIOSH/MSHA-approved respirator.
· **Protection of hands:**

  Chemical resistant gloves (i.e. nitrile, or equivalent).

· **Eye protection:** *Safety glasses*
· **Body protection:** *Protective work clothing (lab coat).*

USA

(Contd. on page 3)

FIGURE 4-8, cont'd

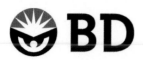 **BD**

Material Safety Data Sheet
acc. to ISO/DIS 11014

Date Prepared: 02/16/2009   *Reviewed On: 12/21/2007*

Product name: Streptococus pneumoniae Antibody-Coated Latex
(Pneumoslide Test Kit)

(Contd. of page 2)

9 Physical and chemical properties:

· **General Information**

Form:	*Solid.*
Color:	*According to product specification*
Odor:	*Characteristic*

· **Change in condition**
  Melting point/Melting range: *Not determined*
  Boiling point/Boiling range: *Not determined*

· **Flash point:** *Not applicable*

· **Flammability (solid, gaseous)** *Product is not flammable.*

· **Danger of explosion:** *Product does not present an explosion hazard.*

· **Density:** *Not determined*

· **Solubility in / Miscibility with**
  Water: *Insoluble*

· **Solvent content:**

· **Solids content:** *100.0 %*

10 Stability and reactivity

· **Thermal decomposition / conditions to be avoided:** *No decomposition if used according to specifications.*
· **Dangerous reactions** *No dangerous reactions known*
· **Dangerous products of decomposition:** *No dangerous decomposition products known.*

11 Toxicological information

· **Acute toxicity:**
· **Primary irritant effect:**
· **on the skin:** *No irritating effect.*
· **on the eye:** *No irritating effect.*
· **Sensitization:** *No sensitizing effects known.*
· **Additional toxicological information:**
  The product is not subject to OSHA classification according to internally approved calculation methods for preparations.
  When used and handled according to specifications, the product does not have any harmful effects according to our experience and the information provided to us.
  This product or product container contains natural rubber latex which may cause allergic reactions. People with known or suspected allergies to latex should use appropriate safety precautions when handling.

12 Ecological information:

· **Ecotoxical effects:**
· **Other information:**
  The ecological effects have not been thoroughly investigated, but currently none have been identified.

(Contd. on page 4)
— USA —

FIGURE 4-8, cont'd

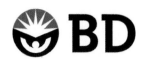

Material Safety Data Sheet
acc. to ISO/DIS 11014

Date Prepared: 02/16/2009   Reviewed On: 12/21/2007

Product name:Streptococus pneumoniae Antibody-Coated Latex
(Pneumoslide Test Kit)

(Contd. of page 3)

· **General notes:** *Generally not hazardous for water.*

13 Disposal considerations

· **Product:**
· **Recommendation**
Smaller quantities can be disposed of with solid waste.
Dispose of material in accordance with federal (40 CFR 261.3), state and local requirements.
This product is not considered a RCRA hazardous waste.

· **Uncleaned packagings:**
· **Recommendation:** *Disposal must be made according to state and federal regulations.*
· **Recommended cleansing agent:** *Water, if necessary with cleansing agents.*

14 Transport information

· **DOT regulations:**

· **Hazard class:**   -

· **Land transport ADR/RID (cross-border)**
· **ADR/RID class:**   -

· **Maritime transport IMDG:**
· **IMDG Class:**   -
· **Marine pollutant:** *No*

· **Air transport ICAO-TI and IATA-DGR:**
· **ICAO/IATA Class:** -

· **Transport/Additional information:**
If a dashed line appears in the Hazard Class section for the type of transportation, this indicates the product is
not regulated for transportation.

15 Regulations

· **SARA Section 355 (extremely hazardous substances)**

None of the ingredients is listed.

· **SARA Section 313 (specific toxic chemical listings)**

None of the ingredients is listed.

· **TSCA (Toxic Substances Control Act)**

	2-methyl-4-isothiazolin-3-one
30007-47-7	5-Bromo-5-nitro-1,3-dioxane

· **California Proposition 65 - Chemicals known to cause cancer**

None of the ingredients is listed.

· **California Proposition 65 - Chemicals known to cause reproductive toxicity for females:**

None of the ingredients is listed.

(Contd. on page 5)
— USA —

FIGURE 4-8, cont'd

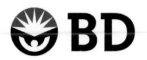

Material Safety Data Sheet
acc. to ISO/DIS 11014

Date Prepared: 02/16/2009   *Reviewed On: 12/21/2007*

Product name: Streptococus pneumoniae Antibody-Coated Latex
(Pneumoslide Test Kit)

(Contd. of page 4)

· **California Proposition 65 - Chemicals known to cause reproductive toxicity for males:**

None of the ingredients is listed.

· **California Proposition 65 - Chemicals known to cause developmental toxicity:**

None of the ingredients is listed.

· **Carcinogenicity categories**

· **IARC (International Agency for Research on Cancer)**

None of the ingredients is listed.

· **NTP (National Toxicology Program)**

None of the ingredients is listed.

· **TLV (Threshold Limit Value established by ACGIH)**

None of the ingredients is listed.

· **Product related hazard information:**
Observe the general safety regulations when handling chemicals
The product is not subject to identification regulations pertaining to regulations on hazardous materials.

---

16 Other information:

To the best of our knowledge, the information contained herein is accurate. However, neither Becton, Dickinson and Company or any of its subsidiaries assumes any liabilities whatsoever for the accuracy or completeness of the information contained herein. Final determination of suitability of any material is the sole responsibility of the user. All materials may present unknown hazards and should be used with caution. Although certain hazards are described herein, we can not guarantee that these are the only hazards that exist.

· **Department issuing MSDS:**
Safety and Environment Department
MSDS created by Michael J. Spinazzola
· **Contact:** *Technical Service Representative*

— USA —

FIGURE 4-8, cont'd

Contain: Close doors to contain fire and smoke.

Extinguish: Use the properly rated fire extinguisher on small fires (Table 4-5). If the situation is out of control, the best course of action is to evacuate.

The fire evacuation plan must be posted, and employees should be familiar with fire exit locations and evacuation procedures. Periodic fire drills should be conducted to ensure that all personnel react quickly and efficiently in case of a real fire emergency. The drills should include both exit and nonexit procedures. Exit drills familiarize personnel with the escape routes and location of fire doors and stairwells. Nonexit procedures alert personnel to the potential for evacuation if the fire is located elsewhere in the building. The laboratory should be kept free of clutter, and exits should remain clear of obstructions.

TABLE 4-5 Classes of Fire Extinguishers

Symbol	Class	Use
Ⓐ	A	Fires in ordinary combustible materials, such as wood, cloth, paper, rubber, and many plastics; contains water or dry chemical to cool
Ⓑ	B	Fires in flammable liquids, gases, and greases; contains CO_2 or dry chemical to smother
Ⓒ	C	Fires involving electrical equipment, for which the electrical nonconductivity of the extinguishing media is important; contains CO_2 or dry chemical to smother without damaging the equipment

WARNING SIGNS AND SYMBOLS	POTENTIAL DANGER
	Flammable
	Toxic hazard Poisonous
	Carcinogenic Cancer-causing agent
	Corrosive Harmful to mucous membranes, skin, eyes, or tissues
	Radiation Radioactive material present

FIGURE 4-9 Miscellaneous warning signs and symbols.

Thermal Injuries

Personnel should be warned of any hot surface or situation in which the potential for burns is present. Use of long thermal gloves that extend to the shoulder is recommended when reaching into autoclaves or hot-air ovens. Signs should be posted warning employees about hot instruments or flasks that have just been sterilized. Burns may also come from extremely low temperatures found with use of liquid nitrogen or freezers that maintain temperatures less than −70° C.

Storage of Compressed Gases

Flammable and nonflammable gas cylinders in use in the laboratory must be properly restrained or stored and secured in vented areas, and well away from open flames and other heat sources. Because a leaking pressurized gas cylinder is a potential "missile," care must be taken to avoid accidental breakage or removal of the pressure valve on top. The metal cap that protects this valve on top of the cylinder must be kept in place when the cylinder is not in use.

Electrical Safety

Today's microbiology laboratories contain many instruments. Each instrument must undergo regular preventive maintenance to ensure that it is functioning properly and in the best repair. Electrical cords should be checked for fraying. All cords should have grounded (three-pronged) plugs. The College of American Pathologists, an organization that provides accreditation to laboratories, requires electrical grounding and leakage checks on instruments before they are put in use, after repairs or modifications, and when there is a suspected problem. Electrical equipment should never be placed near safety showers because of the risk of electrocution.

Miscellaneous Safety Considerations

Back Safety

The best way to care for the back is to prevent back injuries. Carrying heavy trays of culture plates, lifting heavy loads into and out of the autoclaves, and sitting or standing improperly can all contribute to back stress or injury. The following are some ways to prevent back injuries:

- Use the legs to lift, not the back.
- Ask for assistance or use a cart when a load is too heavy.
- Use good posture.
- Stay physically fit.

First Aid Training

All personnel should be trained in cardiopulmonary resuscitation (CPR) and other lifesaving first aid so that they will be able to act quickly in an emergency involving either fellow workers or patients.

Immunizations

OSHA requires that the hepatitis B vaccination be offered free of charge to all personnel who are at risk for exposure to blood-borne pathogens. Microbiology personnel working with sputum specimens or mycobacterial cultures should be screened for exposure to *M. tuberculosis* with an annual tuberculosis skin test.

Safety Training

All clinical laboratories must offer their employees safety training, and this training must be documented. The training must include the following safety issues:

- *Fire*: Knowledge of how and when to report fires, the location of the nearest alarm box and fire extinguishers, how to use fire extinguishers in small fires, and blocking of fire doors
- *Hazardous materials management*: How to use MSDSs
- *Proper storage of gases*
- *Blood-borne pathogens program*: Appropriate practice of infection control, how to handle sharps, compliance with exposure control plan, and handling of biologic spills

Safety training programs for microbiology personnel should be conducted annually to keep safe techniques fresh in everyone's mind. New personnel should be thoroughly trained in safety procedures. It is a good idea to focus on one safety topic at a time and to make the training sessions enjoyable. Safety is each employee's responsibility.

BIOTERRORISM AND THE CLINICAL MICROBIOLOGY LABORATORY

Clinical microbiology laboratorians are critical players in the early detection of a bioterrorism event. In the September 2001 anthrax incident, laboratorians performed the testing that identified the infectious agent. The CDC has developed a program that identifies how health care workers and other public health officials should respond to an event. This program (the Emergency Preparedness and Response Program) addresses biologic agents and diseases, laboratory information, training, preparedness and planning, and surveillance.

Laboratory Response Network

The CDC developed the **Laboratory Response Network** (LRN) in 1999. This program developed a network of laboratories that could respond quickly and effectively to biological and chemical terrorism. The LRN developed three levels of laboratories: (1) sentinel laboratories, (2) reference laboratories, and (3) national laboratories. The roles and responsibilities of each of these levels are defined in order to provide for the rapid and safe identification of biologic agents during a bioterrorism event.

Sentinel Laboratories

Sentinel laboratories comprise most of the hospital-based microbiology laboratories and are divided into two levels. The Advanced Sentinel Clinical Laboratories function at the front lines and have the most capability. The role of these sentinel laboratories is to recognize possible bioterrorism agents and to perform basic testing to rule out these agents and/or to refer suspicious specimens or isolates to the LRN reference lab. The Basic Sentinel Clinical Laboratories have fewer analytical capabilities but may handle suspect samples and would refer these specimens to an LRN reference laboratory. The key to the success of this level of the LRN is the rapid recognition of a bioterrorism event. The American Society for Microbiology has published laboratory guidelines for the infections agents that could be used in a bioterrorism event. Laboratorians must be aware of what organisms are on this list and be familiar with the guidelines established when dealing with these agents.

The potential infectious agents of bioterrorism are divided into the following categories:

Category A agents are those that pose the greatest public health threat because they are easily transmitted and are highly infectious. Examples of category A agents are those that cause smallpox, anthrax, and tularemia.

Category B agents have moderate morbidity and low mortality and are not as easily transmitted as those in category A. Examples of category B agents are those that cause Q fever, melioidosis, and typhus fever.

Category C organisms are classified as emerging pathogens; for example, those that cause yellow fever, dengue, and hemorrhagic fever.

Reference Laboratories and National Laboratories

The role of the reference laboratories and the national laboratories in the LRN is to perform confirmatory testing. Currently more than 100 laboratories are members of the reference laboratory category. The national laboratories in the LRN are the CDC, the U.S. Army Medical Research Institute of Infectious Diseases (USAMRIID), and the Naval Medical Research Center (NMRC).

Safety During a Possible Bioterrorism Event

The agents in categories A and B have been associated with laboratory-acquired infections. The biggest threat with handling these agents is not recognizing the risk associated with these infectious agents and not following the safety procedures instituted in the laboratory for protection. Specimen processing of samples from a possible bioterrorism event should occur within a Class II BSC. However, it is likely that the first patients seen in an event will not be identified as victims of bioterrorism. Therefore the cultures from these patients could cause the greatest risk to laboratorians.

The agents that pose the greatest risk are those that are transmitted by aerosols, and all laboratorians must remember that many of the procedures that are performed in the laboratory create aerosols, such as pipetting, flaming loops, streaking blood plates, and centrifugation. Once a bioterrorism agent is suspected, all manipulations of the culture should be performed using BSL-3 guidelines. Sentinel laboratories should *not* accept environmental samples for testing because of the unknown nature of the sample. As soon as an agent has been identified as a possible select agent, the sample should be referred to the appropriate LRN reference laboratory. For more information on the responsibilities of a sentinel laboratory, visit the American Society for Microbiology Web site.

Packaging and Shipping of Infectious Substances

Laboratory personnel who are involved in the packaging and shipping of infectious materials must be trained and certified before shipping infectious material. Personnel must also be retrained on a regular basis. The International Air Transport Association, the International Civil Aviation Organization (ICAO), and the United States Department of Transportation (DOT) regulations must be followed when packaging and shipping infectious agents. Laboratory personnel must be aware of what agencies will transport these materials to the identified LRN reference or national laboratory.

BIBLIOGRAPHY

American Society for Clinical Microbiology: *Sentinel laboratory guidelines for suspected agents of bioterrorism: clinical laboratory bioterrorism readiness plan*, 2006.

American Society for Microbiology: *Sentinel laboratory guidelines for suspected agents of bioterrorism and emerging infectious diseases: packaging and shipping infectious substances*, 2008.

American Society for Microbiology: *Sentinel level clinical microbiology laboratory guidelines*. Available at: www.asm.org. Accessed October 29, 2008.

Clinical Laboratory Standards Institute: *Clinical laboratory waste management*, Approved Guideline, GP5-A2, Wayne, Pa, 2002.

College of American Pathologists, Commission on Laboratory Accreditation: *Laboratory general checklist*, 2007. Available at: www.cap.org. Accessed October 20, 2008.

Department of Health and Human Services, Centers for Disease Control and Prevention: *Biosafety in microbiological and biomedical laboratories*, ed 5, 2007. Available at: www.cdc.gov. Accessed October 28, 2008.

Department of Health and Human Services, Centers for Disease Control and Prevention: *Exposure to blood: what healthcare personnel need to know 2003*. Available at: www.cdc.gov. Accessed October 29, 2008.

Department of Health and Human Services, Centers for Disease Control and Prevention: *Guideline for isolation precautions: preventing transmission of infectious agents in healthcare settings 2007*. Available at: www.cdc.gov. Accessed October 29, 2008.

Department of Health and Human Services, Centers for Disease Control and Prevention: *Laboratory network for biological terrorism*. Available at: emergency.cdc.gov. Accessed October 29, 2008.

Department of Health and Human Services, Centers for Disease Control and Prevention: *Standard Precautions*. Available at: www.cdc.gov. Accessed October 29, 2008.

Department of Health and Human Services, Centers for Disease Control and Prevention: *Universal precautions for prevention of transmission of HIV and other bloodborne infections*. Available at: www.cdc.gov. Accessed October 29, 2008.

Forbes BA, Sahm DE, Weissfeld AS, editors: *Bailey and Scott's diagnostic microbiology*, ed 12, St Louis, 2007, Elsevier.

Kimman TG, Smit E, Klein MR: Evidence-based biosafety: a review of the principles and effectiveness of microbiological containment measures, *Clin Microbiol Rev* 21:403, 2008.

Kruse RH: *Microbiological safety cabinetry (monograph)*. Lexington, Ky, September 1981, Medico-Biological Environmental Development Institute.

Kruse RH, Puckett WH, Richardson JH: Biological safety cabinetry, *Clin Microbiol Rev* 4:207, 1991.

Mortland KK, Mortland D: Clearing the air: the selection, location, and use of hoods, *Clin Leadership Management Rev* (Jan/Feb):44, 2003.

Murray PR et al, editors: *Manual of clinical microbiology*, ed 9. Washington, DC, 2007, ASM Press.

Natural Research Council: *Prudent practices in the laboratory: handling and disposal of chemicals*, Washington, DC, 1995, National Academy Press.

Sewell DL: Laboratory-acquired infections: are microbiologists at risk, *Clinical Microbiology Newsletter* 28:1, 2006.

Sewell DL: Laboratory safety practices associated with potential agents of biocrime or bioterrorism, *J Clin Microbiol* 41:280, 2003.

Snyder JW: Role of the hospital-based microbiology laboratory in preparation for and response to a bioterrorism event, *J Clin Microbiol* 41:1, 2003.

U.S. Department of Labor. Occupational Safety and Health Administration (OSHA): *Bloodborne pathogens standard*, 29CFR1910.1030, 1991. Available at: www.osha.gov. Accessed October 30, 2008.

U.S. Department of Labor. Occupational Safety and Health Administration (OSHA): *Emergency action plans*, 29CFR 1910.38, 2002. Available at: www.osha.gov. Accessed October 30, 2008.

U.S. Department of Labor. Occupational Safety and Health Administration (OSHA): *Hazard communications: foundation of workplace chemical safety programs*, 2008. Available at: www.osha.gov. Accessed October 30, 2008.

U.S. Department of Labor. Occupational Safety and Health Administration (OSHA): *Hazard communication*, 29CFR1910.1200, 1996. Available at: www.osha.gov. Accessed October 30, 2008.

U.S. Department of Labor. Occupational Safety and Health Administration (OSHA): *Occupational exposure to bloodborne pathogens; needlestick and other sharps injuries; final rule—66:5317-5325*, 2001. Available at: www.osha.gov. Accessed October 30, 2008.

U.S. Department of Labor. Occupational Safety and Health Administration (OSHA): *Occupational exposure to hazardous chemicals in laboratories*, 29CFR1910.1450, 2006. Available at: www.osha.gov. Accessed October 30, 2008.

U.S. Environmental Protection Agency: *Environmental management guide for small laboratories*, 2000. Available at: www.epa.gov. Accessed October 30, 2008.

U.S. Environmental Protection Agency: *Medical Waste Tracking Act of 1988*. Available at: www.epa.gov. Accessed October 30, 2008.

Washington WC et al, editors: *Koneman's color atlas and textbook of diagnostic microbiology*, ed 6, Baltimore, 2006, Lippincott Williams & Williams.

World Health Organization: *Laboratory biosafety manual*, ed 3, 2004. Available at: www.who.int. Accessed October 28, 2008.

Points to Remember

- Major sources of biologic hazards come from patient samples during processing and handling of actively growing culture materials.
- Protective equipment should be used appropriately.
- Safety policies and procedures should always be followed.
- The microbiology safety program includes proper and safe disposal of infectious waste material.
- OSHA regulations for blood-borne pathogen protection should be followed.
- Chemical and fire safety hazards must be identified and measures to prevent chemical spills should be employed.
- Continuing education programs to train laboratory personnel in all aspects of laboratory safety and exposure control should be in place.

Learning Assessment Questions

1. By requiring their employers to offer the hepatitis B vaccine free of charge, OSHA seeks to protect employees who are at risk for exposure to hepatitis B. True or false?

2. Material Safety Data Sheets are important to employees because they contain information relating to which of the following?
   a. Blood-borne pathogens
   b. Fume hoods
   c. Chemical safety
   d. Fire extinguishers

3. Which of the following would be a correct definition of Standard Precautions?
   a. Wearing only gloves to handle blood and body fluids
   b. Viewing all specimens as potentially infectious and using the appropriate protective equipment

   c. Delaying testing of blood and body fluids pending results of HIV and hepatitis B antigen testing

   d. Flagging only those specimens that come from patients who are known HIV carriers for "extra precautions"

4. What type of filter does a Class II biologic safety cabinet use to filter out infectious agents?
   a. Millipore filters
   b. HEPA filters
   c. Dust filters
   d. Charcoal filters

5. Infectious agents can enter the body through which of the following routes?
   a. Inhalation
   b. Ingestion
   c. Inoculation
   d. All of the above

6. Employees can remember the steps to take in case of a fire by remembering which of the following acronyms?
   a. RUSH
   b. REST
   c. RACE
   d. RISK

7. How often must safety training for laboratory employees be conducted for compliance with OSHA regulations?
   a. Annually
   b. Quarterly
   c. At time of employment only
   d. No set requirement

8. Briefly describe the NFPA hazard-rating diamond found on all chemical containers to warn employees of potential hazards associated with that chemical.

9. Washing hands frequently, disinfecting work areas, using needle-resheathing devices, wearing gloves, and using other forms of barrier protection when handling specimens are examples of which of the following?
   a. Universal Precautions
   b. Safe work habits
   c. Responsible methods of fire safety
   d. Chemical hygiene

10. List four hazardous chemicals commonly found in a microbiology laboratory.

Performance Improvement in the Microbiology Laboratory

A. Quality Issues in Clinical Microbiology

Sarojinii Misra

■ **GENERAL GUIDELINES FOR ESTABLISHING QUALITY CONTROL**
Temperatures
Thermometer Calibration
Equipment Quality Control
Media Quality Control
Reagent Quality Control
Antimicrobial Susceptibility Quality Control
Personnel Competency
Use of Stock Cultures
Quality Control Manual

■ **PERFORMANCE IMPROVEMENT**
Vision and Mission Statements
Indicators of Process Improvement: Process versus Outcome
Establishing Performance Monitors
Problem/Action Form
The Customer Concept
Fixing the Process
Benchmarking
Commercially Purchased Monitors

OBJECTIVES

After reading and studying this chapter, you should be able to:

1. Define *quality control* (QC) as it applies in the clinical microbiology laboratory.

2. Discuss the general guidelines for establishing a QC program, describing the way to monitor equipment maintenance and performance, culture media and reagent performance, personnel competency, use of stock cultures, and the development and updating of procedure manuals.

3. Describe proper documentation and institution of appropriate corrective action.

4. Define *performance improvement* (PI) and how it differs from QC.

5. Discuss the 10-step plan for establishing quality monitors.

6. Describe the customer concept.

7. Define *benchmarking*.

Case in Point

A night-shift technologist prepared a cerebrospinal fluid smear by cytocentrifugation by adding 2 drops of albumin to the cyto-centrifuge funnel before adding the specimen. The sample was spun down for 5 minutes at 2000 rpm and the smear was then air-dried, fixed in methanol, and Gram stained. When reading the smear, the technologist observed rare white blood cells and few gram-positive cocci. The physician was promptly notified. After 24-hour incubation, the culture had failed to exhibit growth. All processes involved in smear preparation were reviewed for possible sources of error or contamination.

Issues to Consider

After reading the case history, consider the following:

■ All the intricate processes involved in quality assurance
■ The purpose of QC of media and reagents
■ The steps necessary to ensure continuous quality improvement

KEY TERMS

Analytical activity

Benchmarking

Clinical Laboratory Improvement Act of 1988 (CLIA)

Clinical and Laboratory Standards Institute (CLSI)

College of American Pathologists (CAP)

Competency

Continuing education (CE)

Cross-functional teams

Customer concept

Facilitator

Focused monitors

The Joint Commission (TJC)

ORYX

Outcome monitors

Performance improvement (PI)

Postanalytical activity

Preanalytical activity

Preventive maintenance

Process monitors

Proficiency testing

Q-Probes

Quality control (QC)

TABLE 5-1 Three Stages of Activities That Affect Outcome of Laboratory Testing Activities

Stage	Activities
Preanalytical	Test ordering
	Order transcription
	Patient preparation
	Specimen collection
	Specimen identification
	Specimen transport
Analytical	Sample testing
Postanalytical	Result transcription
	Result delivery
	Result review
	Action taken on basis of result

The issue of quality in the laboratory is complex. The emphasis and the terminology have changed tremendously in recent years. Laboratories have always taken measures to control the testing performed on patient specimens. This effort has been termed **quality control (QC);** it is defined as the measures designed to ensure the medical reliability of laboratory data. Examples are checking media and reagents with specific organisms to determine whether expected results are obtained and documenting that the instrumentation meets all operating parameters before it is used on patient samples.

Laboratory professionals now realize that QC is only a small part of the issue of quality. Even when the laboratory has effectively controlled media, reagents, and instruments, the quality of the test result will be poor if the specimen has degraded before arriving in the laboratory but is tested regardless. Suppose a specimen contained the wrong patient name; again, the media can be top quality, the incubator temperature accurate, and the technologist very competent, but if the results are recorded on the wrong patient chart, quality patient care management does not exist for the intended patient. The actual laboratory testing is called an **analytical activity.** It is now important to realize that **preanalytical,** analytical, and **postanalytical activities** all affect quality. An outcome can be interrupted or destroyed at any point in the process. Table 5-1 attempts to clarify these three stages by giving examples of each kind of activity.

Quality assurance involves taking measures to ensure high-quality patient care. This process involves monitoring all the components of a system or procedure (preanalytical, analytical, and postanalytical) and implementing changes when suboptimal performance is identified. Quality assurance is measured by patient outcome; hence patient care might be adversely affected before problems are identified.

In 1995 **The Joint Commission (TJC)** underwent a change in philosophy. Individual disciplines and departments were replaced with functions critical to patient care. New regulations placed accreditation emphasis on the organization's performance of these functions, thereby making them everyone's responsibility. This new process, called **performance improve-**

ment (PI), replaced quality assurance as a more proactive process of ensuring the quality of health care.

The current TJC accreditation process called *Shared Visions—New Pathway* became effective in January 2004 and focuses on performance measurement of organizational systems that are critical to patient safety, quality of care, treatment, and services. This new initiative involves the use of **ORYX** (an acronym for *Outcome Research Yields Excellence*), a new TJC requirement for the submission and evaluation of performance measurement data. Unlike past accreditation processes, which provided "snapshot" views of an organization's performance, this new requirement allows organizations to have an ongoing view of their performance, thus providing continuous opportunities for quality improvements. (Learn more about ORYX at www.jointcommission. org/PerformanceMeasurement/PerformanceMeasurement systems/comm._guidelines_08.htm.)

In the ever-changing health care arena, the pursuit of quality continues with concepts that integrate all aspects of health care. These concepts, called *total quality management* (TQM) and *continuous quality improvement* (CQI), are continuous, incremental improvement processes that reflect the organization-wide philosophy that quality is everybody's business. Quality control is a small but important part of TQM/CQI, and as such it contributes to the organizational goal of providing quality patient care. This section presents two major quality issues—applications of QC and PI.

GENERAL GUIDELINES FOR ESTABLISHING QUALITY CONTROL

All QC activities that take place must be recorded to prove their existence. All record sheets must list tolerance limits, when applicable, so that the person recording the results will always know whether the value being recorded is acceptable. Corrective action must also be recorded when any measurement falls outside a tolerance limit. The responsibility for QC may rest mainly with one person, but in reality everyone must participate if a program is to be successful. A QC program for a laboratory must include procedures for control of the following items: temperatures, equipment, media, reagents, susceptibility testing, and personnel.

Temperatures

Daily temperature checks are required on all temperature-dependent equipment:

- Incubators
- Heating blocks
- Water baths
- Refrigerators
- Freezers

Incubator and refrigerator thermometers are easier to read if they are permanently immersed in glycerol. This helps prevent temperature fluctuations when the door is opened to read the thermometer. Before use, each thermometer must be checked against a reference thermometer from the National Institute of Standards and Technology (NIST), formerly the National Bureau of Standards (NBS). The most efficient method is to check a large batch of thermometers at the same time and at the temperature ranges likely to be used. A common practice in clinical microbiology is to test all thermometers at −20° C, 2° to 8° C, 37° C, and 56° C. The NIST thermometer comes with certification papers that list correction factors to be used at various temperature ranges. These correction factors are applied to all values obtained on individual laboratory thermometers. Laboratories arbitrarily determine the acceptable temperature variance. For most routine work, thermometers that vary by 1° C or more from the reference thermometer are discarded.

Thermometer Calibration

Thermometers are calibrated by batch on arrival to the laboratory. (Procedure 5-1 outlines the calibration procedure.) Once the thermometer has passed calibration and is placed in use, repeat calibration of the thermometer should not be necessary. Alternatively, thermometers already checked against an NIST thermometer can be purchased. Certificates of calibration should be kept for the life of the thermometer or until the expiration date on the certificate; after that date, the thermometer can be recalibrated or discarded. For environmental and safety reasons, thermometers with no mercury are recommended. Mineral spirits with nontoxic red-dyed alcohol are used in place of the mercury. Thermometers should be checked daily to ensure that gas bubbles have not been introduced into the liquid, making reading the temperature difficult. Gas bubbles can be eliminated by centrifugation or by placing the thermometer at high or low temperature.

Equipment Quality Control

Equipment used in the clinical microbiology laboratory must be tested for proper performance at intervals that are appropriate for each piece. This process may involve checking the percentage of CO_2 in an incubator daily or measuring the revolutions per minute (rpm) of a centrifuge twice a year. Sometimes frequency of testing is dictated by a regulatory agency, and other times it is arbitrary. Table 5-2 gives examples of some laboratory equipment, the type of testing done, and the frequency of testing.

A **preventive maintenance** program must be established as an additional control measure. Preventive maintenance performed on equipment generally involves tasks such as oiling

---

PROCEDURE 5-1
Thermometer Calibration

LABELING

1. Create a calibration log sheet.
2. Etch a number on the back of each thermometer using a diamond-tipped marker.

CALIBRATION METHOD

1. Place the reference thermometer and the thermometer(s) to be calibrated in an ice bath.
2. When the reference thermometer reads 0° C, take the reading of all thermometer(s) being calibrated, and record the readings on the log sheet.
3. Repeat steps 1 and 2 at all other applicable temperatures, such as 37° C and 56° C.

CALCULATION OF CORRECTION FACTOR

1. Correct for the difference in readings between the reference thermometer (reference temperature) and that of each thermometer being calibrated by subtracting the higher reading from the lower reading. If the thermometer being calibrated reads less than the reference thermometer, assign a plus (+) sign to the result of the subtraction step. This value must be added to the thermometer reading to equal the reading that would be taken from the reference thermometer. Conversely, if the reading of the thermometer being calibrated is greater than the reference thermometer, assign a minus (−) sign to the result. This value must then be subtracted from that thermometer's reading to equal the reference value.
2. Correct for the difference between the reading of the reference thermometer and the "real" temperature using the process just described. Add the correction factor for the reference thermometer to the correction factor calculated in Step 1 for each thermometer being calibrated.
3. Determine the correction factor at each temperature for each thermometer, and record it on the log sheet for the thermometer. The log sheet should be kept for the life of the thermometer.
4. Tolerance limits are set by each laboratory but are usually 1° C. Discard all thermometers that exceed the established tolerance limit.
   Examples of correction factors are shown below.

"Real" Reference	Correction Temperature	Temperature Factor
0° C	+0.1° C	+0.1
37° C	36.9° C	+0.1
56° C	55.9° C	+0.1

---

and cleaning, replacing filters, and recalibrating instruments. Keeping an instrument in top shape and functioning at the proper level will increase its lifetime and help control the quality of the results. Figure 5-1 shows an example of a preventive maintenance log sheet.

TABLE 5-2 Frequency of Equipment Testing

Equipment	Test Type	Frequency
Incubator	Temperature, CO_2	Daily
GasPak jar	Anaerobiasis, catalyst heated	Each use
Anaerobe chamber	Anaerobiasis, humidity, temperature	Daily
Biohazard hood	Airflow (done by specialist)	Annually or any time hoods are moved
Centrifuge	rpm check	Every 6 months
Microscope	Cleaned and adjusted	Four times per year or as needed
Autoclave	Temperature	Each load
	Spore testing	Weekly
Balance	Accuracy of weights	Annually

rpm, Revolutions per minute.

Media Quality Control

All prepared media must be quality controlled to document their performance and sterility. Records must be maintained for 2 years. The criteria are established by the **Clinical and Laboratory Standards Institute (CLSI),** formerly the National Committee for Clinical Laboratory Standards (NCCLS), and listed in document M22-A2. Commercial media are always tested by the manufacturer. The laboratory must obtain a statement of QC from the manufacturer for all media the laboratory will not retest. This certificate must be retained for as long as the laboratory uses the specified media. Only certain kinds of media must be retested by the user, usually because of complexity or history of failure rate. Media that require retesting are chocolate agar, selective media for pathogenic *Neisseria*, and *Campylobacter* media. Figure 5-2 lists specialty commercial media that have been retested by the laboratory.

MEDIA, REAGENTS, AND SMALL EQUIPMENT	JANUARY	FEBRUARY	MARCH
MEDIA, REAGENTS:			
1. Check refrigerators and freezers for outdated material.	1/21/09 AF	2/24/09 LH	3/28/09 DS
2. Check for "received" and "opened" dating.	1/21/09 AF	2/24/09 LH	3/28/09 DS
THERMOMETERS: Calibrate by batch on arrival.			
PIPETTORS: Calibrate.			3/10/09 MS
pH METER: (Rooms 337 and 354)			
1. Clean the exterior.	1/21/09 AF	2/24/09 LH	3/28/09 DS
2. Replace water in the electrode holder.	1/21/09 AF	2/24/09 LH	3/28/09 DS
3. Check the AgCl level of the electrode.	1/21/09 AF	2/24/09 LH	3/28/09 DS
EYEWASHES: Flush.			
(Rooms 332, 337, 339, 342, 351[2], 354)	1/21/09 AF	2/24/09 LH	3/28/09 DS
STAINING SINK: Clean.	1/20/09 AF	2/24/09 LH	3/28/09 DS
GROUNDING: Check annually.			
REVIEWED BY: M Rausch Page 1 of 5			
YEAR: 2009			
Preventive maintenance is to be performed in the months highlighted for each item listed.			

FIGURE 5-1 Preventive maintenance log sheet.

MEDIUM TESTED	MFG	LOT NUMBER	EXP. DATE	STERILITY	TEST ORGANISMS	RESULT	ACTION TAKEN	DATE	TECH.
Chocolate II	BD	L3RTP0	5/23/09	OK	H. influenzae N. meningitidis	Pass	None	3/8/09	MR
GC-Lect	BD	–							
Jembec-Neiss.	BD	A 3NENC	4/3/09	OK	N. gonorrhoeae N. meningitidis S. epidermidis C. albicans E. coli	Pass	None	3/8/09	MR
Campy bld	BD	LINDHK	4/28/09	OK	C. jejuni E. coli	Pass	None	3/8/09	LM
Campy thio	BD	H4E0AJ	2/1/09	OK	C. jejuni E. coli	Pass	None	3/8/09	LM

Reviewed by: _____ Date: _____

FIGURE 5-2   Commercial media that have been retested by the laboratory. Result: Pass/Fail.

A list of all media requiring retesting can be found in the CLSI document M22-A2.

Media not quality controlled by the laboratory must still undergo observation for moisture, sterility, breakage, and appearance with every lot or shipment received:
- Moisture: Plates should be free of moisture before use but should never show signs of drying around the edges.
- Sterility: Plates should be free of contaminants.
- Breakage: Petri dishes should not be cracked or broken.
- Appearance: Blood-based plates should not show signs of hemolysis, and any other plate that deviates from the normal color should not be used.

Results of media observations must be recorded and include lot numbers. Figure 5-3 shows an example of a media observation log, which helps to ensure that good-quality media are used on all patient samples. Corrective action must be taken when a medium does not meet standards. This can be documented on a separate record known as a *media failures log* (Table 5-3).

When a medium needs to be quality controlled because it was prepared "in-house" (in the laboratory) or because it is complex, several basic rules must be followed:
- All media must be tested before use.
- Each medium must be tested with organisms expected to grow or give a positive reaction as well as with organisms expected either not to grow or to produce a negative reaction.
- The medium should be tested for sterility and pH.
- The organisms selected for QC should represent the most fastidious organisms for which the medium was designed.

- Testing techniques should be different for primary plating media from that for biochemical or subculture media. Primary plating media should be tested with dilute suspensions of organisms, whereas biochemical media can be tested with undiluted organisms.
- QC testing should be performed according to CLSI recommendations.
- Expiration dates must be established.

Figure 5-4 shows a log sheet used for testing media prepared in-house.

Reagent Quality Control

With few exceptions, reagents should be tested on each day of use with both positive and negative controls. Reagents that are documented to have consistent and dependable results may be tested less frequently. Some reagents may be tested more than once a day. Reagents that are opened and used repeatedly, such as albumin, should be checked daily for sterility. Always examine the manufacturer's package insert for recommended QC requirements. Examples of reagents that should undergo QC in microbiology are as listed:
- All stains
- Bacitracin
- β-lactamase
- Catalase
- Coagulase
- Gelatin
- Germ tube
- Hippurate
- Kovac
- Nitrate

DATE	MEDIUM	LOT NUMBER	MOISTURE	STERILITY	APPEARANCE	BREAKAGE	INITIALS
3/4/09	BAP	A2RUWO	✔	✔	✔	✔	MR
3/4/09	MAC	A4RUUH	✔	✔	✔	✔	MR
3/4/09	CHOC	A4RUUX	✔	✔	✔	✔	MR
3/4/09	CNA	A1RUWB	✔	✔	✔	✔	MR
3/4/09	HE	AZRCUF	✔	✔	✔	✔	MR
3/4/09	CIN	AZNEJE	✔	✔	✔	✔	MR
3/4/09	PD	OSU PREP: 1/6/09	✔	✔	✔	✔	MR
3/4/09	GC-LECT	K3RTNZ	✔	✔	✔	✔	MR
3/4/09	SCH	A4NETG	✔	✔	✔	✔	MR
3/4/09	SCH-GV	A3NENN	✔	✔	✔	✔	MR
3/4/09	CDC ANA	AZRWAW	✔	✔	✔	✔	MR
3/4/09	SMAC	OSU PREP: 2/15/09	✔	✔	✔	✔	MR

FIGURE 5-3   Media observation log. A check in each column indicates that the medium is acceptable.

TABLE 5-3 Media Failures Log

Date	2/14/09
Media	TMS slants
Lot #	In-house preparation 2/13/09
Expiration date	6 months from preparation
Quantity	2 racks
Failure	Failure to give proper reaction with *S. epidermidis*; *S. aureus* and other coagulase-neg. staphs are OK
Action taken	QC repeated; *S. epidermidis* failed; memo sent to all techs and all tubes discarded; new TMS prepared
Technologist	MAR

TMS, Trimethylsilyl esters.

TABLE 5-4 Recommended Control Organisms for Susceptibility Testing

Organism	Susceptibility Test(s)
Escherichia coli	Gram-negative drugs
Escherichia coli	β-Lactamase–inhibitor drugs
Staphylococcus aureus	Gram-positive drugs—Kirby-Bauer test
Staphylococcus aureus	Gram-positive drugs—minimal inhibitory concentration
Pseudomonas aeruginosa	Monitors Ca^{++}, MG^{++} content*
Enterococcus faecalis	Monitors thymidine[†]

*As Ca^{++} and Mg^{++} concentrations increase, *P. aeruginosa* becomes more resistant to the aminoglycosides.
[†]Increases in thymidine cause false resistance to certain drugs, such as sulfonamides, trimethoprim, and trimethoprim/sulfamethoxazole.

- Optochin
- Oxidase
- L-Pyro glutamyl-β-naphthylamine
- Typing sera
- Voges-Proskauer
- X and V strips

Figure 5-5 shows a variety of testing that might be performed daily at an individual workstation.

Antimicrobial Susceptibility Quality Control

The CLSI provides guidelines for control of susceptibility testing. The recommended control organisms are specific strains from the American Type Culture Collection (ATCC; Table 5-4). In addition to the organisms listed in Table 5-4, fastidious organisms such as *Haemophilus influenzae* and *Neisseria gonorrhoeae* are tested to ensure that the best possible results are obtained when testing the same type of isolates recovered from patient samples.

In any susceptibility system, many variables can affect the accuracy of results, including the following:

- Antibiotic potency
- Agar depth (Bauer-Kirby test)
- Evaporation (microtiter dilution)
- Cation content
- pH

DATE	MEDIA AND LOT NUMBER	ORGANISM PLATED	QC PLATED DATE	QC READ DATE	QC PASSED/FAILED	INITIALS
3/8/09	TMA	S. aureus S. epidermidis	3/9/09	3/10/09	Pass	MR
3/8/09	Beta toxin	S. agalactiae ⊕ S. pyogenes ⊖	3/9/09	3/9/09	Pass	MR
3/8/09	PSE	E. faecalis	3/9/09	3/10/09	Pass	MR
3/8/09	TSI	P. aeruginosa C. freundii	3/9/09	3/10/09	Pass	MR

FIGURE 5-4   Log sheet for testing media prepared in house.

BLOOD CULTURE WORKSTATION QUALITY CONTROL

Month _____ March _____

Year _____ 2009 _____

DATE	INITIALS	GASPAK JAR Anaerobic	HEAT CATALYST	CHANGE DESICCANT Date (weekly)	ACRIDINE ORANGE Pos	ACRIDINE ORANGE Neg	NaDesoxy/ WELLCOGEN Pos	NaDesoxy/ WELLCOGEN Neg	HEATING (35°- 37° C) #20	BLOCKS (35°- 37° C) #17
1	LM	OK	✔		N	D	+	−	35°	36°
2	AD	OK	✔		N	D	+	−	35°	36°
3	AD	OK x 2	✔		N	D	N	D	35°	36°
4	MCl	OK	✔		+	−	N	D	36°	36°
5	MCl	OK	✔		N	D	N	D	35°	36°
6	LH	OK x 2	✔		N	D	N	D	35°	36°
7	AD	OK x 2	✔	✔	N	D	+	−	36°	36°
8	AD	OK x 2	✔		N	D	+	−	36°	37°
9	LH	OK	✔		N	D	+	−	36°	36°
10	AD	OK	✔		N	D	N	D	36°	36°
11	Cl	OK	✔		+	−	N	D	36°	36°
12	MG	OK	✔		+	−	+	−	36°	36°
13	DS	OK x 2	✔		N	D	N	D	36°	36°
14	DS	OK	✔	✔	N	D	N	D	36°	35°

REVIEWED BY: Mbtt

DATE: 4/4/05

FIGURE 5-5   Various testing methods that can be performed daily at an individual workstation. Example of a 2-week workstation quality control. *ND,* Not done.

- Thymidine content
- Instrument failure
- Inoculum concentration
- Temperature
- Moisture (Bauer-Kirby test)
- Difficulty in determining endpoints

Careful storage of degradable supplies and precision in implementation of recommended procedures are mandatory to obtain accurate and reproducible susceptibility results.

Susceptibility testing of control organisms is usually conducted daily until precision can be demonstrated with 20 or 30 consecutive days of susceptibility testing using CLSI guidelines. The control organism results must be evaluated before determining endpoints on patient isolates. Minimal inhibitory concentration (MIC) values must be within one log dilution of the expected MIC based on CLSI guidelines. Once the 20- or 30-day evaluation has been accomplished, QC organisms may be tested weekly instead of daily. All results from the 20- or 30-day evaluation should be kept as long as the antimicrobial agent is used or for at least 2 years after discontinuation of the agent.

Personnel Competency

Personnel **competency** is determined by using a variety of techniques such as direct observation, review of work sheets, or written examination. A popular technique used to determine competency is **proficiency testing,** in which carefully designed samples are given to technologists as "unknowns" for the purpose of identifying them. Proficiency samples may be purchased commercially or prepared internally. All tests performed on patients must be subjected to proficiency testing twice a year, even if commercial proficiency testing is not available. Proficiency samples should not receive any "special" treatment and should be tested in the same manner as patient samples.

Another form of personnel QC is to see that each technologist's results are reviewed by another technologist, thereby ensuring mistakes are likely to be caught before results are released. Employee competency has always played a large role in quality. The **Clinical Laboratory Improvement Act of 1988 (CLIA)** has mandated that the competency of each employee be determined and verified upon employment. Reverification must take place annually. Proof of competency must be maintained in each employee's personnel file. A person may be qualified to prepare a slide for staining but may not be able to stain it, or a person may be qualified to prepare and stain a slide but not to read or interpret the smear. As part of CLIA requirements, all tests or analyses have been assigned a complexity rating. In microbiology, all tests are either moderately complex or highly complex. Personnel must meet certain educational requirements before being permitted to perform at each level of complexity.

In addition to meeting educational requirements, a person's competency must be observed and documented for each test performed. The many agencies involved in accreditation and inspection have different requirements and interpretations of competency verification, making this a complicated task for all laboratories. An example of a competency check-off form is shown in Figure 5-6.

The requirement for ongoing **continuing education (CE)** programs for all employees is yet another form of QC. These programs may teach theory or new techniques, present case studies, or simply provide training on new instrumentation. Documentation that all CE programs have been completed is essential. Training for new instrumentation should also be documented in the individual employee's personnel competency file.

Use of Stock Cultures

To operate a QC program, stock cultures must be maintained by all laboratories. They are available from many sources:
- Commercial sources
- Proficiency testing isolates
- Patient isolates
- ATCC

When QC testing appears to have failed, it is usually the stock culture rather than the test itself that has failed. Organisms may mutate with repeated subculturing. For best results, a stock culture should be grown in a large volume of broth and then divided among enough small freezer vials to last a year. With this technique, a new vial can be removed from the freezer weekly so that organisms do not have to be continually subcultured. An organism should be subcultured twice after thawing to return it to a healthy state. Media selection for freezing is at the discretion of individual laboratories but should not contain sugars. If organisms use sugars while being maintained, the acid products that result might kill the organisms with time. The following are popular media choices for stock cultures:
- Schaedler broth with glycerol
- Skim milk
- Chopped meat (anaerobes)
- Tryptic soy agar deeps (at room temperature)
- Cysteine-tryptic agar without carbohydrates

Another popular method of storage is the use of storage beads. Storage beads are contained in a vial containing 1 mL of thioglycollate broth. After the vial has been inoculated with the organism, the broth is removed and the vial with the beads is stored at −70° C. The advantage of this system is that a single bead can be removed without thawing the entire vial. Although this form of storage is more convenient, it is probably more expensive than those previously mentioned, and therefore cost should be taken into consideration. Organisms stored in a freezer should be kept at −70° C; alternative storage methods include freezing in liquid nitrogen and lyophilization.

Quality Control Manual

All rules and procedures for QC should be available to employees at the workstation in written form in a QC manual. The manual must be reviewed and signed at least annually and revised as needed by a supervisor.

PERFORMANCE IMPROVEMENT

Accrediting agencies such as TJC and the **College of American Pathologists (CAP)** emphasize PI in their accreditation checklists. The CLIA also mandates the use of written performance

Employee name: *Carol Johnson*   Year *2009*

Demonstrates following abilities:	Work station		
	#1 Respiratory	#2 Urines	#3 O & Ps
1. Handles specimens safely during testing, storing, and discarding	✔	✔	✔
2. Prepares specimens for analysis according to laboratory policies and procedures (parasitology and special procedure areas)	—	—	✔
3. Analyzes specimens according to laboratory procedures for the workstation; knows theory and principles of the tests being performed	✔	✔	✔
4. Clearly records all work done so that another person could take over the work station	✔	✔	✔
5. Reports results accurately and in a timely manner	✔	✔	✔
6. Makes appropriate critical value and courtesy calls	✔	✔	✔
7. Consistently performs and records quality control and documents all remedial action	✔	✔	✔
8. Remedial action necessary (yes or no)	No	No	No

Remedial actions:_____

_____

_____

_____

_____

Date remediation completed:_____

Evaluator signature *A Holbrook*   Date *2/11/09*   (Work station 1)

Evaluator signature *L Creme*   Date *6/9/09*   (Work station 2)

Evaluator signature *S Young*   Date *8/27/09*   (Work station 3)

Employee signature *Carol Johnson*   Date *8/28/09*

FIGURE 5-6   Competency documentation.

improvement policies in laboratories that include all three phases of testing. Every laboratory must have a plan for improvement. To improve quality effectively, all employees must understand the plan and take active roles.

Vision and Mission Statements

Creating a short vision or mission statement for all employees to learn can be an effective tool for uniting everyone behind the same cause. It can be as simple as the vision statement used by Wilford Hall Medical Center, "The AFMS Flagship—Comprehensive Health-care … On Time … On Target," or the mission statement used at The Ohio State University Medical Center, "Working Together for a Healthy America." An organization's vision and mission statements must be clearly emphasized so that all employees become involved and understand that each and every one of them has a role in the mission and they must strive to make PI part of their everyday life to achieve the organization's vision. Problems are not to be viewed as true problems but as opportunities for improvements and a chance to excel.

Indicators of Performance Improvement: Process versus Outcome

Many types of monitors or indicators can be incorporated into a quality improvement program. Accrediting agencies generally check to be sure that a variety of types are used. Some monitors are ongoing data collections, not instituted in regard to suspected problems. Results are compiled and evaluated routinely. This procedure establishes a trend and makes problems easy to detect when they do occur because they appear as disruptions in the trend. These are often referred to as **process monitors.**

Outcome monitors are measurements of the result of a process. An example is the complications a patient experiences as the result of a process. Other monitors may be created in response to a suspected problem. Data may be collected for a short period to resolve a specific issue. These monitors are called **focused monitors.**

Establishing Performance Monitors

The Joint Commission makes recommendations as an accrediting agency for establishing performance monitors. The components of the recommendation are to plan, design, measure, assess, and improve.

Plan: The plan is not expected to be a single-department approach. Rather, it should be a coordinated, organization-wide approach to improving patient outcomes that includes interdisciplinary collaborative actions.

Design: Clear objectives are needed to describe a new process, component, or service.

Measure: Systematic data collection is necessary either for improvements or for ongoing measurements. (See Box 5-1 for suggested measurable processes.)

Assess: A review of the collected data should be systematic, interdisciplinary, and interdepartmental, as well as statistically based using analytical tools. Internal comparisons or comparisons to similar processes in other organizations are appropriate. Guidelines for assessments

---

BOX 5-1 Measurable Processes

Patient preparation
Specimen handling
    Collection
    Labeling
    Preservation
    Transportation
Communications processes
    Transfer of information
    Completeness of requisitions
    Reporting timeliness
    Report accuracy
Test appropriateness
Patient needs/expectations
Risk management activities
Quality control activities

---

might be accreditation standards, practice guidelines, or legal and regulatory requirements.

Improve: Current processes or a design of new processes may need to be redesigned. Because more opportunities are usually identified than can be acted on, priorities must be established. Priorities are often based on risk, frequency, or high-volume processes.

Problem/Action Form

A simpler approach to monitoring or documenting quality issues is a problem/action form. This approach is most commonly used to document issues that are quickly resolved, but it could also be used for long-term monitor summation. The form is a brief statement consisting of the following information:

- Date
- Problem
- Evaluation
- Corrective action
- Outcome

The form may be signed by the person submitting it, and additional documentation may be attached as necessary. Table 5-5 illustrates the use of the problem/action form.

Customer Concept

Laboratories must focus on the **customer concept.** Who are the customers, and what is a customer's perception of quality? Patients are not the only customers. Anyone who looks to the laboratory for a service is a customer. Doctors, nurses, insurers, and patients are all customers. Each customer may view quality differently and may have different expectations. Laboratory workers may judge quality in terms of accuracy, whereas a physician views it as turnaround time, the patient as compassion and relief from pain, and the insurance company as cost-effectiveness. Customer satisfaction must be surveyed to determine perceptions.

Fixing the Process

When patient outcome is less than desirable, the process must be evaluated and corrected. The focus is on the process, not on an individual. The primary rule to follow is to refrain from finger-pointing or fault-finding. Preanalytical and postana-

TABLE 5-5 Clinical Microbiology Problem/Action Report

Date	11/15/09
Problem	A blood culture was required from a patient at the urgent care facility, but no staff member was trained to draw blood cultures. The patient had to drive from the urgent care facility to the hospital to have the blood drawn by a phlebotomist who was trained in the appropriate techniques.
Evaluation	No employees at the urgent care facility have been trained to collect blood cultures. The same is true of the Clinic Outpatient Lab. This is the second occurrence in about 2 months.
Corrective action	Seriously ill patients should not have to travel from one facility to another to have their blood drawn. Laboratory Administration was informed of this situation.
Outcome	All outpatient sites will receive training and written instructions for the proper collection of blood for culture. Patients will no longer have to drive to the hospital for this service if they are already at an outpatient facility.

Submitted by M. Rausch
Attached documentation? No

---

lytical activities usually take place outside the laboratory and require **cross-functional teams** to evaluate and correct the process. Department representatives can easily become defensive and territorial. Barriers to cooperation must be removed. Cross-functional teams must include a trained **facilitator.** Facilitators are most effective when they have no vested interest in the process being evaluated. The facilitator's role on the team is to use problem-solving training and experience to help the team brainstorm and stay on track. In the formation of a cross-functional team, the people "in the trenches" must be represented; the team should not consist solely of supervisory personnel. If the issue is transportation of specimens, at a minimum the team should include a transporter, a specimen processor, a staff nurse, a medical student or physician representative, appropriate supervisory personnel, and a facilitator. The most accurate and meaningful brainstorming ideas usually come from the people who perform the tasks, not from those who designed the process.

When is a process fixed? It is not fixed just because the reason something went wrong is explained. It is fixed only when the problem is prevented from happening again. For example, a laboratory result was never recorded on a patient's chart. Investigation determined that the patient was transferred to another unit while the report was being generated. This explanation does not suffice to fix the problem. To fix the problem, a process must be established to ensure that charting follows every patient in a timely manner every time.

Benchmarking

A benchmark is a reference point. **Benchmarking** is seeking an industry's or profession's best practices to imitate and improve. Benchmarking was initially practiced in business and industry but has now become an important part of hospital quality management programs. It is done willingly and openly. A hospital may join a large group of other hospitals that all share operating statistics. Productivity and cost-effectiveness are two large categories commonly used in a benchmarking comparison. The best performers in a group of hospitals are highlighted. Hospitals can individually and anonymously see where they are by comparison with other hospitals' statistics and then contact the best performers to evaluate their differences. A code of conduct is followed when benchmarking includes both ethics and etiquette. Although hospitals generally benchmark other hospitals, they eventually incorporate lessons from other successful industries.

Commercially Purchased Monitors

The CAP has put together a national PI assessment program called **Q-Probes.** Laboratories throughout the country subscribe to an annual series of monitors. At least one of these monitors each year has a microbiology focus. Q-Probes have covered topics such as adequacy of sputum cultures, turnaround time for spinal fluid Gram stain results, blood culture contamination rates, and appropriateness of ordering patterns for stool specimens. The method of data collection is precisely outlined, and all worksheets and data forms are provided. Information is returned to subscribers in a manner that enables institutions to benchmark.

BIBLIOGRAPHY

August MJ et al, editors: *Quality control and quality assurance practices in clinical microbiology,* Cumitech 3A, Washington, DC, 1990, American Society for Microbiology.

Clinical and Laboratory Standards Institute (CLSI): *Methods for dilution antimicrobial susceptibility tests for bacteria that grow aerobically* (Approved Standard; M7-A2), vol 23, No. 2, Wayne, Pa, 2003, CLSI.

Clinical and Laboratory Standards Institute (CLSI): *Methods for dilution antimicrobial susceptibility tests for bacteria that grow aerobically,* ed 8 (Approved Standard; M7-A8), Wayne, Pa, 2008 CLSI.

Clinical and Laboratory Standards Institute (CLSI): *Performance standards for antimicrobial disk susceptibility tests* (Approved Standard; M2-8), vol 23, No. 1, Wayne, Pa, Jan 2003, CLSI.

Clinical and Laboratory Standards Institute (CLSI): *Performance standards for antimicrobial susceptibility testing,* ed 10 (Approved Standard; M2-A10), Wayne, Pa, 2008 CLSI.

Clinical and Laboratory Standards Institute (CLSI): *Performance standards for antimicrobial susceptibility testing* (Nineteenth Informational Supplement), Wayne, Pa, 2008 CLSI.

Clinical and Laboratory Standards Institute (CLSI): *Performance standards for antimicrobial susceptibility testing, M100-S15,* Wayne, Pa, 2005, CLSI.

Clinical Laboratory Improvement Act of 1988: Rules and regulations, *Federal Register,* Feb 28, 1992 www.cms.hhs.gov/CLIA.

College of American Pathologists: *Laboratory accreditation program,* Northfield, Ill, 2004, College of American Pathologists.

Eisenberg HD, editor: *Clinical microbiology procedures handbook,* sec 14, Washington, DC, 2004, American Society for Microbiology.

Joint Commission on Accreditation of Healthcare Organizations (JCAHO): *2004 Automated Hospitals*, Oakbrook Terrace, Ill, 2004, The Joint Commission.

Kelvin JF, Houston K: Improving organizational performance: an introduction to the 1995 Joint Commission on Accreditation of Healthcare Organizations Standard, *Cancer Pract* 4:88-95, 1996.

Locock L: Healthcare redesign: meaning, origins, and application, *Qual Saf Health Care* 12:53-57, 2003.

National Committee for Clinical Laboratory Standards (NCCLS): *Quality assurance for commercially prepared microbiological culture media*, ed 2 (Approved Standard; M22-A2), Wayne, Pa, 1996, NCCLS.

Sewell DL, MacLowry JD: Laboratory management. In Murray PR et al, editors: *Manual of clinical microbiology*, ed 8, Washington, DC, 2007, American Society for Microbiology.

Points to Remember

- Quality patient care is directly attributed to the quality of all the processes involved in that care.
- The laboratory can ensure reliability of laboratory data through the implementation of an active quality control (QC) program.
- Personnel competency must be ascertained through the use of techniques that encompass all processes involved in specimen testing.
- Performance improvements and performance measurement allow organizations to monitor their performance continually and to provide opportunities to improve.
- The use of vision and mission statements allows an organization to state expected goals and unite all employees behind a common goal.
- Customers must be taken into account in quality assurance because each customer will have his or her own perception of what quality means.
- When outcomes are less than desirable, the whole process must be reviewed and may require cross-functional teams and a trained facilitator to achieve the desired outcome.
- *Quality* is defined as a degree of excellence and must be constantly monitored and improved to ensure that it is the best we can achieve.

Learning Assessment Questions

1. Which of the following terms refers to checking media and reagents with specific organisms to determine whether expected results are obtained?
   a. Preventative maintenance
   b. Quality control (QC)
   c. Performance improvement (PI)
   d. Total quality management (TQM)

2. Which of the following describes the process of performance improvement?
   a. It involves only preanalytical activities.
   b. It is measured by patient outcome.
   c. It singles out individuals with poor performance.
   d. It is enhanced by understanding customer perception.

3. The laboratory must perform QC on all of the following media except:
   a. All media obtained from a commercial source
   b. Complex media
   c. Media with a history of failure
   d. Media made by the laboratory

4. Which of the following describes the correct way to select organisms for QC?
   a. They should represent the most fastidious organisms for which the media was designed.
   b. They should be organisms that will grow most easily.
   c. They should be immediately removed from the freezer.
   d. They should be streaked only once after removal from the freezer.

5. Susceptibility tests must be quality controlled daily except when which of the following is the case?
   a. An automated system is in use.
   b. Controls have been in an acceptable range for 6 months.
   c. Precision is demonstrated for 20 or 30 consecutive days.
   d. A new antibiotic is added.

6. Which of the following mandates annual employee competency testing?
   a. Clinical and Laboratory Standards Institute (CLSI)
   b. Clinical Laboratory Improvement Act of 1988 (CLIA)
   c. National Institute of Standards and Technology (NIST)
   d. American Type Culture Collection (ATCC)

7. A problem/action form should contain which of the following information?
   a. Date and problem
   b. Evaluation and corrective action
   c. Outcome
   d. All of the above

8. What is the term for PI monitors that are created in response to a specific issue?
   a. Focused monitors
   b. Process monitors
   c. Outcome monitors
   d. Multitask monitors

9. Who is defined as a customer in the laboratory?
   a. The patient
   b. The doctor and nurse
   c. The insurance company
   d. All of the above

10. What is the new TJC initiative to monitor performance measurement?
    a. TQM
    b. Continuous quality improvement (CQI)
    c. PI
    d. ORYX

B. Putting the Laboratory Test to the Test

*Frederic J. Marsik**

- ■ ANALYTICAL ANALYSIS OF TESTS
  Analytical (Technical) Sensitivity
  Analytical (Technical) Specificity
  Accuracy
- ■ CLINICAL ANALYSIS OF TESTS
  Clinical (Diagnostic) Sensitivity
  Clinical (Diagnostic) Specificity

- ■ OPERATIONAL ANALYSIS OF TESTS
  Incidence of Disease
  Prevalence of Disease
  Predictive Values of Tests
  Efficiency of Tests
  Other Concepts
- ■ CHOOSING A LABORATORY METHOD
- ■ TEST VALIDATION

OBJECTIVES

After reading and studying this chapter, you should be able to:

1. Define and differentiate *analytical sensitivity* and *specificity* and *clinical sensitivity* and *specificity.*

2. Define *prevalence* and *incidence of disease* and discuss the importance of prevalence in computing predictive values of tests.

3. Discuss predictive values of tests and show how they are computed.

4. Apply the concepts of predictive values of tests to several clinical examples.

Case In Point

A 5-year-old girl was complaining of a sore throat. A low-grade fever (99° F [37° C]) was noted when the girl was seen in the physician's office. Her pharynx was red, exudates were present, and her tonsils were swollen. The physician requested that a group A streptococcal direct antigen test be performed; the test came back positive for group A streptococci. An antibiotic was prescribed for the patient.

Issues to Consider

- How the sensitivity and specificity of the laboratory test is used in clinical diagnosis of a disease
- How the prevalence of a disease in a population might affect the predictive value of tests
- Why it is important to constantly validate methods and procedures used in the laboratory

KEY TERMS

Analytical sensitivity	Incidence
Analytical specificity	Negative predictive value (NPV)
Accuracy	
Bayes' theorem	Positive predictive value (PPV)
Bias	Precision
Clinical (diagnostic) sensitivity	Predictive value
Clinical (diagnostic) specificity	Prevalence
Detection limit	Test validation

*This section was prepared by F.J. Marsik in his private capacity. No official support or endorsement by the FDA is intended or implied.

New diagnostic tests under development in clinical microbiology are directed more toward the detection of antigens rather than toward the detection of antibodies. Although culture still remains the gold standard for diagnostic purposes, the newer, noncultural antigen detection tests offer simplicity and speed for detection of the etiologic agent. In addition, the immune status of the patient does not affect test results. These noncultural antigen detection tests are being designed for physician's office use and, as such, are easily performed by nonlaboratory personnel. Because the test results are available quickly, the physician can make an informed decision regarding patient management.

These tests can be misused or their results misinterpreted. Tests with a high sensitivity and specificity may be promoted as extremely reliable diagnostic tests. In certain clinical situations, however, such tests may not add meaningful information to the diagnosis. This section reviews the pertinent definitions related to evaluating tests and presents several clinical examples to illustrate the basic concepts.

ANALYTICAL ANALYSIS OF TESTS

The following terms relate to the actual test and are not used in the critical evaluation of a test in the clinical setting. Analytical sensitivity and specificity should not be confused with clinical sensitivity and specificity.

Analytical (Technical) Sensitivity

The **analytical sensitivity** of a test refers to its ability to detect a particular analyte or a small change in its concentration. Analytical sensitivity is usually defined at the 0.95 confidence level (±2 standard deviations [SD]) and may be referred to as the **detection limit.** In microbiology the detection limit may be correlated to the number of colonies in the culture or to the lowest quantity of antigen or antibody a test can detect. For example, the enzyme immunoassay (EIA) is more sensitive than the precipitation test in detecting antibody. The EIA can detect lower concentrations of antibody.

Analytical (Technical) Specificity

A test's **analytical specificity** refers to its ability not to react with substances other than the analyte of interest.

Accuracy

The degree of conformity of a measurement to a standard or a true value is **accuracy.** It is a measure of analytical capability. For example, with the performance standards for antimicrobial disk susceptibility tests, a mean value of several observations is compared with a predetermined standard value or range. If the mean (or range) of control limits found in standard tables is exceeded, a technical systematic error (variation) exists that might lead to misinterpretation of test results.

Accuracy is a function of two characteristics: precision and bias. **Precision** is the measure of exactness or the degree of refinement with which a test is performed. It is the dispersion of repeated observations caused by random errors. The precision (reproducibility) of a test is usually monitored by means of the range (maximum minus minimum) within sets of observations. **Bias** is the mean difference of test results from an accepted reference method caused by systematic errors.

Typically precision and bias are determined by studies wherein several investigators or laboratories perform repeated testing of several specimens of known values. Then the test results are analyzed by statistical methods to determine the test's precision and bias within and among laboratories.

CLINICAL ANALYSIS OF TESTS

Clinical (Diagnostic) Sensitivity

Clinical (diagnostic) sensitivity is the proportion of positive test results obtained when a test is applied to patients known to have the disease; thus it is the frequency of positive test results in patients with the disease (true-positive results). For example, if 100 patients who have gonorrhea are tested for that disease and the test yields positive results in 95 and is negative in the other 5, then the sensitivity of the test is 95%. Five of these 100 patients had false-negative test results.

The highest clinical sensitivity is desired when a disease is serious and when false-positive results will not lead to serious clinical or economic problems. Sensitivity is expressed as a percent:

$$\frac{\text{Number of true-positive results}}{\text{Number of true-positive plus false-negative results}} \times 100$$

The sensitivity of a particular test does not change if the test is performed correctly. The sensitivity is determined by multicenter clinical trials whereby the test results, obtained by performing the test according to a specific protocol, are compared with a gold standard. In microbiology the standard is usually culture, which in many cases is not absolute. Thus the reported sensitivity for a certain test may vary among laboratories. Evaluating new diagnostic tests is difficult because of these imperfect standards.

Clinical (Diagnostic) Specificity

Clinical (diagnostic) specificity is the proportion of negative results obtained when a test is applied to patients known to be free of the disease. Thus it is the frequency of negative test results in patients without the disease (true-negative results). For example, if 100 patients without gonorrhea are tested for that disease and the test yields negative results in 90 and is positive in the other 10, then the specificity of the test is 90%. Ten of these 100 patients had false-positive test results.

The highest clinical specificity is desired when the disease is serious but not treatable, when disease absence has either psychological or public health value, or when false-positive results might cause serious clinical or economic problems. Specificity is expressed as a percent:

$$\frac{\text{Number of true-negative results}}{\text{Number of true-negative plus false-negative results}} \times 100$$

As with sensitivity, the specificity does not change if the test is performed correctly. The specificity is also determined by clinical trials whereby the test results are confirmed by a more definitive test or procedure.

OPERATIONAL ANALYSIS OF TESTS

Although sensitivity and specificity do not change for a given test, the prevalence of the disease and the positive and negative predictive values of a test do change. In clinical medicine these parameters are extremely important to know when evaluating a particular test result.

Incidence of Disease

Incidence is the number of new cases of a disease over a period of time (e.g., months, year) and is a measure of events. The incidence rate is most often calculated by dividing the number of infections acquired during a given period (e.g., month, year) by the population at risk for that same time. The relation between prevalence (P) and incidence (I) can be seen in the equation $P = I \times D$, where D is duration of disease from onset (diagnosis) to termination. For chronic diseases, such as cancer, the prevalence is greater than the incidence; for acute diseases, such as gonorrhea, the prevalence is less than the incidence.

Prevalence of Disease

Prevalence is the frequency of a disease at a designated single point in time in the population being tested. For example, during influenza season the prevalence of "strep" throat in children attending daycare centers will be higher than the prevalence in children who do not attend such centers. The role prevalence plays in determining the positive and negative predictive values of a test can be seen in the formulas below. To interpret test results properly, the clinician must have an understanding or estimate of the prevalence of the disease in the population being tested. Prevalence can be estimated on the basis of clinical experience and information provided by the local and state health departments as well as information periodically provided by the Centers for Disease Control and Prevention (CDC).

Predictive Values of Tests

A test can have both a positive and a negative predictive value. The following three elements are needed to compute the positive and negative predictive values of a test:

- Sensitivity of the test
- Specificity of the test
- Prevalence of the disease being tested

Although predictive value theory has only recently been used in clinical medicine, the formulas and concepts are not new. The formulas for calculating positive and negative predictive values are commonly referred to as **Bayes' theorem,** which was published posthumously in 1763.

The **predictive value** of a test is the probability that a positive result **(positive predictive value [PPV])** accurately indicates the presence of an analyte or a specific disease or that a negative result **(negative predictive value [NPV])** accurately indicates the absence of an analyte or a specific disease. Predictive values vary significantly with the prevalence of the disease or analyte unless the test is 100% sensitive (for NPV) or specific (for PPV).

Positive Predictive Value

The PPV can be computed as follows:

Number of true-positive results = $(P)(Se)$:

$$PPV \frac{(P)(Se)}{(P)(Se)+(1-P)(1-Sp)} \times 100$$

The number of true-positive results plus false-positive results = $(P)(Se) + 1(1-P)(1-Sp)$:
where:

PPV = positive predictive value of test
P = prevalence of the disease being tested
Se = sensitivity of test
Sp = specificity of test

Negative Predictive Value

The negative predictive value can be computed as follows:

Number of true-negative results = $(1-P)(Sp)$:

$$NPV \frac{(1-P)(Sp)}{(1-P)(Sp)+(1-Se)(p)} \times 100$$

The number of true-negative results plus true-positive results = $(1-P)(Sp) + (1-Se)(p)$:
where:

NPV = negative predictive value of test
P = prevalence of the disease being tested
Se = sensitivity of test
Sp = specificity of test

Example

To illustrate the concepts of predictive values, consider a certain diagnostic test that has a sensitivity (Se) of 95% and a specificity (Sp) of 95%. In a primary care hospital where the prevalence of the disease being tested for is 1%, the PPV of the test is only 16%. This is calculated using the PPV equation as follows:

$$PPV \frac{(0.01)(0.95)}{(0.01)(0.95)+(1-0.01)(1-0.95)} \times 100 = 0.16 \text{ or } 16\%$$

The clinician has only a 16% certainty that a patient with a positive test result actually has the disease. If, however, the same test is used in a tertiary care hospital where the prevalence of the disease is 50%, the PPV increases to 95% (calculated using the same equation). The clinician in this case has a 95% certainty that a patient with a positive test result actually has the disease. Therefore the prevalence of the disease has a great influence on the predictive value of a test.

Clinical Applications of Positive and Negative Predictive Values

Group A Streptococcus Testing of Throat Samples. Acute pharyngitis is one of the most common conditions seen by primary care physicians. Although most of the infections are caused by viruses, 5% to 15% of cases have a bacterial etiology; usually group A β-hemolytic streptococci *(Streptococcus pyogenes)*. To test these organisms, 28 to 36 million throat cultures are performed annually in the United States.

Noncultural tests have been developed and approved for use in the private office setting to evaluate patients with acute pharyngitis for the presence of group A streptococci. The reported sensitivities and specificities of these tests vary considerably, however, ranging from the low 60s to the high 90s. Although speculative, explanations for such variations may be the difficulty in obtaining an adequate throat sample, especially in children, and the use of imperfect culture methods as standards.

Assuming that a certain test for streptococci has reported sensitivity and specificity of 90% and 98%, respectively, and that the estimated prevalence for streptococcal infection in acute pharyngitis cases is 5%, the PPV and NPV would be 70.3% and 99.5% respectively. With a positive test result, approximately a 30% chance exists that the patient does not have a streptococcal infection. If the test result is negative, a greater than 99% chance exists that the patient is not infected. If the prevalence in the population being tested increases to 15%, the PPV increases to 88.8%, but the NPV decreases slightly to 98.2%.

Usually negative test results are more reliable in predicting the absence of disease than positive test results are in predicting the presence of disease. In this example, a negative result would indicate the absence of group A β-hemolytic streptococci with a high degree of certainty, and the patient could be spared the administration and cost of penicillin. Although clinical judgment is important, these tests can be helpful to clinicians in the proper evaluation and management of patients with acute pharyngitis.

Direct Detection of *Chlamydia trachomatis* in Urethral and Cervical Specimens. Chlamydia is the most prevalent sexually transmitted disease (STD) in the United States, with estimates of 3 to 10 million new cases occurring annually. Many of the individuals infected are asymptomatic, and proper diagnosis and treatment are essential to prevent the spread of disease and associated complications.

The growth cycle of the bacterium *C. trachomatis* is unique because it is an obligate intracellular parasite that requires living cells for cultivation. Several days are necessary to obtain results, and the sensitivity of the culture is only about 85%. As a result, newer noncultural methods have been developed and tested. Several tests are now available, including tests using the EIA, the immunofluorescence (IF), and DNA probes. Each has a considerable variance in reported sensitivities and specificities, most likely because of the nature of the organism and the imperfect culture standard with which the results are compared. In addition, each test requires specialized equipment that must be maintained and calibrated.

Table 5-6 shows the PPVs and NPVs for the IF and DNA probe tests applied directly to cervical samples in a population of patients in an obstetrics and gynecology clinic in whom the prevalence of chlamydial cervicitis is estimated to be 5%. The sensitivities and specificities for the two tests are similar, but the PPV is better for the DNA probe test. Thus patients with positive results of the DNA probe test are more likely to have chlamydial cervicitis than are those with positive results of the IF test. On the other hand, both tests identify patients with negative test results as not having chlamydial cervicitis with a high degree of certainty (99.5%).

Table 5-6 also shows the predictive values if the same tests are used in an STD clinic where the prevalence of chlamydial cervicitis is estimated to be 30%. The PPVs increase significantly, especially for the IF test, and both tests would function well as diagnostic tools. The NPVs drop for both tests, however, to 95.8%. Thus approximately 4% of patients with negative test results could be infected with *C. trachomatis*; this rate may not be acceptable given the nature of the disease.

Efficiency of Tests

The efficiency of a test indicates the percentage of patients who are correctly classified as having disease or not having disease. The efficiency is calculated using the following equation:

$$\text{Efficiency} \frac{(TP + TN)}{(TP + FP + RN + FN)} \times 100$$

where:

TP = number of patients with true-positive results
TN = number of patients with true-negative results
FP = number of patients with false-positive results
FN = number of patients with false-negative results

Other Concepts

Additional concepts, such as the medical decision-making analysis of tests, "benefit-cost analysis," combination testing, and nondisease factors affecting laboratory test results, are beyond the scope of this discussion.

CHOOSING A LABORATORY METHOD

Once an institution has made the decision to offer a new test, the next step generally is for the laboratory to select the method (Figure 5-7). The following are some steps that may be followed when deciding on the method:

1. Define the purpose for which the method is used. Common purposes for tests are as follows:
   - **Screening** is used for testing large populations of patients. Generally, screening tests have high clinical sensitivity and NPV. Positive results with such tests generally require confirmation by a more specific test.
   - **Confirmation** is used after obtaining a positive screening result to ensure the accuracy of the initial result. Specificity and PPV are generally the considerations for such tests.
   - **Diagnosis** is used for the evaluation of persons suspected of having a given disease state or characteristic.
2. Decide which type of analyte (e.g., organism, antigen, nucleic acid) is to be detected.
3. In conjunction with the end user of the test (e.g., the physician) and information from steps 1 and 2, determine the medical usefulness of the test (e.g., to improve patient care, to shorten hospital time).
4. Survey the technical and medical literature for performance claims of various methods. When reviewing the literature, confirm that the method described is actually the test to be evaluated in the laboratory.
5. Other considerations are as follows:
   - Cost
   - Practicality

TABLE 5-6 Comparison of the IF and DNA Probe Tests to Detect Chlamydial Cervicitis in Patient Populations with 5% and 30% Prevalences of the Disease*

Test	Sensitivity	Specificity	5% Prevalence		30% Prevalence	
			PPV	NPV	PPV	NPV
IF probe	90.0	98.0	70.3	99.5	95.1	95.8
DNA probe	89.8	99.5	90.4	99.5	98.7	95.8

*PPV and NPV were computed using equations (see text). All values are given in percentages.
IF, Immunofluorescence; *NPV,* negative predictive value; *PPV,* positive predictive value.

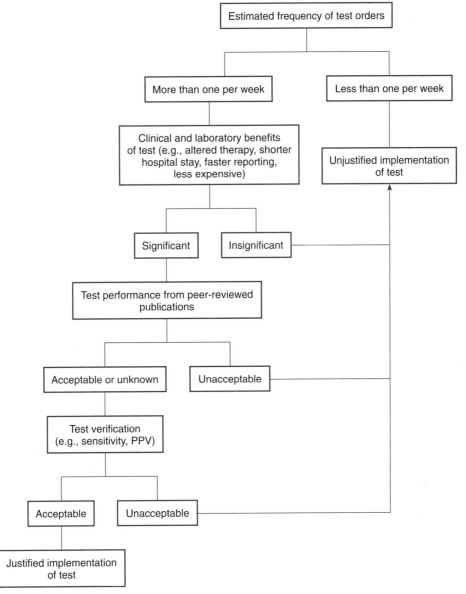

FIGURE 5-7 Choosing a laboratory method. *PPV,* Positive predictive value. (Modified from McCurdy B, editor: *Verification and validation of procedures in the clinical microbiology laboratory,* Cumitech 31, Washington, DC, 1997, American Society for Microbiology.)

- Specimen requirements
- Quantities of reagents and controls needed for test
- Shelf life of reagents and controls before and after opening
- Availability of supplies, service, and technical support
- Possible safety hazards
- Whether the reference range is appropriate for that test and how it will be determined for that institution

6. Perform an in-house verification. Verification of a test serves to establish that the performance parameters of the test are satisfactory. The result of test verification should indicate one of three possibilities:

- The test is acceptable for routine use.
- Further verification studies are required.
- The test is unsuitable for routine use until its performance parameters can be verified.

Test verification records must be kept for at least 2 years. However, it is good laboratory practice to maintain the records for as long as the test is in use.

TEST VALIDATION

Verification of a test does not provide ongoing assurance that the test is continually performing as expected. **Test validation** is the ongoing process providing information that a test is performing correctly. The components of validation are quality control, proficiency testing, verification of employee competency, and instrument calibration. The results of the validation indicate one of three possibilities:

1. The test continues to be acceptable.
2. Further investigation is warranted.
3. Immediate corrective action must be undertaken, and the test must be considered unsuitable for routine use until it can be validated.

Lot numbers and expiration dates should be documented for all reagents and materials used in the validation process. Records of validation should be kept for at least 2 years.

Validation should be done frequently enough to ensure the continual correct performance of tests. In most cases, following the manufacturer's guidelines and the requirements of the regulatory or accrediting agencies will provide this assurance.

New laboratory tests as well as old ones should always be validated. Understanding and using the concepts of predictive values and the effect of prevalence on those values are important for the proper use of a test and interpretation of the results. The development of rapid noncultural tests for the detecting of infectious diseases makes the use of these concepts even more important. A test result can no longer be considered simply "positive" or "negative" but must be interpreted in view of the concepts presented in this discussion. When test results are interpreted properly, better patient care is achieved.

BIBLIOGRAPHY

Clinical and Laboratory Standards Institute (CLSI): *Specifications for immunological testing for infectious diseases* (Approved Guideline I/LA18-A2), Wayne, Pa, 2001, CLSI.

Clinical and Laboratory Standards Institute (CLSI): *Continuous quality improvements: integrating five key quality system components* (Approved Guideline GP22-A2), Wayne, Pa, 2004, CLSI.

Clinical and Laboratory Standards Institute (CSLI): *Quality control for commercially prepared microbiological culture media* (Approved Standard M22-A3), CLSI, Wayne, Pa, 2004, CLSI.

Clinical and Laboratory Standards Institute (CLSI): *Training and competence assessment* (Approved guidelines GP21-A2), Wayne, Pa, 2004, CLSI.

Gullen WH, Bearman JE: Put laboratory tests to the test! *Patient Care* Feb 15, 74-93, 1980.

Healthcare Financing Administration: Medicare, Medicaid, and CLIA programs: regulations implementing the Clinical Laboratory Improvement Amendments of 1988 (CLIA), *Fed Regist* 57:7002, 1992.

Ilstrup DM: Statistical methods in microbiology, *Clin Microbiol Rev* 3:219, 1990.

Jenkins SG: Evaluation of new technology in the clinical microbiology laboratory, *Diagn Microbiol Infect Dis* 23:53, 1995.

McCurdy B, editor: *Verification and validation of procedures in the clinical microbiology laboratory*, Cumitech 31, Washington, DC, 1997, American Society for Microbiology.

Radetsky M, Todd JK: Criteria for the evaluation of new diagnostic tests, *Pediat Infect Dis* 3:461, 1984.

Vecchio TJ: Predictive value of a single diagnostic test in unselected populations, *N Engl J Med* 274:1171, 1966.

Wiegert HT, Wiegert O: The impact of disease prevalence on the predictive value of laboratory tests in primary care, *J Fam Pract* 8:1199, 1979.

Points to Remember

- Analytical sensitivity is the detection limit of a test, usually defined at the 0.95 confidence level (±2 SD).
- Analytical specificity of a test is its ability to not react with substances other than the analyte of interest.
- Clinical or diagnostic sensitivity is the proportion of positive test results in patients with disease (true-positive results).
- Clinical or diagnostic specificity is the proportion of negative test results in patients without the disease (true-negative results).
- Incidence is the number of new cases of a disease over a period; prevalence is the frequency of a disease at a designated single point in time.
- Predictive values are influenced by the prevalence of the disease or analyte unless the test is 100% sensitive (for negative predictive value) or specific (for positive predictive value).
- Laboratory tests must be consistently validated to ensure the constant correct performance of tests.

Learning Assessment Questions

1. Which of the following refers to the ability of a test to detect a particular analyte?
   a. Analytical specificity
   b. Analytical sensitivity
   c. Efficiency of tests
   d. Test validation

2. The sensitivity of a test influences which of the following factors?
   a. Positive predictive value (PPV)
   b. Negative predictive value (NPV)
   c. Efficiency of the test
   d. Method validation

3. Using the formula provided in the chapter, determine the PPV for the chlamydia test in a population where the prevalence of the disease is 15%. The sensitivity and specificity of the test are 95% and 98%, respectively.

4. If 100 individuals without syphilis were tested for the disease and 95 tested negative, what is the diagnostic specificity of the test?

5. What parameter would be used to determine the percentage of patients who are appropriately classified as having the disease or not having the disease?

Specimen Collection and Processing

Lauren Roberts

■ **BASIC PRINCIPLES OF SPECIMEN COLLECTION**
Fundamentals
Collection Procedures
Patient-Collected Specimens
Labeling and Requisitions
Safety

■ **PRESERVATION, STORAGE, AND TRANSPORT OF SPECIMENS**
Specimen Storage
Preservatives
Anticoagulants
Holding or Transport Media
Shipping Infectious Substances

■ **SPECIMEN RECEIPT AND PROCESSING**
Specimen Priority
Unacceptable Specimens and Specimen Rejection
Macroscopic Observation
Microscopic Observation
Primary Inoculation
Specimen Preparation
Isolation Techniques
Incubation

■ **CULTURE WORKUP**
Nonroutine Specimens

■ **COMMUNICATION OF LABORATORY FINDINGS**

OBJECTIVES

After reading and studying this chapter, you should be able to:

1. Identify the role of specimen management in the preanalytical laboratory process.

2. Describe the fundamentals of specimen collection.

3. State the goal of specimen preservation, storage, and transport to the laboratory.

4. Identify the need for preservatives and anticoagulants and describe the appropriate conditions for storage of specific specimen examples.

5. Explain the prioritization guidelines used during processing to prevent degradation of the specimen.

6. Identify situations in which specimens are unacceptable and describe the action to be taken.

7. List the characteristics that can be noted from a macroscopic observation of the specimen.

8. Describe the purposes of a direct microscopic examination and identify specimen sources in which this technique is not performed.

9. Distinguish between the categories of media used in clinical microbiology and explain how media is selected.

10. Explain the different forms of isolation techniques used in the inoculation of solid media.

11. Identify the appropriate temperature and atmospheric conditions for incubation of routine specimens and to recover fastidious bacteria.

12. Describe the steps involved in the culture workup and interpretation.

13. List examples of nonroutine specimens and describe the thought process used to determine methods for processing.

14. Describe the significance of the communication of microbiology findings and the role of the laboratory in the postanalytical process.

Case in Point

Specimens were delivered to the microbiology laboratory from a physician's office. In the specimen receipt area, it was noted that one of the specimens was a cervical sample that was submitted on a JEMBEC (agar plates for transporting cultures of gonococci) plate. The microbiology technologist began to streak through the area of inoculation on the plate and noted that the medium appeared dry. Further evaluation revealed that the medium was expired.

Issues to Consider

After reading the patient's case history, consider the following:
- The role of the laboratory in assessing the acceptability of specimens received
- The consequences of processing inadequate specimens
- The steps that must be taken in rejection of specimens

Key Terms

Aerobe	Expectorated sputum
Anaerobe	Homogenization
Anaerobic transport system	Induced sputum
Broth media	Isolation streak
Capnophile	JEMBEC system
Cary-Blair transport media	Macroscopic observation
Clean-catch midstream urine specimen	Microaerophile
	Nonselective media
Differential media	Quantitative isolation
Direct microscopic examination	Selective media
	Sodium polyanethol sulfonate (SPS)
Enriched media	
Enrichment broth	Suboptimal specimen
Etiologic agent	Transport media

A major goal of the microbiology laboratory is to aid in the diagnosis of infectious diseases. Appropriate specimen selection, collection, and transportation are critical if laboratory results are used to provide information that establishes a diagnosis and successful treatment. The microbiology technologist does not usually perform this preanalytical portion of the laboratory testing process, and yet it directly affects the outcome. The data generated by the laboratory are influenced by the quality of the specimen and its condition when received. A poor specimen may result in failure to detect the infectious agent responsible for the patient's condition. Furthermore, it may result in the administration of inappropriate therapy if treatment is given for a contaminant organism. Thus it is the responsibility of the laboratory practitioner to ensure that appropriate specimen management is performed. The laboratory should establish policies for specimen management, and these policies must be distributed to all users and clients of microbiology laboratory services. A well-written handbook should be available at every patient care unit and should specify the policies for specimen collection and transport as well as test ordering. Training and education, such as in-service classes taught by the microbiology technologist, should be provided to the individuals collecting the specimens. The microbiology technologist must recognize and reject suboptimal specimens and educate other members of the medical team. Open communication between the microbiology technologist and other members of the medical support team is a necessity for quality patient care. This chapter introduces you to the concepts of specimen collection and processing. The steps to ensuring specimen quality are discussed along with the procedures to follow when suboptimal specimens are received. This chapter addresses the steps that follow specimen receipt and are involved in completing the processing for microbiology workup.

BASIC PRINCIPLES OF SPECIMEN COLLECTION

The laboratory can make accurate and useful determinations only if a specimen has been collected properly. The specimens to be analyzed are likely to contain living organisms; the goal of the specimen collector must be to maintain the viability of these organisms with minimal contamination.

Fundamentals

The following basic principles of specimen collection are fundamental to ensuring appropriate specimen management:
- If possible, collect the specimen in the acute phase of the infection and before antibiotics are administered.
- Select the correct anatomic site for collection of the specimen.
- Collect the specimen using the proper technique and supplies with minimal contamination from normal biota (normal flora).
- Collect the appropriate quantity of specimen.
- Package the specimen in a container designed to maintain the viability of the organisms and avoid hazards that result from leakage.
- Label the specimen accurately with the specific anatomic site and the patient information.
- Transport the specimen to the laboratory promptly or make provisions to store the specimen in an environment that will not degrade the suspected organism(s).

Collection Procedures

Specimens for microbiology cultures should be collected in sterile containers, except for stool specimens, which can be collected in clean, leakproof containers. In general, swabs are not recommended for collection because they do not provide sufficient quantity, are easily contaminated, and can become dried out, leading to a loss of organisms. Swabs are appropriate for specimens from the upper respiratory tract, external ear, eye, and genital tract. The tips of swabs may contain cotton, Dacron, or calcium alginate. Cotton-tipped swabs tend to have excessive fatty acids, which may be toxic to certain bacteria. Dacron or polyester swabs have a wide range of uses. Swab collection systems are available that provide **transport media** and protect the specimen from drying.

Lesions, wounds, and abscesses present many problems to the microbiology laboratory. The term *wound* is not an appropriate specimen label, and the exact anatomic site must be provided. The specimen is collected from the advancing margin of the lesion and should be collected by needle aspiration rather than by swab. Before the specimen is collected, the area should be cleansed to eliminate as much of the commensal flora as possible. Aspirated material should be placed into a sterile tube or transport vial and not "squirted" onto a swab. Table 6-1 lists specimen collection procedures.

TABLE 6-1 Specimen Collection Guidelines

Specimen	Patient Preparation	Container/Minimum Quantity
Blood culture	Disinfect skin with alcohol and iodine	Blood culture media set (aerobic and anaerobic bottles) or Vacutainer tube with SPS/adults 20 mL per set; children 5 to 10 mL per set
Body fluids (abdominal, amniotic, ascites, bile, joint, pericardial, pleural)	Disinfect skin before needle aspiration	Sterile, screw-cap tube or anaerobic transport system/≥1 mL
Catheter tips, IV (Foley catheters not cultured)	Disinfect skin before removal	Sterile, screw-cap container
Cerebrospinal fluid	Disinfect skin before aspiration	Sterile, screw-cap tube/bacteria ≥1 mL, fungi ≥2 mL, AFB ≥2 mL, virus ≥1 mL
Ear		
Inner	Clean ear canal with mild soap, aspirate fluid with needle if eardrum intact; use swab if eardrum ruptured	Sterile, screw-cap tube or anaerobic transport system
Outer	Remove debris or crust from ear canal with saline-moistened swab; rotate swab in outer canal	Swab transport system
Eye		
Conjunctiva	Sample both eyes; use separate swabs moistened with sterile saline	Swab transport system
Corneal scrapings	Instill local anesthetic, scrape with sterile spatula and inoculate directly to agar	Agar available at bedside
Feces	Collect directly into container, avoid contamination with urine	Clean, leakproof container or enteric transport system
Fungal scrapings	Wipe nails or skin with alcohol	Clean, screw-cap container
Hair/nails/skin	*Hair:* 10-12 hairs with shaft intact *Nails:* Clip affected area *Skin:* Scrape skin at outer edge of lesion	
Genitalia		
Cervix/vagina	Remove mucus before collection; do not use lubricant on speculum; swab endocervical canal or vaginal mucosa	Swab transport system or JEMBEC transport system
Urethra	Flexible swab inserted 2-4 cm into urethra for 2-3 sec or collect discharge	Swab transport system or JEMBEC transport system
Lesion/wound/abscess	Wipe area with sterile saline or alcohol	
Superficial	Swab along outer edge	Swab transport system
Deep	Aspirate with needle and syringe	Anaerobic transport system
Respiratory tract: lower bronchial specimens		
Sputum	Rinse mouth or gargle with water, instruct to cough deeply into container	Sterile, screw-cap container
Respiratory tract: upper		
Nasal	Insert premoistened swab with sterile saline 1 inch into nares	Swab transport system
Nasopharynx	Insert flexible swab through nose into posterior nasopharynx, rotate for 5 sec	Swab transport system or direct inoculation to media
Throat	Swab posterior pharynx, tonsils, and inflamed areas	Swab transport system
Tissue	Disinfect skin; do not allow tissue to dry out; if necessary, moisten with sterile saline	Anaerobic transport system or sterile screw-cap container
Urine		
Clean-catch midstream	Clean external genitalia; begin voiding and after several mL have passed; collect midstream without stopping flow of urine	Sterile, screw-cap container or urine transport kit 2-3 mL
Catheter	Clean urethral area, insert catheter, and allow first 15 mL to pass; then collect remainder	Sterile, screw-cap container or urine transport kit
Indwelling catheter	Disinfect catheter collection port, aspirate 5-10 mL with needle and syringe	Sterile, screw-cap container or urine transport kit
Suprapubic aspirate	Disinfect skin, aspirate with needle and syringe through abdominal wall into full bladder	Sterile, screw-cap container or anaerobic transport system

AFB, Acid-fast bacilli; *IV,* intravenous; *JEMBEC,* agar plates for transporting cultures of gonococci; *SPS,* sodium polyanethol sulfonate.

Patient-Collected Specimens

Certain specimens are collected by the patients themselves. Ideally, this should be done with assistance from medical personnel following thorough instructions. It should never be assumed that the patient knows how to collect a particular type of specimen. Attaching printed instructions in multiple languages to a collection device does not ensure that patients will read them or understand them. The most effective method is to provide verbal and written instructions. It may be necessary to read the instructions to the patient. The instructions should be written using simple language and pictures to help the patient understand the procedure as it is verbally explained. The specimens commonly obtained by the patient are urine, sputum, and stool.

Urine

Instructions for urine collection must include an explanation of the **clean-catch midstream urine specimen.** A first morning specimen is preferred because it provides a more concentrated sample. The patient collects this specimen following cleansing of the external genitalia to reduce the presence of indigenous flora. Patients are asked to void without collecting the first portion of the urine flow and instead to collect the middle portion. The first portion of the urine flow washes contaminants from the urethra, and the midstream portion is more representative of that in the bladder. Personnel who collect catheterized specimens should also use this technique to eliminate organisms carried up the urethra during catheterization.

Sputum

Sputum specimens are often collected for the diagnosis of bacterial pneumonia. Lower respiratory tract specimens are among the most difficult specimens to collect adequately because they are contaminated with oropharyngeal flora. For this reason, they are one of the least clinically relevant specimens received for culture. Other specimens, such as blood or a bronchoalveolar lavage, may be more accurate in detecting the **etiologic agent** (i.e., the microorganism causing the disease).

Collection of a quality sputum sample requires thorough patient education and medical personnel oversight of the process. The first early morning specimen is preferred. The patient needs to understand the difference between sputum and spit. The patient should rinse the mouth with water and expectorate with the aid of a deep cough directly into a sterile container **(expectorated sputum).** Patients with dentures should remove the dentures first. A single specimen should be adequate for detection of bacterial lower respiratory tract infection. If fungal or mycobacterial infections are possible, three separate early morning specimens (collected on successive days) are appropriate.

Respiratory therapy technicians may assist patients who are unable to expectorate a respiratory specimen. These specimens may be collected through aerosol-induction in which the patient breathes aerosolized droplets of a solution that stimulates cough reflex **(induced sputum).** When sputum specimens are submitted to microbiology, the laboratory should be informed of whether the specimen is expectorated or induced.

Stool

The specimen of choice for the detection of gastrointestinal pathogens is stool. A rectal swab can be submitted for bacterial culture but it must show feces. A single specimen is not usually sufficient to exclude bacteria or parasites. If a bacterial infection is suspected, three specimens should be collected, one a day for 3 days. If parasites are suspected, three specimens collected within 10 days should be sufficient for microscopic detection of ova and parasites. Some laboratories offer an initial parasite screening for *Giardia lamblia* and *Cryptosporidium* spp. The newer methods detect parasite antigens, and one sample is usually sufficient. If the screen is negative, the physician can then decide whether to perform complete parasite studies.

Patients should be instructed to excrete directly into the collection device. Specimens should never be taken from the toilet and should not be contaminated with urine. Commercial systems are available with preservatives for bacteria and parasites. The appropriate ratio of stool to preservative is 1:3, and the patient must understand that if this ratio is not met, the test will be invalid. In addition, the patient needs to be told that the specimen must be thoroughly mixed with the preservative. Specimens for parasite microscopic studies should be performed before any barium studies are done. If this is not feasible, the patient must delay specimen collection until the barium is cleared (4 to 5 days). Barium will appear as a white chalky substance in the specimen and mask the appearance of parasites under the microscope.

Labeling and Requisitions

It is important that correct patient identification be put on the specimen and the requisition. The specimen label must contain sufficient information in order for the specimen and requisition to be matched up when received in the laboratory. The laboratory loses valuable time when specimens are unlabeled or mislabeled. Resolution requires making phone calls and filling out additional paperwork, and it ultimately delays processing the specimen or requires that a new specimen be collected. This ultimately may delay the diagnosis.

Proper identification of each specimen includes a label firmly attached to the container with the following information:

- Name
- Identification number
- Room number
- Physician
- Culture site
- Date of collection
- Time of collection

To perform quality laboratory analysis, the laboratory needs specific information regarding the patient and the specimen. All that the laboratory knows about the patient is learned from the requisition form. The less information that is provided, the more difficult it is for the laboratory to provide good patient care. Incomplete information on the requisition is often a weak link in the specimen management process. The requisition form should provide the following information:

- Patient's name
- Patient's age (or date of birth) and gender
- Patient's room number or location
- Physician's name and address
- Specific anatomic site
- Date and time of specimen collection
- Clinical diagnosis or relevant patient history
- Antimicrobial agents (if the patient is receiving)
- Name of individual transcribing orders

Complete and thorough requisitions can often lead the microbiology technologist to suspect certain pathogens based on the diagnosis or patient history. This will allow use of specific media or making certain adjustments to the incubation to maximize recovery of the pathogen.

Computer-based ordering is performed at many institutions. Ideally, the microbiology technologist should design the test-ordering process. This will enable the laboratory to elicit the necessary information. These systems should be designed to provide key fields that must be completed to submit the request transaction.

It is important for the microbiology technologist to recognize that the individual ordering the test does not have a complete knowledge of what are and are not appropriate tests for each specimen. If the test requested is not recommended, it is the responsibility of the laboratory to communicate with the physician to determine exactly what needs to be done.

Safety

It is imperative that specimens collected for microbiology not pose a safety hazard to those who handle them. Leaking containers and specimens with needles attached present the greatest hazards. All specimens must be transported in leak-proof secondary containers. Because the specimen should be kept separate from any paperwork, plastic bags with permanent seals and separate pouches on the outside for requisitions are recommended.

Transporting personnel should refuse to transport specimens without the protection of a secondary container. Refusing to accept syringes with needles attached is also appropriate. A needle must be replaced with a tight-fitting rubber stopper or a stopcock to put resistance on the plunger. The aspirated material could also be transferred to another sterile container with a tight lid or to an **anaerobic transport system.**

Laboratory personnel must also adhere to strict safety guidelines as they begin to work with the patient's specimen. All individuals handling patient specimens must wear protective clothing, and specimens should be opened only in a biologic safety cabinet.

PRESERVATION, STORAGE, AND TRANSPORT OF SPECIMENS

Specimen transport is another essential component of the preanalytical process of microbiology testing. Whether the specimen comes from within the hospital or clinic or from an outpatient facility or doctor's office across town, the goal is the same. The primary goal in the transportation of speci-

mens to the laboratory is to maintain the specimen as near to its original state as possible with minimal deterioration and to prevent risk to the specimen handler. If specimen deterioration results in death to the infectious agent present or increased growth, the specimen is no longer representative of the disease process.

Specimens should be transported to the laboratory ideally within 30 minutes of collection, preferably within 2 hours. Adverse environmental changes in oxygen, pH, and temperature can prevent the recovery of certain microorganisms and allow overgrowth of others.

If transport to the laboratory is delayed, or if the specimen will not be processed as it is received in the laboratory, the specimen can be maintained by storage under certain conditions or with the use of preservatives, anticoagulants, transport or holding medium, and even culture medium.

Specimen Storage

Some specimens that will not be transported or processed immediately can be maintained by being stored under certain conditions. The individual responsible for storing the specimen needs to be informed as to the best storage environment for each specimen type. Some specimens, such as urine, stool, sputum, swabs (not for anaerobes), foreign devices such as catheters, and viral specimens can be maintained at refrigerator temperature (4° C) for 24 hours. Pathogens that are cold sensitive may be found in other specimens, and those specimens should be kept at room temperature if culture is to be performed. This includes samples that might contain anaerobic bacteria as well as most other sterile body fluids, genital specimens, and ear and eye swabs. If cerebrospinal fluid is not processed immediately, it can be stored in a 35° C incubator for 6 hours. Table 6-2 lists specimen storage guidelines.

Preservatives

Two specimen types in which preservatives can be used are urine and stool. Boric acid is used in commercial products to maintain accurate urine colony counts. The systems are designed to maintain the bacterial population in the urine at

TABLE 6-2 Specimen Storage Guidelines

Refrigerate	Room Temperature
Catheter tips (IV)	Abscess, lesion, wound
CSF for viruses	Body fluids
Ear: outer	CSF for bacteria
Feces (unpreserved)	Ear: inner
Feces for *Clostridium difficile* toxin (up to 3 days; >3 days store at −70° C)	Feces (preserved)
Sputum	Genital
Urine (unpreserved)	Nasal, N/P, throat
	Tissue
	Urine (preserved)

CSF, Cerebrospinal fluid; *IV,* intravenous; *N/P,* nasopharynx.

room temperature for 24 hours and thus are useful for collection of urine specimens at distant locations. Stool specimens for bacterial culture that are not transported immediately to the laboratory can be refrigerated, but if the delay is longer than 2 hours, the specimen can be added to **Cary-Blair transport media.** Stools for *Clostridium difficile* toxin assay should be collected without a preservative and can be refrigerated; if the delay will be longer than 48 hours, the specimen should be frozen at −70° C. Preservatives for ova and parasite (O & P) examinations maintain the morphology of trophozoites and cysts. Laboratories often use a two-vial system in which one vial contains formalin for concentration and the other vial contains a fixative for preparing stained slides, such as modified polyvinyl alcohol (PVA) with zinc.

Anticoagulants

Anticoagulants are used to prevent clotting of specimens, including blood, bone marrow, and synovial fluid. This is necessary because organisms bound up in clotted material are difficult to isolate. The type of anticoagulant used and the concentration are important because some anticoagulants have antimicrobial properties. **Sodium polyanethol sulfonate (SPS)** is the most common anticoagulant used for microbiology specimens. The concentration of SPS must not exceed 0.025% (wt/vol) because some *Neisseria* spp. and certain anaerobes are inhibited by higher concentrations. The ratio of specimen to SPS is important; therefore different sizes of tubes must be available to accommodate adult and pediatric blood specimens and bone marrow or synovial fluid. Heparin is another acceptable anticoagulant and is often used for viral cultures and for isolation of *Mycobacterium* spp. from blood. Citrate and ethylenediamine tetracacetic acid (EDTA) should not be used for microbiology specimens.

Holding or Transport Media

Another way to maintain the integrity of the specimen from the time of specimen collection until laboratory processing of the sample is with the use of holding or transport media. These usually contain substances that do not promote multiplication of microorganisms but ensure their preservation and are available in swab collection systems. Stuart's or Amie's transport medium are commonly used. Some transport systems contain charcoal to absorb fatty acids given off by the swab that can be detrimental to the survival of *Neisseria gonorrhoeae* and *Bordetella pertussis.*

In certain situations, direct inoculation to culture media at the time of specimen collection (bedside inoculation) is optimal for isolation of the pathogen. Blood is usually placed into a broth culture medium immediately after collection. Synovial and peritoneal fluids also can be inoculated into blood culture broth bottles at the bedside. Additional specimen also should be sent to the laboratory in a container besides the blood culture bottles for Gram stain preparation. Specimens for *N. gonorrhoeae* can be placed directly onto a commercial transport system such as the **JEMBEC system.** This system contains selective agar and a CO_2-generating tablet. Nasopharyngeal swabs for the isolation of *B. pertussis* also can be inoculated directly onto selective agar as they are collected. Specimens collected from the eye, especially cornea

scrapings, also are inoculated directly to appropriate media as they are collected.

It is important to recognize that specimens collected at the bedside are more susceptible to contamination. Anytime culture media is taken outside of the laboratory, there is a possibility that it can become contaminated. The individual collecting the specimen needs to be informed as to the appropriate way to manipulate the media. In some situations the microbiology technologist is asked to assist in the collection and can monitor the appropriate application of the specimen to the culture media. In other situations media are maintained at the outpatient facility and the culture is sent to the laboratory already inoculated with the specimen. It is the responsibility of the microbiology laboratory to ensure that the culture media is of good quality when it is received to isolate the pathogens involved in the infection.

Shipping Infectious Substances

The shipment of clinical specimens and cultures of microorganisms is governed by a complex set of national and international guidelines issued by the U.S. Department of Transportation (DOT) and the U.S. Postal Service. International air shipment is regulated by the International Civil Aviation Organization (ICAO). The U.S. Congress requires the Secretary of Transportation to prescribe regulations for the safe transportation of hazardous material in commerce to ensure public safety and minimize risks in transportation. The regulations specify the way potentially infectious substances must be packaged to prevent leaks or spills and how packages must be labeled to caution handlers and other parties about their hazardous content. The goal is to safeguard employees in the transportation industry and the general public. The duty of the laboratory is to use the appropriate packaging for each material being shipped and to label the package properly. Laboratories can purchase packaging materials specifically designed for transporting laboratory specimens.

Infectious substances are considered a hazardous material and must meet the requirements of the DOT's Hazardous Material Regulations as published in the Federal Register Title 49 Code of Federal Regulations (CFR) Parts 171-180 before being transported by rail, water, air, or highway (http://www.phmsa.dot.gov/hazmat). The DOT defines an *infectious substance* as a material known to contain or suspected of containing a pathogen that causes disease in humans or animals. An infectious substance is assigned to a risk group with a number from 1 (low risk) to 4 (high risk). Risk group assignment represents the ability of the microorganism to cause injury through disease to an individual and community based on its severity, mode and ease of transmission, and reversibility through available agents and treatment. Patient specimens or culture isolates must be triple packaged before being shipped. The material is placed into a primary receptacle that must be watertight. Absorbent material is placed around the primary receptacle, and it is then placed into a secondary container that is also watertight. The secondary package is sealed and placed into a sturdy outer container constructed of fiberboard. Specific instructions must be followed for labeling the container as "Hazardous Material." Specimens that are shipped by air require specific labeling and

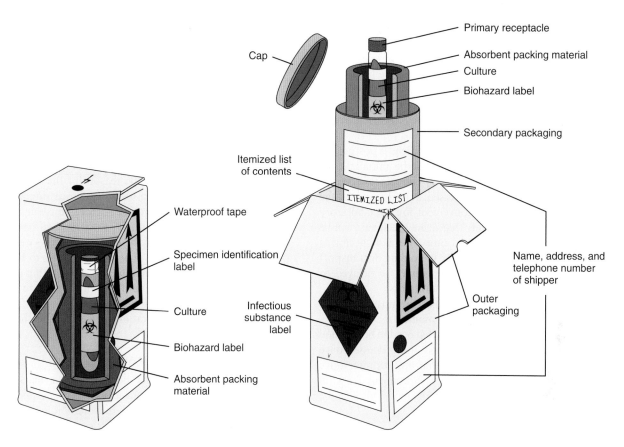

FIGURE 6-1 Packaging infectious substances for shipping. (Modified from Garcia LS: *Clinical laboratory management*, Washington, DC, 2004, ASM Press.)

shipping documents. Figure 6-1 demonstrates the packaging of infectious materials for shipping.

Every employee who packages specimens and infectious materials for shipment must be appropriately trained. Training must include the DOT and International Air Transportation Association (IATA) regulations; retraining should occur every 2 years if shipping by air or every 3 years if only shipping by ground unless there are significant changes in the regulations.

SPECIMEN RECEIPT AND PROCESSING

Specimen Priority

Specimens require prompt processing after arrival in the laboratory. Processing every specimen as soon as it is received is often impossible. Laboratory staffing and specimen load may have a significant impact on timely processing. Appropriate specimen management should include guidelines for prioritizing the handling of specimens. A four-level scheme of prioritization may be used based on the critical nature of the specimen or potential for specimen degradation. Table 6-3 lists clinical samples and the ways each can be prioritized in a four-level system.

Level 1 specimens are classified as critical because they represent a potentially life-threatening illness and are from an

TABLE 6-3   Levels of Specimen Prioritization

Level	Description	Specimens
1	Critical/invasive	Amniotic fluid Blood Brain Cerebrospinal fluid Heart valves Pericardial fluid
2	Unpreserved	Body fluids (not listed for level 1) Bone Drainage from wounds Feces Sputum Tissue
3	Quantitation required	Catheter tip Urine Tissue for quantitation
4	Preserved	Feces in preservative Urine in preservative Swabs in holding medium (aerobic and anaerobic)

invasive source. They require immediate processing. Level 2 specimens are unprotected and may quickly degrade or have overgrowth of contaminating flora. The microbiology technologist must quickly provide an optimal growth environment for the fastidious organisms that may be found in these specimens. Level 3 specimens require quantitation. Delay in processing level 3 specimens may adversely affect the accuracy of quantitation.

If processing of level 2 and level 3 specimens is postponed, appropriate storage or preservation must be initiated. For example, urine and sputum specimens can be refrigerated until a spinal fluid specimen is processed. A refrigerator at the site of specimen processing is convenient for the laboratory worker and makes it more likely that urine specimens will be refrigerated during peak workload times. Level 4 specimens are those that arrive in the laboratory in holding or transport media. Processing of level 4 specimens may be delayed to process specimens of a more critical nature first.

In general, batch processing is not used for most specimens in microbiology; however, in a few situations, it is appropriate. Specimens for acid-fast bacillus (AFB) that need to be digested and decontaminated can be refrigerated and processed once per day. Stool specimens for O & P that are in preservative also can be processed in batch format. Specimens for viral culture that are collected in viral transport media also can be batched.

Unacceptable Specimens and Specimen Rejection

The analytical phase of the laboratory testing process begins as the specimen is received in the laboratory. Upon receipt in the laboratory, the specimen needs to be examined to ensure that it has been properly selected, collected, and transported. Performing tests on specimens that are of poor quality will yield misleading information that might result in misdiagnosis and inappropriate therapy. The microbiology laboratory must establish and publish the criteria for specimen rejection. The following situations are examples of **suboptimal specimens** that must be rejected:

- The information on the requisition does not match the information on the specimen label. If the patient name or source does not match, the specimen should be collected again.
- The specimen is not submitted in the appropriate transport container or the container is leaking.
- The quantity of the specimen is not adequate to perform all tests requested.
- The specimen transport time is more than 2 hours and the specimen has not been preserved.
- The specimen is received in a fixative such as formalin. Stools for ova and parasites are exceptions.
- An anaerobic culture is requested on a specimen in which anaerobes are indigenous.
- Microbiology processing of a particular specimen results in questionable data (Foley catheter tip).
- Specimen is dried up.
- More than one specimen from the same source was submitted from the same patient on the same day, except for blood cultures.

- One swab was submitted with multiple requests for various organisms.
- Expectorated sputum in which the Gram stain reveals fewer than 25 white blood cells (WBCs) and more than 10 epithelial cells per low-power field (LPF) and mixed bacterial flora.

All rejected specimens require a phone call to the person in charge of collecting the specimen. The laboratory should never discard an unacceptable specimen before contacting a member of the health care team. The laboratory must document the situation indicating the reason for the rejection of the specimen. If the physician insists on processing an inadequate specimen, the laboratory report must include a comment explaining the potentially compromised results.

In certain situations it may be necessary to process a suboptimal specimen. Specimens that are impossible to recollect or that would require the patient to undergo another invasive procedure (bone marrow, spinal fluid, or surgery) may need to be processed regardless of the situation. Again, the final report needs to include a notation indicating that the specimen was compromised.

Macroscopic Observation

Processing patient specimens begins with a **macroscopic observation.** The gross appearance of the specimen may provide useful information to both the microbiologist and the physician. The physical characteristics of the specimen should be documented so that if different technologists work on the sample, they all will know the results of the gross examination.

Notations from the macroscopic observation should include the following:

- Swab or aspirate
- Stool consistency (formed or liquid)
- Blood or mucus present
- Volume of specimen
- Fluid: clear or cloudy

The gross examination also allows the processor to determine the adequacy of the specimen and the need for special processing. Areas of blood and mucus are selected for culture and direct microscopic examination. Anaerobic cultures may be indicated if gas, foul smell, or sulfur granules are present. The diagnosis is evident if adult helminths or tapeworm proglottids are present in the specimen.

Microscopic Observation

A **direct microscopic examination** is a useful tool that provides rapid information. In critical situations, such as meningitis, the direct microscopic examination can be used to guide therapy choices when therapy must be initiated before culture results are available. This useful tool serves several purposes: (1) It can be used to determine the quality of the specimen. Sputum specimens that represent saliva rather than lower respiratory secretions can be determined by the quantitation of WBCs or epithelial cells. (2) It can give the microbiology technologist and the physician an indication of the infectious process involved. Gram stain of a sputum specimen revealing WBCs and gram-positive diplococci is indicative of *Streptococcus pneumoniae*. (3) The routine culture workup can be guided by the results of the smear. The technologist can correlate the bacterial isolates with the types detected in the smear. This may alert the technologist to the presence of additional organisms not yet growing, such as anaerobes. (4) It can dictate the need for nonroutine or additional testing. The presence of fungal elements in a specimen for bacterial culture will alert the technologist to notify the physician to request a fungus culture. Specimens may be received in many forms. Preparation of the direct smear depends on the type of material received. Techniques vary according to whether the specimen is a tissue, swab, or fluid. See Chapter 7 for a detailed explanation of the preparation and staining of smears.

In certain specimen types, the direct microscopic examination does not provide useful information and therefore is not appropriate. This includes throat and nasopharyngeal specimens. Gram stains for *N. gonorrhoeae* on specimens from the vagina, cervix, and anal crypts are not recommended because these sites contain other bacteria that can have the same morphology, although Gram stain direct smears are recommended to diagnose bacterial vaginosis. Gram stains on stool specimens are not usually routine, although they can be useful to determine whether the patient has an inflammatory diarrhea based on the presence of white blood cells.

Although a direct Gram stain on a urine specimen provides useful information, many laboratories do not perform them routinely because they are time-consuming and preliminary culture results are available within 24 hours. Physicians can always request that a direct Gram stain be performed.

Primary Inoculation
Types of Culture Media

Culture media may be divided into categories defined by the ability to support bacterial growth. **Nonselective media** support the growth of most nonfastidious microbes. Sheep blood agar is the standard nonselective medium used in the United States. **Selective media** support the growth of one type or group of microbes but not another. A selective medium may contain inhibitory substances such as antimicrobials, dyes, or alcohol. MacConkey agar is selective for enteric gram-negative bacilli, and CNA (Columbia agar with colistin and nalidixic acid) is selective for gram-positive organisms. **Differential media** allow grouping of microbes based on different characteristics demonstrated on the medium. Media may be differential and nonselective (e.g., sheep blood agar is nonselective but differentiates organisms on the basis of hemolysis). Media can be differential and selective (e.g., MacConkey agar inhibits gram-positives and differentiates gram-negative bacilli on the basis of lactose fermentation).

Enriched media contain growth enhancers that are added to nonselective agar to allow fastidious organisms to flourish. Chocolate agar is an enriched medium. **Enrichment broth** is a liquid medium designed to encourage the growth of small numbers of a particular organism while suppressing other flora present. Enrichment broths are incubated for a certain period and then must be subcultured to isolate the particular

organism. Lim broth is used to enhance the growth of group B streptococci. **Broth media** can be used as a supplement to agar plates to detect small numbers of most aerobes, anaerobes, and microaerophiles. Thioglycollate broth (THIO) is an example of a supplemental broth media.

Culture Media Selection

The selection of media to inoculate is based on the type of specimen submitted for culture and the organisms likely to be involved in the infectious process. Specimens in which fastidious pathogens are more likely involved require media with appropriate nutrients to aid in their recovery. Specimens that are collected from a site containing normal biota will require types of media to diminish the normal biota while allowing the pathogens to be detected.

Selection of primary culture media is somewhat standardized for the routine bacterial culture. Individual laboratories may prefer one medium to another, however, on the basis of past experience, patient population, or other special circumstances. A table of media to be inoculated for each specimen should be available in the specimen processing area. In some laboratories, the computer generates labels for media as the specimen is accessioned. Some specimens require a single plate, whereas others will require a battery of several plates. If several plates will be inoculated, the labeled media should be arranged in order, beginning with the most enriched medium and progressing to the most selective. The specimen can then be applied to each culture media and inhibitory substances will not be carried over from one agar to another.

The routine primary plating media include the following items:

- Nonselective agar plate
- Enriched medium for fastidious organisms for normally sterile body fluids or a site in which fastidious organisms are expected
- Selective and differential medium for enteric gram-negative bacilli for most routine bacterial cultures
- Selective medium for gram-positive organisms for specimens in which mixed gram-positive and gram-negative bacteria are found
- Additional selective media or enrichment broths for specific pathogens as needed
- Broth medium may be used as a supplement with specimens from sterile body fluids, tissues, lesions, wounds, and abscesses

Table 6-4 contains a selection of primary media for specific anatomic sites. Equivalent media may be substituted.

Specimen Preparation

Most specimens arrive in the laboratory in one of three forms: swab, tissue, or fluid. Specimens such as sterile body fluids, pus, urine, and sputum are inoculated directly onto selected media. Large volumes of sterile body fluids (peritoneal, pleural, continuous ambulatory peritoneal dialysis [CAPD]) are concentrated to increase the recovery of bacteria. Centrifugation or filtration are methods for concentration. If the volume of fluid is greater than 1 mL, the specimen can be centrifuged for 20 minutes at $3000 \times g$. The sediment is then used to inoculate media and to prepare smears. If the speci-

TABLE 6-4 Direct Gram Stain and Selection of Media for Bacterial Cultures

Specimen	Gram Stain	BAP	CHOC	MAC or EMB	ANA	THIO	TM	Other
Aqueous/vitreous	X	X	X	X		X		
Blood								Blood culture bottles
Body fluids								
Amniotic	X	X	X	X	X	X	X	Blood culture bottles if sufficient volume of fluid
Bile	X	X		X		X		
Bone marrow	X	X	X			X		
Pericardial	X	X	X	X	X	X		
Peritoneal	X	X	X	X		X	X	
Pleural	X	X	X			X		
Synovial	X	X	X			X		
Catheter tips		X						
CSF	X	X	X			X		Cytocentrifuge recommended for Gram stain
Ear								
Inner	X	X	X	X		X		
Outer	X	X	X	X				
Eye	X	X	X	X		X		
Gastrointestinal								
Duodenal aspirate	X	X	X	X				CNA
Feces		X		X				HE or XLD, CAMPY, SMAC
Gastric aspirate	X	X	X	X				
Genital								
IUD	X					X		
Vagina/cervix	X	X	X	X			X	
Urethra	X	X	X				X	
Genital screens								
Neisseria gonorrhoeae			X				X	
Group B beta strep		X						Lim broth* or carrot broth
Lesion/wound/abscess	X	X	X	X	X	X		CNA if Gram suggests mixed Gram positive and negative
Respiratory tract: lower								
Bronchial (brush, wash, lavage)	X	X	X	X				
Sputum	X	X	X	X				
Respiratory tract: upper								
Nasal/nasopharynx		X	X					
Sinus aspirate	X	X	X	X	X	X		
Throat		X						
Tissue	X	X	X	X	X	X		
Urine								
Catheter/void		X		X				
Suprapubic aspirate	X	X		X	X	X		

*Lim broth, selective Todd Hewitt broth with CNA.
BAP, Sheep blood agar; *CHOC,* chocolate agar; *MAC,* MacConkey agar; *EMB,* eosin-methylene blue agar; *ANA,* anaerobic culture media (anaerobic blood agar, *Bacteroides* bile esculin agar, kanamycin-vancomycin laked blood agar, anaerobic CNA or PEA, phenylethyl alcohol agar); *THIO,* thioglycollate broth; *TM,* Thayer-Martin or other *Neisseria*-selective agar; *CSF,* cerebrospinal fluid; *CNA,* Columbia Colistin-Nalidixic acid agar; *HE,* Hektoen-enteric agar; *XLD,* xylose-lysine-deoxycholate agar; *CAMPY, Campylobacter*-selective blood agar; *SMAC,* sorbitol-MacConkey agar;; *IUD,* intrauterine device.

men consistency is thin enough to avoid filter clogging, filtration with a Nalgene filter unit can be performed. Following filtration, the filter is removed and placed on the surface of an agar plate. Specimens received on swabs can be inoculated directly to culture media. The specimen should be submitted on two swabs; one is used for the culture media, and the other is used to make the direct smear. Some laboratories place the swab into 0.5 to 1.0 mL of broth or saline and then vortex the specimen to loosen material from the swab and produce an even suspension of organisms. A sterile pipette is then used to dispense the inoculum onto plates and broth. Tissues can be prepared for culture by **homogenization,** in which the tissue is ground in a tissue grinder. Because homogenization can destroy certain organisms, in some situations the tissue is minced with sterile scissors and forceps into small pieces suitable for culture.

Isolation Techniques

Specimens can be inoculated to agar plates by using a general-purpose **isolation streak** to yield a semiquantitative estimate of growth. The specimen is applied by rolling the swab or placing a drop of liquid specimen onto a small area at the edge of the plate. Broth media can be inoculated by placing a few drops of the liquid specimen into the tube of broth or placing the swab into the broth. The inoculating loop is sterilized and allowed to cool thoroughly before streaking the agar. The cooled loop is passed back and forth through the inoculum in the first quadrant several times. The first quadrant should be at least one quarter of the plate, and the streak lines should be close together. The plate is turned, and quadrant two is streaked by passing the loop through the edge of the first quadrant a few times and then streaking the rest of the area. The plate is turned again, and the loop is passed through the edge of quadrant two a few times and into the rest of the third quadrant, finally passing the loop over the final area of the agar streaks the fourth quadrant. It may be necessary to flame the loop or turn the loop over in between quadrants, depending on the number and type of bacteria present in the specimen. Laboratory personnel must adjust their technique as necessary. When more than one agar plate is used, the loop is flamed in between plates to prevent carryover of a possible contaminant from one plate to another. Figure 6-2 shows a diagram of this technique.

The general-purpose isolation streak is useful for most specimens. The relative number of organisms can be esti-mated based on the extent of growth beyond the original area of inoculum. Growth in the first quadrant can be graded as 1+, or light growth; growth in the second or third quadrant can be graded as 2+ to 3+, or moderate; and growth in the third or fourth quadrant can be considered 4+, or heavy growth. Some specimens require a quantitative technique to determine the number of bacteria present. Urine specimens are inoculated using a **quantitative isolation.** Plates are inoculated using a calibrated loop to deliver a specified volume. The urine is mixed well, and the calibrated loop (0.01 or 0.001 mL) is inserted into the urine and transferred to the culture media by making a single streak down the center of the plate. Without flaming, the loop is streaked back and forth through the original inoculum. Figure 6-3 provides a diagram of this technique.

Incubation

Once the medium is inoculated, incubation conditions must be considered. This includes both temperature and environmental atmosphere and is determined by the type of specimen and the pathogens that may be detected. The laboratory processing area should contain a chart or table stipulating where each medium should be placed for incubation. Most bacteria cultures are incubated at 35° to 37° C. **Aerobes** grow in ambient air, whereas **anaerobes** cannot grow in the presence of oxygen and require an anaerobic atmosphere. Laboratories can achieve an anaerobic environment through the use of jars, bags, or a chamber. Some bacteria are **capnophiles** and require an increased concentration of CO_2. This can be achieved by a candle jar, a CO_2 incubator, jar, or bag. **Microaerophiles** grow with reduced oxygen and increased CO_2 and can be isolated using jars or bags. The length of incubation varies for individual organisms. Most routine bacterial cultures are held for 48 to 72 hours. Cultures for anaerobes and broth cultures may be held for 5 to 7 days. Unusual organisms may require special medium or conditions beyond the routine. It is helpful

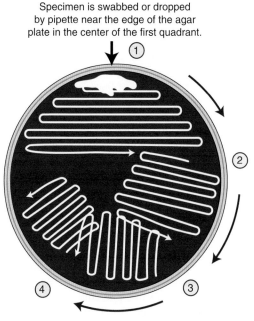

FIGURE 6-2 General-purpose isolation streak.

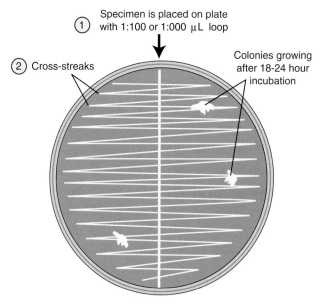

FIGURE 6-3 Quantitative isolation technique.

TABLE 6-5 Isolation of Unusual or Fastidious Bacteria

Organism	Specimens	Media	Comments
Bacillus anthracis	Blood Skin lesion Sputum	Blood agar	Incubate 35°-37° C, ambient air; hold plates at least 3 days
Bordetella pertussis	Nasopharyngeal swab	Regan-Lowe or Bordet-Gengou agar	Bedside inoculation. Incubate 35°-37° C, ambient air; hold plates 6-7 days; DFA used in conjunction with culture
Brucella spp.	Blood Bone marrow	Commercial blood culture systems	Class III pathogen, process all specimens in biohazard hood with protective equipment; incubate at 35°-37° C; most commercial systems detect growth in 7 days; conventional blood bottles should be held 30 days and subcultured at 7, 14, and 30 days
Corynebacterium diphtheriae	Throat Nasopharyngeal Skin	Blood agar Loeffler agar slant Tinsdale or cystine-tellurite blood agar	Incubate 35°-37° C, ambient air, toxigenicity testing necessary to confirm pathogenicity
Francisella tularensis	Eye Lymph node aspirate Skin ulcer Sputum Throat	Glucose cystine agar	Class III pathogen, highly infectious by aerosol or penetration of unbroken skin; recommended that specimens be sent to laboratory equipped to handle
Haemophilus ducreyi	Genital lesion Lymph node aspirate	Supplemented chocolate agar	Incubate 33°-35° C, 3%-5% CO_2 with high humidity; hold for 5 days
Helicobacter pylori	Gastric biopsy	Skirrow Chocolate agar Modified Thayer-Martin	Incubate 35°-57° C, microaerophilic atmosphere with humidity; hold for 5 days, direct smear with silver or Giemsa stain may be diagnostic
Legionella spp.	Blood Lung Pleural fluid Sputum	BCYE agar Selective BCYE	Incubate 35°-37° C, ambient air; hold for at least 7 days, DFA available
Nocardia spp.	Brain Sputum Subcutaneous aspirate Tissue	Blood agar BHI agar (brain heart infusion) SDA BCYE	Incubate 35°-37° C, 3%-5% CO_2; hold for 2-3 wk
Streptobacillus moniliformis	Blood Lymph node Joint fluid	Serum-supplemented medium	Inhibited by SPS, citrate used as anticoagulant; incubate 35°-37° C, 3%-5% CO_2; hold for at least 7 days
Vibrio spp.	Blood Feces Lesion Tissue	Blood agar MacConkey agar TCBS agar Alkaline peptone water (enrichment for feces)	Selective agar (TCBS) only needed for fecal specimens; incubate 35°-37° C, ambient air; hold for 3 days

DFA, Direct fluorescent antibody; *BCYE,* buffered charcoal yeast extract; *BHI,* brain–heart infusion; *SDA,* Sabouraud dextrose agar; *SPS,* sodium polyanethol sulfonate; *TCBS,* thiosulfate-citrate-bile salts-sucrose.

if the clinician indicates to the laboratory that an unusual organism is suspected. Table 6-5 lists unusual or fastidious organisms, recommended media, and incubation requirements.

CULTURE WORKUP

The next part of the microbiology analysis is reading and interpreting the cultures. The microbiology technologist examines the culture media and uses considerable skill and judgment in the interpretation. This interpretive judgment is the fundamental means of arriving at a result that is accurate and clinically relevant. The following questions are asked as each specimen is examined:

- What is the specimen source?
- Does this source have normal biota, or is it a sterile source?
- If normal biota is present, what bacteria are found and what do these colonies look like?
- What are the most likely pathogens in this specimen?
- What is the colonial morphology of these pathogens?
- Which media is demonstrating growth, and what is the purpose of the media?

This evaluation requires professional training to be able to recognize and distinguish the normal biota from the pathogens. The microbiology technologist must have knowledge of which organisms are pathogens in various body sites to perform a clinically relevant workup.

Identification and antimicrobial susceptibility testing (when indicated) are performed on clinically relevant isolates. A challenging issue confronting microbiology technologists is the extent of the identification required. The microbiology technologist can ultimately save the patient money by providing an accurate diagnosis in a timely fashion using a cost-effective strategy. Although definitive identification is the standard for quality patient care, microbiologists have incorporated limited identification procedures into their daily practice. These limited procedures will help keep the laboratory testing cost effective while providing optimal patient care. Each laboratory must establish the protocol for the identification of various organisms.

Nonroutine Specimens

Routine specimens have standardized processing procedures that are well established in the microbiology laboratory. However, the microbiology laboratory may be requested to process nonroutine specimens for which no processing procedures are established. In these situations, where standardized procedures do not exist, the laboratory must use a standardized thought process to ensure that these specimens can be cultured in an appropriate fashion. This process begins by considering the following issues:

- Is the specimen likely to contain low numbers or high numbers of organisms? If there are low numbers of organisms, the concentration of the specimen is advantageous. When few organisms are anticipated, large amounts of specimen yield better results.
- If the number of organisms is extremely low, is it important to enhance them?
- Some specimens are being checked for sterility, and the presence of even one organism is significant. Use of a broth is important when growth must be enhanced.
- Are the organisms to be found in a specific specimen likely to be fastidious or nonfastidious? The choice of medium, temperature(s), atmosphere, and length of incubation depends on whether the organisms are fastidious or nonfastidious.
- Is any normal biota associated with the specimen? The presence of normal biota might make special collection techniques important. It also dictates rapid or protected transportation and timely processing.
- Does the specimen contain any preservatives or growth inhibitors that must be counteracted? Sometimes the effects of a preservative can be eliminated or reduced by dilution or use of a specific medium.
- What is a reasonable amount to culture? Are all areas of the specimen homogeneous, or will the portion chosen for culture affect the results? A 12-cm piece of vein received for culture may contain plaque on only a relatively small portion. Sampling one spot may not be representative of the whole. Sampling and grinding small pieces from multiple sites may be necessary.
- Is the objective to select a single agent from a mixed culture? An enriched or selective medium is helpful for this type of isolation.
- Is there a need to culture both external and internal surfaces? The surface to be cultured becomes important

in devising beneficial methods of culturing catheters and other inanimate objects.

Nonroutine specimens may include vein grafts, multiple-lumen catheters, heart valves, implant soak solutions, perfusates, water samples, and equipment. A description of the processing of some of these follows.

- *Implant soak solutions:* A large volume of soak solution and concentration is required because even one organism may be important. A broth with heavy inoculation, cytocentrifuge smear, and a large volume of filtered specimen placed on a chocolate agar plate should enable detection of low numbers of organisms.
- *Water sterility specimens:* Water from sources such as whirlpools, stills, and reagent water also requires concentration. The Millipore Sampler (Millipore Corp., Billerica, Mass.) is designed for this purpose and uses 18 mL of water.
- *Intrauterine devices (IUD):* Intrauterine devices are usually cultured for the detection of *Actinomyces* spp. A Gram stain of the material should identify the presence of this bacterium.
- *Vascular catheter tips:* Vascular catheter tips are submitted for culture to aid in the diagnosis of catheter-related infection. The Maki roll technique is used in many laboratories. Using sterile forceps, a 5- to 7-cm segment of the catheter is rolled across the surface of a blood agar plate. Following incubation, the laboratory performs identification and susceptibility tests on each organism that produces 15 or more colonies.

COMMUNICATION OF LABORATORY FINDINGS

The postanalytical phase of the laboratory testing process is the communication of laboratory findings. The microbiology technologist has a professional responsibility to the patient to communicate the laboratory results to the health care professional treating the patient. The laboratory must strive to provide accurate and timely information. In some situations preliminary results are communicated as they become available. The physician can then take action on the results to provide effective patient care.

The report should clearly interpret the results and be free of microbiology jargon or abbreviations. The clinician may not be familiar with the laboratory procedures or the taxo-

---

BOX 6-1 Examples of Critical Values in Microbiology

- Positive blood culture
- Positive cerebrospinal fluid Gram stain or culture
- Positive cryptococcal antigen test or culture
- Positive blood smear for malaria
- *Streptococcus pyogenes* from a sterile site
- Positive acid-fast smears or positive mycobacterium culture
- *Streptococcus agalactiae* or herpes simplex virus (HSV) from genital site of woman at term
- Detection of significant pathogen (i.e., *Bordetella pertussis*, *Brucella* sp., *Legionella* sp.)

nomic status of the organisms involved, and thus it may be necessary to include interpretive statements to aid in their understanding.

Some microbiology results are considered critical and must be reported to the physician immediately. Critical values may indicate a life-threatening situation that needs to be acted upon promptly. The microbiology director, in consultation with the medical staff, should establish a list of these critical values. Box 6-1 provides an example of critical values.

BIBLIOGRAPHY

Bekeris LG et al: Urine culture contamination: a College of American Pathologists Q-Probes study of 127 laboratories, *Arch Pathol Lab Med* 132:913, 2008.

Forbes BA, Sahm DF, Weissfeld AS: *Bailey & Scott's diagnostic microbiology*, ed 12, St Louis, 2007, Mosby.

Fuller DD et al: Comparison of BACTEC Plus 26 and 27 media with and without fastidious organism supplement with conventional methods for culture of sterile body fluids, *J Clin Microbiol* 32:1488, 1994.

Garcia LS: *Clinical laboratory management*, Washington, DC, 2004, American Society for Microbiology.

Gile TJ: A safe voyage, *Adv Med Lab Prof* 16:22, 2004.

Isenberg HD: *Essential procedures for clinical microbiology*, Washington, DC, 1998, American Society for Microbiology.

Isenberg HD: *Clinical microbiology procedures handbook*, ed 2, Washington, DC, 2004, American Society for Microbiology.

Leonard MK Jr, Kourbatova E, Blumberg HM: How many sputum specimens are necessary to diagnose pulmonary tuberculosis? *Am J Infect Control* 34:328, 2006

Maki DG, Weise CE, Sarafin HW: A semiquantitative culture method for identifying intravenous–catheter-related infection, *N Engl J Med* 296:1305, 1977.

Miller JM: *A guide to specimen management in clinical microbiology*, ed 2, Washington, DC, 1999, American Society for Microbiology.

Miller JM: The impact of specimen management in microbiology, *MLO Med Lab Obs* 30:28, 1998.

Morris AJ et al: Cost and time savings following introduction of rejection criteria for clinical specimens, *J Clin Microbiol* 34:355, 1996.

Murray PR et al: *Manual of clinical microbiology*, ed 9, Washington, DC, 2007, American Society for Microbiology.

Raad II, Hanna HA: Intravascular catheter-related infections: new horizons and recent advances, *Arch Intern Med* 162:871, 2002.

Saubolle MA, McKellar PP: Laboratory diagnosis of community-acquired lower respiratory tract infection, *Infect Dis Clin North Am* 15:1025, 2001.

Schofield CB: Preventing errors in the microbiology lab, *MLO Med Lab Obs* 38:10, 2006.

Sewell DL: *Cumitech 40: Packing and shipping of diagnostic specimens and infectious substances*, Washington, DC, 2003, American Society for Microbiology.

Stoner KA, Rabe LK, Hillier SL: Effect of transport time, temperature, and concentration on the survival of group B streptococci in amies transport medium, *J Clin Microbiol* 42:5385, 2004.

U.S. Department of Transportation, Office of Hazardous Materials Safety, Research and Special Programs Administration: *Hazardous materials regulations,* Title 49 CFR, Parts 171-180, 2004.

Watterson SA, Drobniewski FA: Modern laboratory diagnosis of mycobacterial infections, *J Clin Pathol* 53:727, 2000.

Weissfeld AC: *Cumitech 2B: Laboratory diagnosis of urinary tract infections,* Washington, DC, 1998, American Society for Microbiology.

Points to Remember

- The microbiology laboratory must take responsibility for specimen management in the preanalytical laboratory process by ensuring that specimens are appropriately selected, collected, and transported.
- The collection of specimens for microbiology must include the use of proper technique and containers, adequate quantity, accurate labels, and prompt transportation or provisions to maintain specimen integrity.
- Shipping of patient specimens or cultures of microorganisms must be performed according to the regulations of the DOT Hazardous Material Regulations.
- The microbiology laboratory must prioritize the processing of specimens as they are received in the laboratory based on the critical nature of the infection and the potential for specimen deterioration.
- Performing microbiology analysis on suboptimal specimens provides misleading results. The laboratory must publish guidelines for specimen rejection, and when a specimen is rejected the laboratory must communicate this information to the person responsible for the patient.
- Macroscopic observation of the specimen allows the processor to determine the adequacy of the specimen and the need for special processing. A direct microscopic examination is useful in determining the quality of the specimen, detecting the etiologic agent, and alerting the technologist for special procedures.
- The selection of culture media for each specimen is based on the anatomic site and the organisms likely to be involved in infection at that site. Specimens with fastidious pathogens require enriched media; specimens with an abundance of normal biota require selective media.
- If several plates are inoculated with a specimen, the media should be arranged in order, beginning with the most enriched medium and progressing to the most selective.
- The general-purpose isolation streak yields a semiquantitative estimate of growth, whereas the quantitative isolation technique will determine the number of bacteria present in a certain volume of the specimen.
- Most bacteria cultures are incubated at 35° to 37° C. The atmosphere will vary depending on the pathogens involved and may involve room air, CO_2, microaerophilic, or anaerobic conditions.
- Microbiology cultures are interpreted using skills to discriminate between normal biota and potential pathogens. The microbiology technologist must have knowledge of which organisms are pathogens in various body sites to perform a clinically relevant workup.
- The microbiology technologist performs definitive identification using accepted limited identification procedures to maintain cost-effective testing while providing optimal patient care.
- The microbiology laboratory contributes to effective patient management by communicating accurate and timely results.

Learning Assessment Questions

1. Why is the specimen in the case presented unacceptable? What are the consequences of processing this specimen? What steps should be taken?

2. A patient has a subcutaneous infection and the specimen is submitted on a swab. Explain why this is an unacceptable collection method. How should the sample be collected?

3. Which of the following anticoagulants is appropriate for use in microbiology?
   a. Citrate dextrose
   b. EDTA
   c. SPS
   d. Sodium citrate

4. Which of the following specimens requires immediate processing when received in the microbiology laboratory?
   a. Urine
   b. Cerebrospinal fluid
   c. Sputum
   d. Stool

5. Which of the following are reasons to reject a specimen for culture?
   a. The specimen is preserved in formalin.
   b. Information on the requisition does not match information on the specimen label.
   c. A second stool sample is submitted from the same patient on the same day.
   d. All of the above.

6. In which of the following specimens is a direct microscopic examination not useful?
   a. Throat swab
   b. Sputum
   c. Urine
   d. Leg abscess

7. Chocolate agar is an example of which of the following?
   a. Nonselective media
   b. Selective media
   c. Differential media
   d. Enriched media

8. Which of the following is an example of a selective and differential media?
   a. Blood agar
   b. Chocolate agar
   c. MacConkey agar
   d. Modified Thayer-Martin

9. Which of the following specimens should not be refrigerated?
   a. Urine
   b. Urogenital swab
   c. Throat swab
   d. Sputum

10. Which of the following specimens is cultured using a quantitative isolation technique?
    a. Urine
    b. Sputum
    c. Blood
    d. Stool

Microscopic Examination of Infected Materials

Leona W. Ayers

OBJECTIVES

After reading and studying this chapter, you should be able to:

1. List the modifications in compound light microscopes that expand their use for direct examination of infected material.

2. Given a list of stains commonly used in the medical diagnostic laboratory, select the stain type for determining whether a microbe is a bacillus, fungus, mycobacterium, or viral inclusion.

3. Given a Gram-stained direct smear of infected material, describe the local material, contaminating material, purulence, and associated microorganisms using the descriptive terminology presented.

4. List the common species associated with the following morphology:

- Gram-negative bacilli, small, pleomorphic

- Gram-positive cocci, groups

- Yeast and pseudohyphae

- Hyphae, septate, branched 45-degree angle

- Enlarged cell with intranuclear and cytoplasmic inclusions

5. Explain the application of quality control and quality improvement activities in the laboratory to the results of the direct microscopic examination and culture.

Case in Point

A 75-year-old man with a history of chronic obstructive pulmonary disease, heavy smoking, and alcohol abuse came to his physician with a fever, chills, and a productive cough. Sputum samples were collected and sent to the laboratory for direct smear and culture. Blood cultures also were drawn three times within 24 hours of admission to the hospital. The direct smear was Gram stained (see Plate 14). The sputum culture produced a heavy growth of α-hemolytic colonies. Blood cultures yielded similar results after 24 hours of incubation.

Issues to Consider

After reading the patient's case history, consider the following:

- What is the role of the Gram stain and microscopic morphology in identification?

- Is there evidence of purulence (inflammation) in the direct smear of the specimen?

- Is there evidence of contamination by normal (resident) microbial flora?

- Is the suspected organism "real," or is it an artifact?

- In a properly performed Gram-stain direct smear, the cells—for example, polymorphonuclear cells, red blood cells, and epithelial cells—should be stained pink.

Key Terms

Acid-fast	Gram stain
Amorphous debris	Microbial morphotype
Colony-forming unit (CFU)	Monomicrobial
Curschmann's spiral	Polymicrobial
Cytocentrifugation	Probe-mediated stain
Differential stain	Purulence
Gram-negative bacteria	Simple stain
Gram-positive bacteria	

Direct microscopy for visualization of microorganisms has been possible for just more than 200 years, but it was not a practical reality until Koch established the germ theory of disease in the 1880s. By 1880 a Scottish surgeon had published his direct observations of cluster-forming cocci in **purulence** from human disease. He named these cocci *Staphylococcus*. In 1884, Christian Gram developed the **Gram stain,** which today allows us to examine a pus specimen directly for the gram-positive cocci *Staphylococcus*. Differential staining and microscopy underpin the laboratory diagnosis of infectious diseases.

This underpinning in the diagnostic microbiology laboratory, as in the Case in Point, is the ability to combine the rapid response of direct specimen examination with culture isolation and antibiotic susceptibility testing to achieve the following:

- Confirm that the material submitted for study is representative.
- Identify the cellular components and debris of inflammation and thereby establish the probability of infection.
- Identify specific infectious agents using direct visual detection of characteristic shape, size, and Gram stain reaction.
- Augment visual identification of microbes by use of specific stains, including antibody or gene-directed probes.
- Provide antibiotic susceptibilities of isolated pathogens to guide treatment.
- Develop epidemiologic data.

In more than 88% of instances, the physician has a correct idea about the diagnosis after taking a patient history and performing a physical examination. In the remaining instances in which the diagnosis is not evident, assistance comes from laboratory or radiologic studies. With infectious diseases the physician has an idea of the likely etiology from the rate of symptom progression and is able to evaluate the extent of the infectious process. The physician is greatly pressured to begin immediate treatment of symptomatic patients. Specimens are collected and sent to the laboratory to confirm the physician's

idea about the patient's illness. The ability of the laboratory to respond to the physician in a timely manner with useful results is the key to keeping the treatment moving in the correct direction or changing treatment direction if the physician's presumptive diagnosis proves incorrect. The diagnostic microbiology laboratory has the opportunity to respond to the physician during the treatment decision-making process or early in presumptive therapy. Direct viewing of pathogens becomes primary or direct evidence to confirm or refute the physician's initial clinical impression. If this impression is incorrect, reconsideration is facilitated, and additional studies can be undertaken as needed. Culture results usually are received too late to alter presumptive therapy. At best they confirm the correctness of the therapeutic choices already made and implemented.

PREPARATION OF SAMPLES

The preparation of samples for routine bright-field microscopy has the objective of preparing material in a manner that facilitates adequate examination within a reasonable time. For smears, specimens should be examined grossly to determine the best approach (Table 7-1). Both thick, but not opaque, and thin (monolayer) smear areas should be produced by the smear process chosen.

Smears from Swabs

Smears should not be prepared from a swab after it has been used to inoculate culture media. Ideally, if the sample can be collected only on swabs, two swabs are submitted. Smears from swabs are prepared by rolling the swab back and forth over contiguous areas of the glass slide to deposit a thin layer of sample material (Figure 7-1). This preserves the morphology and relationships of the microorganisms and cellular elements. The swab should never be rubbed back and forth across the slide because important material on the opposite

TABLE 7-1 Preparing Infected Materials for Visual Examination

Preparation	Specimen or Organism Type
For gross examination	
Wet preparation	Parasites
	Materials >1 mm in size
For microscopic examination	
Wet preparation (direct or sedimented)	Fluids or semisolids
Cytocentrifuged (direct or presedimented)	Clear or slightly turbid fluids
Smear	Clear or slightly turbid fluids
1. Drop	Pus or fluid
	Tissue homogenate
	Swab rinse
2. Pellet	Blood culture
	Dilute specimen
3. Rolled	Swabbed material
4. Imprint (touch preparation)	Tissue

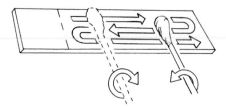

FIGURE 7-1 Smear preparation of a sample collected on a swab. The swab should be rolled back and forth across the slide to deposit the sample completely.

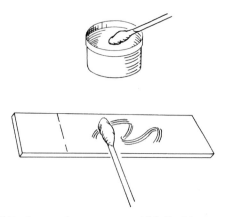

FIGURE 7-2 Smears from opaque thick liquids or semisolids, such as stool, can be made using a swab to sample and smear the material.

side of the swab might not be deposited and smear elements could be broken up.

Smears from Thick Liquids or Semisolids

Swabs also can be used as the tool for preparation of smears from thick liquid or semisolid specimens such as feces (Figure 7-2). The swab is immersed in the specimen for several seconds and then used to prepare a thin spread of material on the glass slide for staining and viewing. This swab method of preparation is adequate but may produce less desirable results than other methods.

Smears from Thick, Granular, or Mucoid Materials

Opaque material must be thinly spread so that a monolayer of material is deposited in some areas. It is most desirable to have both thick and thin areas. Granules within the material must be crushed so that their makeup can be assessed. A better presentation of granules is possible if granules or grains are "fished" from the surrounding materials and crushed on a separate slide using the technique shown in Figure 7-3. Granules that are too hard to crush between two glass slides probably do not represent infectious materials. More likely, they are small stones or foreign bodies. Examination using a dissecting microscope may help to characterize the nature of hard granules.

The following steps should be used to prepare a smear from thick, granular, or mucoid materials:

1. Place a portion of the sample on the labeled slide and press a second slide, with the label down, onto the sample to flatten or crush the components.
2. Rotate the two glass surfaces against each other so that the shear forces break up the material.
3. Once the material is flattened and sufficiently thinned, pull the glass slides smoothly away from each other to produce two smears.
4. If the material is still too thick, repeat the first three steps with another (third) glass slide. The best smear or both smears can be retained for staining.

Slides of material from difficult sample sites, scant samples, or patients with critical illnesses should not be discarded until the culture evaluation is complete.

Smears from Thin Fluids

"Thin" specimens of fluids such as urine, cerebrospinal fluid (CSF), and transudates should be dropped but not spread on the slide. The area of sample drop should be marked on the reverse side of the slide using a wax pencil or placed within the circle or well of a premarked slide. **Cytocentrifugation** is preferred for this type of specimen, if available.

Thin fluid can be prepared by drawing up a small quantity of the fluid or a resuspended sediment of the fluid into a pipette and depositing it as a drop of fluid onto a clearly marked area on the slide (Figure 7-4). The material may not be grossly visible after staining because of a low protein or cell count. The fluid should not be spread over a larger area of the slide unless it is turbid. Turbid or thick fluids can be more efficiently prepared by the previously described method.

Cytocentrifuge Preparations

Cytocentrifugation is an excellent method for preparing non-viscous fluids such as CSF and bronchoalveolar lavage fluids. The cytocentrifugation process deposits cellular elements and microorganisms from the specimen onto the surface of a glass slide as a monolayer. The cellular elements are deposited within a discrete area for easy viewing (Figure 7-5). The protein is dissipated into a filter pad, leaving the background clearer for viewing gram-negative morphotypes. Cell morphology is good, and the concentrating effect shortens viewing time and increases the volume of cellular material reviewed.

Cytocentrifuge Technique

A cytocentrifuge with a closed bowl is preferred for microbiology. The bowl can be loaded and unloaded within a biohazard chamber to avoid possible infectious aerosols. The steps of the technique are as follows:

1. Small aliquots of fluid (0.1 to 0.2 mL) are placed in the cytocentrifuge holders.
2. The material is spun for 10 minutes.
3. The slide is removed. If the deposit of cells is too heavy, a portion of the cellular deposition can be smeared (see Figure 7-5).
4. The sediment is fixed and decontaminated in 70% alcohol for 5 minutes.

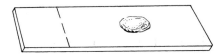

Drop or place the sample onto the surface of a labeled glass slide.

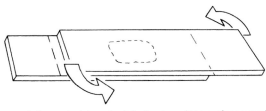

Place the second slide face down over the material.

Press to flatten or crush the material, and rotate the two glass surfaces against each other.

Pull to spread.

FIGURE 7-3   Preparation of smears from thick, granular, or mucoid samples.

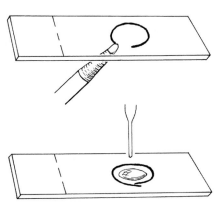

FIGURE 7-4   Smears from thin fluids can be prepared by placing a single drop of fluid or resuspended fluid sediment on a well-marked area of the slide.

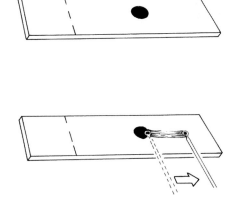

FIGURE 7-5   Cytocentrifuge preparations deposit the concentrated sample within a limited area for viewing. If the deposit is too heavy, a portion of the material may be smeared to produce a thin area.

STAINS

Staining imparts an artificial coloration to the smear materials that allows them to be inspected using the magnification provided by a microscope. There are many types of stains, each with specific applications. Stains can be categorized as **simple stains, differential stains,** and **probe-mediated stains.**

Simple stains are directed toward coloring the forms and shapes present, differential stains are directed toward coloring specific components of those elements present, and diagnostic antibody or DNA probe–mediated stains are directed specifically at identification of an organism. Stains most commonly used in the diagnostic laboratory are listed in Table 7-2. Four of the stains—Gram, **acid-fast,** calcofluor white, and rapid modified Wright-Giemsa—should be available in all diagnostic microbiology laboratories (Procedures 7-1 to 7-4). Most other stains are directed toward specific organism groups and should be available where needed.

MICROSCOPES

Examination of specimens should begin with gross visual inspection and then proceed to the level of magnification needed to identify the pathogen or determine that no pathogen is present. The ordered tests provide a guide to the

TABLE 7-2 Stains for Infected Materials

Stains	Applications
General Morphology	
Wright-Giemsa	Bronchoalveolar lavages
	Tzanck preparations
	Samples with complex cellular back-grounds (visualizes bacteria, yeast, parasites, and viral inclusions)
Selected Morphology	
Leifson	Flagella
Methylene blue	Metachromatic granules of *Corynebacterium diphtheriae*
Acid-fast stains	
Ziehl-Neelsen	Sediments for mycobacteria (concentrated smears)
	Partial acid-fastness of *Nocardia* spp.
Fluorochrome	Sediments for mycobacteria (concentrated smears, auramine, and rhodamine)
	Preferred acid-fast stain
Kinyoun	Acid-fast stain modification of Ziehl-Neelsen method for cryptosporidia and cyclospora parasites in stool specimens
Calcofluor white stain	Bronchoalveolar fungi and some parasitic cysts
	Differentiates them from background materials of similar morphology
Gram stain	
Traditional	Routine stain for diagnostic area
	Yeast differentiated from all other organisms
Enhanced	Provides the same differential staining but enhances red-negative organisms by staining the background material green to gray-green
Genus (Species)-Specific Stains	
Antibody or DNA probe stains	Used for the specific identification of selected pathogens, such as *Chlamydia trachomatis, Bordetella pertussis, Legionella pneumophila*; herpes simplex virus, varicella-zoster virus, cytomegalovirus, adenovirus, and respiratory viruses

---

PROCEDURE 7-1
Gram Stain

PRINCIPLES

The following Gram staining method was developed empirically by the Danish bacteriologist Christian Gram in 1884. The sequential steps provide for crystal violet (hexamethyl-*p*-rosanaline chloride) to color all cells and background material a deep blue and for Gram's iodine to provide the larger iodine element to replace the smaller chloride in the stain molecule. Bacteria with thick cell walls containing teichoic acid retain the crystal violet–iodine complex dye after decolorization and appear deep blue; they are **gram-positive bacteria.** Other bacteria with thinner walls containing lipopolysaccharides do not retain the dye complex; they are **gram-negative bacteria.** The alcohol-acetone decolorizer damages these thin lipid walls and allows the stain complex to wash out. All unstained elements are subsequently counterstained red by safranin dye. The differential ability of the Gram stain makes it useful in microbial taxonomy. The quickness and ease with which the method can be performed make it an ideal choice for the clinical laboratory setting.

APPLICATION

The Gram stain is used routinely and as requested in the clinical microbiology laboratory for the primary microscopic examination of specimens submitted for smear and culture. It is ideally suited for those specimen types in which bacterial infections are strongly suspected, but it may be used to characterize any specimen. Cerebrospinal fluid, sterile fluids, expectorated sputum or bronchoalveolar lavages, and wounds and exudates are routinely stained directly. Urine and stool may not be routinely stained directly. Samples sent for focused screening cultures usually are not stained. The Gram stain is regularly used to characterize bacteria growing on culture media.

PROCEDURE

1. Dry the material on the slide so that it does not wash off during the staining procedure. Adherence can be improved by fixation in 70% to 95% alcohol or by gently warming the slide to remove all water from the material.

2. Place the smear on a staining rack, and overlay the surface of the material to be stained with the stains in sequence as shown in the figures.
3. Place the smear in an upright position in a staining rack, allowing the excess water to drain off and the smear to dry. Never blot a critical smear. Never put immersion oil on a smear until it is completely dry.
4. Examine the stained smear using the low-power objective, and then select an area to examine more closely using a 40 to 60 oil objective. Suspicious areas are evaluated using the 100 oil objective of the microscope.

RESULTS

Gram-positive bacteria stain dark blue to blue-black. All other elements stain safranin red. Individual structures absorb a different amount of safranin, so some will have prominent staining (strong avidity) and others will be weakly stained (low avidity). Among the gram-negative bacteria the enterics have strong avidity and stain bright red; pseudomonads are less avid and stain moderately well. Anaerobic bacilli and other thin-walled gram-negative organisms, such as *Borrelia, Legionella,* and *Spirillum* spp., stain weakly. Always check the quality of the stain before moving to interpretation.

PRECAUTIONS

The Gram-stain reaction may vary from the expected in a number of well-recognized circumstances. If the crystal violet is rinsed too vigorously before it is complexed with the iodine, it will wash away and leave poor or no staining of gram-negative organisms. If the decolorization is too vigorous or prolonged, the gram-positive complex will be removed and the normally gram-positive organisms will not stain. If the decolorization is insufficient, organisms may be falsely gram-positive, and organisms in the thicker areas of the sample may be obscured. If the safranin is left on the slide for a prolonged period (minutes), the gram-positive complex will be leached from the positive cells; however, failure to leave the safranin in place for sufficient time will result in failure to stain gram-negative bacteria and background materials. Gram-stain characteristics may be atypical in antibiotic-treated and dead or degenerating organisms. Typical morphotypes should be sought. Any sample that raises questions about quality of stain or method should be restained.

The crystal violet stain is not tied into the organism until the iodine is added. Any rinsing between the crystal violet and the iodine steps must be very brief.

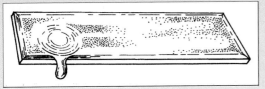

Flood the slide with crystal violet and allow it to stand for 30 seconds.

The dilute iodine solution can be used to wash away the crystal violet, and no water rinse is employed.

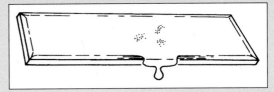

Flood with Gram's iodine and allow it to stand for 30 to 60 seconds.

Acetone is a more rapid decolorizer and may give better results, but the reaction must be stopped with water as soon as the purple color disappears.

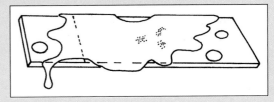

Decolorize the slide with acetone or absolute alcohol or a mixture of the two decolorizers, and wash immediately with water.

The counterstain must not be left in place too long. Anaerobes may stain better at 1 minute or with dilute carbolfuchsin.

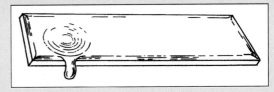

Flood with safranin or dilute carbolfuchsin or neutral red for 30 seconds to 1 minute (anaerobes). Rinse very lightly with water.

Check the staining reactions before proceeding with smear interpretation.

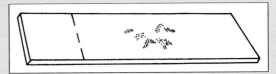

PROCEDURE 7-2
Acid-Fast Staining of Mycobacteria

PRINCIPLES

The primary stain binds to mycolic acid in the cell walls of the mycobacteria and is retained after the decolorizing step with acid alcohol. The counterstain does not penetrate the mycobacteria to affect the color of the primary stain.

APPLICATION

The direct smear examination is a valuable diagnostic procedure for the detection of mycobacteria in clinical specimens.

MATERIALS

TB auramine-rhodamine T stain
Carbolfuchsin stain (prepared by laboratory)
0.5% acid alcohol (0.5% HCl in 70% ethanol)
2% acid alcohol (prepared by laboratory)
1% sulfuric acid (partial acid-fast)
0.5% aqueous potassium permanganate solution
0.3% aqueous methylene blue solution (prepared by laboratory)
Microscope slides 1 × 3 inches
Sterile water

PROCEDURE

Fluorescent Stain

1. Cover smears with Difco TB auramine-rhodamine T stain, and stain for 25 minutes.
2. Wash in running tap water.
3. Move slides to slide rack on acid alcohol collection container.
4. Flood smears with 0.5% acid alcohol, and decolorize for 2 minutes.
5. Wash smears in running tap water.
6. Move slides to original staining rack.
7. Flood smears with potassium permanganate counterstain for 4 minutes.
8. Wash smears in running tap water.
9. Air dry.
10. Examine smears with the 16× and 40× objectives of the fluorescent microscope equipped with a filter system comparable to a BG-12 exciter filter and an OG-1 barrier filter. Examine each smear for 3 to 5 minutes.

Kinyoun Stain

1. Cover smears with carbolfuchsin, and stain for 5 minutes.
2. Wash slides with running tap water.

3. Move slides to staining rack on acid alcohol collection container.
4. Decolorize with acid alcohol until no more color appears in the washings.
5. Wash slides with running tap water, and move them to original staining rack.
6. Flood slides with methylene blue counterstain for 1 minute.
7. Wash with running tap water, drain, and air dry.
8. Examine smears with 100 oil immersion lens.

Modified Kinyoun Stain (Partial Acid-Fast)

1. Flood the slides with carbolfuchsin stain for 5 minutes.
2. Rinse with running tap water.
3. Flood slides with 70% ethanol, and rinse with tap water. Repeat until excess red dye is removed.
4. Move slides to rack on acid collection container.
5. Continuously drop 1% sulfuric acid on the smear until the washing becomes colorless.
6. Rinse with running tap water.
7. Move slides to original staining rack.
8. Counterstain with methylene blue for 30 seconds.
9. Rinse with running tap water, and air dry.
10. Examine smears with 100× oil immersion objective.

Ziehl-Neelsen Stain

1. Cover smear with a piece of filter paper cut slightly smaller than the slide.
2. Layer filter paper with carbolfuchsin stain. With a Bunsen burner, heat the smears gently until steaming occurs. Stain for 5 minutes without additional heating.
3. Proceed as for Kinyoun method, beginning with Step 2.

RESULTS

Fluorescent Stain

Mycobacteria stain bright orange. Count the number of acid-fast bacilli seen on the smear and report as follows

No. of Acid-Fast Bacilli	Report
1 to 20	Number seen
21 to 80	Few
81 to 300	Moderate
300+	Numerous

Kinyoun and Ziehl-Neelsen Stains

Mycobacteria stain red, whereas the background material and non–acid-fast bacteria stain blue.

examination, but a routine approach to specimen management should include an examination procedure that will discover unexpected pathogens. In most diagnostic microbiology laboratories, this procedure consists of visual inspection at the time of smear and culture preparation and microscopic examination of a gram-stained preparation for structures too small to be seen with the unaided eye.

Microscopes vary both in their ability to resolve small structures and in their modifications. Microscopes are divided into two basic types: compound light microscopes, with common resolving limits of 1 to 10 μm and enlargements up to 2000×; and electron microscopes with enlargements greater than 1,000,000× (Table 7-3). The microbiology laboratory uses several modifications of the compound light microscope,

PROCEDURE 7-3
Calcofluor White Stain/Fungi-Fluor Kit*

PRINCIPLE

Calcofluor white is a colorless dye that binds to cellulose and chitin. It fluoresces when exposed to long-wavelength ultraviolet and short-wavelength visible light. Special filters are required for optimal use.

APPLICATION

Calcofluor white may be used as a specific stain for rapid screening of clinical specimens for fungal elements. This stain may be useful when morphology is ambiguous and the nonspecific staining of other techniques such as Grocott-Gomori methenamine-silver (GMS) gives confusing results.

MATERIALS

Stock Solution

A 1% (wt/vol) aqueous solution of calcofluor white is prepared by dissolving the powder in distilled water with gentle heating. The stock solution is stable for 1 year at room temperature.

Working Solution

0.1% calcofluor white containing 0.01% to 0.08% Evans blue as a counterstain.

PROCEDURE

1. Add 1 to 2 drops of working calcofluor white solution or solution A (Fungi-Fluor) to fixed smear or imprint for 1 to 2 minutes.
2. Coverslip or rinse and dry.
3. Examine specimen on fluorescent microscope using the following set of filters: G 365, LP 450, and FT 395.
4. Add Fungi-Fluor solution B if quenching of nonspecific staining is desired. (The quenching with solution B may be excessive [1:4 dilution preferred].)

RESULTS

Yeast cells, pseudohyphae, and hyphae display a bright apple-green or blue-white fluorescence. The central body of the *Pneumocystis* cyst also fluoresces; with quenching (Fungi-Fluor solution B), the cysts of *Pneumocystis* are visible.

*Polysciences, Washington, Penn.

PROCEDURE 7-4
Rapid Modified Wright-Giemsa Stain

PRINCIPLE

The Wright-Giemsa stain is available in a modification that requires only 1 to 3 minutes. This neutral dye is a combination of basic thiazine dyes and acid eosin that attach to oppositely charged sites on proteins. The results are metachromatic.

APPLICATION

Wright-Giemsa (modified) is a rapid stain for smears and imprints to stain fully background materials and cells and a wide variety of microorganisms.

PRECAUTIONS

Avoid getting reagents in eyes or on skin or clothing; if this does occur, flush with copious quantities of water. Use with adequate ventilation. If stain is discarded into sink, flush with large volumes of water to prevent azide buildup, which may react with lead and copper plumbing to form highly explosive metal azides.

PROCEDURE

1. Prepare smear or imprint. Fix with alcohol.
2. Dip slide in fixative solution five times for 1 second each time. Allow excess to drain.
3. Dip slide in solution I five times for 1 second each time. Allow excess to drain.
4. Dip slide in solution II five times for 1 second each time. Allow excess to drain.
5. Rinse slide with tap water.
6. Allow to dry. Examine.

NOTE: The intensity of each stain may be altered by increasing or decreasing dips in solutions I and II. Never use fewer than three dips of 1 full second each.

RESULTS

Blood cells stain as with Wright stain. The cytoplasm is basophilic. The chromatin of white cells is purple. Bacteria are blue. Parasitic protozoan nuclei are red.

---

but the workhorse of the laboratory is the bright-field microscope.

TERMINOLOGY FOR DIRECT EXAMINATIONS

The microscopist must have a consistent vocabulary for the description of materials seen in samples. This vocabulary must be shared by the microbiology and medical communities so that when observations are reported everyone will be able to understand the implications of the descriptions. Common observations can be coded so that they are consistent among observers. The use of computers for recording coded observations and generating reports of the findings further extends the need for uniform terminology. Only unusual findings should be individually described in a report.

The background of the sample being evaluated should be described in sufficient detail to convey the composition of the material. The presence of cells representing a response to injury supports the probability of infection and directs attention toward specific types of pathogens. Common morphotype descriptions and the most prevalent associated species are listed in Table 7-4. Examples of useful descriptive phrases with quantitation are listed in Table 7-5.

Microorganisms can be described in such a way that, based on prevalence, the description implies the identification of the

TABLE 7-3 Observing Microbial Pathogens

Tools	Magnification (×)	Application
Eyes	0	Gross examination
Magnifying glass	5	Gross examination
Dissecting microscope	2.5 to 30	Gross detailed examination and manipulation
Compound light microscope		
Bright-field	10 to 2000	Cells stained
Dark-field	10 to 400	Cells not readily stained for bright-field microscopy
Phase-contrast	10 to 400	Living or unstained cells
Fluorescence	10 to 400	Preparations using fluorochrome stains, which can directly stain cells or be connected to antibodies that attach to cells
Electron microscopes		
Transmission electron	150 to 10 million	Determine ultrastructure of cell organelles
Scanning electron	20 to 10,000	Determine surface shapes and structures

organism. For example, the observation of a gram-negative bacillus, small and pleomorphic, from the spinal fluid of an infant implies that *Haemophilus influenzae* is the infecting agent.

EXAMINATION OF PREPARED MATERIAL

A limited number of microbial pathogens from commonly sampled infected sites are regularly encountered by the technologist or microbiologist. The simple Gram stain or acid-fast stain is the fastest and least expensive method for presumptive diagnosis in these common clinical settings. Organisms are readily seen because more than 105 **colony-forming units (CFUs)** of infecting organisms per milliliter are commonly present in clinically evident infections.

Two types of infection are important to distinguish, those caused by a *single species,* or **monomicrobial,** and those caused by *multiple species,* or **polymicrobial.** The single agents of infection or those causing classic infections are easily recognized by microscopy and require limited interpretations. Infections caused by common single species, or by classic infectious agents, include *Streptococcus pneumoniae* pneumonia, *Staphylococcus aureus* abscesses or pyodermas, *H. influenzae* tracheobronchitis or meningitis in infants, *Clostridium perfringens* gas gangrene, *Nocardia* spp. lung abscesses, and gonococcal urethritis.

Polymicrobial presentations in smears require more interpretation and must take into account smear background, the morphology of the organisms, and the anatomic location of the suspected infection as well as accompanying clinical symptoms. Polymicrobial infections usually arise from displaced normal or altered flora, and culture will yield the same species that can be isolated in culture from uninfected but

contaminated specimens. These infections usually represent displacement of environmental, skin, oropharyngeal, gastrointestinal, or vaginal flora into tissues, with subsequent infection. Commonly encountered infections of this type are surgical wound (skin flora) infection, aspiration (oropharyngeal flora) pneumonia, perirectal (fecal flora) abscesses, and tuboovarian (vaginal flora) abscess.

Characterization of Background Materials

The laboratory professional always should look at the slide material with the unaided eye before beginning the microscopic examination. The distribution and consistency of the material should be noted. The microscope's low-power objective (2.5× to 10×) should be used first to evaluate the general content of the material on the slide. Specimens can be homogeneous or heterogeneous and may contain pathogens evenly distributed throughout the specimen or limited to one visual field. A mental inquiry checklist should be followed until the habit of searching a slide systematically is developed. Items that should be included in such a checklist appear here and on following pages in **bold italic** type preceded by a bullet (•).

- *Is there evidence of contamination by normal (resident) microbial flora?* The laboratory professional should look for squamous epithelial cells, bacteria without the cells of inflammation, food, or other debris. Does this material constitute the entire sample, or is a representative sample also available in a manner that can be recognized? Contamination of specimens not collected from sterile sites diminishes the value of culture studies.

- *Is necrotic (amorphous) debris in the background?* Infection with organisms such as *C. perfringens* and *Nocardia* spp. may elicit few polymorphonuclear neutrophils (PMNs). The inflammatory cells that do migrate into the area of infection can be lysed. Patients with leukopenia also may have few inflammatory cells within their inflammatory debris. **Amorphous debris** usually is the remains of tissue mixed with the breakdown products or fluids of acute inflammation and always should be searched for organisms. *Mycobacterium tuberculosis* organisms stain poorly as beaded grampositive bacilli or not at all with Gram stain; they can appear within necrotic debris as negative images.

- *Are unexpected structures present?* The characteristic coiled structure of a **Curschmann's spiral** is more easily recognized on low power. This structure must not be confused with parasitic larvae, which also can be found in sputum using low-power magnification. Large granules, grains, or fungal forms such as spherules or fungal mats can best be recognized at low power.

Search for Microorganisms

After the full extent of the material has been examined on low power, a representative area should be selected for viewing with the oil immersion lens. A 40× or 60× lens is preferred for scanning, and a 100× lens is used for final evaluation. In infection the organism will be intimate with the purulence of necrotic debris. All grains or granules and the background should be examined carefully. The delicate gram-positive

TABLE 7-4 Gram Stain Morphology and Associated Organisms

Morphotype Description	Most Common Organisms
Bacteria	
Cocci	
Gram-positive cocci	*Aerococcus, Enterococcus, Leuconostoc, Pediococcus, Planococcus, Staphylococcus, Stomatococcus, Streptococcus* spp.
Gram-positive cocci	
Pairs	*Staphylococcus, Streptococcus, Enterococcus* spp.
Tetrads	*Micrococcus, Staphylococcus, Peptostreptococcus* spp.
Groups	*Staphylococcus, Peptostreptococcus, Stomatococcus* spp.
Chains	*Streptococcus, Peptostreptococcus* spp.
Clusters, intracellular	Microaerophilic *Streptococcus* spp., viridans streptococci, *Staphylococcus* spp.
Encapsulated	*Streptococcus pneumoniae, Streptococcus pyogenes* (rarely), *Stomatococcus mucilaginosus*
Gram-positive diplococci (lancet-shaped)	*Streptococcus pneumoniae*
Gram-negative diplococci	Pathogenic *Neisseria* spp., *Moraxella catarrhalis*
Bacilli	
Gram-positive bacilli	
Small	*Listeria monocytogenes, Corynebacterium* spp.
Medium	*Lactobacillus,* anaerobic bacilli
Large	*Clostridium, Bacillus* spp.
Diphtheroid	*Corynebacterium, Propionibacterium, Rothia* spp.
Pleomorphic, gram-variable	*Gardnerella vaginalis*
Beaded	Mycobacteria, antibiotic-affected lactobacilli, and corynebacteria
Filamentous	Anaerobic morphotypes, antibiotic-affected cells
Filamentous, beaded, branched	*Actinomycetes, Nocardia, Nocardiopsis, Streptomyces, Rothia* spp.
Bifid or V forms	*Bifidobacterium* spp., brevibacteria
Gram-negative coccobacilli	*Bordetella, Haemophilus* spp. (pleomorphic)
Masses	*Veillonella* spp.
Chains	*Prevotella, Veillonella* spp.
Gram-negative bacilli	
Small	*Haemophilus, Legionella* (thin with filaments), *Actinobacillus, Bordetella, Brucella, Francisella, Pasteurella, Capnocytophaga, Prevotella, Eikenella* spp.
Bipolar	*Klebsiella pneumoniae, Pasteurella* spp., *Bacteroides* spp.
Medium	Enterics, pseudomonads
Large	Devitalized clostridia or bacilli
Curved	*Vibro, Campylobacter* spp.
Spiral	*Campylobacter, Helicobacter, Gastrobacillum, Borrelia, Leptospira, Treponema* spp.
Fusiform	*Fusobacterium nucleatum*
Filaments	*Fusobacterium necrophorum* (pleomorphic)
Yeast, Fungi, and Algae	
Yeast	
Small	*Histoplasma, Torulopsis* spp.
Medium	*Candida* spp.
With capsules	*Cryptococcus neoformans*
Thick-walled, broad-based bud	*Blastomyces* spp.
Hyphae	
Septate	Fungi
Aseptate	Zygomycetes
With arthroconidia	*Coccidioides* spp.
With branches at 45-degree angle	*Aspergillus* spp.
Pseudohyphae	*Candida* spp.
Spherule (endospores)	*Coccidioides* spp.
Sporangia with endospores	*Protothecae* spp.
Viruses	
Single or multinuclear cells with intranuclear inclusions	Herpes virus, measles virus
Enlarged cells with intranuclear inclusions or cytoplasmic inclusions	Cytomegalovirus
Cells with dark, "smudged" nuclei	Adenovirus

TABLE 7-5 Descriptions of Background Material

Cells and Structures	Associations
Amorphous debris (light, moderate, or heavy)	Necrosis, heavy protein fluid
Black particulate debris	Smoke inhalation, crack cocaine
Charcot-Leyden crystals	Eosinophils
Epithelials with contaminating bacteria	Passage of specimen through contaminated area during collection
Curshmann's spirals present (sputum)	Bronchospasm, obstruction, asthma
Epithelial cells (light, moderate, or heavy)	Epithelial surface involved or adjacent to collection site
Intracellular organisms	Inferred association in infection
Local material (light, moderate, or heavy)	Reflection of collection site
Mononuclear cells present	Chronic inflammation
Mucus (light, moderate, or heavy)	Irritation of glandular surface
Purulence (none, light, moderate, or heavy)	Acute inflammation, exudation
Red blood cells	Trauma, hemorrhage

filaments of *Nocardia* spp. may blend into the background. *H. influenzae* may be present in large numbers, hidden within the mucus, in acute exacerbations of chronic bronchitis. Intracellular and extracellular forms should be noted. Strict criteria for **microbial morphotypes** should be maintained. The examiner must not be distracted by precipitated gram-positive stain, keratohyaline granules, or other artifacts. Organisms should be evaluated for shape, size, and Gram reaction. Because cell wall–damaged bacteria, antibiotic-treated bacteria, or dead bacteria may appear falsely gram-negative, their shapes and sizes are critical "co-characteristics." The classic misleading smear example is the observation of gram-negative, lancet-shaped diplococci mixed with the predominant gram-positive forms. The inexperienced observer might misinterpret this as mixed infection rather than as the simple presence of dead pneumococci in a classic infection.

- *Examine more than one area of the smear.* More than one organism should be found if possible. It is rare not to be able to find more than one because in infection organisms are usually distributed throughout the specimen. Care should be taken in the interpretation of very low numbers of bacteria, especially in the absence of inflammation or necrosis and in specimens from nonsterile sites. Small numbers of organisms in samples from sterile sites must be seriously considered. However, additional smears can be made and examined if the likelihood of contamination is high.
- *Do not overinterpret the findings.* Specific diagnosis should be limited to a small number of instances in which the smear is classic in its presentation and the extent of infection is not an issue. If acid-fast bacteria are suspected, the acid-fast stain should be performed before an opinion is rendered. If a fungal element is not clearly gram-positive, a calcofluor stain should be

performed. Both of these follow-up stains can be performed on the decolorized, Gram-stained preparation.

Evaluation of Choice of Antibiotic

The symptomatic patient with suspected infection most likely will be treated with antibiotics. The physician expects the laboratory to affirm or reject the antibiotic choice made after the presumptive diagnosis. Antibiotic choice should be kept in mind as the smear is viewed. There are a number of important observations.

- *Is there evidence of purulence?* Remember that purulence with red blood cells (RBCs), neutrophils, protein background, and necrosis reflects acute inflammation. Mononuclear cells, including lymphocytes, monocytes, and macrophages, reflect chronic inflammation. Patients who are cytopenic do not have the cellular response seen in normal individuals. Purulence, blood, and necrosis can be present if traumatic tissue damage occurs in the absence of infection.
- *Is there a single most probable etiologic microorganism?* If so, is the morphology sufficiently characteristic to presume identification? Is there a specified antibiotic for treatment of infections with this agent? Will antibiotic susceptibility testing be necessary, or will identification of the suspected pathogen be sufficient?
- *Is the infection monomicrobial or polymicrobial?* Are morphotypes present that characterize the source of the organisms? Can the mixture of organisms be characterized?
- *If antibiotics are to be used, will the suspected pathogens be susceptible?* Specific considerations should be made about the likelihood of the following:
  1. Penicillinase or β-lactamase producers such as *S. aureus, Haemophilus* spp., and the gonococci
  2. Enterococci, which have limited susceptibility to antibiotics and therefore may require synergistic antibiotic action for killing
  3. Species resistant to aminoglycosides, penems, and cephems, such as the *Bacteroides fragilis* group and *Pseudomonas aeruginosa*
  4. Fungal organisms, which will be unresponsive to antibacterial antibiotics

Direct Examination Summary

Once this stepwise evaluation of the smear has been completed, the information yielded, along with the clinical setting, allows for reasonable management of infected patients until the subsequent steps of culture isolation, susceptibility testing, or antibody or antigen detection can take place.

Initiation of Special Handling for Unsuspected or Special Pathogens

The direct microscopic examination of infected materials, along with specimen site and historical information, may suggest modifications in routine culture techniques to allow isolation of a suspected pathogen. Modifications might involve ordering other culture tests, adding special media, increasing incubation time, or changing incubation temperature or atmosphere. If recognition or suspicion of such pathogens does not occur from smear or history, the isolation of certain pathogens will not be made, and diagnosis will be delayed or missed.

Some pathogens will not grow in culture and are usually unsuspected. A common one is the nematode parasite *Strongyloides stercoralis,* which can be seen in the sputum and bronchoalveolar fluid of patients with a hyperinfestation syndrome. Visual recognition can lead to a request for stool examination for parasite load and prompt treatment. Untreated hyperinfestations are associated with the death of the patient.

Other pathogens that will grow in culture but not in routine bacterial culture can be recognized on smear and redirected for appropriate culture. Organisms such as *Legionella* spp., *Mycobacterium* spp., viruses, and *Bartonella* spp. must be placed on appropriate media for culture confirmation of infection.

GRADING OR CLASSIFYING MATERIALS

Microscopic examination also immediately discloses that a specimen is unlikely to be helpful in diagnosis or culture management. The specimen may be just blood rather than infected material, or it may be oropharyngeal surface debris or some other normal surface material. Processing and culture interpretation of such nonrepresentative specimens may lead to delayed treatment because of a falsely negative culture or to inappropriate antibiotic treatment owing to a false-positive culture from growth of normal biota (normal flora) or antibiotic-altered flora.

Several grading or classification systems have been derived to aid the technologist in arriving at decisions relating to culturing the specimen or interpretation of growth from culture of a specimen. Most evaluations are aimed at specimens such as sputum, for which collection is complicated by contamination with throat and mouth flora because culture alone can be misleading. The objective is to separate the representative sample from the contaminated sample before culture or culture evaluation. Bartlett's method for scoring sputum and the Murray-Washington method for contamination assessment document the association of 10 to 20 squamous epithelial cells (SECs) per 10× microscopic field with unacceptable specimens and 10 to 25 PMNs per 10× field with significant specimens. Heineman's method emphasizes the ratio between the SECs and PMNs.

Many diagnostic microbiology laboratories use the documented observations related to SECs and PMNs but attempt to coordinate observations related to background materials, which consist of local materials, contaminating materials, and purulence, and to describe the relationship of microorganisms to these background materials. The body site of the sample and the classification of the smear together determine the extent of culture evaluation.

Contaminating Materials

Contaminating materials (Plate 1) are recognized as those not coming from the collection site, not contributed by the inflammatory response from the tissues, or not likely to contain the infecting organism. They usually have been added to the specimen in the course of collection from or through a nonsterile area. The most bothersome contaminating materials are those containing microorganisms that will grow in culture and potentially confuse the culture evaluation. Expectorated sputum, which collects in the lower lung airways and is expelled through the mouth, is the most common contaminated specimen managed by the clinical laboratory.

Criteria

Fewer than 25 PMN cells per low-power field (LPF) and more than 10 epithelial cells or mixed bacteria per LPF must be present.

Gram Smear Report

Quantitate the contaminating materials as 1+ (light), 2+ (moderate), 3+ (moderately heavy), or 4+ (heavy).

Culture Identification Guidelines

"New culture" using careful collection technique should be requested. If a culture is requested, organism identification should be limited to brief evaluation for *S. aureus,* streptococci or viridans streptococci, *Lactobacillus*, diphtheroids, and β-hemolytic streptococci. Gram-negative rods are reported as enterics (coliforms, nonlactose fermenters, or *Proteus* spp. [spreading colonies]), pseudomonads (oxidase-positive), pathogenic *Neisseria* spp. (identified), *Haemophilus* spp. (smear only), yeast (note only), and any primary pathogen.

Antibiotic Susceptibility Testing

No such testing is appropriate except on primary pathogens.

Local Materials
Criteria

Fewer than 25 PMN leukocytes (white blood cells [WBCs]) per LPF and fewer than 10 contaminating epithelial cells per LPF are seen, along with cellular and fluid elements local to the area sampled.

The local constituents may vary as follows:
- Respiratory secretions (Plate 3), including mucus, alveolar pneumocytes (macrophages), ciliated columnar cells, goblet cells, and occasionally metaplastic epithelial cells (smaller than normal squamous epithelial cells)
- CSF (Plate 5) cellular elements
- Cavity fluid (Plate 8) macrophages, a few mixed WBCs, mesothelial cells, and proteinaceous fluid
- Wounds—blood and proteinaceous fluids
- Amniotic fluid (Plate 2) anucleate squamous cells and heavy proteinaceous fluid
- Cervix—mucus, columnar epithelial cells, goblet cells, metaplastic SECs, and leukocytes (vary with menstrual cycle)
- Prostatic secretions or semen—spermatozoa and mucus

Gram Smear Report

Quantitate local microbial flora as 1+ to 4+ (see Contaminating Materials).

Culture Identification Guidelines

The designation "usual flora" or a brief presumptive description of "colony-type growth" may be used (see Contaminating Materials).

Antibiotic Susceptibility Testing

No such testing is appropriate.

Purulence

Criteria

Fewer than 25 PMN leukocytes (WBCs) per LPF and none or few (i.e., fewer than 10) epithelial cells with mixed bacteria per LPF are seen. Mucus or heavy proteinaceous material may be present.

Gram Smear Report

Quantitate only organisms intimately associated with the WBCs, mucus, or proteinaceous exudate. Use the following system: 1+ (rare organisms per oil immersion field [OIF]), 2+ (few organisms per OIF), 3+ (moderate number per OIF), and 4+ (many per OIF). Quantitate contaminating materials separately—should be 1+ (none or few).

Culture Identification Guidelines

Correlate colony growth with Gram-stained smear, as in the case in point. Identify *S. pneumoniae* from viridans streptococci, β-hemolytic streptococci (Lancefield groups A, B, and D; C, F, and G, if indicated clinically), *S. aureus* (inventory for epidemiology), *H. influenzae*, *Haemophilus parainfluenzae* (test for β-lactamase production), *Haemophilus aphrophilus*, pathogenic *Neisseria* spp., gram-negative bacilli, yeast (*Cryptococcus neoformans* only; note the presence of other genera), filamentous fungi (transparent tape preparation in biosafety hood), and other organisms as indicated by smear findings.

Antibiotic Susceptibility Testing

Check for *S. aureus*, gram-negative nonfastidious bacilli, and other organisms as appropriate or specifically requested.

Mixed Materials

Mixed materials consist of purulent exudate, contaminating materials, and local materials in a single smear.

Criteria

Fewer than 25 PMN leukocytes (WBCs) per LPF and fewer than 10 epithelial cells or contaminating bacteria per LPF are seen. Local secretions may also be present.

Gram Smear Report

For mixed materials, quantitate only those organisms intimately associated with purulent exudate. Also quantitate the amounts of other elements, contaminating materials, and local materials.

Culture Identification Guidelines

A "new culture" may be requested for mixed specimens. A new specimen must be requested if the specimen shows the presence of purulence and the culture results cannot be interpreted. If a new culture specimen cannot be obtained, evaluation should proceed as for contaminating materials.

Antibiotic Susceptibility Testing

Use purulence guidelines for testing organisms that appear significant.

REPORTS OF DIRECT EXAMINATIONS

Reports of the results of direct specimen examination should be made available as soon as they are completed. The availability of computer-managed reporting using direct physician access through computer terminals in patient care areas, as well as paper reporting, facilitates immediate reporting of results. Reports of direct examinations should be simple and include all information elements needed by the physician to understand the report. The report lists the type of material submitted and clearly states whether the observed microbes are of significance. The format for computer-managed microscopic reports from direct specimen examinations at Ohio State University is shown in the samples given in Box 7-1.

Only elements useful in characterizing the specimen should be included in the report. Interpretative comments also may be included when, on the basis of specimen type, background materials, and organism morphology, there is little doubt about the nature of the process or the offending infectious agent. All telephone reports of direct examinations should be recorded in the report.

EXAMPLES OF SAMPLE OBSERVATIONS AND REPORTS

Study the examples of direct observations and the associated reports and comments given in Plates 1 to 111. Practice to determine whether one can make a similar report using only the observation provided. Then read each report to see whether you obtain similar impressions of the specimen and pathogen from the observation and written report.

BOX 7-1 Sample Reports of Direct Microscopic Examinations

Respiratory culture	Acc. no. XXXX
Source:	Sputum: expectorated
Microscopic	Purulence heavy
	Contaminating bacteria, yeast and epithelials heavy
	Gram-positive diplococci: consistent with pneumococci
Called to Dr. Doe at 8:00 PM 4/13/10	
Respiratory culture	Acc. no. XXXXX
Source:	Sinus: ethmoid contents
Microscopic	Purulence moderate
	Local materials light
	Red blood cells present
	Gram-negative bacilli: consistent with pseudomonas
Called to Dr. Doe at 11:35 AM 4/5/10	

QUALITY CONTROL IN DIRECT MICROSCOPIC INTERPRETATIONS

Quality control (QC) issues, such as the quality of specimens submitted and the adequacy of culture interpretation, can be monitored using the results of direct examination. Quality control practice that monitors both the smear and culture interpretation should be an ongoing work activity. Correlation between the two results should be made for each patient. Explanations for discrepant results should be sought within the work material. This repeated inspection of results enables each observer to practice self-education and improve observation skills. Review of these QC activities allows corrections to be made in specimen collection, specimen management, and culture management.

Quality improvement activities often are suggested by the results of quality control monitoring of direct specimen examination. For example, it may be documented that sputum specimens of poor quality are consistently submitted from certain doctors' offices, clinics, or nursing stations in the hospital. This observation becomes the basis for planning corrections that move outside the laboratory to involve the community of patients served.

BIBLIOGRAPHY

Agerer F, Waeckerle S, Hauck CR: Microscopic quantification of bacterial invasion by a novel antibody-independent staining method, *J Microbiol Methods* 59:23, 2004.

Bartlett RC: *Medical microbiology: quality, cost, and clinical relevance*, New York, 1974, John Wiley & Sons.

Bottone EJ, Cho KW: Mycobacterium chelonae keratitis: elucidation of diagnosis through evaluation of smears of fluid from patient's contact lens care system, *Cornea* 24:356, 2005.

Broaddus C et al: Bronchoalveolar lavage and transbronchial biopsy for the diagnosis of pulmonary infections in the acquired immunodeficiency syndrome, *Ann Intern Med* 102:747, 1985.

Cali A et al: Corneal microsporidioses: characterization and identification, *J Protozool* 38:215s, 1991.

Chan-Tack KM, Johnson JK: An unusual Gram stain finding, *Clin Infect Dis* 40:1649, 2005.

Chapin-Robertson K, Dahlver SE, Edberg SC: Clinical and laboratory analyses of cytopsin-prepared Gram stains for recovery and diagnosis of bacteria from sterile body fluids, *J Clin Microbiol* 30:377, 1992.

Cordonnier C et al: Diagnostic yield of bronchoalveolar lavage in pneumonitis occurring after allogeneic bone marrow transplantation, *Am Rev Respir Dis* 132:1118, 1985.

Davis KA et al: Ventilator-associated pneumonia in injured patients: do you trust your Gram's stain? *J Trauma* 58:462, 2005.

Forbes B et al, editors: *Bailey & Scott's diagnostic microbiology*, ed 12, St Louis, 2007, Mosby.

Golden JA et al: Bronchoalveolar lavage as the exclusive diagnostic modality for *Pneumocystis carinii* pneumonia, *Chest* 90:18, 1986.

Goswitz JJ et al: Utility of slide centrifuge Gram's stain versus quantitative culture for diagnosis of urinary tract infection, *Am J Clin Pathol* 99:132, 1993.

Hautala T et al: Blood culture Gram stain and clinical categorization based empirical antimicrobial therapy of bloodstream infection, *Int J Antimicrob Agents* 25:329, 2005.

Heineman HS, Chawla JK, Lofton WM: Misinformation from sputum cultures without microscopic examination, *J Clin Microbiol* 6:518, 1977.

Huang M, Wang JH: Gram stain as a relapse predictor of bacterial vaginosis after metronidazole treatment, *J Microbiol Immunol Infect* 38:137, 2005.

Inglis TJ et al: Comparison of diagnostic laboratory methods for identification of *Burkholderia pseudomallei*, *J Clin Microbiol* 43:2201, 2005.

Ison CA, Hay PE: Validation of a simplified grading of Gram stained vaginal smears for use in genitourinary medicine clinics, *Sex Transm Infect* 78:413, 2002.

Kokoskin E et al: Modified technique for efficient detection of microsporidia, *J Clin Microbiol* 32:1074, 1994.

Kullavanijaya P et al: Analysis of eight different methods for the detection of *Helicobacter pylori* infection in patients with dyspepsia, *J Gastroenterol Hepatol* 19:1392, 2004.

La Scolea LJ Jr, Dryja D: Quantitation of bacteria in cerebrospinal fluid and blood of children with meningitis and its diagnostic significance, *J Clin Microbiol* 19:187, 1984.

Laupland KB, Church DL, Gregson DB: Validation of a rapid diagnostic strategy for determination of significant bacterial counts in bronchoalveolar lavage samples, *Arch Pathol Lab Med* 129:78, 2005.

Lewis JF, Alexander J: Microscopy of stained urine smears to determine the need for quantitative culture, *J Clin Microbiol* 4:372, 1976.

Magee CM et al: A more reliable Gram staining technique for diagnosis of surgical infections, *Am J Surg* 130:341, 1975.

Mengel M: The use of the cytocentrifuge in the diagnosis of meningitis, *Am J Clin Pathol* 84:212, 1985.

Murphy P, et al, editors: *Manual of clinical microbiology*, ed 9, Washington, DC, 2007, American Society for Microbiology.

Murray PR, Washington JA: Microscopic and bacteriologic analysis of expectorated sputum, *Mayo Clin Proc* 50:339, 1975.

Musher DM: The usefulness of sputum gram stain and culture, *Arch Intern Med* 165:470, 2005.

Niederman MS: The clinical diagnosis of ventilator-associated pneumonia, *Respir Care* 50:788, 2005.

Ognibene FP et al: The diagnosis of *Pneumocystis jiroveci* pneumonia in patients with the acquired immunodeficiency syndrome using subsegmental bronchoalveolar lavage, *Am Rev Respir Dis* 129:929, 1984.

Olson ML et al: The slide centrifuge Gram stain as a urine screening method, *Am J Clin Pathol* 96:454, 1991.

Procop GW et al: Detection of *Pneumocystis jiroveci* in respiratory specimens by four staining methods, *J Clin Microbiol* 42:3333, 2004.

Ryan NJ et al: A new trichrome-blue stain for detection of microsporidial species in urine, stool, and nasopharyngeal specimens, *J Clin Microbiol* 31:3264, 1993.

Shanholtzer CJ, Schaper PJ, Peterson LR: Concentrated Gram stain smears prepared with a Cytospin centrifuge, *J Clin Microbiol* 16:1052, 1982.

Smith JW, Barlett MS: Laboratory diagnosis of pneumocytosis, *Clin Lab Med* 11:957, 1991.

Southern PM Jr, Colvin DD: Pseudomeningitis again: association with cytocentrifuge funnel and Gram-stain reagent contamination, *Arch Pathol Lab Med* 120:456, 1996.

Spengler M et al: The Gram stain—the most important diagnostic test of infection, *JACEP* 7:434, 1978.

Stover DE et al: Bronchoalveolar lavage in the diagnosis of diffuse pulmonary infiltrates in immunosuppressed host, *Ann Intern Med* 101:1, 1984.

Thrall M, Cartwright CP: Fungal conidiospores in a peritoneal fluid gram stain, *Arch Pathol Lab Med* 129:123, 2005.

Van Scoy RE: Bacterial sputum cultures: a clinician's viewpoint, *Mayo Clin Proc* 52:39, 1977.

Wang H, Murdoch DR: Detection of *Campylobacter* species in faecal samples by direct Gram stain microscopy, *Pathology* 36:343, 2004.

Zarakolu P et al: Reliability of interpretation of gram-stained vaginal smears by Nugent's scoring system for diagnosis of bacterial vaginosis, *Diagn Microbiol Infect Dis* 48:77, 2004.

Points to Remember

Direct microscopy of materials submitted to the laboratory for identification of infectious organisms offers the first, last, and best opportunity to:

- Confirm probable infection.
- Confirm the diagnostic quality of specimen submitted.
- Recognize "classic" organism morphotypes associated with infection.
- Recognize pathogens that will not grow in culture or the culture type requested, thus requiring a different diagnostic approach.
- Provide a "stat" laboratory response to serious infection.

Learning Assessment Questions

1. Direct smear examination of clinical samples is a rapid means to identify presumptively the etiologic agents of infectious disease. True or false?

2. The presence of an infectious disease process can be assessed on a direct smear based on which of the following?
   a. The presence of numerous inflammatory cells
   b. Morphology of the bacteria present
   c. Types of bacteria present
   d. The presence of numerous epithelial cells

3. Which of the following stains may be used for direct smear examination?
   a. Gram stain
   b. Acid-fast stain
   c. Wright or Giemsa stain
   d. Calcofluor-white stain
   e. All of the above

4. Which of the following stains is best used to detect mycobacterial organisms in clinical samples?
   a. Gram stain
   b. Giemsa stain
   c. Acid-fast stain
   d. Lacto-phenol-cotton blue stain

5. Calcofluor white is a colorless dye that binds with which of the following structures?
   a. Cell wall containing mycolic acid
   b. Chitin
   c. Peptidoglycan layer
   d. Metachromatic granules

6. Cytocentrifugation is an excellent method for which of the following types of samples?
   a. Heavily contaminated
   b. Nonviscous fluids
   c. Thick purulent material
   d. Filled with mucous

7. A monobacterial type of infection can be immediately suspected based on the direct microscopic examination of the clinical sample. True or false?

8. In a Wright-Giemsa stained smear, bacteria would appear as which of the following colors?
   a. Red
   b. Blue
   c. Purple
   d. Orange

DIRECT EXAMINATION SHOWING LOCAL AND CONTAMINATING MATERIALS

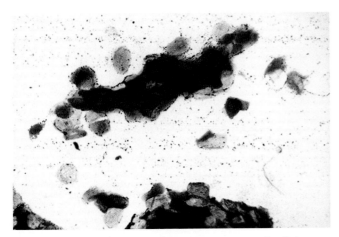

PLATE 1 Expectorated sputum, smear, Gram stain, light microscopy, low-power view (LPV). Purulence, none. Contaminating bacteria and epithelial cells, heavy. No pathogens seen. A carefully collected sample of lower respiratory tree material should be submitted. The sample is saliva, not sputum. There could be several reasons for submission of this sample to the laboratory. The patient could have been poorly directed and simply "spit" into the collection container, or the patient's cough might not be productive of sputum.

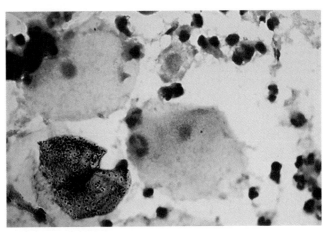

PLATE 2 Amniotic fluid, cytocentrifuge preparation, Gram stain, light microscopy, medium-power view (MPV). Purulence, moderate. Local materials, moderate. No organisms seen. The presence of purulence (neutrophils or "polys") indicates a process suspicious for infection. The absence of organisms in this normally sterile fluid is a critical observation. Squamous epithelial cells are local to this specimen type and confirm that the sample is amniotic fluid. The blue keratohyalin granules must never be mistaken for bacteria.

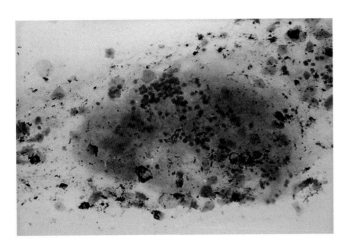

PLATE 3 Expectorated sputum, smear, Gram stain, light microscopy, LPV. Purulence, none. Local materials, moderate. Contaminating bacteria and epithelials, heavy. No pathogens seen. The bolus of sputum, consisting of mucus with entrapped alveolar macrophages, confirms that lower respiratory tree material is present. There is no evidence of an infectious process. The sputum is heavily coated by contaminating materials from the oropharynx or mouth. Contaminating organisms will grow in a routine sputum culture.

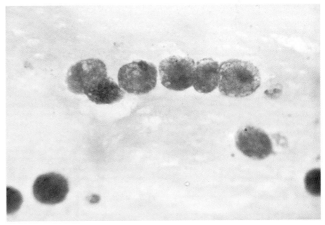

PLATE 4 Aspirated sputum, smear, Gram stain, light microscopy, high-power view (HPV). Purulence, none. Local materials, moderate. No organism seen. The alveolar macrophages and mucus (pink-stained background) are the local materials from the tracheobronchial tree. This smear confirms that sputum was sampled and there is no suspicion for infection and no evidence of significant contamination. Routine culture of this specimen can grow insignificant oral flora because culture is more sensitive than direct examination.

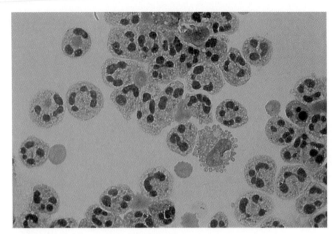

PLATE 5 Cerebrospinal fluid (CSF), cytocentrifuge preparation, Gram stain, light microscopy, HPV. Purulence, moderate. No organisms seen. CSF is a sterile fluid and normally does not have purulence. The presence of neutrophils is critical. Careful observation for bacteria is mandatory. Acridine orange stain may be helpful in clinical settings in which bacteria are low in number and gram-negative. Cytocentrifuged sediments commonly have a concentration of organisms sufficient for routine microscopy (105/mL or greater).

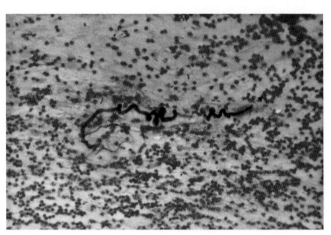

PLATE 6 Expectorated sputum, smear, Gram stain, light microscopy, MPV. Purulence, heavy. Local materials, Curschmann's spiral. No organisms seen. The Curschmann's spiral is material local to the tracheobronchial tree but is not normal, so it is specifically reported. This spiral may present in a variety of sizes depending on the size of bronchus involved. Spirals can be particularly prominent following an asthmatic episode with bronchial constriction.

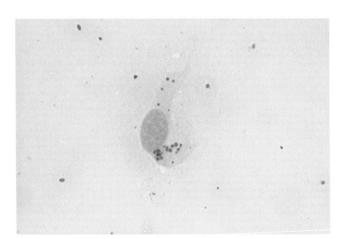

PLATE 7 Trauma eye, vitreous aspirate, smear, Gram stain, light microscopy, HPV. Purulence, none. No organisms seen. Local materials, light. The light protein background and the pigment-containing cell are normal material local to the vitreous of the eye. This local material confirms that the sample is representative. The ability to see this brown pigment cell in smear material is related to the eye trauma. The important emphasis is the absence of purulence.

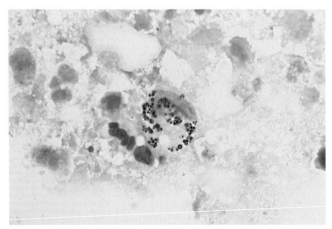

PLATE 8 Eye, vitreous aspirate, smear, Gram stain, light microscopy, HPV. Purulence, light. Amorphous debris, moderate. Local materials, light. No organisms seen. This smear suggests that there has been an injury. The pigment has undergone phagocytosis and is seen within a large macrophage. Pigment must never be mistaken for bacteria, and bacteria must never be overlooked if mixed with local materials, such as pigment granules.

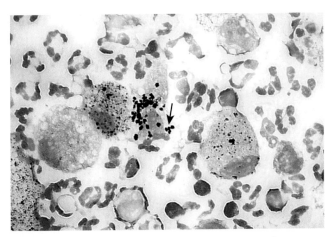

PLATE 9 Bronchoalveolar lavage (BAL), cytocentrifuge smear, Gram stain, light microscopy, HPV. Purulence, heavy. No organisms seen. Local materials, black particulate debris (BPD). This size and type of carbon particle is commonly seen in respiratory samples in small amounts and is usually not noted in a smear report.

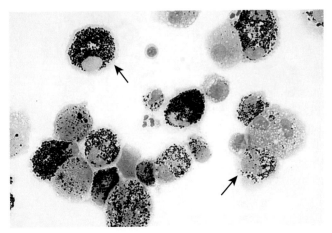

PLATE 10 BAL, cytocentrifuge smear, Gram stain, light microscopy, HPV. Purulence, none. No organisms seen. Local materials, heavy BPD. This small-size carbon particle seen prominently in respiratory samples can be associated with smoking crack cocaine. The gross sample usually has a gray appearance. BPD should not be confused with gram-positive cocci.

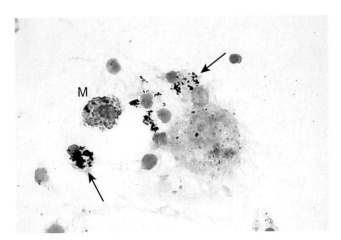

PLATE 11 BAL, cytocentrifuge smear, Gram stain, light microscopy, HPV. Purulence, none. No organisms seen. Local materials, BPD moderate. This BPD is irregular in shape and usually varies in size. This type of carbon debris is commonly associated with smoke inhalation from house or other types of fires. In the early phase of smoke inhalation, much of the BPD will be extracellular. Later much of the debris will be intracellular within phagocytes. The golden-colored macrophage present contains yellow material associated with cigarette smoking.

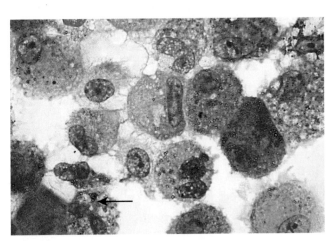

PLATE 12 BAL, cytocentrifuge smear, Gram stain, light microscopy, HPV. Purulence, none. No organisms seen. Local materials, alveolar macrophages containing very small, light to golden yellow, refractile but not polarizing particles. These small, fine particles can be hemosiderin, sometimes deposited as small particles or other fine particles from the environment. Such refractile particles are not usually reported except in response to specific questions from the patient's physician.

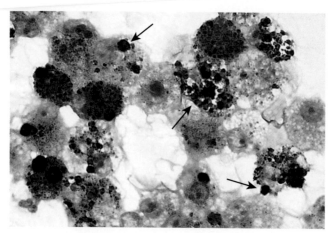

PLATE 13 BAL, cytocentrifuge smear, Gram stain, light microscopy, HPV. Purulence, none. No organisms seen. Local materials, alveolar macrophages containing golden yellow to Gram's safranin-colored chunky, irregular particles consistent with hemosiderin. This type of large particle hemosiderin deposition within lung phagocytes is commonly associated with blood in the lung as seen in heart failure or aspirated blood from large-volume nosebleeds. Blood and hemosiderin in a Gram-stained smear make smear viewing more difficult.

DIRECT EXAMINATION IN COMMON BACTERIAL INFECTIONS

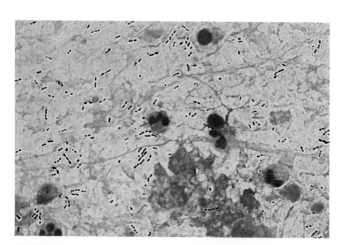

PLATE 14 Expectorated sputum, smear, Gram stain, light microscopy, MPV. Purulence, light. Amorphous debris, moderate. Gram-positive diplococci, encapsulated, extracellular. *Impression:* pneumococcal disease.

This is a typical smear presentation for early pneumococcal pneumonia. The pneumococci have proliferated to high numbers, and the lung is responding with increased mucus and fluid release. There is early migration of the neutrophils, but phagocytosis of the diplococci is limited. Routine bacterial culture of this sample should yield a heavy growth of *Streptococcus pneumoniae.*

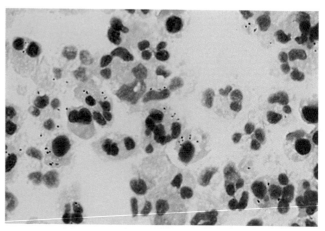

PLATE 15 Expectorated sputum, smear, Gram stain, light microscopy, HPV. Purulence, heavy. The presence of gram-positive diplococci, intracellular morphology suggest antibiotic effect. *Impression:* pneumococcal disease.

This is a typical smear presentation of a treated but unresolved pneumococcal pneumonia. Neutrophils cover the field, the diplococci are largely intracellular and partially digested, and the background amorphous material is gone. Routine bacterial culture of this sample may be negative for typical colonies of *S. pneumoniae.* A few colonies may be found by a careful search among the contaminating normal biota colonies.

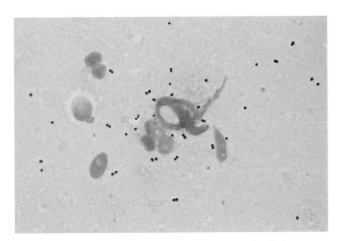

PLATE 16 Aspirated sputum, smear, Gram stain, light microscopy, MPV. Purulence, light. Amorphous debris, heavy. Gram-positive cocci, pairs, encapsulated, extracellular. Initial antibiotic therapy can be directed toward streptococci and staphylococci *(Stomatococcus)*. Routine bacterial culture isolated a pure growth of an encapsulated strain of *Streptococcus pyogenes*. The heavy amorphous background is protein-rich edema fluid from the capillary bed damaged by *S. pyogenes* toxins. The patient subsequently died of the infection despite correct antibiotic therapy and a correct diagnosis.

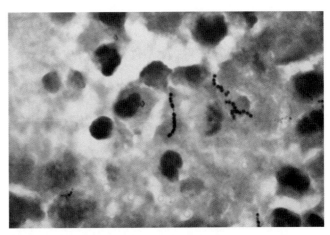

PLATE 17 Wound, smear, Gram stain, light microscopy, MPV. Purulence, moderate. Amorphous debris, moderate. Gram-positive cocci, chains, extracellular. *Impression:* streptococcal disease.

The presence of typical chains of *Streptococcus* on a background showing purulence with poorly preserved "polys" and amorphous debris is suggestive of hemolytic streptococci with tissue cytotoxicity. Routine bacterial culture yielded a pure growth of *S. pyogenes*.

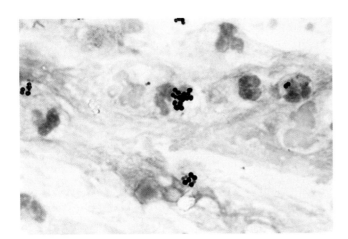

PLATE 18 Expectorated sputum, smear, Gram stain, light microscopy, MPV. Purulence, light. Local materials, moderate. Gram-positive cocci, pairs, groups, intracellular and extracellular. *Impression:* staphylococcal disease.

Smear morphology is typical for staphylococci, but no staphylococcal colonies were present on the culture plates. *Stomatococcus mucilaginosus* colonies were present in high numbers. Careful correlation between direct and culture examinations demonstrated this organism to be the probable cause of infection. The presumptive report implying or suggesting staphylococci followed by a negative culture report without explanation raises doubts about the competence of the laboratory.

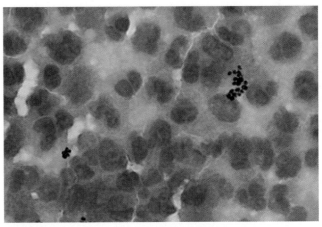

PLATE 19 Abscess aspirate, smear, Gram stain, light microscopy, MPV. Purulence, heavy. Gram-positive cocci, groups, extracellular. *Impression:* staphylococcal disease.

Aerobic and anaerobic culture plates were negative at 24 hours. There was culture isolation of *Staphylococcus aureus* from this same abscess 5 days previously. The patient was being treated with clindamycin. Because the cocci in the smear did not appear antibiotic damaged, another species of gram-positive coccus was sought. The anaerobic culture grew *Peptostreptococcus* organisms, which are clindamycin resistant.

DIRECT EXAMINATION IN GRAM-POSITIVE BACILLARY INFECTIONS

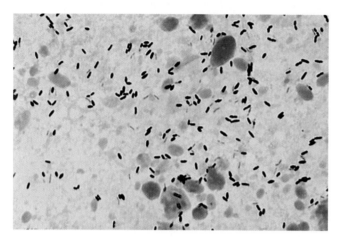

PLATE 20 Amniotic fluid, cytocentrifuge, Gram stain, light microscopy, MPV. Purulence, light. Local materials, moderate. Gram-positive bacilli, small. Morphology consistent with *Listeria monocytogenes*. *Impression:* congenital listeriosis.

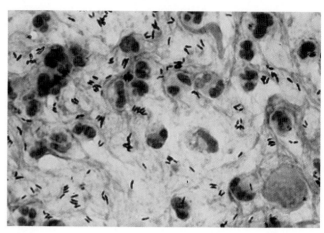

PLATE 21 Expectorated sputum, smear, Gram stain, light microscopy, MPV. Purulence, moderate. Local materials, moderate. Gram-positive bacilli, diphtheroid. Morphology suggests coryneform infection. Routine bacterial culture grew *Corynebacterium pseudodiphtheriticum*.

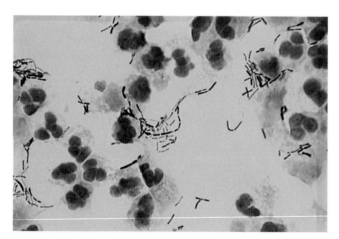

PLATE 22 Urine, cytocentrifugation, Gram stain, light microscopy, MPV. Purulence, moderate. Gram-positive bacilli, medium, long, chaining. Morphology consistent with *Lactobacillus* spp. *Impression:* cystitis.

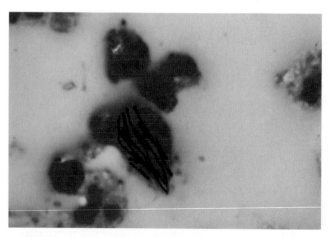

PLATE 23 Amniotic fluid, cytocentrifuge preparation. Gram stain, light microscopy, HPV. Purulence, light. Local materials, moderate. Gram-positive bacilli, medium, long, intracellular. Morphotype consistent with *Lactobacillus* spp. *Impression:* amnionitis.

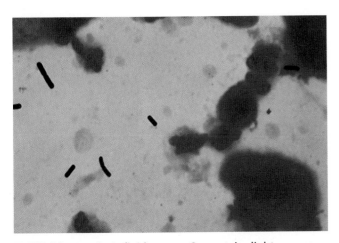

PLATE 24   Amniotic fluid, smear, Gram stain, light microscopy, MPV. Purulence, light. Local materials, moderate. Gram-positive bacilli, large. Morphology consistent with *Clostridium perfringens*. *Impression:* amnionitis.

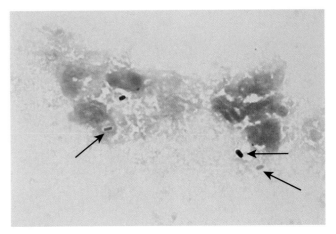

PLATE 25   Wound cellulitis, smear, Gram stain, light microscopy, MPV. Purulence, none. Amorphous debris, moderate. Gram-positive bacilli, large. Gram-negative bacilli, large. Morphology consistent with *Clostridium* spp. *Impression:* gas gangrene. Note that the growth rate of this organism is rapid and that both viable (gram-positive) and nonviable (gram-negative) bacilli can be present in the smear material.

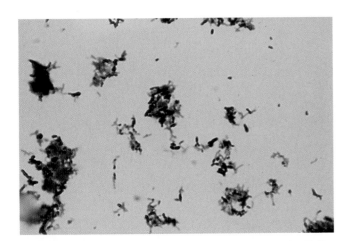

PLATE 26   Colony from blood agar, smear, Gram stain, light microscopy, HPV. Gram-positive bacilli, diphtheroid, variably Gram staining. Morphotype consistent with *Gardnerella vaginalis* (see Plate 27).

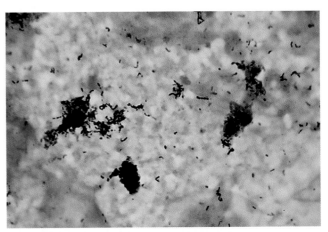

PLATE 27   Amniotic fluid, smear, Gram stain, light microscopy, HPV. Local materials, heavy. Gram-positive bacilli, diphtheroid, variably Gram staining. Morphotype consistent with *G. vaginalis*. *Impression:* amnionitis.

DIRECT EXAMINATION IN UNCOMMON GRAM-POSITIVE BACILLI

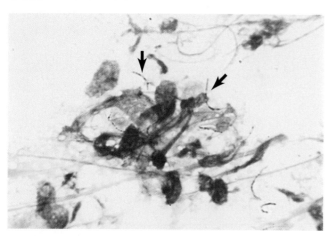

PLATE 28   Abscess aspirate, smear, Gram stain, light microscopy, HPV. Purulence, moderate. Amorphous debris; light. Gram-positive bacilli, beaded. Suspect mycobacteria: initiate additional testing (see Plate 29).

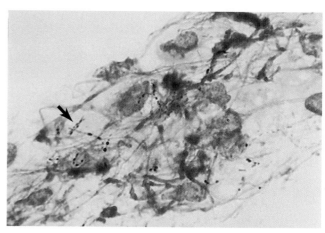

PLATE 29   Abscess aspirate, smear, acid-fast stain (Ziehl-Neelsen), light microscopy, MPV. Purulence, moderate. Acid-fast bacilli, numerous. Mycobacterial cultures grew *Mycobacterium kansasii*.

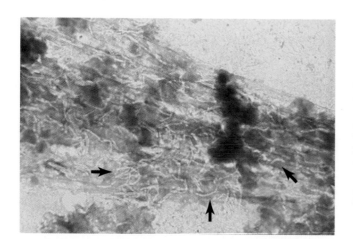

PLATE 30   Expectorated sputum, smear, Gram stain, light microscopy, MPV. Amorphous debris, heavy. Bacillary shapes, negative image. Oil removed from smear, decolorized with acid alcohol, and immediately restained with Ziehl-Neelsen acid-fast stain. Acid-fast bacilli, numerous. Specimen recovered; acid-fast culture requested by laboratory. Suspicious for tuberculosis.

PLATE 31   Expectorated sputum, concentrated smear, fluorochrome acid-fast stain, fluorescent microscopy, MPV. Typical acid-fast bacteria, numerous. *Impression:* mycobacterial disease.

The patient had been placed in respiratory isolation following physical examination and history and was immediately begun on antituberculosis therapy following receipt of the direct examination report. *Mycobacterium tuberculosis* was identified from culture.

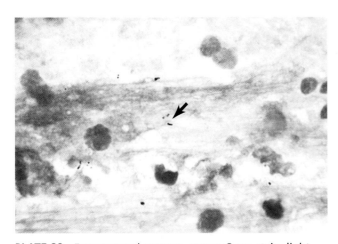

PLATE 32   Expectorated sputum, smear, Gram stain, light microscopy, MPV. Purulence, light. Local materials, light. Amorphous debris, moderate. Gram-positive bacilli, medium, beaded. Follow-up acid-fast stain positive. Chest radiograph with right upper lobe mass. Culture isolation of *Rhodococcus equi.*

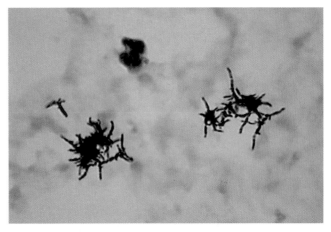

PLATE 33   Blood culture, sediment smear, Gram stain, light microscopy, MPV. Blood. Gram-positive bacilli, branched, beaded. Morphology consistent with *Actinomyces* or *Propionibacterium* spp. Culture isolation of *Actinomyces israelii.*

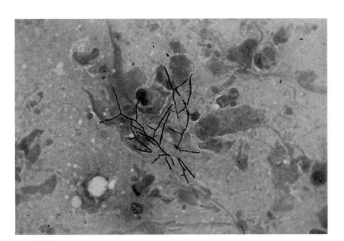

PLATE 34   Expectorated sputum, smear, Gram stain, light microscopy, MPV. Purulence, light. Local materials, light. Amorphous debris, moderate. Gram-positive bacilli, branched, beaded. Morphotype consistent with *Nocardia* or *Actinomyces.*

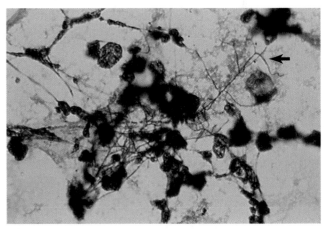

PLATE 35   Expectorated sputum, smear, partial acid-fast stain, light microscopy, MPV. Partially acid-fast bacilli, branched, beaded. Morphology consistent with *Nocardia* spp. *Impression*: nocardiosis.

DIRECT EXAMINATION IN GRAM-POSITIVE BACILLI WITH FILAMENTS AND BRANCHES

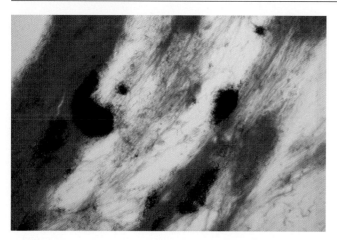

PLATE 36   Jaw abscess aspirate, smear, Gram stain, light microscopy, LPV. Purulence, heavy. Granules present. Suspicious for *Actinomyces* (see Plate 37).

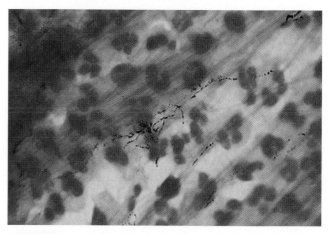

PLATE 37   Jaw abscess aspirate, smear, Gram stain, light microscopy, HPV. Purulence, heavy. Gram-positive bacilli, filamentous, beaded, branched, partial acid-fast stain negative. Morphology consistent with *Actinomyces* spp. *Impression:* actinomycosis (lumpy jaw).

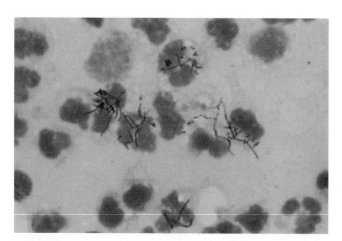

PLATE 38   Cutaneous sinus tract aspirate, smear, Gram stain, light microscopy, HPV. Purulence, heavy. Gram-positive bacilli, filamentous, beaded, branched, partial acid-fast stain negative. Morphology consistent with *Actinomyces* spp. (see Plate 39). *Impression:* actinomycosis.

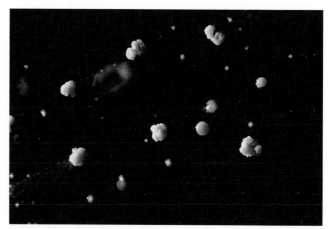

PLATE 39   Cutaneous sinus tract aspirate, colonies on anaerobic blood agar plate. Mixed colony morphotypes. Molar tooth colonies. Morphology consistent with *Actinomyces israelii. Impression:* mixed anaerobic infection: actinomycosis.

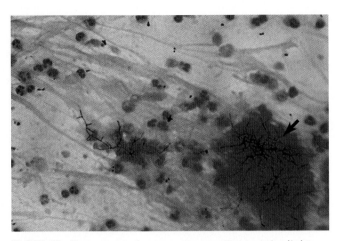

PLATE 40 Expectorated sputum, smear, Gram stain, light microscopy, HPV. Purulence, heavy. Local materials, moderate. Grain present. Gram-positive bacilli, filamentous, beaded, branched. Suspicious for *Nocardia* or *Actinomyces* (see Plate 41).

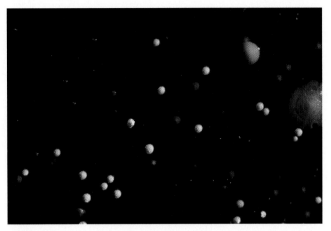

PLATE 41 Expectorated sputum, chalky white colonies on plate with 5% sheep's blood agar at 5 days' incubation. Routine sputum culture. Morphology consistent with *Nocardia*, *Nocardiopsis*, or *Streptomyces* spp.

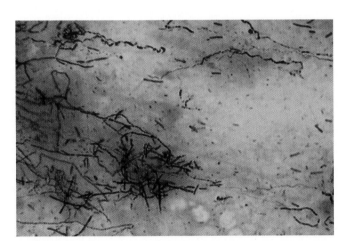

PLATE 42 Sinus-tract granule, crush-pull smear, Gram stain, light microscopy, HPV. Amorphous debris, moderate. Gram-positive bacilli, filamentous, beaded, branched, partial acid-fast negative. Gram-positive bacilli, regular. Gram-negative bacilli, small. Gram-positive cocci. Morphology suggests mixed anaerobic infection with actinomycetes. *Impression:* actinomycosis. Culture isolation of *Actinomyces naeslundii*.

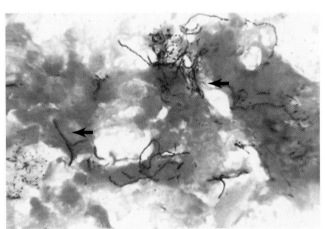

PLATE 43 Surgical biopsy of abnormal area in jawbone, smear, Gram stain, light microscopy, HPV. Amorphous debris, heavy. Gram-positive bacilli, filamentous, beaded, branched, partial acid-fast stain negative. Morphology suggests actinomycete. Aerobic and anaerobic cultures negative.

DIRECT EXAMINATION IN SELECTED GRAM-NEGATIVE BACTERIAL INFECTIONS

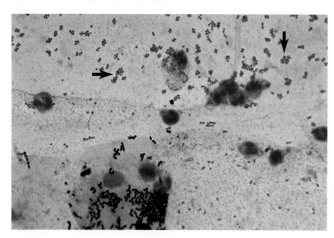

PLATE 44 Expectorated sputum, smear, Gram stain, light microscopy, MPV. Mixed materials, type I, layered. Contaminating bacteria and epithelial cells, moderate. Purulence, light. Gram-negative diplococci. Morphology suggests pathogenic *Neisseria* or *Moraxella* spp. Routine bacterial culture isolated *Moraxella catarrhalis*.

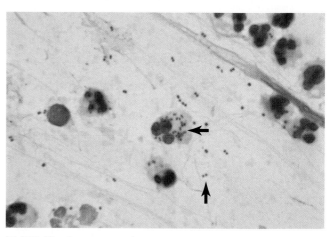

PLATE 45 Expectorated sputum, smear, Gram stain, light microscopy, MPV. Purulence, moderate. Local materials, moderate. Gram-negative diplococci, intracellular, extracellular. Morphology suggests pathogenic *Neisseria* or *Moraxella* spp. Routine bacterial culture isolated *Neisseria meningitidis*.

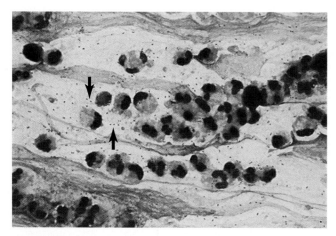

PLATE 46 Expectorated sputum, smear, Gram stain, light microscopy, HPV. Purulence, moderate. Local materials, heavy. Mucus present. Gram-negative coccobacilli, intracellular, extracellular. Morphology consistent with *Haemophilus influenzae*.

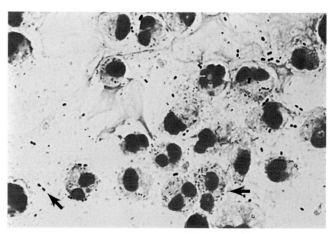

PLATE 47 Expectorated sputum, smear, Gram stain, light microscopy, HPV. Purulence, heavy. Local materials, moderate. Gram-negative bacilli, small, pleomorphic, intracellular, extracellular. Gram-positive diplococci, encapsulated, intracellular, extracellular. Morphology consistent with *H. influenzae* and *S. pneumoniae*. *Impression:* polymicrobial infection.

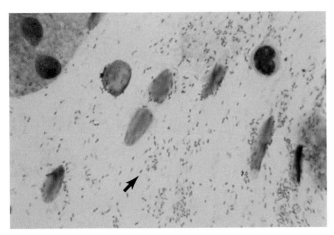

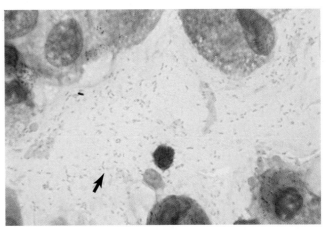

PLATE 48   Bronchoalveolar lavage, cytocentrifuge preparation, Wright-Giemsa stain, light microscopy, HPV. Purulence, none. Lymphocytes present. Local materials, moderate. Small bacilli, numerous (see Plate 49).

PLATE 49   Bronchoalveolar lavage, cytocentrifuge preparation, Gram stain, light microscopy, HPV. Purulence, none. Lymphocytes present. Local materials, moderate. Gram-negative bacilli, small (see Plate 50).

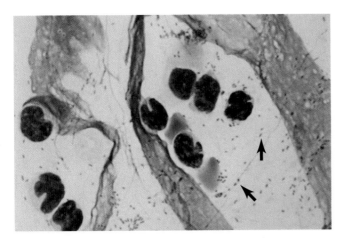

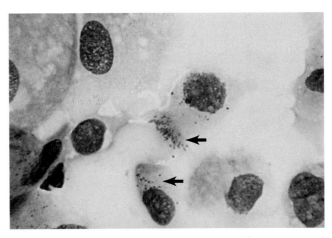

PLATE 50   Bronchoalveolar lavage, cytocentrifuge preparation, Wright-Giemsa stain, light microscopy, HPV. Purulence, none. Lymphocytes present. Local materials, moderate. Gram-negative bacilli, small (see Plate 51).

PLATE 51   Bronchoalveolar lavage, cytocentrifuge preparation, Wright-Giemsa stain, light microscopy, HPV. Purulence, none. Lymphocytes present. Local materials, moderate. Ciliated columnar epithelial cells with numerous small bacilli adherent to cilia. Morphology consistent with *Bordetella pertussis. Impression:* whooping cough.

DIRECT EXAMINATION IN SELECTED GRAM-NEGATIVE BACILLARY INFECTIONS

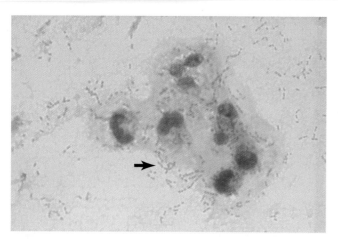

PLATE 52 Cerebrospinal fluid, drop smear, Gram stain, light microscopy, HPV. Purulence, moderate. Gram-negative coccobacilli, chains. Morphotype suggests *Bacteroides* spp. *Impression:* gram-negative bacillary meningitis.

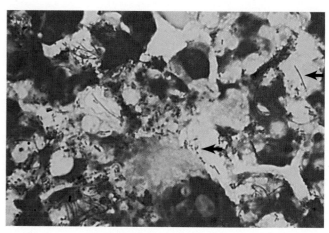

PLATE 53 Amniotic fluid, cytocentrifuge preparation, Gram stain, light microscopy, HPV. Purulence, moderate. Local materials, moderate. Gram-negative coccobacilli. Gram-negative bacilli, filamentous, medium, fusiform. Morphology suggests gram-negative bacillary anaerobic infection. *Impression:* amnionitis, mixed anaerobic bacteria.

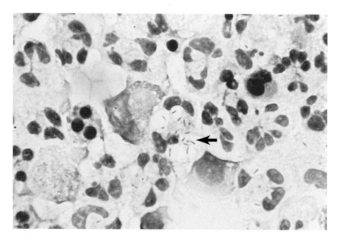

PLATE 54 Bronchoalveolar lavage, cytocentrifuge preparation, Gram stain, light microscopy, HPV. Purulence, moderate. Local materials, light. Gram-negative bacilli, small, intracellular within phagocytic vacuoles (see Plate 55).

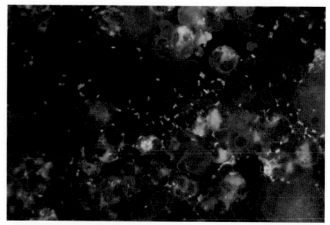

PLATE 55 Bronchoalveolar lavage, cytocentrifuge preparation, direct fluorescent antibody (DFA). *Legionella pneumophila*, polyvalent antisera, fluorescent microscopy, HPV. Immunofluorescence positive. *Impression:* Legionnaires' disease.

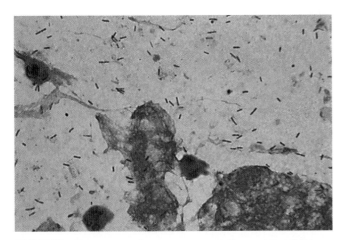

PLATE 56   Expectorated sputum, smear, Gram stain, light microscopy, MPV. Purulence, light. Local materials, light. Mucus moderate. Gram-negative bacilli, medium. *Impression:* enteric bacillary infection.

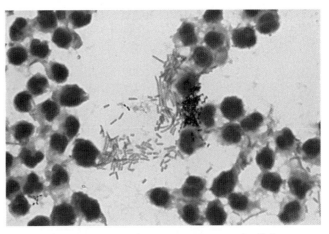

PLATE 57   Urine, direct drop smear, Gram stain, light microscopy, MPV. Purulence, heavy. Gram-negative bacilli, medium. Gram-positive cocci. Urine culture grew *Escherichia coli* and *Enterococcus faecalis.* The smear is consistent with a bacterial density of 105 colony-forming units (CFU) per milliliter of urine.

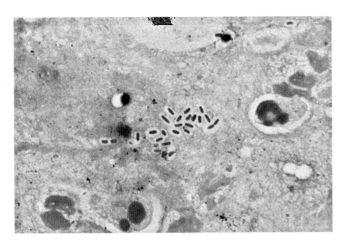

PLATE 58   Decubitus skin ulcer, smear, Gram stain, light microscopy, HPV. Purulence, moderate. Amorphous debris, heavy. Gram-negative bacilli, medium, encapsulated. Yeast. Morphology suggests *Klebsiella pneumoniae*. *Impression*: enteric bacillary disease.

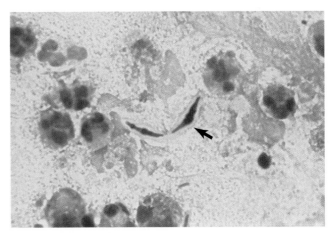

PLATE 59   Expectorated sputum, smear, Gram stain, light microscopy, HPV. Purulence, moderate. Mucus, moderate. Gram-negative bacilli, aberrant, encapsulated. Morphology suggests antibiotic-affected *Klebsiella pneumoniae.* *Impression*: enteric bacillary disease, partially treated.

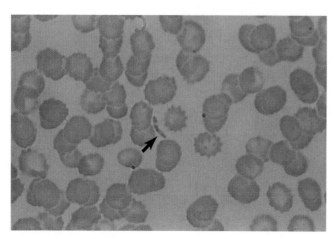

PLATE 60 Peripheral blood, smear, Wright-Giemsa stain, light microscopy MPV. Bacilli, medium, bipolar staining (see Plate 61).

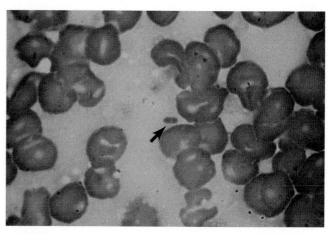

PLATE 61 Peripheral blood, smear, Gram stain, light microscopy, HPV. Local materials, moderate. Gram-negative bacillus, medium, with prominent bipolar staining. Suspicious for *Yersinia pestis*. *Impression*: bubonic plague.

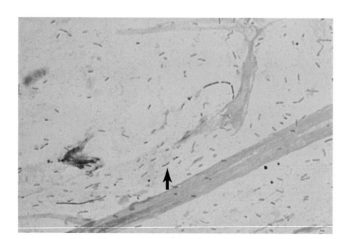

PLATE 62 Expectorated sputum, smear, Gram stain, light microscopy, HPV. Purulence, none. Local materials, none. Mucus present. Gram-negative bacilli, regular, chains. Morphotype suggests *Pseudomonas aeruginosa*. *Impression*: pseudomonas infectious disease.

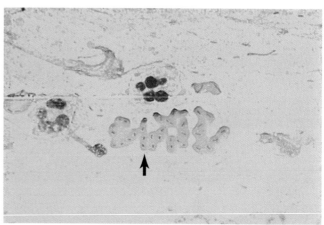

PLATE 63 Expectorated sputum, smear, Gram stain, light microscopy, HPV. Purulence, light. Local materials, none. Mucus present. Gram-negative bacilli, regular, enveloped in prominent slime layer. Morphotype suggests mucoid *P. aeruginosa*. *Impression*: pseudomonas infectious disease.

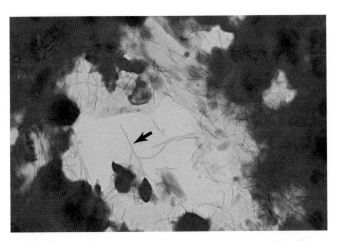

PLATE 64   Amniotic fluid, cytocentrifuge preparation, Gram stain, light microscopy, HPV. Purulence, light. Local material, moderate. Gram-negative bacilli, fusiform. Morphology suggests *Fusobacterium nucleatum*. *Impression*: amnionitis anaerobic bacteria.

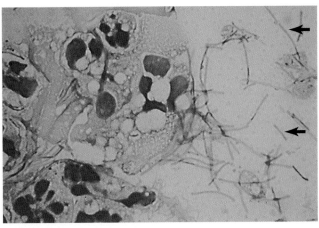

PLATE 65   Amniotic fluid, cytocentrifuge preparation, Gram stain, light microscopy, HPV. Purulence, moderate. Local material, moderate. Gram-negative bacilli, medium and long forms. Morphology suggests *Fusobacterium* spp. *Impression*: amnionitis, anaerobic bacteria.

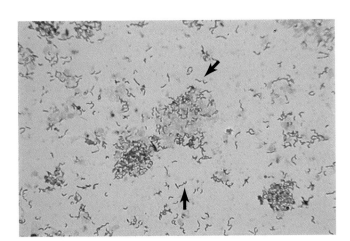

PLATE 66   Colonies on blood agar medium, subculture from blood culture, smear, Gram stain, light microscopy, HPV. Local material, light. Gram-negative bacilli with spirals, gull wings. Morphology suggests *Campylobacter* spp.

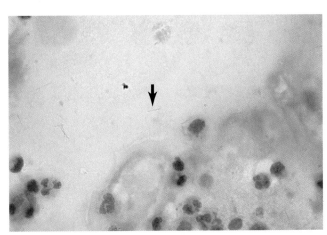

PLATE 67   Amniotic fluid, drop smear, Gram stain, light microscopy, HPV. Purulence, moderate. Local materials, moderate. Gram-negative bacilli, spiral. *Impression*: amnionitis.

DIRECT EXAMINATION IN POLYMICROBIAL INFECTIONS

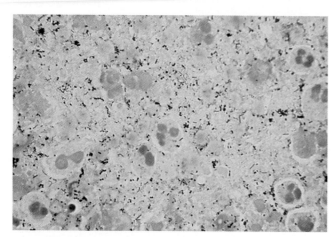

PLATE 68   Buccal space abscess, smear, Gram stain, light microscopy, HPV. Purulence, heavy. Gram-positive cocci, pairs, chains. Gram-positive bacilli, small, diphtheroid, medium, branched. Gram-negative coccobacilli. Morphology suggests polymicrobial infection from mouth flora. *Impression:* polymicrobial infection, oropharyngeal flora.

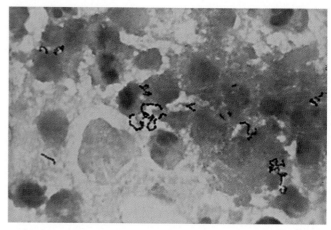

PLATE 69   Maxillary sinus aspirate, smear, Gram stain, light microscopy, HPV. Purulence, heavy. Gram-positive cocci, chains. Gram-negative coccobacilli, large masses. Morphotype suggests mixed infection with streptococci and anaerobic gram-negative coccobacilli. *Impression:* polymicrobial infection, aerobic and anaerobic species.

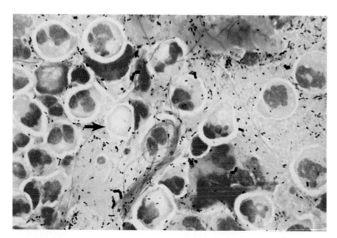

PLATE 70   Cervix, smear, conventional Gram stain, light microscopy, MPV. Purulence, heavy. Gram-positive cocci, pairs. Gram-negative coccobacilli. Gram-negative filaments. Trichomonads (*arrow; Trichomonas vaginalis;* compare with Plate 71). *Impression:* trichomoniasis with mixed aerobic and anaerobic bacterial flora.

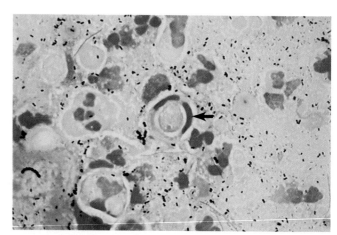

PLATE 71   Cervix, smear, enhanced Gram stain, light microscopy, MPV. Purulence, heavy. Gram-positive cocci, pairs. Gram-negative coccobacilli. Gram-negative filaments. Trichomonads (*arrow; T. vaginalis*). *Impression:* trichomoniasis with mixed aerobic and anaerobic bacterial flora.

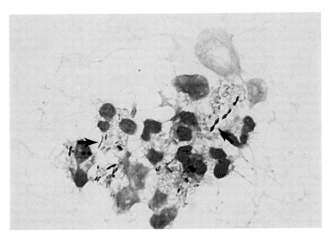

PLATE 72 Eye, vitreous aspirate, smear, Gram stain, light microscopy, MPV. Purulence, moderate. Gram-positive diplococci, encapsulated, lancet-shaped. Gram-negative bacilli, small, pleomorphic. Morphotype suggests mixed infection with *S. pneumoniae* and *H. influenzae*. *Impression:* vitritis, mixed infection.

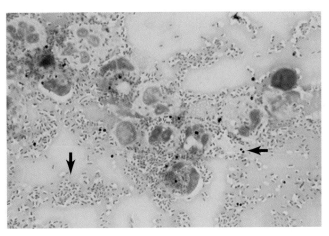

PLATE 73 Wound, smear, Gram stain, light microscopy, MPV. Purulence, heavy. Gram-negative bacilli, medium. Gram-positive cocci, pairs. *Impression:* enteric bacillary infectious disease.

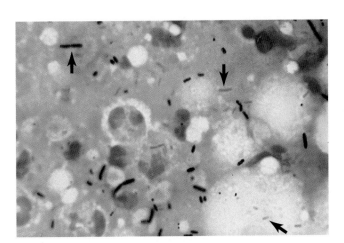

PLATE 74 Drainage, ruptured appendix, smear, light microscopy, HPV. Purulence, heavy. Gram-positive bacilli, large and medium forms. Gram-negative bacilli, small, bipolar. Gram-positive cocci. Morphology suggests polymicrobial infection with fecal flora. *Impression:* polymicrobial infection, fecal flora.

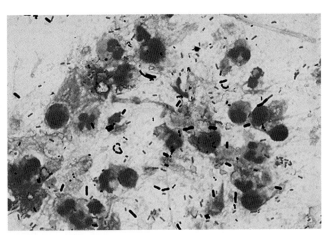

PLATE 75 Aspirated sputum, smear, Gram stain, light microscopy, MPV. Purulence, light. Local materials, light. Gram-positive bacilli, large. Gram-negative bacilli, medium, intracellular. Gram-positive cocci, pairs, chains. Morphology suggests polymicrobial infection with fecal flora. *Impression:* polymicrobial infection, fecal flora.

DIRECT EXAMINATION IN FUNGAL INFECTIONS

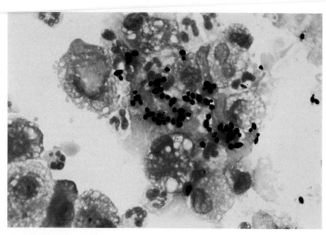

PLATE 76 BAL, cytocentrifuge preparation, Gram stain, microscopy, HPV. Purulence, light. Local materials, moderate. Gram-positive yeast with buds. Morphotype consistent with *Candida* spp. *Impression:* candidiasis.

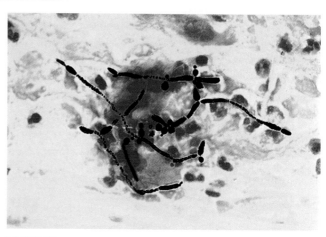

PLATE 77 Expectorated sputum smear, Gram stain, light microscopy, HPV. Purulence, light. Local materials, moderate. Gram-positive pseudohyphae. Morphotype consistent with *Candida* spp. *Impression:* candidiasis.

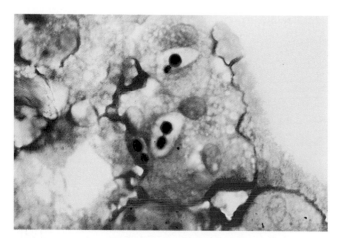

PLATE 78 BAL, cytocentrifuge preparation, Gram stain, light microscopy, HPV. Local materials, moderate. Red blood cells present. Gram-variable yeast with capsules. Morphology suggests *Cryptococcus* (see Plate 79).

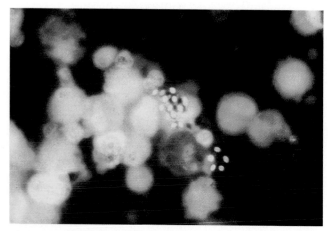

PLATE 79 BAL, cytocentrifuge preparation, calcofluor-white stain, fluorescence microscopy, HPV. Fluorescent yeast, small, with capsules. Morphology suggests *Cryptococcus neoformans*. *Impression:* cryptococcosis.

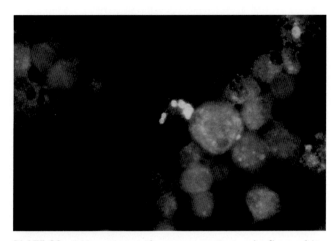

PLATE 80   BAL, cytocentrifuge preparation, calcofluor white stain, light microscopy, HPV. Fluorescent yeast (2 to 4 μm), small, budding. Morphology suggests *Histoplasma capsulatum*. *Impression:* histoplasmosis.

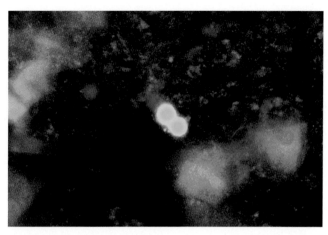

PLATE 81   Expectorated sputum, smear, calcofluor white stain, fluorescence microscopy, MPV. Yeast (8 to 20 μm), round, thick-walled, broad-based bud. Morphology suggests *Blastomyces dermatitidis*. *Impression:* blastomycosis.

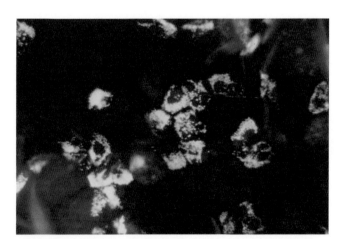

PLATE 82   Expectorated sputum, smear, calcofluor white stain, fluorescence microscopy, MPV. Eosinophils. These cells are another component that stains with calcofluor white. The granules from ruptured eosinophils stain brightly and should not be interpreted as remnants of fungi or parasites.

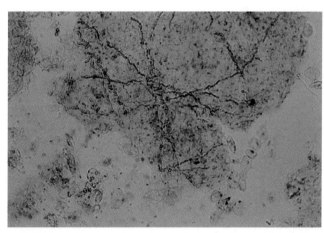

PLATE 83   Skin scales, scrapings, potassium hydroxide (KOH) wet preparation, light microscopy, HPV. Hyphae present, septate, thin. Morphology suggests dermatophyte.

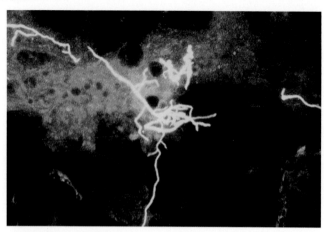

PLATE 84 Skin scales from scrapings, calcofluor white stain, fluorescence microscopy, HPV. Hyphae, thin. Morphology suggests dermatophyte. *Impression:* dermatophytosis.

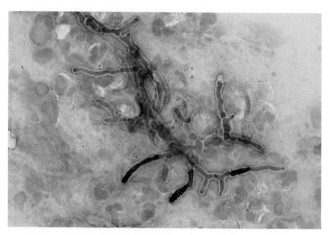

PLATE 85 Expectorated sputum, smear, Gram stain, light microscopy, HPV. Purulence, light. Local materials, heavy. Gram-variable hyphae present (3 to 10 μm), septate, branched 45-degree angle. Morphology suggests *Aspergilus* spp. (see Plate 86).

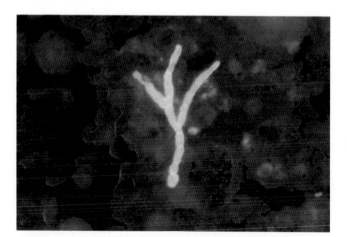

PLATE 86 Expectorated sputum, smear, calcofluor white stain, fluorescence microscopy, MPV. Fungal hyphae present (3 to 10 μm), septate, branched 45-degree angle. Morphology suggests *Aspergillus* spp. *Impression:* aspergillosis.

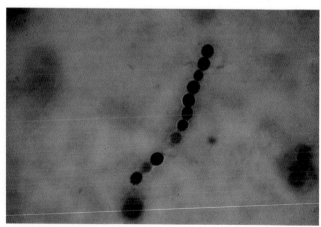

PLATE 87 Expectorated sputum, smear, Gram stain, light microscopy, HPV. Purulence, none. Local materials, moderate. Gram-positive conidia (2 to 4 μm), in chain. Morphotype suggests *Aspergillus* spp. in cavity with air interface. *Impression:* cavitary aspergillosis. Care must be taken not to mistake these conidia for streptococci or for yeast (see Plate 88).

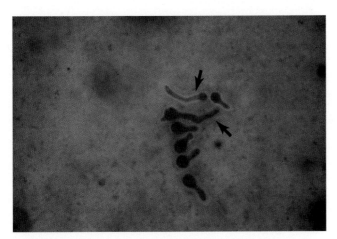

PLATE 88   Expectorated sputum, smear, Gram stain, light microscopy, HPV. Purulence, none. Local materials, moderate. Gram-negative conidia (2 to 4 μm), sporulating. Care must be taken not to confuse these conidia with yeast germ tubes.

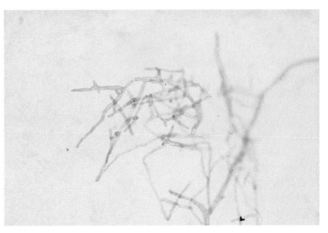

PLATE 89   Brain abscess, smear, toluidine blue stain, light microscopy, MPV. Fungal hyphae present (3 to 10 μm), septate, branched 45-degree angle. Morphology suggests *Aspergilus* spp. *Impression:* cerebral aspergillosis.

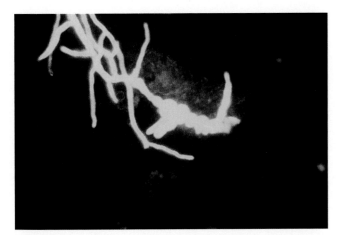

PLATE 90   Soft tissue abscess, smear, calcofluor white stain, fluorescence microscopy, HPV. Fungal hyphae, septate, branched chlamydospores. *Impression:* Mycosis.

These hyphae were not clearly visible on the Gram stain smear but stain brightly here. A dermatophyte was isolated in culture.

DIRECT EXAMINATION IN PARASITIC INFECTIONS

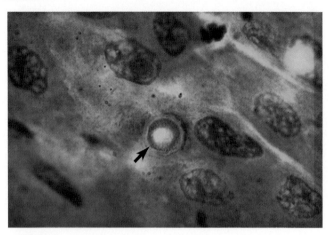

PLATE 91 Cornea, scraping, Wright-Giemsa stain, light microscopy, HPV. Purulence, none. Local materials, moderate. Parasitic precyst (13 μm). Morphology consistent with *Acanthamoeba* spp.

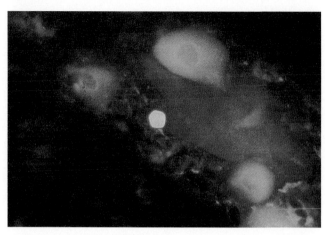

PLATE 92 Cornea, scraping from Plate 91, calcofluor white stain, fluorescence microscopy, MPV. Polyhedral parasitic cyst (13 μm). Morphology consistent with *Acanthamoeba* cyst. *Impression: Acanthamoeba* keratitis.

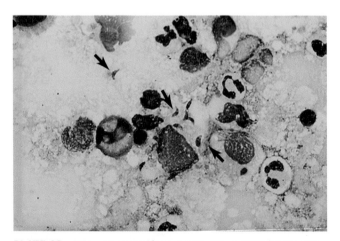

PLATE 93 BAL, cytocentrifuge preparation, Wright-Giemsa stain, light microscopy, HPV. Purulence, light. Local materials, light. Amorphous debris light. Crescent-shaped cells with central nucleus (see Plate 94).

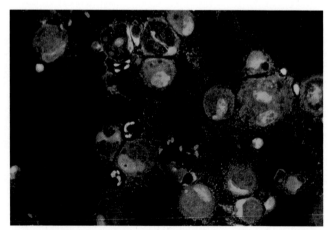

PLATE 94 BAL, cytocentrifuge preparation, acridine orange stain, fluorescence microscopy, HPV. Crescent-shaped cells composed of RNA. Morphology consistent with trophozoites (tachyzoites) of *Toxoplasma gondii*. *Impression:* toxoplasmosis.

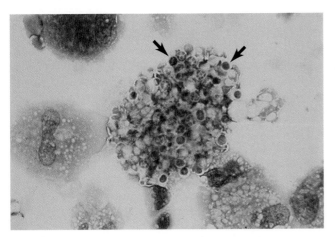

PLATE 95 BAL, cytocentrifuge preparation, Gram stain, light microscopy, HPV. Purulence, none. Local materials, moderate. Alveolar cast composed of gram-negative matrix and intracystic bodies. Morphology consistent with *Pneumocystis jiroveci* (carinii) (see Plate 96).

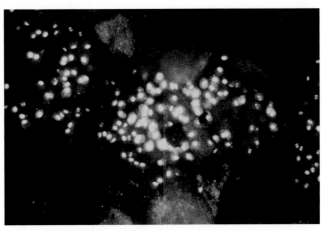

PLATE 96 BAL, cytocentrifuge preparation, calcofluor white stain, fluorescence microscopy, HPV. Fluorescent cysts with coccoid bodies. Morphology consistent with *P. jiroveci* (carinii). *Impression:* pneumocystosis.

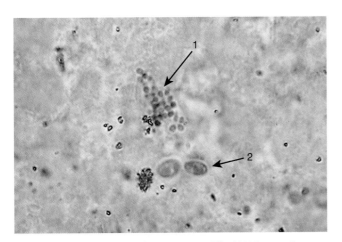

PLATE 97 Diarrheic stool, smear, modified Weber stain, light microscopy, 2000× oil. Purulence, none. Parasite spores, small (1.5 × 0.9 μm). Morphology consistent with enterocytozoon (*arrow 1*) (see Plate 98). Compare with size of the yeast (*arrow 2*).

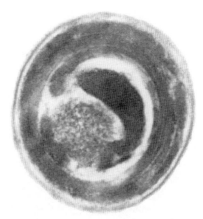

PLATE 98 Diarrheic stool from concentration, transmission electron microscopy, 57,000×. Endospore layer and polar tubes present. Morphology consistent with *Enterocytozoon bieneusi. Impression:* intestinal microsporidiosis.

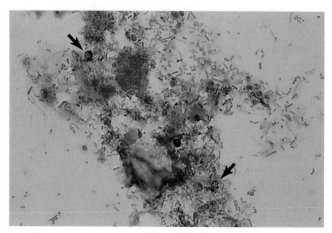

PLATE 99 Watery, frothy diarrheic stool, smear, acid-fast stain, MPV. Purulence, none. Local materials, heavy. Acid-fast oocysts (4 to 6 μm) (see Plate 100). The measurement is taken to clearly separate this oocyst from the 8 to 10 μm oocysts of *Cyclospora* spp.

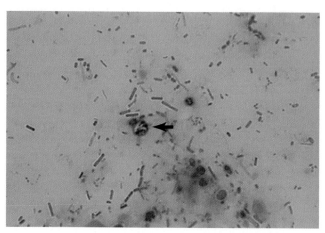

PLATE 100 Watery, frothy diarrheic stool from Plate 99, smear, acid-fast stain, HPV. Acid-fast oocysts (4 to 6 μm). Sporulated oocysts containing four sporozoites. Morphology consistent with *Cryptosporidium parvum. Impression:* cryptosporidiosis.

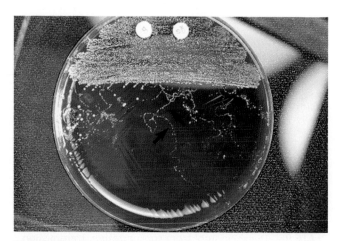

PLATE 101 Five-percent sheep blood agar plate inoculated with expectorated sputum, 24-hour incubation with 5% CO_2 in air. Note the heavy bacterial growth in the area of primary inoculation with thin trails of colonies lacing the surface of the agar (see Plate 102).

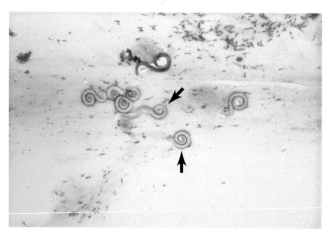

PLATE 102 Aspirated sputum, Gram stain, light microscopy, LPV. Purulence, none. Local materials, moderate. Mucus present. Coiled nematode larvae. Morphology consistent with *Strongyloides stercoralis. Impression: Strongyloides* hyperinfestation syndrome.

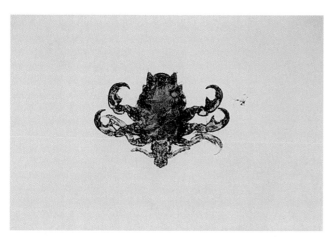

PLATE 103 Parasite, pubic hair from surgical patient, unstained mount, light microscopy, LPV. Three pairs of legs are identified with characteristic claws at tips. Morphology consistent with *Phthirus pubis* (crab louse). *Impression:* louse infestation.

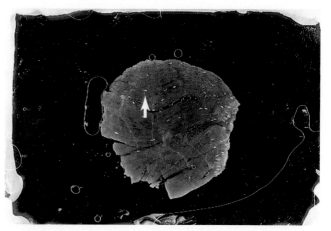

PLATE 104 Muscle tissue, directly viewed. Encysted calcified larvae. Morphology consistent with *Trichinella spiralis*. *Impression:* trichinosis.

DIRECT EXAMINATION IN VIRAL INFECTIONS

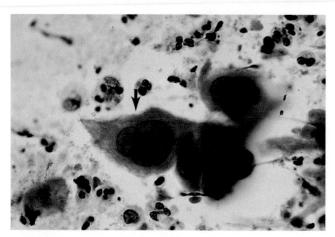

PLATE 105   Skin, vesicle fluid, Tzanck preparation, hematoxylin and eosin (H&E) stain, light microscopy, MPV. Purulence, moderate. Local materials, light. Multinucleated epithelial cells present. Intranuclear inclusions present. Morphology consistent with herpes viral inclusions. Impression: herpes simplex infection.

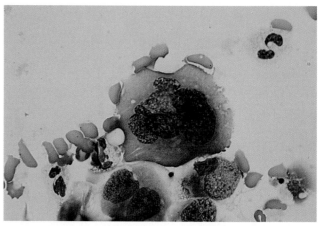

PLATE 106   BAL, cytocentrifuge preparation, rapid Wright-Giemsa stain, light microscopy, MPV. Purulence, light. Local materials, light. Red blood cells present. Multinucleated epithelial cells present. Intranuclear inclusions present. Morphology consistent with herpes viral inclusions. *Impression:* herpes simplex infection. Compare with Plate 105. Note the change in appearance of the herpes-infected cells with the change in the type of fixation and stain. The H&E stain more clearly shows the "ground-glass" appearance of the nuclear inclusion rimmed by the cell nuclear chromatin. The rapid Wright's stain provides an adequate visual presentation and is more time efficient.

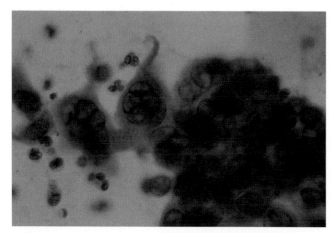

PLATE 107   Skin, vesicle fluid, Tzanck preparation, Wright-Giemsa stain, light microscopy, HPV. Purulence, light. Multinucleated epithelial cells present. Intranuclear inclusions present. Morphology consistent with herpes viral inclusions. *Impression:* varicella-zoster infection.

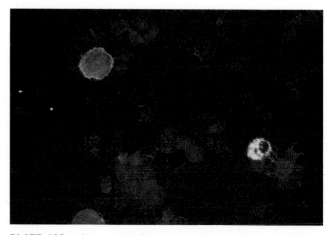

PLATE 108   Skin, vesicle fluid, Tzanck preparation, antibody stain for herpes simplex virus, fluorescent microscopy, MPV. Immunostaining positive. Herpes simplex infection, confirmed.

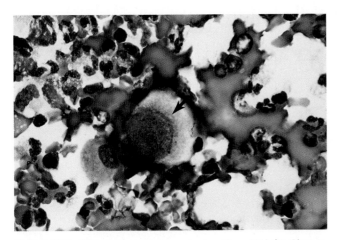

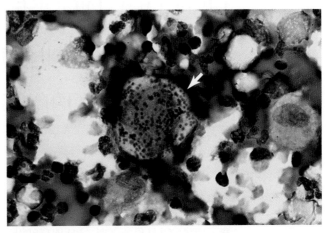

PLATE 109 BAL, cytocentrifuge preparation, Wright-Giemsa stain, light microscopy, MPV. Purulence, light. Blood, moderate. Local materials, light. Enlarged pneumocyte with intranuclear inclusion. Morphology consistent with cytomegalovirus. Observe the characteristic nuclear changes for cytomegalovirus. The cell and the nucleus are enlarged, the nucleus is granular, and the nuclear membrane is indistinct. Blood is an indication of capillary damage. *Impression:* cytomegalovirus disease.

PLATE 110 BAL, cytocentrifuge preparation, Wright/Giemsa stain, light microscopy, MPV. Purulence, light. Blood, moderate. Local materials, light. Enlarged pneumocyte with intracytoplasmic inclusions. Morphology consistent with cytomegalovirus. The large, regular-sized, magenta cytoplasmic viral inclusions, when present, are characteristic of this virus. *Impression:* cytomegalovirus disease.

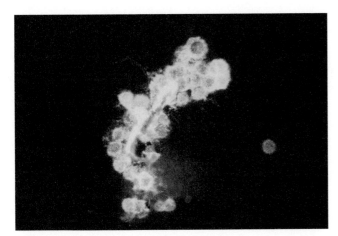

PLATE 111 BAL, cytocentrifuge preparation, immunofluorescent antibody adenovirus stain, fluorescence microscopy, HPV. Prominent specific fluorescent staining of infected cells. *Impression:* adenovirus infection. The necrosis and cellular debris associated with adenovirus within the bronchi can be easily overlooked because the necrotic, virus-infected "smudge" cells may not be recognized. Specific immunostaining should be performed on the basis of clinical suspicion and compatible background material.

Use of Colonial Morphology for the Presumptive Identification of Microorganisms

George Manuselis

- ■ IMPORTANCE OF COLONIAL MORPHOLOGY AS A DIAGNOSTIC TOOL
- ■ INITIAL OBSERVATION AND INTERPRETATION OF CULTURES
- ■ GROSS COLONY CHARACTERISTICS USED TO DIFFERENTIATE AND PRESUMPTIVELY IDENTIFY MICROORGANISMS
  Hemolysis
  Size

Form or Margin
Elevation
Density
Color
Consistency
Pigment
Odor

- ■ COLONIES WITH MULTIPLE CHARACTERISTICS
- ■ GROWTH OF ORGANISMS IN LIQUID MEDIA

OBJECTIVES

After reading and studying this chapter, you should be able to:

1. Describe how growth on blood, chocolate, and MacConkey agars is used in the preliminary identification of isolates.

2. Differentiate α-hemolysis from β-hemolysis.

3. Describe how gross colony characteristics are used in the presumptive identification of microorganisms.

4. Using colonial morphology, differentiate among the following microorganisms:

- ■ Staphylococci and streptococci
- ■ *Streptococcus agalactiae* and *Streptococcus pyogenes*
- ■ α-Hemolytic *Streptococcus* spp. and *Streptococcus pneumoniae*
- ■ *Neisseria* spp. and staphylococci
- ■ Yeast and staphylococci
- ■ "Diphtheroids" and staphylococci
- ■ Lactose fermenters from lactose nonfermenters
- ■ "Swarming" *Proteus* species from other Enterobacteriaceae

Case in Point

An exudate from a sacral decubital ulcer on a 65-year-old hospital inpatient was cultured on blood agar plate (BAP), chocolate, and MacConkey (MAC) agars. Direct smear examination showed many white blood cells, a moderate number of gram-positive cocci in pairs and clusters, and a few gram-negative bacilli. After overnight incubation, three colony morphotypes were visible on the BAP. The first was a moderate growth of a medium-sized β-hemolytic, which was yellowish white and creamy-buttery looking. The second colony was also β-hemolytic but larger, mucoid, and gray. The third type of colony was large, gray, and mucoid like the second but was nonhemolytic. The MAC agar showed two colony morphotypes, a light growth of dark pink, dry-looking colonies with a surrounding pink precipitate and a few clear nonlactose fermenting colonies. Based on the Gram stain results and colonial characteristics of the isolates, appropriate biochemical tests and antibiotic susceptibilities were performed to identify the causative agents of the ulcer.

Issues to Consider

After reading the patient's history, consider the following:

- The role of colony morphology in the presumptive identification of microorganisms
- How each component of colony morphology can help differentiate between pathogenic and nonpathogenic microorganisms

Key Terms

α-Hemolysis
β-Hemolysis
Brittle
Butyrous
Colonial morphology
Consistency
Creamy
Density
Elevation
Escherichia/Citrobacter-like organisms
Fastidious
Filamentous
Form
Hemolysis
Klebsiella/Enterobacter-like organisms

Lactose fermenter
Margin
Nonlactose fermenter (NLF)
Opaque
Pigment
Rhizoid
Smooth
Streamers
Swarming
Transillumination
Translucent
Transparent
Turbidity
Umbilicate
Umbonate

The mastery of **colonial morphology** (colony characteristics and **form**) and interpretation of Gram-stained smears from clinical specimens and microbial colonies cannot be overemphasized. Although Gram-stained smears provide initial identification of microorganisms by microscopic characterization, the physical growth characteristics of microorganisms on certain types of laboratory media facilitate description of colonial morphology for their identification processes.

Close your eyes and imagine the physical characteristics of a parent, relative, or friend. The height, weight, shape, color or style of hair, eyes, freckles, color of skin, and even the voice or laugh may make people distinctive even in a crowd or when their backs are facing you. In the same manner, many specific microorganisms have characteristics that distinguish them in a crowd of other genera or species.

This chapter explains how the characterization of colonies on culture media facilitates presumptive identification of commonly isolated organisms. It discusses the characteristics that are used to describe colony morphology of certain groups of organisms and how these characteristics are used to differentiate one species from a closely related species and one genus from another.

IMPORTANCE OF COLONIAL MORPHOLOGY AS A DIAGNOSTIC TOOL

In many ways, the usefulness of colonial morphology extends the capabilities of the microbiologist and, ultimately, the clinical laboratory. The ability to provide a presumptive identification by colonial morphology may include the following:

- **Provide a presumptive identification to the physician.** Even in this age of rapid identification systems, incubation times and procedures can be protracted. In a critical situation, the microbiologist makes an educated judgment about the presumptive identity before performing diagnostic procedures.
- **Enhance the quality of patient care through rapid reporting of results and by increasing this cost-effectiveness of laboratory testing.** This may best be illustrated by using sputum cultures as an example. Because the upper respiratory tract contains many indigenous organisms, to identify every organism in culture would be a time-consuming, cost-prohibitive, and insurmountable task. Microbiologists must be able to differentiate potential pathogens from the "usual" inhabitants of the upper respiratory tract and direct the diagnostic workup toward only potential pathogens. Moreover, potential pathogens are presumptively identified by colonial characteristics, and preliminary reporting initiates immediate therapy.
- **Play a significant role in quality control, especially of automated procedures and other commercially available identification systems.** When commercial and automated systems are used, a mixed inoculum (polymicrobic/containing more than one genus and species or both) will produce biochemical test results or erroneous interpretation of reactions that significantly alters the identification (see Chapter 9). The ability of the microbiologist to determine whether the inoculum is mixed and to ascertain whether the results generated by a commercial or automated system correlate with the suspected identification of the organism is an important component of quality control that is accomplished by recognizing organisms by their colonial characteristics.

INITIAL OBSERVATION AND INTERPRETATION OF CULTURES

Generally, microbiologists observe the colonial morphology of organisms isolated on primary culture after 18 to 24 hours of incubation. Incubation time may certainly vary according to when the specimen is received and processed in the laboratory, which may affect the "typical" morphology of a certain isolate. For example, young cultures of *Staphylococcus aureus* may appear smaller and may not show the distinct β-hemolysis that older cultures produce. In addition, the microbiologist must be aware of factors that may significantly alter the colonial morphology of growing microorganisms. These factors include the medium's ingredients, its inhibitory nature, and antibiotics present in the medium.

The interpretation of primary cultures, commonly referred to as *plate reading,* is actually a comparative examination of microorganisms growing on a variety of culture media. Many specimens, such as sputum and wounds that arrive in the clinical laboratory, are plated on blood agar (BAP), chocolate agar (CHOC), and MacConkey (MAC). Each type of agar plate is examined in relationship to the other. Therefore, as a culture set from a specimen, growth on these three culture media illustrates the comparative colonial examination of plate reading.

First, the ability to determine which organisms grow on selective and nonselective media aids the microbiologist in making an initial distinction between gram-positive and gram-negative isolates. The BAP and CHOC support the growth of a variety of **fastidious** (hard to grow, requires additional growth factors) and nonfastidious organisms, gram-positive bacteria, and gram-negative bacteria. As illustrated in the Case in Point, three colony morphotypes were observed on BAP. Because the gram-stained smear showed both gram-positive and gram-negative bacteria, three types of organisms should be observed on a nonselective medium such as BAP.

Generally, organisms that grow on BAP will also grow on CHOC, but not all organisms that grow on CHOC will grow on BAP. Although BAP supports fastidious organisms, highly fastidious species such as *Haemophilus* species and *Neisseria gonorrhoeae* do not grow on it. Chocolate agar provides nutritional growth requirements to support highly fastidious organisms such as *Haemophilus* species and *N. gonorrhoeae*. Therefore a gram-negative bacillus that grows on CHOC but not on BAP or MAC will be suspected to be *Haemophilus* species, whereas gram-negative diplococci with the same growth pattern will be suspected to be *N. gonorrhoeae* (Figure 8-1). The microbiologist then is able to provide a presumptive identification and determine how to proceed in identifying the isolated organisms.

Second, MAC agar, which inhibits gram-positive organisms and some fastidious gram-negative organisms, such as *Haemophilus* and *Neisseria* species, supports most gram-negative rods, especially the Enterobacteriaceae. Growth on BAP and CHOC but not on MAC, therefore, is indicative of a gram-positive isolate or of a fastidious gram-negative bacillus or coccus.

Gram-negative rods are better described on MAC agar because these organisms produce similar-looking colonies on

BAP and CHOC media: large, gray, and mucoid. Remember true hemolysis is not seen on CHOC. MAC is best used, however, to differentiate **lactose fermenters** from **nonlactose fermenters** (NLFs). Lactose fermenters are easily detected by the color change they produce on the media; as the pH changes when lactose is fermented, the organisms produce pink, dark pink, or red colonies (Figure 8-2, *A*). Again, in the Case in Point presented, dry, dark pink colonies were observed on MAC agar, indicating the presence of a lactose-fermenting, gram-negative rod. Colonies of nonfermenters remain clear and colorless (Figure 8-2, *B*). This differentiation is particularly important in screening for enteric pathogens from stool cultures. Most enteric pathogens do not ferment lactose.

Certain enteric pathogens produce a characteristic colony on MAC that is helpful in presumptive identification. *Escherichial Citrobacter*-**like organisms,** as seen in the Case in Point, produce a dry, pink colony with a surrounding "halo" of pink, precipitated bile salts (Figure 8-3). *Klebsiellal Enterobacter-*

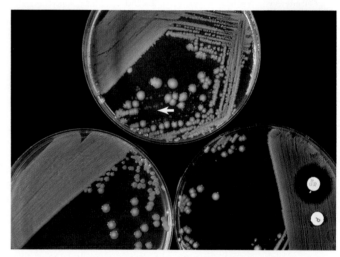

Figure 8-1 Clockwise from the top: chocolate agar (CHOC), blood agar (BAP), MacConkey agar (MAC). The large colonies growing on all three plates are gram-negative rods (enterics). These gram-negative rods grow larger, gray, and mucoid on BAP and CHOC. Notice the smaller grayish-brown fastidious colonies of *Haemophilus* organisms growing on CHOC *(arrow)*, which are not growing on BAP or MAC.

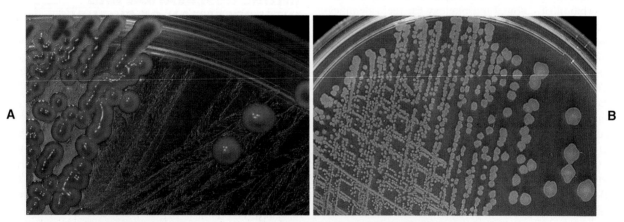

Figure 8-2 **A,** Example of lactose-fermenting gram-negative rods producing pink colonies on MacConkey agar (MAC). **B,** Example of nonlactose-fermenting gram-negative rods producing colorless colonies on MAC.

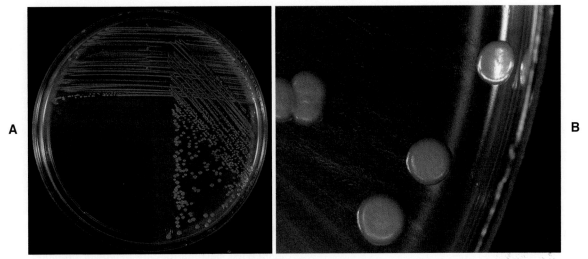

Figure 8-3   A, Lactose-fermenting *Escherichia/Citrobacter*-like organisms growing on MacConkey agar (MAC). Notice the dry appearance of the colony and the pink precipitate of bile salts extending beyond the periphery of the colonies. **B,** Close-up of dry, flat *Escherichia/Citrobacter*-like lactose fermenters growing on MAC. Compare with Figure 8-4, *B*.

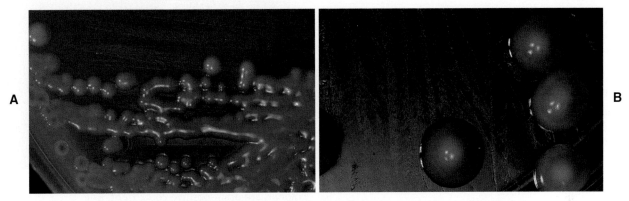

Figure 8-4   A, *Klebsiella/Enterobacter*-like lactose fermenters growing on MacConkey agar (MAC). Notice the pink, heaped, mucoid appearance. **B,** Close-up of *Klebsiella/Enterobacter*-like colonies on MAC. Notice the mucoid, heaped appearance and the slightly cream-colored center after 48 hours' growth.

like organisms produce large, mucoid pink colonies that occasionally have cream-colored centers (Figure 8-4).

Microorganisms grow on culture media in the same proportion or concentration in which they are present in the clinical specimen. Because many specimens are polymicrobic, this trait can be beneficial in identifying different colony types. The reader should remember that this is a comparative analysis of the growth on the three types of culture media.

GROSS COLONY CHARACTERISTICS USED TO DIFFERENTIATE AND PRESUMPTIVELY IDENTIFY MICROORGANISMS

By observing the colonial characteristics of the organisms that have been isolated, the microbiologist is able to make an educated guess regarding the identification of the isolate. The following descriptions are routinely used to examine colony characteristics. It is important to remember that many of the following colony characteristics may vary among species and strains of the same genus.

Hemolysis

On blood agar, **hemolysis** (Gr: *lysis,* dissolution or break apart; *hemo,* pertaining to red blood cells [RBCs]) is a reaction caused especially by enzymatic or toxin activity of bacteria, observed in the media immediately surrounding or underneath the colony. Often the colony has to be removed with a loop to visualize the hemolytic pattern. Hemolysis on blood agar is helpful in the presumptive identification, particularly of streptococci. Hemolysis (e.g., α, β, or no hemolysis with other colony characteristics) can be variable for streptococci and *Enterococcus* (see Chapter 15). It is important to determine whether true hemolysis is present or whether discoloration of the media is the result of growth of the organism on the plate. Proper technique requires the passing of bright light through the bottom of the plate **(transillumination)** to determine whether the organism is hemolytic (Figure 8-5). Many organisms have no lytic effect on the RBCs in

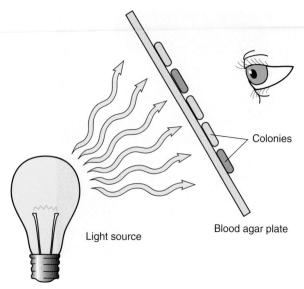

Figure 8-5 The use of transillumination to determine whether the colonies are hemolytic. The technique can be used for MacConkey agar also to see slight color differences in nonlactose fermenters.

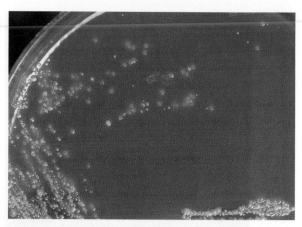

Figure 8-6 Chocolate agar (CHOC) does not display true hemolysis because the red cells in the medium have already been lysed. Bacteria that are hemolytic on blood agar plate usually are green around the colony on CHOC.

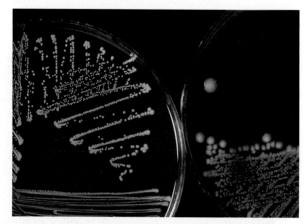

Figure 8-7 *Left,* Blood agar plate (BAP): small white colonies are gram-positive cocci; *right,* BAP: large, gray, mucoid colonies are enteric gram-negative rods.

the BAP and are referred to as *gamma (γ)-hemolytic* or *-nonhemolytic.* Although there are many types of hemolysis, only α-hemolysis and β-hemolysis are illustrated in this chapter.

α-Hemolysis

α-Hemolysis is partial lysing of erythrocytes in a BAP around and under the colony that results in a green discoloration of the medium. Examples of organisms that produce α-hemolysis include *Streptococcus pneumoniae* and certain viridans streptococci. (For a comparison of the colonial morphology of these two organisms, see Figure 8-24.)

β-Hemolysis

β-Hemolysis is complete clearing of erythrocytes in a BAP around or under the colonies because of the complete lysis of RBCs. Certain organisms, such as group A β-hemolytic streptococci *(Streptococcus pyogenes),* produce a wide, deep, clear zone of β-hemolysis, whereas others, such as group B β-hemolytic streptococci *(Streptococcus agalactiae)* and *Listeria monocytogenes* (a short, gram-positive rod) produce a narrow, diffuse zone of β-hemolysis close to the colony. These features are helpful hints in the identification of certain species of bacteria. (For a comparison of the colonial characteristics of group A and group B streptococci, see Figure 8-25.) Chocolate agar does not display true hemolysis, because the red cells in the medium have already been lysed. Organisms that are α-hemolytic or β-hemolytic on BAP usually show a green coloration around the colony on CHOC (Figure 8-6). This coloration, however, should not be mistaken for a hemolytic characteristic.

Size

Colonies are described as large, medium, small, or pinpoint. Rarely, however, does a microbiologist take a ruler and actually measure a colony. Size is generally a visual comparison

between genera or species. For example, gram-positive bacteria, in general, produce smaller colonies than gram-negative bacteria. *Staphylococcus* species are usually larger than *Streptococcus* species. Figure 8-7 shows colonies of gram-negative rods in comparison with gram-positive cocci.

Form or Margin

The edge of the colonies should be observed and the form, or **margin,** described as **smooth, filamentous,** rough or **rhizoid,** or irregular (Figure 8-8). Colonies of *Bacillus anthracis* on visual examination are described as "Medusa heads" because of the filamentous appearance. Certain genera such as *Proteus* species (especially the species *Proteus mirabilis* and *Proteus vulgaris*), may swarm on nonselective agar such as blood or chocolate. **Swarming** is a hazy blanket of growth on the surface that extends well beyond the streak lines. Figure 8-9 shows swarming colonies of *Proteus* spp. Diphtheroids produce colonies that have rough edges (Figure 8-10), whereas certain yeast produce colonies that are described as stars or colonies with feet or pedicles. (For a comparison of the colonial morphology of yeast and staphylococci, see Figure 8-26.)

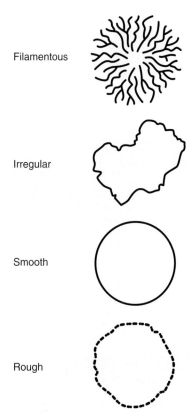

Filamentous

Irregular

Smooth

Rough

Figure 8-8   Illustration of form or margin to describe colonial morphology.

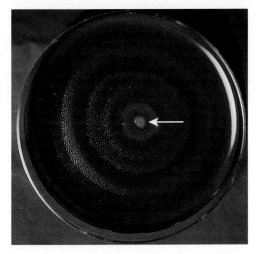

Figure 8-9   Swarming colonies of *Proteus* spp. The organism was inoculated in the middle of the blood agar plate (*arrow*).

Elevation

The **elevation** should be determined by tilting the culture plate and looking at the side of the colony (Figure 8-11). Elevation may be raised, convex, flat, **umbilicate** (depressed center, concave, an "innie"), or **umbonate** (raised or bulging center, convex, an "outie"). *S. pneumoniae* typically produces umbilicate colonies unless the colonies are mucoid because of the presence of polysaccharide capsule. *S. aureus* typically pro-

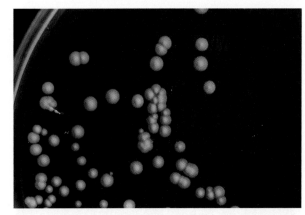

Figure 8-10   "Diphtheroid" colonies with rough edges, dry appearance, and umbonate center growing on blood agar.

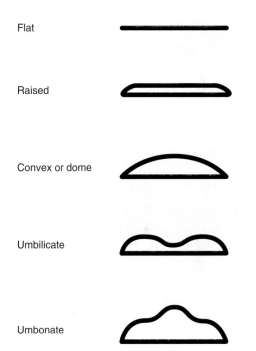

Flat

Raised

Convex or dome

Umbilicate

Umbonate

Figure 8-11   Illustration of elevations to describe colonial morphology.

duces convex colonies. In comparison, β-hemolytic streptococci generally produce flat colonies.

Density

The **density** of the colony can be **transparent, translucent,** or **opaque.** To see the differences in the density of colonies, it is useful to look through the colony while using transillumination. Translucent colonies allow some light to pass through the colony, and opaque colonies do not (Figure 8-12). β-Hemolytic streptococci, except group B *(S. agalactiae),* are described as translucent. *S. agalactiae* produces colonies that are semi-opaque, with the organisms concentrated at the center of the colony, sometimes described as a bull's-eye colony. Staphylococci and other gram-positive bacteria are usually opaque. Most gram-negative rods are also opaque.

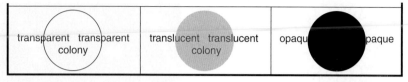

Figure 8-12 Density.

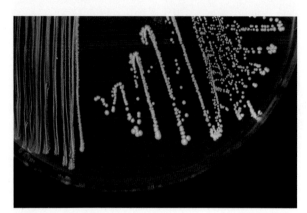

Figure 8-13 Example of white colonies of coagulase-negative staphylococci on blood agar.

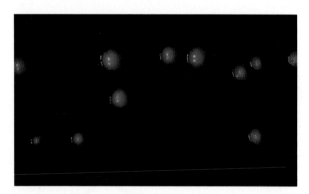

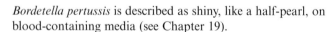

Figure 8-14 Example of the yellow colonies characteristic of certain nonpathogenic species of *Neisseria* organisms on blood agar.

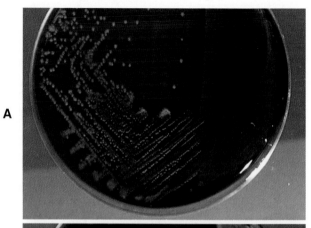

A

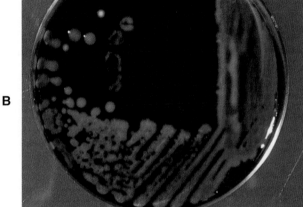

B

Figure 8-15 **A,** *Pseudomonas aeruginosa* illustrating the metallic sheen and green pigmentation of colonies on blood agar plate (BAP). **B,** Not all strains of the same organism have the same colonial appearance. This is a mucoid strain of *P. aeruginosa* on BAP.

Bordetella pertussis is described as shiny, like a half-pearl, on blood-containing media (see Chapter 19).

Color

Color, in contrast to pigmentation, is a term used to describe in general a particular genus. Colonies may be white, gray, yellow, or buff. Coagulase-negative staphylococci are white (Figure 8-13), whereas *Enterococcus* spp. may appear gray. Certain Micrococcus species and *Neisseria* (nonpathogenic) species are yellow or off-white (Figure 8-14). "Diphtheroids" are buff. Most gram-negative rods are gray on BAP.

Consistency

Consistency is determined by touching the colony with a sterile loop. Colony consistency may be **brittle** (splinters), **creamy (butyrous),** dry, or waxy; occasionally, the entire colony adheres (sticks) to the loop. *S. aureus* is creamy, whereas certain *Neisseria* spp. are sticky. *Nocardia* spp. produce colonies that are brittle, crumbly, and wrinkled, resembling bread crumbs on a plate. Diphtheroid colonies are usually dry and waxy. Most β-hemolytic streptococci are dry (except for mucoid types), and when pushed by a loop, the whole colony remains intact.

Pigment

Pigment production is an inherent characteristic of a specific organism confined generally to the colony. Examples of organisms that produce pigment include the following:

- *P. aeruginosa*—green, sometimes a metallic sheen (Figure 8-15)
- *Serratia marcescens*—brick-red (Figure 8-16), especially at room temperature

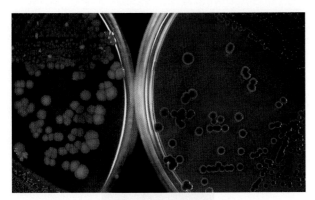

Figure 8-16 Brick-red pigment of *Serratia marcescens*, which is evident on the MacConkey agar (*right*). This brick-red pigment should not be confused with lactose fermentation. The pigment is slightly visible on chocolate agar (*left*). Additional incubation at room temperature enhances the brick-red pigmentation.

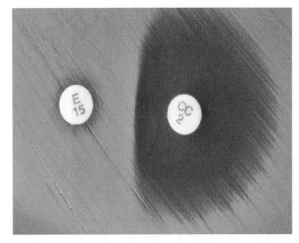

Figure 8-17 Large, rough, greenish-appearing, hemolytic colonies of *Bacillus cereus* on blood agar plate.

- *Kluyvera* spp.—blue
- *Chromobacterium violaceum*—purple
- *Prevotella melaninogenica*—brown-black (anaerobic)
  Pigment production for these organisms is variable.

Odor

Odor should be determined when the lid of the culture plate is removed and its odor dissipates into the surrounding environment. Never inhale directly from the plate. Examples of microorganisms that produce distinctive odors include the following:

- *S. aureus*—old sock (stocking that has been worn continuously for a few days without washing); this odor is evident when growing on mannitol salt agar
- *P. aeruginosa*—fruity or grape-like
- *P. mirabilis*—putrid
- *Haemophilus* spp.—musty basement, "mousy" or "mouse nest" smell
- *Nocardia* spp.—freshly plowed field

The Case in Point illustrates the sequential deductive reasoning that occurs during "plate reading" of the culture, the direct smear of the clinical specimen, and colony morphology. Both techniques play an important role in the presumptive identification required in plate reading. The first step is to examine the direct smear of the specimen for important clues, for example, the presence of white blood cells (WBCs; an inflammatory process) and specific Gram-stain morphology. Gram-positive cocci in pairs and clusters in the direct smear are suggestive of staphylococci (see Chapter 7), whereas the enteric gram-negative bacilli are difficult to distinguish between. The β-hemolytic, which is white with a light yellow tinge, creamy-butter–looking, medium colonies on BAP are highly suggestive of *S. aureus* (see Figure 8-26, *B*). *S. aureus* would be inhibited by MAC and would not grow, leaving the other two colony types to identify. The lactose fermenter (pink) on MAC with a halo of pink precipitate surrounding the colonies is indicative of *Escherichia/Citrobacter*-like organisms. Of these two, *Escherichia coli* can be β-hemolytic on BAP (see Chapter 19). The NLF is the third type of colony

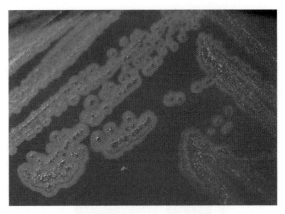

Figure 8-18 Small, "fuzzy-edged," umbonate center-appearing colony of *Eikenella corrodens* on chocolate agar. This organism has the tendency to "pit" the agar.

present in the clinical specimen. Both the lactose fermenters and nonlactose fermenters are growing on the BAP because this medium is noninhibitory but is best differentiated on MAC.

COLONIES WITH MULTIPLE CHARACTERISTICS

In addition to the organisms already mentioned, other bacteria fit in multiple descriptive categories of colonial morphology. *Bacillus cereus* forms large, rough, greenish, hemolytic colonies on BAP (Figure 8-17). *Eikenella corrodens* forms a small, "fuzzy-edged" colony with an umbonate center on BAP or CHOC (Figure 8-18).

GROWTH OF ORGANISMS IN LIQUID MEDIA

Important clues to an organism's identification can also be detected by observing the growth of the organism in liquid media such as thioglycollate. **Streamers** or vines and puffballs

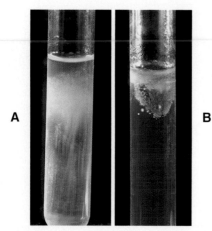

Figure 8-19 **A,** "Vine" or "streamer" effect exhibited by certain species of streptococci when growing in thioglycollate. Notice that the effect is more prevalent toward the bottom of the tube. **B,** Example of the "puffed balls" effect exhibited by certain streptococcal species when growing in thioglycollate.

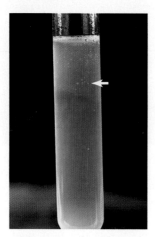

Figure 8-20 Turbidity produced by enterics when growing in thioglycollate. Notice the gas bubbles at the surface of and in the middle of the medium *(arrow)*.

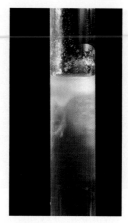

Figure 8-21 Production of "scum" by yeast at the surface of the thioglycollate.

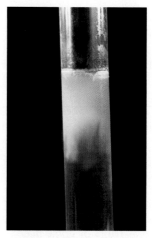

Figure 8-22 Illustration of *Pseudomonas* organisms producing surface "scum" at the sides of the thioglycollate. Occasionally *Pseudomonas aeruginosa* produces a diffusible green pigment and a metallic sheen at the surface.

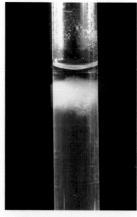

Figure 8-23 Yeast growing in the microaerophilic area of thioglycollate.

are associated with certain species of streptococci (Figure 8-19). **Turbidity,** which refers to as cloudiness of the medium resulting from growth (and usually gas if the media contains glucose), is produced by many Enterobacteriaceae (Figure 8-20). Yeast and *Pseudomonas* species produce scum at the sides of the tube (Figures 8-21 and 8-22). In addition, yeast occasionally grows below the surface, in the microaerophilic area of the media (Figure 8-23).

Figures 8-24, *A* and *B* (*S. pneumoniae,* and α-hemolytic streptococci); 8-24, *C* (*Enterococcus* spp., see Chapter 15); 8-25 (*S. pyogenes* and *S. agalactiae*); and 8-26 (staphylococci and yeast) show the differences between various organisms by colonial morphology.

Differentiation of **streptococcus pneumoniae,** α-hemolytic viridans streptococci, and Enterococcus by colonial morphology

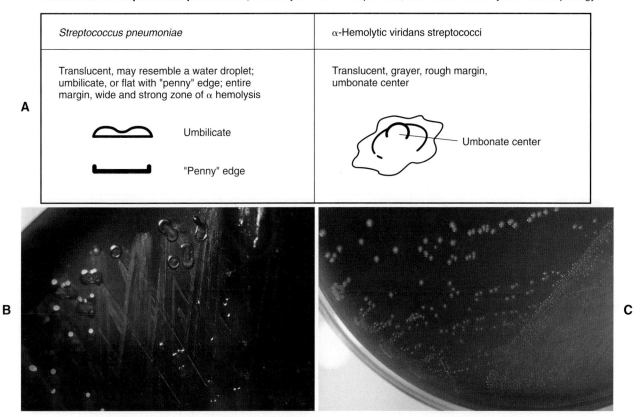

Streptococcus pneumoniae	α-Hemolytic viridans streptococci
Translucent, may resemble a water droplet; umbilicate, or flat with "penny" edge; entire margin, wide and strong zone of α hemolysis	Translucent, grayer, rough margin, umbonate center

A

Umbilicate

"Penny" edge

Umbonate center

B

C

Figure 8-24   A, Differentiation of *Streptococcus pneumoniae* and α-hemolytic viridans streptococci by colonial morphology. **B,** *S. pneumoniae* growing on blood agar plate (BAP). Notice the strong zone of α-hemolysis, umbilicate center, and wet (mucoid) appearance of the colonies. **C,** *Enterococcus* growing on BAP. It does not have an umbilicate or umbonate center, but it is more heaped and gray-appearing than *S. pneumoniae.* Enterococci have larger colonies, and a smooth, darker margin, unlike many strains of α-hemolytic streptococci. The green color on the plate is not hemolysis but is a characteristic of growth.

Microbiologists might become frustrated when changes in colony morphology, Gram staining, and biochemical reactions occur in microorganisms that produce characteristic features. Many times, organisms exhibit characteristics far different from those previously described for them. The ability to recognize these differences and changes in characteristics makes this discipline a challenge.

BIBLIOGRAPHY

LeBeau LJ: Effective lighting systems for photography of microbial colonies, *J Biol Photogr Assoc* 44:4, 1976.

Points to Remember

- The colonial morphology described in this chapter is not infallible. Variations do occur quite frequently. Therefore the morphologies described are general characteristics for any given organism.
- The identification process must include Gram stain and biochemical reactions in addition to colonial morphology.

- Gram stain of the colony from the culture plate may look different from the direct smear from the specimen itself. Competition, crowding, and metabolic byproducts may alter the Gram stain microscopic morphology. For example, in contrast to the direct smear or liquid media, streptococci may not appear as positive cocci in chains from the colony.

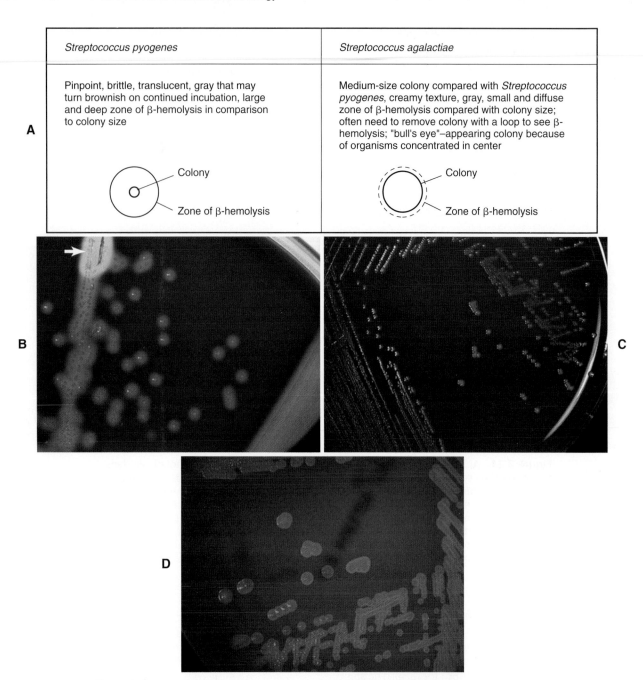

Streptococcus pyogenes	Streptococcus agalactiae
Pinpoint, brittle, translucent, gray that may turn brownish on continued incubation, large and deep zone of β-hemolysis in comparison to colony size	Medium-size colony compared with Streptococcus pyogenes, creamy texture, gray, small and diffuse zone of β-hemolysis compared with colony size; often need to remove colony with a loop to see β-hemolysis; "bull's eye"–appearing colony because of organisms concentrated in center

Figure 8-25 A, Differentiation of *Streptococcus pyogenes* and *Streptococcus agalactiae* by colonial morphology. **B,** Pinpoint colony of *S. pyogenes* exhibiting large, deep zone of β-hemolysis on blood agar plate (BAP). **C,** Colonies of *S. agalactiae* growing on BAP. This organism produces a larger colony and a smaller, more diffuse zone of hemolysis than *S. pyogenes.* Notice that the hemolysis is not evident in this photograph. Compare with **B. D,** Colonies of *S. agalactiae* growing on BAP. Through the use of transillumination, the hemolytic pattern is now evident; hemolysis is diffuse, and it remains close to the periphery of the colony. The same colonial morphology is produced by *Listeria monocytogenes*, a gram-positive rod. Compare with **B.** *Arrow: S. pyogenes* produces two hemolysins; one is oxygen stabile (S), and the other is oxygen labile (O). Stabbing the medium with an inoculating loop carries the organism into areas where anaerobic conditions are more prevalent, allowing the enhanced hemolysin (O) to be seen.

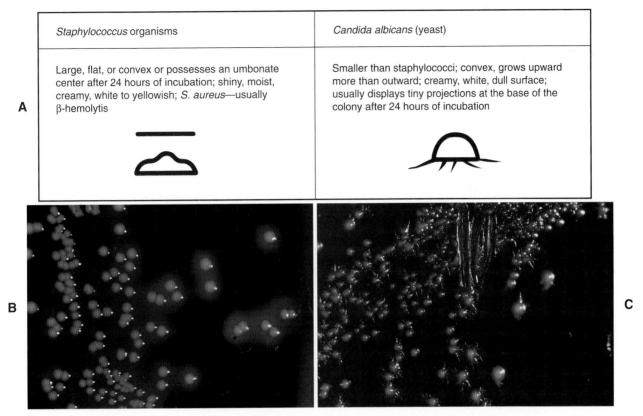

Staphylococcus organisms	Candida albicans (yeast)
A Large, flat, or convex or possesses an umbonate center after 24 hours of incubation; shiny, moist, creamy, white to yellowish; *S. aureus*—usually β-hemolytis	Smaller than staphylococci; convex, grows upward more than outward; creamy, white, dull surface; usually displays tiny projections at the base of the colony after 24 hours of incubation

Figure 8-26   A, Differentiation between staphylococci and *Candida albicans* (a yeast) by colonial morphology. **B,** Large, white, convex, shiny, moist, β-hemolytic colonies of *Staphylococcus aureus* growing on blood agar plate (BAP). **C,** "Heaped" or convex, white, dull appearance and butyrous texture of *Candida albicans* on BAP. Notice the tiny projections or "feet" at the edge of the colonies.

Learning Assessment Questions

1. What do the dark pink colonies on MacConkey (MAC) agar indicate?

2. Why were there three colony types that grew on the blood agar plate (BAP) but only two on the MAC agar?

3. What genus of bacteria would you suspect if you were to find α-hemolytic colonies from a respiratory sample?

4. How would you describe the colonies produced on MAC by nonfermenting gram-negative bacilli?

5. How would you differentiate β-hemolysis from α-hemolysis?

6. What would you suspect if you noticed "puffballs" growing in the broth medium?

7. "Swarming" colonies is a characteristic of which genus of bacteria?

8. A moderate growth of a heaped, dry-appearing, white organism is isolated from a patient with "thrush." The colony has tiny projections or "feet" projecting out along the edge of its margin. A presumptive identification of this organism would be:
   a. *Staphylococcus aureus*
   b. *Staphylococcus epidermidis*
   c. *Neisseria* spp.
   d. *Candida albicans*

9. Moderate growth of a β-hemolytic, gray colony is seen on a vaginal culture from a 25-year-old pregnant female. The colonies are growing on the BAP and chocolate agar (CHOC), but the MAC is negative for growth. The colonies are described as large with small, diffuse zones of β-hemolysis. This type of hemolysis is noticed when a colony is removed with a loop. A presumptive identification of this organism would be:
   a. *Streptococcus pyogenes* (group A)
   b. *Staphylococcus aureus*
   c. *Streptococcus agalactiae* (group B)
   d. *Streptococcus pneumoniae*

10. If a smear of an individual colony from the BAP (question 9) indicated a regular, short, gram-positive bacilli, the organism would have a presumptive identification as a:
    a. *Streptococcus agalactiae* (Group B)
    b. *Listeria monocytogenes*
    c. *Streptococcus pneumoniae*
    d. *Staphylococcus epidermidis*

Biochemical Identification of Gram-Negative Bacteria

Donald C. Lehman

OBJECTIVES

After reading and studying this chapter, you should be able to:

1. Explain the difference between phenotyping and genotyping.
2. Discuss the utilization of lactose by bacteria.
3. Compare the differences between oxidation and fermentation.
4. Explain the different reactions that may be observed in the triple sugar iron (TSI) agar.
5. Describe the reactions involved and the products of metabolism tested in each of the following:
   - ONPG (ortho-nitrophenyl β-D-galactopyranoside) test
   - Methyl red and Voges-Proskauer test
   - Decarboxylase, dihydrolase, and deaminase tests
   - Citrate utilization
   - DNase test
   - Gelatin liquefaction test
   - Indole test
   - Malonate utilization
   - Motility test
   - Nitrate and nitrite reduction tests
   - Oxidase test
   - Urease test
   - Lysine iron agar

- Motility-indole-ornithine agar
- Sulfide-indole-motility agar

6. Discuss the advantages of multitest systems.

7. Describe the significance of rapid reporting of bacterial identification.

8. Describe how established manual methods have been designed for the rapid identification of isolates.

9. Compare the automated methods for rapid identification of bacteria.

10. Discuss the evaluation of identification systems.

Case in Point

A 36-year-old man went to a local emergency department complaining of diarrhea that had persisted for approximately 1 week. The patient reported recently spending about 45 days in India. He claimed to have eaten a strictly vegetarian diet and some well-cooked indigenous foods and he drank only bottled water. He became acutely ill on the last day of his trip when he experienced headache, fever, chills, and 6 to 8 episodes of diarrhea per day. He reported that his stool did not appear bloody. A few days before today's visit, the patient had been diagnosed with *Giardia*, *Endolimax*, and *Blastocystis hominis* infection at another hospital. He had been given ciprofloxacin but was not responding to treatment. Bacterial cultures were ordered from stool, urine, and blood specimens. No pathogens were noted in the stool or urine cultures; however, a gram-negative bacillus was isolated from the blood cultures. The positive blood culture bottles were inoculated onto chocolate, sheep blood, and MacConkey agar plates. Medium-sized, gray colonies were seen on the chocolate and sheep blood agar plates. The colonies were nonhemolytic on sheep blood agar. On MacConkey agar, oxidase-negative, clear colonies were seen. Additional testing revealed the following: triple sugar iron, alkaline over acid with a black precipitate; glucose broth, acid no gas; indole, negative; urease, negative; and lysine, positive.

Issues to Consider

After reading the patient's case history, consider:
- What might be significant about this patient's travel to India?
- What are the principles of the biochemical tests?

Key Terms

Asaccharolytic	Indole test
β-galactosidase	Kligler iron agar (KIA)
β-galactoside permease	Lysine iron agar (LIA)
Chromogenic substrate	Malonate test
Citrate test	Methyl red test
Deaminase	Moeller decarboxylase base medium
Decarboxylase	
DNase	Motility-indole-ornithine (MIO) agar
Fermentation	
Fluorogenic substrate	Nitrate reduction test
Gelatinase	Numeric codes
Genotype	O/F basal medium

o-Nitrophenyl-β-D-galactopyranoside	Sulfide-indole-motility (SIM) medium
Oxidase test	Triple sugar iron (TSI) agar
Oxidation	Urease test
Phenotype	Voges-Proskauer test
Serotyping	

Historically, the identification of bacteria has been based on colony morphology, Gram staining, and biochemical testing. These methods are based on the **phenotype** of microorganisms, detecting observable or measurable characteristics. Biochemical testing was originally done in test tubes. Although this method was accurate, it required a lot of time to inoculate the multiple tubes of media and required lots of space in incubators. Over time, many of the biochemical tests were miniaturized and multitest systems were developed, resulting in time and space savings. More recently, automated systems have been developed; after inoculation, a computerized system records the test results and provides a printout identifying the organism. The automated systems can provide preliminary identification and antimicrobial susceptibility patterns in a few hours. **Serotyping** or serogrouping, another example of phenotypic testing, is used with biochemical testing for identifying different strains of bacteria within a species. Serotyping uses antibodies to detect specific antigens on the surface of bacteria.

Clinical microbiology is now using the next generation of test systems for the identification of bacteria: molecular biology assays. These methods, based on nucleic acid sequences, are highly sensitive, specific, and rapid, thereby providing accurate results in a few hours or less. Nucleic acid assays are based on the **genotype** of the organism, and this is believed to be more accurate than examining the phenotype. Genotyping involves characterizing genes. This chapter discusses the principles of biochemical tests commonly used in the identification of gram-negative bacteria. Box 9-1 lists some of these traditional biochemical tests. Microscopic examination and colony morphology are discussed in previous chapters. Serotyping is mentioned in Chapter 10 and molecular diagnostics is covered in Chapter 11.

CARBOHYDRATE UTILIZATION

Among bacteria there is great diversity in the ability to use carbohydrates; however, determining lactose utilization is the

Embden-Meyerhof Pathway   **Entner-Doudoroff Pathway**

One molecule glucose   One molecule glucose

↓   ↓

Glucose 6-phosphate   Glucose 6-phosphate

↓   ↓

Fructose 6-phosphate   6-Phosphogluconic acid

↓   ↓

Fructose 1,6-diphosphate   2-Keto-3-deoxy-6-
phosphogluconic acid

↓   ↓

Two molecules glyceraldehyde   Glyceraldehyde 3-phosphate
3-phosphate   and pyruvic acid

↓

Two molecules pyruvic acid

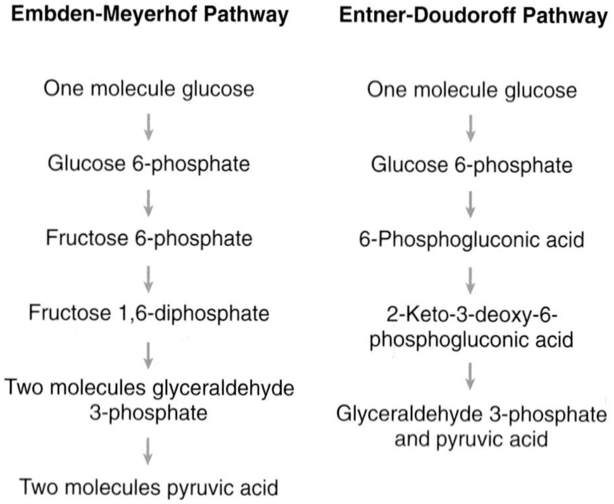

FIGURE 9-1 Two pathways for glucose degradation.

carbohydrate determination test that is the most important. Lactose degradation has been used initially to differentiate those bacterial species able to ferment lactose (lactose fermenters [LFs]) from those that are nonlactose fermenters (NLFs). Lactose is a disaccharide consisting of glucose and galactose connected by a galactoside bond.

Two enzymes are necessary for a bacterium to take up lactose and to cleave it into monosaccharides. These enzymes are **β-galactoside permease** (lactose permease), which serves as a transport enzyme that facilitates entry of the lactose molecule across the bacterial plasma membrane, and **β-galactosidase,** the enzyme that hydrolyzes lactose into glucose and galactose. After lactose is hydrolyzed, glucose is available for metabolism primarily through the Embden-Meyerhof pathway, also referred to as *glycolysis* (Figure 9-1). Alternatively, bacteria can use the Entner-Doudoroff pathway. Certain bacterial species may be able to use carbohydrates only in their simplest form, glucose, and are not able to attack the disaccharide lactose. Similarly, those bacterial species incapable of fermenting glucose cannot use lactose.

By definition, LFs possess both β-galactoside permease and β-galactosidase, and NLFs do not possess either enzyme.

Some bacterial species lack β-galactoside permease but possess β-galactosidase. These bacterial species, termed *late* or *delayed lactose fermenters* (dLFs), eventually are able to cleave the lactose molecule.

Numerous other carbohydrates—monosaccharides, disaccharides, and polysaccharides—can be used by bacteria. Frequently these carbohydrates are ultimately converted into glucose for entry into glycolysis. Examples of sugars used to differentiate bacteria include lactose, maltose, rhamnose, sucrose, raffinose, and arabinose. The polyhydric alcohols (which end in "ol"), collectively called *sugars*, include adonitol, dulcitol, mannitol, and sorbitol. Bacteria can utilize carbohydrates either by **oxidation** (aerobically), fermentatively (anaerobically), or both. Bacteria that can grow either aerobically or anaerobically are called *facultative anaerobes.* Some bacteria are **asaccharolytic.** They do not use any carbohydrate; instead they use other organic molecules for energy and carbon sources.

Oxidation-Fermentation Tests

Determining a bacterium's oxidation-fermentation (O/F) pattern is an important test in the identification of bacteria. In particular it is helpful in differentiating members of the family Enterobacteriaceae, glucose fermenters, from the aerobic pseudomonads and similar gram-negative bacteria, which are nonfermenters. Carbohydrate fermentation tests determine the ability of a microorganism to ferment a specific carbohydrate incorporated into a basal medium. During **fermentation,** glucose enters the glycolysis pathway, resulting in the formation of pyruvic acid, which can be further oxidized to other acids. The end product of carbohydrate fermentation is acid or acid with gas. Acid formation is detected with pH indicators added to the medium. Some bacteria produce primarily a single acid, such as the streptococci, which are homolactic acid fermenters. Other bacteria produce several different acids, including lactic acid, propionic acid, and succinic acid. These organisms are referred to as *mixed acid fermenters.*

Oxidation also begins by glucose entering the glycolysis pathway; however, the pyruvic acid formed from glycolysis is further oxidized to CO_2. Oxidation requires oxygen (aerobic respiration) or another inorganic molecule (anaerobic respiration), such as nitrate (NO_3) as a terminal electron acceptor. Higher acidity is produced during fermentation than during oxidation. The same medium is used for both oxidative and fermentative tests.

Characteristically, oxidizers and fastidious fermenters often produce either weak or small amounts of acids from carbohydrates. In media that contain large amounts of peptones (2.0%), such as **triple sugar iron (TSI) agar,** whatever acids produced are neutralized or masked by the alkaline reaction from peptone utilization. To detect small amounts of acids produced, whether fermentatively or oxidatively, Hugh and Leifson developed an **O/F basal medium** (OFBM) that contains the same concentration of carbohydrates (1%) found in the TSI medium but a lower concentration of peptones (0.2%). The pH indicator is bromthymol blue. Uninoculated medium is green; in an acid environment the indicator is yellow, and it is blue in an alkaline environment (Figure 9-2).

TABLE 9-1 Biochemical Reactions Characteristic of Gram-Negative Bacilli on TSI, KIA, and OFBM Media

	TSI Agar	KIA	Hugh-Leifson OFBM
Carbohydrates (concentration)	Glucose (0.1%)	Glucose (0.1%)	Glucose or other carbohydrate being tested (1%)
	Lactose (1%)	Lactose (1%)	
	Sucrose (1%)		
Peptone	2%	2%	0.2%
Fermenter	Acid butt	Acid butt	Open tube: acid
	Acid or alkaline slant	Acid or alkaline slant	Sealed tube: acid
Nonfermenter			
Oxidizer	Alkaline butt	Alkaline butt	Open tube: acid
	Alkaline slant	Alkaline slant	Sealed tube: no acid
Nonoxidizer (asaccharolytic)	Alkaline butt	Alkaline butt	Open tube: no acid
	Alkaline slant	Alkaline slant	Sealed tube: no acid

TSI, Triple sugar iron; *KIA,* Kligler iron agar; *OFBM,* oxidation-fermentation basal medium.

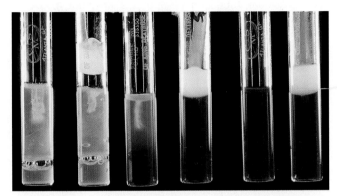

FIGURE 9-2 Reactions in oxidative fermentation media. *Left to right:* Fermenter: open and sealed tubes positive for acid production; nonfermenter: open tube positive for acid production, sealed tube negative for acid production; nonfermenter/nonoxidizer: open and sealed tubes negative for acid production.

Table 9-1 shows the differences in reactions among different groups of organisms. When O/F tests are performed, two tubes of Hugh-Leifson OFBM are inoculated; one is overlayed with sterile mineral oil to create an anaerobic environment (closed), and the other tube is left aerobic (open), without mineral oil overlay. When acid is produced in both tubes, the isolate is an oxidizer and fermenter. The presence of acid only in the closed tube indicates only that the organism is a fermenter, whereas the presence of acid in the open tube indicates an oxidizer. The open tube may or may not show acidity. No acid production in the open tube may indicate that the organism is a nonoxidizer; in fact many nonoxidizers will produce an alkaline reaction from peptone utilization.

Triple Sugar Iron Agar

Triple sugar iron agar and **Kligler iron agar (KIA)** are highly useful in the presumptive identification of gram-negative enteric bacteria, particularly in screening for intestinal pathogens. The formulas for TSI agar and KIA are identical except that TSI contains sucrose in addition to glucose and lactose. Lactose is present in a concentration 10 times that of glucose

(1% lactose and 0.1% glucose). In TSI agar, sucrose is also present in a 1% concentration. Ferrous sulfate and sodium thiosulfate are added to detect the production of hydrogen sulfide gas (H_2S). Phenol red is used as the pH indicator, which is yellow below the pH of 6.8. Uninoculated medium is red because the pH is buffered at 7.4. Both TSI agar and KIA are useful in detecting the ability of the microorganism to ferment carbohydrates, glucose and lactose in KIA and glucose, lactose, or sucrose in TSI agar; to produce gas from the fermentation of sugars; and to detect the production of H_2S.

Both TSI agar and KIA are poured on a slant. The slant portion is aerobic; the butt, or deep portion, is anaerobic. To inoculate TSI agar or KIA, the laboratory scientist should pick a well-isolated colony with an inoculating needle and stab the butt almost all the way to the bottom of the tube. Then the laboratory scientist moves the needle back and forth, known as *fish tailing,* across the surface of the slant. The cap is replaced loosely to allow oxygen to enter the tube, and the medium is incubated in a non-CO₂ incubator for 18 to 24 hours. The reaction patterns are written with the slant results first, followed by the butt reaction, separated by a slash (slant reaction/butt reaction), and it is important that the reactions be read within an 18- to 24-hour incubation period; otherwise, erroneous results are possible.

Reactions on TSI Agar or KIA

1. *No fermentation: Alkaline slant/alkaline butt (ALK/ALK or K/K) or alkaline slant/no change (ALK/no change or K/ NC).* These reactions are typical of organisms that are not members of the family Enterobacteriaceae. Although unable to ferment either lactose or glucose, these organisms can degrade the peptones present in the medium aerobically or anaerobically, resulting in the production of alkaline byproducts in the slant or deep, respectively, changing the indicator to a deep red color.

2. *Glucose fermentation only, no lactose (or sucrose in TSI) fermentation: Alkaline slant/acid butt (K/A).* TSI agar and KIA contain glucose in a 0.1% concentration. The acid produced from this concentration of glucose is enough to change the indicator to yellow initially throughout the medium. After about 12 hours, however, the glucose will

be consumed, and bacteria on the slant will utilize the peptones aerobically, producing an alkaline reaction, which changes the indicator to a deep red color. Fermentation of glucose (anaerobic) in the butt produces larger amounts of acid, overcoming the alkaline effects of peptone degradation; therefore the butt remains acidic (yellow). Reading the results after fewer than 12 hours of incubation gives the false appearance of an organism capable of fermenting glucose and lactose (or sucrose in the case of TSI agar). For this reason, TSI agar or KIA must be incubated for 18 to 24 hours.

3. *Lactose (and/or sucrose) fermentation: acid/acid (A/A).* Glucose fermenters will attack the simple sugar glucose first and then the lactose or sucrose. The acid production from the fermentation of the additional sugar(s) is sufficient to keep both the slant and the butt acid (yellow) when examined at the end of 18 to 24 hours. If the medium is incubated beyond 24 hours, however, it is possible that the lactose or sucrose could be consumed and an alkaline slant be formed. It is important that the TSI and KIA tests are not read after 24 hours of incubation.

4. *Hydrogen sulfide production: alkaline slant/acid butt, H_2S in butt (K/A, H_2S) or acid slant/acid butt, H_2S in butt (A/A H_2S).* Two indicators are present in the medium to detect H_2S formation: sodium thiosulfate and ferrous sulfate. The H_2S production is a two-step process. In the first step, H_2S is formed from sodium thiosulfate. Because H_2S is a colorless gas, the second indicator, ferrous sulfate, is necessary to visually detect its production. In some cases, the butt of the tube will be completely black, obscuring the yellow color from carbohydrate fermentation. Because H_2S production requires an acid environment, even if the yellow color cannot be seen, it is safe to assume glucose fermentation.
    a. Bacterium (acid environment) + Sodium thiosulfate → H_2S gas
    b. H_2S + Ferric ions → Ferrous sulfide (black precipitate)

5. *Gas production (aerogenic) or no gas production (nonaerogenic).* The production of gas results in the formation of bubbles or splitting of the medium in the butt or complete displacement of the medium from the bottom of the tube. Figure 9-3 illustrates the reactions on TSI agar.

Ortho-Nitrophenyl-β-D-Galactopyranoside Test

Organisms that are dLFs appear as nonfermenting colonies on primary isolation medium. When placed on TSI or KIA slants, these species produce similar results after 18 to 24 hours of incubation. The *o-nitrophenyl-β-D-galactopyranoside* (ONPG) and the *p*-nitrophenyl-β-D-galactopyranoside (PNPG) tests determine whether the organism is a dLF (one that lacks the enzyme β-galactoside permease but possesses β-galactosidase) or a true NLF. ONPG is structurally similar to lactose, but ONPG is more easily transported through the bacterial plasma membrane and does not require β-galactoside permease. β-Galactosidase hydrolyzes ONPG, a colorless compound, into galactose and *o*-nitrophenol, a yellow com-

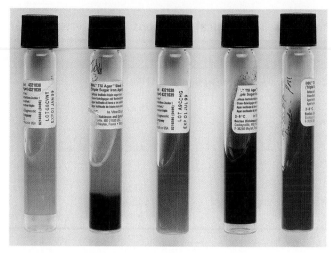

FIGURE 9-3 Triple sugar iron agar reactions. *Left to right:* Tube 1, A/A gas; tube 2, A/A H_2S; tube 3, K/A; tube 4, K/A H_2S; tube 5, K/K.

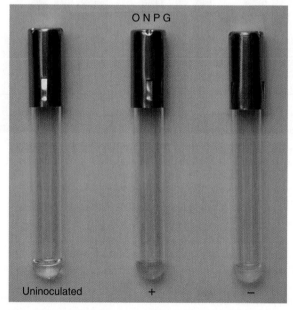

FIGURE 9-4 Ortho-nitrophenyl β-D-galactopyranoside test. (Courtesy American Society for Clinical Laboratory Science, Education and Research Fund, Inc., 1982.)

pound. ONPG remains colorless if the organism is an NLF (Figure 9-4).

The test can be performed by making a heavy suspension of bacteria in sterile saline and adding commercially prepared ONPG disks or tablets. The suspension is incubated at 37° C, and positive results can generally be seen within 6 hours. Because β-galactosidase is an inducible enzyme, the gene is expressed only if lactose or a similar substrate is present; therefore bacteria should be taken from lactose-containing media. Bacteria producing a yellow pigment should not be tested because of the risk of a false-positive result.

GLUCOSE METABOLISM AND ITS METABOLIC PRODUCTS

Glucose metabolized via the Embden-Meyerhof pathway produces several intermediate byproducts, including pyruvic acid. Further degradation of pyruvic acid can produce mixed acids as end products. However, enterics take two separate pathways: the mixed acid fermentation pathway or the butylene glycol pathway. The **methyl red** (MR) and **Voges-Proskauer** (VP) **tests** detect the end products of glucose fermentation. Each test detects products from a different pathway. The MR and VP tests are part of the IMViC reactions: indole, methyl red, Voges-Proskauer, and citrate.

Methyl Red Test

Bacteria are incubated in a broth medium containing glucose. Most commercial MR media are a modification of Clark and Lubs medium. The broth should be incubated 3 to 5 days. After incubation, approximately half the broth is transferred to a clean tube for the VP test. If glucose is metabolized by the mixed acid fermentation pathway, stable acid end products are produced, which results in a low pH. A red color develops after addition of the pH indicator methyl red (Figure 9-5). MR negative cultures will remain yellow after addition of the pH indicator (pH 6.0).

Glucose → Pyruvic acid → Mixed acid fermentation (pH 4.4)
↓
Red color with methyl red indicator

Voges-Proskauer Test

In some bacteria, acids formed during fermentation can be further metabolized to 2, 3-butanediol through the intermediate acetoin. After incubation, first α-naphthol is added as a catalyst or color intensifier. Next 40% KOH or NaOH is added, and the tube is gently shaken to increase oxygenation. Under these conditions, acetoin is oxidized to diacetyl. Diacetyl in the presence of potassium hydroxide and α-naphthol forms a red complex. The pH remains relatively neutral. Figure 9-5 illustrates the MRVP test. Bacteria tend to be positive for either MR or VP, but not both. Some bacteria are negative for both tests.

Glucose → Pyruvic acid → Acetoin → Diacetyl + KOH + α-Naphthol → Red complex → 2,3 Butanediol

AMINO ACID UTILIZATION

Decarboxylase and Dihydrolase Tests

Many bacteria have the ability to use amino acids as energy and carbon sources. **Decarboxylase** tests determine whether the bacterial species possess enzymes capable of decarboxylating (removing the carboxyl group, COOH) specific amino acids in the test medium. Two amino acids commonly used to test for decarboxylase activity are lysine and ornithine. The products of decarboxylation are amine or diamine molecules

and CO_2, with resulting alkalinity. Degradation of the amino acids and their specific end products are shown in the following reaction:

Degradation of amino acids and their specific end products

Lysine (amino acid) → Lysine decarboxylase → Cadaverine (amine) + CO_2

Ornithine → Ornithine decarboxylase → Putrescine

Arginine → Arginine dihydrolase → Citrulline → Ornithine → Putrescine

Lysine is decarboxylated by the enzyme lysine decarboxylase to cadaverine, a diamine, and CO_2. Ornithine is cleaved by ornithine decarboxylase to putrescine, a diamine, and CO_2. Both cadaverine and putrescine are stable in anaerobic conditions. Arginine can be decarboxylated in a two-step process. In the first step, arginine undergoes decarboxylation by arginine decarboxylase to form agmatine and CO_2. Then agmatine is further metabolized to putrescine and urea. If the bacteria also produce urease, the urea will be degraded to ammonia (NH_3) and CO_2. Arginine can also be degraded by arginine dihydrolase forming citrulline, ammonia, and inorganic phosphate. In the next step, citrulline undergoes phosphorolytic cleavage to yield ornithine. If the bacteria also possess ornithine decarboxylase, ornithine will be converted to putrescine.

The test to detect decarboxylation uses **Moeller decarboxylase base medium.** This is a broth containing glucose; peptones; two pH indicators, bromcresol purple and cresol red; and the specific amino acid at a concentration of 1%. The medium has an initial pH of 6.0. Having glucose in the medium is important because decarboxylases are inducible enzymes produced in an acid pH. The uninoculated medium is purple; metabolism of the small amount of glucose drops the pH to about 5.5, turning the medium yellow. For decarboxylation to take place, two conditions must be met: an acid pH and an anaerobic environment. A control tube containing only the base medium without the amino acid is inoculated to determine the viability of the organism. The control tube also determines whether sufficient acid is produced. Both tubes are inoculated with the test organism; are overlayed with a layer of sterile mineral oil, which creates anaerobic conditions; and then are incubated at 35° C.

During the first few hours of incubation, organisms attack the glucose first, changing the pH to acid. If the organism produces the specific decarboxylase and the amino acid in the medium is attacked, release of the amine products causes an alkaline pH shift. This results in a purple (positive result) color in the medium. If the organism does not possess the specific decarboxylase, the medium remains yellow (negative result). The control tube remains yellow. Results can usually be recorded in 24 hours; however, bacteria with weak decarboxylase activity may take up to 4 days to be positive. Modifications of the decarboxylase test to detect other biochemical reactions are also routinely used. Examples of these include the motility-indole-ornithine (MIO) and lysine iron agar (LIA) tests (Figure 9-6).

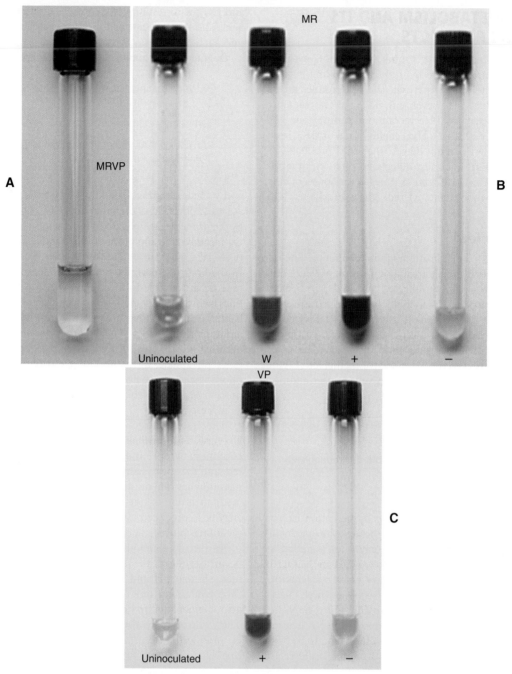

FIGURE 9-5 **A**, The methyl red–Voges-Proskauer test is inoculated and incubated overnight. Then it is split equally into two parts: one part for the methyl red test, the other for the Voges-Proskauer test. **B**, Methyl red test. **C**, Voges-Proskauer test. (Courtesy American Society for Clinical Laboratory Science, Education and Research Fund, Inc., 1982.)

Deaminase Test

Amino acids can be metabolized by **deaminases** that remove an amine (NH_2) group. The phenylalanine deaminase (PAD) test determines whether an organism possesses the enzyme that deaminates phenylalanine to phenylpyruvic acid. The test medium is an agar slant containing a 0.2% concentration of phenylalanine. The surface of the slant is inoculated with a bacterial colony. After incubation, addition of a 10% ferric chloride ($FeCl_3$) reagent results in a green color if phenylpyruvic acid is present. This test is helpful in initial differentiation of *Proteus*, *Morganella*, and *Providencia* organisms, which are positive, from the rest of the Enterobacteriaceae (Figure 9-7).

Deamination of Phenylalanine

Phenylalanine → Phenylalanine deaminase →
Phenylpyruvic acid + ($FeCl_3$) Green

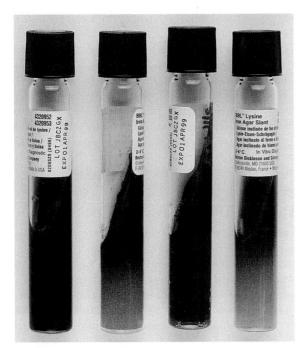

FIGURE 9-6 Lysine iron agar reactions. *Left to right:* K/K (positive decarboxylation without H$_2$S), K/A H$_2$S (negative decarboxylation with H$_2$S), K/K H$_2$S (positive decarboxylation with H$_2$S), R/Y (negative decarboxylation, positive deamination without H$_2$S).

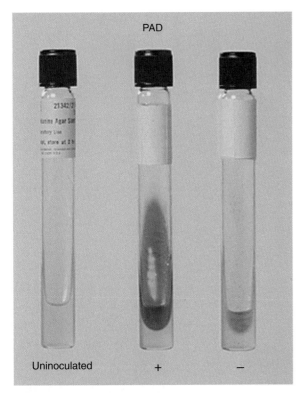

FIGURE 9-7 Phenylalanine deaminase test. (Courtesy American Society for Clinical Laboratory Science, Education and Research Fund, Inc., 1982.)

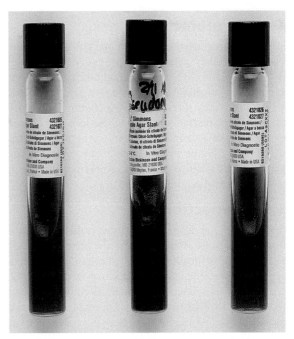

FIGURE 9-8 Citrate utilization test. *Left,* Uninoculated; *middle,* positive result; *right,* negative result.

MISCELLANEOUS TESTS

Citrate Utilization

The **citrate test** determines whether an organism can use sodium citrate as a sole carbon source. Simmons citrate medium is frequently used to determine citrate utilization. In addition to citrate, the test medium contains ammonium salts as the sole nitrogen source. Bacteria able to use citrate will use the ammonium salts, thereby releasing ammonia. The alkaline pH that results from use of the ammonium salts changes the pH indicator (bromthymol blue) in the medium from green to blue. It is important to use a light inoculum because dead organisms can be a source of carbon, producing a false-positive reaction (Figure 9-8). Christensen citrate medium is an alternative test medium. This medium incorporates phenol red (as the pH indicator) and organic nitrogen. At an alkaline pH, the indicator turns from yellow to pink.

DNase

DNA is a polynucleotide composed of repeating purine and pyrimidine mononucleotide monomeric units. Most bacterial **DNases** are endonucleases cleaving internal phosphodiester bonds resulting in smaller subunits. Extracellular DNase can be produced by a number of bacteria such as *Staphylococcus aureus* and *Serratia marcescens*. DNase test medium usually contains 0.2% DNA. A heavy inoculum of bacteria is streaked onto the surface of the medium in a straight line; several organisms can be tested at once. The plate is incubated at 35° C for 18 to 24 hours, and then 1N HCl is added to the surface of the plate. Unhydrolyzed DNA is insoluble in HCl and will form a precipitate. Oligonucleotides formed from the action of DNase will dissolve in the acid, forming a clear zone (halo) around the inoculum.

Gelatin Liquefaction

Gelatin is a protein derived from animal collagen. A number of bacteria produce **gelatinases**—proteolytic enzymes that break down gelatin into amino acids. Gelatinase activity is detected by loss of gelling (liquefaction) of gelatin. Gelatinase activity is affected by several factors, including the size of the inoculum and incubation temperature. Some bacteria produce larger amounts of gelatinase at room temperature compared with 35° C. It may be necessary to incubate media several weeks to detect a positive reaction. Several methods are available for detecting gelatinase.

Indole Production

Indole is one of the degradation products of the amino acid tryptophan. Organisms that possess the enzyme tryptophanase are capable of deaminating tryptophan, with formation of the intermediate degradation products of indole, pyruvic acid, and ammonia. Bacteria are inoculated into tryptophan or peptone broth. Most commercial peptone broth contains enough tryptophan for a positive reaction; tryptophan can be added to obtain a final concentration of 1%. After inoculation, the broth should be incubated at 35° C for 48 hours. After incubation, one of two methods can be used to detect indole. In the Ehrlich **indole test,** the indole is extracted from the broth culture by the addition of 1 mL of xylene. After the xylene is added, the tube is shaken well. After waiting a few minutes for the xylene to rise to the top, 0.5 mL of Ehrlich reagent, containing para-dimethylaminobenzaldehyde (PDAB), is added. If indole is present, a red color develops after the addition of PDAB (Figure 9-9). Alternatively,

Kovac reagent, which also contains PDAB, can be used. This method does not use a xylene extraction. Approximately 5 drops of Kovac's reagent is added directly to the broth culture. The tube is shaken, and if indole is present, a red color develops. The Ehrlich method is more sensitive than Kovac reagent and is preferred with nonfermentative bacteria. If indole-nitrate (trypticase nitrate) medium is used, the indole test can be performed from the same broth culture as a nitrate test. Before adding any reagents, the broth is divided in half, one aliquot for the indole test and the other for the nitrate test. A rapid indole test utilizing *p*-dimethylaminocinnamaldehyde is available.

Malonate Utilization

The **malonate test** determines whether the organism is capable of using sodium malonate as its sole carbon source. Malonate broth normally contains bromthymol blue as a pH indicator. Bacteria able to use malonate as a sole carbon source will also use ammonium sulfate as a nitrogen source. A positive test results in increased alkalinity from utilization of the ammonium sulfate, changing the indicator from green to blue (Figure 9-10).

Motility

Motility can be determined by microscopic examination of bacteria or by observing growth in a semisolid medium. Motility test media have agar concentrations of 0.4% or less to allow for the free spread of microorganisms. A single stab into the center of the medium is made. Best results are obtained if the stab is made as straight as possible. After incubation, movement away from the stab line or a hazy

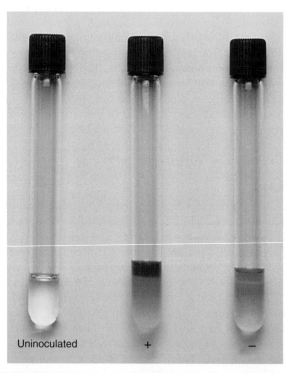

FIGURE 9-9 Indole broth. (Courtesy American Society for Clinical Laboratory Science, Education and Research Fund, Inc., 1982.)

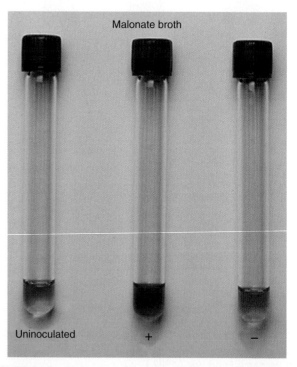

FIGURE 9-10 Malonate test. (Courtesy American Society for Clinical Laboratory Science, Education and Research Fund, Inc., 1982.)

appearance throughout the medium indicates a motile organism. Incubation temperature is important. Some bacteria are motile only at room temperature, but this temperature may not be optimal for growth. It is suggested that two motility tubes be inoculated, one incubated at room temperature and the other at 35° C. Comparing inoculated with uninoculated tubes may help in interpreting results.

Nitrate and Nitrite Reduction

The **nitrate reduction test** determines whether the organism has the ability to reduce nitrate to nitrite and further reduce nitrite to nitrogen gas (N_2). The organism is inoculated into a nutrient broth containing a nitrogen source. After 24 hours of incubation, N,N-dimethyl-α-naphthylamine and sulfanilic acid is added. A red color indicates the presence of nitrite.

Nitrate reduction test reaction

Nutrient broth with 0.1% potassium nitrate $\rightarrow$
Nitrate reductase $\rightarrow$ Nitrite + Sulfanilic acid +
N,N-Dimethyl-α-naphthylamine $\rightarrow$ Diazo red dye

If no color develops, this may indicate that nitrate has not been reduced or that nitrate has been further reduced to N_2, nitric oxide (NO), or nitrous oxide (N_2O), which the reagents will detect. Adding a small amount of zinc dust will help to determine whether the test has produced a true-negative result or whether the lack of color production was due to reduction beyond nitrite. Zinc dust reduces nitrate to nitrite. Therefore development of a red color after the addition of zinc confirms a true-negative test result. Alternatively, a small glass tube, called a *Durham tube,* can be inserted into the broth upside down when the medium is aliquoted into test tubes. During incubation, if nitrogen gas is produced, it will be trapped in the inverted Durham tube.

Oxidase

The **oxidase test** determines the presence of the cytochrome oxidase system that oxidizes reduced cytochrome with molecular oxygen. The oxidase test is helpful in differentiating between the Enterobacteriaceae, oxidase negative, and the pseudomonads, which are oxidase positive. The oxidase test is also useful in identifying *Neisseria* organisms, which are oxidase positive. A modified oxidase test is used to distinguish *Staphylococcus* from *Micrococcus*. Several methods for performing an oxidase test are available. Kovac oxidase test uses a 0.5% or 1% aqueous solution of tetramethyl-p-phenylenediamine dihydrochloride. A drop of the reagent is added to filter paper, and a wooden applicator stick is used to rub a colony onto the moistened filter paper. The development of a lavender color within 10 to 15 seconds is a positive reaction. p-Aminodimethylaniline oxalate is less sensitive than tetramethyl-p-phenylenediamine dihydrochloride, but it is cheaper and more stable. Commercial forms of oxidase reagent are available in glass ampules and on filter paper disks.

Urease

The **urease test** determines whether a microorganism can hydrolyze urea, releasing a sufficient amount of ammonia to

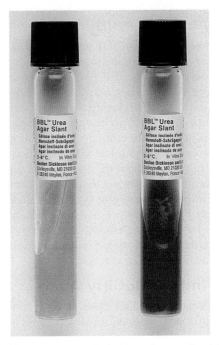

FIGURE 9-11 Urease test. *Left,* Negative result; *right,* positive result.

produce a color change by a pH indicator. Urease hydrolyzes urea to form ammonia, water, and CO_2. Different formulations of urea agar are available, but Christensen urea agar is generally preferred. The surface of the agar slant is inoculated but not stabbed. The medium contains phenol red as the pH indicator. The resulting alkaline pH from hydrolysis of urea is indicated by a bright pink color (Figure 9-11).

Lysine Iron Agar Slant

The **lysine iron agar** (LIA) test is a tubed agar slant. It contains the amino acid lysine, glucose, ferric ammonium citrate, and sodium thiosulfate. The pH indicator is bromcresol purple. LIA is used primarily to determine whether the bacteria decarboxylate or deaminate lysine (see Figure 9-6). Hydrogen sulfide production is also detected in this medium. LIA is inoculated in the same manner as a TSI agar slant. LIA is most useful in conjunction with TSI in screening stool specimens for the presence of enteric pathogens, differentiating *Salmonella* (lysine positive) from *Citrobacter* species (lysine negative). Decarboxylation only occurs anaerobically; the presence of a dark purple butt is positive for lysine decarboxylation. The production of H_2S can mask the purple color in the butt of the tube. Because H_2S production in LIA occurs only in an alkaline environment, a black precipitate indicating H_2S is also a positive result for decarboxylation. LIA is also useful in differentiating *Proteus, Morganella,* and *Providencia* species from most other members of Enterobacteriaceae. This group of enterics deaminates (attacks the NH_2 group instead of the carboxyl group) amino acids. In the LIA slant, deamination of lysine turns the original light purple color slant to a plum or reddish-purple color; the butt turns yellow because of glucose fermentation.

Motility-Indole-Ornithine Agar

Motility-indole-ornithine (MIO) agar is a semisolid agar medium used to detect motility and indole and ornithine decarboxylase production. MIO is useful in differentiating *Klebsiella* spp. from *Enterobacter* and *Serratia* spp. The medium is inoculated by making a straight stab down the center of the medium with an inoculating needle. Motility is shown by a clouding of the medium or spreading growth from the line of inoculation. Ornithine decarboxylation is indicated by a purple color throughout the medium. Because MIO is a semisolid medium, it does not have to be overlayed with mineral oil to provide anaerobic conditions. Indole production is detected by the addition of Kovac reagent; a pink to red color is formed in the reagent area if the test result is positive. Ornithine decarboxylase and motility should be read first before addition of Kovac reagent.

Sulfide-Indole-Motility Agar

Sulfide-indole-motility (SIM) medium is a semisolid agar helpful in differentiating gram-negative bacteria in the family Enterobacteriaceae. An inoculating needle is used to make a straight stab down the center of the medium. Cloudiness spreading from the inoculation line is positive for motility. The production of H_2S is indicated by a black precipitate, and a pink to red color after the addition of Kovac reagent is positive for indole.

MANUAL MULTITEST SYSTEMS

Principles of Identification

Commercial identification systems fall into one of five categories or a combination thereof: pH-based reactions, enzyme-based reactions, utilization of carbon sources, visual detection of bacterial growth, or detection of volatile or nonvolatile fatty acids by gas chromatography. Identification of bacteria and yeast can be facilitated by the use of automated or packaged kit systems by which organisms are identified with computer-assisted or computer-derived books of **numeric codes.** These numeric codes are generated based on the metabolic profiles of each organism. Each metabolic reaction, or phenotype, is translated into one of two responses: plus (+) for positive reactions and minus (−) for negative reactions. These plus-minus sequences are catalogued as binary numbers and stored in a computer database. Binary codes are computer converted into code profile numbers that represent the identifying phenotype of specific organisms. Once metabolic profiles have been translated into numbers, a percent probability of correct identification is assigned based on the comparison of the unknown profile to known profiles within the database. As more organisms are included in the database, the genus and species designations and probabilities become more precise. With all the name changes that occur, it is sometimes difficult to maintain the current taxonomy in a database. For example, from the early 1960s to 2003, the number of genera of Enterobacteriaceae increased from 10 to 31, and the number of species increased from 24 to 130. All commercial suppliers of multicomponent biochemical test systems provide users with one or more of the following: a computer with profile number database, a computer-derived code book or compact disk, access to a Web site, or access to a telephone inquiry center to facilitate matching profile numbers with species.

Analytical Profile Index

The Analytical Profile Index (API; bioMérieux Vitek, Hazelwood, Mo.) was released in 1970. The system for identification of gram-negative fermentative bacteria (the family Enterobacteriaceae) is called the API 20E. This system has a series of 20 cupules attached to a plastic strip. Inside the cupules are lyophilized, pH-based substrates. A bacterial suspension made in saline is used to rehydrate the reagents in the cupules. The principles of the tests are the same or similar to the principles of tests performed in test tubes. Some of the cupules, such as those for amino acid deaminases and dehydrolase, require a mineral oil overlay. The strip is incubated 18 to 24 hours, and reagents are added to some of the cupules. Results are recorded, and a seven-digit code profile number is determined. The last test used to determine the profile number is the oxidase test, which is not part of the API strip.

After determining the code profile number, a database provided by the manufacturer is consulted, providing the most probable identification. If the identification is in question, nitrate reduction and motility are supplemental tests that can be used to obtain an additional digit for the profile number. The API system has been a standard product in many clinical microbiology laboratories and has remained unchanged. Accuracy for commonly isolated Enterobacteriaceae, such as *Escherichia coli, Klebsiella pneumoniae,* and *Proteus mirabilis,* has been reported to be 87.7% at 24 hours of incubation. For less commonly isolated Enterobacteriaceae, the accuracy drops to 78.7% at 24 hours. BioMérieux markets a number of multitest systems, including those for gram-positive cocci, nonfermentive gram-negative bacilli (20NE), and a rapid system for identification of the Enterobacteriaceae in 4 hours (RapID 20E).

Other multitest systems include the Crystal E/NF (BD Diagnostic Systems, Sparks, Md.), the RapID NF Plus (Remel, Lenexa, Kan.), the Microbact (Oxoid, Ltd., Basingstoke, United Kingdom), the Enterotube II (BD Diagnostic Systems), Uni-N/F-Tek plate (Remel), Micro-ID (Remel), and the GN2 MicroPlate (Biolog, Inc., Hayward, Calif.). Biolog offers the MicroLog 1 and 2, manually read systems; the MicroLog MicroStation, a semiautomated system; and the OmniLog ID, a fully automated system. The Biolog database is one of the largest, with more than 500 species or taxa.

RAPID AND AUTOMATED IDENTIFICATION SYSTEMS

Until the late 1970s, microbiologists relied on the growth and isolation of bacteria in broth culture and agar media. Once bacteria are cultured in vitro, their biochemical or metabolic characteristics can be used for identification. Isolation of the infectious agent from clinical samples typically requires 24 to 48 hours. Identification protocols often require another 24 hours of incubation in the presence of specific biochemical substrates. Rapid diagnosis of infectious disease therefore remains a major challenge for the clinical microbiology laboratory. The clinical outcome of rapid and accurate reporting of results should directly affect patient care in two ways: (1) early diagnosis and (2) subsequent selection of appropriate antimicrobial therapy. When these outcomes are achieved, the clinical microbiology laboratory will have a proactive, rather than retrospective, effect on patient management.

Rapid reporting also becomes increasingly important in light of today's diagnostic challenges. Newly emerging pathogens, recognition of old pathogens in different clinical settings, world travel, increasing nosocomial infections, and the prevalence of multidrug-resistant organisms all contribute to the need for the design and development of new identification capabilities. Some of the major concepts and applications of rapid methods and automation currently available for the identification of clinically significant microorganisms are listed in the following sections. Although not exhaustive, the principles of most rapid identification technologies found in the clinical microbiology laboratory have been included. Other specific identification methods are discussed in greater detail in subsequent chapters in association with specific organism descriptions.

The Term *Rapid*

Direct microscopic examination of body fluids provides results within 15 to 30 minutes; these results are often valuable in patient management. For example, Gram stain results from a cerebrospinal fluid specimen along with blood and spinal fluid chemistry (glucose and protein) and hematology (complete blood count and differential) may be critical in establishing the cause of infectious meningitis. Chapter 7 discusses the microscopic examination of clinical samples.

For decades microbiologists relied on the ability of an organism to ferment sugars, degrade amino acids, and produce unique end products for identification purposes. Diagnosis of an infectious disease has been a complex, laborious, and frequently slow process. In the late 1950s and 1960s, traditional biochemical tests became miniaturized. Smaller test tubes and molded plastic vessels were introduced. These changes made testing more convenient but did not improve turnaround times in reporting results. In the 1970s, microbiologists began to rely on computerized databases so that numerous results could be considered simultaneously and the most statistically probable result could be regarded as the identification of the unknown organism. This development improved reliability of the results but still did not improve reporting turnaround times. In the mid to late 1970s, automated instruments for identification and susceptibility testing gradually appeared. In many laboratory settings, they shortened turnaround times, yielded greater precision, improved productivity, and provided accurate test results.

The phrase *rapid method* encompasses a wide variety of procedures and techniques and has been loosely applied to any procedure affording results faster than the conventional method. Rapid methods exist for microscopy, biochemical identification, antigen detection, and antibody detection. *Rapid* is a relative term used to describe time and depends on the procedures being compared. For example, a 3-hour enzyme immunoassay method to detect *Clostridium difficile*

toxin is rapid compared with a 48-hour cell culture cytotoxicity assay. On the other hand, the fluorescent quenching–based oxygen sensor detection of *Mycobacterium tuberculosis* within 2 weeks with the BACTEC 9000 MB (BD Diagnostic Systems) is rapid compared with 6 weeks required to grow the organism on agar slants.

Microscopic procedures using common stains and fluorescent antibody to detect specific organisms are rapid methods; so are some conventional procedures used for initial differentiation or presumptive identification of certain groups of organisms. These procedures have been modified to provide immediate results that may lead to presumptive identification. Rapid identification of clinical isolates often involves commercially packaged identification kits or fully automated instruments. These manufactured kits are usually miniaturized test systems that employ chromogenic or **fluorogenic substrates** to assess preformed enzymes. **Chromogenic substrates** are colorless; when cleaved by a microbial enzyme, a colored compound is produced. Fluorogenic substrates are nonfluorescent until cleaved by microbial enzymes. Reaction endpoints may be reached after 2 to 6 hours of incubation, although some may require an overnight incubation. The capabilities of these kits and systems vary widely. Certain systems may still require manual reading by the laboratory scientist, whereas others may use mechanized reading through spectrophotometry, numeric coding, and computerized databases. Some of these instruments also incubate, read, and interpret the enzymatic test results.

Rapid Biochemical Tests Performed on Isolated Colonies

Table 9-2 summarizes the principles, modes of action, and applications of certain established manual procedures for quick presumptive differentiation between groups of organisms or presumptive identification to bacterial species. Often more than one test must be performed for a presumptive identification. These tests may also provide direction about additional tests needed for definitive identification. Further discussion of these and other similar rapid biochemical methods is included in subsequent chapters as they apply to specific organism identification.

Identification Systems Relying on Carbohydrate Utilization or Chromogenic Substrates

Rapid tests for detection of end products resulting from carbohydrate metabolism or enzymatic tests using chromogenic substrates produce reaction endpoints in minutes to hours. Plastic cupules, reaction chambers, or filter paper strips contain desiccated or dehydrated reagents or substrates. In general a suspension of bacterial cells or a loopful of an isolated colony is added to the system or rubbed off to a reaction area. A positive reaction is measured by enzymatic activity and color change.

Multitest kits using conventional carbohydrate metabolism take advantage of one test inoculum distributed to multiple reaction sites to yield more than one result. To obtain more rapid results, conventional methods have been modified by decreasing the test substrate medium volume and increas-

TABLE 9-2 Rapid Biochemical Tests Performed on Isolated Colonies

Test	Bacterial Enzyme	Mode of Action	Applications
Spot indole	Tryptophanase	Organism from blood agar or any tryptophan-containing medium is placed on a swab and reagent is added Hydrolysis of tryptophan to indole is indicated by the production of blue to blue-green color upon addition of DMAC	Positive reaction identifies *Escherichia coli*, *Proteus vulgaris;* aids in the identification of anaerobes
ONPG	β-Galactosidase	An ester linkage of orthonitrophenyl moieties to various carbohydrates Hydrolysis results in release of yellow ortho-nitrophenol	Determines lactose fermentation (yellow color) in slow lactose fermenters Differentiates *Neisseria lactamica* from pathogenic *Neisseria* sp.
Oxidase	Cytochrome C oxidase	A blue compound is produced when tetramethyl-para-phenylenediamine reacts with cytochrome c	Differentiation of nonfermenters; aids in the identification of *Neisseria* sp., *Aeromonas* sp., *Vibrio* sp., and *Campylobacter* sp.
Catalase	Catalase	Breakdown of hydrogen peroxide into oxygen and water, resulting in rapid production of bubbles	Differentiation of staphylococci from streptococci and of *Listeria* sp. from streptococci
Bile solubility		Autocatalyzes colony in the presence of the surfactant sodium deoxycholate (bile salt)	Presumptive identification of *Streptococcus pneumoniae* in sputum, blood, and CSF cultures
PYR	L-Pyroglutaml-aminopeptidase	Hydrolysis of amide substrate with formation of the free β-naphthylamide, which combines with DMAC to form a bright red color	Identification of group A streptococci; differentiates *Enterococcus* from group D streptococci
Rapid urease	Urease	Rapid hydrolysis of urea by urease releases ammonia; the alkalinity causes the phenol red indicator to change from yellow to red	Screening test for *Cryptociccus* spp., *Proteus* spp., *Klebsiella* spp., and *Yersinia enterocolitica*
Rapid hippurate hydrolysis	Hippuricase	Enzymatic hydrolysis of hippurate visualized by addition of ninhydrin (triketohydrindine)	Speciation of *Streptococcus agalactiae*, *Campylobacter jejuni*, *Listeria* spp.
MUG	β-Glucuronidase	Hydrolysis of substrate to the fluorescent compound 4-methylumbelliferyl-β-D-glucuronide, which fluoresces blue under long-wave UV light	Presumptive identification of *E. coli* and *Streptoccus anginosus* group; enterohemorrhagic *E. coli* is negative
LAP	Leucine aminopeptidase	LAP hydrolyzes the substrate to leucine and α-naphthylamine, which reacts with DMAC to form a red color	Presumptive identification of catalase negative, gram-positive cocci

DMAC, p-dimethylaminocinnamaldehyde; *ONPG*, orthonitrophenyl galactoside; *CSF*, cerebrospinal fluid; *PYR*, l-pyrrolidonly-β-naphthylamide; *MUG*, 4-methylumbelliferyl-β-D-glucuronide; *UV*, ultraviolet; *LAP*, leucine aminopeptidase.

ing the concentration of bacteria in the inoculum. Methods based on enzyme substrates have certain advantages over conventional methods. Because enzymatic methods involve preformed enzymes, they do not require multiplication of the organism (growth independent). Therefore endpoints are reached in minutes to a few hours. The tests are very sensitive for the presence of the enzyme although not always specific for genus and species identification; however, sensitivity does depend on the concentration and stability of the substrate, the enzyme, and the age of the inoculum. Several of the rapid modifications of conventional methods for bacterial and yeast identification are listed in Table 9-3. Remel markets a series of RapID panels that can provide an identification in about 4 hours (Figure 9-12).

Automated Identification Systems

Several automated identification systems are currently available; most of these systems use turbidity, colorimetry, or fluo-

rescent assay principles. Panels of freeze-dried or lyophilized reagents are provided in microtiter trays or sealed cards. Fully automated systems incubate and read the reactions, and computer software interprets the results and provides the identification. An advantage of automated systems includes an interface to laboratory information systems, leading to decreased turnaround times for reporting of results. Other advantages include statistical prediction of correct identification, increased data acquisition and epidemiologic analysis, and automated standardization of identification profiles that can reduce analytical errors. If these systems are used in conjunction with automated susceptibility testing, these data may be linked to the pharmacy for patient management applications. Theoretically early reporting of results can shorten length of hospital stay, augment therapeutic management of appropriate antimicrobial agents, and therefore also cut hospital costs.

Whether using manual multitest (as discussed previously) or automated systems, laboratories use an incubated "purity"

TABLE 9-3 Commercially Available Manual and Automated Systems for Microbial Identification

Name	Manufacturer	Principle	Organism(s) Identified
Manual			
API	bioMérieux[1]	Carbohydrate utilization/ chromogenic substrate	Enterobacteriaceae, other GN bacilli, *Staphylococcus, Streptococcus, Enterococcus, Neisseria,* GP bacilli, yeast, anaerobes
Crystal E/NF	BD Diagnostic Systems[2]	Carbohydrate utilization/ chromogenic substrate	Enterobacteriaceae, other GN bacilli, *Neisseria, Haemophilus,* GP cocci, GP bacilli
Enterotube II	BD Diagnostic Systems	Carbohydrate utilization/ chromogenic substrate	Enterobacteriaceae, other GN bacilli
GN2 Microplate	Biolog[4]	Carbohydrate utilization	GP, GN, yeasts, anaerobes
Gonochek	EY Laboratories[6]	Chromogenic substrate	*Neisseria/Moraxella*
Micro-ID (RapID)	Remel[3]	Carbohydrate utilization/ chromogenic substrate	Enterobacteriaceae, other GN bacilli, *Neisseria, Haemophilus,* streptococci, enterococci, yeast, anaerobes, UTI, GP bacilli
MicroScan (TouchScan)	Siemens Healthcare Diagnostics[5]	Carbohydrate utilization/ chromogenic substrate	GP, GN, urinary tract, *Haemophilus, Neisseria*
Oxi-Ferm II	BD Diagnostic Systems	Carbohydrate utilization	Nonfermenter GN bacteria
Plate	Remel	Chromogenic substrate	*Neisseria/Moraxella, Escherichia coli, Streptococcus,* yeasts
Uni-N/F-Tek	Remel	Carbohydrate utilization	Nonfermenters, yeast
Automated			
BD Phoenix	BD Diagnostic Systems	Carbohydrate utilization/ chromogenic substrate/fluorogenic substrate	Enterobacteriaceae, other GN bacilli, GP
MicroScan (Autoscan, WalkAway)	Siemens Healthcare Diagnostics	Carbohydrate utilization/ chromogenic substrate/fluorogenic substrate	Enterobacteriaceae, other GN bacilli, *Neisseria, Haemophilus,* streptococci, enterococci, staphylococci, GP bacilli, yeast, anaerobes
Sensititre	TREK Diagnostic Systems[7]	Carbohydrate utilization/ chromogenic substrate	GN, GP, anaerobes
Sherlock Microbial Identification System	MIDI[8]	Fatty acid analysis of microbial cells	GN, GP, *Mycobacterium,* yeasts
Vitek (AMS)	bioMérieux	Carbohydrate utilization/ chromogenic substrate	Enterobacteriaceae, other GN bacilli, *Neisseria, Haemophilus,* streptococci, enterococci, staphylococci, GP bacilli, yeast, anaerobes

API, Analytical Profile Index; *GN,* gram-negative organisms; *UTI,* urinary tract infection; *AMS,* AutoMicrobic System.
[1]Hazelwood, Mo.
[2]Sparks, Md.
[3]Lenexa, Kan.
[4]Hayward, Calif.
[5]Deerfield, Ill.
[6]San Mateo, Calif.
[7]Cleveland, Ohio.
[8]Newark, Del.

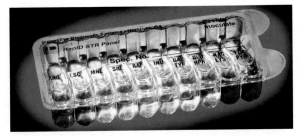

FIGURE 9-12 A RapID cartridge containing various substrates. (Courtesy Remel, Lenexa, Kan.)

plate of the inoculum to accompany the identification procedure. Because many specimens are polymicrobic, a purity plate ensures that the inoculum was pure and was not mixed with another microorganism that would produce erroneous results. With the threat of biologic terrorism, automated systems address the rapid, accurate identification of biothreat level A organisms. Many of these organisms, such as *Bacillus anthracis, Francisella tularensis,* and *Yersinia pestis,* are rarely seen in clinical microbiology laboratories. Manufacturers of identification systems have responded by including updated data on biothreat level A organisms in their identification databases.

MicroScan System

The MicroScan System (Siemens Healthcare Diagnostics, Deerfield, Ill.) consists of plastic standard-sized 96-well microtiter trays in which as many as 32 reagent substrates are included for the identification of bacteria and yeasts. Three systems are available: TouchScan, Autoscan, and WalkAway. Some trays, called *combo trays,* include broth microdilutions of various antimicrobial agents for performing susceptibility tests along with biochemical tests for identification. MicroScan panels containing dehydrated substrates are supplied. Dehydrated panels are more convenient than frozen panels for shipping and allow for room temperature storage and a longer shelf-life. The wells are inoculated with a heavy suspension of the organism to be tested and incubated at 35° C. Most panels are incubated a minimum of 16 hours up to about 20 hours. With the TouchScan system, reagents are added to some wells, and the panels are interpreted visually. Biochemical results are recorded with a computer by manually touching a probe near wells with positive reactions, after which the biochemical results are converted into a seven- or eight-digit biotype number. The number is compared with a database, and the computer provides the most likely identification of the microorganism.

With antimicrobial susceptibility testing, the endpoints in the microtiter plates are determined by the laboratory scientist and recorded by the computer, and a printout provides the minimal inhibitory concentration for each antimicrobial agent. Alternatively an automated tray reader, such as the Autoscan system, can be used to detect bacterial growth or color changes by differences in light transmission. As with other automated systems, the organism identification is accomplished electronically by collating the readings and matching them to the system's software database for final identification. The MicroScan WalkAway is fully automated with capabilities to incubate more than one panel, automatically add reagents to conventional panels when required, read and interpret panel results, and print results, all without operator intervention (Figure 9-13).

In a comparison of the Neg Combo type 12 panel for nonglucose fermenting, gram-negative bacteria with conventional biochemical tests, the WalkAway system correctly identified 215 of 301 isolates (71.8%). In addition to the conventional MicroScan panels, rapid fluorescence panels are available for use in the WalkAway instrument. The rapid panels, such as the Rapid ID type 3, use fluorescent labeled compounds and require only a 2-hour incubation period for bacterial identification. Fluorometric reactions detect changes in pH as a result of carbohydrate fermentation. The resultant acid production causes a drop in pH and a decrease in fluorescence. The Rapid ID type 3 panel does not require mineral overlay for amino acid reactions and has a reported accuracy for Enterobacteriaceae of 88.5% and for nonfermenting gram-negative bacilli of 78.8%.

Sensititre System

The Sensititre System (TREK Diagnostic Systems, Cleveland, Ohio) offers two automated systems: the Sensititre Auto-

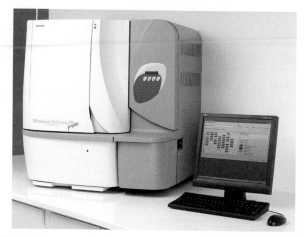

FIGURE 9-13 WalkAway® 96 *plus* System featuring the test platform and automated data management system. (Courtesy Siemens Healthcare Diagnostics, Inc., Deerfield, ILL.)

reader and the fully automated Sensititre ARIS2X identification system. Both systems use the same gram-negative intracellular diplococci (GNID) panel for the identification of gram-negative bacteria. The Sensititre system uses fluorescent technology to detect bacterial growth and enzyme activity. The system comprises 32 biochemical tests, including selected classic biochemical media reformulated to yield a fluorescent signal. The biochemical test medium, along with an appropriate fluorescent indicator, is dried into the individual wells of the Sensititre plate. Each biochemical reaction is repeated three times in the 96-well plates; therefore each plate is designed to test three separate organisms. All tests are read on the Sensititre Autoreader for the presence or absence of fluorescence. The results are transmitted to a computer for analysis and identification.

Vitek System

The Vitek AutoMicrobic System (AMS; bioMérieux Vitek) was first introduced in the 1980s. The Enterobacteriaceae Biochemical Card (EBC) provided automatic identification of the Enterobacteriaceae within 8 hours of incubation. By 1982 the EBC+ card was introduced, and it could identify nonenteric gram-negative bacteria and provide results in as soon as 4 hours. Additional 30-microwell cards contain substrates for the identification of numerous gram-positive and gram-negative bacteria and yeasts and also can perform antimicrobial susceptibility testing. A suspension of the organism is prepared in saline, and the card is attached to the bacterial suspension by a transfer tube and placed in the filling module of the instrument. The card is inoculated by a vacuum-release method. The card is then placed in the reader-incubator module of the instrument, where it is optically scanned and read on a periodic basis. The computer software collates the readings and matches them to the automated database for final identification. The GNI+ card has 30 wells and is used for the identification of Enterobacteriaceae, Vibrionaceae, and nonglucose-fermenting gram-negative bacilli. The card can provide identification within 4 to 12 hours.

Compared with conventional biochemical testing of nonglucose-fermenting gram-negative bacilli, the GNI+ card correctly identified 216 of 301 isolates (71.8%). The Vitek 2 was introduced in 1999. This system included new hardware, software, and increased automation, resulting in less hands-on time. The Vitek 2 can process 60 or 120 cards at one time. In 2004 the colorimetric 2GN card was released. This is a 64-well card used for the identification of fermenting and nonfermenting gram-negative bacilli. Compared with the API 20E, the 2GN card had an accuracy rate of 97.6%.

BD Phoenix 100 System

The BD Phoenix 100 (BD Diagnostic Systems), released in 2003, is the latest automated system. Once the panels are inoculated, it is a totally hands-off system that can hold 99 panels at one time. Panels are read every 20 minutes for up to 16 hours. Results are generally available in 8 to 12 hours. The gram-negative identification (NID) panel for gram-negative bacteria contains dried enzymatic substrates, carbohydrate substrates, and growth and inhibition tests. Compared with the API 20E, the accuracy rate is 92.5%; compared with the API 20NE, it had a reported accuracy of 96.3%. An accuracy rate of 94.6% was found when 500 strains of Enterobacteriaceae were tested and compared with conventional biochemical tests. Gram-positive cards and cards for antimicrobial susceptibility are also available. Compared with the agar dilution method, susceptibility cards had 100% concordance for determining susceptibility to the majority of antimicrobial agents for staphylococci, enterococci, and Enterobacteriaceae. A concordance of less than 90% was reported only for ciprofloxacin susceptibility of enterococci (84.6%) and gram-negative nonfermenters (88.5%) and for trimethoprim-sulfamethoxazole susceptibility of *Stenotrophomonas maltophilia* (80.0%).

Sherlock Microbial Identification System

The Sherlock Microbial Identification System (MIDI, Newark, Del.) takes a totally different approach; identification is based on the 9- to 20-carbon fatty acid composition of microorganisms (Figure 9-14). The Sherlock system examines which fatty acids are present as well as their relative concentration (percentage). Fatty acids are located in the plasma membrane of bacteria and are modified by the bacteria, depending on environmental conditions. For this reason it is important that growth conditions are well standardized for accurate identification. The standard incubation conditions for most aerobic bacteria are tryptic soy agar incubated at 28° C for 24 hours. After incubation, a loopful of bacteria is suspended in a methanolic base and heated for 30 minutes in a boiling water bath. During this step the cells are lysed, and the fatty acids are cleaved from the lipids and converted into the sodium salt. After cooling the sample is mixed with a solution of methanol and hydrochloric acid to methylate the fatty acids to fatty acid methyl esters. The fatty acid methyl esters are extracted, washed, and injected into a high-

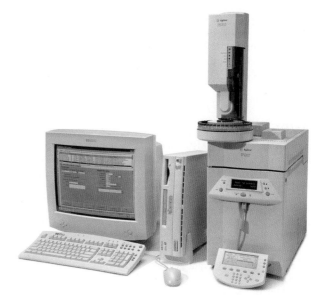

FIGURE 9-14   Sherlock Microbial Identification System incorporates Agilent gas chromatograph; model #6850. (Courtesy Agilent Technologies, Inc., Palo Alto, Calif.)

resolution gas chromatograph (GC). The fatty acid esters are separated by the column in the GC, and a chromatogram is created. The size of the molecule and degree of saturation determine the retention time in the column. The fatty acids are identified by their retention time compared with standards, and the height of the peak determines the concentration. MIDI also markets a high-performance liquid chromatography system for the identification of *Mycobacterium* spp.

The Sherlock system compares the fatty acid profile of the unknown with the database and determines a similarity index. The similarity index is a numeric value expressing how close the unknown organism's fatty acid profile is to the mean profile of an organism suspected of being a match. The similarity index is a measure of relative distance from the mean and not a probability match used in many other systems. A similarity index of 1.000 is an exact match, and a similarity index less than 0.300 indicates the unknown is not in the database.

Evaluation of Identification Systems

Most rapid and automated procedures are designed to provide results with greater speed and precision than traditional methods. Many automated systems are highly accurate and can provide results in as soon as 2 to 4 hours. Whether greater efficiency and productivity are achieved depends largely on the laboratory and the institution(s) that it supports. Therefore both manual and automated systems should be evaluated onsite before changing or augmenting current protocols. The best studies are prospective, side-by-side comparisons of the current in-house or reference procedure to the new system for accuracy, cost effectiveness, and effect on work flow. These systems often provide decreased sensitivity and specificity for the identification of the biochemically inert bacteria and some fastidious organisms. Therefore supplemental and differential media and conventional biochemicals must still be kept on hand to support the identification of these organisms.

BIBLIOGRAPHY

Carroll KC, Weinstien MP: Manual and automated systems for detection and identification of microorganisms. In Murray PR, Baron EJ, Jorgensen JH, et al, editors: *Manual of clinical microbiology*, ed 9, Washington, DC, 2007, ASM Press, p 192.

Endimiani A et al: Identification and antimicrobial susceptibility testing of clinical isolates of nonfermenting gram-negative bacteria by the Phoenix Automated Microbiology System, *Microbiologica* 25:323, 2002.

Funke G et al: Evaluation of VITEK 2 system for rapid identification of medically relevant gram-negative rods, *J Clin Microbiol* 36:1948, 1998.

MacFaddin JF: *Biochemical tests for identification of medical bacteria,* ed 3, Philadelphia, 2000, Lippincott Williams & Williams.

Maquelin K et al: Idntification of medically relevant microorganisms by vibrational spectroscopy, *J Microbiol Methods* 51:255, 2002.

O'Hara CM: Manual and automated instrumentation for identification of Enterobacteriaceae and other aerobic gram-negative bacilli, *Clin Microbiol Rev* 18:147, 2005.

Stefaniuk E et al: Evaluation of the BD Phoenix automated identification and susceptibility testing system in clinical microbiology laboratory practice, *Eur J Clin Microbiol Infect Dis* 22:479, 2003.

Sung LL et al: Evaluation of autoSCAN-W/A and the Vitek GNI+ AutoMicrobic system for identification of non-glucose-fermenting gram-negative bacilli, *J Clin Microbiol* 38:1127, 2000.

Willis MS, So SG: Acute diarrhea in a young traveler, *Lab Med* 33:775, 2002.

Points to Remember

- In many laboratories, identification of gram-negative bacteria is still based on biochemical testing.
- Phenotyping, serotyping, and genotyping all have important uses in the identification of bacteria.
- Molecular biology assays, such as nucleic acid amplification tests, provide accurate identification more rapidly than conventional biochemical testing.
- Bacteria can utilize carbohydrates oxidatively, fermentatively, or not at all.
- Triple sugar iron and Kligler iron agars are useful in determining bacteria's ability to utilize certain carbohydrates and to produce H_2S.
- The methyl red and Voges-Proskauer (MRVP) tests are used to determine the end products of glucose fermentation.
- Decarboxylase, dihydrolases, and deaminases are enzymes used by bacteria to metabolize amino acids.
- A number of tests, such as citrate, DNase, indole, nitrate reduction, oxidase, and urease, are important in the identification of gram-negative bacteria.
- Manual multitest systems improved the identification of bacteria by simplifying inoculation of many different biochemical tests and producing numeric codes that can be compared with numbers in a database.

- Rapid tests often use chromogenic or fluorogenic substrates to assay for preformed bacterial enzymes.
- Automated microbial identification systems offer accurate, rapid, identifications with less hands-on time by laboratory scientists.

Learning Assessment Questions

1. Which of the following tests detects the production of mixed acids as a result of subsequent metabolism of pyruvate?
   a. Methyl red test
   b. Voges-Proskauer test
   c. Citrate test
   d. Indole test

2. The metabolism of glucose to pyruvate by members of the family Enterobacteriaceae is via the Embden-Meyerhof pathway. The subsequent metabolism of pyruvate shows this reaction:

   Glucose → Pyruvate → Acetylmethylcarbinol (acetoin) → 2,3 Butanediol

   This reaction is the basis for the:
   a. Oxidase reaction
   b. Methyl red test
   c. Indole test
   d. Voges-Proskauer test

3. An oxidase-negative, gram-negative bacillus that produces an acid slant and acid butt on triple sugar iron (TSI) agar is able to ferment which of the following carbohydrates?
   a. Glucose only
   b. Glucose and lactose and/or sucrose
   c. Lactose only
   d. Lactose and sucrose, but not glucose

4. Why is an oil overlay used when testing carbohydrate utilization?
   a. Minimizes the risk of airborne contamination
   b. Provides a nutrient source
   c. Creates an anaerobic environment
   d. Enhances activity of pH indicator

5. Tryptophan broth is inoculated and incubated 24 hours. After incubation, Kovac reagent is added. A red color develops at the surface of the broth. What product of metabolism was formed?
   a. Mixed acids
   b. Malonate
   c. Phenylpyruvate
   d. Indole

6. In the citrate utilization test, a positive result is determined by:
   a. Increase in pH from peptone metabolism
   b. Increase in pH from urease activity
   c. Decrease in pH from citrate utilization
   d. Decrease in pH from nitrate reduction

7. Lysine deaminase:
   a. Cleaves the carboxy group from lysine
   b. Cleaves the amino group from lysine
   c. Adds an amino group to lysine
   d. Adds a carboxy group to lysine

8. A TSI agar slant is inoculated with an oxidase-negative, gram-negative bacillus. After incubation, the slant is red and the butt (deep) is black. Explain the biochemical reactions that have occurred.

9. How do bacteria that are able to rapidly ferment lactose differ from bacteria that are delayed lactose fermenters?

10. After 24-hour incubation of a nitrate broth with visible growth, N,N-dimethyl-α-naphthylamine and sulfanilic acid are added. No color change is noted. What are two possible explanations concerning the reduction of nitrate? What should you do next to determine which explanation is correct?

Immunodiagnosis of Infectious Diseases

Donald C. Lehman

■ **ANTIBODIES IN SEROLOGIC TESTING**
Antigens
Acute and Convalescent Antibody Titers
Monoclonal Antibodies
Antibody Specificity and Cross-Reactivity
False-Negative and False-Positive Serologic Results
Population Studies
Immune Status Testing
Congenital Infections

■ **ANTIGEN DETECTION**

■ **PRINCIPLES OF IMMUNOLOGIC ASSAYS**
Precipitation Assays
Agglutination Assays
Neutralization Assays
Labeled Immunoassays

■ **USE OF SEROLOGIC TESTING IN SPECIFIC DISEASES**
Serologic Testing of Syphilis
Serologic Testing for Streptococcal Infections
Serologic Diagnosis of Toxoplasmosis
Serologic Diagnosis of Viral Diseases
Serologic Diagnosis of Fungal Infections

■ **DIRECT ANTIGEN DETECTION ASSAYS**
Respiratory Tract Infections
Bacterial Meningitis and Sepsis
Infections in Immunocompromised Patients
Gastrointestinal Tract Infections
Sexually Transmitted Diseases
Human Immunodeficiency Virus

OBJECTIVES

After reading and studying this chapter, you should be able to:

1. Describe antigens.

2. Compare immunoglobulin G and immunoglobulin M antibodies.

3. Discuss the importance of acute and convalescent antibody titers.

4. Interpret significant antibody titer results.

5. Compare polyclonal and monoclonal antibodies.

6. Discuss the causes of false-negative and false-positive immunologic test results.

7. Recognize the significance of serologic tests in the following situations:

- Population studies

- Immune status testing

- Congenital infections

- Infections beyond the newborn period

8. Describe the principles and applications of each of the following immunologic methods:

- Precipitation assays

- Agglutination assays

- Neutralization assays

- Immunofluorescent assays

- Enzyme immunoassays

- Complement fixation

- Western blotting

- Immunoblotting

9. Compare direct agglutination passive agglutination, and reverse passive agglutination. Describe the clinical applications of antibody detection for the following diseases:

- Syphilis

- *Streptococcus pyogenes* infection

- Toxoplasmosis
- Rubella
- Infectious mononucleosis
- Cytomegalovirus infection
- Hepatitis
- Human immunodeficiency virus infection
- Fungal infections

10. Describe the current clinical applications of direct antigen detection methods in each of the following infectious diseases:

- Respiratory tract infections
- Bacterial meningitis and sepsis
- Infections in immunocompromised patients
- Gastrointestinal tract infections
- Sexually transmitted diseases
- Human immunodeficiency virus infection

Case in Point

A 3-year-old girl awoke one morning complaining that she was "not feeling well" and that her "head hurt." The child started vomiting and was feverish. Case history also revealed that the child and her family had recently moved to the United States from Mexico. A week before this presentation, the child was seen at the primary care clinic for a viral respiratory syndrome but seemed to have been recovering well. On examination by the physician, the child was lethargic, and her condition had worsened. Subsequent laboratory tests included urinalysis, which produced no abnormal findings, complete blood count (CBC) with differential, and blood cultures. The CBC revealed an elevated white blood cell (WBC) count, predominantly polymorphonuclear cells. Based on these findings and clinical presentation, a lumbar puncture was performed. The cerebrospinal fluid appeared cloudy, with a WBC count of 1500 cells/mm^3, protein level of 150 mg/dL, and glucose level of 45 mg/dL. The serum glucose was 88 mg/dL (reference range: 70 to 105 mg/dL). The direct smear of the fluid showed numerous WBCs, but no organisms were visible. Culture and direct antigen detection for microbial pathogens were requested.

Issues to Consider

After reading the patient's case history, consider:

- The importance of the patient's case history and laboratory results
- The significance of the family being from Mexico
- The role of cultures and direct antigen detection in the diagnosis of infectious diseases

Key Terms

Acute-phase
Anamnestic immune response
Antibody titer
Antigens
Avidity
Chemiluminescent immunoassay (CLIA)
Coagglutination
Cold-agglutinating antibodies
Complement fixation
Conjugate
Convalescent-phase
Cytopathic effect (CPE)
Direct fluorescent antibody (DFA)
Epitopes
False-negative
False-positive
Fluorochrome
Heterophile antibodies
Hybridoma
Immune complex
Immunodiffusion
Immunogen
Indirect agglutination
Indirect fluorescent antibody (IFA)
Indirect sandwich immunoassays
Monoclonal antibody
Polyclonal
Polyclonal antibody
Postzone
Precipitation
Prozone
Reagin antibodies
Reverse passive agglutination
Rheumatoid factor
Seroconversion
Serology
Specificity
Zone of equivalence

The phenomenon of bacterial agglutination in human sera was discovered as early as 1896 and was quickly recognized as a powerful tool by bacteriologists. Not only could sera be used to identify and differentiate bacteria (serotyping), but the sera from infected patients could be tested for the ability to agglutinate a known microorganism. The reaction of patients' sera with bacteria was indicative of prior exposure to the organism and of the level of immune response and protection against the infectious agent. The proteins in human sera causing bacterial agglutination, called *antibodies,* form as a result of infection by microorganisms and viruses.

Serology is the study of antibodies and their reaction to **antigens,** molecules that bind specifically to antibodies or T-cell receptors, in the diagnosing of infectious diseases. Immunologic assays based on the principles of antibody-antigen reactions are also used to detect and quantify analytes, such as serum proteins, hormones, and drugs, in clinical chemistry. Perhaps the greatest advantage of serologic testing is that it is an excellent means for detecting infectious agents that are either difficult or impossible to culture. Certain infectious agents, such as viruses or some sexually transmitted bacteria, are difficult to culture, usually because of either their specific growth requirements or previous antimicrobial therapy that decreases the number of viable organisms. Fungi and mycobacteria, for example, take an extremely long time to grow. In addition, many organisms are not grown because of significant risk to laboratory workers. Not only are serologic tests used under these conditions, but they also can be used for prognostic information and in the monitoring of therapy, such as with chronic hepatitis.

As powerful as immunologic tests are, using serologic procedures in diagnosis has disadvantages. The most significant problem is that, to measure the host immune response to an organism, 10 to 14 days must pass after the onset of an infection. In some cases (e.g., human immunodeficiency virus [HIV], hepatitis B [HBV] and C viruses [HCV]), weeks to months must pass before antibody levels are detectable. Immunocompromised patients can have an antibody response that is either diminished or nonexistent, thereby impairing the ability to use any serologic procedure. Also, the antibody being detected may actually have been produced against another organism and a **false-positive** test is observed.

Reactions and cross-reactions of antisera prepared against proteins, both animal and plant, have shown that immune responses can be applied to the study of taxonomic relationships and even in forensics. However, nucleic acid sequencing is thought to be the most important assay for taxonomic studies. The discovery that immune hemolysis could be mediated by antierythrocyte antibodies in the presence of complement and could be titrated added a new approach to the diagnosis of infectious diseases. The blood of patients could be examined for the presence of antibodies that do not agglutinate or precipitate their respective antigens but do fix complement. This serologic method became known as **complement fixation** and is a very sensitive assay for detecting antibodies to their corresponding antigens.

The first practical laboratory tests for newly discovered infectious agents are still generally based on serology. The types of tests available continue to increase dramatically, allowing the diagnosis of many new infections. For example, acquired immunedeficiency syndrome (AIDS), hepatitis, and Lyme disease are most frequently diagnosed in the laboratory with serologic tests. These three diseases are all caused by infectious agents that are difficult to cultivate in routine clinical laboratories. Although currently available serologic tests for these and other agents are not perfect, improvements have resulted from advancements in preparation of antibodies and antigens of high purity. A wide variety of commercial kits of high quality are available. Immunologic tests are also used to detect antigens that are detectable earlier than antibodies; however, they are not available for as many organisms as the classic antibody detection tests. This chapter discusses the aspects of using immunologic assays to diagnose infectious disease—by detecting either antibodies or antigens in patient samples.

ANTIBODIES IN SEROLOGIC TESTING

Antigens

Antigens are relatively high–molecular-weight substances, usually proteins or polysaccharides (less commonly, lipids or nucleic acids either alone or complexed to proteins or polysaccharides), that can combine specifically with antibody molecules. Antigens that are recognized as foreign substances by a host are said to be *immunogenic,* capable of eliciting an immune response. Often, the terms *antigen* and **immunogen** are used interchangeably, but the former term really refers to the antibody-binding properties of the molecule, whereas the latter term refers to the antibody-eliciting property of the molecule.

The typical immune response to a large complex antigen, such as a bacterium or a virus, results in the stimulation of many different lymphocytes with differing **specificity** to all of the available antigenic determinants **(epitopes).** Refer to Chapter 2 for a detailed explanation of antibody formation. Most natural antigens are extremely large. Therefore the response generated to these molecules is **polyclonal,** resulting in a mixture of antibodies recognizing different antigens and epitopes with different binding affinities. **Polyclonal antibody** is a mixture of multiple antibody molecules derived from multiple cells against multiple epitopes found on an antigen. For instance, when an animal or person is exposed to any bacterium, different antibody molecules are made to each of the numerous epitopes found on the bacterium.

Microorganisms contain a wide array of molecules capable of eliciting an immune response in the host. Immunogenic substances may be structural or nonstructural components of the microorganism. For example, many bacteria have polysaccharide capsules that coat the organism. Because these capsules are located on the cell surface, they are often the first antigenic determinants recognized by the host. Additional structural antigenic components are the bacterial cell wall, membrane proteins, and pili proteins. Nonstructural antigens include bacterial enzymes and toxins that may be found within the cell or released into host tissues. Because many bacterial components are "hidden" deep within the cell, antibody responses to some of them may not develop until the cell has been partially degraded by the host's natural immunity (e.g., phagocytic cells, complement). Thus a single infecting bacterial species might stimulate the production of a large number of antibodies with different specificities.

Acute and Convalescent Antibody Titers

In serologic assays, patient's serum is tested for antibodies reactive to specific antigens taken from an infectious agent. If the antibodies are present, this indicates an infection. It is possible to semiquantitate the amount of antibody by making serial twofold (doubling) dilutions of the serum, producing progressively lower concentrations of antibody (1:2, 1:4, and so on). A standard amount of antigen from an infectious agent is mixed with each antibody dilution. The antibody-antigen reactions are then detected in some manner. A positive result is reported as an **antibody titer,** which is the reciprocal of the highest dilution of serum showing reactivity. This type of serial dilution method, however, is not very precise, and the difference of only one tube dilution is not considered significant in determining the presence of a recent infection. Antibody tests for a wide variety of infectious agents are commercially available (Table 10-1). Antigen-antibody (immune complex) detection methods, along with specific diagnostic applications, are discussed later in this chapter.

An individual's first exposure to an infectious agent primarily results in the production of immunoglobulin M (IgM). A subsequent exposure to the same antigen elicits a secondary or anamnestic immune response, characterized by a rapid increase in immunoglobulin G (IgG) antibody associated with higher levels, a prolonged elevation, and a more gradual decline (Figure 10-1). IgM antibody synthesis plays a minor role in a secondary immune response. Serologic tests that are designed to separately detect IgG and IgM antibodies take advantage of the differences in IgM production between a primary and a secondary immune response. Thus a positive test result for IgM antibody is considered indicative of a primary, current, or very recent infection, whereas the presence of IgG antibody alone suggests a previous infection or exposure. Similarly, the presence of significant levels of IgM antibody (with or without IgG) in a newborn suggests in utero infection. IgM can be synthesized by the fetus and cannot cross the placenta from mother to fetus, whereas the presence of IgG antibody only in the newborn is indicative of passive maternal transfer of IgG across the placenta, not in utero infection.

Several methods are available for removal or inactivation of serum IgG. One of the most popular methods for physical removal of IgG uses miniature ion-exchange chromatography columns to trap IgM while allowing IgG to be washed through with a buffer solution. The IgM antibody is then collected by elution from the column with a lower-pH buffer; these columns are available commercially. Another method of removing IgG from whole serum uses adsorption to protein A found in the cell wall of staphylococci. Protein A binds most subclasses of human IgG, thus facilitating their removal. Also, anti–human IgG inactivates or removes (requires precipitation and centrifugation) IgG for IgM specific assays. This method has the additional advantage of removing rheumatoid factor, because the latter will bind to the IgG–anti-IgG complexes.

Unless a serologic test is designed to measure IgM-specific antibody in a single serum specimen, serodiagnosis of an infectious disease requires measurement of total antibody concentration in both acute-phase and convalescent-phase serum specimens. Specific IgG antibody is usually not detected in serum collected during the acute phase of the illness (within 1 week of manifestation of symptoms). A significant rise in IgG detected during the convalescent (recovery) phase, usually 2 weeks later, is diagnostic for infection and is referred to as seroconversion. Although seroconversion usually occurs within 2 to 3 weeks after onset of illness, it may be delayed in certain patients or types of infection.

Because some IgG antibody may already be present in a patient's acute-phase serum specimen, it is generally necessary to quantify the concentration of antibody in both the acute-phase and convalescent-phase specimens. A relatively high titer of IgG does not necessarily indicate a current infection. Sera are generally tested as twofold dilutions in a series of tubes. A fourfold rise (two doubling dilutions) in antibody titer between acute phase (acute antibody titer) and convalescent-phase (convalescent antibody titer) serum specimens is considered diagnostic for a current infection. It is important that both sera be tested at the same time, because most serologic tests have an inherent variability that can alter the titer by at least twofold. Testing the sera at the same time reduces this variability.

TABLE 10-1 Examples of Commercially Available Serologic Tests for the Diagnosis of Infectious Disease

Organisms	Serologic Test Methods Available
Blastomyces dermatitidis	CF, ID, EIA
Bordetella pertussis	EIA
Borrelia burgdorferi	IFA, EIA, WB
Cytomegalovirus	EIA, LA, IFA
Epstein-Barr virus	HA, LA
Helicobacter pylori	EIA
Hepatitis virus A, B	EIA
Hepatitis C virus	EIA, dot blot
Herpes simplex virus	EIA, LA, IFA
Human immunodeficiency virus types 1, 2	EIA, IFA, ICT, WB
Histoplasma capsulatum	CF, ID, EIA
Influenza virus A, B	EIA
Legionella pneumophila	IFA, EIA
Mycoplasma pneumoniae	EIA, IFA
Respiratory syncytial virus	EIA
Rubella virus	EIA, IFA, HAI
Streptococcus pyogenes	NT, IHA
Toxoplasma gondii	EIA, IFA, LA
Treponema pallidum	IFA, EIA, flocculation

CF, Complement fixation; *ID,* immunodiffusion; *IFA,* indirect fluorescent antibody; *EIA,* enzyme immunoassay; *WB,* Western blot; *HA,* hemagglutination; *LA,* latex agglutination; *ICT,* immunochromatographic test; *HAI,* hemagglutination inhibition; *NT,* neutralization; *IHA,* indirect hemagglutination; *LA,* latex agglutination.

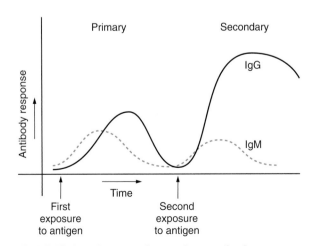

FIGURE 10-1 Primary and secondary antibody responses.

In practice, it is not uncommon to test a single serum specimen for IgG antibody to attempt to diagnose current or recent infection. In many cases, the presence of IgG antibody is difficult or impossible to evaluate; it may represent past infection, either clinically apparent or subclinical (without overt symptoms). In certain other cases, however, such as infections that are rare (e.g., rabies) or will have been present a relatively long time when symptoms first appear (e.g., AIDS), the presence of IgG antibody in a single serum specimen may be diagnostic.

More and more commercial diagnostic tests are designed without needing to perform serial dilution and establishment of titers. Instead, undiluted serum or a single serum dilution is tested. In these situations, the determination of a single positive result suggests, but does not always prove, current infection. Generally, if serologic diagnosis of current infection on a single serum specimen is to be attempted, an IgM assay as well as an IgG-specific assay should be done. If both assays are negative, the patient has probably not been infected. If both assay results are positive, or just IgM antibody is detected, the patient has probably been recently infected. If just IgG antibody is present, the patient has probably been infected in the past and does not have a current infection. It is very important that laboratory scientists completely understand all the performance characteristics of a commercial serologic test system.

Monoclonal Antibodies

When an animal is exposed to a single antigen, antibodies to different epitopes on the antigen can be produced. These antibodies are called *polyclonal antibodies* because each antibody was derived from a different clone of plasma cells. In serologic testing, antibodies can be used to detect antigens in patient samples. The problems with polyclonal antibody are low specificity, because the antibody solution contains multiple antibodies, and a high level of cross-reactivity for the same reason.

The problems with polyclonal antibody can be minimized through the use of **monoclonal antibody.** This antibody is derived from one cell initially, which has been exposed to one epitope. This cell then divides and produces an antibody specific to this one epitope. Monoclonal antibodies are rarely naturally occurring and are usually associated with some type of abnormal immune disease process. The production of monoclonal antibody in the laboratory has become commonplace. It is used extensively in serologic testing, where the identification or quantification of an antigen is the primary goal. These antibodies have strong binding kinetics to specific epitopes on antigens **(avidity)** and have the ability to discriminate between closely related antigenic determinants (specificity). Monoclonal antibodies, however, can be too specific. If a bacterial population contains an altered or mutated form of an antigen, it may not react to the monoclonal antibody, resulting in a **false-negative** test result.

Monoclonal antibodies are purified antibodies from a single clone of cells. In 1975, George Kohler developed the technique for producing monoclonal antibodies in the laboratory. This technique allows a scientist to inject a crude antigen mixture into a mouse and then select a clone, producing a specific antibody against a single cell surface antigen. This process of producing a monoclonal antibody may take as long as 3 to 6 months. The process involves fusing a single antibody-producing lymphocyte to a myeloma cell to form a hybrid. This hybrid then proliferates to form a cell line called a *hybridoma* (Figure 10-2).

Antibody Specificity and Cross-Reactivity

Most antigen-antibody reactions show high specificity; that is, the antigen-binding sites on the antibody molecule react with specific epitopes and not with other antigens containing different epitopes. Some antigens from different microorganisms are similar, however, and a host may respond by producing antibody, not only to the invading organism but also to antigenetically similar organisms. These antibodies are said to *cross-react,* which may lead to misinterpretation of serologic tests. Antibodies produced in response to one molecule that also react against an antigen from an unrelated source are called **heterophile antibodies.** Because of antibody cross-reactivity, it is often best to perform a battery of serologic tests using the organisms known to show cross-reactivity and to do so with paired sera. An example of this type of testing would be a fungal battery consisting of tests for histoplasmosis, blastomycosis, and coccidioidomycosis.

False-Negative and False-Positive Serologic Results

An ideal serologic test should have 100% diagnostic accuracy; that is, it should be positive on all specimens from patients with the infection and negative on all specimens from patients without the infection by the specific agent. In practice, serologic tests, like other laboratory tests, fall short of this ideal. The accuracy of diagnostic tests is measured in terms of sensitivity, specificity, positive predictive value, and negative predictive value. See Chapter 5 for a discussion of these terms.

A *false-negative serologic test* is defined as a negative result for a patient who really is infected. It may occur for a number of reasons. For example, a patient may be immunocompromised and therefore may not be able to respond to an immunogenic stimulus. This might be the case in an individual with a congenital or acquired immunodeficiency disease or in a patient receiving either immunosuppressive therapy after organ transplantation or cancer chemotherapy. In addition, neonates may not always respond to an infectious agent because of an immature immune system. For some infections, such as Lyme disease and Legionnaires disease, antibody titers may not rise until months after acute infection, thus leading to apparent false-negative serologic test results on serum samples collected too early in the course of the infection. It is important to remember that not all individuals react the same way to immunogenic stimuli, owing to the inherent genetic differences in the immune system among individuals.

A different type of false-negative result may occur in assays designed specifically to detect IgM antibody. It might be a result of competition for antigen-binding sites between IgG and IgM antibodies in a serum specimen from a patient with high levels of IgG and relatively low levels of IgM (Figure 10-3, *B*). For example, IgM antibody tests are sometimes

1. INOCULATION

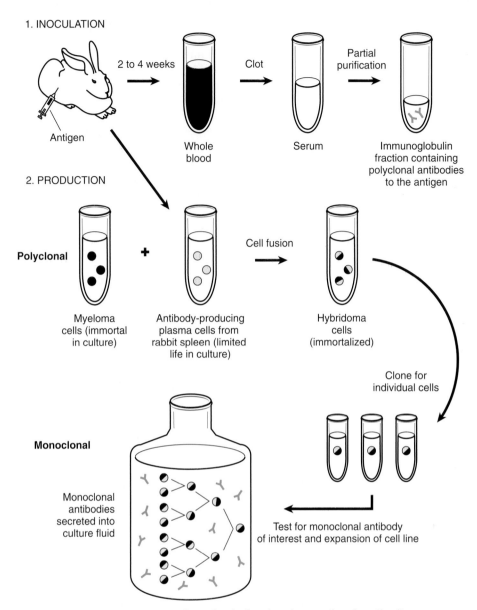

FIGURE 10-2 Preparation of polyclonal and monoclonal antibodies.

performed on the serum of a newborn to diagnose a suspected in utero infection. A newborn's serum specimen might contain maternal IgG to a specific infectious agent as well as low levels of fetal IgM. The IgG antibody molecules bind to antigen in the assay and block IgM binding, thus producing a false-negative IgM result. Most assays designed to detect IgM antibody include some initial procedure to physically separate IgG from IgM or to "capture" IgM in the assay and then remove IgG.

A false-positive serologic test result is a positive result for a patient who is not infected by the specific agent for which the test is designed. It might occur from the production of cross-reacting antibody, as discussed previously, or from the reactivation of a latent organism due to infection by a different organism. For example, influenza A virus infection may cause reactivation of latent cytomegalovirus (CMV) with a concomitant rise in CMV antibody. False-positive IgM anti-

body assays may also occur. These are due to the presence of rheumatoid factor activity in the serum. Rheumatoid factor is IgM antibody, which is produced in some individuals, that binds to the Fc region of the individual's own IgG. IgM rheumatoid factor cannot be readily differentiated from organism-specific IgM in some serologic tests. Thus if both organism-specific IgG and rheumatoid factor (but not organism-specific IgM) are present in a patient's serum specimen, the serologic test result may be falsely positive for organism-specific IgM antibody (Figure 10-3, *C*). Finally, individuals receiving intravenous immunoglobulin, a product prepared by pooling large quantities of plasma from multiple volunteer donors, may show specific antibody to a variety of infectious agents because of passive transfer, not active infection. Laboratory personnel must be aware of this and any therapy that may be of significance in interpreting serologic test results for a specific patient specimen.

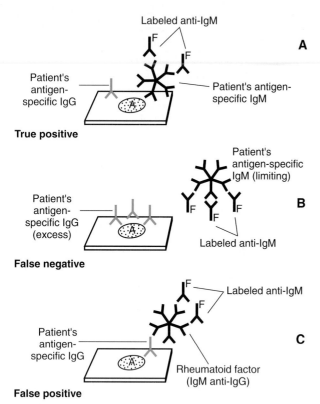

FIGURE 10-3 Causes of false-positive and false-negative immunoglobulin M (IgM) assays. **A,** True-positive IgM assay. **B,** False-negative IgM assay. Excess antigen-specific immunoglobulin G (IgG) inhibits antigen-specific IgM from binding. **C,** False-positive IgM assay. Rheumatoid factor (RF) binds to antigen-specific IgG and is detected with labeled anti-IgM antibody.

Population Studies

Serologic tests for a specific infectious agent or a battery of agents may be performed to determine the percentage of individuals previously exposed or infected with the agent(s) in a geographic area. This information provides epidemiologists and public health officials with information about how widespread an infectious agent is in a given area. For example, such studies have shown that the fungus *Histoplasma capsulatum,* which causes histoplasmosis, is widely distributed in the Ohio River Valley and that the bacterium *Borrelia burgdorferi,* which causes Lyme disease, is common in the Upper Midwest, New England, and Middle Atlantic states. Similarly, serologic studies performed on animals that are reservoirs for human disease may alert public health officials that the disease (e.g., West Nile virus) may be active in the area and may pose a threat to humans.

Immune Status Testing

In several situations, it may be important to determine whether an individual is immune (through either previous infection or immunization) to a specific infectious disease. For example, health care facilities may require prospective employees to show evidence of immunity to varicella-zoster virus, which causes chickenpox. This is because if infected, they may transmit the virus during the incubation period (before symptoms develop) to susceptible patients. Infection with varicella-zoster virus in a newborn or immunosuppressed patient may be life threatening. Similarly, women considering pregnancy should be screened for rubella and cytomegalovirus (CMV) antibodies; both agents may cause morbidity or mortality to the developing fetus if contracted during pregnancy. It is generally recommended that all women of child-bearing age be tested for their rubella immune status and, if it is negative, that they be vaccinated before considering pregnancy.

An additional situation in which immune status testing might be considered is organ or bone marrow transplantation. CMV may reside latently in leukocytes of donor tissue and may cause significant disease in a nonimmune recipient. Thus it is recommended that a CMV-negative transplant recipient receive tissue and blood products from a CMV-negative donor.

Congenital Infections

Serologic testing is often used to attempt to diagnose congenital infections (acquired in utero) in a newborn; some infectious agents have the ability to cross the placenta and cause infection of the fetus. Such infections may cause only minimal symptoms in the mother during pregnancy and thus may go undiagnosed at the time. If the mother is nonimmune, however, the infection may be significant to the fetus. The agents most commonly found by testing are the TORCH agents—*Toxoplasma gondii* (which causes toxoplasmosis), rubella virus, CMV, and herpes simplex virus—and *Treponema pallidum* subspecies *pallidum* (which causes syphilis).

Testing the mother's serum for IgG antibody is useless unless she was screened prenatally or early in pregnancy and antibody test results were negative. Because the TORCH agents are common infectious agents, many individuals have antibody remaining from previous infections. Similarly, testing for IgG antibody in the newborn is of no value, because maternal IgG crosses the placenta and is present in neonatal serum. Testing for maternal IgM antibody is likewise of little value (unless infection occurred near the time of delivery), because it may be undetectable by 1 or 2 months following infection. Thus, as previously discussed, IgM antibody detection on neonatal serum is the method of choice for serologic diagnosis of congenital infection by one of the TORCH agents.

ANTIGEN DETECTION

Antibody testing requires a certain amount of time to become positive. Direct antigen-based tests are generally considered to be less sensitive than culture; however, they are able to yield diagnostic information much sooner. This is extremely important in treatments that require the documentation of the presence of a specific organism. In the Case in Point, a direct antigen detection test could be used to identify *Haemophilus influenzae* serotype b, allowing appropriate antimicrobial therapy before the organism would be recovered in culture.

A large number of infectious agents produce antigens that can be identified from almost any body fluid (serum, urine, sputum, cerebraspinal fluid [CSF], or exudates) or cellular material. The modern era of direct antigen detection began

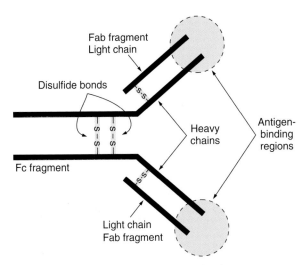

FIGURE 10-4 Structure of an antibody monomer.

in the mid-1970s. Since then, physicians have become increasingly interested in the rapid diagnosis of infectious diseases. The capability to produce large quantities of highly specific monoclonal antibodies has led to a sharp increase in production of rapid diagnostic products. Direct microbial antigen detection is the process by which microbial antigens such as capsular polysaccharide or cell wall components are identified in specimens obtained from an infected host. These antigens can be recognized by and can combine specifically with antibody molecules to form stable complexes.

The basic process of antigen detection involves reacting a clinical specimen with an antibody preparation specific for the antigen of interest. If the microbial antigen is present in the specimen, an antigen-antibody interaction occurs, forming an immuno-complex. This complex can then be detected by a number of techniques. Some methods take advantage of the fact that antibody molecules are polyvalent—they have two or more antigen-binding sites—and can combine with two or more antigens (Figure 10-4). Many techniques use indicator molecules such as enzyme substrate, fluorochrome excitation, or chemiluminescence. The tests used to detect these proteins (antigens) are similar to those used in the detection of antibody.

PRINCIPLES OF IMMUNOLOGIC ASSAYS

Precipitation Assays

The **precipitation** reaction is found in assays involving the diffusion of soluble antigen and antibody. At a critical point, when the concentrations are optimal, a visible precipitate forms, which is composed of an insoluble complex of antigens and antibodies. Precipitation reactions are most stable when performed in an agarose gel. Precipitation methods with diagnostic significance for infectious diseases are double **immunodiffusion,** radial immunodiffusion, and flocculation tests.

Double Immunodiffusion

Antibody-antigen reactions in agarose are performed in the clinical laboratory by a technique called *double immunodiffusion* or *Ouchterlony gel diffusion* (Figure 10-5). In this tech-

nique, cylindric holes or wells are cut out of an agarose gel, spaced appropriately, in a small Petri dish. For antibody detection, a known crude or purified antigen extract of a microorganism is placed in one well of the agar plate, and patient's serum is added to an adjacent well. The antigen and antibody molecule in solution diffuse out of the wells and through the porous agarose. If antibody specific for the antigen is present, the two components combine at a point of optimal concentration called the **zone of equivalence** and produce a visible precipitin band, or line of precipitation. Because the test relies on passive diffusion of molecules, diffusion is slow and is not generally amenable to rapid diagnosis. Reactions may take 48 to 72 hours to develop. It is most commonly used to detect fungal exoantigens or serum antibodies. Double immunodiffusion is commonly used to detect antibody to a battery of fungal pathogens, including *H. capsulatum*, *Blastomyces dermatitidis*, and *Coccidioides immitis*.

Single Radial Immunodiffusion

With single **radial immunodiffusion** (RID), known antibody is evenly distributed in agar placed into a plastic dish. Wells are cut in the agar and a sample is added to the wells that may contain antigen recognized by the antibody. The antigen passively diffuses through the agar and, at the zone of equivalence with the antibody, forms a precipitate. The diameter of the zone of precipitation is directly proportional to the concentration of the antigen. This technique is used to quantify antigen concentration.

Flocculation

Flocculation tests are a variation of precipitation tests that also have some properties of agglutination assays. In these tests, because of the chemical nature of the antigen (not a truly soluble antigen), the antigen-antibody reaction forms a macroscopically or microscopically visible clump or precipitate of fine particles that remain in suspension. The most important applications for flocculation tests in antibody detection relate to syphilis serology. Following infection with *T. pallidum*, the body reacts by developing two different classes of antibodies: (1) specific or treponemal antibodies, directed against *T. pallidum* antigens, and (2) nonspecific or nontreponemal antibodies, directed against normal host tissue. These nontreponemal antibodies are also referred to as **reagin antibodies.** Syphilis serology is discussed later in this chapter.

Agglutination Assays

Agglutinating antibodies react with antigens on the surface of microscopic particles to form visible clumps. Agglutination tests can be performed in test tubes, but they are generally performed on the surface of glass, plastic, or cardboard slides. Agglutination tests for antibody detection can be classified as either direct (natural particle) or indirect (artificial carrier particle) agglutination. **Indirect agglutination** is also referred to as *passive agglutination*. **Reverse passive agglutination** uses antibody attached to a particle to detect antigen. Unlike precipitation reactions, with agglutination reactions either the antigen or the antibody is bound to a particulate carrier before forming an immune complex.

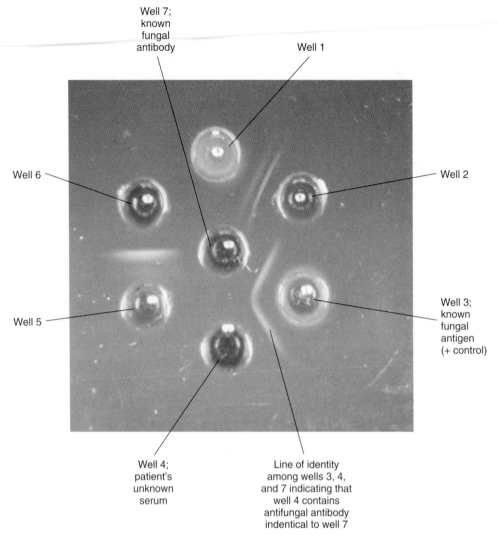

Well 7;
known
fungal
antibody

Well 1

Well 6

Well 2

Well 5

Well 3;
known
fungal
antigen
(+ control)

Well 4;
patient's
unknown
serum

Line of identity
among wells 3, 4,
and 7 indicating that
well 4 contains
antifungal antibody
indentical to well 7

FIGURE 10-5 Ouchterlony plate. A serum specimen containing an unknown antibody is placed in one well (e.g., well 4), a known antigen of interest is placed in an adjacent well (well 3—positive control), and a known antisera to the antigen (well 7—positive control) is placed in another adjacent well. The antigen and antibody molecules in the solution diffuse from the wells and through the porous agarose. If the unknown serum contains antibody to the known antigen, a precipitin band forms at a point of optimal concentration of each component. This precipitin band is called a *line of identity.*

Serologic tests based on direct particle agglutination take advantage of antigens that are naturally occurring on biologic cells. Most commonly, these cells are whole bacteria or erythrocytes. In whole bacterial cell agglutination, surface antigens that make up the bacterial cell wall or capsule allow cross-linking and visible agglutination of the cells in the presence of specific antibody. The so-called febrile agglutinin tests, for the detection of antibodies to *Brucella* spp., *Salmonella,* and *Francisella tularensis*, are based on bacterial agglutination. In some cases, an organism different from the suspected infectious agent may carry a chemically related antigen and may be more easily used in agglutination tests than the actual infectious agent. This approach is used in the Weil-Felix test to determine infection resulting from certain rickettsial agents by testing for agglutinating antibodies to various bacteria in the genus *Proteus*. Both febrile agglutinin and Weil-Felix agglutinin tests have been generally replaced in the United States by more sensitive and specific methods of diagnosis. However, because of their low cost, they are still used in some countries.

Latex Agglutination

A variety of antigens can be passively or chemically coupled to naturally occurring particles such as erythrocytes or to synthetic particles such as latex (polystyrene) beads. These beads, usually about 1 micron in diameter (Figure 10-6), enhance the visibility of agglutination reactions. In this arrangement, the particle can then be agglutinated by specific antibody found in a patient's serum specimen. The antigen-coated latex beads form a homogeneous milky suspension, which when mixed with a specimen containing specific antibody, results in antigen-antibody binding. However, this

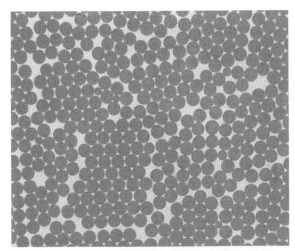

FIGURE 10-6 Transmission electron micrograph of a latex suspension. Each latex bead is about 1 micron in diameter. (Courtesy Molecular Probes, Invitrogen Detection Technologies, Eugene, Ore.)

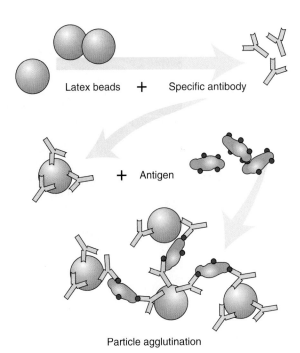

Particle agglutination

FIGURE 10-7 Alignment of antibody molecules bound to the surface of a latex particle and latex agglutination reaction.

primary binding between antigen and antibody molecules does not produce a visible agglutination (clumping) reaction. The antibody must interact with antigen on two different latex beads (secondary binding) to produce agglutination.

In reverse passive agglutination, each latex bead can contain thousands of antibody molecules. Monoclonal or polyclonal antibody molecules can be attached to the latex beads. When mixed with a specimen that contains antigen specific for the antibody on the latex beads, antigen-antibody binding results. However, only if the antigen molecules contain multiple epitopes, as is common for high–molecular weight polysaccharides, proteins, or microorganisms, will antigen molecules be cross-linked by the antibody-coated latex beads. It is this secondary cross-linking of antigen and antibody, resulting in a macromolecular lattice, which produces a visible agglutination reaction (Figure 10-7).

Latex agglutination (LA) assays are generally conducted on a treated cardboard or glass slide using liquid specimen and latex volumes of about 50 µL each (Figure 10-8). The reagents are mixed thoroughly. Then the slide is rocked or rotated by hand or with a mechanical device for 2 to 3 minutes before being read using appropriate lighting and the naked eye. The reaction depends on many variables; therefore standardization is imperative. Variables include latex particle size, avidity of antibody, isotype of antibody (IgM or IgG), reaction temperature, pH, ionic strength, and concentration of antigen in the specimen. IgM is a pentamer and is therefore a more effective agglutinin than IgG. Levels of detection of microbial polysaccharide or protein can be as low as 0.1 ng/mL.

The strength and rapidity of the reaction varies depending on the test conditions and, most importantly, on the concentration of antigen in the specimen. With high antigen concentration in the test sample, a maximum agglutination reaction (4+ on a 1+ to 4+ scale) may occur in only a few seconds. In the absence of specific antigen, the latex suspension remains homogeneous and milky; that is, no agglutination is seen. Although most applications of LA use white latex beads,

colored latexes are also available to enhance visual detection.

Controls must accompany the testing of patient specimens (Table 10-2). These controls include (1) a positive antigen control (a solution containing the known antigen of interest), (2) a negative antigen control (a solution not containing the antigen), and (3) a control latex suspension to detect the presence of nonspecific agglutination reactions. The control latex involves testing the patient specimen with latex beads coated with an immunoglobulin whose specificity is not directed to the test antigen. This nonimmune serum is generally obtained from the same animal species in which the specific antibody was made. A nonspecific agglutination reaction occurs when the patient's specimen reacts with both the test and the control latex. When such reactions occur, the test is uninterpretable. A positive test result requires that the test latex, but not the control latex, agglutinate the patient specimen.

Latex agglutination assays for microbial antigens, like other laboratory tests, are subject to false- negative and false-positive reactions when compared with culture. False-negative reactions (negative antigen test result, positive culture) may be due to the presence of antigen in the specimen at concentrations below the test detection limit. **Prozone** occurs when the relative concentration of antibody exceeds the concentration of antigen. In this situation, each antigen combines with one or two antibody molecules, and cross-linking between antigen and antibody does not occur. In addition, false-negative reactions can occur with antigen excess—**postzone.** When the concentration of antigen exceeds the relative con-

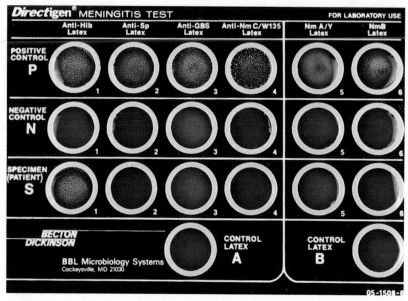

FIGURE 10-8 Commercial latex agglutination test slide showing reaction of controls and a patient's cerebrospinal fluid with latex reagents specific for *Haemophilus influenzae* serotype b (Hib). *Streptococcus pneumoniae* (Sp), group B *Streptococcus* (GBS), and five different serogroups (groups C and W135, groups A and Y, and group B) of *Neisseria meningitidis* (Nm). Note the positive reactions with each test latex reagent and positive control (P), as well as the positive reaction with the patient's specimen and Hib test latex. (Courtesy and © BD Diagnostic Systems, Inc, Sparks, Md.)

TABLE 10-2 Interpretation of Latex Agglutination Test Controls and Patient Specimens

		Agglutination Reaction		
Reaction Number	Test Specimen	Test Latex	Control Latex	Interpretation
1	Positive antigen control	+	0	Control OK
2	Negative antigen control	0	0	Control OK
3	Patient A	+	0	Positive test
4	Patient B	0	0	Negative test
5	Patient C	+	+	Nonspecific agglutination

+, Agglutination; 0, no agglutination.

centration of antibody, cross-linking between antigen and antibody does not occur and a proper lattice does not develop. Some test kits require all negative results be retested with a diluted sample to rule out postzone.

False-positive reactions (positive antigen test result, negative culture) are more difficult to explain; they may be due to the presence of cross-reacting antigens or nonviability of organisms in the original specimen. It is important to remember that antigen detection tests do not require viable microbes. Antibody-coated latex suspensions can agglutinate viable or nonviable organisms, microbial components such as cell wall or membrane fragments, or soluble antigen such as bacterial capsular polysaccharide. Thus an apparent false-positive latex test result may really represent a true-positive result for disease in a patient with a negative culture.

A number of specimen pretreatment procedures can be used to eliminate or minimize nonspecific agglutinations, presumably by removing or inactivating factors in the specimen responsible for these reactions. These procedures include specimen centrifugation to remove particulate material, boiling to inactivate protein constituents (acceptable when test antigen is a heat-stable polysaccharide), and passing the specimen through a membrane filter. Some specimens, such as urine, may be concentrated by centrifugation or membrane filtration before testing. Filters typically hold back or exclude high–molecular-weight antigenic materials while allowing water and small compounds to pass through. These concentration methods increase the sensitivity of the test. As commercial latex kits have become more specific and sensitive, pretreatments are less frequently required.

The advantages of LA tests are the availability of good quality reagents in complete kit form, good sensitivity, relative rapidity, and ease of performance. Disadvantages include subjectivity in reading endpoints and nonspecific reactions resulting from interfering substances in clinical samples. Still, the LA test is one of the most widely used antigen detection

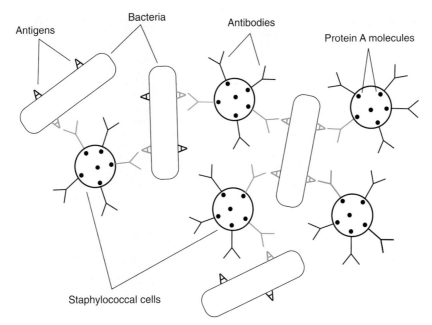

FIGURE 10-9 Diagram of coagglutination reaction with whole bacterial cell antigen. *A*, Antigen.

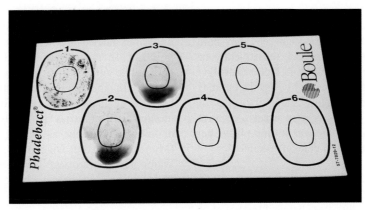

FIGURE 10-10 Commercial coagglutination test card showing positive *(1)* and negative *(2 and 3)* reactions. The blue color is an indicator dye added to make the agglutination reaction easier to read against a white background.

methods in the clinical laboratory. In many clinical laboratories, detection of *Cryptococcus neoformans* in serum or CSF, detection of bacteria causing meningitis in CSF, and serogroup identification of the β-hemolytic *Streptococcus* spp. from culture plates or throat swabs are routinely performed using LA test kits. Commercial serologic tests based on LA are available for a number of viral infections, including CMV, rubella, and infectious mononucleosis (heterophile antibody), as well as a few bacterial (streptococcal, mycoplasmal antibodies), fungal (candidal antibody), and parasitic (toxoplasmal antibody) infections.

Staphylococcal Coagglutination

Similar to LA, staphylococcal coagglutination, or simply **coagglutination,** uses particle-bound antibody to enhance the visibility of antigen-antibody reactions. Instead of a latex

bead, intact formalin-killed *Staphylococcus aureus* cells (typically Cowan 1 strain) are used. The cell wall of this strain of *S. aureus* contains a large amount of protein A, which can bind the Fc portion (base of the heavy immunoglobulin chain) of the IgG antibody molecule. This leaves the antigen-binding sites of the molecule (Fab portion) available to react with specific antigens (Figures 10-9 and 10-10). It has been estimated that each staphylococcal cell has about 80,000 antibody binding sites. The actual number of antibody molecules bound to the staphylococcal cell is limited by stearic hindrance. Coating is sufficient, however, to render the product of clinical utility in direct antigen tests.

Most of the observations made regarding LA are also true for coagglutination. Reactions are prepared by mixing antibody-sensitized staphylococcal cells with a solution containing the antigen of interest on a slide or card (Figure 10-10).

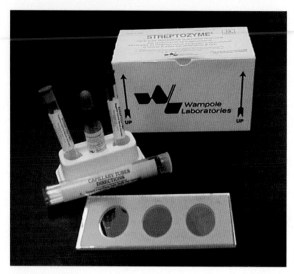

FIGURE 10-11 Streptozyme test (Wampole Laboratories, Cranbury, NJ) for the detection of antibodies to streptococcal products.

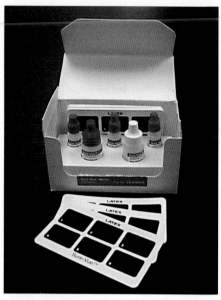

FIGURE 10-12 Sure-Vue, Mono test kit (Biokit) for the detection of heterophile antibodies produced during the disease infectious mononucleosis.

Coagglutination procedures appear more susceptible to non-specific agglutination reactions, and thus specimen preparation is important. This is particularly true for testing serum specimens, probably because staphylococcal cells may bind human IgG in test serum specimens and subsequently be agglutinated by the presence of rheumatoid factor (anti-IgG IgM) in the serum. Coagglutination is highly specific but may be less sensitive than LA in detecting small quantities of antigen. Therefore these reagents are often used to confirm the identification of bacterial colonies on culture plates, but not for rapid antigen detection from clinical specimens.

Hemagglutination

In passive or indirect hemagglutination (IHA), microbial antigens are attached to erythrocytes after chemical treatment of the cells with tannic acid, chromic chloride, glutaraldehyde, or another substance that promotes cross-linking of the antigens. The sensitized cells can then be reacted with patient's serum to detect agglutinating antibody. One example of an IHA test is the Streptozyme kit (Wampole Laboratories, Cranbury, N.J.) for the detection of antibodies to streptococcal extra-cellular antigens (Figure 10-11). In this assay, aldehyde-fixed sheep erythrocytes are sensitized with group A streptococcal exoantigens. When patient's serum containing specific antibody is reacted with the cells on a slide, an agglutination reaction occurs.

A special kind of natural particle agglutination test, known as *hemagglutination*, detects antibodies to naturally occurring antigens present on the surface of erythrocytes. During infection with *Mycoplasma pneumoniae*, for example, antibodies that can agglutinate human erythrocytes at 4° C but not at 37° C develop in some patients. These **cold-agglutinating antibodies,** which rise very quickly, may suggest *M. pneumoniae* infection, but the test lacks sensitivity and specificity. Testing for cold-agglutinating antibodies to diagnose *M. pneumoniae* infections has been replaced by more specific assays.

Another example of a direct hemagglutination test is the detection of heterophile antibodies in the acute stage of infectious mononucleosis, resulting from Epstein-Barr virus (EBV) infection. In the case of infectious mononucleosis, human heterophile antibody reacts with horse, ox, and sheep erythrocytes. In the appropriate setting, heterophile antibody testing is diagnostically very useful and is still commonly used in clinical laboratories. It may be performed as a tube test or, more commonly, as a slide or card agglutination test (Monospot, Ortho Diagnostics, Raritan, NJ; Mono-Test, Wampole Laboratories). Newer assays are based on heterophile antigens attached to latex particles (Sure-Vue; Biokit USA, Lexington, Mass.; Figure 10-12).

Hemagglutination Inhibition

A serologic test that has great historical significance to diagnostic serology, particularly to viral serology, is the hemagglutination inhibition (HI) test. This test takes advantage of the fact that a number of viral agents, including rubella and influenza viruses, have surface antigens that can agglutinate erythrocytes from certain mammalian species. Antibodies present in sera can bind to the virus and inhibit this agglutination reaction. The HI antibody titer is the highest dilution of the patient's serum that completely inhibits agglutination of the erythrocytes by the virus. Most HI tests have been replaced by other methods for determining viral antibodies, particularly enzyme immunoassays.

Liposome-Mediated Agglutination

One of the newer developments in agglutination technology, liposome-mediated agglutination, involves the use of liposomes, single-lipid bilayer membranes that form closed vesicles under appropriate conditions. In their manufacture, antigen or antibody molecules may be incorporated into the surface of the membrane and thus be available for interaction

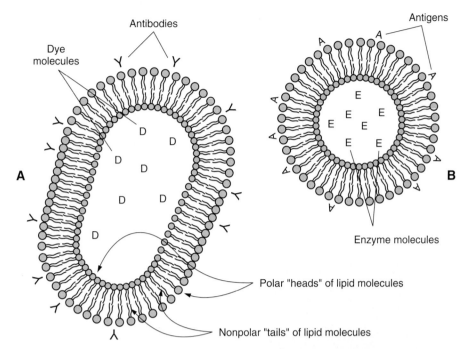

FIGURE 10-13 Diagram of liposome particles showing bilipid layer structure. Either antibody **(A)** or antigen **(B)** can be attached to the surface of the liposome. The interior of the liposome can carry reporter molecules (e.g., dyes, enzymes).

TABLE 10-3 Comparison of Particle Agglutination Methods

Agglutination Method	Particle Type	Nature of Antibody-Binding to Particle	Diagnostic Utility
Latex agglutination	Latex beads	Nonspecific absorption or chemical coupling	Most widely used agglutination method for direct detection
Staphylococcal coagglutination	Formalin-fixed staphylococci	Fc portion of immunoglobulin G molecule combines with protein A on staphylococcal cell wall	Used for antigenic identification of bacteria in culture
Liposome-mediated agglutination	Liposomes	Chemical coupling	Newer method; limited applications of commercial tests

with the corresponding molecule (Figure 10-13). In addition, the liposome vesicle may be constructed with a chemical dye or bioactive molecule trapped in the interior. The colored dye allows easy visual detection of lattice formation and agglutination between liposome-bound antibody and antigen. Alternatively, combining dye-containing liposomes and latex beads, both of which contain the reactive antibody on the surface, may increase the sensitivity of LA. Perhaps the greatest potential advantage of liposome technology is in its application to immunoassays other than particle agglutination that make use of the ability of the liposome to carry reactive chemicals. Liposomes have yet to reach their full potential as diagnostic reagents in the clinical laboratory. A comparison of particle agglutination methods is found in Table 10-3.

Neutralization Assays

Neutralization assays for antibody detection are based on the interaction of a biologically active antigen with antibodies that can block or inactivate the biologic activity of the antigen.

These neutralizing antibodies may play an important role not only in serologic tests but also in functioning as protective antibodies in vivo. For example, immunity to a number of viruses depends on circulating antibodies that may neutralize, or destroy the infectivity of, viruses that reach the bloodstream. Neutralization probably occurs because the antibody binds to the viral particle and blocks subsequent attachment of the virus to receptor sites on target cells. Neutralizing antibodies to viruses can be measured in vitro by the use of cell cultures.

In viral neutralization, a patient's serum sample is serially diluted, and each dilution is mixed with a standard amount of a known virus suspected of causing disease in the patient. The virus–serum mixtures are then inoculated to a series of cell culture tubes or flasks. If the patient's serum contains neutralizing antibody to the virus, the antibody will block viral infection and prevent **cytopathic effect (CPE)** on the cells. CPE is the visual changes occurring in cell monolayers caused by viruses or toxins. The neutralizing antibody titer is the highest dilution of the patient's serum to completely block

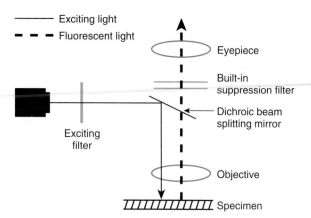

—— Exciting light
- - - Fluorescent light

Eyepiece

Built-in suppression filter

Dichroic beam splitting mirror

Exciting filter

Objective

Specimen

FIGURE 10-14 Light path of incident light microscope.

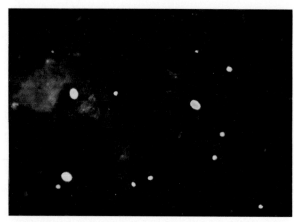

FIGURE 10-15 Direct fluorescent antibody–stained cells of *Giardia lamblia* (three larger apple-green, oval cells) and *Cryptosporidium* sp. (smaller cells) in stool. (Courtesy Meridian Bioscience, Cincinnati, Ohio.)

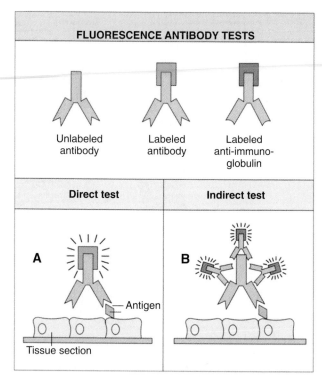

FLUORESCENCE ANTIBODY TESTS

Unlabeled antibody

Labeled antibody

Labeled anti-immuno-globulin

Direct test	Indirect test

A

Antigen

B

Tissue section

FIGURE 10-16 The fluorescence antibody test for identification of tissue antigens or their antibodies. **A,** Direct fluorescent antibody (DFA) test. The antigen-specific–labeled antibody is applied to the fixed specimen, incubated, washed, and visualized with a fluorescent microscope. **B,** Indirect fluorescent antibody (IFA). A second fluorochrome-labeled antibody specific for the first unlabeled antibody is applied. (From Goering R et al: *Mims Medical microbiology,* ed 4, London, 2008, Mosby.)

CPE. For diagnosis of current disease, acute-phase and convalescent-phase sera should be tested.

Viral neutralization assays are highly sensitive and specific, but they are also technically demanding and require the use of active virus and cell culture. They are not commonly used serologic tests today, but neutralization tests are valuable in identifying an unknown virus with known antibody. Other examples of a neutralization assays are the HI assay (previously discussed) and the anti-streptolysin-O (ASO) neutralization test to detect antistreptococcal antibodies.

Labeled Immunoassays
Immunofluorescent Assays

Immunofluorescent assays are a popular method for rapid antigen and antibody detection in the clinical laboratory. When specific monoclonal or polyclonal antibodies are conjugated with fluorescent dyes *(fluorochromes)*, they can be visualized with a fluorescent microscope. Fluorochromes are chemicals that absorb light of one wavelength and emit light of a different wavelength. The fluorescent microscope utilizes an epiluminescent (incident) light system of vertical illumination, wavelength filters, and a dichroic mirror (Figure 10-14).

The dichroic mirror allows passage of light at an excitation wavelength from the light source to the specimen. The mirror also allows passage of the emission (longer) wavelength light from the labeled source to the objective lens. This emitted, or excited, wavelength light appears as a bright color depending on the dye. A very commonly used fluorochrome is fluorescein isothiocyanate (FITC), which, when excited, emits a bright apple-green fluorescence (Figure 10-15).

Detection techniques may be direct or indirect. In the **direct fluorescent antibody (DFA)** test, the clinical specimen containing the antigen of interest is fixed onto a glass slide with formalin, methanol, ethanol, or acetone. Fixation renders mammalian cell membranes permeable to the stains. The antigen-specific–labeled antibody is applied to the fixed specimen, incubated, washed, and examined with a fluorescent microscope. If the antigen was present in the clinical specimen, the labeled antibody **(conjugate)** will bind to the antigen and fluorescence will be seen (Figure 10-16, *A*). Immunofluorescent staining allows for rapid visualization of infected tissue, cell culture, body fluids, and swab specimens.

When the infectious agent does not produce enough free antigen for detection in body fluids, testing cells directly must be considered. The use of specific antibody for the infectious agent enables the detection of the agent inside the infected cells. Direct immunofluorescent techniques are the assay of choice under these conditions. The DFA test is commonly used to detect *Bordetella pertussis, Legionella pneumophila, Giardia lamblia, Cryptosporidium* spp., *Pneumocystis (carinii) jiroveci,* herpes simplex virus, CMV, varicella-zoster virus, and most of the commonly isolated respiratory viruses such as parainfluenza virus, influenza virus, adenovirus, and respiratory syncytial virus (RSV) in clinical specimens.

In the **indirect fluorescent antibody (IFA)** test for antibody, whole microbial cells (bacteria, fungi, protozoan parasites) or virus-infected mammalian cells are washed and then fixed at a given density to glass slides. Frequently with commercially prepared assays, cells are placed into small wells on the glass slide, and different patient samples are added to individual wells. Fixation is usually accomplished with methanol, ethanol, or acetone.

The patient's serum can be serially diluted, applied to the fixed-cell preparations, and incubated for a short time (10 to 30 minutes) at 22° to 37° C in a humid environment to prevent drying; this procedure allows antigen-antibody binding to occur. The slides are then washed with a buffered solution to remove unbound antibody, and a second, antihuman IgG and/or IgM antibody, which is fluorescently labeled and reactive with human immunoglobulin, is applied. The labeled second antibody is frequently referred to as the conjugate. The slides are incubated again, and then washed, air-dried, and viewed using a microscope fitted with a light source and filters to excite the fluorochrome (see Figure 10-16, *B*). If specific antibody to the microbial antigen is present in the patient's serum, the antibody will bind and secondary binding by the conjugate will occur. The cells will fluoresce and be scored on a semiquantitative scale as positive (1+ to 4+) or negative. The titer is the reciprocal of the highest dilution of the patient's serum giving a minimum level of fluorescence (often at 2+ or greater).

The IFA assay remains the method of choice for serologic diagnosis of a number of infectious diseases such as the TORCH agents, EBV, *L. pneumophila, B. burgdorferi, Rickettsia rickettsii,* and *M. pneumoniae.* The detection of *T. pallidum* antibodies using the fluorescent treponemal antibody absorption (FTA-ABS) test (discussed later in this chapter) was the most widely used application of IFA tests. The FTA-ABS test, however, is gradually being replaced by assays that are easier to perform.

The IFA test is also useful in detecting IgM- or IgG-specific antibody, by using a FTIC-labeled second antibody highly specific for human IgM or IgG, respectively. As discussed previously, IgM-specific assays are particularly important in several clinical settings. As with any IgM test, IFA for IgM is subject to false-negative results owing to excess IgG and to false-positive results owing to rheumatoid factor. To avoid these problems, IgG should be physically removed or functionally inactivated for IgM-specific assays.

The utility of the IFA test is limited by a number of factors, including the labor-intensive nature of the procedures, the requirement for a fluorescent microscope, and the significant subjective interpretation involved in reading the slides. The procedure may not be very rapid (1 to 4 hours) and is not easily amenable to automation. Finally, fluorescence fades over time. Therefore antibodies have been conjugated to other

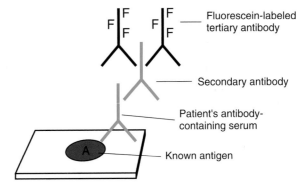

FIGURE 10-17 Double indirect fluorescent antibody tests for antibody detection.

markers besides fluorochromes. Colorimetric labels use enzymes, such as horseradish peroxidase, alkaline phosphatase, and avidin-biotin, to detect the presence of immune complexes by converting a colorless substrate into a colored end product. These products do not fade with storage and can be detected with a simple light microscope. The ability to visualize and evaluate reactions, however, gives a high level of certainty to the procedure. Thus newer serologic assays are often evaluated with IFA procedures. The IFA test is also quickly adaptable to studying serologic response to newly discovered infectious agents.

A number of variations of the IFA test have been developed. The basic objective in most of these procedures has been to increase sensitivity while maintaining specificity of the assay. One example of such a procedure is the double IFA test (Figure 10-17). This method uses a second, unlabeled antihuman IgG and/or IgM antibody to bind to microbial-specific antibody in the patient's serum. The FITC-labeled antibody is directed at the second antibody. The additional step amplifies the reaction, because multiple molecules of the second antibody can bind to the patient's antibody, thus providing additional binding sites for the FITC-labeled antibody.

Another example of enhanced immunofluorescent assay sensitivity uses a biotin-labeled second antibody. The binding of this reagent to the patient's antibody is detected using FITC-labeled avidin. Each biotin molecule binds four avidin molecules, thus increasing the total amount of bound FITC and, ultimately, the sensitivity of the assay. These and other microscopic techniques using fluorescent as well as enzymatic labels will continue to play an important role in serologic diagnosis of infectious diseases.

Enzyme Immunoassays

Enzyme immunoassay (EIA) provides an alternative to immunofluorescent assays for detecting antigens and antibodies in clinical samples. Instead of labeling an antibody with a fluorochrome, EIA depends on the fact that enzyme molecules can be conjugated to specific antibodies in such a way that both enzymatic and antigen-binding activities are preserved. The enzymes used are often alkaline phosphatase or horseradish peroxidase. When the appropriate substrate is added to the antigen-conjugated antibody complex, the enzyme cata-

A　　　　　　　　　　　　　　**B**

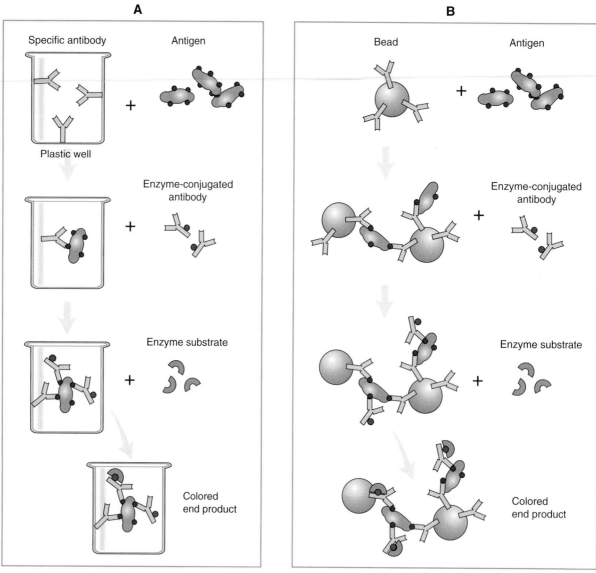

FIGURE 10-18 Principle of direct solid-phase immunosorbent assay. **A,** Solid phase is microtiter well. **B,** Solid phase is bead.

lyzes the production of a visible (colored) end product that can be quantified spectrophotometrically. EIA procedures can detect either antigen or antibody and are very amenable to automation and testing large numbers of samples.

Enzyme immunoassays are widely used for the serologic diagnosis of infectious diseases. They have become popular for a number of reasons. These include (1) the availability of commercial EIA kits for a large number of infectious agents; (2) the adaptability of EIA tests to automation, thus allowing more tests to be performed in shorter times; and (3) the objective interpretation of test results with colored end products that can be read spectrophotometrically. Many commercial products are tailored to suit high-volume laboratories; others are designed for single-use applications on individual patient specimens.

Most commercially developed EIA systems for detection of infectious agents require physical separation of the specific antigens from nonspecific complexes found in clinical samples.

Such systems are called *solid-phase immunosorbent assays (SPIAs)*. Separation is achieved through binding the antigen-specific antibody to a solid phase or matrix. A variety of solid matrix platforms are commercially available that include individual wells of polystyrene microtiter trays (Figure 10-18, *A*), spheric plastic beads, or magnetic beads (see Figure 10-18, *B*). The solid matrix allows for separation, or washing, of the sample and reagent to decrease nonspecific binding or background activity.

When performing an EIA to detect an antigen, a clinical sample is added to the solid matrix. If the antigen of interest is present in the sample, it will form a stable complex with the antibody (capture antibody) bound to the matrix. Unbound sample is removed by washing, and a second antibody specific for the antigen is added. In the direct method for antigen detection, this second antibody is conjugated to an enzyme. In the indirect method, a second nonconjugated antibody is added and washed, and then a third antibody specific for the

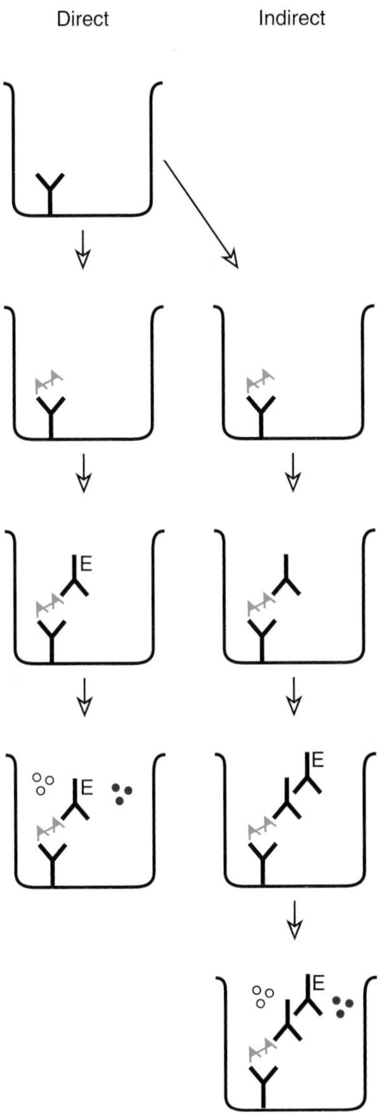

Direct   Indirect

FIGURE 10-19 Principle of various enzyme immunoassays for antigen. Both methods (direct and indirect sandwich immunoassays) start with specific antibody bound to the solid phase. Arrows (→) separate steps in the procedures where washing of the solid phase takes place. *Y,* Antibody; *A-A,* antigen; *E,* enzyme; o, enzyme substrate; •, enzyme product.

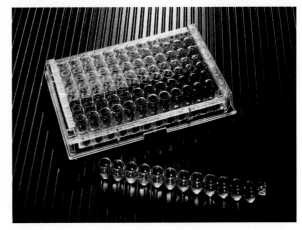

FIGURE 10-20 Enzyme immunoassay test in microtiter plate *(top)* and strip *(bottom)* showing wells with product of enzymatic reaction before *(blue)* and after *(yellow)* addition of an acidic stop solution.) (Courtesy Meridian Bioscience, Cincinnati, Ohio.)

second is added. The third antibody is conjugated to the enzyme and is directed against the Fc portion of the unlabeled second antibody.

In either method, once the conjugate is added and washed, the specific substrate is added. The amount of colored end product is directly proportional to the amount of enzyme-bound conjugate, and therefore antigen present in the original clinical sample. Both methods of detection are described in a step-by-step manner in Figure 10-19. The methods just described are often called *direct sandwich* and indirect sandwich immunoassays. The advantage of the indirect sandwich immunoassay is the need for only one enzyme conjugated anti-immunoglobulin antibody (third antibody) that can be used in different assays to detect a variety of antigens. A

disadvantage is that heterophile antibodies can produce false-positive or falsely increased results. The heterophile antibody can behave like the antigen binding to both the capture and signal antibodies.

Commercial companies have produced good-quality EIA kits for detection of a variety of microbial antigens. Conjugates can be inexpensively prepared, are stable for as long as 6 months, and have reasonably good sensitivity in most applications. The use of microtitration plates and instrumentation for dispensing reagents, wash procedures, and automated optical reading of reactions has greatly facilitated EIA methods to allow large volumes to be batch tested (Figure 10-20). Some methods are time consuming, however, and may not be practical for low-volume laboratories or STAT runs. Thus they cannot always be considered rapid tests when compared with other procedures such as latex agglutination. EIA are commonly used for rapid detection of *Chlamydia trachomatis, L. pneumophila, Clostridium difficile* toxins, *G. lamblia,* and *Cryptosporidium* spp.

Immunoassays for the detection of serum antibody are performed in a manner similar to immunoassays for microbial antigen detection, except that the roles of antigen and antibody are reversed (Figure 10-21). Most serum antibody assays are performed as SPIAs using antigen-coated tubes or wells. Ninety-six–well microtiter plates have become popular for this purpose because of the large number of tests that can be performed and the small serum volume required. Single-test, single-serum dilution cassettes are also available from commercial sources for the low-volume or infrequent test setting. In either case, patient antibody is bound to the microbial antigen–coated surface, and the antibody is detected using an enzyme-labeled antihuman immunoglobulin, or conjugate. Enzyme immunoassays or, more specifically, solid-phase EIAs (enzyme-linked immunosorbent assay [ELISA]), are the most popular types of immunoassay in use today.

Many laboratories are using some form of ELISA testing for antibody detection. In this test, results are reported not as

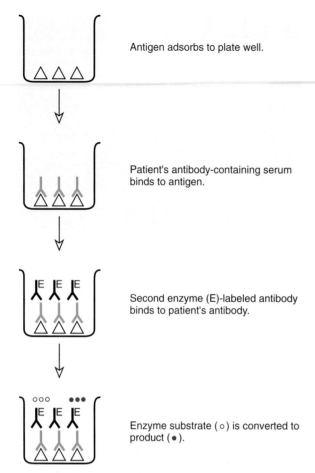

Antigen adsorbs to plate well.

Patient's antibody-containing serum binds to antigen.

Second enzyme (E)-labeled antibody binds to patient's antibody.

Enzyme substrate (o) is converted to product (•).

FIGURE 10-21 Principle of indirect solid-phase enzyme immunoassay for antibody detection.

antibody titer but as the results relate to the relative amount of signal generated by the patient's serum when compared with that of a known, weakly positive serum. Results are usually reported as either relative units with a numeric reference range (U/mL) or as a ratio of results in the sample to the low positive control (e.g., patient 15 U/mL, control 10 U/mL, ratio 1.5). It is impossible to compare the results of serial dilution methods with those of ELISA because of the variation from test to test. There is, however, a linear relationship in each individual assay between the amounts of antibody present. This means that a doubling in the result yields a two-fold rise in the amount of antibody.

One approach to detecting IgM antibody is referred to as *IgM antibody capture ELISA* (Figure 10-22). In this procedure, the solid phase is first coated with animal antibody specific for human IgM. The patient's serum is added and incubated, and then the tube or plate is washed. At this point, IgM antibody molecules, regardless of antigen specificity, should be bound to the solid phase, and antibodies of other immunoglobulin classes should be washed away. The next step in the IgM capture assay involves adding the antigen of interest and can be performed in one of two ways. The antigen can be directly labeled with an enzyme or can be added unlabeled. In either case, the antigen is bound to the solid phase if specific IgM antibody was present. With labeled antigen, the assay is completed by adding enzyme substrate and measuring

the colored product. Alternatively, unlabeled antigen bound to IgM is detected by adding a secondary enzyme-labeled antibody directed against the specific antigen, followed by addition of enzyme substrate. The amount of colored product is directly proportional to the amount of specific IgM captured on the solid phase.

The IgM antibody capture assay has the advantage of eliminating the need for separation of IgG that might compete with IgM and yield false-negative results. The capture assay may be susceptible to false-positive results because of IgM rheumatoid factor bound to the solid phase. Modifications of the assay can be employed to reduce the possibility of this problem. Another way to distinguish between IgG and IgM is to use IgG- and IgM-specific conjugates.

A variation of enzyme labeling involves coupling a reactive molecule such as biotin to the primary antibody. Binding of antibody to specific antigen is then detected by reacting with enzyme-labeled streptavidin, which binds very tightly and specifically to biotin by one of four reactive sites on each streptavidin molecule. The avidin-biotin interaction takes the place of primary antibody-secondary antibody interaction. This method tends to increase the amount of signal detected (increased sensitivity) for the following reasons: (1) multiple biotin molecules may be bound to the primary antibody and (2) each avidin molecule has four reactive sites to biotin. In combination, avidin-biotin interactions allow for multiple complexes with enzyme to bind and cleave substrate.

Membrane-Bound Enzyme Immunoassay

The flow-through and large surface area characteristics of nitrocellulose, nylon, or other membranes have been demonstrated to enhance the speed and sensitivity of EIA reactions. The improvements associated with membrane-bound EIAs are largely the result of immobilizing antibody onto the surface of porous membranes. This modification of SPIA uses a disposable plastic cassette consisting of the antibody-bound membrane and a small chamber to which the antigen-containing clinical sample can be added (Figure 10-23). An absorbent material is placed below the membrane to pull, or wick, the liquid reactants through the membrane. This helps to separate nonreacted components from the antigen-antibody complexes of interest bound to the membrane and thus simplify washing steps. Incubation times are also decreased because the rate of antigen binding is proportional to its concentration in solution near the membrane surface; this action increases the rate and extent of binding. Membrane-bound EIA tests are commonly used for the rapid detection of rotavirus, respiratory syncytial virus, *C. difficile* toxins, influenza A and B viruses, and group A *Streptococcus* (Figure 10-24).

Lateral flow ELISAs, also called *immunochromatographic* (ICT) tests, are based on a similar principle. This assay can be used to detect antibody or antigen. To detect antigen in a clinical specimen, a capture rabbit antibody with specificity for the antigen in question is applied in a line (called the *sample* or *test*) to the membrane. Above the test line, a line of goat anti-rabbit antibody (control) is attached. Below the test line on the membrane is rabbit antibody with specificity for the antigen in question labeled with a dye or colloidal gold. The clinical specimen is placed in a buffer diluent, and the

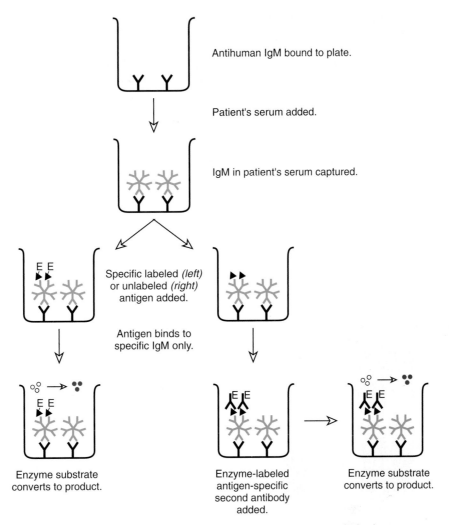

Antihuman IgM bound to plate.

Patient's serum added.

IgM in patient's serum captured.

Specific labeled *(left)* or unlabeled *(right)* antigen added.

Antigen binds to specific IgM only.

Enzyme substrate converts to product.

Enzyme-labeled antigen-specific second antibody added.

Enzyme substrate converts to product.

FIGURE 10-22   Immunoglobulin M (IgM) antibody capture enzyme-linked immunosorbent assay using labeled antigen *(left)* or unlabeled antigen; a secondary enzyme-labeled antibody is added later *(right)*.

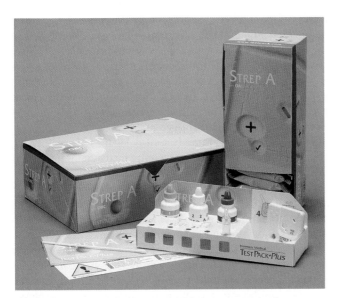

FIGURE 10-23   TestPack Strep A kit components of membrane-bound enzyme immunoassay test for group A streptococcal polysaccharide antigen. (Courtesy Inverness Medical Professional Diagnostics–BioStar, Inc., Louisville, Colo.)

membrane is inserted into the buffer. The buffer is carried up the membrane by capillary action. The labeled rabbit antibody is suspended in the buffer. If antigen is present in the clinical specimen, it will combine with the labeled antibody.

As the buffer continues to migrate upwards, the antigen-antibody complex will bind to the capture antibody affixed to the membrane. Enough of the complex will bind to form a visible color on the test line. The control line is an internal control that must be positive for results to be valid. The control line will capture any labeled rabbit antibody and will be positive in specimens with or without the antigen. The control line ensures that the buffer has migrated past the test line and confirms a negative test result.

In an ICT assay to detect antibody, such as anti-HIV (OraQuick, OraSure Technologies, Bethlehem, Pa.), staphylococcal protein A, labeled with a red dye, in the kit binds to the Fc portion of IgG in the clinical specimen. The complex is carried to the test line, which contains HIV antigens. If anti-HIV antibody is present in the clinical specimen, it will bind to the antigens, and a red line will develop. The control line contains antihuman antibody that will bind other IgG molecules present in the specimen, producing a red line (Figure 10-25).

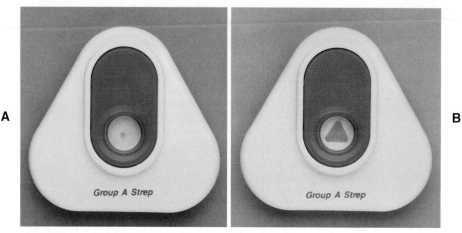

FIGURE 10-24 Color PAC devices showing negative **(A)** and positive **(B)** reactions of liposome enhanced membrane-bound enzyme immunoassay for group A streptococcal polysaccharide antigen. (Courtesy and © Becton, Dickinson and Company, Sparks, Md.)

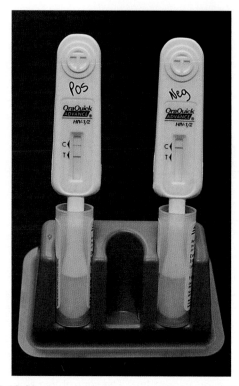

FIGURE 10-25 Immunochromatographic test. The OraQuick test is a rapid assay for the detection of antibody to human immunodeficiency virus types 1 and 2. Formation of a red line in the test area is a positive reaction.

Optical Immunoassays

Optical immunoassay (OIA) relies on the interaction of antigen-antibody complexes on inert surfaces. Specific antigen-antibody interaction actually alters the thickness of the reactants on the test surface. Light reflecting off the surface film containing antibody only is viewed as one color. However, when specific antigen is bound to antibody, it increases the thickness of the film. This causes the surface to appear a different color to the naked eye. An OIA is available to detect group A *Streptococcus* in pediatric populations (Figure 10-26). An OIA has also been approved by the Food and Drug Administration (FDA) for the detection of influenza A virus.

Complement Fixation Test

Complement fixation tests are versatile assays that can be used for both antibody and antigen detection. They are broadly applicable for a variety of infectious agents and have been used for many years, particularly for antibody detection. CF tests have gradually been replaced by more rapid and sensitive assays; however, they are still used in reference and public health laboratories for certain agents.

Although a discussion of the serum complement protein system is beyond the scope of this chapter (see Chapter 2), it is important to note that the system plays a vital role in a number of immunologic functions. The proteins involved in the complement system are usually found in an inactive form; however, once activated, the proteins become involved in an enzymatic cascade that involves production of proteins with a variety of biologic activities. Activation of complement occurs by the classical pathway when specific IgG or IgM antibody combines with antigen and exposes a complement-binding site on the antibody molecule. It is the cell-lysing ability of activated complement components that is important in CF tests.

The CF test requires both an indicator system and a test system (Figure 10-27). The indicator system typically consists of a combination of sheep erythrocytes, rabbit antibody to sheep erythrocytes, and guinea pig complement. When these three components are present and active, the rabbit antibody first combines with the sheep erythrocytes, and complement is subsequently bound (fixed) to the antibody-antigen complex, resulting in activation of complement by the classical pathway; this results in lysis of the sheep erythrocytes. The test system consists of a mixture of known antigen and the patient's heat-inactivated serum that may or may not contain

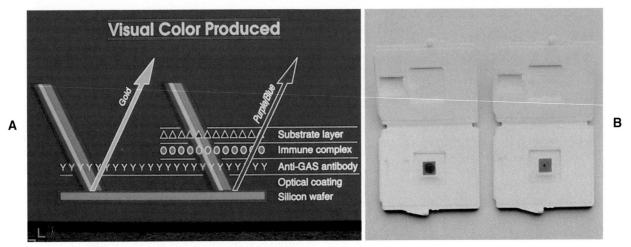

FIGURE 10-26 Optical ImmunoAssay (OIA) for group A streptococcus. **A,** Principle of Biostar OIA Strep A test showing color change from gold to purple following attachment of immune complex containing group A streptococcal antigen. **B,** Test cassettes showing a positive reaction on the left and negative on the right. (Courtesy Inverness Medical Professional Diagnostics–BioStar, Inc., Louisville, Colo.)

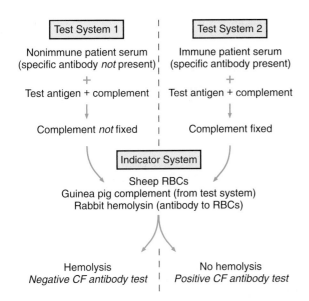

FIGURE 10-27 Principles of complement fixation (CF) test. *RBCs,* Red blood cells.

specific antibody to the antigen. Heating the patient sample is necessary to inactivate complement present in human sera.

The CF test is performed as a two-step procedure. The patient's serum is serially diluted in test tubes, and each dilution is mixed with a known amount of antigen (test system). A fixed amount of complement is then added to each tube, and the mixture is incubated. Next, the sheep erythrocytes and rabbit antibody are added to each tube, and the tubes are incubated again. If the patient's serum had specific antibodies to the test antigen, complement would be fixed by the test system and would not be available to lyse the erythrocytes of the indicator system. If the patient's serum did not have specific antibody to the test antigen, complement would be fixed by the indicator system, resulting in erythrocyte lysis. The CF

antibody titer is considered the highest dilution of patient serum resulting in 100% hemolysis. It is usually read spectrophotometrically.

Western Blotting

Although serologic test methods for detecting antibody such as IFA assays and EIAs provide excellent sensitivity and specificity in most clinical applications, they are limited in their ability to resolve the complex antibody response occurring during infection by most infectious agents. Because most antigens used in these assays are crude microbial and viral extracts, a positive result may represent an antibody response to one or to many antigens. The EIA test can be designed to detect antibody to a number of individual antigens, but this requires the expensive and labor-intensive process of purifying antigens and running multiple EIAs. As an alternative, the technique of Western blotting is used. This technique allows for characterization of multiple antibodies to an infectious agent by first electrophoretic separation of the microbial or viral antigens and transfer to a nitrocellulose membrane. Western blotting has gained importance and is extensively used to confirm antibodies to human immunodeficiency virus type 1 (HIV-1) in patients whose sera have been repeatedly reactive in EIA tests.

It is also applied to serologic diagnosis of Lyme disease and other infections in which the development of antibody to a specific microbial antigen or antigens has diagnostic significance. In the Western blotting procedure, a crude antigen preparation (e.g., a partially purified virus preparation) is first heated with a detergent such as sodium dodecyl sulfate (SDS). The SDS releases individual polypeptides from complex proteins. The polypeptides are then separated according to their molecular weight by polyacrylamide gel electrophoresis with SDS (SDS-PAGE). The separated polypeptides form invisible protein "bands" in the gel. The protein bands are transferred to an inert filter membrane support, usually made of nitrocellulose. The nitrocellulose membrane thus becomes a solid

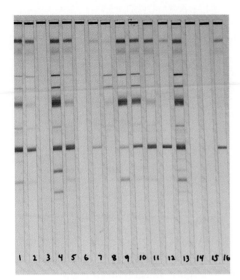

FIGURE 10-28 Western blot for the detection of antibody to HIV-1. Strips 1 and 4 are high-positive strips; strips 2 and 5 are low-positive; strips 3 and 6 are negative controls. Strips 7 through 13 and strip 16 are positive reactions of patient sera. Strips 14 and 15 are negative reactions of patient sera. Gp160 represents a viral glycoprotein with a molecular weight of 160,000 daltons; gp41 and p24 represent other viral proteins. (Courtesy bioMérieux, Inc., Durham, N.C.)

matrix to which the separated protein antigens tightly adhere and upon which an antibody-antigen reaction can occur and be visualized—much like a microtitration plate well with an ELISA.

A number of commercial kits for Western blotting contain nitrocellulose membrane strips on which the protein antigens of interest have already been electrophoretically separated. For analysis, the nitrocellulose membrane is immersed in a patient's serum sample (usually diluted) and allowed to incubate. Specific antibodies in the sample, if present, will bind to unique epitopes in the protein bands. After incubation, the nitrocellulose membrane is thoroughly washed to remove unbound antibody, and a labeled antihuman immunoglobulin (secondary antibody) is allowed to react with the membrane. The secondary antibody is commonly labeled with an enzyme or biotin. The detection of an antigen-antibody reaction at any protein band is accomplished by the addition of enzyme substrate (or enzyme-labeled streptavidin followed by enzyme substrate) and final wash (Figure 10-28).

Western blotting has added a new dimension of versatility and specificity to immunoassays. It has helped to resolve false-positive EIA results (particularly for HIV-1 infection) owing to antibodies cross-reacting to other viruses, autoimmune disorders, technical error, and other undetermined reasons. It has also helped to dissect and analyze the antibody response to individual proteins in complex mixtures. Western blotting is a procedure that must be well controlled and interpreted using strict criteria. It should also be recognized that antibodies detected by other methods may not be detected by Western blotting techniques, because the polypeptide antigens used are not native, intact proteins (SDS treatment denatures the proteins), and some antigens may not be transferred well to the

membranes. Western blotting is a qualitative assay; antibody titers cannot be determined. Despite these drawbacks, Western blotting will continue to play an important role in immunoserology of selected infectious agents.

Immunoblots

Immunoblots, or dot blots, are similar to Western blots except the protein antigens are not electrophoretically separated and transferred to a solid surface. Instead, the proteins are purified and directly applied (blotted) to specific locations on the solid surface. In the case of the strip immunoblot assay (SIA) for HCV (RIBA-3.0 HCV; Chiron Corp., Emeryville, Calif.), four HCV proteins are produced and applied to a nitrocellulose filter strip along with two internal positive controls and a negative control. Patient serum is added to the strip, and if antibody is present to the any of the four proteins, they will bind. An enzyme- labeled antihuman antibody is added, followed by the enzyme's substrate to detect binding of patient antibody. The strips can be read manually. Chiron also markets an automated processing system that reads the intensity (density of reflectance) of the test bands and compares them with the intensity of the internal controls calculating the relative intensity.

Other Labeled Immunoassays

Besides enzymes and fluorochromes, other labels can be used to detect in vitro antigen-antibody reactions, including radioimmunoassay (RIA) and chemiluminescent immunoassay (CLIA). The principles are similar to EIA, except a label other than an enzyme is used. Radionucleotides (usually ^{125}I or ^{14}C) are substituted for enzymes in RIA. Although RIA was once the key method for antigen detection of numerous infectious agents, especially hepatitis B virus, it has largely been replaced by EIA, which does not require use of radioactive substances. The CLIA uses chemicals, such as luminol, acridium esters, and ruthenium derivatives that emit light. Instrumentation is required to read CLIAs.

USE OF SEROLOGIC TESTING IN SPECIFIC DISEASES

As the sensitivity, specificity, and ease of use improved, serologic tests became a mainstay in clinical laboratories. Manufacturers produce kits for screening large number of samples and kits for confirming positive or negative screening results. In addition, some kits are single use, designed for low test volume, whereas other kits lend themselves to large-volume testing and can be automated. Table 10-1 lists commonly used, commercially available serologic tests to detect antibodies and the organisms identified. This section discusses some important diseases diagnosed by antibody detection. The following section examines direct antigen detection in the diagnosis of infectious diseases.

Serologic Testing of Syphilis

Sexually transmitted diseases (STDs) are some of the most common infectious diseases in the United States. The most common of these diseases are genital warts, chlamydia, and genital herpes; however, it is syphilis that is one of the most dangerous if left untreated. *T. pallidum* subsp. *pallidum*, the spirochete that causes syphilis, may be identified from a lesion or chancre. However, serologic testing for syphilis is the most common method of diagnosis. Two forms of testing exist for syphilis: screening tests and confirmatory tests. The confirmatory tests use treponemal antigens and are very sensitive and specific, but they are not suited for testing large numbers of individuals (screening), because they are technically demanding and time consuming and, like other diagnostic tests, they would result in decreased diagnostic accuracy if applied to a large population with a disease of low prevalence. Approximately 1% of the population will give a false-positive result. Confirmatory tests also cannot be used to monitor therapy. Examples of confirmatory assays are the FTA-ABS test and the *T. pallidum* particle agglutination (TP-PA) test (Fujirebio America, Fairfield, N.J.), which has generally replaced the microhemagglutination assay for *T. pallidum* (MHA-TP) test. In this test, specific treponemal antibodies are detected using treponemal antigen-coated erythrocytes.

Nontreponemal antigen tests are technically easier and more rapid to perform; therefore they are the tests of choice for syphilis screening. The most commonly used nontreponemal tests today are the Venereal Disease Research Laboratory (VDRL) and the rapid plasma reagin (RPR) tests. The VDRL test, named after the laboratory that developed it, is a microscopic flocculation test using heat-inactivated serum and performed on glass slides. The test detects reaginic antibodies (reagin) that bind to an alcoholic solution of cardiolipin-lecithin-cholesterol particles. The RPR test uses the same antigen as the VDRL test; however, carbon particles have been added so that the flocculation reaction can be more clearly seen. The RPR assay can be performed on unheated serum or plasma and is read macroscopically (Figure 10-29). The VDRL and RPR tests detect both IgM and IgG and may be performed as both qualitative and quantitative tests. Because of the extreme attention to reagent preparation and quality control required and the difficulty in reading results, the VDRL test has been replaced by the RPR test in most clinical laboratories. However, the VDRL assay can be used to test CSF for diagnosing neurosyphilis and to follow antibody titers in a newborn to diagnose congenital syphilis.

The VDRL and RPR tests are very sensitive, but a patient may not have antibodies until 3 to 4 weeks after infection. Because screening tests do not use treponemal antigens, they are subject to false-positive results that may be as high as 10% to 30% for all sera tested. These screening tests detect antibodies to lipoprotein-like material and possibly cardiolipin from the spirochetes. The antilipoidal antibody can be produced as a result of infections, autoimmune diseases, pregnancy, and other conditions. False-positive results occur most commonly in autoimmune disorders (lupus erythematosus, rheumatic fever), infectious diseases (infectious mononucleosis, hepatitis, malaria, AIDS, tuberculosis), pregnancy, cardiovascular disease, and old age. It is imperative that positive VDRL or RPR test results be followed by confirmatory treponemal antibody tests.

Commonly used confirmatory tests for a reactive screening test include the FTA-ABS and the TP-PA. Both of these tests detect antibodies specific to *T. pallidum*. The FTA-ABS is an indirect immunofluorescent assay. *T. pallidum* spirochetes, Nichols strain, grown in laboratory animals are fixed to wells in a glass microscope slide. Patient sera are first absorbed with antigens from the Reiter strain of *Treponema*; this step is performed to remove antibodies to nonpathogenic spirochetes that could produce false-positive results. Next, sera from different patients are placed into separate wells on the slide. After washing to remove nonspecific antibody binding, a fluorescent-labeled antihuman antibody is added. If the patient serum has antibodies to *T. pallidum,* they will bind to the spirochetes on the slide, and then the antihuman antibody will bind to the patient's antibodies. The presence of yellow-green fluorescence under an ultraviolet microscope is indicative of a positive result. Results are reported as reactive, reactive minimal (1+), or nonreactive.

The TP-PA uses gelatin particles coated (sensitized) with *T. pallidum* antigens; an absorption step is not needed. The assay is performed in a microtiter plate on patient sera diluted 1:20. After addition of the coated gelatin particle solution, the final serum dilution is 1:40. If treponemal antibodies are

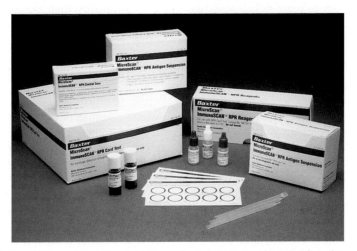

FIGURE 10-29 RPH card test for detection of nontreponemal antibodies. (Courtesy Baxter U.S. Distribution, Division of Baxter Healthcare, Inc., Deerfield, Ill.)

present, a mat of agglutinated particles will form in the wells. Results are recorded as reactive (1+ to 4+), nonreactive, or inconclusive. Because of ease of use, less technical time, and lack of an absorption step and fluorescent microscope, the TP-PA test is gradually replacing the FTA-ABS assay.

At least nine EIA tests have been developed for diagnosing syphilis. The assays use sonicated spirochetes or recombinant proteins as antigens. EIAs include the Captia Syphilis-G test (Trinity Biotech, Dublin, Ireland; Biorad, Richmond, Calif.; and Wapole Laboratories, Princeton, N.J.) and the Trep-Chek test (Phoenix Bio-Tech Corp., Mississauga, Ontario), which are designed as confirmatory tests.

Serologic Testing for Streptococcal Infections

Antistreptolysin-O Test

Streptococcus pyogenes, or group A *Streptococcus* (GAS), causes a number of acute, common pyogenic (associated with pus or neutrophil response) infections, including pharyngitis and skin infections. In addition, the organism is responsible for certain nonsuppurative (nonpyogenic) diseases, such as acute rheumatic fever and poststreptococcal glomerulonephritis, which occur weeks after the acute infectious process and are thought to be autoimmune-mediated diseases; that is, the damage is due to the host's immune response. Although the pyogenic infections are best diagnosed by isolation of the organism in culture, the nonsuppurative diseases occur at a time when the organism may no longer be present; thus serologic diagnosis is usually performed. In addition, it may be necessary to diagnose infections by serology after antimicrobial therapy has been initiated.

The ASO antibody test is commonly used to demonstrate serologic response to *S. pyogenes*. One method to detect ASO is to measure the ability of the patient's serum to neutralize the erythrocyte-lysing (hemolytic) ability of the streptococcal enzyme (streptolysin O). The patient's serum is mixed with a standard concentration of streptolysin-O. If antibody to streptolysin-O is present, it will bind to the hemolysin neutralizing it. Then when red blood cells (RBCs) are added, the RBCs will not be lysed. If antibody to streptolysin-O was not present in the serum sample, then the hemolysin will not be neutralized, and the RBCs will be lysed. An immunonephelometry assay is also available. In this method, antibody in a patient's sample combines with antigen (streptolysin-O), forming aggregates that scatter light. The amount of light scattered is measured in a nephelometer and is proportional to the amount of antibody present in the sample.

Antibody titers are based on comparison of the patient sample to known standards. Antibody titers are reported as Todd units, which were named after E.W. Todd, who discovered streptolysins. High titers of ASO antibody develop in about 85% of the cases of rheumatic fever, but the titers and percentages of patients with streptococcal wound infections and poststreptococcal glomerulonephritis who develop ASO antibodies are significantly lower. Thus when these diseases are suspected in patients who do not show an elevation in ASO titers, additional serologic tests directed at other strep-

tococcal enzymes should be performed; antibody to DNase-B is the most valuable. DNase-B is present in the greatest amounts among the four DNase isoenzymes (A, B, C, and D) produced by *S. pyogenes*. It is important to use two different assays when screening for antibodies to *S. pyogenes*.

Because serodiagnosis is usually attempted late after acute infection, it may be difficult to show seroconversion in streptococcal neutralization tests. Thus "upper limit of normal" titers have been established; these vary by patient age and geographic location. The upper limits should not discourage an attempt to show seroconversion, however.

Streptozyme

As mentioned earlier, the Streptozyme Test is an IHA assay detecting antibodies to five different streptococcal proteins: (1) streptolysin-O, (2) DNase-B, (3) hyaluronidase, (4) streptokinase, and (5) nicotinamide adenine dinucleotidase (NADase). A high antibody titer to any one of these antigens will produce agglutination. Streptozyme is a screening test; any negative result should be confirmed with an ASO or anti–DNase-B test. Discrepancies have been reported between the Streptozyme and ASO tests.

Serologic Diagnosis of Toxoplasmosis

The protozoan *T. gondii* causes the disease toxoplasmosis. Because domestic cats are the natural host, pregnant women should be careful about handling cat feces and cat litter and should especially avoid stray cats. Symptoms of the disease in humans may be fatigue, fever, and lymph gland swelling. If passed to a fetus during pregnancy, toxoplasmosis can cause severe neurologic damage and eye problems.

Toxoplasmosis can be treated with drugs and is usually not serious in adult patients unless they are immunocompromised, such as patients with AIDS. Toxoplasmosis in an immunosuppressed patient may be serious or even fatal unless treated early. In otherwise healthy adults, toxoplasmosis can resemble infectious mononucleosis (caused by EBV) and infections caused by CMV. For optimal treatment, it is important to differentiate among these diseases. Infants infected in utero typically have IgM antibody to *T. gondii*; in addition, infants may have an increased IgG titer resulting from transfer of antibodies from the mother. Detecting antibodies to *T. gondii* is part of the TORCH profile discussed previously in this chapter.

Serologic Diagnosis of Viral Diseases

Rubella

Rubella (German measles) is normally insignificant except in pregnant women. This disease may cause a miscarriage, or it may cause congenital heart disease, cataracts, deafness, and brain damage in the fetus. Therefore it is extremely important to determine whether women who may become pregnant have immunity to rubella. Serologic testing is generally by EIA for either IgM or IgG antirubella antibodies. Women who are not immune or have a low antibody titer should be vaccinated before becoming pregnant. Rubella vaccine is part of the trivalent measles, mumps, rubella vaccine most children in developed countries receive.

Infectious Mononucleosis

The heterophile antibody titer is one of the tests used to diagnose infectious mononucleosis caused by EBV. Recall that *heterophile antibody* refers to an antibody with an affinity to an antigen from more than one group or species. Humans rarely have antibodies to sheep RBCs. However, many patients with infectious mononucleosis have been shown to develop antibodies that will agglutinate sheep, bovine, and horse RBCs. A number of commercial diagnostic kits are available to help diagnose infectious mononucleosis. These kits are generally known as *spot tests* and use a saline suspension of antigen derived from the RBCs of horses. Mixing of the test material with a drop of the patient's serum causes a coarse granulation if the patient has infectious mononucleosis. These tests are very rapid and sensitive for screening; however, they do not positively identify EBV infection. Because EBV antigens are not used, other factors may increase heterophile antibody titers; therefore the test is not specific. Other tests are often needed to confirm active infectious mononucleosis. Tests for the Epstein-Barr nuclear antigen (EBNA) as well as for antibodies to the viral capsid antigen (VCA) are used. Some diagnostic kits place EBV antigens on carrier particles—RBCs or latex beads. Either IgM or IgG antibodies can be identified by these methods.

Cytomegalovirus

Cytomegalovirus can be found in almost all body fluids. The virus can cross the placenta and may be transfused in blood and blood products. Most adults have been exposed to the virus and have some level of immunity. Nonimmune, pregnant women should be concerned about potential damage to the fetus such as cerebral malformation (microencephalopathy) and necrosis of brain tissue. Patients who are immunosuppressed are highly susceptible to CMV infection. Patients who have AIDS and acquire an acute CMV infection may have eye damage and blindness as well as cerebral damage.

The risk to health care workers is minimal because healthy individuals have active immune systems. CMV infections in immunocompetent individuals are typically mild and can resemble infectious mononucleosis. Infection from CMV is considered positive with a fourfold rise in titer between acute and convalescent patient samples. A single IgM-specific titer of more than 1:8 is evidence of an acute infection. Patients with CMV infection will have a negative heterophile test for infectious mononucleosis.

Hepatitis

Hepatitis is an inflammation of the liver. A number of agents, including chemicals and infectious agents, can cause hepatitis; however, most cases of hepatitis have a viral etiology. Several different viruses have been linked to hepatitis. Hepatitis A virus (HAV), HBV, and HCV, are the most common agents diagnosed. HBV was discovered as early as 1965. The blood of an infected patient is infectious; the disease can also be sexually transmitted.

A number of HBV serologic markers, both antibodies and antigens, are present in patients' sera. Serologic assays are often performed as a profile or battery of tests. One of the earliest markers detected in infections is the hepatitis B surface antigen (HBsAg). Although the virus has numerous antigens, HBsAg is highly antigenic and easy to detect. Additional antigen assays include detection of hepatitis B core antigen (HBcAg) and hepatitis B e antigen (HBeAg). The detection of HBsAg in a patient's serum signifies that the patient either is ill with the disease or is a carrier and is potentially infectious. The laboratory can also test for antibodies to the various antigens: anti-HBsAg antibody, anti-BcAg antibody, and anti-HBeAg antibody. The presence of anti-HBsAg indicates immunity.

Hepatitis A virus is generally spread by the fecal-oral route and by food handlers and children. The tests most commonly used for diagnosis are the anti-HAV-IgM and anti-HAV-IgG. A positive IgM-anti-HAV test is suggestive of acute infection, whereas a positive IgG-anti-HAV test is indicative of past exposure. Patients diagnosed with acute infection should not be allowed to handle or prepare food for others.

In the 1980s, a gene associated with an HCV protein was cloned. This protein was then used to develop a test to detect antibodies to HCV in the blood. This was the first time that a viral genome was used to develop a serologic test without first isolating the causative agent. Research has determined that the primary agent in non-A non-B transfusion hepatitis is HCV. In 1990, the FDA approved the first test kits for the detection of HCV. Blood units are now routinely screened for HCV with multiantigen assays detecting antibodies and with nucleic acid amplification tests (see Chapter 11).

Many patients with HCV infection are asymptomatic. However, even asymptomatic cases can progress to chronic hepatitis and cirrhosis—requiring a liver transplant. Both HBV and HCV have been associated with liver cancer. In chronic cases, the only clue to HCV infection may be an elevated liver enzyme known as *alanine aminotransferase* (ALT), although this test is not specific for viral hepatitis. Detection of anti-HCV antibody is commonly used for the diagnosis of HCV infection, although the most effective tests may be the nucleic acid amplification tests.

Human Immunodeficiency Virus

The detection of anti-HIV antibodies has generally used two tests: ELISA for screening and the Western blot for confirmation. The Western blot test is highly sensitive and specific and remains the standard confirmatory test for HIV infection. Numerous screening tests based on different methods are available. Second-generation kits use recombinant or synthetic viral proteins instead of purified viral lysates. The double-antigen sandwich (DAGS) assay, referred to as a *third-generation test,* uses recombinant antigen to capture antibody in patients' sera. One of the antibody's antigen-binding sites binds to recombinant antigen on a solid surface. A second labeled antigen is added that binds to another antigen-binding site on the antibody and is subsequently detected.

A problem with HIV infection is that antibody development has a wide variation, depending on the patient, the infective dose, and the phenotype of the virus. With 95% certainty, seroconversion occurs an average of 45 days after infection. For this reason, other tests that identify specific HIV proteins (antigens) such as p24, a core protein, or gp41, a glycoprotein on the envelope of the virus, may be preferred. These tests are discussed later in this chapter. Screening kits detecting both antibody and antigen, referred to as *fourth-generation tests,* are some of the most sensitive screening tests. Nucleic acid probes and the polymerase chain reaction may also be used in the identification of viral RNA. Assays vary in their sensitivity, specificity, and diagnostic utility and should be individually tested before use in a clinical laboratory.

Because a number of individuals are asymptomatic and unaware they are infected with HIV, health professionals encourage people in high-risk groups to be tested. To facilitate testing, several rapid tests and a home collection assay have been developed. Rapid tests can be performed in about 30 minutes without expensive laboratory equipment. These assays are useful in clinics where patients may not return to receive laboratory results and in assessing the risk of HIV transmission after a needlestick. Some tests, such as the Ora-Quick (discussed earlier), are single step, whereas others, Reveal (MedMira, Halifax, Nova Scotia) and Multispot (BioRad, Hercules, Calif.), are multistep. The sensitivity of these assays varies from 90% to 100%, and specificity varies from 95% to 100%. The OraQuick received FDA approval in 2002 and, despite concerns by laboratorians about potential false-positive and false-negative results, received Clinical Laboratory Improvement Act of 1988 (CLIA)-waived status. The OraQuick test, which uses blood collected by a finger-stick, has a reported sensitivity and specificity to be 99.6% and 100%, respectively.

A home collection kit has received FDA approval. Blood is collected at home by a finger-stick and sent to a diagnostic laboratory for testing. If the sample is reactive, additional tests can be performed on the same sample. Some home testing kits, assays performed by the consumer, are available on the Internet, but as of yet, these kits have not been approved for use in the United States, and several organizations have issued warnings about their use. The FDA has approved some kits for testing on samples other than blood, such as saliva and urine.

Serologic Diagnosis of Fungal Infections

The laboratory can identify antibodies that occur in response to fungal disease by the use of complement fixation or immunodiffusion techniques. The primary fungal diseases diagnosed by these means are histoplasmosis and coccidioidomycosis. Histoplasmosis is found primarily in the Ohio Valley and coccidioidomycosis, or valley fever, is primarily seen in the San Joaquin Valley of California. One fungal titer is not enough to be diagnostic, because the people who live in an endemic area may have positive serologic tests from past exposure. A fourfold rise in titer is evidence of current infection. A travel history is mandatory when fungal disease is suspected, however.

Skin testing and cultures may also be used in the identification of the organism causing a systemic infection. A positive skin test does not, however, indicate a current infection because the immune response could be due to a past exposure. The conversion of a skin test from a negative to a positive is the most diagnostically significant. Skin tests should be started only after the blood is drawn for serologic testing, because the skin test itself can cause the serologic test to be falsely positive.

DIRECT ANTIGEN DETECTION ASSAYS

The importance of antigen detection for organisms that are difficult or impossible to culture ensures the diagnostic use of these technologies. Table 10-4 lists some of the infectious diseases that can be diagnosed by detecting antigens in clinical specimens. Other techniques developed for similar reasons, such as nucleic acid amplification, are discussed in Chapter 11. As with any test procedure, all laboratories must evaluate the tests for their situations.

Respiratory Tract Infections
Streptococcal Pharyngitis

One of the most widely used applications of direct antigen tests, popularized in the 1980s, is for the detection of GAS in throat swab specimens for the diagnosis of streptococcal pharyngitis. The main advantage of rapid direct antigen testing for GAS over a standard throat culture is that results are available while the patient is in the physician's office. Also,

TABLE 10-4 Some Representative Infectious Diseases and the Direct Antigen Detection Methods Commercially Available to Detect Them

Type of Infection	Test Methods
Bacterial	
Group A streptococcal pharyngitis	LA, EIA, liposome-enhanced immunoassay, OIA
Bacterial meningitis*	LA, CoA
Clostridium difficile colitis	LA, EIA
Chlamydial urethritis	EIA, FA
Pertussis	FA
Legionnaires' disease	FA
Fungal	
Cryptococcal meningitis	LA, EIA
Parasitic	
Giardiasis	FA, EIA
Cryptosporidiosis	FA, EIA
Pneumocystis pneumonia	FA
Trichomonas vaginitis	FA
Viral	
Rotavirus gastroenteritis	LA, EIA
Hepatitis B infection	EIA
Respiratory virus infection†	FA, EIA
Herpes simplex virus infection	FA, EIA
Cytomegalovirus infection	FA
Human immunodeficiency virus infection	EIA

CoA, Coagglutination; *EIA,* enzyme immunoassay; *FA,* fluorescent antibody test; *LA,* latex agglutination test; *OIA,* optical immunoassay.
*Includes *Haemophilus influenzae* b, *Streptococcus pneumoniae, Neisseria meningitidis,* and *Streptococcus agalactiae.*
†Includes influenza, parainfluenza, and respiratory syncytial viruses.

antimicrobial therapy can be given immediately instead of waiting 24 to 48 hours for culture results. This is more convenient for both the physician and patient. Although antimicrobial treatment is critical for prevention of poststreptococcal pharyngitis syndromes such as rheumatic fever and glomerulonephritis, early antimicrobial administration may also shorten the illness. In addition, early treatment may reduce secondary infections to close contacts, allowing the patient to return to work or school sooner. The most important reason for diagnosing and treating GAS pharyngitis is to prevent the nonsuppurative sequelae. Delay in initiation of therapy for a few days (while awaiting culture results) will not increase the patient's risk of developing such complications.

Currently, more than 20 manufacturers produce diagnostic test kits for direct GAS antigen detection. The majority of these kits use either LA or some version of SPIA. Generally, both types of tests contain reagents to perform an initial extraction of the group A carbohydrate antigen from the cell wall of the organism. This is most commonly achieved by exposing the sample to nitrous acid, but it can be accomplished by enzymatic digestion (pronase). Once the solubilized antigen preparation has been pH adjusted in a buffer solution, the specimen is tested according to the specific procedure of the manufacturer. A number of EIA tests have become popular, particularly those that use membrane-bound antibody to speed up the reaction and facilitate the washing procedure. Because of the colored product, they are generally easier to read than LA tests. One variation of the membrane-bound EIA for GAS uses colored, dye-filled liposomes bound to antibody as the detection reagent. As previously mentioned, a highly sensitive and specific OIA is commercially available.

A number of tests like the LINK2 Strep A Rapid Test (BD Diagnostic Systems, Sparks, Md.) are CLIA-waived. The LINK2 Strep A Rapid Test is a rapid, lateral-flow, two-site sandwich immunoassay for detection of group A streptococcal antigen directly from throat swabs. It consists of a membrane strip precoated with rabbit anti-group A *Streptococcus* antibody on the test band region and goat anti-rabbit antibody on the control band region. A colored rabbit anti-group A *Streptococcus* antibody-colloidal gold conjugate pad is placed at the end of the membrane. Visible, easy-to-read results are available in as little as 1 minute. The manufacturer reports an overall accuracy of 95.8%.

Numerous studies have compared the performance of direct GAS tests with one another and against the gold standard—throat culture. Sensitivity and specificity of GAS antigen tests are in the ranges of 75% to 90% and 90% to 95%, respectively. Values vary by manufacturer, individual performing the test, quality of the specimen, and accuracy of the throat culture procedure used for comparison. Despite their accuracy, false-negative results do occur, presumably from low numbers of bacteria in the clinical specimen. Another source of false-negative results is uneven distribution of bacteria in the specimen.

Several health organizations, such as the American Academy of Pediatrics, recommend that all negative rapid antigen tests for GAS pharyngitis be backed up with a culture. The sensitivity of a rapid test with culture backup is about 95%. If a low concentration and uneven distribution of antigen can produce false-negative results, then increasing the inoculum could improve the sensitivity. For example, using two swabs in the extraction step instead of one increased the sensitivity from 80% to 94%, although the specificity was lower, 81.5% compared with about 90%.

Legionnaires' Disease

Legionella pneumophila and other *Legionella* spp. cause acute lobar pneumonia with multisystem involvement, known as *Legionnaires' disease*. Early diagnosis and therapy are important, particularly in immunosuppressed patients. Disease may occur as community-acquired individual cases or outbreaks and as nosocomial infections. A variety of antigen detection methods have been evaluated and compared with culture isolation. The DFA test is commonly performed on respiratory specimens, although the sensitivity (25% to 75%) is much lower than for culture.

Monoclonal antibody (e.g., MONOFLUO; Bio-Rad Laboratories, Redmond, Wash.) is usually directed against *L. pneumophila* serogroup (SG) 1, whereas polyclonal antibody may include other serogroups and, in some cases, other *Legionella* spp. Specificity has been a problem with some reagents, owing to antigens shared with other gram-negative rods. Cross-reactions with both the polyvalent and monovalent sera have been reported with *Bacteroides fragilis, Pseudomonas* spp., and *Stenotrophomonas maltophilia*.

A number of immunoassays are available for detecting soluble urinary antigen. Two EIA kits are the Binax EIA (Binax, Portland, Me.) and Bartels EIA (Issaquah, Wash.). These assays have sensitivities in the 75% to 85% range, with a specificity of 95% or more. An RIA kit (the Binax RIA) is also available. Concentrating the urine by centrifugation or ultrafiltration can increase the sensitivity. The EIA tests primarily detect *L. pneumophila* SG 1; therefore a negative test does not rule out legionellosis caused by other serogroups or species. Binax has also produced an ICT test called Binax NOW. The sensitivity is reported to be about 80% with a specificity of 97%.

Respiratory Viral Infections

A number of respiratory viruses can be directly detected in both upper respiratory and lower respiratory specimens. The use of flocked swabs to collect respiratory tract specimens increases the sensitivity of these assays. Flocked swabs have short stiff nylon fibers extending from the shaft and act like a mini-brush. This improves the quality of the specimen collected. Fluorescent antibody is a technique used for detecting RSV, influenza A and B viruses, parainfluenza viruses 1, 2, and 3, and adenovirus. These assays may be used for direct detection or to confirm viral isolation in conventional cell culture tubes or shell vials. When used for direct detection, these reagents are between 80% and 95% sensitive and are 90% to 99% specific.

Of particular importance is the direct detection of RSV by fluorescent antibody or membrane-bound EIA in nasopharyngeal samples. Rapid direct detection is important because RSV causes serious lower respiratory tract disease (bronchiolitis and pneumonia) in young children, often requiring hospitalization. Rapid results can help in making cohorting decisions upon hospital admission. Also, it is difficult to maintain viral viability during transport, and therefore it can be difficult to recover RSV in culture.

Influenza is another respiratory tract infection in which a rapid diagnosis is important for treatment. A number of direct antigen tests are available for detecting both influenza A and B viruses, including the Directigen FluA+B (BD Diagnostic Systems). These tests in general have very good sensitivities and specificities. Two CLIA-waived point-of-care tests are the QuickVue Influenza test (Quidel Corp., San Diego, Calif.) and the FLU OIA (ThermoBioStar). These tests can be performed on a number of clinical specimens such as nasal, nasopharyngeal, and throat swabs. The sensitivities and specificity vary depending on the clinical specimen. The QuickVue test has a reported sensitivity slightly less than that of the FLU OIA, although it has a greater specificity.

Bacterial Meningitis and Sepsis

For approximately 25 years, clinical laboratories have regularly used antigen detection testing of CSF and other body fluids to detect organisms causing bacterial meningitis. Techniques have included countercurrent immunoelectrophoresis (popular in the 1970s), EIA, and coagglutination. Today, clinical laboratories typically use LA assays when performing rapid antigen testing for bacterial meningitis. The bacterial agents detected in commercially available kits include *H. influenzae* type b, *Neisseria meningitidis*, *Streptococcus pneumoniae*, and *Streptococcus agalactiae* (group B *Streptococcus*). Although antibodies in each kit vary, they are all designed to detect capsular polysaccharide antigens of the organisms. When these organisms cause infection, the antigens are shed by growing bacterial cells into the body tissues and fluids.

These organisms often cause a bacteremia before they invade the central nervous system. Thus the organism and antigens may be detected in the serum before or at the same time they are found in the CSF in cases of meningitis. Furthermore, circulating organisms and soluble antigens are trapped, degraded, and released by phagocytic cells of the liver and spleen. These products are cleared from the body by filtration in the kidney and excreted in the urine; thus urine can be examined for the presence of antigen in addition to CSF in suspected cases of meningitis. Urine is also useful as a test specimen either alone or in addition to serum in cases of bacteremia and focal infections other than meningitis. It may be concentrated by ultrafiltration to increase test sensitivity. It should be mentioned that with the advent of *H. influenzae* type b vaccine, the incidence of invasive *H. influenzae* infection has declined by greater than 95% in countries routinely using the vaccine. Fortunately, no other microorganism seems to have filled this potential niche.

The clinical utility of antigen tests for diagnosing meningitis varies with a number of factors, including the manufacturer of the kit, the specific organism, and the type of specimen tested. In many clinical laboratories, the use of these tests is reserved for very specific diagnostic testing requirements. In most situations, the Gram stain is sufficiently sensitive to detect bacterial meningitis. However, as in the Case in Point, the Gram-stained direct smear was negative. The responsible

organism could be detected by a direct antigen test. Gram stains and/or antigen detection tests must always be performed along with appropriate culture. Most importantly, appropriate antimicrobial treatment should never be withheld pending culture results in patients with negative antigen test results (unlike the situation with antigen testing for group A streptococci). The greatest clinical utility of these antigen tests probably occurs when testing specimens from patients who have received antimicrobial therapy before cultures were collected and in whom the Gram stain was negative. In this situation, the likelihood of recovering the organism in culture is dramatically decreased.

Infections in Immunocompromised Patients

Cryptococcus neoformans, CMV, and *P. jiroveci* are important pulmonary pathogens in transplant, cancer, and AIDS patients. Cryptococcosis is a devastating systemic infection generally limited to immunocompromised persons. Infection occurs initially in the lungs and rapidly disseminates to the brain and meninges. Before the advent of AIDS, disseminated cryptococcal infection rarely occurred. Traditionally the diagnosis of cryptococcosis meningitis has been based on culture of CSF or the presence of encapsulated yeast cells in India ink preparations of CSF. Antigen testing of CSF, commonly performed by LA, is considerably more sensitive than India ink direct examination of CSF. Antigen detection methods use polyclonal or monoclonal antibodies to the capsular (polysaccharide) antigen and are easy to perform. Quantitative antigen detection, which consists of titrating CSF antigen by performing serial dilutions, is an important prognostic indicator of clinical response to antifungal therapy.

The Cryptococcal Antigen Latex Agglutination System (CALAS, Meridian Diagnostics, Cincinnati, Ohio) uses rabbit polyclonal IgG. This assay is prone to false-positive results from rheumatoid factor, but it is more sensitive than the assays using monoclonal antibodies. The Murex Cryptococcus Test (Murex Diagnostics, Norcross, Ga.) uses mouse monoclonal IgM; this assay is not subject to false-positive results by rheumatoid factor. The Premier EIA (Meridian Diagnostics, Inc.) has the advantage of fewer false-positive results, does not react with rheumatoid factor, and can be run on a large number of samples at once.

Early CMV structural proteins can be monitored by the CMV antigenemia assay. In this procedure, buffy coats from whole blood specimens are stained by fluorescent antibody and the number of positive polymorphonuclear (PMN) cells per 100,000 cells is counted. Increased numbers of fluorescently stained PMN nuclei are indicative of increased risk of developing CMV pneumonia or other end-stage organ disease.

A fluorescent antibody procedure for *P. jiroveci* is approved for use on induced sputum and bronchoscopy specimens (Figure 10-30). In patients with high probability of pneumocystic pneumonia, a negative fluorescent antibody on induced sputum should be followed by a fluorescent antibody on a bronchoscopically obtained specimen. *P. jiroveci* culture is not widely available, making fluorescent antibody assays the only

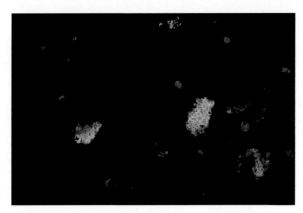

FIGURE 10-30 Bronchoalveolar lavage showing *Pneumocystis jiroveci* using fluorescent antibody test.

reliable method for its detection in the clinical microbiology laboratory.

Gastrointestinal Tract Infections

Clostridium difficile–Associated Disease

Direct microbial detection methods have been applied to the diagnosis of bacterial, viral, and parasitic agents of gastrointestinal tract infections. *C. difficile,* an anaerobic gram-positive rod, causes pseudomembranous colitis and antibiotic-associated diarrhea. These diseases typically occur in hospitalized patients receiving antimicrobial agents that alter bowel flora. The organism produces two exotoxins, toxins A and B, that are involved in pathogenesis. Toxin A functions as an enterotoxin causing inflammation, increased vascular permeability, and fluid secretion. Toxin B is a cytotoxin that causes mucosal damage with 10-fold more potency than toxin A and causes hemorrhagic colitis and cytopathic effects.

Two gold-standard laboratory tests exist for *C. difficile.* One is a cell culture cytotoxicity and neutralization test, which is a primary indicator of toxin B presence. The other method is culture on selective media in anaerobic conditions followed by testing isolates for toxin production. Both procedures require 24 to 96 hours for final identification. A large number of EIA tests for toxin A and/or B have been evaluated. Results vary considerably; sensitivities range from 34% to 100% and specificities range from 88% to 100%. Most EIA kits use microtiter plates, whereas others use a membrane. The membrane assays tend to give quicker results, but the microtiter plate-based assays have greater sensitivity and specificity. *C. difficile* isolates can be toxin A–/B+; therefore assays detecting both toxins are generally preferred over toxin A specific tests.

Shiga-Toxin–Producing *Escherichia coli*

Food-borne outbreaks of shiga-toxin–producing *E. coli* (STEC), also referred to as *enterohemorrhagic E. coli* (EHEC), are being reported with increased frequency. EHEC strains, such as O157:H7 and others, secrete a verotoxin that causes endothelial injury that can result in the development of hemolytic uremic syndrome (HUS). Many rapid tests are available for detection of verotoxin and/or specific EHEC strains

directly from stool samples. Principles used include EIA, immunomagnetic beads, latex slide agglutination, and tube agglutination. Rapid identification may prove useful in identifying exposed individuals in an outbreak situation. Those individuals can then be carefully watched for progression to systemic disease including HUS.

Viral Gastroenteritis

The most important identifiable agents of viral gastroenteritis are human rotaviruses, enteric adenoviruses, caliciviruses, and the noroviruses (formerly the Norwalk and Norwalk-like viruses). These agents are either difficult or impossible to grow in cell culture, and detection by electron microscopy is rarely cost efficient in a clinical microbiology laboratory. Therefore antigen detection methods are very important for diagnosis.

Rotaviruses are the most important agents in this group for a number of reasons. They commonly infect very young infants, often in daycare settings, causing vomiting and diarrhea, resulting in dehydration. Rotavirus disease can also be severe and long lasting, whereas gastroenteritis due to these other viruses is usually much shorter in duration. Both EIA and LA tests using either polyclonal or monoclonal antibodies are available for rotavirus detection in stool specimens; EIA is generally more sensitive than LA. In either case, soluble antigen must be extracted from the particulate matter in stool before testing. This is generally accomplished by mixing the stool with extract buffer solution. At least two EIA kits are available for detection of enteric adenoviruses and one kit for astrovirus. No rapid tests for Norwalk virus or caliciviruses are commercially available.

Giardiasis and Cryptosporidiosis

The classical workup for ova and parasites (O & P) requires chemical extraction, concentration, and microscopic examination of stool specimens. These methods are technically demanding and time consuming and require trained personnel. In settings not including areas of endemicity for certain parasites (e.g., the United States), a number of studies have suggested that 95% of all clinically important parasites detected are either *G. lamblia* or *Cryptosporidium parvum.* Several DFA, EIA, and ICT kits are available for detection of antigen directly from stool. These kits generally have sensitivities and specificities in excess of 90%. Some formats include one monoclonal antibody to detect one organism; other formats use separate monoclonal antibodies for both organisms. When testing by DFA assays (see Figure 10-15), the difference in size between these two parasites allows the laboratory scientist to visually distinguish the two organisms when using both antibodies in one procedure. Many laboratories offer these tests to screen the immunocompetent outpatient population.

A problem with antigen detection assays is that only one or two organisms can be detected; other clinically significant intestinal parasites could be missed that might have been detected by microscopic examination. Testing algorithms usually are established so that only those patients with a history of travel or immunosuppression require a full O & P workup when the screening test is negative. DFA assays can also be used to check municipal water supplies for *G. lamblia* cysts; however, polymerase chain reaction assays are more sensitive and are being used more frequently instead.

The Triage parasite panel (BIOSITE Biodiagnostics, San Diego, Calif.) offers an ICT test for the detection of *G. lamblia, Cryptococcus,* and *Entamoeba histolytica/dispar. E. histolytica* causes some of the most severe gastrointestinal parasitic infections. *E. histolytica* should be differentiated from the morphologically identical but nonpathogenic *E. dispar.* TechLab (Blacksburg, Va.) offers an EIA *E. histolytica*–specific kit using monoclonal antibody against the Gal/GalNAc-specific lectin.

Sexually Transmitted Diseases

Chlamydial Infections

Chlamydia trachomatis, an obligate intracellular bacterium, infects the genital tract, causing urethritis, cervicitis, and other infections. In addition, neonates born to infected mothers are at risk for developing conjunctivitis and pneumonia. Although isolation in cell culture is still considered the gold standard for diagnosis, a large number of direct antigen detection assays are commercially available. Most of these assays are based on EIA or fluorescent antibody. The EIAs use either polyclonal or monoclonal antibody to chlamydial lipopolysaccharide. The numerous published evaluations of these products suggest moderately good sensitivity and very good specificity (about 97%) when they are used on symptomatic patients at high risk for infection (e.g., patients visiting an STD clinic). The tests do not, however, perform as well when used in low-prevalence populations or asymptomatic patients (e.g., OB-GYN clinics). In addition, they are not approved for use in children in whom evidence of chlamydial infection subsequent to sexual abuse is being sought. Confirmatory tests are available that can increase the specificity to 99.5%. Nucleic acid amplification assays are generally more sensitive than antigen detection methods and are preferred by many laboratories.

Human Immunodeficiency Virus

Although diagnosis of HIV infection is generally accomplished by antibody detection, EIA for the viral p24 antigen is used to detect active viral replication in blood. Its greatest value is in the diagnosis during early infection, before antibodies are detectable, and in neonates in whom serologic diagnosis is of little value because of maternal anti-HIV IgG from a seropositive mother. Detection of p24 antigen is generally performed by capture EIA using monoclonal antibody. One problem with this assay occurs during seroconversion. As the patient begins making antibodies to p24 antigen, immune complexes can form, which prevents the antigen and antibody from reacting with in vitro assays. This can result in false-negative results for both antigen and antibody detection assays.

Another problem with p24 antigen detection has been low sensitivity. This issue has been reduced by modification of the procedure, such as boiling the serum before testing to release immune complexes. In addition, combining antigen detection with antibody detection (fourth-generation assays) also increases the sensitivity of diagnosing a patient with HIV

infection. Although p24 antigen detection assays are easy to perform, their sensitivity remains less than that of nucleic acid amplification tests. Blood units for transfusion are typically screened for antibodies to HIV, and a nucleic acid amplification test is performed for detecting viral RNA.

BIBLIOGRAPHY

Aldeen WE et al: Comparison of nine commercially available enzyme-linked immunosorbent assays for detection of *Giardia lamblia* in fecal specimens, *J Clin Microbiol* 36:1338, 1998.

Berzofsky JA et al: Antigen-antibody interactions and monoclonal antibodies. In *Fundamental immunology,* ed 4, Philadelphia, 2008, Lippincott,Williams & Wilkins.

Carpenter AB: Immunoassays for the diagnosis of infectious diseases. In Murray PR et al, editors: *Manual of clinical microbiology,* ed 9, Washington, DC, 2007, ASM Press.

Chan KH et al: Evaluation of the Directigen FluA+B test for rapid diagnosis of influenza virus type A and B infections, *J Clin Microbiol* 40:1675, 2002.

Dean D et al: Comparison of performance and cost-effectiveness of direct fluorescent-antibody, ligase chain reaction, and PCR assays for verification of chlamydial enzyme immunoassay results for populations with a low to moderate prevalence of *Chlamydia trachomatis* infection, *J Clin Microbiol* 36:94, 1998.

Domínguez J et al: Assessment of a new test to detect *Legionella* urinary antigen for the diagnosis of Legionnaires' disease, *Diagn Microbiol Infect Dis* 41:199, 2001.

Essig A et al: *Chlamydia* and *Chlamydophila.* In Murray PR et al, editors: *Manual of clinical microbiology,* ed 9, Washington, DC, 2007, ASM Press.

Fabrizi F et al: Automated RIBA HCV strip immunoblot assay: a novel tool for the diagnosis of hepatitis C virus infection in hemodialysis patients, *Am J Nephrol* 21:104, 2001.

Farkas T, Jiang X: Rotaviruses, caliciviruses, astroviruses, and other diarrheic viruses. In Murray PR et al, editors: *Manual of clinical microbiology,* ed 9, Washington, DC, 2007, ASM Press.

Gerna G et al: Standardization of the human cytomegalovirus antigenemia assay by means of in vitro–generated positive peripheral blood polymorphonuclear leukocytes, *J Clin Microbiol* 36:3585, 1998.

Gieseker KE et al: Comparison of two *Streptococcus pyogenes* diagnostic tests with a rigorous culture standard, *Pediatric Infect Dis J* 21:922, 2002.

Gieseker KE, et al: Evaluating the American Academy of Pediatrics diagnostic standard for *Streptococcus pyogenes* pharyngitis: backup culture versus repeat rapid antigen testing, *Pediatrics* 111:666, 2005.

Griffith BP et al: Human immunodeficiency viruses. In Murray PR et al, editors: *Manual of clinical microbiology,* ed 9, Washington, DC, 2007, ASM Press.

Helbig JH et al: Detection of *Legionella pneumophila* antigen in urine samples by the BinaxNOW immunochromatographic assay and comparison with both Binax *Legionella* urinary enzyme immunoassay (EIA) and Biotest Legionella urine antigen EIA, *J Med Microbiol* 50:509, 2001.

Johnson EA et al: Clostridium. In Murray PR et al, editors: *Manual of clinical microbiology,* ed 9, Washington, DC, 2007, ASM Press.

Kiely PR et al: Anti-HCV confirmatory testing of voluntary blood donors: comparison of the sensitivity of two immunoblot assays, *Transfusion* 42:1053, 2002.

Kurtz B et al: Importance of inoculum size and sampling effect in rapid antigen detection for diagnosis of *Streptococcus pyogenes* pharyngitis, *J Clin Microbiol* 38:279, 2000.

Leber AL, Novak-Weekley S: Intestinal and urogenital amebae, flagellates, and ciliates. In Murray PR et al, editors: *Manual of clinical microbiology,* ed 9, Washington, DC, 2007, ASM Press.

McNeely M: Antibodies: the laboratory depends on them but they can let us down, *Lab Med* 11:873, 2002.

Nataro JP et al: *Escherichia, Shigella,* and *Salmonella.* In Murray PR et al, editors: *Manual of clinical microbiology,* ed 9, Washington, DC, 2007, ASM Press.

Needham CA et al: Streptococcal pharyngitis: impact of a high-sensitivity antigen test on physician outcome, *J Clin Microbiol* 36:3468, 1998.

Okada C et al: Cross-reactivity and sensitivity of two *Legionella* urinary antigen kits, Biotest EIA and Binax NOW, to extracted antigens form various serogroups of *L. pneumophila* and other *Legionella* species, *Microbiol Immunol* 14:51, 2002.

Poehling KA et al: Bedside diagnosis of influenza virus infections in hospitalized children, *Pediatrics* 110:83, 2002.

Pope V et al: *Treponema* and other human host-associated spirochetes. In Murray PR et al, editors: *Manual of clinical microbiology,* ed 9, Washington, DC, 2007, ASM Press.

Stanley J: *Essentials of immunology and serology,* Albany, NY, 2002, Thomson Delmar Learning.

Stringer J et al: A new name *(Pneumocystis jiroveci)* for *Pneumocystis* from humans, *Emerg Infect Dis* 8:891, 2002.

Tanyuksel M, Petri WA: Laboratory diagnosis of amebiasis, *Clin Microbiol Rev* 16:713, 2003.

Tucker SP et al: A flu optical immunoassay (ThermoBioStar's FLU OIA): a diagnostic tool for improved influenza management, *Phil Trans R Soc London B* 356:1915, 2001.

Turgeon ML: *Immunology and serology in laboratory medicine,* ed 4, St Louis, 2009, Mosby.

Yeo SF, Wong B: Current status of nonculture methods for diagnosis of invasive fungal infections, *Clin Microbiol Rev* 15:465, 2002.

Points to Remember

- Although the words *antigen* and *immunogen* are often used interchangeably, an immunogen is a molecule stimulating an immune response, whereas an antigen is a molecule capable of binding to a specific antibody or T-cell receptor.
- Using antibodies to diagnose infectious diseases requires either demonstrating a fourfold rise in titer or distinguishing between IgG and IgM.
- Although monoclonal antibodies have the advantage of being more specific than polyclonal antibodies in detecting antigens, polyclonal antibodies can be more sensitive.
- False-negative tests for antibodies to specific antigens can occur if the serum sample is collected too soon in the course of the infection, the patient is immunocompromised, or antibody concentration is extremely high (prozone phenomenon).
- False-positive tests for antibody can be caused by a number of situations including the presence of heterophile antibodies or rheumatoid factor.

- Precipitation reactions are based on the insolubility of immune complexes formed following the binding of soluble antigen to a soluble antibody.
- Agglutination assays use particulate substances, such as latex, to form visible clumps to detect immune complexes.
- Antigens or antibodies can be labeled with a number of markers, such as fluorochromes or enzymes, to detect antigen-antibody binding in vitro.
- In syphilis serology, screening tests use nontreponemal antigens, whereas confirmatory tests use spirochete antigens.
- *Streptococcus pyogenes* produces several exotoxins that can induce antibody formation. Detection of these antibodies is sometimes important in diagnosing infections.
- Direct antigen detection methods offer accurate, rapid alternatives to culturing infectious agents.

Learning Assessment Questions

1. What is the significance of a high titer of IgM to cytomegalovirus in a neonate?

2. Many diagnostic kits for detecting antigens in clinical specimens use monoclonal antibodies. What are the advantages and disadvantages of using monoclonal antibodies instead of polyclonal antibodies?

3. List some of the causes of false-negative serologic test results.

4. How does double immunodiffusion differ from single radial immunodiffusion?

5. How does passive agglutination differ from reverse passive agglutination?

6. Serial twofold dilutions of a patient's serum sample are prepared. The dilutions are tested for the presence of antistreptolysin-O (ASO) antibody in a neutralization assay. Dilutions 1:1 through 1:16 show no hemolysis, whereas dilutions 1:32 through 1:128 exhibit hemolysis. How should the results be reported?

7. In the indirect immunofluorescent assay for detecting antibody, what is the conjugate?

8. Western blots are generally regarded as confirmatory tests. What advantage does the Western blot assay have over many other serologic tests?

9. A patient's serum sample was reported as reactive in a rapid plasma reagin (RPR) test. What should be done next? Why?

10. The presence of antibodies that agglutinate sheep and horse red blood cells is suggestive of what disease?

Applications of Molecular Diagnostics

Steven D. Mahlen

- ■ **NUCLEIC ACID HYBRIDIZATION TECHNIQUES**
  Hybridization Reaction Variables
  Probe Selection
  Hybridization Formats
  Applications of Nucleic Acid Hybridization
    Techniques
- ■ **NUCLEIC ACID AMPLIFICATION PROCEDURES**
  Introduction to Nucleic Acid Amplification
    Procedures
  Polymerase Chain Reaction
  Other Nucleic Acid Amplification Reactions

- ■ **STRAIN TYPING AND IDENTIFICATION**
  Nonamplified Typing Methods
  Amplified Typing Methods
- ■ **THE FUTURE OF MOLECULAR DIAGNOSTICS
  TESTING IN THE CLINICAL MICROBIOLOGY
  LABORATORY**
  Sequencing
  Pyrosequencing
  Nanobiotechnology
  DNA Microarrays and Nanoarrays
  Proteomics

OBJECTIVES

After reading and studying this chapter, you should be able to:

1. Provide a synopsis of the different molecular diagnostics applications in the clinical microbiology laboratory.
2. Describe the concept of nucleic acid hybridization and how the different formats are used in the clinical microbiology laboratory.
3. Discuss what nucleic acid probes are and how they are used in molecular diagnostics techniques.
4. Explain the concept of nucleic acid amplification reactions and how these techniques may be used in the clinical microbiology laboratory.
5. Describe the advantages and disadvantages of using nucleic acid amplification procedures.
6. Discuss the theory and components of the polymerase chain reaction (PCR).
7. List and describe the methods of detecting PCR products.
8. Provide an overview of real-time PCR and the various real-time PCR detection methods.
9. Discuss the alternative types of PCR assays and their uses in the clinical microbiology laboratory.
10. Describe the different non-PCR–based amplification procedures and how they are employed.
11. Give an overview of strain typing procedures that are used in microbiology.
12. Compare the various strain typing methodologies and discuss their advantages and disadvantages.
13. Discuss sequencing techniques, large-scale genomics, nanotechnology, and proteomics assays.

Case in Point

One day, a 26-year-old man noticed a small "pimple" on his right flank. The pimple developed into a boil (an infection of one of his hair follicles) in a few days. The area around the boil became inflamed—the skin was red, the area around the boil began to swell, and the whole area was painful. In another day, the man became nauseated, started vomiting, and had a low-grade fever when he presented to the emergency department. He was ill enough to be admitted to the hospital.

The boil, a type of abscess, was drained, and the pus was sent to the microbiology laboratory. Gram-positive cocci in clusters were observed in a Gram stain of the purulent material. The

following day, creamy-white, β-hemolytic colonies were observed on culture media. The colonies were catalase-positive and positive by latex agglutination for coagulase. A preliminary report of "*Staphylococcus aureus* present, susceptibilities to follow" was entered into the hospital's laboratory information system.

A real-time polymerase chain reaction (PCR) assay was run to determine whether the *S. aureus* isolate carried the *mecA* gene, the determinant of methicillin resistance in many staphylococci. The real-time PCR assay took less than 2 hours to determine that the patient's isolate was positive for presence of the *mecA* gene, meaning that the patient had a methicillin-resistant *S. aureus* infection. An internal control for a *S. aureus*-specific gene was also used in the assay, further confirming the etiologic agent of disease. The patient was treated with appropriate antibiotics and recovered.

Issues to Consider

After reading the patient's case history, consider:

- The patient's symptoms and presentation that may indicate the identity of the agent
- The use of rapid molecular diagnostic techniques that may aid in identification of an etiologic agent and in treatment of disease
- The potential benefits to patient care that may result from using molecular diagnostics techniques
- The length of time that standard microbiologic methods take compared to molecular diagnostics assays

Key Terms

Agarose gel electrophoresis

Amplicon

Anneal

Branched DNA (bDNA) detection

Cycling probe technology

Denaturation

Dendrogram

Deoxynucleotide triphosphates (dNTPs)

DNA microarrays

DNA polymerase

Dual-probe FRET

5′ Nuclease assay

Fluorescence resonance energy transfer (FRET)

Fluorophore

Housekeeping genes

Hybrid capture

Insitu amplification (ISA)

Insitu hybridization (ISH)

Melting curve analysis

Melting temperature (T_m)

Metagenomics

Molecular beacon

Multilocus enzyme electrophoresis (MLEE)

Multilocus sequence typing (MLST)

Multilocus variable number of tandem repeat analysis (MLVA)

Multiplex PCR

Nanobiotechnology

Nested PCR

Northern blot

Nucleic acid hybridization

Nucleic acid sequence based amplification (NASBA)

Oligonucleotide

Plasmid profile analysis

Plasmids

Polymerase chain reaction (PCR)

Primer annealing

Primer extension

Primer-dimers

Primers

Probe

Proteomics

Pulsed-field gel electrophoresis (PFGE)

Pyrosequencing

Random amplified polymorphic DNA (RAPD)

Real-time PCR

Repetitive palindromic extragenic elements PCR (Rep-PCR)

Restriction enzyme

Reverse transcription-PCR (RT-PCR)

Ribonuclease H (RNase H)

Ribotyping

Scorpion primers

Sequencing

Southern blot

SYBR green

Target

Template

Thermal cycler

Transcript

Transcription-mediated amplification (TMA)

Uracil-*N*-glycosylase (UNG)

olecular diagnostics is one of the most recent innovations in the clinical microbiology laboratory over the past several years and is probably the fastest-growing section or department in many clinical laboratories. Molecular biologic techniques are now used to aid in the diagnosis of infectious diseases and are gaining acceptance as viable testing options for clinicians. This is partly because of the increased sensitivity and specificity that molecular-based assays now provide. Molecular diagnostics tests provide rapid detection of certain microorganisms and are particularly useful for microorganisms that are difficult to culture or take a long time to grow on culture media. Molecular diagnostics assays are used to give clinicians rapid answers for treatment options, thereby saving valuable time in cases of life-threatening infections.

The types of assays used in molecular diagnostics for infectious disease testing include nucleic acid hybridization techniques, nucleic acid and signal amplification techniques, and assays that aid in epidemiologic investigations. This chapter discusses these molecular-based techniques and their applications in a modern clinical microbiology laboratory.

NUCLEIC ACID HYBRIDIZATION TECHNIQUES

Nucleic acid hybridization is a technique that was first described in 1961 by Marmur and Doty. Most molecular diagnostics testing procedures use the basic concept of nucleic acid hybridization. Conceptually, nucleic acid hybridization refers to the formation of hydrogen bonds between nucleotides of single-stranded DNA and/or RNA molecules that are complementary to each other. This forms a stable double-stranded nucleic acid molecule under the right conditions. The resulting double-stranded hybrids may be DNA:DNA, DNA:RNA, or RNA:RNA, as depicted in Figure 11-1. This hybridization process is also called *duplex formation*. This coupling of complementary single-stranded molecules is a key component for many of the tests discussed in the rest of this chapter, including blotting methods, the **polymerase chain reaction (PCR)**, and other molecular-based techniques.

A
GTTTATCGTATAAAG
CAAATAGCATATTTC

B
GTTTATCGTATAAAG
CAAAUAGCAUAUUUC

C
GUUUAUCGUAUAAAG
CAAAUAGCAUAUUUC

FIGURE 11-1 Three different oligonucleotide hybrids. **A,** DNA:DNA hybrid. **B,** DNA:RNA hybrid. The top strand is DNA and the bottom strand is RNA; note the "U"s instead of "T"s. **C,** RNA:RNA hybrid.

The two single-stranded nucleic acid molecules used in hybridization techniques are referred to by different terms. One of the strands is known as the **target**. The target strand is the DNA or RNA sequence that will be identified by the employed molecular diagnostics method. The target nucleic acid molecule typically is either immobilized on a solid support mechanism or suspended in solution. The target is also referred to as the **template**. The other strand involved in hybridization methods is called the **probe**. The probe is usually a single-stranded DNA or RNA **oligonucleotide** that is labeled with an attached reporter chemical or a radionucleotide that can be detected visually, by film, or by an instrument. In essence, the probe is used to detect the target nucleic acid molecule. In most currently used molecular-based methods, the probe is produced synthetically to detect a specific target nucleic acid sequence of a given microorganism. Often, probes are available for purchase from manufacturers in kits designed to detect a specific target sequence. Probes are used in detection of microbial pathogens in many different types of samples, gene expression analysis, identification of gene rearrangements and chromosomal translocations, detection of point mutations, and other clinical applications.

Hybridization Reaction Variables

Several variables affect the outcome of a given hybridization reaction. These variables include the temperature, nucleotide base composition of the probe, the length of the probe, probe concentration, degree of complementarity between the target and the probe, ionic strength (salt concentration), and pH. When one or more of these variables is not optimized for a hybridization assay, the hybrids may not efficiently form.

Temperature

Temperature is a variable that is probably the most easily controlled during hybridization. The stability of a given hybrid can be calculated by determining the **melting temperature (T_m)** of a probe. The T_m is the temperature at which 50% of hybrids have formed and 50% of the single-stranded nucleic acid molecules are still dissociated. The T_m may be calculated by various methods; companies that synthetically manufacture probes typically calculate the T_m for the customer. For the most part, the T_m is dependent on the nucleotide composition of the probe, particularly on the percentage of guanine (G) and cytosine (C) nucleotides in the probe. This is often referred to as the *G+C composition*, or the *G+C ratio*, of the probe. The T_m is dependent on the G+C ratio because three hydrogen bonds form between G and C, instead of the two hydrogen bonds that form between adenine (A) and thymine (T); the G/C bond pair is more thermodynamically stable than the A/T bond pair.

Length of Probe

Another aspect that affects the T_m is the length of the probe; in general the T_m is lower for a shorter probe. Hybridization reactions tend to occur more rapidly for shorter probes than for longer probes. Furthermore, all of the other factors that affect hybridization reactions become more influential for shorter probes than for longer probes.

Probe Concentration

The probe concentration also affects hybridization reactions. Higher probe concentrations typically lower the reaction time by saturating all of the available probe target sequences. However, excessive probe concentrations promote nonspecific binding of the probe to nontarget sequences. The optimal probe concentration may be determined by testing several different reactions with different probe concentrations, if this has not been determined already. In general, probes labeled with radioactive isotopes require lower concentrations than do probes labeled with nonisotopic molecules.

Degree of Target and Probe Complementarity

Many hybridization assay conditions are based on the expectation that a probe has exact or near-exact complementarity to the target nucleic acid. This will not always be the case, in that different strains of microorganisms can develop slightly different target sequences through point mutations. When conditions are stringent, exact matches between the probe and target will hybridize first, whereas mismatches form duplexes more slowly. High temperatures (e.g., the T_m temperature), in fact, may even inhibit the formation of hybrids. The short oligonucleotides that are most often used as probes can be highly affected by mismatches; very long probes are not nearly as affected. A lower temperature than the T_m will help alleviate stringency and allow mismatches to form duplexes more readily.

Salt Concentration

The concentration of salt (the ionic strength) may affect the stringency of a given hybridization reaction. The rate of a hybridization reaction will increase as the salt concentration increases, up to a threshold; past 1.2 M NaCl, the rate of the reaction becomes constant.

pH

pH affects the stability of double-stranded nucleic acid molecules in solution. An alkaline pH promotes dissociation of double-stranded molecules, whereas acidic pH solutions can depurinate probes and target nucleic acid molecules. Thus a neutral pH is preferable for most hybridization reactions. Usually, the pH of most hybridization reactions conducted in the clinical microbiology laboratory does not have to be adjusted because manufacturer-supplied reagents and probes are provided with buffers at the proper pH.

Probe Selection

Selection of the proper probe for nucleic acid hybridization reactions is just as important as the hybridization reaction method itself. Essentially, the function of the probe is to form a duplex with every complementary sequence available in the reaction, and the probe must be suited for the particular hybridization reaction that will be used. Probes may be either DNA- or RNA-based and are either radiolabeled or nonisotopically labeled. At one time, nucleic acid probes typically carried a radionucleotide label. The radiolabeled probe often had to be prepared by the user, and success of a hybridization reaction depended on the efficient incorporation of the radionucleotide label into the probe. Now, radiolabeled probes are rarely, if ever, used in the clinical microbiology laboratory. Isotopes that are used for labeling probes include ^{32}P, ^{35}S, ^{3}H, and occasionally ^{33}P. Most of these isotopes have short half-lives and thus have little clinical utility; in addition, undesirable radioactive waste is generated and radioisotopes must be handled with care. Radiolabeled probes have been replaced for the most part by nonisotopic labels, including biotin, digoxigenin (DIG), and fluorescein. Generally, nonisotopic labels have resolution and sensitivity that approaches, matches, or even exceeds that of radionucleotide labels, depending on the manufacturer and process used. In addition, nonisotopic labels do not require special handling and specialized waste disposal.

A probe may also be end-labeled or continuously labeled. An end-labeled probe has the label attached to either the 5′ or the 3′ end of the nucleic acid sequence. A 5′ end-labeled probe may be synthesized by transfer of the probe via a kinase reaction, whereas a 3′ end-labeled probe can be synthesized by using a terminal transferase enzyme. A continuously labeled probe has the label incorporated at intervals along the length of the nucleic acid sequence. Continuously labeled probes may be synthesized by using PCR or by other methods.

Hybridization Formats

Hybridization reactions may occur on a solid support mechanism, in situ, or in solution.

Solid Support Hybridization

Solid support hybridization reactions have been used for several years, although in-solution hybridization formats are more commonly used in clinical microbiology laboratories now. In solid support hybridization (a technique often called *blotting*) the target nucleic acid is transferred and immobilized to a membrane, composed of either nitrocellulose or nylon. The solid membrane is often pretreated to reduce nonspecific probe binding to the membrane itself. Labeled probe is then hybridized to the immobilized nucleic acid, and washing steps are used to remove excess probe and clarify the signal. Detection is based on the type of probe used; colorimetric probes enable visual determination of positive and negative reactions, whereas chemiluminescent and radiolabeled probes require film and/or a detection system. Two examples of solid support hybridization techniques are the Southern blot and the Northern blot.

Southern Blot

The **Southern blot** was first described in 1975 by E.M. Southern; he described a technique whereby chromosomal DNA could be separated by **agarose gel electrophoresis,** then transferred and immobilized to a nitrocellulose membrane. Usually, this method is used after the chromosomal DNA has been digested with a **restriction enzyme.** The DNA is first digested because chromosomal DNA is too large to separate in an agarose gel. Once the DNA has been separated and immobilized onto a solid membrane, labeled probe is hybridized to the specific target DNA sequence and detected, as depicted in Figure 11-2. Southern blotting is somewhat labor intensive,

often takes more than 1 day to perform, and is not often used anymore in clinical microbiology laboratories. Southern blotting can be used to identify microorganisms, to detect mutations, to type strains for epidemiologic investigations, and for other purposes.

Northern Blot

A **Northern blot** is used to detect RNA molecules, which are nearly always **transcript.** The procedure to blot RNA onto a solid support mechanism was first described by Alwine et al. in 1977; this technique was not named after a person named "Northern." Northern blots may be used to determine the size of particular RNA molecules and to semiquantitate the amount of a particular RNA transcript. The actual procedure of the Northern blot is similar to that of the Southern blot—RNA is separated in an agarose gel, transferred to a membrane, immobilized, and detected with a probe that hybridizes to the RNA species of interest. Detection is also accomplished to the type of label on the probe. One difference between Southern blotting and Northern blotting is that a restriction enzyme is not used to digest RNA before separation; RNA molecules are small enough to separate efficiently by agarose gel electrophoresis. Like Southern blotting, Northern blotting is not often used in clinical microbiology laboratories.

In-situ Hybridization

In-situ hybridization (ISH), first described in 1969 by Pardue and Gall, is also not often used in clinical microbiology laboratories. This is a method of hybridization wherein DNA or RNA transcript can be detected directly in tissue with labeled probes. This technique is often performed directly in tissue that has been embedded in paraffin. ISH can also detect nucleic acids in intact cells and chromosomal genetic material. In microbiology, ISH may be used to detect low levels of viruses in tissue specimens, such as human papillomavirus (HPV). Some laboratories will couple an amplification procedure such as PCR with ISH to increase sensitivity and specificity. This technique is called **insitu amplification (ISA).** Like ISH, ISA is not often used in clinical microbiology laboratories, but it may be used to detect viruses in tissue specimens.

In-Solution Hybridization

In-solution hybridization is the type of hybridization reaction most often used by clinical microbiology laboratories. Several manufacturers have developed useful assays that promote hybridization between a labeled probe and target nucleic acids in a liquid solution in tubes or in microtiter wells. Generally, detection methods for these commercial systems are chemiluminescent-based. Labeled probes are used during in-solution hybridization for confirming culture-based identifications of bacteria and fungi and to rapidly identify infectious disease organisms.

Applications of Nucleic Acid Hybridization Techniques
Culture Confirmation Probe Applications

The Gen-Probe AccuProbe system uses nucleic acid hybridization to confirm suspicious cultures for several different

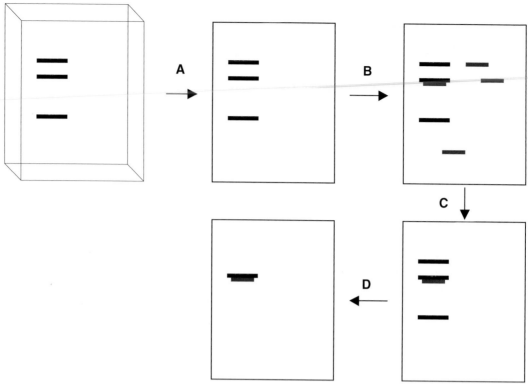

FIGURE 11-2 Southern blot. **A,** Chromosomal DNA fragments separated in an agarose gel are transferred to a solid membrane. **B,** Labeled probe specific for a nucleic acid target is incubated with the separated DNA on the membrane. **C,** Excess probe is washed from the membrane, leaving probe bound only to the appropriate target DNA. **D,** The probe:target DNA hybrid is detected.

organisms, including various mycobacteria, fungi, and bacteria. Regardless of the particular application, all of the AccuProbe tests use the same technology principle. A single-stranded, chemiluminescent-labeled DNA probe is designed to hybridize to the target organism's ribosomal RNA (rRNA), forming a DNA:RNA duplex. A detector called a *luminometer* is used to detect these labeled duplexes. The luminometer gives a reading in relative light units (RLU), and the RLU result for a suspicious culture is compared to a positive cutoff RLU value; any reading above the cutoff value is positive, and readings below are negative. The RLU cutoff value can change from assay run to assay run. These assays can be used from cultures obtained in either solid or liquid media. The sensitivity and specificity for most of these assays approaches 100%, and most of these tests take about an hour to perform. Table 11-1 shows the various organisms and their sensitivities and specificities of available AccuProbe assays from Gen-Probe.

Probe-Based Assays That Identify Microorganisms Directly from Specimens

Many assays use labeled probes for direct detection of microbial nucleic acid from specimens. ENZO Diagnostics, Inc. (Plymouth Meeting, Pa.), for example, has several chemiluminescent-labeled probes under their product line BioProbe Labeled Probes, which may be used to detect nucleic acid from infectious disease agents by Southern blotting, Northern blot-

ting, or ISH. Box 11-1 lists the various microorganisms that may be detected in this manner. ENZO Diagnostics, Inc., also has labeled probes that detect HPV by ISH as part of their PathoGene and Bio-Pap systems. The PathoGene system can also be used to detect the microorganisms listed in Box 11-1 by ISH.

In addition, Gen-Probe, Inc., also offers a few different systems for the detection of *Chlamydia trachomatis* and *Neisseria gonorrhoeae* from clinical specimens. One system, the PACE 2 system (and its predecessor, PACE), has been used for several years in many clinical microbiology laboratories. The PACE 2 system tests for both *C. trachomatis* and *N. gonorrhoeae* from a single endocervical or male urethral swab specimen. PACE 2 uses chemiluminescent-labeled DNA probes that target specific rRNA sequences from these microbes and form DNA:RNA hybrids (as with the AccuProbe assays). A luminometer is used to detect the hybrids. An initial test tells the laboratory whether either microorganism's nucleic acid is present in the sample; a confirmatory test is then performed to determine actual identity. Although popular and inexpensive, the PACE 2 system is primarily a manual procedure, and many clinical microbiology laboratories with high *C. trachomatis* and *N. gonorrhoeae* test volumes use the Gen-Probe, Inc., Aptima system now, an automated, **transcription-mediated amplification (TMA)** assay that is discussed later.

TABLE 11-1 Organisms Identified by AccuProbe*

	Sensitivity (%)	Specificity (%)
Mycobacterial Identification		
Mycobacterium avium complex	99.9	100
Mycobacterium avium	99.3	100
Mycobacterium intracellulare	100	100
Mycobacterium gordonae	98.8	99.7
Mycobacterium kansasii	92.8	100
Mycobacterium tuberculosis complex	99.2	99.0
Fungal Identification		
Blastomyces dermatitidis	98.1	99.7
Coccidioides immitis	98.8	100
Histoplasma capsulatum	100	100
Bacterial Identification		
Campylobacter spp.[†]	100	99.7
Enterococcus spp.[‡]	100	100
Haemophilus influenzae	97.1	100
Listeria monocytogenes	100	99.7
Neisseria gonorrhoeae	100	100
Staphylococcus aureus	100	100
Streptococcus agalactiae	97.7	99.1
Streptococcus pneumoniae	100	100
Streptococcus pyogenes	99.0	99.7

*Gen-Probe, Inc., San Diego, Calif.
[†]Includes *Campylobacter jejuni*, *C. coli*, and *C. lari*.
[‡]Includes *Enterococcus avium*, *E. casseliflavus*, *E. durans*, *E. faecalis*, *E. faecium*, *E. gallinarum*, *E. hirae*, *E. mundtii*, *E. pseudoavium*, *E. malodorous*, and *E. raffinosus*.

BOX 11-1 Infectious Disease Agents Detectable by BioProbe Labeled Probes from ENZO Diagnostics, Inc.*

Adenovirus
BK virus
Cytomegalovirus
Epstein-Barr virus
Hepatitis A virus
Herpes simplex virus
JC virus
SV 40

*Plymouth Meeting, Pa.

NUCLEIC ACID AMPLIFICATION PROCEDURES

Introduction to Nucleic Acid Amplification Procedures

Even though labeled probes can be used in nucleic acid hybridization assays to detect microorganisms in the clinical microbiology laboratory, amplification assays probably have more clinical utility. Amplification may be used to increase the target microorganism's nucleic acid in a sample in a short amount of time. This increase of the nucleic acid can be detected by various methods. Amplification is also used in some assays to increase the amount of signal after hybridizing a probe to an organism's nucleic acid. Both types of amplification assays are discussed. Amplification procedures have many advantages over standard microbiologic methods and over direct nucleic acid hybridization procedures. Many amplification assays combine rapid detection times with high sensitivity and high specificity. In general, amplification assays are more sensitive than their nucleic acid hybridization counterparts because target nucleic acid sequences may not be present in high enough numbers for direct hybridization assays to detect. Amplification tests can also be used to detect target nucleic acid in clinical specimens in some cases, and they present the advantage of speed over standard culture identification methods. Some amplification techniques also provide quantitative data and are useful to track the progress of a disease or to provide the number of copies of microbial nucleic acid present in a sample.

Disadvantages of amplification procedures include expense, the need for specialized testing and detection equipment, dedicated space to reduce contamination, and specially trained technicians. In addition, a given amplification procedure may provide a rapid response and provide an accurate identification of a given microorganism present in a disease state, but that answer does not mean that other microorganisms may not be present as well. Also, some amplification techniques are so specific that nucleic acid from an organism may be detected at low levels even if that organism is not responsible for a current infection. The standard amplification procedure that is used by most laboratories is PCR or a derivation of it; other amplification procedures include nucleic acid sequence based amplification (NASBA), transcription-mediated amplification (TMA), branched DNA (bDNA) detection, hybrid capture, and cycling probe technology.

Polymerase Chain Reaction

The introduction of PCR was one of the greatest recent breakthroughs in the chemical and biologic sciences, if not one of the greatest advances ever in these fields. The technique of synthesizing DNA was first described in 1971 by Kleppe et al., although Kary B. Mullis and others at the Cetus Corporation in California developed PCR into the current application in the early 1980s. Mullis eventually received the Nobel Prize in Chemistry for PCR, and the advent of PCR initiated a revolution in molecular biology and several other fields, including microbiology. PCR is valuable because it is simple, sensitive, and powerful. PCR can amplify a single copy of target DNA into an exponential amount of nucleic acid product over the course of 25 to 40 reaction cycles. As shown in Table 11-2, each cycle consists of three steps: (1) **denaturation** of target DNA, (2) **primer annealing** to the target sequence, and (3) **primer extension**. PCR requires several components, including an enzyme commonly called **DNA polymerase** (properly called *DNA-dependent DNA polymerase*), a buffer for the polymerase, **primers** (oligonucleotides that anneal specifically to target DNA and prime, or start, the synthesis of new DNA strands), the four **deoxynucleotide triphosphates** (**dNTPs**: dA, dC, dG, and dT), and a source of

TABLE 11-2 Three Basic Steps of Polymerase Chain Reaction

Step	Purpose
Denaturation	Separates double-stranded DNA
Primer annealing	Anneals primers to target DNA
Primer extension	Synthesizes new strands of DNA

template DNA (the target). An instrument called a **thermal cycler** is also required.

The original described method of PCR was labor intensive and used two separate heat blocks and the Klenow fragment from *Escherichia coli* as the DNA polymerase. Target DNA is denatured at temperatures greater than 90° C, so one heat block was set to 95° C. The other heat block was set to 30° C (the temperature at which the Klenow fragment from *E. coli* functioned best) to anneal primers. The amplification reaction then proceeded by manually transferring the reaction tube from heat block to heat block for several cycles; in addition, new Klenow fragment had to be added after every cycle, because it denatures at 95° C. In 1986, an instrument called the *thermal cycler* was developed; it was basically a heat block that cycled between temperatures, such that individual heat blocks were not required. In 1988, a heat-stable (thermostable) DNA polymerase from the thermophilic bacterium *Thermus aquaticus* was used in PCR. This was a major breakthrough for PCR, in that the polymerase only had to be included at the beginning of the reaction and did not have to be added after every cycle. Several variations of standard PCR have been described, including very useful applications such as **reverse transcription-PCR (RT-PCR), multiplex PCR,** and **nested PCR.**

The Mechanism of Polymerase Chain Reaction

As described earlier, PCR amplifies DNA in three basic steps: denaturation, primer annealing, and primer extension. The target DNA is exponentially amplified over many (25 to 40) cycles of these three reaction steps. Figure 11-3 shows one cycle of PCR.

Denaturation. Single-stranded DNA targets are necessary for PCR assays. The target double-stranded DNA (dsDNA) is separated into single strands during the denaturation step. Once the target dsDNA is separated, primers anneal to the single strands. The bonds in dsDNA separate at temperatures above 90° C, so most PCR protocols denature at 94° C or 95° C. The time required for denaturation is variable, usually depending on the type of PCR performed. During standard PCR assays, 15 to 30 seconds is often used for denaturation. Most PCR assays will also denature the target DNA for a few minutes before the actual cycles begin to ensure proper separation before PCR cycles begin. It is very important that all DNA be denatured; PCR product will not be obtained in high quantity if complete denaturation is not obtained. Incomplete denaturation may occur if the temperature is too low or if the denaturation period is too short.

Primer Annealing. The goal of this step is to hybridize, or anneal, oligonucleotide primers to the denatured, single-stranded target DNA strands. A pair of primers is used in standard PCR, one for each strand of dsDNA. The 5' ends of these primers frame the amplification region of the target DNA. Thus the 5' ends of the primer pair define the eventual size of the PCR product. Primer annealing occurs best within a temperature range that is usually defined by the T_m. The temperature in the reaction tube should not rise above the T_m; otherwise, proper hybridization of primers to target DNA will not occur. In most PCR reactions, the primer-annealing temperature used is a few degrees below the melting temperature; some laboratories use a formula such as $T_a = T_m - 5°$ C, where T_a is the annealing temperature and T_m is the melting temperature. Primer-annealing temperatures usually range from about 45° C to about 65° C for about 30 seconds to 2 minutes. Higher annealing temperatures can increase annealing specificity, so primers are often designed to have annealing temperatures on the high end of the scale.

Primer Extension. The purpose of primer extension is to produce the PCR products. The addition of the thermostable *Taq* DNA polymerase in 1988 supported primer extension at elevated temperatures, such that this step can be accomplished at 68° to 72° C, the temperature range at which this polymerase functions best. Furthermore, *Taq* DNA polymerase, as well as other thermostable DNA polymerases, survives the high heat of the denaturation step. During this step, the DNA polymerase takes the individual dNTPs and adds them to the 3' end of each primer that is annealed to the target DNA strands. The target DNA strands act as reference strands for the polymerase. This reaction usually is allowed to proceed for 1 to 2 minutes. Once this step is completed, the cycles begin again. The yield of PCR product is initially low over the first several cycles; however, after about 20 cycles the yield is high and generates most of the PCR product, or **amplicon.** After all PCR cycles are completed, many PCR protocols include a final 2- to 10-minute extension to ensure that all of the primer extension reactions have been completed and that all DNA in the reaction tube is double-stranded. After the final extension is completed, PCR amplicons can be either stored at –20° C or analyzed immediately.

Polymerase Chain Reaction Components

Polymerase chain reaction, with its extremely high sensitivity, has drawbacks. One drawback is that the reaction conditions must be set up properly; otherwise, nonspecific amplification may occur, or no amplification may occur. As discussed earlier, several components are necessary for a successful PCR assay, including template DNA, oligonucleotide primers, a thermostable DNA polymerase, magnesium, a buffer for the polymerase, and deoxynucleotides. In addition, a thermal cycler is required. Table 11-3 lists these components and their uses.

Template DNA. The amount and quality of template DNA is important for a successful PCR assay. Target DNA is usually obtained by isolating nucleic acid from samples. At one time, the isolation of nucleic acid was a laborious technique that could take several hours or even more than 1 day.

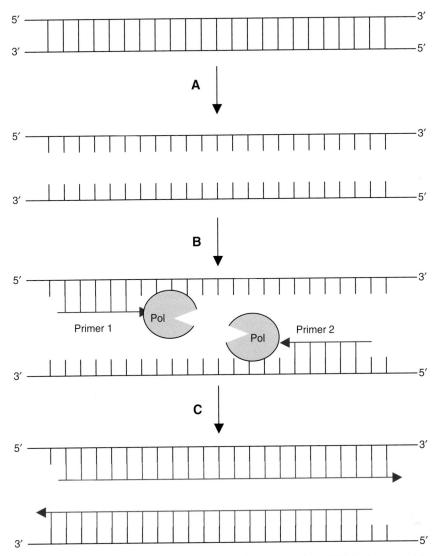

FIGURE 11-3 One polymerase chain reaction cycle. **A,** Template DNA is denatured by heat to yield two single-stranded DNA strands. **B,** The temperature of the reaction is cooled and the two single-stranded primers (Primer 1 and 2, in blue) anneal to the template DNA strands. DNA polymerase (blue spheres, labeled *Pol*). **C,** The temperature of the assay is heated to 72° C, and DNA polymerase adds nucleotides to the primers to synthesize new double-stranded DNA molecules (new DNA in red) in the primer extension step. The new DNA is then used for the next cycle.

Now, numerous commercial kits are available to isolate nucleic acid from many different sources, such as clinical specimens and environmental samples. Nucleic acid isolation kits are commercially available for specific types of microorganisms as well, such as kits for viral nucleic acid. Also, automated nucleic acid isolation systems, such as the MagNA Pure Compact or LC system (Roche Diagnostics Corp., Indianapolis, Ind.), are available for high-volume laboratories. The use of kits and/or automated extraction systems is highly recommended so that high-quality, pure-template nucleic acid can be obtained in as high a concentration as possible. Total DNA in a concentration of 0.1 to 1 μg is often used for many PCR protocols, although a standard volume of DNA is generally used after extraction with a kit. High amounts of template DNA can increase the chances of forming nonspecific PCR products.

Oligonucleotide Primers. A pair of primers is used in standard PCR assays, wherein one primer is homologous to the left flanking region of the target and the other is homologous to the right flanking region. Automated instruments are available to synthesize primers; however, in most cases, laboratories will have primers synthesized for them. Published primer sequences are available for many microbial targets, including antibiotic-resistance genes. Some laboratories design their own primer sequences, and when this is done, several parameters should be followed. The primers should not be complementary to each other so that **primer-dimers** (primers that anneal to each other during PCR) do not form,

TABLE 11-3 Polymerase Chain Reaction Components

Component	Purpose
Template DNA	Serves as target for PCR
Oligonucleotide primers	Used to start synthesis new strands of DNA
Thermostable DNA	Synthesizes new strands polymerase of DNA
Magnesium	Required by DNA polymerase
Buffer	Ensures proper conditions and pH for DNA polymerase
Deoxynucleotides	Used by DNA polymerase to synthesize new DNA
Thermal cycler	Instrument that heats and cools PCR cycle steps

PCR, Polymerase chain reaction.

and the primers should be as specific for the target of interest as possible. The G+C content of the primers should be 40% to 60%, and the two primers should have similar G+C contents. Also, avoid a group of three or more *G*'s or *C*'s at the 3′ ends of primers, because this could increase the chances of nonspecific PCR products. Primers used in PCR are typically 15 to 30 nucleotides in length. Primers that are smaller than this have increased chances of nonspecifically annealing to other DNA sequences, while the annealing time may be increased for longer primers. As discussed earlier, manufacturers who synthesize probes and primers will usually calculate T_m for the consumer. For primers that are less than 25 nucleotides long, the formula $T_m = 4(G+C) + 2(A+T)$ may be used to derive a rough T_m calculation. For example, a 20-base primer with a 50% G+C content would have a T_m of $4(10) + 2(10)$ or 60° C. This calculation is invalid if the determined T_m is greater than 68° C. For primers and probes longer than 25 nucleotides, computers should be used to calculate T_m. Most PCR assays are designed to form relatively small PCR amplicons, often less than 1000 base pairs (bp). In fact, many PCR assays produce amplicons of approximately 100 bp. PCR assays can be faster for small amplicons, and the DNA polymerase has a smaller chance of making an error.

Thermostable DNA Polymerase. Various thermostable DNA polymerases have been isolated and characterized from thermophilic bacteria. Of these, *Taq* DNA polymerase was described first for use in PCR and is still most commonly used. There are many available *Taq* DNA polymerases on the market. By now, many are recombinant enzymes produced in bacteria (e.g., *E. coli*) and are highly purified. *Taq* DNA polymerase does make occasional errors during primer extension, although many commercially available DNA polymerases are now enzyme blends that have reduced error rates. In addition, the commercially available *Taq* DNA polymerases may have different rates by which they add free dNTPs to synthesize new strands of DNA; a rate of about 100 dNTPs added per second under the correct conditions has been reported for many *Taq* DNA polymerases.

Magnesium. A divalent cation, usually Mg^{2+} in the form of $MgCl_2$, is required for the proper function of *Taq* DNA polymerase. A typical $MgCl_2$ concentration range is 1 to 2 mM; many DNA polymerase buffers are supplied with 1.5 mM $MgCl_2$. A low yield of PCR products will result if the concentration of magnesium is too low. If the concentration is too high, then nonspecific products and misincorporation of nucleotides may result. Also, Mg^{2+} will bind to some of the PCR components, including free dNTPs, the template DNA, and primers, so there should be a slight excess of $MgCl_2$ in the final reaction mixture. High concentrations of Mg^{2+} may even inhibit the DNA polymerase. The concentration of $MgCl_2$ may have to be optimized for a particular PCR assay.

Buffer. An optimized buffer is needed to generate proper reaction conditions for *Taq* DNA polymerase. Standard *Taq* DNA polymerase buffers used in PCR are composed of Tris-HCl and a salt, such as KCl, at a pH of 8.3. The buffer is often supplied with the manufacturer's DNA polymerase and is usually supplied as a 10× concentrated solution. The buffer is diluted by a factor of 10 in the final PCR mixture. Some buffers are available with $MgCl_2$. This is fine if the PCR assay works correctly with the supplied concentration of $MgCl_2$, but many laboratories prefer to use buffer without $MgCl_2$ and add $MgCl_2$ as a separate component to optimize the PCR assay.

Deoxynucleotides. Individual deoxynucleotides are added to the 3′ end of annealed primers by DNA polymerase during primer extension. Nearly all PCR assays use a final concentration of 200 μM for each of the dNTPs. It is important that the same concentration of each dNTP be used so that misincorporation of incorrect dNTPs does not occur. If the concentration of each dNTP is too high, the error rate of *Taq* DNA polymerase may be increased.

Thermal Cycler. A thermal cycler is essentially a programmable heat block used to cycle PCR assays. Most thermal cyclers heat and cool efficiently and cycle between temperatures rapidly so that reactions occur quickly. There are many different types of thermal cyclers, and many accept different sizes of PCR tubes.

Contamination Prevention

Because PCR is so sensitive, small amounts of extracted nucleic acid or carryover amplicons from previous PCR assays can contaminate future PCR assays. This may result in false-positive results. When contamination occurs, all equipment and work surfaces must be thoroughly cleaned, and usually new reagents (including primers) must be used. In addition, patient care may be compromised if false-positive PCR results are generated in a clinical microbiology laboratory. This can also lead to reduced confidence in future results from hospital staff members. Thus it is very important to prevent contamination in a laboratory that performs PCR. Laboratories that perform PCR and other amplification methods should, if possible, use separate rooms for template extraction, PCR reagent preparation, and amplification. If this is not possible, use different benchtops and work spaces of the laboratory for each function. In any case, sample nucleic acid and PCR amplicon should never be placed in the room or work space reserved for reagent preparation. Work should always flow from the cleanest room to the dirtiest room. For example,

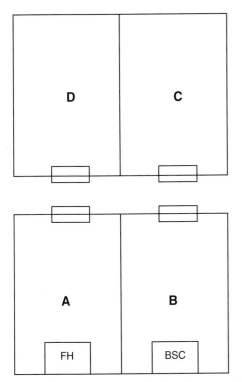

FIGURE 11-4 Work flow diagram for a polymerase chain reaction (PCR) laboratory. *Room A:* Reagent preparation room for PCR components; this is a clean room with a laminar flow hood where no template nucleic acid is allowed. *Room B:* Nucleic acid extraction room with a biologic safety cabinet for clinical specimens and contamination control. *Room C:* Thermal cycling room where specimens are amplified. *Room D:* Agarose gel electrophoresis detection room, if necessary. *BSC,* Biologic safety cabinet; *FH,* flow hood.

and unknown samples if not used carefully. It is prudent to set up positive controls after all unknown samples have been set up. Negative controls should be extensively used to ensure that the PCR process is not contaminated. Many laboratories use a "sample, no template control" (SNTC) that has all reagents except for DNA template added to it. If amplification occurs from this tube, contamination is probably present.

Some laboratories take routine samples from work spaces and equipment to determine contamination. Such contamination screenings should be adopted in the laboratory's quality control program. The samples are used as template in PCR assays; screening can occur at a rate (e.g., on a quarterly basis) determined by the laboratory.

Last, **uracil-*N*-glycosylase (UNG)** has been used very successfully to reduce carryover from PCR assays. Some laboratories employ dUTP instead of dTTP in standard PCR assays; nonproofreading polymerases such as *Taq* DNA polymerase will position the dUTP nucleotides where dTTP nucleotides should be placed, with no apparent affect on specificity or sensitivity. Thus PCR amplicon is produced normally, but with uracil substituted for thymine. The enzyme UNG prevents replication of uracil-containing DNA. PCR reagents can be preincubated with UNG to ensure that amplicon carryover does not contaminate the reagents.

Polymerase Chain Reaction Product Analysis

Analysis of PCR amplicons may be accomplished by different ways. In the past, analysis by agarose gel electrophoresis was very popular and used by many laboratories. Now this amplicon detection technique is being overtaken by **real-time PCR** in popularity, particularly for clinical microbiology laboratories.

Agarose Gel Electrophoresis. Electrophoresis is a technique used to separate biologic macromolecules, such as nucleic acids and proteins. Electrophoresis separates such molecules based on size, charge, and shape. Agarose is a compound made from seaweed, and agarose gel electrophoresis is used to separate RNA and DNA. The nucleic acids are moved through an agarose matrix—basically a molecular sieve—by an electric current. RNA and DNA possess a net negative charge in solution because of their phosphate backbones, so an electric field will force these molecules from a negative to a positive electric pole. Large nucleic acid molecules move more slowly through the agarose matrix than smaller molecules do, so smaller nucleic acids move faster through the agarose gel.

To perform agarose gel electrophoresis, powdered agarose is mixed with a buffer and heated to a boil to get the agarose in solution. Many laboratories melt agarose in a microwave; care must be taken to avoid superheating, which can cause the agarose to boil over and cause burns. The melted agarose is allowed to cool briefly and the mixture is poured into a casting tray with a plastic comb placed in a gel box. The casting tray is sealed on the ends with either tape or rubber gaskets, and the agarose solidifies when allowed to cool for 20 to 30 minutes. The plastic comb is removed from the solidified agarose, and this leaves several wells in the agarose gel. Then, running buffer is poured over the solidified agarose gel so that the gel is completely submerged. Nucleic acid samples are

tubes with PCR reagents should be moved into the area reserved for target nucleic acid extraction and finally to the area where PCR cycling takes place. Laboratory equipment, including pipettors, lab coats, and supplies, should not leave their designated areas; thus each area should have dedicated equipment. If possible, reagent setup should be performed in a laminar flow hood, and nucleic acid extraction should be performed in a biosafety cabinet. Exposing work spaces to ultraviolet (UV) light greatly reduces the chances of contamination. Do not expose PCR reagents and extracted nucleic acids to UV light, because the light might damage them. Figure 11-4 provides a work flow diagram.

In addition, aerosol-resistant pipette tips should always be used for all amplification procedures, and safe pipetting should be practiced. Always wear gloves, and change them frequently as required. Dedicated lab coats should be used in each work area as well. All sample and reagent tubes should be capped when they are not being handled. All laboratory equipment and work surfaces must be cleaned after each use, either with a fresh solution of 10% bleach or with products available from various manufacturers designed to eliminate contaminating nucleic acids. Another way to reduce contamination is to limit the number of positive controls used in each PCR assay. Positive controls can easily contaminate solutions then mixed with a loading buffer that serves two purposes: (1) it contains a dense reagent (e.g., sucrose or glycerol) that increases the density of the nucleic acid sample, and (2) it contains a colored dye, such as bromophenol blue and/or xylene cyanol, that may be used to measure the progress of the samples through the agarose gel. The loading buffer, sometimes referred to as *sample buffer* or *blue juice*, can be purchased premade from several manufacturers. Next, the nucleic acid samples are pipetted into the wells in the gel, the lid is placed over the gel box, and the voltage source is connected, set, and turned on. The dense reagent in the loading buffer keeps the samples from floating out of the wells and into the gel running buffer. The time and voltage used when separating nucleic acid fragments depends on the concentration of the agarose gel and the anticipated size of the RNA or DNA molecules.

Large nucleic acid fragments (generally greater than 1000 bp for DNA or 1000 bases for RNA) are typically separated best in low-percentage agarose gels, such as 0.8% to 1%. Smaller nucleic acid fragments (less than 1000 bp or bases) are separated best in 1.5% to 2% agarose gels. The movement of sample nucleic acids can be tracked by monitoring the flow of the loading buffer through the gel. Bromophenol blue will usually run at approximately 100 bp of DNA, depending on the agarose gel concentration. Many laboratories run gels at approximately 70 to 100 volts for 1 to 2 hours. The voltage may be increased to speed separation, although voltages greater than 100 volts can heat the agarose and cause uneven separation of nucleic acids. When the gel is finished running, the samples can be visualized by staining. Figure 11-5 depicts the migration of DNA samples in an agarose gel.

The most common nucleic acid stain used after separation by agarose gel electrophoresis is ethidium bromide. This compound will bind to nucleic acids by intercalating between bases. When ethidium bromide is irradiated with UV light, it fluoresces bright orange. This fluorescence can be visualized

with the naked eye by holding a UV lamp over the gel, or with an imaging instrument that shines UV light up through the bottom of the gel. Most laboratories use imaging systems for agarose gels, because images of fluorescent nucleic acids can be captured and subsequently analyzed by computers. Many laboratories pipette ethidium bromide at a concentration of 0.5 to 1 µg/mL into molten agarose so that the nucleic acids are stained as they travel through the gel matrix. Otherwise, the gel must be bathed in a solution of ethidium bromide for staining before visualization can occur. Nucleic acids appear as bands on gels. Care must be taken with ethidium bromide, because it is a powerful mutagen. It should always be handled with gloves, and stained gels should never be touched with bare hands. All ethidium bromide waste should be treated as toxic waste and must be disposed of properly. For this reason, many laboratories are switching to alternative staining dyes, such as **SYBR green,** which is less mutagenic than ethidium bromide (although it still has mutagenic properties and should be handled and disposed of with care as well) and is considered to be more sensitive than ethidium bromide.

There are two types of SYBR green. SYBR green I is used to stain DNA; SYBR green II is used to stain RNA. Both fluoresce green after exposure to UV light. The addition of SYBR green to molten agarose gels tends to cause wavy nucleic acid bands. For this reason, most gels are stained in a solution of SYBR green after electrophoresis is finished.

A size standard, often called a *ladder,* is also used when separating nucleic acids by agarose gel electrophoresis. There are many commercially available nucleic acid size standards. A ladder is used to determine the approximate size of nucleic acid bands in an agarose gel. Usually, one of the lanes of the gel is reserved for the size standard, and the ladder is electrophoresed with the samples. Because many PCR amplicons are less than 1000 bp long, many laboratories use a 1000-bp standard to look for the expected size of the PCR product. The size of the PCR amplicon should be known, because the primers can be used to calculate the expected size. Figure 11-6 shows an image of ethidium bromide–stained PCR products in an agarose gel visualized with a UV lamp. Figure 11-7 shows a picture of ethidium bromide–stained PCR products separated by agarose gel electrophoresis visualized with an imaging system.

As stated earlier, many clinical laboratories no longer use agarose gel electrophoresis to analyze PCR amplicons. Agarose gel electrophoresis takes 1 to 2 hours to separate PCR products, generates hazardous waste, and requires an imaging system. Now, many clinical laboratories are switching to a PCR technique called *real-time PCR* to analyze PCR products.

Real-Time Polymerase Chain Reaction. Real-time PCR was a major breakthrough for detection of PCR products. The method was developed in the early 1990s by Higuchi et al. Other names for real-time PCR include *kinetic PCR* and *homogenous PCR.* PCR amplicons are assayed as they accumulate during real-time PCR after each cycle, as opposed to standard PCR, where amplicons are detected at the end of the entire procedure. A positive result can thus be observed quickly, often while the assay is still running. This technique does not use an agarose gel, it usually does not accumulate

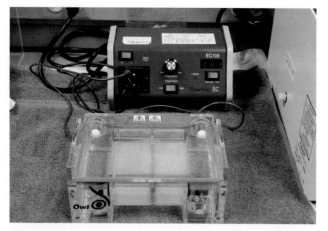

FIGURE 11-5 Agarose gel electrophoresis. An agarose gel is shown submerged in running buffer in a gel box; next to the gel box is a voltage source that supplies the electric current to separate nucleic acids. The blue loading dye is visible in individual samples after migrating partway through the agarose gel matrix. Wells are visible at the top of the gel (at left in this image) for loading samples.

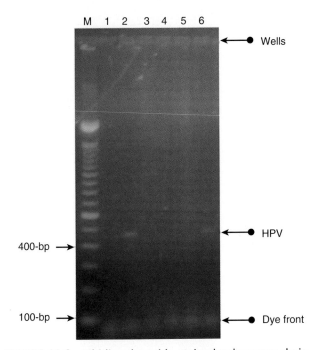

FIGURE 11-6 Ethidium bromide–stained polymerase chain reaction (PCR) amplicons separated in an agarose gel. The image was obtained with an ultraviolet (UV) lamp. PCR was used to amplify a gene from unknown human papillomavirus (HPV) from clinical samples. Lane M is a 100-bp ladder; the 100-bp and 400-bp bands are indicated by arrows to the left of the image. Wells in which the samples were loaded are indicated by the arrow on the top right of the image, and the loading buffer dye front is indicated at the bottom right. *Lane 1:* Negative control (dH2O instead of template DNA). *Lane 2:* HPV-positive control. *Lanes 3 to 6:* Unknown samples. The unknown sample in lane 6 was positive for HPV. Nonspecific amplicons can be observed in lanes 3 and 5.

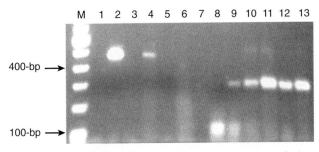

FIGURE 11-7 Ethidium bromide–stained polymerase chain reaction (PCR) amplicons separated in an agarose gel. The image was obtained with an imaging system. PCR was used to amplify a gene from unknown human papillomavirus (HPV) from clinical samples. Lane M is a 100-bp ladder; the 100-bp and 400-bp bands are indicated by arrows to the left of the image. Lanes 1 to 6 were assayed for HPV; lanes 8 to 13 were assayed for β-actin, an internal control that should be present in all human specimens. *Lanes 1 and 8:* Negative control (dH2O instead of template DNA). *Lanes 2 and 9:* HPV-positive control (also a positive control for β-actin). *Lanes 3 to 6 and 10 to 13:* Unknown samples. *Lane 7:* Empty lane. The unknown sample in lane 4 was positive for HPV. β-Actin was present in all unknown samples.

hazardous waste, and the imaging system is a part of the real-time instrumentation. Another major benefit to real-time PCR is that the reactions occur in closed tubes that do not have to be opened for detection. Thus there is a much smaller chance that amplicon from a real-time PCR assay will contaminate equipment, reagents, and work spaces. Real-time PCR is also used to quantitate nucleic acids, which is useful for monitoring the progress of certain diseases, such as human immunodeficiency virus (HIV), hepatitis, and infections caused by cytomegalovirus. Real-time PCR uses a fluorescent reporter dye (often in the form of labeled probes or beacons, sometimes called a **fluorophore**), a thermal cycler that uses a UV light source to excite the reporter, and a camera controlled by a computer system. Real-time PCR instruments have the ability to measure increases in reporter fluorescence as PCR product accumulates, leading to accurate results. Fluorescent peaks are recorded by the computer system as fluorescence intensity versus PCR cycle number. Figure 11-8 shows a real-time PCR fluorescence curve.

Fluorescence is measured by either directly monitoring an increase in fluorescence or indirectly by a process called **fluorescence resonance energy transfer (FRET)**. FRET is the transfer of energy from a donor dye molecule to an acceptor dye molecule; FRET also occurs between a fluorescent dye and a quenching molecule that keeps emitted light low until the fluorescent dye is released from the quencher. For FRET to occur, the two molecules must be in close proximity—within about one to five nucleotides of each other.

Some real-time PCR platforms can provide a **melting curve analysis** to determine assay results or to verify the purity of the PCR product and to determine whether primer-dimers are present. All dsDNA molecules have a T_m at which 50% of hybrids melt, or become single stranded. This is determined by the length and GC content of the dsDNA hybrid. When a fluorescent dye is bound to the PCR product or attached to a probe bound to the PCR product, a fluorescent signal is detected by the real-time PCR platform. However, when the temperature is increased and reaches the T_m, the amount of fluorescence suddenly decreases as the probes and/or fluorescent dye dissociates from the PCR product. This sudden decrease in fluorescence can be measured as a peak.

Among the several commercially available real-time PCR systems are the LightCycler (Roche Diagnostics, Indianapolis, Ind., shown in Figure 11-9), the SmartCycler (Cepheid Instruments, Sunnyvale, Calif., shown in Figure 11-10), the GeneAmp 5700 and Prism 7700 (Applied Biosystems, Foster City, Calif.), the iCycler iQ (BioRad), the MX4000 (Stratagene, La Jolla, Calif.), the R.A.P.I.D. and Rapid-Cycler 2 (Idaho Technology, Inc., Salt Lake City, Utah), and the Rotor Gene (Corbett Research, Sydney, Australia). Rapid thermocycling is used by these platforms because they use rapid air exchange or rapid thermal conductivity around the reaction vessel; they also have a high surface-to-volume ratio of the PCR reagent mixture. Thus, in addition to the advantages of real-time PCR compared to standard PCR discussed above, real-time PCR is extremely rapid. Many real-time PCR assays yield positive results in 30 to 40 minutes, compared with about 4 to 5 hours for standard PCR. For example, denaturation time for real-time PCR is usually a few seconds, compared

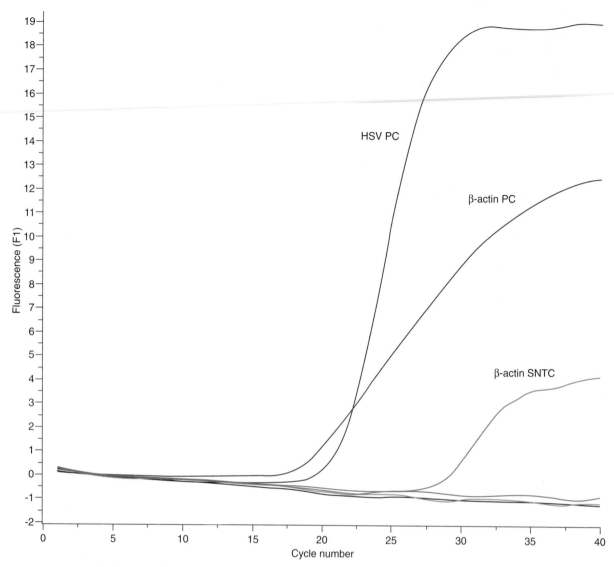

FIGURE 11-8 Real-time PCR data analysis for herpes simplex virus (HSV) from a human specimen. Fluorescent peaks are depicted as fluorescence intensity (Y-axis) versus PCR cycle number (X-axis). A positive control (HSV PC) was assayed along with an internal control, β-actin, which should be present in all human samples. The HSV PC and the β-actin positive control (β-actin PC) have fluorescent peaks, as does the β-actin assay from the unknown specimen. The unknown specimen did not have a peak for HSV. In addition, a sample no template control (SNTC) was assayed for both HSV and β-actin, and there are no fluorescent peaks for either.

with 15 to 30 seconds for standard PCR. Also, many real-time PCR procedures use primers with a T_a of around 72° C, so that annealing and primer extension occur at the same temperature. This saves considerable time.

Real-time PCR platforms use different detection variations, including the 5′ *nuclease assay* (sometimes called the *Taqman assay*), **dual-probe FRET,** the **molecular beacon** method, **Scorpion primers,** and intercalating dyes such as SYBR green detection of accumulated products.

5′ Nuclease Assay (Taqman). The 5′ nuclease assay uses the 5′ exonuclease activity of some *Taq* polymerases (e.g., Gold DNA polymerase, Applied Biosystems, Inc.) and Taqman probes (Roche Molecular Systems, Inc.). Taqman probes are oligonucleotides about 18 to 22 bases long that are

usually labeled on the 5′ end with a fluorescent reporter dye and the 3′ end with a quencher dye. Figure 11-11 illustrates the principle of 5′ nuclease assay. Fluorescence from the reporter dye is kept to a low background level because of the close proximity of the quencher dye by FRET (due to the conformation of the probe), where the fluorophore donates energy to the quencher dye. The Taqman probe for a specific PCR assay is designed to complement part of the internal region of the PCR amplicon during the primer-annealing step. During primer extension, the *Taq* DNA polymerase extends from the primers and replicates the template to which the Taqman probe is annealed. The reporter dye is released by the 5′ nuclease activity of the polymerase first, and then the entire probe is released. Fluorescence increases as the fluo-

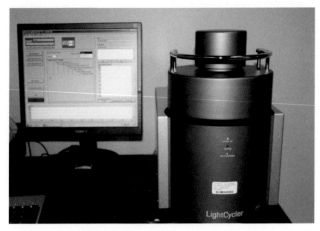

FIGURE 11-9 The LightCycler (Roche Diagnostics), a real-time polymerase chain reaction system.

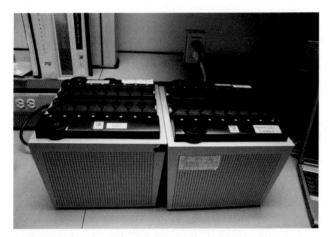

FIGURE 11-10 The SmartCycler (Cepheid Instruments), another real-time polymerase chain reaction platform.

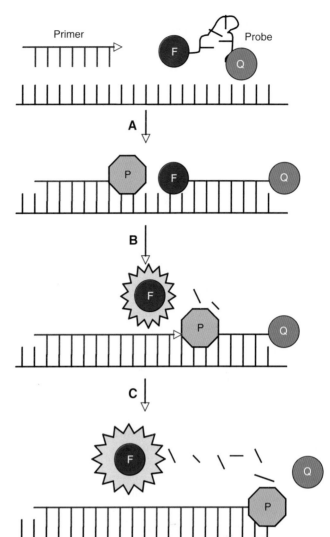

FIGURE 11-11 The 5′ nuclease assay (Taqman). **A,** Primer and probe are annealed to template DNA. DNA polymerase *(P)* starts to extend from the primer. **B,** DNA polymerase cleaves the fluorescent dye *(F)* from the probe and from the quencher. Fluorescence is observed. **C,** As DNA polymerase continues to extend and synthesize a new strand of DNA, the probe is fragmented, and the fluorescent dye and the quencher are fully released from each other. Fluorescence accumulates as fluorescent dye molecules are released.

rophore is removed from the immediate vicinity of the quencher dye. Fluorescence thus increases on a linear scale as more PCR product is synthesized during subsequent PCR cycles. Advantages of the 5′ nuclease method include the following: only specific PCR products are detected, standard PCR protocols can be used, and the hybridization and cleavage reactions do not interfere with production of PCR product. One disadvantage is that specific probes must be designed and/or purchased for specific targets, and fluorescent-labeled probes are expensive compared with unlabeled oligonucleotides. Another disadvantage is that melting curve analysis cannot be performed when Taqman probes are used, because these probes are hydrolyzed during the amplification process.

Dual-Probe FRET. This method is sometimes called the *dual-oligonucleotide FRET method* or simply the *FRET technique.* Dual-probe FRET uses two labeled probes, as shown in Figure 11-12. One probe is labeled on the 3′ end with a donor fluorescent dye, and the other probe is labeled at the 5′ end with an acceptor fluorescent dye. The probes are designed to anneal head-to-tail to PCR products. When this occurs, the

two fluorescent dyes are brought into close proximity to each other, and FRET occurs. The light source emitted by the real-time PCR platform excites the dye on the first probe, and this dye then gives off a fluorescent light at a longer wavelength. The energy given off by the 3′ dye then excites the fluorescent dye on the second probe, because the two dyes are so close together. This dye then emits fluorescent light at a longer wavelength than before and is measured by the instrument. The intensity of fluorescent emitted light is proportional to the amount of PCR product amplified during the reaction. Emission is only detected when the two probes anneal to their respective complementary sequences on the PCR amplicons. It is important to note that detection of fluorescence occurs only after the two probes have hybridized, so measurement

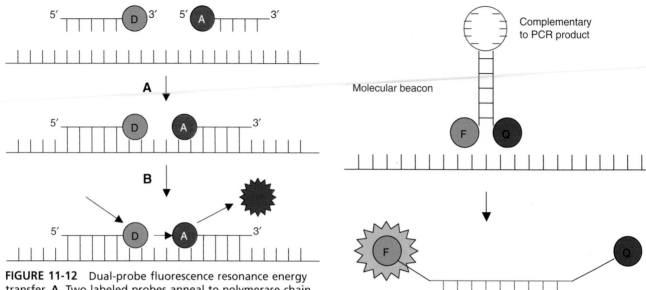

FIGURE 11-12 Dual-probe fluorescence resonance energy transfer. **A,** Two labeled probes anneal to polymerase chain reaction (PCR) product as it accumulates. One probe is labeled with a donor fluorescent dye *(D)* on the 3' end, while the other probe is labeled on the 5' end with an acceptor dye *(A)*. The two probes anneal to the PCR product head-to-tail. A single strand of PCR product is shown in this diagram after denaturation has occurred. **B,** The light source from the real time-PCR platform excites the donor fluorescent dye. The donor then transfers this energy to the acceptor dye. The acceptor dye is excited and emits fluorescent light that is read by the instrument. Fluorescence increases as PCR product accumulates.

FIGURE 11-13 Molecular beacons. The molecular beacon probe is a complementary hairpin loop structure. A fluorescent dye is bound to the 5' end of the hairpin and a quencher is attached to the 3' end. A loop structure at the top of the molecule is complementary to formed polymerase chain reaction (PCR) product. When the denaturation step of PCR occurs, PCR product and molecular beacon probes dissociate; a single strand of a PCR amplicon is shown here. The beacon anneals to formed PCR product, then the fluorescent dye is removed from the quencher molecule. Fluorescence increases as PCR product accumulates.

occurs during the primer-annealing step. When the temperature is raised for the primer extension step, the two probes are displaced by *Taq* DNA polymerase, and FRET stops because the probes are not in close proximity anymore. The next measurement occurs after the primer-annealing step in the next cycle. This is a specific technique that also allows for melting curve analysis of resulting PCR amplicons. However, the technique is expensive and requires probe design skill. The LightCycler system uses dual-probe FRET for several assays. The first probe is labeled at the 3' end with the donor fluorescein and the second probe is labeled with the acceptor dye LightCycler Red 640 at the 5' end. The LightCycler Red 640 releases a red fluorescent light that is measured by the instrument as PCR product increases.

Molecular Beacons. The molecular beacon technique uses short segments of DNA with dyes attached to the 5' and 3' ends. A fluorescent-labeled reporter dye is attached to the 5' end of the DNA segment and a quencher dye is attached to the 3' end of the beacon, as Figure 11-13 shows. The molecular beacon is designed to have complementary DNA bases on each end so that they can base-pair with each other and form a hairpin structure with a loop; this is the natural form of the molecular beacon. The loop portion of the hairpin molecule is complementary to one of the PCR amplicon strands. Fluorescence from the reporter dye is quenched by FRET while the beacon is in the hairpin structure because the two dyes are held together in close proximity. As PCR proceeds, the denaturation step separates template DNA,

PCR product DNA (if present), and the molecular beacon. When the temperature cools for the primer-annealing step, a beacon DNA strand anneals to PCR amplicon if present, and the quencher dye and the reporter dye are no longer in close proximity. Fluorescence is observed in a linear fashion as PCR product accumulates. Molecular beacon molecules that do not anneal to PCR amplicons re-form hairpin structures, and fluorescence is not observed.

Scorpion Primer. A Scorpion primer uses a single oligonucleotide to prime a specific sequence and to detect accumulation of PCR product. Figure 11-14 illustrates Scorpion primers and their mechanism. Structurally, Scorpion primers are somewhat similar to molecular beacons, in that the non-hybridized form of the Scorpion primer is a complementary hairpin loop. Scorpion primers have a fluorophore probe with a PCR blocker linked to the 5' end and a quencher attached to the 3' end of the hairpin loop structure; FRET reduces fluorescence. In addition, a stem on the 3' end of the hairpin loop is complementary to a specific sequence of the target DNA. DNA polymerase extends from this stem, so that at the end of the first round of PCR the Scorpion primer is linked to the synthesized product. At the start of the second cycle, the hairpin structure of the Scorpion primer denatures along with the template DNA in the assay. The hairpin probe sequence then hybridizes to the product that was just synthesized. When this occurs, the fluorophore and the quencher

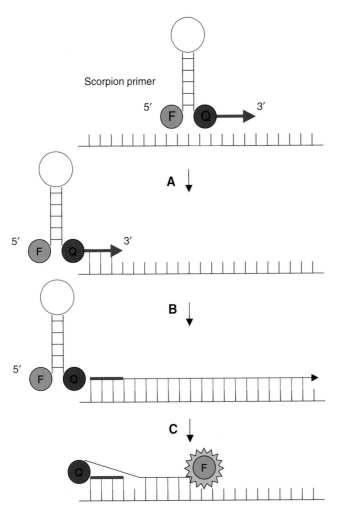

Scorpion primer

FIGURE 11-14 Scorpion primer mechanism. **A,** A Scorpion primer is a probe and a primer in one molecule. It is a hairpin molecule labeled on the 5′ end with a fluorophore and on the 3′ end with a quencher. A short priming sequence is attached to the 3′ end also. The priming sequence anneals to the target DNA. **B,** DNA polymerase synthesizes a new strand of DNA from the short priming sequence. **C,** Denaturation occurs, and the newly formed DNA and the Scorpion primer dissociate. An internal portion of the Scorpion primer is complementary to the product just formed. This portion anneals to the PCR product and separates the fluorophore from the quencher; fluorescence then accumulates.

molecule become separated, and accumulation of fluorescence indicates accumulation of PCR product.

SYBR Green Detection of Real-Time Polymerase Chain Reaction Products. As described earlier, SYBR green is a fluorescent dye that binds to nucleic acids. SYBR green I binds nonspecifically to dsDNA. The end result of most real-time PCR applications is DNA amplicon, so SYBR green I is most often used. Fluorescence increases as PCR product accumulates. During the denaturation step, SYBR green I does not bind to DNA because of high temperatures and because DNA molecules are single-stranded. Some dye molecules begin binding to DNA during the primer-annealing phase, resulting in low-level background fluorescence. The dye

then quickly binds to dsDNA during the primer extension step. As the cycles begin anew, fluorescence drops back to low background levels when the temperature is increased and denaturation occurs again. Thus detection by the real-time PCR platform occurs after every PCR cycle. Using SYBR green is cheaper than using labeled probes, and it may be used for melting curve analysis. However, the dye binds to any nonspecific PCR products that may form during assays and binds to primer-dimers as well. Indeed, melting curve analysis should be performed after SYBR green detection is used to determine whether primer-dimers or nonspecific PCR products have formed; the melting curve temperature for primer-dimers and nonspecific products will be different than that for the amplified PCR products.

Applications of Polymerase Chain Reaction in the Clinical Microbiology Laboratory

With the advent of real-time PCR and the commercial availability of real-time platforms and assays, standard PCR using agarose gel electrophoresis is not used in many clinical microbiology laboratories anymore. Many laboratories and reference laboratories use PCR methods to diagnose bacterial, viral, fungal, or parasitic infections. There are many described assays for antibiotic resistance mechanisms as well. In short, PCR assays have been described for nearly every organism possible. Several companies produce kit-based assays called *analyte specific reagents (ASRs).* ASRs are basically the active ingredient of an in-house test and are used by laboratories to establish and perform in-house (or "home brew") PCR tests. The manufacturer registers the product with the Food and Drug Administration (FDA), and laboratories use the ASRs in assays. Laboratories that use ASRs must establish and maintain performance of the PCR test and the reagents. Polymerase chain reaction assay patient results obtained with the use of ASRs may be reported in a diagnostic setting; ASRs fall into a class of reagents that does not require the approval of the FDA. Laboratories that report results with ASRs must include a statement with the results, such as:

> This assay, and the test's performance characteristics, was developed by [insert laboratory name]. This test has not been cleared or approved by the U.S. Food and Drug Administration (FDA). The FDA has determined that such clearance or approval is not necessary. This test is used for clinical purposes. It should not be regarded as investigational or for research. This laboratory is regulated under the Clinical Laboratory Improvement Amendments of 1988 (CLIA-88) as qualified to perform high complexity clinical laboratory testing.

Box 11-2 lists some of the companies that supply ASRs and/or FDA-approved kits for their respective instrument systems for various organisms or antibiotic-resistance genes.

Other Polymerase Chain Reaction Procedures

Many different variants of PCR have been published in the literature or developed by companies. Many of these PCR variations are used for specific purposes. Some of the more common variant PCR procedures are discussed, including reverse transcription-PCR (RT-PCR), multiplex PCR, and nested PCR.

Reverse Transcription-PCR. The most sensitive technique available for detecting and quantifying messenger RNA (mRNA, or transcript) is RT-PCR, also called *reverse transcriptase-PCR* and *RNA PCR*. The technique is so sensitive that evaluation of transcript from a single cell is possible. The method uses an enzyme called *reverse transcriptase* (properly, RNA-dependent DNA polymerase) to synthesize a complementary strand of DNA (complementary DNA, or cDNA) from an RNA template. The resulting cDNA is then used as template in a PCR assay, using DNA polymerase as described earlier. Most clinical microbiology laboratories use RT-PCR assays to detect RNA viruses from clinical specimens.

High-quality template RNA is important for RT-PCR. Numerous kits are available on the commercial market for extraction of RNA from clinical specimens, including specific kits for viruses and other microorganisms. Usually, clinical laboratories isolate total RNA from specimens, although mRNA is actually used as the template by reverse transcriptase. Kits are available for just mRNA extraction. However, mRNA constitutes only about 1% to 4% of the total RNA of a cell, so it is generally easier to isolate total RNA and use that for RT-PCR. Automated nucleic acid extraction systems can be used to isolate RNA. The integrity of the RNA template can be assessed by agarose gel electrophoresis, by UV spectrophotometry, or by the use of proper controls during the RT-PCR assay. Generally, RNA extracted with the use of commercial kits is of high quality, so most clinical laboratories use controls to assess quality and integrity of RNA specimens. Genomic DNA in a specimen may contaminate the RNA template, so laboratories should treat RNA with a DNase—an enzyme that hydrolyzes DNA—before the RNA is used in RT-PCR. Many RNA extraction kits include a DNase step.

Internal controls are commonly employed during RT-PCR. When clinical laboratories assay for RNA viruses from human clinical specimens, an internal control for a human RNA species is most often used to assess integrity and quality of a specimen. Internal controls for these assays include transcripts from human genes such as β-actin, glyceraldehyde phosphate dehydrogenase (GAPDH), 18S rRNA, and others. Each clinical specimen must be positive during an RT-PCR assay for one of these internal controls, or else the assay is not valid.

PCR products that result from RT-PCR assays may be assayed in clinical microbiology laboratories by agarose gel electrophoresis or by real-time PCR. As for standard PCR, most laboratories now use real-time PCR to analyze RT-PCR amplicons. Some commercially available kits include all of the components used for RT-PCR assays, and most of these are either designed for real-time PCR or are readily amenable to real-time PCR. In addition, some kits and ASRs are available for detection of particular organisms by RT-PCR. Two general types of RT-PCR assays are used by both clinical and research laboratories: one-step and two-step RT-PCR. One-step RT-PCR uses a single tube to conduct both the reverse transcriptase step and subsequent PCR cycling of the cDNA. Two-step RT-PCR uses a single tube for the reverse transcriptase step, followed by transfer of cDNA into a second tube (or series of tubes) for the ensuing PCR steps. One of the key advantages of using one-step RT-PCR is that it minimizes potential carryover of amplicons to the working environment, equipment, and other assay reagents. Tube-to-tube variation is reduced, because potential errors are not induced by removing amplicon from the first tube and pipetting into other tubes. An advantage of two-step RT-PCR is that resulting cDNA can be used in many different types of subsequent reactions, especially if a laboratory attempts to optimize a reaction. Two-step RT-PCR is also useful for detection of more than one type of transcript from a sample. For example, cDNA template could be removed from the first tube and added to a second tube with primers specific for one type of transcript. At the same time, the same cDNA template could be added to a different second tube with other primers specific for a different transcript. Use of two-step RT-PCR requires careful pipetting; clinical laboratories should use a flow hood to reduce the risk of carryover when opening the first cDNA tube.

The initial step of RT-PCR entails synthesizing a cDNA complementary to RNA transcript with reverse transcriptase. This is not a specific reaction—cDNA is synthesized from all transcripts in a tube. Several types of reverse transcriptase are available, including avian myeloblastosis virus (AMV) reverse transcriptase, Moloney murine leukemia virus reverse transcriptase, and *rTth* reverse transcriptase from *Thermus thermophilus,* among others. Many commercial reverse transcriptases are blended enzymes that have different properties, including enzymes that have both reverse transcriptase and DNA polymerase assets. Thus the same enzyme can be used in one-tube RT-PCR. Many reverse transcriptases function best at 42° C, so the first step of many RT-PCR assays is incubation at 42° C for 30 minutes. Following this step, the temperature is raised to 95° C for 1 to 5 minutes to denature DNA and, for several commercial enzymes, inactivate the reverse transcriptase function of the enzyme. Raising the temperature also activates the DNA polymerase function of blended enzymes. Then, standard PCR cycling is performed and PCR products are analyzed.

As described previously, RT-PCR is often used in clinical microbiology laboratories to detect RNA viruses from clinical specimens. RT-PCR can be used to quantify the amount of viruses in clinical specimens as well; this is performed for HIV and hepatitis C virus with the Roche Amplicor System. Other applications of RT-PCR include quantitative analysis of gene expression, detection of human genes involved in diseases, and detection of cancers from human specimens.

Multiplex Polymerase Chain Reaction. Some laboratories use multiplex PCR to simultaneously detect two (or perhaps more than two) different targets from one PCR tube. This technique uses two different primer sets and is often used to detect an internal control in the same tube as the target of interest. For example, a PCR assay designed to detect the methicillin-resistance *(mecA)* gene in *S. aureus* may use an internal control primer set to ensure that the organism is *S. aureus* and a primer pair for the *mecA* gene in one tube. This technique can be adapted for real-time PCR or analyzed by agarose gel electrophoresis. If the internal control is not detectable, then the assay results are not dependable and the test should be repeated. If the internal control is detected and the target of interest is not detected, then it can be reasonably assumed that the target of choice is not present. However, the PCR assay conditions for multiplex PCR must be carefully optimized. The primer sets should all have a similar T_m, and this is not always easy to design. Also, other reaction conditions have to be optimized, such as concentrations of all reagents and denaturation, annealing, and extension times. In some cases, mixing primers causes interference. Setting up an efficient multiplex PCR assay can take a lot of work and development time. In place of this, many laboratories use one tube for the internal control reaction and one tube for the target of interest. Figure 11-15 shows multiplex PCR products separated by agarose gel electrophoresis and visualized with an imaging system.

Nested Polymerase Chain Reaction. Nested PCR is a highly sensitive and specific PCR technique. The assay itself basically serves as a form of internal control and ensures specificity. Nested PCR consists of two different, consecutive PCR assays. The first reaction is a standard PCR assay using one set of PCR primers. The amplicon produced from this first reaction is then used as the target in a subsequent PCR assay. The second primer pair is complementary to an internal region of the amplicon derived from the first PCR assay.

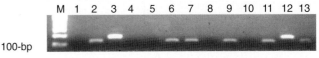

FIGURE 11-15   Multiplex polymerase chain reaction (PCR) products separated by agarose gel electrophoresis. Multiplex PCR for the *ermA* (139-bp) and *ermC* (190-bp) genes from unknown *Staphylococcus aureus* isolates. Lane M is the 100-bp ladder; the 100-bp band is indicated by an arrow to the left of the image. *Lane 1:* Negative control (dH₂O as the template). *Lane 2: ermA*-positive control (cloned PCR product). *Lane 3: ermC*-positive control (cloned PCR product). *Lanes 4 to 13:* Unknown MRSA isolates. Unknown isolates from lanes 6, 7, 9, 11, and 13 were positive for *ermA,* whereas the isolate from lane 12 was positive for *ermC.*

Amplicon is only synthesized during this second PCR assay if amplicon was produced from the first reaction, so this internal control mechanism serves as a marker of specificity. Some clinical laboratories use nested PCR when the amount of starting template DNA is very low, so that the first reaction generates template DNA that is then further amplified to a detectable amount. Also, some laboratories use a primer pair specific for a genus or for a viral family. If amplicon is present as determined by either agarose gel electrophoresis or real-time PCR, then primers that determine species, strain, or type from a subsequent reaction are used. For example, the first PCR assay could be used to ascertain whether a human herpevirus is present in a sample. If present, then primers specific for either human herpevirus type 1 or 2 could be used to determine actual identity. One of the main drawbacks to nested PCR is that it is not a closed system, in that the first assay tube must be opened, so there is potential for contamination.

Other Nucleic Acid Amplification Reactions

In the previous discussion of the many variations of PCR, several different nucleic acid amplification variations are also described. Two of these nucleic acid amplification variants include NASBA and TMA.

Nucleic Acid Sequence Based Amplification

Nucleic acid sequence based amplification is an isothermic procedure, which means that it does not require a thermal cycler and amplification proceeds at one temperature (usually 41° C). NASBA is also referred to as *self-sustained sequence replications* (3SR). The original method was first described in 1989, but the method described then was not isothermal; instead it used heat to denature the hybrids that form during the procedure.

NASBA, in its current form, uses three enzymes: AMV reverse transcriptase, **ribonuclease H (RNase H),** and T7 RNA polymerase. The amplification procedure results in multiple copies of RNA from the target sequence, as opposed to PCR, which results in multiple copies of DNA from the target sequence. The target nucleic acid can be either DNA or RNA, although NASBA is most often used for RNA viruses, such as for HIV detection. During amplification, primers are used

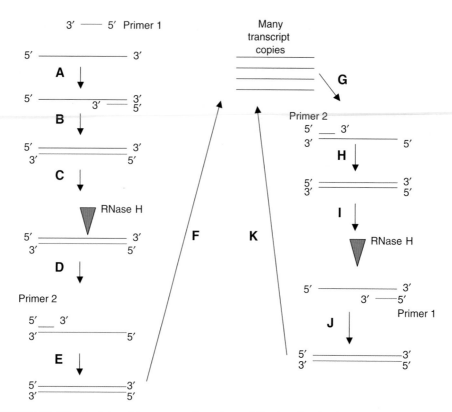

FIGURE 11-16 Nucleic acid sequence based amplification (NASBA). **A,** Primer 1 anneals to target RNA. **B,** Reverse transcriptase synthesizes a DNA copy of the RNA template. **C,** RNase H degrades the original RNA template. **D,** Primer 2 anneals to the DNA copy. **E,** Reverse transcriptase synthesizes another DNA strand, resulting in double-stranded DNA (dsDNA). **F,** T7 RNA polymerase synthesizes many copies of transcript using the dsDNA as template. **G,** Primer 2 anneals to the synthesized transcripts. **H,** Reverse transcriptase makes a DNA copy of the transcripts. **I,** RNase H degrades the transcript copies and primer 1 anneals to the DNA copies. **J,** Reverse transcriptase synthesizes new DNA strands, again resulting in dsDNA. **K,** The many copies of dsDNA are then used as template by T7 RNA polymerase, which synthesizes even more transcript. This process continues in a loop.

to anneal to the target nucleic acid. One of the primers has a T7 RNA polymerase promoter built into it, and this primer initially anneals to the target sequence (Figure 11-16). The reverse transcriptase generates a cDNA copy of the target, which results in a DNA:RNA hybrid. Then, the RNase H enzyme degrades the RNA, leaving the cDNA copy of the target; RNase H only degrades RNA from DNA:RNA hybrids. The second primer then anneals to the cDNA strand. Double-stranded DNA of the target is produced by the DNA-dependent DNA polymerase activity of AMV reverse transcriptase. The original primer with the T7 RNA polymerase promoter is integrated into this dsDNA copy of the original target nucleic acid. The T7 RNA polymerase enzyme then generates large amounts of transcript of the dsDNA. The transcript can then be used again as template for further amplification; instead, at this point, the second primer anneals to the generated transcript and the DNA-dependent DNA polymerase activity of AMV reverse transcriptase once again makes a cDNA copy of these transcripts. The RNase H once again degrades the RNA, and the first primer with the T7 RNA polymerase promoter anneals to the cDNA copies. The

reverse transcriptase once again synthesizes dsDNA, and then the T7 RNA polymerase makes even more transcript. Thus amplification is a continuing process, and transcript on the order of 10^9 is produced. The same methodology is used for DNA targets, although an initial denaturation step is required before NASBA can begin. NASBA is used to detect many types of organisms from clinical samples. bioMérieux offers the NucliSens system of detection, which uses NASBA for either detection or quantification of organisms such as HIV-1 and cytomegalovirus. bioMérieux also offers a basic NASBA kit that can be used to design testing for any organism that has known sequences.

Transcription-Mediated Amplification

Transcription-mediated amplification is a similar process to NASBA. TMA was developed by Gen-Probe, Inc. (San Diego, Calif.). TMA targets rRNA sequences of various microorganisms and produces large numbers of transcript using the same enzymatic processes as NASBA. Resulting amplified transcript is detected by Gen-Probe's Hybrid Protection Assay. TMA is used by many clinical laboratories to detect

C. trachomatis and *N. gonorrhoeae* from clinical specimens. The Aptima system marketed by Gen-Probe automates the TMA method for laboratories that have a high enough volume of specimens.

Signal Amplification Reactions

Several methods have been described and are currently in use in clinical microbiology laboratories that exploit signal amplification for detection, rather than amplification of target nucleic acid. One such amplification procedure was the ligase chain reaction (LCR). This technique used DNA ligase to seal a gap between two probes annealed to target DNA. The sealed probe was then used in subsequent amplification steps as template, and probe amplification would occur. This technique was used to identify *C. trachomatis* and *N. gonorrhoeae* from clinical specimens. However, subsequent problems with the assay have taken LCR off the market for detection of these organisms. Other signal amplification procedures that are in use include branched DNA (bDNA) detection, hybrid capture, and cycling probe technology (CPT).

Branched DNA Detection. Branched DNA detection is a sensitive signal amplification technique that has been used most often to quantify viral nucleic acids from clinical specimens. The technique was first described in 1991, and commercial assays are available for quantification of RNA from hepatitis C virus and HIV and quantification of DNA from hepatitis B virus. This method uses oligonucleotide capture probes that hybridize target nucleic acid to a solid support mechanism, such as a microtiter tray, as depicted in Figure 11-17. Other probes, the target probes, anneal to a different region of the target nucleic acid than the capture probes. The target probes also hybridize to preamplifier probes. Amplifier probes then bind to the preamplifier probes, and this forms a branched DNA structure. Finally, probes labeled with alkaline phosphatase (AP) are added and hybridized to the complex; the complex is large, and many AP probes can hybridize to the bDNA structure. When the AP substrate is added, chemiluminescence results and light emission is collected by an analyzer and reported as light units. The amount of light signal is related to the amount of nucleic acid present

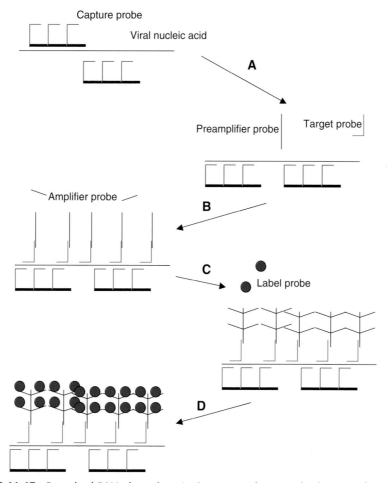

FIGURE 11-17 Branched DNA detection. **A,** Capture probes attached to a surface anneal to target nucleic acid. **B,** Target probes anneal to nucleic acid and to preamplifier probes. **C,** Amplifier probes anneal to preamplifier probes, forming a branched DNA (bDNA) structure. **D,** Label probes (with bound alkaline phosphatase [AP]) anneal to the bDNA structure. A large, amplified signal is detected enzymatically when the AP substrate is added.

in the sample. Standards are used with known concentrations of target nucleic acid, so that a standard curve is established in light units during each bDNA assay. Unknown samples are then compared with the standard curve to determine concentration. In addition to FDA-approved bDNA assays on the market, basic bDNA kits are available on the marketplace to tailor bDNA detection for a particular target for which a laboratory wishes to test. These kits are compatible with most starting materials, including paraffin-embedded tissue, fresh tissue, cells, and other specimens.

Hybrid Capture. The hybrid capture method was developed by Digene in 1995 to detect HPV from clinical specimens. The initial assay, the Hybrid Capture I test, detected human papilloma virus (HPV) in two risk groups for cervical cancer based on the type of HPV detected (high-risk HPV types and low-risk HPV types). Testing was performed in tubes, and the method was a liquid hybridization assay. The Hybrid Capture II method also tests for HPV high-risk and low-risk types, *C. trachomatis*, and *N. gonorrhoeae*. All three organisms can be detected from a single clinical sample in a microtiter plate format, although currently it is FDA-approved for Pap smear specimens. Thus the test is used for female patients. Hybrid Capture II has been automated, and the Rapid Capture System offered by Digene uses this technology for detection of the three organisms described. Target nucleic acid is first released from clinical samples with an alkaline agent. This process denatures DNA in the specimen and destroys RNA. Then, as Figure 11-18 shows, an RNA probe specific for the target DNA is added to the sample, and a DNA:RNA hybrid forms. A capture antibody is used to bind the hybrid onto the microtiter wells. At this point antibodies conjugated to AP are added to detect the captured hybrids. Multiple AP-antibodies bind to each hybrid, resulting in

signal amplification of approximately 3000-fold after a chemiluminescent substrate is added for AP. A luminometer reads light signals as relative light units (RLU).

Cycling Probe Technology. Cycling probe technology (CPT) proceeds under isothermal conditions. The technique uses a chimeric probe, composed of DNA and RNA, usually in a sequence of DNA-RNA-DNA (Figure 11-19). A fluorescent dye is attached to the 5′ end of the probe, while a quencher is connected to the 3′ end. As long as the probe is intact, only a low background fluorescence is emitted because of the action of the quenching molecule. The chimera probe anneals to its target sequence and forms a hybrid. Then the enzyme RNase H is used to cleave the RNA in the probe. This cleavage separates the fluorophore from the quencher, and fluores-

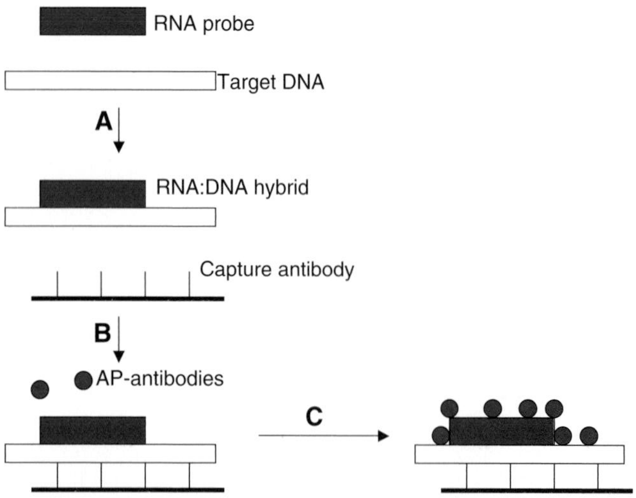

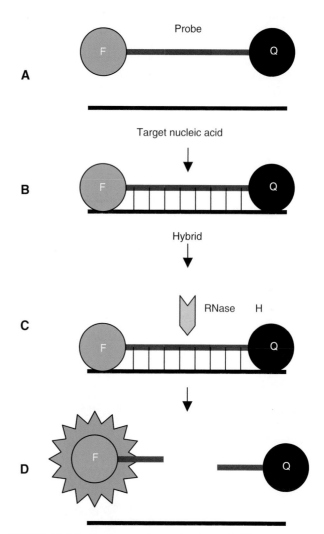

FIGURE 11-19 Cycling probe technology. **A,** The DNA:RNA:DNA chimeric probe with a 5′ fluorescent dye (*F*, in green) and a 3′ quenching molecule (*Q*, in black) is incubated with the target nucleic acid; DNA is in red whereas RNA in the probe is in blue. **B,** The probe anneals to the target nucleic acid and forms a hybrid. **C,** RNase H digests the RNA in the chimeric probe. **D,** Digestion of the RNA releases the fluorescent dye from the vicinity of the quencher, resulting in fluorescence. A new probe molecule will then anneal to the same target nucleic acid molecule, and the process continues. Signal amplification results.

FIGURE 11-18 Hybrid capture. **A,** RNA probes are annealed to target DNA, resulting in RNA:DNA hybrids. **B,** The hybrids are bound to capture antibodies attached to a solid support mechanism. **C,** Several alkaline-phosphatase (AP)–conjugated antibodies bind to hybrids. The substrate is added for the AP, and resulting light emission is captured by a luminometer.

cence increases. The target nucleic acid is then free of probe, and a new chimera probe hybridizes to it. This probe is also cleaved, resulting in even more fluorescence. The reaction proceeds in this manner, resulting in signal amplification. The CPT method has been marketed by ID Biomedical Corporation and has been used for *mecA* detection for methicillin resistance in *S. aureus*.

STRAIN TYPING AND IDENTIFICATION

With the rise of large numbers of antibiotic resistance isolates of many microorganisms, increases in the rates of toxin-producing bacteria, and the spread of pathogenic microbes across the world, there is a need for accurate epidemiologic surveillance of these organisms. Standard techniques in clinical microbiology laboratories do not often provide the necessary resolution to distinguish types and strains from each other. Instead, more refined techniques that separate related organisms from each other at the genetic level are necessary for epidemiologic investigations. Many typing methods have been described to determine genetic relatedness among bacteria, fungi, and parasites, and some provide better resolution than others. These techniques, often called *DNA* or *genetic fingerprinting*, are based on the mutations that accumulate in biologic organisms over time.

Strain typing techniques are often used to compare local strains to determine whether a local outbreak is due to a single strain type or to multiple strains. A single strain that is responsible for a disease outbreak may have a point source that can be then targeted by the local public health service. Strain typing methods are also used to compare local isolates with worldwide isolates, which can show long-term spread of a strain or strains (clonality). Whether testing local isolates or isolates from many locales, the technique chosen should have high discriminatory power or the ability to finely resolve different strains. Genetic fingerprinting techniques comprise both nonamplified and amplified methods. Nonamplified strain typing methods usually involve analysis of restriction enzyme fragments of chromosomal DNA. As strains diverge genetically over time, restriction enzyme sites on the chromosomal DNA will also change as point mutations accumulate. When chromosomal DNA from different strains is digested with one restriction enzyme and separated by agarose gel electrophoresis, fragments of different sizes will be observed. These fragments are referred to as *restriction fragment length polymorphisms (RFLP)*. Comparisons of these RFLP patterns lead to strain typing, and evolutionary ancestors can be derived from the RFLP patterns of strains. Similar RFLP patterns imply genetic relatedness. Nonamplified typing techniques include Southern blotting, **plasmid profile analysis,** restriction enzyme analysis of chromosomal DNA, **pulsed field-gel electrophoresis (PFGE),** and **multilocus enzyme electrophoresis (MLEE).** Amplified DNA fingerprinting methods use PCR. Either known primers or arbitrary primers are used, depending on the particular technique. Amplified methods that are commonly used include arbitrarily primed PCR (AP-PCR), also called **random amplified polymorphic DNA (RAPD), repetitive palindromic extragenic elements PCR (Rep-PCR),** and **multilocus sequence typing (MLST).**

Nonamplified Typing Methods
Southern Blotting

Southern blotting, as described earlier, is sometimes used in epidemiologic investigations to analyze RFLP patterns. Chromosomal DNA is digested with a restriction enzyme, and the resulting fragments are separated by agarose gel electrophoresis. These fragments are transferred from the agarose gel to a nylon or nitrocellulose membrane, and a labeled probe is used to identify a specific target. One of the most popular targets is the DNA that codes for rRNA in microorganisms. When rRNA RFLP patterns are detected by Southern blotting, the technique is called **ribotyping.** The genes that code for rRNA are conserved in different species of organisms and appear in conserved positions of a species chromosome. For this reason, ribotyping displays excellent reproducibility and discriminatory power. A fully automated ribotyping platform that uses Southern analysis methodology is the RiboPrinter Microbial Characterization System (Dupont Qualicon, Wilmington, Del.). The instrument automates the entire process, including lysing cells and data processing. Unknown patterns are compared with known patterns to identify strains. Some reports indicate that other methods, such as PFGE and RAPD, have greater discriminatory power than automated ribotyping. However, automated ribotyping is advantageous for high-volume laboratories that evaluate large numbers of isolates. Other targets for Southern analysis are insertion sequences and transposons that often contain genes involved in virulence and antibiotic resistance. However, insertion sequences are not present in all strains of bacteria, so some strains are nontypeable.

Plasmid Profile Analysis

This technique was one of the first methods used to type strains of bacteria. **Plasmids** are extrachromosomal, circular pieces of DNA found in variable number in the cytoplasm of many bacteria. Many bacteria carry antibiotic-resistance genes, virulence genes, and other targets of interest on plasmids. The theory behind this technique is that a given strain with a plasmid profile will be unique from other strains with other plasmids. When a plasmid profile of different isolates is the same, it is possible then that these strains are identical.

Plasmid DNA is extracted from bacteria being investigated and separated by agarose gel electrophoresis. Unfortunately, because plasmids are extrachromosomal genetic elements, they are readily lost by bacteria. Some plasmids also contain transposons, or "jumping genes," that are readily transferred to other bacteria. In addition, plasmids can exist in different forms in bacterial cells. Plasmids that have been cut or nicked will have different sizes on agarose gels than uncut plasmids. All of these factors can readily change the plasmid profile of a given bacterial isolate. Thus this technique is not often used and is not considered very reproducible.

Restriction Enzyme Analysis of Chromosomal DNA

This technique is similar to Southern blotting. Chromosomal DNA is extracted from isolates of interest and digested with a restriction enzyme (or more than one restriction enzyme).

The enzyme used for digestion should cut the chromosomal DNA in several places so that small and large fragments are produced. The resulting RFLP pattern is analyzed by agarose gel electrophoresis; transfer to a membrane and subsequent use of a probe to identify a specific sequence is not performed. The discriminatory power of this method is not high, and many of the fragments overlap and are difficult to distinguish from each other.

Pulsed-Field Gel Electrophoresis

Schwartz and Cantor developed PFGE in the early 1980s. The technique is extremely popular and is perhaps the most well-known epidemiologic investigation method. It also may be the most used of the strain typing and identification techniques. A restriction enzyme is used to digest chromosomal DNA at a small number of sites along the chromosome. This results in large DNA fragments that are difficult to resolve by standard agarose gel electrophoresis. During PFGE, these large fragments are separated in a low-percentage, low-melt agarose gel by an angled electrical field that periodically changes orientation. These changes in electrical field orientation are pulses that successfully "force" the large DNA fragments through the agarose gel and separate them by size. A low-percentage agarose gel is used for the large DNA fragments, and low-melt agarose enables large fragments to migrate easier. Relatively simple RFLP patterns result from this process, so comparison is easy in most circumstances. PFGE is also very reproducible and can theoretically be used on any organism. Figure 11-20 shows representative PFGE patterns

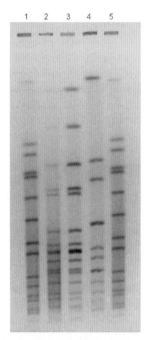

FIGURE 11-20 Example of pulsed field gel electrophoresis (PFGE) analysis of *Staphylococcus aureus* strains. Lanes 1 and 5 are known control strains of a *S. aureus* isolate. Lanes 2 to 4 are unknown strains from different patients with *S. aureus* isolates. Lanes 2 and 3 have the same banding pattern after PFGE and are the same strains. The lane 4 isolate is an unrelated strain.

from different *S. aureus* strains. Special equipment that can provide electrical pulses is necessary to run PFGE. Generally, a system must be obtained specifically for PFGE. Most PFGE assays take several hours (up to overnight) to efficiently separate the large DNA fragments produced in the restriction enzyme reaction. Most PFGE systems incorporate a chilling module within the system to cool the electrophoresis buffer and circulate it to improve separation. Without circulation and a chilling unit, the buffer will get very warm when separation proceeds for several hours—warm enough to potentially degrade the low-melt agarose gels used in PFGE. The warm temperatures also can produce wavy and difficult-to-interpret RFLP patterns. Among the various PFGE systems available is the GenePath Strain Typing System (Bio-Rad Laboratories, Inc., Hercules, Calif.).

Multilocus Enzyme Electrophoresis

Unlike the other typing techniques described in this section, MLEE analyzes gene expression polymorphism. Analysis of protein polymorphisms by electrophoresis has been studied since the 1970s. MLEE involves the extraction of proteins from isolates of interest, followed by electrophoretic separation and selective staining of these proteins. The expression of the protein's genotype is reflected in the position of the stained band, according to the protein's mobility. Mobility is determined by the net charge of the protein and by the structure of the protein. Two bands of the same protein in different positions after separation suggests two different conformations of the protein—two alleles of the same gene. MLEE is considered to be an excellent strain typing method. Unfortunately, the DNA sequence of the proteins separated during MLEE cannot be directly assumed, because different DNA sequences can result in the same protein due to the redundancy of the genetic code. In addition, two completely different proteins could have the same mobility and could be interpreted to be the same proteins. Another problem is that interlaboratory comparisons are difficult. Because of these potential problems with MLEE, MLST was eventually developed.

Amplified Typing Methods
Random Amplified Polymorphic DNA

The RAPD technique, also called *arbitrarily primed PCR,* was first described in 1990 by two different groups (Welsh and McClelland; Williams et al.). This is a popular method of DNA fingerprinting. Small primers (about 10 nucleotides in length) with random sequences are used during RAPD. These primers thus do not have a specific target. Instead, the random primers indiscriminately amplify chromosomal DNA during PCR cycles. This results in fragments of varying lengths after separation by agarose gel electrophoresis. A particular strain will have a different fragmentation pattern than other strains.

RAPD is a simple DNA fingerprinting method capable of providing high resolution and discriminatory power, particularly when more than three different random primers are used. A single primer can be used in a RAPD PCR assay, because the single random oligonucleotide can prime random targets on either strand of template DNA. However, the discriminatory power of just one primer is low with RAPD. The discriminatory power increases if three or more primers are used, although this increases the assay time. Many laboratories use eight or more primers for RAPD DNA fingerprinting. One potential problem of RAPD is interlaboratory agreement and reproducibility; this method typically provides excellent intralaboratory reproducibility. RAPD often yields some minor amplicons that exhibit low reproducibility in the same laboratory. Some researchers believe that PFGE has higher discriminatory power than RAPD analysis.

Repetitive Palindromic Extragenic Elements PCR

The Rep-PCR technique is an amplification strain typing method that was first described in 1991 by Versalovic et al. All organisms have repetitive DNA sequences—the repetitive palindromic extragenic elements—that repeat throughout the genome. The unique DNA sequences that lie in between these palindromic repeats are amplified during Rep-PCR using primers specific for the repeat DNA. Rep-PCR results in fragments of varying size, depending on the locations of the palindromic repeats. The amount of DNA in between the repeats varies from strain to strain.

The discriminatory power of Rep-PCR is thought to be a little lower than for PFGE, although results seem to correlate well between the methods; some studies suggest that Rep-PCR has superior discriminatory power. The technique is easy to use and can be scaled up for several isolates, although RAPD assays are somewhat easier to perform. As always, a given laboratory should evaluate the methods to determine the most feasible DNA fingerprinting procedure for the number of expected isolates and for the type of equipment and expertise available.

The DiversiLab System (Bacterial Barcodes, Inc., Athens, Ga.) is an automated rep-PCR instrument on the market that uses proprietary rep-PCR primers for different organisms (such as *C. difficile* and *S. aureus*). The system uses a microfluidic chip that evaluates rep-PCR products. As many as thirteen different isolates can be evaluated on one chip. Rep-PCR product fragments are analyzed with the Web-based DiversiLab software to determine strain relatedness. Strain patterns can also be compared with the patterns obtained by other labs that use the DiversiLab System.

Multilocus Variable Number of Tandem Repeat Analysis

Like Rep-PCR, **multilocus variable number of tandem repeat analysis (MLVA)** takes advantage of repetitive DNA sequences in genomes. MLVA amplifies regions of DNA that contain repeats. Repeated sequences in genomes tend to be unstable, so a given bacterial strain may have more repeats at one locus than a different bacterial strain of the same species. When there are different numbers of repeated sequences at a given locus, it is referred to as a *variable number of tandem repeats* (VNTR). MLVA maps VNTRs among bacterial strains by using PCR. This is a useful typing method because it produces quantitative data, is easy to perform, is reproducible, and is easy to interpret.

Multilocus Sequence Typing

Multilocus sequence typing (MLST) is a derivation of MLEE, described in 1998 by Maiden et al., that analyzes the sequences of genes. Specifically, MLST is used to identify alleles by determining the internal sequences of **housekeeping genes.** Housekeeping genes are genes that code for proteins necessary for basic functions for cells. Housekeeping genes are constitutive genes (i.e., they are almost always turned on), so they are almost always being expressed. Both eukaryotic and prokaryotic organisms have housekeeping genes. Human housekeeping genes include the β-actin gene and the glyceraldehyde-3 phosphate dehydrogenase gene. Bacterial housekeeping genes include the 16S rRNA gene and dihydrofolate reductase. Because housekeeping genes are nearly always turned on, they also make excellent controls for many molecular methods.

For a typical MLST assay, several loci are chosen representing different internal regions of housekeeping genes. Polymerase chain reaction is used to amplify the DNA at each locus; primers are designed to complement to highly conserved regions of the housekeeping genes. Once amplicon is obtained, it is sequenced with an automated sequencer and given a unique number based on the sequence. Strains of a particular species can then be compared using the same loci. High resolution between strains is possible by comparing these DNA sequences (or the numbers representing these sequences). In addition, the method has achieved excellent interlaboratory comparisons; other laboratories merely need to use published primers for loci of the same species to compare data and determine the spread of strains. The method is achieving global recognition, and a Web-based database of strain type exists (www.mlst.net), the Multi Locus Sequence Typing home page. The Web site provides protocols, information, and software for sequence analysis. A drawback of MLST is that a laboratory requires an automated sequencer, and the method is expensive compared with PFGE. However, of all the methods described in this chapter for DNA fingerprinting of strains, MLST probably has the highest resolution and the greatest chance of interlaboratory agreements.

THE FUTURE OF MOLECULAR DIAGNOSTICS TESTING IN THE CLINICAL MICROBIOLOGY LABORATORY

As molecular testing procedures become cheaper, easier to use, and more available, more clinical microbiology laboratories will use them for clinical specimens. Several companies offer ASRs now, and more organism-specific ASRs will be available in the near future. The genomes of many microorganisms have been fully or partially sequenced, and these data provide potential to develop screening and confirmation tests based on organism sequence; see the National Center for Biotechnology Information Web site (www.ncbi.nlm.nih.gov) for a list of organism sequences and associated links. A trend is developing toward standardization of molecular diagnostics methods as ASRs and kit-based detection of microorganisms becomes available. As standardization increases, so will the number of laboratories using molecular diagnostics procedures. New technology improvements and methodologies also continuously occur. There are now automated nucleic acid extraction systems and automated amplification platforms. The increase in automation also makes molecular diagnostics techniques more attractive to the clinical microbiology laboratory. Automation also aids standardization with other laboratories.

As more sequences of clinically significant microbes and automation of molecular diagnostics procedures have become available, more clinical labs are starting to use DNA sequencing procedures to either identify microbes from clinical samples or to confirm identifications of bacterial isolates. Usually, 16S rDNA sequencing is employed by these laboratories, and this technique is becoming an important tool in modern clinical microbiology laboratories. A newer sequencing technique called **pyrosequencing** has also been used to identify microorganisms and to detect antibiotic resistance mutations.

In addition, large-scale screening of nucleic acids and proteins is available now, especially as organism genome sequencing has increased. The information obtained from sequencing an organism's genome allows for comprehension of cellular processes, protein associations, and interrelatedness of biological activities. Genomics research, coupled with the use of **nanobiotechnology,** has stimulated the invention of methods such as DNA microarray analysis and proteomics. Techniques such as **DNA microarrays** (and nanoarrays), **proteomics,** and **metagenomics** possess the capacity to revolutionize the analysis of microorganism populations and disease interpretation and treatment. These methods are not ready for routine use in clinical microbiology laboratories yet; they are primarily research tools at this time. Nevertheless, they are interesting methods with great potential.

Sequencing

Sequencing is determining the order of nucleotides in a fragment of DNA. Usually, the chain termination method devised by Frederick Sanger is used. DNA sequencing has been used for years; initially, the technique was somewhat labor intensive and was usually used to identify the sequence of genes. Now, sequencing is automated and has been applied on large-scale processes such as whole genome sequencing. The human genome has been sequenced, as have the genomes of several other eukaryotic and prokaryotic organisms. Whole genome sequencing is not a technique that clinical laboratories typically perform; however, clinical laboratories have started employing smaller-scale sequencing techniques to identify microorganisms. Many clinical microbiology laboratories now perform 16S rRNA gene sequencing to confirm the identity of problematic bacterial isolates. Other genes may also be sequenced to determine identity, such as *rpoB* (RNA polymerase B), which is often used to identify mycobacteria. To identify fungi by sequencing, a variety of targets have been used, usually within the rRNA gene complex, encompassing the 18S, 5.8S, and 28S rRNA genes, the external transcribed spacer regions 1 and 2 (ETS1 and ETS2) that flank the rRNA genes, and the variable internal transcribed spacer regions 1 and 2 (ITS1 and ITS2).

There are different ways to perform sequencing. In one popular method, a pair of primers is hybridized to template DNA prepared from bacterial cells and PCR is performed to amplify a 500- to 1500-bp product. The PCR products are then purified with a commercial kit to remove excess primers and template DNA. Two reactions are performed during the next step, called *cycle sequencing;* one reaction utilizes a forward primer, and the other reaction uses a reverse primer. In each reaction, the purified PCR products from the previous PCR are used as DNA template. In the cycle sequencing reactions, the four standard deoxynucleotide bases (A, C, G, T) are included in the reaction mix along with low concentrations of chain terminating nucleotides of each dNTP. These chain terminating nucleotides are often called *dideoxynucleotide nucleotides* (ddNTPs). Each ddNTP is labeled with a different fluorescent dye (thus they are often also called *dye terminators*). When a labeled ddNTP is incorporated into the growing complementary strand of DNA, it terminates that particular strand—dNTPs cannot be added at this point. Thus a series of related DNA fragments is synthesized, which are terminated at the position where the labeled ddNTP was incorporated. Fragments of every size are generated during this process. The generated fragments are purified to remove unincorporated dye terminators and are then separated by capillary electrophoresis in an automated analyzer. The sequence is thus generated based on fragment size, and a fluorimeter that determines the particular dye on the end of each fragment. Each ddNTP has a different color fluorophore, making identification of what ddNTP is on the end of each fragment easier.

Once the sequence has been determined, software can be used to compare the generated sequence with a database of known sequences. A most likely identity can then be obtained. When examining the relatedness of different species and strains of bacteria by sequencing, dendrograms are often used. There are different methods of generating dendrograms, including neighbor-joining (NJ), unweighted pair group of method with arithmetic averages (UPGMA), and weighted pair group method with arithmetic averages (WPGMA). Generally, these different methods produce comparable results.

To determine the most likely identity of the unknown sequence, the software user chooses similar organisms for comparison. For example, if the unknown isolate that was sequenced is an oxidase-positive, nonfermenting gram-negative rod, several *Pseudomonas* species and related organisms may be chosen from the software database to compare with the unknown isolate. In addition, an outgroup is chosen—this is a sequence against which all of the other similar sequences are compared. The outgroup should be somewhat related to the other chosen organisms, but still outside the group being studied. Once the dendrogram is generated, a horizontal line with a percentage is produced by the software at the top of the dendrogram next to the method used to generate it. This horizontal line can be used as a rough measure of the degree of relatedness or difference between isolates in the dendrogram. To determine relatedness, add the two horizontal lines of the two isolates in question, and compare with the top horizontal line percentage. Although this method is not really

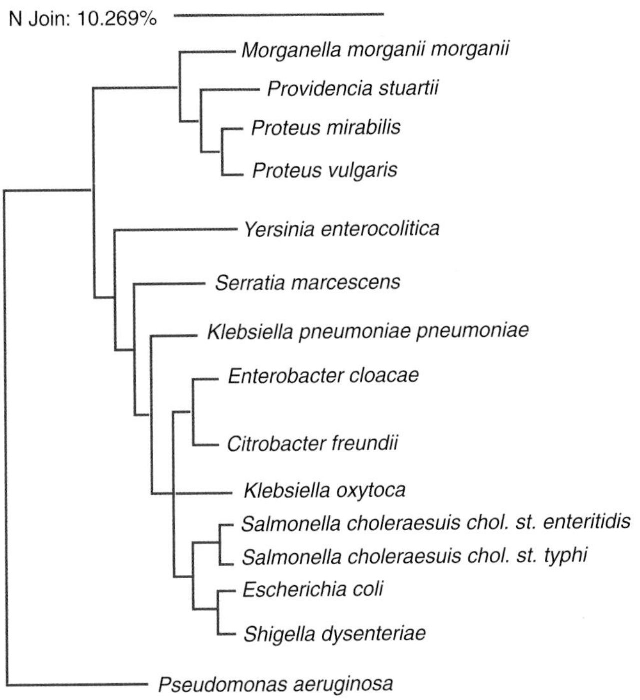

N Join: 10.269%

— Morganella morganii morganii
— Providencia stuartii
— Proteus mirabilis
— Proteus vulgaris
— Yersinia enterocolitica
— Serratia marcescens
— Klebsiella pneumoniae pneumoniae
— Enterobacter cloacae
— Citrobacter freundii
— Klebsiella oxytoca
— Salmonella choleraesuis chol. st. enteritidis
— Salmonella choleraesuis chol. st. typhi
— Escherichia coli
— Shigella dysenteriae
— Pseudomonas aeruginosa

FIGURE 11-21 Example of a dendrogram showing the genetic relationships among different Enterobacteriaceae based on 16S rRNA gene sequencing.

all that accurate, it does give a useful estimate of relatedness. See Figure 11-21 for a depiction of a dendrogram of different Enterobacteriaceae species, generated with the MicroSeq software package. *Pseudomonas aeruginosa* was chosen as the outgroup for this dendrogram.

Pyrosequencing

Pyrosequencing is a sequencing-by-synthesis technique that does not require labeled nucleotides or primers and also does not require a postreaction electrophoresis step. It is a rapid sequencing technique that generates approximately 20- to 50-base long sequences per primer; thus this technique is best used for short sequences. Conventional sequencing is the best choice for longer DNA fragments.

Pyrosequencing utilizes the enzymes DNA polymerase, ATP sulfurylase, luciferase, and apyrase, and the substrates adenosine 5′ phosphosulfate (APS) and luciferin. A sequencing primer is hybridized to single-stranded DNA template and incubated with the enzyme/substrate mix. Then, the four different nucleotides are added one at a time in a defined order. If the added nucleotide base-pairs to the DNA template, the DNA polymerase will incorporate the nucleotide with the release of pyrophosphate (PPi). In the presence of the substrate APS, ATP sulfurylase converts PPi to adenosine triphosphate (ATP). Luciferase then uses the newly formed ATP to convert luciferin to oxyluciferin, which also releases light. The released light is detected with a charge-coupled device (CCD) camera. This is a quantitative and real-time process; each light signal indicates that a nucleotide has been incorporated by DNA polymerase. The generated light is visualized as a peak, and the height of the peak indicates how many

nucleotides were incorporated. The enzyme apyrase degrades excess nucleotide. After degradation, a new nucleotide is added, and the process begins again. The nucleotide sequence of interest is thus determined from the light peaks that occur during the nucleotide-addition and incorporation process.

Pyrosequencing was initially used to determine sequences in mutation analyses of human DNA. However, the technique has also been used to identify microorganisms and has also been used to detect various antibiotic resistance mutations in *Mycobacterium tuberculosis*.

There is an automated pyrosequencing analyzer on the market, the PSQ 96 System (Biotage AB, Uppsala, Sweden). This system can cheaply and simultaneously perform as many as 96 pyrosequencing reactions at one time in a microwell plate format.

Nanobiotechnology

The use of nanotechnology has offered new clinical diagnostics options, and applications of this form of technology will greatly increase in the coming years. Although there are different definitions of nanotechnology, it is useful to consider it as a technology that uses atomic and/or molecular properties to build structures starting at the molecular level, at the nanometer scale (a nanometer is a billionth of a meter). The use of nanotechnology (sometimes called *nanobiotechnology* when used for biologic purposes) in molecular diagnostics is also called *nanomolecular diagnostics*. There are many nanomolecular diagnostics applications, including detection of microorganisms, drug discovery and development, and monitoring treatment of patients with new methods such as gene therapy.

DNA Microarrays and Nanoarrays

The term *DNA microarray* refers to a grouping at the micron level of DNA molecules attached to a solid support mechanism. Silicon chips, glass, or plastic have been used as the solid surfaces to support an array. DNA microarray is sometimes referred to as *DNA chip*, or *genechip*. A DNA microarray gives investigators the potential to evaluate gene expression from an entire organism, or even from several organisms. DNA microarrays are often used to analyze transcriptional levels of genes during a particular disease state. This technique has been used for many purposes, such as determining mutations, identifying new genes, monitoring response after treatment, determining binding sites for transcription factors, and identifying pathogens. A DNA microarray, for example, could be used to simultaneously detect nearly all pathogens. This could be applied to pathogens of interest in clinical medicine, in veterinary medicine, for public health issues, and for homeland security (e.g., screening for all potential biothreat agents on one DNA chip).

A DNA microarray is constructed with special microinstruments, capable of placing microscopic spots of DNA on a solid surface. Thousands—or more—can be placed on one chip. These spots of DNA are commonly called *reporters*. Fluorescently labeled DNA or RNA strands from a specimen of interest are incubated with the DNA on the chip. A scanner reads fluorescence that occurs only when a hybrid occurs. The hybrid that fluoresces is matched to the known map of the DNA chip. For example, an investigator may have a DNA microarray constructed with single-stranded DNA sequence from every known pathogenic bacterium. RNA is extracted from a patient sample, and reverse transcriptase is used to prepare large amounts of cDNA from each transcript. A fluorescent probe is enzymatically attached to the produced cDNA. The tagged cDNA is then incubated with the DNA on the chip and analyzed by a screener. A fluorescent signal from one DNA spot would indicate a hybrid and could implicate a disease role for a particular organism. Amplification procedures can also be coupled to DNA microarrays for a potentially even more powerful identification and analytical tool.

As the use of nanotechnology has increased in recent years, *nanoarrays* (nanochips) have also been developed. A nanoarray has molecules placed on a surface at defined locations with nanometer spatial resolution. Like microarrays, nanoarrays are being developed for genomics and proteomics applications, such as organism detection. Nanotechnology applied to a chip does not need coupled reporters, as DNA microarrays do, and can screen more molecules, so nanoarrays will be more sensitive.

Proteomics

Genomic sequencing has also led to an increased understanding of protein interrelationships and expression in cells. Proteomics is the study of proteins on a cellular level. Like genomics, proteomics is a large-scale process, but it is probably more complicated than analysis at the gene and transcriptional levels. Protein expression changes, for example, from cell to cell, from disease state to disease state, during the life cycle of a cell, and during responses to changing environmental conditions. In addition, proteins with the same genetic origin can be vastly different after post-translational modification and alternative splicing. The genome of an organism is the sum of the genetic material; the proteome of an organism is the sum of proteins found during all changing conditions for a cell. Thus the proteome is often larger and more complex than the genome. Proteomics is used to determine protein expression in disease conditions, such as cancers, genetic diseases, and other diseases to include microbial infections. For example, proteins identified in a certain disease state may become targets for new laboratory tests. In another example, therapy for a given condition may be based on the protein expression involved in another disease state.

Metagenomics

It is estimated that only about 1% of all prokaryotes from most environments on our planet are culturable in the laboratory. Understanding the complexity and interactions of mixed microbial populations may yield valuable information that can affect human health and our association with the environment. Metagenomics was developed as a means to identify nonculturable microorganisms; it is the identification of microbial genomes from mixed populations using molecular techniques. Both sequencing and gene expression methods have been used in metagenomics. This method has great application in environmental studies; for example, metage-

nomics has been applied to study microbial populations from soil, biofilms, and the Sargasso Sea. Metagenomics has also been used to study populations of microorganisms from the human body, such as bowel or urogenital tract flora. Many human infections are polymicrobial, and it is possible that many of the bacteria that play a role in infectious processes are not cultivable in the laboratory. In short, the potential application of metagenomics is limited only by the imagination.

BIBLIOGRAPHY

Alwine JC et al: Method for detection of specific RNAs in agarose gels by transfer to diazobenzyloxymethyl-paper and hybridization with DNA probes, *Proc Natl Acad Sci USA* 74:5350, 1977.

Atkins SD, Clark IM: Fungal molecular diagnostics: a mini review, *J Appl Genet* 45:3, 2004.

Bretagne S: Molecular diagnostics in clinical parasitology and mycology: limits of the current polymerase chain reaction (PCR) assays and interest of the real-time PCR assays, *Clin Microbiol Infect* 9:505, 2003.

Call DR: Challenges and opportunities for pathogen detection using DNA microarrays, *Crit Rev Microbiol* 31:91, 2005.

Clarridge JE III: Impact of 16S rRNA gene sequence analysis for identification of bacteria on clinical microbiology and infectious diseases, *Clin Microbiol Rev* 17:840, 2004.

Eckert KA, Kunkel TA: High fidelity DNA synthesis by the *Thermus aquaticus* DNA polymerase, *Nucleic Acids Res* 18:3739, 1990.

Gall JG, Pardue ML: Formation and detection of RNA-DNA hybrid molecules in cytological preparations, *Proc Natl Acad Sci USA* 63:378, 1969.

Gingeras TR et al: Fifty years of molecular (DNA/RNA) diagnostics, *Clin Chem* 51:1, 2005.

Haase AT et al: Amplification and detection of lentiviral DNA inside cells, *Proc Natl Acad Sci USA* 87:4971, 1990.

Higuchi R et al: Simultaneous amplification and detection of specific DNA sequences, *Biotechnology* 10:413, 1992.

Higuchi R et al: Kinetic PCR: real time monitoring of DNA amplification reactions, *Biotechnology* 11:1026, 1993.

Kleppe K et al: Studies on polynucleotides. XCVI. Repair replication of short synthetic DNAs as catalyzed by DNA polymerases, *J Mol Biol* 56:341, 1971.

Kwoh DY et al: Transcription-based amplification system and detection of amplified human immunodeficiency virus type I with a bead-based sandwich hybridization format, *Proc Natl Acad Sci USA* 86:1173, 1989.

Lukinmaa S et al: Application of molecular genetic methods in diagnostics and epidemiology of food-borne bacterial pathogens, *APMIS* 112:908, 2004.

Maiden MCJ et al: Multilocus sequence typing: a portable approach to the identification of clones within populations of pathogenic microorganisms, *Proc Natl Acad Sci USA* 95:3140, 1998.

Marmur J, Doty P: Thermal renaturation of deoxyribonucleic acids, *J Mol Biol* 3:585, 1961.

Pardue ML, Gall JG: Molecular hybridization of radioactive DNA to the DNA of cytological preparations, *Proc Natl Acad Sci USA* 64:600, 1969.

Resing KA, Ahn NG: Proteomics strategies for protein identification, *FEBS Lett* 579:885, 2004.

Saiki RK et al: Primer-directed enzymatic amplification of DNA with a thermostable DNA polymerase, *Science* 239:487, 1988.

Saiki RK et al: Enzymatic amplification of β-globin genomic sequences and restriction site analysis for diagnosis of sickle cell anemia, *Science* 230:1350, 1985.

Schwartz DC, Cantor CR: Separation of yeast chromosome-sized DNAs by pulsed field gradient gel electrophoresis, *Cell* 37:67, 1984.

Soll DR et al: Laboratory procedures for the epidemiological analysis of microorganisms. In Murray PR, et al, editors: *Manual of clinical microbiology*, ed 8, Washington, DC, 2003, ASM Press, p 139.

Urdea MS et al: Branched DNA amplification multimers for the sensitive, direct detection of human hepatitis viruses, *Nucleic Acids Symp Ser* 24:197, 1991.

van Belkum A: Molecular diagnostics in medical microbiology: yesterday, today, and tomorrow, *Curr Opin Pharmacol* 3:497, 2003.

Vernet G: Molecular diagnostics in virology, *J Clin Virol* 31:239, 2004.

Versalovic J et al: Distribution of repetitive DNA sequences in eubacteria and application to fingerprinting of bacterial genomes, *Nucleic Acids Res* 19:6823, 1991.

Welsh J, McClelland M: Fingerprinting genomes using PCR with arbitrary primers, *Nucleic Acids Res* 18:7213, 1990.

Whitcombe DJ et al: Detection of PCR products using self-probing amplicons and fluorescence. *Nat Biotechnol* 17:804, 1999.

Williams JG et al: DNA polymorphisms amplified by arbitrary primers are useful genetic markers, *Nucleic Acids Res* 18:6531, 1990.

Wu DY, Wallace RB: The ligation amplification reaction (LAR)—amplification of specific DNA sequences using sequential rounds of template dependent ligation, *Genomics* 4:560, 1989.

Points to Remember

- The three basic molecular diagnostics applications used in clinical microbiology laboratories are (1) nucleic acid hybridization assays, (2) amplification techniques, and (3) strain typing techniques.

- Nucleic acid hybridization assays detect nucleic acid targets with labeled probes. These assays can occur on a solid support, in situ, or in a solution. Solid support nucleic acid hybridization techniques include Southern and Northern blots and ISH. In-solution nucleic acid hybridization procedures are frequently performed in clinical microbiology laboratories to detect target nucleic acid in specimens.

- Amplification procedures exponentially increase either the amount of target nucleic acid or the signal that binds to the target nucleic acid. Amplification procedures include PCR and derivations of PCR (e.g., RT-PCR, multiplex PCR, and nested PCR), NASBA, TMA, bDNA detection, hybrid capture, and cycling probe technology.

- PCR is frequently used in laboratories and consists of three basic steps: denaturation of target DNA, primer annealing, and primer extension. These basic steps are repeated in several cycles to increase the amount of target DNA to levels high enough for easy detection. PCR amplicons are detected by either agarose gel electrophoresis or real-time PCR.

- Real-time PCR is a popular detection technique that is used to view PCR products as they accumulate. The technique is also used to quantitate DNA. Several varieties of real-time PCR are used for detection, including the 5′ nuclease assay, dual-probe FRET, molecular beacons, Scorpion primers, and SYBR green.

- RT-PCR is used to study target RNA. The initial step of RT-PCR produces cDNA copies of transcript with reverse transcriptase. The cDNA is then amplified by PCR. RT-PCR, like standard PCR, is often analyzed by RT-PCR.

- Multiplex PCR uses more than one primer set during PCR. One of the primer sets is often targeted at an internal control gene, while the other primer set is used to amplify the target gene. Multiplex PCR is useful because essentially two reactions can be run from one tube; however, the method is difficult to optimize.

- Nested PCR is essentially two different PCR assays run one after the other. The first assay uses a primer pair that amplifies target DNA. The PCR product then is used as DNA template for the second PCR assay. The second assay primers are internal to the first PCR product. Nested PCR is sensitive but is more time consuming than most PCR assays.

- NASBA and TMA are performed at a single temperature and produce large amounts of RNA copies of the target nucleic acid. These techniques use three enzyme activities, reverse transcriptase, RNase H, and T7 polymerase. Both techniques have been automated and are used in many clinical microbiology laboratories for detection of sexually transmitted disease organisms.

- bDNA detection uses several different probes to amplify signal instead of nucleic acid sequence. A branched probe that allows many detection probe molecules to bind to it is used to amplify the signal.

- Hybrid capture uses an RNA probe to bind to target DNA and form an RNA:DNA hybrid. A capture probe is added that binds the hybrid to a solid support. Detection probes are then added that amplify signal.

- CPT uses a fluorescently labeled chimeric DNA:RNA:DNA probe that anneals to target DNA. The fluorescent dye on the probe is held to low fluorescence because of a nearby quencher molecule. RNase H is used to cleave the probe, and fluorescence results when the fluorescent dye is released from the quencher. A new chimeric probe binds to the target DNA, and the process continues to amplify signal.

- Strain typing methods are used for epidemiologic purposes. Either nonamplifiable methods or amplifiable methods are used to detect different strain types. Nonamplifiable methods include Southern blotting, plasmid profile analysis, restriction enzyme digestion of chromosomal DNA, PFGE, and MLEE. Amplified methods include RAPD, Rep-PCR, and MLST.

- Of the nonamplified strain typing procedures, PFGE is probably most used by clinical microbiology laboratories. Chromosomal DNA from strains of interest is digested with a restriction enzyme and separated by an electrophoresis system that electrically pulses the large fragments of DNA through an agarose gel. Strains will have unique banding patterns. The method has excellent intralaboratory reproduction but is difficult to normalize with other laboratories.

- RAPD-PCR, Rep-PCR, and MLVA are used fairly often to type strains. RAPD-PCR uses random primers to anneal to random sequences in the genome of a given strain. After amplification by PCR, strains will have unique patterns. Rep-PCR uses primers that anneal to repeating palindromic sequences in a genome. The DNA in between the palindromic sequence repeats is amplified by PCR, resulting in unique patterns for strains. MLVA amplifies variable numbers of repeats in bacterial genomes. All of these techniques produce excellent intralaboratory results but, like PFGE, they are difficult to correlate with other laboratories.

■ MLST identifies mutations in genes by sequencing different loci from strains after PCR amplification. The technique produces excellent intralaboratory and interlaboratory comparisons, although the technique is expensive and requires sequencing equipment.

Learning Assessment Questions

1. Which of the following is true regarding Southern blotting?
   a. Southern blotting detects transcript after restriction enzyme digestion and separation by agarose gel electrophoresis.
   b. Southern blotting detects a DNA target after restriction enzyme digestion and separation by agarose gel electrophoresis.
   c. Southern blotting detects protein polymorphisms after separation by electrophoresis.
   d. Southern blotting is an amplification technique that analyzes a particular DNA target.

2. Which of the following is not a component of standard polymerase chain reaction (PCR)?
   a. Deoxynucleotides
   b. Primers
   c. Restriction enzymes
   d. Magnesium

3. Branched DNA detection:
   a. is a signal amplification method that uses capture, target, preamplifier, amplifier, and label probes.
   b. is a form of PCR that analyzes transcript.
   c. is a signal amplification method that uses RNA probes, capture probes, and alkaline phosphatase labeled probes.
   d. is a target amplification method that uses reverse transcriptase, RNase H, and T7 RNA polymerase.

4. Which of the following is true of agarose gel electrophoresis?
   a. Nucleic acids are separated in an electrical field because they have a net positive charge.
   b. Large nucleic acid molecules migrate through the agarose gel faster than smaller molecules.
   c. Nucleic acids are separated in agarose by shape, charge, and size.
   d. Agarose is a dye that intercalates in double-stranded DNA.

5. Which of the following procedures does not use FRET?
   a. 5′ nuclease assay
   b. Scorpion primers
   c. Molecular beacons
   d. Transcription-mediated amplification

6. Reverse transcription-PCR:
   a. uses reverse transcriptase to produce cDNA from transcript.
   b. uses T7 RNA polymerase to produce transcript from cDNA.
   c. uses T7 RNA polymerase to produce cDNA from transcript.
   d. uses RNase H to degrade RNA in DNA:RNA hybrids.

7. Which of the following is not a factor that influences hybridization reactions?
   a. Degree of complementarity between the probe and target nucleic acid
   b. pH
   c. Length of the target's genome
   d. Temperature

8. The strain typing procedure that probably has the greatest interlaboratory agreement is
   a. Multilocus enzyme electrophoresis
   b. Multilocus sequence typing
   c. Pulsed field gel electrophoresis
   d. Random amplified polymorphic DNA

9. Which of the following is not true about the 5′ nuclease assay?
   a. It is also referred to as the Taqman assay.
   b. The method uses a probe with a 5′ fluorophore and a 3′ quencher that gets degraded by the action of DNA polymerase.
   c. The method uses FRET to keep background fluorescence low.
   d. The method uses a hairpin-shaped probe with a fluorophore on the 5′ end and a quencher on the 3′ end.

10. Which of the following is incorrect about primers?
    a. Primers are generally at least 100 nucleotides long.
    b. Primers are usually 15 to 30 nucleotides long.
    c. Primers should have a GC percentage of 40% to 60%.
    d. Primers should anneal to a specific target.

Antibiotic Mechanisms of Action and Resistance

Patrick F. McDermott, David G. White

- ■ **ANTIBIOTIC TARGETS AND MECHANISMS OF ACTION**
  Inhibition of Bacterial Cell Wall Biosynthesis
  Inhibition of Folate Synthesis
  Interference of DNA Replication
  Interference of DNA Transcription
  Interference of mRNA Translation

- ■ **MECHANISMS OF ANTIBIOTIC RESISTANCE**
  Origins of Antibiotic Resistance
  Intrinsic (Chromosomal) Mechanisms of Resistance
  Acquired Mechanisms of Resistance

- ■ **DISSEMINATION**

OBJECTIVES

After reading and studying this chapter, you should be able to:

1. Describe the mechanism of action of the different classes of antimicrobials.

2. Describe the targets of the different antibiotic classes.

3. Describe and distinguish differences between intrinsic and acquired mechanisms of antibiotic resistance.

4. Discuss the mechanisms used by microorganisms to disseminate resistant determinants.

Case in Point

A nosocomial outbreak of bacteremia occurred in an adult oncology unit, and active surveillance for the presence of the causative pathogen was instituted by monitoring stools and perianal cultures of patients. *Enterococcus faecium* was isolated from stools in patients with bacteremia and 22 noninfected carriers. The stool isolates of bacteremic patients were found to be closely related to the respective blood isolates as determined by DNA typing techniques, in this case pulsed-field gel electrophoresis. Prior treatment with an aminoglycoside and high-dose ampicillin in some bacteremia patients proved to be ineffective. Therefore, to determine appropriate antimicrobial therapy for the treatment of the nosocomial *E. faecium* outbreak isolate, susceptibility testing was performed. Because prior therapy with aminoglycoside and high-dose ampicillin failed, molecular and genetic studies were performed to characterize the mechanisms of resistance and their possible means of dissemination.

Issues to Consider

After reading the patient's case history, consider:

- The role of empirical therapy in the treatment of disease
- Whether prior antibiotic treatment failure provides insight to possible mechanisms of resistance

- How the bacterial targets of the different antibiotic classes differ
- Whether antibiotics affect more than one bacterial antibiotic target
- Which antibiotic mechanisms of resistance can produce the same resistance phenotype
- Which mechanism of resistance is most likely to produce cross-resistance to multiple classes of antibiotics
- The separate role of intrinsic and acquired mechanisms of resistance in antibiotic therapy
- How acquired mechanisms of resistance are transmitted between microorganisms

Key Terms

Acquired resistance
Aminoglycosides
Antibiotic
Antimicrobial agents
β-Lactam antibiotics
β-Lactamases
Biofilms
DNA replication
DNA transcription

Efflux pumps
Glycopeptide
Glycylcycline
Insertion sequences
Integrons
Intrinsic resistance
Linezolid
Macrolides
mRNA translation

Narrow spectrum	Porins
Oxazolidinone	Streptogramin
Quinolones	Sulfamethoxa zole
Penicillin-binding proteins	Tetracycline
Peptidoglycan	Transcription
Plasmids	Transposons

The discovery of potent, relatively nontoxic antimicrobial therapeutic agents was perhaps the foremost medical advance of the twentieth century. **Antimicrobial agents** include antiseptics, antibiotics, preservatives, sterilants, and disinfectants; all have the capacity to kill or suppress the growth of microorganisms. Antimicrobial agents are an essential component of the practice of medicine. They are used to treat, prevent and control the dissemination of bacterial pathogens in and on animal tissue and nonliving materials. The term **antibiotic** has been traditionally reserved for compounds that are naturally produced by living microorganisms such as bacteria and fungi. The term has come to be more widely applied to any natural, semisynthetic, or synthetic molecule that is used to treat or prevent disease. Antibiotics target anabolic cellular processes such as cell wall synthesis, DNA replication, RNA transcription, and messenger RNA (mRNA) translation. Although numerous antibiotic classes have been discovered with different modes of action, bacteria evolve and adopt numerous strategies to counteract the action of antibiotics.

Antibiotic resistance was observed soon after the discovery of antibiotics. It is a natural consequence of drug exposure and results from both the use and overuse of antimicrobial agents. Antibiotic use presents a selection pressure, allowing only the fittest and least susceptible bacterial populations to thrive and displacing susceptible populations. Over time, and with the use of multiple antimicrobial agents, resistant strains predominate and often acquire multiple drug resistance (MDR). The continuous development of new antimicrobial classes of compounds historically has helped medical science stay ahead of developing resistances. The pace of discovery has slowed, making antibiotic resistance and its associated clinical failure an issue of global public health concern.

In the context of antimicrobial resistance, bacteria display three fundamental phenotypes: susceptibility, intrinsic resistance, or acquired resistance. **Intrinsic resistance** is natural to all members of a species, is a result of the biochemical makeup of the wild-type organism, and is passed vertically to progeny cells. For example, some gram-negative bacteria are intrinsically resistant to the activity of macrolides because these agents either are too large to traverse the cell wall (impermeability) or are pumped out of the cell before gaining access to the cytoplasmic target (constitutive drug efflux). Alternatively, a bacterium may lack the target of the drug altogether. Intrinsic resistance limits the spectrum of antimicrobial activity.

This is in contrast to **acquired resistance,** which is present in only certain isolates of a species that are distinct from the parental strain. Acquired resistance typically arises as a result of chromosomal mutations, or by the horizontal transfer of preexisting resistance genes that may impart resistance to one or more antimicrobial classes. Acquired resistance is usually expressed phenotypically as efflux, modification or acquisition of target sites, and enzymatic modification or degradation of the antibiotic.

Not only have bacteria acquired the mechanisms necessary to withstand the toxic effects of antibiotics, they have also acquired elaborate mechanisms to mobilize and disseminate these successful strategies via plasmids, transposons, **insertion sequences,** integrons, and other mechanisms. The adaptive strategies used by microorganisms to survive the hostile antibiotic environment are remarkable in their evolution and complexity. DNA sequence data show that many different resistance determinants can amass in linked clusters on plasmids or the chromosome, such that antimicrobials of a different class, including substances such as disinfectants or heavy metals, may select for MDR bacteria. Although resistance, in particular MDR, appears to be most serious in certain bacterial species, this situation may be shifting as large mobile MDR elements spread to new hosts in different environs. This chapter provides an introduction to these strategies, using select members of antibiotic classes to illustrate mechanisms of action and resistance. Intrinsic and acquired mechanisms that facilitate resistance to important therapeutic regimens are included. Many of these resistance mechanisms may be generalized to other pathogens. Furthermore, multiple mechanisms of resistance may be present simultaneously in a microorganism, resulting in the MDR phenotypes frequently observed in clinical settings.

ANTIBIOTIC TARGETS AND MECHANISMS OF ACTION

Approximately 23 unique classes and 18 subclasses of clinically useful antibiotics representing approximately 100 antibiotics are used in clinical medicine. Although the classification scheme and number of antibiotics is complex and continues to expand as new classes emerge or existing classes are modified, their mechanisms of action target bacterial cell wall biosynthesis, folate synthesis, DNA replication, RNA transcription, and **mRNA translation.** These are logical targets critical to the survival of the microorganism and are sufficiently distinct from eukaryotic cells to permit selective toxicity. In addition, understanding of the mechanisms of action of antibiotics allows insight into strategies used by microorganisms to evade their toxic effects. Figure 12-1 shows the primary cellular process of antibacterial action for major classes of antimicrobial agents.

Inhibition of Bacterial Cell Wall Biosynthesis

Many antibacterial agents function by targeting bacterial cell wall synthesis. Cell walls are not found in mammalian cells and differ in composition between various bacterial species. Therefore cell wall synthesis provides a number of potential therapeutic targets for anti-infective drugs.

Gram-positive and gram-negative bacteria have a multilayered cell wall structure composed of an inner cytoplasmic membrane, a **peptidoglycan** layer; and in gram-negative bac-

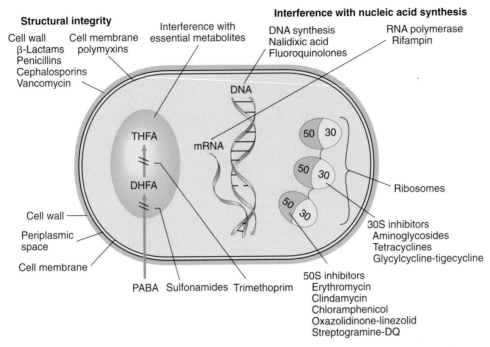

FIGURE 12-1   Primary sites of antibacterial action for major classes of antimicrobial agents. *THFA,* Tetrahydrofolic acid; *DHFA,* dihydrofolic acid; *PABA, para-*aminobenzoic acid.

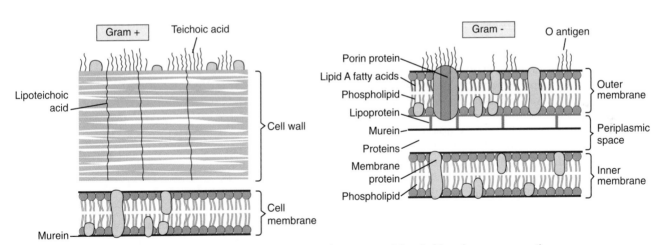

FIGURE 12-2   The cell envelope structure of a gram-positive *(left)* and a gram-negative *(right)* bacterium.

teria, a second outer membrane (Figure 12-2). The cytoplasmic membrane, composed of phospholipids and proteins, surrounds the cytoplasm, acts as an osmotic barrier, and is the location of the electron transport chain responsible for energy production. Peptidoglycan (murein) is a unique mucopolysaccharide constituent of the bacterial cell wall. The quantity of this polymer and its location within the cell envelope is different between gram-negative and gram-positive bacteria. The peptidoglycan layer is made up of chains of alternating disaccharide subunits of *N*-acetyl-D-glucosamine (NAG) and *N*-acetyl-D-muramic acid (NAM) (Figure 12-3).

The NAM subunit has a short peptide chain attached, which mediates cross-linking of parallel glycan molecules in mature peptidoglycan. This peptide consists of L- and D-amino acids, which typically end in D-alanyl-D-alanine (D-Ala-D-Ala). Cross-links between neighboring peptide side chains impart mechanical strength to the molecule, as well as presenting opportunities for biochemical diversity in the types of cross-links within and between different bacterial species. In gram-positive bacteria, the peptidoglycan layer is substantially thicker and more multilayered than in gram-negative bacteria. The outer membrane of gram-negative bacteria is composed

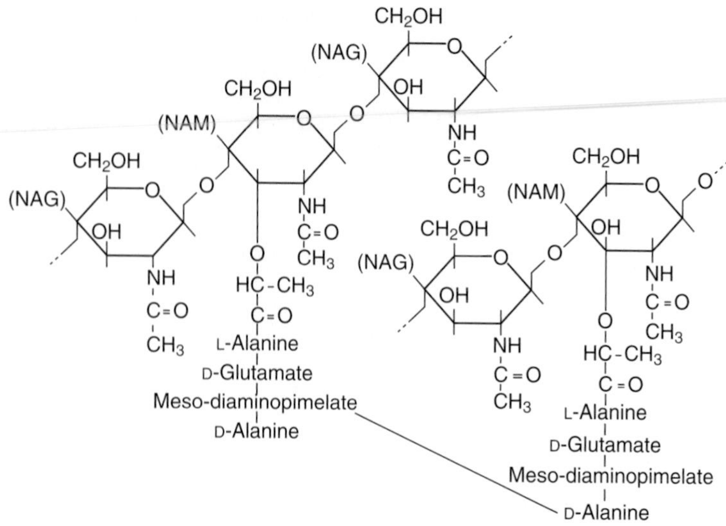

FIGURE 12-3 A diagram that demonstrates the structure of the peptidoglycan layer in the cell wall of *Escherichia coli*. The amino acids in the cross-linking tetrapeptides may vary among species. *NAG*, N-acetyl-D-glucosamine; *NAM*, N-acetyl-D-muramic acid. (From Neidhardt FC et al: *Physiology of the bacterial cell: a molecular approach*, Sunderland, Mass., 1990, Sinauer Associates.)

of lipopolysaccharides, phospholipids, and porin proteins and is separated from the cytoplasmic membrane by the periplasmic space.

Peptidoglycan biosynthesis has four major stages: (1) synthesis of precursors in the cytoplasm; (2) transport of lipid-bound precursors across the cytoplasmic membrane; (3) insertion of glycan units into the cell wall; and (4) transpeptidation linking and maturation. D-cycloserine and bacitracin inhibit the first two steps, respectively. The most commonly used inhibitors of cell wall biosynthesis, β-lactams and glycopeptides, act on processes in stages 3 and 4. Under normal growing conditions, peptidoglycan synthesis proceeds by the ligase-mediated formation of D-ala-D-ala, a precursor used to form UDP-NAM-acetyl-muramyl-pentapeptide (see Figure 12-3). This precursor molecule elongates peptidoglycan by undergoing transglycosylation of the glycan strands, and elongation of the peptide strands occurs by transpeptidation.

The **β-lactam antibiotics** include the penicillins and cephalosporins. These closely related compounds act by forming covalent complexes with enzymes that generate the mature peptidoglycan molecule. Because the functions of these enzymes were studied in the context of penicillin binding and resistance, they are known collectively as the **penicillin-binding proteins** (PBPs). In gram-negative cells, the β-lactams must pass through cell wall porin channels to reach the target PBPs. The effects of drug binding on cell growth differ depending on the agent and PBP involved. Some inhibit cell division, leading to long filamentous forms, whereas others lead to the formation of cell wall deficient types that readily lyse under osmotic pressure.

β-Lactam antibiotics, such as penems, cephems, carbapenems, and monobactams, act by binding to PBPs, which are bifunctional transpeptidase/transglycosylase enzymes that mediate peptidoglycan cross-linking (Table 12-1).

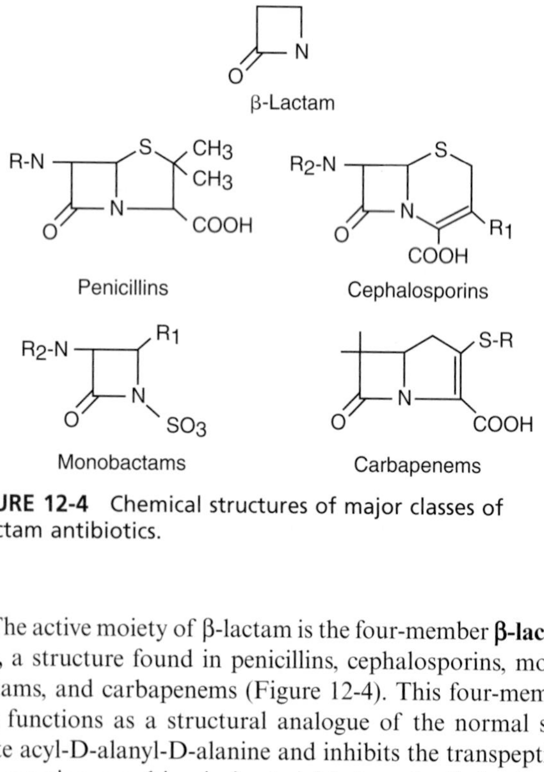

FIGURE 12-4 Chemical structures of major classes of β-lactam antibiotics.

The active moiety of β-lactam is the four-member **β-lactam ring,** a structure found in penicillins, cephalosporins, monobactams, and carbapenems (Figure 12-4). This four-member ring functions as a structural analogue of the normal substrate acyl-D-alanyl-D-alanine and inhibits the transpeptidation reaction, resulting in bacterial lysis and cell death. The narrow to broad-spectrum antimicrobial activity, safety, and efficacy properties of β-lactam antibiotics are typically enhanced by modification of moieties attached to the penicillin and cephalosporin ring structures (see Figure 12-4).

Glycopeptides, such as vancomycin, dalbavancin, teicoplanin, and the investigational drugs ortivancin and televancin, act by binding to the terminal D-ala-D-ala of the pentapeptidyl-glycosyl peptidoglycan intermediates (see

TABLE 12-1 Examples of Penems, Cephems, Carbapenems, and Monobactam β-Lactam Antibiotics

Class	Subclass	Category	U.S. Adopted Name
Penems	Penicillin	Narrow spectrum	Penicillin G, penicillin V
		Penicillinases—sensitive	Methicillin, oxacillin
		Penicillinases—resistant	Amoxicillin, ampicillin
		Broad spectrum	Carbenicillin, ticarcillin
		Aminopenicillins	Piperacillin
		Antipseudomonals	Amoxicillin-clavulanate
		Extended spectrum	Ampicillin-sulbactam
		Penem-β-lactamase combinations	
Cephems	Cephalosporin I	Narrow spectrum first generation	Cephalothin, cefazolin
	Cephalosporin II	Expanded spectrum second generation	Cefonicid, cefuroxime
	Cephalosporin III	Broad spectrum third generation	Cefoperazone, ceftazidime
	Cephalosporin IV	Extended spectrum fourth generation	Cefepime
	Cephamycin		Cefmetazole, cefoxitin
	Oxacephem		Moxalactam
	Carbacephem		Loracarbef
Carbapenems			Ertapenem, imipenem, meropenem
Monobactams			Aztreonam

Figure 12-3). This prevents their incorporation into the peptidoglycan chain by blocking the transpeptidation step in cell wall biosynthesis. Glycopeptides bind to the substrate of the transpeptidation enzyme while penicillins bind to the enzyme mediating the transpeptidation reaction. Because they cannot cross the outer membrane of gram-negative bacteria, the clinical spectrum of glycopeptides is limited to gram-positive microorganisms; thus they are mainly used to treat aerobic clinical infections caused by staphylococci, streptococci, and enterococci in the United States.

Inhibition of Folate Synthesis

Antibiotics are also capable of interfering with intracellular anabolic processes. The folic acid pathway provides the essential precursor molecules needed in DNA biosynthesis. The pathway is mediated by two key enzymes: dihydropteroate synthase and dihydrofolate reductase, which mediate the formation of tetrahydrofolate (THF) from dihydrofolate (Figure 12-5).

Sulfamethoxazole (SMZ) blocks the step leading to the formation of 7,8-dihydropteroate by competitively inhibiting the binding of the structural analogue *para*-aminobenzoic acid with dihydropteroate synthase. Trimethoprim blocks the step leading to formation of THF by preventing the dihydrofolate reductase–mediated recycling of folate coenzymes. Unlike other members of the current antibiotic classes, sulfamethoxazole (SMZ) and trimethoprim (TMP) are completely synthetic molecules that do not exist in and never have existed in nature. The spectrum of activity of folate pathway inhibitors, especially when provided in combination, provides a broad spectrum of activity against the Enterobacteriaceae that cause urinary tract infections.

Interference of DNA Replication

The prokaryotic cell cycle consists of **DNA replication** followed immediately by cell division. In microorganisms such

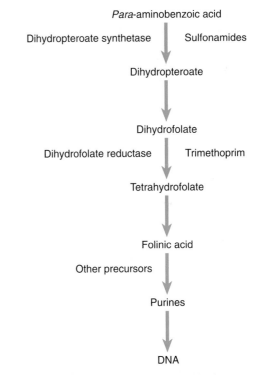

FIGURE 12-5 Sites of action of sulfonamides and trimethoprim and their effects on synthesis of essential amino acids and nucleic acids.

as *Escherichia coli* that divide in approximately 30 minutes under ideal growth conditions, DNA replication must be initiated and completed to ensure that each DNA duplex is delivered to each daughter cell. The enzymes necessary for DNA replication are topoisomerases I, II, III, and IV. **Quinolones** are antibiotics that affect DNA replication by targeting topoisomerases II (DNA gyrase) and IV, enzymes considered important in controlling DNA topology, replication, and decatenation at the end of bacterial DNA replicative cycle. DNA gyrase and topoisomerase IV are tetrameric molecules composed of dimeric A and B subunits. The subunits of DNA gyrase are encoded by *gyrA* and *gyrB*, while the subunits of topoisomerase IV are encoded by *parC* and *parE*. The tetramers of DNA gyrase and topoisomerase IV are highly homologous, with gyrA homologous to parC and gyrB homologous to parE. Interestingly, the targets of quinolones appear to be selective, targeting DNA gyrase in gram-negative bacteria and topoisomerase IV in gram-positive bacteria, but newer quinolones appear to have high affinity for both targets. Analyses of mechanism of action suggest that quinolones interact with DNA gyrase–DNA complexes and topoisomerase IV–DNA complexes to trap the enzymes as stabilized reaction intermediates forming barriers to further DNA replication. The quinolones and fluoroquinolones are used to treat the Enterobacteriaceae, pseudomonads, and other non-Enterobacteriaceae, staphylococci, enterococci, neisseria, and streptococci species other than *Streptococcus pneumoniae*.

Interference of DNA Transcription

DNA transcription is the process by which a template DNA strand is copied into a functional RNA sequence, resulting in mature mRNA or structural RNA. The **transcription** of DNA into RNA is mediated by RNA polymerase; bacterial RNA polymerase is a core tetramer composed of an α subunit, two β subunits (ββ'), a γ subunit, and a dissociable σ subunit that controls transcription of particular gene classes. Rifampin, a synthetic derivative of rifamycin B, is used in combination with other antibiotic classes to treat *Mycobacterium tuberculosis* by targeting transcription of DNA. The target of rifampin in *M. tuberculosis* is the RNA polymerase β subunit at an allosteric site, with the subsequent blocking of RNA chain elongation. As a result, RNA transcription is aborted at the initiation step. Aerobic species treated with rifampin include staphylococci, enterococci, *Haemophilus* spp., and *S. pneumoniae*.

Interference of mRNA Translation

The cellular machinery of living organisms decodes mRNA into functional protein, a process called *mRNA translation*. Protein biosynthesis requires the sequential binding of the 30S and 50S ribosomal subunits to mRNA leading to translation of the genetic message. The initiation phase commences with initiation factors, proteins that bind to the 30S subunit, and the initiator transfer ribonucleic acid (tRNA), formylmethionyl tRNA, which binds to the P site of the 30S ribosomal subunit. This 30S subunit helps the bound initiator tRNA scan and find the start codon on mRNA. Next, the 50S subunit binds to form the preinitiation complex. The codon immediately following the initiation codon dictates binding of the next tRNA to the ribosomal A site. Because protein synthesis is central to cellular function, it is an excellent target for antibiotic drug product development. Thus the bacteria ribosome is a primary target of numerous antibiotics with some targeting the 30S ribosomal subunit (i.e., aminoglycosides, tetracyclines, glycylcyclines) and others the 50S ribosomal subunit (e.g., macrolides, oxazolidinones, streptogramins; see Figure 12-1).

Aminoglycosides are cationic carbohydrate-containing molecules, and their positive charge provides the basis for their interaction with a specific region of the 16S ribosomal ribonucleic acid (rRNA) in the 30S ribosomal subunit. The 30S subunit provides a high-affinity docking site mediated by hydrogen bonding to the various substituents in the aminoglycoside cyclitol ring. Binding of the aminoglycosides to the A-binding site on the 30S subunit prevents the docking of aminoacyl-tRNA, resulting in mistranslation and subsequent production of aberrant proteins. The incorporation of aberrant proteins into the cell wall also results in cell leakage and enhanced cellular penetration of additional antibiotic.

Tetracycline compounds are members of the polyketide class of antibiotics and are represented by tetracycline, doxycycline, and minocycline. As shown in Figure 12-1, the tetracyclines target the 30S ribosomal subunit. Tetracyclines reversibly inhibit protein synthesis by binding to 16S ribosomal RNA near the amino-acyl tRNA acceptor (A) site, thus inhibiting the rotation of bound tRNA into the A site during translation. This physical blocking by tetracycline results in premature release of tRNA and termination of peptide bond formation.

Macrolides such as erythromycin, clarithromycin, and azithromycin target the 50S subunit specifically by binding to the peptidyltransferase cavity in the proximity of the A and P loops, near adenine 2058 of 23S rRNA. By blocking the exit tunnel of the elongating peptides, premature release of peptidyl-tRNA intermediates occurs and polypeptide translation ceases. Macrolides also prevent assembly of the 50S ribosomal subunit by binding to 23S rRNA. As shown in Figure 12-1, lincosamide and chloramphenicol also target the 50S ribosomal subunit, thus inhibiting mRNA translation and subsequently protein synthesis. Macrolides and tetracyclines allow initiation and mRNA translation to begin but act by inhibiting peptide elongation. The most recently approved classes of antibiotics targeting protein synthesis are **oxazolidinone** represented by linezolid, a streptogramin represented by quinupristin-dalfopristin, and a glycylcycline represented by tigecycline. Linezolid is thought to bind to the 50S ribosomal subunit of prokaryotes, preventing formation of the preinitiation complex with the 30S ribosomal subunit containing bound initiation factors. The 50S ribosomal target appears to be the ribosomal P site in the peptidyltransferase center, and by blocking this site, the first peptide-forming step is prevented and protein synthesis is terminated.

Linezolid differs from other protein synthesis inhibitors by blocking the initiation step while macrolides and tetracyclines block peptide chain elongation. **Streptogramin** antibiotics are composed of a mixture of two classes of distinct molecules designated *streptogramin A* and *streptogramin B*. Dalfopristin-quinupristin is a combination of these two streptogramins in a ratio of 70:30. Dalfopristin is a polyunsaturated macrolactone classified as a type A streptogramin, and quinupristin is a peptide macrolactone classified as a type B streptogramin. Streptogramins disrupt translation of mRNA into protein by binding to the peptidyltransferase domain of the bacterial ribosome. Dalfopristin interferes with the elongation of the polypeptide chain by preventing binding of aminoacyl-tRNA to the ribosome and the formation of peptide bonds. Quinupristin stimulates the dissociation of the peptidyl-tRNA and is thought to interfere with the release of the completed polypeptide by blocking the exit tunnel through which it normally leaves the ribosome. Dalfopristin and quinupristin act synergistically as a result of the enhanced affinity of quinupristin for the ribosome. Dalfopristin induces a conformational change such that quinupristin binds with greater affinity. The natural streptogramins are produced as mixtures of dalfopristin and quinupristin, the combination of which is a more potent antibacterial agent than either type of compound alone.

Glycylcycline is represented by tigecycline, which carries a glycylamido moiety attached to the 9-position of minocycline. Tigecycline inhibits protein translation in bacteria by binding to the 30S ribosomal subunit and blocking entry of aminoacyl tRNA molecules into the A site of the ribosome, thus preventing incorporation of amino acid residues into elongating peptide chains.

MECHANISMS OF ANTIBIOTIC RESISTANCE

Resistance to antibiotics is conveniently divided into mechanisms that are either intrinsic to the microorganism or acquired. *Intrinsic* mechanisms of resistance are innate characteristic of the microorganism and are transmitted to progeny vertically. *Acquired* mechanisms of resistance are those that result from the acquisition of DNA by transformation and recombination or by acquisition of extrachromosomal DNA and are transmitted horizontally. The latter includes acquisition of mobile genetic elements such as plasmids and transposons capable of disseminating resistant determinants. Where feasible, this section uses members of the antibiotic classes previously discussed to exemplify intrinsic or acquired mechanisms of resistance.

Origins of Antibiotic Resistance

Resistance genes and transfer mechanisms existed long before the discovery and use of modern therapeutic antimicrobials. For example, antimicrobial resistant bacteria estimated at being more than 2000 years old have been recovered from glacial samples obtained from the Canadian Arctic Archipelago, whereas a more recent study detected β-lactamases from a metagenomic library of cold-seep sediments of deep-sea Edison seamount (near Papua New Guinea) estimated to be about 10,000 years old. In addition, plasmids found in gram-negative bacteria that were isolated before antibiotics were introduced into clinical practice were very similar to currently described plasmids, except that the early isolates did not possess any resistance genes.

Resistance to natural antimicrobial agents, synthetic derivatives, and completely synthetic antimicrobials has been recently observed in a collection of soil-dwelling actinomycetes, with some displaying resistance mechanisms not traditionally observed in clinical bacterial pathogens. Most soil isolates display resistance to at least six to eight different antimicrobial agents and, in some cases, as many as 20. The use of novel resistance mechanisms by these organisms, coupled with the fact that these soil microbes are not as intensively exposed to antimicrobial selective pressures as are the clinical pathogens, emphasizes the fact that resistance is natural part of microbial ecosystems and highlights the evolutionary possibilities for novel antimicrobial resistance determinants.

If bacterial antimicrobial resistance is not a new phenomenon, where did it originate? One popular belief is that antibiotic resistance mechanisms arose within antibiotic-producing microorganisms as a mechanism to protect them against the action of their own antibiotic (autotoxicity). This has been substantiated by the finding of aminoglycoside-modifying enzymes in aminoglycoside-producing organisms that display marked homology to modifying enzymes found in aminoglycoside-resistant bacteria. Also, the essential genetic determinants associated with resistance to vancomycin, *vanA, vanH,* and *vanX,* appear to be very similar to the self-protection mechanism employed in the vancomycin producing *Actinomyces* strains. In addition, some antibiotic preparations employed for human and animal use were found to be contaminated with chromosomal DNA of an antibiotic-producing organism, including antimicrobial resistance gene sequences. It has been postulated that this presence of DNA encoding antimicrobial resistance in antibiotic preparations has been a factor in the rapid development of multiple resistance, by providing the resistance sequences that can then be taken up by the causative pathogen.

Intrinsic (Chromosomal) Mechanisms of Resistance

Bacteria differ widely in cell wall composition and thus their intrinsic susceptibility or resistance to antibiotics. Intrinsic resistance of bacteria to the action of antibiotics depends on the hydrophobic or hydrophilic nature of the antibiotic and on impermeability of the cell wall to the antibiotic. Thus intrinsic resistance mediated by impermeability is exemplified by cell wall composition, formation of biofilms, and efflux. Intrinsic resistance is also due to chromosomally mediated enzymatic inactivation of antibiotics that penetrate the cell wall.

Impermeability

For antibiotics to affect internal cellular processes, they must penetrate the cell wall of bacteria to reach their target. Influx of antibiotics through the cell wall depends on the chemical nature of the antibiotic and the structural characteristics of the cell wall (see Figure 12-2). There are two fundamental structures of the cell wall leading to clinically relevant resistance owing to impermeability: (1) lipopolysaccharide (LPS) composition, and (2) the structure and expression of outer membrane proteins (Omps) called *porins*. Resistance to the glycopeptide antibiotic vancomycin is an example of intrinsic impermeability resulting in its **narrow spectrum** of activity for gram-positive bacteria (previously discussed under Inhibition of Bacterial Cell Wall Biosynthesis). Intrinsic resistance of gram-negative bacteria is mediated by porins. **Porins** naturally serve as outer membrane channels that permit the influx of nutrients and efflux of waste products. They also serve to restrict the influx of antibiotics and maintain low intracellular concentration. In addition, alterations leading to either decreased porin production or changes in the structure of porins that reduce their affinity for an antibiotic can alter a resistance phenotype. Common Omps in *E. coli* are OmpF, OmpC, and OmpE. OmpF is the major channel in *E. coli* through which many molecules diffuse, and the alteration of this porin can result in decreased susceptibility to a number of different antimicrobial agents. Nosocomial pathogens showing decreases or loss of porin synthesis are often observed in combination with other resistance mechanisms, resulting in MDR pathogens.

Molecular analysis of gram-negative bacteria reveals that the strongly negatively charged core region of the LPS functions as a selective permeability barrier for negatively charged antibiotics, resulting in decreased susceptibility to these compounds. Mutations in the O-antigen side chains of the LPS can change the shape and overall charge of the cell wall, decreasing the binding efficiency of some cationic antibiotics. Mutations in the LPS genes have been shown in conjunction with increasing antibiotic selective pressure. Thus the cell wall, in part, accounts for the intrinsic resistance of bacteria to antibiotics. It is usually only clinically significant in the context of other resistance mechanisms, such as efflux (see later discussion), which work synergistically to mediate survival of the organism.

Biofilms

Biofilms are sessile bacterial communities that are irreversibly attached to a substrate and embedded in an **exopolysaccharide matrix.** Bacterial biofilms are prevalent in the clinical setting, occurring on numerous environmental surfaces and indwelling medical devices. Biofilms can be made up of single or multiple bacterial species, with as many as 500 different bacterial taxa in some cases, such as dental biofilms. Bacterial biofilms are highly resistant to antibiotic exposure, which can lead to serious challenges in antibacterial therapy. The mechanisms of biofilm-associated antimicrobial resistance seem to be multifactorial, involving a complex system of cell-cell chemical communication that varies from organism to organism. Resistance exhibited by bacteria when they grow in biofilms is not attributed to typically acquired genetic mechanisms (i.e., gene mutation, mobile acquisition), but is instead determined by chemical and physical characteristics of biofilm formation.

The genetic mechanisms of biofilm antibiotic resistance appear to fall into two general classes: **innate** resistance factors and **induced** resistance factors. Innate mechanisms are activated as part of the biofilm developmental pathway, the factors being integral parts of biofilm structure and physiology (e.g., decreased penetration of antibiotics through the biofilm matrix, decreased oxygen and nutrient availability accompanied by altered metabolic activity, and formation of persister cells). **Persister cells** can be described as subpopulations of bacteria deep in the biofilm which can differentiate into a phenotypically resistant state (e.g., slow or nongrowing bacteria). Induced resistance factors include those resulting from induction by the antimicrobial agent itself, resulting in differential resistance gene expression throughout the biofilm community. Thus biofilm antibiotic resistance can be viewed as a complex combination of innate anabolic metabolism and

induced genetic mechanisms, many of which still need to be elucidated. Because of the extreme nature of biofilm associated antibiotic resistance, numerous investigators are focusing on the development of novel anti-biofilm therapies aimed at disrupting biofilms and killing the constituent bacteria.

Efflux

Intrinsic resistance of bacteria to certain antibiotics is explained by the activity of efflux systems and impermeability (Figure 12-6). **Efflux pumps** are found in gram-positive and gram-negative bacteria and function as transporter proteins involved in the removal of toxic substances from the interior of the cell to the external environment. Efflux pumps are naturally occurring and are present in both susceptible and resistant microorganisms. Efflux mechanisms can confer resistance to a particular antimicrobial agent, a class of agents, or a number of unrelated antimicrobials resulting in multidrug resistance.

Five major efflux pump protein families that mediate resistance to antibiotics are (1) the major facilitator subfamily (MFS), (2) the resistance nodulation cell division subfamily (RND), (3) the small multidrug regulator subfamily (SMR), (4) the adenosine triphosphate (ATP)-binding cassette (ABC) family, and (5) the multidrug and toxic effects (MATE) family. A proton motive force mediated by the counterflow of protons drives the MFS, RND, MATE, and SMR subfamilies. The ABC family uses the hydrolysis of ATP by ATPase to provide the energy for active transport of antibiotics and other toxic molecules. Intrinsic efflux mechanism of resistance is chromosomally located and is activated by environmental signals or by mutation in regulatory genes.

In the RND superfamily, the *mexAB-oprM* operon in *Pseudomonas aeruginosa* regulates porin and pump genes. This genetic locus plays a major role in the intrinsic resistance of pseudomonads and is a major reason that infections caused by members of this genus are difficult to treat. Mutations in

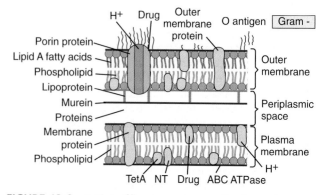

FIGURE 12-6 Active efflux in gram-negative bacteria mediated by transmembrane proteins located in cytoplasmic and outer membrane. *Emr/Mex,* Multidrug transporter efflux system; *ABC ATPase,* ATP-binding cassette family pumps; *ATP,* adenosine triphosphate; *ADP,* adenosine diphosphate; *Tet A,* tetracycline specific transporter pump; *H⁺,* efflux pumps driven by proton motive force mediated by the counterflow of protons.

the repressor protein encoded by the *mexR* gene results in reduced affinity for the promoter target and up-regulation of the *mexAB-oprM* operon, resulting in increased expression of the porin pump. This three-component efflux pump provides an exit portal for numerous antibiotics including quinolones, tetracyclines, macrolides, chloramphenicol, β-lactams, and meropenem, but not imipenem. Cross-resistance of bacteria to multiple antibiotics can be mediated by efflux pumps capable of using various substrates. Exposure of a microorganism possessing an efflux pump to any one substrate belonging to a similar or different substrate profile used by that pump results in overexpression and consequent cross-resistance to all other substrates. Antibiotics are no exception; in the *mexAB* system of *P. aeruginosa*, mutants that overproduce MexAB are less susceptible to fluoroquinolones, β-lactams, chloramphenicol, trimethoprim, and the antiseptic triclosan. Efflux-mediated resistance to the oxazolidinone and streptogramin antibiotics has been identified in gram-negative bacteria and *Enterococcus faecalis*, respectively. *E. faecalis* appears to be intrinsically resistant to dalfopristin, a streptogramin component of the quinupristin-dalfopristin antibiotic. The efflux mechanism designated *lsa* for "lincosamide and streptogramin A resistance" shows similarities to members of the superfamily of transporter proteins known as *ABC transporters* and influences resistance to quinupristin-dalfopristin and clindamycin. Most bacteria possess numerous efflux pumps; however, only a few per species appear to contribute resistance to antibiotics used in clinical practice.

Enzymatic Inactivation

β-Lactam antibiotics are the most commonly used class of agents used to treat bacterial infections. They consist of four major groups: penicillins, cephalosporins, monobactams, and carbapenems (see Table 12-1). As shown in Figure 12-4, all four groups have a four-member β-lactam ring represented by the β-lactam structure and are susceptible to the hydrolytic activity of β-lactamases, the most widespread mechanism of bacterial resistance to this class of antibiotics (Figure 12-7). Thus this antibiotic class is used to discuss intrinsic enzymatic chromosomal mechanisms of resistance.

β-Lactamases hydrolyze β-lactam antibiotics using two distinct mechanisms: (1) a metallo-based mechanism of action and (2) a serine-based mechanism of action. These mechanisms of action allow classification of β-lactamases into four major classes with class B β-lactamases exhibiting metallo-based mechanisms of action and classes A, C, and D containing active-site serine enzymes (Table 12-2).

β-Lactam antibiotics act by binding to PBPs, bifunctional transglycosylases/transpeptidases responsible for cross-linking of glycan strands and backbone peptide strands, respectively. The similarities of class A, C, and D β-lactamases to mechanistic and architectural structures of PBPs suggest that the serine-based enzymes evolved from PBPs. Because of their structural similarity, both PBPs and β-lactamases can serve as receptors for β-lactam antibiotics entering the cell. It is the binding equilibrium between PBP, β-lactamases, as well as the β-lactam antibiotic, that determines the fate and ultimate survival of the microorganism. In addition, the observation that β-lactamases compete with PBPs for the antibiotic leads to the logical conclusion that development of structural analogues of the β-lactam that bind the β-lactamase would enhance the activity of the β-lactam antibiotic. This observation led to the development of the β-lactamase inhibitors clavulanic acid, sulbactam, and tazobactam. The β-lactamase inhibitors are structural analogues of the β-lactam antibiotics and function as substrates for β-lactamase, thus reducing their detrimental effects on the β-lactam antibiotic. When used jointly with β-lactam antibiotics, these inhibitors enhance the in vitro microbiologic and clinical activity of the antibiotic.

Class A and C β-lactamases are considered the most clinically important, with class A enzymes primarily found on plasmids and constitutively expressed, whereas class C enzymes are usually chromosomally located and inducible by exposure to β-lactams. In gram-negative bacteria, the β-lactamases are localized to the periplasmic space where they act on incoming β-lactam antibiotics. In gram-positive bacteria, β-lactamases are secreted as exoenzymes and offer less protection to the microorganism. Virtually all gram-negative bacteria mediate intrinsic (chromosomal) resistance by enzymatic inactivation of penicillin class antibiotics exemplified by the class C β-lactamases. For example, *Citrobacter freundii, Enterobacter aerogenes,* and *P. aeruginosa* are clinically important nosocomial pathogens encoding chromosomal versions of class C β-lactamases. Most class B metallo-dependent enzymes are chromosomally encoded cephalosporinases and their expression can be either constitutive or inducible. These

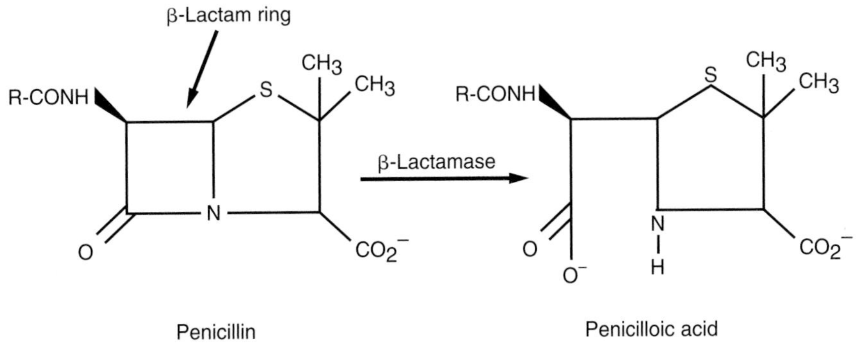

FIGURE 12-7 β-Lactamase hydrolyzes the β-lactam ring portion of the penicillin molecule. The hydrolysis results in the formation of penicilloic acid, which does not have antibacterial activity.

TABLE 12-2 Current Major β-Lactamase Functional and Molecular Classification Scheme

MOA	Molecular Class	Functional Group	Major Subgroup	Clavulanic Inhibition	Main Attributes
Serine-based	A	2	2a	+	Confers high-level resistance to penicillins; includes staphylococcal and enterococcal penicillinases
			2b	+	Broad-spectrum β-lactamases found primarily in gram-negative bacteria
			2be	+	Extended-spectrum β-lactamases conferring resistance to monobactams and oxyimino-cephalosporins
			2br	−	Broad-spectrum β-lactamases with reduced binding to clavulanic acid and sulbactam; called inhibitor-resistant *TEM (IRT)*
			2c	+	Carbenicillin-hydrolyzing enzyme
			2e	+	Cephalosporinases
			2f	+	Carbapenem-hydrolyzing enzyme
	C	1		−	Chromosomal mediated cephalosporinases in gram-negative bacteria; emerging plasmid-encoded bacterial populations; confers resistance to all β-lactams except carbapenems
Metallo-based	D	2	2d	+/−	Oxacillin-hydrolyzing enzyme
			3a	−	β-Lactamases conferring resistance to all
	B	3	3b	−	β-Lactam classes, carbapenems, but not
			3c	−	monobactams
	Unknown	4			Unsequenced enzymes not fitting into other molecular classes

Modified from Bush K: New β-lactamases in gram-negative bacteria: diversity and impact on the selection of antimicrobial therapy, *Clin Infect Dis* 32:1085, 2001.
MOA, mode of action.

β-lactamases are usually expressed in clinically important nosocomial pathogens such as *Stenotrophomonas maltophilia*, *Klebsiella pneumoniae*, and *P. aeruginosa*. Although these enzymes are commonly found on the chromosome, they can escape to plasmids and become transmissible, as has occurred for the class C enzyme encoded by bla_{CMY}, which is widespread in enteric bacteria.

Acquired Mechanisms of Resistance

As mentioned previously, the resistance mechanisms and the genes that mediate resistance have presumably evolved in organisms that produce antibiotics such that the antibiotic produced is not effective against the producing organism. Furthermore, organisms that co-evolved with antibiotic-producing organisms may have acquired new functions in normal housekeeping genes to help detoxify antibiotics. Thus, by the process of natural selection, target organisms may acquire, evolve, and disseminate resistance determinants and use multiple combinations of intrinsic and acquired antibiotic resistance strategies to survive toxic environments. This section focuses on acquired mechanisms such as efflux, modification of existing antibiotic targets, acquisition of new targets, and production of enzymes that inactivate the antibiotic.

Efflux

Although efflux plays a major role in intrinsic resistance, changes in these cell wall proteins can also result in novel acquired traits. In addition, some efflux pumps have translo-cated to plasmids, which can be acquired by horizontal gene exchange. The *acrAB* in gram-negative bacteria is an efflux pump conferring intrinsic resistance. An efflux pump encoded by the *mef* gene in *Streptococcus* is an example of an acquired trait that encodes macrolide resistance. The genetic element carrying *mefA* appears to be widely disseminated in *S. pneumoniae* and is transferable to other streptococcal species and various other genera. *S. pneumoniae* isolates with efflux resistance are susceptible to clindamycin and usually have erythromycin minimum inhibitory concentrations (MICs) ranging from 1 to 16 μg/mL. Because the *mef* phenotype demonstrates resistance to erythromycin but susceptibility to clindamycin, surveillance studies monitoring *S. pneumoniae* susceptibility patterns of erythromycin and clindamycin reveal that the most prevalent mechanism of macrolide resistance in the United States is efflux mediated.

Target Site Modification

Modification of a target can reduce the binding affinity of the antibiotic to the target. Modification of target sites occurs primarily by chromosomal mutation, as is observed with the quinolone and oxazolidinone antimicrobials, and by enzymatic alteration of macrolide, glycopeptide, and β-lactam antibiotic target sites.

Chromosomal Mutation. Quinolones target DNA gyrase and topoisomerase IV. While there are plasmid-mediated quinolone resistance genes (termed *qnr*), the primary mechanism of resistance to this antimicrobial class is modification by mutations encoding single amino acid changes in the genes encoding these DNA topoisomerases. Mutations are generally localized to the amino terminal domains of GyrA and ParC, termed the *quinolone resistance–determining region* (QRDR). These mutations occur equally in both the *gyrA* and *gyrB* subunits, but isolates from clinical settings usually demonstrate an exclusive prevalence for mutations in *gyrA*. In *E. coli,* alterations in *gyrA* resulting in amino acid substitutions occur predominantly in the QRDR between positions 67 and 106. Although the presence of a single mutation in the QRDR of *gyrA* usually results in high-level resistance to nalidixic acid, the presence of additional mutations in *gyrA* and/or in another target such as *parC* is required to produce high levels of resistance to fluoroquinolones. Conversely, in gram-positive bacteria, first-step mutations leading to fluoroquinolone resistance occur in *parC* or *parE* subunits of topoisomerase IV and second-step mutations occur in *gyrA*. Interestingly, first-step mutations in *gyrA* do not cause elevated MICs in *S. aureus*, suggesting that the primary target of the quinolone is topoisomerase IV.

β-Lactam antibiotics kill *S. pneumoniae* by targeting endogenous high–molecular-weight penicillin-binding proteins PBP1A, 1B, 2A, 2B, and 2X. Mutations in these PBPs confer low-level to high-level resistance to β-lactam antibiotics depending on the number of mutations and PBPs involved. Mutations in PBP2 or PBP2X mediated by amino acid changes in close proximity to the active-site region of the PBP result in low-level resistance. Mutations in any of these transpeptidases/transglycosylases result in elevated MICs, and high-level resistance is the result of mutation in all five PBPs. In *S. pneumoniae*, evidence suggests that PB2B and 2X high-level resistance is also mediated by horizontal acquisition of DNA fragments via transformation and by homologous recombination of these fragments with the coding sequences of the PBP proteins. Resistance to oxazolidinone and streptogramin antibiotics is also mediated by changes in target site leading to reduced affinity of the antibiotic for its target. In vancomycin-resistant *E. faecalis,* resistant mutants contain amino acid changes in domain V of the peptidyltransferase center of 23S rRNA. The most frequently encountered change is a transversion from guanine to uracil in position 2576—a mutation previously described in *E. faecium* isolated from patients who developed oxazolidinone resistance while on therapy. Resistance to the streptogramin antibiotic quinupristin-dalfopristin in *S. aureus* clinical isolates reveals that ribosomal proteins also lead to reduced affinity of the streptogramin for its target. Evaluation of the resistant mutants revealed the presence of insertions or deletions in the β hairpin structure that is part of the conserved C terminus of the L22 protein that interacts with 23S rRNA in the 50s ribosomal subunit. The presence of the mutant proteins reduces the affinity of quinupristin for its target but does not affect the activity of dalfopristin; therefore the MIC susceptibility of pathogens containing this mutation increase and there is a corresponding loss in the combined action of both antibiotics.

Enzymatic Target Site Alteration. Enzymatic alterations of antibiotic targets result in reduced affinity of antibiotics for their microbial targets and are exemplified by erythromycin ribosomal methylase and by reprogramming of the peptidoglycan termini. Macrolides such as erythromycin bind the 50S subunit of the ribosome at the peptidyltransferase cavity in the proximity of the A and P loops, and near adenine 2058 of 23S rRNA. Monomethylation or dimethylation of the amino group in the adenine residue of 23S rRNA results in reduced affinity of the macrolide for its target site and in elevated MICs. Resistance to macrolides is mediated by an erythromycin ribosome methylase (ERM) found on plasmids and transposons that allow broad dissemination to many bacterial species. Methylation does not affect the function of the adenine residue other than to help the organism become less susceptible to the macrolide class of antibiotics. Methylation of the 23S rRNA also results in cross-resistance to the lincosamide family and streptogramin B class of antibiotics. Cross-resistance to all three antibiotics groups is known as the *macrolide-lincosamide-streptogramin B (MLS$_B$) resistance phenotype.* The ERM gene conferring the MLS$_B$ may be constitutively or inducible expressed. Alteration of target site to the streptogramin quinupristin-dalfopristin has been observed for the individual components of the combination resulting in loss of microbiologic synergy between the components. The most commonly known mechanism of resistance to the streptogramin B antibiotics is mediated by erythromycin-resistant methylase (MLS$_B$), as previously discussed. This phenotype does alter the affinity of dalfopristin, a streptogramin B antibiotic, for its ribosomal target, but because quinupristin is not affected by the MLS$_B$ mechanism of resistance, it maintains bacteriostatic activity.

The glycopeptide vancomycin is used to treat enterococcal infections, in particular endocarditis, and is the drug of choice for the treatment of methicillin-resistant *S. aureus*. In an attempt to avoid the overuse and subsequent emergence of resistance to vancomycin, vancomycin was used sparingly during its introduction. Unfortunately this strategy did not prevent widespread use and resulted in the emergence of **vancomycin-resistant enterococci (VRE)** isolates in health care settings. Currently there are two choices approved for the treatment of VRE, synercid and linezolid, and several approved for cases of vancomycin-susceptible infections (e.g., daptomycin and tigecycline).

Proteins encoded by the *vanA* and *vanB* genes confer resistance to vancomycin in clinically important enterococcal species. *Enterococcus* spp. containing the VanA phenotype are highly resistant to vancomycin (MICs greater than or equal to 64 μg/mL) and teicoplanin (MICs greater than or equal to 16 μg/mL). *vanA* is resident on plasmids and on transposons that mediate spread of the determinant. Conversely, the VanB phenotype exhibits a range of susceptibilities and resistance to vancomycin but remains susceptible to teicoplanin. The *vanB* determinant appears to be on large chromosomal elements. *vanA* can be induced by vancomycin and teicoplanin, which is controlled by *vanS* and *vanR* genes, a regulatory pair that combine sensor and response regulators responsible for control and expression of inducible vancomycin resistance. The transmissibility of *vanA* is of great concern in the medical community, particularly transmission to methicillin-resistant *Staphylococcus aureus* (MRSA) because vancomycin is the treatment of choice for MRSA. The recent emergence and subsequent genetic analysis of a high-level vancomycin resistant *S. aureus* isolate (MIC 1024 µg/mL) of clinical origin revealed the presence of a multiresistant conjugative plasmid harboring transposon Tn 1546 *(vanA)*. Potential spread of this strain in health care settings would have grave consequences for the continued therapeutic usefulness of vancomycin. Molecular and genetic analysis of the *vanA* determinant demonstrates the presence of five genes in tandem array, three of which are involved in target modification.

The product of the *vanH, vanA,* and *vanX* genes sequentially modifies the peptidoglycan termini, N-acyl-D-Ala-D-Ala, involved in cross-linking to *N*-acyl-D-Ala-D-lactate. The non–cross-linked peptidoglycan termini result in resistance to vancomycin. *vanH* codes for a D-hydroxy acid dehydrogenase that synthesizes the D-lactate used by VanA, a ligase that mediates the preferential production of D-Ala-D-lac. In addition, the Van X protein acts specifically to cleave the natural peptidoglycan termini D-Ala-D-Ala, preventing its incorporation into and production of vancomycin-susceptible peptidoglycan. Other Van-type phenotypes exist that mediate resistance to vancomycin using analogous mechanisms.

Acquisition of New Targets

Microorganisms also adapt become resistant by acquiring cellular targets with reduced affinity for the antibiotic. **Methicillin-resistant *S. aureus* (MRSA)** emerged soon after the introduction of methicillin into clinical medicine in the 1960s and exemplifies the acquisition of a new target by a pathogen to solve exposure to the toxic effects of the antibiotic. *S. aureus* evaded the antimicrobial activity of methicillin by acquiring a mobile element carrying a staphylococcal cassette chromosome mec (SCCmec), which confers resistance to methicillin. The mobile DNA element encodes a triad of genes: *mecR1-mecI-mecA. mecA* is the gene responsible for methicillin resistance and encodes a penicillin-binding protein, PBP2A (also PBP2A′), a bifunctional transglycosylase/transpeptidase with reduced affinity for β-lactam antibiotics including penicillins, cephalosporins, carbapenems, and penems. The origin of the *mecA* gene remains unknown, as does the molecular basis of its nonsusceptibility to β-lactams.

Target site substitution operates in resistance to folate pathway inhibitors. Sulfonamides competitively compete for the (dihydropteroate synthetase) enzyme active site and block the formation of nucleotide precursors. Resistance in both gram-negative and gram-positive bacteria is usually due to the acquisition of a new enzyme that is unaffected by sulfonamides.

Enzymatic Inactivation of Antibiotics

The acquisition of enzymes that inactivate antibiotics directly is one of the first mechanisms of resistance identified in bacteria and is a successful strategy used by numerous microorganisms to survive the action of many antibiotic classes. Several of the best studied classic examples are enzymes that mediate hydrolysis of the β-lactam ring of β-lactam antibiotics and modification of structural moieties of aminoglycoside antibiotics. The substrate of β-lactamases is the β-lactam ring structure, which the β-lactamases selectively hydrolyze to form the microbiologically inactive penicilloic acid (see Figure 12-7). The β-lactam antibiotics make up the largest group of

antibiotics, consisting of penicillins, cephalosporins, monobactams, and carbapenems (see Table 12-1). They differ from each other in the basic ring structure and moieties attached to the rings (see Figure 12-4). Because numerous β-lactamases with varying enzymatic characteristics have been discovered that hydrolyze these β-lactam antibiotics, attempts have been made to classify them using both biochemical and functional characteristics, or using molecular methods allowing comparison of nucleotide and amino acid sequence homologies. The latter method allows classification of the β-lactamases into four major groups: class A, C, and D, which act by serine-based mechanisms, and Class B β-lactamases, which require zinc for their action and are described as metallo-based enzymes. Class A β-lactamases are primarily penicillinases produced by gram-negative and gram-positive bacteria capable of hydrolyzing penicillin class antibiotic substrates. They are also structural analogues of PBPs and act as receptors for β-lactam antibiotics. The most important clinical class A β-lactamases are TEM-1 and SHV-1, usually found in gram-negative bacteria. TEM-1 is typically found in *E. coli, K. pneumoniae, E. aerogenes,* and *Haemophilus influenzae* and is typically located on transmissible plasmids. SHV-1 is usually found in clinical isolates of *K. pneumoniae* and appears to be the most common of the chromosomal β-lactamases found in this species.

With the emergence of plasmid-mediated β-lactamase resistance, concern regarding the possible widespread transmission of these resistance mechanisms led to the development of new oxyimino-β-lactam parenteral antibiotics resistant to the hydrolysis of class A β-lactamases. Although these parenterally administered cephalosporins and monobactams are excellent therapies, their continued use provided selection pressure for variants of existing β-lactamases that could hydrolyze these new antibiotics. These extended-spectrum β-lactamases (ESBLs) are now known to be derivatives of the common TEM, SHV, and OXA type B β-lactamases that differ by one or more amino acid substitutions near the reactive site of the enzyme. The modified amino acid sequence yields a protein capable of extending substrate utilization and greater affinity for the antibiotic target molecule. Interestingly, the enhanced spectrum of the ESBLs also makes them better substrates for β-lactamase inhibitors. Also, ESBLs have specific sets of penicillins, cephalosporins, and monobactams that they can hydrolyze, and not all ESBLs are capable of hydrolyzing all cephalosporins equally well.

In addition to degradation, enzyme-mediated resistance mechanisms may exert their effects by modification of the drug. As previously discussed, amino and hydroxy radicals of aminoglycoside antibiotics form hydrogen bonds with the 30S ribosomal subunit, thus preventing mRNA translation. Resistance to aminoglycosides is mediated by efflux, changes in target site, impermeability, or enzymatic modification of the amino and hydroxy moieties appended to the cyclitol rings. The most clinically relevant is enzymatic modification, which prevents recognition of the 16S binding sites and subsequent inhibition of mRNA translation.

Enzymatic modification of aminoglycosides results from N-acetylation, O-phosphorylation, and O-adenylation. To aid in the development of a classification system for aminoglycoside-modifying enzymes, their modifying reaction, their specificity on the aminoglycoside ring structure, and their specific isozyme sequence are considered. The classification system incorporates the type of enzyme mediating the reaction (e.g., N-acetyltransferase [ACC], O-adenyltransferase [ANT], O-phosphotransferase [APH]), recognition of the specific site modified using the aminoglycoside ring numbering convention, and the distinct phenotype exhibited by the modification. Thus APH (3″) Ib is an O-phosphotransferase that phosphorylates the 3″ position of the double-prime ring, resulting in resistance to streptomycin. Inactivation of the aminoglycoside by the aminoglycoside-modifying enzymes is a result of the transfer of a functional group to the aminoglycoside: AAC transfers the acetyl group from acetyl-CoA to the NH_2 group, ANT transfers the nucleotide triphosphate, and APH transfers the phosphoryl group from ATP to the OH or NH_2 group.

Recent evidence also demonstrates that the most recently approved streptogramin A, quinupristin, used in combination with streptogramin B, dalfopristin, is a target for enzymatic modification by acetyltransferases encoded by the *vat* genes found in staphylococcal and enterococcal pathogens. *E. faecium* isolates displaying resistance to virginiamycin, a streptogramin used in animal husbandry as a growth promoter, are also resistant to quinupristin, and the mechanism mediating resistance is either of two genes encoding an acetyltransferase, *vat(D)* or *vat(E)*. Characterization of *E. faecium* isolates from retail meat samples resistant to virginiamycin contained numerous allelic variations of *vat(E)*, but there is no correlation between the number of base changes observed and quinupristin-dalfopristin MICs.

Finally, a recently discovered example of enzymatic alteration of a synthetic antimicrobial involves a plasmid-borne variant of an aminoglycoside acetyltransferase (AAC(6′)-Ib) that acetylates fluoroquinolones and reduces their activity. Because fluoroquinolones are fully synthetic, naturally evolving antimicrobial resistance genes have not been considered a threat in the reduction of their activity. This variant enzyme acts against some fluoroquinolones and effects resistance to aminoglycosides, raising the implication that plasmids bearing this gene may co-select for multiple resistance.

DISSEMINATION

Resistance is an evolutionary strategy that allows microorganisms to survive chemically hostile environments such as those posed by antibiotic exposure. However, the evolution and vertical transfer of these resistance determinants to progeny is only part of the survival strategy used by microorganisms. They have evolved efficient mechanisms to exchange resistance determinants that evolved in other genera or species through evolutionary processes. The elements of transmission or dissemination that evolved to enhance the horizontal and vertical dissemination of genetic material are plasmids, transposons, insertions sequences, and integrons. **Plasmids** are circular DNA elements that replicate independently of the chromosome. They partition to daughter cells during cell division and can be donated to suitable recipient cells by conjugation following direct contact. Plasmid-encoded traits are typically not essential to survival, but carry genes that impart some selective advantage to the host bacterium, such as virulence determinants, adhesions, and antibiotic resistance genes. Plasmids also acquire and exchange information with the chromosome and other host-resident plasmids, including antibiotic resistance genes. Plasmids may be conjugative and self-transmissible or nonconjugative and require mobilization by conjugative plasmids.

Transposons (Tn) are DNA elements that encode transposition and excision functions and can transpose from one place on the chromosome and/or plasmid to another. Transposase, an enzyme that facilitates nonhomologous recombination, mediates the transposition event. Much like plasmids, transposons are also capable of carrying antibiotic resistance genes and function as shuttles, carrying these determinants among plasmids and between plasmids and the chromosome. Some transposons are conjugative and mediate their own transfer. Plasmid NR1 isolated from *Shigella flexneri* is the archetype plasmid responsible for the dissemination of antibiotic resistance in this species utilizing these elements. NR1 is a 94.5-kb multiple antibiotic-resistant plasmid that carries the genes for self-transmissibility and autonomous replication. NR1 also carries a resistance-determining region bound by direct repeats and is self-transmissible as Tn2670. Nested within Tn2670 is Tn21, a transom of particular interest not only because it exhibits the transpositional characteristic of transposons and the presence of resistance determinants, but also because it contains a potentially mobile DNA element, the integron.

Integrons are genetic elements capable of integrating resistance genes (**cassettes**) by an integron-encoded site-specific recombinase. The integron in Tn21 does not code for its own mobilization but can be moved when transposition proteins are provided in *trans*. It is bound by imperfect terminal inverted repeats, and it contains the *aadA1* resistant determinant on a cassette. The integron also contains a promoter that directs transcription of any cassette inserted into the 5′ conserved sequence of the integron. Gene cassettes contain a 59-base element recombination site that is recognized by the integron-encoded, site-specific recombinase and mediates insertion into the integron. In various bacteria, multiple gene cassettes can be arranged in tandem, and more than 60 distinct cassettes have been identified. Cassette-associated genes have been shown to confer resistance to beta-lactams, aminoglycosides, phenicols, trimethoprim, streptothricin, sulfonamides, and quaternary ammonium compounds.

NR1 also carries Tn10, which confers resistance to tetracycline and is bound by insertion sequences IS10L and IS10R. Insertion sequences (ISs) are transposons found in bacteria that carry genes only for the enzymes needed to promote their own transposition. Insertion sequence elements can form composite transposable genetic elements, such as Tn10, with the IS elements forming the proximal and distal ends and genetic material that codes for antibiotic resistance located in between. As stated previously, vancomycin is an important antibiotic used to treat infections caused by MRSA. Recently, an MRSA isolate of clinical origin was found to express phenotypic resistance to one of the few antimicrobials remaining effective in its treatment, vancomycin. This clinical isolate was found to contain a conjugative multidrug-resistant plasmid that encoded resistance to vancomycin, trimethoprim, β-lactams, aminoglycosides, and hospital disinfectants. Genetic analysis revealed the presence of a multiresistant conjugative plasmid harboring Tn 1546 (VanA). A Tn-1546–like transposable genetic element encoding for transposition, regulation of VanA expression, and resistance is also found in enterococci. The data suggest the interspecies transfer of Tn1546 from a co-resident isolate of *E. faecalis* to MRSA. Resistance to vancomycin can be spread by the transposition of the Tn-1547 to a conjugative plasmid and transferred by conjugation to recipient strains, or by excision and circularization of the transposons followed by conjugation.

Until recently, quinolone resistance was believed to arise solely from chromosomal mutations in genes encoding target enzymes or via active efflux. It is now clear that plasmid-mediated quinolone resistance (PMAR) occurs and is conferred by unusual resistance determinants including *qnr, aac(6′)-Ib-cr,* and *qepA* (an efflux pump belonging to the major facilitator subfamily). *Qnr* was discovered in a *K. pneumoniae* isolate from Birmingham, Alabama, collected in 1994 and was found in an integron-like structure on the MDR plasmid, pMG252. Qnr, the gene product, is a member of the pentapeptide repeat family of proteins and has been shown to block the action of ciprofloxacin on purified DNA gyrase and topoisomerase IV. Subsequently, *qnr* plasmids have been reported from clinical isolates of *E. coli, Citrobacter freundii, Enterobacter* spp., *K. pneumoniae, Providencia stuartii,* and *Salmonella* species from across the globe. The different *qnr* genes reported to date include *qnrA, qnrB, qnrC,* and *qnrS,* and a total of 6 *qnrA,* 4 *qnrS,* and 20 *qnrB* variants have been described in the literature.

The plasmid-encoded Qnr proteins derived from *E. coli, Klebsiella oxytoca,* and *K. pneumoniae* isolates recovered from different geographic sources (China, Europe, and the United States) show almost identical amino acid residues, indicating that these proteins likely have common origins. There is also evidence supporting a role for these plasmids in linking resistance to quinolones and extended-spectrum β-lactams. This is especially troubling given the importance of fluoroquinolones and β-lactams in clinical medicine.

In addition to self-transmissible mobile DNA elements, antimicrobial resistance determinants can be spread among bacteria via uptake of naked DNA from the surrounding environment **(transformation)** or upon infection with a bacteriophage carrying resistance genes **(transduction).** Transformation was the first mechanism of DNA transfer to be discovered among prokaryotes and involves DNA scavenging by a bacterium after the death and deterioration of a nearby bacterium. The DNA in a dead bacterium degrades and is broken into fragments released into the surrounding milieu, which can be taken up by transformation-competent recipients. If antibiotic resistance genes are included in the degraded DNA, they can be taken up by a nearby bacterium and incorporated into the bacterial genome. Genetic exchange via transduction involves **bacteriophage** infection of a bacterium, phage replication, packaging of some of the bacterial DNA with the phage DNA (which may include resistance determinants), and lysis of that bacterium and infection of subse-

quent bacteria. Upon subsequent infection, those resistance determinants may be transferred to the infected bacterium. The contribution of transformation and transduction in the evolution of multidrug resistance is difficult to assess, but laboratory demonstrations indicate that it theoretically plays a role in antimicrobial resistance development.

BIBLIOGRAPHY

Abbanat D, Morrow B, Bush K: New agents in development for the treatment of bacterial infections, *Curr Opin Pharmacol* 8:582-592, 2008.

Anderson GG, O'Toole GA: Innate and induced resistance mechanisms of bacterial biofilms, *Curr Top Microbiol Immunol* 322:85, 2008.

Arias CA, Murray BE: Emergence and management of drug-resistant enterococcal infections, *Expert Rev Anti Infect Ther* 6:637, 2008.

Boucher HW, Talbot GH, Bradley JS, Edwards JE, Gilbert D, Rice LB, Scheld M, Spellberg B: Bad bugs, no drugs: no ESKAPE! An update from the Infectious Diseases Society of America. *Clin Infect Dis* 48(1):1-12, 2009 Jan 1.

Bartlett J: Bad bugs, no drugs: no ESKAPE! An update from the Infectious Diseases Society of America. *Clin Infect Dis* 48(1):1-12, 2009 Jan 1.

Bush K: Extended-spectrum beta-lactamases in North America, 1987-2006, *Clin Microbiol Infect* 14(Suppl 1):134-143, 2008.

Davies D: Understanding biofilm resistance to antibacterial agents, *Nat Rev Drug Discov* 2:114, 2003.

Davies JA: Origins, acquisition, and dissemination of antibiotic resistant determinants. In Chadwick DJ, Goode J, editors: *Antibiotic resistance: origins, evolution, and spread,* New York, 1997, Wiley.

Davin-Regli A et al: Membrane permeability and regulation of drug "influx and efflux" in enterobacterial pathogens, *Curr Drug Targets* 9:750, 2008.

D'Costa VM et al: Sampling the antibiotic resistome, *Science* 311:374, 2006.

Depardieu F et al: Modes and modulations of antibiotic resistance gene expression, *Clin Microbiol Rev* 20:79, 2007.

Drlica K et al: DNA gyrase, topoisomerase IV, and the 4-quinolones, *Microbiol Mol Biol Rev* 61:377, 1997.

French GL: What's new and not so new on the antimicrobial horizon? *Clin Microbiol Infect* 14(Suppl 6):19, 2008.

Hong HJ, Hutchings MI, Buttner MJ; Biotechnology and Biological Sciences Research Council, UK: Vancomycin resistance VanS/VanR two-component systems, *Adv Exp Med Biol* 631:200, 2008.

Hooper D: Target modification as a mechanism of antimicrobial resistance. In Lewis K et al, editors: *Bacterial resistance to antimicrobials,* New York, 2002, Marcel Dekker.

Ito T et al: Structural composition of three types of staphylococcal cassette chromosome mec integrated in the chromosome of methicillin-resistant *Staphylococcus aureus, Antimicrob Agents Chemother* 45:1323, 2001.

Jacobs MR: Antimicrobial-resistant *Streptococcus pneumoniae:* trends and management, *Expert Rev Anti Infect Ther* 6:619, 2008.

Jacoby GA: AmpC beta-lactamases, *Clin Microbiol Rev* 22:161, 2009.

Kiran MD et al: Suppression of biofilm related, device-associated infections by staphylococcal quorum sensing inhibitors, *Int J Artif Organs* 31:761, 2008.

Lee C: Therapeutic challenges in the era of antibiotic resistance, *Int J Antimicrob Agents* 32(Suppl 4):S197, 2008.

Li XZ, Nikaido H: Efflux-mediated drug resistance in bacteria, *Drugs* 64:159, 2004.

Liebert CA et al: Transposon Tn21, flagship of the floating genome, *Microbiol Molecular Biol Rev* 63:507, 1999.

Luna VA et al: A variety of gram-positive bacteria carry mobile *mef* genes, *J Antimicrob Chemother* 44:19, 1999.

Lundstrom TS et al: Antibiotic for gram-positive bacterial infections: vancomycin, quinupristin-dalfopristin, linezolid, and daptomycin, *Infect Dis Clin North Am* 18:651, 2004.

Macgowan AP; BSAC Working Parties on Resistance Surveillance: Clinical implications of antimicrobial resistance for therapy, *J Antimicrob Chemother* 62(Suppl 2):ii105, 2008.

Martinez JL et al: A global view of antibiotic resistance, *FEMS Microbiol Rev* 33:44-65, 2009.

Martínez-Martínez L et al: Plasmid-mediated quinolone resistance, *Expert Rev Anti Infect Ther* 6:685, 2008.

Pagès JM et al: The porin and the permeating antibiotic: a selective diffusion barrier in Gram-negative bacteria, *Nat Rev Microbiol* 6:893, 2008.

Pallecchi L et al: Antibiotic resistance in the absence of antimicrobial use: mechanisms and implications, *Expert Rev Anti Infect Ther* 6:725, 2008.

Patterson JE: Extended-spectrum beta-lactamases, *Semin Respir Infect* 15:299, 2000.

Pietras Z et al: Structure and mechanism of drug efflux machinery in Gram negative bacteria, *Curr Drug Targets* 9:719, 2008.

Rodríguez-Baño J, Pascual A: Clinical significance of extended-spectrum beta-lactamases, *Expert Rev Anti Infect Ther* 6:671, 2008.

Schairer J et al: Methicillin-resistant *Staphylococcus aureus* infection with intermediate sensitivity to vancomycin: a case report and literature review, *J Intensive Care Med* 23:338, 2008.

Spellberg B, Bartlett J: Bad bugs, no drugs: no ESKAPE! An update from the Infectious Diseases Society of America, *Clin Infect Dis* 48:1, 2009.

Webb V, Davies J: Antibiotic preparations contain DNA: a source of drug resistance genes? *Antimicrob Agents Chemother* 37:237, 1993.

Werner G et al: Acquired vancomycin resistance in clinically relevant pathogens, *Future Microbiol* 3:547, 2008.

White PA et al: Integrons and gene cassettes in the Enterobacteriaceae, *Antimicrob Agents Chemother* 45:2685, 2001.

White DG et al, editors: *Frontiers in antimicrobial resistance: a tribute to Stuart B. Levy*, Washington, DC, 2005, American Society for Microbiology.

Yoshida H et al: Quinolone resistance-determining region in the DNA gyrase *gyrA* gene of *Escherichia coli*, *Antimicrob Ag Chemother* 34:1271, 1990.

Points to Remember

- Although resistance to antibiotics may be genetically intrinsic or acquired, both genetic types can be found in the same pathogen.
- Impermeability and efflux mechanism of resistance can produce multidrug resistance phenotypes.
- A single organism may acquire multiple mechanisms of resistance, including different mechanisms conferring resistance to the same compound.
- Antibiotic mechanisms of resistance and their dissemination are not static processes.

Learning Assessment Questions

1. Which characteristic describes the origin of antibiotics?
   a. They are natural molecules.
   b. They are synthetic molecules.
   c. They are semisynthetic molecules.
   d. All of the above.

2. Microorganisms can exhibit antibiotic resistance due to which of the following?
   a. Intrinsic
   b. Acquired
   c. Both
   d. Neither

3. Which mechanisms of antibiotic resistance are intrinsic and acquired?
   a. Efflux
   b. Enzymatic
   c. Biofilm
   d. Acquisition of new targets
   e. a and b
   f. a and c

4. Plasmids can contain which of the following?
   a. Transposons
   b. Insertion sequences
   c. Integron cassettes
   d. All of the above
   e. a and c

5. Transposons do not contain:
   a. Cytoplasmic membranes
   b. Transposase
   c. Excision proteins
   d. Antibiotic resistance determinants
   e. Conjugative functions

6. Which of the following characteristics apply to efflux pumps?
   a. They are found in gram-positive and gram-negative bacteria.
   b. They are transporter proteins.
   c. They have single or multiple substrates.
   d. a and c.
   e. All of the above.

7. Which does not apply for antibiotic resistance due to target site modification?
   a. Chromosomal mutation of target site
   b. Quinolone resistance determining region
   c. SCCmec
   d. Erythromycin resistance methylase

8. Enzymatic modification of aminoglycosides is not due to which of the following?
   a. N-acetylation
   b. Dimethylation
   c. O-phosphorylation
   d. O-adenylation
   e. All of the above

9. Which is not a characteristic of integrons?
   a. Potentially mobile element
   b. Gene cassettes
   c. 59–base-pair element
   d. All of the above
   e. Peptidoglycan

10. Serine-based β-lactamases appear to have evolved from the PBPs of bacteria. True or false?

Antimicrobial Susceptibility Testing

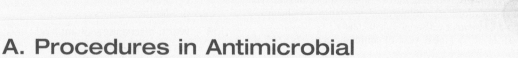

A. Procedures in Antimicrobial Susceptibility Testing

Frederic J. Marsik*

- **REASONS AND INDICATIONS FOR PERFORMING ANTIMICROBIAL SUSCEPTIBILITY TESTS**
  Factors to Consider When Determining Whether Testing Is Warranted
- **SELECTING ANTIMICROBIAL AGENTS FOR TESTING AND REPORTING**
  Selection of Test Batteries
  Reporting of Susceptibility Test Results
- **TRADITIONAL ANTIMICROBIAL SUSCEPTIBILITY TEST METHODS**
  Inoculum Preparation and Use of McFarland Standards
  Dilution Susceptibility Test Methods
  Disk Diffusion Testing
  Modified Methods for Testing Slow-Growing or Fastidious Bacteria
  Additional Organism and Antimicrobial Agent Testing Concerns

- **AUTOMATED ANTIMICROBIAL SUSCEPTIBILITY TEST METHODS**
  Principles of Technologies Used
  Currently Available Automated Systems
  Nonautomated Antimicrobial Susceptibility Test Method: Etest
- **INTERPRETATION OF IN VITRO ANTIMICROBIAL SUSCEPTIBILITY TEST RESULTS**
- **METHODS OF DETECTING ANTIMICROBIAL-INACTIVATING ENZYMES**
  β-Lactamase Tests
- **QUALITY CONTROL OF ANTIMICROBIAL SUSCEPTIBILITY TESTS**
- **SELECTING AN ANTIMICROBIAL SUSCEPTIBILITY TEST METHOD**

OBJECTIVES

After reading and studying this chapter, you should be able to:

1. Explain the rationale behind the performance of antimicrobial susceptibility tests.
2. Describe the method for selection of specific drugs in testing and reporting.
3. Define *minimal inhibitory concentration* (MIC) and the methods that are used for determination of MICs.
4. Explain how zone interpretive criteria used with the disk diffusion test are established.
5. List the variables that must be controlled when antimicrobial susceptibility tests are performed.
6. Describe test modifications for antimicrobial susceptibility testing of *Campylobacter* spp., *Streptococcus* spp. (including *Streptococcus pneumoniae*), *Haemophilus* spp., *Neisseria gonorrhoeae, Neisseria meningitidis,* and anaerobes.
7. Explain the principles behind automated antimicrobial susceptibility test methods.
8. Discuss several commercially available antimicrobial susceptibility test systems in current use.
9. List the organisms for which β-lactamase testing is useful.
10. Explain the reliable methods for detection of methicillin-resistant *Staphylococcus aureus,* vancomycin-intermediate *S. aureus,* and vancomycin-resistant *S. aureus.*
11. Discuss use of the D-zone test.
12. Describe the significance of high-level aminoglycoside resistance in enterococci.

---

*This chapter was originally prepared and written by Janet Fick Hindler and James H. Jorgenson.

13. Explain extended-spectrum β-lactamases and how organisms that produce these enzymes are detected in the clinical laboratory.

14. Discuss quality control procedures for antimicrobial susceptibility tests.

15. Describe how antibiograms can be used to help verify the accuracy of results generated by testing patient isolates.

16. Discuss situations in which cumulative antibiograms may help to guide antimicrobial therapy.

17. Explain how to select a particular susceptibility test method for routine use.

18. Explain the meanings of *nonsusceptible, susceptible, intermediate,* and *resistant* as applied to antimicrobial susceptibility test results.

Case in Point

The microbiology laboratory supervisor was reviewing patient reports that the "floating" technologist had generated earlier in the day. She saw a susceptibility report for *Staphylococcus aureus* isolated from a patient's wound; this report included the following results from disk diffusion testing: cefazolin-S, cefoxitin-R, clindamycin-R, erythromycin-R, penicillin-R, and vancomycin-S, but there was no result for oxacillin. The supervisor realized that the technologist who had reported these results might have forgotten about the new method for detecting methicillin-resistant staphylocorcus areus (MRSA) that was implemented a few months earlier and the reporting rules for β-lactam agents and MRSA. She went to the technologist and reminded her of the special testing methods and reporting rules, and the technologist corrected and re-released the report, which was as follows: cefazolin-R, clindamycin-R, erythromycin-R, oxacillin-R, penicillin-R, and vancomycin-S.

Issues to Consider

After reading the patient's case history, consider:

- Use of surrogate antimicrobial agents to test for resistance or susceptibility for the drug actually reported
- Editing certain susceptible results to resistant when bacteria with specific types of resistance are encountered
- Modifications of standard tests that might be necessary to detect specific types of emerging resistance

Key Terms

Agar-dilution MIC

β-lactamases

Borderline–oxacillin-resistant isolates

Breakpoint (cutoff)

Breakpoint panel

Broth-macrodilution MIC

Broth-microdilution MIC

Chromosomally mediated–resistant *Neisseria gonorrhoeae* (CMRNG)

Clinical and Laboratory Standards Institute (CLSI)

Cumulative antibiogram

D-zone test

Etest

Extended-spectrum β-lactamase (ESBL)

Food and Drug Administration (FDA)

Heteroresistant

High-level aminoglycoside resistance

Intermediate

Kirby-Bauer test

McFarland turbidity standards

mecA gene

Methicillin-resistant *Staphylococcus aureus* (MRSA)

Minimal inhibitory concentration (MIC)

Nonsusceptible

Oxacillin screen plate

Penicillinase-producing *Neisseria gonorrhoeae* (PPNG)

Penicillinase-resistant penicillins

Population analysis profiles (PAP)

Resistant

Selective reporting

Skipped wells

Susceptible

Trailing

Tube-dilution MIC

Vancomycin agar screen plate

Vancomycin-intermediate *Staphylococcus aureus* (VISA)

Vancomycin-resistant enterococci (VRE)

Vancomycin-resistant *Staphylococcus aureus* (VRSA)

Zone of inhibition

Antimicrobial susceptibility testing is performed on bacteria isolated from clinical specimens to determine which antimicrobial agents might be effective in treating infections caused by the bacteria. Only bacteria that are likely to be contributing to an infection should be tested. Testing bacteria that are not involved in the infection would be misleading to the physician and could lead to a more serious infection with development of antimicrobial resistance. One of the major challenges in clinical microbiology is the identification of the bacterium or bacteria that are the cause of infections. Often these bacteria need to be distinguished from the flora that may reside at the site of the infection normally, although in some situations the microbial flora that reside at the site of the infection may be contributing to the infection. Therefore it is important to realize that thought needs to go into determining which bacterium or bacteria from a specimen will be tested for susceptibility to antimicrobials. Most microbiology laboratories have guidelines for determining when susceptibility testing will be done and on which bacteria the susceptibility testing will be done. When in doubt about the significance of a bacterium or bacteria from a specimen, it is best to discuss the situation with the attending physician.

In clinical laboratories, susceptibility testing is usually performed by either disk diffusion or a dilution (**minimal inhibitory concentration [MIC]**) method. Standards that describe these methods are published and frequently updated by the **Clinical and Laboratory Standards Institute (CLSI,** formerly the National Committee for Clinical Laboratory Standards

[NCCLS]). Clinical laboratories can perform testing according to recommendations in the CLSI standards or use one of several different types of commercial manual or automated antimicrobial susceptibility test systems. In all cases, it is important to maintain an awareness of which antimicrobial agents it would be appropriate to test, the reliability of various test systems for detecting antimicrobial resistance, and strategies for effectively communicating results on laboratory reports.

REASONS AND INDICATIONS FOR PERFORMING ANTIMICROBIAL SUSCEPTIBILITY TESTS

Antimicrobial susceptibility testing should be performed on a bacterial isolate from a clinical specimen if the isolate is determined to be a probable cause of the patient's infection and the susceptibility of the isolate to particular antimicrobial agents cannot be reliably predicted. Susceptibility tests are not performed on bacteria that are predictably susceptible to the antimicrobial agents commonly used to treat infections caused by these bacteria. Group A β-hemolytic *Streptococcus,* for example, is not routinely tested because it is universally susceptible to penicillin, the drug of choice in treating infections caused by this bacterium. In contrast, the recommended agent for treating *Staphylococcus aureus* infections is oxacillin, but *S. aureus* may or may not be susceptible to oxacillin. Consequently, susceptibility testing is indicated for an *S. aureus* isolate that is the suspected cause of an infection.

Factors to Consider When Determining Whether Testing Is Warranted

In addition to the unpredictable susceptibility of a potential pathogen, other important factors must be considered when determining whether antimicrobial susceptibility testing is warranted; these factors include the following:
- The body site from which the organism was isolated
- The presence of other bacteria and the quality of the specimen from which the organism was grown
- The host's status

Body Site

Susceptibility tests are not routinely performed on bacteria that are isolated from an anatomic site for which they are normal inhabitants. For example, *Escherichia coli* are normal biota in the lower gastrointestinal tract and therefore would not be tested when isolated from stool; however, *E. coli* from a blood culture would be tested because blood should be sterile. Similarly, viridans group streptococci represent normal biota in throat specimens and would not be routinely tested. Coagulase-negative staphylococci isolated from multiple blood cultures would be tested. However, because coagulase-negative staphylococci are commonly found on skin surfaces, these organisms would not be tested when isolated from superficial wound specimens. Testing of normal biota isolates or isolates likely to represent contamination or colonization should be avoided because reporting of antimicrobial susceptibility results may encourage a physician to treat a normal condition and refrain from further investigation of the true cause of the patient's problem.

Presence of Other Bacteria and Quality of Specimen

The isolation of an organism in pure culture is less likely to represent contamination than a mixed culture. The presence of more than two species at greater than 10^5 colony-forming units (CFU) per milliliter isolated from urine suggests contamination, and these organisms may not require susceptibility testing; however, a pure culture of *E. coli* at greater than 10^5 CFU per milliliter would likely represent true infection and would be tested. A few *Klebsiella pneumoniae* organisms in the presence of many normal biota in a sputum culture may not be significant. In the absence of normal biota, however, a few colonies of this species, particularly if noted on a Gram stain of the sputum, may be significant and warrant testing of the isolates.

Host Status

The host status of the patient often influences susceptibility testing decisions. Species usually viewed as normal biota might be responsible for an infection and therefore at times might require testing in immunosuppressed patients. Additionally, in patients who are allergic to penicillin and who have a group A β-hemolytic streptococcal infection, erythromycin (or another macrolide) is the drug of choice, and β-hemolytic streptococci are occasionally resistant to this agent. Consequently, testing of erythromycin is warranted on isolates from penicillin-allergic patients.

SELECTING ANTIMICROBIAL AGENTS FOR TESTING AND REPORTING

Approximately 50 antimicrobial agents are in use presently for treating bacterial infections, and many of these have comparable clinical efficacy. Each laboratory must determine which agents are appropriate for routine testing against various organisms (or organism groups) in its particular setting. Laboratory workers should not formulate testing and reporting protocols without input from drug prescribers. Representatives from the infectious diseases service and other services, the institution's pharmacy, and the therapeutics committee must provide input regarding the clinical utility of various agents in an institution. The antimicrobial package inserts written by the U.S. **Food and Drug Administration (FDA)** should be consulted for information concerning the dosing and indications for which the antimicrobial was approved and the performance of the antimicrobial agent during initial clinical trials.

It is important that the drugs tested by the laboratory match as closely as possible the institutional formulary. From the laboratory perspective, the limiting factor for the numbers of drugs tested is usually the number that can be practically tested with a particular method. For example, the standard disk diffusion test uses a 150-mm agar plate, which can accommodate no more than 12 disks. In the case of MIC test panels, 12 to 15 antimicrobials can be tested on one panel. Depending on the format of the panel, some commercial antimicrobial susceptibility systems can test more drugs.

The patient population must be considered in the choice of antimicrobial agents to be tested. Some agents are contraindicated in pediatric patients (e.g., fluoroquinolones, which may impair cartilage development, and tetracycline, which damages developing teeth). Emphasis should be placed on testing oral agents when dealing with outpatient specimens. Additional guidelines for developing a testing and reporting strategy are found within the CLSI documents for disk diffusion or MIC testing. These documents include tables (Box 13-1 and Table 13-1) that list primary and secondary agents appropriate for testing against various organism groups. Also listed are drugs that should be reported on urine isolates only. An example of a listing for Enterobacteriaceae is shown in Box 13-1.

Selection of Test Batteries

Generally a laboratory will define a battery of 10 to 15 antimicrobial agents for routine testing against the Enterobacteriaceae, *Pseudomonas* spp., nonfastidious gram-negative bacilli (e.g., *Acinetobacter* spp., *Stenotrophomonas maltophilia*, and *Burkholderia cepacia*), staphylococci, and enterococci. Sometimes a separate battery is performed for urine isolates, representing drugs appropriate for treating urinary tract infections (UTIs). A supplemental battery that contains antimicrobial agents with enhanced activity may be included by laboratories that encounter a significant number of organisms resistant to the more commonly used antimicrobials.

Reporting of Susceptibility Test Results

Because the identity of the bacterial isolate is often unknown at the time the susceptibility test is performed, some drugs may be tested on an isolate that may be inappropriate for reporting. In such instances, a drug should not be indiscriminately reported because results may be misleading. Some drugs may appear active against certain species in vitro but are inappropriate for clinical use (e.g., cephalosporins and trimethoprim-sulfamethoxazole against enterococci). The final reporting decision should be made once the identity of

---

BOX 13-1 Suggested Groupings of Antimicrobial Agents with FDA Clinical Indications That Should Be Considered for Routine Testing and Reporting by Clinical Microbiology Laboratories for Enterobacteriaceae

Group A Primary Test and Report
Ampicillin[a]
Cefazolin[b]
Cephalothin[b]
Gentamicin
Tobramycin

Group B Primary Test Report Selectively
Amikacin
Amoxicillin-clavulanic acid
Ampicillin/sulbactam
Piperacillin-tazobactam
Ticarcillin-clavulanic acid
Cefonicid or cefuroxime
Cefepime
Cefotetan
Cefoxitin
Cefotaxime[a,c,d] or ceftriaxone[a,c,d]
Ciprofloxacin[a]

Levofloxacin[a]
Ertapenem
Imipenem
Meropenem
Piperacillin
Trimethoprim-sulfamethoxazole[a]

Group C Supplemental Report Selectively
Aztreonam
Ceftazidime
Aztreonam and ceftazidime are helpful indicators of extended spectrum β-lactamases[d]
Chloramphenicol[a,e]
Tetracycline[f]

Group U Supplemental for Urine Only
Lomefloxacin or ofloxacin
Nitrofurantoin
Sulfisoxazole
Trimethoprim

Modified from Clinical and Laboratory Standards Institute (CLSI) publication M100-S19, *Performance standards for antimicrobial susceptibility testing: nineteenth informational supplement.* Copies of the current edition may be obtained from CLSI, 940 West Valley Road, Suite 1400, Wayne, Pa., 19087-1898.

[a]When fecal isolates of *Salmonella* and *Shigella* spp. are tested, only ampicillin, a fluoroquinolone, and trimethoprim-sulfamethoxazole should be tested and reported routinely. In addition, chloramphenicol and a third-generation cephalosporin should be tested and reported for extraintestinal isolates of *Salmonella* spp.

[b]Cephalothin can be used to represent cephalothin, cephapirin, cephradine, cephalexin, cefaclor, and cefadroxil. Cefazolin, cefuroxime, cefpodoxime, and cefprozil (urinary isolates only) may be tested individually because some isolates may be susceptible to these agents when resistant to cephalothin.

[c]Cefotaxime or ceftriaxone should be tested and reported on isolates from cerebrospinal fluid in place of cephalothin and cefazolin.

[d]Strains of *Klebsiella* spp. and *Escherichia coli* that produce extended spectrum β-lactamases (ESBLs) may be clinically resistant to therapy with penicillins, cephalosporins, or aztreonam, despite apparent in vitro susceptibility to some of these agents. Some of these strains will show zones of inhibition below the normal susceptible population but above the standard breakpoint for certain extended-spectrum cephalosporins or aztreonam; such strains may be screened for potential ESBL production by using the screening breakpoints listed in Table 13-1. Other strains may test intermediate or resistant by standard breakpoints to one or more of these agents. In all strains with ESBLs, the zone diameters for one or more of the extended-spectrum cephalosporins should increase in the presence of clavulanic acid. For all ESBL-producing strains, the test interpretation should be reported as resistant for all penicillins, cephalosporins, and aztreonam.

[e]Not routinely reported on organisms isolated from the urinary tract.

[f]Organisms that are susceptible to tetracycline are also considered susceptible to doxycycline and minocycline. However, some organisms that are intermediate or resistant to tetracycline may be susceptible to doxycycline or minocycline or both.

TABLE 13-1 Examples of Antimicrobial Agents Reported Following a Selective Reporting Protocol, as Suggested in Table 1, CLSI M100-S19*

	Drug	Result
Escherichia coli (source: urine)	Ampicillin	S
	Cephalothin	S
	Gentamicin	S
	Nitrofurantoin	S
	Trimethoprim/sulfamethoxazole	S
E. coli (source: urine)	Ampicillin	R
	Ampicillin/sulbactam	R
	Cefoxitin	S
	Cephalothin	R
	Ciprofloxacin	S
	Gentamicin	S
	Nitrofurantoin	S
	Trimethoprim/sulfamethoxazole	R
Enterobacter cloacae (source: blood)	**Amikacin**	S
	Ampicillin	R
	Ampicillin/sulbactam	R
	Cefepime	S
	Cefoxitin	R
	Cefotaxime	S
	Gentamicin	R
	Trimethoprim-sulfamethoxazole	R

Modified from Clinical and Laboratory Standards Institute (CLSI) publication M100-S19: *Performance standards for antimicrobial susceptibility testing: nineteenth informational supplement.* Copies of the current edition may be obtained from CLSI, 940 West Valley Road, Suite 1400, Wayne, Pa., 19087-1898.
R, Resistant; *S,* susceptible.
*Primary agents (group A) are in plain type and secondary agents (group B) are in bold type.

the isolate is known (sometimes a preliminary identification is sufficient), and the overall susceptibility results and specimen source must be taken into consideration.

As mentioned previously, reporting protocols should be developed following discussion with infectious disease clinicians, pharmacists, and others who have clinical experience with the antimicrobial therapy practices of the particular institution. A primary tenet of antimicrobial therapy is to use the least toxic, most cost-effective, and most clinically effective agents and to refrain from costly, broader-spectrum agents. Achieving physician compliance with this objective is often difficult. Sometimes all drugs tested are reported, and the mechanism of control for inappropriate prescribing is then outside the laboratory's purview. Alternatively the laboratory may assist in discouraging inappropriate antimicrobial prescribing by refraining from reporting broad-spectrum agents if narrower-spectrum agents are active in vitro. The CLSI provides guidance for development of such a selective-reporting or cascade-reporting protocol.

For several organism groups, CLSI categorizes antimicrobial agents into four groups (see Box 13-1). As a general guideline, it is suggested that within a particular antimicrobial class, primary (group A) agents be reported first and that secondary (group B) agents be reported only if one of the following conditions exists:

- The isolate is resistant to the primary agents.
- The patient cannot tolerate the primary agents.
- The infection has not responded to the primary agents.
- A secondary agent would be a better clinical choice for the particular infection (e.g., meningitis).
- The patient has organisms isolated from another site, and a secondary agent might be useful for treating both organisms.

For example, a primary cephalosporin, such as cefazolin (a first-generation cephalosporin), would be a reasonable choice for a susceptible *E. coli,* and secondary cephalosporins, such as cefuroxime (a second-generation cephalosporin) or cefotaxime (third-generation cephalosporin), would generally not be required. An exception would occur with meningitis because third-generation cephalosporins cross the blood-brain barrier much more effectively than their first-generation counterparts. Gentamicin is usually the aminoglycoside of choice for treating serious infections caused by gentamicin-susceptible *Pseudomonas aeruginosa,* and tobramycin or amikacin may be considered for gentamicin-resistant isolates. Aminoglycosides are not effective for treating meningitis because they do not readily cross the blood-brain barrier.

A secondary agent may be reported also if the patient has a polymicrobial infection, and a secondary (but not a primary) agent would be more likely to be effective against all pathogens present. Similarly, a secondary agent may be reported if the patient has a disseminated infection, and a secondary (but not a primary) agent would be more likely to be effective at all sites. Agents with very broad-spectrum activity or increased potency (group C) may be tested and reported for the reasons listed for secondary agents. In addition, group C agents would be considered for routine testing if a particular institution encounters large numbers of isolates resistant to group A and group B agents. Finally, agents with activity only in the urinary tract should be reported only on isolates from urine because these drugs are clinically ineffective in treating other infections. Examples of reports generated following a **selective reporting** protocol are shown in Table 13-1; CLSI Table 1 (see Box 13-1) was used to determine whether agents are considered primary or secondary.

TRADITIONAL ANTIMICROBIAL SUSCEPTIBILITY TEST METHODS

Inoculum Preparation and Use of McFarland Standards

Inoculum Preparation

Inoculum preparation is one of the most critical steps in any susceptibility test. Inocula are prepared by adding cells from four to five isolated colonies of similar colony morphology to a broth medium and then allowing them to grow to the log phase. Four to five colonies, rather than a single colony, are selected to minimize the possibility of testing a colony that might have been derived from a susceptible mutant. Inocula can also be prepared directly by suspending colonies grown overnight on an agar plate directly in broth or saline. This direct inoculum suspension preparation technique is preferred for bacteria that grow unpredictably in broth (e.g., fastidious bacteria). Because it does not rely on growth in an inoculum broth, the use of fresh (16- to 24-hour) colonies is imperative.

McFarland Turbidity Standards

The number of bacteria tested must be standardized regardless of the susceptibility method used. False-susceptible results may occur if too few bacteria are tested, and false-resistant results may be the outcome of testing too many bacteria. The most widely used method of inoculum standardization involves **McFarland turbidity standards.** McFarland standards can be prepared by adding specific volumes of 1% sulfuric acid and 1.175% barium chloride to obtain a barium sulfate solution with a specific optical density. The most commonly used is the McFarland 0.5 standard, which contains 99.5 mL of 1% sulfuric acid and 0.5 mL of 1.175% barium chloride. This solution is dispensed into tubes comparable with those used for inoculum preparation, which are sealed tightly and stored in the dark at room temperature. The McFarland 0.5 standard provides turbidity comparable with that of a bacterial suspension containing approximately 1.5×108 CFU/mL. Recently, suspensions of latex particles have been used as a simpler, more stable alternative to barium sulfate to achieve turbidity comparable with that of the McFarland standard.

Inoculum Standardization

To standardize the inoculum, the inoculated broth or direct suspension is vortexed thoroughly; then, under adequate lighting, the tube is positioned side by side with the 0.5 McFarland standard against a white card containing several horizontal black lines (Figure 13-1). The turbidities are compared by looking at the black lines through the suspensions. The suspension is too dense if it is more difficult to see the lines through the inoculum suspension than through the McFarland 0.5 standard. In such a case the inoculum would be diluted with additional sterile broth or saline. If the test suspension is too light, more organisms are added or the suspension is reincubated (depending on the inoculum preparation protocol) until the turbidity reaches that of the McFarland standard. Once standardized, the inoculum suspensions should be used within 15 minutes of preparation. A convenient and more precise alternative to visual adjustment to match the McFarland standard is the use of a nephelometric or spectrophotometric device. Several simple, commercially available benchtop instruments are available for more objective standardization of bacterial inocula in the clinical laboratory (Figure 13-2).

Dilution Susceptibility Testing Methods

Principle

Dilution antimicrobial susceptibility test methods are used to determine the MIC, or the lowest concentration of antimicrobial agent required to inhibit the growth of a bacterial isolate. Varying concentrations of an antimicrobial agent are added to broth or agar media. Generally serial twofold-dilution con-

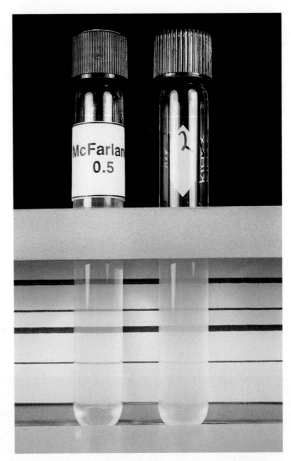

FIGURE 13-1 The tube on the left is a McFarland 0.5 turbidity standard. The tube on the right is a test bacterial suspension that has turbidity greater than that of the McFarland standard; it is more difficult to see the black lines through the test suspension than through the McFarland standard. Sterile saline or broth must be added to the test suspension to dilute it until the turbidity matches that of the McFarland standard.

centrations are tested (expressed in μg/mL), and these approximate concentrations that are attainable in vivo following standard dosages for the respective antimicrobial agent. Because the concentrations attainable in vivo vary with different agents, the ranges of concentrations tested vary also. For example, sustained concentrations greater than 8 μg/mL for gentamicin and tobramycin cannot be safely attained in the patient, and therefore the concentrations tested are generally in the range of 0.25 to 8.0 μg/mL. In contrast, much higher levels of the extended-spectrum penicillin piperacillin are attainable in vivo, and a range of 4 to 128 μg/mL might be tested. Once the MIC is determined, the organism is interpreted as either **nonsusceptible, susceptible, intermediate,** or **resistant** to each agent with the use of a table provided in the CLSI dilution testing document or in the FDA-approved package insert for the antimicrobial. Both the FDA and CLSI are involved in determining antimicrobial interpretive criteria for MIC test results. An example is shown in Table 13-2. Note that for some antimicrobial agents, different MIC interpretive criteria exist for different organisms or organism groups. For

TABLE 13-2 Minimal Inhibitory Concentration Interpretive Standards (μg/mL) for Several Organism Groups

Antimicrobial Agent	Susceptible	Intermediate	Resistant
Ampicillin			
When testing Enterobacteriaceae	≤8	16	≥32
When testing staphylococci	≤0.25	—	≥0.5
When testing enterococci	≤8	—	≥16
When testing *Haemophilus* spp.	≤1	2	≥4
When testing viridans group streptococci	≤0.25	0.5-4.0	≥8
When testing *Listeria monocytogenes*	≤2	—	—
Gentamicin			
When testing Enterobacteriaceae	≤4	8	≥16
When testing *Pseudomonas aeruginosa*	≤4	8	≥16
When testing staphylococci	≤4	8	≥16
Oxacillin			
When testing *Staphylococcus aureus*	≤2	—	≥4
When testing coagulase-negative staphylococci	≤0.25	—	≥0.5

Modified from Clinical and Laboratory Standards Institute (CLSI) publication M100-S19: *Performance standards for antimicrobial susceptibility testing: nineteenth informational supplement.* Copies of the current edition may be obtained from CLSI, 940 West Valley Road, Suite 1400, Wayne, Pa., 19087-1898.

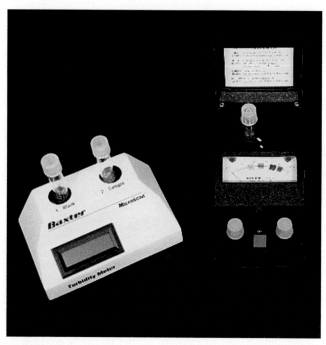

FIGURE 13-2   Three benchtop nephelometric-type devices can be used to standardize the turbidity of a test inoculum suspension to match that of a McFarland 0.5 (or other) turbidity standard.

each antimicrobial agent, the MIC breakpoint separates susceptible from resistant results. Organisms with MICs at or below the breakpoint are susceptible, and those with MICs above that breakpoint are intermediate or resistant. The CLSI documents describe the details of performing MIC tests by broth macrodilution, broth microdilution, and agar dilution methods. These methods are briefly summarized in the following sections.

Antimicrobial Stock Solutions

Antimicrobial stock solutions used in MIC tests must be prepared from reference standard antimicrobial powders, not from the pharmaceutical preparations administered to patients. Details of preparation are found in the CLSI protocols. Stock drug solutions must be stored frozen in non–frost-free freezers. Temperatures at or below −60° C are optimal and necessary for more temperature-labile drugs such as imipenem and clavulanic acid; however, −20° C storage is acceptable for some agents. Antimicrobial solutions must not be refrozen after thawing.

Broth-Macrodilution (Tube-Dilution) Tests

Broth dilution MIC tests performed in test tubes are referred to as **broth-macrodilution MIC** or **tube-dilution MIC** tests. Generally a twofold serial dilution series, each containing 1 to 2 mL of antimicrobial agent, is prepared. Mueller-Hinton broth is the medium recommended for broth dilution MIC tests of nonfastidious bacteria. A standardized suspension of test bacteria is added to each dilution to obtain a final bacterial concentration of 5×10^5 CFU/mL. A growth-control tube (broth plus inoculum) and an uninoculated control tube (broth only) are used with each test. After overnight incubation at 35° C, the MIC is determined visually as the lowest concentration that inhibits growth, as demonstrated by the absence of turbidity.

Broth macrodilution is impractical for use as a routine method when several antimicrobial agents must be tested on an isolate or if several isolates must be tested. Some laboratories use broth macrodilution when it is necessary to test drugs not included in their routine system or for fastidious bacteria that require special growth media. Additionally, this method can be used when minimum bactericidal concentration (MBC) endpoints are to be subsequently determined. The MBC test is discussed later in this chapter.

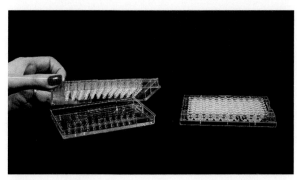

FIGURE 13-3 Broth-microdilution minimal inhibitory concentration (MIC) tray shown with inoculum reservoir trough. Diluted inoculum suspension is placed in the reservoir trough. Then the prongs are dipped into the suspension, raised, and subsequently lowered into the wells of the broth-microdilution MIC tray to inoculate all wells simultaneously.

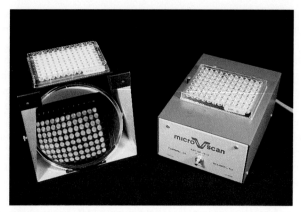

FIGURE 13-4 Tray-reading stand with magnifying mirror *(left)* and a light box *(right)*. Following incubation, either of these devices is used to examine growth in the broth-microdilution minimum inhibitory concentration (MIC) trays. A tray is placed on the tray-reading stand, and wells are examined by looking into the magnifying mirror. A tray is placed over the hole in the light box, and light is allowed to shine through the tray to facilitate close examination of the wells.

Broth-Microdilution Tests

The broth-macrodilution test has been miniaturized and adapted to multiwell microdilution trays (Figure 13-3) for **broth-microdilution MIC** testing. Plastic trays containing between 80 and 100 (usually 96) wells are filled with small volumes (usually 0.1 mL) of twofold dilution concentrations of antimicrobial agent in broth. Because of the large number of wells, several dilutions of as many as 12 to 15 antimicrobial agents can be contained in a single tray that subsequently will be inoculated with one bacterial isolate. The inoculum suspension is prepared and standardized, as described previously. An intermediate dilution of this inoculum suspension is prepared in water or saline, and a multipronged inoculator or other type of inoculating device is used to inoculate the wells to obtain a final concentration of approximately 5×10^5 CFU/mL (5×10^4 CFU per 0.1-mL well). The actual dilution factor used for preparation of the intermediate dilution depends on the volume of inoculum delivered to each well by the inoculating device and the organism being tested. An example of this calculation is illustrated in Table 13-3. A growth- control well and uninoculated control well are included on each tray. After overnight incubation at 35° C, the tray is placed on a tray-reading device to facilitate visual examination of each well (Figure 13-4). Provided growth is adequate in the growth-control well, the MIC for a particular drug is the lowest concentration showing no obvious growth. Growth may be seen as turbidity, a haze, or a pellet in the bottom of the well. Results for quality control organisms should be read prior to reading results for patient isolates to determine whether the test performed correctly.

Some laboratories have dispensing devices that are used to prepare broth microdilution panels, but most laboratories purchase commercially prepared panels, either frozen or freeze-dried. Frozen panels are stored at –20° to –70° C until used. They are thawed at room temperature just before inoculation. For dried panels, the dried or lyophilized drugs in the wells are reconstituted at the same time as the panels are inoculated. In addition to the panels, all commercial companies sell other materials needed for testing (e.g., inoculum

TABLE 13-3 **Example of Calculations Representing Dilution Schema for Preparation of Inocula for Broth Microdilution Minimal Inhibitory Concentration (MIC) Tests***

Step	Resulting Organism Concentration
1. Standardize suspension to McFarland 0.5	1.5×10^8 CFU/mL
2. Add 0.75 mL from step 1 to 25 mL water diluent (1:33 dilution)	$4\text{-}5 \times 10^6$ CFU/mL
3. Use inoculator prong set to inoculate wells of MIC tray (each prong delivers 0.01 mL, which results in an additional 1:100 dilution)	$4\text{-}5 \times 10^4$ CFU/100-μL well
	$4\text{-}5 \times 10^5$ CFU/mL

*Calculations shown here are based on use of inoculator prong set (each prong delivers 0.01 mL). Dilutions in step 2 vary, depending on the number of organisms in the initial suspension and the volume delivered to each well by the inoculating device.

broths, inoculum diluents, panel inoculators, reading devices). Usually a variety of panels containing different drugs are available for testing various organism groups (e.g., gram-positive, gram-negative), and some panels are designed to include wells containing various biochemical reagents so that organism identification and antimicrobial susceptibility testing can be done simultaneously in a single panel. Some companies have automated or semiautomated devices to facilitate inoculation and reading, and these are discussed in the following sections.

Breakpoint (Cutoff) MIC Panels. A variation of the standard broth microdilution MIC panel is the **breakpoint panel,** in which only one or a few concentrations of each antimicrobial agent are tested on a single panel. **Breakpoint (cutoff)** is the term applied to the concentration of an antimicrobial agent that coincides with a susceptible or intermediate MIC breakpoint for a particular drug. When two concentrations are tested and no growth is present in either well, the isolate is susceptible. When there is growth in the low concentration but no growth in the high concentration, the isolate has intermediate susceptibility and a resistant isolate grows in both wells. The qualitative interpretation—nonsusceptible, susceptible, intermediate, or resistant—rather than an MIC is reported. The primary advantage of breakpoint panels is that numerous drugs can be tested on a single panel (often in combination with biochemical tests). The primary disadvantage of breakpoint panels is that a precise MIC is not obtained because most results are either equal to or lower than the lowest concentration tested or greater than the highest concentration tested. Additionally, performing relevant quality control on breakpoint panels is difficult.

Trailing Growth and Skipped Wells. Dilution methods sometimes produce an MIC endpoint that is not clear-cut, and growth in the wells may demonstrate trailing or skipped wells. **Trailing** involves heavy growth at lower concentrations followed by one or more wells that show greatly reduced growth in the form of a small button or a light haze. This commonly occurs with sulfonamides, trimethoprim, and trimethoprim-sulfamethoxazole; the mode of action of the agents allows the bacterial cells to grow through several generations before inhibition. In this case, the trailing is ignored, and the endpoint is read as an 80% reduction in growth compared with the growth control. Trailing with most other drugs may represent contamination and should not be ignored unless it is known that trailing commonly occurs with the particular antimicrobial agent–organism combination.

Skipped wells involve growth at higher concentrations and no growth at one or more of the lower concentrations. This may occur as a result of contamination, improperly inoculated wells, improper concentrations of antimicrobial agent in the wells, the presence of unusual resistance with the test isolate (e.g., a small resistant subpopulation), or a combination of two or more of these factors. As with trailing, each skipped-well occurrence must be evaluated individually to determine whether results are reportable. If any doubt exists with regard to the validity of the results, they should not be reported and the test should be repeated.

One shortcoming of the broth microdilution MIC method is its inability to produce a penicillin MIC that is consistently within the resistant range for staphylococci that are low-level β-lactamase producers. If the penicillin MIC is 0.03 μg/mL or less, the isolate may be reported as penicillin susceptible; a result of 0.25 μg/mL or higher is considered resistant. An induced β-lactamase test must, however, be performed on isolates with penicillin MICs of 0.06 to 0.12 μg/mL. If the β-lactamase test result is positive, the isolate is reported as penicillin resistant; if the result is negative, the isolate is reported as penicillin susceptible.

Agar-Dilution Tests

An MIC test can also be performed using an **agar-dilution MIC** method. Specific volumes of antimicrobial solutions are

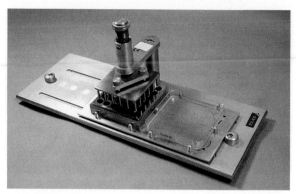

FIGURE 13-5 Steer's replicator. The inoculator prongs are positioned above a 36-well seed trough that contains 36 different standardized inoculum suspensions. The handle on top of the prong unit is pressed to lower the prongs into all suspensions simultaneously, and when the prongs are raised, each contains a standardized volume of inoculum. The agar plate containing a defined concentration of antimicrobial agent is positioned under the prongs (steel plate holding agar plate slides back and forth), and the prongs are carefully lowered to the agar, at which point the inocula are deposited on the agar surface. This process is repeated until all antimicrobial-containing and control agar plates (without antimicrobial agent) have been inoculated.

dispensed into premeasured volumes of molten and cooled agar, which is subsequently poured into standard Petri dishes. Mueller-Hinton agar is recommended for testing aerobic isolates; however, this can be supplemented with sheep's blood (to a final concentration of 5% sheep blood) or other nutrients for testing fastidious bacteria. A series of plates containing varying concentrations of each antimicrobial agent and growth-control plates without antimicrobial agent are prepared. The agar is allowed to solidify, and then a standard number of test bacteria (10^4 CFU for aerobes) are "spot" inoculated onto each plate using a multipronged replicating device (Figure 13-5). As many as 32 different isolates can be simultaneously inoculated onto each 100-mm round Petri dish; 100-mm square plates generally accommodate 36 isolates. After overnight incubation, the MIC is read as the lowest concentration of antimicrobial agent that inhibits the visible growth of the test bacterium (one or two colonies are ignored).

The shelf life of agar-dilution plates is only 1 week for most antimicrobial agents because plates must be stored at 2° to 8° C, and many drugs are labile at this temperature. Because plate preparation is laborious and this procedure is practical only if large numbers of isolates are tested, agar dilution is generally performed only in research settings, although it is currently considered the reference method for antimicrobial susceptibility testing of anaerobes and *Neisseria gonorrhoeae*.

Disk Diffusion Testing

Principle

The disk diffusion test, also commonly known as the **Kirby-Bauer test,** has been widely used in clinical laboratories since

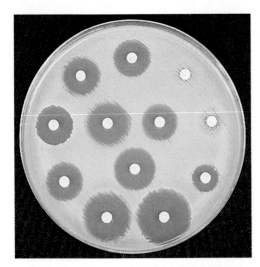

FIGURE 13-6 *Enterobacter aerogenes* tested by the disk diffusion method. Zone measurements confirm that the isolate is susceptible to all agents tested except ampicillin (at the 1-o'clock position) and cefazolin (at the 2-o'clock position). No zones are present for either of these agents.

1966, when the first standardized method was described. Briefly a McFarland 0.5 standardized suspension of bacteria is swabbed over the surface of a Mueller-Hinton agar plate, and paper disks containing specific concentrations of each antimicrobial agent are placed onto the inoculated surface. After overnight incubation, the diameters of the zones produced by antimicrobial inhibition of bacterial growth are measured and the isolate is interpreted as either nonsusceptible, susceptible, intermediate, or resistant to a particular drug according to preset criteria. A photograph of an isolate of *Enterobacter aerogenes* tested by disk diffusion is shown in Figure 13-6.

Establishing Zone-Diameter Interpretive Breakpoints

The disk diffusion test depends on the formation of a gradient of antimicrobial concentrations as the antimicrobial agent diffuses radially into the agar. The drug concentration decreases at increasing distances from the disk. At a critical point the amount of drug at a specific location in the medium is unable to inhibit the growth of the test organism, and a **zone of inhibition** is formed.

The zones of inhibition are related to MICs, and it is this relationship that has been used to determine the breakpoints for interpreting a particular zone measurement as indicating that the isolate is nonsusceptible, susceptible, intermediate, or resistant. To establish breakpoints for a single agent, the first step is to determine the optimum concentration of drug to incorporate into the disk, which takes into consideration the drug's pharmacokinetic properties as well as some of the biochemical properties (e.g., molecular size, solubility, diffusibility in agar). Next a sample of 150 to 200 isolates with comparable growth rates and varying susceptibility to the agent are tested by both the standard disk diffusion test and a standard dilution MIC test, and results are plotted on a graph. For each isolate the observed MIC value is expressed

in logarithmic form ($\log_2$) and plotted on the *y* axis, and the corresponding zone measurement is plotted on the *x* axis on an arithmetic scale (scattergram; Figure 13-7). Zone-diameter breakpoints are then selected based on a comparison of the susceptible, intermediate, and resistant MIC breakpoints with the zone diameters. The zone-diameter breakpoints are chosen best to categorize isolates correctly with minimal interpretive errors.

The CLSI and the FDA are involved in developing zone interpretive criteria, and the procedure just described has been performed for every antimicrobial agent for which zone interpretive criteria exist. With some of the newer, extremely potent drugs, resistant isolates may not presently exist, such that only a susceptible criterion is defined; no intermediate- or resistant-zone interpretive criteria are specified. Further tests, possibly in a reference laboratory, should be performed on any isolate that is interpreted as other than susceptible (nonsusceptible) when only susceptible OR nonsusceptible criteria are specified by the CLSI for the particular antimicrobial agent-organism combination.

Test Performance

Disk Storage. Most clinical laboratories follow the protocol specified by the CLSI for disk diffusion testing, and the CLSI document contains explicit details for test performance. Only FDA-approved disks should be used; they must be stored properly to ensure that the drugs maintain their potency. For long-term storage, disks are stored at –20° C or below in a non–frost-free freezer. A working supply of disks can be stored in a refrigerator at 2° to 8° C for at least 1 week. Disks should always be stored in a tightly sealed container with desiccant. The container should be allowed to warm to room temperature before it is opened to prevent condensation from forming on the disks when warm room air contacts the cold disks.

Inoculation and Incubation. Inoculum suspensions are prepared using either a log-phase or direct-colony suspension standardized to match the turbidity of a McFarland 0.5 standard, as previously described. A sterile cotton swab is dipped into the suspension, pressed and rotated firmly against the side of the tube to express excess liquid, and then swabbed evenly across the surface of a Mueller-Hinton agar plate. Usually a plate 150 mm in diameter is used; it can accommodate testing of as many as 12 different antimicrobial disks with most organisms (placement of more than 12 disks on the plate may result in overlapping zones, which are difficult to measure and may produce erroneous results). Within 15 minutes of inoculation, the antimicrobial disks are applied to the agar with a multiple-disk dispenser (Figure 13-8). The disks are pressed firmly to ensure contact with the agar. Within 15 minutes of disk placement, plates are inverted and placed in a 35° C ambient air incubator for 16 to 18 hours. Mueller-Hinton agar containing 5% sheep blood is used for testing streptococci that do not grow adequately on unsupplemented Mueller-Hinton agar. Although incubation in an atmosphere of increased CO_2 is recommended for testing some fastidious bacteria, this should not be done with most organisms. Incubation in CO_2 results in a decreased pH, which affects the activity of some antimicrobial agents.

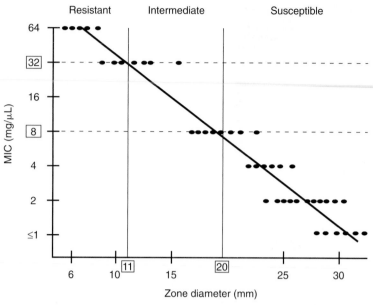

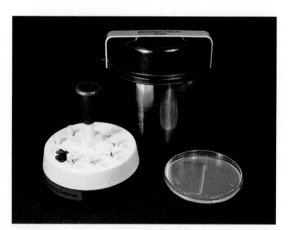

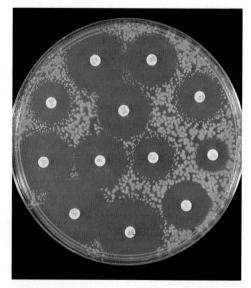

FIGURE 13-7 Example of scattergram and regression analysis plot used to determine disk diffusion zone diameter interpretive breakpoints for hypothetical drug "X." Based on clinical response data, isolates with minimum inhibitory concentration (MIC) 8.0 μg/mL or less are considered susceptible. As derived from this scattergram, corresponding zones of 20 mm or more would be interpreted as susceptible. Isolates with MICs of 32.0 μg/mL or more and zones of 11 mm or less are resistant. The intermediate designation is used for isolates whose values fall between the susceptible and the resistant MICs (16 μg/mL) and zone interpretive breakpoints (12 to 19 mm).

FIGURE 13-8 Cartridges containing antimicrobial susceptibility test disks are inserted into the dispenser *(left).* The dispenser (which can hold up to 12 different cartridges of disks) is positioned over an inoculated plate, and light pressure is applied to the handle to simultaneously deposit one of each type of disk onto the plate. The tight-sealing container in the background contains a desiccant packet and is used for storage (at 2° to 8° C) of the dispenser containing a working supply of disks.

FIGURE 13-9 *Escherichia coli* tested by the disk diffusion method. The lawn of growth following overnight incubation shows individual colonies, representing unsatisfactory growth. The most likely explanation for the scanty growth is the use of an inoculum that either is too light or contains too many nonviable cells, resulting in larger than normal zones and potentially false susceptible results.

Reading Plates and Test Interpretation. After incubation the plate is examined to make certain the test organism has grown satisfactorily. The lawn of growth must be confluent or almost confluent, and the appearance of individual colonies is unacceptable (Figure 13-9). Quality control plates should be read prior to reading results of patient isolates to determine whether the test was performed correctly. Provided growth is satisfactory, the diameter of each inhibition zone is measured using a ruler or calipers. Plates are placed a few inches above a black, nonreflecting surface, and zones are

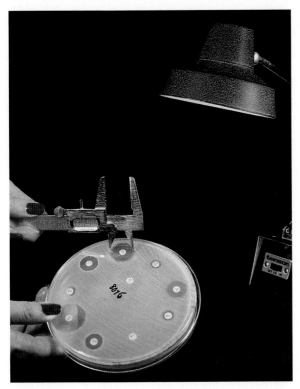

FIGURE 13-10   Routine disk diffusion tests are examined by placing the plate on or 2 to 3 inches above a black, nonreflecting surface. Reflected light is used to illuminate the plate.

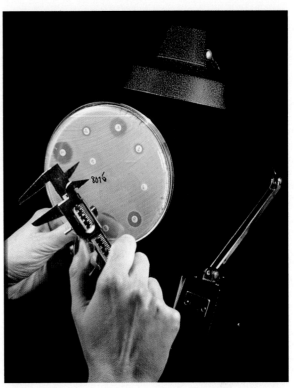

FIGURE 13-11   Disk diffusion tests for staphylococci with oxacillin (or methicillin or nafcillin) and vancomycin and for enterococci with vancomycin are examined by holding the plate up to a light source (transmitted light) for zone examination. Any growth within the zone is significant.

examined from the back side (agar side) of the plate illuminated with reflected light (Figure 13-10). Tiny colonies at the zone edge and the swarm of growth into the zone that often occurs with swarming *Proteus* spp. are ignored; the obvious zone is measured. As with dilution tests, the endpoint for the sulfonamides, trimethoprim, and trimethoprim-sulfamethoxazole is an 80% reduction of growth. Obvious colonies within a clear zone should not be ignored. These colonies may occur as a result of contamination or testing of a mixed culture; however, these colonies sometimes represent a minority resistant subpopulation. When such colonies are noted, the original isolate should be retested. If repeat testing of the original isolate produces the same results, the isolate should be reported as resistant.

Transmitted light (plate held up to light source; Figure 13-11) rather than reflected light will improve the accuracy of tests with the **penicillinase-resistant penicillins,** linezolid, and vancomycin when testing staphylococci and for vancomycin when testing enterococci. Tests performed on media containing blood are examined from the top of the plate with the lid removed. For plates containing blood, it is important to read the zone of inhibition of growth and not the zone of inhibition of hemolysis.

Once zone measurements have been made, the millimeter reading for each antimicrobial agent is compared with that specified in the interpretive tables of the CLSI documents and results are interpreted as susceptible, nonsuceptible, intermediate, or resistant. An excerpt from the chart is shown in Table

13-4. The equivalent MIC breakpoints that are used to define resistance and susceptibility are also shown. Note that as with MIC interpretive criteria, several sets of interpretive criteria may exist for some antimicrobial agents, which are specific for various organisms or organism groups. A summary of the variables that must be carefully controlled in the performance of disk diffusion and broth microdilution MIC tests is listed in Table 13-5.

Modified Methods for Testing Slow-Growing or Fastidious Bacteria

Mueller-Hinton broth and agar are the standard media used for routine dilution and disk diffusion susceptibility tests. These media, however, do not support the growth of all bacteria that require testing; consequently, routine methods must be modified for testing fastidious bacteria that require supplemental nutrients, modified incubation conditions, or both.

Streptococcus pneumoniae and *Streptococcus* Species

Streptococcus pneumoniae and *Streptococcus* spp. require a more nutritious medium for antimicrobial susceptibility testing; they will not grow satisfactorily on unsupplemented Mueller-Hinton medium. Broth-dilution tests are performed in Mueller-Hinton broth that has been supplemented with 2% to 5% lysed horse blood. Agar dilution and disk diffusion tests are performed using Mueller-Hinton agar supplemented with 5% sheep blood.

TABLE 13-4 Zone Diameter Interpretive Standards and Equivalent Minimal Inhibitory Concentration Breakpoints for Several Organism Groups

Antimicrobial Agent	Disk Content (mcg)	Zone Diameter, nearest whole mm			Equivalent MIC Breakpoints (mcg/mL)	
		Resistant	Intermediate	Susceptible	Resistant	Susceptible
Ampicillin						
When testing Enterobacteriaceae	10	≤13	14-16	≥17	≥32	≤8
When testing staphylococci	10	≤28	—	≥29	β-lactamase	≤0.25
When testing enterococci	10	≤16	—	≥17	≥16	≤8
When testing *Haemophilus* spp.	10	≤18	19-21	≥22	≥4	≤1
When testing β-hemolytic streptococci	10	—	—	≥24	—	≤0.25
Gentamicin						
When testing Enterobacteriaceae	10	≤12	13-14	≥15	≥8	≤4
When testing *Pseudomonas aeruginosa*	10	≤12	13-14	≥15	≥8	≤4
When testing staphylococci	10	≤12	13-14	≥15	≥8	≤4
Oxacillin						
When testing *Staphylococcus aureus*	1	≤10	11-12	≥13	≥4	≤2
When testing coagulase-negative staphylococci	1	≤17	—	≥18	≥0.5	≤0.25
When testing *Streptococus pneumoniae* (non-pneumonia isolates) for penicillin susceptibility	1	≤19	—	≥20	—	≤0.06

Modified from Clinical and Laboratory Standards Institute (CLSI) publication M100-19: *Performance standards for antimicrobial susceptibility testing: nineteenth informational supplement.* Copies of the current edition may be obtained from CLSI, 940 West Valley Road, Suite 1400, Wayne, Pa., 19087-1898.

TABLE 13-5 Primary Variables That Must Be Controlled in Performance of Routine Disk Diffusion and Broth Microdilution Minimal Inhibitory Concentration Tests

Variable	Standard	Comments
Inoculum	Disk diffusion: 1.5×10^8 CFU/mL Broth microdilution: 5×10^5 CFU/mL (final concentration)	Use "adequate" McFarland turbidity standard (0.5 for disk diffusion) When preparing direct suspensions (without incubation), do not use growth from plates more than 1 day old
Media		
Formulation	Mueller-Hinton	Prepare in-house or purchase from reliable source Perform media quality control to verify acceptability before use for patient tests
Ca^{2+}, Mg^{2+} content	25 mg/L Ca^{2+}, 12.5 mg/L Mg^{2+}	Increased concentrations result in decreased activity of aminoglycosides against *Pseudomonas aeruginosa* and decreased activity of tetracyclines against all organisms (decreased concentrations have the opposite effect)
Thymidine content	Minimal or absent	Excessive concentrations can result in false resistance to sulfonamides and trimethoprim
pH	7.2-7.4	Decreased pH can lead to decreased activity of aminoglycosides, erythromycin, and clindamycin and increased activity of tetracyclines (increased pH has the opposite effect)
Agar depth (disk diffusion)	3-5 mm	Possibility for false susceptibility if less than 3 mm or false resistance if more than 5 mm
Incubation		
Atmosphere	Humidified ambient air	CO_2 incubation decreases pH, which can lead to decreased activity of aminoglycosides, erythromycin, and clindamycin and increased activity of tetracyclines
Temperature	–35° C	Some MRSA may go undetected if more than 35° C
Length	Disk diffusion: 16-18 hr Broth microdilution: 16-20 hr	Some MSRA may go undetected if less than 24 hr Some vancomycin-resistant enterococci may go undetected if less than 24 hr with disk diffusion

TABLE 13-5 **Primary Variables That Must Be Controlled in Performance of Routine Disk Diffusion and Broth Microdilution Minimal Inhibitory Concentration Tests—cont'd**

Variable	Standard	Comments
	24 hr for staphylococci with oxacillin* and vancomycin and for enterococci with vancomycin and gentamicin HLAR; 48 hr enterococci with streptomycin HLAR; 24 hr sometimes needed for fastidious bacteria	Some HLAR (gentamicin) enterococci may go undetected if less than 24 hr (broth microdilution) Some HLAR (streptomycin) enterococci may go undetected if less than 48 hr (broth microdilution)

Antimicrobial Agents

Variable	Standard	Comments
Disks	Used disks containing appropriate FDA/CLSI-defined concentration of drug	Check CLSI publication or FDA package insert (accompanying disks) for specifications
	Proper storage	For long-term storage, use non–frost-free freezer at –20° C or less in tightly sealed, desiccated container
		For short-term storage (at least 1 week), maintain temperature at 2° to 8° C in tightly sealed, desiccated container
		Allow to warm to room temperature before opening container
	Proper placement on agar	Place 12 or fewer disks per 150-mm plate (no overlapping zones)
Solutions	Prepared from reference standard powders	Pharmacy-grade antimicrobial agents are unacceptable (they may not show antimicrobial activity in vitro)
	Proper storage	Store in non–frost-frost freezer, optimally at –70° C or less
		Never refreeze

Endpoint Measurement

Variable	Standard	Comments
Disk diffusion	Reflected light (except for staphylococci with oxacillin* and vancomycin, and for enterococci with vancomycin) and plate held against black background	Lawn must be confluent or almost confluent Ignore faint growth of tiny colonies at zone edge
	Zones measured from back of plate	Trimethoprim and sulfonamide endpoint at 80% or more inhibition Ignore swarm within obvious zone for swarming *Proteus* spp. Retest when colonies within zone (except for staphylococci with oxacillin, and for enterococci with vancomycin)
	Transmitted light used for staphylococci with oxacillin* and vancomycin, and for enterococci with vancomycin	Call "resistant" if *any* growth within zone (unless possibly artifactual or contaminated) Reproducibility of zone measurements is within ±2 mm
Broth microdilution	Adequate lighting and reading device	MIC is the lowest concentration that inhibits growth (turbidity, haze, or pellet) Sulfonamides and trimethoprim may trail (ignore trailing less than 2 mm buttons) Justify "skip wells" or repeat Staphylococci and penicillin: perform induced β-lactamase test if MIC is 0.06-0.12 μg/mL Reproducibility should be within ±1 twofold dilution

Modified from Hindler JA, Mann LM: Principles and practices for the laboratory guidance of antimicrobial therapy. In Tilton RC et al, editors: *Clinical laboratory medicine*, St Louis, 1992, Mosby.

*Includes all penicillinase-resistant penicillins (oxacillin, methicillin, nafcillin, and dicloxacillin).

FDA, U.S. Food and Drug Administration; *CLSI*, Clinical and Laboratory Standards Institute; *HLAR*, high-level aminoglycoside resistance; *MRSA*, methicillin-resistant *Staphylococcus aureus*; *MIC*, minimal inhibitory concentration.

Penicillins and cephalosporins remain the drugs of choice for treating pneumococcal infections; however, resistance to penicillin as well as to other potentially useful agents has become widespread. Penicillin resistance is due to the presence of altered penicillin-binding proteins (drug targets in the cell wall). The disk diffusion test can be used to determine the susceptibility of pneumococci to a variety of antimicrobial agents. The standard disk diffusion procedure uses Mueller-Hinton agar with 5% sheep blood incubated in 5% to 7% CO_2.

It is possible to screen for penicillin susceptibility in *S. pneumoniae* using an oxacillin disk (1 μg). A penicillin disk should not be used because it is less accurate. If the oxacillin zone of inhibition is 20 mm or larger, the isolate can be safely reported as penicillin (not oxacillin) susceptible (penicillin MIC of 0.06 μg/mL or less). If the oxacillin zone is 19 mm or smaller, a penicillin (not oxacillin) MIC test must be performed to determine the degree of resistance (Figure 13-12).

Streptococcus pneumoniae isolates from nonmeningitis sites with penicillin MICs of 0.06 μg/mL or less are interpreted as susceptible, 0.12 to 1.0 μg /mL are intermediate, and 2.0 μg/mL or more are resistant when oral penicillin V is to be used for treatment. When parenteral penicillin is to be used for treatment of isolates from nonmeningitis sources (e.g., isolates from sputum), the isolate is considered susceptible when the MIC is 2 μg /mL or less, intermediate when the MIC is 4 μg/mL, and resistant when the MIC is 8 μg/mL or more.

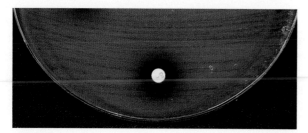

FIGURE 13-12 An oxacillin (1-μg) disk is used to screen for penicillin susceptibility in *Streptococcus pneumoniae* isolated from specimens other then sputum. If the oxacillin zone of inhibition is 20 mm or more, the isolate is reported as penicillin susceptible. If the oxacillin zone is 19 mm or less, a penicillin minimal inhibitory concentration (MIC) test must be performed. The isolate pictured has an oxacillin zone of approximately 15 mm, so a penicillin MIC test must be performed.

If the *S. pneumoniae* isolate is from cerebrospinal fluid (CSF), the isolate is considered susceptible to penicillin when the MIC is 0.06 μg/mL or less, and resistant when the MIC is 0.12 μg/mL or more. Determining the degree of penicillin resistance is important because the recommended therapy may be different for penicillin intermediate and resistant strains. It is important to test penicillin-resistant isolates with other clinically relevant antimicrobial agents, such as cefotaxime or ceftriaxone (by an MIC method, not disk diffusion), erythromycin, a fluoroquinolone, vancomycin, and perhaps clindamycin or a tetracycline.

Methods for testing nonpneumococcal streptococci are the same as those for *S. pneumoniae;* however, separate breakpoints for this group of bacteria have been defined. β-hemolytic streptococci remain universally susceptible to penicillin, the drug of choice for treating infections caused by these organisms. Consequently, routine susceptibility testing on β-hemolytic streptococci is generally not necessary. For highly penicillin-allergic patients, alternative agents for therapy include a macrolide (e.g., erythromycin) or clindamycin. In contrast to penicillin, some β-hemolytic streptococci are resistant to erythromycin only or to both erythromycin and clindamycin. Isolates that appear erythromycin resistant and clindamycin susceptible may have inducible or constitutive resistance to clindamycin. Before reporting clindamycin as susceptible in these cases, a **D-zone test** must be performed as described for staphylococci. Accurate penicillin susceptibility results are needed for viridans streptococci isolated from serious infections such as bacteremia or endocarditis. If the isolate has a penicillin MIC of 0.12 μg/mL or less, penicillin alone is often prescribed; however, higher penicillin MICs (0.25 to 2.0 μg/mL) suggest the need for concomitant therapy with an aminoglycoside. Isolates with penicillin MICs greater than 2.0 μg/mL are highly resistant, and for these vancomycin rather than penicillin is generally prescribed. Because of the critical nature of penicillin results, the disk diffusion test is not recommended in these situations, and MIC tests should be performed. As with *S. pneumoniae,* penicillin resistance in viridans streptococci is due to altered penicillin-binding proteins.

Haemophilus influenzae and Haemophilus parainfluenzae

Haemophilus test medium (HTM), which consists of Mueller-Hinton medium base supplemented with X (hematin) and V (nicotinamide adenine dinucleotide [NAD]) factors, has been standardized for testing *Haemophilus influenzae* and *Haemophilus parainfluenzae*. HTM broth can be used for broth-dilution tests, and HTM agar is used for disk diffusion tests. The test procedures for *Haemophilus* spp. are identical to those described for nonfastidious bacteria with the exception that the disk diffusion test with HTM is incubated in an atmosphere of 5% to 7% CO_2. The CLSI has established zone diameter and MIC interpretive criteria that are unique for this genus. For some agents, such as cefotaxime, only a susceptible range is defined because cefotaxime-resistant *Haemophilus* spp. have not been identified. In those cases where the determined MIC is greater than what would make the organism cefotaxime susceptible, the organism is reported as "nonsusceptible." In these cases the organism should be reidentified and the MIC redetermined. If the same results are obtained after re-testing, the organism should be submitted to a reference laboratory such as a state health laboratory.

Ampicillin or amoxicillin is often effective in treating localized, less serious *H. influenzae* infections; however, 25% to 50% of *H. influenzae* produce a β-lactamase that inactivates these agents. β-Lactamase–producing strains can be quickly identified by using a rapid β-lactamase test. *H. influenzae* also may be resistant to ampicillin and amoxicillin because of altered penicillin-binding proteins. These isolates are referred to as *β-lactamase-negative ampicillin-resistant* (BLNAR). This resistance occurs in less than 1.0% of clinical isolates. Very small proportions of isolates possess both resistance caused by altered penicillin-binding proteins and production of β-lactamase and are referred to as β-lactamase-positive amoxicillin-clavulanate-resistant (BLPACR) isolates. Both the BLNAR and BLPACR are only detectable by in vitro susceptibility testing. There are no rapid detection methods for these types of resistance.

Because most ampicillin-resistant (amoxicillin-resistant) *H. influenzae* produce β-lactamase, and because *H. influenzae* are often susceptible to alternative agents currently recommended, some laboratories may perform only a β-lactamase test or test only ampicillin and trimethoprim-sulfamethoxazole by the disk diffusion or MIC methods but may test additional agents (e.g., fluoroquinolones) if the isolate is from nonrespiratory sources or if requested by the clinicians.

Neisseria gonorrhoeae and Neisseria meningitidis

Neisseria gonorrhoeae and *Neisseria meningitidis* are organisms of public health significance that may be isolated by clinical laboratories with varying frequencies. Therapy of disseminated meningococcal infections and various types of gonococcal infections are generally empiric and based on recommendations from the Centers for Disease Control and Prevention (CDC) and various professional groups. Most often clinical microbiology laboratories are not required to perform antimicrobial susceptibility testing of these two species. Public health laboratories, on the other hand, may test them on a periodic or consistent basis. The CLSI has described both MIC and disk diffusion methods that may be used to test these species.

Although for many years penicillin was the drug of choice for treating uncomplicated gonorrhea, the increased incidence of penicillin-resistant isolates and more recently fluoroquinolone-resistant isolates has led to the use of ceftriaxone or cefixime as first-line therapy. Penicillin resistance in *N. gonorrhoeae* may be due to production of a β-lactamase similar to that produced by ampicillin-resistant *H. influenzae*, and this resistance can be readily detected with a rapid β-lactamase test. β-lactamase–producing isolates are also referred to as **penicillinase-producing *Neisseria gonorrhoeae* (PPNG).** Some *N. gonorrhoeae* are penicillin resistant because of an altered penicillin-binding protein; this resistance can be detected only with conventional dilution or disk diffusion tests. The production of altered penicillin-binding proteins is chromosomally mediated, and *N. gonorrhoeae* with altered penicillin-binding proteins are often referred to as **chromosomally mediated–resistant *Neisseria gonorrhoeae* (CMRNG).** Because current therapeutic recommendations do not include penicillin and because virtually all *N. gonorrhoeae* are currently susceptible to ceftriaxone or cefixime, testing is rarely needed, except for public health surveillance purposes.

Gonococcal (GC) agar base is supplemented with various nutrients for testing *N. gonorrhoeae*. Dilution tests are performed using agar dilution because this species has a tendency to lyse in broth media, resulting in false-susceptible results. Disk diffusion tests are performed on the same agar, and all tests are incubated in an atmosphere containing 5% to 7% CO_2. The CLSI has specified interpretive criteria unique for this species. For several agents, resistant isolates have not yet been encountered, so only susceptible criteria are available. Except for very rare isolates that have been shown to produce β-lactamase, *N. meningitidis* is usually susceptible to penicillin; however, in the United States, ceftriaxone or cefotaxime is most often the drug of choice for treating invasive meningococcal infections. Isolates with elevated penicillin MICs (penicillin-intermediate) have been reported, although their significance is minimized through the more extensive use of third-generation cephalosporins for therapy. Meningococci are often resistant to sulfonamides (including trimethoprim-sulfamethoxazole) and are occasionally resistant to rifampin. For these reasons, a fluoroquinolone (e.g., ciprofloxacin) is most often administered prophylactically to individuals in close contact with patients who have meningococcal meningitis. The CLSI has described MIC and disk diffusion methods for testing meningococci that are the same as those used for testing the streptococci, except that broth microdilution tests with meningococci require CO_2 incubation. If needed, breakpoints for determining susceptibility or resistance in meningococci for a number of agents can be found in the latest CLSI tables.

Helicobacter pylori

The susceptibility of *Helicobacter pylori* to antimicrobials can be determined by agar dilution testing using Mueller-Hinton agar to which 5% aged (2 or more weeks old) sheep blood is added. Susceptibility test plates need to be incubated in a microaerobic environment and read at 3 days of incubation.

CLSI has described the method by which the testing can be done as well the QC strain to use and interpretive criteria for specific antimicrobials.

Susceptibility Testing of Agents of Bioterrorism

With the occurrence of the terrorism attacks in the United States on "9/11," the more eminent threat of the use of bacteria and other microorganisms as agents of bioterrorism was given heightened attention. Before 9/11 there were no standardized methods for testing the susceptibility of *Bacillus anthracis, Yersinia pestis, Burkholderia mallei, Burkholderia pseudomallei, Francisella tularensis,* and *Brucella* spp. to antimicrobials. In addition, little was known about the use of antimicrobials to prevent or treat infections caused by these organisms. Since that time the CLSI has standardized the methods for doing susceptibility testing of these bacteria against a variety of antimicrobials and has established interpretive criteria for the results of these tests. Also a great deal more information is now available on the use of antimicrobials that can be used to prevent infections with these organisms and to treat infections if they do occur. However, these organisms are an eminent danger when being tested in the laboratory, and work with these organisms should be conducted only in biosafety level 2 (BSL2) or higher facilities by trained individuals. This limitation applies even to routine susceptibility tests. As soon as it is suspected either that a specimen may contain one of these bacteria or that one of these bacteria has been isolated, all work with the specimen or isolate must cease, the specimen or isolate must be quarantined, and the proper officials must be alerted. All laboratories should establish contingency plans to deal with a situation in which agents of bioterrorism have appeared in the laboratory.

Anaerobes

The reference method described by the CLSI for testing anaerobic bacteria is an agar dilution method, and the recommended medium is supplemented *Brucella* laked sheep blood agar. As previously mentioned, however, agar dilution is not practical for use in the routine clinical laboratory, and a broth microdilution method is more often used. The CLSI broth microdilution procedure is similar to that used for testing aerobes except that *Brucella* broth with lysed horse blood is used for testing the *B. fragilis* group of anaerobes. Additionally, the number of organisms in the test inoculum is 0.5 log_{10} higher (10^6 CFU/mL) than that for testing aerobes, and panels are incubated anaerobically at 35° C for 48 hours. As with tests for aerobic bacteria, the CLSI has defined susceptible, intermediate, and resistant criteria for interpretation of MICs for anaerobes. Several commercial companies produce broth microdilution MIC panels for testing anaerobes. The **Etest,** discussed in detail later, has been shown to perform satisfactorily for susceptibility testing of anaerobes and is used in some clinical laboratories.

Infrequently Encountered or Fastidious Bacteria

A new CLSI publication, M45, focuses on infrequently encountered or fastidious bacteria not addressed in the standard MIC and disk diffusion documents. When clinically indicated, isolates of *Corynebacteria* (and some other gram-positive bacilli), *Aeromonas, Vibrio, Pasteurella, Moraxella catarrhalis*, members of the HACEK (*Haemophilus, Actinobacillus, Cardiobacterium, Eikenella, Kingella*) group of gram-negatives, and *Abiotrophia/Granulicatella* may be tested using various standard CLSI methods and media, and the results are interpreted using the CLSI tables specific for the particular organism. This publication also contains information on suscaptibility testing of agents of bioterrorism.

Additional Organism and Antimicrobial Agent Testing Concerns

Special procedures must be used to detect clinically significant resistance in some nonfastidious bacteria.

Detection of Oxacillin (Methicillin) Resistance in Staphylococci

Oxacillin and other penicillinase-resistant penicillins, such as methicillin, nafcillin, cloxacillin, and dicloxacillin, constitute the drug class of choice for treating staphylococcal infections. Oxacillin has been the class representative most commonly used to detect resistance in staphylococci and has produced more reliable results than testing one of the other agents. When an isolate shows resistance to one of the penicillinase-resistant penicillins, it must be considered resistant to the entire group. Staphylococcal resistance to the penicillinase-resistant penicillins is due to the presence of a unique penicillin-binding protein (PBP2a or PBP2′) in the cell wall. The penicillin-binding protein, which has a low affinity for binding all β-lactam drugs, is encoded by the ***mecA* gene.** Isolates of oxacillin-resistant *S. aureus* are commonly referred to as **methicillin-resistant *Staphylococcus aureus* (MRSA)** for historical reasons. Detecting oxacillin resistance in isolates that possess the *mecA* gene has sometimes proven difficult under standard susceptibility testing conditions because some staphylococci exhibit heteroresistance or heterogeneous expression of resistance to oxacillin. In **heteroresistant** strains, all cells in the test population have the genetic element (the *mecA* gene) for oxacillin resistance, but not all the cells express this resistance by virtue of PBP2a production. Consequently, in the oxacillin susceptibility test, some cells may appear resistant and some appear susceptible. If too few cells appear resistant, an oxacillin-resistant strain may not be detected.

In vitro testing conditions can be modified to enhance the expression of oxacillin resistance; they are as follows:

- Preparation of inocula using the direct inoculum suspension procedure
- Incubation of tests at temperatures no greater than 35° C
- Making final test readings after a full 24 hours of incubation
- Supplementation of Mueller-Hinton broth or agar with 2% NaCl for dilution tests

The extended incubation allows the more slowly growing resistant subpopulation sufficient time to grow to detectable numbers. In addition, test plates should always be examined very closely. For oxacillin disk diffusion tests, zones of inhibition must be examined by using transmitted light (holding the plate up to the light source; see Figure 13-11), and any growth

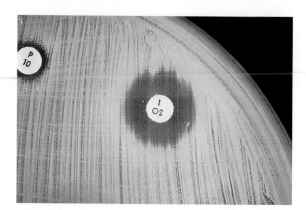

FIGURE 13-13 The oxacillin zone for heteroresistant oxacillin-resistant *Staphylococcus aureus* often shows a haze of growth within the zone of inhibition. This haze is significant, and the isolate here is oxacillin resistant.

is considered significant. A "haze" of growth within the inhibition zone for oxacillin-resistant isolates is sometimes observed (Figure 13-13).

An **oxacillin screen plate** that contains Mueller-Hinton agar supplemented with 4% NaCl and 6 µg/mL oxacillin has been used to detect MRSA. To perform the oxacillin screen test, a McFarland 0.5 suspension is prepared as for the disk diffusion test. A swab is dipped into this suspension and streaked over an area of approximately 2 × 5 cm or deposited as a "spot" on the agar surface. After overnight incubation at 35° C, growth (more than one colony) is an indication that the isolate is oxacillin resistant. This method does not reliably detect oxacillin-resistant coagulase-negative staphylococci. Testing a surrogate marker of resistance (i.e., cefoxitin) may provide a more accurate indication of oxacillin resistance than testing oxacillin itself. This is because cefoxitin serves to induce greater expression of PBP2a in *mecA*-containing strains of staphylococci and also functions as a test reagent to detect resistance. Carefully conducted studies have shown that performing a disk diffusion test with cefoxitin and using the specific cefoxitin breakpoints recommended by the CLSI provides sensitivity and specificity equivalent to testing oxacillin (by both disk diffusion and MIC methods) with *S. aureus* and greater sensitivity and specificity of cefoxitin when testing coagulase-negative staphylococci. Despite equivalent performance with *S. aureus*, however, cefoxitin disk diffusion test results are more easily interpreted than disk diffusion tests using oxacillin. For these reasons, cefoxitin disk diffusion testing is now recommended by the CLSI as the preferred method for detection of oxacillin resistance in both *S. aureus* and coagulase-negative staphylococci. In relation to the coagulase-negative organism *Staphylococcus lugdunensis*, even though it is coagulase-negative because of its characteristics similar to *S. aureus*, the results of the cefoxitin screen test should be interpreted using *S. aureus* interpretive criteria. It is important to report the findings from the cefoxitin disk diffusion test as indicative or either oxacillin susceptibility or resistance; cefoxitin results should not be reported.

Sometimes oxacillin-resistant staphylococci can appear susceptible in vitro to other β-lactam agents, such as the cephalosporins; however, these are clinically ineffective. Consequently all oxacillin-resistant staphylococci must be reported as resistant to all β-lactam agents (including cephalosporins, β-lactam/β-lactamase inhibitor combinations, and carbapenems) if those agents are tested, regardless of the in vitro test results. For practicality, it is better simply to perform the cefoxitin disk diffusion test and to deduce susceptibility to other β-lactam agents based on whether a staphylococcal isolate is oxacillin-susceptible or resistant. MRSA has emerged as a significant cause of community-associated infections in recent years and requires that all clinical microbiology laboratories pay particular attention to accurate detection of resistance in *S. aureus*. In prior years, health care–associated strains of MRSA were often resistant to several other drug classes in addition to the β-lactams. Although the majority of recent community-associated MRSA isolates often have been resistant only to the macrolides (e.g., erythromycin) in addition to various β-lactams, an increasing number of MRSA isolates from the community have the same antimicrobial resistance profile as hospital-acquired MRSA isolates.

Rare *S. aureus* isolates have a more subtle and less common type of oxacillin resistance that is unrelated to the presence of the *mecA* gene. The resistance mechanism in these isolates is due to either hyperproduction of β-lactamase or the presence of altered normal penicillin-binding proteins (not PBP2a). These isolates generally have MICs right above (or zones of inhibition right below) the breakpoint for oxacillin susceptibility, and they are sometimes referred to as **borderline–oxacillin-resistant isolates.** Isolates with borderline oxacillin resistance generally do not grow on oxacillin screen plates. The clinical response of isolates with borderline oxacillin resistance to penicillinase-resistant penicillins as well as to other β-lactam agents has not been clearly defined.

Vancomycin Resistance or Diminished Susceptibility in *Staphylococcus aureus*

Between 2002 and 2005, five different isolates of MRSA were detected for the first time with vancomycin resistance. All these isolates had apparently acquired a plasmid containing the *vanA* vancomycin-resistance genes from vancomycin-resistant enterococci. The MRSA isolates demonstrated various levels of resistance to vancomycin. Some were obviously resistant by routine susceptibility testing methods, and others were initially missed by routine testing methods. This important emerging resistance followed recognition in 1996 of the first MRSA isolate with more subtle diminished susceptibility to vancomycin. Shortly thereafter several similar isolates were encountered that all had vancomycin MICs of 8 µg/mL. These isolates of *S. aureus* with reduced susceptibility to vancomycin have been called **vancomycin-intermediate *Staphylococcus aureus* (VISA)** or glycopeptide-intermediate *S. aureus* (GISA). Although still uncommon, both **vancomycin-resistant *S. aureus* (VRSA)** and VISA isolates are of great concern because vancomycin is one of the most proven agents for treating serious MRSA infections. The CLSI recommends use of either the broth microdilution test or the vancomycin agar screen recommended for enterococci as the best methods for detection of either VRSA or VISA. The vancomycin disk diffusion test has not uniformly detected these isolates, and some of the commercial susceptibility testing instruments have likewise not

always provided reliable detection of these strains. The use of the macro Etest method, a modification of the standard Etest discussed later, has proven to be of value in detecting heteroresistant vancomycin intermediate resistant *S. aureus* (hVISA) because the test uses a higher concentration of organisms (approximately 1×10^8 bacteria/mL) than is used routinely for susceptibility testing, thus enhancing the probability of detecting the small number of these organisms in the overall population of cells. **Population analysis profiles (PAP)** of both *S. aureus* and coagulase-negative staphylococci has been used to detect hVISA. This is done by plating increasing numbers of these organisms on plates containing various concentrations of vancomycin and then dividing the number by the area under the curve. Both the Etest method and PAP can be used for detecting heteroresistance in other organisms to other antimicrobials. Because the PAP technique is labor intensive, it is not suitable for most clinical laboratories.

Inducible Clindamycin Resistance in Staphylococci

Two different resistance mechanisms confer macrolide (e.g., erythromycin) resistance in staphylococci. The *erm* gene codes for methylation of the 23S rRNA, which results in resistance to erythromycin and either inducible or constitutive resistance to clindamycin. The *msrA* gene codes for an efflux mechanism, which results in resistance to erythromycin but susceptibility to clindamycin. Consequently, when an erythromycin resistant and clindamycin susceptible staphylococcal isolate is encountered, a D-zone test for inducible clindamycin resistance must be performed before clindamycin is reported to be susceptible. For the D-zone test, an erythromycin disk is placed adjacent to a clindamycin disk (15 to 26 mm edge to edge) as part of a standard disk diffusion test. Following overnight incubation, flattening of the clindamycin zone between the two disks (Figure 13-14) indicates the isolate has inducible clindamycin resistance because of *erm*. No flattening indicates the isolate is erythromycin resistant only (due to *msrA*). When an isolate demonstrates inducible resistance, clindamycin is reported as resistant.

Enterococci

Ampicillin or penicillin is effective in treating uncomplicated enterococcal infections (e.g., urinary tract infections) by most *Enterococcus* spp. (*Enterococcus faecium* is the exception). These cell wall–active agents are only bacteriostatic against enterococci and, when administered alone, are inadequate for treating very serious infections, such as endocarditis, that require bactericidal therapy. To obtain a bactericidal effect, ampicillin or penicillin (or vancomycin in the penicillin-allergic patient or with *Enterococcus faecium*) must be given in combination with an aminoglycoside, usually gentamicin or sometimes streptomycin.

Detection of High-Level Aminoglycoside Resistance in Enterococci. Enterococci are inherently resistant to low concentrations of aminoglycosides, precluding their use as single agents for treatment of enterococcal infections. This low-level resistance is caused by poor drug uptake by the enterococcal cells. For isolates with low-level aminoglycoside resistance, a synergistic interaction occurs when an aminogly-

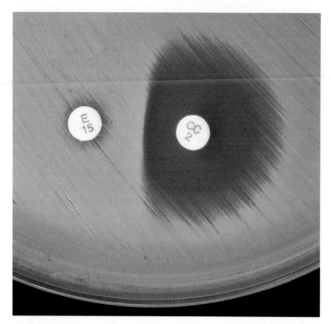

FIGURE 13-14 D-zone testing of *Staphylococcus aureus* that has *erm*-mediated inducible clindamycin resistance. The positive reaction is noted by a flattening of the zone around the clindamycin disk in the area where there has been diffusion of both erythromycin and clindamycin molecules.

TABLE 13-6 Aminoglycosides Represented When High Concentrations of Gentamicin and Streptomycin Are Tested to Determine High-Level Aminoglycoside Resistance in Enterococci

Agent Tested	Aminoglycoside(s) Represented
Gentamicin*	Gentamicin
	Amikacin
	Kanamycin
	Tobramycin
Streptomycin†	Streptomycin

*An isolate that has high-level resistance to gentamicin also has high-level resistance to the other aminoglycosides listed; enzymes that modify gentamicin also modify the other agents.
†An isolate that has high-level resistance to streptomycin has high-level resistance to this agent only, unless it also has high-level resistance to gentamicin as indicated by testing high concentrations of gentamicin.

coside is administered together with a cell wall–active agent such as ampicillin, penicillin, or vancomycin. Sometimes, however, enterococci develop high-level aminoglycoside resistance, in which the particular aminoglycoside does not demonstrate synergism with the cell wall–active agent (ampicillin, penicillin, or vancomycin). **High-level aminoglycoside resistance** in enterococci is usually the result of enzymatic inactivation of the drugs, and the enzymes that destroy gentamicin also destroy tobramycin, amikacin, and kanamycin, as shown in Table 13-6. Consequently none of these agents is used in treating serious infections caused by enterococci with high-level gentamicin resistance. If the isolate does not have concomitant high-level streptomycin resistance, however, streptomycin could be used, although some isolates have high-level resistance to both gentamicin and streptomycin.

In vitro tests for detection of high-level aminoglycoside resistance include broth, agar, or disk diffusion methods. For screening, gentamicin is tested at concentrations of 500 μg/mL and streptomycin at 2000 μg/mL (agar) or 1000 μg/mL (broth). The tests are performed as described for routine dilution tests, and growth at the high concentration indicates that the isolate has high-level resistance to the agent tested. Disk diffusion tests have also been described that use special disks containing high concentrations of gentamicin (120 μg) or streptomycin (300 μg).

Detection of Vancomycin Resistance in Enterococci. The incidence of vancomycin resistance in enterococci increased sharply in the 1990s and the early part of the decade of 2000s. *E. faecium* is the most common species demonstrating vancomycin resistance among clinical isolates, followed by *E. faecalis*. Isolates that are highly resistant to vancomycin can be readily detected as vancomycin resistant when tested by conventional antimicrobial susceptibility test methods. Some isolates, however, may have a more subtle type of vancomycin resistance whereby MICs or inhibition zone measurements are just slightly above or below, respectively, the susceptible breakpoints. Hence dilution tests must be viewed closely, and inhibition zones in disk diffusion testing must be examined using transmitted (rather than reflected) light; any growth within the zone should be considered significant. The **vancomycin agar screen plate** contains brain-heart infusion (BHI) agar supplemented with 6 μg/mL vancomycin and is very useful in screening for vancomycin resistance. The same vancomycin agar screen plate can be used both for testing enterococci and *S. aureus* for vancomycin resistance or diminished susceptibility.

Low-level vancomycin resistance is intrinsic in the motile enterococcal species, *Enterococcus gallinarum* and *Enterococcus casseliflavus*. These differ from true **vancomycin-resistant enterococci (VRE)** for infection-control purposes. Additionally, *Leuconostoc* spp., *Pediococcus* spp., and *Lactobacillus* spp. also demonstrate intrinsic, high-level vancomycin resistance, and these bacteria must be carefully separated from the morphologically similar enterococci.

Extended Spectrum β-Lactamases

Most *K. pneumoniae*, *Klebsiella oxytoca*, and many *E. coli* are resistant to ampicillin because of production of a plasmid-mediated β-lactamase known as TEM-1 or SHV-1. Most isolates are susceptible to later-generation cephalosporins and aztreonam; however, spontaneous mutations occur that may result in novel **β-lactamases** that can inactivate extended-spectrum cephalosporins, penicillins, and aztreonam. These β-lactamases are known as **extended-spectrum β-lactamases (ESBLs).** The enzymes are characterized and numbered based on their relationship to the parent enzymes. There are now more than 130 TEM-derived ESBLs and more than 60 derived from SHV-1. In addition, other novel β-lactamases have been designated as CTX-M or OXA that are not a result of mutations of the TEM or SHV parent enzymes. Some of these β-lactamases give rise to subtle or difficult-to-detect resistance among cephalosporins, penicillins, or aztreonam. Recently these enzymes have been found in other genera and species including *Proteus mirabilis, Salmonella* spp., and *Enterobacter* spp. most notably.

Strategies for laboratory detection of ESBL-producing *E. coli, Klebsiella* spp., and *P. mirabilis* include testing of drugs that are most likely to indicate the presence of an ESBL (the "indicator" drugs). These include, in decreasing order of sensitivity for detection, cefpodoxime, ceftazidime, cefotaxime, ceftriaxone, aztreonam, and use of special screening zone or MIC breakpoints to facilitate recognition of ESBL production. Indicator drugs have been selected based on the likelihood of their being readily hydrolyzed by one of the many types of ESBLs. The use of more than one antimicrobial agent increases the sensitivity of detection. Once an ESBL-producing isolate is presumptively detected, confirmatory testing must be performed. Because ESBL activity is inhibited by β-lactamase inhibitor agents such as clavulanic acid, this property forms the basis of the confirmatory tests. If the activity of either cefotaxime or ceftazidime or both is restored when tested in combination with clavulanic acid by disk diffusion or a MIC test, the resistance is due to ESBL production. Figure 13-15 shows an ESBL confirmatory test performed using the disk diffusion method. Resistance in ESBL-producing strains to various β-lactam agents is not always predicted by in vitro tests performed using standard inoculum density. For example, a confirmed ESBL-producing *K. pneumoniae* isolate may appear susceptible to cefotaxime by disk diffusion or MIC tests; however, cefotaxime is hydrolyzed at a high inoculum density and is ineffective in treating infections caused by such strains. Consequently, when an ESBL-producing isolate is identified, it should be reported as clinically resistant to all cephalosporins, penicillins, and aztreonam, despite the in vitro test results. The carbapenems (imipenem, meropenem, ertapenem) are active against ESBL-producing strains, as are the

cephamycins (cefoxitin and cefotetan). ESBL-producing isolates show variable susceptibility to aminoglycosides, fluoroquinolones, and trimethoprim-sulfamethoxazole, although many isolates are multiply resistant to those agents.

Carbapenemases

***Klebsiella pneumoniae* Carbapenemase.** *Klebsiella pneumoniae* carbapenemases (KPC), although initially identified in *K. pneumoniae,* have now been recognized in a variety of other Enterobacteriaceae. Organisms possessing these enzymes are often resistant to one or more of the carbapenems. In vitro susceptibility testing of Enterobacteriaceae containing KPC may indicate that the isolate is susceptible to carbapenems, but therapeutically the carbapenems antimicrobial may not work. Currently no reliable in vitro method exists for identifying these organisms. However, if an isolate possess ESBL and the MIC for a carbapenems is 2 or 4 µg/mL, there is a possibility that it may produce KPC-type or some other carbapenemase. Because these organisms are resistant to carbapenems, infections often are treated with colistin or polymyxin antimicrobials with mixed results.

AUTOMATED ANTIMICROBIAL SUSCEPTIBILITY TEST METHODS

Principles of Technologies Used

The automated susceptibility testing instruments that are currently available represent a choice of several different levels of automation. One instrument interprets growth endpoints of broth-microdilution panels only when they are placed into an automated reader device, whereas certain other instruments provide hands-off incubation and reading functions for microdilution trays or special cards in an incubator-reader device. The instruments that offer the highest level of automation accomplish these tasks through the use of robotics to move the panels or cards in the instrument during the incubation-reading sequences or to add reagents to certain test wells for biochemical tests.

Current instruments employ one of two optical approaches for examining the test wells of the antimicrobial-containing panels or cards. Most current instruments use the principle of turbidimetric detection of bacterial growth in a broth medium by use of a photometer to examine the test wells. The determination of antimicrobial susceptibility based on lack of development of turbidity (suppression of growth) or, conversely, an indication of resistance based on an increase in turbidity in the presence of an antimicrobial agent is the same principle as that used when manual interpretation of growth endpoints is performed. The second means of growth detection is the detection of hydrolysis of a fluorogenic growth substrate incorporated in a special test medium. With this technology, growth is detected by a fluorometer as emission of a fluorescent signal when a microorganism consumes fluorophore-labeled substrate in the test medium during growth.

Instruments for antimicrobial susceptibility testing may function to provide assistance in the interpretation of test results after a conventional overnight incubation period, or they may allow results to be determined in a shortened analy-

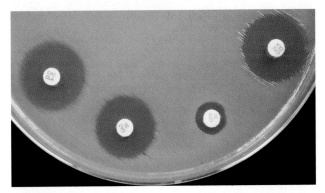

FIGURE 13-15 Extended spectrum β-lactamase (ESBL) phenotypic confirmatory testing of *Klebsiella pneumoniae.* The standard disk diffusion test is performed with both cefotaxime and ceftazidime with and without clavulanic acid. The diameter of the zone around cefotaxime-clavulanic acid (4-o'clock position) is greater than 5 mm larger than the zone around cefotaxime (5-o'clock position), which indicates a positive reaction as clavulanic acid restores the activity of cefotaxime. Although the zones for ceftazidime and ceftazidime-clavulanic acid are comparable, only one "set" of drugs needs to be positive to confirm an isolate as an ESBL producer.

sis period of 5 to 15 hours. Instrumentation may allow the interpretation of antimicrobial susceptibility test endpoints sooner than manual readings because of the greater sensitivity of the instruments' optical systems in the detection of subtle increases in microbial growth. All the instruments rely heavily on microprocessor-controlled functions and use personal computer hardware to provide final printed reports and to store and retrieve data on antimicrobial susceptibility. Most of the instruments also may be used to perform identifications of gram-negative or gram-positive bacteria and to merge and print identification and antimicrobial susceptibility results into a single report or to transfer the information to a laboratory information system (LIS) using a unidirectional or bidirectional interface.

Currently Available Automated Systems

Reader Devices for Broth Microdilution Susceptibility Tests

Every commercial manufacturer of broth microdilution antimicrobial susceptibility testing panels offers a view box or mirror device to facilitate manual reading of results after incubation. Products that feature freeze-dried antimicrobial panels also offer a mechanized device to simplify hydration and inoculation of panels. In addition, TREK Diagnostic Systems (Cleveland, Ohio) offers an instrument-assisted reader, the Sensititre SensiTouch, that allows the technologist to record the results of manual readings of the panels by use of a touch-sensitive template that overlies the microdilution panel. A similar instrument, the MicroScan TouchScan, is available from Siemans Healthcare Diagnostics (Sacramento, Calif.) and can be used with the MicroScan system. Siemans Healthcare Diagnostics also manufacturers an automated reader, the autoSCAN-4, that interprets growth patterns in panels by turbidimetric analysis following placement of individual panels into the device. These instruments are configured with personal computers for report printing and long-term data storage.

Automated Instrument Systems

Currently four instruments are available that are capable of generating rapid (5 to 15 hours) or overnight (16 to 24 hours) susceptibility test results.

BD Phoenix System. The newest automated susceptibility-testing instrument is the BD Phoenix Automated Microbiology System (BD Diagnostic Systems, Sparks, Md.). It has been marketed in Europe, Japan, Canada, and the United States. The Phoenix consists of an upright instrument with a built-in keyboard and bar-coding station that can accommodate 100 test panels simultaneously, along with a separate printer (Figure 13-16). The specially designed test cartridges contain 136 small wells (Figure 13-17) to test as many as 16 to 25 different antimicrobial agents, either alone or in combination with wells containing biochemical substrates for simultaneous identification of common gram-positive or gram-negative bacteria, including streptococci. The test panels are inoculated manually by a simple gravity-fed transfer of inoculated medium throughout the disposable cartridge

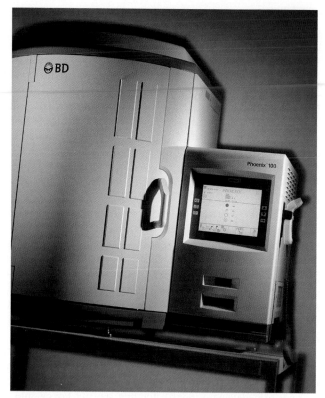

FIGURE 13-16 BD Phoenix Automated Microbiology System. (Courtesy BD Diagnostic Systems, Sparks, Md.)

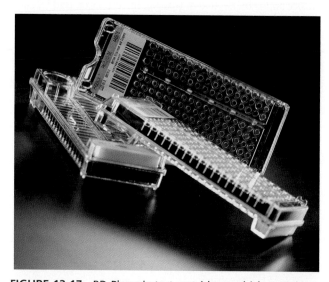

FIGURE 13-17 BD Phoenix test cartridges, which contain 136 wells of antimicrobial agents or biochemical tests.

after pouring inoculated broth through an opening in the test device. The Phoenix employs a redox indicator system (similar to resazurin) to measure bacterial growth in the susceptibility test wells. The indicator is added to the broth at the time of organism inoculation. This approach allows susceptibility determinations following approximately 6 to 8 hours of incubation. The Phoenix instrument includes a rules-based expert system (BDXpert) and can be purchased with a data management personal computer (PC) and software package called *BD EpiCenter,* which allows networking with other BD microbiology instruments and a bidirectional interface for connection with an LIS.

MicroScan WalkAway SI. The MicroScan WalkAway SI (Siemans Healthcare Diagnostics, Sacramento, Calif.) consists of a large, self-contained incubator-reader unit with capacities for either 40 or 96 test panels and a PC with video display terminal and printer (Figure 13-18). The WalkAway uses microdilution panels that are hydrated and inoculated with a hand-operated inoculator device (Figure 13-19). Panels are then placed in one of the positions in the large incubator module. The type of test to be performed is indicated on an instrument-readable bar-code label located on the end of each panel. The instrument incubates the panels for the appropriate period (depending on the type of panel and organism), robotically positions the trays to add reagents if needed, and moves them under the central photometer station to perform the final readings of growth endpoints at the conclusion of the tests.

Standard dried panels are read turbidimetrically by the WalkAway after an overnight incubation period. The instru-

ment offers the possibility of early, "read when ready" interpretations of the standard panels in 4.5 to 6.5 hours if an isolate is unequivocally susceptible or highly resistant. Organisms with inducible or slow to be expressed resistance are automatically extended to overnight incubation. MIC or breakpoint panels are available for testing of gram-positive and gram-negative bacteria as well as special "combo" panels that allow simultaneous susceptibility and organism identification in the same panel. With the standard dried panels, it is possible to read the panels visually in the case of an instrument malfunction. MicroScan rapid panels that use fluorogenic substrates have been available for some time, but now such panels are only available for testing gram-negative bacteria. Results are available in 3.5 to 15 hours. This older, rapid technology, however, is being phased out in favor of the "read when ready" approach. MicroScan also provides panels containing lysed horse blood for testing streptococci that are incubated offline and read manually. MicroScan LabPro software contains rules to alert users of any susceptibility profile on an individual isolate that requires attention and also contains a component for epidemiologic analyses of stored data.

TREK Sensititre. The Sensititre Automated Incubator Reader (ARIS 2X, TREK Diagnostic Systems) was the first system to be marketed in the United States that used a fluorometric detection system for detecting growth endpoints of common, rapidly growing bacteria using MIC or breakpoint formats with either a 5- or 18-hour incubation period. Subsequent experience using rapid fluorogenic substrate detection of growth with this system and one other system demonstrated that some resistance mechanisms cannot be accurately detected in a 5-hour period. For this reason, TREK has FDA clearance for only the 16- to 24-hour incubation version of the instrument in the United States for susceptibility testing.

The Sensititre ARIS 2X (Figure 13-20) is a fully automatic, benchtop incubating and reading system. It fits onto the AutoReader and uses an internal bar-code scanner to identify each plate type and assign the appropriate incubation time; when the assigned time has elapsed, the plate is then trans-

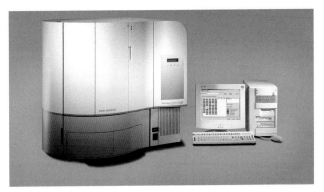

FIGURE 13-18 MicroScan WalkAway *SI.* (Courtesy Siemens Healthcare Diagnostics Inc. Sacramento, Calif.)

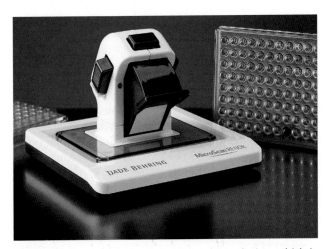

FIGURE 13-19 MicroScan Renok inoculator device, which is used to reconstitute and inoculate dried antimicrobial agents or biochemical tests in the test panels. A test panel is also shown.

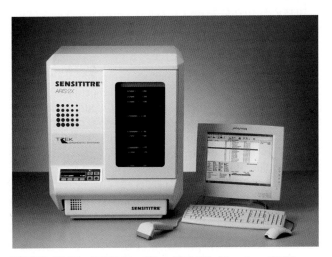

FIGURE 13-20 TREK Sensititre ARIS 2X. (Courtesy TREK Diagnostic Systems, Cleveland, Ohio.)

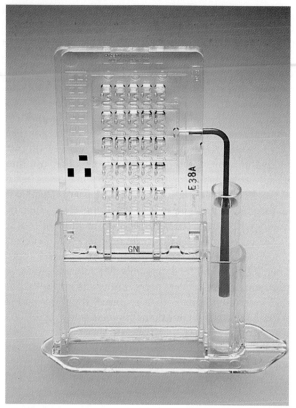

FIGURE 13-21 Vitek test card containing dried antimicrobials connected by a transfer straw to a tube containing a standardized inoculum suspension of bacteria to be tested. These are placed into an evacuating chamber, which allows the inoculum to be transferred into the card. All wells containing varying concentrations of various antimicrobial agents are reconstituted during this inoculation process. Finally, the inoculated cards are placed into the Vitek instrument for processing.

ported to the AutoReader for fluorescence measurement with no manual intervention. The AutoReader holds as many as 64 plates.

VITEK 1, VITEK 2, and VITEK 2 Compact. The VITEK System (bioMérieux Vitek, Hazelwood, Mo.) was originally designed for use in the United States space exploration efforts of the 1970s as an onboard test system for spacecraft exploring other planets for life. Because of its original design intention, it was highly automated and relatively compact. Small plastic reagent cards (similar in size to a credit card; Figure 13-21) contain microliter quantities of various concentrations of antimicrobial agents in 45 wells for susceptibility testing. The VITEK (now called the VITEK 1) can be configured to accommodate 30, 60, 120, or 240 cards. The susceptibility cards allow quantitative MIC results accompanied by susceptible, intermediate, or resistant results interpretations for most rapidly growing gram-positive and gram-negative aerobic bacteria in a period of 4 to 18 hours. Owing in part to its aerospace design heritage, the VITEK 1 has proven to be a highly reliable instrument. VITEK 1 hardware consists of a

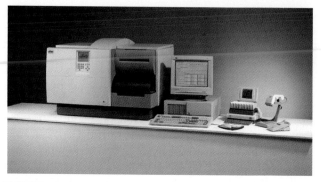

FIGURE 13-22 VITEK 2 System. (Courtesy bioMérieux Vitek, Hazelwood, Mo.)

filling module for inoculation of the cards, an incubator-reader module that incorporates a carousel to hold the test cards, a robotic system to manipulate the cards, a photometer for turbidimetric measurement of growth once per hour, and a computer module with video display terminal and printer for viewing and printing results. VITEK 1 also offers an information management system for storing and retrieving test data for a variety of statistical reports.

A newer and more automated instrument is the VITEK 2 (Figure 13-22), which automates the initial sample processing steps to a greater degree than the VITEK 1. It facilitates adjustment of the inoculum density, the transfer of inoculum suspension to the cards, and the sealing of the cards in a single instrument module. The VITEK 2 cards are slightly thicker than those of the previous VITEK and contain 64 wells to allow testing of more drugs in a single card. The VITEK 2 incorporates bar-code labeling of cards and storage of isolate data programmed by the "smart carrier" work-station in a computer chip imbedded in a cassette that moves the cards through the instrument. The VITEK 2 can be configured to accommodate 60 to 120 cards in the instrument, and a larger version, the VITEK 2 XL will allow testing of 180 to 240 cards. The VITEK 2 cards are read turbidimetrically every 15 minutes and analyzed according to several computer algorithms specific to each drug and organism. The VITEK 2 can test *S. pneumoniae* in addition to the nonfastidious aerobic gram-positive and gram-negative bacteria. The VITEK 2 offers one of the highest levels of automation currently available in microbiology instrumentation.

The newest instrument from bioMérieux is the VITEK 2 Compact. It represents a less automated version of the VITEK 2 that uses the same cards but without the smart carrier and programmed cassette for specimen handling automation available in the VITEK 2. It includes a compact, self-contained vacuum chamber and card sealer similar to the separate modules of the VITEK 1. The instrument is available in a 30- or 60-card size and represents a more compact, simpler, and less expensive option for laboratories that do not require the level of automation provided by the smart carrier of the VITEK 2.

All three of the VITEK instruments use kinetic measurements of growth in the presence of antimicrobial agents to

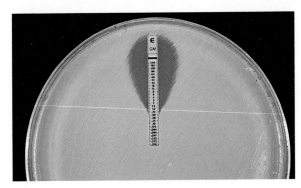

FIGURE 13-23 *Escherichia coli* tested with an Etest gentamicin strip. The gentamicin minimal inhibitory concentration (where the ellipse crosses the gradient) is 0.75 μg/mL.

provide analysis of growth curves, leading to computer algorithm–derived MIC values. All three instruments include either a rules-based expert system (VITEK 1) or an Advanced Expert System (VITEK 2 and Compact) to assist in controlling common technical errors and to facilitate detection of unusual resistance mechanisms before results are reported.

Nonautomated Antimicrobial Susceptibility Test Method: Etest

A product that differs slightly in principle from the test methods described thus far is Etest (AB Biodisk, Solna, Sweden), which employs the principle of establishing an antimicrobial density gradient in an agar medium as a means of determining antimicrobial susceptibility. The Etest uses thin plastic test strips that are impregnated on the under surface with an antimicrobial concentration gradient and are marked on the upper surface with a concentration index or scale. The strips may be placed in a radial fashion on the surface of an agar plate that has been inoculated in a manner similar to that for a disk diffusion test. After overnight incubation the test results are read by viewing the plates from the top side with the lids removed. The antimicrobial gradient that forms in the agar around the Etest strips gives rise to elliptic inhibitory areas with each strip. The MIC is determined where the growth ellipse intersects the Etest strip (Figure 13-23). The Etest shares with the disk diffusion test the intrinsic flexibility of drug selection and testing because selected strips are applied to the surface of test plates. The cost of Etest strips is much greater than that of disks, however, and represents one of the main limitations of this product. Published studies have indicated in general that MICs determined using the Etest compare favorably (within one twofold-dilution interval) with those determined by conventional broth- or agar-dilution methods.

The Etest can be especially useful for testing fastidious organisms such as *S. pneumoniae*, other streptococci, *H. influenzae*, and anaerobic bacteria, in part because the strips can be placed on special enriched media or in a special incubation atmosphere (e.g., increased CO_2 or anaerobic) and the fact

that relatively few antimicrobial agents may need to be tested against fastidious organisms. Consequently the relatively high cost of the Etest strips could be minimized.

INTERPRETATION OF IN VITRO ANTIMICROBIAL SUSCEPTIBILITY TEST RESULTS

Several elements are important in performing any in vitro antimicrobial susceptibility test. This chapter described the methods for several types of tests. The procedural steps of each method must be followed explicitly to obtain reproducible results. A susceptibility test should never be performed using an inoculum that is not standardized or a mixed culture. For that reason, direct susceptibility tests that incorporate the use of a patient's infected body fluid cannot be recommended, even to obtain a presumptive result.

The results of a susceptibility test must be interpreted in the laboratory before a report is communicated to a patient's physician. In the case of a disk diffusion test, the inhibition zone size must be interpreted using a table of values that relates the diameter of the zone to a category of susceptibility, which is sometimes related to the identity of the isolate for correct interpretation. The table used for such interpretations must represent the most up-to-date criteria that have been reviewed and accepted by the CLSI. It is important to recognize that the CLSI documents are updated frequently, usually once per year. Use of old or outdated CLSI tables could represent a serious shortcoming in the reporting of patients' results.

The inhibition zone size and MIC interpretive criteria published by the CLSI and the FDA are established by careful analysis of three kinds of data: (1) microbiologic data (e.g., a comparison of MICs versus zone sizes on a large number of bacterial strains, including those with known resistance mechanisms), (2) pharmacokinetic data (e.g., serum, cerebrospinal fluid [CSF], urine, and other secretion and tissue levels of an antimicrobial agent), and (3) results of clinical studies obtained during the phase before FDA approval and marketing of an antimicrobial agent. Thus MIC interpretive criteria are not based simply on a comparison of serum levels of an antimicrobial agent and MIC values. Zone-diameter interpretive criteria are, however, based in large part on direct correlations of MICs and zone sizes.

Whether based on determination of an MIC or on interpretation of a disk diffusion zone diameter, the four categories of susceptibility should be interpreted in the same manner. If the MIC or zone size is interpreted as susceptible using the most recent interpretive criteria, the clinical interpretation of the result is that the patient's infecting organism should respond to therapy with that antimicrobial agent using the recommended dosage for the site of infection. Conversely an MIC or zone size interpreted as resistant is unlikely to be inhibited by the usually achievable concentrations of the antimicrobial agent based on the dosages normally used with that drug. An intermediate result indicates that a microorganism falls into a range of susceptibility in which the MIC approaches or exceeds the level of antimicrobial agent that can ordinarily

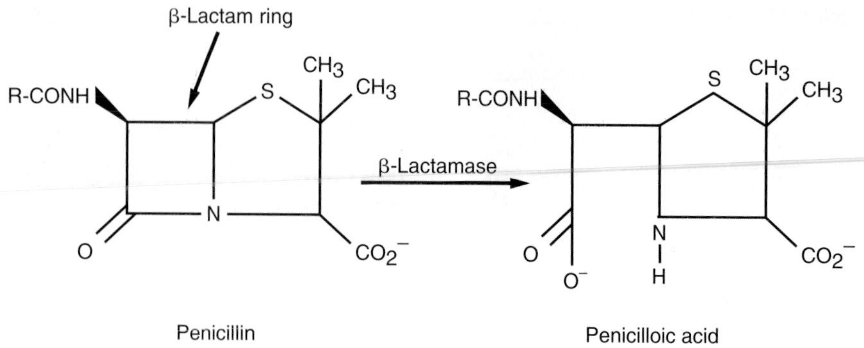

FIGURE 13-24 β-Lactamase hydrolyzes the β-lactam ring portion of the penicillin molecule. The hydrolysis results in the formation of penicilloic acid, which does not have antibacterial activity.

be achieved and for which clinical response is likely to be less than with a susceptible strain. Exceptions can occur if the antimicrobial agent is highly concentrated in a body fluid, such as urine, or if a higher-than-normal dosage of the antimicrobial agent can be safely administered (e.g., some penicillins and cephalosporins). At times the intermediate result means that certain variables in the susceptibility test may not have been well controlled and the values have fallen into a "buffer zone" separating susceptible from resistant strains.

Another category that may be used for reporting is "nonsusceptible." This category is used when there are no *intermediate* or *resistant* interpretive criteria, only a *susceptible* interpretive criteria, and the MIC or disk diffusion zone size for classifying the organism as susceptible is not achieved. In these cases the identity of the organism should be confirmed and the susceptibility testing repeated. If the results are still nonsusceptible, it may be appropriate to send the organism to a reference laboratory. The *nonsusceptible* category commonly occurs with newer antimicrobials because during drug development and initial clinical trials, no organisms were found that were resistant to the antimicrobial. The category nonsusceptible does not necessarily mean that the organism is resistant to the antimicrobial.

Certain other specific aspects of susceptibility test reporting are detailed in the CLSI tables, such as refraining from reporting results for antimicrobial agents that do not penetrate into the CSF on isolates from patients who have meningitis. Additionally, results for antimicrobial agents that are only useful for treating UTIs must not be reported on isolates from specimens other than urine.

Lastly, no objective evidence suggests that the reporting of an MIC result is any more clinically relevant than the reporting of a category (*S, I, R*) result in the majority of infections. Perhaps the reporting of MIC results could aid a physician in selecting from among a group of similar drugs for therapy of infective endocarditis or osteomyelitis, in which therapy is likely to be protracted. For virtually all other infections, however, category results provide the clinician with the information necessary to select appropriate therapy. Only physicians trained in infectious diseases are likely to be familiar with expected MICs for the multitude of antimicrobial agents

currently available. Thus, if MIC results are to be reported, inclusion of appropriate interpretive criteria with the results is essential.

METHODS OF DETECTING ANTIMICROBIAL-INACTIVATING ENZYMES

β-Lactamase Tests

The β-lactamases are enzymes that chemically inactivate β-lactam molecules by disrupting the β-lactam ring component of the molecule (Figure 13-24). Production of β-lactamase is a significant mechanism contributing to resistance to some β-lactams in certain organisms, such as *H. influenzae, N. gonorrhoeae, M. catarrhalis, Staphylococcus* spp., and some *Bacteroides* spp. Simple β-lactamase tests can be performed in the clinical laboratory to identify β-lactamase production in these organisms, and a positive reaction means that the β-lactam agent(s) commonly used to treat infections caused by the organism (primarily the penicillins ampicillin, amoxicillin, and penicillin) would be ineffective. Although many other organisms, such as members of the Enterobacteriaceae family and the *Pseudomonas* spp., produce a variety of different types of β-lactamases, the currently available direct β-lactamase tests cannot predict resistance to the newer β-lactam agents that might be used for these organisms, and thus β-lactamase testing should not be performed on them.

Several methods are available for detection of β-lactamase production, the most common of which uses the chromogenic cephalosporin nitrocefin. Cefinase disks represent a commercial product available from BD Diagnostic Systems (Sparks, Md.). The product consists of filter paper disks impregnated with nitrocefin. A disk is moistened with water or saline and a loopful of organisms is applied directly onto the disk. Within 10 minutes (or within 60 minutes for staphylococci), the area where the organisms were applied will turn red in the case of a β-lactamase–producing organism. No color change occurs with β-lactamase–negative organisms (Figure 13-25).

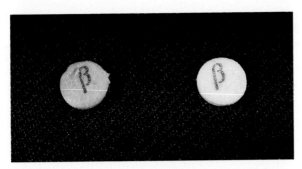

FIGURE 13-25 Cefinase β-lactamase disk test. Cells from several colonies of *Haemophilus influenzae* were applied to a moistened disk. This photo shows results following testing of two different isolates. Within 10 minutes, the disk on the left turned brown-red (positive), and that on the right maintained a light yellow color (negative).

Other types of β-lactamase tests include penicillin-based acidimetric and iodometric tests that detect production of penicilloic acid from hydrolysis of penicillin by a β-lactamase. The acidimetric method uses citrate-buffered penicillin and phenol red as a pH indicator. When colonies of a β-lactamase–producing organism are added to the solution, the penicilloic acid results in a drop in pH, causing a color change from red to yellow. In the iodometric method, a solution of phosphate-buffered penicillin and starch-iodine complex is used. With β-lactamase–positive organisms, penicilloic acid reduces iodine and prevents it from combining with starch. A positive reaction is colorless, and a negative reaction is purple.

All the species mentioned previously in this section, except staphylococci, produce β-lactamase constitutively, meaning that the same amount of enzyme is produced regardless of exposure to an inducing agent. Production of β-lactamase in staphylococci is inducible, and exposure to an inducing agent (another β-lactam agent) is often required to obtain enough concentrations of the enzyme for detection with conventional β-lactamase tests.

Testing organisms (e.g., staphylococci) that have been exposed to an inducing agent can be accomplished by using growth from the periphery of a zone surrounding a β-lactam disk (e.g., oxacillin; Figure 13-26). The bacterial cells at the zone edge have been stimulated to express their β-lactamase. Alternatively the test can be performed on bacteria growing in a well of a broth microdilution panel that contains a sub-inhibitory concentration (i.e., a low concentration that does not inhibit visual growth) of a β-lactam agent. The rapidity of β-lactamase tests makes them attractive as a means for direct detection of one important resistance determinant. A positive reaction indicates resistance to ampicillin, amoxicillin, and penicillin; and a negative reaction indicates that the test organisms do not produce β-lactamase, although they may be resistant to these agents through another mechanism. Resistance related to other mechanisms may be detected only with conventional dilution or disk diffusion tests. With organisms in which the rate of resistance associated with β-lactamase production is the predominant mechanism of resistance (e.g., *M. catarrhalis*), other testing may not be necessary for routine patient care.

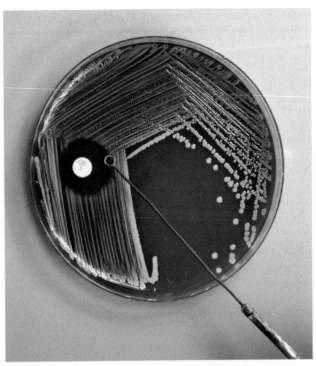

FIGURE 13-26 *Staphylococcus aureus* grown on a blood agar plate to which an oxacillin disk has been applied. Cells around the periphery of the zone have been exposed to oxacillin molecules as they diffused into the agar, and these cells are used for the β-lactamase test. Oxacillin is a good inducer of staphylococcal β-lactamase and will induce the strain to produce larger quantities of β-lactamase. Consequently, strains that are penicillin susceptible (minimal inhibitory concentration 0.06 to 0.12 µg/mL) are tested for β-lactamase production following exposure to an inducing agent to determine whether they are β-lactamase positive and thus penicillin resistant.

QUALITY CONTROL OF ANTIMICROBIAL SUSCEPTIBILITY TESTS

Quality control (QC) of antimicrobial susceptibility tests involves testing standard reference strains that have defined antimicrobial susceptibility (or resistance) to the drugs tested. It is important to use QC strains that represent the types of patient isolates tested in the respective laboratory. Additionally the QC strains should represent varying degrees of susceptibility (or resistance). Ideal QC strains for MIC tests have what is known as *on-scale MIC endpoints* for the drugs tested. An on-scale endpoint falls within the range of concentrations tested compared with off-scale endpoints where the MIC is less than the lowest or greater than the highest concentration tested.

The CLSI has identified American Type Culture Collection (ATCC) strains that are useful for QC testing (Table 13-7). The CLSI documents also include tables that define acceptable results (zone measurements for disk diffusion tests or MICs for dilution tests) for these strains; examples are shown in Tables 13-8 and 13-9, respectively. The procedure followed in testing QC reference strains must be identical to

TABLE 13-7 Strains Commonly Used for Quality Control of Routine Antimicrobial Susceptibility Tests

Test	QC Strains Used	Comments
Antimicrobial susceptibility of gram-positive organisms	*Staphylococcus aureus* ATCC 25923	β-lactamase negative for disk diffusion tests
	S. aureus ATCC 29213	β-lactamase positive for MIC tests
Oxacillin salt agar screen for *S. aureus*	*S. aureus* ATCC 43300	Oxacillin resistant
Vancomycin BHI screen, synergy screen for enterococci and *S. aureus*	*Enterococcus faecalis* ATCC 29212	Susceptible to vancomycin and susceptible to high levels of gentamicin and streptomycin (synergy screen tests negative)
	E. faecalis ATCC 51299	Resistant to vancomycin and resistant to high levels of gentamicin and streptomycin (synergy screen tests positive)
Antimicrobial susceptibility of gram-negative organisms	*Escherichia coli* ATCC 25922	
	Pseudomonas aeruginosa ATCC 27853	
	E. coli ATCC 35218	β-Lactamase positive for testing β-lactam/β-lactamase inhibitor combination agents only
ESBL test	*Klebsiella pneumoniae* ATCC 700603	ESBL screen test and ESBL confirmatory test positive
Antimicrobial susceptibility of *Haemophilus* spp.	*Haemophilus influenzae* ATCC 49247	Ampicillin resistant, non–β-lactamase producing
	H. influenzae ATCC 49766	Ampicillin susceptible
	H. influenzae ATCC 10211	Used by media manufacturers to assess growth-supporting capabilities of the medium
Antimicrobial susceptibility of *Neisseria gonorrhoeae*	*N. gonorrhoeae* ATC 49226	β-Lactamase negative
Antimicrobial susceptibility testing of *S. pneumoniae* and other streptococci	*Streptococcus pneumoniae* ATCC 49619	Penicillin-intermediate
Antimicrobial susceptibility of anaerobes	*Bacteroides fragilis* ATCC 25285 *Bacteroides thetaiotamicron* ATCC 29741 *Eubacterium lentum* ATCC 43055	
Assessment of acceptability of medium (low thymine and thymidine content) for testing sulfonamides, trimethoprim, and trimethoprim-sulfamethoxazole	*E. faecalis* ATCC 29212	

ATCC, American Type Culture Collection; *BHI,* brain–heart infusion; *ESBL,* extended-spectrum β-lactamase; *MIC,* minimal inhibitory concentration; *QC,* quality control.

TABLE 13-8 Acceptable Limits for Quality Control Strains Used to Monitor Accuracy of Disk Diffusion Testing of Nonfastidious Organisms (Using Mueller-Hinton Medium Without Blood or Other Supplements)

Antimicrobial Agent	Disk Content (mcg)	*Escherichia coli* ATCC 25922	*Staphylococcus aureus* ATCC 25923	*Pseudomonas aeruginosa* ATCC 27853	*Escherichia coli* ATCC 35218
Ampicillin	10	16-22	27-35	—	6
Amoxicillin/clavulanic acid	20/10	18-24	28-36	—	17-22
Cefazolin	30	21-27	29-35	—	—
Gentamicin	10	19-26	19-27	16-21	—

Modified from Clinical and Laboratory Standards Institute (CLSI) publication M100-S19: *Performance standards for antimicrobial susceptibility testing: nineteenth informational supplement.* Copies of the current edition may be obtained from CLSI, 940 West Valley Road, Suite 1400, Wayne, Pa., 19087-1898. *ATTC,* American Type Culture Collection.

that used for testing patient isolates. If results with QC strains do not fall within the defined acceptable limits, corrective action must be taken to determine the reason for the out-of-control observation before reporting of any patient results. Quality control testing is recommended each day that patient tests are performed; however, the frequency of QC testing can be reduced to weekly if a laboratory can demonstrate acceptable performance with the QC strains. This consists of obtaining results that are within acceptable limits for each antimicrobial agent-QC strain combination for 20 or 30 consecutive test days. Quality control procedures must always be performed when new lots of materials are put into use, and

TABLE 13-9 Acceptable Limits for Quality Control Strains Used to Monitor Accuracy of MICs (mcg/mL) of Nonfastidious Organisms (Using Cation-Adjusted Mueller-Hinton Medium Without Blood or Other Nutritional Supplements)

Antimicrobial Agent	Escherichia coli ATCC 25922	Staphylococcus aureus ATCC 29213	Pseudomonas aeruginosa ATCC 27853	Escherichia coli ATCC 35218
Ampicillin	2-8	0.5-2	—	—
Amoxicillin/clavulanic acid	2/1-8/4	0.12/0.06-0.5/0.25	—	4/2-16/8
Cefazolin	1-4	0.25-1	—	—
Gentamicin	0.25-1	0.12-1	0.5-2	—

Modified from Clinical and Laboratory Standards Institute (CLSI) publication M100-S19: *Performance standards for antimicrobial susceptibility testing: nineteenth informational supplement.* Copies of the current edition may be obtained from CLSI, 940 West Valley Road, Suite 1400, Wayne, Pa., 19087-1898.
MICs, Minimal inhibitory concentrations.

TABLE 13-10 Examples of Typical Antibiograms for Several Gram-Negative Species*

Antimicrobial Agent	Escherichia coli	Enterobacter cloacae	Proteus mirabilis	Pseudomonas aeruginosa	Stenotrophomonas maltophilia
Amikacin	S	S	S	S	R
Ampicillin	S	R	S	R	R
Ampicillin/sulbactam	S	R	S	R	R
Cephalothin	S	R	S	R	R
Cefoxitin	S	S-R	S	R	R
Cefotaxime	S	S-R	S	S-R	R
Ceftazidime	S	S	S	S	S-R
Ciprofloxacin	S	S	S	S	R
Gentamicin	S	S	S	S	R
Imipenem	S	S	S	S	R
Piperacillin	S	S	S	S	R
Nitrofurantoin	S	S	R	R	R
Tobramycin	S	S	S	S	R
Trimethoprim-sulfamethoxazole	S	S	S	R	S

R, Resistant; *S,* susceptible; *S-R,* variable result.
*Results indicated represent the typical response found in the majority of clinical isolates; however, these can vary significantly.

test materials must never be used beyond their stated expiration dates.

There are other less obvious components of a QC program for antimicrobial susceptibility testing. Supplemental QC strains may be periodically tested to validate acceptable performance of specific antimicrobial agent-organism combinations that may be only modestly controlled with the routine reference strains. An MRSA strain could be included to ensure that the test system can detect heteroresistant strains. Similarly, ampicillin-resistant *Enterobacter cloacae* might be included to ensure that the system can detect ampicillin resistance. Supplemental QC strains are sometimes used for troubleshooting specific problems or training new employees. Another component of a QC program involves the inclusion of mechanisms to ensure that personnel performing testing are proficient in their tasks. Self-assessment checklists and supervisory review of reported results are examples of such mechanisms. Satisfactory performance on proficiency survey specimens and the use of relevant testing strategies are also QC parameters.

The most widely used supplemental QC measure is the use of antibiograms to verify results generated on patient isolates.

An antibiogram is the overall antimicrobial susceptibility profile of a bacterial isolate to a battery of antimicrobial agents. Certain species have "typical" antibiograms, which can be used to verify the identification as well as the susceptibility results generated on the isolate (Table 13-10). For example, *P. aeruginosa* is typically resistant to ampicillin, cefazolin (and other first- and second-generation cephalosporins), and trimethoprim-sulfamethoxazole; however, it is often susceptible to gentamicin (and other aminoglycosides), extended-spectrum penicillins (e.g., piperacillin), and ciprofloxacin. In contrast, *E. coli* is generally susceptible to all the aforementioned antimicrobial agents. Table 13-11 shows several atypical antibiograms suggesting the result highlighted is erroneous. The CLSI now provides a listing of those results that should be verified because they (1) have never been encountered, (2) are uncommon, or (3) represent results that could easily occur as a result of technical errors and might have significant clinical consequences. One list includes susceptibility test results for certain genera or species that should be verified by all laboratories, and another reflects results that need not be verified in facilities where the results are common. An excerpt from these listings is shown in Table 13-12.

TABLE 13-11 Examples of "Problem" Antibiograms Suggestive of Technical Errors

Antimicrobial Agent	Escherichia coli*	Enterobacter cloacae†	Pseudomonas aeruginosa‡	Stenotrophomonas maltophilia§
Amikacin	R	S	S	R
Ampicillin	S	R	S	R
Cephalothin	S	S	R	R
Cefoxitin	S	R	R	R
Cefotaxime	S	R	S-R	R
Gentamicin	S	S	S	R
Tobramycin	S	S	S	R
Trimethoprim-sulfamethoxazole	S	S	R	R

R, Resistant; *S*, susceptible; *S-R*, variable result.

*It is very unusual for an isolate to be resistant to amikacin and susceptible to gentamicin and tobramycin because amikacin is typically the most active of these three aminoglycosides.

†Third-generation cephalosporins (e.g., cefotaxime) are usually more active than second-generation cephalosporins (e.g., cefoxitin), which in turn are more active than first-generation cephalosporins (e.g., cephalothin) against the Enterobacteriaceae. In addition, *E. cloacae* are typically resistant to cephalothin. Consequently, this antibiogram is unusual.

‡Ampicillin does not produce activity against *P. aeruginosa*, and this antibiogram is unusual.

§*S. maltophilia* is usually susceptible to trimethoprim-sulfamethoxazole, which is the drug of choice for infections caused by this very resistant species. This antibiogram is unusual.

TABLE 13-12 Suggestions for Verification of Antimicrobial Susceptibility Test Results and Confirmation of Organism Identification

Organism or Group	Category I Verify at All Laboratories	Category II Verify: Institution Specific
Klebsiella spp.	Ampicillin-S	ESBL confirmed positive
Streptococcus pneumoniae	Fluoroquinolone-R	Penicillin-R
	Linezolid-NS	Third-generation
	Vancomycin-NS	cephalosporin-R

ESBL, Extended-spectrum β-lactamase; *S*, susceptible; *R*, resistant; *NS*, not susceptible.

Modified from Clinical and Laboratory Standards Institute publication M100-S19, *Performance standards for antimicrobial susceptibility testing: nineteenth informational supplement.* Copies of the current edition may be obtained from Clinical and Laboratory Standards Institute, 940 West Valley Road, Suite 1400, Wayne, Pa., 19087-1898.

When atypical antibiograms are encountered, the results must be verified. Verification procedures include the following:

- Reexamination of the disk diffusion plate, MIC tray, and other components to ensure that results were properly interpreted and that the materials were not overtly defective (e.g., empty well in tray)
- Checking earlier reports to see whether the particular patient previously had an isolate with an atypical antibiogram (that was verified)
- Repeating the test, if necessary (sometimes it is necessary to repeat the identification tests as well as the antimicrobial susceptibility tests to verify the atypical results; sometimes testing with an alternative method is useful)

With emerging resistance and nosocomial transmission of resistant organisms, there is now more variability in susceptibility profiles among individual clinical isolates than was pre-viously noted. In contrast to what was seen a decade ago, it would not be uncommon for a particular facility to now see a high percentage of isolates that are resistant to multiple antimicrobial agents.

Cumulative antibiograms are generated by analysis of individual susceptibility results on isolates from a particular institution in a defined period; this analysis represents the percentage of isolates of a given species that is susceptible to the antimicrobial agents commonly tested against the species (e.g., the percentage of *E. coli* isolates that are susceptible to ampicillin). Cumulative antibiograms are generally compiled annually for the purpose of guiding physicians in empiric therapy decisions. If a physician were treating a patient with a suspected infection caused by *P. aeruginosa* and the culture and susceptibility test results were not yet available, the physician could review the cumulative antibiogram to see the percentage of *P. aeruginosa* in that facility susceptible to various antipseudomonal agents. This information could assist the physician in designing the empiric therapy regimen pending completion of culture and susceptibility testing. Cumulative antibiogram data also might be used for infection-control purposes. An increase in the incidence of MRSA from 25% in the first quarter of 2007 to 60% in the second quarter of 2008 might suggest a problem with nosocomial transmission of MRSA among the patients in that facility. An investigation by infection-control personnel into the reason behind such observations would be warranted.

SELECTING AN ANTIMICROBIAL SUSCEPTIBILITY TEST METHOD

Clinical microbiology laboratories can choose from several manual or instrument-based methods to perform their routine antimicrobial susceptibility testing: the disk diffusion (or Kirby-Bauer) test, broth microdilution (with or without use of an instrument for panel readings), and rapid automated instrument methods. The Etest also can be useful for certain fastidious or anaerobic bacteria.

The Kirby-Bauer test provides the greatest flexibility and cost-effectiveness. A frequently mentioned problem with commercial microdilution or automated systems is the inflexibility of the standard antimicrobial agent batteries or test panels. With the current availability of more than 50 antimicrobial agents in the United States and the diversity that exists among antimicrobial agent formularies in different hospitals, it is impossible for manufacturers to provide standard test panels that fit every hospital's needs. Thus the inherent flexibility of the disk diffusion test allows a laboratory to test any 12 antimicrobial agents that are considered appropriate on a 150-mm Mueller-Hinton agar plate. Other assets of the disk diffusion procedure are that it is one of the longest standardized methods and that its performance is continually updated by the CLSI. The interpretive category results (i.e., nonsusceptible, susceptible, intermediate, resistant) of the disk diffusion test should be readily understandable by all physicians; that is frequently not the case with MIC results. In fact, MIC results without attached interpretations may be misinterpreted by many physicians.

As stated previously, commercial microdilution susceptibility test products have become the most popular among United States clinical laboratories. Advantages of this method include its quantitative nature (i.e., an MIC rather than a strict category result); the fact that MICs may be determined with some organisms for which the disk test may not be standardized; and the attraction of automated panel readers. In addition, the computerized data management systems that accompany some of the instruments may be helpful to some laboratories for storage and calculation of cumulative antibiograms and other susceptibility statistics. An MIC method should not be chosen, however, on the grounds that MICs are more valuable to physicians. As stated previously, many physicians who are not infectious diseases specialists are not familiar with MIC values for the myriad of contemporary antimicrobial agents.

A laboratory may perform automated antimicrobial susceptibility testing to generate test results more rapidly than can be accomplished by manual methods or to reduce the amount of labor required for susceptibility tests. Provision of important laboratory results one day sooner than by conventional methods is a logical advancement in patient care. Only a few studies have managed to document a decrease in patient morbidity or mortality, however, as well as demonstrating substantial cost savings. If physicians are aware of critical susceptibility data on patients' isolates, an opportunity exists for improving the quality of care and for realizing cost savings in a particular institution.

One of the previous shortcomings of rapid susceptibility testing methods has been some sacrifice in the ability to detect certain inducible or otherwise subtle antimicrobial resistance mechanisms. Manufacturers have made significant strides toward correcting these problems. In some cases this has meant reformulating the test devices or improving the software used to interpret the susceptibility testing results, which may be aided in part by the use of computer expert systems that have the ability to detect common technical errors and explain some newer resistance mechanisms. Nevertheless, it is important for microbiologists to scrutinize carefully all susceptibility results before issuing final patient reports.

The concept that automated susceptibility instruments reduce labor requirements through greater efficiency has been realized only partially. Some time savings can be achieved when using panels that allow antimicrobial susceptibility testing and organism identification on the same panel. In addition, some of the newer instruments have mechanized or simplified panel inoculation and reading to achieve some labor savings. The magnitude of the labor savings realized in clinical chemistry or hematology through automation has yet to be achieved in clinical microbiology. If a serious mechanical failure occurs, only tests from instruments that utilize conventional microdilution trays normally interpreted after overnight incubation can be completed by manual incubation and interpretation. The instrument methods that incorporate rapid test interpretation or that use fluorogenic substrate analysis cannot be manually interpreted. Therefore laboratories must have access to a backup testing procedure, such as disk diffusion or manual overnight broth microdilution testing, to avoid delays in generating patients' results.

BIBLIOGRAPHY

Bauer AW et al: Antibiotic susceptibility testing by a standardized single disk method, *Am J Clin Pathol* 45:493, 1966.

Clinical and Laboratory Standards Institute/NCCLS: *Development of in vitro susceptibility testing criteria and quality control parameters: approved guideline M23-A3*, Wayne, Pa, 2008, CLSI.

Clinical and Laboratory Standards Institute/NCCLS: *Methods for antimicrobial susceptibility testing of anaerobic bacteria: approved standard M11-A8*, Wayne, Pa, 2009, CLSI.

Clinical and Laboratory Standards Institute: *Analysis and presentation of cumulative antimicrobial susceptibility test data: approved guideline M39-A2*, Wayne, Pa, 2008, CLSI.

Clinical and Laboratory Standards Institute: *Methods for antimicrobial dilution and disk susceptibility testing of infrequently isolated or fastidious bacteria, approved guideline M45-A*, Wayne, Pa, 2005, CLSI.

Clinical and Laboratory Standards Institute: *Methods of dilution antimicrobial susceptibility testing for bacteria that grow aerobically: approved standard M7-A7*, Wayne, Pa, 2006, CLSI.

Clinical and Laboratory Standards Institute: *Performance standards for antimicrobial susceptibility testing, eighteenth informational supplement M100-S18*, Wayne, Pa, 2008, CLSI.

Clinical and Laboratory Standards Institute: *Performance standards for antimicrobial disk susceptibility tests: approved standard M2-A9*, Wayne, Pa, 2009, CLSI.

Hindler JF, Munro S, editors (section): Antimicrobial susceptibility testing. In Isenberg HD, editor: *Clinical microbiology procedures handbook*, ed 2, Washington, DC, 2004, ASM Press.

Jorgensen JH et al: Susceptibility test methods: Dilution and disk diffusion methods. In Murray PR et al, editors: *Manual of clinical microbiology*, ed 9, Washington, DC, 2007, ASM Press.

Livermore DM et al: Interpretative reading: recognizing the unusual and inferring resistance mechanisms from resistance phenotypes, *J Antimicrob Chemother* 48:87, 2001.

Lorian V, editor: *Antibiotics in laboratory medicine: making a difference*, ed 5, Philadelphia, 2005, Lippincott Williams & Wilkins.

Moellering RC Jr, Eliopooulos G: Principles of anti-infective therapy. In Mandell GL et al, editors: *Principles and practice of infectious diseases*, ed 6, Philadelphia, PA, 2005, Elsevier.

Richter SS, Ferraro MJ: Susceptibility testing instrumentation and computerized expert systems for data analysis and interpretation. In Murray PR et al, editors: *Manual of clinical microbiology*, ed 9, Washington DC, 2007, ASM Press.

Turnidge JD et al: Susceptibility test methods: General considerations. In Murray PR, et al, editors: *Manual of clinical microbiology*, ed 9, Washington, DC, 2007, ASM Press.

Turnidge J, Paterson DL: Setting and revising antibacterial susceptibility breakpoints, *Clin Microbiol Rev* 20:391, 2007.

Points to Remember

- Antimicrobial susceptibility testing should be performed only on bacteria likely to be causing an infection.
- The Clinical and Laboratory Standards Institute (CLSI, formerly NCCLS) produces standards for antimicrobial susceptibility testing and reporting in clinical laboratories.
- The U.S. Food and Drug Administration (FDA) has the regulatory authority for setting susceptibility test interpretive criteria and quality control parameters.
- Antimicrobial susceptibility testing protocols describing what, when, and how to test and report should be developed with input from clinicians, pharmacists, and others who have clinical experience with the antimicrobial therapy practices of the particular institution.
- *Selective reporting* basically refers to reporting broader-spectrum agents only in select situations such as when the patient's isolate is resistant to narrower spectrum agents.
- Several variables must be controlled when performing any type of antimicrobial susceptibility test, and inoculum standardization is one of the most important of these. Testing too few or too many bacteria can yield erroneous results.
- The disk diffusion, broth microdilution minimal inhibitory concentration (MIC), and automated MIC tests represent the most common methods used for antimicrobial susceptibility testing in clinical laboratories.
- The disk diffusion, or Kirby-Bauer, test represents a qualitative method, and results are reported as susceptible, intermediate, or resistant.
- The MIC test represents a semiquantitative method and the concentration (μg/mL) of a drug required to inhibit the growth of bacterial isolate is reported together with a susceptible, intermediate, or resistant interpretation (e.g., ampicillin MIC = 8 μg/mL susceptible).
- Routine antimicrobial susceptibility test methods can be modified for testing fastidious bacteria that require supplemental nutrients, modified incubation conditions, or both.
- An oxacillin disk (1 μg) can be used to screen for penicillin susceptibility in *S. pneumoniae*.
- β-hemolytic streptococci remain universally susceptible to penicillin, the drug of choice for treating infections caused by these organisms, and usually does not require susceptibility testing.
- β-lactamase testing is performed on *H. influenzae* to determine whether the isolate is resistant to ampicillin and amoxicillin.
- The third-generation cephalosporins ceftriaxone and cefotaxime are often used to treat meningococcal meningitis because *N. meningitidis* is always susceptible to these agents and they have good penetration into cerebrospinal fluid.

- The CLSI reference method described for testing anaerobic bacteria is agar dilution; however, a broth microdilution method can be used for less fastidious species of anaerobes such as *Bacteroides* spp.
- *MecA* is the gene responsible for oxacillin-resistance in staphylococci.
- The cefoxitin disk performs better than the oxacillin disk in detecting oxacillin-resistant staphylococci by the disk diffusion method.
- Oxacillin-resistant staphylococci should be considered resistant to all β-lactam agents, despite any susceptible result for these in vitro.
- The D-zone test is used to detect inducible clindamycin resistance in staphylococci and β-streptococci.
- Either vancomycin broth-microdilution MIC or vancomycin agar screen is recommended to detect VISA or VRSA, and some test methods are unable to detect these strains.
- Special tests for high-level aminoglycoside resistance and routine tests with cell-wall active agents such as penicillin are performed on enterococci to determine whether combination therapy would be effective in treating serious enterococcal infections, such as endocarditis.
- Vancomycin-resistant enterococci (VRE) are important nosocomial pathogens; however, low-level vancomycin resistance is intrinsic in *E. gallinarum* and *E. casseliflavus*. These differ from true VRE for infection control purposes.
- ESBL-producing bacteria should be considered resistant to all cephalosporins, penicillins, and aztreonam, despite any susceptible result for these in vitro.
- Most automated instruments for antimicrobial susceptibility testing are based on either turbidimetric detection of bacterial growth or detection of hydrolysis of a fluorogenic growth substrate.
- Quality control of antimicrobial susceptibility tests is performed with standard reference strains that have defined antimicrobial susceptibility (or resistance) to the drugs tested.
- Certain species have "typical" antibiograms, which can be used to verify the identification as well as the susceptibility results generated on the isolate.
- Cumulative antibiograms represent the percentage of isolates of a given species susceptible to the antimicrobial agents commonly tested against the species.
- "Nonsusceptible" does not necessarily mean the organism is resistant to the antimicrobial.

Learning Assessment Questions

1. Why would it be inappropriate to perform antimicrobial susceptibility tests on viridans streptococci isolated from a throat culture?

2. The turbidity of a 0.5 McFarland standard corresponds to approximately _____ bacteria per milliliter.

3. The _____ disk cannot be used to screen for penicillin susceptibility in *Streptococcus pneumoniae* from sputum.

4. Which method does CLSI suggest is most reliable for detecting oxacillin resistance in staphylococci?
   a. Oxacillin disk diffusion test
   b. Cefoxitin disk diffusion test
   c. Cefoxitin MIC test
   d. Penicillin MIC test
   e. Oxacillin agar screen

5. What does the *mecA* gene code for in staphylococci?
   a. β-lactamase and penicillin resistance
   b. ESBLs and cephalosporin resistance
   c. Penicillin binding protein 2a and oxacillin resistance
   d. Altered penicillin binding protein and vancomycin resistance
   e. β-lactamase and oxacillin resistance

6. *S. aureus* or β-streptococci with which of the following profiles should be subjected to D-zone testing?
   a. Oxacillin resistant
   b. Erythromycin resistant and clindamycin susceptible
   c. Erythromycin resistant and clindamycin resistant
   d. Penicillin resistant
   e. Oxacillin and penicillin resistant

7. An ampicillin-susceptible *Enterococcus faecalis* from a blood culture has high-level resistance to the aminoglycoside gentamicin. Which of the following statements is true?
   a. Ampicillin and gentamicin will be synergistic.
   b. Ampicillin and gentamicin will not be synergistic.
   c. Penicillin and gentamicin will be synergistic.
   d. Cefazolin and gentamicin will be synergistic.
   e. Ampicillin and tobramycin will be synergistic.

8. ESBL-producing isolates should be considered resistant to which of the following agents?
   a. Cephalosporins, penicillins, and aztreonam
   b. Cephalosporins, penicillins, and aminoglycosides
   c. Cephalosporins, penicillins, and β-lactamase inhibitors
   d. Penicillins and aminoglycosides
   e. Cefotaxime-clavulanic acid and ceftazidime-clavulanic acid

9. Which of the following organisms is commonly tested for β-lactamase production?
   a. *Neisseria meningitidis*
   b. *Klebsiella pneumoniae*
   c. *Streptococcus pneumoniae*
   d. *Haemophilus influenzae*
   e. *Escherichia coli*

10. Which of the following is true about quality control (QC) testing?
    a. A laboratory must perform QC every day patient isolates are tested.
    b. A laboratory can perform weekly QC if the lab performs fewer than 10 tests daily.
    c. A laboratory can perform weekly QC once accurate performance of 20 to 30 days of daily quality control is documented.
    d. A laboratory does not have to perform QC if an automated test antimicrobial susceptibility test system is used.
    e. Testing materials can be used beyond their expiration date if they look satisfactory.

11. Mark each of the following statements as true or false.
    a. Ampicillin susceptibility in *P. aeruginosa* is unusual.____
    b. Many *S. aureus* are vancomycin resistant. ____
    c. Penicillin is the drug of choice for treating gonorrhea. ____
    d. *S. maltophilia* are usually susceptible to trimethoprim-sulfamethoxazole. ___
    e. *E. coli* are always resistant to all aminoglycosides. ____

12. Which of the following statements is true?
    a. An organism that is reported as "nonsusceptible" to an antimicrobial is definitely resistant to the antimicrobial.
    b. The term *nonsusceptible* is used when the interpretive categories of "intermediate" and "resistant" do not apply.

B. Special Antimicrobial Susceptibility Tests

*Frederic J. Marsik**

- ■ MINIMUM BACTERICIDAL CONCENTRATION TEST
  Controlling Test Variables
  Interpretation Concerns
- ■ TIME-KILL ASSAYS
- ■ SYNERGY TESTS
- ■ SERUM BACTERICIDAL TEST

- ■ MOLECULAR PROBES FOR IDENTIFYING DETERMINANTS OF ANTIMICROBIAL RESISTANCE
- ■ MEASUREMENT OF ANTIMICROBIAL AGENTS IN SERUM AND BODY FLUIDS
  Biologic Assays
  Immunoassays
  Chromatographic Assays

OBJECTIVES

After reading and studying this chapter, you should be able to:

1. Describe the minimum bactericidal concentration (MBC) test and list the indications for performing this test.

2. Define *synergism, antagonism,* and *indifference* as related to testing combinations of antimicrobial agents.

3. Describe the serum bactericidal test, and list the indications for performing this test.

4. Explain how molecular probes might be used to detect antimicrobial resistance.

5. Discuss methods used for measuring concentrations of antimicrobial agents in serum and body fluids, and indicate when such tests are used.

Case in Point

Viridans group streptococcus was isolated from six of six blood culture bottles submitted for a patient with suspected bacterial endocarditis. The isolate was susceptible to penicillin (minimal inhibitory concentration [MIC] 0.03 or less µg/mL), but the physician was concerned about the bactericidal activity of penicillin alone. The laboratory performed minimum bactericidal concentration (MBC) testing and reported an MBC result of 32 µg/mL. The physician considered this information in conjunction with clinical observations of the patient and documentation in the literature of previous experiences with patients with similar conditions. This patient was continued on a therapeutic regimen of penicillin and gentamicin.

Issues to Consider

After reading the patient's case history, consider:

- ■ Circumstances when it might be appropriate to do more than a disk diffusion or minimal inhibitory concentration (MIC) test on a clinical isolate
- ■ Factors that might contribute to the MBC being five twofold dilutions greater than the MIC
- ■ Rationale for adding a second agent (gentamicin) to treat the infection

Key Terms

Antagonism
Antimicrobial assay
Indifference
MBC endpoint
Minimal inhibitory concentration (MIC)
Minimum bactericidal concentration (MBC)

Paradoxic (Eagle) effect
Persister
Serum bactericidal test (SBT)
Synergism
Time-kill assay
Tolerance

Clinical microbiology laboratories that perform bacterial cultures generally perform antimicrobial susceptibility tests using either a disk diffusion or minimal inhibitory concentration (MIC) method. These tests assess the ability of antimicrobial agents to inhibit the growth of bacteria and are sufficient for guiding antimicrobial therapy in most situations. In very select cases, a physician may wish to determine how well specific antimicrobial agents kill bacteria or how the activity of a combination of antimicrobial agents compares with that of a single agent. Unlike disk diffusion and MIC tests, tests for bactericidal activity (e.g., minimum bactericidal concentration [MBC], serum bactericidal tests) and antimicrobial synergism are not highly stan-

*This section was originally prepared and written by Janet Fick Hindler.

TABLE 13-13 Special Antimicrobial Susceptibility Tests

Test	Purpose
Antimicrobial concentration test (assay)	Measure the amount of antimicrobial agent in serum or body fluid
Minimum bactericidal concentration (MBC) test	Measure of the lowest concentration of antimicrobial agent that kills a bacterial isolate
Serum bactericidal test (SBT)	Measure of the highest dilution or titer of a patient's serum that is inhibitory to the patient's own infecting bacterium and the highest dilution or titer that is bactericidal
Synergy test	Measure of the susceptibility of a bacterial isolate to a combination of two or more antimicrobial agents
Time-kill assay	Measure of the rate of killing of bacteria by an antimicrobial agent as determined by examining the number of viable bacteria remaining at various intervals after exposure to the agent

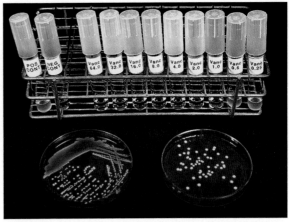

FIGURE 13-27 Broth-macrodilution test showing vancomycin and *Staphylococcus aureus*. The minimal inhibitory concentration (MIC) is 1.0 µg/mL. The purity plate shows a pure culture. The colony count plate shows 53 colonies, which means that 5.3×10^5 colony-forming units (CFU)/mL of bacteria were in the test tubes immediately after inoculation of the MIC test. For the colony count plate, immediately after inoculation the growth control tube was diluted 1:1000, and 0.1 mL was plated. Now 0.01 mL will be plated from each clear tube (tubes containing 1.0 through 128 µg/mL of vancomycin) for the minimum bactericidal concentration determination. Because it was shown that the actual colony count in the MIC test was 5.3×10^5 CFU/mL, growth of five or fewer colonies would indicate a 3 $\log_{10}$ decrease or 99.9% killing. By definition the concentration of drug in the respective tube would be considered bactericidal.

dardized. Molecular assays for *mecA*, the gene that codes for oxacillin resistance in staphylococci, are used in some clinical laboratories. Lack of association between other resistance genes and clinical resistance has limited the development of additional gene assays. When patients are prescribed antimicrobial agents that have a low toxic-to-therapeutic ratio, it may be necessary to monitor the concentrations of drug in the patient's serum to avoid excessive concentrations that may be harmful. Various methods are used for **antimicrobial assays.** Several special antimicrobial susceptibility tests are generally performed only in specialized laboratories and are used in only a few defined clinical settings. They are listed in Table 13-13.

MINIMUM BACTERICIDAL CONCENTRATION TEST

Minimal inhibitory concentration (MIC) tests identify the amount of antimicrobial agent required to inhibit the growth or multiplication of a bacterial isolate. If a concentration of antimicrobial agent that is the same or preferably exceeds the MIC is attained at the infection site for an appropriate amount of time, the drug generally inhibits multiplication of the bacteria so that the patient's immune defense mechanisms are no longer overwhelmed. The immune defense mechanisms (e.g., phagocytic cells, antibody) work in concert with antimicrobial agents to eradicate infecting bacteria; for this reason, inhibitory concentrations of the drug at the infection site are generally sufficient for treating most infections.

In immunosuppressed patients and patients with serious infections such as endocarditis, meningitis, and osteomyelitis, the immune defense mechanisms are suboptimal. Inhibitory concentrations of the drug may not be sufficient, and obtaining bactericidal concentrations of antimicrobial agents at the infection site is important in achieving a cure. For many types

of infections, the bactericidal capacity of a specific antimicrobial regimen can be predicted on the basis of previous experience. For example, most β-lactam antimicrobial agents are bactericidal for *Escherichia coli*, provided their MIC is in the susceptible range. On the other hand, the bactericidal activity of β-lactams and other cell wall–active agents (e.g., vancomycin) against *Staphylococcus aureus* is less predictable. In very select circumstances when a serious *S. aureus* infection occurs in a patient with poor immune defense mechanisms, an in vitro determination of the amount of antimicrobial agent required to kill as well as inhibit the isolate may be helpful; the **minimum bactericidal concentration (MBC)** test can be used for this purpose. The CLSI has described several procedures for assessing bactericidal activity; however, unlike disk diffusion and MIC tests, a standardized MBC test has not been in use for a sustained period. In the past numerous methodologic variations compromised the use of the test results.

The MBC test is performed in conjunction with a broth macrodilution or broth microdilution MIC test. The antimicrobial agent concentrations that show inhibition (at and above the MIC) may or may not have killed the bacteria in the test inoculum (Figure 13-27). After the MIC determination, a 0.01-mL aliquot of each clear tube or well is subcultured to an agar medium to determine the MBC or the lowest concentration of antimicrobial agent needed to kill the test bacterium. The numbers of colonies that grow on subculture are compared with the actual number of organisms inoculated into the MIC test tubes or wells to determine the extent of bactericidal activity at each antimicrobial concentration. If the numbers of colonies on a subculture plate total less than 0.1% of the initial inoculum (indicating 99.9% or more killing), a bactericidal effect has by definition been achieved.

As described previously, the final number of bacteria in each tube (or well) immediately after inoculation of the MIC test is approximately 5×10^5 colony-forming units (CFU)/mL. For the MBC test, however, an actual colony count must be performed on the test inoculum at the time the MIC test is inoculated. A small aliquot from the growth control tube or well is diluted in saline or broth to obtain a countable number of colonies; the final dilution is plated to an agar medium. Generally a 1:1000 dilution is performed (0.01 mL from the growth control tube is diluted in 10 mL), and 0.1 mL is spread over the surface of an agar plate. Following overnight incubation, the number of colonies that have grown on the colony count plate is noted. Because this count represents a 1:10,000 dilution, the count is multiplied by 10^4 to determine the number of bacteria in the original growth control (and antimicrobial agent) solutions. A calculation is performed to determine the number of colonies representing 99.9% of the test inoculum in the MIC test because the **MBC endpoint** is defined as the lowest concentration of antimicrobial agent that kills 99.9% of the test bacteria.

In the example shown in Figure 13-27, the actual count on the colony count plate is 53; therefore the number of bacteria in each tube of the MIC test immediately after inoculation was 5.3×10^5 CFU/mL (calculated by multiplying 53 times the dilution factor, which is 10^4). A 99.9% killing (or 0.1% survival) would be accomplished if five or fewer colonies grow on subculture of each clear well or tube after reading of the MIC test (Figure 13-28). In this example, subcultures from all tubes containing 2.0 µg/mL vancomycin or more grew fewer than five colonies. Consequently the MBC is 2.0 µg/mL. The

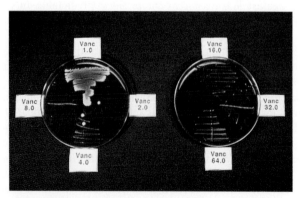

FIGURE 13-28 Subculture plates from the minimal inhibitory concentration test of vancomycin and *Staphylococcus aureus* shown in Figure 13-27. Subcultures from tubes containing 8.0 to 128 µg/mL of vancomycin show no growth. Subcultures from the tubes containing 2.0 µg/mL and 4.0 µg/mL show one and two colonies, respectively, indicating a greater than 99.9% killing. More than five colonies have grown from the 1.0 µg/mL tube, so the minimum bactericidal concentration is 2.0 µg/mL.

99.9% endpoint (or three $\log_{10}$ reduction in growth of the original inoculum) is an arbitrary value with 95% confidence limits, although its clinical relevance has not been rigorously confirmed.

Controlling Test Variables

Minimum bactericidal concentration tests are subject to more technical pitfalls than MIC tests, and several variables must be rigidly controlled during MBC testing. The first involves inoculum. Because many antimicrobial agents exert a bactericidal effect only on growing cells, bacteria in the mid-logarithmic phase of growth must be used as the inoculum to prevent falsely elevated MBCs. The inoculum preparation methods described for MIC tests that use stationary phase growth are unacceptable for MBC tests.

Second, during inoculation for MIC tests, care must be taken to ensure that all bacteria in the test inoculum are deposited directly into the antimicrobial solution. If this is not done, bacteria may stick to the wall of the tube or well above the meniscus of the antimicrobial solution and may remain viable during incubation of the MIC portion of the test. These cells (which have not been exposed to antimicrobial agent) may then be inadvertently transferred during the subculture step, ultimately resulting in falsely elevated MBCs.

Third, the volume subcultured following reading of the MIC test must be large enough to contain sufficient inoculum but small enough to prevent carryover of large amounts of antimicrobial agent to continue to exert an antibacterial effect. Usually 10 µl (0.01 mL) is recommended.

Interpretation Concerns

Several interpretive problems, most common with β-lactam agents, have been associated with MBC tests, and they relate to technical or biologic issues. Sometimes more colonies are growing on subcultures at higher drug concentrations than at lower concentrations. This decreased bactericidal activity at higher concentrations is referred to as a **paradoxic (Eagle) effect.** Sometimes small numbers (but slightly greater than 0.1% of the test inoculum) of bacteria grow on several subculture plates (**persisters**). This may occur if some bacteria are metabolically inactive at the times of testing; however, when the persisting colonies are retested, their MICs are comparable with those originally obtained. Finally, tolerance to the intrinsic bactericidal effect of an antimicrobial agent is demonstrated when the numbers of colonies growing on subculture plates exceed the 0.1 cutoff for several successive drug concentrations above the MIC. **Tolerance** is generally defined as an MBC:MIC ratio of 32 or greater. Tolerance has been associated with a defect in bacterial cellular autolytic enzymes.

TIME-KILL ASSAYS

Bactericidal activity of antimicrobial agents also can be assessed by performance of in vitro **time-kill assays.** Briefly, test bacteria in the mid-logarithmic growth phase are inoculated into several tubes of broth containing varying concentrations of antimicrobial agent and a growth control tube without drug. These tubes are incubated at 35° C. Then small aliquots are removed at specific time intervals (e.g., at 0, 4, 8, and 24 hours), diluted to obtain countable numbers of colonies, and plated to agar for colony count determinations. The number of bacteria remaining in each sample is plotted over time to determine the rate of antimicrobial agent killing. Generally, a three or more $\log_{10}$ reduction in bacterial counts in the antimicrobial suspensions as compared with the growth control indicates an adequate bactericidal response. Because this test is quite labor intensive, it is usually performed only in research settings.

SYNERGY TESTS

Some types of infections require therapy with a combination of two or more antimicrobial agents. Enterococcal endocarditis, for example, requires use of a penicillin (or vancomycin) and an aminoglycoside for reliable killing of the organism. A broad-spectrum cephalosporin and an aminoglycoside are often prescribed for gram-negative sepsis in neutropenic patients. Goals of combination therapy are to obtain broad-spectrum coverage, enhance antibacterial activity through synergistic interactions, and minimize resistance development. For most infections requiring combination therapy, single-agent MIC results and previous experience in treating similar types of infections are sufficient to guide the selection of an antimicrobial agent. In unusual situations, however, when the patient is not responding to what would appear to be an adequate regimen, unusual organisms or resistance properties are encountered, or host factors preclude the use of certain agents, in vitro synergy tests may be warranted.

In vitro synergy tests may be performed using a broth dilution checkerboard method or time-kill assays. The checkerboard assay is a type of two-dimensional test; all steps are performed as for single agents, but two agents are tested in each well or tube.

Checkerboard synergy tests are usually performed in broth microdilution MIC trays. A wide variety of combinations of concentrations is tested by dispensing drugs in a two-dimensional checkerboard format, and each drug tested in the combination is also tested by itself. A combination is said to show **synergism** if its antibacterial activity is significantly greater than that of the single agents—that is, when the MIC for each drug in the combination is less than or equal to one fourth of the single-agent MICs. Conversely, **antagonism** is defined as the activity of the combination less than (and MICs are greater than) that of the single agents. For **indifference** the activity of the combination is equal to that of the single agents (Figure 13-29).

Time-kill assays also can be used to study synergistic interactions by testing a combination of drugs in a single tube and each drug individually in additional tubes. Several drug concentrations alone and in combination are usually examined. If subsequent colony counts reveal a two or more $\log_{10}$ reduction in the combination tube counts at 24 hours compared with the most active single-agent tube count, synergy has been demonstrated (Figure 13-30). A change of less than tenfold (increase or decrease) in colony counts from the combination tube compared with the most active single-agent tube represents indifference. The Clinical and Laboratory Standards Institute (CLSI) has not addressed synergy testing, and numerous methodologic variations exist.

SERUM BACTERICIDAL TEST

In the late 1940s, Schlichter and MacLean described a test that measured the effectiveness with which penicillin in serum killed bacteria associated with endocarditis. This test was subsequently modified slightly and standardized; it is now referred to as the **serum bactericidal test (SBT)**. The CLSI has published procedures for serum bactericidal tests, including broth-macrodilution and broth-microdilution methods. Some clinical data available support the use of the SBT to evaluate specimens from patients with serious bacterial infections such as endocarditis, osteomyelitis, and gram-negative bacteremia.

The SBT is similar to the MIC/MBC test in that both inhibitory and bactericidal parameters are evaluated. The patient's serum and the bacterial isolate responsible for the patient's infection are required. Serial twofold dilutions of the patient's serum are prepared, and then a standardized inoculum of the patient's bacterial isolate is added to each dilution. Following overnight incubation, the tubes or wells are examined to determine the greatest dilution of patient's serum that inhibits the bacteria. Subsequently, as with the MBC tests, all tubes or wells showing inhibition are subcultured to an agar medium to determine the highest dilution that kills the bacteria. All the potential technical pitfalls mentioned for the MBC test also apply to the SBT test. The SBT results relate to the amount of antimicrobial agent and any other antibacterial factors (e.g., antibody, opsonins, complement) present in the patient's serum. Timing the collection of serum is critical, and generally both trough and peak titers are tested (Box 13-2). Older literature holds that a peak bactericidal titer of 1:8 or greater indicates that therapy is adequate. The CLSI states that a trough bactericidal titer of 1:32 or greater and a peak bactericidal titer of 1:64 or greater correlates with bacteriologic cure in patients with endocarditis. The CLSI interpretive guidelines are applicable only if CLSI methods are followed in performing the test. As with the MBC tests, technical complexity limits the widespread use of the SBT.

BOX 13-2 Guidelines for Obtaining Serum Specimens for the Serum Bactericidal Test and Antimicrobial Assays

Trough*	Obtain 0-30 min before next dose
Peak*	Obtain per one of the following: • 30-60 min after completion of a 30-min intravenous infusion • 60 min after an intramuscular injection • 90 min after an oral dose (varies by specific drug)

*Ideally, trough and peak specimens should be collected for the same dose.

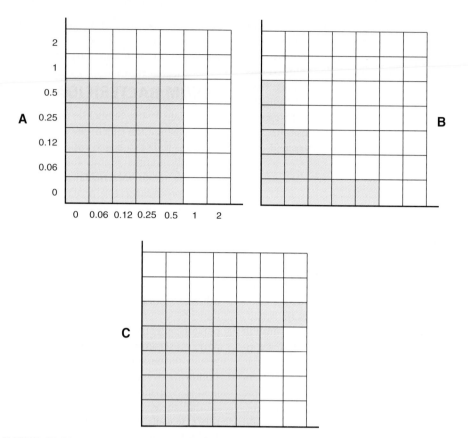

FIGURE 13-29 Assessment of antimicrobial combinations with the checkerboard method. Panels **A, B,** and C depict the results of testing combinations of two drugs (diluted in geometric twofold increments along the *x* and *y* axes; *drug A* along the *x* axis and *drug B* along the *y* axis). Shading indicates visible growth, and concentrations are expressed as multiples of the minimum inhibitory concentration. **A,** Indifference; **B,** synergism; C, antagonism. (Modified from Pillai SK, Moellering RC Jr, Eliopoulos GM: Antimicrobial combinations. In Lorian V, editor: *Antibiotics in laboratory medicine: making a difference,* ed 5, Philadelphia, 2005, Lippincott Williams & Wilkins.)

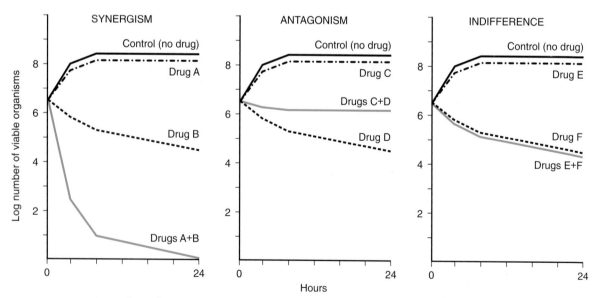

FIGURE 13-30 Effects of antimicrobial combinations as measured with the killing-curve method. A + B = synergism; C + D = antagonism; E + F = indifference. (Modified from Pillai SK, Moellering RC Jr, Eliopoulos GM: Antimicrobial combinations. In Lorian V, editor: *Antibiotics in laboratory medicine: making a difference,* ed 5, Philadelphia, 2005, Lippincott Williams & Wilkins.)

MOLECULAR PROBES FOR IDENTIFYING DETERMINANTS OF ANTIMICROBIAL RESISTANCE

Molecular methods are being used with increasing frequency throughout the clinical microbiology laboratory to identify certain microorganisms. Molecular methods for detection of antimicrobial resistance genes are limited to those organism/antimicrobial combinations in which only a few genes are associated with the resistance and the resistance has a high degree of clinical significance. Consequently molecular tests most widely used for resistance detection are for oxacillin (methicillin) resistance in staphylococci. As mentioned, the *mecA* gene codes for oxacillin (methicillin) resistance in staphylococci and PBP2a is the *mecA* gene product. Probes (without amplification) and amplification using methods such as the polymerase chain reaction (PCR) have been developed to detect *mecA*. In addition, there are agglutination tests that use a latex antibody directed toward PBP2a. Depending on the method, testing can be done on isolated colonies, on broth cultures, or in some cases directly on clinical specimens.

Probes directed toward genes responsible for other resistance mechanisms (e.g., β-lactamases, aminoglycoside-modifying enzymes, tetracycline resistance factors, vancomycin resistance factors) also have been described; however, these have been used only in research settings. A concern about using probes to confirm resistance involves the ability of some bacteria to contain specific resistance genes that may not be expressed. In these cases, the clinical significance of the presence of the resistance genes is questionable.

MEASUREMENT OF ANTIMICROBIAL AGENTS IN SERUM AND BODY FLUIDS

The amount of antimicrobial agent in serum or other body fluid can be measured by a variety of antimicrobial assay procedures. Antimicrobial assays are performed for antimicrobial agents in which the therapeutic concentration is close to the toxic concentration. Assay results often lead to modification of subsequent doses to prevent accumulation of excessive drug concentrations that might be harmful to the patient. A patient's renal and hepatic status greatly influences in vivo levels of some antimicrobial agents. The antimicrobial agents with the greatest toxic risks and those most commonly monitored are the aminoglycosides, vancomycin, and chloramphenicol. For evaluation of antimicrobial levels, both trough and peak samples should be assayed as for the serum bactericidal test (see Table 13-13).

Biologic Assays

Antimicrobial assays were initially performed by a biologic assay method; bioassays are still sometimes used today when the focus is on the amount of biologically active drug present rather than the amount of "chemical" present. The bioassays use a specific strain of bacteria (indicator organism) that is susceptible to the drug to be assayed, and the test is performed in either broth or agar. The antibacterial activity of the patient's specimen against this bacterium is compared with

that of solutions containing defined concentrations of the antimicrobial being assayed to determine the concentration in the patient's specimen through use of standard dose-response curves.

Immunoassays

Radioimmunoassay (RIA), fluorescent immunoassay, fluorescent polarization immunoassay, and enzyme immunoassay (EIA) procedures have all been used to measure antimicrobial agents in serum and other body fluids. The basic principles of these assays are similar in that they all use antibodies directed against the specific antimicrobial agents to be assayed. Because of the nature of these tests, they are often performed in the chemistry or therapeutic drug-monitoring sections of the laboratory. Several commercial manufacturers offer various types of immunoassay kits for performing gentamicin, tobramycin, amikacin, vancomycin, and chloramphenicol assays.

Chromatographic Assays

Various chromatographic methods, including gas-liquid, thin-layer, and paper chromatography, have been used on occasion for antimicrobial assays. The most widely used chromatographic method, however, has been high-performance liquid chromatography (HPLC). Chromatographic methods are used primarily to measure levels of antimicrobial agents for which commercial immunoassay kits are not available. These tests are usually performed in research settings.

BIBLIOGRAPHY

Baddour LM et al: Infective endocarditis: diagnosis, antimicrobial therapy, and management of complications: a statement for healthcare professionals from the Committee on Rheumatic Fever, Endocarditis, and Kawasaki Disease, Council on Cardiovascular Disease in the Young, and the Councils on Clinical Cardiology, Stroke, and Cardiovascular Surgery and Anesthesia, American Heart Association: endorsed by the Infectious Diseases Society of America, *Circulation* 111:e394, 2005.

Berenbaum MC: A method for testing synergy with any number of agents, *J Infect Dis* 137:122, 1978.

Clinical and Laboratory Standards Institute/NCCLS: *Methodology for the serum bactericidal test: approved guideline M21-A*, Wayne, Pa, 1999, CLSI.

Clinical and Laboratory Standards Institute/NCCLS: *Methods for determining bactericidal activity of antimicrobial agents: approved guideline M26-A*, Wayne, Pa, 1999, CLSI.

Klein RD, Edberg SC: Applications, significance of, and methods for the measurement of antimicrobial concentrations in human body fluids. In Lorian V, editor: *Antibiotics in laboratory medicine: making a difference*, ed 5, Philadelphia, 2005, Lippincott Williams & Wilkins.

Leven M: Molecular methods for the detection of antibacterial resistance genes. In Lorian V, editor: *Antibiotics in laboratory medicine: making a difference*, ed 5, Philadelphia, 2005, Lippincott Williams & Wilkins.

Moody J: Synergism tests. In Isenberg HD, editor: *Clinical microbiology procedures handbook*, ed 2, Washington, DC, 2004, ASM Press.

Moody J, Knapp C: Tests to assess bactericidal activity. In Isenberg HD, editor: *Clinical microbiology procedures handbook*, ed 2, Washington, DC, 2004, ASM Press.

Pankey GA, Sabath LD: Clinical relevance of bacteriostatic versus bactericidal mechanisms of action in the treatment of Gram-positive bacterial infections, *Clin Infect Dis* 38:864, 2004.

Pillai SK, Moellering RC Jr, Eliopoulos GM: Antimicrobial combinations. In Lorian V, editor: *Antibiotics in laboratory medicine: making a difference*, ed 5, Philadelphia, 2005, Lippincott Williams & Wilkins.

Schlichter JG, MacLean H: A method for determining the effective therapeutic level in the treatment of subacute bacterial endocarditis with penicillin, *Am Heart J* 34:209, 1947.

Points to Remember

- Minimum bactericidal concentration (MBC) testing or serum bactericidal testing may be useful in very select situations, such as for patients who are immunosuppressed, patients with serious infections, or where infection is at a site where immune mechanisms are not optimal.
- MBC testing is performed following completion of a broth-dilution minimal inhibitory concentration (MIC) test and the endpoint is 99.9% killing of the test bacteria.
- Although there are CLSI guidelines for MBC and serum bactericidal tests, these tests are not as standardized as disk diffusion or MIC tests.
- Synergism testing is performed using either a time-kill or checkerboard assay in very select situations, and there is no CLSI guideline or standardized method for synergism testing.
- Serum bactericidal testing requires the use of the patient's serum obtained at appropriate times surrounding dosing of the antimicrobial agent(s) and the bacterium causing the patient's infection.
- Some clinical laboratories use a *mecA* assay to determine oxacillin susceptibility or resistance in staphylococci.
- When obtaining serum samples for serum bactericidal or antimicrobial assay, both trough and peak specimens are usually obtained.

Learning Assessment Questions

1. Why is a bactericidal drug regimen necessary for treating patients with bacterial endocarditis?
2. The minimum bactericidal concentration (MBC) endpoint is the lowest concentration of antimicrobial agent that kills _____ of the test bacteria.
3. It is important to test bacteria in the _____ phase of growth when performing tests to assess bactericidal activity.
4. True or false?____
   Antimicrobial agents categorized as having bactericidal activity always kill 100% of the test bacteria when the bacteria are exposed to concentrations of the agent greater than or equal to the minimal inhibitory concentration (MIC).

5. Which of the following definitions best defines synergism?
   a. The activity of the drug combination is greater than that of the individual agents.
   b. The activity of the drug combination is less than that of the individual agents.
   c. The activity of the drug combination is equal to that of the individual agents.
   d. The test organism is susceptible to both drugs in the combination.
   e. The test organism is resistant to both drugs in the combination.
6. Another name for the serum bactericidal test is the _____ test.
7. Which of the following factors contribute to results in the serum-cidal test?
   a. Antibody, opsonins, complement
   b. Opsonins
   c. Antibody
   d. Complement
   e. None of the above
8. When are serum specimens obtained for serum bactericidal and antimicrobial assays?
   a. Trough 1 hour before dose; peak 1 hour after intravenous (IV) dose
   b. Trough 1 hour after dose; peak 3 hours before intramuscular (IM) dose
   c. Trough 30 minutes before dose; peak 60 minutes after IM dose
   d. Trough 30 minutes before dose; peak 12 hours after IV dose
   e. Trough 1 hour before dose; peak 8 hours after oral dose
9. Use of molecular assays to detect antimicrobial resistance genes is limited because
   a. Genes are not responsible for most types of antimicrobial resistance.
   b. Genes may be present but may not be expressed; therefore the presence of the gene does not always correlate with resistance.
   c. Researchers have been unable to identify genes for antimicrobial resistance.
   d. Large numbers of genes are responsible for all clinically important resistance.
   e. Testing is too expensive.
10. Which of the following classes of antimicrobial agents pose the greatest toxicity risks and therefore are frequently monitored using antimicrobial assays?
    a. Penicillins
    b. Cephalosporins
    c. Sulfonamides
    d. Aminoglycosides
    e. Tetracyclines

PART II

Laboratory Identification of Significant Isolates

Staphylococci

Linda S. Monson

- **GENERAL CHARACTERISTICS**
- **CLINICALLY SIGNIFICANT SPECIES**
  Staphylococcus aureus
  Staphylococcus epidermidis
  Staphylococcus saprophyticus
  Staphylococcus lugdunensis
  Other Coagulase-Negative Staphylococci

- **LABORATORY DIAGNOSIS**
  Specimen Collection and Handling
  Microscopic Examination
  Isolation and Identification
- **ANTIMICROBIAL SUSCEPTIBILITY**
  Methicillin-Resistant Staphylococci
  Vancomycin-Resistant Staphylococci
  Macrolide Resistance

OBJECTIVES

After reading and studying this chapter, you should be able to:

1. Describe the general characteristics of the genus *Staphylococcus*.
2. Compare the characteristics of the staphylococci to other gram-positive cocci.
3. Describe the virulence factors associated with staphylococci.
4. Compare the clinical infections associated with various staphylococcal species.
5. Develop an algorithm of key tests to differentiate among the clinically relevant *Staphylococcus* species.
6. Discuss the characteristics that should be utilized to identify a *Staphylococcus*-like organism isolated from a clinical sample.
7. Explain why methicillin and vancomycin resistance is a serious clinical problem.

Case in Point

A 51-year-old healthy male received a minor abrasion at a local physical fitness center that resulted in a raised hard lesion on his thigh. He visited his primary care physician, who drained the lesion and prescribed an oral first-generation cephalosporin commonly used for skin infections and lesions. The patient was asked to drain the lesion daily and wipe the affected area with disposable clindamycin medicated pads. He was instructed to keep the infected area covered with a clean dry bandage and to not participate in any athletic activity unless he could keep the wound dry and covered. He was also told to practice good personal hygiene after cleaning the wound and to avoid using any shared items. A culture was performed, and catalase-positive, coagulase-positive, gram-positive cocci were isolated. Automated antimicrobial susceptibility testing showed the isolate to be penicillin, oxacillin, and erythromycin resistant and clindamycin susceptible. Further testing by a double-disk–diffusion susceptibility D test showed the isolate was positive for inducible clindamycin resistance.

Issues to Consider

After reading the patient's case history, consider:

- The identity of the isolate described in the case study
- Which species of staphylococci are most frequently associated with disease
- The importance of susceptibility testing
- Risk factors associated with acquiring this organism

Key Terms

α-Hemolysin
β-Hemolysin
β-Lactamase
Borderline oxacillin-resistant
  Staphylococcus aureus
  (BORSA)
Bullous impetigo
Carbuncles
Catalase

Clumping factor
Coagulase test
Coagulase-negative
  staphylococci (CoNS)
Community-associated MRSA
  (CA-MRSA)
Cytolytic toxins
D test
Enterotoxin

Exfoliative toxin

Folliculitis

Furuncle

Hospital-associated MRSA
(HA-MRSA)

Impetigo

Methicillin-resistant
Staphylococcus aureus
(MRSA)

Methicillin-resistant
Staphylococcus
epidermidis (MRSE)

Nosocomial

Novobiocin susceptibility

Osteomyelitis

Panton-Valentine leukocidin
(PVL)

Penicillin-binding protein
(PBP)

Protein A

Ritter disease

Scalded skin syndrome (SSS)

Small-colony variants

Toxic epidermal necrolysis
(TEN)

Toxic shock syndrome (TSS)

Toxic shock syndrome toxin-1
(TSST-1)

Vancomycin-intermediate
Staphylococcus aureus
(VISA)

Vancomycin-resistant
Staphylococcus aureus
(VRSA)

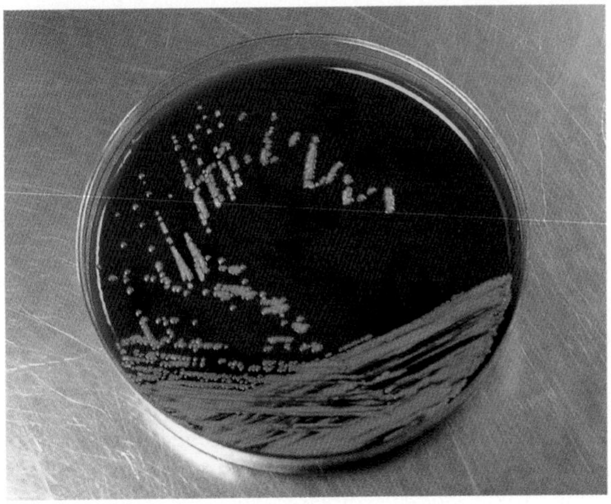

FIGURE 14-1 Micrococcus growing on sheep blood agar showing yellow pigment.

GENERAL CHARACTERISTICS

Gram-positive cocci are common isolates in the clinical microbiology laboratory. Although most are members of the indigenous microbial biota, some species are causative agents of serious infectious disease. This chapter discusses the most commonly encountered staphylococci, their characteristics, the infections they produce, and their laboratory identification. Infections caused by *Staphylococcus aureus*, *S. epidermidis*, *S. saprophyticus*, *S. lugdunensis*, and *S. haemolyticus* are emphasized.

The staphylococci are **catalase**-producing, gram-positive cocci. On stained smears they exhibit spherical cells (0.5 to 1.5 μm) that appear singly, in pairs, and in clusters. The genus name, *Staphylococcus*, is derived from the Greek term *staphle*, meaning "bunches of grapes." Although the Gram stain can be characteristic of staphylococci, microscopy alone will not differentiate staphylococci from other gram-positive cocci.

Although members of the family Bacillaceae, the staphylococci resemble some members of the family Micrococcaceae, which includes the genera *Planococcus*, *Stomatococcus*, and *Micrococcus*. Micrococci are catalase-producing, coagulase-negative, gram-positive cocci found in the environment and as residents of the indigenous skin biota. They are often recovered with staphylococci and can easily be differentiated from coagulase-negative staphylococci with the characteristics found in Table 14-1. Some micrococci have a tendency to produce a yellow pigment (Figure 14-1). Other gram-positive cocci that are occasionally recovered with staphylococci include *Rothia* spp., *Aerococcus* spp., and *Alloiococcus otitis* (recovered from human middle-ear fluid).

The staphylococci are nonmotile, non–spore-forming, and aerobic or facultatively anaerobic, except for *S. saccharolyticus*, which is an obligate anaerobe. Colonies produced after 18 to 24 hours of incubation are medium sized (4 to 8 mm) and appear cream-colored, white, or rarely light gold and

TABLE 14-1 Differentiation Between Staphylococci and Micrococci in the Routine Laboratory

Test	Staphylococci	Micrococci
Modified oxidase	−	+
Anaerobic acid production from glucose	+	−*
Growth on Furoxone-Tween 80-oil red 0 agar	−	+
Anaerobic acid production form glycerol in the presence of erythromycin	+	−
Resistance to bacitracin (0.04 units)	R†	S
Lysosome (50-mg disk)	R	S
Lysostaphin test	S†	R

Modified from Schumacher-Perdreau F: Clinical significance and laboratory diagnosis of coagulase-negative staphylococci, *Clin Microbiol Newsl* 13:97, 1991.
R, Resistant; *S*, sensitive.
Micrococcus krisinae and *Micrococcus varians* are positive.
†Some strains show opposite reaction.

"buttery-looking." Rare strains of staphylococci are fastidious requiring CO_2, hemin, or menadione for growth. These so-called **small-colony variants** grow on media containing blood, forming colonies about one tenth the size of wild type strains after at least 48 hours' incubation. Some species are β-hemolytic. Staphylococci are common isolates in the clinical laboratory and are responsible for several suppurative types of infections. These organisms are normal inhabitants of the skin and mucous membranes of humans and other animals.

Species of staphylococci are initially differentiated by the **coagulase test;** a positive test is a clot formed in plasma. Staphylocoagulase is the active enzyme in this test. The staphylocoagulase-producing (coagulase-positive) staphylococci are *S. aureus*, *S. intermedius*, *S. delphini*, *S. lutrae,* and some strains of *S. hyicus*. Isolates such as *S. lugdunensis* and *S. schleiferi* can also be occasionally confused as coagulase-positive staphylococci because of the presence of **clumping factor.** Clumping factor causes bacterial cells to agglutinate in plasma. The principles of these tests are discussed later. With the exception of *S. aureus*, these are often animal-associated species and are infrequently isolated from human specimens. Consequently, for the vast majority of clinical laboratory situations, coagulase-positive isolates from human sources are considered to be *S. aureus*. A review of the patient history and antimicrobial susceptibility pattern can be helpful in differentiating these less frequently isolated staphylococci from *S. aureus*.

S. aureus causes cutaneous infections such as **folliculitis,** boils, **carbuncles, impetigo,** and purulent abscesses. These cutaneous infections can progress to deeper abscesses involving other organ systems and progress to septicemia and bacteremia. Toxin-induced diseases such as food poisoning, **scalded skin syndrome (SSS),** and **toxic shock syndrome (TSS)** are also associated with this organism.

Staphylococci that do not produce coagulase are referred to as **coagulase-negative staphylococci (CoNS).** The most clinically and commonly recovered significant species in this group are *S. epidermidis* and *S. saprophyticus*. *S. haemolyticus* and *S. lugdunensis* are also recovered occasionally and can be significant pathogens. *S. epidermidis* has been known to cause various hospital-acquired infections, whereas *S. saprophyticus* is associated mainly with urinary tract infections (UTIs), predominantly in female adolescents and young women. *S. haemolyticus* is a CoNS occasionally recovered in septicemia and wound, urinary tract, and native valve infections. *S. lugdunensis* is also a CoNS, but it can occasionally be confused with *S. aureus* if only a traditional slide coagulase method using plasma is performed. *S. lugdunensis* is more aggressive than other CoNS in its ability to be infective and has been associated with catheter-related bacteremia and endocarditis. Because of reporting criteria, it may need to be identified to the species level to provide the correct treatment options when reporting antimicrobial susceptibilities. More than 40 recognized species of CoNS exist. Most of these species have been isolated from humans, usually from the skin and mucous membranes, and some of these are listed in Table 14-2. Certain species are found in very specific sites such as the head *(S. capitis)* or ear *(S. auricularis)*. Others have been isolated from animals and animal products.

CLINICALLY SIGNIFICANT SPECIES

Staphylococcus aureus

Staphylococcus aureus is the most clinically significant species of staphylococci. It is responsible for a number of infections both relatively mild and life-threatening. *S. aureus* can be recovered from almost any clinical specimen and is an important cause of **nosocomial** or hospital-acquired infections. Increasing drug resistance is an important concern with this common isolate.

Virulence Factors

The pathogenicity of *S. aureus* can be attributed to a number of virulence factors, including enterotoxins, cytolytic toxins,

TABLE 14-2 Groups of Coagulase-Negative Staphylococci and Their Clinical Source and Significance

Staphylococcus Species	Source
S. epidermidis group	
S. epidermidis	Human,* animal
S. haemolyticus	Human*
S. hominis	Human
S. capitis subsp. *capitis*	Human
S. capitis subsp. *ureolyticus*	Human
S. caprae	Human, animal
S. articularis	Human
S. saccharolyticus	Human
S. warneri	Human, animal
S. pasteri	Animal, human
S. saprophyticus group	
S. saprophyticus	Human*
S. cohnii subsp. *cohnii*	Animal, human
S. cohnii subsp. *urealyticum*	Animal, human
S. xylosus	Animal
S. arlettae	Animal
S. equorum	Animal, human
S. gallinarum	Animal
S. kloosii	Animal
S. lentus	Animal
S. simulans group	
S. simulans	Animal, human
S. carnosus	Animal
S. intermedius group	
S. schleiferi subsp. *Schleiferi*	Animal,* human
S. sciuri group	
S. sciuri	Animal, human
S. lentus	Animal, human
S. vitulinus	Animal
S. hyicus group	
S. chromogenes	Animal*
Unspecified sp. group	
S. caseolyticus	Animal
S. felis	Animal
S. hyicus	Animal
S. lugdunensis	Human,* animal
S. muscae	Animal
S. piscifermentans	Animal

Courtesy Leona W. Ayers.
*Common human or veterinary disease.

and cellular components such as protein A. Several cytolytic toxins and exfoliative toxins have been identified. Despite these virulence factors, innate resistance to *S. aureus* is fairly high, and the organism is regarded as an opportunistic pathogen.

Enterotoxins. Staphylococcal **enterotoxins** are heat-stable exotoxins that cause a variety of symptoms including diarrhea and vomiting. Nine serologically distinct enterotoxins have been identified that fall into the following groups, A to E and G to J. These toxins are produced by 30% to 50% of *S. aureus* isolates. Because the enterotoxins are stable at 100° C for 30 minutes, reheating contaminated food will not prevent disease. Staphylococcal food poisoning is most commonly caused by enterotoxins A, B, and D. Enterotoxins B and C and sometimes G and I are associated with TSS. Enterotoxin B has been linked to staphylococcal pseudomembranous enterocolitis. These toxins, along with **toxic shock syndrome toxin-1 (TSST-1),** are superantigens that have the ability to interact with many T cells, activating an aggressive immune response.

Toxic Shock Syndrome Toxin-1. Toxic shock syndrome toxin-1 causes nearly all cases of menstruating-associated TSS. Previously referred to as *enterotoxin F,* this chromosomal-mediated toxin is also associated with approximately 50% of the nonmenstruating-associated TSS cases. TSST-1 is a superantigen that stimulates T cell proliferation and the subsequent production of a large amount of cytokines that are responsible for the symptoms. At a low concentration, TSST-1 causes leakage by endothelial cells, and at a higher concentration, it is cytotoxic to these cells. TSST-1 is absorbed through the vaginal mucosa, permitting the systemic effects seen in TSS.

Exfoliative Toxin. Produced by phage group II, **exfoliative toxin** is also known as *epidermolytic toxin.* It causes the epidermal layer of the skin to slough off and is known to cause staphylococcal SSS, sometimes referred to as **Ritter disease.** This toxin has also been implicated in bullous impetigo.

Cytolytic Toxins. *Staphylococcus aureus* produces other extracellular proteins that affect red blood cells (RBCs) and leukocytes. These hemolysins and leukocidins are **cytolytic toxins** with properties different from those of previously described toxins. *S. aureus* produces four hemolysins: alpha, beta, gamma, and delta. α-**Hemolysin,** in addition to lysing erythrocytes, can damage platelets and macrophages and cause severe tissue damage. β-**Hemolysin** (sphingomyelinase C) acts on sphingomyelin in the plasma membrane of erythrocytes and is also called the "hot-cold" lysin. The "hot-cold" feature associated with this toxin is seen as an enhanced hemolytic activity on incubation at 37° C and subsequent exposure to cold (4° C). This hemolysin is exhibited in the Christie, Atkins, and Munch-Petersen (CAMP) test sometimes performed in the laboratory to identify group B streptococci. δ-Hemolysin, although found in a higher percentage of *S. aureus* stains and some CoNS, is considered less toxic to cell structure than either α- or β-hemolysins. γ-Hemolysin is often only found associated with **Panton-Valentine leukocidin (PVL).**

Staphylococcal leukocidin, PVL, is an exotoxin lethal to polymorphonuclear leukocytes. It has been implicated as contributing to the invasiveness of the organism by suppressing phagocytosis and has been associated with severe cutaneous infections and necrotizing pneumonia. Although produced by relatively few strains of *S. aureus,* it is often associated with community-acquired staphylococcal infections.

Enzymes. Several enzymes are produced by staphylococci. Examples are coagulase, protease, hyaluronidase, and lipase. Staphylocoagulase is produced mainly by *S. aureus.* Although the exact role of coagulase in pathogenicity remains uncertain, it is considered a virulence marker. Many strains of *S. aureus* produce hyaluronidase. This enzyme hydrolyzes hyaluronic acid present in the intracellular ground substance that makes up connective tissues, permitting the spread of bacteria during infection. Lipases are produced by both coagulase-positive and coagulase-negative staphylococci. Lipases act on lipids present on the surface of the skin, particularly fats and oil secreted by the sebaceous glands. Protease, lipase, and hyaluronidase are capable of destroying tissue and may facilitate the spread of infection to adjoining tissues.

Protein A. **Protein A** is one of several cellular components that have been identified in the cell wall of *S. aureus.* Probably the most significant role of protein A in infections caused by *S. aureus* is its ability to bind the Fc portion of immunoglobulin G (IgG). Binding IgG in this manner neutralizes IgG and can block phagocytosis.

Epidemiology

The primary reservoir for staphylococci is the nares, with colonization also occurring in the axillae, vagina, pharynx, and other skin surfaces. Nasal carriage in patients admitted to the hospital is common. Because close contact among patients and hospital personnel is not unusual, transfer of organisms often takes place. Consequently, increased colonization in patients and hospital workers frequently occurs. Hospital outbreaks may develop in nurseries and burn units and among patients who have undergone surgery or other invasive procedures. Transmission of *S. aureus* may occur by direct contact with unwashed, contaminated hands and by inanimate objects (fomites). Both hospital- and community-acquired infections caused by **methicillin-resistant *Staphylococcus aureus* (MRSA)** have become a major health care concern.

Infections Caused by *Staphylococcus aureus*

As with most infections, the development of staphylococcal infection is determined by the virulence of the strain, size of the inoculum, and status of the host's immune system. Infections are initiated when a breach of the skin or mucosal barrier allows staphylococci access to adjoining tissues or the bloodstream. Any event that compromises the host's ability to resist infection encourages colonization and infection. Individuals with normal defense mechanisms are able to combat the infection more easily than those with impaired immune systems. Once the organism has crossed the initial barriers, it activates the host's acute inflammatory response, which leads to the proliferation and activation of polymorphonuclear cells. However, the organisms are able to resist the action of inflammatory cells by the production of toxins and enzymes, thereby establishing a focal lesion.

Skin and Wound Infections. Infections caused by *S. aureus* are suppurative. Typically the abscess is filled with pus and surrounded by necrotic tissues and damaged leukocytes. Some of the common skin infections caused by *S. aureus* are folliculitis, **furuncles,** carbuncles, and bullous impetigo. These opportunistic infections usually occur as a result of previous skin injuries such as cuts, burns, and surgical wounds. Folliculitis is a relatively mild inflammation of a hair follicle or oil gland; the infected area is raised and red. Furuncles (boils), which can be an extension of folliculitis, are large, raised, superficial abscesses. Carbuncles occur when larger, more invasive lesions develop from multiple furuncles, which may progress into deeper tissues. Unlike furuncles, patients with carbuncles often present with fever and chills, indicating systemic spread of the bacteria. **Bullous impetigo** caused by S. aureus is different from streptococcal nonbullous impetigo in that staphylococcal pustules are larger and surrounded by a small zone of erythema. Bullous impetigo is a highly contagious infection that is easily spread by direct contact, fomites, or autoinoculation.

Staphylococcal infections can also be secondary to skin diseases of different etiologies. Dry, irritated skin combined with poor personal hygiene encourages the development of infection. Some of these infections are manifested because of increased colonization of the organisms in blocked hair follicles, sebaceous glands, and sweat glands. Immunocompromised individuals—particularly those who are receiving chemotherapy, are debilitated by chronic illnesses, or have invasive devices—are predisposed to developing staphylococcal infections.

Scalded Skin Syndrome. Scalded skin syndrome, or Ritter disease, is an extensive exfoliative dermatitis that occurs primarily in newborns and previously healthy young children. This syndrome is caused by staphylococcal exfoliative or epidermolytic toxin produced by S. aureus phage group II, which is probably present at a lesion distant from the site of exfoliation. The disease has also been recognized in adults. Cases of SSS in adults occur most commonly in patients with chronic renal failure and in those with compromised immune systems. Although the mortality rate is low (0% to 7%) in children, the rate in adults is as high as 50%.

The severity of the disease varies from being a localized skin lesion in the form of bullous impetigo to a more extensive generalized condition. Bullous impetigo manifests as a localized lesion that contains purulent material. This lesion may progress to the generalized form, which is characterized by cutaneous erythema followed by profuse peeling of the epidermal layer of the skin. The typical pattern in which the erythema occurs is origination from the face, neck, axillae, and groin and then extension to the trunk and extremities. The duration of the disease is brief, about 2 to 4 days. The incidence of spontaneous recovery among children is high. The toxin is metabolized and excreted by the kidneys. Investigators believe this may be why the incidence of SSS is higher among children younger than 5 years old and among adults with chronic renal failure and impaired immune systems.

Toxic Shock Syndrome. Toxic shock syndrome is a rare but potentially fatal, multisystem disease characterized by a sudden onset of fever, chills, vomiting, diarrhea, muscle aches, and rash, which can quickly progress to hypotension and shock. It was first described in children by Todd in 1978 and was later associated with highly absorbent tampon use, although some cases appeared in men, children, and nonmenstruating women. The two categories of TSS are menstruating-associated and nonmenstruating-associated. Although nonmenstruating TSS has been associated with nearly any staphylococcal infection, many cases have been seen with postsurgical infections and secondary to influenza virus infections. During 1979 and 1980, 91% of TSS cases were menstruating-associated; during 1987 to 1996, this percentage declined to

59%. The number of TSS cases has decreased from 482 cases being reported to the Centers for Disease Control and Prevention (CDC) in 1984 to only 87 confirmed cases in 2007, although underreporting may be occurring because of misdiagnosis or failure to meet the CDC case criteria.

Staphylococcal TSS generally results from a localized infection by S. aureus; only the toxin TSST-1 is systemic. The initial clinical presentation of TSS consists of high fever, rash, and signs of dehydration, particularly if the patient has had watery diarrhea and vomiting for several days. In extreme cases, patients may be severely hypotensive and in shock. The rash is found predominantly on the trunk but can spread over the entire body. Laboratory findings include an elevated leukocyte count, with the differential blood count showing an increase in band forms and metamyelocytes. The number of platelets is decreased, and although there is no evidence of bleeding, disseminated intravascular coagulation is likely to occur. The effects of dehydration on the kidneys are manifested by elevations in serum creatinine and urea. Cultures of focal lesions may yield S. aureus, but blood cultures are usually negative. S. aureus does not need to be isolated to confirm the diagnosis of TSS. Supportive therapy to replace vascular volume loss is given, along with appropriate antimicrobial therapy. Most patients with TSS recover, although 2% to 5% of the cases may be fatal. Preventive measures, such as the use of minimum absorbency tampons and warning-label requirements by the U.S. Food and Drug Administration (FDA) for tampon products have greatly decreased the risk of TSS.

Toxic Epidermal Necrolysis. **Toxic epidermal necrolysis (TEN)** is a clinical manifestation with multiple causes; it is most commonly drug induced, but some cases may have been linked to infections and vaccines. The cause is unknown, but symptoms appear to be due to a hypersensitivity reaction. Although it has a very similar initial presentation to that of SSS, treatments differ. Whereas TEN can be resolved by the administration of steroids early in the initial stages of presentation, steroids aggravate SSS. The mortality rate associated with TEN is high, and administration of suspected offending drugs should be stopped as soon as possible.

Food Poisoning. Staphylococcus aureus enterotoxins, most commonly A (78%), D (38%), and B (10%), have been identified and associated with gastrointestinal disturbances. The source of contamination is usually an infected food handler. Staphylococcal food poisoning is a type of intoxication resulting from ingestion of a preformed toxin. Disease occurs when food becomes contaminated with enterotoxin-producing strains of S. aureus by improper handling and is then improperly stored, which allows growth of the bacteria and resulting toxin production. An individual then ingests the food contaminated with enterotoxin.

Foods that are often incriminated in staphylococcal food poisoning include salads, especially those containing mayonnaise and eggs, meat or meat products, poultry, egg products, bakery products with cream fillings, sandwich fillings, and dairy products. Foods kept at room temperature are especially susceptible to higher levels of toxin production when contaminated with toxin-producing staphylococci and are more commonly associated with food poisoning. The enterotoxins do not cause any detectable odor or change in the appearance or taste of the food. Symptoms appear rapidly (approximately 2 to 8 hours after ingestion of the food) and resolve within 24 to 48 hours. Although no fever is associated with this condition, nausea, vomiting, abdominal pain, and severe cramping are common. Diarrhea and headaches may also occur. Death from staphylococcal food poisoning is rare, although such cases have occurred among elderly patients, infants, and severely debilitated persons.

Other Infections. Staphylococcal pneumonia has been known to occur secondary to influenza virus infection. Although rare, staphylococcal pneumonia has a high mortality rate. The pneumonia, which develops as a contiguous, lower respiratory tract infection or a complication of bacteremia, is characterized by multiple abscesses and focal lesions in the pulmonary parenchyma. Infants and immunocompromised patients, such as elderly patients and those receiving chemotherapy or immunosuppressants, are most affected.

Staphylococcal bacteremia leading to secondary pneumonia and endocarditis has been observed among intravenous (IV) drug users. The organisms gain entrance to the bloodstream via contaminated needles or from a focal lesion present on the skin or in the respiratory or genitourinary tract. Staphylococcal **osteomyelitis** occurs as a manifestation secondary to bacteremia. The infection develops when the organism is present in a wound or other focus of infection and gains entrance into the blood. Bacteria may lodge in the diaphysis of the long bones and establish an infection. Symptoms include fever, chills, swelling, and pain around the affected area. Septic arthritis is frequently caused by *S. aureus* in children, especially with trauma to the extremities, and can occur in patients with a history of rheumatoid arthritis or IV drug abuse. The organisms may or may not be recovered from aspirated joint fluid.

Staphylococcus epidermidis

The role of *S. epidermidis* as an etiologic agent of disease has become increasingly evident. Infections caused by *S. epidermidis* are predominantly hospital acquired. Some of the predisposing factors are instrumentation procedures such as catheterization, medical implantation, and immunosuppressive therapy. *S. epidermidis* is probably the most common cause of hospital-acquired UTIs. Prosthetic valve endocarditis is most commonly caused by *S. epidermidis*, although other CoNS such as *S. lugdunensis* have also been recovered in these cases. *S. epidermidis* infections have been associated with intravascular catheters, cerebrospinal fluid shunts, and other prosthetic devices. Septicemia has been reported in immunocompromised patients.

Infections associated with the use of implants, such as indwelling catheters and prosthetic devices, are often caused by isolates shown to produce a biofilm. Biofilm production is a key component in bacterial pathogenesis and is a complex interaction between host, indwelling device, and bacteria (see Chapter 31). One of the bacterial factors involved in adherence of *S. epidermidis* may be poly-gamma-DL-glutamic acid, which provides a protective advantage against host defenses.

Staphylococcus saprophyticus

Staphylococcus saprophyticus has been associated with UTIs in young women. This species adheres more effectively to the epithelial cells lining the urogenital tract than other CoNS. It is rarely found on other mucous membranes or skin surfaces. When present in urine cultures, *S. saprophyticus* may be found in low numbers (less than 10,000 colony forming units/mL) and still be considered significant.

Staphylococcus lugdunensis

Staphylococcus lugdunensis is another CoNS, although it can give a positive clumping factor test result, but it will have a negative tube coagulase reaction. It can cause both community associated and hospital acquired infections. This organism is of note in that it can be more virulent and can clinically mimic *S. aureus* infections. *S. lugdunensis* has been known to contain the gene *mec*A that encodes oxacillin resistance. It is an important pathogen in infective endocarditis, septicemia, meningitis, skin and soft tissue infections, urinary tract infections and septic shock. Endocarditis due to *S. lugdunensis* is particularly aggressive, frequently requiring valve replacement, and infections have a high mortality rate.

Other Coagulase-Negative Staphylococci

Species less commonly seen but that have established themselves as opportunistic pathogens are *S. warneri, S. capitis, S. simulans, S. hominis,* and *S. schleiferi.* A wide range of infections have been associated with these organisms; for example, endocarditis, septicemia, and wound infections. Other species of CoNS are found as normal biota in humans and animals. Although they are uncommonly seen as pathogens, their role in some infections is well established. Therefore they cannot be automatically discarded as contaminants in all cases. *S. haemolyticus* is a commonly isolated CoNS. It has been reported in wounds, bacteremia, endocarditis, and UTIs. Of notable interest is the existence of vancomycin resistance in some *S. haemolyticus* isolates.

LABORATORY DIAGNOSIS

Specimen Collection and Handling

Proper specimen collection, transport, and processing are essential elements in the correct diagnosis and interpretation of any bacterial culture result. Clinical materials collected from infected sites should be transported to the laboratory without delay to prevent drying, maintain the proper environment, and minimize the growth of contaminating organisms. Although the recovery of staphylococci requires no special procedures, specimens should be taken from the site of infection after appropriate cleansing of the surrounding area to avoid contamination by the skin microbiota.

Microscopic Examination

Microscopic examination of stained smears prepared directly from clinical samples (Figure 14-2) provides information that

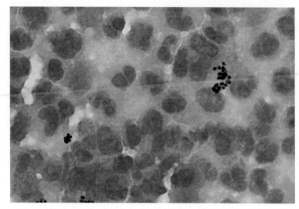

FIGURE 14-2 Numerous gram-positive cocci in clusters, with many polymorphonuclear cells from an aspirated abscess in staphylococcal disease.

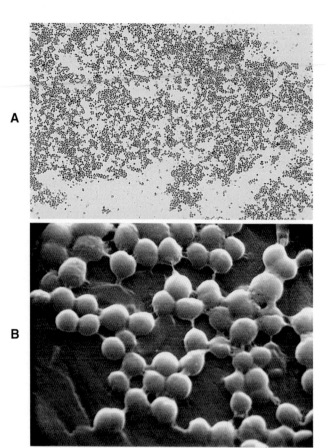

FIGURE 14-3 **A,** Microscopic morphology of *Staphylococcus* sp. on Gram stain. Gram-negative–looking cells show how older cells easily decolorize. **B,** Scanning electron micrograph showing the typical "clusters" of staphylococci.

is helpful in the early diagnosis and treatment of the infection and should always be performed on appropriate specimens. Numerous gram-positive cocci, along with polymorphonuclear cells in purulent exudates, joint fluids, aspirated secretions, and other body fluids, are easily seen when these sites are infected with staphylococci. A culture should be done regardless of the results of the microscopic examination, because the genus or species cannot be appropriately identified by microscopic morphology alone (Figure 14-3). An aspirate is the best sample, whereas a single swab will be less satisfactory for both culture and smear results. Optimally, clinicians should send two swabs when requesting a Gram stain and culture.

Isolation and Identification

Staphylococci grow easily on routine laboratory culture media, particularly sheep blood agar (SBA). A selective medium such as mannitol salt agar (MSA), Columbia colistin–nalidixic acid (CNA) agar, or phenylethyl alcohol (PEA) agar can be used for heavily contaminated specimens. The high NaCl concentration (7.5%) in MSA makes this medium selective. Chromagar Staph aureus (BD Diagnostic Systems, Sparks, Md.) is a proprietary selective and differential medium for isolation of *S. aureus*.

Cultural Characteristics

Staphylococci produce round, smooth, white, creamy colonies on SBA after 18 to 24 hours of incubation at 35° to 37° C. *S. aureus* may produce hemolytic zones around the colonies (Figure 14-4) and may exhibit pigment production (yellow) with extended incubation. *S. epidermidis* colonies are usually small- to medium-sized, nonhemolytic, white to gray colonies (Figure 14-5). Some may be weakly hemolytic. *S. saprophyticus* forms slightly larger colonies, with about 50% of the strains producing a yellow pigment. *S. haemolyticus* produces medium-sized colonies, with moderate or weak hemolysis and variable pigment production. Colonies of *S. lugdunensis* are often hemolytic and medium-sized, although small colony variants can occur. Identification of staphylococci on the basis of colony morphology should not be done.

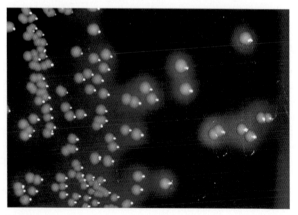

FIGURE 14-4 *Staphylococcus aureus* growing on sheep blood agar showing β-hemolytic, creamy, buttery-looking colonies.

Identification Methods

Staphylococci have been traditionally differentiated from micrococci on the basis of oxidation-fermentation (O/F) reactions produced in O/F glucose medium. Staphylococci ferment glucose, whereas micrococci fail to produce acid under anaerobic conditions. However, the O/F tests do not sufficiently discern certain weak acid producers such as *Micrococcus*

TABLE 14-3 Differentiation Among Staphylococci and Other Gram-Positive Cocci

Characteristic	Staphylococci	Enterococci	Streptococci	Aerococci	Alloiococci	Planococci	Stomatococci	Macrococci	Micrococci	*Rothia*
Strict aerobe	–	–	–	–	+	+	–	±	+	–
Facultative anaerobe	d	+	+	+	–	–	+	±	–	+
Motility	–	d	–	–	–	+	–	–	–	–
Growth on NaCl agar										
5% NaCl	+	+	d	+	+	+	–	+	+	
6.5% NaCl	+	+	d	+	+	+	–	+	+	
12% NaCl	d	(±)	–	+	ND	+	–	±	d	–
Catalase	+	–	–	–	±	+	±	+	+	±
Benzidine test	+	–	–	–	±	+	+	+	+	+
Anaerobic acid from glucose	d	+	+	(+)	ND	–	+	–	–	+
Lysostaphin (200 mg/mL)	–	+	+	+	ND	+	+	–	+*	+
Erythromycin (0.04-unit disk)	+	+	–	ND	ND	ND	ND	+	–†	ND
Bacitracin (0.04-unit disk)	+	+	d	–	ND		–	+	–	–

Modified from Bannerman TL: Staphylococcus, micrococcus, and other catalase: positive cocci that grow aerobically. In Murray PR et al, editors: *Manual of clinical microbiology*, ed 9, Washington, DC, 2007, ASM Press.
+, 90% or more species or strains positive; ±, 90% or more species or strains weakly positive; –, 90% or more species or strains negative; d, 11% to 89% of species or strains positive; (), delayed reaction; *ND*, not determined.
*Some strains of *M. luteu*, *M. roseus*, and *M. sedentarius* demonstrate susceptibility to lysostaphin, presumably because of contaminating levels of endo-β-*N*-acetylglucosaminidase activity.
†A few *Micrococcus* strains demonstrate high-level (minimal inhibitory concentration equal to or greater than 50 μg/mL) erythromycin resistance.

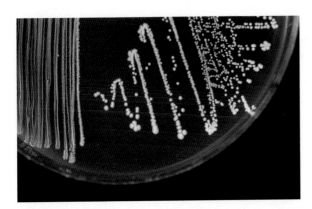

FIGURE 14-5 Coagulase-negative staphylococci growing on sheep blood agar, revealing nonhemolytic, white, creamy colonies.

kristinae, and those staphylococci that fail to grow or produce acid anaerobically: *S. saprophyticus*, *S. auricularis*, *S. hominis*, *S. xylosus*, and *S. cohnii*. Tests to differentiate micrococci from staphylococci are shown in Table 14-1. A modified oxidase test such as the Microdase disk (Remel, Lenexa, Kan.) can be used to rapidly differentiate staphylococci from micrococci. Most staphylococci will be negative, whereas micrococci will be positive. Table 14-3 outlines key characteristics for differentiating staphylococci from other gram-positive cocci. Many commercial multitest systems have incorporated these traditional biochemical tests. In addition, molecular testing, plasmid typing, and fatty acid analysis have been used for species and strain identification.

S. aureus is often identified by the **coagulase tests.** Clumping factor, formerly referred to as *cell-bound coagulase*, causes agglutination in human, rabbit, or pig plasma and is considered an important marker for *S. aureus*. Clumping factor on the surface of the bacterial cells directly converts fibrinogen to fibrin, which precipitates onto the cell surface, causing agglutination. Clumping factor is easily detected by the slide coagulase test and is used to screen catalase-positive colonies that morphologically resemble *S. aureus*. A heavy suspension of the suspected organism is prepared on a glass slide in water or saline and is mixed with a drop of plasma. If agglutination occurs, the isolate can be identified as *S. aureus*. However, some strains of *S. lugdunensis* and *S. schleiferi* are also positive for clumping factor.

Because about 5% of *S. aureus* organisms do not produce clumping factor, any negative slide coagulase test result must be confirmed with the tube method, which detects staphylocoagulase, or free coagulase. Staphylocoagulase is an extracellular molecule that causes a clot to form when bacterial cells are incubated with plasma (Figure 14-6). Staphylocoagulase reacts with a thermostable, thrombin-like molecule called *coagulase-reacting factor* (CRF) to form coagulase-CRF complex. The complex resembles thrombin and indirectly converts fibrinogen to fibrin. The clot formed in the tube may have a tendency to undergo autolysis (because of fibrinolysin), giving the appearance of a negative result. Clinical laboratorians should look for clot formation after 4 hours of incubation at 37° C. If no clot appears, the tube should be left at room temperature and checked the following day. Fibrinolysin activity is enhanced at 37° C which might result in a false negative result. Table 14-4 lists the coagulase-positive staphylococci and identifies their clinical source and significance. The clinical laboratorian must be aware that staphylococci other than *S. aureus* produce clumping factor or staphylocoagulase (Table 14-5).

Testing for pyrrolidonyl arylamidase activity can be used to differentiate *S. aureus* (negative) from *S. lugdun-* ensis, *S. intermedius*, and *S. schleiferi* (positive). The substrate, pyroglutamyl-β-naphthylamide (L-pyrrolidonyl-β-naphthylamide; PYR), is hydrolyzed to L-pyrrolidone and β-naphthylamine, which combines with *p*-dimethylaminocinnamaldehyde to form a red compound. Some laboratorians get more reliable results differentiating *S. aureus* (positive) from *S. intermedius* (negative) with the Voge-Proskauer (VP) test. In the VP test, a positive result is the formation of acetoin from glucose or pyruvate. *S. intermedius* is an animal pathogen, and most human infections are associated with

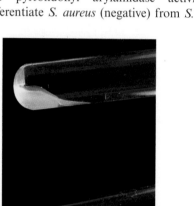

FIGURE 14-6 Tube coagulase test detects extracellular enzyme "free coagulase." Top tube is coagulase positive.

TABLE 14-4 Groups of Coagulase-Positive Staphylococci and Their Clinical Source and Significance

Staphylococcus Species	Source
S. aureus group	
S. aureus	Human,* animal
S. aureus subsp. anaerobius	Animal
S. hyicus group	
S. hyicus	Animal*
S. intermedius group	
S. intermedius	Animal*
S. schleiferi subsp. coagulans	Animal*
S. delphini	Animal

Courtesy Leona W. Ayers.
*Common in human or veterinary disease.

TABLE 14-5 Key Test for Identification of the Most Clinically Significant *Staphylococcus* Species

Test	S. aureus	S. epidermidis	S. haemolyticus	S. lugdunensis	S. saprophyticus	S. schleiferi	S. simulans
Colony pigment	+	−	d	d	d	−	−
Staphylocoagulase	+	−	−	−	−	−	−
Clumping factor	+	−	−	(+)	−	−	−
Heat-stable nuclease	+	−	−	−	−	+	−
Alkaline phosphatase	+	+*	−	−	−	+	−
Pyrrolidonlyl arylamidase	−	−	+	+	−	+	(d)
Ornithine decarboxylase	−	(d)	−	+	−	−	+
Urease	d	+	−	d	+	−	+
β-Galactosidase	−		(d)	−	+	(+)	+
Acetoin production	+	+	+	+	+	+	d
Novobiocin resistance	S	S	S	S	R	S	S
Polymyxin B resistance	R	R	S	(d)	S	S	S
Acid (aerobically from)							
D-Trehalose	+	−	+	+	+	d	d
D-Mannitol	+	−	d	−	d	−	+
D-Mannose	+	(+)	−	+	−	+	d
D-Turanose	+	(d)	(d)	(d)	+	−	−
D-Xylose	−	−	−	−	−	−	−
D-Cellubiose	−	−	−	−	−	−	−
Maltose	+	+	+	+	+	−	(±)
Sucrose	+	+	+	+	+	−	+

Modified from Bannerman TL: Staphylococcus, micrococcus, and other catalase: positive cocci that grow aerobically. In Murray PR, et al, editors: *Manual of clinical microbiology*, ed 9, Washington, DC, 2007, ASM Press.
+, 90% or more strains positive; ±, 90% or more strains weakly positive; −, 90% or more strains negative; *d*, 11% to 89% of strains positive; (d), delayed reaction; *R*, resistant; *S*, sensitive.
*, *A low but significant number (6% to 15%) of clinical isolates are alkaline phosphatase negative.*

animal bites. *S. lugdunensis, S. haemolyticus,* and *S. schleiferi* are also VP positive.

Isolates that do not produce either clumping factor or staphylocoagulase are reported as coagulase-negative staphylococci. Urine isolates that are coagulase negative are further tested to identify *S. saprophyticus.* Presumptive identification of *S. saprophyticus* is accomplished by testing for **novobiocin susceptibility** using a 5-μg novobiocin disk (Figure 14-7). *S. saprophyticus* is resistant to novobiocin, whereas most other coagulase-negative staphylococci are susceptible. Isolates producing a zone of inhibition of ≤16 mm are considered resistant. Figure 14-8 shows the schema for the identification of clinically significant staphylococci. Although *S. epidermidis* and *S. saprophyticus* are the most clinically significant species of CoNS, other species, such as *S. lugdunensis* and *S. haemolyticus,* are becoming more important clinically. Table 14-5 outlines some key tests for the identification of the clinically significant species of *Staphylococcus,* including coagulase-negative isolates.

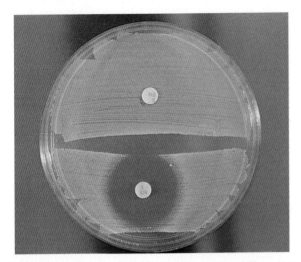

FIGURE 14-7 Novobiocin susceptibility test to differentiate coagulase-negative staphylococci isolated from urine samples. *Staphylococcus saprophyticus* (*top*) is resistant to novobiocin, indicated by the lack of a zone of inhibition around the disk.

Rapid Methods of Identification

Numerous rapid agglutination test kits are on the market for differentiating *S. aureus* from the CoNS. Among these are the BBL Staphyloslide (BD Diagnostic Systems), Staphaurex (Remel, Lenexa, Kan.), BactiStaph (Remel; Figure 14-9), and Prolex (Pro-Lab Diagnostics; Cheshire, United Kingdom). These kits use plasma-coated carrier particles, such as latex. The plasma detects both clumping factor (with fibrinogen) and protein A in the cell wall of *S. aureus* (with IgG). These kits often have a higher specificity and sensitivity than the traditional plasma slide test and are commonly used in clinical laboratories. They are particularly useful for the identification of MRSA that is often weakly or negative in the slide

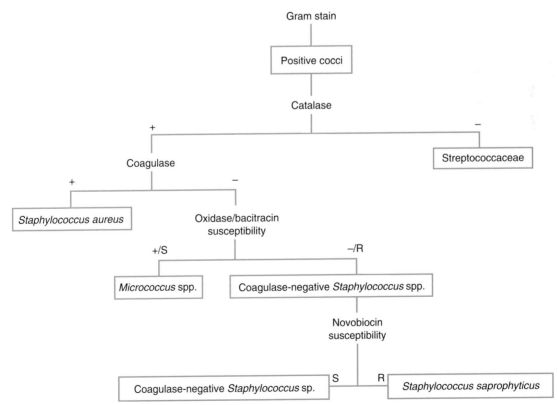

FIGURE 14-8 Schema for the identification of staphylococcal species. NOTE: Other *Staphylococcus* spp. that are coagulase positive besides *S. aureus* include *S. schleiferi* and *S. lugdunensis* (which can be slide-test positive), *S. intermedius,* and *S. hyicus* (tube positive and slide positive).

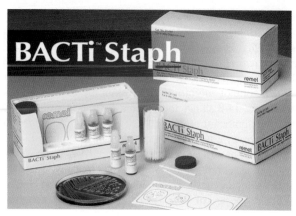

FIGURE 14-9 Slide coagulase test (BactiStaph), a latex agglutination method commercially available for the detection of both clumping factor and protein A. (Courtesy Remel, Lenexa, Kan.)

coagulase test. Users should be aware that some strains of *S. saprophyticus, S. sciuri, S. lugdunensis,* and *Micrococcus* spp. may produce positive tests with the latex-coated assays, but they would be tube coagulase negative on further testing. Careful consideration of source, colony morphology, and susceptibility pattern can eliminate most errors.

Although numerous automated and rapid multitest systems for the identification of staphylococci are available, their accuracy varies. Most systems are able to identify *S. aureus,* most *S. epidermidis,* and *S. saprophyticus* strains accurately as well as some of the other staphylococcal species such as *S. capitis, S. haemolyticus, S. simulans, S. lugdunensis,* and *S. intermedius.* However, the accuracy varies with less frequently recovered staphylococci.

ANTIMICROBIAL SUSCEPTIBILITY

Routine testing of staphylococcal isolates can be easily performed in the laboratory using standard guidelines issued by the Clinical and Laboratory Standards Institute (CLSI), formally known as the *National Committee for Clinical Laboratory Standards* (NCCLS). When using commercial tests, laboratories need to adhere to the manufacturers' recommended procedures.

Testing of CoNS depends on source and determination if the isolate is a contaminant or a likely pathogen. Current CLSI guidelines do not require routine reporting of susceptibilities on *S. saprophyticus.* Serious infections with *S. aureus* require susceptibility testing. Because of the production of **β-lactamase**s (penicillinases), which break down the β-lactam ring of many penicillins, most *S. aureus* isolates are resistant to penicillin. Increasing resistance to alternative antimicrobial agents is a major concern.

Methicillin-Resistant Staphylococci

Penicillin-resistant strains require treatment with penicillinase-resistant penicillins, such as nafcillin or oxacillin. Even though methicillin is no longer used in the United States, isolates that are resistant to nafcillin or oxacillin have been traditionally termed *methicillin-resistant staphylococci;* for

example, *S. aureus* being called **MRSA** and *S. epidermidis* referred to as **MRSE (methicillin-resistant *Staphylococcus epidermidis*).** The incidence of MRSA has been on the rise for the past several decades. In addition, since the 1990s **community-associated MRSA (CA-MRSA)** infections have risen and can be found in patients who lack traditional health care–associated risk factors such as recent hospitalization, long-term care, dialysis, or indwelling devices. CA-MRSA infections and outbreaks have been reported among athletes, correctional facility inmates, military recruits in close contact environments, pediatric patients, and tattoo recipients. All of these MRSA infections, whether **hospital-associated MRSA (HA-MRSA)** or CA-MRSA, are costly and pose a serious threat to health institutions. Control of MRSA requires strict adherence to infection-control practices such as barrier protection, contact isolation, and handwashing compliance. The use of vancomycin for MRSA remains the treatment of choice, but concerns with rising resistance to glycopeptides call for the restrictive use of these drugs and selective reporting by the laboratory.

In the past, oxacillin was generally used for detection of methicillin resistance for staphylococci species. The latest CLSI M100 document recommends cefoxitin be used to detect methicillin resistance. Cefoxitin is a better inducer of *mecA*-mediated resistance. At a minimum, the laboratory should report susceptibilities for penicillin and cefoxitin. Recently *S. lugdunensis* has been given the same minimal inhibitory concentration breakpoints as *S. aureus,* which are different from other CoNS.

MRSA populations are often heterogenous in resistance to β-lactams, meaning one subpopulation is sensitive whereas another is resistant to methicillin. Even though nearly all cells possess the genetic information to be resistant, only a small fraction (1 in 10^4 or 10^8 cells) expresses the resistance phenotype. Growth of the resistant subpopulation is enhanced at a neutral pH, NaCl concentration of 2% to 4%, cooler incubation temperature (30° to 32° C), and prolonged incubation (up to 48 hours).

The use of an oxacillin-salt agar plate can be used to screen for MRSA in clinical samples or as a way to differentiate MRSA isolates from those that are hyperproducers of β-lactamase, known as **borderline oxacillin-resistant *S. aureus* (BORSA)** strains, which will not grow on these plates. Oxacillin-salt agar is not recommended to screen for CoNS. Chromogenic selective, differential media, such as MRSA Select (Biorad Laboratories; Hercules, Calif.), Spectra MRSA (Remel), and CHROMagar MRSA (BD Diagnostic Systems) have the ability to identify MRSA directly from nasal samples. Antimicrobial compounds such as cefoxitin are incorporated in the media and inhibit non-MRSA isolates. After 24 or 48 hours of incubation, MRSA isolates will produce a colored colony, whereas methicillin-susceptible *S. aureus* and most other organisms will be inhibited or produce a non-colored colony.

Most oxacillin resistance is due to the gene *mecA,* which codes for an altered **penicillin-binding protein (PBP)** called PBP2a, also designated PBP2′. The altered PBP does not bind oxacillin, thereby rendering the drug ineffective. Latex agglutination tests are available to detect these altered PBPs, and they provide an alternative method for testing and confirmation of oxacillin resistance. This test can be performed on both CoNS and *S. aureus*. This assay may be the preferred method if *S. lugdunensis* is suspected but the laboratory is unable to perform identification to the species level, because *S. lugdunensis* has separate breakpoints from the CoNS in the current CLSI guide on susceptibility testing.

The "gold standard" for MRSA detection is the detection of the *mecA* gene by using nucleic acid probes or polymerase chain reaction (PCR) amplification. A number of systems are available for direct detection from anterior nare swabs, such as the BD GeneOhm MRSA assay and the Cepheid Xpert MRSA (Sunnyvale, Calif.) using the GeneXpert system, both of which use real-time PCR and produce results within the same day. This type of test, with a decreased time to detection, has the potential to reduce unnecessary transmission of both HA-MRSA and CA-MRSA within the hospital setting. These assays are moderate- and/or high-complexity testing at the moment, but CLIA-waived versions may be available as point-of-care testing in the future and could be used in nursing homes and long-term health care facilities. In addition, some novel PCR assays are able to identify the most common CA-MRSA strains, designated as USA 300 and USA 400, which have a high mortality and morbidity rate and often carry the PVL genes. Although CA-MRSA can cause nosocomial infections, this might have an important implication in treatment and epidemiology. The Joint Commission, an accreditation agency for health care facilities, recently proposed safety goals for a laboratory-based alert system to identify MRSA, and a number of states already have legislation in place that includes either enacted or pending MRSA screening laws.

Vancomycin-Resistant Staphylococci

Vancomycin is the drug of choice, and sometimes the only drug available, for serious staphylococcal infections, and thus the development of vancomycin resistance has been a serious concern for the medical community. In 1996 the first **vancomycin-intermediate *S. aureus* (VISA)** strains were recovered in Japan. In 2002 isolates of true **vancomycin-resistant *S. aureus* (VRSA)** were reported in the United States, isolated from patients undergoing long-term vancomycin treatment. Automated antimicrobial susceptibility testing methods may not be reliable in detecting these isolates. The disk diffusion procedure also has limitations in detecting resistance. Screening using a vancomycin agar plate as described by the CLSI performance guidelines should enhance detection of VISA and VRSA. Detection of these isolates should be confirmed by a reference method, and reporting should follow CDC guidelines. Adherence to infection-control practices and CDC guidelines for vancomycin resistance may limit the emergence of this highly resistant organism.

Macrolide Resistance

Resistance to other categories of antimicrobials such as macrolides might not always be readily apparent by routine testing. Clindamycin, a macrolide, is frequently used in staphylococcal skin infections; additional testing using a modified double-disk diffusion test **(D test)** might be useful when dis-

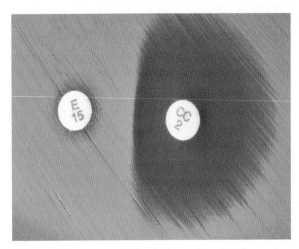

FIGURE 14-10 D test positive isolate, showing flattening of the clindamycin *(CC)* zone adjacent to the erythromycin *(E)* disk and the characteristic D-like pattern.

crepant macrolide test results are obtained (e.g., erythromycin resistant and clindamycin susceptible). Erythromycin and clindamycin susceptibility results are normally the same. However, staphylococcal resistance to clindamycin is occasionally inducible, meaning it is only detectable in vitro when the bacteria are also exposed to erythromycin. Inducible clindamycin resistance can be detected by disk diffusion by placing an erythromycin disk near a clindamycin disk and using the latest performance standards for susceptibility testing. If an isolate possesses inducible clindamycin resistance, the bacteria will grow around the erythromycin disk and in the area of the agar where the two drugs overlap. However, a zone of inhibition will be observed on the side of the clindamycin disk farther away from the erythromycin disk (Figure 14-10). It is important for laboratories to keep up with the latest trends in antimicrobial resistance and to be aware of limitations that can occur with susceptibility testing.

BIBLIOGRAPHY

Association for Professionals in Infection Control & Epidemiology, Inc, MRSA Laws and Pending Legislation. Available at: www.apic.org/AM/images/maps/mrsa_map.gif. Accessed August 11, 2008.

Balaban N, Rasooly A: Staphylococcal enterotoxins, *Int J Food Microbiol* 61:1, 2000.

Bannerman TL, Peacock SJ: *Staphylococcus, Micrococcus*, and other catalase-positive cocci. In Murray PR, Baron EJ, Jorgensen JH et al, editors: *Manual of clinical microbiology*, ed 9, Washington, DC, 2007, ASM Press.

Bascomb S, Manafi M: Use of enzyme tests in characterization and identification of aerobic and facultatively anaerobic gram-positive cocci, *Clin Microbiol Rev* 11:318, 1998.

Centers for Disease Control and Prevention: *Toxic shock syndrome*. Available at: www.cdc.gov/ncidod/dbmd/diseaseinfo/toxicshock_t.htm. Accessed August 11, 2008.

Centers for Disease Control and Prevention: *Algorithm for testing S. aureus with vancomycin*. Available at: www.cdc.gov/ncidod/dhqp/pdf/ar/VISA_VRSA_algo06v7.pdf. Accessed August 11, 2008.

Centers for Disease Control and Prevention: *Notifiable diseases/deaths in selected cities weekly information*. Available at: www.cdc.

gov/mmwr/preview/mmwrhtml/mm5718md.htm#tab1. Accessed August 11, 2008.

Clinical and Laboratory Standards Institute: *Approved Standard M100-S18, Performance standards for antimicrobial susceptibility testing, nineteenth informational supplement*, January 2008, Clinical and Laboratory Standards Institute.

Costa AM, Kay I, Palladino S et al: Rapid detection of *mecA* and *nuc* genes in staphylococci by real-time multiplex polymerase chain reaction, *Diagn Microbiol Infect Dis* 51:13, 2005.

De Paulis AN, Predari SC, Chazarreta CD et al: Five-test simple scheme for species-level identification of clinically significant coagulase-negative staphylococci, *J Clin Microbiol* 41:1219, 2003.

Dinges MM, Orwin PM, Schlievert PM: Exotoxins of *Staphylococcus aureus*, *Clin Microbiol Rev* 13:16, 2000.

Fischetti VA et al: The gram-positive cell wall. In Fischetti VA et al, editors: *Gram-positive pathogens*, Washington DC, 2006, ASM Press.

Hanakawa Y et al: Molecular mechanisms of blister formation in bullous impetigo and staphylococcal scalded skin syndrome, *J Clin Invest* 110:53, 2002.

The Joint Commission: *Draft 2009 National patient safety goals for hospital and critical access hospitals*. Available at: www.jointcommission.org/NR/rdonlyres/5928FA30-6BAB-4017-8DF6-5545E5470154/0/09_Hospital_NPSG_FR.pdf. Accessed August 11, 2008.

Kocianova S et al: Key role of poly-γ-DL-glutamic acid in immune evasion and virulence of *Staphylococcus epidermidis*, *J Clin Invest* 115:688, 2005.

Lusky K: Mitigating MRSA, steps ahead of the law, *CAP Today* May 22(5), 2008.

McCormick JK et al: Toxic shock syndrome and bacterial superantigens: an update, *Annu Rev Microbiol* 55:77, 2001.

Naimi TS et al: Comparison of community- and health care–associated methicillin-resistant *Staphylococcus aureus* infection, *JAMA* 290:2976, 2003.

Patel R et al: Frequency of isolation of *Staphylococcus lugdunensis* among staphylococcal isolates causing endocarditis; a 20-year experience, *J Clin Microbiol* 38:4262, 2000.

Smith TL et al: Emergence of vancomycin resistance in *Staphylococcus aureus*, *N Engl J Med* 340:493, 1999.

Spanu T et al: Use of the VITEK 2 system for rapid identification of clinical isolates of staphylococci from bloodstream infections, *J Clin Microbiol* 41:4259, 2003.

Srinivasan A, Dick JD, Peri TM: Vancomycin resistance in staphylococci, *Clin Microbiol Rev* 15:430, 2002.

Swensen JM et al: Special phenotypic methods for detecting antibacterial resistance. In Murray PR et al, editors: *Manual of clinical microbiology*, ed 9, Washington, DC, 2007, ASM Press.

Tenover FC et al: Vancomycin-resistant *Staphylococcus aureus* isolate from a patient in Pennsylvania, *Antimicrob Agents Chemother* 48:275, 2004.

Todd J et al: Toxic-shock syndrome associated with phage-group-1 staphylococci, *Lancet* 312:116, 1978.

Warren DK et al: Detection of methicillin-resistant *Staphylococcus aureus* directly from nasal swab specimens by a real-time PCR assay, *J Clin Microbiol* 42:5578, 2004.

Wen WS et al: *Staphylococcus lugdunensis* carrying the *mecA* gene causes catheter-associated bloodstream infection in premature neonate, *J Clin Microbiol* 41:519, 2003.

Zhang K et al: Novel multiplex PCR assay for simultaneous identification of community-associated methicillin-resistant *Staphylococcus aureus* strains USA300 and USA400 and detection of *mecA* and Panton-Valentine leukocidin genes, with discrimination of *Staphylococcus aureus* from coagulase-negative staphylococci, *J Clin Microbiol* 46:1118, 2008.

Zinderman et al: Community-acquired methicillin-resistant *Staphylococcus aureus* among military recruits, *Emerg Infect Dis* 10:941, 2004.

Points to Remember

- The staphylococci are catalase-positive, gram-positive cocci.
- *Staphylococcus aureus* is the primary pathogen within this genus, and the isolation of *S. aureus* from any source can usually be considered clinically significant.
- *S. aureus* produces a number of virulence factors including protein A, enterotoxins, toxic shock syndrome toxin-1, exfoliative toxin, cytolytic toxins, and numerous exoenzymes.
- *S. aureus* is associated with a number of infections including skin infections, scalded skin syndrome, toxic shock syndrome, food poisonings, osteomyelitis, and pneumonia.
- *S. epidermidis* and other CoNS have been linked to important nosocomial infections, often associated with foreign body implants.
- CoNS recovered from sterile sites, and those sites associated with indwelling devices, should be considered potential pathogens.
- HA-MRSA and CA-MRSA are important and costly health care concerns.
- *S. saprophyticus* is an important cause of urinary tract infections. The identification of *S. saprophyticus* from urine specimens should be made, especially if they are predominant, because even low numbers can be significant.
- *S. aureus* is frequently separated from less pathogenic species by being coagulase positive.
- Novobiocin susceptibility testing is used to identify *S. saprophyticus*.
- Increasing antimicrobial resistance to compounds such as oxacillin and vancomycin is a problem with the staphylococci, particularly *S. aureus*.

Learning Assessment Questions

1. In what population(s) do(es) *Staphylococcus aureus* cause infection?
2. What types of infections are associated with *S. aureus*?
3. How does protein A contribute to the virulence of *S. aureus*?
4. What toxin causes toxic shock syndrome?
5. What type of toxin is associated with scalded skin syndrome?
6. What toxins are involved in staphylococcal food poisoning?
7. In what clinical condition would coagulase-negative staphylococci be significant?
8. Which coagulase-negative staphylococci are considered more significant and might need to be identified to the species level?
9. What are the two types of coagulase produced by *S. aureus*, and how is each type detected in the clinical laboratory?

10. How is *S. aureus* differentiated from other similar isolates?

11. What test is used to identify *Staphylococcus saprophyticus*?

12. What is the significance of a *S. aureus* isolate being oxacillin resistant?

13. Describe some of the risk factors associated with HA-MRSA and CA-MRSA.

14. What new recommendations have been described for detecting oxacillin, clindamycin, or vancomycin resistance?

15. A staphylococcal isolate is positive for clumping factor but negative for coagulase. Which species should you suspect and why?

Streptococcus, Enterococcus, and Other Catalase-Negative Gram-Positive Cocci

Donald C. Lehman, Connie R. Mahon,* Kalavati Suvarna*

- **GENERAL CHARACTERISTICS**
  Cell Wall Structure
  Hemolysis
- **CLINICALLY SIGNIFICANT STREPTOCOCCI AND STREPTOCOCCUS-LIKE ORGANISMS**
  Streptococcus pyogenes
  Streptococcus agalactiae
  Groups C and G Streptococci

  Streptococcus pneumoniae
  Viridans Streptococci
  Enterococcus
  Streptococcus-like Organisms
- **LABORATORY DIAGNOSIS**
  Classification Schemes
  Noncultural Identification
  Susceptibility Testing

OBJECTIVES

After reading and studying this chapter, you should be able to:

1. Compare the general characteristics of the streptococci and similar organisms.
2. Explain the Lancefield classification of the streptococci.
3. Apply the knowledge of hemolytic patterns on sheep blood agar in the identification of streptococcal isolates.
4. Contrast the significance of the streptococci commonly isolated in the clinical laboratory, both those that occur as normal biota and those that are potential pathogens.
5. Compare the virulence factors associated with the Streptococcaceae.
6. Explain how infections caused by the Streptococcaceae are established.
7. Give the characteristic morphology of streptococci in direct smears and from culture.
8. Given the microscopic and colony morphology of an organism isolated from a clinical sample, use the appropriate biochemical tests for presumptively identifying the organism.
9. State the principle and purpose of each differential test used in the identification of the Streptococcaceae.
10. Discuss the major serologic tests used to detect antibodies that are produced after recent streptococcal infections.

Case in Point

A 9-year-old boy complained of fever and sore throat over a 3-day period. On examination by his physician, the patient's pharynx was red and both tonsils were swollen. Pronounced cervical lymphadenopathy was present. A swab of the tonsillar area was taken and inoculated to a sheep blood agar plate. After 24 hours of incubation, small, shiny, translucent colonies showing β-hemolysis were noted.

Issues to Consider

After reading the patient's case history, consider:
- The most likely causative agent
- Key tests to be performed on the bacterial isolate for identification
- Nonculture assays available for the rapid identification of the isolate

*This chapter was prepared by C.R. Mahon and K. Suvarna in their private capacities. No official support or endorsement by the FDA is intended or implied.

Key Terms

Acute glomerulonephritis (AGN)

α-Hemolysis

β-Hemolysis

Bile solubility

CAMP test

Capnophilic

Cellulitis

Empyema

Erysipelas

Hippurate hydrolysis test

Hyaluronidase

Impetigo

Lancefield classification system

Leucine aminopeptidase (LAP)

M protein

Necrotizing fasciitis (NF)

Optochin test

Pharyngitis

Pyogenic streptococci

Pyrrolidonyl-α-naphthylamide (PYR) hydrolysis

Rheumatic fever

Scarlet fever

Streptolysin O (SLO)

Streptolysin S

Voges-Proskauer (VP) test

I n the last two decades, DNA homology and DNA sequencing studies have led to numerous taxonomic changes to the family Streptococcaceae. The enterococci, formerly known as group D streptococci, have been classified in their own genus, *Enterococcus*. Similarly, lactococci, previously classified as group N streptococci, now belong in the genus *Lactococcus*. Although traditional phenotypic characteristics such as hemolysis and Lancefield classification (antigen serogrouping) are still useful toward presumptive identification, nucleic acid studies have provided more information on the genetic relationships among different phenotypes of the members of the family Streptococcaceae. This chapter presents the role of the *Streptococcus* and *Enterococcus* spp. in human disease, characteristics of the members in each genus, and how isolates are identified in the clinical microbiology laboratory. Other gram-positive cocci that resemble streptococci, including *Aerococcus, Lactococcus, Leuconostoc,* and *Pediococcus* spp., are also discussed.

GENERAL CHARACTERISTICS

Streptococcus and *Enterococcus* spp. belong to the family Streptococcaceae. Members of both genera are catalase-negative, gram-positive cocci that are usually arranged in pairs or chains (Figure 15-1). A negative catalase test result differentiates the streptococci and enterococci from the staphylococci. Weak false-positive catalase reactions can be seen when growth is taken from media containing blood. Compared with other gram-positive cocci, the cells of enterococci and some streptococci appear somewhat more elongated than spherical. The streptococcal cells are more likely to appear in chains when grown in broth cultures.

Most members of the genera *Streptococcus* and *Enterococcus* behave like facultative anaerobes. Because they grow in the presence of oxygen but are unable to use oxygen for respiration, they may be considered *aerotolerant anaerobes*. Carbohydrates are metabolized fermentatively with lactic acid as the major end product; gas is not produced. Some species are **capnophilic,** requiring increased concentration of CO_2, whereas the growth of others is stimulated by increased CO_2 but is not required. Growth is poor on nutrient media such as trypticase soy agar. On media enriched with blood or serum, however, growth is more pronounced. The colonies are usually small and somewhat transparent.

Cell Wall Structure

The streptococci possess a typical gram-positive cell wall consisting of peptidoglycan and teichoic acid. Most streptococci, except for many of the viridans group, have a group or

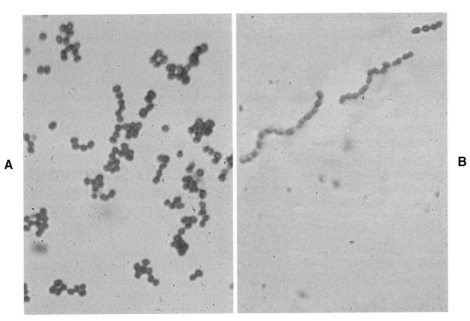

A

B

FIGURE 15-1   Gram stain of *Streptococcus*. **A,** Solid medium. **B,** Liquid medium.

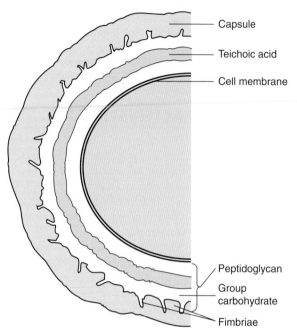

FIGURE 15-2 Schematic representation of streptococcal cell wall.

TABLE 15-1 Types of Hemolysis

Hemolysis	Description
Alpha (α)	Partial lysis of red blood cells around colony
	Greenish discoloration of area around colony
Beta (β)	Complete lysis of red blood cells around colony
	Clear area around colony
Nonhemolytic	No lysis of red blood cells around colony
	No change in agar
Alpha-prime (α′) or wide zone	Small area of intact red blood cells around colony surrounded by a wider zone of complete hemolysis

common C carbohydrate (polysaccharide), which can be used to classify an isolate serologically. This classification scheme was developed in the 1930s by Rebecca Lancefield. After first recognizing the antigen in β-hemolytic streptococci, Lancefield was able to divide the streptococci into serologic groups, designated by letters. Organisms in group A possess the same antigenic C carbohydrate; those in group B have the same C carbohydrate, and so on. A schematic diagram of the streptococcal cell wall is shown in Figure 15-2. Some species can produce a type-specific polysaccharide capsule as well.

Hemolysis

The streptococci and similar organisms can produce a number of exotoxins that damage intact red blood cells (RBCs). The types of hemolysis are described in Table 15-1. When lysis of RBCs in the agar surrounding the colony is complete, the resulting area is clear; this is termed **β-hemolysis** (Figure 15-3). Partial lysis of the RBCs results in a greenish discoloration

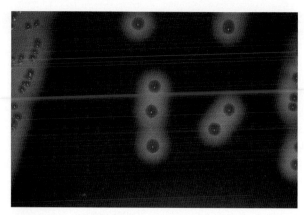

FIGURE 15-3 A β-hemolytic streptococcal colony on sheep blood agar.

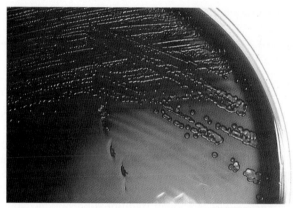

FIGURE 15-4 An α-hemolytic streptococcal colony on sheep blood agar.

of the area surrounding the colony and is termed **α-hemolysis** (Figure 15-4).

When the RBCs immediately surrounding the colony are unaffected, the bacteria are described as nonhemolytic. Some references term this result γ-*hemolysis*. Because no lysis of the RBCs occurs, however, the term γ-*hemolysis* is confusing and is not recommended. Some isolates belonging to the viridans group produce what is called wide-zone or α-prime hemolysis. The colonies are surrounded by a very small zone of no hemolysis and then a wider zone of β-hemolysis. This reaction may be mistaken for β-hemolysis at first glance. The use of a dissecting microscope or handheld lens reveals the narrow zone of intact RBCs and the wider zone of complete hemolysis.

CLINICALLY SIGNIFICANT STREPTOCOCCI AND *STREPTOCOCCUS*-LIKE ORGANISMS

The role of the streptococci and enterococci in disease has been known for more than 100 years. The range of infections caused by these organisms is wide and well studied. As we have seen with other organisms, the previously unknown or poorly characterized species and the saprobes are playing more prominent roles in disease. Some of the clinically important species and the diseases they cause are listed in Table

TABLE 15-2 Classification of *Streptococcus* and *Enterococcus*

Species	Lancefield Group Antigen	Hemolysis Type(s)	Common Terms	Disease Association(s)
S. pyogenes	A	β*	Group A strep	Rheumatic fever, scarlet fever, pharyngitis, glomerulonephritis, pyogenic infections
S. agalactiae	B	β*	Group B strep	Neonatal sepsis, meningitis, puerperal fever, pyogenic infections
S. dysgalactiae, S. equi	C	β	Group C strep	Pharyngitis, impetigo, pyogenic infections
S. bovis group	D	α, none	Nonenterococcus. member of viridans strep	Endocarditis, urinary tract infections, pyogenic infections
E. faecalis, E. faecium	D	α, β, none	*Enterococcus*	Urinary tract infections, pyogenic infections
S. pneumoniae	—	α	Pneumococcus	Pneumonia, meningitis, pyogenic infections
Anginosus group, mutans group, mitis group, salivarius group	A, C, F, G, N, or —	β, α, none	Viridans strep (all four groups referred to as viridans strep)	Pyogenic infections, endocarditis, dental caries, abscesses in various tissues

*Occasionally isolates are found that are nonhemolytic.

15-2. The clinically isolated streptococci have historically been separated into the β-hemolytic streptococci and the species that are non-β-hemolytic. The β-hemolytic streptococci often isolated from humans include *S. pyogenes, S. agalactiae, S. dysgalactiae* subsp. *equisimilis,* and *S. anginosus* group (some species are α-hemolytic or nonhemolytic).

Streptococcus pyogenes

Antigenic Structure

Streptococcus pyogenes has a cell-wall structure similar to that of other streptococci and gram-positive bacteria. The group antigen is unique, placing the organism in Lancefield group A. **M protein** is attached to the peptidoglycan of the cell wall and extends to the cell surface. The M protein is essential for virulence.

Virulence Factors

The best-defined virulence factor in *S. pyogenes* is M protein, encoded by the *emm* genes. More than 80 different serotypes of M protein exist, identified as M1, M2, and so on. Resistance to infection with *S. pyogenes* appears to be related to the presence of type-specific antibodies to the M protein. This means that an individual with antibodies against M5 is protected from infection by *S. pyogenes* with the M5 protein but remains unprotected against infection with the roughly 80 remaining M protein serotypes. The M protein molecule causes the streptococcal cell to resist phagocytosis and also plays a role in adherence of the bacterial cell to mucosal cells.

Additional virulence factors associated with group A streptococci are fibronectin-binding protein (protein F); lipoteichoic acid; hyaluronic acid capsule; and extracellular products, including hemolysins, toxins, and enzymes. Lipoteichoic acid and protein F are adhesion molecules that mediate adherence to host epithelial cells. Lipoteichoic acid, which is affixed to proteins on the bacterial surface, in concert with M proteins and fibronectin binding protein, secures the attachment of streptococci to the oral mucosal cells. The hyaluronic acid capsule of *S. pyogenes* is weakly immunogenic. The capsule prevents opsonized phagocytosis by neutrophils or macrophages. The capsule also allows the bacterium to mask its antigens and remain unrecognized by its host.

Other products produced by *S. pyogenes* are streptolysin O, streptolysin S, deoxyribonuclease (DNase), streptokinase, hyaluronidase, and erythrogenic toxin. Although all of these products have been postulated to play a role in virulence, the exact role each has in infection is not clear. *S. pyogenes* secretes four different DNases: A, B, C, and D. All strains produce at least one DNase; the most common is DNase B. These enzymes are antigenic, and antibodies to DNase can be detected following infection.

A hemolysin responsible for hemolysis on sheep blood agar (SBA) plates incubated anaerobically is **streptolysin O (SLO).** The *O* refers to this hemolysin being oxygen labile. It is active only in the reduced form, which is achieved in an anaerobic environment. SLO lyses leukocytes, platelets, and other cells as well as RBCs. SLO is highly immunogenic, and the infected individual readily forms antibodies to the hemolysin. These antibodies can be measured in the antistreptolysin-O (ASO) test to determine whether an individual has had a recent infection with *S. pyogenes*. Streptolysin S is oxygen stable, lyses leukocytes, and is nonimmunogenic. The hemolysis seen around colonies that have been incubated aerobically is due to **streptolysin S.**

Group A streptococci cause the lysis of fibrin clots through the action of streptokinase on plasminogen. The plasminogen is converted into a protease (plasmin), which lyses the fibrin clot. Antibodies to streptokinase can be detected following infection but are not specific indicators of group A infection because groups C and G also form streptokinase. **Hyaluronidase,** or spreading factor, is an enzyme that solubilizes the ground substance of mammalian connective tissues (hyaluronic acid). It was postulated that the bacteria use this enzyme to separate the tissue and then spread the infection; however, no real evidence to support this hypothesis exists.

Some strains of *S. pyogenes* cause a red spreading rash, referred to as *scarlet fever*, caused by streptococcal pyrogenic exotoxins (Spes), formerly called erythrogenic toxins. The three immunologically distinct exotoxin types are SpeA, SpeB, and SpeC. These toxins function as superantigens. Streptococcal superantigens belong to a family of highly mitogenic proteins secreted individually or in combinations by many *S. pyogenes* strains. These proteins share the ability to stimulate T-lymphocyte proliferation by interaction with class II major histocompatibility complex (MHC) molecules on antigen-presenting cells and specific variable β-chains of the T-cell receptor. This interaction results in the production of interleukin-1, tumor necrotizing factor, and other cytokines that appear to mediate the disease processes associated with these toxins.

Clinical Infections

Infections resulting from *S. pyogenes* include pharyngitis, scarlet fever, skin or pyodermal infections, and other septic infections. In addition, rheumatic fever and acute glomerulonephritis may occur as a result of infection with *S. pyogenes*.

Bacterial Pharyngitis. The most common clinical manifestations of group A streptococcal infection are **pharyngitis** and tonsillitis. Most cases of bacterial pharyngitis are due to *S. pyogenes*. Other groups, particularly C and G, have the capability to produce significant acute pharyngitis but are less commonly seen.

"Strep throat" is most often seen in children between 5 and 15 years of age. After an incubation period of 1 to 4 days, an abrupt onset of illness ensues, with sore throat, malaise, fever, and headache. Nausea, vomiting, and abdominal pain are not unusual. The tonsils and pharynx are inflamed. The cervical lymph nodes are swollen and tender. The disease ranges in intensity, and these symptoms may not be seen. In fact, in a child with fever and complaint of only a mild sore throat, it is not unusual to isolate a nearly pure culture of *S. pyogenes* from the throat. The symptoms subside within 3 to 5 days unless complications, such as peritonsillar abscesses, occur. The disease is spread by droplets and close contact. Although clinical criteria have been proposed, the diagnosis of streptococcal sore throat relies on a throat culture or direct antigen detection. About one third of those complaining of sore throat have a throat culture positive for *S. pyogenes*.

Pyodermal Infections. Skin or pyodermal infections with group A streptococci result in the syndrome of impetigo, cellulitis, erysipelas, wound infection, or arthritis. **Impetigo,** a localized skin disease, begins as small vesicles that progress to weeping lesions. The lesions crust over after several days. Impetigo is usually seen in young children (2 to 5 years) and affects exposed areas of the skin. Inoculation of the organism occurs through minor abrasions or insect bites. **Erysipelas** is an uncommonly seen infection of the skin and subcutaneous tissues most frequently occurring in elderly patients. It is characterized by an acute spreading skin lesion that is intensely

erythematous with a plainly demarcated but irregular edge. **Cellulitis** may develop following deeper invasion by streptococci. The infection can be serious, even life threatening, with bacteremia or sepsis. In patients with peripheral vascular disease or diabetes, cellulitis may lead to gangrene.

Infection with strains of *S. pyogenes* that produce Spes may result in **scarlet fever.** Strains of *S. pyogenes* infected with the temperate bacteriophage T12 produce streptococcal pyrogenic exotoxins. Scarlet fever, which appears within 1 to 2 days following bacterial infection, is characterized by a diffuse red rash that appears on the upper chest and spreads to the trunk and extremities. The rash disappears over the next 5 to 7 days and is followed by desquamation.

Necrotizing Fasciitis. Group A streptococcus has been associated with necrotizing fasciitis (NF), an invasive infection characterized by a rapidly progressing inflammation and necrosis of the skin, subcutaneous fat, and fascia. Although relatively uncommon, NF is a life-threatening infection. Morbidity and mortality may be prevented if early intervention is instituted; the mortality rate may reach greater than 70% if left untreated. Many different bacteria can cause destruction of the soft tissue in this manner, a clinical feature that has been described as "flesh-eating disease." Depending on which organisms are cultured, NF may be categorized as type 1, 2, or 3. A polymicrobial infection from which aerobic and anaerobic bacteria are recovered is categorized as type 1 NF. Type 2 NF consists of only group A streptococci. Type 3 is gas gangrene or clostridial myonecrosis. A variant of NF type 1 is saltwater NF, in which an apparently minor skin wound is contaminated with saltwater containing a *Vibrio* sp.

Cases of NF were described as far back as the eighteenth century, but the term was not conceived until 1952. In addition to flesh-eating bacteria syndrome, other terms for NF have included *suppurative fasciitis, hospital gangrene,* and *necrotizing erysipelas.* NF may occur as a result of trauma, such as burns and lacerations. In most cases NF occurs in an individual with an underlying illness who has suffered trauma to the skin. The break in the skin may become the portal of entry for the bacteria. NF infections caused by group A streptococci, however, occur in young, healthy individuals, and in many cases, a break in the skin that served as portal of entry is not found.

Streptococcal Toxic Shock Syndrome. An increase in streptococcal toxic shock syndrome (STSS) cases has been reported in recent years. STSS is a condition in which the entire organ system shuts down, leading to death. The exact portal of infection is unknown for most STSS cases, although minor injuries or surgeries have been implicated. The initial streptococcal infection is often severe (e.g., pharyngitis, peritonitis, cellulitis, wound infections), and the symptoms that develop are similar to those of staphylococcal toxic shock syndrome. Patients are often bacteremic and have NF. Group A streptococcus associated with STSS produce an Spe, notably SpeA. It has been proposed that these toxins play a major role in the pathogenesis of this disease. Other virulence factors, such as SLO and various cell-wall antigens, can also cause toxic shock.

Post-Streptococcal Sequelae. Two serious complications of group A streptococcal disease are **rheumatic fever** and

acute glomerulonephritis (AGN). Rheumatic fever is a complication that typically follows *S. pyogenes* pharyngitis. It is characterized by fever and inflammation of the heart, joints, blood vessels, and subcutaneous tissues. Attacks usually begin within a month after infection. The most serious result is chronic, progressive damage to the heart valves. Repeated infections may produce further valve damage. By 1980 many clinicians considered rheumatic fever eradicated. A resurgence of rheumatic fever occurred during the late 1980s; however, it is once again rare in most developed countries. It is no longer a reportable disease in the United States. Acute rheumatic fever and its chronic sequela, rheumatic heart disease, remain problematic in developing countries and in some poor populations in industrialized countries.

The pathogenesis of rheumatic fever is poorly understood. Several theories have been proposed, including antigenic cross-reactivity between streptococcal antigens and heart tissue, direct toxicity resulting from bacterial exotoxins, and actual invasion of the heart tissues by the organism. Most evidence favors cross-reactivity as being responsible for the effects.

Acute glomerulonephritis sometimes occurs after a cutaneous or pharyngeal infection. It is more common in children than in adults. The pathogenesis appears to be immunologically mediated. Circulating immune complexes are found in the serum of patients with AGN, and it is postulated that these antigen-antibody complexes deposit in the glomeruli. Complement is subsequently fixed, and an inflammatory response causes damage to the glomeruli, resulting in impairment of kidney function.

The group A streptococci are susceptible to penicillin, which remains the drug of choice for treatment. For patients allergic to penicillin, erythromycin can be used. For patients who have a history of rheumatic fever, prophylactic doses of penicillin are given to prevent any recurrent infections that might cause additional damage to the heart valves.

Laboratory Diagnosis

An essential step in the diagnosis of streptococcal pharyngitis is proper sampling. The tongue should be depressed and the swab rubbed over the posterior pharynx and each tonsillar area. If exudate is present, it should also be touched with the swab. Care should be taken to avoid the tongue and uvula. Examination of Gram stains of upper respiratory specimens or skin swabs is of little value because these areas have considerable amounts of gram-positive cocci as part of the normal bacterial biota.

Transport media are not required for normal conditions. The organism is resistant to drying and can be recovered from swabs several hours after collection. An SBA plate is inoculated and streaked for isolation. Incubation should be at 35° C either in ambient air or under anaerobic conditions. Studies have shown that the normal respiratory microbiota tend to overgrow the β-hemolytic streptococci when incubated in increased CO_2. Several selective media, such as SBA containing sulfamethoxazole (SXT), have been recommended for better recovery of β-hemolytic streptococci from throat cultures. The plate is observed after 24 hours for the presence of β-hemolytic colonies. If none are found, incubation should

continue for an additional 24 hours before the culture is reported as negative.

Colonies of *S. pyogenes* on SBA are small, transparent, and smooth with a well-defined area of β-hemolysis. A Gram stain will reveal gram-positive cocci with some short chains. Suspect colonies can be Lancefield-typed using serologic methods, which will give a definitive identification, or biochemical tests can be performed. The correlation between the presumptive identification using biochemical methods and the rapid definitive serologic method is high. Key tests that can be done are bacitracin susceptibility or **pyrrolidonyl-α-naphthylamide (PYR) hydrolysis.** *S. pyogenes* is susceptible to bacitracin and hydrolyzes PYR, whereas most other β-hemolytic groups are resistant to bacitracin and are PYR negative. The best way to differentiate groups C and G from group A streptococci is Lancefield typing. The group C streptococci are generally bacitracin sensitive. The group G streptococci may be bacitracin resistant or sensitive.

When the origin of an isolate is not the throat (i.e., blood or sputum), additional tests should be part of the early identification scheme. In this case, hippurate hydrolysis, the CAMP test, bile esculin test, and growth in 6.5% NaCl broth should be included. The reactions of some of the catalase-negative, gram-positive cocci in various biochemical tests are outlined in Table 15-3. Some immunologic tests used to detect infection with *S. pyogenes* include ASO, anti-DNase, antistreptokinase, and antihyaluronidase titers.

Streptococcus agalactiae

Antigenic Structure

All strains of *S. agalactiae* have the group B–specific antigen, an acid-stable polysaccharide located in the cell wall. Additionally, there are several capsular polysaccharide serotypes: Ia, Ia/c, Ib/c, II, IIc, and III to VIII. These type-specific antigens can be detected by precipitin tests. The terminal position in the repeating unit is composed of sialic acid.

Virulence Factors

The capsule is an important virulence factor in group B streptococcal infections. Antibodies against the type-specific antigens protect mice against strains of *S. agalactiae* with the homologous polysaccharide in the capsule. The capsule prevents phagocytosis but is ineffective after opsonization. Sialic acid appears to be the most significant component of the capsule and a critical virulence determinant. Studies with mutant strains of *S. agalactiae* showed that loss of capsular sialic acid was associated with loss of virulence. It is postulated that the sialic acid on the surface of the bacterial cell inhibits activation of the alternative pathway of complement. Other products produced by *S. agalactiae* include a hemolysin, CAMP factor, neuraminidase, DNase, hyaluronidase, and protease. No evidence exists that any of these products plays a role in the virulence of this organism.

Clinical Infections

Group B streptococci have been known for many years as the cause of mastitis in cattle. It was not until Lancefield defined streptococcal classification that their role in human disease

TABLE 15-3 Biochemical Identification of *Streptococcus* and Similar Organisms

Characteristic	S. pyogenes	S. agalactiae	Other β-hemolytics*	Enterococcus	Group D Streptococci	S. pneumoniae	Viridans Streptococci	Aerococcus	Pediococcus	Leuconostoc
Hemolysis type	β	β	β	α, β, none	α, none	α	α, none	α, none	α, none	α, none
Susceptibility to										
Vancomycin	S	S	S	S(R)	S	S	S	S	R	R
Bacitracin	S	R†	R†	R	R	S	R†	S		
SXT	R	R	S	R	V	S	S			
Optochin	R	R	R	R	R	S	R			
Hydrolysis of										
Hippurate	−	+	−	−†	−	−	−†	+		
PYR	+	−	−	+	−	−	−	+	+	−
CAMP	−	+	−	−	−	−	−	−	−	−
Leucine aminopeptidase	+	+	+	+	+	+	+	−	+	−
Bile esculin	−	−	−	+	+	−	−†	V	+	V
Growth in 6.5% NaCl	−	−	−	+	−	−	−	+	V	V

R, Resistant; *S*, susceptible; *S(R)*, greater percentage susceptible; *V*, variable; +, present; −, absent; *SXT*, sulfamethoxazole; *PYR*, pyrrolidonyl-α-naphthylamide.
*β-Hemolytic groups other than A, B, and D.
†Exceptions may occur.

was recognized. *S. agalactiae* is a significant cause of invasive disease in the newborn. Two clinical syndromes are used to describe neonatal group B streptococcal disease: early-onset infection (less than 7 days old) and late-onset infection (at least 7 days old). Early-onset disease accounts for about 80% of the clinical cases in newborns and is caused by vertical transmission of the organism from the mother. Colonization of the vagina and rectal area with group B streptococci is found in 10% to 30% of pregnant women.

Most infections of infants occur in the first 3 days after birth, usually within 24 hours. This infection is commonly associated with obstetric complications, prolonged rupture of membranes, and premature birth. Infection often presents as a pneumonia or meningitis with bacteremia. The mortality rate is high, and death usually occurs if treatment is not started quickly. The most important determining factor seems to be the presence of group B streptococci in the vagina of the mother. It is recommended that all pregnant women be screened for group B streptococci at 35 to 37 weeks' gestation. Screening methods are discussed below. Late-onset infection occurs between 1 week and 3 months after birth and usually presents as meningitis. This infection is uncommonly associated with obstetric complications. Also, the organism is rarely found in the mother's vagina prior to birth. The mortality rate is considerably less than that of early-onset disease, but it is high enough to be of serious concern.

The incidence of group B streptococcal infections drops dramatically after the neonatal period. In adults, the infection affects two types of patients. The first is young, previously healthy women who become ill after childbirth or abortion; endometritis and wound infections are most common. The second type of patient is the elderly person with a serious underlying disease or immunodeficiency.

The drug of choice for treating group B streptococci infections is penicillin, although this group is less susceptible to penicillin than are group A streptococci. The clinical response to antimicrobial therapy is often poor despite the heavy doses given. Some clinicians recommend a combination of ampicillin and an aminoglycoside for treating group B streptococci infections.

Laboratory Diagnosis

The group B streptococci grow on SBA as grayish white mucoid colonies surrounded by a small zone of β-hemolysis (Figure 15-5). These organisms are gram-positive cocci that form short chains in clinical specimens and longer chains in culture. Presumptive identification is based on biochemical reactions. The most useful tests are hippurate hydrolysis and the CAMP test. These tests enable the organism to be readily differentiated from other β-hemolytic streptococcal isolates. Figure 15-6 demonstrates how bacitracin and the CAMP test can be used to differentiate *Streptococcus* spp. The definitive identification can be made by extracting the group antigen and reacting it with specific anti-group B antisera in an agglutination procedure.

Detection of group B streptococci in expectant women is done by collecting vaginal and rectal material with swabs between 35 and 37 weeks of gestation. Samples are inoculated into selective broth such as Todd-Hewitt broth containing

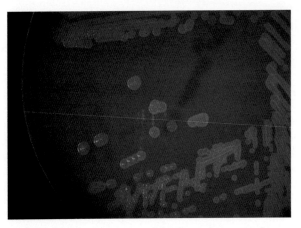

FIGURE 15-5 *Streptococcus agalactiae* colony growing on sheep blood agar.

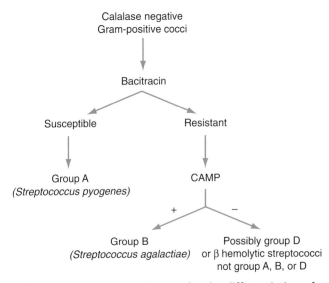

FIGURE 15-6 Schematic diagram for the differentiation of group A from group B streptococci.

10 μg/mL of colistin and 15 μg/mL nalidixic acid (BBL Lim broth; BD Diagnostic Systems, Sparks, Md.). Gentamicin, 8 μg/mL, and 15 μg/mL nalidixic acid may also be used. The inoculated media are incubated at 35° C for 18 to 24 hours before being subcultured to SBA. Cultures are examined for colonies resembling group B streptococci after 24 hours of incubation at 35° C in an incubator containing 5% CO_2. Cultures that do not show colonies resembling group B streptococci are incubated for an additional 24 hours.

StrepB Carrot Broth (SCB; Hardy Diagnostics, Santa Maria, Calif.) was recently shown to have improved diagnostic value and efficiency. β-Hemolytic group B streptococci produce an orange or red pigment in SCB after as little as 6 hours incubation. Vaginal/rectal swabs are placed into SCB and incubated 18 to 24 hours at 35° C. Broths that turn orange or red are reported as positive for group B streptococci. Further identification is not necessary. Isolates that are nonhemolytic will not produce a color change, requiring that the broth be subcultured.

Groups C and G Streptococci

In the most recent classification of β-hemolytic streptococci, isolates from humans that belong to Lancefield groups A, C, or G are subdivided into large- and small-colony forms. The large-colony–forming isolates with groups A (S. pyogenes), C, and G antigens are classified with the **pyogenic streptococci.** The large-colony–forming β–hemolytic isolates with groups C and G antigens belong to the subspecies S. dysgalactiae subsp. equisimilis. However, there have been reports of blood culture isolates in which S. dysgalactiae subsp. equisimilis exhibited group A antigen and not group C or G antigens. The small-colony–forming β–hemolytic isolates with groups C and G antigens belong to the S. anginosus group, which are included in the viridans streptococci discussed below.

Clinical infections from groups C and G streptococci have been reported in the literature, although these are uncommon human pathogens. S. dysgalactiae subsp. equisimilis isolates were recovered from the upper respiratory tract, vagina, and skin of humans and are thought to be uncommon in domestic animals. The spectrum of infections resembles S. pyogenes: upper respiratory tract infections, skin infections, soft tissue infections, and invasive infections such as NF. Because several antigenic groups (C, G, L, and A) are included within the species, serotyping of S. dysgalactiae to determine species is complex. S. equi subsp. zooepidemicus is primarily an animal pathogen rarely isolated from humans. It has been associated with cases of glomerulonephritis and rheumatic fever following infections.

Streptococcus pneumoniae

Antigenic Structure

Also known as pneumococcus, S. pneumoniae is isolated from a variety of infections. The cell wall of S. pneumoniae contains an antigen, referred to as C substance, which is similar to the C carbohydrate of the various Lancefield groups. A β-globulin in human serum, called the C-reactive protein (CRP), reacts with C substance to form a precipitate. This is a chemical reaction and not an antigen-antibody combination. The amount of CRP increases during inflammation and infection.

The pneumococcus can express one of approximately 80 different capsular types based on chemical variations of the capsular polysaccharide. Antibody directed against the capsular antigen is protective. Isolates from certain sources—for example, cases of lobar pneumonia—show a predominance of particular capsular types. The capsule is antigenic and can be identified with appropriate antisera in the Neufield test. In the presence of specific anticapsular serum, the capsule swells (Quellung reaction). This reaction not only allows for identification of S. pneumoniae but also serves to serotype the isolate specifically.

Virulence Factors

The characteristic of S. pneumoniae that is clearly associated with virulence is the capsular polysaccharide. Laboratory strains that have lost the ability to produce a capsule are nonpathogenic. In addition, opsonization of the capsule renders the organism avirulent. Several toxins are produced including a hemolysin, an immunoglobulin A protease, neuraminidase, and hyaluronidase. None of these have been shown to have a role in disease production.

Clinical Infections

Streptococcus pneumoniae is a common isolate in the clinical microbiology laboratory. It is an important human pathogen that causes pneumonia, sinusitis, otitis media, bacteremia, and meningitis. S. pneumoniae is the most frequently encountered isolate in children under the age of 3 years with recurrent otitis media. S. pneumoniae, the number one cause of bacterial pneumonia, is especially prevalent in elderly persons and in patients with underlying disease. Of the more than 80 capsular serotypes, about a dozen account for most pneumococcal pneumonia cases.

For an individual to contract pneumococcal pneumonia, the organism must be present in the nasopharynx and the individual must be deficient in the specific circulating antibody against the capsular type of the colonizing strain of S. pneumoniae. Pneumonia resulting from S. pneumoniae is not usually a primary infection but rather a result of disturbance of the normal defense barriers. Predisposing conditions such as alcoholism, anesthesia, malnutrition, and viral infections' of the upper respiratory tract can lead to pneumococcal disease in the form of lobar pneumonia. Pneumococcal pneumonia is characterized by sudden onset with chills, dyspnea, and cough. The infection begins with aspiration of respiratory secretions, which often contain pneumococci. The infecting organisms in the alveoli stimulate an outpouring of fluid, which serves to facilitate the spread of the organism to adjacent alveoli. The process stops when the fluid reaches fibrous septa that separate the major lung lobes. This accounts for the "lobar" distribution of the infection—hence the name. Most isolates from pneumococcal lobar pneumonia are capsular serotypes 1, 2, and 3.

Pneumonia may be complicated by a pleural effusion that is usually sterile **(empyema).** The laboratory may receive fluid from a pleural aspirate for culture. An infected effusion contains many white blood cells and pneumococci, which are visible on Gram stain. Even with antimicrobial therapy, mortality is relatively high (5% to 10%); without therapy, however, the mortality rate approaches 50%. Pneumococcus causes bacterial meningitis in all age groups. Meningitis usually follows other S. pneumoniae infections such as otitis media or pneumonia. The course of the disease is rapid, and the mortality rate is near 40%. Direct smears of the cerebrospinal fluid (CSF) often reveal leukocytes and numerous gram-positive cocci in pairs. Pneumococci may also be involved in other infections such as endocarditis, peritonitis, and bacteremia. Bacteremia often occurs during the course of a serious infection. Consequently samples for blood culture are often taken simultaneously with sputum or a fluid aspirate.

Two pneumococcal vaccines are available. One is composed of purified polysaccharides of seven serotypes conjugated to a diphtheria protein, the heptavalent pneumococcal conjugate vaccine (PCV7), approved for use in children. The PCV7 vaccine is part of the routine pediatric immunization schedule. The other vaccine is composed of 23 purified capsular polysaccharides, the 23-valent vaccine (PS23), and is used for adults. Vaccination is recommended for those at risk of developing pneumococcal disease (e.g., asplenic individuals, elderly patients with cardiac or pulmonary disease). The vaccine has been successful in reducing the incidence and severity of pneumococcal disease.

Laboratory Diagnosis

The cells characteristically seen on Gram stain appear as gram-positive cocci in pairs (diplococci). The ends of the cells are slightly pointed, giving them an oval or lancet shape (Figure 15-7). The cocci may occur singly, in pairs, or in short chains but most often are seen as pairs. As the culture ages, the Gram stain reaction becomes variable, and gram-negative cells are seen. The capsule can be demonstrated by using a capsule stain.

The nutritional requirements of *S. pneumoniae* are complex. Media such as brain-heart infusion agar, trypticase soy agar with 5% sheep RBCs, or chocolate agar are necessary for good growth. Some isolates require increased CO_2 for growth during primary isolation. Isolates produce a large zone of α-hemolysis on SBA surrounding the colonies. Young cultures have a round, glistening, wet, mucoid, dome-shaped appearance (Figure 15-8). As the colonies become older, autolytic changes result in a collapse of each colony's center, giving it the appearance of a coin with a raised rim. The tendency of *S. pneumoniae* to undergo autolysis can make it difficult to keep isolates alive. Clinical isolates and stock cultures require frequent subculturing (every 1 to 2 days) to ensure viability.

The colonies may closely resemble those of the viridans streptococci, but a presumptive differentiation is not difficult to make. The greatest concern in the laboratory diagnosis is distinguishing *S. pneumoniae* from the viridans streptococci. Procedures used to accomplish this are optochin susceptibility and bile solubility; optochin susceptibility is the more commonly used procedure. Optochin susceptibility takes advantage of the fact that *S. pneumoniae* is susceptible to optochin, whereas other α-hemolytic species are resistant. The bile solubility test evaluates the ability of *S. pneumoniae* to lyse in the presence of bile salts. It correlates with optochin susceptibil-ity; that is, *S. pneumoniae* isolates are optochin susceptible and bile soluble.

Antimicrobial Resistance

Because most isolates are susceptible, pneumococcal infections are usually treated with penicillin. Over the last three decades, however, *S. pneumoniae* has become increasingly resistant to penicillin, and these isolates are generally treated with erythromycin or chloramphenicol. Moreover, penicillin-resistant pneumococci are reported to show resistance to other classes of drugs such as β-lactams, macrolides, and tetracyclines. The susceptibility of *S. pneumoniae* to penicillin and macrolides has varied over time, geographic region, and country. Resistance to extended-spectrum cephalosporins such as ceftriaxone and cefotaxime has also been on the rise, although these agents have been used successfully in the treatment of serious infections caused by penicillin-resistant pneumococci.

Multidrug-resistant *S. pneumoniae*, defined as pneumococcal isolates resistant in vitro to two or more classes of antimicrobial agents, has been reported and can occur in the presence or absence of penicillin resistance. Pneumococcal strains that exhibit resistance to various antimicrobial agents such as erythromycin, tetracycline, chloramphenicol, and trimethoprim-sulfamethoxazole have emerged.

Viridans Streptococci

The viridans streptococci are constituents of the normal microbiota of the upper respiratory tract, the female genital tract, and the gastrointestinal tract. The term *viridans* means "green," referring to the α-hemolysis many species exhibit. However, β-hemolytic and nonhemolytic species are also classified as viridans streptococci. Viridans streptococci are fastidious, with some strains requiring CO_2 for growth.

More than 30 species are now recognized. The current classification assigns streptococci species in the viridans group to one of five groups: (1) *S. mitis group* (*S. mitis, S. sanguis, S. parasanguis, S. gordonii, S. cristatus, S. infantis, S. oralis,* and *S. peroris*); (2) *S. mutans group* (*S. mutans* and *S. sobrinus*); (3) *S. salivarius group* (*S. salivarius, S. vestibularis,* and *S. thermophilus*); (4) *S. bovis group* (*S. equinus, S. gallolyticus,*

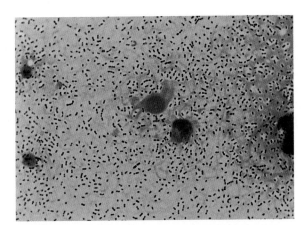

FIGURE 15-7 Gram stain of *Streptococcus pneumoniae*. Direct smear of sputum from a patient with pneumonia caused by *S. pneumoniae*. Note the clear, nonstained area around the organism that represents the capsule.

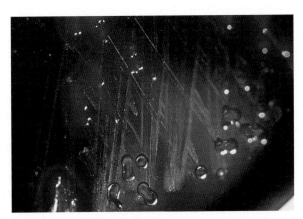

FIGURE 15-8 *Streptococcus pneumoniae* colonies on sheep blood agar. The colonies demonstrate a characteristic mucoid appearance and a concave center.

S. infantarius, and *S. alactolyticus*), and (5) *S. anginosus group* (*S. anginosus, S. constellatus,* and *S. intermedius*). Organisms of the anginosus group may possess Lancefield group A, C, F, G, or N antigen and in some instances may not be groupable. The organisms may also cross-react with other grouping sera. Thus identification using the Lancefield sera is of little value. However, a small-colony–forming streptococcus positive for group F antigen isolated from a human specimen is likely a member of the *S. anginosus* group.

The *S. bovis* group and the enterococci possess the group D antigen. *S. bovis* is no longer a valid species name. DNA studies found that *S. bovis* and *S. equinus* were the same species. The earlier species name, *S. equinus,* was adopted. Until the mid-1980s, the group D streptococci were subdivided into the enterococcal and nonenterococcal groups, with the understanding that those found in the intestinal tract were part of the enterococcal group. Both groups were bile esculin positive, but the nonenterococcal organisms would not grow in a nutrient broth with 6.5% NaCl. As more became known about the molecular characteristics of each of these subgroups, the enterococcal group was placed into a new genus, *Enterococcus,* but the nonenterococcal group remained part of the group D streptococci.

Clinical Infections

The viridans streptococci are oropharyngeal commensals that are regarded as opportunistic pathogens. Although their virulence is low, they cause disease if host defenses are compromised. Viridans streptococci are the most common cause of subacute bacterial endocarditis. Transient bacteremia is associated with endocarditis. Viridans streptococcal bacteremia is more common in children than in adults and is usually more prevalent in patients with hematologic malignancies. Fatal cases have been characterized by fulminant cardiovascular collapse or meningitis. Generally the course of endocarditis is very slow; symptoms may be present for weeks or months. Individuals whose heart valves have been damaged by rheumatic fever are especially susceptible to endocarditis resulting from viridans streptococci.

Besides bloodstream infections, oral infections such as gingivitis and dental caries (cavities) are caused by viridans streptococci. They have also been implicated in meningitis, abscesses, osteomyelitis, and empyema. Although viridans streptococci are frequently isolated in association with other bacteria from bronchial brushing, their role in bacterial pneumonia is unclear. Viridans streptococci infections are treated with penicillin. Although some resistant strains have been reported, most remain susceptible.

Most members of the *S. anginosus* group are considered part of the normal oral and gastrointestinal microbiota; however, they have been associated with abscess formation in the oropharynx, brain, and peritoneal cavity. Members of the *S. anginosus* group have been isolated from bacteremic patients associated with invasive pyogenic infections with the tendency to form abscesses. *S. constellatus* subsp. *pharyngis* has been linked to pharyngitis.

The *S. mitis* group is normally found in the oral cavity, gastrointestinal tract, and female genital tract. Members can also be found as transient normal microbiota of the skin.

Although they can be isolated from the blood of asymptomatic individuals, they are the most common isolates associated with bacterial endocarditis in native valves and, less frequently, in prosthetic valve infections. *S. salivarius* and *S. vestibularis* have been isolated from human specimens. *S. salivarius* has been linked to bacteremia, endocarditis, and meningitis, whereas *S. vestibularis* has not been associated with disease.

Members of the *S. bovis* group are often encountered in blood cultures of patients with bacteremia, septicemia, and endocarditis. The presence of *S. gallolyticus* subsp. *gallolyticus* in blood cultures has a high correlation with gastrointestinal carcinoma. *S. mutans* group is the most commonly isolated among the viridans group. They are usually isolated from the oral cavity. *S. mutans* is the primary contributor to dental caries. It is also the most common member of the mutans group associated with bacteremia.

Virulence Factors

Virulence factors that characterize the pathogenicity of viridans streptococci have not been well established. A polysaccharide capsule and cytolysin have been identified in some members of the anginosus group. Besides these, extracellular dextran and cell surface–associated proteins (adhesins) have been implicated in adherence and colonization of these organisms in endocarditis. The groups C and G streptococci possess M proteins with similarity to group A streptococci. Some of them also produce extracellular enzymes such as streptolysin O, hyaluronidase, and DNase.

Laboratory Diagnosis

It is extremely difficult to identify isolates of the viridans group to the species level; clinical laboratories should be satisfied to place isolates into one of the five groups. All members are PYR negative and leucine aminopeptidase (LAP) positive. Viridans streptococci show typical *Streptococcus* characteristics on Gram stain. Colonies are small and are surrounded by a zone of α-hemolysis; some isolates are β-hemolytic or nonhemolytic. The lack of β-hemolysis separates the viridans streptococci from groups A, B, C, and G. The differentiation of α-hemolytic viridans streptococci from *S. pneumoniae,* also α-hemolytic, is based on optochin sensitivity and bile solubility tests.

The ability to ferment sugars, Voges-Proskauer (VP) reaction, β-D-glucuronidase activity, and hippurate hydrolysis are used for rapid differentiation of species within the viridans group. Some commercial multitest kits are able to identify the more commonly isolated species; however, not all species are part of the manufacturers' databases. The hemolytic patterns and some of the biochemical tests that distinguish members of the viridans group are shown in Table 15-4.

S. anginosus is composed of strains that may have A, C, F, G, or no Lancefield antigen. These are minute colony types showing α-, β-, or no hemolysis. When they are β-hemolytic, the zone size is several times the size of the colony. When they are growing in pure culture or in high concentration, a characteristic sweet odor of honeysuckle or butterscotch may be present.

Two groups that might be confused with each other are the genus *Enterococcus* and the group D streptococci. Members

TABLE 15-4 Characteristics of the Viridans Streptococci*

	Mannitol	Sorbital	Voges-Proskauer	Hydrolysis or Arginine	Hydrolysis of Esculin	Urease	Hemolytic Pattern
Anginosus group	–/v	–	+	+	+	–	α, β, Non
Bovis group	v	–	+	–	+	–	α, Non
Mitis group	–	–/v	–	+/–/v	+/–/v	–	α
Mutans group	+	+	+	–	+	–	α, β, Non
Salvarius group	–	–	+/v	–	+/v	+/v	α

Data from Spellerberg B, Brandt C. In Murray PR et al, editors: *Manual of clinical microbiology,* ed 9, Washington, DC, 2007, ASM Press.
+, Positive test result; –, negative test result; *v,* variable test result; *Non,* nonhemolytic.
*All viridans streptococci species are leucine aminopeptidase (LAP) positive and PYR negative.

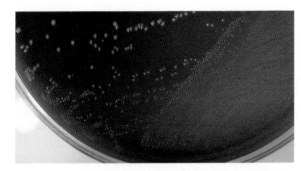

FIGURE 15-9 *Enterococcus* sp. growing on sheep blood agar.

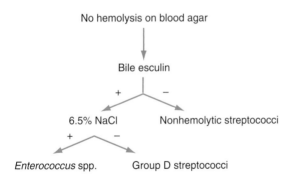

FIGURE 15-10 Schematic diagram for identification of nonhemolytic streptococci.

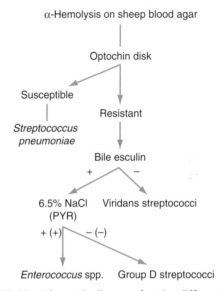

FIGURE 15-11 Schematic diagram for the differentiation of α-hemolytic streptococci from *Enterococcus.*

of the *S. bovis* group express the D antigen. Both group D streptococci and enterococci are usually nonhemolytic (Figure 15-9), although on occasion enterococcal isolates can be α- or β-hemolytic. The differentiation of nonhemolytic streptococci is outlined in Figure 15-10. Both the enterococci and group D streptococci are bile esculin positive. Growth in 6.5% NaCl broth differentiates the *Enterococcus* from the viridans streptococci that fail to grow (Figure 15-11). In addition, group D streptococci can be separated from *Enterococcus* with the PYR test; group D is negative, whereas *Enterococcus* is positive. It is important to distinguish the group D streptococci from *Enterococcus* because group D is susceptible to penicillin, whereas *Enterococcus* is usually resistant. Some strains of *S. salivarius* can be misidentified as *S. bovis* group

because a significant number of *S. salivarius* isolates are bile esculin positive.

Enterococcus

Enterococci were previously classified as group D streptococci. This group consists of gram-positive cocci that are natural inhabitants of the intestinal tracts of humans and animals. The commonly identified species in clinical specimens are *E. faecalis* and *E. faecium.* Other species such as *E. durans, E. avium, E. casseliflavus, E. gallinarum,* and *E. raffinosus* are observed occasionally. All species produce the cell wall–associated group D antigen in the Lancefield classification system.

Most enterococci are nonhemolytic or α-hemolytic, although some strains show β-hemolysis. It should be noted that enterococci sometimes exhibit a pseudocatalase reaction—weak bubbling in catalase test. Identification of the different species is based on biochemical characteristics. Unlike streptococci, enterococci have the ability to grow under extreme conditions, for example, in the presence of bile or 6.5% NaCl or at 45° C or alkaline pH. The ability of enterococci to hydrolyze PYR is useful for differentiating them from the group D streptococci (Figure 15-12).

Virulence Factors

The virulence factors that contribute to the pathogenicity of enterococci are not completely understood. The enterococci have a survival advantage over other organisms in that they can grow in extreme conditions and are resistant to multiple antimicrobial agents. The extracellular surface protein, extracellular serine protease, and gelatinase of *E. faecalis* are thought to play a role in the colonization of the species and adherence to heart valves and renal epithelial cells. *E. faecalis* also produces a two-subunit toxin, termed *cytolysin*. This toxin shows similarity to bacteriocins produced by gram-positive bacteria and is expressed by a quorum-sensing mechanism.

Clinical Infections

Enterococci are frequent causes of nosocomial infections. Of these, UTIs are the most common, followed by bacteremia. UTI is often associated with urinary catheterization or other urologic manipulations. Prolonged hospitalization is a risk factor for acquiring enterococcal bacteremia. Bacteremia is often observed in hemodialysis patients, immunocompromised patients with a serious underlying disease, or patients who have undergone a prior surgical procedure. Endocarditis from enterococci is seen mainly in elderly patients with prosthetic valves or valvular heart disease. Enterococci account for about 5% to 10% of infections in patients with bacterial endocarditis.

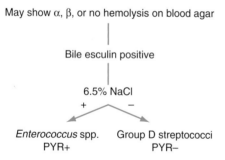

May show α, β, or no hemolysis on blood agar

Bile esculin positive

6.5% NaCl

\+   −

Enterococcus spp.   Group D streptococci
PYR+   PYR−

FIGURE 15-12 Schematic diagram for the differentiation of group D streptococci from *Enterococcus*.

Although frequently isolated from intraabdominal or pelvic wound infections, their role in these infections remains contentious. In burn patients, enterococcal wound infection and sepsis resulting from contaminated xenografts have been reported. Rare cases of enterococcal infection of the central nervous system in patients who have had neurosurgery or head trauma and in immunosuppressed patients with enterococcal bacteremia have been reported. Respiratory tract infections from enterococci are also rare and have been reported in severely ill patients who have had prolonged antimicrobial therapy.

Laboratory Diagnosis

Standard procedures for collecting and transporting of blood, urine, or wound specimens should be followed. The specimens should be cultured as soon as possible with minimum delay. Trypticase soy or brain-heart infusion agar supplemented with 5% sheep blood is routinely used to culture enterococci. Enterococci grow well at 35° C in the presence of CO_2 but do not require a high level of CO_2 for growth. If the clinical specimen is obtained from a contaminated site or is likely to contain gram-negative organisms, selective media containing bile esculin azide, colistin-nalidixic acid, phenylethyl alcohol chromogenic substrates, or cephalexin-aztreonam-arabinose agar should be used for isolation of enterococci.

Enterococcus spp. are identified based on their ability to (1) produce acid in carbohydrate broth, (2) hydrolyze arginine, (3) tolerate 0.04% tellurite, (4) utilize pyruvate, (5) produce acid from methyl-α-d-glucopyranoside (MGP), (6) growth around 100-μg efrotomycin acid disk, and (7) exhibit motility. Table 15-5 shows the differentiation of the enterococci species based on these phenotypic and biochemical characteristics. *E. faecalis* is easily identified by its ability to be grown in the presence of tellurite. Commercially available multitest kits may be useful for identification of *E. faecalis*, but they are not adequate for other enterococci. Molecular typing methods, such as pulsed-field gel electrophoresis, contour-clamped homogeneous electric-field electrophoresis, ribotyping and PCR-based typing methods have been used mainly to type enterococcal species in epidemiologic studies and investigations of vancomycin-resistant enterococci (VRE).

TABLE 15-5 Phenotype and Biochemical Characteristics of Enterococcal Species

Enterococcus Species	MOT	MAN	SOR	ARA	RAF	TEL	ARG	PYU	MGP
E. faecalis	−	+*	−	−	−	+	+*	+	−
E. faecium	−	+*	−	+	V	−	+	−	−
E. durans	−	−	−	−	−	−	+	−	−
E. avium	−	+	+	+	−	−	−	+	+
E. casseliflavus	+*	+	−	+	+	−*	+*	V	+
E. gallinarum	+*	+*	−	+	+	−	+*	−	+
E. raffinosus	−	+	+	+	+	−	−	+	+

Data from Teixeira LM et al: *Enterococcus.* In Murray PR et al, editors: *Manual of clinical microbiology,* ed 9, Washington, DC, 2007, ASM Press.
MOT, Motility; *MAN,* mannitol; *SOR,* sorbose; *ARA,* arabinose; *RAF,* raffinose; *TEL,* tellurite; *ARG,* arginine; *PYU,* pyruvate; *MGP,* methyl α-D-glucopyranoside; +, positive test; −, negative test; *v,* variable test.
*Occasional exceptions occur.

Antimicrobial Resistance

Enterococci show resistance to several of the commonly used antimicrobial agents, so differentiation from *Streptococcus* and susceptibility testing are important. Enterococci have intrinsic or acquired resistance to several antimicrobial agents, including aminoglycosides, β-lactams, and glycopeptides. Resistance of enterococci to glycopeptides such as vancomycin and teicoplanin were first described in the late 1980s. Of the six vancomycin-resistance phenotypes (VanA to VanE and VanG), VanA and VanB phenotypes are most frequently encountered. The VanA phenotype is inducible, carried on a transposon (Tn1546), and characterized by high-level resistance to vancomycin (minimal inhibitory concentration [MIC] greater than 32 μg/mL) and teicoplanin (MIC greater than 16 μg/mL), whereas the VanB phenotype is chromosomal mediated and characterized by variable levels of resistance to vancomycin and susceptibility to teicoplanin.

VanC phenotype is characterized by low levels of resistance to vancomycin (MIC 8 to 16 μg/mL) and susceptibility to teicoplanin and has been described in only one strain of *E. gallinarum*. VanD phenotype has been described in a few strains of *E. faecium* and is characterized by low-level resistance to vancomycin with susceptibility or intermediate resistance to teicoplanin. VanE phenotype has been described in two *E. faecalis* strains, and VanG phenotype has been described in a few *E. faecalis* strains from Australia and Canada. The VanE and VanG phenotypes are similar to VanC in that they are characterized by low levels of vancomycin resistance. Vancomycin-containing agar has been used for screening of VRE colonization and for infection control in hospitals. Susceptibility testing of the enterococcal isolate should be performed only if the isolate is clinically significant.

Streptococcus-like Organisms

The genera *Aerococcus, Gemella, Lactococcus, Leuconostoc,* and *Pediococcus* consist of organisms that resemble viridans streptococci. These bacteria have been isolated in clinical specimens and are associated with infections similar to those caused by enterococci and streptococci. These organisms are frequently identified when antimicrobial susceptibility testing of a "streptococcal" isolate reveals it to be vancomycin resistant. The vancomycin-resistant, gram-positive cocci are likely to be *Leuconostoc* or *Pediococcus*. *Aerococcus* is normally susceptible to vancomycin.

Abiotrophia and *Granulicatella*

Abiotrophia and *Granulicatella* spp., formerly known as the nutritionally variant streptococci (NVS), were first described in 1961. These bacteria grow as satellite colonies around other bacteria and require sulfydryl compounds for growth. These organisms are part of the human oral and gastrointestinal microbiota. Phylogenetic analysis using 16S rRNA revealed that NVS were genetically distinct from streptococci and warranted separate species names. Most of the species are not groupable by the Lancefield system; however, strains with group antigens A, F, H, L, and N have been reported.

Abiotrophia and *Granulicatella* spp. are a significant cause of bacteremia, endocarditis, and otitis media. Endocarditis

resulting from these organisms is difficult to treat because of their increased tolerance to antimicrobial agents. Surgery is usually required to achieve a cure. *Abiotrophia* and *Granulicatella* spp. have been linked to a few cases of osteomyelitis, endophthalmitis after cataract extraction, brain abscess, chronic sinusitis, septic arthritis, meningitis and breast implant–associated infections. *Abiotrophia* and *Granulicatella* should be suspected when gram-positive cocci resembling streptococci are observed in positive blood cultures that subsequently fail to grow on subculture. It would be appropriate to use an SBA plate with an *S. aureus* streak and examine it for satellitism. Alternatively, media can be supplemented with 10 mg/L pyridoxal hydrochloride. Biochemical characteristics that differentiate species within the genera *Granulicatella* and *Abiotrophia* spp. (*G. adiacens, G. elegans, G. balaenopterae, A. defective,* and *A. adjacens*) are production of α-and β-galactosidase, production of β-glucuronidase, hippurate hydrolysis, arginine hydrolysis, and acid production from trehalose and starch.

Aerococcus

Aerococcus sp. is a common airborne organism. It is a widespread, opportunistic pathogen associated with bacteremia, endocarditis, and UTIs in immunocompromised patients. Aerococci resemble viridans streptococci on culture but are microscopically similar to staphylococci in that they occur as tetrads or clusters. These organisms sometimes show a weak catalase or pseudocatalase reaction. They grow in the presence of 6.5% NaCl and can easily be confused with enterococci. Two species *A. viridans* and *A. urinae* have been associated with infection. Some strains of *A. viridans* are bile esculin positive and PYR positive. *A. urinae* is bile esculin negative and is PYR negative.

Gemella

Gemella spp. are similar in colony morphology and habitat to the viridans streptococci; they produce α-hemolysis or are nonhemolytic. The bacteria easily decolorize on Gram staining and therefore appear as gram-negative cocci in pairs, tetrads, clusters, or short chains. *Gemella* spp. have been isolated from cases of endocarditis, wounds, and abscesses. Four species have been associated with clinical infections: *G. haemolysans, G. morbillorum* (formerly *Streptococcus morbillorum*), *G. bergeriae,* and *G. sanguinis.*

Lactococcus

Lactococcus spp. are gram-positive cocci that occur singly, in pairs, or in chains and are physiologically similar to enterococci. On SBA these organisms produce α-hemolysis or are nonhemolytic. These organisms were previously classified as group N streptococci. *Lactococcus* spp. have been isolated from patients with UTIs and endocarditis. Production of acid from carbohydrates is useful in distinguishing *Lactococcus* spp. from enterococci. These microorganisms also do not react with the genetic probe in the AccuProbe *Enterococcus* Culture Confirmation test (Gen-probe, San Diego, Calif.).

Leuconostoc

The genus *Leuconostoc* consists of catalase-negative, gram-positive microorganisms with irregular coccoid morphology

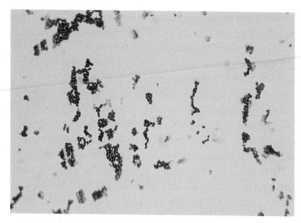

FIGURE 15-13 Gram stain of *Leuconostoc* sp.

FIGURE 15-14 *Leuconostoc* sp. colonies growing on sheep blood agar. *Leuconostoc* spp. may produce α-hemolysis and can resemble viridans streptococci.

(Figure 15-13). These organisms share several phenotypic and biochemical characteristics with *Lactobacillus*, viridans streptococci (Figure 15-14), *Pediococcus*, and *Enterococcus* spp. and are sometimes misidentified. Some species cross-react with the Lancefield group D antiserum. These microorganisms are intrinsically resistant to vancomycin. In nature they are frequently found on plant surfaces, on vegetables, and in milk products. They are recognized as opportunistic pathogens in patients who are immunocompromised or treated for underlying disease with vancomycin. These microorganisms have been isolated from cases of meningitis, bacteremia, UTIs, and pulmonary infections. Species associated with infection include *L. citreum, L. cremoris, L. dextranicum, L. lactis, L. mesenteroides,* and *L. pseudomesenteroides.* Biochemical identification is based on the absence of catalase, PYR and LAP activities, hydrolysis of esculin in the presence of bile, growth in the presence of 6.5% NaCl, and production of gas from glucose.

Pediococcus

Members of the genus *Pediococcus* are facultatively anaerobic, gram-positive cocci (arranged in pairs, tetrads, and clusters) that can grow at 45° C. They may be misidentified as viridans streptococci or enterococci. Like *Leuconostoc* spp.,

Pediococcus spp. are intrinsically resistant to vancomycin. The following species have been associated with infection: *P. acidilactici, P. damnosus, P. dextrinicus, P. parvulus,* and *P. pentasaceus. Pediococcus* spp. have been associated with patients who have underlying gastrointestinal abnormalities or who have previously undergone abdominal surgery. The organisms have also been associated with bacteremia, abscess formation, and meningitis. Biochemical characteristics used to identify them include a positive bile esculin, the presence of LAP activity, and absence of PYR activity. The organisms do not produce gas from glucose. Some of the strains are able to grow in the presence of 6.5% NaCl.

In addition to the preceding genera, a few species of *Globicatella, Helcococcus,* and *Alloiococcus* have been reported to cause clinically significant infections. *Globicatella* and *Helcococcus* resemble *Aerococcus. Globicatella sanguinis* has been associated with sepsis, meningitis, bacteremia, and UTIs. *G. sanguis* is α-hemolytic, PYR positive, LAP negative, and vancomycin susceptible. *Helcococcus kunzii* has been isolated from wound infections and is frequently misidentified as *A. viridans. Alloiococcus otitidis* has been associated with otitis media in children. Alloiococci are nonhemolytic but may show α-hemolysis after prolonged incubation. These organisms are PYR and LAP positive but grow slowly in the presence of 6.5% NaCl.

LABORATORY DIAGNOSIS

Classification Schemes

Several different approaches to the classification of the catalase-negative, gram-positive cocci have been used. Four commonly used classification schemes are (1) hemolytic pattern on sheep red blood cell agar; (2) physiologic characteristics; (3) serologic grouping or typing of C carbohydrate (Lancefield classification), capsular polysaccharide, or surface protein, such as the M protein of *S. pyogenes*; and (4) biochemical characteristics. The identification process for a streptococcal isolate in the clinical laboratory may use features from each scheme.

Hemolytic Patterns

The laboratory scientist often makes an initial classification of the streptococci based on the hemolytic pattern of the isolate grown on SBA. Although hemolysis patterns can be helpful during the initial workup of an isolate, it must be kept in mind that many species of streptococci show variable hemolytic patterns. The types of hemolysis possible are outlined in Table 15-1.

Physiologic Characteristics

Streptococci have been classified according to physiologic characteristics. This classification divides the species into four groups: pyogenic streptococci, lactococci, enterococci, and viridans streptococci. The pyogenic streptococci are those that produce pus; these organisms are mostly β-hemolytic and constitute the majority of the Lancefield groups. The lactococci are nonhemolytic organisms with Lancefield group N antigen and are often found in dairy products. The enterococci comprise species found as part of the normal biota of the human intestine.

The viridans streptococci are widely found as normal biota in the upper respiratory tract of humans. Most strains lack a C carbohydrate and are not part of the Lancefield classification; however, some have A, C, F, G, or N antigen. The viridans streptococci are α-hemolytic or nonhemolytic and are often seen as opportunistic pathogens. For the most part, this physiologic classification is historical. Nevertheless, the terms *enterococci* and *viridans streptococci* remain and are still used to describe clinical isolates.

Lancefield Classification Scheme

The **Lancefield classification system** is the most commonly used scheme. The classification system is based on extraction of C carbohydrate from the streptococcal cell wall by placing the organisms in dilute acid and heating for 10 minutes. The soluble antigen is used to immunize rabbits to obtain antisera to the various C carbohydrate groups. The Lancefield serologic grouping has been most significant in classifying and identifying β-hemolytic streptococci. During the past several decades, however, since DNA relatedness has been applied to the classification and identification of α-hemolytic streptococcal species, investigators have found no correlation between genetic relationships and streptococcal group antigens. Con-

trary to group B β-hemolytic streptococci, in which only one species is identified, α-hemolytic streptococci as a whole are phenotypically and genotypically diverse and therefore difficult to characterize.

The C carbohydrate is also present in streptococcal species other than those that produce β-hemolysis. Some are found as normal biota in animals or as animal pathogens, and others may be found in both humans and animals. These species belong to Lancefield groups A, B, C, D, F, G, and N, although not all members of these groups cause human infection. The classification of *Streptococcus* and *Enterococcus* species is shown in Table 15-2.

Biochemical Identification

Biochemical identification can be performed even by small laboratories. Although definitive identification requires a large number of biochemical characteristics or perhaps serologic methods, presumptive identification can be accomplished relatively easily with a few key tests and characteristics (Figure 15-15). Initial biochemical tests performed are often selected based on the hemolytic reaction of the isolate. Presumptive identification, in the great majority of cases, possesses a high enough rate of accuracy to be useful to the clinician and does not require the exhaustive additional tests that are needed to meet the criteria for definitive identifica-

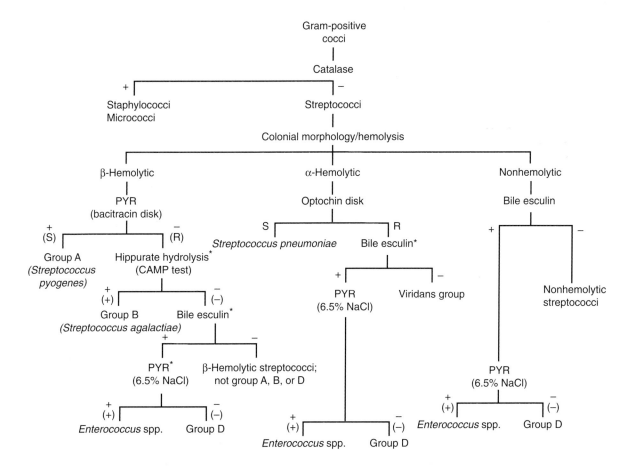

*Perform additional tests if isolate is from nonrespiratory source.

FIGURE 15-15   Schematic diagram for the presumptive identification of gram-positive cocci. *S,* Susceptible; *R,* resistant.

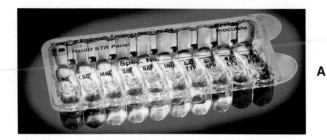

A

REMEL/IDS RapID STR Color Guide

Test	Cavity	Positive Reactions	Negative Reactions	Comments
				Without the addition of any reagents, read cavities 1-10 and record results:
ARG	1	● ●	○ ○	**Cavity 1:** Development of a red or dark orange color is a positive test; a yellow or yellow-orange color is a negative test.
ESC	2	●	○ ○ ○	**Cavity 2:** Development of a black color is a positive test; a clear, tan, or a light brown color is a negative test.
MNL	3			
SBL	4	○ ○	● ●	**Cavities 3-5:** Development of a yellow or yellow-orange color is a positive test; a red or orange color is a negative test.
RAF	5			
INU	6	○ ○	●	**Cavity 6:** Development of a yellow or orange color is a positive test; a red color is a negative test.
GAL	7			
GLU	8	○	○	**Cavities 7-10:** Development of a significant yellow color is a positive test; a very pale or clear color is a negative test.
NAG	9			*Add RapID STR Reagent to cavities 7-10. Allow at least 30 seconds but no longer than 3 minutes for color development.*
PO4	10			
TYR	7	● ●	○ ○ ○	**Cavities 7-8:** Development of a purple color, without regard to intensity, is a positive test; a clear, tan, or yellow color is a negative test.
HPR	8			
LYS	9	● ●	○ ○ ○	**Cavities 9-10:** Development of a very dark purple color is a positive test; a light to medium purple color is a negative test.
PYR	10			

B

Note: The RapID Color Guides are intended as an educational aid to be used in conjunction with the Technical Insert for the product. The reaction colors shown in the charts represent the typical shades of positive and negative colors.

800-447-3641 or **800-225-5443**
(Technical Service)
PRINTED IN U.S.A. 3/98

FIGURE 15-16 RapID Streptococci panel for the identification of *Streptococcus* spp. **A,** The commercial test well cartridge containing appropriate substrates. **B,** The interpretive color guide to reactions. (Courtesy Remel, Lenexa, Kan.)

tion, especially for species in groups A, B, and D and also *Streptococcus pneumoniae* and *Enterococcus*. Speciation of the viridans streptococci, however, does require a considerable increase in the number of tests.

The biochemical tests used for identification of the streptococci include (1) bacitracin susceptibility, (2) CAMP, (3) hippurate hydrolysis, (3) PYR hydrolysis, (e) leucine aminopeptidase (LAP), (5) Voges-Proskauer (VP), (6) β-D-glucuronidase, (7) bile esculin and salt tolerance, (8) optochin susceptibility, and (9) bile solubility. Some of these tests are described in Appendix A. Table 15-3 outlines the biochemical characteristics used to presumptively identify selected members of the family Streptococcaceae and similar organisms. Several multitest commercial kits are available, such as

Remel's IDS RapID STR (Lenexa, Kan.) shown in Figure 15-16. Some clinical laboratories forgo biochemical testing and identify streptococci by detection of the group antigen. In selecting an identification scheme or kit, the laboratory scientist must evaluate the needs of the clinicians and patient population served, the cost of an expanded identification scheme, the resources and abilities of the laboratory, and the usefulness of the data obtained.

Bacitracin Susceptibility. Historically bacitracin susceptibility has been used as an inexpensive test to presumptively identify *S. pyogenes* (group A streptococci). This method is helpful in screening for group A streptococci in throat cultures. The throat swab is used to inoculate SBA containing SXT, and a bacitracin disk is placed directly onto the agar.

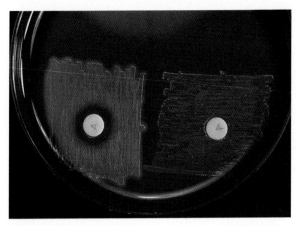

FIGURE 15-17 Group A *Streptococcus* on sheep blood agar showing susceptibility to bacitracin. *Left,* Susceptible; *right,* resistant.

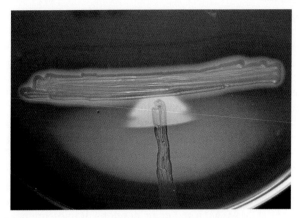

FIGURE 15-18 The CAMP test for presumptive identification of group B streptococci. *Streptococcus agalactiae* shows the classic arrow shape near the streptococcal streak.

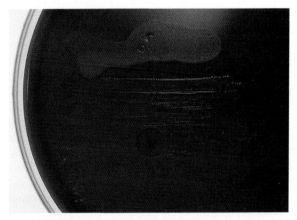

FIGURE 15-19 A modification of the CAMP test showing the enhanced hemolysis produced by *Streptococcus agalactiae* when a drop of extracted β-lysin is placed on the colony.

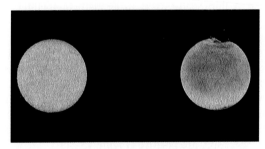

FIGURE 15-20 The PYR test for *Streptococcus pyogenes* and *Enterococcus. Left,* Negative; *right,* positive.

Growth of most interfering respiratory microbiota will be inhibited by SXT, but *S. pyogenes* and *S. agalactiae* will grow. Those β-hemolytic colonies that grow and are susceptible to bacitracin are presumptively identified as *S. pyogenes* (Figure 15-17). See Appendix D for the bacitracin susceptibility test procedure. The pattern shown by *S. pyogenes* (group A) is susceptibility to bacitracin and resistance to SXT. The pattern shown by *S. agalactiae* (group B) is resistance to both bacitracin and SXT. The PYR test, discussed later, is a more specific rapid test for group A streptococcus.

CAMP Test. The **CAMP test** is used to presumptively identify group B streptococci. "CAMP" is an acronym from the first letters of the surnames of the individuals who first described the reaction: Christie, Atkins, and Munch-Petersen. The CAMP test can be performed three ways. One is with the use of a β-lysin–producing strain of *Staphylococcus aureus*; another is with the use of a disk impregnated with the β-lysin. Both methods take advantage of the enhanced hemolysis occurring when the β-lysin and the hemolysin produced by group B streptococci are in contact.

In the assay utilizing *S. aureus,* the unknown streptococcal isolate is inoculated perpendicularly to the *S. aureus* inoculum. See Appendix D for the CAMP procedure. The result is a characteristic arrowhead-shaped hemolysis pattern (Figure 15-18). When a disk containing β-lysin is used, the enhanced hemolysis is not a typical arrowhead shape because the disk is round. A third method, the rapid CAMP test (or spot CAMP test), involves placing a drop of extracted β-lysin on the area of confluent growth of the suspected group B streptococci. After incubation at 35° C for at least 20 minutes, enhanced hemolysis is observed (Figure 15-19).

Hippurate Hydrolysis. A useful test for differentiating *S. agalactiae* from other β-hemolytic streptococci is the **hippurate hydrolysis test**. *S. agalactiae* possess the enzyme hippuricase (also called *hippurate hydrolase*), which hydrolyzes sodium hippurate to form sodium benzoate and glycine. A 2-hour rapid test is available to detect the presence of hippurate hydrolase; See Appendix for the hippurate hydrolysis test procedure.

PYR Hydrolysis. The **pyrrolidonyl-α-naphthylamide (PYR) hydrolysis** test provides a high probability for the

presumptive identification of the β-hemolytic group A streptococci and the nonhemolytic group D (Figure 15-20). The only species of *Streptococcus* PYR positive is *S. pyogenes.* Other genera that are PYR positive include *Enterococcus, Aerococcus,* and *Gemella.* The PYR test detects the activity of L-pyrrolidonyl arylamidase, also called *pyrrolidonyl aminopeptidase.* The PYR test takes advantage of the fact that

S. pyogenes and *Enterococcus* spp. are able to hydrolyze the substrate PYR. Several commercial systems are available. The specificity of this test for *Enterococcus* spp. is similar to that of the bile esculin and salt tolerance tests (see Bile Esculin and Salt Tolerance later in this chapter). The PYR test is more specific for *S. pyogenes* than bacitracin. See Appendix D for the PYR hydrolysis test procedure.

Leucine Aminopeptidase. Leucine aminopeptidase **(LAP)** is a peptidase that hydrolyzes peptide bonds adjacent to a free amino group. Because LAP reacts most quickly with leucine, it is called *leucine aminopeptidase*. The substrate, leucine-β-naphthylamide, is hydrolyzed to β-naphthylamine. After the addition of para-dimethylaminocinnamaldehyde reagent (DMACA), a red color develops. Rapid commercial tests that use filter paper disks impregnated with the substrate are available. The LAP test is often used with the PYR test and is most helpful in differentiating *Aerococcus* and *Leuconostoc* spp. from other gram-positive cocci. *Streptococcus,* *Enterococcus,* and *Pediococcus* spp. are LAP positive, and *Aerococcus* and *Leuconostoc* spp. are LAP negative.

Voges-Proskauer Test. The **Voges-Proskauer test** is used to distinguish the small-colony–forming β-hemolytic anginosus group containing groups A or C antigens from large-colony–forming pyogenic strains with the same antigens. The VP test detects acetoin production from glucose. In the modified VP test, a heavy suspension of bacteria is made in 2 mL of VP broth. After about 6 hours of incubation at 35° C, a few drops of 5% α-naphthol and 40% potassium hydroxide are added. The tube is shaken vigorously to increase the concentration of dissolved oxygen, and the broth is incubated at room temperature for 30 minutes. The formation of a red or pink color is a positive reaction. Members of the anginosus group are positive.

β-D-Glucuronidase. The β-D-glucuronidase (BGUR) test detects the action of BGUR, an enzyme found in isolates of large-colony–forming β-hemolytic groups C and G streptococci but not in the small-colony–forming β-hemolytic anginosus group. Several commercially prepared rapid assays are available. A fluorogenic assay using methylumbelliferyl-β-D-glucoronide has also been described.

Bile Esculin and Salt Tolerance. The two tests that have been mainstays in identification schemes for the nonhemolytic, catalase-negative, gram-positive cocci are the bile esculin hydrolysis test (see Appendix D) and the salt-tolerance test (see Appendix D). The bile esculin test is a two-step test detecting growth of bacteria in the presence of 40% bile and the ability to hydrolyze esculin. Group D streptococci and *Enterococcus* spp. are positive (Figure 15-21).

Organisms positive for bile esculin are separated into group D streptococci or *Enterococcus* by the salt-tolerance test. Growth in 6.5% sodium chloride broth is used to identify *Enterococcus* and *Aerococcus* organisms. Some species of *Pediococcus* and *Leuconostoc* grow in 6.5% NaCl broth when incubated for 24 hours. Group D streptococci, however, do not grow in a 6.5% NaCl broth.

Optochin Susceptibility. In the **optochin test,** a filter paper disk containing optochin (ethylhydrocuprein hydrochloride) is added to the surface of an SBA plate that has just been inoculated with an α-hemolytic streptococcus. The plate

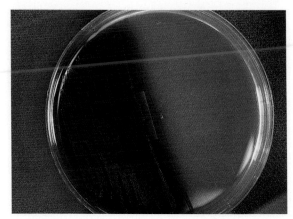

FIGURE 15-21 The bile esculin test. A positive test *(left)* shows blackening of the agar. Right side is negative.

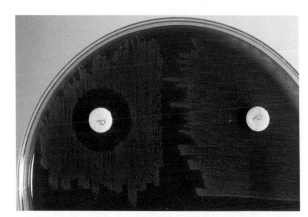

FIGURE 15-22 *Streptococcus pneumoniae* on blood agar showing susceptibility to optochin. *Left,* Susceptible *S. pneumoniae; right,* resistant viridans streptococci.

is incubated overnight at 35° C in a CO_2 incubator. A zone of inhibition greater than 14 mm with a 6-mm disk or a zone of inhibition greater than 16 mm with a 10-mm disk is considered susceptible and a presumptive identification of *S. pneumoniae* (Figure 15-22). Isolates producing smaller zones should be tested for bile solubility to confirm their identity.

Bile Solubility. A characteristic that correlates well with optochin susceptibility is **bile solubility.** The test for bile solubility takes advantage of the very active *S. pneumoniae* autocatalytic enzyme amidase. Under the influence of a bile salt or detergent, the organism's cell wall lyses during cell division. A suspension of *S. pneumoniae* in a solution of sodium deoxycholate lyses, and the solution becomes clear. Other α-hemolytic organisms do not undergo lysis, and the solution remains cloudy. Suspensions of bacteria made in saline serve as negative controls.

Noncultural Identification

Immunoassays

Identification of streptococci, particularly group A, can be made by the detection of the group-specific antigen from either isolated colonies or, in some cases, a direct clinical

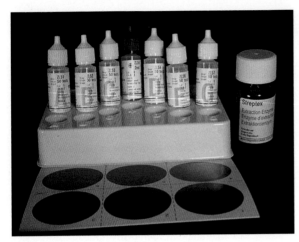

FIGURE 15-23 Slide agglutination test for grouping streptococci.

specimen such as a throat swab. Identification from isolated colonies can be accomplished by extracting the C carbohydrate by means of acid or heat. The extract containing the specific group carbohydrate is then used in a capillary precipitin or a slide agglutination test. In the capillary precipitin test, antiserum to the specific group carbohydrate is overlayed with the solution containing the streptococcal extract. After 5 to 10 minutes the interface between the extraction solution and the antiserum is examined carefully for a white precipitate, which indicates a positive reaction. Each extract can be tested with a number of antisera specific to the various group antigens.

An easier-to-perform alternative method is the slide agglutination test that uses a carrier particle, such as latex, for the group-specific antibody. When an antibody-antigen reaction occurs, it is seen macroscopically as agglutination of the particles (Figure 15-23). These immunoassays give a definitive identification as to the Lancefield group the isolate belongs to; however, when the group comprises several species, the methods do not give a species identification. Of course if the results indicate that the isolate belongs to group B, it can be identified as *S. agalactiae.* The cost of these methods is higher than that of the standard cultural approaches; however, the results are often quicker and more accurate.

More than two dozen different antigen-detection products are commercially available, many of which use slide agglutination or an enzyme-linked immunosorbent assay (ELISA) system to detect group A streptococci from throat swabs. These are designed primarily for use in a clinic or physician's office. Although a positive finding allows the primary care provider to treat for *S. pyogenes* infections without waiting for culture results, a negative result necessitates a throat culture because the sensitivity of direct detection methods for group A streptococci is not high enough to ensure that the negative result is not a false-negative. Additionally, the cost of using direct detection methods can be significantly higher than that of culture only. The direct detection method for group A streptococci can be a valuable diagnostic tool in the right context; however, the cost and sensitivity must be weighed carefully.

Nucleic Acid Probes

Nucleic acid probe assays are commercially available and offer rapid results and increased specificity compared with conventional identifications methods. However, nucleic acid probe assays are more costly. The LightCycler (Roche Applied Science, Indianapolis, Ind.) is a real-time polymerase chain reaction (PCR) instrument that can identify group A and group B streptococci as well as groups C and G. The assay detects the *cfb* gene, which encodes the CAMP-factor protein of group B streptococci and the *pts*I (phosphotransferase) gene of group A streptococci. Groups C and G have a *pts*I gene sequence similar to group A streptococci, but the instrument is able to distinguish among the three groups. Compared with bacterial throat cultures for group A streptococci, the LightCycler has a sensitivity of 93% and a specificity of 98%. It should be noted that the LightCycler had more positive results (58 of 384) than cultures (55 of 384) in one study.

The AccuProbe pneumococcus test (Gen-Probe, San Diego, Calif.) uses a DNA probe to detect the 16s rRNA sequence of *S. pneumoniae.* The less than 1% difference in the rRNA sequence between *S. pneumoniae* and *S. oralis* and *S. mitis* raises questions about the specificity of this assay. The Smart Cycler (Cepheid, Sunnyvale, Calif.) real-time PCR instrument also provides kits for the detection of streptococci. This instrument has four-channel optics, allowing the detection of several targets in one sample (multiplex).

Susceptibility Testing

Despite widespread use, penicillin remains the drug of choice in treating most streptococcal infections. However, penicillin-resistant *S. pneumoniae* and viridans group isolates have been reported worldwide, and the incidence of penicillin-resistant *S. pneumoniae* seems to be increasing. Erythromycin and narrow-spectrum cephalosporins are alternatives, although erythromycin resistance appeared in the early 1990s. Multiple-drug–resistant pneumococci have also been reported.

Vancomycin is an effective antimicrobial for treating infections caused by gram-positive organisms. Until the mid-1980s resistance to vancomycin was rarely seen in clinical isolates. Vancomycin resistance is now more commonly seen, although it is still not widespread. Gram-positive isolates are generally routinely tested for vancomycin susceptibility. Table 15-3 lists the usual patterns of vancomycin susceptibility for a number of gram-positive cocci. In particular, *Pediococcus* and *Leuconostoc* spp. are resistant to vancomycin. Some streptococci and a significant number of enterococci demonstrate resistance to this antimicrobial agent as well.

Because of the fastidious nature of the streptococci, antimicrobial susceptibility testing is not normally performed. As their susceptibility patterns have become less predictable, however, more laboratories have been forced to offer antimicrobial susceptibility testing. Fastidious bacteria do not grow well in most standardized procedures for antimicrobial susceptibility testing. In the case of *S. pneumoniae* and other streptococci, the Clinical and Laboratory Standards Institute (CLSI), formerly the National Committee for Clinical Laboratory Standards (NCCLS), has established procedures for both disk diffusion and broth dilution assays. Commercial methods including the Etest (AB Biodisk, Solna, Sweden) are available. It should be noted that elevated MICs may be observed with the Etest for some antimicrobial agents, possibly due to CO_2 incubation conditions.

BIBLIOGRAPHY

Carapetis JR et al: Acute rheumatic fever, *Lancet* 366:155, 2005.

Church DL et al: Evaluation of StrepB carrot broth versus Lim broth for detection of group B *Streptococcus* colonization status of near-term pregnant women, *J Clin Microbiol* 46:2780, 2008.

Christensen JJ, Facklam RR: *Granulicatella* and *Abiotrophia* species from human clinical specimens, *J Clin Microbiol* 39:3520, 2001.

Coburn PS et al: *Enterococcus faecalis* senses target cells and in response expresses cytolysin, *Science* 306:2270, 2004.

Collins MD: The genus *Gemella*. In Dworkin M et al, editors: *Procaryotes: a handbook on the biology of bacteria: bacteria, firmicutes, and cyanobacteria*, ed 3, New York, NY, 2006, Springer Press.

Diekema DJ et al: Antimicrobial resistance in viridans group streptococci among patients with and without the diagnosis of cancer in the USA, Canada and Latin America, *Clin Microbiol Infect* 7:152, 2001.

Facklam RR: What happened to the streptococci: overview of taxonomy and nomenclature changes, *Clin Microbiol Rev* 15:613, 2002.

Golden SM et al: Evaluation of a real-time fluorescent PCR assay for rapid detection of group B streptococci in neonatal blood, *Diag Microbiol Infect Dis* 50:7, 2004.

Korman TM et al: Fatal case of toxic shock-like syndrome due to group C *Streptococcus* associated with superantigen exotoxin, *J Clin Microbiol* 42:2866, 2004.

Leclercq R, Courvalin P: Resistance to macrolides and related antibiotics in *Streptococcus pneumoniae*, *Antimicrob Agents Chemother* 46:2727, 2002.

MacFaddin JF: *Biochemical tests for identification of medical bacteria*, ed 3, Philadelphia, 2000, Lippincott Williams & Wilkins.

Mahajan VK, Sharma NL: Scarlet fever, *Indian Pediatr* 42:829, 2005.

Pontes T, Antunes H: Group A beta-hemolytic streptococcal toxic shock, *Acta Med Port* 17:395, 2004.

Reynolds PE, Courvalin P: Vancomycin resistance in enterococci due to synthesis of precursors terminating in D-alanyl-D-serine, *Antimicrob Agents Chemother* 49:21, 2005.

Ruoff KL et al: *Aerococcus, Abiotrophia*, and other aerobic catalase-negative, gram-positive cocci. In Murray PR et al, editors: *Manual of clinical microbiology*, ed 9, Washington, DC, 2007, ASM Press.

Spellerberg B, Brandt C: In Murray PR et al, editors: *Manual of clinical microbiology*, ed 9, Washington, DC, 2007, ASM Press.

Teixeira LM et al: *Enterococcus*. In Murray PR et al, editors: *Manual of clinical microbiology*, ed 9, Washington, DC, 2007, ASM Press.

Trent JT, Kirsner RS: Diagnosing necrotizing fasciitis, *Advances in Skin & Wound Care* May/Jun 2002. Available at: www.findarticles.com/p/articles/mi_qa3977/is_200205/ai_n9033539. Accessed November 10, 2008.

Uhl JR et al: Comparison of LightCycler PCR, rapid antigen immunoassay and culture for detection of group A streptococci from throat swabs, *J Clin Microbiol* 41:242, 2003.

Vandamme P et al: Taxonomic study of Lancefield streptococcal C, G, and L (*Streptococcus dysagalactiae*) and proposal of *S. dysagalactiae* subsp. *equisimilis* subsp. *nov*, *Int J Syst Bacteriol* 46:774, 1996.

Vieira VV et al: Genetic relationships among the different phenotypes of *Streptococcus dysagalactiae* strains, *Int J Syst Bacteriol* 48:1231, 1998.

Points to Remember

- The organisms included in the family Streptococcaceae and the *Streptococcus*-like organisms are gram-positive cocci usually arranged in pairs or chains that are catalase negative.
- Hemolysis on sheep blood agar is often a starting point for the identification of streptococci and similar organisms.
- Many streptococci can be categorized based on Lancefield group antigens.
- Key tests for the identification of the streptococci and similar organisms include bacitracin susceptibility, CAMP test, hippurate hydrolysis, PYR hydrolysis, leucine aminopeptidase, Voges-Proskauer, BGUR, bile esculin, salt tolerance, optochin susceptibility, and bile solubility.
- Group A *Streptococcus* remains an important pathogen that causes acute bacterial pharyngitis, skin and soft tissue infections, and invasive infections, including necrotizing fasciitis.
- Emerging resistance of *S. pneumoniae* to numerous antimicrobials is becoming a major health concern.
- Viridans streptococci, although usually nonpathogenic, may cause bacteremias, abscesses, and oral infections such as gingivitis and dental caries.
- Nutritionally variant streptococci are classified within the genera *Granulicatella* and *Abiotrophia*.
- Enterococci cause approximately 5% to 10% of the infection in patients with bacterial endocarditis.
- *Streptococcus agalactiae* is a significant cause of invasive disease in newborns.
- Groups C and G streptococci are important human pathogens associated with infections such as endocarditis, meningitis, primary bacteremia, necrotizing fasciitis, or myositis.

Learning Assessment Questions

1. Name three tests that could be performed on an isolate or initial swab to give the presumptive identity of the isolate described in the Case in Point.

2. A β-hemolytic, catalase-negative, gram-positive coccus is found to be resistant to bacitracin and sulfamethoxazole. Which of the following is a likely presumptive identification?
   a. Group A streptococci
   b. Group B streptococci
   c. Group D streptococci
   d. Enterococci

3. The CAMP test is based on enhanced hemolysis between CAMP factor and β-lysin from:
   a. *Streptococcus agalactiae*
   b. *Staphylococcus epidermidis*
   c. *Staphylococcus aureus*
   d. *Enterococcus*

4. A nonhemolytic, catalase-negative, gram-positive coccus is PYR-positive. You should also expect the isolate to be:
   a. Bile esculin positive
   b. Salt tolerant
   c. Bile soluble
   d. Both a and b

5. The optochin test is most valuable in the identification of:
   a. α-streptococci
   b. β-streptococci
   c. Nonhemolytic streptococci
   d. Both a and b

6. What antimicrobial agent is most commonly used to treat infections like the one presented in the Case in Point?

7. *Streptococcus pyogenes* has been associated with what invasive infection(s)?

8. Which streptococcal species is the most common cause of community-acquired bacterial pneumonia?

9. What is the clinical significance of group B streptococci isolated from a vaginal culture of a pregnant woman?

10. How would you recover nutritionally variant streptococci from clinical samples such as blood?

Aerobic Gram-Positive Bacilli

Steven D. Mahlen, Amanda T. Harrington

■ **NON–SPORE-FORMING, NONBRANCHING CATALASE-POSITIVE BACILLI**
Corynebacterium
Rothia
Undesignated CDC Coryneform Groups

■ **NON–SPORE-FORMING, NONBRANCHING CATALASE-NEGATIVE BACILLI**
Erysipelothrix rhusiopathiae
Arcanobacterium
Gardnerella vaginalis

■ **NON–SPORE-FORMING, BRANCHING AEROBIC ACTINOMYCETES**
Nocardia
Other *Actinomycetes*

■ **SPORE-FORMING, NONBRANCHING CATALASE-POSITIVE BACILLI**
Bacillus

OBJECTIVES

After reading and studying this chapter, you should be able to:

1. Compare the general characteristics of the aerobic gram-positive bacilli discussed in this chapter.
2. Compare the clinical significance of the aerobic gram-positive bacilli and describe how the infections they cause are acquired.
3. Describe the types of clinical specimens that are likely to contain the aerobic gram-positive bacilli discussed in this chapter.
4. Describe the microscopic morphology and colony appearance of the aerobic gram-positive bacilli discussed in this chapter.
5. Describe the general characteristics of the genus *Corynebacterium*.
6. Describe the clinical infections associated with *Corynebacterium diphtheriae*.
7. Discuss the differential procedures used to diagnose infections caused by *Corynebacterium* spp.
8. Compare the culture and identifying characteristics of *Listeria monocytogenes* to *Streptococcus agalactiae* (group B *Streptococcus*).
9. Differentiate *L. monocytogenes* from other non–spore-forming gram-positive bacilli and streptococci.
10. Describe the motility patterns of *L. monocytogenes* in hanging drop and semisolid medium.
11. Differentiate *Erysipelothrix rhusiopathiae* from other non–spore-forming gram-positive bacilli.
12. Differentiate *Arcanobacterium haemolyticum* from other non–spore-forming gram-positive bacilli and β-hemolytic streptococci.
13. Differentiate *Gardnerella vaginalis* from other non–spore-forming gram-positive bacilli.
14. Describe the clinical infections associated with *Nocardia*, *Actinomadura*, and *Streptomyces*.
15. Differentiate infections caused by *Nocardia*, *Actinomadura*, *Streptomyces*, *Gordonia*, *Tsukamurella*, and *Rhodococcus* from those caused by fungal agents.
16. Describe *Tropheryma whipplei* and Whipple disease.
17. Describe the general characteristics of the genus *Bacillus*.
18. Describe the clinical infections associated with *Bacillus anthracis*.
19. Compare the relationship among the three exotoxin proteins of *B. anthracis*.
20. Describe the differential tests used to identify *B. anthracis*.
21. Discuss the clinical significance of *Bacillus* spp. other than *B. anthracis*.
22. Differentiate *B. anthracis* from other *Bacillus* spp.

Case in Point

A 76-year-old woman, receiving corticosteroid therapy for a malignant tumor, complained to her physician of fever and headache of 7 days' duration. Her headache had become progressively worse, and her temperature was elevated. A complete blood count was performed and showed a slightly elevated white blood cell count (WBC) with normal distribution. A lumbar puncture was performed with the following laboratory results:

250 WBC/mm^3
Glucose 30 mg/dL (serum glucose was 105 mg/dL)
Protein 180 mg/dL

No bacteria were observed on a Gram-stained smear of the cerebrospinal fluid (CSF). The CSF was inoculated onto sheep blood and chocolate agars. Two days later, β-hemolytic colonies grew on the sheep blood agar. Similar colony growth was present on the chocolate agar. Gram stain morphology revealed a pleomorphic, gram-positive, non–spore-forming bacillus. The isolate had the following biochemical characteristics:

- Catalase positive
- Esculin hydrolysis positive
- Hippurate hydrolysis positive
- Motile at room temperature but not at 35° C
- Christie, Atkins, Munch-Peterson (CAMP) test positive (block shape)

Issues to Consider

After reading the patient's case history, consider:
- What key tests differentiate the non–spore-forming gram-positive bacilli
- What factors increase an individual's risk for infection by the non–spore-forming gram-positive bacilli
- The distribution in nature of non–spore-forming gram-positive bacilli and the species that constitute the normal bacterial biota of humans

KEY TERMS

Actinomycotic mycetomas	Eumycotic mycetomas
Anthrax	Human blood bilayer Tween (HBT) agar
Babès-Ernst granules	
Bacterial vaginosis (BV)	Lethal factor (LF)
Cold enrichment	Loeffler medium
Cystine-tellurite blood agar (CTBA)	Medusa head
	Pleomorphic
Diphtheria	Protective antigen (PA)
Diphtheria toxin	Sulfur granules
Edema factor (EF)	Tumbling motility
Elek test	Whipple disease
Eschar	Woolsorter's disease

This chapter discusses a large group of bacteria commonly encountered in the clinical microbiology laboratory. Most species are found in the environment easily isolated from water and soil. The majority of these organisms are not highly pathogenic but are being isolated from clinical infections with increasing frequency. Bacteria that belong to the gram-positive aerobic bacilli group include the spore-forming genus *Bacillus*; the non–spore-formers, including the genera *Corynebacterium*, *Arcanobacterium*, *Rhodococcus*, *Listeria*, *Erysipelothrix*, and *Gardnerella*; and the branching, non–spore-forming aerobic actinomycetes, including *Nocardia*. Figure 16-1 shows a schematic diagram for the presumptive identification of aerobic gram-positive bacteria, including spore formers, non–spore formers, and the branching aerobic actinomycetes.

A wide range of clinical conditions result from infection with these organisms. Although several of these organisms are frequently isolated in the clinical laboratory, they are typically considered contaminants or commensals (e.g., *Bacillus* and *Corynebacterium*). Several of these organisms are rarely encountered but cause significant disease (*Listeria*, *Erysipelothrix*, *Corynebacterium diphtheriae*, and *Bacillus anthracis*). For some species, the frequency of isolation is increasing, and new clinical syndromes are being established especially in immunocompromised patients. As genetic and biochemical tools progress, the diversity of many of these genera is being identified (e.g., *Nocardia*, *Corynebacterium*) and clinical correlations are still being made.

NON–SPORE-FORMING, NONBRANCHING CATALASE-POSITIVE BACILLI

Corynebacterium

General Characteristics

The genus *Corynebacterium* is a large diverse group of bacteria that includes animal and human pathogens as well as saprophytes and plant pathogens. There are more than 60 species in the genus, and at least 40 are thought to be clinically significant. The majority of the species are found as normal biota on skin and mucous membranes of humans and animals. Some species are found worldwide in the environment. The corynebacteria are closely related to the mycobacteria and nocardiae. The cell walls of corynebacteria contain meso-diaminopimelic acid (m-DAP) as the diamino acid, as well as short-chained mycolic acids. The medically significant corynebacteria are all catalase positive and nonmotile. In addition, the corynebacteria can be divided into nonlipophilic and lipophilic species. Lipophilic corynebacteria are often considered fastidious and grow slowly on standard culture media; cultures must often be incubated at least 48 hours before growth is detected. If lipids are included in the culture medium, however, growth is enhanced.

Upon Gram staining, corynebacteria are slightly curved, gram-positive rods with unparallel sides and slightly wider ends, producing the described "club shape" or coryneform. The term *diphtheroid*, meaning "diphtheria-like," is sometimes used in reference to this Gram staining morphology. The classification of the diphtheroids is not well characterized. Consequently, there is a low rate of identification for clinical isolates. Even when sent to a reference laboratory, 30% to 50%

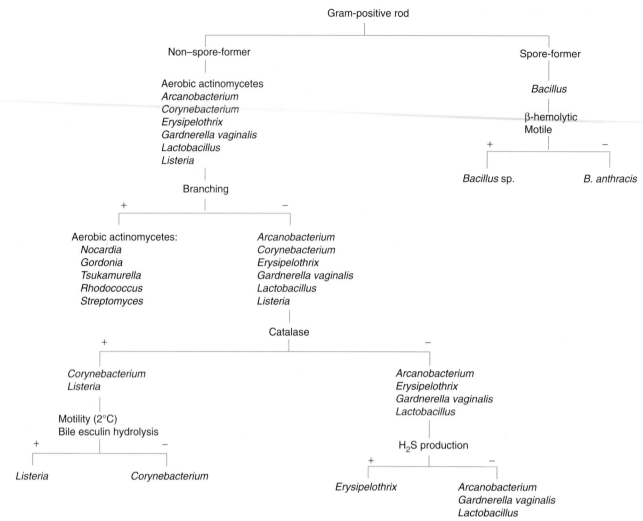

FIGURE 16-1 Schematic diagram for the identification of gram-positive bacteria. *Lactobacillus* sp. is an aerotolerant anaerobe discussed in Chapter 22.

of the coryneform-like isolates are unable to be identified to the species level without 16S rRNA gene sequencing.

Although they are typically dismissed as contaminants, the nondiphtheria corynebacteria are frequently isolated from clinical specimens. As with many previously deemed nonpathogenic organisms, however, the coryneforms are isolated from a variety of body sites, especially in immunocompromised patients. The most significant pathogen of the group, *C. diphtheriae,* has been extensively studied and is well characterized. Disease caused by *C. diphtheriae* is referred to as **diphtheria.** Other species that produce disease in humans include, but are not limited to, *C. bovis, C. ulcerans, C. xerosis, C. jeikeium, C. pseudodiphtheriticum,* and *C. pseudotuberculosis.*

Corynebacterium diphtheriae

Virulence Factors. **Diphtheria toxin** is the major virulence factor associated with *C. diphtheriae.* This toxin is produced by strains of *C. diphtheriae* infected with a lysogenic β-phage, which carries the *tox* gene for diphtheria toxin. Nontoxigenic strains can be converted to *tox*+ by infection with the appropriate β-phage. Only toxin-producing *C. diphtheriae* causes

diphtheria; however, *C. ulcerans* and *C. pseudotuberculosis,* which belong to the "*C. diphtheriae* group," may also produce the toxin when they become infected with the *tox*-carrying β-phage.

Diphtheria toxin is a protein of 62,000 daltons. It is composed of two fragments, A and B, which are linked together by a disulfide bridge. The toxin is exceedingly potent and is lethal for humans in amounts of 130 ng/kg of body weight. The toxicity of the toxin is due to its ability to block protein synthesis in eukaryotic cells. The toxin is secreted by the bacterial cell and is nontoxic until exposed to trypsin. Trypsinization cleaves the toxin into the two fragments. Both fragments are necessary for cytotoxicity. Fragment A is responsible for the cytotoxicity, and fragment B binds to receptors on the eukaryotic cells and mediates the entry of fragment A into the cytoplasm. On reaching the cytoplasm, fragment A disrupts protein synthesis. Fragment A splits nicotinamide adenosine dinucleotide (NAD) to form nicotinamide and adenosine diphosphoribose (ADPR). ADPR binds to and inactivates elongation factor 2 (EF-2), an enzyme required for elongation of polypeptide chains on ribosomes.

Production of the toxin in vitro depends on a number of environmental conditions: an alkaline pH (7.8 to 8.0), oxygen, and, most importantly, the iron concentration in the medium. The amount of iron needed for optimal toxin production is less than the amount needed for optimal growth. The toxin is released in significant amounts only when the available iron in the culture medium is exhausted.

Clinical Infections. *Corynebacterium diphtheriae* causes two different forms of disease in humans: respiratory and cutaneous diphtheria. Respiratory diphtheria is found worldwide but is uncommon in North America and Western Europe. Diphtheria has been uncommon in the United States since universal vaccination began in the 1940s; those cases that occur are invariably in nonimmunized populations. Epidemic diphtheria emerged in the New Independent States of the former Soviet Union in the 1990s, probably due to inadequate mass vaccination strategies. To prevent the spread of diphtheria, the Centers for Disease Control and Prevention (CDC) recommends that international travelers ensure that they are up-to-date on all vaccinations. Individuals vaccinated as children who have not been revaccinated as adults are susceptible to infection. Humans are the only natural hosts for *C. diphtheriae.*

C. diphtheriae is carried in the upper respiratory tract and spread by droplet infection or hand-to-mouth contact. The incubation period averages 2 to 5 days. The illness begins gradually and is characterized by low-grade fever, malaise, and a mild sore throat. The most common site of infection is the tonsils or pharynx. The organisms rapidly multiply on the epithelial cells, and the toxigenic strains of *C. diphtheriae* produce toxin locally, causing tissue necrosis and exudate formation triggering an inflammatory reaction. This combination of cell necrosis and exudate forms a tough gray to white pseudomembrane, which attaches to the tissues. It may appear on the tonsils and then spread downward into the larynx and trachea. There is the potential for suffocation if the membrane blocks the air passage or if it is dislodged, perhaps as the result of sampling for a throat culture.

The toxin also is absorbed and can produce a variety of systemic effects involving the kidneys, heart, and nervous system, although all tissues possess the receptor for the toxin and may be affected. Death often is a result of cardiac failure. Another effect of the toxin is a demyelinating peripheral neuritis, which may result in paralysis following the acute illness.

Other nonrespiratory sites may be infected, although much less often than the upper respiratory tract. In the cutaneous form of diphtheria, which is prevalent in the tropics, the toxin also is absorbed systemically, but systemic complications are less common than from upper respiratory infections. Cutaneous diphtheria consists of nonhealing ulcers with a dirty gray membrane. Although this form is unusual in the United States, there have been outbreaks of cutaneous diphtheria in Native Americans and in homeless individuals.

Diphtheria is treated by prompt administration of antitoxin. Commercial diphtheria antitoxin is produced in horses. Approximately 10% of patients who receive the antitoxin develop an allergic reaction to the horse serum. Consequently, hypersensitivity to horse serum precludes its administration. Antimicrobial agents have no effect on the toxin that is already circulating, but they do eliminate the focus of infection as well as prevent the spread of the organism. The drug of choice is penicillin; erythromycin is used for penicillin-sensitive individuals.

Laboratory Diagnosis

Microscopy. *Corynebacterium diphtheriae* is a highly **pleomorphic** (many shapes) gram-positive bacillus that appears in palisades or as individual cells lying at sharp angles to another in V and L formations. Although it may be demonstrated by other *Corynebacterium* spp., club-shaped swellings and beaded forms are common (Figure 16-2). The organisms often stain

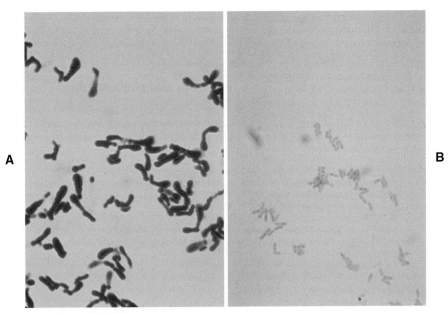

FIGURE 16-2 A, Microscopic Gram stain of diphtheroid. **B,** Microscopic Loeffler methylene blue stain of *Corynebacterium* spp. (Courtesy Cathy Bissonette.)

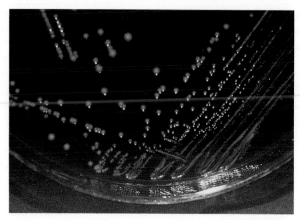

FIGURE 16-3 *Corynebacterium diphtheriae* growing on sheep blood agar. (Courtesy Cathy Bissonette.)

irregularly, especially when stained with methylene blue, giving them a beaded appearance. The metachromatic areas of the cell, which stain more intensely than other parts, are called **Babès-Ernst granules.** They represent accumulation of polymerized polyphosphates. The presence of the Babès-Ernst granules indicates the accumulation of nutrient reserves and varies with the type of medium and the metabolic state of the individual cells.

Culture Characteristics. The diphtheria bacillus, like most other corynebacteria, is a facultative anaerobe. It grows best under aerobic conditions and has an optimal growth temperature of 37° C, although multiplication occurs within the range of 15° to 40° C. Growth requirements are complex, requiring eight essential amino acids. Although *C. diphtheriae* will grow on nutrient agar, better growth is usually obtained on a medium containing blood or serum, such as Loeffler serum or Pai agars. Characteristic microscopic morphology is demonstrated well when organisms are grown on **Loeffler medium.** On sheep blood agar (SBA) (Figure 16-3), the organism may have a very small zone of β-hemolysis.

Cystine-tellurite blood agar (CTBA), a modification of Tinsdale medium, contains sheep red blood cells, bovine serum, cystine, and potassium tellurite. CTBA is both a selective and differential medium. The potassium tellurite inhibits many non-coryneform bacteria. When grown on CTBA, corynebacteria form black or brownish colonies from the reduction of tellurite. This appearance, however, is not unique for *C. diphtheriae,* so care must be taken not to presumptively identify other genera that produce black colonies (e.g., *Staphylococcus* and *Streptococcus*) as *Corynebacterium.* A brown halo surrounding the colony, due to cystinase activity, is a useful differentiating feature, because only *C. diphtheriae, C. ulcerans,* and *C. pseudotuberculosis* produce a brown halo on CTBA.

Identification. The biochemical identification of medically important corynebacteria is outlined in Table 16-1. All of the medically important corynebacteria are catalase positive and nonmotile. CTBA medium is useful for differentiating corynebacteria because only *C. diphtheriae, C. ulcerans,* and *C. pseudotuberculosis* form a brown halo. *C. diphtheriae* is distinguished from the other two species by its lack of urease production. *C. diphtheriae* ferments glucose and

maltose, producing acid but not gas, and reduces nitrate to nitrite. A schematic diagram to presumptively identify *C. diphtheriae* is shown in Figure 16-4.

Test for Toxigenicity. The identification of an isolate as *C. diphtheriae* does not mean that the patient has diphtheria. Diagnosis of diphtheria is established by also demonstrating that the isolate produces diphtheria toxin. The growth medium and conditions markedly affect toxin production. The iron content of the medium must be growth rate–limiting for full toxin production. The addition of iron to iron-starved cultures inhibits toxin production very quickly. Toxin detection can be done either by in vivo or by in vitro testing. However, in vivo testing is rarely done because the in vitro methods are reliable, less expensive, and free from the need to use animals.

The in vitro diphtheria toxin detection procedure is an immunodiffusion test first described by Elek. In the **Elek test,** organisms (controls and unknowns) are streaked on medium of low iron content. Each organism is streaked in a single straight line parallel to each other and 10 mm apart. A filter paper strip impregnated with diphtheria antitoxin is laid along the center of the plate on a line at right angles to the inoculum lines of control and unknown organisms (Figure 16-5). The plate is then incubated at 35° C and examined after 18, 24, and 48 hours. Lines of precipitation are best seen by transmitted light against a dark background. The white precipitin lines start about 4 to 5 mm from the filter paper strip and are at an angle of about 45 degrees to the line of growth. If an isolate is positive for toxin production, and it is placed next to the positive control, the toxin line of the positive control should join the toxin line of the positive unknown to form an arch of identity.

The Elek test requires that reagents and antisera be carefully controlled and titrated. For this reason, and because of the difficulty of the test, it is performed only in certain reference laboratories. Rapid enzyme-linked immunosorbent assays (ELISA) and immunochromatographic strip assays are also available for the detection of diphtheria toxin. In addition, procedures for detecting the *C. diphtheriae tox* gene by the polymerase chain reaction (PCR) have been developed. The PCR assay can also be applied directly to clinical specimens.

Other Corynebacteria

Corynebacterium jeikeium. *Corynebacterium jeikeium,* named after Johnson and Kaye, who first linked this organism with human infections, appears to be part of the normal skin microbiota. Infections are typically limited to patients who are immunocompromised, have undergone invasive procedures, or have a history of intravenous drug abuse. The presence of catheters or prosthetic devices also contributes to infection with *C. jeikeium,* and it is also the most common cause of diphtheroid prosthetic valve endocarditis in adults. *C. jeikeium* causes septicemia, meningitis, and prosthetic joint infections in addition to endocarditis. Many patients develop skin complications such as rash and subcutaneous nodules.

The organism is lipophilic and a strict aerobe that is nonhemolytic, urease positive, and reduces nitrate. *C. jeikeium* has been reported to be resistant to a wide range of antimicrobials including penicillins, cephalosporins, and aminoglycosides,

TABLE 16-1 Identification of Corynebacteria

Characteristic	Corynebacterium diphtheriae	Corynebacterium ulcerans	Corynebacterium pseudotuberculosis	Corynebacterium xerosis	Corynebacterium jeikeium	Corynebacterium urealyticum	Corynebacterium pseudodiphtheriticum	Corynebacterium striatum
Tinsdale halo	+	+	+	−	−	−	−	−
Catalase	+	+	+	+	+	+	+	+
β-Hemolysis	V	V	+	−	−	−	−	−
Nitrate reduction	+	−	V	+	−	−	+	+
Urease	−	+	+	−	−	+	+	−
Hydrolysis								
Gelatin	−	+*	−	−	−	−	−	−
Esculin	−	−	−	−	−	−	−	−
Carbohydrate fermentation								
Glucose	+	+	+	+	+	−	−	+
Maltose	+	+	+	+	V	−	−	−
Sucrose	−	−	−	+	−	−	−	+

+, Present or positive; −, absent or negative; V, variable.
*25° C.

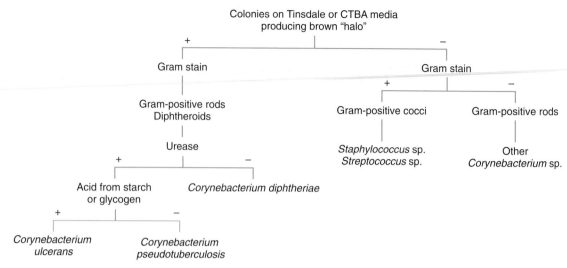

FIGURE 16-4 A schematic diagram of the presumptive identification of *Corynebacterium diphtheriae*. CTBA, Cystine-tellurite blood agar.

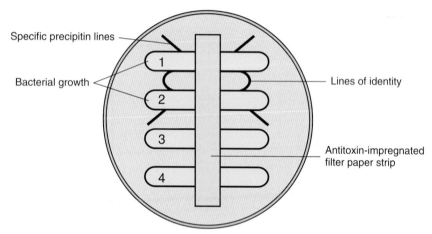

FIGURE 16-5 Elek test for toxin-producing stains of *Corynebacterium diphtheriae*. *1*, Positive control; *2*, unknown (toxigenic); *3*, negative control; *4*, unknown (nontoxigenic).

and they are inducibly resistant to macrolides such as erythromycin. The drug of choice for treating *C. jeikeium* infections is vancomycin. Multidrug resistance cannot be used as the only identifying characteristic because CDC group G may also demonstrate this characteristic.

Corynebacterium pseudodiphtheriticum. Part of the normal biota of the human nasopharynx, *C. pseudodiphtheriticum* very rarely causes infection, but when infection occurs, it often takes the form of respiratory tract infections in immunocompromised individuals. In addition, *C. pseudodiphtheriticum* causes endocarditis, urinary tract infections, and cutaneous wound infections in immunosuppressed patients, including those with acquired immunodeficiency syndrome (AIDS). *C. pseudodiphtheriticum*, unlike other corynebacteria, does not show the characteristic pleomorphic morphology. The cells stain evenly and often lie in parallel rows (palisades). The species grows well on standard laboratory media, reduces nitrate, and hydrolyzes urea.

Corynebacterium pseudotuberculosis. Like *C. ulcerans* discussed later, *C. pseudotuberculosis* is primarily a veteri-

nary pathogen. Human infections have typically been associated with contact with sheep and are rare. *C. pseudotuberculosis* causes a granulomatous lymphadenitis in humans. The organism produces a dermonecrotic toxin that causes death of a variety of cell types, and it can produce diphtheria toxin. Like *C. diphtheriae*, *C. pseudotuberculosis* also produces a brown halo on CTBA. On SBA, *C. pseudotuberculosis* forms small yellowish-white colonies. It is urease positive and gelatin negative. The organism is susceptible to penicillin and erythromycin.

Corynebacterium striatum. In addition to being found in the nasopharynx, *C. striatum* is normal human skin biota and is a rare cause of true infections in humans. The organism is a frequent isolate in clinical microbiology laboratories and is usually considered a contaminant or a colonizer. Nosocomial infections have been reported. The organism is nonlipophilic and pleomorphic, and it often produces small, shiny, convex colonies in about 24 hours. *C. striatum* is resistant to penicillins but is sensitive to other β-lactams and to vancomycin.

Corynebacterium ulcerans. A veterinary pathogen causing mastitis in cattle and other domestic and wild animals, *C. ulcerans* has been isolated from patients with diphtheria-like illness. A significant number of isolates produce the diphtheria toxin; however, the amount of toxin elaborated is much less than by *C. diphtheriae*. Human infections usually are acquired through contact with animals or by ingestion of unpasteurized dairy products. The organism has been isolated from skin ulcers and exudative pharyngitis. It grows well on Loeffler agar and produces a brown halo around the colonies on CTBA. The organisms grow well on SBA and produce a narrow zone of β-hemolysis. Unlike *C. diphtheriae*, *C. ulcerans* does not reduce nitrate. It is gelatin positive at room temperature.

Corynebacterium urealyticum. *Corynebacterium urealyticum* is one of the most frequently isolated clinically significant corynebacteria. It has been described primarily as a urinary pathogen. Urine isolates with pinpoint, nonhemolytic, white colonies that have characteristic diphtheroid microscopic morphology are likely *C. urealyticum*. This species is lipophilic and is a strict aerobe. For a presumptive identification, the isolate should be catalase positive and rapidly urease positive, within minutes following inoculation on a Christensen urea slant. In addition, *C. urealyticum* does not ferment glucose. It also has shown resistance to a wide variety of antimicrobials, such as the β-lactams, aminoglycosides, and trimethoprim-sulfamethoxazole. Some isolates are also resistant to fluoroquinolones, macrolides, and tetracycline. The drug of choice for *C. urealyticum* infections is vancomycin.

Corynebacterium xerosis. *Corynebacterium xerosis* is commonly found on skin and mucocutaneous sites. Opportunistic infections associated with this organism include prosthetic valve endocarditis, bacteremia associated with intravenous catheters, postsurgical wound infections, and pneumonia. Human infection with *C. xerosis* is rare, and affected patients are invariably immunosuppressed. This organism grows well on SBA and forms dry, pigmented (yellow to tan) colonies. Isolates are generally susceptible to most antimicrobial agents.

Identification of Coryneform Bacteria

Coryneform bacteria should be identified to the species level (1) if they are isolated from normally sterile sites, particularly from two or more blood cultures; (2) if they are the predominant organism from properly collected clinical material; (3) from urine samples if they are the predominant organism and the total colony count is greater than 10^5/mL or if they are the sole isolate with a colony count of greater than 10^4/mL.

In addition to conventional biochemical testing, commercial identification systems presently available include the RapID CB Plus system (Remel, Lenexa, Kan.), API Rapid Coryne System (bioMérieux, Durham, N.C.), the Microscan Panel (Sieman, Deerfield, Ill.), and the BBL Crystal GP System (BD Diagnostics Sparks, Md.), among others. Although these systems have short incubation times ranging from a few hours to 48 hours, users should keep in mind their limitations. The test systems perform best with species that grow rapidly in air and do not require nutritional supplements. Despite the small number of substrates in the panels and infrequently updated databases, commercial systems coupled with Gram stain and colony morphologies can provide relevant data for identification. Clinically significant, unidentifiable coryneform bacteria should be sent to a reference laboratory for complete characterization. Many reference laboratories now use 16S rDNA gene sequencing to identify species of corynebacteria and other coryneform bacteria, although methods such as thin-layer chromatography, gas chromatography, mass spectrometry, or high-performance liquid chromatography have been previously used.

Rothia

A member of the normal human oropharyngeal microbiota, *Rothia dentocariosa* may be found in saliva and supragingival plaque. It has been isolated from patients with endocarditis. Microscopically, this organism resembles the coryneform bacilli, forming short gram-positive bacilli but also branching filaments that resemble those of facultative actinomycetes. When placed in broth, however, the species produces coccoid cells, a characteristic differentiating it from the actinomycetes. *Rothia* is nitrate positive, nonmotile, esculin hydrolysis positive, and urease negative. Approximately two thirds of the isolates are catalase positive.

Undesignated CDC Coryneform Groups

Several coryneform bacilli are unnamed and remain designated with CDC group numbers and letters while awaiting proper species designation. These organisms have been isolated from a wide range of clinical samples, and they should be regarded as potential nosocomial pathogens or opportunistic pathogens in the immunocompromised patient. CDC group G, for example, has been associated with bacteremia, endocarditis, wound infections, eye infections, and other infections. In addition, this group of corynebacteria has a similar antimicrobial resistance profile to *C. jeikeium*.

Listeria monocytogenes

General Characteristics. The genus *Listeria* comprises six species, of which only *L. monocytogenes* and *L. ivanovii* are considered pathogenic. *L. monocytogenes* is an important human pathogen, whereas *L. ivanovii* is primarily an animal pathogen. *L. monocytogenes* is widespread in the environment and has been recovered from soil, water, vegetation, and animal products, such as raw milk, cheese, poultry, and processed meats. It also has been isolated from crustaceans, flies, and ticks. *L. monocytogenes* has long been known to cause illness in many species of wild and domestic animals including sheep, cattle, swine, horses, dogs, cats, rodents, birds, and fish, and it can be isolated from both human and animal asymptomatic carriers. Listeriosis is recognized as an uncommon but serious infection primarily of neonates, pregnant women, the elderly, and immunocompromised hosts. Infection may also occur in healthy individuals.

Virulence Factors. *Listeria monocytogenes* produces a number of products that have been proposed as virulence factors. These include hemolysin (listeriolysin O), catalase, superoxide dismutase, phospholipase C, and a surface protein (p60). Protein p60 induces phagocytosis through increased adhesion and penetration into mammalian cells. Listeriolysin O damages the phagosome membrane, effectively preventing killing of the organism by the macrophage. The correlation between listeriolysin O production and virulence is strong. Nonhemolytic isolates are found to be avirulent and demonstrate no intracellular spread of the organism.

Clinical Infections. The infectious dose and portal of entry of listeriosis have not been determined, but animal studies as well as analysis of human outbreaks seem to indicate that the ingestion of contaminated food with subsequent systemic spread through the intestine is likely. *L. monocytogenes* appears to have a tropism for the central nervous system (CNS), and a high mortality rate (20% to 50%) is seen in patients with CNS infections. The clinical manifestations of listeriosis differ among patient groups. Infections of newborns and immunocompromised adults are the most common, but disease in healthy individuals, particularly in pregnant women, also occurs.

Disease in Pregnant Women. During pregnancy, listeriosis is most commonly seen during the third trimester. It has been postulated that *L. monocytogenes* is responsible for spontaneous abortion and stillborn neonates. A pregnant woman with listeriosis may experience a flulike illness with fever, headache, and myalgia. At this point, the organism is in the bloodstream and has seeded the uterus and fetus. It may progress and result in premature labor or septic abortion within 3 to 7 days. It appears that the infection often is self-limited, because the source of the infection is eliminated when birth occurs.

Disease in the Newborn. Infection of the neonate with *L. monocytogenes* is extremely serious; fatality rates approach 50% if the fetus is born alive. Like *Streptococcus agalactiae* neonatal disease, there are two forms of neonatal listeriosis: early onset and late onset. Early-onset listeriosis results from an intrauterine infection that can cause illness at or shortly after birth. The result is most often sepsis. Early-onset disease may be associated with aspiration of infected amniotic fluid. Late-onset disease occurs several days to weeks after birth. Affected infants generally are full term and healthy at birth. The disease is most likely to manifest as meningitis. The fatality rate is lower than in early-onset infection, although it also is a very serious, often fatal infection.

Disease in the Immunosuppressed Host. Invasive listeriosis most commonly occurs in persons who are immunosuppressed or in older adults, and particularly in patients receiving chemotherapy, as demonstrated in the Case in Point. Young children are also at risk for infection. In older adults and immunocompromised persons, the fatality rate is high. The most common manifestations are CNS infection and endocarditis. Diagnosis is made by culturing *L. monocytogenes* from the blood or cerebrospinal fluid (CSF).

Infection of apparently healthy individuals may occur through the intestinal tract when they eat food contaminated with *L. monocytogenes*. Outbreaks have occurred as a result of eating contaminated cheese, coleslaw, and chicken. Contaminated ice cream, hot dogs, and luncheon meats have served as vehicles for this food-borne disease. The penicillans, aminoglycosides, and macrolides have been effectively used to treat listeriosis. Ampicillin is usually the preferred drug. Resis-

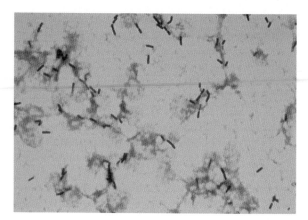

FIGURE 16-6 Gram stain of *Listeria monocytogenes* in the blood. (Courtesy Cathy Bissonette.)

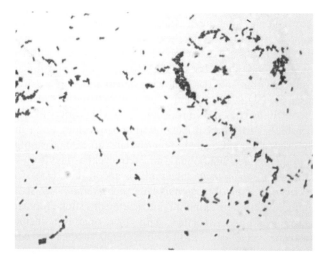

FIGURE 16-7 Gram stain of *Listeria monocytogenes* from a culture. (Courtesy Steve Mahlen and Amanda Harrington.)

tance is not common, although some strains are resistant to one or more agent.

Laboratory Diagnosis

Microscopy. In direct smears (Figure 16-6), *L. monocytogenes* appears as a gram-positive coccobacillus. With subculturing, it tends to appear as coccoid forms (Figure 16-7). Older cultures often appear gram-variable. Cells may be found singly, in short chains, or in palisades. Depending upon the cultural conditions, *L. monocytogenes* may resemble *Streptococcus* when found in the coccoid form and *Corynebacterium* when the bacillus forms prevail. Organisms are not usually seen on the CSF smear.

Cultural Characteristics. *Listeria monocytogenes* grows well on SBA and chocolate agar, as well as on nutrient agars and in broths such as brain–heart infusion and thioglycolate. The organism prefers a slightly increased CO_2 tension for isolation. The colonies are small, round, smooth, and translucent. They are surrounded by a narrow zone of β-hemolysis, which may be visualized only if the colony is removed. The colonies and hemolysis resemble those seen with *S. agalactiae* (Figure 16-8, *A*).

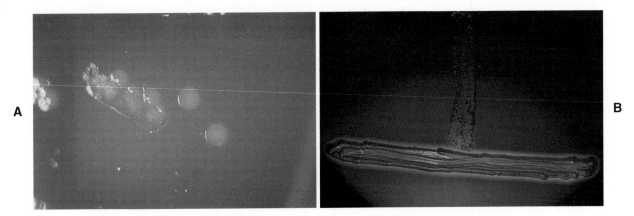

FIGURE 16-8 A, β-Hemolysis: *Listeria* on sheep blood agar (SBA) plate. *Listeria monocytogenes* growing on SBA with colony morphology similar to that of group B β-hemolytic streptococci. **B,** Conventional CAMP test with *L. monocytogenes* showing "block" hemolysis at the junction with the *Staphylococcus aureus* inoculum.

TABLE 16-2 Differentiation of *Listeria monocytogenes* and Other Gram-Positive Bacteria

Organism	Catalase	Esculin Hydrolysis	Motility	β-Hemolysis	Growth in 6.5% NaCl
Listeria monocytogenes	+	+	+	+	+
Corynebacterium spp.	+	−	V	V	V
Streptococcus agalactiae	−	−	−	+	V
Enterococcus spp.	−*	+	−	V	+

+, Present or positive; −, absent or negative; *V*, variable.
*May be weak.

The optimal growth temperature for *L. monocytogenes* is 30° to 35° C, but growth occurs over a wide range (0.5° to 45° C). Because *L. monocytogenes* grows at 4° C, a technique called **cold enrichment** may be used to isolate the organism from clinical specimens. This technique calls for inoculation of the specimen into broth and incubation at 4° C for several weeks. Subcultures are made at weekly intervals and examined for *L. monocytogenes*. The length of time required for isolation using this method lessens its importance in the clinical setting, because treatment must begin early in the infectious process.

Identification. The diagnosis of listeriosis depends upon isolating *L. monocytogenes* from blood, CSF, or swabs taken from lesions. Table 16-2 lists the characteristics of *L. monocytogenes* and bacteria with similar colony morphologies. *L. monocytogenes* is catalase-positive and motile at room temperature, which, along with β-hemolysis, excludes the corynebacteria. In wet mount preparations, *L. monocytogenes* exhibits tumbling (end-over-end motility) when viewed microscopically. In motility medium, the characteristic "umbrella" pattern is seen when the organism is incubated at room temperature (22° to 25° C) but not at 35° C (Figure 16-9).

L. monocytogenes is hippurate hydrolysis and bile esculin hydrolysis positive and produces a positive CAMP reaction. A more pronounced CAMP reaction is seen with *L. monocytogenes* when *Rhodococcus equi* is used in place of *Staphylococcus aureus*. *L. monocytogenes* produces a "block" type hemolysis with the CAMP test. This type of hemolysis is in

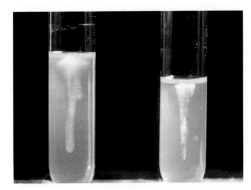

FIGURE 16-9 Umbrella motility: *Listeria*. Motility test for *Listeria monocytogenes* showing the typical "umbrella" pattern, which occurs toward the surface of the medium when this organism is incubated at room temperature. Tube on left is positive; tube on right is negative control.

contrast to the "arrowhead" type produced by *S. agalactiae* (group B *Streptococcus*), see Figure 16-8, B. The positive CAMP reaction distinguishes *L. monocytogenes* from the other *Listeria* spp., which are CAMP negative. *L. monocytogenes* is differentiated from *S. agalactiae* and the enterococci by a positive catalase test and motility. A presumptive identification can be made based on the results of a Gram stain, tumbling motility, positive catalase, and esculin hydrolysis. Confirmatory tests are acid production from glucose and positive Voges-Proskauer and methyl red reactions.

NON–SPORE-FORMING, NONBRANCHING CATALASE-NEGATIVE BACILLI

Erysipelothrix rhusiopathiae

General Characteristics

There are three species in the genus *Erysipelothrix*: *E. rhusiopathiae*, *E. tonsillarum*, and *E. inopinata*. *E. rhusiopathiae* is the only species in the genus known to cause disease in humans. It is a gram-positive, catalase negative, non–spore-forming, pleomorphic rod that has a tendency to form long filaments. It is found worldwide and is a commensal or a pathogen in a wide variety of vertebrates and invertebrates including domestic swine, birds, and fish. Human cases typically result from occupational exposure. Those individuals whose work involves handling fish and animal products are most at risk. The usual route of infection is through cuts or scratches on the skin. The organism is resistant to salting, pickling, and smoking and survives well in environmental sources such as water, soil, and plant material.

Clinical Infections

Erysipelothrix rhusiopathiae produces three types of disease in humans: erysipeloid, which is a localized skin disease; septicemia, which is often associated with endocarditis; and a generalized, diffuse cutaneous infection. The incidence of *E. rhusiopathiae* infections is low. Systemic infection is uncommon and rarely develops from erysipeloid. Endocarditis has been seen in patients who have had valve replacements but also in individuals with apparently normal heart valves. Risk factors for endocarditis include having had a previous history of heart disease and/or a history of alcohol abuse. Endocarditis caused by *E. rhusiopathiae* has a 38% mortality rate, and approximately one third of patients who develop endocarditis must get a valve replacement.

Erysipeloid, the most common infection caused by *E. rhusiopathiae* in humans, is a localized skin infection that resembles streptococcal erysipelas. The lesions usually are seen on the hands or fingers because the organisms usually are inoculated through work activities. The incubation period is 2 to 7 days. The infected area is painful and swollen and gives rise to a characteristic lesion—a sharply defined, slightly elevated, purplish-red zone that spreads peripherally as discoloration of the central area fades. Low-grade fever, arthralgia, lymphangiitis, and lymphadenopathy may occur. Erysipeloid is a self-limiting infection that normally heals within 3 to 4 weeks, but may continue for months. Relapses are known to occur. Symptoms can resemble erysipelas caused by *Streptococcus pyogenes*.

The generalized, diffuse cutaneous disease caused by *E. rhusiopathiae* is rare and presents as an exacerbation of the erysipeloid lesion. This cutaneous disease tends to last longer than erysipeloid and also relapses. Antimicrobial therapy is effective for treating *E. rhusiopathiae* infections, with penicillins, cephalosporins, erythromycin, and clindamycin being useful. Penicillin is the drug of choice for both cutaneous and systemic infections.

Laboratory Diagnosis

Microscopy. *Erysipelothrix rhusiopathiae* is a thin, rod-shaped, gram-positive organism that may form long filaments (Figure 16-10). It is arranged singly, in short chains, or in a V shape. The latter arrangement is similar to that seen with the corynebacteria. Also, *E. rhusiopathiae* decolorizes easily, so it may appear gram-variable.

Culture Characteristics. Typical specimens received for the isolation of *E. rhusiopathiae* include tissue biopsy or aspirates from skin lesions. These should be inoculated to a nutrient broth with 1% glucose and incubated in 5% CO_2 at 35° C. The organism will also grow on standard culture media such as SBA and chocolate agar. Subcultures from both should be inoculated daily to SBA plates. On SBA, the colonies are usually nonhemolytic and pinpoint after 24 hours of incubation. A comparison of the colonies of *E. rhusiopathiae* and *L. monocytogenes* is shown in Figure 16-11, *A* and *B*. After 48 hours of incubation, two distinct colony types are seen. A smaller, smooth form is transparent, glistening, and convex with entire edges. The larger, rough colonies are flatter with a matte surface, curled structure, and irregular edges. The colonies often appear α-hemolytic after a few days of growth. In

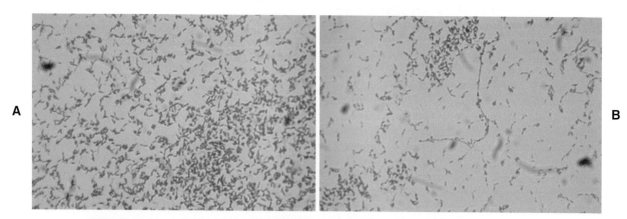

FIGURE 16-10 **A,** Gram stain of *Erysipelothrix rhusiopathiae* at 24 hours. **B,** Gram stain of *E. rhusiopathiae* at 72 hours showing the tendency to form long filaments, which are easily decolorized. (Courtesy Cathy Bissonette.)

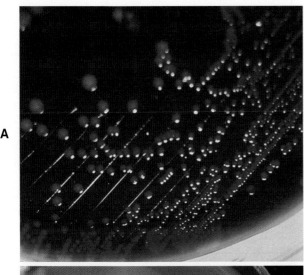

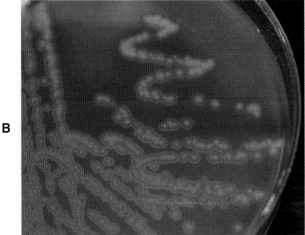

FIGURE 16-11   Comparison of colony morphology of *Listeria* **(A)** and *Erysipelothrix* **(B)** growing on sheep blood agar after 24 hours of incubation. (Courtesy Cathy Bissonette.)

addition, *E. rhusiopathiae* will grow in blood culture media from systemic infections.

Identification. Table 16-3 lists the characteristics of *Erysipelothrix* and similar gram-positive bacilli. A catalase-negative, nonmotile, pleomorphic, aerobic or facultatively anaerobic gram-positive rod that is H_2S-positive is suspicious for *E. rhusiopathiae*. In addition, the organism is urease-negative, Voges-Proskauer-negative, and does not hydrolyze esculin. Growth of *E. rhusiopathiae* in a gelatin stab culture yields a highly characteristic "test tube brush-like" pattern at 22° C.

Arcanobacterium

The genus *Arcanobacterium* contains six species, three of which are medically important: *A. haemolyticum* (formerly *Corynebacterium haemolyticum*), *A. pyogenes*, and *A. bernardiae*. *A. haemolyticum* has been recovered from 10- to 20-year-old patients with pharyngitis and therefore must be distinguished from *C. diphtheriae* and *C. ulcerans* as well as group A *Streptococcus*. Pharyngitis caused by *A. haemolyticum* can be mild or severe and is often clinically indistinguishable from pharyngitis caused by β-hemolytic streptococci. Most patients develop cervical lymphadenopathy, and approximately 50% of patients develop a pruritic, scarlatiniform rash and desquamation of the skin of the hands and feet. In addition, *A. haemolyticum* has been associated with soft tissue infections, sepsis, endocarditis, and other infections.

All three medically relevant *Arcanobacterium* spp. are catalase negative. *A. haemolyticum* produces small colonies on SBA that demonstrate a narrow zone of β-hemolysis after 24 to 48 hours of incubation similar in appearance to the β-hemolytic streptococci (Figure 16-12). Frequently, a black opaque dot is observed on the agar when the colony is scraped away. Pitting of the agar beneath the colony has also been reported. A Gram stain of the isolated colony quickly eliminates the possibility of group A streptococci. Many of the rods are pleomorphic, and some cells may demonstrate rudimentary branching (Figure 16-13). *A. haemolyticum* is both lipase and lecithinase positive. It exhibits a reverse CAMP reaction (CAMP inhibition reaction) because the hemolysis

TABLE 16-3 **Characteristics of *Listeria*, *Corynebacterium*, *Erysipelothrix*, and Other Similar Gram-Positive Bacilli**

Organisms	Catalase Production	Motility	Esculin Hydrolysis	Acid from Glucose	H_2S from TSI Agar	Hemolysis Type	Nitrate Reduction	Urease Production
Corynebacterium spp.	+	−	V	V	−	V	V	V
Listeria monocytogenes	+	+*	+	+	−	β	−	−
Erysipelothrix rhusiopathiae	−	−	−	+	+	None, α	−	−
Arcanobacterium haemolyticum	−	−	−	+	−	β	−	−
Gardnerella vaginalis	−	−	−	+	−	None†	V	+
Rhodococcus spp.	+	−	−	−	−	None	V	+
Rothia dentocariosa	+	−	+	+	−	None	+	−
Oerskovia	+	+	+	+	−	None	V	V

+, Present or positive; −, absent or negative; *V*, variable; *TSI*, triple-sugar iron.
*Motile at 25° C.
†β–Hemolytic on human blood agar, but nonhemolytic on SBA.

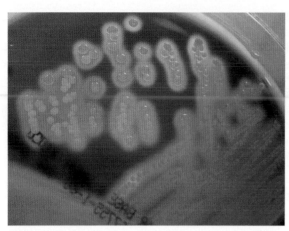

FIGURE 16-12 *Arcanobacterium haemolyticum* growing on sheep blood agar. (Courtesy Steve Mahlen and Amanda Harrington.)

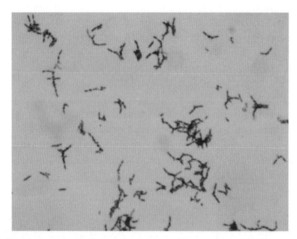

FIGURE 16-13 Gram stain of *Arcanobacterium haemolyticum* from a colony. (Courtesy Steve Mahlen and Amanda Harrington.)

TABLE 16-4 Nugent Scoring System for Gram-Stained Vaginal Smears

Lactobacillus Morphotypes (boxy, gram-positive bacilli)		*Gardnerella* and *Bacteroides* Morphotypes (pleomorphic, gram-variable and gram-negative, short bacilli)		*Mobiluncus* Morphotypes (curved, gram-variable bacilli)	
Quantity	Points	Quantity	Points	Quantity	Points
4+	0	0	0	0	0
3+	1	1+	1		
2+	2	2+	2	1+ to 2+	1
1+	3	3+	3		
0	4	4+	4	3+ to 4+	2

Modified from Nugent RP et al: Reliability of diagnosing bacterial vaginosis is improved by a standardized method of Gram stain interpretation, *J Clin Microbiol* 29:297, 1991.
Interpretation: 0-3, normal vaginal microbiota; 4-6, indeterminate for bacterial vaginosis; 7-10, bacterial vaginosis.

ism can be isolated from as many as 40% of women without BV. More than likely, BV is a polymicrobial disease in which *G. vaginalis* and other bacteria such as *Prevotella* spp., *Peptostreptococcus* spp., *Porphyromonas* spp., *Mobiluncus* spp., *Atopobium vaginae*, and *Mycoplasma hominis* are involved. BV is characterized by a malodorous discharge and vaginal pH greater than 4.5. In general, BV results from a reduction in the *Lactobacillus* population in the vagina, followed by a rise in vaginal pH. This results in overgrowth by *G. vaginalis* and other BV-associated organisms. *G. vaginalis* may also play a role in urinary tract infections in both men and women. The organism has rarely been isolated from other clinical sources such as blood cultures or wounds. The drug of choice to treat BV is metronidazole, although clindamycin is also often used.

Laboratory Diagnosis

Microscopy. *Gardnerella vaginalis*, as described previously, often appears as a pleomorphic, gram-variable coccobacillus or short rod. The cells often stain gram-negative and are 1.5 to 2.5 μm in length. In addition, they can be visualized in wet mounts of vaginal fluid when BV is suspected. The observation of "clue cells," large squamous epithelial cells with gram-positive and gram-variable bacilli and coccobacilli clustered on the edges, aids the diagnosis of BV, particularly if *Lactobacillus* rods are absent in the wet mount. The Nugent scoring system for Gram-stained vaginal smears is a more accurate means of diagnosing BV than cultures (Table 16-4). Stained smears are examined and scored for the presence of *Lactobacillus*, *Gardnerella*, and *Mobiluncus* spp. morphotypes.

Culture Characteristics. Vaginal discharge collected from suspected BV cases is the most common specimen used for the isolation of *G. vaginalis*. Because it is part of the urogenital microbiota, the organism can also be isolated from urine. Because *G. vaginalis* can be found as normal vaginal biota and its role in BV is questionable, cultures for *G. vaginalis* are infrequently performed. It often takes longer than 24 hours to develop visible colonies, and *G. vaginalis* grows best

produced by a β-lysin–producing *S. aureus* is inhibited by a phospholipase D excreted by *A. haemolyticum*. Erythromycin is the drug of choice for treatment; *A. haemolyticum* is penicillin resistant.

Gardnerella vaginalis

General Characteristics

Gardnerella vaginalis is a short, pleomorphic gram-positive rod or coccobacillus that often stains gram-variable or gram-negative. *G. vaginalis* has a gram-positive type of cell wall; however, the peptidoglycan layer is thinner than that found in other gram-positive bacteria, such as *Corynebacterium* and *Lactobacillus*. *G. vaginalis* is the only species in the genus and was first described in 1953. It is found as normal biota in the human urogenital tract.

Clinical Infections

Gardnerella vaginalis is primarily known for its association with **bacterial vaginosis (BV)** in humans. For years *G. vaginalis* was thought to be the only cause of BV. However, the organ-in 5% to 7% CO_2 at a temperature of 35° to 37° C. *G. vaginalis* grows on SBA as pinpoint, nonhemolytic colonies. It will also grow on chocolate agar. The medium of choice for *G. vaginalis*, however, is **human blood bilayer Tween (HBT) agar.** When cultured on human blood, colonies are β-hemolytic, small, gray, and opaque. *G. vaginalis* will also produce β-hemolytic colonies on media made with rabbit blood.

Identification. Table 16-3 lists some key biochemical characteristics of *G. vaginalis* and other gram-positive bacilli. *G. vaginalis* is catalase-negative, oxidase-negative, and hippurate hydrolysis positive. β-Hemolytic colonies on HBT agar should be suspected as *G. vaginalis*. Some laboratories utilize 16S rRNA gene sequencing to definitively identify *G. vaginalis*.

NON–SPORE-FORMING, BRANCHING AEROBIC ACTINOMYCETES

Nocardia

General Characteristics

The organisms in this genus are aerobic, branched, beaded gram-positive bacilli. The beads are not usually spaced at consistent intervals. In many instances, finely beaded, branching rods are a primary clue that a clinical sample contains *Nocardia* spp. Although *Nocardia* spp. are, strictly speaking, gram-positive, organisms may not stain with Gram stain (Figure 16-14, *A*). In addition, *Nocardia* spp. are weakly acid fast, using weak acid as the decolorizer during acid-fast staining (Figure 16-14, *B*). This characteristic is also referred to as modified acid fast positive. The acid-fast stain is used to visualize the mycobacteria and is discussed in Chapter 26.

The colony and microscopic morphology, as well as the types of infections caused, sometimes resemble those of the fungi, but these organisms are true bacteria. *Nocardia* spp. grow on standard nonselective media; however, growth may take a week or more. The taxonomy of the genus is confusing and has been revised greatly in the past decade, based primarily on 16S rRNA gene sequencing. Most *Nocardia* spp. are commonly found in soil, and several have been implicated in human infections. Generally, infections caused by *Nocardia* occur in immunocompromised patients. However, reports of infection in patients with no apparent illness or immunosuppressive therapy are increasing. The most commonly encountered species are *N. asteroides, N. brasiliensis, N. farcinica,* and *N. nova*. Less commonly encountered species include *N. otitidiscaviarum, N. pseudobrasiliensis, N. abscessus, N. africana,* and *N. transvalensis*.

Virulence Factors

The role of factors such as toxins and extracellular proteins in nocardiosis is unclear. No virulence factors have been identified, although virulence has been correlated with alterations in the components in the cell wall. The precise role of the various cell wall molecules in virulence is unknown. Nocardiae produce superoxide dismutase and catalase that may provide resistance to oxidative killing by phagocytes. They

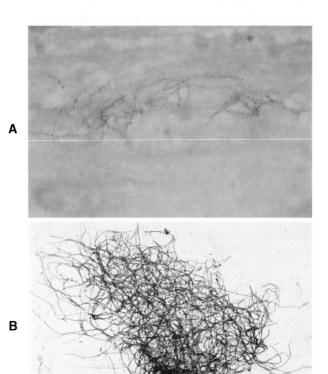

FIGURE 16-14 A, Gram stain of *Nocardia* sp. demonstrating irregular staining. **B,** Acid-fast stain of *Nocardia* showing partially acid-fast appearance. (Courtesy Steve Mahlen and Amanda Harrington.)

also produce an iron-chelating compound called *nocobactin*. A correlation has been reported between the amount of nocobactin produced by the organism and its virulence.

Clinical Infections

Nocardia spp. are found worldwide in soil and on plant material. Infection occurs by two routes: pulmonary and cutaneous. Pulmonary infection by *Nocardia* occurs from the inhalation of the organism present in dust or soil. The disease appears to be associated with impaired host defenses, because most individuals with nocardiae infections have an underlying disease or compromised immune defenses. Even so, approximately 10% of *Nocardia* infections occur in seemingly healthy patients with no obvious immune impairment. Infection with *Nocardia* spp. can be serious. Approximately 40% of the diagnoses are made at autopsy. The mortality rate is high, and those who survive often suffer significant tissue damage.

Pulmonary Infections. The majority of pulmonary infections are caused by the *N. asteroides* complex. The most common manifestation of infection is a confluent bronchopneumonia that is usually chronic but may be acute or relapsing. The disease generally progresses more rapidly than tuberculosis and is measured in months rather than years. In the acute form, which is often seen in patients with underlying immune defects, the time course is a matter of weeks.

The initial lesion in the lung is a focus of pneumonitis that advances to necrosis. The abscesses that form may extend into

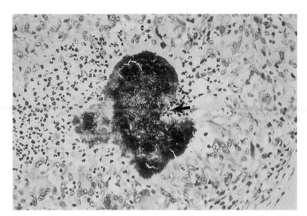

FIGURE 16-15 Appearance of sulfur granule collected from draining sinus tracts. These granules contain masses of filamentous organisms with pus materials.

the tissue and coalesce with each other. Extensive tissue involvement and damage result. Unlike some pneumonias, there is little inflammatory response or scarring, no encapsulation of the abscesses, and no granuloma formation occurs. The sputum is thick and purulent. Unlike infection by the anaerobic actinomycetes, no **sulfur granules** (masses of filamentous organisms bound together by calcium phosphate) or sinus tract formation occurs. Dissemination to other organs, especially the brain, may occur, with reports of involvement of virtually every organ.

Cutaneous Infections. Cutaneous infection occurs following inoculation of the organism into the skin or subcutaneous tissues. *N. brasiliensis* is the most frequent cause of this form of nocardiosis, which is usually seen in the hands and feet as a result of outdoor activity. The trauma most likely is minor, such as from a thorn or wood sliver.

The infection begins as a localized subcutaneous abscess that is invasive and quite destructive of the tissues and underlying bone. These lesions are termed **actinomycotic mycetomas.** Some species of fungi also cause mycetomas; mycetomas caused by bacteria are called *actinomycotic mycetomas,* whereas those caused by fungi are known as **eumycotic mycetomas.** Mycetomas are characterized by swelling, draining sinuses, and granules. About half of the mycetomas seen clinically are caused by the actinomycetes, and the remaining half are caused by fungi. As the infection progresses, burrowing sinuses open to the skin surface and drain pus. The pus may be pigmented and contain "sulfur granules" (Figure 16-15). They often appear yellow or orange and have a distinct granular appearance, hence the term *sulfur granules.*

Laboratory Diagnosis

Microscopy. The gram-positive, beaded branching filaments characteristic of *Nocardia* are often seen in sputum and exudates or aspirates from skin or abscesses. The specimen often contains coccobacillary bodies as well. The beaded appearance of *Nocardia* may be confused by laboratory scientists as chains of gram-positive cocci; however, the beads do not usually touch each other and are not as regular as cocci. Presumptive identification of *Nocardia* can be made based on observation of a filamentous, branching isolate that is par-

tially acid-fast upon staining with carbolfuchsin and decolorizing with a weak acid (0.5% to 1% sulfuric acid) compared with 3% HCl in the stain for mycobacteria. Additional testing is needed for speciation and to distinguish *Nocardia* spp. from *Streptomyces* spp.

Wet mounts should also be performed on clinical specimens. Tissue and pus from the draining sinuses are the specimens of choice for direct examination. Granules may be seen in specimens from cutaneous infection. The granules may be visualized by separating them from the pus with an inoculating needle and then washing in sterile saline. The granules of *N. asteroides, N. brasiliensis,* and *N. otitidiscaviarum* are soft, white to cream colored, and 0.5 to 1 mm in size. They may be crushed between two glass slides to visualize the branching and cellular morphology comprised of gram-positive, thin (0.5 to 1.0 μm in diameter), interwoven filaments. The granules may also be used to inoculate the appropriate growth media. The granules of a eumycotic mycetoma are composed of broad, interwoven, septate hyphae that are wider (2 to 5 μm) than those of actinomycotic mycetoma.

Culture Characteristics. The growth requirements of *Nocardia* spp. are not as well defined as those of many other medically important bacteria. These organisms show an oxidative-type metabolism, and as a genus, they use a wide variety of carbohydrates. They do not require specific growth factors as do *Haemophilus* and *Francisella* spp. *Nocardia* spp. grow well on most common nonselective laboratory media incubated at temperatures between 22° and 37° C, although 3 to 6 days or longer may pass before growth is seen. In fact, *Nocardia* spp. grow on simple media containing a single organic molecule as a source of carbon. Media containing antimicrobial agents used for isolating fungi should not be used because *Nocardia* spp. are susceptible to many of the agents used in these media. Selective media, such as Thayer-Martin, may enhance recovery of *Nocardia* spp. by inhibiting the growth of contaminating organisms. *Nocardia* spp. will grow on the nonselective buffered-charcoal yeast extract (BCYE) agars.

Colonies of *Nocardia* spp. might have a chalky, matte, or velvety appearance and might be pigmented. They can have a dry, crumbly appearance likened to that of breadcrumbs (Figure 16-16). Table 16-5 outlines the colony appearance and tentative identification and differentiation of the aerobic actinomycetes. Examination of colonies with a dissecting microscope may reveal the presence of aerial hyphae. These macroscopic and microscopic phenotypic colony morphologies provide the first clues to the identity of the organism as belonging to the genus *Nocardia.*

Identification. An isolate showing beaded, branching filaments that are gram-positive and partially acid fast should be suspected of belonging to the genus *Nocardia* (see Figure 16-14). Phenotypic tests have been used in identification of clinically relevant *Nocardia.* Methods employed for identification include (1) substrate hydrolysis (casein, tyrosine, xanthine, and hypoxanthine), (2) other substrate and carbohydrate utilization (arylsulfatase, gelatin liquefaction, and carbohydrate utilization), (3) antimicrobial susceptibility profile, and (4) fatty acid analysis by high-performance liquid chromatography. However, the most reliable method for the identifica-

TABLE 16-5 Gram Stain Morphology, Colony Appearance, and Preliminary Grouping of Aerobic Actinomycetes

Genus	Gram Stain Morphology	Colony Appearance on Routine Agar	Partially Acid-Fast	Nitrate	Urea	Lysozyme Resistance
Actinomadura	Moderate, fine, intertwining branching with short chains or spores, fragmentation	White-to-pink pigment, mucoid, molar tooth appearance after 2 weeks', incubation; sparse aerial hyphae	−	+	−	−
Gordonia	Short rods	Somewhat pigmented; *G. sputi* smooth, mucoid, and adherent; *G. bronchialis* dry and raised	±	+	+	−
Mycobacterium	Refractile or nonvisible	Dry, buff colored; some species are pigmented; smooth or rough colonies	Strongly acid-fast	±	±	Not performed
Nocardia	Branching, fine, intertwining, delicate filaments with fragmentation	Extremely variable; some isolates are β-hemolytic on SBA; wrinkled; often dry, chalky-white appearance to orange-tan pigment; crumbly; may produce spores from aerial hyphae	+	+	+	+
Rhodococcus	Diphtheroid-like with minimal branching or coccobacillary; colony growth appears as coccobacilli in "zigzag" configuration	Nonhemolytic; round; often mucoid with orange to red, salmon-pink pigment developing within 4 to 7 days; pigment may vary widely	±	±	±	±
Streptomyces	Extensive branching with chains and spores; does not fragment easily	Glabrous or waxy heaped colonies; variable morphology; wide range of pigmentation from cream to brown-black; white aerial hyphae	−	±	±	−
Tsukamurella	Mostly long bacilli that fragment, no spores or aerial hyphae	May have rhizoid edges, dry, white to creamy to orange	±	−	+	+

Modified from Howard BJ et al, editors: *Clinical and pathogenic microbiology*, St Louis, 1987, Mosby; Conville PS, Witebsky FG: *Nocardia, Rhodococcus, Gordonia, Actinomadura, Streptomyces,* and other aerobic actimomycetes. In Murray PR et al, editors: *Manual of clinical microbiology*, ed 9, Washington DC, 2007, ASM Press.
+, Predominantly positive; −, predominantly negative; ±, predominantly positive with some negative isolates; *SBA*, sheep blood agar.

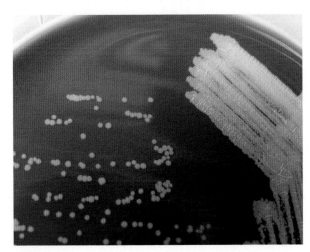

FIGURE 16-16 Colony morphology of *Nocardia* sp. on chocolate agar. (Courtesy Steve Mahlen and Amanda Harrington.)

tion of *Nocardia* spp. is 16S rRNA gene sequencing, which is typically beyond the capabilities of most clinical laboratories. If routine tests used do not result in identification, confirmation of the identity can be confirmed by a reference laboratory with experience in identification of such organisms.

Treatment. Treatment of nocardiosis often involves drainage and surgery along with antimicrobials. The organisms are resistant to penicillin but susceptible to sulfonamides. Antifungal agents, of course, have no activity against *Nocardia* spp. This fact underscores the importance of laboratory diagnosis, because many of the clinical manifestations of pulmonary and cutaneous infection are shared with other organisms, including fungi. The *Nocardia* spp. represent a classic example of a situation in which laboratory results are absolutely essential for proper antimicrobial treatment.

Other Actinomycetes

Actinomadura

The aerobic actinomycetes of clinical importance belonging to the genus *Actinomadura* include *A. madurae* and *A. pelletieri*, formerly classified as members of the genus *Nocardia*. They are etiologic agents of mycetomas, which are identical to those caused by *Nocardia*. The microscopic and colony morphology of *Actinomadura* spp. are very similar to that of the *Nocardia* spp. (see Table 16-5). Differentiation can be made using metabolic variations. *A. madurae* is cellobiose and xylose positive, whereas the *Nocardia* spp. do not produce acid from these two carbohydrates. Treatment parallels that for infections with *Nocardia*.

Streptomyces

The genus *Streptomyces* is a large diverse group of bacteria. *Streptomyces* spp. are primarily saprophytes found as soil inhabitants and resemble the other aerobic actinomycetes with regard to morphology and the diseases they cause. *S. somaliensis* is an established human pathogen associated with actinomycotic mycetoma in many countries. More recently, *S. anulatus* (formerly *S. griseus*) has been increasingly isolated from a number of clinical specimens including sputum, wound, blood, and brain. Table 16-5 compares the colony morphology and metabolic characteristics of *Streptomyces* spp. with those of other members of the aerobic actinomycetes. Isolates from this genus may need to be identified by reference laboratories.

Gordonia

Members of the genus *Gordonia* are aerobic, catalase positive, gram-positive to gram-variable, partially acid fast, and nonmotile. They grow with mycelial forms that fragment into rod-shaped or coccoid elements, hence the term "nocardioform." Members are distinguished from similar organisms by simple biochemical tests. They differ from rapidly growing mycobacteria by their weak acid fastness and the absence of arylsulfatase. They are distinguished from the genus *Nocardia* by their ability to reduce nitrate and the absence of mycelia.

The colony morphology of *Gordonia* spp. varies from slimy, smooth, and glossy to irregular and rough; it may even differ within a single species depending on the medium used for growth. Distinguishing these organisms from the closely related *Rhodococcus* may be difficult due to shared morphological and biochemical features. As is the case with many members of closely related genera, 16s rRNA gene sequencing, and previously fatty acid analysis with high-pressure liquid chromatography have been shown to be reliable for identification of *Gordonia* spp. Such techniques are not available in most laboratories.

Gordonia spp. are typically isolated from environmental sources, but some human infections do occur. So far, reports of human infections are rare in comparison to infections caused by *Rhodococcus* or *Nocardia*. In almost all cases, patients were immunosuppressed after underlying diseases, and infections by *Gordonia* spp. occurred only secondarily. Most reported cases of infections were caused by *G. bronchialis* and included postsurgical sternal wounds, coronary artery infection, and central venous catheters. *Gordonia* spp. are susceptible to several antimicrobial agents including many β-lactams, quinolones, aminoglycosides, macrolides, and other agents active against gram-positive organisms. In absence of clear guidelines, treatment should be guided by susceptibility test results.

Tsukamurella

Similar to related genera, such as *Nocardia*, *Gordonia*, and *Rhodococcus*, members of the genus *Tsukamurella* are gram-positive, aerobic, catalase positive, and partially acid-fast. Because of similar morphologic features, differentiation of these organisms from others and speciation within the genus usually requires extensive physiological, biochemical, and other laboratory tests. 16S rRNA gene sequencing and fatty acid analysis have been used to provide correct identification and speciation.

Several *Tsukamurella* spp. have been reported to cause infections in humans. Most infections reported in the literature have been due to *T. paurametabola* and include chronic lung infection, subcutaneous abscess, cutaneous lesions, catheter-related bacteremia, peritonitis associated with continuous ambulatory peritoneal dialysis, knee prosthesis infection, and conjunctivitis. *Tsukamurella* spp. are generally susceptible to several antimicrobial agents including β-lactams and the aminoglycosides.

Rhodococcus

Rhodococcus equi (formerly *Corynebacterium equi*) is found in soil and causes respiratory tract infections in animals. Human infection is rare, although an increased incidence in immunosuppressed patients, particularly patients with AIDS, has been reported. On Gram stain, *R. equi* may demonstrate filaments, some with branching. *R. equi* may be partially acid-fast or acid-fast. On SBA, the colonies resemble *Klebsiella* and can form a salmon-pink pigment upon prolonged incubation, especially at room temperature. Biochemical identification is difficult because it does not ferment carbohydrates and shows a variable reaction to a number of characteristics (e.g., nitrate reduction, urease). Key features for the identification of *Rhodococcus* is the salmon-pink pigment and a Gram stain showing characteristic diphtheroid gram-positive rods with traces of branching.

Tropheryma whipplei

Tropheryma whipplei is the agent of **Whipple disease**. *T. whipplei* is a facultative intracellular pathogen first identified by PCR from a duodenal biopsy in 1991. Phylogenetic analysis has revealed that *T. whipplei* is a gram-positive actinomycete, most closely related to the genera *Rothia*, *Rhodococcus*, *Arthrobacter*, and *Streptomyces*. *T. whipplei* has been detected in human feces, saliva, and gastric secretions and is apparently ubiquitous in the environment. The organism has been cultivated in stable cell lines and has been adapted to an axenic culture medium supplemented with essential amino acids; however, these techniques are not easily performed in the clinical microbiology laboratory. Typically, *T. whipplei* is identified by PCR or 16S rRNA gene sequencing. In addition, rod-shaped bacteria can be observed in macrophages from infected tissues.

Whipple disease was first described in 1907 and was first successfully treated in the 1950s with antimicrobials. If untreated. this is a uniformly fatal disease, with typical symptoms of diarrhea, weight loss, malabsorption, arthralgia, and abdominal pain. Neurologic and sensory changes often occur.

Whipple disease is more common in middle-aged men. Trimethoprim-sulfamethoxazole is the treatment of choice and must be maintained for at least 1 year for proper treatment. Tetracycline has also been used to treat Whipple disease but has also been associated with serious relapses.

SPORE-FORMING, NONBRANCHING CATALASE-POSITIVE BACILLI

Bacillus

General Characteristics

Members of the genus *Bacillus* stain gram-positive or gram-variable; they are aerobic or facultative anaerobic bacilli that form endospores. There are more than 100 species within the genus, and all are widely distributed in the soil and the environment. Members of the genus *Bacillus* are metabolically diverse, and some species are thermophiles that grow best at 55° C or higher. The survival of *Bacillus* spp. in nature is aided by the formation of spores, which are resistant to conditions to which vegetative cells are intolerant.

Most species grow well on SBA and other commonly used enriched media. Colony characteristics vary considerably among the species and are often influenced by the type of media used. Most species form nonpigmented colonies. They are catalase positive and form endospores under aerobic and anaerobic conditions. Members of the genus *Bacillus* can be confused with aerotolerant strains of the other primary endospore-forming genus, *Clostridium*. *Clostridium* spp. are typically catalase negative, although some strains may form trace amounts. In addition, *Bacillus* spp. form endospores aerobically, whereas *Clostridium* spp. form endospores only anaerobically. The *Bacillus* spp. are divided into groups based on genetic identity and morphologic features. The *B. cereus* group, consisting of *B. anthracis*, *B. cereus*, *B. thuringiensis*, and *B. mycoides*, is the most medically relevant group. The four species in the *B. cereus* group are so closely related genetically that they are considered to be variants of a single species.

Many *Bacillus* spp. are commonly isolated as laboratory contaminants. As such, most laboratories do not identify *Bacillus* spp. to the species level. Several species are described as insect and plant pathogens, and some species are associated with human infections, including *B. anthracis* and *B. cereus*. Robert Koch, in the development of Koch's postulates, showed that *B. anthracis* caused **anthrax** in cattle and helped to prove the germ theory of disease. Historically, *B. anthracis* has been the most important member of this genus; however, anthrax is rarely reported in the United States. Because *B. anthracis* is considered to be a potential bioterrorism agent, it is important for clinical laboratories to rule this organism out when *Bacillus* spp. are isolated.

Bacillus anthracis

Virulence Factors. The virulence of *B. anthracis* depends on a glutamic acid capsule and a three-component protein exotoxin. The genes that code for the toxin and the enzymes responsible for capsule production are carried on plasmids. If a virulent isolate is repeatedly subcultured in vitro, the plasmids can be lost, and the organism is no longer virulent. The capsule, which protects the organism from phagocytosis, is a polypeptide of D-glutamic acid. This particular isomer of glutamic acid is resistant to hydrolysis by host proteolytic enzymes because it is the "unnatural" form of the amino acid. Although the capsule is necessary for virulence, antibodies against the capsule do not confer immunity. Anthrax toxin consists of three proteins called **protective antigen (PA), edema factor (EF),** and **lethal factor (LF),** each of which individually is nontoxic but which together act synergistically to produce damaging effects.

Protective antigen serves as a necessary binding molecule for EF and LF, permitting their attachment to specific receptors on the host cell's surface. The effect of EF and LF is seen when either is combined with PA. Edema results from the combination of PA with EF, whereas death occurs when PA and LF combine. EF is an adenylate cyclase that increases the concentration of cyclic adenosine monophosphate (cAMP) in host cells. LF is a protease that kills host cells by disrupting the transduction of extracellular regulatory signals.

Clinical Infections. Anthrax is a common disease in livestock worldwide when the vaccine is not used. The disease is not spread from animal to animal but rather by animals feeding on plants contaminated with the spores. Humans are infected primarily as a result of accidental or occupational exposure to animals or animal products. Human anthrax in the United States is rare; generally, fewer than three cases per year are reported. In 2006, there was one case of anthrax in the United States, a resident of New York City who acquired the first case of natural inhalation anthrax since 1976. In 2001, however, 11 cases of inhalation and 11 cases of cutaneous anthrax occurred in the United States. Investigations into these cases revealed that they were bioterrorism-related, and a suspect in the case was recently identified. Cases mostly occurred among postal workers as a result of exposure to spore-tainted material (powder in or on envelopes) sent through the mail, although for some cases, the actual source remains unknown. Refer to Chapter 30 for a discussion of *B. anthracis* as an agent of bioterrorism.

Worldwide, however, cases of anthrax number several thousand per year. The disease is enzootic in many parts of the world, including Africa, Central America, and South America. The largest outbreak of largely cutaneous anthrax occurred in Zimbabwe in the early 1980s, with approximately 10,000 cases. A number of names have been given to infections with *B. anthracis*. The majority refer to occupational associations. Terms such as *woolsorter's disease* and *ragpicker's disease* were used to describe infection with the spores of *B. anthracis* as a result of handling contaminated animal fibers, hides, and other animal products. Three forms of anthrax are recognized in humans: cutaneous, inhalation or pulmonary, and gastrointestinal. Infection results from wound contamination, inhalation, or ingestion of spores, which germinate within the host tissue.

Cutaneous Anthrax. Cutaneous anthrax can occur when wounds are contaminated with anthrax spores acquired through skin cuts, abrasions, or insect bites. The overwhelming majority of anthrax cases in the world are cutaneous. In this form of anthrax, a small pimple or papule appears at the site of inoculation 2 to 3 days after exposure. A ring of vesicles develops, and then the vesicles coalesce to form an erythematous ring. A small dark area appears in the center of the ring and eventually ulcerates and dries, forming a depressed black necrotic central area known as an **eschar** or black eschar. The lesion is sometimes referred to as a *malignant pustule,* even though it is not a pustule and is not malignant. The lesion is painless and does not produce pus, unless it becomes secondarily infected with a pyogenic organism. The eschar is normally 1 to 3 cm in diameter, although it may be more extensive. The eschar begins to heal after 1 to 2 weeks. The lesion dries, separates from the underlying base, and falls off, leaving a scar. Usually the infection remains localized, but regional lymphangitis and lymphadenopathy appear. If septicemia occurs, symptoms of fever, malaise, and headache are seen. Normally, in uncomplicated cases, no systemic symptoms are present.

Inhalation Anthrax. Inhalation anthrax, also called **woolsorter's disease,** is acquired when spores are inhaled into the pulmonary parenchyma. The infection begins as a nonspecific illness consisting of mild fever, fatigue, and malaise 2 to 5 days after exposure to the spores. It resembles an upper respiratory tract infection such as that seen with colds and "flu." This initial, mild form of the disease lasts 2 to 3 days. It is followed by a sudden severe phase in which respiratory distress is common. The severe phase of the disease has a high mortality rate. The respiratory problems (dyspnea, cyanosis, pleural effusion) are followed by disorientation, then coma, and death. The course of the severe phase (onset of respiratory symptoms to death) may last only 24 hours.

Gastrointestinal Anthrax. Gastrointestinal anthrax occurs when the spores are inoculated into a lesion on the intestinal mucosa following ingestion of the spores. The symptoms of gastrointestinal anthrax include abdominal pain, nausea, anorexia, and vomiting. Bloody diarrhea may also occur. Because this form of the disease is difficult to diagnose, the fatality rate is higher than in the cutaneous form. Gastrointestinal anthrax accounts for less than 1% of the total cases worldwide; it has never been reported in the United States.

Complications. Approximately 5% of patients with anthrax (cutaneous, inhalation, or gastrointestinal) develop meningitis. The symptoms are typical of any bacterial meningitis and develop rapidly. Unconsciousness and death, if they occur, follow 1 to 6 days after initial exposure. Recovery from infection appears to confer immunity. An effective vaccine is available for those who are at risk for occupational exposure. In addition, vaccines are available for veterinary use.

Laboratory Diagnosis

Microscopy. *Bacillus anthracis* is a large (1.0 to 1.5 μm × 3.0 to 5.0 μm), square-ended, gram-positive or gram-variable rod found singly or in chains (Figure 16-17). When in chains, the ends of the single cells fit snugly together. This, together with the unstained central spore, gives the appearance of bamboo rods. Young cultures stain gram-positive; as the cells become older, or if they are under nutritional stress, they become gram-variable. In Gram stain preparations of clinical samples,

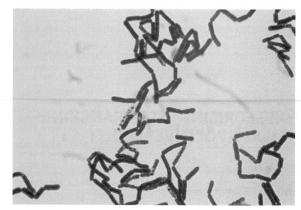

FIGURE 16-17 Gram stain of *Bacillus* sp. (Courtesy Cathy Bissonette.)

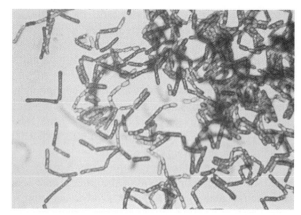

FIGURE 16-18 Spore stain of *Bacillus* sp. Vegetative cells are red; spores are green. (Courtesy Cathy Bissonette.)

vegetative cells can appear with clear zones around the cells, representing the presence of a capsule. The presence of large encapsulated gram-positive rods in the blood is strongly presumptive for *B. anthracis* identification. As the bacteria are subcultured, capsule production will cease. To stimulate capsule production, cultures can be incubated in an atmosphere containing increased CO_2. This is an important characteristic for laboratory identification. The spores are generally not present in clinical samples but can sometimes be seen as unstained areas within the cells. Spores can be observed with a spore stain. With this technique, vegetative cells stain red while the spores stain green (Figure 16-18).

Cultural Characteristics. On SBA, colonies of *B. anthracis* are nonhemolytic, large (2 to 5 mm), gray, and flat with an irregular margin because of outgrowths of long filamentous projections of bacteria that can be seen with a dissecting microscope. The term **Medusa head** has been used to describe the colony morphology of *B. anthracis*. Colonies have a tenacious consistency, holding tightly to the agar surface, and when the edges are lifted with a loop, they stand upright without support. This has been described as having the appearance or characteristic of beaten egg whites. While *B. anthracis* is nonhemolytic on SBA, weak hemolysis may appear under areas of heavy growth after prolonged incuba-

---

TABLE 16-6 Differentiation of *Bacillus anthracis* and *Bacillus cereus*

Characteristic	B. anthracis*	B. cereus*
Hemolysis on sheep blood agar	−	+
Motility	−	+
Penicillin susceptibility	S	R
Lecithinase production	+	+
Fermentation of salicin	−	+/−
Growth in penicillin (10 U/mL) agar	−	+
"String of pearls" reaction	+	−
Gelatin hydrolysis	−	+
Growth on phenylethyl alcohol agar	−	+

Modified from Braude AI et al, editors: *Infectious diseases and medical microbiology*, Philadelphia, 1986, Saunders.
S, Sensitive; *R,* resistant.
*All cultures were incubated at 36° to 37° C.

tion. This should not be confused with β-hemolysis. Many other *Bacillus* spp. are hemolytic.

Because *B. anthracis* would typically be isolated from normally sterile sites, such as blood, lung tissue, and CSF, selective media are not usually needed for recovery. However, it should be noted that while some strains of *B. anthracis* will grow on phenylethyl alcohol (PEA) medium, growth is usually weak. The current CDC level A testing protocol for the presumptive identification of anthrax recommends using PEA agar for stools suspected of containing *B. anthracis*, in addition to SBA and other commonly used media.

Identification. *B. anthracis* is catalase positive and will grow aerobically or anaerobically. It is nonmotile, distinguishing it from most other members of the genus *Bacillus*. Although *B. anthracis* ferments glucose, it fails to ferment mannitol, arabinose, or xylose. *B. anthracis* produces lecithinase; therefore an opaque zone can be seen around colonies growing on egg-yolk agar. This species grows in high salt (7% NaCl) and low pH (<6). Unlike *B. cereus*, *B. anthracis* is generally susceptible to penicillin (10 U/mL). Characteristics important to differentiate *B. anthracis* from the closely related *B. cereus* are listed in Table 16-6.

The CDC and the Association of Public Health Laboratories established the Laboratory Response Network (LRN) in August 1999 to help the public health system be better prepared for chemical and biological attacks. Currently, the LRN consists of three levels: sentinel, reference, and national laboratories. The role of sentinel laboratories is to recognize, rule out, and refer. See Chapter 30 for a discussion of the LRN. In order to rule out *B. anthracis*, the CDC has established basic diagnostic protocols. These protocols include a minimum number of common tests; the protocols can be found on the CDC Web site (emergency.cdc.gov/agent/anthrax/index.asp).

Caution should always be used in working with an isolate suspected of being *B. anthracis*. Work should be performed in a biological safety cabinet, and the area should be disinfected when the work is completed. Approved tests to be performed by sentinel laboratories include Gram stain, colony morphology, catalase, motility, and capsule detection. The Gram stain can be performed directly on clinical specimens or on culture isolates. If the microscopic and colony morphologies of the isolate are compatible with *B. anthracis*, additional tests need to be performed. *B. anthracis* is catalase positive, nonhemolytic, and nonmotile. Motility can be tested by either wet mount preparation or inoculation into motility test medium. Lack of motility is unusual among the *Bacillus* spp.; *B. mycoides* is also nonmotile. Capsule production by *B. anthracis* can be detected by the India ink stain on blood or CSF specimens, or on cells isolated in media supplemented with sodium bicarbonate. As mentioned previously, growth in increased CO_2 also stimulates capsule production.

If the laboratory cannot rule out *B. anthracis*, then the isolate is sent to a reference laboratory, usually a state laboratory, for confirmation. The reference laboratory will likely perform direct fluorescent antibody assays for a cell wall polysaccharide and a capsule antigen. The presence of both antigens is confirmation for *B. anthracis*. Antimicrobial susceptibility testing will be performed by reference or national laboratories. A test of historical importance is performed by inoculating the suspected isolate onto agar containing penicillin (0.05 to 0.5 U/mL). After incubation for 3 to 6 hours at 37° C, the areas of inoculation are examined microscopically for the presence of large spherical bacilli in chains. This phenomenon is referred to as a "string of pearls." Species identification of bacilli can be accomplished by the combined use of the API 20E and 50CH systems (bioMérieux, Inc., Hazelwood, Mo). Nucleic acid amplification tests have been developed, but such applications for diagnosis and identification of *B. anthracis* remain useful in special situations and at specialized laboratories.

Treatment. Most isolates of *B. anthracis* are susceptible to penicillin, but resistance can occur due to β-lactamase production; thus penicillin should not be used alone in treatment. The organism is often susceptible to many broad-spectrum antimicrobial agents including gentamicin, erythromycin, tetracycline, and chloramphenicol. In 2000, ciprofloxacin was approved by the U.S. Food and Drug Administration for management of postexposure inhalation anthrax based on data from animal models. According to the CDC recommendations and based on studies in nonhuman primates and other animal and in vitro data, ciprofloxacin or doxycycline should be used for initial intravenous therapy until antimicrobial susceptibility results are known. Current recommendations for initial therapy of pulmonary and cutaneous anthrax include ciprofloxacin or doxycycline plus one or two additional antimicrobial agents depending on disease severity. In addition, the CDC recommends oral treatment with either ciprofloxacin or doxycycline for postexposure prophylaxis for pulmonary anthrax.

Bacillus cereus

Bacillus cereus is a relatively common cause of food poisoning and opportunistic infections in susceptible hosts. Food poisoning caused by *B. cereus* takes two forms: diarrheal and emetic. The diarrheal syndrome, usually associated with ingestion of meat or poultry, is characterized by an incuba-

TABLE **16-7** Comparison of Enterotoxins Produced by *Bacillus cereus*

	Type of Enterotoxin	
Characteristic	Diarrheal	Emetic
Clinical syndrome		
Incubation period	8 to 16 hours	1 to 5 hours
Diarrhea	Very common	Fairly common
Vomiting	Occasional	Very common
Duration of illness	12 to 24 hours	6 to 24 hours
Foods implicated	Meat products, soups, vegetables, puddings, sauces	Fried or boiled rice
Enterotoxin		
Molecular weight	ca. 50,000	<5000
Stability to heat	−	+
Fluid accumulation in ligated rabbit ileal segment	+	−
Increases vascular permeability in guinea pig or rabbit skin	+	−
Lethal for mice after intravenous injection	+	−
Stimulation of adenylate cyclase–cAMP system in intestinal epithelial cells	+	−
Response when fed to rhesus monkey	Diarrhea	Vomiting

Modified from Braude AI et al, editors: *Infectious diseases and medical microbiology*, Philadelphia, 1986, Saunders.
cAMP, Cyclic adenosine monophosphate.

tion period of 8 to 16 hours. Afflicted individuals suffer abdominal pain and diarrhea. About 25% of individuals experience vomiting; fever is uncommon. The average duration of the illness is 24 hours. The diarrheal form is clinically indistinguishable from the diarrhea caused by *Clostridium perfringens*.

The emetic form has the predominant symptoms of abdominal cramps and vomiting. Diarrhea is present in about one third of those affected. This form has been associated with ingestion of fried rice, particularly when prepared in Asian restaurants. The average duration of the illness is 9 hours. For both the diarrheal and emetic forms of *B. cereus* food poisoning, the illness is usually mild and self-limiting. The two forms of illness are caused by two distinct enterotoxins. A comparison of the enterotoxins is shown in Table 16-7.

Bacillus cereus is similar to *B. anthracis* in many ways—morphologically and metabolically. Differentiation of the two species is outlined in Table 16-6. *B. cereus* can be grown aerobically at 37° C on SBA. A β-hemolytic frosted glass–appearing colony (Figure 16-19) containing spore-forming, gram-positive bacilli that are motile, able to ferment salicin, and lecithinase positive is likely *B. cereus*. *B. cereus* is biochemically identical to *B. thuringiensis*, except that *B. thuringiensis*, an insect pathogen, typically produces parasporal crystals that can be observed by phase-contrast microscopy or by spore staining.

Culture of suspected food from a food poisoning incident may be done to quantify and isolate *B. cereus*. If more than 10^5 *B. cereus* cells per gram of food are present and other pathogens are absent, then food poisoning by this organism is confirmed. Although the organism can be part of the normal fecal biota, the stool of patients with food poisoning may also be examined for *B. cereus*. To confirm the organism

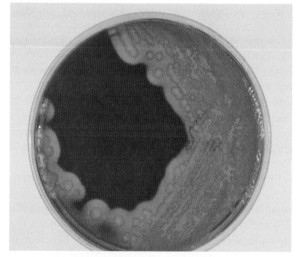

FIGURE 16-19 *Bacillus cereus* on sheep blood agar. (Courtesy Cathy Bissonette.)

as the cause of the disease, viable counts from the stool should also be at least 10^5 cells per gram. Because *B. cereus* may be found in small numbers in a significant proportion of healthy people, quantitative cultures must be done.

B. cereus eye infections are the most common type of nongastrointestinal infection caused by this organism; these include endophthalmitis, panophthalmitis, and keratitis with abscess formation. *B. cereus* infection in penetrating ocular trauma cases is nearly always associated with a poor visual outcome. This organism has also been documented as a cause of meningitis, septicemia, endocarditis, osteomyelitis, and a number of other types of infections. Although rare, these serious, nongastrointestinal infections occur more frequently in intravenous drug abusers, neonates, and immunosuppressed and postsurgical patients. In addition, there have been a few reports of *B. cereus* strains carrying the *B. anthracis* toxin genes. In these cases, *B. cereus* caused severe pneumonia clinically similar to pulmonary anthrax.

Most food poisoning cases caused by *B. cereus* do not require antimicrobial treatment. However, treatment, may be indicated in other *B. cereus* infections. Unlike *B. anthracis*, *B. cereus* is resistant to penicillin and all of the other β-lactam antibiotics except for the carbapenems. Treatment with vancomycin or clindamycin with or without an aminoglycoside has been successful.

Other *Bacillus* Species

Infections by other members of the genus are rare; these include, but are not limited to, infections caused by *B. subtilis, B. licheniformis, B. circulans, B. pumilus,* and *B. sphaericus.* These organisms have been reported to cause food poisoning, bacteremia, meningitis, pneumonia, and other infections. They are more commonly seen, however, as contaminants.

BIBLIOGRAPHY

Arenskötter M et al: Biology of the metabolically diverse genus *Gordonia, Appl Environ Microbiol* 70:3195, 2004.

Avashia SB et al: Fatal pneumonia among metalworkers due to inhalation exposure to *Bacillus cereus* containing *Bacillus anthracis* toxin genes, *Clin Infect Dis* 44:414, 2007.

Bernard K: *Corynebacterium* species and coryneforms: an update on taxonomy and diseases attributed to these taxa, *Clin Microbiol Newsl* 27:9, 2005.

Bernard K et al: Characteristics of rare or recently described *Corynebacterium* species recovered from human clinical material in Canada, *J Clin Microbiol* 40:4375, 2002.

Bille J: *Listeria* and *Erysipelothrix.* In Murray PR et al, editors: *Manual of clinical microbiology,* ed 9, Washington, DC, 2007, ASM Press.

Brown-Elliott BA et al: Clinical and laboratory features of the *Nocardia* spp. based on current molecular taxonomy, *Clin Microbiol Rev* 19:259, 2006.

Brouqui P, Rauoult D: Endocarditis due to rare and fastidious bacteria, *Clin Microbiol Rev* 14:177, 2001.

Centers for Disease Control and Prevention: Approved tests for the identification of *Bacillus anthracis* in the laboratory response network (LRN). Available at: www.bt.cdc.gov/agent/anthrax/labtesting/approvedlrntests.asp. Accessed September 1, 2008.

Centers for Disease Control and Prevention: Diphtheria epidemic—new independent states of the former Soviet Union, 1990-1994, *MMWR* 44:177, 1995. Available at www.cdc.gov/mmwr/preview/mmwrhtml/00036527.htm. Accessed September 22, 2008.

Centers for Disease Control and Prevention: Fatal respiratory diphtheria in a U.S. traveler to Haiti—Pennsylvania, 2003, *MMWR* 52:1285, 2004. Available at www.cdc.gov/mmwr/preview/mmwrhtml/mm5253a3.htm. Accessed September 22, 2008.

Cockerill FR 3rd, Smith TF: Response of the clinical microbiology laboratory to emerging (new) and reemerging infectious diseases, *J Clin Microbiol* 42:2359, 2004.

Conville PS, Witebsky FG: *Nocardia, Rhodococcus, Gordonia, Actinomadura, Streptomyces,* and other aerobic actinomycetes. In Murray PR et al, editors: *Manual of clinical microbiology,* ed 9, Washington, DC, 2007, ASM Press.

Corti ME, Villafane-Fioti MF: Nocardiosis: a review, *Int J Infect Dis* 7:243, 2003.

Funke G, Bernard KA: Coryneform gram-positive rods. In Murray PR et al, editors: *Manual of clinical microbiology,* ed 9, Washington, DC, 2007, ASM Press.

Jernigan DB et al: Investigation of bioterrorism-related anthrax, United States, 2001: epidemiologic findings, *Emerg Infect Dis* 8:1019, 2002. Available at www.cdc.gov/ncidod/EID/vol8no10/02-0353.htm. Accessed September 22, 2008.

Lederman ER, Crum NF: A case series and focused review of nocardiosis: clinical and microbiologic aspects, *Medicine (Baltimore)* 83:300, 2004.

Limjoco-Antonio et al: *Arcanobacterium haemolyticum* sinusitis and orbital cellulites, *Pediatr Infect Dis J* 22:465, 2003.

Logan NA et al: *Bacillus* and other aerobic endospore-forming bacteria. In Murray PR et al, editors: *Manual of clinical microbiology,* ed 9, Washington, DC, 2007, ASM Press.

Meyerhoff A et al: US Food and Drug Administration approval of ciprofloxacin hydrochloride for management of postexposure inhalational anthrax, *Clin Infect Dis* 39:303, 2004.

Mohammed MJ et al: Antimicrobial susceptibility testing of *Bacillus anthracis*: comparison of results obtained by using the National Committee for Clinical Laboratory Standards broth microdilution reference and Etest agar gradient diffusion methods, *J Clin Microbiol* 40:1902, 2002.

National Committee for Clinical Laboratory Standards: *Susceptibility testing of mycobacteria, nocardiae, and other aerobic actinomycetes*; M24-A, Wayne, Pa, National Committee for Clinical Laboratory Standards, 2003.

Oncu S et al: Anthrax—an overview, *Med Sci Monit* 9:RA276, 2003.

Patel JB et al: Sequence-based identification of aerobic actinomycetes, *J Clin Microbiol* 42:2530, 2004.

Ross MJ et al: *Corynebacterium jeikeium* native valve endocarditis following femoral access for coronary angiography, *Clin Infect Dis* 32:e120, 2001.

Saubolle MA, Sussland D: Nocardiosis: review of clinical and laboratory experience, *J Clin Microbiol* 41:4497, 2003.

Schneider T et al: Whipple's disease: new aspects of pathogenesis and treatment, *Lancet Infect Dis* 8:179, 2008.

Siegman-Igra Y et al: *Listeria monocytogenes* infection in Israel and review of cases worldwide, *Emerg Infect Dis* 8:305, 2002. Available at: www.cdc.gov/ncidod/EID/vol8no3/01-0166.htm. Accessed December 2, 2009.

Smith H: Discovery of the anthrax toxin: the beginning of studies of virulence determinants regulated in vivo, *Int J Med Microbiol* 291:411, 2002.

Vazquez-Boland JA et al: *Listeria* pathogenesis and molecular virulence determinants, *Clin Microbiol Rev* 14:584, 2001.

Points to Remember

- *Corynebacterium diphtheriae* causes serious disease in populations for which the diphtheria vaccine is not available.
- *Listeria monocytogenes* can be differentiated from streptococci and enterococci on the basis of Gram stain morphology, catalase reaction, and motility.
- *Erysipelothrix rhusiopathiae* differs from *L. monocytogenes* in catalase reaction, H₂S production, and its lack of ability to grow at 4° C.
- *Arcanobacterium haemolyticum* can be differentiated from other non–spore-forming gram-positive bacilli and β-hemolytic streptococci by Gram stain morphology, catalase activity, and the CAMP inhibition reaction.
- *Gardnerella vaginalis* is part of the normal biota of the urogenital tract. It is weakly β-hemolytic on HBT agar and stains as a gram-variable rod.
- The aerobic actinomycetes are generally soil inhabitants. They are weak pathogens sometimes associated with wounds following traumatic implantation into subcutaneous tissue.
- *Nocardia* spp. are gram-positive filamentous organisms that can grow on nutritionally simple media and are partially acid fast.
- *Tsukamurella* and other related organisms, such as *Streptomyces*, *Gordonia*, and *Rhodococcus*, have similar morphologic features.
- Differentiation or speciation of the actinomycetes usually requires 16s rRNA gene sequencing to provide accurate identification and speciation of the actinomycetes but is not available in most laboratories.
- Members of the genus *Bacillus* are aerobic, gram-positive, catalase positive, rod-shaped organisms that form endospores.
- Many of the aerobic gram-positive spore-forming bacilli are rarely associated with human infections. The most important pathogen in this group is *Bacillus anthracis*.
- *B. anthracis* is generally susceptible to penicillin and is nonmotile and nonhemolytic on sheep blood agar features important to differentiate the organism from *B. cereus*.
- *B. cereus* is a common cause of food poisoning and opportunistic infections. Food poisoning caused by *B. cereus* takes two forms: diarrheal and emetic.

Learning Assessment Questions

1. An isolate with the appropriate colony and microscopic morphology may be suspected of being *Bacillus anthracis* if it is:
   a. β-Hemolytic on sheep blood agar
   b. Nonmotile
   c. Catalase negative
   d. Gram-negative, non–spore former

2. An aerobic, gram-positive, spore-forming bacillus was isolated from raw vegetables that were associated with an outbreak of gastroenteritis. The organism produced β-hemolysis, was catalase positive, and was motile. The most likely organism is:
   a. *Bacillus anthracis*
   b. *Nocardia asteroides*
   c. *Bacillus cereus*
   d. *Tsukamurella* spp.

3. Describe the appearance of spore-forming bacteria seen with the spore stain.

4. The biochemical tests performed on a gram-positive bacillus were consistent with *Corynebacterium diphtheriae*. As a definitive test, the laboratory scientist should now:
   a. Perform an Elek test to determine whether the organism produces exotoxin.
   b. Subculture the organism to cystine-tellurite agar and examine for black colonies.
   c. Prepare a methylene blue stain and examine for metachromatic granules.
   d. Gram stain the isolate and observe for its pleomorphic morphology.

5. A commercial fisherman who was complaining of red sores on his hands was seen by his physician. One of the lesions was biopsied and cultured. The culture grew an organism with the following characteristics:
   - Nonhemolytic on sheep blood agar
   - Gram-positive bacilli, no spores observed
   - Catalase negative
   - H₂S production positive
   - Growth in gelatin resembled a test-tube brush
   This organism is most likely:
   a. *Rhodococcus equi*
   b. *Listeria monocytogenes*
   c. *Lactobacillus acidophilus*
   d. *Erysipelothrix rhusiopathiae*

6. Which phenotypic test is **not** useful for the identification and differentiation of *Nocardia* and aerobic actinomycetes?
   a. Casein hydrolysis
   b. Spore test
   c. Fatty acid analysis by HPLC
   d. Antimicrobial susceptibility profile

7. What other organisms may give similar clinical and laboratory findings as *Listeria monocytogenes*? How are these organisms differentiated from *L. monocytogenes*?

8. A 17-year-old male is admitted to the minor medical clinic with a history of multiple episodes of febrile pharyngitis followed in 10 to 14 days with extensive desquamation of his hands and feet. The reoccurrences have followed several courses of antimicrobial therapy including amoxicillin and cephalosporins. Both rapid group A *Streptococcus* screens and cultures have been consistently negative for *Streptococcus pyogenes*. A specimen with a request for an alternative agent was

submitted to a reference laboratory. The following results were observed:

- SBA: dry, wrinkled, slightly hemolytic colony, which at 48 hours is a dark spot sunken in the agar
- Catalase negative
- Nitrate negative
- Reverse CAMP test positive

The patient was subsequently treated with erythromycin, and he recovered. The etiologic agent was identified as:

a. *Corynebacterium diphtheriae*
b. *Arcanobacterium haemolyticum*
c. *Listeria monocytogenes*
d. *Rhodococcus equi*

9. *Bacillus cereus* is most noted for causing:
a. Food poisoning
b. Meningitis
c. Sexually transmitted disease
d. Urinary tract infections

10. A sample is sent to the laboratory from a female patient suspected of having bacterial vaginosis. Which of the following would be an appropriate medium for this specimen?
a. Loeffler medium
b. Human blood bilayer Tween agar
c. Cystine-tellurite blood agar
d. Buffered charcoal yeast extract agar

Neisseria Species and Moraxella catarrhalis

Karen S. Long, George Manuselis

■ **GENERAL CHARACTERISTICS**

■ **PATHOGENIC *NEISSERIA* SPECIES**
  Neisseria gonorrhoeae
  Neisseria meningitidis
  Moraxella catarrhalis

■ **NONPATHOGENIC *NEISSERIA* SPECIES**
  Identification
  Neisseria cinerea

Neisseria flavescens
Neisseria lactamica
Neisseria mucosa
Neisseria polysaccharea
Neisseria sicca
Neisseria subflava
Neisseria elongata
Neisseria weaveri

OBJECTIVES

After reading and studying this chapter, you should be able to:

1. List the general characteristics of the genus *Neisseria*.

2. Discuss the function of pili (fimbriae) and polysaccharide capsules as virulence factors of pathogenic *Neisseria* species.

3. Compare and contrast gonorrhea in male and female patients.

4. Discuss potential complications of asymptomatic gonococcal infections in women.

5. Define and discuss ophthalmia neonatorum.

6. Discuss specimen collection, transport, and processing for *N. gonorrhoeae* culture.

7. Compare and contrast the usefulness of the direct Gram stain in the diagnosis of gonorrhea in men and women.

8. List two selective media for *N. gonorrhoeae* and *N. meningitidis* and describe their components.

9. Compare nonculture detection methods available for the identification of *N. gonorrhoeae*.

10. Develop an identification flowchart (algorithm) for the identification of the pathogenic *Neisseria*.

11. Discuss criteria required for identification of *N. gonorrhoeae* in sexual abuse cases.

12. Discuss modes of antimicrobial resistance in *N. gonorrhoeae* isolates and current recommendations for therapy.

13. List risk groups for epidemic meningococcal meningitis and discuss the usefulness of the meningococcal vaccine.

14. Discuss the clinical findings in meningococcemia.

15. Discuss the pathogenic significance of *Moraxella catarrhalis* in children and adults.

16. Differentiate between the pathogenic and nonpathogenic *Neisseria* spp.

Case in Point

An 18-year-old, sexually active college student on the women's gymnastics team visited student health services complaining of pain, redness, and swelling of both wrist joints and the left elbow. She gave a history of casual, unprotected sexual intercourse with "three or four" men during the past 4 months. She denied any vaginal discharge or abdominal pain, but recalled having had a rash recently on both her arms. An aspirate from the left wrist was sent to the laboratory for culture and Gram stain. The direct smear stain of the aspirate was reported as

"Several polymorphonuclear white blood cells, several intracellular and extracellular gram-negative diplococci seen." The fluid was plated to sheep blood agar (SBA), chocolate (CHOC) agar, MacConkey agar, and CDC anaerobic blood agar and incubated appropriately. At 24 hours, many small, tan colonies were visible on the CHOC agar, with no growth on sheep blood, CDC anaerobic, or MacConkey agars. The β-lactamase test on the organism was negative. The organism was identified according to routine laboratory protocol.

Issues to Consider

After reading the patient's case history, consider:
- The identity of the organism causing the patient's infection
- Risk factors for acquisition of the organism
- Types and consequences of sequelae of untreated primary infection in females and males
- Importance of definitive identification of the microorganism

Key Terms

Capnophilic

Fitz-Hugh-Curtis syndrome

Gonorrhea

Ophthalmia neonatorum

Pelvic inflammatory disease (PID)

Penicillinase-producing *Neisseria gonorrhoeae* (PPNG)

Waterhouse-Friderichsen syndrome

The family Neisseriaceae currently contains the genus *Neisseria,* as well as *Kingella, Eikenella, Simonsiella,* and *Alysiella. Moraxella catarrhalis* is in the family Moraxellaceae with other *Moraxella* spp. and *Acinetobacter.* Because of its similarities to the *Neisseria, M. catarrhalis* is included in this chapter. Characteristics of the family Neisseriaceae and differential characteristics of these genera are shown in Figure 17-1. At present, the genus *Neisseria* contains 12 species and biovars that can be isolated from humans. This chapter discusses only the morphologically and biochemically similar *Neisseria* spp. and *M. catarrhalis.* The genera *Eikenella* and *Kingella* are discussed in Chapter 18.

GENERAL CHARACTERISTICS

Essentially all *Neisseria* spp. are aerobic, nonmotile, non–spore-forming, cytochrome oxidase- and catalase-positive, gram-negative diplococci. *Neisseria elongata,* which is catalase negative and rod shaped, and *Neisseria weaveri,* which is catalase positive and rod shaped, are the only known exceptions to being gram-negative diplococci. Many *Neisseria* spp. are **capnophilic,** requiring CO_2 for growth, and have optimal growth in a humid atmosphere. They can grow anaerobically if alternate electron acceptors (e.g., nitrites) are available. The natural habitat of *Neisseria* spp. is the mucous membranes of the respiratory and urogenital tracts. Table 17-1 shows the pathogenicity and host range of *Neisseria* spp. and *M. catarrhalis.*

N. gonorrhoeae and *N. meningitidis* are the primary human pathogens of the genus. *N. gonorrhoeae* is always pathogenic. It is not considered to be part of the normal biota, but *N. meningitidis* may be found as a commensal inhabitant of the upper respiratory tract of carriers. Pathogenic *Neisseria* spp. are fastidious organisms, requiring enriched media for optimal recovery. Both *N. gonorrhoeae* and *N. meningitidis* require iron for growth. They compete with their human hosts by binding human host transferrin to their specific surface receptors.

Their ability to bind transferrin may be a primary reason that they are strict human pathogens. *N. weaveri,* which is a commensal in the upper respiratory tract of dogs, has been isolated from dog bites in humans. All other *Neisseria* spp. are considered opportunistic pathogens. These opportunists must be recognized and differentiated from *N. gonorrhoeae* and *N. meningitidis* in isolates from clinical specimens.

PATHOGENIC *NEISSERIA* SPECIES

Neisseria gonorrhoeae

Humans are the only natural host for *N. gonorrhoeae,* the agent of **gonorrhea.** Gonorrhea is an acute pyogenic infection of nonciliated columnar and transitional epithelium; infection may be established at any site where these cells are found. Gonococcal infections are primarily acquired by sexual contact and occur primarily in the urethra, endocervix, anal canal, pharynx, and conjunctiva. Disseminated infections from the primary site may also occur, as seen in the Case in Point.

The first use of the term *gonorrhea,* meaning a "flow of seed," was in the second century when the urethral discharge was mistaken for semen. For centuries thereafter, the diseases syphilis and gonorrhea were confused because the two were often present together in the same infected individual; this still occurs. In 1530, it was thought that gonorrhea was an early symptom of syphilis. The issue was further confused in 1767 because of a classic blunder by a physician who inoculated himself intentionally with pus from a patient with symptoms of gonorrhea. The pus gave the physician syphilis instead. Gonorrhea was also called the "clap" from the French word *clapoir* meaning "brothel."

Virulence Factors

The pathogenic *Neisseria* spp. have several characteristics that contribute to their virulence, including the following:
- Receptors for human transferrin
- Capsule
- Pili (fimbriae)
- Cell membrane proteins
- Lipooligosaccharide (LOS) or endotoxin; lipid A moiety and core LOS that differentiates it from the lipopolysaccharide (LPS) found in most gram-negative bacilli and is loosely attached to the underlying peptidoglycan
- Immunoglobulin A (IgA) protease that cleaves IgA on mucosal surfaces

N. gonorrhoeae is divided into five morphologically distinct colony types. Types T1 through T5 are based on the presence or absence of pili, the fine hairlike projections that are important in the initial attachment of the organism to host tissues. Pili also inhibit phagocytosis of the organism by neutrophils and aid in the exchange of genetic material between cells. Types T1 and T2, which possess pili, are virulent forms, whereas T3 through T5, devoid of pili, are avirulent strains. Piliated organisms usually predominate when first isolated from uncomplicated urogenital tract infections, but on subculture, pili are lost and colony types T3 through T5 appear.

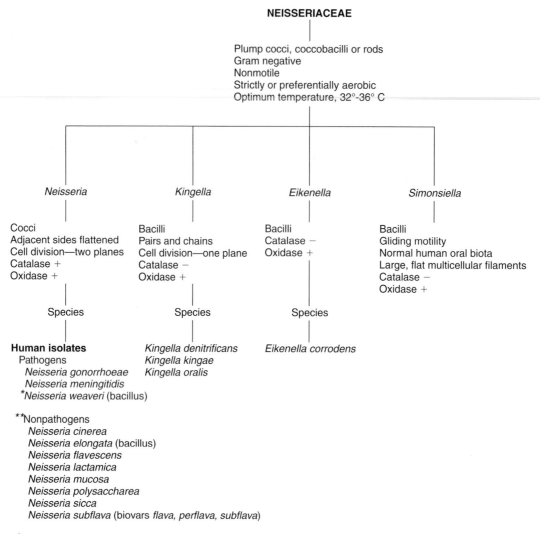

NEISSERIACEAE

Plump cocci, coccobacilli or rods
Gram negative
Nonmotile
Strictly or preferentially aerobic
Optimum temperature, 32°-36° C

| *Neisseria* | *Kingella* | *Eikenella* | *Simonsiella* |

Neisseria
Cocci
Adjacent sides flattened
Cell division—two planes
Catalase +
Oxidase +

Kingella
Bacilli
Pairs and chains
Cell division—one plane
Catalase −
Oxidase +

Eikenella
Bacilli
Catalase −
Oxidase +

Simonsiella
Bacilli
Gliding motility
Normal human oral biota
Large, flat multicellular filaments
Catalase −
Oxidase +

Species

Human isolates
Pathogens
  Neisseria gonorrhoeae
  Neisseria meningitidis
  Neisseria weaveri (bacillus)

**Nonpathogens
  Neisseria cinerea
  Neisseria elongata (bacillus)
  Neisseria flavescens
  Neisseria lactamica
  Neisseria mucosa
  Neisseria polysaccharea
  Neisseria sicca
  Neisseria subflava (biovars *flava, perflava, subflava*)

Species

Kingella denitrificans
Kingella kingae
Kingella oralis

Species

Eikenella corrodens

*Normal oral biota of dogs, wounds from dog bites. **May cause opportunistic infections in human hosts.

FIGURE 17-1 Characteristics of the family and the six genera. *Moraxella catarrhalis,* although morphologically and biochemically similar to the *Neisseria* spp., is no longer a member of the family Neisseriaceae, so it is not included here.

TABLE 17-1 Pathogenicity and Host Range for Species of *Neisseria* and *Moraxella*

Species	Pathogenicity	Infected Host
N. gonorrhoeae	Primary pathogen	Humans only
N. meningitidis	Primary pathogen	Humans only
N. lactamica	Opportunistic pathogen	Warm-blooded animals
N. sicca	Opportunistic pathogen	Warm-blooded animals
N. subflava	Opportunistic pathogen	Warm-blooded animals
N. mucosa	Opportunistic pathogen	Warm-blooded animals
N. flavescens	Opportunistic pathogen	Warm-blooded animals
N. cinerea	Opportunistic pathogen	Warm-blooded animals
N. polysaccharea	Opportunistic pathogen	Warm-blooded animals
N. elongata	Opportunistic pathogen	Warm-blooded animals
M. catarrhalis	Opportunistic pathogen	Humans only

The capsule, cell outer membrane proteins I, II, and III, and the LOS not only serve as protective devices of the organism but are also important in antigenic variation. Moreover, the LOS endotoxin is a major in vivo virulence factor that mediates damage to body tissues and elicits the inflammatory response. The organism releases outer membrane fragments called "blebs." During periods of rapid growth, these blebs contain LOS. The major outer membrane porin protein (Por), or protein I, forms channels for nutrients to pass into and waste products to exit the cell. They are coded for by two genes: *por*A and *por*B. Both genes are expressed in *N. meningitidis,* but only *por*B is expressed in *N. gonorrhoeae.* PorB is also protective against the host's inflammatory response and serum complement mediated killing. Protein II (Opa, for opacity) is a group of proteins that facilitate the adherence to phagocytic and epithelial cells. Protein III (reduction modified protein [Rmp]) blocks host serum bactericidal (IgG) action against the organism. A schematic diagram of the cellular structure of *N. gonorrhoeae* is shown in Figure 17-2.

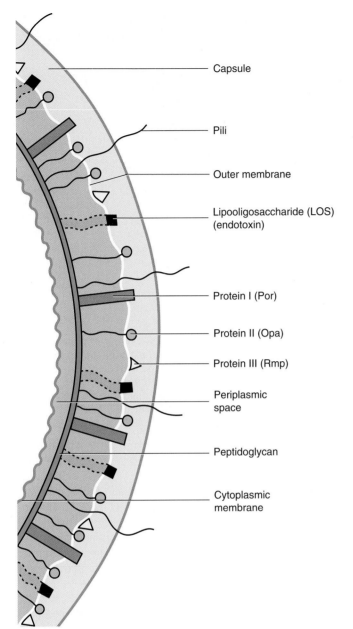

FIGURE 17-2 Cellular structure of *Neisseria gonorrhoeae*.

Capsule

Pili

Outer membrane

Lipooligosaccharide (LOS) (endotoxin)

Protein I (Por)

Protein II (Opa)

Protein III (Rmp)

Periplasmic space

Peptidoglycan

Cytoplasmic membrane

Epidemiology

Neisseria gonorrhoeae infections are most commonly transmitted by sexual contact. The primary reservoir is the asymptomatic carrier. Gonorrhea is a national reportable disease; therefore all culture confirmed cases must be reported to state health laboratories. Gonorrhea is second to *Chlamydia trachomatis* in the number of confirmed sexually transmitted bacterial infections in the United States. However, human papillomavirus (HPV), is estimated to be the most common cause of sexually transmitted disease in the United States. There were 355,991 cases of gonorrhea reported in 2007, an increase of 6% from the previous year. Actual numbers of infected individuals are probably much higher than reported, due to a large reservoir of asymptomatic carriers and other unreported cases. Reported cases increased steadily through

the 1960s and 1970s, but declined steadily through the mid-1980s and 1990s. As noted earlier, cases have risen in the past few years; sexually active teens and young adults have the highest rates of infection. In women, most cases are seen in ages 15 to 19 years; the highest rates in men occur in the ages 20 to 24 years. Overall, the highest rates are seen in the southeastern United States and in high-density, urban areas where individuals are more likely to have multiple partners and unprotected sexual intercourse.

Clinical Infections

Gonorrhea has a short incubation period of approximately 2 to 7 days. In men, acute urethritis, usually resulting in purulent discharge and dysuria (painful urination), is the common manifestation. Asymptomatic gonococcal infection in men is uncommon; only 3% to 5% of cases may be asymptomatic, whereas 95% show acute infections. *N. gonorrhoeae* strains with a nutritional requirement for arginine, hypoxanthine, and uracil (AHU strains) are often isolated from asymptomatic men. Complications in males include ascending infections such as prostatitis and epididymitis.

The endocervix is the most common site of infection in women, resulting in cervical discharge and dysuria; however, as many as 50% of cases in women may be asymptomatic. Symptoms of infection, when present, include dysuria, cervical discharge, and lower abdominal pain. Untreated gonococcal cervicitis is a major cause of **pelvic inflammatory disease (PID)** in women, which may cause sterility, ectopic pregnancy, or perihepatitis **(Fitz-Hugh-Curtis syndrome).**

Blood-borne dissemination of *N. gonorrhoeae* occurs in less than 1% of all infections, resulting in purulent arthritis and rarely septicemia. The organism will not be recovered from routine blood cultures, however, because growth of *N. gonorrhoeae* is inhibited by sodium polyanethol sulfonate, the anticoagulant in blood culture media. Fever and a rash on the extremities may also be present. The majority of disseminated gonococcal infections is attributed to the AHU strains and occurs in women.

Other conditions associated with *N. gonorrhoeae* include anorectal and oropharyngeal infections. Infections in these sites are more common in males who have sex with males but can also occur in women. Most infections are asymptomatic or have nonspecific symptoms. Pharyngitis is the chief complaint in symptomatic oropharyngeal infections, whereas discharge, rectal pain, or bloody stools may be seen in rectal gonorrhea. Approximately 30% to 60% of females with genital gonorrhea have concurrent rectal infection.

Newborns can acquire **ophthalmia neonatorum,** a gonococcal eye infection, during vaginal delivery through an infected birth canal. This condition, which can result in blindness if not treated immediately, is rare in the United States because application of antimicrobial eyedrops, generally erythromycin, is legally required at the birth of every infant. Ocular infections can occur in adults due to inoculation of the eye with infected genital secretions or, rarely, as a result of a laboratory accident.

Laboratory Diagnosis

Specimen Collection and Transport. Specimens collected for the recovery of *N. gonorrhoeae*, as noted previously, may

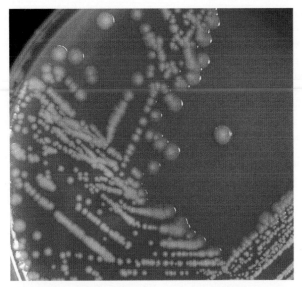

FIGURE 17-3 Virulent *Neisseria gonorrhoeae* after 24 hours of growth on modified Thayer-Martin (MTM) agar.

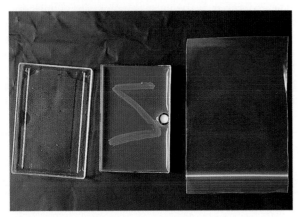

FIGURE 17-4 Twenty-four hour growth of *Neisseria gonorrhoeae* on a JEMBEC plate streaked in a characteristic Z pattern.

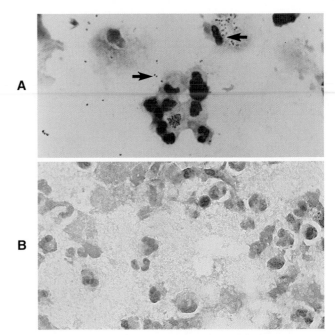

FIGURE 17-5 **A,** Direct Gram-stained smear of male urethral discharge showing intracellular and extracellular, gram-negative diplococci, which is diagnostic of *Neisseria gonorrhoeae*. **B,** A direct smear with more than five polymorphonuclear neutrophils per field, but no bacteria, may suggest nongonococcal urethritis.

come from genital sources or from other sites such as the rectum, pharynx, and joint fluid. The laboratory should be notified when cultures for *N. gonorrhoeae* from sites other than the genital tract are requested, because normal laboratory protocols for such specimens would not recover the organism.

The specimen of choice for genital infections in males is the urethra, and in females, the endocervix. In males, purulent discharge can be collected directly onto swab for culture. When no apparent discharge is present, the swab is inserted 2 to 3 cm into the anterior urethra and slowly rotated to collect material. Swabs for rectal culture should be inserted 4 to 5 cm into the anal canal. Disinfectants should be avoided in preparing the patient for collection of the specimen.

Because *N. gonorrhoeae* is extremely susceptible to drying and temperature changes, direct plating of the specimen to gonococcal-selective media gives optimal results (Figure 17-3). Calcium alginate and cotton swabs are inhibitory *to N. gonorrhoeae*, so Dacron or rayon swabs are preferred. Inocu-

lated swabs should be placed in a transport system such as Amies medium with charcoal, transported to the laboratory immediately, and plated within 6 hours. Several commercial transport systems, such as James E. Martin Biological Environmental Chamber (JEMBEC) plates (Figure 17-4), Bio-Bag, Gono-Pak, and Transgrow, contain selective media and a carbon dioxide atmosphere to provide optimal conditions until the specimen reaches the laboratory. These systems are especially useful when the clinic or physician's office is some distance from the laboratory.

Direct Microscopic Examination. Smears for direct Gram stains should be prepared from urogenital specimens when the culture is collected. A Gram stain is not recommended for pharyngeal specimens because commensal *Neisseria* spp. can be present. Demonstration of gram-negative intracellular diplococci, appearing as kidney or coffee bean shaped, from a symptomatic male with discharge correlates at a rate of 95% with culture and is evidence of gonococcal infection (Figure 17-5, *A*). Many times avirulent forms (lacking pili) of the organism are seen as extracellular, gram-negative diplococci in the direct smear of the clinical specimen.

Because women have vaginal commensal microbiota that resemble gonococci, direct Gram stain correlates in only 50% to 70% of cases with culture. The direct Gram stain may be helpful in a symptomatic woman with discharge, but culture is necessary for confirmation. A Gram stain with more than five polymorphonuclear neutrophils (PMNs) per field but no bacteria (Figure 17-5, *B*) may suggest nongonococcal urethritis with organisms such as *C. trachomatis* or *Ureaplasma urealyticum*.

TABLE 17-2 Selective Media for the Isolation of *Neisseria gonorrhoeae* and *Neisseria meningitidis*

Selective Medium	Inhibitory Agents	Suppressed Organisms
Thayer-Martin	Vancomycin	Gram-positive
	Colistin	Gram-negative
	Nystatin	Yeast
Modified Thayer-Martin	Vancomycin	Gram-positive
	Colistin	Gram-negative
	Nystatin	Yeast
	Trimethoprim	Swarming *Proteus* spp.
Martin-Lewis	Vancomycin	Gram-positive
	Colistin	Gram-negative
	Anisomycin	Yeast
	Trimethoprim	Swarming *Proteus* spp.
New York City	Vancomycin	Gram-positive
	Colistin	Gram-negative
	Amphotericin B	Yeast
	Trimethoprim	Swarming *Proteus* spp.
GC-LECT	Vancomycin	Gram-positive
	Lincomycin	Gram-positive
	Colistin	Gram-negative
	Amphotericin B	Yeast
	Trimethoprim	Swarming *Proteus* spp.
		Capnocytophaga spp.

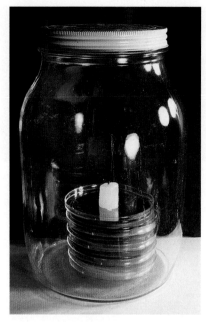

FIGURE 17-6   Candle extinction jar with inoculated modified Thayer-Martin agar plates.

Culture. Cultivation of *N. gonorrhoeae* requires the use of chocolate (CHOC) agar, but this enriched medium also supports the growth of many other organisms found as commensals in specimens collected for recovery of gonococci. To prevent overgrowth of the normal biota and to enhance the recovery of the pathogenic species, a selective medium containing inhibitors for gram-negative and gram-positive organisms and yeast is used. Commonly used selective media are described in Table 17-2.

New York City (NYC) medium, a transparent agar, has the added advantage of supporting the growth of possible urogenital pathogens *Mycoplasma hominis* and *U. urealyticum*. Over the past several years, as many as 10% of *N. gonorrhoeae* strains have been reported as sensitive to vancomycin, an antimicrobial agent used in most selective media for *N. gonorrhoeae*. To recover these vancomycin-sensitive strains, including a nonselective CHOC agar plate as a primary plating medium is good practice. Several other bacteria will grow on selective gonococcal media. Some of these are *Acinetobacter* spp., *Capnocytophaga* spp., and *Kingella denitrificans*. These are differentiated from *N. gonorrhoeae* by the oxidase and catalase tests.

All specimens received in the laboratory for recovery of *Neisseria* spp. should be held at room temperature and plated as soon as possible. Because *Neisseria* spp. are susceptible to cold, media should be warmed to room temperature before inoculation. Specimens on swabs should be rolled in a Z pattern on the media and cross-streaked with a loop to facilitate growth of isolated colonies.

Incubation. Inoculated plates should be incubated at 35° C in a 3% to 5% CO_2 atmosphere. This is accomplished by use of a candle extinction jar (Figure 17-6) or a CO_2 incubator. Sufficient humidity is provided by the moisture evaporating from the media in a closed jar; most CO_2 incubators are automatically humidified, or a pan of water can be placed in the bottom. Scented or colored candles may be inhibitory to the gonococci, so only white wax candles are used in the candle extinction jar.

Presumptive Identification

Microscopic Morphology. The Gram stain must be performed on all suspected *Neisseria* isolates to verify the appearance of gram-negative diplococci. Some gram-negative rods, such as *Kingella* and *Acinetobacter* spp., are occasionally able to grow on gonococcal selective media. To differentiate these from the gram-negative diplococci, the organism can be streaked to a plate with a 10-unit penicillin disk added (Figure 17-7). After growth, the edge of the zone of inhibition is stained to visualize the morphology.

Colony Morphology. Cultures are examined daily for growth and held for 72 hours. Colonies of *N. gonorrhoeae* on CHOC or selective agars are small, tan, translucent, and raised after 24 to 48 hours of incubation. As noted previously, five colony types of *N. gonorrhoeae* have been described: T1 and T2 have pili and are considered virulent types; these colonies are smaller and raised and they appear bright in reflected light. Types T3 through T5 do not have pili and usually grow as larger, flatter colonies. The AHU strains produce smaller colonies and grow more slowly; they are often more difficult to identify with biochemical methods. The gonococci can produce autolytic enzymes that may make the isolate nonviable, so primary plates should not be incubated once sufficient growth is obtained. A fresh subculture should be used for identification tests.

Oxidase Test. The filter paper or direct plate oxidase test must be done on all isolates. In the filter paper method,

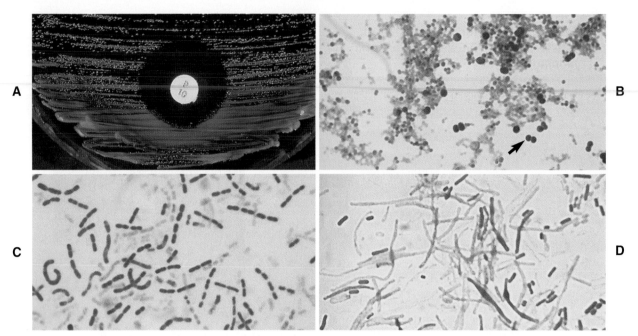

FIGURE 17-7 **A,** To differentiate some gram-negative rods from the gram-negative diplococci, the organism can be streaked to a plate and a 10-unit penicillin disk added. After growth, the edge of the zone of inhibition is stained to visualize microscopic morphology. **B,** The microscopic morphology of *Neisseria gonorrhoeae* remains gram-negative diplococci using the 10-unit penicillin disk. **C,** The gram-negative rod microscopic morphology of *Kingella* spp. after the penicillin disk test. **D,** The elongated gram-negative rod microscopic morphology of *Acinetobacter* spp. after the penicillin disk test.

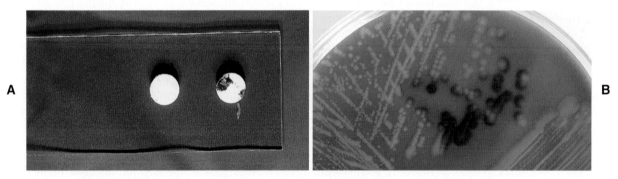

FIGURE 17-8 **A,** The oxidase disk test. The negative control is on the left and the positive reaction (purple) is on the right. **B,** Example of a positive oxidase reaction when the reagent is dropped directly on the colony.

oxidase reagent (1% dimethyl-*p*-phenylenediamine dihydrochloride or tetramethyl-*p*-phenylenediamine dihydrochloride) is placed on filter paper, and a colony from the plate is rubbed onto the reagent with an applicator stick or a nonnichrome needle. In a positive reaction on a fresh isolate, purple color should develop within 10 seconds (Figure 17-8, *A*). Alternatively, the oxidase reagent may be dropped directly onto a colony. In a positive reaction, the colony turns pink, then black (Figure 17-8, *B*). If subculture of the positive colony is needed, it must be done while the colony is still pink; when black, the organism is no longer viable.

Definitive Identification. A presumptive diagnosis of gonorrhea was once acceptable if an oxidase-positive, gram-negative diplococcus was recovered on gonococcal-selective media; this presumptive diagnosis is no longer acceptable. Oxidase-positive, gram-negative diplococci, such as *N. cinerea*, *N. meningitidis*, and *M. catarrhalis* can grow on selective media from sites where *N. gonorrhoeae* is expected. These organisms would be incorrectly reported as *N. gonorrhoeae* if no further identification were performed. Many different methods are currently used for the speciation of *Neisseria* and *Moraxella* species or for confirmation only of *N. gonorrhoeae* isolates. Both culture and nonculture tests are available for the detection of *N. gonorrhoeae* and are listed by type in Tables 17-3 and 17-4. All have advantages and disadvantages, and the selection of a particular method depends on the demo-

TABLE 17-3 Selected Culture-Based Test Methods for Identification of *Neisseria* and Related Species

Method Type and Name	Manufacturer	Principle	Comments
Conventional			
Cystine trypticase agar with 1% carbohydrates	Various	Acid production from carbohydrate utilization	Require pure culture; must be incubated 24-72 hr; no longer recommended
Chromogenic substrate			
Gonochek II	EY Laboratories[1]	Detects enzyme production	Confirms isolates only from selective media
BactoCard *Neisseria*	Remel, Inc.[2]		
Coagglutination			
Phadebact Monoclonal GC	Bactus AB[3]	Monoclonal antibodies used to detect *N. gonorrhoeae*	Does not require pure or viable culture
GonoGen II	BD Diagnostic Systems[4]		
Modified conventional/chromogenic enzyme			
BBL Crystal *Neisseria/Haemophilus* ID Kit	BD Diagnostic Systems	Multitest systems—combines enzyme substrate with other biochemical tests; speciates *Neisseria* and *Haemophilus* species	Isolates from selective or nonselective media
CarboFerm *Neisseria* Test	Hardy Diagnostics[5]		
Neisseria-Haemophilus Identification	bioMérieux[6]		
RapID NH System	Remel, Inc.		
Microscan HNID Panel	Siemens Healthcare Diagnostics[7]		
API NH	bioMérieux		
FA monoclonal antibody			
Microtrak *Neisseria gonorrhoeae* culture confirmation test	Trinity Biotech[8]	Fluorescent-labeled monoclonal antibodies to detect *N. gonorrhoeae*	Does not require pure culture; requires ultraviolet microscope

[1]San Mateo, Calif.
[2]Lenexa, Kan.
[3]Huddinge, Sweden.
[4]Sparks, Md.
[5]Santa Maria, Calif.
[6]Hazelwood, Mo.
[7]Deerfield, Ill.
[8]Bray, Ireland.

graphic profile of the patients, sensitivity and specificity of the method with low- or high-prevalence groups, cost of materials and technical time, and number of tests performed.

Carbohydrate Utilization. The traditional method for the identification of *Neisseria* spp. has been by carbohydrate utilization in cystine trypticase agar (CTA), containing 1% of the individual carbohydrate and phenol red as a pH indicator. If the organism uses the particular carbohydrate, then acid, characterized by a yellow color, is produced in 24 to 72 hours. Many problems are associated with this method, however, and it has been replaced by rapid, more accurate methods (see Tables 17-3 and 17-4).

The rapid carbohydrate degradation tests require pure cultures but can be read in 2 to 4 hours rather than the 24 to 72 hours needed for the CTA carbohydrate test. These rapid tests also detect acid production from various carbohydrates, but they are based on the presence of preformed enzymes for carbohydrate utilization rather than on bacterial growth.

Problems noted with these methods, however, include the following:

- Weak acid production from glucose by certain strains of *N. gonorrhoeae*
- Misidentification of sucrose-negative strains of *N. subflava* as *N. meningitidis*
- Strains of *N. cinerea* that give positive glucose reactions

Chromogenic Substrates. Chromogenic substrate tests detect enzymes that hydrolyze colorless substrates and produce colored end products. Only strains that are isolated on selective media should be tested. The advantage of these tests is the identification of *Neisseria* spp. strains with aberrant carbohydrate utilizations. Problems noted with these tests include misidentification of nonpathogenic species, such as *N. cinerea*, *N. sicca*, *N. subflava*, and *N. mucosa*, as *N. gonorrhoeae* or *N. meningitidis*. The multitest conventional-chromogenic enzyme methods combine enzyme substrate tests with other biochemical tests and allow identification of strains isolated on selective or nonselective media. These tests can also speciate other

TABLE 17-4 Selected Nonculture Test Methods for Identification of *Neisseria gonorrhoeae* and Other Species

Method Type and Name	Manufacturer	Principle	Notes
Nucleic acid hybridization, nonamplified			
Neisseria gonorrhoeae PACE 2	Gen-Probe[1]	DNA probe for direct detection of gonococcal rRNA from specimen	Chemiluminescent labeled, single-strand DNA probe used to detect species-specific rRNA
PACE 2 C	Gen-Probe		Used to detect both *N. gonorrhoeae* and *Chlamydia trachomatis*
AccuProbe *Neisseria* Culture Confirmation Test	Gen-Probe	Nucleic acid hybridization for confirmation of *N. gonorrhoeae*	Chemiluminescent labeled, single-strand DNA probe used to detect species-specific rRNA
Digene HC2 CT/GC DNA Test	Qiagen[2]	RNA hybridization for probes specific for DNA sequences of *N. gonorrhoeae* and *C. trachomatis*	
Nucleic acid amplification tests			
Roche AMPLICOR CT/NG Test	Roche Diagnostics[3]	Thermophilic amplification of target gene; for *N. gonorrhoeae* and *C. trachomatis*	Specimens include urogenital and male and female urine
Roche Cobas AMPLICOR CT/ NG Test	Roche Diagnostics		
BD ProbeTec ET	BD Diagnostic Systems[4]	Stand displacement amplification	
Gen-Probe APTIMA ACG	Gen-Probe	Transcription-mediated amplification	For *N. gonorrhoeae* only
Gen-Probe APTIMA Combo2	Gen-Probe	Multi-test systems—combines enzyme substrate with other biochemical tests; speciates *Neisseria* and *Haemophilus* species	For *N. gonorrhoeae* and *C. trachomatis*

[1]San Diego, Calif.
[2]Gaithersburg, Md.
[3]Indianapolis, Ind.
[4]Sparks, Md.

genera, such as *Haemophilus* (see Chapter 18). Characteristics of clinically significant species of *Neisseria*, *Moraxella*, and *Kingella* are listed in Table 17-5. Key differentiating reactions of the major pathogens include use of glucose only by *N. gonorrhoeae*, whereas *N. meningitidis* uses glucose and maltose. *M. catarrhalis* is asaccharolytic but, unlike the *Neisseria* spp., is DNase and butyrate esterase positive.

Immunologic Assays. Immunologic methods employ monoclonal antibodies for the identification of *N. gonorrhoeae*. These methods do not require pure or viable organisms and can be done from the primary plates. Immunologic methods include coagglutination and fluorescent antibody testing. The coagglutination tests use monoclonal antibodies directed against *N. gonorrhoeae* attached to killed *Staphylococcus aureus* cells; agglutination is a positive reaction. No reported cross-reaction with *N. cinerea* exists, but rare isolates of *N. lactamica* have been reported as *N. gonorrhoeae*.

The fluorescent antibody (FA) method uses monoclonal antibodies that recognize epitopes on the principal outer membrane protein (Por) of *N. gonorrhoeae*. The method is extremely sensitive and specific; no demonstrated cross-reactivity with *N. cinerea* or other *Neisseria* spp. has been reported. The FA method also microscopically confirms the diplococci's morphologic appearance.

Nucleic Acid Assays. Alternatives to culture for *N. gonorrhoeae* are available. These methods detect gonococcal antigen or nucleic acid directly in cervical, urine, and/or urethral exudates. Nucleic acid detection methods include both nonampli-

fied and amplified probe technologies (see Table 17-4). One nucleic acid probe test is a nonisotopic chemiluminescent DNA probe that hybridizes specifically with ribosomal RNA (rRNA) of *N. gonorrhoeae*. Nucleic acid detection methods are rapid and sensitive but they do have some drawbacks. Some disadvantages of the nucleic acid probes include the following:

- Nonamplified probe tests are only marginally more sensitive than cervical culture in females; used in high-risk populations only
- Not approved for pharyngeal or rectal specimens; not used in children or sexual abuse cases
- Cannot identify an *N. gonorrhoeae* infection produced by a β-lactamase–producing strain
- Do not allow for recovery of an organism to be used for susceptibility testing

Nucleic acid amplification tests (NAATs) amplify a specific nucleic acid sequence (e.g., polymerase chain reaction [PCR]), before detecting the target sequence with a probe. Other methodologies rely on an amplified signal after a specific probe binds to the target sequence. NAATs are extremely sensitive and do not require viable organisms. Because urine can be used in these procedures, self-collection of the specimen is possible and pelvic examination or intraurethral swabs are not required. These methods have the additional advantage of being less sensitive to transport and storage conditions than is culture. NAATs can also detect both *N. gonorrhoeae* and *C. trachomatis* in the same specimen. Disadvantages of NAATs include the following:

TABLE 17-5 Characteristics of Significant Species of *Neisseria*, *Moraxella*, and *Kingella*

Characteristic	N. gonorrhoeae	N. meningitidis	N. lactamica	N. cinerea	N. sicca	N. flavescens	Moraxella	Kingella
Pigment on nutrient agar	−	−	−	−	+	+	−	−
Catalase (3% H_2O_2)	+	+	+	+	+	+	+	−
Superoxol (30% H_2O_2)	+	−	−	−	−	−	−	−
Growth on								
MTM, ML, NYC	+	+	+	d	−	−	d	+
Nutrient medium at 35° C	−	−	+	+	+	+	+	−
Acid production from								
Glucose	+	+	+	+*	+	−	−	+
Maltose	−	+	+	−	+	−	−	−
Sucrose	−	−	−	−	+	−	−	−
Lactose	−	−	+	−	−	−	−	−
Fructose	−	−	−	−	+	−	−	−
DNase	−	−	−	−	−	−	+	−
Reduction of								
NO_3	−	−	−	−	−	−	+	+
NO_2[†]	−	d	d	+	+	+	+	−
Tributyrin hydrolysis	−	−	−	−	−	−	+	NT
Enzymes produced								
β-*D*-Galactosidase	−	−	+	−	−	NT	−	−
γ-Glutamylaminopeptidase	−	+	−	−	−	NT	−	−
Hydroxyprolylaminopeptidase	+	−	−	+	NT	+	−	+

+, Most strains (>90%) positive; −, most strains (>90%) negative; *d*, some strains positive, some negative; *MTM*, modified Thayer-Martin agar; *ML*, Martin-Lewis agar; *NYC*, New York City medium; *NT*, not tested.
*Occasional strains may give weak glucose reactions in some rapid carbohydrate tests.

- False-negative results may occur if the specimen contains inhibitors of amplification; amplification controls are important in eliminating this problem.
- Because amplification is highly sensitive, strict attention to procedural factors and quality control is mandatory, including prescribed work areas, specimen handling to avoid cross-contamination, and positive and negative controls.

Probe technology and amplification methods can be expensive. These methods are probably not cost-effective if they are the only probe or amplification test used in the laboratory or if low volumes of *N. gonorrhoeae* tests are requested. Added to the expense is the need to repeat the test after equivocal results are obtained.

Additional Methods. Additional tests such as superoxol can aid in the identification of *N. gonorrhoeae*. The superoxol test uses 30% H_2O_2 and is performed in the same way as the catalase test. Colonies of *N. gonorrhoeae* produce immediate, vigorous bubbling. *N. meningitidis* and *N. lactamica* produce weak delayed bubbling in this reagent. Other *Neisseria* spp. produce weak delayed bubbling or none at all.

Some strains of *N. gonorrhoeae* have a specific need for one or more nutritional factors to be included in artificial media for growth to occur. These strains are called *auxotypes;* of the approximately 30 known auxotypes, the most common is AHU, which requires arginine, hypoxanthine, and uracil. The AHU strains are usually highly susceptible to penicillin, commonly recovered from patients with disseminated gonococcal infection, and can cause asymptomatic urethral infection in males. The auxotyping procedure is labor intensive; for this reason, it is not recommended for the routine clinical microbiology laboratory.

In low-prevalence populations, such as children, or in cases of suspected sexual assault/abuse, nonculture detection methods must not be used. The isolation of the gonococcus from children beyond the neonatal period is indicative of sexual abuse. The specimens should be cultured onto selective gonococcal media. Isolates must exhibit typical colony morphology, microscopic morphology of gram-negative diplococci, and be oxidase and catalase positive. Isolates must be identified to species level by the use of two biochemical, enzymatic, or serologic procedures with different principles. The organism should also be frozen in case further testing is needed. With various methods, isolates such as *N. cinerea, M. catarrhalis,* and *K. denitrificans,* all of which closely resemble *N. gonorrhoeae* biochemically, have been incorrectly reported as *N. gonorrhoeae.* Potentially serious medical, social, and legal ramifications could obviously result.

Antimicrobial Resistance

Until 1976, almost all strains of *N. gonorrhoeae* in the United States were susceptible to penicillin. The first plasmid-mediated **penicillinase-producing *Neisseria gonorrhoeae* (PPNG)** strains were isolated in that year, largely imported from Southeast Asia or Africa. By 1980, more than half of the reported PPNG cases were of domestic origin. The Gonococcal Isolate Surveillance Project (GISP) reported that PPNG has decreased in the United States from its peak of 11% in

TABLE 17-6 Resistance of *Neisseria gonorrhoeae* in the United States

Type	Acronym	First Observed	Mechanism
Plasmid-mediated penicillin resistance	PPNG	1976	Plasmid codes for β-lactamase production
Chromosome-mediated resistance	CMRNG	1983	Selection of mutants for low-level penicillin and tetracycline resistance
Plasmid-mediated, high-level tetracycline resistance	TRNG	1985	Plasmid codes for tetracycline resistance
Chromosome-mediated spectinomycin resistance	—	1981	Mutation causes high-level resistance
Chromosome-mediated fluoroquinolone resistance	QRNG	1991	Mutation causes resistance

PPNG, Penicillinase-producing *N. gonorrhoeae*; CMRNG, chromosomally mediated resistant *N. gonorrhoeae*; TRNG, tetracycline-resistant *N. gonorrhoeae*; QRNG, quinolone-resistant *N. gonorrhoeae*.

1991 to 0.4% in 2006. In addition to plasmid-mediated penicillin resistance, in which the organism acquires a plasmid with genes for β-lactamase production, *N. gonorrhoeae* can exhibit chromosome-mediated penicillin resistance (PenR), which was initially noted in the United States in 1983. These isolates are β-lactamase negative. Resistance in these strains is due to a combination of mutations at several chromosomal loci resulting in altered penicillin-binding proteins. The incidence of PenR increased from 0.5% in 1988 to 5.7% in 1999 and then decreased to 1.2% in 2006.

In addition to penicillin resistance, *N. gonorrhoeae* exhibits plasmid-mediated resistance as well as chromosomally mediated resistance to tetracycline, spectinomycin, and fluoroquinolones (e.g., ciprofloxacin). Chromosomally mediated resistance to both penicillin and tetracycline (CMRNG) increased from 3% in 1989 to 9.3% in 2006. Spectinomycin resistance, first reported in the United States in 1981, is due to a chromosomal mutation resulting in high-level resistance to the antimicrobial agent. Only five spectinomycin-resistant isolates of *N. gonorrhoeae* were reported by GISP in 2003 and none in 2006. Fluoroquinolone resistance was less than 1% in 1990. In 2006, 15.1% of *N. gonorrhoeae* isolates were intermediate resistant or resistant to ciprofloxacin. The mechanisms of resistance of *N. gonorrhoeae* are summarized in Table 17-6. In 2005, the Clinical and Laboratory Standards Institute (CLSI) issued performance standards for antimicrobial disk susceptibility testing (Document M100-S15) of organisms including *N. gonorrhoeae*.

Treatment

Because of the widespread increase in fluoroquinolone resistance throughout the United States, the Centers for Disease Control and Prevention (CDC) issued a recommendation in 2007 that fluoroquinolones no longer be used as therapy for gonorrhea and associated gonococcal infections. One class of drug, the cephalosporins (e.g., ceftriaxone, cefixime), is currently recommended. Because coinfection with *C. trachomatis* is fairly common in patients with gonorrhea, dual therapy is frequently prescribed. One of the primary therapies for *N. gonorrhoeae* is used, plus azithromycin or doxycycline for *C. trachomatis*. Routine use of dual therapy can be cost effective, can decrease the prevalence of chlamydial infection, and may reduce the development of resistant strains of *N. gonorrhoeae*.

Neisseria meningitidis

Neisseria meningitidis can be found in the nasopharynx and oropharynx of 3% to 30% of asymptomatic individuals, and it is an important etiologic agent of endemic and epidemic meningitis, meningococcemia, and rarely pneumonia, purulent arthritis, or endophthalmitis. *N. meningitidis* has also been recovered from urogenital and rectal sites as a result of oral-genital contact. Meningococcal carriage, usually involving nonencapsulated strains, may cause an increase in protective antibody against the pathogenic strains. In one study of university students, nasopharyngeal carriage increased significantly during the first few weeks of the academic year.

Virulence Factors

With few exceptions, *N. meningitidis* exhibits the same cellular structural characteristics as *N. gonorrhoeae*: the virulence factors pili, polysaccharide capsule, the cellular membrane proteins (Por, Opa, Rmp), and LOS endotoxin. PorA and PorB are both produced in the meningococcus, whereas only PorB is expressed in the gonococcus. Many virulent meningococcal strains produce IgA1 protease, an enzyme that aids invasiveness. As in the gonococcus, the outer membrane structures, or blebs, are seen during rapid growth.

Of the 13 meningococcal encapsulated serogroups, strains A, B, C, Y, and W-135 are most often associated with epidemics. Group A strains are often incriminated in pandemics. Serogroups B and C are most common in the United States, with group B frequently being involved in community-acquired disease. Serogroup Y primarily causes meningococcal pneumonia, whereas W-135 is often responsible for invasive disease. In the United States, the highest rates of meningococcal disease occur in infants, with most cases due to serogroup B. Eighteen-year-olds have the next highest rate; 75% of cases in this age group are caused by the serogroups (A, C, Y. W-135) included in the current *N. meningitidis* vaccine (Menactra; Sanofi Pasteur, Inc., Swiftwater, Pa.).

Clinical Infections

The primary sources of epidemic meningitis are oral secretions or, less efficiently, respiratory droplets from asymptomatic carriers, especially among close contacts in closed populations such as college dormitories and military barracks. Epidemic meningitis most often occurs in young adults.

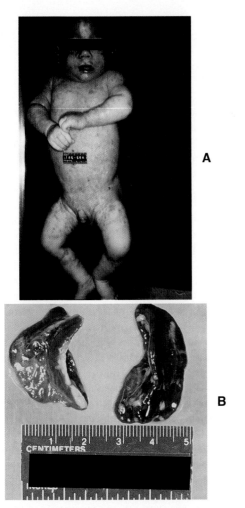

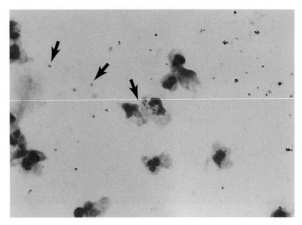

FIGURE 17-10 Direct Gram-stained smear of cerebrospinal fluid illustrating intracellular and extracellular gram-negative diplococci of *Neisseria meningitidis.*

FIGURE 17-9 A, Petechial skin rash associated with meningococcemia in a baby. **B,** Waterhouse-Friderichsen syndrome illustrating hemorrhage (dark red areas) in the adrenal glands.

It is characterized by abrupt onset of frontal headache, stiff neck (nuchal rigidity), and sometimes fever. The fatality rate is 10% to 15%; an additional 10% to 20% will have sequelae such as neurologic complications or seizures.

When *N. meningitidis* enters the bloodstream, two main diseases can occur: fulminant meningococcemia or meningitis. Meningococcemia, or sepsis, may occur with or without meningitis and carries a 25% mortality rate, even if treated. Purpura (hemorrhaging of blood into the skin and mucous membranes producing bruises) with petechial skin rash (pinpoint red spot caused by hemorrhage; Figure 17-9, *A*), tachycardia, and hypotension can develop during bacteremia, and thrombosis is common. In some cases, the disease becomes fulminant and spreads rapidly, causing disseminated intravascular coagulation (DIC), septic shock, or hemorrhage in the adrenal glands (**Waterhouse-Friderichsen syndrome;** Figure 17-9, *B*). Death may occur in 12 to 48 hours from onset. Individuals with a deficiency in complement components C5 to C8 are at increased risk of meningococcemia. Meningococcal pneumonia usually affects older individuals with underlying pulmonary problems.

Laboratory Diagnosis

Specimen Collection and Transport. Culture specimens for *N. meningitidis* may come from a wide variety of sterile and nonsterile sites. These include cerebrospinal fluid (CSF), blood, nasopharyngeal swabs and aspirates, and less commonly, sputum and urogenital sites. Collection and transport should be performed as specified by the laboratory for the various specimen types. When commercial blood culture systems are used, data from the manufacturer should be consulted to determine whether *N. meningitidis* can be routinely recovered or whether techniques such as blind subculture (subculture to CHOC agar from bottle with no apparent visual growth) are required.

Direct Microscopic Examination. On Gram-stained smears from specimens such as CSF, the meningococci appear as intracellular and extracellular gram-negative diplococci (Figure 17-10). Encapsulated strains can have a halo around the organisms. The highest yield of positive CSF Gram stains is obtained when specimens are concentrated. A number of investigators have reported that concentration by cytocentrifugation is superior to that by traditional centrifugation and has the potential to increase Gram stain detection by tenfold to 100-fold. In a patient with disseminated meningococcemia who has petechiae from hemorrhage of surface blood vessels, an impression Gram stain smear is often positive for gram-negative diplococci.

Culture. Selective and nonselective media for the isolation of *N. meningitidis* should, like cultures for *N. gonorrhoeae*, be incubated under increased CO_2. *N. meningitidis* and the commensal *Neisseria* spp. will grow on sheep blood agar (SBA) and CHOC agar. *N. meningitidis* grown on SBA under CO_2 produce bluish-gray colonies. *N. meningitidis* will grow on gonococcal selective agars and will produce small, tan, sometimes mucoid, convex colonies on CHOC agar (Figure 17-11). *N. lactamica*, generally a nonpathogenic species that may mimic *N. meningitidis*, can also grow on selective media. The lactose-positive characteristic of *N. lactamica* may be delayed or nonexistent. A rapid *o*-nitrophenyl-β-d-galactopyranoside (ONPG) test, which detects lactose utilization, is usually posi-

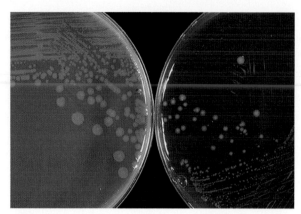

FIGURE 17-11 Growth of *Neisseria meningitidis* after 48 hours on chocolate (CHOC) agar on the left and sheep blood agar (SBA) on the right. Of the classic *Neisseria* pathogens, only the meningococcus grows on SBA and CHOC agar.

tive in 30 minutes for *N. lactamica*. See Chapter 9 for a description of the ONPG test.

Identification. The oxidase and catalase tests should be performed on all isolates. Any of the carbohydrate utilization tests described earlier can be used to speciate *N. meningitidis*. Optimal results in these tests are obtained when a fresh subculture of the organism is used. Serogrouping of the meningococci is most commonly done by slide agglutination.

Although rare, glucose-negative, maltose-negative, asaccharolytic strains of *N. meningitidis* have been isolated. Maltose-negative strains could be misidentified as *N. gonorrhoeae*, especially if recovered from genital or other unusual sites. Maltose-negative strains may lack the maltose phosphorylase pathway; this occurs mainly in serogroup B but also rarely in groups C and Y. To avoid misidentification of maltose-negative strains, other means of identification in addition to carbohydrate utilization should be used. These include the use of chromogenic substrate confirmation tests and serogrouping. One useful test included in some identification systems is γ-glutamyl aminopeptidase, which is usually positive in *N. meningitidis* and negative in *N. gonorrhoeae, N. lactamica,* and *M. catarrhalis.*

Immunologic methods such as latex agglutination are commercially available in kits and are used to detect the group-specific surface antigens of *N. meningitidis*. These bacterial antigen tests, when performed on CSF, blood, or urine, often allow more rapid detection of a causative organism, but due to lack of sensitivity, they should not replace culture, Gram stain, and conventional identification.

Laboratory-Acquired Disease

In 2000, two cases of fatal laboratory-acquired meningococcal disease were reported to the CDC. Both clinical microbiologists had examined plates, performed Gram stains, subcultured, and/or performed slide agglutination serogrouping on patient isolates on the open bench. Isolates recovered from the laboratory scientists were identical to patient organisms. A retrospective survey identified 16 probable laboratory-acquired meningococcal infections worldwide from 1996 to

2001. Because exposure to *N. meningitidis* aerosols increases risk of infection, the CDC recommends use of a biosafety level-2 cabinet for manipulation of suspected isolates of *N. meningitidis* from sterile sites.

Treatment

The drug of choice for treatment of confirmed *N. meningitidis* meningitis is penicillin, but rifampin or a sulfonamide is recommended as prophylaxis for close contacts. Patients with meningococcemia are best treated with third-generation cephalosporins.

Vaccine

In January 2005, the U.S. Food and Drug Administration (FDA) approved the polysaccharide diphtheria toxoid conjugate vaccine (Menactra), a new meningococcal vaccine for use in people 11 to 55 years of age. This vaccine, like the previous quadrivalent vaccine, contains polysaccharide antigens to serogroups A, C, Y, and W-135. In Menactra, however, these antigens are conjugated to diphtheria toxoid protein; this conjugate vaccine is expected to provide long-term immunity. This vaccine, like its predecessor, does not protect against meningitis caused by serogroup B, one of the more common serotypes causing infection in the United States, because group B polysaccharide is a very poor immunogen in humans.

The Advisory Committee on Immunization Practices recommends Menactra to be administered to students 11 to 12 years of age. If not previously vaccinated, those entering high school (15 years of age) and college freshmen living in dormitories should receive Menactra. Meningococcal vaccine is also recommended for military recruits, asplenic patients more than 2 years of age, and travelers to areas with epidemic disease. In October 2005, the FDA and the CDC issued a health advisory for Menactra. Five cases of Guillain-Barré syndrome (GBS), a serious neurologic syndrome, were reported following vaccination. It is unknown whether the GBS was associated with the vaccine or was just coincidental.

Moraxella catarrhalis

Moraxella catarrhalis is in the family Moraxellaceae, which contains three genera: *Moraxella, Acinetobacter,* and *Psychrobacter*. Isolated only from humans, *M. catarrhalis* is a commensal of the upper respiratory tract.

Clinical Infections

Moraxella catarrhalis has become an opportunistic pathogen and is recognized as a cause of upper respiratory tract infection in otherwise healthy children and the elderly. It also can cause lower respiratory infections, especially in adults with chronic obstructive pulmonary disease. Predisposing factors in the pathogenesis include advanced age, immunodeficiency, neutropenia, and chronic debilitating diseases. *M. catarrhalis* has been reported as the third most common cause of acute otitis media and sinusitis in children. Infections include life-threatening systemic diseases such as endocarditis, meningitis, and bacterial tracheitis (Figure 17-12, *A*). Severe infections are seen in immunocompromised hosts; hospital outbreaks of

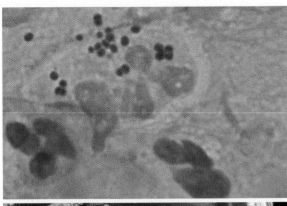

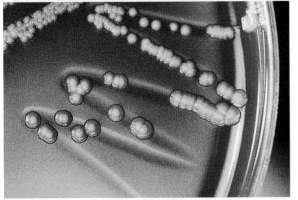

FIGURE 17-12   **A,** Direct smear of an otitis media specimen illustrating intracellular, gram-negative diplococci. The organism was identified biochemically as *Moraxella catarrhalis* from cultures. **B,** Growth of *M. catarrhalis* after 48 hours, illustrating the wagon-wheel appearance on chocolate agar.

M. catarrhalis respiratory infections have occurred. The presence of intracellular, gram-negative diplococci in these specimens may alert the microbiologist to possible infection with *M. catarrhalis.* Most isolates produce β-lactamase, making them resistant to ampicillin and amoxicillin, which are commonly used to treat otitis media.

Laboratory Diagnosis

Specimen Collection and Identification. Specimen collection for *M. catarrhalis* should be determined by the laboratory according to the various specimen types. The organism will grow on both SBA and CHOC agar, producing smooth, opaque, gray to white colonies (Figure 17-12, *B*). The term *hockey puck* has been used to describe the colony because it remains intact when pushed across the plate with a loop. Unlike other *Neisseria* spp. that have an optimal growth temperature of 35° to 37° C, strains of this organism can tolerate lower temperatures and grow well at 28° C. *M. catarrhalis* is usually inhibited on gonococcal selective agars by colistin in the media, but some species resistant to this antimicrobial may grow. Like *Neisseria* species, *M. catarrhalis* is oxidase and catalase positive. The organism is asaccharolytic, and it may be differentiated from *Neisseria* spp. by positive DNase and butyrate esterase reactions. Tributyrin is used as the substrate to detect butyrate esterase activity.

TABLE 17-7   **Infections Reported to Be Caused by *Neisseria* Species Other Than *N. gonorrhoeae* and *N. meningitidis***

Infection	*Neisseria* species
Meningitis	*N. lactamica*
	N. sicca
	N. subflava
	N. mucosa
	N. flavescens
Endocarditis	*N. sicca*
	N. subflava
	N. mucosa
Prosthetic valve infection	*N. sicca*
Bacteremia	*N. lactamica*
	N. flavescens
	N. cinerea
Pneumonia	*N. sicca*
Empyema	*N. mucosa*
Bacteriuria	*N. subflava*
Osteomyelitis	*N. sicca*
Ocular infection	*N. mucosa*
Dog bite	*N. weaveri*

NONPATHOGENIC *NEISSERIA* SPECIES

Other *Neisseria* spp. exist as normal inhabitants of the upper respiratory tract. Referred to as *commensals, saprophytes,* or *nonpathogens,* these species are occasionally isolated from the genital tract. The commensal *Neisseria* spp. rarely cause disease, but they have sporadically been implicated in meningitis, endocarditis, prosthetic valve infections, bacteremia, pneumonia, empyema, bacteriuria, osteomyelitis, and ocular infections (Table 17-7). Many rapid tests for the identification of *N. gonorrhoeae* test for a limited number of characteristics, which may be shared by one or more nonpathogenic *Neisseria* spp. One must keep in mind that the incidence of infections caused by the commensal *Neisseria* spp. is extremely low and that the main reason for the microbiologist to be familiar with these organisms is to accurately separate them from the pathogenic species.

Identification

Table 17-8 lists the colony morphology and primary isolation sites of the *Neisseria* spp. and related organisms. Table 17-9 lists the traditional and additional tests used to identify the *Neisseria* spp. and some related genera. These organisms are divided into three groups:

Group 1: Traditional pathogens
Group 2: Commensal *Neisseria* spp. that can grow on selective medium
Group 3: Commensal *Neisseria* spp. that do not usually grow on selective medium

Groups 2 and 3 are further divided on the basis of their activities toward carbohydrates. Saccharolytic organisms are able to metabolize carbohydrates, whereas asaccharolytic organisms are unable to do so.

TABLE 17-8 Colony Morphology and Primary Isolation Sites of *Neisseria* and Related Organisms

Organism	Colony Morphology*	Primary Isolation Sites
N. gonorrhoeae	Small (0.5-1 mm), grayish white, translucent, raised with entire edge Usually easily emulsified Smaller than *N. meningitidis* Up to 5 different colony morphologies from primary culture	Male: urethra Female: endocervix Laboratory should be notified to look for this organism from other sites so that appropriate media can be used
N. meningitidis	1-2 mm, bluish gray or tan (serogroup 6 may be yellowish) Serogroup A and C may be mucoid, translucent, and convex with smooth glistening surface; may be greenish cast in agar around colonies Usually easily emulsified	Nasopharynx and oropharynx (carriers) Spinal fluid: meningitis Blood: meningococcemia Lower respiratory tract: meningococcal pneumonia
N. polysaccharea	Small, gray (sometimes yellowish), translucent, raised Resembles *N. gonorrhoeae* colony	Nasopharynx of infants and children
N. lactamica	Small, grayish white (often with a yellow ring), translucent, slightly butyrous Resembles *N. meningitidis* but smaller	Nasopharynx of infants and children Rarely found in adults
N. cinerea	Small (1-1.5 mm), grayish white, translucent, raised with entire edge and slightly granular Resembles *N. gonorrhoeae*	Nasopharynx
N. mucosa	Large (up to 4 mm), grayish to buff yellow, translucent and mucoid, smooth surface, entire edge Viscous (sticky) consistency	Nasopharynx
N. sicca	Large (up to 3 mm), grayish white, opaque, deeply wrinkled, dry, irregular (breadcrumb) colony Firmly adherent, difficult to impossible to emulsify	Nasopharynx, saliva, sputum
N. subflava biovars	0.5-2 mm, pale greenish yellow to yellow, smooth surface with entire edge Often adherent	Nasopharynx
N. flavescens	Colonies similar to *N. meningitidis* but with golden yellow pigment	Pharynx (not often isolated from clinical specimens)
N. elongata	Large (up to 3 mm), grayish white with yellowish tinge, low convex to almost flat Corroding of agar may occur Claylike colony, difficult to emulsify	Nasopharynx
N. weaveri	Small, semiopaque with a smooth appearance	Wounds from dog bites
Kingella denitrificans	Small (1-2 mm), gray, semitransparent, convex, may pit the agar Colonial morphology of those that do not pit the agar similar to *N. gonorrhoeae*	Upper respiratory tract
Moraxella catarrhalis	3-5 mm, grayish white, opaque 48-hr colony may have elevated center, thinner wavelike periphery (wagon wheel) Often granular, difficult to emulsify Colony can be swept across plate intact (hockey puck)	Upper respiratory tract

*On chocolate agar at 24 to 48 hours.

In the clinical laboratory, when isolated from respiratory specimens, the commensal *Neisseria* spp. are usually identified only by Gram stain and gross colony morphology and are called *Neisseria* spp. or "usual oral flora." Further identification by biochemical tests is not done. When they are isolated from selective agar medium or sterile body sites, differentiation from the pathogenic *Neisseria* may be required. Common laboratory tests and observations do not always adequately differentiate all the commensal species from one another or from the pathogens. In addition, insufficient test parameters and equivocal carbohydrate reactions have led to confusion between the pathogenic and commensal *Neisseria* spp. Additional tests used to help further differentiate these organisms include growth on nutrient agar at 35° C, growth on SBA or CHOC agar at 22° C, and the reduction of nitrate and nitrite.

Neisseria cinerea

Neisseria cinerea was first described in 1906 but was subsequently misclassified as a subtype of *M. catarrhalis* (*Neisseria pseudocatarrhalis*). It was named *N. cinerea* in 1939. The organism has received considerable attention in the past few years because of its misidentification as *N. gonorrhoeae* in some commercial identification systems. Although *N. cinerea* is glucose negative in CTA sugars, in some commercial kits the glucose was read as positive, making it biochemically identical to *N. gonorrhoeae*.

The colony morphology of *N. cinerea* is also similar to the T3 colonies of *N. gonorrhoeae* on CHOC agar. *N. cinerea* also grows on SBA (Figure 17-13). Colistin susceptibility is a helpful test in differentiating *N. cinerea* from *N. gonorrhoeae*.

TABLE 17-9 Differential Tests for Commensal *Neisseria* and Related Genera

Organism	Traditional Tests									Additional Tests			
	Growth on ML, MTM, or NYC	Catalase	Oxidase	Acid Produced from					Growth on Blood or Chocolate Agar at 22° C	Growth on Nutrient Agar at 35° C	Reduction of		DNase
				Glucose	Maltose	Lactose (ONPG)	Sucrose	Fructose			Nitrate	Nitrite	
Group 1: traditional pathogens													
N. gonorrhoeae	+	+	+	+	−	−	−	−	−	−	−	−	−
N. meningitidis	+	+	+	+	+	−	−	−	−	−	−	V	−
Group 2: Commensal species—possible growth on selective agar media													
Saccharolytic													
K. denitrificans	V	−	+	(+)	−	−	−	−	+	+	+	V	−
N. lactamica	+	+	+	+	+	+	−	−	V	+	−	V	−
N. polysaccharea	+	+	+	+	+	−	V	−	−	+	−	V	−
Asaccharolytic													
N. cinerea	V	+	+	−	−	−	−	−	−	+	−	+	−
M. catarrhalis	V	+	+	−	−	−	−	−	V	+	+	+	+
Group 3: Commensal species—no growth on selective agar media													
Saccharolytic													
N. mucosa	−	+	+	+	+	−	+	+	+	+	+	+	−
N. sicca	−	+	+	+	+	−	+	+	+	+	+	+	−
N. subflava biovars													
subflava	−	+	+	+	+	−	−	−	+	+	−	V	−
flava	−	+	+	+	+	+	−	+	+	+	−	V	−
perflava	−	+	+	+	+	−	+	+	+	+	−	V	−
Asaccharolytic													
N. flavescens	−	+	+	−	−	−	−	−	+	+	−	+	−
N. elongata	−	−	+	−	−	−	−	−	+	+	−	+	−
N. weaveri	−	+	+	−	−	−	−	−	+	+	−	+	−

+, Positive; −, negative; (+), positive (delayed); *ML*, Martin-Lewis agar; *MTM*, modified Thayer-Martin agar; *NYC*, New York City medium; *V*, variable.

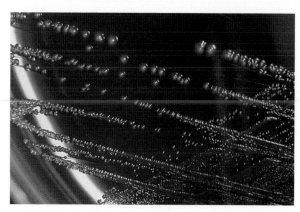

FIGURE 17-13 Colony morphology of *Neisseria cinerea* on sheep blood agar (48-hour culture).

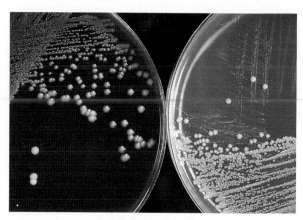

FIGURE 17-14 Culture of *Neisseria lactamica* after 48 hours on blood agar *(left)* and chocolate agar *(right)*. This organism resembles *Neisseria meningitidis*.

A suspension of the organism is swabbed onto an SBA or CHOC agar plate, a 10-μg colistin disk is applied to the inoculum, and the plate is incubated in CO_2 for 18 to 24 hours. *N. cinerea* is susceptible (10 mm or more zone of inhibition) to colistin, whereas *N. gonorrhoeae* is resistant. Useful tests for differentiation of *N. cinerea* from *M. catarrhalis* are reduction of nitrate and negative DNase reaction. Useful observation for differentiation from *N. flavescens* is lack of yellow pigment production.

Neisseria flavescens

Neisseria flavescens (*flavescens* means "yellow") is a yellow-pigmented *Neisseria* species that is asaccharolytic. It can be differentiated from *N. cinerea* by its ability to grow on SBA or CHOC agar at 22° C and its yellow colonies.

Neisseria lactamica

Neisseria lactamica was reported as early as 1934 but did not become widely recognized as being separate from *N. meningitidis* until 1968. It is commonly found in the nasopharynx of infants and children and, like *N. polysaccharea*, is commonly encountered in meningococcal carrier surveys. The carriage rate of this species in children appears to peak at about 2 years of age and then steadily declines. It is rarely isolated from adults. It is the only *Neisseria* species that uses lactose, thus its species designation *lactamica*.

    N. lactamica can be misidentified as *N. meningitidis* because of its similar colony morphology (*N. lactamica* is slightly smaller; Figure 17-14), its ability to grow on selective media (e.g., MTM), its carbohydrate reactions (glucose and maltose positive), and some cross-reaction with meningococcal typing sera. The definitive test for differentiation from *N. meningitidis* and all other *Neisseria* spp. is lactose utilization or positive ONPG reaction; however, *N. lactamica* can exhibit delayed lactose utilization.

Neisseria mucosa

Colonies of *N. mucosa* are large, often adherent to the agar, and very mucoid, giving the species its name. It is usually isolated from the nasopharynx of children or young adults. It has also been isolated from the airways of dolphins. This organism has been documented to cause pneumonia in chil-

dren. It has the same carbohydrate pattern as *N. sicca* and *N. subflava* biovar *perflava*, but it differs from these species in its ability to reduce nitrite to nitrogen gas, its colony morphology, and its lack of pigment production.

Neisseria polysaccharea

Neisseria polysaccharea was first described in 1974 by French investigators who isolated the organism from throats of healthy children while conducting meningococcal carriage rate surveys. The organism produces large amounts of extracellular polysaccharide when grown in media containing 1% or 5% sucrose; thus the species name. The colony morphology and carbohydrate utilization (glucose and maltose; rarely sucrose positive) of *N. polysaccharea* have led to its misidentification as the pathogenic *N. meningitidis*. Tests to separate *N. polysaccharea* from *N. meningitidis* are the ability to grow on nutrient agar at 35° C and production of polysaccharide from 1% or 5% sucrose. Additional differential tests to separate *N. polysaccharea* from *N. subflava* biovar subflava are growth on SBA or CHOC agar at 22° C and lack of yellow pigment production.

Neisseria sicca

The colonies of *N. sicca* are usually dry, wrinkled, adherent, and breadcrumb like (Figure 17-15). The word *sicca* in Latin means "dry." *N. sicca* and *N. subflava* biovar perflava are usually the two most common *Neisseria* spp. found in the respiratory tract of adults. Differentiation of this organism from *N. mucosa* and *N. subflava* biovar *perflava* has been discussed.

Neisseria subflava

The species name for *N. subflava* means "less yellow" (Figure 17-16). The organism is considered to be part of the upper respiratory microbiota. It consists of three biovars that differ from one another by their carbohydrate utilization patterns. Although it is considered to be a nonpathogen, it has been reported to cause serious infections, such as bacteremia, meningitis, and septicemia. Its clinical description may resemble *N. meningitidis* infection, including septic shock, petechial hemorrhage, and purpura. Differentiation of this species from

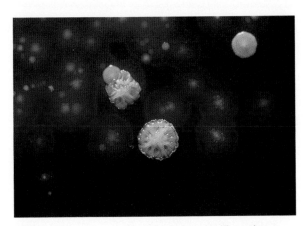

FIGURE 17-15 Dry, wrinkled, breadcrumb-like colony morphology of *Neisseria sicca* on sheep blood agar (48-hour culture).

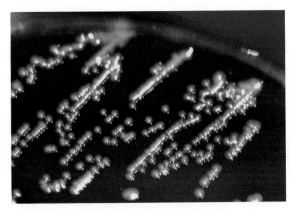

FIGURE 17-16 Yellow pigmentation of *Neisseria subflava* on sheep blood agar (48-hour culture).

N. polysaccharea is through its ability to grow on SBA or CHOC agar at 22° C and its yellow pigmentation.

Neisseria elongata

Neisseria elongata and *N. weaveri* are unique among the members of the genus *Neisseria* in that they are rods. *N. elongata* contains three subspecies, *elongata*, *glycolytica*, and *nitroreducens*. Tests used to differentiate the three subspecies are catalase, acid production from glucose, and reduction of nitrate. *N. elongata* subsp. *elongata* is catalase and nitrate reduction negative but nitrite reduction positive. *N. elongata* subsp. *glycolytica* is catalase positive and a weak acid producer from glucose. *N. elongata* subsp. *nitroreducens* is catalase negative, but nitrate and nitrite positive. The catalase test for this group of subspecies is weakly positive or negative compared with the other *Neisseria* spp. All three subspecies are commensals in the upper respiratory tract and therefore are considered opportunistic pathogens.

Neisseria weaveri

Neisseria weaveri is normal oral microbiota in dogs and can be found in humans in infections following dog bites. It is catalase positive and does not produce acid from any of the carbohydrates traditionally used to identify the *Neisseria* spp.

N. weaveri is a gram-negative rod that does not reduce nitrate but does reduce nitrite to gas. It is also weakly phenylalanine deaminase positive. This organism is usually sensitive to penicillin.

BIBLIOGRAPHY

Abuhammour WM et al: *Neisseria subflava* septicemia and meningitis, *Int Pediatr* 18:100, 2003.

American Society of Health Care Professionals: Next generation meningococcal vaccine approved. Available at: www.ashp.org/import/news/HealthSystemPharmacyNews/newsarticle.aspx?id=1772. Accessed November 19, 2008.

Association for Molecular Pathology: FDA-approved molecular diagnostic tests. Available at: www.amp.org/FDATable/FDATable.doc. Accessed November 19, 2008.

Bruce MG et al: Risk factors for meningococcal disease in college students, *JAMA* 286:688, 2001.

Centers for Disease Control and Prevention: Prevention and control of meningococcal disease. Recommendations of the Advisory Committee on Immunization Practices (ACIP), *MMWR* 54 (No. RR-7):1, 2005. Available at: www.cdc.gov/mmwr/PDF/rr/rr5407.pdf. Accessed November 19, 2008.

Centers for Disease Control and Prevention: Laboratory-acquired meningococcal disease—United States, 2000, *MMWR* 51:141, 2002. Available at: www.cdc.gov/mmwr/preview/mmwrhtml/mm5107a1.htm. Accessed November 19, 2008.

Centers for Disease Control and Prevention: Screening tests to detect *Chlamydia trachomatis* and *Neisseria gonorrhoeae* infections—2002, *MMWR* 51(No. RR15):1, 2002. Available at: www.cdc.gov/mmwr/preview/mmwrhtml/rr5115a1.htm. Accessed November 19, 2008.

Centers for Disease Control and Prevention: Sexually transmitted diseases treatment guidelines, 2006, *MMWR* 55(No. RR11):1, 2006. Available at: http://www.cdc.gov/std/treatment/2006/rr5511.pdf. Accessed November 19, 2008.

Centers for Disease Control and Prevention: Sexually transmitted disease surveillance 2006 supplement: Gonococcal Isolate Surveillance Project (GISP) Annual Report 2006 Department of Health and Human Services, April, 2008. Available at: http://www.cdc.gov/std/gisp2006/GISPSurvSupp2006Short.pdf. Accessed November 19, 2008.

Centers for Disease Control and Prevention: Update to CDC's sexually transmitted diseases treatment guidelines, 2006: Fluoroquinolones no longer recommended for treatment of gonococcal infections, *MMWR* 56:332, 2007. Available at: www.cdc.gov/mmwr/preview/mmwrhtml/mm5614a3.htm. Accessed November 19, 2008.

Centers for Disease Control and Prevention: Summary of notifiable diseases—United States 2006, *MMWR* 55:1, 2008. Available at: www.cdc.gov/mmwr/preview/mmwrhtml/mm5553a1.htm. Accessed November 19, 2008.

Centers for Disease Control and Prevention: CDC changes recommendations for gonorrhea treatment due to drug resistance, Press Release. Available at: www.cdc.gov/media/pressrel/2007/r070412a.htm. Accessed November 18, 2008.

Centers for Disease Control and Prevention: Gonorrhea laboratory information. Available at: www.cdc.gov/std/gonorrhea/lab/default.htm. Accessed November 18, 2008.

Clinical and Laboratory Standards Institute: Performance standards for antimicrobial susceptibility testing, *Eighteenth informational supplement M100-MS18* 28:1, 2008.

Janda WM, Gaydos CA: *Neisseria*. In Murray PR et al, editors: *Manual of clinical microbiology*, ed 9, Washington, DC, 2007, ASM Press.

Murray PR et al: *Neisseria* and related genera. In *Medical microbiology*, ed 5, St Louis, 2005, Mosby.

Verduin CM et al: *Moraxella catarrhalis*: from emerging to established pathogen, *Clin Microbiol Rev* 15:125, 2002.

van Deuren M et al: Update on meningococcal disease with emphasis on pathogenesis and clinical management, *Clin Micro Rev* 13:144, 2000.

Willus M et al: Neck pain and rash in an 18 year old student, *Lab Med*, 36:418, 2005.

Yazdankhah SP, Caugant DA: *Neisseria meningitidis*: an overview of the carriage state, *J Med Microbiol* 53:821, 2004.

Points to Remember

- The majority of *Neisseria* spp. are gram-negative diplococci that occur in pairs, tetrads, or short chains with adjacent sides flattened.
- Species of the genus *Neisseria* are oxidase-positive, aerobic organisms that grow best in CO_2 and increased humidity.
- *N. gonorrhoeae* and *N. meningitidis* are the primary human pathogens of the genus.
- All other *Neisseria* are considered opportunistic pathogens and must be differentiated from *N. gonorrhoeae* and *N. meningitidis*.
- Pathogenic species are fastidious organisms requiring enriched and selective media for optimal recovery.
- Growth of the primary human pathogens on selective media, such as MTM or NYC agars, is not considered confirmatory. Gram stain of the colony, oxidase, and additional laboratory tests must be performed in order to confirm the identification.
- Incidence of infections caused by commensal *Neisseria* is very low. They are not usually identified unless found in a specimen from a sterile site.
- *M. catarrhalis* is asaccharolytic, and it is differentiated from the *Neisseria* spp. by being tributyrin hydrolysis positive.

Learning Assessment Questions

1. What other organism should be considered as a possible cause of the arthritis in the patient in the Case in Point?
   a. *Neisseria lactamica*
   b. *N. meningitidis*
   c. *N. sicca*
   d. *Moraxella catarrhalis*

2. What risk factor(s) did the patient in the Case in Point likely have for acquiring this infection?
   a. Unprotected intercourse
   b. Multiple sexual partners
   c. Excessive stress on the joints
   d. Both a and b

3. What tests should be performed to identify the isolate in the Case in Point?
   a. Catalase and nitrate reduction
   b. Gram stain and oxidase test
   c. Gram stain, oxidase, and superoxol test
   d. Gram stain, oxidase, rapid carbohydrate degradation

4. What is the optimal specimen to collect for the diagnosis of gonorrhea by culture in males?
   a. Pharyngeal swab
   b. Rectal swab
   c. Urethral swab
   d. Urine

5. At what temperature should specimens for *Neisseria* spp. be transported and held in the laboratory until plated?
   a. Refrigerator temperature (4° C)
   b. Room temperature (22° C)
   c. 37° C
   d. 42° C

6. Colonies of a gram-negative diplococcus produces vigorous bubbling after the addition of 30% H_2O_2. Which of the following should you suspect?
   a. *N. gonorrhoeae*
   b. *N. lactamica*
   c. *N. meningitidis*
   d. *M. catarrhalis*

7. Which organism is a relatively common cause of otitis media in children?
   a. *N. lactamica*
   b. *N. meningitidis*
   c. *N. sicca*
   d. *M. catarrhalis*

8. A young boy is playing "fetch" with his neighbor's dog. As he attempts to take the ball out of the dog's mouth, the dog accidentally bites him on his index finger. Within 24 hours, the wound shows the classic signs of inflammation, including redness, pain, swelling, and an exudate leaking from the wound. He is taken to a pediatric hospital where a culture is performed. The direct smear indicates many polymorphonuclear neutrophils with moderate amount of intracellular and extracellular gram-negative rods. The subsequent isolate is oxidase and weak catalase positive but does not produce acid from glucose, maltose, sucrose, or lactose, and it is nitrate negative and nitrite positive. Which of the following would be the probable etiologic agent?
   a. *N. elongata* subsp. *elongata*
   b. *N. elongata* subsp. *nitroreducens*
   c. *N. weaveri*
   d. *M. catarrhalis*

9. Why is the Gram stain not recommended for diagnosing pharyngeal gonorrhea?

10. Define pelvic inflammatory disease (PID) and name possible consequences of PID. What microorganisms are the major cause of PID?

Haemophilus and Other Fastidious Gram-Negative Bacilli

A. *Haemophilus*, HACEK Group, and Similar Microorganisms

George Manuselis

- **HAEMOPHILUS**
  General Characteristics
  Haemophilus influenzae
  Infections Associated with Other *Haemophilus* Species
  Laboratory Diagnosis
  Treatment
- **HACEK GROUP**
  Haemophilus species*
  Aggregatibacter aphrophilus

*Aggregatibacter actinomycetemcomitans**
Cardiobacterium hominis
Eikenella corrodens
Kingella
- **CAPNOCYTOPHAGA**
- **PASTEURELLA**
- **BRUCELLA**
- **FRANCISELLA**

OBJECTIVES

After reading and studying this chapter, you should be able to:

1. Characterize each of the bacterial species in this section by colony and microscopic morphology, habitat, and nutritional requirements.
2. Compare the modes of transmission of each of the organisms discussed.
3. Explain the clinical significance of these organisms when isolated in the clinical laboratory.
4. Name the appropriate specimens for the recovery of these organisms.
5. Determine the appropriate culture media required for isolation of each of the organisms.
6. List the genus and species of the organisms included in the acronym HACEK and the major diseases they cause.
7. Identify the most common animal reservoir for the members of the genera *Pasteurella*, *Brucella*, and *Francisella*.
8. Compare the methods of identification currently used to diagnose infections caused by the organisms discussed in this section.

Case in Point

A 59-year-old female stroke victim was confined temporarily to a respite nursing home because her immediate family was on a short vacation. Upon admission, she complained of a slight respiratory ailment. Three days later she awoke with a stiff neck and a severe headache. Because of a high fever and other signs and symptoms of meningitis, she was transported to a nearby hospital emergency department, where a spinal tap was performed. The cerebrospinal fluid (CSF) was sent to the laboratory. The specimen was cloudy, had a high protein concentration and a low glucose concentration, and more than 420 white blood cells (WBCs)/mL were noted; 92% were polymorphonuclear cells. The Gram-stained direct smear revealed many WBCs and many small, gram-negative bacilli; some appeared coccobacillary with clear halos around them. Cultures of the CSF and blood produced heavy bacterial growth on chocolate agar but not on sheep blood or MacConkey agars.

*Some members of the HACEK group are currently under taxonomic review for nomenclature changes; for example, *Actinobacillus actinomycetemcomitans*. The newly proposed terminology is used in this chapter.

Issues to Consider

After reading the patient's case history, consider:

- The factors that would have predisposed the patient to meningitis
- Whether a vaccine is available for the etiologic agent in question
- The primary causes of meningitis in this age group
- The characteristics of the microscopic morphology and growth patterns on laboratory media that help provide a presumptive identification

Key Terms

Bipolar staining	Porphyrin
Buboes	Satellitism
Capnophilic	Select biological agent
Chancroid	Suppurative
Delta-aminolevulinic acid (ALA)	V factor (NAD)
	X factor (hemin or hematin)
Genital ulcer disease (GUD)	Zoonoses
HACEK	

This chapter describes fastidious, miscellaneous, pleomorphic (many shapes), small, gram-negative bacilli. Most of these organisms require special nutrients and environmental growth factors for isolation and identification. *Haemophilus* spp. are facultative anaerobes and obligate parasites primarily adapted to the respiratory tract of humans and animals. One major exception is *Haemophilus ducreyi*, which causes the sexually transmitted disease (STD) **chancroid.** The genera *Haemophilus, Actinobacillus,* and *Pasteurella* and the newly proposed genus *Aggregatibacter* belong to the family Pasteurellaceae. Pasteurellaceae are characteristically gram-negative, pleomorphic, coccoid- to rod-shaped cells that are nonmotile and facultatively anaerobic. They form nitrites from nitrates and are oxidase and catalase positive. Specific species of the genera *Haemophilus, Aggregatibacter (Actino-*

bacillus*), Cardiobacterium, Eikenella,* and *Kingella* have been grouped together to form the acronym **HACEK** (first letter of each genus). They reside in the human oral cavity, and some species have an enhanced capacity to cause endocarditis.

Other fastidious, gram-negative bacilli, including *Capnocytophaga, Brucella,* and *Francisella,* are also discussed in this chapter. Members of these genera are also facultative anaerobes and fastidious, gram-negative bacilli. Currently, there are seven species of *Capnocytophaga,* five of which inhabit the human oral cavity. The remaining two species are primarily normal inhabitants of the oral cavities of dogs and cats. Many members of the genera *Pasteurella, Brucella,* and *Francisella* cause zoonoses (animal diseases that are transmitted to humans from its primary animal host). Figure 18-1 depicts the prevalence of some of these fastidious organisms in relation to other gram-negative bacilli found in clinical specimens.

HAEMOPHILUS

General Characteristics

The genus *Haemophilus* consists of gram-negative, pleomorphic coccobacilli or rods that may vary microscopically from small coccobacilli in direct smears of clinical material to long filaments occasionally seen in stained smears of colony growth. They are nonmotile and facultatively anaerobic, ferment carbohydrates, are generally oxidase and catalase positive, reduce nitrates to nitrites, and are obligate parasites on the mucous membranes of humans and animals. There are currently 13 species of *Haemophilus.* The species associated with humans are *H. influenzae, H. parainfluenzae, H. haemolyticus, H. parahaemolyticus, H. aphrophilus, H. paraphrophilus, H. paraphrohaemolyticus, H. pittmaniae, H. aegyptius, H. segnis,* and *H. ducreyi.*

Based on multilocus sequence analysis, three *Haemophilus* species have been combined and placed, under taxonomic review, in the genus *Aggregatibacter* with the organism formerly named *Actinobacillus actinomycetemcomitans. H. aphrophilus* and *H. paraphrophilus* are now considered to be

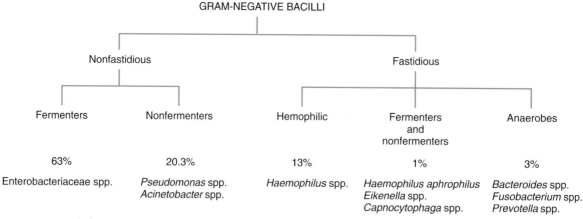

FIGURE 18-1 Prevalence of gram-negative bacilli isolated from cultures in a large tertiary hospital. Data on *Pasteurella, Brucella, Legionella,* and *Bordetella* are not included. (Data from Clinical Microbiology Laboratory, OSU Medical Center, 2000-2003.)

a single species known as *Aggregatibacter aphrophilus; H. segnis* is reclassified as *Aggregatibacter segnis*. The *Aggregatibacter* spp., especially *A. actinomycetemcomitans*, will be discussed later in the chapter. There are formal obstacles to the taxonomy changes: differences in pathogenicity, growth requirements, and other characteristics. The reader should be aware of these proposed taxonomy changes because they are seen currently in the scientific literature. The proposed new nomenclature will be used in this chapter.

Most members of the genus *Haemophilus* are nonpathogenic or produce opportunistic infections. They constitute approximately 10% of the microbiota of the healthy upper respiratory tract. The emphasis of this section is on the major pathogenic species: *H. influenzae, H. aegyptius,* and *H. ducreyi. Haemophilus* is derived from the Greek words meaning "blood-lover." As the name implies, *Haemophilus* organisms require preformed growth factors present in blood: **X factor** (hemin or hematin; "X for unknown") and/or **V factor** (nicotinamide-adenine dinucleotide [NAD], "V for vitamin"). Traditionally, a small, gram-negative bacillus (coccobacillus) is assigned to this genus based on its requirements for X and/or V factor. *Haemophilus* species with the prefix *para* only require V factor for growth.

The production of hemolysis on 5% horse or rabbit blood agar is an important differential characteristic. Although certain species are also hemolytic on sheep blood agar (SBA), the organisms will not grow in pure culture on this medium. Both X and V factors are found within red blood cells; however, only X factor is directly available. Most laboratories use SBA prepared by commercial sources. *Haemophilus* spp. that are V factor dependent do not grow because the red blood cells are still intact and the sheep red blood cells contain enzymes (NADases) that hydrolyze V factor. To alleviate this problem, clinical laboratories use chocolate (CHOC) agar for the recovery of *Haemophilus* spp. from clinical specimens. The lysing of the red blood cells by heat in the preparation of CHOC agar releases both the X and the V factors and inactivates NADases.

A phenomenon that helps in the recognition of *Haemophilus* spp. that require V factor is **satellitism.** Satellitism occurs when an organism such as *Staphylococcus aureus, Streptococcus pneumoniae,* or *Neisseria* spp. produces V factor as a byproduct of metabolism. The *Haemophilus* isolate obtains X factor from the SBA and V factor from one of these organisms. On SBA plates, tiny colonies of *Haemophilus* may be seen growing around the V factor–producing organism. Figure 18-2 illustrates *H. influenzae* satellitism around colonies of *S. aureus.* Except for *H. ducreyi,* all clinically significant *Haemophilus* spp. require V factor for growth and display this unusual growth pattern.

The indigenous microbiota of the healthy upper respiratory tract consists of many different genera and species of organisms (see Chapters 2 and 32). Approximately 10% of this normal bacterial biota in adults consists of *Haemophilus* spp., with the majority of the organisms being *H. parainfluenzae* and, to a lesser extent, nonencapsulated *H. influenzae.* Colonization begins in infancy with encapsulated strains and average 2% to 6% throughout childhood. In selected populations, such as children who attend daycare centers, coloniza-

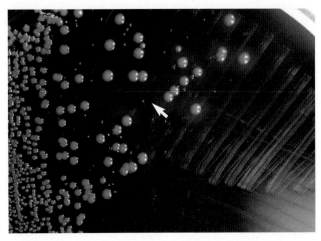

FIGURE 18-2 *Haemophilus influenzae* satellitism around and between the large, white, hemolytic staphylococci. The small, gray glistening colony is *H. influenzae (arrow).*

tion may reach as high as 60%. Nonencapsulated strains of *H. influenzae* in healthy children average 2% of the normal bacterial biota.

Haemophilus influenzae

Historical Perspective

Influenza, commonly referred to as the *flu,* is a viral disease characterized by acute inflammation of the upper airways. Symptoms often progress to intense inflammation of the mucous membranes lining the nose (coryza), headache, bronchitis, and severe generalized muscle pain (myalgias). *H. influenzae* was erroneously named during the influenza pandemic that ravaged the world between 1889 and 1890. The basis for this assumption was the frequent isolation of this bacillus from the nasopharynx of influenza patients and from postmortem lung cultures (viral isolation methods were not available). After viral culture techniques were developed, it became apparent that influenza was caused by a virus and that the actual role of *H. influenzae* was that of a secondary (opportunistic) invader.

Virulence Factors

Haemophilus influenzae, the major pathogen within the genus, has a wide range of pathogenic potential. The following virulence factors play a role in the initiation of infection and the invasiveness of this organism:

- Capsule
- Immunoglobulin A (IgA) proteases
- Adherence by fimbriae and other structures
- Outer membrane proteins and lipopolysaccharide (LPS)

Capsule. Of all the virulence factors, the capsule, if present, plays the most significant role. The serologic grouping of *H. influenzae* into six antigenically distinct types, a, b, c, d, e, and f, is based on differences of the capsular polysaccharide. Before widespread use of a vaccine, most invasive infections were caused by encapsulated strains of *H. influenzae* belonging to serotype b (Hib) and occurred primarily in young children. Currently, serotype b strains are rarely seen in children in countries using the vaccine; however, occasional serious invasive infections are seen in adults. In unvaccinated children, type b is a leading cause of meningitis. In contrast with the other serotypes, the serotype b capsule is a unique polymer composed of ribose, ribitol, and phosphate (polyribitol phosphate [PRP]). The capsule plays a significant role in the pathogenesis of invasive disease. Evidence suggests that the antiphagocytic property and anticomplementary activity of the type b capsule are important factors in virulence. Not all strains of *H. influenzae* are encapsulated.

IgA Proteases. Secretory IgA is present on human mucosal surfaces of the respiratory tract, areas for which *H. influenzae* has a predilection. *H. influenzae* is the only member of the genus that produces IgA protease. Because this enzyme has the ability to cleave secretory IgA, its production can contribute to the organism's virulence.

Adherence Mechanisms. The role of adherence mechanisms as virulence factors is not well defined. Studies indicate that most nonencapsulated strains are adherent to human epithelial cells, whereas most serotype b strains are not. The lack of this adherent capability in type b organisms may explain the tendency for type b strains to cause systemic infections. The presence of this adherent capability by nonencapsulated strains may explain the tendency for these strains to cause more localized infections.

Outer Membrane Components. Although the role of outer membrane proteins and LPS is not well defined, antibody directed against these antigens may play a significant role in human immunity. Each one of these components may be responsible for a specific activity, such as invasiveness, attachment, and antiphagocytic function. LPS has been shown to have a paralyzing effect on the sweeping motion of ciliated respiratory epithelium.

Clinical Manifestations of *Haemophilus influenzae* Infections

Two patterns of disease are attributed to *H. influenzae*. The first is invasive disease caused by encapsulated strains, in which bacteremia plays a significant role. Examples of invasive disease include septicemia, meningitis, arthritis, epiglottitis, tracheitis, and pneumonia. The second pattern of disease is a more localized infection caused by the contiguous spread of nonencapsulated strains and occurs within or in close proximity to the respiratory tract. Examples of localized infection include conjunctivitis; sinusitis; and otitis media with effusion (middle ear infections), the second most prevalent cause after *Streptococcus pneumoniae*. Nonencapsulated strains are also occasionally associated with invasive diseases such as bronchitis and pneumonia in older patients. Unlike encapsulated strains of *H. influenzae*, the nonencapsulated strains may enter the central nervous system by direct extension through infected sinuses, otitis media, and head trauma. Exceptions to the diseases caused by the encapsulated and nonencapsulated strains do occur. Nonencapsulated strains can cause meningitis in the adult population, especially in an immunocompromised or debilitated person, and they can cause neonatal sepsis.

Before the advent of the Hib vaccine, the other serotypes rarely caused invasive disease in humans. Reports of infec-

TABLE 18-1   Infections Caused by *Haemophilus influenzae*

Encapsulated Strains	Nonencapsulated Strains
Septicemia	Otitis media with effusion
Septic arthritis	Conjunctivitis
Meningitis	Sinusitis
Osteomyelitis	Bacteremia
Cellulitis	Pneumonia*
Pericarditis	
Pneumonia	
Epiglottitis	

*Nonencapsulated strains cause lower respiratory tract infections primarily in elderly patients and individuals with underlying respiratory tract problems including cystic fibrosis.

tions with these serotypes have included pneumonia and bacteremia caused by serotypes a, d, and f in immunocompromised adults and neonatal sepsis caused by serotype c. Because of the widespread use of the Hib vaccine, hospital laboratories are reporting a significant decrease in invasive disease among children, and those that do occur are generally caused by serotypes other than b. The rate of invasive *H. influenzae* infection in children younger than 5 years of age declined 99% from 1990 to 2000. Encapsulated serotypes c and f and nonencapsulated strains are currently responsible for most *H. influenzae* diseases in the United States. Type b accounts for fewer than 100 invasive *H. influenzae* infections annually. However, in developing countries where there is a lack of vaccination, serotype b is still the leading cause of bacterial pneumonia deaths and meningitis in children. *H. influenzae* still remains a problem in the older and debilitated populations who have not been vaccinated. Table 18-1 summarizes infections caused by *H. influenzae*.

Meningitis. Before widespread use of the Hib vaccine, virtually all cases of meningitis due to *H. influenzae* in children between the ages of 3 months and 6 years were caused by serotype b. Bloodstream invasion and bacteremic spread follow colonization, invasion, and replication of this organism in the respiratory mucous membranes. Headache, stiff neck, and other meningeal signs are usually preceded by mild respiratory disease.

Epiglottitis. The manifestations of epiglottitis include rapid onset, acute inflammation, and intense edema that may cause complete airway obstruction, requiring an emergency tracheostomy. To avoid causing further possible damage, the area is not swabbed for culture, but is treated empirically based on signs and symptoms. The peak incidence occurs in children between 2 and 4 years of age. Maintenance of a secure airway is the most important aspect of treatment.

Bacterial Tracheitis. Like epiglottitis, bacterial tracheitis is a serious life threatening disease in young children. It can arise after an acute, viral respiratory infection. The child begins with a mild to moderate illness for approximately 2 to 7 days, then progresses rapidly. Use of broad-spectrum antimicrobial agents during the early stages of the disease is imperative because thick secretions can occlude the trachea; therefore the disease must be differentiated from epiglottitis.

Infections Associated with Other *Haemophilus* Species

Haemophilus aegyptius

Haemophilus aegyptius (Koch-Weeks bacillus) is genetically related to *H. influenzae*. Because of their similar identifying characteristics, it is difficult to differentiate *H. influenzae* from *H. aegyptius* and *H. influenzae* biogroup aegyptius in the clinical laboratory. *H. aegyptius* was observed in conjunctivitis exudates from Egyptians by Koch in 1883, hence the species name. *H. aegyptius* is associated with an acute, contagious conjunctivitis, commonly referred to as "pinkeye" (see Chapter 41).

Haemophilus influenzae Biogroup aegyptius

Haemophilus influenzae biogroup aegyptius and *H. aegyptius* both can cause conjunctivitis, primarily in pediatric populations. Despite being nonencapsulated, *H. influenzae* biogroup aegyptius causes a severe systemic disease known as *Brazilian purpuric fever* (BPF) in hot climates. BPF is characterized by recurrent or concurrent conjunctivitis, high fever, vomiting, petechial/purpural rash, septicemia, shock, and vascular collapse. The mortality rate for BPF may reach as high as 70% within 48 hours after onset.

Haemophilus ducreyi

Haemophilus ducreyi, a strict human pathogen, is the causative agent of chancroid, a highly communicable sexually transmitted **genital ulcer disease (GUD).** It infects mucosal epithelium, genital and nongenital skin, and regional lymph nodes. Chancroid is commonly referred to as *soft chancre,* in contrast to the *hard chancre* of syphilis. Because chancroid facilitates the transmission of other STDs, all patients who have GUD should also be tested for human immunodeficiency virus along with syphilis and herpes virus.

Unlike other *Haemophilus* spp., this organism is not part of the normal microbiota. After an incubation period of approximately 4 to 14 days, a nonindurated, painful lesion with an irregular edge develops, generally on the genitalia or perianal areas. The most common sites of infection are on the penis or the labia or within the vagina. **Suppurative** (pus-forming), enlarged, draining, inguinal lymph nodes **(buboes)** are common in the majority of infected patients (Figure 18-3). Men have symptoms related to the inguinal tenderness and genital lesions, whereas most women are asymptomatic. Although fewer than 5000 cases of chancroid are reported in the United States annually, as with *Neisseria gonorrhoeae* and *Chlamydia trachomatis*, cases are probably underreported. *H. ducreyi* is an important cause of GUD in Latin America, Africa, and Asia.

Miscellaneous Species

Haemophilus parainfluenzae and the other species found in the oral cavity have a very low incidence of pathogenicity and have been rarely implicated as causative agents of endocarditis. *H. parainfluenzae*–related endocarditis has an insidious onset (a progressing disease without marked symptoms before becoming apparent); first symptoms appear approximately 1

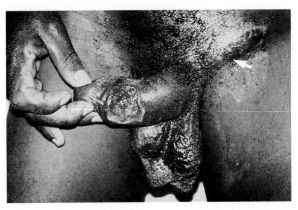

FIGURE 18-3   Lesions of chancroid on the penis, showing draining bubo *(arrow)* in the adjacent groin area. Chancroid is caused by *Haemophilus ducreyi.*

month after routine dental procedures. The mitral valve is the primary site of infection. In the absence of other pathogens, *H. parahaemolyticus* may be a cause of some cases of pharyngitis.

Laboratory Diagnosis

Specimen Processing and Isolation

Haemophilus spp. have been associated with many diseases in humans. Almost any specimen submitted for routine bacteriology examination may harbor these organisms. Common sources include blood, cerebrospinal fluid (CSF), middle-ear exudate, joint fluids, upper and lower respiratory tract specimens, swabs from conjunctivae, vaginal swabs, and abscess drainage. For culture of the lower respiratory tract, bronchial washing is recommended. *Haemophilus* spp. die rapidly in clinical specimens; therefore prompt transportation and processing are vital for their isolation. This is especially true of genital specimens submitted for *H. ducreyi*, which is extremely fastidious. Genital sites should first be cleaned with sterile gauze moistened with sterile saline before specimens are collected for the isolation of this organism. A swab, pre-moistened with sterile phosphate-buffered saline, should then be used to collect material from the base of the ulcer. As an alternative, pus can be aspirated from buboes if they are present. Direct plating on selective media at the bedside is preferred instead of using transport media. Because *Haemophilus* spp. are susceptible to drying, specimen processing in the laboratory should take place soon after collection for maximum recovery.

Because of the lack of one or more growth factors, most conventional media do not support the growth of *Haemophilus* spp. When attempting to isolate *H. influenzae*, CHOC agar is a commonly used medium incubated between 33° C and 37° C in an atmosphere of 5% to 10% CO_2. It has been shown that CHOC agar supplemented with bacitracin (300 mg/L) is an excellent medium for the isolation of *Haemophilus* spp. from respiratory specimens. Bacitracin is added to reduce overgrowth of normal respiratory microbiota. Growth on CHOC agar is usually seen after 18 to 24 hours of incubation.

Because of their fastidious nature, specimens submitted for *H. ducreyi* and *H. aegyptius* must be plated to special media. For *H. aegyptius*, CHOC agar supplemented with 1% IsoVitaleX (BD Diagnostic Systems, Sparks, Md.) or Vitox (Oxoid, Basingstoke, United Kingdom) are required. For *H. ducreyi*, Nairobi biplate medium is commonly used; it consists of GC agar base with 2% bovine hemoglobin and 5% fetal calf serum on one half, and Mueller Hinton agar with 5% chocolatized horse blood on the other. Both sides contain 3 mg/L of vancomycin. The use of GC agar (GIBCO Laboratories, Grand Island, N.Y.) containing 1% hemoglobin, 5% fetal calf serum, 1% IsoVitaleX, and 3 mg/L of vancomycin is reported to be reliable. The use of vancomycin (most *H. ducreyi* are resistant) in this medium helps reduce the growth of commensal biota from genital specimens and improves the detection of *H. ducreyi*. The plates for the recovery of this organism should be incubated in a 5% to 10% CO_2 atmosphere containing high humidity. In contrast to the optimum growth temperature (35° to 37° C) of the other *Haemophilus* spp., *H. ducreyi* grows best at 33° C. Specimens submitted for *H. aegyptius* should be held for at least 4 days, and specimens for *H. ducreyi* should be held for at least 7 days, before reporting a negative result.

Microscopic Morphology

As is common with most of the *Haemophilus* spp., the microscopic morphology varies from small, gram-negative coccobacilli to long filaments. The coccobacillary morphology is the more predominant form found in clinical specimens. Capsules of *H. influenzae* may be observed in Gram-stained direct smears as clear, nonstaining areas ("halos") surrounding the organisms in purulent secretions. Because the organism is small and pleomorphic and often stains a faint pink, it can resemble the amorphous serous material (serum-like or proteinaceous background material) in Gram stains of clinical specimens.

Because of the low specificity and sensitivity of Gram stains, an acridine orange or methylene blue stain of the specimen may help in detecting *Haemophilus*. Figure 18-4 illustrates the microscopic morphology of *H. influenzae* in a direct Gram-stained smear of CSF from a patient with meningitis. Figure 18-5 is an example of a Gram stain of an isolated colony of *H. influenzae*. Gram stains for microscopic morphology of genital lesions or colonies for *H. ducreyi* may show pale staining gram-negative coccobacilli arranged singly, or in groups (clusters) commonly referred to as "school of fish" or "railroad tracks" that are loosely coiled clusters of organisms lined up in parallel, or appearing as "fingerprints."

Colony Morphology

Most clinical specimens are plated onto a variety of culture media and examined after 24 hours of incubation. Usually SBA, CHOC, and MacConkey (MAC) agar plates are inoculated simultaneously from clinical specimens from areas of the human body where *Haemophilus* organisms may be isolated. Colonies of *H. influenzae* on CHOC agar appear translucent, tannish, moist, smooth, and convex, with a distinct "mousy" or bleachlike odor. Figure 18-6 shows the typical colony morphology of *H. influenzae*. The growth of *H. influ-*

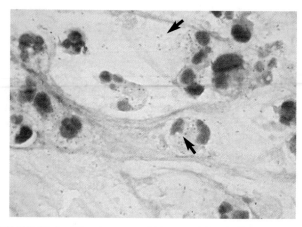

FIGURE 18-4 Direct smear of *Haemophilus influenzae* in cerebrospinal fluid in a case of meningitis. Note the intracellular and extracellular, gram-negative coccobacilli.

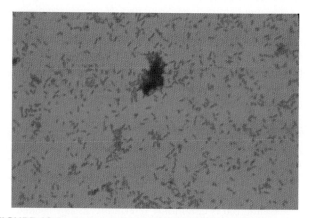

FIGURE 18-5 Gram stain of a *Haemophilus influenzae* colony. Note the slightly more elongated bacilli.

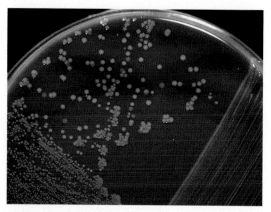

FIGURE 18-6 Example of *Haemophilus influenzae* growing on chocolate agar. Notice the tan mucoid colonies characteristic of encapsulated strains.

enzae biogroup aegyptius resembles *H. influenzae*. Encapsulated strains of *H. influenzae* grow larger and more mucoid than the nonencapsulated strains. *Haemophilus* species will not grow on MAC agar.

On CHOC agar, *H. parainfluenzae* appears tannish and drier with a medium to large size compared to *H. influenzae*.

On CHOC agar, *H. parahaemolyticus* resembles *H. parainfluenzae*; however, when grown on horse or rabbit blood agar, it is β-hemolytic whereas *H. influenzae* is nonhemolytic. *H. ducreyi* appears as small, flat, smooth, nonmucoid, transparent to opaque colonies, or appears tan or yellow on CHOC agar. Individual colonies can be pushed intact using a loop across the agar plate surface. They are difficult to pick up and produce a "clumpy" nonhomogeneous appearance when suspended in saline. Culture media for identification are available commercially, but when used, sensitivity is less than 80%. No U.S. Food and Drug Administration (FDA)-cleared polymerase chain reaction (PCR) test is currently available.

Laboratory Identification

The first clue that an isolate may belong to the genus *Haemophilus* is the growth of gram-negative pleomorphic coccobacilli on CHOC agar, with no growth on SBA and MAC in pure culture. Several tests can be used in the clinical laboratory for the identification of *Haemophilus* isolates. These include testing for growth factors (X and V), traditional biochemicals, hemolysis on media containing rabbit or horse red blood cells, oxidase, and catalase. In place of traditional biochemicals, several manual and automated commercial systems can be used to identify and biotype *Haemophilus* spp. within 4 hours.

X- and V-Factor Requirement. Testing for X- and V-factor requirements using impregnated strips or disks is the traditional approach for identification of *Haemophilus* spp. and some of the *Aggregatibacter* spp. Care must be taken not to transfer any X factor–containing medium to the agar plates used for X factor requirement; carryover may produce erroneous or less than definitive results causing *H. influenzae* to be misidentified as *H. parainfluenzae* (see Appendix D). Figures 18-7, 18-8, and 18-9 illustrate the reactions obtained when testing for X and V factor requirements using impregnated strips. When *Haemophilus* spp are grown anaerobically they do not require heme but still require NAD. If an *H. influenzae* isolate was incubated anaerobically in this test, it could be misidentified as *H. parainfluenzae*. Of all the species that

require V factor, *A. segnis* is the only organism that is oxidase negative.

Porphyrin Test. The **porphyrin** test is an alternative method for differentiating the heme-producing species of *Haemophilus*. The porphyrin test can be performed in agar, in broth, or on a disk. The principle of the test is based on the ability of the organism to convert the substrate **delta-aminolevulinic acid (ALA)** into porphyrins or porphobilinogen, which are intermediates in the synthesis of X factor. After incubation at 35° C for 4 hours, porphobilinogen is detected by the addition of *p*-dimethylaminobenzaldehyde (Kovacs reagent). After the addition of Kovacs reagent, a red color forms in the lower aqueous phase if porphobilinogen is present. Porphyrins can be detected using an ultraviolet light with a wavelength of about 360 nm (Wood's lamp). Porphyrins fluoresce reddish-orange under ultraviolet light.

The main advantage of the porphyrin test is that X factor is not required; therefore the problem of carryover is elimi-

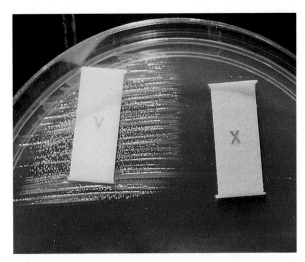

FIGURE 18-8 This organism requires V factor only would be identified as *Haemophilus parainfluenzae*.

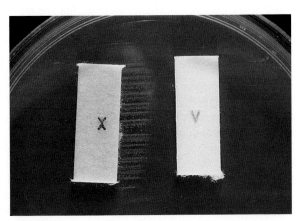

FIGURE 18-7 This organism would be identified as *Haemophilus influenzae* because it requires both X and V factors.

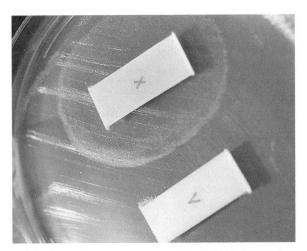

FIGURE 18-9 This organism is positive for X factor only. The probable species is *Aggregatibacter aphrophilus* because this species can appear to be hemin dependent on initial isolation.

TABLE 18-2 Differential Tests for *Haemophilus* and *Aggregatibacter* Species

	Oxidase	Catalase	Hemolysis (Horse, Rabbit Blood)	Carbon Dioxide Enhances Growth	ONPG	Glucose	Sucrose	Mannose
Factor X+, V+, Porphyrin−								
H. influenzae	+	+	−	−	−	+	−	−
H. haemolyticus	+	+	+	−	−	+	−	−
Factor X−, V+, Porphyrin+								
H. parainfluenzae	+	V	−	V	V	+	+	V
H. parahaemolyticus	+	+	+	−	−	+	+	−
H. paraphrohaemolyticus	+	+	+	+	V	+	+	−
A. segnis	−	V	−	−	−	W	W	−
Factor X+, V−, Porphyrin−								
H. ducreyi	−	−	+/−	+/−	−	−	−	−
Factor X−, V−, Porphyrin+								
A. aphrophilus*	+/−	−	−	+	+	+	+	V

+, Greater than 90% positive; −, greater than 90% negative; +/−, more positive than negative; V, variable; W, weak reception.
*On initial isolation, may appear to be hemin dependent.

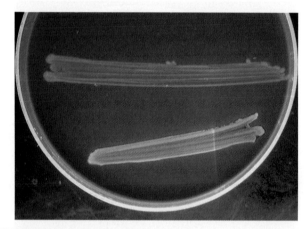

FIGURE 18-10 Under ultraviolet light, the organism on the bottom is exhibiting a positive porphyrin reaction. The organism on the top is porphyrin negative.

nated. The disadvantage is that primary identification is based on a negative test result. In the case of *H. influenzae*, the ultraviolet light test is negative (no fluorescence), and after the addition of Kovacs reagent, no color change occurs. Species that are porphyrin negative cannot synthesize heme and therefore are X factor positive (require hemin) when the impregnated strip is used. *Haemophilus* spp. that can synthesize heme are porphyrin positive (X strip negative, do not require hemin). Figure 18-10 illustrates a positive porphyrin test performed on agar.

The Haemophilus Quad Plate (Remel, Inc., Lenexa, Kan.) can be used to identify *Haemophilus* isolates. The Quad Plate contains four zones: media with X factor only, V factor only, X and V factors, and X and V factors with horse red blood cells. The *Haemophilus* isolate may be identified based on the factors required for growth and the presence of hemolysis. *H. haemolyticus* is generally β-hemolytic on horse blood, whereas *H. influenzae* is negative. Misidentifying *H. haemolyticus* as *H. influenzae* may result in overtreatment, because hemolysis

is the major differentiating characteristic between the two species.

Biochemical Tests. Biochemical tests, such as carbohydrate fermentations, can help further differentiate the *Haemophilus* spp. In addition, indole, urease, and ornithine decarboxylase tests are used to biotype some of the *Haemophilus* spp. A number of commercial multitest systems are available, including the IDS RapID-NH (Remel, Inc.), HNID (Dade Behring, Newark, Del.), Crystal Neisseria/Haemophilus (BD Diagnostic Systems), and NHI Card (bioMérieux, Inc., Hazelwood, Mo.). Table 18-2 lists the differential tests for *Haemophilus* and *Aggregatibacter* spp. Table 18-3 lists the tests that differentiate the *H. influenzae* and *H. parainfluenzae* biogroups. Differentiating the biogroups is generally only necessary in epidemiology studies.

Treatment

The current recommended treatment of life-threatening illness caused by *H. influenzae* is cefotaxime or ceftriaxone. Alternate drugs include trimethoprim-sulfamethoxazole, imipenem, and ciprofloxacin. Also effective is chloramphenicol. Because of the increased resistance to ampicillin and the possibility of resistance to chloramphenicol, combination therapy with ampicillin and chloramphenicol may also be used for initial therapy. Non–life-threatening *H. influenzae* infection may be treated with amoxicillin-clavulanate, an oral second- or third-generation cephalosporin, or trimethoprim-sulfamethoxazole. For the treatment of *H. ducreyi*, erythromycin is the drug of choice, and azithromycin, ceftriaxone or ciprofloxacin is also recommended.

Increased resistance to ampicillin by *Haemophilus* spp. owing to β-lactamase or, to a lesser extent, altered penicillin-binding proteins has been reported. Several rapid tests to detect β-lactamase production are available, including the chromogenic cephalosporin test (Cefinase, BD Diagnostic Systems) and acidometric tests (see Chapter 13). A positive β-lactamase test means that the microorganism is resistant to ampicillin and amoxicillin.

TABLE 18-2 Differential Tests for *Haemophilus* and *Aggregatibacter* Species—cont'd

Fructose	Mannitol	Maltose	Xylose	Lactose	Nitrate	Esculin	Ornithine	Indole	Urea
V	−	−	+	−	+	−	See biotype chart		
V	−	−	V	−	+	−	−	V	+
+	−	+	−	−	+	−			
+	−	+	−	−	+	−	V	−	+
+	−	+	−	−	+	−	−	−	+
W	−	W	−	−	+	−	See biotype chart		
−	−	−	−	−	+	−	−	−	−
+	−	+	−	+	+	−	−	−	−

TABLE 18-3 Differential Tests for *Haemophilus* Biogroups

Haemophilus Biogroups	Ornithine	Indole	Urea	Distribution of Biotypes			
				Meningitis and Epiglottis	Ear Infection	Conjunctivitis	Upper Respiratory Tract
H. influenzae							
Biotype I	+	+	+	••••	••	•	•
Biotype II	−	+	+	•	••	••	•
Biotype III	−	−	+	•	•	••	•
Biotype IV	+	−	+	•	•	•	•
Biotype V	+	+	−	•	•	•	•
Biotype VI	+	−	−	•	•	•	•
Biotype VII	−	+	−	•	•	•	•
Biotype VIII	−	−	−	•	•		•
H. parainfluenzae							
Biotype I	+	−	−				
Biotype II	+	−	+				
Biotype III	−	−	+				

+, Greater than 90% positive; −, greater than 90% negative; • , 0% to 25%; ••, 26% to 50%; •••, 51% to 75%; ••••, 76% to 100%.

In the chromogenic cephalosporin test, a disk impregnated with Nitrocefin is moistened with a drop of water. Using a sterile loop, several colonies are smeared onto the disk surface, or forceps can be used to wipe the moistened disk across the colonies. If the β-lactam ring of Nitrocefin is broken by the β-lactamase enzyme, a red color on the area where the culture was applied develops. The reaction usually occurs within 5 minutes.

In the acidometric test, a strip impregnated with benzyl-penicillin and a pH indicator, bromcresol purple, is moistened with one or two drops of sterile distilled water. Using a sterile loop, several colonies are smeared onto the test strip. If the β-lactam ring of the benzylpenicillin is broken by the β-lactamase, penicilloic acid is formed, causing a drop in pH. This drop in pH is demonstrated by a color change from purple (negative) to yellow (positive) on the strip within 5 to 10 minutes.

HACEK GROUP

HACEK is an acronym consisting of the first initial of each genus represented in the group:

Haemophilus spp., especially *Aggregatibacter aphrophilus*, formerly *H. aphrophilus* and *H. paraphrophilus*

Aggregatibacter actinomycetemcomitans, formerly *Actinobacillus actinomycetemcomitans*

Cardiobacterium hominis

Eikenella corrodens

Kingella spp.

Members of this group of gram-negative bacilli have in common the need for an environment with increased CO_2 (**capnophilic**). Unlike *Haemophilus* spp., the latter four members of the HACEK group are considered to be more dysgonic (slower or poorer growing). Their predilection for attachment to heart valves, usually damaged or prosthetic,

TABLE 18-4 Summary of Key Reactions and Characteristics of HACEK and *Capnocytophaga* Species

	Catalase	Oxidase	Glucose	Maltose	Sucrose	Lactose	Comments
Aggregatibacter aphrophilus Gram stain: small coccobacillus Colony morphology: raised, convex, granular, yellowish	−	V	+	+	+	+	
Aggregatibacter actinomycetemcomitans Gram stain: very small coccobacillus Colony morphology: small colonies that adhere to agar	+	V	+	+	−	−	
Cardiobacterium hominis Gram stain: straight bacilli, spindles, rosettes Colony morphology: smooth, opaque, adherent to agar	−	+	+	+	+	−	Indole+
Eikenella corrodens Gram stain: straight bacilli Colony morphology: usually pits the agar	−	+	−	−	−	−	Smells like bleach Ornithine+
Kingella kingae Gram stain: coccoid to straight bacilli, chains and pairs, square ends Colony morphology: 2 types—spreading and corroding or smooth and convex β-hemolysis under colony	−	+	+	+	−	−	Nitrate−
***Capnocytophaga* spp.** Gram stain: long, thin bacilli; tapered ends Colony morphology: flat colonies, irregular in shape, may appear purple	−	−	+	+	−	V	Esculin V

+, Positive; −, negative; *V*, variable.

makes many of them an important cause of endocarditis. Endocarditis most commonly involves the heart valves; the lesion (referred to as *vegetation*) is composed of fibrin, platelets, polymorphonuclear cells, monocytes, and microorganisms. Additional organisms that make up the majority of cases of endocarditis are the viridans group of streptococci (most common after 1 year of age), *S. aureus, Streptococcus pneumoniae,* the coagulase-negative staphylococci, the so-called nutritionally variant streptococci (*Abiotrophia* spp.), and enterococci.

Members of the HACEK group include both fermentative and nonfermentative, gram-negative bacilli. All members can be normal biota of the oral cavity, allowing for their introduction in the bloodstream and resultant infections. All HACEK organisms are opportunists and generally require a compromised host. Risk factors for infective (bacterial) endocarditis include tooth extraction, history of endocarditis, gingival surgery, heart valve surgery, and mitral valve prolapse. Table 18-4 summarizes the key reactions and characteristics of HACEK and *Capnocytophaga* spp.

Aggregatibacter aphrophilus

Aggregatibacter aphrophilus (Gr. *aphros:* "foam loving" or needing high concentration of CO_2) is the most prevalent species in the HACEK group involved in endocarditis. It is found in dental plaque and gingival scrapings. Infections present commonly with clinical features of fever, heart murmur, congestive heart failure, and embolism. *H. aphrophilus* and *H. paraphrophilus* have been recently reclassified into the single species, *A. aphrophilus.* This species contains V factor dependent (see Figure 18-9) and independent strains

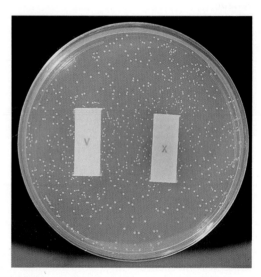

FIGURE 18-11 An *Aggregatibacter aphrophilus* isolate that is not X factor dependent and is growing over the entire surface of a trypticase soy agar plate.

(Figure 18-11). *A. aphrophilus* colonies are convex, granular, and yellow with an opaque zone near the center on CHOC agar. Figures 18-12 and 18-13 illustrate the colony and microscopic morphology of *A. aphrophilus.*

Aggregatibacter actinomycetemcomitans

Aggregatibacter actinomycetemcomitans was formerly in the genus *Actinobacillus.* The remaining members of that genus include animal pathogens or animal endogenous biota that in

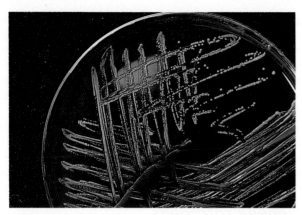

FIGURE 18-12 *Aggregatibacter aphrophilus* growing on sheep blood agar.

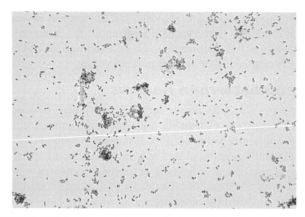

FIGURE 18-14 Gram stain morphology of *Aggregatibacter aphrophilus* (1000×).

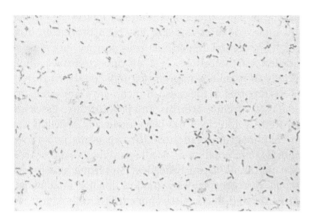

FIGURE 18-13 Gram stain, microscopic morphology of *Aggregatibacter aphrophilus* (1000×).

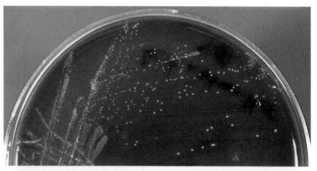

FIGURE 18-15 *Aggregatibacter actinomycetemcomitans* on sheep blood agar. The star-shaped centers of the colonies are not usually evident until after 48 hours of incubation and are best observed using a 100× magnification (light microscope) or a stereomicroscope.

general do not routinely cause infections in humans. Human tissue infections attributed to cattle, sheep, pig, and horse bites, or through contact with these animals have occurred. Six species of *Actinobacillus* have been recovered from humans. The *Actinobacillus* and *A. actinomycetemcomitans* produce small bacilli to coccoid gram-negative bacilli (Figure 18-14) that are nonmotile.

Aggregatibacter actinomycetemcomitans was given the species name because it was isolated with *Actinomyces* in a polymicrobic infection. *A. actinomycetemcomitans* is divided into six serotypes (a-f) based on its surface polysaccharides, of which a, b, and c are the most common. The organism is found as normal oral microbiota in humans. Clinically *A. actinomycetemcomitans* has been isolated from blood, lung tissue, abscesses of the mouth and brain, and sinuses. However, it has been isolated from the blood as the causative agent of subacute bacterial endocarditis with an insidious and protracted presentation. It is a recognized etiologic pathogen in the development of periodontitis. Individuals with juvenile periodontal disease or other dental disease harbor the organism where it can cause destruction of the alveolar bone that supports the teeth. Major virulence factors include collagenase and a leukotoxin that is toxic to polymorphonuclear cells and monocytes.

All members of the HACEK group, including *A. actinomycetemcomitans,* are fastidious, requiring increased CO_2 at least for initial isolation from clinical specimens. *A. actinomycetemcomitans* is a fermenter, although the addition of serum to the carbohydrate containing media is often necessary to demonstrate fermentation. The isolates may require more than 24 hours for visible growth; a distinctive "star shape with 4 to 6 points" in the center of the colonies is often seen at 48 hours. The star shape is best observed after 48 hours by using 100× magnification under a light microscope when subcultured to a clear medium, or a stereomicroscope at the highest magnification available. Figure 18-15 depicts the colony morphology. In broth, the organism is granular and may adhere to the sides of the tube. Isolates are catalase positive and oxidase variable, do not grow on MAC, and are negative for X and V growth factors, urease, indole, esculin, and citrate. *A. actinomycetemcomitans* is typically urease negative, which differentiates it from the members of the genus *Actinobacillus.* Glucose fermentation is positive (with or without gas), and fermentation of xylose, mannitol, and maltose are variable. The isolates do not ferment lactose or sucrose.

A. actinomycetemcomitans demonstrates sensitivity to penicillin in vitro, although this agent is not always successful clinically. In addition, isolates are susceptible to aminoglycosides, third-generation cephalosporins, quinolones, chloramphenicol, and tetracycline. Resistance is common to vancomycin and erythromycin. Usual treatment for endocarditis is with penicillin and an aminoglycoside.

Cardiobacterium hominis

The genus *Cardiobacterium* contains two species, *C. hominis* and *C. valvarum*. *C. hominis*, a pleomorphic, nonmotile, fastidious, gram-negative bacillus, is normal microbiota of the nose, mouth, and throat and may be present in the gastrointestinal tract. Oral infections or dental procedures usually precede the endocarditis. The usual clinical manifestation is that of endocarditis, often presenting with very large vegetations and no demonstrable fever. It infects the aortic valve more frequently than the other HACEK organisms. Rarely, *C. hominis* has been associated with meningitis.

Gram stains of the bacilli often show false gram-positive reactions in parts of the cells. The organisms tend to form rosettes, swellings, long filaments, or in yeast extract, sticklike structures. They grow slowly on SBA and CHOC agar but not at all on MAC agar. Incubation in a humid atmosphere (either aerobic or anaerobic) with 5% CO_2 enhances growth. Figures 18-16 and 18-17 illustrate the colony and microscopic mor-

phology. On agar, "pitting" may be produced. *C. hominis* is a fermenter, but as with *A. actinomycetemcomitans*, reactions may be weak, and serum may be needed. *C. hominis* ferments glucose, mannitol, sucrose (unlike *A. actinomycetemcomitans*), and maltose. Isolates are oxidase positive, catalase negative, and indole positive; the latter two traits help to further differentiate them from *Aggregatibacter* spp. *C. hominis* is negative for urease, nitrate, gelatin, and esculin. Sensitivity can be seen to β-lactams, chloramphenicol, and tetracycline with variable response to aminoglycosides, erythromycin, clindamycin, and vancomycin. Usual therapy includes penicillin and an aminoglycoside.

Eikenella corrodens

Eikenella corrodens is a member of the normal biota of the oral and bowel cavities. Most infections associated with this organism have been mixed and often occur as a result of trauma, especially after human bites or fights (i.e., "clenched fist wounds," or after the skin has been broken by human teeth). Poor dental hygiene or oral surgery has also been associated with infections. It is an opportunistic pathogen, especially in immunocompromised individuals. *E. corrodens* has been reported as the cause of meningitis, empyema, pneumonia, osteomyelitis, arthritis, and postoperative tissue infections. In drug addicts, it has been implicated in cellulitis as a result of direct inoculation of the organisms into the skin after oral contamination of needle paraphernalia (because of licking the needle clean instead of sterilizing and for good luck). *E. corrodens* shows a predilection for attachment to heart valves and thus causes endocarditis, although it is the least common isolate of the HACEK group in adult infectious endocarditis.

E. corrodens isolates are fastidious, gram-negative coccobacilli that grow best under conditions of increased CO_2 with hemin. They are nonmotile, oxidase positive, and asaccharolytic and therefore are very similar to the *Moraxella* spp. Unlike the latter, however, they are catalase negative and often produce a yellow pigment. About 45% of the isolates of *E. corrodens* "pit" (make a depression) or corrode the surface of the agar. Figures 18-18 and 18-19 illustrate the colony and microscopic morphology. Although they are nonhemolytic on

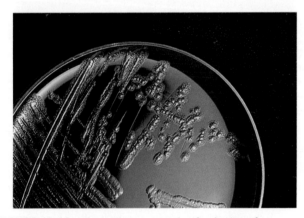

FIGURE 18-16 The 48-hour growth of colonies of *Cardiobacterium hominis* on sheep blood agar.

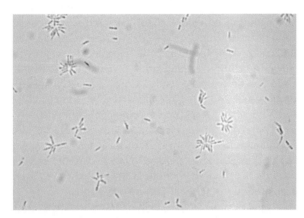

FIGURE 18-17 Gram stain of *Cardiobacterium hominis* showing typical "rosettes" (1000×).

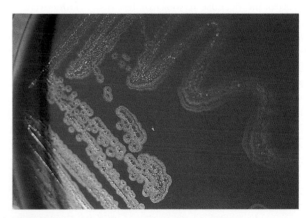

FIGURE 18-18 Growth of *Eikenella corrodens* on chocolate agar. (Compare with Figure 18-21.)

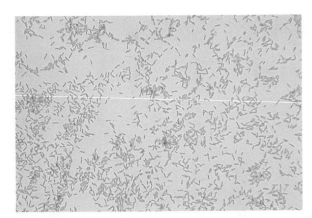

FIGURE 18-19 Gram-stain morphology of *Eikenella corrodens* (1000×).

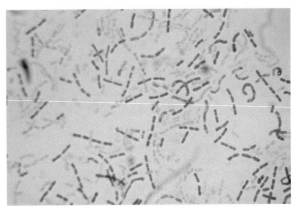

FIGURE 18-20 Gram stain of *Kingella kingae* illustrating the plump bacilli in chains. Compare with the other members of the HACEK group (1000×).

SBA, a slight greening effect due to growth may occur around the colonies. A chlorine bleachlike odor from the agar surface may be obvious. Isolates do not usually grow on MAC or eosin-methylene agar (EMB) media. In broth medium, *E. corrodens* may adhere to the sides of the tube and produce granules. It is lysine and ornithine decarboxylase positive and arginine dehydrolase negative. Typically, *E. corrodens* is resistant to clindamycin and the aminoglycosides. In vitro, isolates demonstrate sensitivity to penicillin, ampicillin, cefoxitin, chloramphenicol, carbenicillin, and imipenem.

Kingella

Members of the genus *Kingella* are coccobacillary to short bacilli with squared ends that occur in pairs or short chains (Figure 18-20). They tend to resist decolorization in the Gram stain. *Kingella* spp. are typically nonmotile. They are nutritionally fastidious, oxidase-positive, catalase-negative, fermenters of glucose and other sugars but with no gas. They colonize the upper respiratory tract, especially the tonsils. Viral infections can be a precursor to infections by these organisms. Poor dental hygiene or oral surgery is associated with infection.

The genus consists of three species: *Kingella kingae, K. denitrificans,* and *K. oralis. Kingella* species may grow on *Neisseria* selective agar (e.g., Thayer-Martin medium) and, if the isolate does not pit the agar as many strains do, can resemble *Neisseria gonorrhoeae.* Gram stain morphology of a rod with square ends and in chains should aid in distinguishing *Kingella* spp. from *N. gonorrhoeae.* Because *Kingella* spp. are usually catalase negative, and *Moraxella* and *Neisseria* are catalase positive, this test should help in differentiation. *K. denitrificans* is positive for glucose fermentation and nitrate reduction and might grow at 42° C. Unlike *Neisseria* gonorrhoeae, *K. denitrificans* is both catalase and superoxol negative. It is negative for urease, indole, esculin, gelatin, and citrate and does not grow on MAC agar. *K. denitrificans* has two types of colonies; a smooth, convex type and a spreading corroding type. This species is rarely isolated as a pathogen but has been associated with bacteremia and abscesses.

Kingella spp, especially *K. kingae,* are recognized as an important pathogen in the pediatric population. *K. kingae*

weakly ferments glucose and maltose but is negative for sucrose. Unlike other *Kingella* spp., it may produce a yellow-brown pigment. *K. kingae* has two types of colony morphologies: a spreading, corroding colony or a smooth, convex, and β-hemolytic colony. The hemolysis may appear beneath the colony or in close proximity after 24 hours. After 48 hours of incubation, the hemolysis is more evident. Isolates have been obtained clinically from blood, bone, joint fluid, urine, and wounds. It is the major gram-negative bacterium isolated from degenerative joint and bone infections (osteoarthritis) in children younger than 3 years old; in adults and school-age children, endocarditis predominates. Isolates of *Kingella* are usually susceptible to most agents, including penicillin.

CAPNOCYTOPHAGA

Capnocytophaga belongs to the family Flavobacteriaceae and includes bacteria previously called DF-1 and DF-2 (dysgonic fermenters). Currently, the genus consists of seven species, five of which are normal microbiota of the oral cavity of humans. *Capnocytophaga* resemble the HACEK in their requirements for CO_2 for enhanced growth and their isolation from blood cultures. *Capnocytophaga* spp. are not as commonly involved in endocarditis as they are in septicemia, notably in patients with neutropenia. *Capnocytophaga* spp. are fastidious, facultatively anaerobic, gram-negative bacilli. They are thin and often fusiform (pointed ends) resembling *Fusobacterium* spp.; spindle-shaped, coccoid, and curved filaments may be also seen.

Although flagella are usually absent, *Capnocytophaga* may produce gliding motility on solid surfaces. On agar, colonies are often adherent and produce a yellow-orange pigment; they can resemble colonies of *E. corrodens.* Most *Capnocytophaga* isolates are nonhemolytic, except for *C. haemolytica* (β-hemolytic). Figures 18-21 and 18-22 depict the colony and microscopic morphology. *Capnocytophaga* spp. ferment sucrose, glucose, maltose, and lactose, although triple sugar iron agar (TSIA) may be negative without enrichment. They are negative for most biochemical reactions, including indole; however, they may reduce nitrates and hydrolyze esculin. The five normal inhabitants of the human oral cavity, *C. ochracea,*

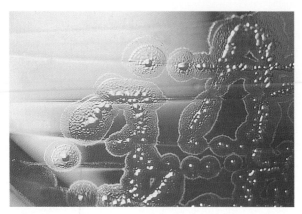

FIGURE 18-21 Growth of *Capnocytophaga* organisms on chocolate agar. Notice the spreading away from the center of the colony. Compare this growth with *Eikenella* (see Figure 18-18).

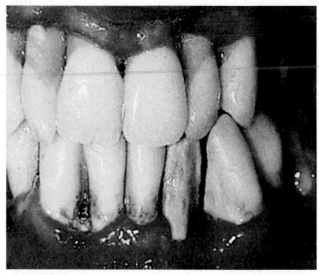

FIGURE 18-23 Advanced periodontitis. Periodontitis is the inflammation of the periodontium caused by a complex reaction initiated when subgingival plaque bacteria are in close contact with the epithelium of the gingival sulcus. (From Murray PR et al: *Medical microbiology,* ed 2, St Louis, 1994, Mosby.)

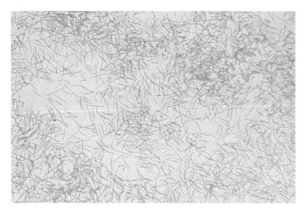

FIGURE 18-22 Gram stain of *Capnocytophaga* organisms (1000×). Notice the thin fusiform bacilli.

C. gingivalis, C. sputigena, C. haemolyticus, and *C. granulosa,* are all oxidase and catalase negative. *C. ochracea, C. gingivalis,* and *C. sputigena* are implicated in periodontitis (Figure 18-23), whereas the remaining two human species have been isolated from dental plaque. Common sites of clinical isolation include blood cultures from neutropenic patients who have oral ulcers (source of the *Capnocytophaga*), juvenile periodontal disease, and endocarditis. *C. ochracea* is the most common clinical isolate.

C. canimorsus and *C. cyodegmi* are normal inhabitants of the oral cavity of dogs and cats and are oxidase and catalase positive. *C. canimorsus* can cause a fulminant, life-threatening infection in humans following a dog or cat bite or through continuous contact. This etiologic agent should be considered in patients with a history of dog bites or saliva transfer with progressive illness. *Capnocytophaga* spp. are susceptible to imipenem, erythromycin, clindamycin, tetracycline, chloramphenicol, quinolones, and β-lactams, but they are resistant to the aminoglycosides. For *C. canimorsus* and *C. cyodegmi* infections, penicillin is the drug of choice.

PASTEURELLA

Pasteurellosis, infection with *Pasteurella* sp., is a **zoonosis**—a disease that humans acquire from exposure to infected animals or products made from infected animals. Although systemic (septicemia, arthritis, endocarditis, osteomyelitis, meningitis) and pneumonic forms are possible, cutaneous infection, frequently resulting from animal bites, is the most common presentation. These wounds can become infected with *Pasteurella* spp. because these organisms often reside in the respiratory tract and oral cavity of birds and mammals. Cutaneous infections can quickly progress resulting in inflammation and exudate production. While *Pasteurella* infections can result from a variety of animal bites, they often occur as the result of feline bites. At least 17 species of *Pasteurella* have been identified; based on DNA hybridization several species are more closely related to other genera such as *Actinobacillus*. *P. multocida* is the most frequently isolated species and includes three sub-species: *multocida, septica,* and *gallicida*. *P. multocida* also consists of five serogroups (A, B, D, E, and F) defined by capsular antigens. *P. canis* (associated with dogs), and *P. stomatis* and *P. dagmatis* (both associated with dogs and cats) are also isolated from humans.

Pasteurella spp. are gram-negative, nonmotile, facultative, anaerobic coccobacilli appearing ovoid, filamentous, or as bacilli. **Bipolar staining** (safety pin appearance when the poles of the cells are more intensely stained) is frequently observed. In biochemical tests, these bacteria are catalase and oxidase (most isolates) positive and ferment glucose with weak to moderate acid production without gas. In TSIA, a weak glucose fermentation reaction appears. All *Pasteurella* spp. will grow on SBA and CHOC agar, producing grayish colonies (Figure 18-24). Conversely, MAC agar will not support

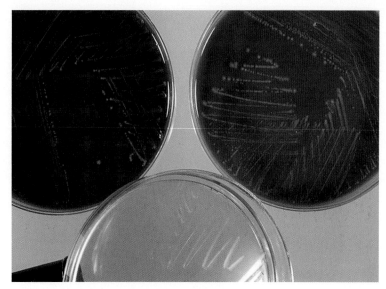

FIGURE 18-24 *Pasteurella multocida* growing on sheep blood agar and chocolate agar. The MacConkey agar plate is negative growth.

the growth of most *Pasteurella* spp. Growth on SBA in the absence of satellitism or in pure culture combined with bipolar staining may differentiate *Pasteurella* from *Haemophilus*. *P. multocida* produces nonhemolytic colonies on SBA that may appear mucoid followed by the production of a narrow green to brown halo around the colony after 24 and 48 hours of incubation at 37° C, respectively. Table 18-5 lists the various growth characteristics and biochemical reactions that can be useful in the differentiation of *Pasteurella* spp. associated with human infections. *P. bettyae* has been obtained from placenta, amniotic fluid, blood, rectal sites, abscesses, and urogenital specimens. Isolates are fastidious, capnophilic coccobacilli and bacilli that are facultatively anaerobic. They ferment glucose and fructose and are catalase positive, oxidase variable, and indole positive. They may grow on MAC and are nonmotile.

BRUCELLA

Brucellosis, infection with bacteria from the genus *Brucella*, is an important zoonotic disease found throughout the world. Due to the potential application in bioterrorism, *Brucella* spp. are considered category B **select biological agents** by the Centers for Disease Control and Prevention (CDC). Category B agents are easy to disseminate and cause moderate morbidity but low mortality. U.S. Federal Code 42CFR72.6 describes the requirements for possession and transfer of select biological agents. For more information about biological threat agents, see Chapter 30. Brucellosis is a CDC reportable disease because diagnosis can have public health implications.

Brucellosis has been described by both the disease course (undulant fever) and geographic locations where cases have occurred (Mediterranean, Crimean, and Malta fevers). Certain subpopulations are at higher risk of contacting brucellosis, such as those exposed to animals and animal products (e.g., veterinarians, hunters) and laboratory workers.

Brucellosis is acquired through aerosol, percutaneous, and oral routes of exposure. Although direct person-to-person transmission is considered rare, cases resulting from sexual contact and breast-feeding have been reported. The resulting clinical presentation appears to be similar for all exposure routes. The three clinical stages of brucellosis are acute, subchronic, and chronic. Symptoms of acute infection are nonspecific (fever, malaise, headache, anorexia, myalgia, and back pain) and usually occur within 8 weeks of exposure. Brucellosis is a systemic, deep-seated disease resulting in various long-term sequelae. The subchronic or undulant form of the disease typically occurs within a year of exposure and is characterized by undulating fevers (characterized by normal temperatures in the morning followed by high temperatures in the afternoon and evening), arthritis, and epididymoorchitis (inflammation of the epididymis and testis) in males. The chronic manifestation commonly presents 1 year after exposure with symptoms such as depression, arthritis, and chronic fatigue syndrome.

The four species that are most commonly associated with human illness are *B. melitensis, B. abortus, B. suis,* and *B. canis*. Two other species are *B. ovis* and *B. neotomae*; in recent years, additional species have been isolated from marine mammals. Brucellae are small gram-negative, aerobic, nonmotile, unencapsulated bacteria that do not form spores and may appear as coccobacilli or bacilli. Under optimal growth conditions on agar, smooth, raised, and translucent colonies will appear (Figure 18-25). The bacteria are facultative intracellular pathogens that can reside within phagocytic cells. It can be difficult to diagnose brucellosis through direct examination of a clinical sample, most often blood or bone marrow, and the ability for direct isolation and culture can vary between acute and chronic manifestations. Whereas 50% to 80% of acute cases yield positive blood cultures, only 5% of chronic cases produce positive cultures. As a result, serologic tests are frequently used, in conjunction with patient history and disease status, to diagnose brucellosis.

TABLE 18-5 Differential Characteristics of *Pasteurella* Species Associated with Human Infections

Species/ Subspecies	Normal Habitat	Hemolysis	Oxidase	Catalase	ODC	Indole	Growth on MacConkey	Urease	Comments
P. multocida subsp. *multocida* subsp. *septica* subsp *gallicida*	Oral cavities of healthy domestic dogs, cats, and other animals (swine, horses, cattle)	-	+	+	+	+	-	+	Most common isolate from human specimens; most infections are associated with dog and cat bites and scratches; can cause respiratory tract infections, including lung abscesses, pneumonia, empyema, and tonsillitis; usually underlying disease present or immune complications Differentiated by acid production from dulcitol and sorbitol; rare clinical isolates, primarily of veterinary interest; subsp. *multocida* is sorbitol+, dulcitol-, *septica* is sorbitol-, dulcitol-, *gallicida* is sorbitol and dulcitol+
P. pneumotropica	Respiratory tract of dogs, cats, and some rodents	-	+	+	+	+	V	+	Human infections acquired mostly through dog and cat bites
P. haemolytica	Severe infections in cattle, sheep, swine, and poultry	+	+	+	V	+	V	+	72% are β-hemolytic of initial isolation but may lose this characteristic on subculture; rare human infections caused by occupational or recreational exposure to animals
P. aerogenes	Oropharyngeal and intestinal biota in swine	-	+	+	V	-	+	+	Human infections caused by bites or occupational exposure
P. dagmatis	Respiratory tracts of dogs and cats	-	+	+	-	+	-	+	Human infections caused by bites and scratches of dogs and cats
P. stomatis	Oropharyngeal biota of dogs and cats	-	+	+	-	+	+	-	Caused by bites
P. canis	Biotype I is found in the oral cavity of dogs	-	+	+	+	V	-	-	Wound infections caused by dog bites
P. bettyae	Isolated from genitourinary tract including vagina, cervix, Bartholin glands, and amniotic fluid	-	V	V	-	+	V	-	Pathogen may be sexually transmitted; formally known as CDC group HB-5
P. caballi	Upper respiratory tract of horses	-	+	-	V	-	-	-	One reported case of a finger lesion in a veterinarian

+, >90% Positive; -, >90% negative; V, 20% to 80% positive.

Brucellae are oxidase and catalase positive and are urease positive within 2 hours. As shown in Table 18-6, *Brucella* spp. can vary in their requirement for CO_2 and production of a positive result for hydrogen sulfide using the lead acetate method. These tests can also differentiate brucellae from similar organisms (e.g., *Bordetella bronchiseptica*, *Acinetobacter* spp., and *H. influenzae*) when combined with growth on SBA, colony morphology, specimen source, and testing for X and V factor requirements (Table 18-7).

Because of the aerosol mode of transmission, *Brucella* spp. should be handled under biosafety level 3 conditions by an appropriately equipped laboratory. Approximately 2% of all reported cases of brucellosis are acquired in the laboratory, illustrating the risk of infection to clinical laboratory personnel. The chance of acquiring an infection from a laboratory exposure varies from 30% to 100% and depends on a range of factors.

FRANCISELLA

According to the current taxonomic classification, there are two species in the genus *Francisella*: *F. tularensis* and *F. philomiragia*, but only *F. tularensis* has been implicated in human disease. *F. tularensis* has four subspecies or biovars: subsp. *tularensis* (type A), subsp. *holarctica* (type B), subsp. *mediasiatica*, and subsp. *novicida*. *F. tularensis* subsp. *tularensis* causes the most severe disease, whereas *F. tularensis* subsp. *novicida* is an opportunistic pathogen, primarily causing disease in immunocompromised individuals. *F. tularensis* subsp. *holarctica* and *mediasiatica* produce a similar disease to *F. tularensis* subsp. *tularensis*, but infections are rarely fatal.

Tularemia, infection with bacteria from the genus *Francisella*, is also a zoonotic disease and has many other names, including rabbit, deerfly and lemming fever, and water rat trappers' disease. Tularemia can be contracted through inges-

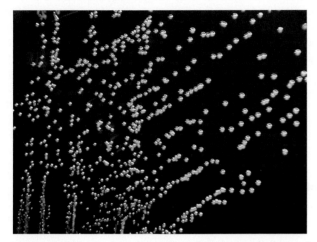

FIGURE 18-25 *Brucella melitensis* colonies on sheep blood agar appear smooth, raised, and translucent. (From the CDC Public Health Image Library. Available at: www.phil.cdc.gov/phil. Courtesy Larry Stauffer, Oregon State Public Health Laboratory.)

TABLE 18-6 Differential Characteristics of *Brucella* Species Associated with Human Infections

Brucella Species	Natural Hosts	Serum Agglutination (Patient Antibodies)	H₂S (Lead Acetate)	Urease	CO₂ (Enhanced Growth)	Growth in Dyes Thionine	Fuchsin
B. melitensis	Goat or sheep	+	−	V	−	−	−
B. abortus	Cattle	+	+	+<2 hours	+/−	+	−
B. suis	Swine	+	+	+<0.5 hour	−	−	+
B. canis	Dogs	−	−	+<0.5 hour	−	−	−

+, >90% Positive; −, >90% negative; +/−, more positive than negative; *V*, variable.

TABLE 18-7 Differential Characteristics for the Identification of *Brucella* from Similar Organisms

Test	*Brucella* spp.	*Bordetella bronchiseptica*	*Acinetobacter* spp.	*Psychrobacter phenylpyruvicus**	*Oligella ureolytica*	*Haemophilus influenzae*
Oxidase	+†	−	−	+	+	V
Motility	−	+	−	−	V	−
Urea hydrolysis	+	+	V	+	+	V
Nitrate reduction	+	+	−	V	+	+
Growth SBA	+	+	+	+	+	−
Cellular morphology	Tiny ccb stains faint	Small ccb, bacilli	Broad ccb	Broad ccb	Tiny ccb	Small ccb
Specimen source	Blood, bone marrow	Respiratory tract	Various sites	Various sites	Urinary tract	Mucous membranes
X or V factor requirement	−	−	−	−	−	+

From CDC: Presumptive *Brucella* spp. Identification and Similar Organisms: www.bt.cdc.gov/documents/PPTResponse/table5brucellaid.pdf.
+, >90% positive; −, >90% negative; *V*, variable (11% to 89% positive); *SBA*, sheep blood agar plate; *ccb*, coccobacillus.
*Formerly *Moraxella phenylpyruvica*.
†*B. abortus*, *B. melitensis*, and *B. suis* are ≥95% positive; *B. canis* is 72% positive.

tion, inhalation, arthropod bite (e.g., ticks, biting flies), or contact with infected tissues. Clinical presentation can assume a variety of forms and is influenced by the route of bacteria exposure. The most common clinical form is ulceroglandular, in which an ulcer forms at the site of inoculation and is followed by an enlargement of the regional lymph nodes. Tularemia can also occur in pneumonic (contracted via the inhalation route), glandular, oropharyngeal, oculoglandular, and typhoidal forms. In the postantimicrobial era, the case-fatality rates for *F. tularensis* subsp. *tularensis* have decreased from 5% to 10% to 1% to 2%. However, mortality rates for untreated pneumonic and typhoidal forms before the introduction of antimicrobial agents were 30% to 60%. *F. tularensis* is a CDC category A select biological agent. Category A agents are described as posing a risk to national security because they can be spread through person-to-person contact or are easily disseminated and result in high mortality rates, leading to a potentially great public health impact and public panic.

Francisella spp. appear as small, nonmotile, non–spore-forming, gram-negative bacilli or coccoid bacteria and are strictly aerobic. Similar to *Brucella* spp., *Francisella* are also facultative intracellular pathogens. *Francisella* spp. may initially grow on SBA, but they are fastidious and require supplementation with cysteine, cystine, or thiosulfate for growth on successive passage. CHOC agar, modified Thayer-Martin, and buffered charcoal yeast extract agars and Mueller-Hinton and tryptic soy broths may be used. MAC and EMB agars will not support *F. tularensis* growth. Due to slow growth rates, *F. tularensis* colonies may not be visible before 48 hours of incubation at 37° C. Once visible, gray-white, raised colonies with a smooth appearance will be seen (Figure 18-26).

F. tularensis is oxidase, urease, and satellite or X and V test negative, and weakly positive for catalase and β-lactamase activity. Additionally, clinical symptoms, patient exposure to geographic locations where tularemia is endemic, and serology are used in the diagnosis of *F. tularemia* infections. A presumptive identification can be made by a positive test result in any one of the following assays: direct fluorescent antibody, immunohistologic staining with monoclonal antibody, PCR, slide agglutination, or single serology test. Confirmation would require culture identification or a fourfold rise in antibody titer. Like brucellosis, tularemia is a CDC reportable disease. *F. tularensis* is a highly infectious agent with as few as 50 organisms causing an infection through the cutaneous (ulceroglandular form) or inhalational (pneumonia) routes and has been the cause of many laboratory-acquired infections. In a recent incident, three Boston University scientists became infected through work unknowingly performed with a fully virulent strain. Laboratory personnel should utilize appropriate laboratory safety techniques and precautions. Biosafety level 3 conditions should be implemented when working with suspected *F. tularensis* samples.

BIBLIOGRAPHY

Al Dahouk S et al: Laboratory-based diagnosis of brucellosis—a review of the literature, part II: serological tests for brucellosis, *Clin Lab* 49:577, 2003.

Brouqui P, Raoult D: Endocarditis due to rare and fastidious bacteria, *Clin Microbiol Rev* 14:177, 2001.

Centers for Disease Control and Prevention: *Kingella denitrificans.* Available at: www.cdc.gov/std/Gonorrhea/lab/Kden.htm. Accessed January 9, 2009.

Centers for Disease Control and Prevention: *Division of Bacterial and Mycotic Diseases, disease information Web site.* Available at: www.cdc.gov/ncidod/dbmd/diseaseinfo/brucellosis_g. htm. Accessed January 9, 2009.

Centers for Disease Control and Prevention: Biological and chemical terrorism: strategic plan for preparedness and response. Recommendations of the CDC Strategic Planning Workgroup, *MMWR* 49:1, 2000. Available at: www.cdc.gov/mmwr/preview/mmwrhtml/ rr4904a1.htm. Accessed January 9, 2009.

Centers for Disease Control and Prevention: Progress toward eliminating *Haemophilus influenzae* type b disease among infants and children—United States, 1998-2000, *MMWR* 51:2234, 2002. Available at: www.cdc.gov/mmwr/preview/mmwrhtml/mm5111a4. htm. Accessed January 9, 2009.

Clinical and Laboratory Standards Institute: *Abbreviated identification of bacteria and yeast.* CLSI document M35-2, Wayne, Pa, 2008.

Clock SA, et al: Outer membrane components of TAD (tight adherence) secreton of *Aggregatibacter actinomycetemcomitans, J Bacteriol* 1990:980, 2008.

Department of Health and Human Services: 45CFR Part 73, Possession, use, and transfer of select agents and toxins, *Fed Reg* 240:76886, 2002.

Ellis J et al: Tularemia, *Clin Microbiol Rev* 15:631, 2002.

Feder H et al: HACEK endocarditis in infants and children: two cases and a literature review, *Pediatric Infect Dis J* 22:557, 2003.

Fiori PL et al: *Brucella abortus* infection acquired in microbiology laboratories, *J Clin Microbiol* 38:2005, 2000.

Foster G et al: A review of *Brucella* sp. infection of sea mammals with particular emphasis on isolates from Scotland, *Vet Microbiol* 90:563, 2002.

Health Protection Agency: Identification of *Haemophilus* species and the HACEK group of organisms. National Standard Method BSOP ID 12. Available at: www.hpa-standardmethods.org.uk/ documents/bsopid/pdf/bsopid12.pdf. Accessed January 10, 2009.

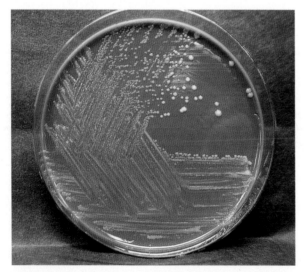

FIGURE 18-26 *Francisella tularensis* colonies grown on chocolate agar. Gray-white, raised colonies with a smooth appearance are visible following 72 hours of incubation. (From the CDC Public Health Image Library. Available at: www.phil.cdc.gov/phil. Courtesy Larry Stauffer, Oregon State Public Health Laboratory.)

Jacobs RF: Tularemia. In *Harrison's principles of internal medicine*, ed 16, New York, 2005, McGraw-Hill.

Jansen A et al: Clinical picture: rabbit's revenge, *Lancet* 3:348, 2003.

Koneman EW et al: *Color atlas and textbook of diagnostic microbiology*, ed 7, Philadelphia, 2006, J Lippincott.

Kilian M: *Haemophilus*. In Murray PR et al, editors: *Manual of clinical microbiology*, ed 9, Washington, DC, 2006, ASM Press.

Lawler A: Boston University under fire for pathogen mishap, *Science* 307:501, 2005.

Letesson JJ et al: Fun stories about *Brucella*: the "furtive nasty bug," *Vet Microbiol* 90:317, 2002.

Lindquist D et al: *Francisella* and *Brucella*. In Murray PR et al, editors: *Manual of clinical microbiology*, ed 9, Washington, DC, 2007, ASM Press.

Madoff L: Infections from bites, scratches, and burns. In *Harrison's principles of internal medicine*, ed 16, New York, 2005, McGraw-Hill.

Mandell GL et al, editors: *Principles and practices of infectious diseases*, ed 3, New York, 2000, Churchill Livingstone.

Mylonakis E, Calderwood S: Infective endocarditis in adults, *N Engl J Med* 345:1318, 2001.

Nørskov-Lauritsen N, Kilian M: Reclassification of *Actinobacillus actinomycetemcomitans*, *Haemophilus aphrophilus*, *Haemophilus paraphrophilus* and *Haemophilus segnis* as *Aggregatibacter actinomycetemcomitans* gen. nov., comb. nov., *Aggregatibacter aphrophilus* comb. nov. and *Aggregatibacter segnis* comb. nov., and emended description of *Aggregatibacter aphrophilus* to include V factor-dependent and V factor-independent isolates, *Int J Syst Evol Microbiol* 56:2135, 2006.

Omer MK et al: Prevalence of antibodies to *Brucella* spp. and risk factors related to high-risk occupational groups in Eritrea, *Epidemiol Infect* 129:85, 2002.

Robichaud S et al: Prevention of laboratory-acquired brucellosis, *Clin Infect Dis* 38:e119, 2004.

Sarinas PSA, Chitkara RK: Brucellosis, *Semin Respir Infect* 18:168, 2003.

Spinola S et al: Immunopathogenesis of *Haemophilus ducreyi* infection (chancroid), *Infect Immun* 70:1667, 2002.

Starnes CT et al: Brucellosis in two hunt club members in South Carolina, *JSC Med Assoc* 100:113, 2004.

Tarnvik A, Berglund L: Tularaemia, *Eur Respir J* 21:361, 2003.

Titball RW et al: Will the enigma of *Francisella tularensis* virulence soon be solved? *Trends Microbiol* 11:118, 2003.

von Graevenitz A et al: *Actinobacillus*, *Capnocytophaga*, *Eikenella*, *Kingella*, *Pasteurella*, and other fastidious or rarely encountered gram negative rods. In Murray PR et al, editors: *Manual of clinical microbiology*, ed 9, Washington, DC, 2007, ASM Press.

Points to Remember

- The genus *Haemophilus* consists of gram-negative pleomorphic coccobacilli or bacilli. They are nonmotile, facultative anaerobes that ferment carbohydrates and are generally oxidase and catalase positive.
- *Haemophilus* spp. require preformed growth factors present in blood: X and V factors. Testing for these factors, with X and V strips, and the porphyrin test are important aspects of laboratory identification procedures.
- The advent of the Hib vaccine has decreased infection by *H. influenzae* in vaccinated children in the United States by 99%, but serotype b remains prevalent in developing

countries. Serotype b continues to pose problems in the unvaccinated, the debilitated, and the immunocompromised adult populations of the United States.

- *H. ducreyi* causes the sexually transmitted disease chancroid. Unlike many other *Haemophilus* spp., it is not considered part of the normal oral biota of humans.
- HACEK is an acronym consisting of the first initial of each genus represented in the group: *Haemophilus*, *Aggregatibacter* (*Actinobacillus*) *actinomycetemcomitans*, *Cardiobacterium hominis*, *Eikenella corrodens*, and *Kingella* spp. The HACEK group is an important cause of endocarditis, specifically related to poor oral hygiene or dental procedures.
- Because of the lack of one or more growth factors, most conventional media do not support the growth of many of the genera discussed in this section; therefore enriched media are needed for isolation. Prolonged incubation time and increased CO_2 also play a role in culture success.
- *Pasteurella*, *Brucella*, and *Francisella* are important causes of zoonotic infections.
- The most common *Pasteurella* sp. isolated from humans, *P. multocida*, most frequently causes wounds following cat or dog bites.
- *Brucella* and *Francisella* are fastidious gram-negative coccobacilli causing zoonoses and are considered potential bioterror agents.

Learning Assessment Questions

1. The organism in the Case in Point was later identified as *Haemophilus influenzae*. Describe the appearance of this organism with the X and V strip testing.

2. The porphyrin test for *H. influenzae* would be _____, because the organism _____ biosynthesize heme. The fluorescence result of the test would be _____.
   a. Negative; cannot; negative
   b. Positive; cannot; positive
   c. Negative; can; positive
   d. Positive; can; negative

3. Infections caused by β-lactamase–positive *H. influenzae* should be treated with which of the following?
   a. Ampicillin
   b. Penicillin
   c. Either of the above
   d. None of the above

4. *Haemophilus ducreyi* is one of the most fastidious species of *Haemophilus*. Describe the optimal growth conditions for the recovery of this organism.

5. Compare the pathogenesis of *H. aegyptius* to *H. influenzae* biogroup aegyptius.

6. A cervical culture for possible gonococcal infection is sent to the microbiology laboratory. After 24 hours of incubation, the Thayer-Martin plate has small opaque

colonies that adhere slightly to the medium. Microscopic examination reveals gram-negative coccobacilli, many with square ends. The organism ferments glucose and is superoxol and catalase negative. The most likely identification is:

a. *Neisseria gonorrhoeae*
b. *Kingella denitrificans*
c. *Moraxella catarrhalis*
d. *Haemophilus ducreyi*

7. A 52-year-old recipient of a recent kidney transplant was admitted to the hospital with a low-grade fever, a heart murmur, and neutropenia. He had a history of periodontal disease and recently had two teeth extracted. Blood cultures were positive after 48 hours. The isolate grew on CHOC agar and SBA in 5% CO_2. The colonies were nonhemolytic, slightly adhered to the surface of the media, and had a slight yellow appearance when removed. The isolate was catalase, indole, and oxidase negative. Microscopic morphology indicated gram-negative fusiform bacilli. The most probable identification is:

a. *Aggregatibacter (Haemophilus) aphrophilus*
b. *Kingella kingae*
c. *Cardiobacterium hominis*
d. *Capnocytophaga* spp.

8. An isolate from a wound infection is oxidase, catalase, ornithine decarboxylase, indole, and urease positive. After 48 hours of incubation at 37° C, growth on SBA was described as mucoid colonies exhibiting a greenish brown halo. A MAC agar plate shows no growth. What organism is the mostly likely cause of the infection?

9. Which microbiologic tests are most useful in differentiating *Brucella melitensis* from *Haemophilus influenzae*?

10. A patient is complaining of a painful cervical lymph node following a case of pharyngitis. Further investigation reveals that the patient consumed a medium-cooked wild rabbit in a restaurant in Germany 2 months earlier. What is the most likely cause of infection?

B. *Legionella*

A. Christian Whelen

- ■ GENERAL CHARACTERISTICS
- ■ CLINICAL SIGNIFICANCE
  - Virulence Factors
  - Infections Caused by *Legionella*
  - Epidemiology

- ■ LABORATORY DIAGNOSIS
  - Specimen Collection and Handling
  - Microscopic Examination
  - Isolation and Identification
  - Serologic Testing
- ■ ANTIMICROBIAL SUSCEPTIBILITY

OBJECTIVES

After reading and studying this chapter, you should be able to:

1. Describe the mode of transmission of *Legionella* spp. from an environmental source to a human host.
2. Compare and contrast Legionnaires' disease and Pontiac fever.
3. Describe the cellular and colony morphology of *Legionella* spp.
4. Determine the appropriate culture media required for isolation of *Legionella* spp. from clinical specimens.
5. Discuss rapid assays useful in the detection of *Legionella* spp.

Case in Point

A group of two dozen retirees from the tobacco industry arranged to go on a 2-week cruise of the Caribbean islands. Typical accommodations included small cabins for couples, three meals a day with a late-night buffet, full bar, and recreation such as casino and floor shows that lasted well into the night. The group booked a block of rooms together and spent time socializing over drinks and cigarettes in the cabins, saunas, and poolside. On the fifth day of the cruise, several members of the party asked to see the ship's doctor because of a worsening cough. Within the next few days, 10 members of the retiree party and several other passengers were acutely ill with pneumonia and required medical evacuation to a hospital. Chest radiographs revealed progressive patchy lobar pneumonia that improved after erythromycin was administered.

Issues to Consider

After reading the patient's case history, consider:

- ■ Risk factors for the retirees for pneumonia
- ■ Causes of community-acquired pneumonia
- ■ Empirical therapy options

Key Terms

Atypical pneumonia	"Ground-glass" appearance
Buffered charcoal yeast extract (BCYE)	Legionnaire's disease
	Pontiac fever

In 1976, during an American Legion convention in Philadelphia, 221 persons became ill with pneumonia, and 34 of them died of a mysterious disease. *Legionella pneumophila*, the agent of this outbreak, became the first named member of the family Legionellaceae. The family most closely resembles the family Coxsiellaceae. Currently, the genus *Legionella* includes 50 species and more than 70 serogroups. The primary human pathogen, *L. pneumophila*, contains 16 serogroups.

The identification of *Legionella* from patient specimens is possible for most microbiology laboratories using commercial media and other diagnostic methods. An understanding of the microscopic and colony morphology of the *Legionella* spp., their nutritional requirements, the pathogenesis of infection, and the capabilities of various commercial laboratory tests enables clinical microbiologists to reliably identify these microorganisms.

GENERAL CHARACTERISTICS

The genus *Legionella* contains 50 known species, 20 of which have been isolated from humans (Box 18-1). They are ubiquitous gram-negative bacilli acquired by humans primarily through inhalation. Infected patients may present with a wide variety of conditions ranging from asymptomatic infection to life-threatening disease. The laboratory diagnosis of *Legionella* infection typically depends on one or more of the following methods:

- • Isolation using special media
- • Urine antigen detection
- • Direct fluorescent antibody
- • Serology

BOX 18-1 Grouping of Clinically Significant *Legionella* Species Based on Colony Autofluorescence*

Yellow-Green
L. birminghamensis
L. cincinnatiensis
L. hackeliae
L. jordanis
L. longbeachae
L. maceachernii
L. micdadei
L. oakridgensis
L. pneumophila[†]
L. sainthelensi
L. wadworthii

Blue-White
L. bozemanii
L. dumofii
L. gormanii
L. lytica
L. parisiensis
L. tusconensis

Blue-White or Yellow-Green
L. anisa

No Color
L. feeleii
L. lansingensis

Data from Edelstein PH: *Legionella*. In Murray PR et al, editors: *Manual of clinical microbiology*, ed 9, Washington, DC, 2007, American Society for Microbiology.
*Colonies are exposed to long-wave ultraviolet light (366 nm).
[†]Very pale yellow-green, young colonies may be negative.

CLINICAL SIGNIFICANCE

Infections caused by *Legionella* spp. produce a spectrum of symptoms, from mild upper respiratory tract infections to pneumonia. *Legionella* are responsible for 2% to 15% of community-acquired pneumonia and result in 8,000 to 18,000 hospitalizations in the U.S. annually. Because not all hospitals routinely test for *Legionella*, the actual incidence is likely higher. These microorganisms are also associated with nosocomial infections. Most human cases of legionellosis are caused by *L. pneumophila*. Other important species are *L. micdadei*, *L. longbeachae*, *L. dumoffi*, and *L. bozemanii*.

Virulence Factors

Differing presentations of *Legionella* spp. infection may be influenced by several factors, including the organism's ability to enter, survive, and multiply within the host's cells, especially bronchoalveolar macrophages, and the ability to produce proteolytic enzymes. *Legionella* spp. cause intracellular infections in humans but also survive in an extracellular environment.

Infections Caused by *Legionella*

Clinical manifestations of *Legionella* infections include febrile disease with pneumonia **(Legionnaire's disease),** febrile disease without pulmonary involvement **(Pontiac fever),** and asymptomatic infection. The mode of transmission and the number of infecting organisms in the inoculum play a role in the clinical features of the infection. In addition, host factors, such as a suppressed immune system, chronic lung disease, alcoholism, and heavy smoking predispose individuals to Legionnaires' disease.

Legionnaire's Disease

Legionnaire's disease typically presents in three major patterns: (1) sporadic cases, which are most common and usually

occur in the community; (2) epidemic outbreaks, characterized by short duration and low attack rates; and (3) nosocomial clusters, occurring in compromised patient populations. Greater than 90% of Legionnaire's disease cases are caused by *L. pneumophila,* and approximately 20% of cases are associated with travel. Pneumonia is the predominant manifestation of legionellosis, and the organisms are among the top four causes of community acquired bacterial pneumonia. *Streptococcus pneumoniae* is the most common cause of bacterial pneumonia. *Mycoplasma pneumoniae, Chlamydophila pneumoniae,* and *Legionella* produce symptoms different from *S. pneumoniae* and cause a disease sometimes referred to as **atypical pneumonia.** The mortality rate for Legionnaire's disease is 15% to 30% and may approach 50% in patients with nosocomial pneumonia if the correct diagnosis is not made early.

Serogroup 1 accounts for most cases (approximately 85%) of infection by *L. pneumophila.* Other *L. pneumophila* serogroups, commonly 4 and 6, and *L. micdadei* are more frequently implicated in clinical infections than the other *Legionella* spp. The incubation period for Legionnaire's disease is 2 to 10 days. Patients typically present with a nonproductive cough, fever, headache, and myalgia. Later, as pulmonary infiltrates develop, sputum may be bloody or purulent. Rales, dyspnea, and shaking chills are clinical manifestations of progressing disease. Dissemination via the circulatory system may lead to extrapulmonary infections with or without pneumonia. Infections of the kidneys, liver, heart, central nervous system (CNS), lymph nodes, spleen, and bone marrow as well as cutaneous abscesses have been described. Bacteremia, renal failure, liver function abnormalities, watery diarrhea, nausea, vomiting, headache, confusion, lethargy, and other CNS abnormalities have been associated with these infections.

Pontiac Fever

The nonpneumonic form of legionellosis, Pontiac fever, usually has a short incubation period of about 2 days. Patients are previously healthy individuals who complain of flulike symptoms of fever, headache, and myalgia that last 2 to 5 days and then subside without medical intervention. The incidence of Pontiac fever in the general population is unknown. *L. pneumophila* is responsible for most cases of this illness.

Epidemiology

Most members of the family Legionellaceae are found worldwide, occurring naturally in aquatic sources such as lakes, rivers, hot springs, and mud. Some species have been recovered only from environmental sources. Because *Legionella* spp. can tolerate chlorine concentrations up to 3 mg/L, they resist water treatment and subsequently gain entry into and colonize human-made water supplies and distribution systems. Hot water systems, cooling towers, and evaporative condensers are major reservoirs. Other sources include cold water systems, ornamental fountains, whirlpool spas, humidifiers, respiratory therapy equipment, and industrial process waters. The factors that contribute to the ability of *Legionella* spp. to colonize these sources include:

- The ability to multiply over the temperature range of 20° to 43° C and survive for varying periods at 40° to 60° C
- The capacity to adhere to pipes, rubber, plastics, and sediment and persist in piped water systems even when flushed
- The ability to survive and multiply within free-living protozoa and in the presence of commensal bacteria and algae

Legionella spp. are transmitted to human hosts from these environmental sources primarily via aerosolized particles, such as those produced by normal tap water pressure. Transmission between humans has not been demonstrated.

LABORATORY DIAGNOSIS

Several methods such as direct examination, culture, and antigen and antibody detection are available for the laboratory diagnosis of infections caused by *Legionella* spp. Legionnaires' disease is best approached using a combination of urine antigen detection and culture. Diagnosis of Pontiac fever is usually limited to serology. Most laboratories utilize more than one method to maximize their diagnostic capabilities.

Specimen Collection and Handling

Specimens for culture and direct examination commonly include sputum, bronchoalveolar lavage, and bronchial washings. It has been recommended that sputum purulence screens not be used. Transtracheal aspiration, lung tissue, blood, wound and abscess material, and pleural, peritoneal, and pericardial fluids may also be submitted. Respiratory secretions and body fluids (except blood) are submitted in sterile, leak-proof containers. Small pieces of tissue may be overlaid with sterile water. Saline or buffer should not be used in processing or transporting specimens because of the inhibitory effects of sodium on *Legionella* spp. Because overgrowth of contaminating microbiota can inhibit growth of *Legionella* spp. when transport of the specimens is prolonged, specimens should be refrigerated if more than 2 hours pass between collection and processing. Transport specimens to a reference laboratory on wet ice, and freeze specimens at −70° C if processing will be delayed for several days.

For blood cultures, the Isolator (Wampole Laboratories, Cranbury, N.J.) system, which uses the lysis centrifugation method, is preferred. Approximately 10 mL of blood is collected in the adult Isolator collecting tube and transported to the laboratory for processing. *Legionella* spp. can also be isolated from Bactec or BacTAlert blood culture bottles (BD Diagnostic Systems). Urine is an important specimen to be collected for antigen detection. Specimens are collected in sterile, leak-proof containers and assayed within 24 hours of collection. If testing is delayed, specimens should be stored at 2° to 8° C or frozen at −20° C. Water from environmental sources may be cultured for epidemiologic investigation.

Microscopic Examination

Legionella spp. are pleomorphic, weakly staining, gram-negative bacilli that are approximately 1 to 2 μm × 0.5 μm in size. Extending the safranin counterstaining time to at least 10

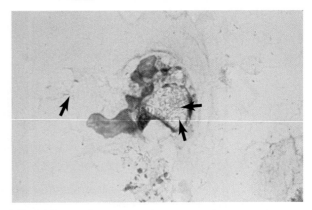

FIGURE 18-27 Gram stain of specimen demonstrating intracellular and extracellular *Legionella pneumophila* (1000×).

minutes can enhance the staining intensity of the organisms. *L. micdadei* is weakly acid-fast in tissue and stains best with the modified Kinyoun procedure (see Chapter 7). Other stains, including Diff-Quik (Baxter Scientific, Kansas City, Mo.) and Giemsa, can be used to facilitate observation of the organisms.

Nonspecific staining methods are most useful for examination of specimens from normally sterile sites. The faint-staining, pleomorphic gram-negative bacilli may be found outside of and within macrophages and segmented neutrophils (Figure 18-27). The modified Kinyoun procedure can be used for tissue if *L. micdadei* is suspected. The direct fluorescent antibody (DFA) test, discussed in the Rapid Methods section, also provides a useful method of confirming that an isolate is a *Legionella* sp. and for identifying the more common species and serogroups of the genus.

Isolation and Identification

Isolation Methods

Acid treatment of specimens contaminated with bacteria before inoculation enhances isolation of *Legionella* spp. (Figure 18-28). In this procedure, an aliquot of the specimen is first diluted 1 : 10 with 0.2 N KCl-HCl and allowed to stand for 5 minutes. Then the medium is inoculated with a portion of the acid-treated specimen. Inoculated medium is incubated at 35° to 37° C in air for at least 7 days. Usually within 3 to 5 days, *Legionella* spp. colonies are visible.

The most important test for Legionnaires' disease is culture of the organism and should always be attempted even when employing a rapid test such as urine antigen detection. *Legionella* spp. are fastidious, aerobic bacteria that will not grow on sheep blood agar (SBA) and require L-cysteine for growth. Tiny colonies may appear on chocolate agar (CHOC) agar that contains L-cysteine; however, **buffered charcoal yeast extract (BCYE)** agar with L-cysteine is best for *Legionella* isolation. BCYE is available commercially as nonselective and semiselective media, and both should be used for optimal isolation. Semiselective BCYE contains polymyxin B, anisomysin, and either vancomycin (PAV) or cefamandole (PAC). Although semiselective medium improves recovery of *Legio-*

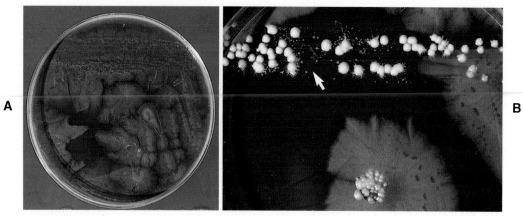

FIGURE 18-28 **A,** Nonselective buffered charcoal yeast extract (BCYE) agar plate inoculated with sputum specimen. Note overgrowth of respiratory flora. **B,** Selective BCYE agar plate inoculated with same sputum specimen, which has been acid-washed before inoculation. Much of the respiratory flora has been eliminated. *Legionella* colonies are the smallest ones in the first quadrant. (Courtesy Richard Brust.)

nella spp. from highly contaminated specimens, it can inhibit growth of some *Legionella* spp.; therefore it should not be used alone.

Colony Morphology

On BCYE medium, colonies appear as grayish-white or blue-green, convex, and glistening, measuring approximately 2 to 4 mm in diameter. When these colonies are viewed with a dissecting microscope illuminated from above, they reveal a characteristic appearance (Figure 18-29). The central portion of young colonies has a **"ground-glass" appearance,** light gray and granular, whereas the periphery of the colony has pink and/or light blue or bottle green bands with a furrowed appearance. Plates should be examined daily because older colonies lose these characteristic features and may be mistaken for other bacteria. Plates with suspicious colonies can also be illuminated with a long-wave ultraviolet light (366 nm) and can be most helpful in distinguishing those colonies that fluoresce bright blue-white from others (see Box 18-1).

Identification Methods

Conventional Methods. The physical and biochemical properties of *Legionella* spp. are listed in Box 18-2. The presumptive identification of suspected colonies as belonging to the genus *Legionella* can be accomplished by demonstrating requirement for L-cysteine, Gram stain, and DFA tests (Figure 18-30). Unfortunately biochemical testing has limited value in the further identification of isolates to the species level. The following protocol can be used to evaluate suspected colonies:

- Gram stain any suspicious colony growing on BCYE medium. *Legionella* spp. are thin, gram-negative bacilli that may show size variation from 2 to 20 μm in length.
- Subculture the isolate to BCYE with L-cysteine and to either SBA or BCYE without L-cysteine. *Legionella* spp. will grow only on BCYE medium supplemented with L-cysteine.

BOX 18-2 **Common Phenotypic Characteristics of *Legionella* Species**

- Slow growth (3 to 5 days)
- Characteristic "ground-glass" colony morphology
- Lightly staining, gram-negative bacillus
- Requires L-cysteine for primary isolation
- No growth on unsupplemented sheep blood agar
- Asaccharolytic
- Catalase or oxidase: weakly positive

- Prepare smears from colonies that require L-cysteine for growth and test with polyvalent and monovalent conjugates to determine specific species and serogroup.

Definitive identification of less-common species is usually performed at reference or public health laboratories, frequently using 16S rRNA sequencing methodology.

Rapid Methods

Urine Antigen Test. The FDA has approved several assay methods, such as radioimmunoassay, microplate enzyme immunoassay, and rapid immunochromographic assay, for *Legionella* antigen detection in urine specimens. The Binax NOW (Binax, Inc., Portland, Me.) is a 15-minute immunochromographic assay that detects soluble antigen from *L. pneumophila* serogroup 1, which is responsible for as many as 85% of the cases of legionellosis. The test has a reported sensitivity of 97.1% and a specificity of about 100%. The antigen can be detected as early as day 3 of the infection and can persist as long as 1 year; consequently the test is of limited value in persons with a recent history of *Legionella* spp. infection.

Enzyme immunoassays are also used by many clinical laboratories. Compared with culture, when using concentrated urine, the assays' sensitivity ranges from 90% to 94% and their specificity ranges from 97% to 100%. With a sensitivity of 95% and a specificity of 95%, the positive predictive value drops to 90.5%, which means 1 of every 10 positive test

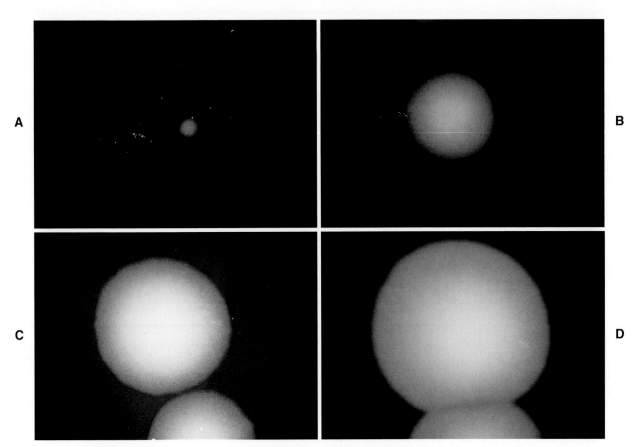

FIGURE 18-29   A, *Legionella pneumophila* colony on buffered charcoal yeast extract (BCYE) agar after 3 days of incubation, viewed with a dissecting microscope (20×). **B,** Same colony after 4 days of incubation. **C,** Same colony after 5 days of incubation. **D,** Same colony after 7 days of incubation.

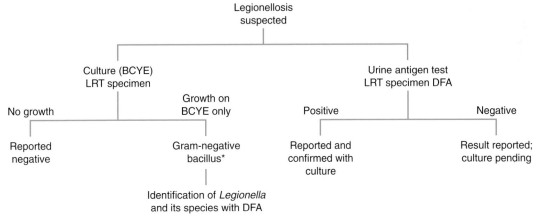

FIGURE 18-30   Schema for identification of *Legionella* organisms. *BCYE,* Buffered charcoal yeast extract; *LRT,* lower respiratory tract; *DFA,* direct fluorescent antibody. *Biohazard precautions; consider organisms such as *Francisella* spp.

results is a false positive. Furthermore, as the prevalence of *Legionella* spp. infections declines, the false-positive rate increases, making it more important to confirm results with culture, especially when determining the dynamics of this organism in a given patient population. In addition to persistent antigenuria following clinical disease mentioned earlier, prolonged secretion has also been associated with immuno-suppression, renal failure, and chronic alcoholism. Conversely, early antimicrobial intervention with macrolides may decrease antigen excretion in some patients. Despite some limitations, these rapid tests represent an important step forward in timely diagnosis of *Legionella* infections.

Direct Fluorescent Antibody Test. The DFA test is a rapid laboratory procedure for detection of the more common

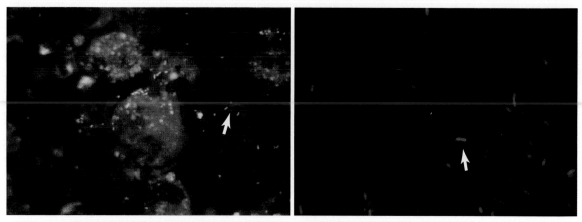

FIGURE 18-31   **A,** *Legionella pneumophila* in specimen smear stained by direct fluorescent antibody (DFA) technique (450×). **B,** *Legionella pneumophila* in specimen smear stained by DFA technique (1000×). Note intense peripheral staining of the organisms.

species of *Legionella* found in clinical samples from the lower respiratory tract. Available are fluorescein isothiocyanate (FITC)–labeled conjugates that detect all known serogroups of *L. pneumophila* (Genetic Systems, Seattle, Wash.) and *L. pneumophila* groups 1 to 7, *L. bozemanii, L. dumoffii, L. gormanii, L. longbeachae* groups 1 and 2, *L. micdadei,* and *L. jordanis.* The conjugate binds to antigens on the cell surface, and the antigen-antibody complexes are detected using a fluorescence microscope. The organisms thus appear as bright yellow to green, short or coccobacillary bacilli with intense peripheral staining (Figure 18-31).

Because of specificity and sensitivity issues, it is recommended that the DFA test should only be performed when specifically requested by the clinician, the Gram stain or special stains reveal suspicious organisms, or a large number of neutrophils are present but no organisms are seen. The microscopist must have experience with the morphologic and staining features of *Legionella* spp. so that atypical organisms will not be misidentified. The specificity of the DFA test has been reported to be 94% to 99%, but some species of *Pseudomonas, Bacteroides, Corynebacterium,* and other bacteria can cross-react with the polyvalent conjugates. Some laboratories prefer not to use polyvalent reagents for direct specimen examination because of these cross-reactions.

The sensitivity of DFA testing for direct specimen examination is approximately 25% to 80% when compared with that of culture, so a negative result does not rule out *Legionella* spp. infection. To visualize organisms, approximately 10,000 to 100,000 organisms/mL of specimen must be present. Other factors such as excessively thick smears, which tend to obscure microorganisms, and the technical skill of the observer may influence the sensitivity of the test. Consequently, DFA should not be the only test used.

DNA Detection.   Several in-house DNA detection systems have been described. The first commercially available DNA test kit (Gen-Probe, San Diego, Calif.) used an ^{125}I-labeled, single-stranded DNA probe that hybridized to the target organism's ribosomal RNA. However, this assay has been

removed from the market. The Probe-Tec ET *Legionella* assay (BD Diagnostic Systems, Sparks, Md) is FDA approved. It has a reported sensitivity of 91% and a specificity of 87% to 100%. Nucleic acid amplification tests such as polymerase chain reaction and strand displacement amplification have demonstrated potential; however, testing is not commonly available for routine clinical use.

Serologic Testing

The indirect fluorescent antibody (IFA) assay is the most common method employed for the serologic diagnosis of Legionnaires' disease, although other methods such as enzyme immunosorbent assay are available. For IFA, heat- or formalin-killed bacteria are fixed to a microscope slide. Higher titers can be seen with heat-treated organisms; however, less cross-reactivity occurs with formalin preparations. Cross-reacting immunoglobulins have been reported in patients with an infection caused by gram-negative bacilli, *Mycoplasma,* or *Chlamydia.* The sensitivity of serologic tests is reported to be 75% to 80%, with a specificity of 90% to 100%. The specificity of the test is enhanced when paired sera from patients with symptoms of legionellosis are tested. A fourfold rise in IFA titer to at least 1:128 from the acute serum phase (obtained within 1 week of onset of symptoms) to the convalescent serum phase (3 to 6 weeks later) is evidence of recent infection. However, patients with disease may not demonstrate a rise in titer for 8 weeks or longer after symptoms commence.

ANTIMICROBIAL SUSCEPTIBILITY

Susceptibility testing of *Legionella* spp. is not standardized or routinely performed. When infections are diagnosed early, they can usually be treated successfully with a macrolide such as azithromycin or a fluoroquinolone. This is particularly important in nosocomial infections, because they usually involve compromised patients and the disease often takes an aggressive course. An alternate drug is doxycycline.

BIBLIOGRAPHY

Centers for Disease Control and Prevention: Surveillance for travel-associated Legionnaires Disease—United States, 2005-2006, *MMWR* 56:1261, 2007. Available at: www.cdc.gov/mmwr/preview/mmwrhtml/mm5648a2.htm. Accessed December 22, 2008.

Domínguez J et al: Assessment of a new test to detect *Legionella* urinary antigen for the diagnosis of Legionnaires' disease, *Diagn Microbiol Infect Dis* 41:199, 2001.

Edelstein PH: *Legionella*. In Murray PR et al, editors: *Manual of clinical microbiology*, ed 8, Washington, DC, 2007, ASM Press.

Fields BS et al: *Legionella* and Legionnaires' disease: 25 years of investigation, *Clin Microbiol Reviews* 15:506, 2002.

Hayden RT et al: Direct detection of *Legionella* species from bronchoalveolar lavage and open lung biopsy specimens: comparison of LightCycler PCR, in situ hybridization, direct fluorescence antigen detection, and culture, *J Clin Microbiol* 39:2618, 2001.

Mandell LA et al: Infectious Diseases Society of America/American Thoracic Society consensus guidelines on the management of community-acquired pneumonia in adults, *Clin Infect Dis* 44(S2):S27, 2007.

Rantakokko-Jalava K, Jalava J: Development of conventional and real-time PCR assays for detection of *Legionella* DNA in respiratory specimens, *J Clin Microbiol* 39:2904, 2001.

Points to Remember

- *Legionella* are pleomorphic, weakly staining gram-negative bacilli that are ubiquitous in aquatic environments and infect humans through the respiratory route.
- *Legionella* spp. are transmitted to humans primarily via aerosolized particles. Sources include contaminated potable water distribution systems, respiratory therapy equipment, and recreational waters. Transmission between humans has not been demonstrated.
- Legionnaires' disease is a febrile disease with pneumonia that is often associated with travel, whereas Pontiac fever is a milder febrile disease without pulmonary involvement.
- On BCYE medium, colonies appear convex and glistening. The central portion of young colonies have a "ground-glass" appearance, light gray and granular, whereas the periphery of the colony has pink and/or light blue or bottle-green bands.
- Using a combination of nonselective and semiselective BCYE agar is the best strategy for *Legionella* isolation. Furthermore, acid treatment of specimens contaminated with other bacteria before inoculation also enhances isolation of *Legionella* spp.
- Rapid assays useful for the detection of *Legionella* are the urine antigen detection test and direct fluorescent antibody test.

Learning Assessment Questions

1. What three bacterial agents are the main causes of community-acquired, atypical pneumonia?
2. What risk factors contribute to the more severe form of legionellosis?
3. What environmental factors contribute to infection caused by *Legionella* spp.?
4. What are the advantages and disadvantages of direct fluorescent antibody testing for *Legionella* spp.?
5. What is the culture medium of choice for the recovery of *Legionella* spp.?
6. What is the best nonrespiratory specimen for rapid detection of *Legionella*?
7. What factors of *Legionella* can contribute to the colonization of human-made water supplies?
8. What presumptive identification methods are currently used to identify *Legionella* spp. in culture?
9. What are common phenotypic characteristics of *Legionella*?
10. Besides respiratory tract specimens, what clinical specimen is useful for the sensitive detection of *Legionella* antigen?
    a. Blood
    b. Stool
    c. Urine
    d. Cerebrospinal fluid

C. Bordetella

A. Christian Whelen

OBJECTIVES

After reading and studying this chapter, you should be able to:

1. Describe the mode of transmission of *Bordetella* spp.

2. Explain the clinical significance of *Bordetella* spp. when isolated in the clinical laboratory.

3. Describe the microscopic and colony morphology of *Bordetella* spp.

4. Determine the appropriate culture media required for isolation of *Bordetella* spp. from nasopharyngeal swabs.

5. Compare the methods of identification currently used to diagnose infections caused by *Bordetella* spp.

Case in Point

A 2-month-old girl was taken to the pediatric clinic after a 6-day history of persistent and worsening cough. The physician believed that the respiratory distress was caused by allergies and pre-scribed Albuterol MicroDiffusion Inhaler, two puffs every 4 hours for a period of 4 to 5 days. After the fifth day, the infant was taken by her parents to the emergency department. She had been coughing with increased severity, resulting in posttussive vomiting with some choking. Upon physical examination, the patient was observed having a paroxysm of cough with an inspiratory whoop. The infant was admitted to the intensive care unit (ICU) for antimicrobial therapy and monitoring of feeding and breathing.

Issues to Consider

After reading the Case in Point, consider:
- The vaccinations that would be appropriate for a child this age
- Why her physicians are concerned enough about feeding and breathing that they would admit her to the ICU

Key Terms

Adenylate cyclase toxin
Bordet-Gengou potato infusion agar
Catarrhal phase
Convalescent phase
Filamentous hemagglutinin (FHA)

Paroxysmal phase
Pertussis
Pertussis toxin (PT)
Regan-Lowe transport medium
Tracheal cytotoxin
Whooping cough

Both *Bordetella pertussis* and *B. parapertussis* are primary human pathogens of the respiratory tract, causing **whooping cough** or **pertussis,** although the latter organism is usually associated with a milder form of the disease. At least five other species are recognized: *B. bronchiseptica, B. avium, B. hinzii, B. holmesii,* and *B. trematum. B. bronchiseptica* and *B. avium* are respiratory tract pathogens of wild and domestic birds and mammals and are generally nonfastidious and recoverable on routine microbiologic culture media. *B. hinzii* appears to be an avian commensal. *B. bronchiseptica* is an opportunistic human pathogen, causing respiratory and wound infections. *B. holmesii* and *B. trematum* have only recently been described as respective agents of immune-compromised bacteremia and wound or ear infection.

GENERAL CHARACTERISTICS

Members of the genus *Bordetella* are small gram-negative bacilli or coccobacilli. All are obligate aerobic bacteria, grow best at 35° to 37° C, do not ferment carbohydrates, oxidize amino acids, are relatively inactive in biochemical test systems, and produce catalase, although this is variable in *B. pertussis*. *B. pertussis* is fastidious and requires special collection and transport systems as well as culture media. *B. pertussis* is inhibited by fatty acids, metal ions, sulfides, and peroxides, constituents found in many media. Therefore media for the isolation of *B. pertussis* requires protective substances such as charcoal, blood, or starch. The other *Bordetella* spp. are less fastidious and will grow on MAC agar or media containing blood. Among the six nonfastidious species, *B. holmesii, B. parapertussis,* and *B. trematum* are oxidase negative, whereas

B. avium, *B. bronchiseptica*, and *B. hinzii* are oxidase positive.

CLINICALLY SIGNIFICANT SPECIES

Bordetella pertussis and *Bordetella parapertussis*

Virulence Factors

Bordetella pertussis possesses a variety of virulence factors that play a role in pathogenesis of disease. **Filamentous hemagglutinin (FHA)** and pertactin (a 69-kDa outer membrane protein) are believed to facilitate attachment to ciliated epithelial cells. **Pertussis toxin (PT)** is a protein exotoxin that produces a wide variety of responses in vivo. The main activity of PT is modification of host proteins by ADP-ribosyl (adenosine diphosphate) transferase, which interferes with signal transduction. *B. parapertussis* and B. *bronchiseptica* contain the structural gene for PT but do not express the complete operon. **Adenylate cyclase toxin** inhibits host epithelial and immune effector cells by inducing supraphysiologic concentrations of cyclic adenosine monophosphate (cAMP). **Tracheal cytotoxin** contributes to pathogenesis by causing ciliostasis, inhibiting DNA synthesis, and promoting cell death. Other virulence factors have been proposed, but their current roles in disease remain unclear.

Clinical Manifestations

Classic pertussis or whooping cough resulting from *B. pertussis* infection occurs following exposure to the organism through the respiratory tract and a 1- to 3-week incubation period, usually 7 to 10 days. The initial **catarrhal phase** symptoms are insidious and nonspecific. These include sneezing, mild cough, runny nose, and perhaps conjunctivitis, although infants can develop apnea and/or respiratory distress. At this stage, the infection is highly communicable because of the large number of organisms in the respiratory tract. However, cultures are not often performed at this stage because the symptoms are nonspecific.

The catarrhal phase is followed by the **paroxysmal phase** of the disease. The hallmark of this phase is the sudden onset of severe, repetitive coughing followed by the characteristic "whoop" at the end of the coughing spell. The whooping sound is caused by the rapid gasp for air following the prolonged bout of coughing. Coughing spells may occur many times a day and are sometimes followed by vomiting. Young children may experience apnea and/or pneumonia and require aid in maintaining a patent airway. Many of these symptoms may be either absent or altered in very young infants, partially immunized children, or adolescents and adults. *B. parapertussis* generally causes a similar disease with milder symptoms. The **convalescent phase** of disease generally begins within 4 weeks of onset with a decrease in frequency and severity of the coughing spells. Complete recovery may require weeks or months.

Epidemiology

Pertussis is a human disease. No known animal reservoir or vector has been found. Infections caused by *Bordetella* spp. are acquired through the respiratory tract via respiratory droplets or direct contact with infectious secretions. Organisms are uniquely adapted to adhere to and replicate on ciliated respiratory epithelial cells. The organisms remain localized to the respiratory tract, but toxins and other virulence factors are produced and have systemic effects.

Pertussis is one of the most highly communicable diseases of childhood; secondary attack rates of 80% occur among susceptible contacts. In fact, of all childhood diseases for which universal vaccination is recommended, only pertussis incidence has increased in recent decades. This increase is also due to expansion of reporting into adolescents and adults, as well as additional diagnostic tools such as polymerase chain reaction (PCR). During 2007, the incidence of pertussis actually decreased to 3.5 cases per 100,000 population after peaking sharply the previous 2 years at 8.9 per 100,000 population. The highest rates were among infants younger than 6 months old, who were too young to be fully vaccinated; however, the greatest number of cases was reported among adolescents (10 to 19 years of age) and adults more than 20 years old. These are the age groups (infants, adolescents, and adults) when immunity from acellular pertussis (aP) vaccine, given in combination with the diphtheria-tetanus toxoids (DTaP), is either immature or waning.

Single-dose booster vaccines, administered in combination with diphtheria and tetanus toxoids, were approved in the United States in 2005 and are now available for use in both adolescents and adults; however, the 2007 decrease was probably due to the cyclic nature of the disease because immunization recommendations were not published until 2006. Even in well-immunized populations such as the United States, periodic outbreaks occur every 3 to 5 years, and isolated cases occur at all times. The childhood vaccination series consists of five doses from age 6 weeks to 6 years, and decreases in immunization rates lead to increased attack rates or major epidemics. For example, from 1990 to 1996, 54% of 10,650 children ages 3 months to 4 years with pertussis and with known vaccine status were not age-appropriately vaccinated. Immunity is short-lived, and *B. pertussis* appears to be maintained in the human population by adults who become transiently colonized. Adults may or may not experience respiratory symptoms, which can range in severity from persistent cough to acute exacerbation of chronic bronchitis. If a child has recovered from confirmed pertussis, additional doses of pertussis vaccine are not necessary.

Miscellaneous Species

The remaining *Bordetella* spp. are either opportunists or not primary human pathogens. *B. bronchiseptica* is a respiratory tract pathogen of a number of animals including dogs, in which it causes kennel cough. Symptomatic *B. bronchiseptica* infections in humans generally present with a nonspecific cough or bronchitis, and often the patients have underlying conditions such as immunosuppression or contact with animals. *B. bronchiseptica* and *B. holmesii* have been infrequently associated with pertussis syndrome and other respiratory tract infections.

LABORATORY DIAGNOSIS

Contemporary laboratory diagnosis of pertussis generally employs culture isolation with or without PCR or direct fluorescent antibody (DFA) testing. Organisms do not survive well outside the host, so culture can lack sensitivity. Rapid detection with DFA is about 60% to 70% sensitive when compared with culture and can lack specificity. Detection of *B. pertussis* DNA by PCR amplification was added to case inclusion criteria in 1995 and has gained considerable use, but a lack of standardization and single target testing has also led to false positives and outbreaks that were mistakenly attributed to pertussis in several states. However, PCR assays are generally regarded as more sensitive than cultures and DFA assays. Currently, no PCR kit is commercially available. Likewise, serologic testing can identify more cases but is not generally used because it has also not been standardized and is not widely available.

Specimen Collection and Handling

Nasopharyngeal aspirates or swabs (calcium alginate or Dacron polyester with a flexible wire shaft) are the specimen of choice for culture, DFA, and PCR testing for *Bordetella*. Throat cultures have a much lower sensitivity and should be discouraged. Generally, two swabs are collected, one through each of the external nares; the swabs should be inserted as far back as possible into the nasopharynx, rotated, held a few seconds, and then gently withdrawn. In practice, swabs are used more commonly than aspiration methods.

Nasopharyngeal swab specimens should be plated directly onto culture media or transferred to an appropriate transport system at the bedside. Fresh media or transport systems and swabs must be available to medical providers on short notice. Transport systems should be selected based on anticipated transport time and test desired. If the transit time is less than 2 hours or DFA is the desired test, the swab can be expressed into a solution of 1% casein hydrolysate (casamino acids) broth. Amies transport medium with charcoal is appropriate for up to 24 hours.

Specimens should be transported at room temperature and transferred to culture media as soon as they arrive at the laboratory. In situations requiring overnight or several day transport, half-strength charcoal agar containing 10% horse blood and 40 mg/L cephalexin (**Regan-Lowe transport medium**) should be used. This medium is prepared in screw-capped containers and is inoculated by streaking the surface and then submerging the swab in the agar and leaving it in place. The inoculated Regan-Lowe medium may be sent to the processing laboratory immediately or incubated at the local laboratory for 1 or 2 days at 35° C. The processing laboratory can test any growth on the transport medium directly for *Bordetella* spp. and use it to subculture for isolation. The CDC Pertussis Laboratory does not recommend incubation of specimens in the transport medium due to overgrowth of commensal biota and decreased yield of *B. pertussis*.

Nucleic Acid Detection

Detection of *Bordetella* spp. nucleic acid by PCR from nasopharyngeal swabs is a primary rapid diagnostic strategy. This methodology can circumvent many of the problems associated with specimen transport and bacterial cultivation; however, laboratories should use at least two DNA targets (e.g., IS*481* and *pxtS*1) and may need to seek confirmation to avoid the mischaracterization of respiratory illness. Presently, laboratories that offer PCR must conduct in-house verification and validation studies because FDA approval of products is limited to analyte-specific reagents. External proficiency testing is available from the College of American Pathologists to assist with the laboratory's overall quality assurance program.

Microscopic Examination

Clinical specimens can only be examined for *Bordetella* spp. microscopically using DFA staining. The DFA test should only be used along with culture because the lack of sensitivity diminishes the clinical utility of a negative result, and false-positive results can occur even in experienced hands. Thus DFA should not be used as a replacement for culture. Slides for DFA testing may be prepared directly from swab specimens or following expression of the material from the swab to a solution of 1% casein hydrolysate. At least two slides should be prepared; slides are dried, heat-fixed, and stained on the same day of collection or stored at −70° C and heat-fixed immediately before staining. Polyclonal fluorescent-labeled conjugates for both *B. pertussis* and *B. parapertussis* are normally used so that each reagent can serve as a negative control for the other. On microscopic examination, the organisms appear as small, fat bacilli or coccobacilli with intense peripheral yellow-green fluorescence and darker centers.

Isolation and Identification

Isolation Methods

Since the original development of **Bordet-Gengou potato infusion agar** with glycerol and horse or sheep blood, few alternative formulations have been as successful. The most successful of these is charcoal agar supplemented with 10% horse blood and 40 mg/L cephalexin. This medium is identical in composition to the transport medium of Regan and Lowe except that it contains agar at full strength. The medium has a shelf life of up to 8 weeks and is commercially available. Care should be taken to ensure the appropriate concentration of cephalexin in the medium. Some strains of *B. pertussis* have been reported to be inhibited at 40 mg/L or above. For this reason, it may be advisable to also plate a medium without cephalexin.

Plates for the recovery of *Bordetella* spp. should be incubated at 35° C in ambient air for a minimum of 7 days. It is important to ensure adequate moisture during this period to prevent plates from drying out. Most isolates of *B. pertussis* are detected in 3 to 5 days, whereas *B. parapertussis* is detected a day or so sooner. A stereomicroscope should be used to detect the colonies before they become visible to the unaided eye.

Colony Morphology

On charcoal–horse blood and Regan-Lowe media, young colonies are smooth, glistening, and silver, resembling mercury

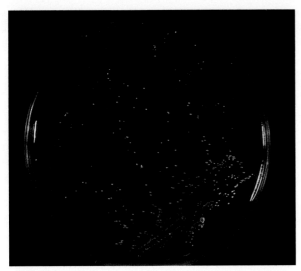

FIGURE 18-32   Five-day-old colonies of *Bordetella pertussis* on charcoal–horse blood agar *(incident light from lower right corner).*

TABLE 18-8 Differential Characteristics of *Bordetella* Species Infecting Humans

Characteristics	B. pertussis	B. parapertussis	B. bronchiseptica
Growth on			
Charcoal–horse blood	+ (3 to 5 days)	+ (2 to 3 days)	+ (1 to 2 days)
Blood agar	–	+	+
MacConkey agar	–	–	+
Catalase	+	+	+
Oxidase	+	–	+
Urease production	–	+ (24 hours)	+ (4 hours)
Nitrate reduction	–	–	+
Motility	–	–	+

droplets (Figure 18-32). Colonies turn whitish-gray as they age. On Bordet-Gengou agar, colonies of *B. pertussis* and *B. parapertussis* are hemolytic.

Identification Methods

On Gram stain of culture isolates, the organisms stain as tiny gram-negative coccobacilli and may become elongated if recovered from media containing cephalexin. It may be necessary to increase the safranin counterstaining time to 2 minutes to see typical morphology. Suspicious colonies should be further screened for *B. pertussis* and *B. parapertussis* using agglutinating or fluorescein-labeled antisera. For the fluorescent antibody test from a plate isolate, slides should be carefully prepared so that organisms are well dispersed on the slide. This ensures that individual cells show characteristic peripheral staining. The agglutination test requires a larger quantity of bacteria, so subculture from the primary isolation plate is sometimes necessary.

When the results of fluorescent staining or agglutination are clear, confirmatory testing is not required. *B. pertussis* and *B. parapertussis* can be adequately identified and separated with these serologic reagents alone. If these tests yield equivocal results, suspicious organisms should be subcultured to charcoal–horse blood agar, Sheep blood agar, and chocolate agar (the last to assess for *Haemophilus* spp. that may have broken through on selective charcoal–horse blood). Growth patterns should be observed, serologic tests repeated, and additional biochemical tests performed (Table 18-8) to confirm the identification. Box 18-3 summarizes the laboratory diagnosis of pertussis by culture.

Serologic Testing

Serologic diagnosis of pertussis can be used to study outbreaks and to document seroconversion following immunization or infection. Unfortunately, the lack of association between antibody levels and immunity to pertussis makes

BOX 18-3 Summary of Laboratory Diagnosis of Pertussis by Culture

1. Using calcium alginate or Dacron flexible wire swabs, collect two pernasal specimens from the posterior pharynx.
2. Transfer to transport system a, b, or below:
   a. 1% casein hydrolysate (1- to 2-hour holding time)
   b. Amies transport medium with charcoal (24-hour holding time)
   c. Half-strength charcoal agar with horse blood and cephalexin (incubate 1 to 2 days at 35° C before transport to laboratory)
3. Prepare two smears for direct fluorescent antibody test for *B. pertussis.*
4. Inoculate charcoal–horse agar (with cephalexin). Incubate in moist chamber (without CO_2) at 35° C for 7 days.
5. Examine plates at 2 days; thereafter for typical colonies use stereomicroscope.
6. Screen *B. pertussis*/*B. parapertussis*–like colonies with Gram stain and fluorescent antibody test or agglutinating antisera.
7. Confirm identification of equivocal results by subculture; repeat antisera tests and biochemical tests.

results of serologic testing difficult to interpret, so tests for routine purposes are not approved for diagnostic use. If serologic assays are to be performed, reference sera available from the Laboratory of Pertussis (U.S. Food and Drug Administration, Bethesda, Md) should be used for quality control.

Optimal diagnostic sensitivity requires paired sera and testing for multiple immunoglobulin class-antigen combinations (e.g., IgG to FHA and PT, along with IgA to FHA). Testing for IgM as an acute-phase antibody has been disappointing and currently is of little assistance. Serology also tends to be retrospective; several weeks are often required to demonstrate a diagnostic response. Enzyme immunoassays for IgG or IgA antibody to FHA from a single serum specimen or from nasopharyngeal aspirates have been developed but have not gained widespread acceptance.

ANTIMICROBIAL SUSCEPTIBILITY

Although a few strains of erythromycin-resistant *B. pertussis* have been reported, erythromycin is still the drug of choice for treatment and prophylaxis of pertussis. Erythromycin is important for eradication of the organism and prevention of secondary cases but has clinical efficacy only if treatment is started during the catarrhal phase of disease. Azithromycin has fewer and milder side effects, has a longer half-life, and requires fewer daily doses and better patient compliance. Trimethoprim-sulfamethoxazole is also an alternative for treatment or prophylaxis. Routine antimicrobial susceptibility testing of *B. pertussis* or *B. parapertussis* is not necessary because of predictable sensitivity to macrolides. The susceptibility of *B. bronchiseptica* is not predictable, and tests should be performed, although the organism is usually susceptible to the aminoglycosides.

BIBLIOGRAPHY

Baughman AL et al: Establishment of diagnostic cutoff points for levels of serum antibodies to pertussis toxin, filamentous hemagglutinin, and fimbriae in adolescents and adults in the United States, *Clin Diagn Lab Immunol* 11:1045, 2004.

Centers for Disease Control and Prevention: *Epidemiology and prevention of vaccine-preventable diseases,* ed 10, 2008. Available at: www.cdc.gov/vaccines/pubs/pinkbook/default.htm. Accessed December 22, 2008.

Centers for Disease Control and Prevention: FDA approval of expanded age indication for a tetanus toxoid, reduced diphtheria toxoid and acellular pertussis vaccine, 2009, *MMWR* 58:374. Available at: www.cdc.gov/mmwr/preview/mmwrhtml/mm5814a5.htm. Accessed September 10, 2009.

Centers for Disease Control and Prevention: Outbreaks of respiratory illnesses mistakenly attributed to pertussis—New Hampshire, Massachusetts, and Tennessee, 2004-6, *MMWR* 56:33, 2007. Available at: www.cdc.gov/mmwr/preview/mmwrhtml/mm5633a1.htm. Accessed December 22, 2008.

Centers for Disease Control and Prevention: Recommended childhood and adolescent immunization schedule—United States, 2006, *MMWR* 54:Q1, 2006. Available at: www.cdc.gov/mmwr/preview/mmwrhtml/mm5451-Immunizationa1.htm. Accessed December 22, 2008.

Centers for Disease Control and Prevention: Summary of Notifiable Diseases—United States, 2007, *MMWR* 56: 2009. Available at: www.cdc.gov/mmwr/PDF/wk/mm5653.pdf. Accessed September 18, 2009.

Langley JM et al: Azithromycin is as effective and better tolerated than erythromycin estolate for the treatment of pertussis, *Pediatrics* 114:e96, 2004.

Loeffelholz MJ et al: *Bordetella*. In Murray PR, et al, editors: *Manual of clinical microbiology*, ed 9, Washington, DC, 2007, ASM.

Winn W Jr et al, editors: *Koneman's color atlas and textbook of diagnostic microbiology*, ed 6, Philadelphia, 2006, Lippincott Williams & Wilkins.

Points to Remember

- Infections caused by *Bordetella* spp. are acquired through the respiratory tract via respiratory droplets or direct contact with infectious secretions.
- *B. pertussis* and *B. parapertussis* cause pertussis, or whooping cough, and are primary human pathogens of the respiratory tract.
- Isolation of *Bordetella* spp. in the clinical laboratory might be the first objective indication of suboptimal vaccination of children, colonization in adults, or waning immunity in adolescents—any of which may set the stage for an explosive outbreak because of the ease with which it is transmitted person-to-person.
- *Bordetella* spp. are tiny gram-negative coccobacilli and might become elongated if recovered from media containing cephalexin. On charcoal–horse blood agar, young colonies are smooth, glistening, and silver, resembling mercury droplets (see Figure 18-32).
- Nasopharyngeal aspirates or swab specimens should be plated directly onto culture media or transferred to an appropriate transport system (1% casein hydrolysate, Amies, or Regan-Lowe transport medium) at the bedside. The medium of choice is charcoal agar supplemented with 10% horse blood with and without 40 mg/L cephalexin.
- Contemporary laboratory diagnosis of pertussis generally employs culture isolation with or without more rapid PCR or DFA testing.
- *B. bronchiseptica* can be part of the normal oral biota of dogs and cats, and infections in humans typically follows bites by these animals.

Learning Assessment Questions

1. Public health infrastructure declined in the former Soviet-bloc countries soon after the collapse of communism. Why was this important in the spread and transmission of pertussis?
2. Are adults immune to *Bordetella pertussis* infection? Explain.
3. What are the clinical samples of choice for the diagnosis of *B. pertussis* infection?
4. What transport media are appropriate for maximum recovery of *B. pertussis*?
5. Which method is preferred for the detection of *Bordetella* in nasopharyngeal smears?
6. What is the preferred laboratory method for rapid detection of *B. pertussis* in respiratory specimens?
7. Describe the colony morphology of *B. pertussis* on charcoal agar supplemented with horse blood after 72 hours incubation.
8. How many immunizations are required for protection against pertussis in children?
9. Compare the diseases caused by *B. pertussis* and *B. parapertussis*.
10. Is serology a good method to identify and respond to pertussis outbreaks in real time?

Enterobacteriaceae

*Kimberly E. Walker, Amy J. Horneman, Connie R. Mahon,
George Manuselis*

■ **GENERAL CHARACTERISTICS**
Microscopic and Colony Morphology
Classification
Virulence and Antigenic Factors
Clinical Significance

■ **OPPORTUNISTIC MEMBERS OF THE FAMILY
ENTEROBACTERIACEAE AND ASSOCIATED
INFECTIONS**
Escherichia coli
Klebsiella
Enterobacter, Cronobacter, and *Pantoea*
Serratia
Hafnia
Proteus
Morganella
Providencia
Edwardsiella
Erwinia and *Pectobacterium*
Citrobacter

■ **PRIMARY INTESTINAL PATHOGENS OF THE FAMILY
ENTEROBACTERIACEAE**
Salmonella
Shigella
Yersinia

■ **OTHER GENERA OF THE FAMILY
ENTEROBACTERIACEAE**
Budivicia
Buttiauxella
Cedecea
Ewingella
Kluyvera
Leclercia
Leminorella
Moellerella
Obesumbacterium
Photorhabdus
Pragia
Rahnella
Tatumella
Trabulsiella
Yokenella

■ **LABORATORY DIAGNOSIS OF
ENTEROBACTERIACEAE**
Specimen Collection and Transport
Isolation and Identification
Screening Stool Cultures for Pathogens
Serologic Grouping

OBJECTIVES

After reading and studying this chapter, you should be able to:

1. List the general characteristics of organisms that belong to the family Enterobacteriaceae.

2. Describe the antigenic structures of this family of organisms and explain how these structures are used for identification.

3. Compare the virulence factors of the *Escherichia coli* strains pathogenic for the gastrointestinal tract and those involved in extraintestinal diseases.

4. Compare the pathogenesis of the three species of *Yersinia* most often recovered from humans.

5. Describe the pathogenesis of the clinically relevant members of the family Enterobacteriaceae.

6. Given the organism's characteristic growth on nonselective and selective differential media, presumptively identify the isolate to the genus level.

7. Given the key reactions for identification, place an unknown organism in its proper tribe, genus, and species.

8. Develop an algorithm using biochemical tests to identify presumptively the clinically significant Enterobacteriaceae.

Case in Point

A 67-year-old diabetic woman hospitalized for an amputation complained of flank pain and a strong urge to urinate, even though she had a urinary catheter placed at the time of the surgery. A urine sample was obtained and plated. After 24 hours of incubation, a MacConkey agar plate showed moderate growth of oxidase negative, nonlactose-fermenting organisms. A sheep blood agar plate showed no isolated colonies, just a "wave" of bacterial growth covering the entire surface of the plate. Biochemical tests to identify the isolate were performed with the following results: triple sugar iron, alkaline over acid with H$_2$S production; IMViC reactions were − − + +; urea was hydrolyzed; ornithine was decarboxylated; and phenylalanine was deaminated.

Issues to Consider

After reading the patient's case history, consider the following:

■ The significance of this patient's health status and medical history
■ The colony morphology feature that provides clues about the identity of the organism
■ The biochemical tests that are the most specific for identification of this organism

Key Terms

Buboes

Diffusely adherent *Escherichia coli* (DAEC)

Enterics

Enteroaggregative *Escherichia coli* (EAEC)

Enterohemorrhagic *Escherichia coli* (EHEC)

Enteroinvasive *Escherichia coli* (EIEC)

Enteropathogenic *Escherichia coli* (EPEC)

Enterotoxigenic *Escherichia coli* (ETEC)

H antigen

K antigen

O antigen

Shiga toxin (Stx)

Traveler's diarrhea

Verotoxin

Vi antigen

The family Enterobacteriaceae includes many genera and species. The last edition of *Bergey's Manual of Systematic Bacteriology* (Vol. 2) describes 176 named species among 44 different genera; however, clinical isolates in general acute-care facilities consist primarily of *Escherichia coli*, *Klebsiella pneumoniae*, and *Proteus mirabilis*. It is nonetheless important to be aware of the other species because they also cause significant infectious diseases.

This chapter is divided into three major areas. The first discusses clinically significant enteric species that cause opportunistic infections, the second covers primary intestinal pathogens and their related human infections, and the third describes methods of identification of these organisms. Among the many organisms in the family Enterobacteriaceae, this chapter focuses on those members that have been associated with human diseases.

GENERAL CHARACTERISTICS

The family Enterobacteriaceae, often referred to as **enterics,** consists of a large number of diverse organisms. The Enterobacteriaceae have several key laboratory features in common, but as DNA studies on each of these organisms progress, classification of the members change. Some are being added (e.g., *Plesiomonas*), and some may eventually be removed

---

> **BOX 19-1 Key Characteristics of the Family Enterobacteriaceae**
>
> • They are gram-negative bacilli/coccobacilli.
> • They do not produce cytochrome oxidase, except *Plesiomonas* (see Chapter 20).
> • They all ferment glucose.
> • They reduce nitrate to nitrite, except for *Photorhabdus* and *Xenorhabdus*.
> • They are all motile at body temperatures, except for *Klebsiella*, *Shigella*, and *Yersinia*.
> • Except for *Klebsiella*, *Proteus*, and some Enterobacter isolates, none has remarkable colony morphology on supportive media. They appear large, moist, and gray on sheep blood agar, chocolate agar, and most nonselective media.

---

from the family. At this time, several characteristics are still used to place an organism in the family Enterobacteriaceae (Box 19-1). Common characteristics also subcategorize members of the Enterobacteriaceae into a number of tribes.

Microscopic and Colony Morphology

Members of the family Enterobacteriaceae are gram-negative, nonspore-forming, facultatively anaerobic bacilli. On Gram-stained smears, they may appear as coccobacilli or as straight rods. Colony morphology on nonselective media, such as sheep blood agar (SBA) or chocolate (CHOC) agar, is of little value in their initial identification. With the exception of certain members (e.g., *Klebsiella* and, sometimes, *Enterobacter*) that produce characteristically large and very mucoid colonies, members of this family produce large, moist, gray colonies on nonselective media and are therefore indistinguishable. However, many isolates of *E. coli* are β-hemolytic.

A wide variety of differential and selective media, such as MacConkey (MAC) agar, and highly selective media, such as Hektoen enteric (HE) agar and xylose-lysine-desoxycholate (XLD) agar, are available for the presumptive identification of enteric pathogens. These media contain one or more carbohydrates, such as lactose and sucrose, which show the ability of the species to ferment specific carbohydrates. Fermentation is indicated by a color change on the medium, which results from a drop in pH detected by a pH indicator incorporated into the medium. Nonfermenting species are differentiated by lack of color change, and colonies retain the original color of the medium. Species that produce hydrogen sulfide (H$_2$S) may be readily distinguished when placed on HE or XLD agar. HE and XLD agars contain sodium thiosulfate and ferric ammonium citrate, which produce blackening of H$_2$S-producing colonies. These features have been used to initially differentiate and characterize certain genera. Definitive identification depends on the biochemical reactions and serologic antigenic structures demonstrated by the particular species.

Classification

The use of tribes in classifying the members in this family was proposed by Ewing in 1963 and has since been continued and extended in subsequent editions of Edwards and Ewing's

TABLE 19-1 Classification of Selected Species Within the Family Enterobacteriaceae

Tribe	Genus	Species	Tribe	Genus	Species
I. Escherichieae	*Escherichia*	coli	V. Klebsielleae, cont'd	*Enterobacter*	aerogenes
		albertii			cloacae
		blattae			gergoviae
		vulneris			cancerogenus (taylorae)
		fergusonii			hormaechei
		hermanii		*Pantoea*	agglomerans
	Shigella	dysenteriae		*Cronobacter*	sakazakii
		flexneri		*Hafnia*	alvei
		boydii		*Serratia*	marcescens
		sonnei			liquefaciens
II. Edwardsielleae	*Edwardsiella*	tarda			rubidaea
		liquefaciens			fonticola
		hoshinae			odorifera
		ictaluri			plymuthica
III. Salmonelleae	*Salmonella*	enterica	VI. Proteeae	*Proteus*	mirabilis
		bongori			vulgaris
IV. Citrobacteriaceae	*Citrobacter*	freundii			penneri
		koseri (C. diversus)			hauseri
		amalonaticus			myxofaciens
		youngae		*Morganella*	morganii
		braakii		*Providencia*	alcalifaciens
		farmeri			rettgeri
V. Klebsielleae	*Klebsiella*	pneumoniae subsp. pneumoniae			stuartii
		pneumoniae subsp. ozaenae	VII. Yersinieae	*Yersinia*	pseudotuberculosis
		pneumoniae subsp. rhinoscleromatis			pestis
		varicola			enterocolitica
		ornitholytica			frederiksenii
					kristensenii
					intermedia
					ruckeri

Modified and revised from Ewing WH: *Edwards and Ewing's identification of Enterobacteriaceae*, ed 4, East Norwalk, Conn, 1986, Appleton & Lange.

Identification of Enterobacteriaceae. In classifying species into tribes, Ewing grouped bacterial species with similar biochemical characteristics. Within the tribes, organisms are further classified into genera and species.

Differentiation of each genus and definitive identification of species are based on biochemical characteristics. Table 19-1 lists the bacterial species in the family Enterobacteriaceae and their respective tribes; Table 19-2 shows the biochemical features that differentiate the tribes. Although the concept of using tribes in the classification of bacteria has not been used in *Bergey's Manual of Systematic Bacteriology*, this classification has been an effective way of placing species in groups based on similar biochemical features and will be employed throughout this chapter.

Virulence and Antigenic Factors

The virulence of the Enterobacteriaceae genera is controlled by a number of factors, such as the ability to adhere, colonize, produce toxins, and invade tissue. Some species harbor plasmids that can provide antimicrobial resistance genes. For example, an increasing number of *E. coli*, *K. pneumoniae*, and *K. oxytoca* clinical strains produce plasmid-mediated extended-spectrum β-lactamases (ESBLs), which can inactivate extended-spectrum cephalosporins (e.g., cefotaxime),

penicillins, and aztreonam. Testing procedures for the detection of ESBLs are described in Chapter 13.

Many members of this family possess antigens that can be used in the identification of different serologic groups. These antigens include the following:
- **O antigen**, or somatic antigen—this is a heat-stable antigen located on the cell wall.
- **H antigen**, or flagellar antigen—this is a heat-labile antigen found on the surface of flagella, structures responsible for motility.
- **K antigen**, or capsular antigen—this is a heat-labile polysaccharide found only in certain encapsulated species. Examples are the K1 antigen of *E. coli* and the **Vi antigen** of *Salmonella enterica* subsp. *enterica* serotype Typhi.

Clinical Significance

Members of the family Enterobacteriaceae are ubiquitous in nature. Additionally, the Enterobacteriaceae, with few exceptions, share a common niche; they reside in the gastrointestinal (GI) tract. Except for *Salmonella*, *Shigella*, and *Yersinia*, they can be resident microbiota if confined to their natural environment. Paradoxically, they are often commensals, causing no harm, and yet can be responsible for a large

TABLE 19-2 Biochemical Characteristics of Tribes of Enterobacteriaceae

Tests or Substrate	Escherichieae	Edwardsielleae	Citrobacteriaceae	Salmonelleae*	Klebsiellae	Proteeae†	Yersiniae
Hydrogen sulfide (TSI agar)	–	+	+ or –	+	–	+ or –	–
Urease	–	–	(+^{w}) or –	–	– or (+)	+ or –	+
Indole	+ or –	+	– or +	–	–	+ or –	+ or –
Methyl red	+	+	+	+	–	+	+
Voges-Proskauer	–	–	–	–	+	–	–
Citrate (Simmons)	–	–	+	+	+	d	–
KCN	–	–	+ or –	–	+	+	–
Phenylalanine deaminase	–	–	–	–	–	+	–
Mucate	d	–		d	+ or –	–	
Mannitol	+ or –	–	+	+	+	– or +	+

Modified from Ewing WH: *Edwards and Ewing's identification of Enterobacteriaceae*, ed 4, East Norwalk, Conn, 1986, Appleton & Lange.
+, ≥90% positive within 1 or 2 days; (+), positive reaction after 3 or more days (decarboxylase tests: 3 or 4 days); –, ≥90% no reaction in 30 days; + or –, most cultures positive, some strains negative; – or +, most strains negative, some cultures positive; d, different reactions, +, (+), –; +^{w}, weakly positive reaction; *TSI*, triple sugar iron; *KCN*, potassium cyanide.
Salmonella serovars Typhi and Paratyphi and some rare serovars fail to use citrate in Simmons medium. Cultures of serovar Paratyphi and some rare serotypes may fail to produce hydrogen sulfide.
†Some cultures of *Proteus mirabilis* may yield positive Voges-Proskauer tests.

number of opportunistic infections. Some species exist as free-living organisms in water, soil, or sewage, and some are plant pathogens.

Based on the clinical infections they produce, members of the family Enterobacteriaceae may be divided into two broad categories: (1) opportunistic pathogens and (2) primary pathogens. The opportunistic pathogens are often a part of the usual intestinal microbiota of both humans and animals. Outside their normal body sites, however, these organisms may produce serious extraintestinal, opportunistic infections, many of which are described in this chapter. For example, *E. coli*, one of the best-studied members of the Enterobacteriaceae, is a member of the normal bowel biota but can cause urinary tract infections (UTIs), septicemia, wound infections in healthy individuals, and meningitis in neonates. Other organisms can be equally devastating in immunocompromised hosts or when introduced to wounds from contaminated soil or water. The primary pathogens, which include *S. enterica*, *Shigella* spp., and *Yersinia* spp., are considered true pathogens; that is, they are not present as commensal biota in the GI tract of humans. These organisms produce infections resulting from ingestion of contaminated food or water, or from other sources, which are discussed in this chapter. Table 19-3 lists some of the diseases associated with members of the family Enterobacteriaceae.

OPPORTUNISTIC MEMBERS OF THE FAMILY ENTEROBACTERIACEAE AND ASSOCIATED INFECTIONS

Escherichia coli

Escherichia coli, the most significant species in the genus *Escherichia*, was first described by Theodore Escherich in 1885. *E. coli* was initially considered a harmless member of the colon resident biota. It is now recognized as an important human pathogen associated with a wide range of clinical syndromes,

TABLE 19-3 Bacterial Species and the Infections They Commonly Produce

Bacterial Species	Diseases
Escherichia coli	Bacteriuria, septicemia, neonatal sepsis, meningitis, diarrheal syndrome
Shigella spp.	Diarrhea, dysentery
Edwardsiella spp.	Diarrhea, wound infection, septicemia, meningitis, enteric fever
Salmonella spp.	Septicemia, enteric fever, diarrhea
Citrobacter spp.	Opportunistic and nosocomial infections (wound, urinary)
Klebsiella spp.	Bacteriuria, pneumonia, septicemia
Enterobacter spp.	Opportunistic and nosocomial infection, wound infections, septicemia, bacteriuria
Serratia spp.	Opportunistic and nosocomial infection, wound infections, septicemia, bacteriuria
Proteus spp.	Bacteriuria, wound infection, septicemia
Providencia spp.	Opportunistic and nosocomial infection, wound infections, septicemia, bacteriuria
Morganella spp.	Opportunistic and nosocomial infections
Yersinia	
pestis	Plague
pseudotuberculosis	Mesenteric adenitis, diarrhea
enterocolitica	Mesenteric adenitis, diarrhea
Erwinia spp.	Wounds contaminated with soil or vegetation
Pectobacterium spp.	Wounds contaminated with soil or vegetation

Modified from Washington J: *Laboratory procedures in clinical microbiology*, ed 2, New York, 1981, Springer-Verlag.

from UTIs, to central nervous system (CNS) infections, to diarrheal diseases. It is so commonly isolated from colon biota that *E. coli* is used as a primary marker of fecal contamination in water purification.

Most strains of *E. coli* are motile and generally possess adhesive fimbriae and sex pili and O, H, and K antigens. *E. coli* O groups have shown remarkable cross-reactivity with O

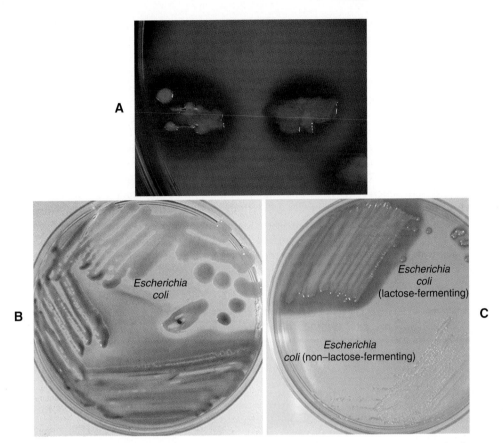

FIGURE 19-1   A, The typical dry, lactose-positive *Escherichia coli* growing on MacConkey (MAC) agar. Note the pink precipitate surrounding the individual colonies. **B,** Mucoid colonies of *E. coli* growing on MAC agar. **C,** Non–lactose-fermenting *E. coli* compared with typical lactose-fermenting *E. coli* on MAC agar. (**B** and **C,** Courtesy Jean Barnishan.)

antigens from other members of the Enterobacteriaceae, most notably the *Shigella*. This is one of the reasons the *Escherichia* and the *Shigella* are grouped together in the tribe Escherichiae. Serotyping for both O and H antigens is often useful in identification of strains, particularly those associated with serious enteric disease. The K antigen often masks the O antigen during bacterial agglutination by specific antiserum. Some *E. coli* K antigens are identical to capsular antigens of other species. The K1 antigen has been found to be identical to the capsular antigen found on *Neisseria meningitidis* group B, suggesting a role for K antigens in virulence.

On certain selective and differential media, such as MAC or eosin-methylene blue (EMB) agars, *E. coli* has a distinctive morphology. It usually presents as a lactose-positive (pink) colony with a surrounding area of precipitated bile salts on MAC agar (Figure 19-1). On EMB agar, it presents with a green metallic sheen and is associated with the following properties:

- Fermentation of glucose, lactose, trehalose, and xylose
- Indole production from tryptophan
- Glucose fermentation by the mixed acid pathway: methyl red positive and Voges-Proskauer negative
- Does not produce H_2S, DNase, urease, or phenylalanine deaminase
- Cannot use citrate as a sole carbon source

Uropathogenic *Escherichia coli*

Escherichia coli is widely recognized as the most common cause of UTIs in humans. The *E. coli* strains that cause UTIs usually originate in the large intestine as resident biota and can exist either as the predominant *E. coli* population or as a small part of the *E. coli* strains in the large intestine. Moreover, strains causing lower UTIs and acute pyelonephritis in immunocompetent hosts are different from those causing disease in the urinary tracts of individuals who are compromised either by urinary tract defects or by instrumentation such as placement of catheters. *E. coli* strains that cause acute pyelonephritis in immunocompetent hosts have been shown to be the dominant resident *E. coli* in the colon. They belong to a few serotypes and are resistant to the antibacterial activity of human serum. Conversely, isolates from immunocompromised hosts consist of a wide variety of strains.

Strains that cause UTIs are able to do so because they produce factors that allow them to attach to the urinary epithelial mucosa. The primary virulence factor associated with the ability of *E. coli* to cause UTIs is the production of pili, which allow uropathogenic strains to adhere to epithelial cells and not be washed out with urine flow. Other factors also contribute to the virulence of uropathogenic *E. coli* (e.g., cytolysins, aerobactins). Cytolysins (often also characterized as hemolysins) can kill immune effector cells and inhibit the phagocytosis and chemotaxis of certain white blood cells. Aerobactin allows the bacterial cell to chelate iron; free iron is generally unavailable within the host for use by bacteria.

Gastrointestinal Pathogens

Escherichia coli may cause several different GI syndromes (Table 19-4). Based on definitive virulence factors, clinical manifestation, epidemiology, and different O and H sero-types, there are five major categories of diarrheagenic *E. coli*: **enterotoxigenic (ETEC), enteroinvasive (EIEC), enteropatho-genic (EPEC), enterohemorrhagic (EHEC),** and enteroadher-ent, which includes the **diffusely adherent (DAEC)** and the **enteroaggregative (EAEC)** strains. These are sometimes col-lectively referred to as the enterovirulent *E. coli*, or diarrhea-genic *E. coli*. The serotypes associated with these categories and the features associated with the intestinal infections pro-duced by these strains are summarized in Chapter 34.

Enterotoxigenic *Escherichia coli.* The ETEC strains are associated with diarrhea of infants and adults in tropical and subtropical climates, especially in developing countries, where it is one of the major causes of infant bacterial diarrhea. In the United States and other Western industrialized nations, ETEC diarrhea is the most common cause of a diarrheal disease, sometimes referred to as **traveler's diarrhea.** Travelers from industrialized countries often become infected with ETEC when they visit developing nations. ETEC infection commonly is spread via consumption of contaminated food or water. Poor hygiene, reduced availability of sources of potable water, and inadequate sanitation are major contribut-ing factors in the spread and transmission of this disease. A high infective dose (10^6 to 10^{10} organisms) is necessary to initi-ate disease in an immunocompetent host. Protective mecha-nisms such as stomach acidity have been described as inhibiting colonization and initiation of disease; those suffer-

TABLE 19-4 Features of Pathogenic *Escherichia coli*

Type	Virulence Factor(s)	Relevant Disease	Relevant Serotypes	Laboratory Tests
Uropathogenic *E. coli*				
UPEC	P pilus/*pap* pili, type 1 fimbriae	UTIs		
DAEC*	Afa/Dr adhesions	UTIs		
Enteric pathogens				
EPEC	Pathogenicity islands	Infantile diarrhea	O55:NM O55:H6 O111:NM O111:H2 O114:NM O114:H2	HeLa cell adherence assay, DNA probes
EHEC	Shiga toxin/verotoxin	Hemorrhagic diarrhea, colitis, HUS	O157:H7 O157:NM O26:H11 O104:H21 O111:H2 O111:H8 O113:H21 O118:H2	SMAC plates, MUG
EIEC	Invasin	Dysentery	O124:H30 O143:NM O164:NM	DNA probes
ETEC	LT, ST	Traveler's diarrhea	O6:NM O6:H16 O8:H9 O25:NM O27:NM O63:H12	Immunoassays for LT or ST
Enteroadherent *E. coli*				
EAEC	AAF fimbriae Afa/Dr adhesions, AIDA-1, pathogenicity islands	Persistent pediatric diarrhea	O44:H18	
DAEC*		Pediatric diarrhea, UTIs		HeLa cell adherence assay, DNA probes
Extraintestinal pathogens				
	Capsule	Septicemia and meningitis	K1	

UPEC, uropathogenic *E. coli*; *UTI*, urinary tract infection; *DAEC*, Diffusely adherent *E. coli*; *EPEC*, enteropathogenic *E. coli*; *NM*, nonmotile; *EHEC*, enterohemorrhagic *E. coli*; *HUS*, hemolytic uremic syndrome; *SMAC*, MacConkey agar containing sorbitol; *MUG*, 4-methylumbelliferyl β-D-glucuronide; *EIEC*, enteroinvasive *E. coli*; *EAEC*, enteroaggregative *E. coli*; *ETEC*, enterotoxigenic *E. coli*; *LT*, labile toxin; *ST*, stable toxin;
*DAEC causes both urinary tract infections and gastrointestinal infections.

ing from *achlorhydria* (deficiency of hydrochloric acid within the stomach) seem to be at higher risk than are normal individuals.

Colonization of ETEC on the proximal small intestine has been recognized as being mediated by fimbriae that permit ETEC to bind to specific receptors on the intestinal microvilli. Once ETEC strains are established, they may release one or both of two toxins into the small intestine. They produce a heat-labile toxin (LT), which is similar in action and amino acid sequence to cholera toxin from *Vibrio cholerae*. LT consists of two fragments (A and B), which follow the A/B model of bacterial toxins, where A is the enzymatically active portion. The B moiety, or binding portion, confers the specificity. The B portion binds to the GM_1 ganglioside of the intestinal mucosa, thereby providing entry for the A portion.

During infection the A portion activates cellular adenylate cyclase, causing a rise in the conversion of adenosine triphosphate (ATP) to cyclic adenosine monophosphate (cAMP). The consequence of accumulation of cAMP is hypersecretion of both electrolytes and fluids into the intestinal lumen, resulting in watery diarrhea similar to cholera. In contrast, the heat-stable toxin (ST) stimulates guanylate cyclase, causing increased production of cyclic guanosine monophosphate (cGMP), accumulation of which also causes hypersecretion.

The usually mild, self-limiting disease caused by ETEC is characterized by watery diarrhea, abdominal cramps, and sometimes nausea, usually with no vomiting or fever. Mucosal penetration and invasion do not appear to be part of ETEC disease. Diagnosis of ETEC infection is made primarily by the characteristic symptoms and the isolation of solely lactose fermenting organisms on differential media. Testing for toxins or colonizing factors is performed by research and reference laboratories, and its use is not justified in the clinical laboratory for diagnostic purposes. Enzyme-labeled oligonucleotide probes have been reported to detect ETEC in fecal specimens, but this method is undergoing further testing to determine its efficacy. ETEC infections must be differentiated, however, from other diarrheal illnesses that may appear similar.

Enteroinvasive *Escherichia coli*. EIEC differs greatly from EPEC and ETEC strains. Enteroinvasive strains produce dysentery with direct penetration, invasion, and destruction of the intestinal mucosa. This diarrheal illness is very similar to that produced by *Shigella* spp. EIEC infections seem to occur in adults and children alike. Direct transmission of EIEC from person to person via the fecal-oral route has been reported. The clinical infection is characterized by fever, severe abdominal cramps, malaise, and watery diarrhea.

The organisms might be easily misidentified because of their similarity to the shigellae. EIEC strains can be nonmotile and generally do not ferment lactose; cross-reaction between shigellae and EIEC O antigens has been reported. EIEC isolates may be mistaken for nonpathogenic *E. coli*; although EIEC do not decarboxylate lysine, more than 80% of *E. coli* strains do decarboxylate lysine. For these reasons, cases of diarrheal illness resulting from EIEC might be underreported.

Although EIEC and *Shigella* spp. are morphologically similar and present similar clinical disorders, the infective dose of EIEC necessary to produce disease is much higher (10^6) than that of the shigellae (as few as 10 bacterial cells). The enteroinvasiveness of EIEC has to be demonstrated for definitive identification. The tests currently available to determine the invasive property of EIEC are not widely performed in most clinical microbiology laboratories. The Sereny test, which determines the organisms' ability to produce keratoconjunctivitis in the guinea pig, was one of the assays previously used to determine the virulence of both shigellae and EIEC. DNA probes to identify EIEC give results comparable to the Sereny test. It is also possible to detect invasiveness using monolayer cell cultures with human epithelial–2 (HEp-2) cells. Recently, DNA probes for EIEC have become commercially available; these kits are used to screen stool samples, eliminating the need for other tests to identify EIEC.

Enteropathogenic *Escherichia coli*. Although the EPEC strain has been known to cause infantile diarrhea since the 1940s, its pathogenic role has remained controversial over the last few decades. Certain O serogroups of EPEC were identified in the late 1960s and 1970s as a cause of diarrhea, but only certain H antigenic types within each O serogroup were connected to the intestinal infections. O serogrouping could not, however, differentiate these *E. coli* strains from strains of normal biota. In 1978, Levine et al. attempted to settle the dispute concerning the pathogenic role of EPEC by challenging volunteers with EPEC strains that lacked the toxins of ETEC and the invasiveness of EIEC. The study showed that these EPEC strains caused distinct diarrhea. Subsequent studies further showed the adhesive property of EPEC strains, a characteristic not seen in ETEC or EIEC strains.

Diarrheal outbreaks caused by EPEC have occurred in hospital nurseries and daycare centers, but cases in adults are rarely seen. The illness is characterized by low-grade fever, malaise, vomiting, and diarrhea. The stool typically contains large amounts of mucus, but apparent blood is not present. Detection of diarrheal illness attributable to EPEC depends primarily on the suspicion of the physician. In cases of severe diarrhea in children younger than 1 year, infection with EPEC should be suspected. Serologic typing with pooled antisera may be performed to identify EPEC serotypes, but this is generally used for epidemiologic studies rather than for diagnostic purposes.

Enterohemorrhagic *Escherichia coli*. In 1982, the O157:H7 strain of *E. coli* was first recognized during an outbreak of hemorrhagic diarrhea and colitis. The EHEC strain serotype O157:H7 has since been associated with hemorrhagic diarrhea, colitis, and hemolytic uremic syndrome (HUS). HUS is characterized by low platelet count, hemolytic anemia, and kidney failure.

The classic illness caused by EHEC produces a watery diarrhea that progresses to bloody diarrhea with abdominal cramps, a low-grade fever, or an absence of fever. The stool contains no leukocytes, which distinguishes it from dysentery caused by *Shigella* spp. or EIEC infections. The infection is potentially fatal, especially in young children and elderly persons in nursing homes. Processed meats, such as undercooked hamburgers served at fast-food restaurants, unpasteurized dairy products and apple cider, bean sprouts, and spinach have all been implicated in the spread of infection. In 2009, EHEC was the cause of a multistate outbreak linked to prepackaged cookie dough. Approximately 80 people in 31 states were affected. Infection was associated with consumption of raw dough.

E. coli O157:H7 produces two cytotoxins: **verotoxin** I and verotoxin II. Verotoxin I is a phage-encoded cytotoxin identical to the **Shiga toxin (Stx)** produced by *Shigella dysenteriae* type I. This toxin produces damage to Vero cells (African green monkey kidney cells)—hence the term *verotoxin*. It also reacts with and is neutralized by the antibody against Stx. In contrast, verotoxin II is not neutralized by antibody to Stx. Verotoxin II is biologically similar to, but immunologically different from, both Stx and verotoxin I. These toxins have also been reported under the name Shiga-like toxins but are most likely to be found in the literature as Shiga toxin I (Stx1) and Shiga toxin 2 (Stx2); *E. coli* strains that produce these toxins are also called Shiga toxigenic *E. coli* (STEC). Several different STEC strains have been identified; O157:H7 is only the first to have been widely reported. Any of the STEC serotypes can cause clinical syndromes similar to that produced by O157:H7 *E. coli*. Table 19-4 lists non-O157:H7 EHEC/STEC isolated from patients with bloody diarrhea, hemorrhagic colitis, or HUS. In the laboratory, verotoxin producing *E. coli* may be identified by one of three methods:

- Stool culture on highly differential medium, with subsequent serotyping
- Detecting the verotoxin in stool filtrates
- Demonstration of a fourfold or greater increase in verotoxin-neutralizing antibody titer

Stool culture for *E. coli* O157:H7 may be performed using MAC agar containing sorbitol (SMAC) instead of lactose. *E. coli* O157:H7 does not ferment sorbitol in 48 hours, a characteristic that differentiates it from most other *E. coli* strains. The use of this differential medium facilitates the primary screening of *E. coli* O157:H7, which ordinarily would not be distinguishable from other *E. coli* strains on lactose-containing MAC or other routine enteric agar. *E. coli* O157:H7 appears colorless on SMAC agar. Although isolation of other nonsorbitol-fermenting organisms may occur in up to 15% of cultures, *E. coli* O157:H7, when present, produces heavy growth. In addition to sorbitol fermentation, the commercially available MUG (4-methylumbelliferyl-β-D-glucuronide) assay is a biochemical test used to screen isolates for *E. coli* O157:H7. *E. coli* O157:H7 rarely produces the enzyme β-glucuronidase, whereas 92% of other strains do produce it. If the enzyme is present, MUG is cleaved and a fluorescent product is formed. Sorbitol-negative and/or MUG negative colonies are subsequently subcultured for serotyping using *E. coli* O157:H7 antiserum.

Enzyme-linked immunosorbent assay (ELISA) or latex agglutination can be used to detect the O157 antigen. In the latex agglutination assay, isolates must be tested with the negative control to detect nonspecific agglutination. The O157 somatic antigen, which is usually the target in the commercial assays, may present a problem with regard to specificity because other enteric bacteria produce false-positive results. It is therefore important to biochemically confirm the identification of MUG-negative or sorbitol-negative colonies

as *E. coli* isolates. A latex test to detect H7 antigen is available as well. When testing colonies taken directly from the SMAC plate, the test for the H7 antigen may be initially negative. It is helpful to grow these isolates in motility media first to enhance flagella production and agglutination with the latex particles.

Following serotyping, isolates are tested for the presence of Stx. Reports have shown that all *E. coli* O157:H7 strains produce high levels of cytotoxins, and STEC strains may be detected using cell culture assays with Vero cells. Because other toxins present in diarrhea stools may produce similar cytopathic effects, this test must be verified with specific antitoxins to Stx1 and Stx2. Free verotoxins present in stool specimens have been detected in samples that yielded negative culture results. It was previously reported that hemorrhagic colitis patients shed the organisms for only brief periods; nevertheless, verotoxins may still be detected in the stool. An approved ELISA test from Meridian Diagnostics, Inc. (Cincinnati, Ohio) is able to detect Stx even in bloody stools, although not all patients have bloody stools. Gene amplification assays like those available in Europe from SY-LAB (Geräte GmbH, Austria) may be useful in detecting STEC strains. A fourfold increase in verotoxin-neutralizing antibody titer has been demonstrated in patients with HUS and in whom verotoxin or verotoxin-producing *E. coli* has been detected.

Enteroadherent *Escherichia coli*. Enteroadherent *E. coli* strains are generally associated with two kinds of human disease: diarrheal syndromes and UTIs. The two types of enteroadherent *E. coli* are DAEC and EAEC. DAEC are associated with both UTIs and diarrheal disease. The uropathogenic DAEC strains are closely associated with cystitis in children and acute pyelonephritis in pregnant women. They also seem to be associated with chronic or recurring UTIs. Several strains of DAEC have been associated with pediatric diarrheal disease, particularly in developing nations.

EAEC causes diarrhea by adhering to the surface of the intestinal mucosa. These strains are found to adhere to HEp2 cells, packed in an aggregative "stacked-brick" pattern on the cells and between the cells by means of fimbriae. These organisms produce watery diarrhea, vomiting, dehydration, and occasionally abdominal pain, mostly in children. The symptoms typically persist for 2 or more weeks.

Extraintestinal Infections

Escherichia coli remains one of the most common causes of septicemia and meningitis among neonates, accounting for about 40% of the cases of gram-negative meningitis. Similar infections resulting from this organism are uncommon in older children. The newborn usually acquires the infection in the birth canal just before or during delivery, when the mother's vagina is heavily colonized. Infection may also result if contamination of the amniotic fluid takes place.

The strains associated with diarrheal disease appear to be distinct from those associated with neonatal sepsis or meningitis. The capsular antigen K1 present in certain strains of *E. coli* is the most documented virulence factor associated with neonatal meningeal infections. *E. coli* K1 is also immunochemically identical to the capsular antigen of *N. meningitidis*

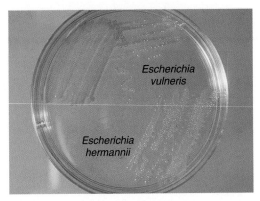

FIGURE 19-2 Comparison of the colony morphology of *Escherichia vulneris* and a yellow-pigmented *Escherichia hermannii* on MacConkey agar. *Escherichia vulneris* may also produce a yellow-pigmented colony, but the yellow is more prevalent in *E. hermannii*. (Courtesy Jean Barnishan.)

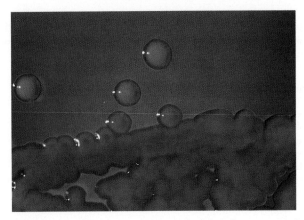

FIGURE 19-3 Mucoid appearance of *Klebsiella pneumoniae* on MacConkey agar.

group B. The association of K1 antigen was established when *E. coli* strains possessing the capsular K1 antigen were isolated from neonates with septicemia or meningitis. Fatality rates for infants with meningitis caused by *E. coli* were higher than those for infants infected with non-K1 strains. In addition to the neonatal population, *E. coli* remains as a clinically significant isolate in blood cultures from adults. *E. coli* bacteremia in adults may result primarily from a urogenital tract infection or from a GI source.

Other *Escherichia* Species

Escherichia hermannii, formerly called *E. coli* atypical or enteric group II, is a yellow-pigmented organism that has been isolated from cerebrospinal fluid (CSF), wounds, and blood. Reports of isolating *E. hermannii* from foodstuffs such as raw milk and beef, the same sources as *E. coli* O157:H7, have been published. However, its clinical significance is not established as yet.

E. vulneris has been isolated from humans with infected wounds. More than half of the strains of *E. vulneris* also produce yellow-pigmented colonies. Figure 19-2 compares the colony morphology of *E. hermannii* with that of *E. vulneris*. The newest species added to this genus, *E. albertii*, is associated with diarrheal disease in children. The other members of the tribe Escherichiae, the shigellae, will be discussed in the enteric pathogens portion of the chapter.

Klebsiella

Members of the genera *Klebsiella, Enterobacter, Serratia, Pantoea, Cronobacter,* and *Hafnia* belong to the tribe Klebsielleae. Members of these genera are usually found in the intestinal tract of humans and animals or free-living in soil, water, and on plants. These microorganisms have been associated with a wide variety of opportunistic and nosocomial infections, particularly pneumonia, wound, and UTIs. Members of these genera demonstrate variable biochemical reactions. Common characteristics include the following:

- Most grow on Simmons citrate and in potassium cyanide broth.
- None produce hydrogen sulfide.

- A few hydrolyze urea slowly.
- All give a negative reaction with the methyl red test and a positive reaction with the Voges-Proskauer test.
- With a few exceptions, indole is not produced from tryptophan.
- Motility is variable.

Usually found in the GI tract of humans and animals, the genus *Klebsiella* consists of several species; namely, *K. pneumoniae* subsp. *pneumoniae, K. oxytoca, K. pneumoniae* subsp. *ozaenae, K. pneumoniae* subsp. *rhinoscleromatis, K. ornitholytica, K. planticola,* and *K. terrigena*. The absence of motility distinguishes *Klebsiella* spp. from most other members of the family Enterobacteriaceae. Differential features of *Klebsiella* spp. are shown in Table 19-5. *K. pneumoniae* is the most commonly isolated species and has the distinct feature of possessing a polysaccharide capsule. The capsule offers the organism protection against phagocytosis and antimicrobial absorption, thus contributing to its virulence. This capsule is also responsible for the moist, mucoid colonies characteristic of *K. pneumoniae*. Occasionally evident in direct smears from clinical materials, this capsule is sometimes helpful in providing a presumptive identification. Figure 19-3 illustrates the mucoid appearance of *K. pneumoniae* on MAC agar.

Colonization of gram-negative bacilli in the respiratory tracts of hospitalized patients, particularly by *K. pneumoniae*, increases with the length of hospital stay. *K. pneumoniae* is a frequent cause of lower respiratory tract infections among hospitalized patients and in immunocompromised hosts such as newborns, elderly patients, and seriously ill patients on respirators. Other infections commonly associated with *K. pneumoniae* involving immunocompromised hosts are wound infections, UTIs, and bacteremia. Reports describe nosocomial outbreaks of *Klebsiella* resistant to multiple antimicrobial agents in newborn nurseries. These outbreaks have been attributed to the plasmid transfer of antimicrobial resistance. Other *Klebsiella* spp. have been associated with a number of infections.

Biochemically, *K. oxytoca* is identical to *K. pneumoniae* except for its production of indole, and there are reports of ornithine-positive isolates as well. *K. oxytoca* produces infections similar to those caused by *K. pneumoniae*. *K. pneumoniae* subsp. *ozaenae* has been isolated from nasal secretions

TABLE 19-5 Differentiation of Common Species within the Genus *Klebsiella*

Test or Substrate	*K. pneumoniae* subsp. *pneumoniae* Sign	% +	(% +)	*K. oxytoca* Sign	% +	(% +)	*K. pneumoniae* subsp. *ozaenae* Sign	% +	(% +)
Urease	+	95.4	(0.1)	+	90		D	0	(14.8)
Indole	−	0		+	99		−	0	
Methyl red	− or +	10		−	20		+	97.7	
Voges-Proskauer	+	98		+	96		−	0	
Citrate (Simmons)	+	98	(0.6)	+	95		D	30	(32.4)
Gelatin (22° C)	−	0	(0.2)	−	0		−	0	
Lysine decarboxylase	+	98	(0.1)	+	99		− or +	40	(6.3)
Malonate	+	92.5		+	98		−	6	
Mucate	+	90		+	93		− or +	25	
Sodium alginate (utilization)	+ or (+)	88.5	(9.2)	nd			− or (+)	0	(11)
Gas from glucose	+	96		+	97		d	50	(9.4)
Lactose	+	98.7	(1)	+	100		d	30	(61.3)
Dulcitol	− or +	30		+ or −	55		−	0	
Organic acid media									
Citrate	+ or −	64.4		nd			− or +	18	
D-Tartrate	+ or −	67.1		nd			− or +	39	

Modified from Ewing WH: *Edwards and Ewing's identification of Enterobacteriaceae*, ed 4, East Norwalk, Conn, 1986, Appleton and Lange.
+, ≥90% positive within 1 or 2 days; (+), positive reaction after 3 or more days (decarboxylase tests: 3 or 4 days); −, ≥90% no reaction in 30 days; + or −, most cultures positive, some strains negative; − or +, most strains negative, some cultures positive; d, different reactions, +, (+), −; *nd,* no data.

and cerebral abscesses. As previously mentioned, these species are highly associated with the presence of plasmid-mediated ESBLs, contributing to the large numbers of nosocomial infections seen today.

K. pneumoniae subsp. *rhinoscleromatis* has been isolated from patients with rhinoscleroma, an infection of the nasal cavity that manifests as an intense swelling and malformation of the entire face and neck. Cases of rhinoscleroma have been reported in Africa and South America. Originally, both *K. ozaenae* and *K. rhinoscleromatis* were considered true species. Based on nucleic acid studies, they have been reclassified as subspecies of *K. pneumoniae*. *K. ornithinolytica* (indole and ornithine decarboxylase positive) and *K. planticola* have been isolated from the urine, respiratory tracts, and blood of humans.

Enterobacter, Cronobacter, and Pantoea

The genus *Enterobacter* is composed of 12 species, one of which consists of two biotypes. Clinically significant *Enterobacter* spp. that have been isolated from clinical samples include *E. cloacae*, *E. aerogenes*, *E. gergoviae*, and *E. hormaechei*. Members of this genus are motile. The colony morphology of many of the species resembles that of *Klebsiella* when growing on MAC. *Enterobacter* spp. grow on Simmons citrate medium and in potassium cyanide broth; the methyl red test is negative and the Voges-Proskauer test is positive. Unlike *Klebsiella*, however, *Enterobacter* spp. usually produce ornithine decarboxylase; lysine decarboxylase is produced by most species but not by *E. gergoviae* or *E. cloacae*.

Enterobacter cloacae and *E. aerogenes* are the two most common isolates from this group. These two species have been isolated from wounds, urine, blood, and CSF. Distinguishing

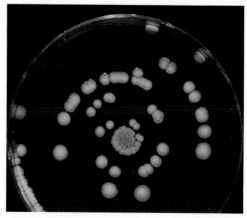

FIGURE 19-4 Yellow-pigmented *Pantoea agglomerans* (formerly *Enterobacter agglomerans*) on a sheep blood agar. (Courtesy Jean Barnishan.)

characteristics among *E. cloacae*, *E. aerogenes*, and *K. pneumoniae* are shown in Table 19-6. *Pantoea (Enterobacter) agglomerans* gained notoriety with a nationwide outbreak of septicemia resulting from contaminated intravenous fluids. Designated early on as *E. agglomerans* complex, it includes species that are lysine, ornithine, and arginine negative or "triple decarboxylases negative." More than 13 hybridization groups (HG) have been described in this complex. *P. agglomerans* HG XIII, which may produce a yellow pigment, is primarily a plant pathogen. Figure 19-4 depicts a yellow-pigmented *P. agglomerans*.

E. gergoviae is found in respiratory samples and is rarely isolated from blood cultures. *Cronobacter (Enterobacter) sakazakii* typically produces a yellow pigment and has been documented as a pathogen in neonates causing meningitis and

TABLE 19-6 Diagnostic Features of *Enterobacter cloacae*, *Enterobacter aerogenes*, and *Klebsiella pneumoniae* subsp. *pneumoniae*

Test or Substrate	E. cloacae			E. aerogenes			K. pneumoniae subsp. pneumoniae		
	Sign	% +	(% +)	Sign	% +	(% +)	Sign	% +	(% +)
Urease	+w or –	65		–	2		+	95.4	(0.1)
Motility	+	95		+	97		–	0	
Lysine decarboxylase	–	0		+	98		+	98	(6.3)
Arginine dihydrolase	+	97	(2)	–	0		–	0	
Ornithine decarboxylase	+	96	(1.3)	+	98	(0.8)	–	0	
Gelatin (22° C)	(+)	0	(94.2)	(+) or –	0	(61.2)	–	0	(0.2)
Adonitol, gas	– or +	21.7	(1.3)	+	94.2		d	84.4	(0.3)
Inositol									
Acid	D	13	(8)	+	96.7		+	97.2	(0.9)
Gas	–	4.1	(1.5)	+	93.4		+	92.5	(1.5)
D-tartrate, Jordan's	– or +	30		+	95		+	95	
Sodium alginate (utilization)	–	0		–	0		+ or (+)	88.9	(8.9)

Modified from Ewing WH: *Edwards and Ewing's identification of Enterobacteriaceae*, ed 4, East Norwalk, Conn, 1986, Appleton & Lange.

+, ≥90% Positive within 1 or 2 days; (+), positive reaction after 3 or more days (decarboxylase tests: 3 or 4 days); –, ≥90% no reaction in 30 days; + *or* –, most cultures positive, some strains negative; – *or* +, most strains negative, some cultures positive; d, different reactions; +, (+), –; +w, weakly positive reaction.

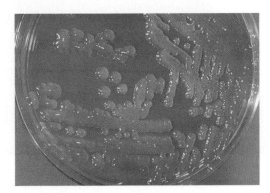

FIGURE 19-5 Mucoid, yellow-pigmented colonies of *Cronobacter (Enterobacter) sakazakii* growing on brain–heart infusion agar. (Courtesy Jean Barnishan.)

bacteremia, often coming from powdered infant formula. It has also been isolated from cultures taken from brain abscesses and respiratory and wound infections. Figure 19-5 illustrates the colony morphology of *C. sakazakii*. *E. hormaechei* has been isolated from human sources such as blood, wounds, and sputum. *E. asburiae* is similar biochemically to *E. cloacae* and has been isolated from blood, urine, feces, sputum, and wounds. *E. dissolvens* and *E. nimipressuralis* are newly recognized species with unknown clinical significance. *E. cancerogenus* (formerly *E. taylorae*) has been associated with osteomyelitis following traumatic wounds.

Serratia

The genus *Serratia* is composed of *S. marcescens*, *S. liquefaciens*, *S. rubidaea*, *S. odorifera*, *S. plymuthica*, *S. ficaria*, *S. entomophila*, and *S. fonticola*. *Serratia* spp. are opportunistic pathogens associated with nosocomial outbreaks. With the exception of *S. fonticola*, *Serratia* spp. ferment lactose slowly

and are positive for the ortho-nitrophenyl galactoside (ONPG) test. They are differentiated from other members of the tribe by their ability to produce extracellular DNase. *Serratia* spp. are also known for their resistance to a wide range of antimicrobials. Susceptibility tests must be performed on each isolate to determine appropriate antimicrobial therapy.

S. marcescens, *S. rubidaea*, and *S. plymuthica* often produce a characteristic pink to red pigment, prodigiosin, especially when the cultures are incubated at room temperature. Figure 19-6 illustrates the pigmentation of *S. marcescens* and *S. rubidaea*. *S. marcescens* is the species considered most clinically significant. It has frequently been found in nosocomial infections of the urinary or respiratory tract and in bacteremic outbreaks in nurseries and cardiac surgery and burn units. Contamination of antiseptic solution used for joint injections has resulted in an epidemic of septic arthritis.

S. plymuthica osteomyelitis was found following a motorcycle accident. *S. odorifera* contains two biogroups and, as the species name implies, emits a dirty, musty odor resembling that of potatoes. *S. odorifera* biogroup 1 is isolated predominantly from the respiratory tract and is positive for sucrose, raffinose, and ornithine. In addition, biogroup 1 may be indole positive (60%). *S. odorifera* biogroup 2 is negative for sucrose, raffinose, and ornithine and has been isolated from blood and CSF. Biogroup 2 may also be indole positive (50%). *S. liquefaciens*, *S. rubidaea*, and *S. fonticola* have also been isolated from human sources.

Hafnia

The genus *Hafnia* is composed of one species, *H. alvei*. However, two distinct biotypes are recognized: *H. alvei* and *H. alvei* biotype 1. Biotype 1 grows in the beer wort of breweries and has not been isolated clinically. *Hafnia* has been isolated from a number of anatomic sites in humans and in the environment. *Hafnia* is not known to cause gastroenteritis but

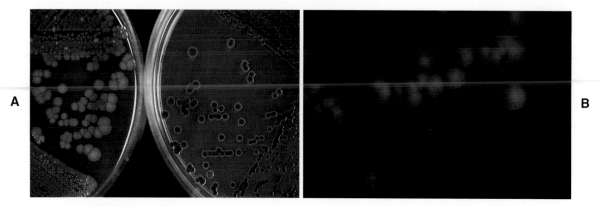

FIGURE 19-6 **A,** *Serratia marcescens* growing on a sheep blood agar plate *(left)* and showing brick-red pigment when grown on MacConkey (MAC) agar *(right)*. **B,** Pinkish red pigmentation of *Serratia rubidaea* growing on MAC.

is occasionally isolated from stool cultures. A delayed positive citrate reaction is a major characteristic of *Hafnia*.

Proteus

The genera *Proteus, Morganella,* and *Providencia* belong to the tribe Proteeae. They are normal intestinal microbiota and are recognized as opportunistic pathogens. The tribe Proteeae is distinguished from the other members of the Enterobacteriaceae by virtue of the ability to deaminate the amino acid phenylalanine. Virtually no other members of the Enterobacteriaceae synthesize the required enzyme, phenylalanine deaminase. None of the members of this tribe ferment lactose.

The genus *Proteus* consists of four species: *P. mirabilis, P. vulgaris, P. penneri,* and *P. myxofaciens. P. mirabilis* and *P. vulgaris* are widely recognized human pathogens. Both species have been isolated from urine, wounds, and ear and bacteremic infections. *Proteus* spp. are responsible for up to 3% of all nosocomial infections in the United States, particularly UTIs, as described in the Case in Point. They ascend the urinary tract, causing infections in both the lower and upper urinary tract. They can infect the proximal kidney tubules and can cause acute glomerulonephritis, particularly in patients with urinary tract defects or catheterization.

P. mirabilis and *P. vulgaris* are easily identified in the clinical laboratory because of their characteristic colony morphology. Both species produce "swarming" colonies on nonselective media, such as SBA (Figure 19-7). This characteristic swarming is a result of a tightly regulated cycle of differentiation from standard vegetative cells (swimmers) to hyperflagellated, elongated, polyploid cells (swarmers) capable of coordinated surface movement. These swarmer cells also produce the distinct odor associated with *Proteus* colonies, sometimes described as "burnt chocolate," and are thought to play a role in the ascending nature of *Proteus*-associated UTIs. Both species also produce hydrogen sulfide and hydrolyze urea. *P. mirabilis* is differentiated from *P. vulgaris* by the indole and ornithine decarboxylase tests; *P. mirabilis* does not produce indole from tryptophan and is ornithine positive, whereas *P. vulgaris* produces indole and is ornithine negative. *P. vulgaris* ferments sucrose and therefore gives an acid/acid reaction in triple sugar iron (TSI) agar.

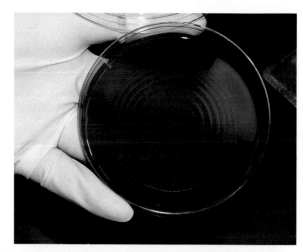

FIGURE 19-7 Example of *Proteus mirabilis* swarming on a sheep blood agar plate. (Courtesy Kimberly Walker and R. Abe Baalness.)

P. penneri can also swarm on nonselective media. *P. penneri* has been isolated from patients with diarrhea, although the organism's role in disease has not been proven. *P. myxofaciens,* a species that has been isolated only from gypsy moths, is characterized by the large amount of slime it produces.

Morganella

The genus *Morganella* currently has only one species, *M. morganii,* with two subspecies: *M. morganii* subsp. *morganii* and *M. morganii* subsp. *sibonii.* Neither subspecies has been implicated in diarrheal illness, but the role they might play as an etiologic agent of diarrheal disease has not been fully examined. *M. morganii* is, however, a documented cause of UTI and has been isolated from other human body sites.

Providencia

The genus *Providencia* consists of five species: *P. alcalifaciens, P. stuartii, P. rettgeri, P. rustigianii,* and *P. heimbachae. P. rettgeri* is a documented pathogen of the urinary tract and

TABLE **19-7** **Differentiating Characteristics of Selected Species of** *Proteus, Providencia,* **and** *Morganella*

Test	Proteus penneri	Proteus mirabilis	Proteus vulgaris	Providencia alcalifaciens	Providencia stuartii	Providencia rettgeri	Morganella morganii
Indole	–	–	+	+	+	+	+
Methyl red	+	+	+	+	+	+	+
Voges-Proskauer	–	– or +	–	–	–	–	–
Simmons citrate	–	+ or (+)	d	+	+	+	–
Christensen urea	+	+ or (+)	+	–	– or +	+	+
H₂S (TSI)	– (70%)	+	+	–	–	–	–
Ornithine decarboxylase	–	+	–	–	–	–	+
Phenylalanine deaminase	+	+	+	+	+	+	+
Acid produced from							
Sucrose	+	d	+	d	d	d	–
Mannitol	–	–	–	–	d	+	–
Salicin	–	–	d	–	–	d	–
Adonitol	–	–	–	+	–	+	–
Rhamnose	–	–	–	–	–	+ or –	–
Maltose	+	–	+	–	–	–	–
Xylose	+	+	+ or (+)	–	–	– or +	–
Arabitol	–	–	–	–	–	+	–
Swarms	+	+	+	–	–	–	–

Modified from Washington J: *Laboratory procedures in clinical microbiology,* ed 2, New York, 1981, Springer-Verlag.
+, 90% or more positive reaction within 1 or 2 days; –, no reaction (90% or more) in 30 days; – or +, most strains negative, some cultures positive; + or (+), most reactions occur within 1 or 2 days; some are delayed; d, different reactions; + or –, most cultures positive, some strains negative; TSI, triple-sugar iron agar.

has caused occasional nosocomial outbreaks. It has also been implicated in diarrheal disease among travelers. Similarly, *P. stuartii* has been implicated in nosocomial outbreaks in burn units and has been isolated from urine cultures. Infections caused by *P. stuartii* and *P. rettgeri,* especially in immunocompromised patients, are particularly difficult to treat because of their resistance to antimicrobials.

P. alcalifaciens is most commonly found in the feces of children with diarrhea; however, its role as a cause of diarrhea has not been proven. *P. rustigianii,* formerly identified as a strain of *P. alcalifaciens,* is rarely isolated, and its pathogenicity also remains unproven, whereas *P. heimbachae* has yet to be isolated from any clinical specimens. Table 19-7 shows the differentiating characteristics of medically important *Proteus, Providencia,* and *Morganella.*

Edwardsiella

The genus *Edwardsiella* is composed of three species: *E. tarda, E. hoshinae,* and *E. ictaluri. E. tarda* is the only recognized human pathogen. Members of this genus are negative for urea and positive for lysine decarboxylase, hydrogen sulfide, and indole and do not grow on Simmons citrate. *E. tarda* is an opportunist, causing bacteremia and wound infections. Its pathogenic role in cases of diarrhea remains controversial. *E. hoshinae* has been isolated from snakes, birds, and water. *E. ictaluri* causes enteric septicemia in fish.

Erwinia and Pectobacterium

Both *Erwinia* and *Pectobacterium* spp. are plant pathogens and are not significant in human infections. *Erwinia* organisms grow poorly at 37° C and fail to grow on selective media, such as EMB and MAC, and other differential media typi-

cally used for the isolation of enterics. Identification of these organisms is more for academic interest than for the evaluation of their significance as causative agents of infection. Most *Erwinia* spp. have been placed in other genera and given new designations.

Citrobacter

Earlier classifications of the family Enterobacteriaceae included the genus *Citrobacter* within the tribe Salmonelleae, which formerly consisted of the genera *Salmonella, Citrobacter,* and *Arizona.* However, changes in the classification and nomenclature of bacterial species belonging to the tribe Salmonelleae have caused the reclassification of the genus *Citrobacter* into its own tribe, Citrobacteriaceae, and of *Arizona* as a subspecies of *Salmonella.* The genus *Citrobacter* currently consists of 11 species that have all been isolated from clinical specimens: *C. freundii, C. koseri (C. diversus), C. amalonaticus, C. farmeri, C. braakii, C. gillenii, C. murliniae, C. rodentium, C. sedlakii, C. werkmanii,* and *C. youngae.* Most *Citrobacter* spp. hydrolyze urea slowly and ferment lactose, producing colonies on MAC agar that resemble those of *E. coli.* All species grow on Simmons citrate medium and give positive reactions in the methyl red test.

C. freundii can be isolated in diarrheal stool cultures, and although it is a known extraintestinal pathogen, its pathogenic role in intestinal disease is not established. *C. freundii* has been associated with infectious diseases acquired in hospital settings; UTIs, pneumonias, and intra-abdominal abscesses have been reported. In addition, *C. freundii* has been associated with endocarditis in intravenous drug abusers. One of the reported cases of *C. freundii* endocarditis required aortic valve replacement when antimicrobial therapy failed.

Because most (80%) *C. freundii* produce hydrogen sulfide and some strains (50%) fail to ferment lactose, the colony morphology of *C. freundii* on primary selective media can be easily mistaken for that of *Salmonella* when isolated from stool cultures. It is therefore important to differentiate *C. freundii* from *Salmonella*. Differentiation can be done by using a minimal number of biochemical tests, such as urea hydrolysis and lysine decarboxylase. Most (70%) *C. freundii* hydrolyze urea, but all fail to decarboxylate lysine, whereas *Salmonella* fails to hydrolyze urea and most isolates decarboxylate lysine. *C. koseri* is a pathogen documented as the cause of nursery outbreaks of neonatal meningitis and brain abscesses. *C. amalonaticus* is frequently found in feces, but no evidence has been found that it is a causative agent of diarrhea. It has been isolated from sites of extraintestinal infections, such as blood and wounds.

PRIMARY INTESTINAL PATHOGENS OF THE FAMILY ENTEROBACTERIACEAE

Salmonella and *Shigella* organisms produce GI illnesses in humans. Salmonellae inhabit the GI tracts of animals. Humans acquire the infection by ingesting the organisms in contaminated animal food products or insufficiently cooked poultry, milk, eggs, and dairy products. Some *Salmonella* infections are transmitted by human carriers.

Infections caused by *Shigella* spp. are associated with human carriers responsible for spreading the disease; no animal reservoir has been identified. *Shigella* dysentery usually indicates improper sanitary conditions and poor personal hygiene. *Yersinia* spp. infections, on the other hand, are transmitted by a wide variety of wild and domestic animals. *Yersinia* infections range from GI disease, to mediastinal lymphadenitis, and to fulminant septicemia and pneumonia.

Salmonella

Members of the genus *Salmonella* produce significant infections in humans and in certain animals. *Salmonella* organisms are gram-negative, facultatively anaerobic bacilli that morphologically resemble other enteric bacteria. On selective and differential media used primarily to isolate enteric pathogens (e.g., MAC), salmonellae produce clear, colorless, nonlactose-fermenting colonies; colonies with black centers are seen if the media (e.g., HE or XLD) contain indicators for hydrogen sulfide production. The biochemical features for the genus include the following:

- In almost every case, they do not ferment lactose.
- They are negative for indole, the Voges-Proskauer test, phenylalanine deaminase, and urease.
- Most produce hydrogen sulfide; a major exception is *Salmonella* Paratyphi A, which does not produce hydrogen sulfide.
- They do not grow in medium containing potassium cyanide.

Classification

Previously the genus *Salmonella* comprised three biochemically discrete species: *S. enteritidis*, *S. choleraesuis*, and *S. typhi*. Genetic studies have shown, however, that bacterial species in the genus *Salmonella* are very closely related and that only two species, *S. enterica* (the type species of the genus) and *S. bongori*, should be designated. *S. bongori* is a rarely isolated species that is named after the town of Bongor in Chad, Africa, and was initially isolated in 1966 from a lizard. It is usually isolated from cold-blooded animals and the environment, but there was a report of 18 cases of human enteritis in Sicily between 1984 and 1997.

Within the species *S. enterica* are six subspecies: *S. enterica* subsp. *enterica* (I), *S. enterica* subsp. *salamae* (II), *S. enterica* subsp. *arizonae* (IIIa), *S. enterica* subsp. *diarizonae* (IIIb), *S. enterica* subsp. *houtenae* (IV), and *S. enterica* subsp. *indica* (VI). A recently published Taxonomic Note by Tindall et al. and an opinion issued from the Judicial Commission of the International Committee on the Systematics of the Prokaryotes in 2005 both clearly support this two-species designation and have placed nearly all former species as serotypes below the level of *S. enterica* subspecies *enterica* (e.g., *S. enterica* subsp. *enterica* serotype Typhi). This is often more simply written as *Salmonella* Typhi (capitalized but not italicized). Table 19-8 shows the characteristic features of *Salmonella* serotype Typhi, *Salmonella* serotype Choleraesuis, and *Salmonella* serotype Paratyphi.

TABLE 19-8 Biochemical Differentiation of Selected Members of the Genus *Salmonella*

Test	*S.* serotype Choleraesuis	*S.* serotype Paratyphi	*S.* serotype Typhi	Other*
Arabinose fermentation	−	+	−	+
Citrate utilization	V	−	−	+
Glucose gas production	+	+	−	+
Hydrogen sulfide (TSI)	V	−	+	+
Lysine decarboxylase	+	−	+	+
Ornithine decarboxylase	+	+	−	+
Rhamnose fermentation	+	+	−	+
Trehalose fermentation	−	+	+	+

Data from Farmer JJ et al: Enterobacteriaceae: introduction and identification. In Murray PR et al, editors: *Manual of clinical microbiology*, ed 9, Washington, DC, 2007, ASM Press.

−, ≤9% of strains positive; +, ≥90% of strains positive; *V*, 10% to 89% of strains positive; *TSI*, triple sugar iron agar.
*Typical strains in serogroups A through E.

Many *Salmonella* serotypes are typically found in cold-blooded animals as well as in rodents and birds, which serve as their natural hosts. Members of the former genus *Arizona*, now subspecies IIIa of *S. enterica*, are found in infections with symptoms identical to those of *Salmonella* infections and may be transmitted to humans from pet turtles, snakes, and fish. A *Morbidity and Mortality Weekly Report* (56:649, 2007) described several outbreaks of human salmonellosis in the United States related to small turtles, despite a 1975 law prohibiting their sale.

Virulence Factors

Factors responsible for the virulence of salmonellae have been the subject of speculation and still remain uncertain. The role of fimbriae in adherence in initiating intestinal infection has been cited. It is apparent that fimbriated strains appear more virulent than nonfimbriated strains. Another factor that contributes to the virulence of salmonellae is their ability to traverse intestinal mucosa. Specific factors that mediate this mechanism have not been established. Enterotoxin produced by certain *Salmonella* strains that cause gastroenteritis has been implicated as a significant virulence factor.

Antigenic Structures

Salmonellae possess antigens similar to those of other enterobacteria. The somatic O antigens and flagellar H antigens are the primary antigenic structures used in serologic grouping of salmonellae. A few strains may possess capsular (K) antigens, designated Vi antigen. The serologic identification of the Vi antigen is important in identifying *Salmonella* serotype Typhi. Figure 19-8 shows the antigenic structures used in serologic grouping and their locations.

The heat-stable O antigen of salmonellae, as is the case with other enteric bacteria, is the lipopolysaccharide (LPS) located in the outer membrane of the cell wall. Many different O antigens are present among the subspecies of *Salmonella;* more than one O antigen may also be found in a particular strain. The O antigens are designated by Arabic numbers.

Unlike the O antigens, flagellar antigen proteins are heat labile. The H antigens of salmonellae occur in one of two phases: phase 1, the specific phase and phase 2, the nonspecific phase. Phase 1 flagellar antigens occur only in a small number of serotypes and determine the immunologic identity of the particular serotype. Phase 1 antigens agglutinate only with homologous antisera. Phase 2 flagellar antigens, on the other hand, occur among several strains. Shared by numerous serotypes, phase 2 antigens react with heterologous antisera. The heat-labile Vi (from the term *virulence*) antigen is a surface polysaccharide capsular antigen found in *Salmonella* serotype Typhi and a few strains of *Salmonella* serotype Choleraesuis. The capsular antigen plays a significant role in preventing phagocytosis of the organism. The Vi antigen often blocks the O antigen during serologic typing but may be removed by heating.

Clinical Infections

In humans, salmonellosis may occur in several forms:
- An acute gastroenteritis or food poisoning characterized by vomiting and diarrhea
- Typhoid fever, the most severe form of enteric fever, caused by *Salmonella* serotype Typhi; and enteric fevers caused by other *Salmonella* serotypes (e.g., *Salmonella* Paratyphi and Choleraesuis)
- Nontyphoidal bacteremia
- Carrier state following *Salmonella* infection

Humans acquire the infection by ingesting the organisms in food, water, and milk contaminated with human or animal excreta. With the exception of *Salmonella* Typhi and *Salmonella* Paratyphi, salmonellae organisms infect various animals that serve as reservoirs, and sources of human infections. *Salmonella* serotypes Typhi and Paratyphi have no known animal reservoirs, and infections seem to occur only in humans. Carriers are often the source of infection.

Gastroenteritis. One of the most common forms of "food poisoning," GI infection caused by salmonellae results from the ingestion of the organisms through contaminated food. The *Salmonella* strains associated with this infection are usually those found in animals; most such strains in the United States are members of *S. enterica* subsp. *enterica*. Consequently the source of the infection has been attributed primarily to poultry, milk, eggs, and egg products as well as to handling pets. Insufficiently cooked eggs and domestic fowl, such as chicken, turkey, and duck, are common sources of infection. More recently in the United States, there has been a series of outbreaks by a variety of *Salmonella* serovars related to the ingestion of foodstuffs such as peanut butter, cantaloupe, puffed rice and wheat cereals, corn and vegetable coated snacks, and raw tomatoes. *Salmonella* Typimurium was responsible for a nationwide outbreak linked to peanut butter-containing products. More than 700 cases in 46 states were identified between September 2008 and March 2009.

Cooking utensils such as knives, pans, and cutting boards used in preparing the contaminated meat can spread the bacteria to other food. Direct transmission from person to person has been reported in institutions. *Salmonella* gastroenteritis, also referred to as *food poisoning,* occurs when a sufficient number of organisms contaminate food that is maintained under inadequate refrigeration, thus allowing growth and multiplication of the organisms. The infective dose necessary to initiate the disease, 10^6 bacteria, is higher than that required for shigellosis. Infections resulting from lower infective doses have been reported.

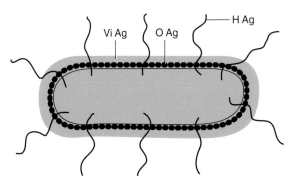

FIGURE 19-8 The antigenic structures of salmonellae used in serologic typing.

The symptoms of intestinal salmonellosis, which may appear 8 to 36 hours after ingestion of contaminated food, include nausea, vomiting, fever, and chills, accompanied by watery diarrhea and abdominal pain. Most cases of *Salmonella* gastroenteritis are self-limiting. Symptoms usually disappear within a few days, with few or no complications. Those who suffer from sickle cell disease and other hemolytic disorders, ulcerative colitis, and malignancy seem to be more susceptible to *Salmonella* spp. infection. The infection may be more severe in very young patients, elderly patients, and those suffering from other underlying disease. Dissemination may occasionally occur; in such cases, antimicrobial therapy is required.

The antimicrobials of choice include chloramphenicol, ampicillin, and trimethoprim-sulfamethoxazole. Nevertheless, susceptibility testing must be performed. However, antimicrobial therapy is usually not indicated in uncomplicated cases. Antimicrobial therapy is believed to prolong the carrier state. Antidiarrheal agents are also restricted in cases of salmonellosis because these agents may encourage adherence and further invasion. In cases of dehydration, fluid replacement therapy may be indicated.

Enteric Fevers. The clinical features of enteric fevers include:

- Prolonged fever
- Bacteremia
- Involvement of the reticuloendothelial system, particularly the liver, spleen, intestines, and mesentery
- Dissemination to multiple organs

Enteric fever caused by *Salmonella* Typhi is known as *typhoid fever,* a febrile disease that results from the ingestion of food contaminated with the organisms originating from infected individuals or carriers. *Salmonella* Typhi does not have a known animal reservoir; humans are the only source of infection. Other enteric fevers include paratyphoid fevers, which may be due to *Salmonella* serotypes Paratyphi A, B, and C, and *Salmonella* serotype Choleraesuis. The clinical manifestations of paratyphoid fevers are similar to those of typhoid fever but are less severe, and the fatality rate is lower.

Typhoid fever occurs more often in tropical and subtropical countries, where foreign travelers are more likely to acquire the infection. Improper disposal of sewage, poor sanitation, and lack of a modern water system have caused outbreaks of typhoid fever when the organisms reach a water source. This is uncommon in the United States and other developed countries, where water is purified and treated and handling of wastes is greatly improved. Carriers, particularly food handlers, are important sources of infection anywhere in the world. Direct transmission through fomites is also possible. Laboratory workers in the microbiology laboratory have contracted typhoid fever while working with the organisms.

Typhoid fever develops approximately 9 to 14 days after ingestion of the organisms. The onset of symptoms depends on the number of organisms ingested; the larger the inoculum, the shorter the incubation period. Characteristically, during the first week of the disease, the patient develops a fever accompanied by malaise, anorexia, lethargy, myalgia, and a continuous dull frontal headache.

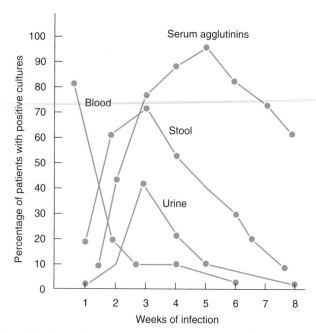

FIGURE 19-9 Culture and serologic diagnosis of typhoid fever. (Modified from Koneman E et al: *Color atlas and textbook of diagnostic microbiology*, ed 3, Philadelphia, 1988, Lippincott.)

When the organisms are ingested, they seem to be resistant to gastric acids and, on reaching the proximal end of the small intestine, subsequently invade and penetrate the intestinal mucosa. At this time, the patient experiences constipation rather than diarrhea. The organisms gain entrance into the lymphatic system and are sustained in the mesenteric lymph nodes. They eventually reach the bloodstream and are further spread to the liver, spleen, and bone marrow, where they are immediately engulfed by mononuclear phagocytes. The organisms multiply intracellularly; later they are released into the bloodstream for the second time. The febrile episode becomes more evident during this release of the organisms into the circulatory system. At this time, the organisms may easily be isolated from the blood. Figure 19-9 shows the course of typhoid fever.

During the second and third weeks of the disease, the patient experiences sustained fever with prolonged bacteremia. The organisms invade the gallbladder and Peyer's patches of the bowel. They also reach the intestinal tract via the biliary tract. "Rose spots" (blanching, rose-colored papules around the periumbilical region) appear during the second week of fever. Involvement of biliary system sites initiates GI symptoms as the organisms reinfect the intestinal tract. The organism now exists in large numbers in the bowel and may be isolated from the stool. The gallbladder becomes the foci of long-term carriage of the organism, occasionally reseeding the intestinal tract and shedding the organisms in the feces. Necrosis in the gallbladder leading to necrotizing cholecystitis and necrosis of the Peyer's patches leading to hemorrhage and perforation of the bowel may occur as serious complications. Pneumonia and thrombophlebitis are other complications that occur in typhoid fever as well as meningitis, osteomyelitis, endocarditis, and abscesses.

Bacteremia. *Salmonella* bacteremia, with and without extraintestinal foci of infection caused by nontyphoidal *Salmonella*, is characterized primarily by prolonged fever and intermittent bacteremia. The serotypes most commonly associated with bacteremia are Typhimurium, Paratyphi, and Choleraesuis. *Salmonella* infection has been observed among two different groups: (1) young children, who experience fever and gastroenteritis with brief episodes of bacteremia and (2) adults, who experience transient bacteremia during episodes of gastroenteritis or develop symptoms of septicemia without gastroenteritis. The latter manifestations were observed among patients who had underlying illnesses, such as malignancies and liver disease. The risk of metastatic complications could be more severe than the bacteremia itself, even in individuals who do not have underlying diseases. Cases of septic arthritis may also occur in patients who had asymptomatic salmonellosis.

Carrier State. Individuals who recover from infection may harbor the organisms in the gallbladder, which becomes the site of chronic carriage. Such individuals excrete the organisms in their feces either continuously or intermittently; nevertheless, they become an important source of infection for susceptible persons. The carrier state may be terminated by antimicrobial therapy if gallbladder infection is not evident. Otherwise, cholecystectomy has been the only solution to the chronic state of enteric carriers.

Shigella

The genera *Shigella* and *Escherichia* are closely related and according to molecular analyses should be a single genus. However, for medical purposes, and because of the useful association of the genus epithet with the distinct disease shigellosis or bacillary dysentery, they remain as separate genera, but both belong to the tribe Escherichieae. *Shigella* spp., however, are not members of the normal GI microbiota, and all *Shigella* spp. can cause bacillary dysentery. The genus *Shigella* is named after the Japanese microbiologist Kiyoshi Shiga, who first isolated the organism in 1896. The organism, descriptively named *Shigella dysenteriae,* caused the enteric disease bacillary dysentery. Dysentery was characterized by the presence of blood, mucus, and pus in the stool. The disease occurred in an epidemic. The following are characteristics of *Shigella* spp.:

- They are nonmotile.
- Except for certain types of *S. flexneri*, they do not produce gas from glucose.
- They do not hydrolyze urea.
- They do not produce hydrogen sulfide.
- They do not decarboxylate lysine.

Unlike *Escherichia* spp., *Shigella* spp. do not utilize acetate or mucate as a source of carbon. Table 19-9 shows the biochemical characteristics of *Shigella* spp. *S. sonnei* is unique in its ability to decarboxylate ornithine; it slowly ferments lactose; that is, one sees a "delayed" positive fermentation of lactose with the formation of pink colonies on MAC agar only after 48 hours of incubation. *S. sonnei* is also ONPG positive, and these two key positive reactions help to distinguish it from the other three species. Figure 19-10 illustrates the growth of *S. sonnei* on MAC after 24 and 48 hours of

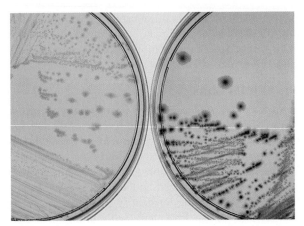

FIGURE 19-10 *Left,* Lactose-negative appearance of *Shigella sonnei* growing on MacConkey (MAC) agar at 18 to 24 hours of incubation. *Right,* Lactose-positive appearance of *S. sonnei* growing on MAC after 48 hours of incubation.

TABLE 19-9 Biochemical and Serologic Differentiation of *Shigella* Species

Test	S. dysenteriae	S. flexneri	S. boydii	S. sonnei
Mannitol fermentation	–	+	+	+
ONPG	V	–	V	+
Ornithine decarboxylase	–	–	–	+
Serogroup	A	B	C	D

From Farmer JJ et al: Enterobacteriaceae: introduction and identification. In Murray PR et al, editors: *Manual of clinical microbiology*, ed 9, Washington, DC, 2007, ASM Press.
–, ≤9% of strains positive; +, ≥90% of strains positive; *ONPG*, orthonitrophenyl galactoside; *V*, 10% to 89% of strains positive.

incubation. On differential and selective media used primarily to isolate intestinal pathogens, shigellae generally appear as clear, nonlactose-fermenting colonies. Shigellae are fragile organisms. They are susceptible to the various effects of physical and chemical agents, such as disinfectants and high concentrations of acids and bile. Because they are susceptible to the acid pH of stool, feces suspected of containing *Shigella* organisms should be plated immediately onto laboratory media to increase recovery of the organism.

Antigenic Structures

The genus consists of four species that are biochemically similar. *Shigella* spp. are also divided into four major O antigen groups and must be identified by serologic grouping. The four species and their respective serologic groups are depicted in Table 19-9.

Several serotypes exist within each species, with the exception of *S. sonnei*, which has only one serotype. All *Shigella* species possess O antigens, and certain strains can possess K antigens. *Shigella* K antigens, when present, interfere with the detection of the O antigen during serologic grouping. The K antigen is heat labile and may be removed by boiling the organism in a cell suspension. The shigellae are nonmotile and therefore lack H antigens.

Clinical Infections

Although all *Shigella* species can cause dysentery, species vary in epidemiology, mortality rate, and severity of disease. In the United States, *S. sonnei* is the predominant isolate, followed by *S. flexneri*. In the United States and other industrialized countries, shigellosis is probably underreported because most patients are not hospitalized and usually recover from the infection without culture to identify the etiologic agent. *S. sonnei* infection is usually a short, self-limiting disease characterized by fever and watery diarrhea.

The demographics of *S. flexneri* infection have changed during recent years, from a disease affecting mostly young children to one producing infections in young adults (approximately 25 years old). This observation was made simultaneously with the recognition of gastroenteritis in men who have sex with men, in which *S. flexneri* has been the leading isolate. Conversely, in developing countries, *S. dysenteriae* type 1 and *S. boydii* are the most common isolates. *S. dysenteriae* type 1 remains the most virulent species, with significant morbidity and high mortality. Reports exist of mortality rates of 5% to 10%, and perhaps even higher, resulting from *S. dysenteriae* type 1, particularly among undernourished children during epidemic outbreaks.

Humans are the only known reservoir of *Shigella* spp. Transmission can occur by direct person to person contact, and spread can take place via the fecal-oral route, with carriers as the source. Shigellae may also be transmitted by flies, fingers, and food or water contaminated by infected persons. Personal hygiene plays a major role in the transmission of *Shigella* organisms. Young children in daycare centers, people living in crowded and less-than-adequate housing, and people who participate in anal-oral sex are most likely affected. Children younger than 10 years of age seem to be most affected, and those 1 year of age and younger are the most susceptible. Most disturbing are the reports of multidrug-resistant *S. sonnei* outbreaks in daycare centers in several states. Multiple *Shigella* outbreaks associated with passengers on cruise ships from various cruise lines have been reported.

Because of the low infective dose required to produce the disease, shigellosis is highly communicable. It has been reported that fewer than 200 bacilli are needed to initiate the disease in some healthy individuals. Bacillary dysentery caused by *Shigella* spp. is marked by penetration of intestinal epithelial cells following attachment of the organisms to mucosal surfaces, local inflammation, shedding of the intestinal lining, and formation of ulcers following epithelial penetration.

The clinical manifestations of shigellosis vary from asymptomatic to severe forms of the disease. The initial symptoms, marked by high fever, chills, abdominal cramps, and pain accompanied by tenesmus, appear approximately 24 to 48 hours after ingestion of the organisms. The organisms, which originally multiply in the small intestine, move toward the colon, where they may be isolated 1 to 3 days after the infection develops. Bloody stools containing mucus and numerous leukocytes follow the watery diarrhea, as the organisms invade the colonic tissues and cause an inflammatory reaction.

In dysentery caused by *S. dysenteriae* type 1, patients experience more severe symptoms. Bloody diarrhea that progresses to dysentery may appear within a few hours to a few days. Patients suffer from extremely painful bowel movements, which contain predominantly mucus and blood. In young children, abdominal pain is quite intense, and rectal prolapse may result from excessive straining. Severe cases of shigellosis may become life-threatening as extraintestinal complications develop. One of the most serious complications is ileus, an obstruction of the intestines, with marked abdominal dilatation, possibly leading to toxic megacolon.

Although *Shigella* spp. infrequently penetrate the intestinal mucosa and disseminate to other body sites, it has been reported that as many as 4% of severely ill hospitalized patients in Bangladesh suffer from bacteremia caused by *S. dysenteriae* type 1. *S. flexneri* bacteremia and bacteremia resulting from other enteric organisms occur, presumably predisposed by ulcers initiated by the shigellae. Other complications of shigellosis include seizures, which may occur during any *Shigella* sp. infection, and HUS, a complication exclusively associated with *S. dysenteriae* type 1 shigellosis. Although the effects of shigella toxin have been implicated as the mechanism responsible for the signs of the disease, the connection between the toxin and the symptoms remains unclear. However, it has been reported that the detectable toxin levels produced by *S. dysenteriae* type 1 are higher than those produced by other *Shigella* spp.

Yersinia

The genus *Yersinia* currently consists of 11 named species. Although most have been isolated from humans, only three species are considered human pathogens. *Y. pestis* is the causative agent of plague, a disease primarily of rodents transmitted to humans by fleas. *Y. pseudotuberculosis* and *Y. enterocolitica* have caused sporadic cases of mesenteric lymphadenitis in humans, especially in children, and generalized septicemic infections in immunocompromised hosts. The DNA relatedness between *Y. pestis* and *Y. pseudotuberculosis* is about 90%. *Y. enterocolitica* produces an infection that mimics appendicitis. It has also been found to be the cause of diarrhea in a number of community outbreaks. The other members of the genus *Yersinia* are found in water, soil, and lower animals; occasionally isolates have been found in wounds and the urine of humans. Evidence that other species, in addition to *Y. enterocolitica*, have caused intestinal disease has not been found. *Y. ruckeri* is well documented as the causative agent of red mouth disease in fish.

Yersinia pestis

The causative agent of the ancient disease plague still exists in areas where reservoir hosts are found. Plague, caused by *Y. pestis*, is a disease primarily of rodents. It is transmitted to humans by bites of fleas, which are its most common and effective vectors. In humans, plague can occur in two forms:

the bubonic, or glandular, form and the pneumonic form. The bubonic form usually results from the bite of an infected flea. Characteristic symptoms appear 2 to 5 days after infection. The symptoms include high fever with painful regional lymph nodes as **buboes** (swollen lymph nodes) begin to appear. Pneumonic plague occurs secondary to the bubonic plague when organisms proliferate in the bloodstream and respiratory tract. Subsequent epidemic outbreaks may arise from the respiratory transmission of the organisms. The fatality rate in pneumonic plague is high if patients remain untreated.

Y. pestis is a gram-negative, short, plump bacillus. When stained with methylene blue or Wayson stain, it shows intense staining at each end of the bacillus, referred to as *bipolar staining,* which gives it a "safety-pin" appearance. *Y. pestis* may be isolated on routine culture medium. Although it grows at 37° C, it has a preferential growth temperature of 25° C to 30° C. A *Y. pestis*–specific DNA probe for plague surveillance has been studied. If this DNA probe is proven successful, it may be applicable for laboratory diagnostic testing. *Y. pestis* is a Class A Bioterrorism Agent, and further information relating to this classification can be found in Chapter 30 on Agents of Bioterror.

Yersinia enterocolitica

Human infections resulting from *Y. enterocolitica* have occurred worldwide, predominantly in Europe, although cases in the northeastern United States and Canada have been reported. It is the most commonly isolated species of *Yersinia.* The organisms have been found in a wide variety of animals, including domestic swine, cats, and dogs. The infection can therefore be acquired from contact with household pets. The role of pigs as a natural reservoir has been greatly emphasized in Europe. Other animal reservoirs, however, have also been identified, and cultures from environmental reservoirs, such as water from streams, have yielded the organism.

Human infections have also been reported following the ingestion of contaminated food (oftentimes pork and vacuum-packed meat) and possibly chocolate milk and water. There are several reports of gastroenteritis, especially in infants who were infected by caretakers who had improperly handled raw pork chitterlings (pork intestines) during food preparation procedures. A major concern regarding the potential risk of transmitting infection with this organism is its ability to survive in cold temperatures; food refrigeration becomes an ineffective preventive measure. In addition, *Y. enterocolitica* sepsis associated with the transfusion of contaminated packed red blood cells has been reported.

Y. enterocolitica infections manifest in several forms: an acute enteritis, an appendicitis-like syndrome, arthritis, and erythema nodosum. The incidence of generalized infection is higher among adults with underlying diseases, such as liver cirrhosis, diabetes, acquired immunodeficiency syndrome, leukemia, aplastic anemia, and other hematologic conditions. Cases of liver abscess and acute infective endocarditis caused by *Y. enterocolitica* have also been reported. Acute enteritis, the most common form of the infection, is characterized by acute gastroenteritis with fever accompanied by headaches, abdominal pain, nausea, and diarrhea. Stools may contain

blood. This form of infection, which often afflicts infants and young children between the ages of 1 and 5 years, is usually mild and self-limiting.

The clinical form that mimics acute appendicitis occurs primarily in older children and adults. It presents with severe abdominal pain and fever; the abdominal pain is concentrated in the right lower quadrant. Enlarged mesenteric lymph nodes and inflamed ileum and appendix are common findings in cases of *Y. enterocolitica* infections. Arthritis is a common extraintestinal form of *Y. enterocolitica* infection, usually following a GI episode or an appendicitis-like syndrome. This form of yersiniosis has been reported more often in adults than in children. The arthritic form resembles the arthritis seen in other bacterial infections; that is, in infections with *Shigella* spp., *Salmonella* spp., and *Neisseria gonorrhoeae* and in acute rheumatic fever. Erythema nodosum is an inflammatory reaction caused by *Y. enterocolitica* characterized by tender, red nodules that may be accompanied by itching and burning. The areas involved include the anterior portion of the legs; some patients have reported nodules on their arms. The reported cases have shown the syndrome to be more common in female patients than in male ones.

Y. enterocolitica morphologically resembles other *Yersinia* spp., which appear as gram-negative coccobacilli with bipolar staining. The organism also grows on routine isolation media, such as SBA and MAC agar. It has an optimal growth temperature of 25° C to 30° C. *Y. enterocolitica* grows better with cold enrichment, and motility is clearly noted at 25° C but not at 35° C. Appropriate cultures on a specific *Yersinia* media at 25° C should be performed in diarrheal outbreaks of unknown etiology. For cold enrichment, fecal samples suspected of containing this organism are inoculated into isotonic saline and kept at 4° C for 1 to 3 weeks, with weekly subculturing to selective agar for *Yersinia.*

Cefsulodin-igrasan-novobiocin (CIN) agar, a selective medium to detect the presence of *Y. enterocolitica,* incorporates cefsulodin, irgasan, novobiocin, bile salts, and crystal violet as inhibitory agents. This medium, which inhibits normal colon microbiota better than MAC agar, provides more opportunities to recover *Y. enterocolitica* from feces. This selective medium has since been modified, and manufacturers such as BD Diagnostic Systems (Sparks, Md.) have added a differential property to the medium, named *Yersinia*-selective agar (YSA) base, by adding mannitol. Fermentation of mannitol results in a drop in pH around the colony, causing the pH indicator, neutral red, to turn red at the center of the colony and the bile to precipitate. Nonfermentation of mannitol produces a colorless, translucent colony. A slightly modified formulation of the original CIN medium, known as CIN II, can be used to simultaneously isolate most *Aeromonas* spp. from stool samples.

Yersinia pseudotuberculosis

Yersinia pseudotuberculosis, like *Y. pestis,* is a pathogen primarily of rodents, particularly guinea pigs. In addition to farm and domestic animals, birds are natural reservoirs; turkeys, geese, pigeons, doves, and canaries have yielded positive cultures for this organism. *Y. pseudotuberculosis*

TABLE 19-10 Differentiation of Selected Species within the Genus *Yersinia*

Test	*Y. pestis*	*Y. enterocolitica*	*Y. pseudotuberculosis*
Indole	−	d	−
Methyl red	+	+	+
Voges-Proskauer			
25° C	−	d	−
37° C	−	−	−
Motility			
25° C	−	+	+
37° C	−	−	−
β-Galactosidase	+	+	+
Christensen urea	−	+	+
Phenylalanine deaminase	−	−	−
Ornithine decarboxylase	−	+	−
Acid produced from			
Sucrose	−	+	−
Lactose	−	−	−
Rhamnose	−	− or +*	+
Melibiose	−	− or +*	+
Trehalose	−	+ or −	+
Cellobiose	−	+	−

Modified from Washington J: *Laboratory procedures in clinical microbiology*, ed 2, New York, 1985, Springer-Verlag.
+, 90% or more positive reaction within 1 or 2 days; −, no reaction (90% or more) in 30 days; − *or* +, most strains negative, some cultures positive; + *or* (+), most reactions occur within 1 or 2 days, some are delayed; d, different reactions; + *or* −, most cultures positive, some strains negative.
*Test results at 25° C.

causes a disease characterized by caseous swellings called *pseudotubercles*. The disease is often fatal in animals.

Human infections, which are rare, are associated with close contact with infected animals or their fecal material or ingestion of contaminated drink and foodstuff. When the organisms are ingested, they spread to the mesenteric lymph nodes, producing a generalized infection. The clinical manifestations include septicemia accompanied by mesenteric lymphadenitis, a presentation similar to appendicitis. *Y. pseudotuberculosis* appears as a typical-looking plague bacillus. It can be differentiated from *Y. pestis* by its motility at 18° to 22° C, production of urease, and ability to ferment rhamnose. Table 19-10 shows differentiating characteristics among *Yersinia* spp.

OTHER GENERA OF THE FAMILY ENTEROBACTERIACEAE

Budivicia

Based on DNA hybridization, *Budivicia aquatica* is a group of closely related organisms. They are not as closely related to the other members of Enterobacteriaceae, but they do qualify to belong to the family. These organisms are usually found in water; however, they occasionally occur in clinical specimens.

Buttiauxella

The genus *Buttiauxella* consists of seven species isolated from water. Only *B. agrestis* and *B. noackiae* have been isolated from human specimens. Biochemically these organisms are similar to both *Citrobacter* and *Kluyvera* species, but DNA hybridization distinctly differentiates *Buttiauxella* from both genera.

Cedecea

The genus *Cedecea* is composed of five species: *C. davisae*, *C. lapagei*, *C. neteri*, and *Cedecea* species types 3 and 5. Most have been recovered from sputum, blood, and wounds. Of the five, *C. davisae* is the most commonly isolated species.

Ewingella

Ewingella americana is the only species of this genus. Most isolates have come from human blood cultures or respiratory specimens. *Ewingella* was first thought to be related to *Cedecea*; however, DNA hybridization confirmed the finding of a new genus.

Kluyvera

The genus *Kluyvera* is composed of three closely related species: *K. ascorbata*, *K. cryocrescens*, and *K. georgiana*. They have been found in respiratory, urine, and blood cultures and may produce a blue-violet pigment, usually but not exclusively on nonblood-containing media. All species resemble *E. coli* colonies growing on MAC agar. Figure 19-11 illustrates the colony characteristics of *Kluyvera* spp. Cephalothin and carbenicillin disk susceptibility tests separate the first two species; *K. cryocrescens* shows large zones of inhibition, and *K. ascorbata* has small zones. In addition, *K. ascorbata* does not ferment glucose at 5° C, whereas *K. cryocrescens* ferments glucose at this temperature. *K. georgiana* is very similar to the other two species but is negative for gas production during the fermentation of glucose.

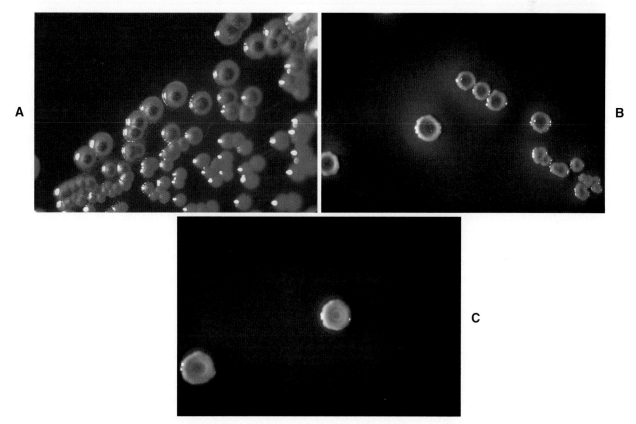

FIGURE 19-11 **A,** Blue-violet pigment of *Kluyvera* spp. growing on sheep blood agar. This *Kluyvera* sp. resembles the colony morphology of *Escherichia coli* growing on MacConkey (MAC) agar. **B,** Appearance of *K. cryocrescens* growing on MAC. **C,** Appearance of *K. ascorbata* growing on MAC agar.

Leclercia

The name *Leclercia* was proposed in 1986 for 58 isolates from human clinical specimens, including blood, urine, sputum, and feces and 27 isolates from nonhuman sources. The single species is *L. adecarboxylata,* which can have a yellow pigment, but only on initial isolation. Although it has similar IMViC reactions to *E. coli,* it is negative for lysine and ornithine decarboxylase and arginine dihydrolase (i.e., triple decarboxylase negative).

Leminorella

Leminorella was proposed as a genus for the Enteric Group 57, with two species: *L. grimontii* and *L. richardii.* These organisms produce hydrogen sulfide and have shown weak reactions with *Salmonella* antisera. However, complete biochemical tests will differentiate *Leminorella* from *Salmonella; Leminorella* spp. are relatively inactive. The clinical significance of these organisms is unknown; however, they have been isolated from urine, feces, and water.

Moellerella

The genus *Moellerella* contains one species, *M. wisconsensis. Moellerella* is positive for citrate, methyl red, lactose, and sucrose. It is negative for lysine, ornithine, arginine decarboxylase, and indole, and it resembles *E. coli* growing on enteric media. The clinical significance of this organism has not been established, although it has been isolated from feces in two cases of diarrhea, infected gallbladders, and a bronchial aspirate.

Obesumbacterium

Obesumbacterium proteus biogroup 2 is more closely related to *Escherichia blattae* than to other members of the family Enterobacteriaceae. These isolates are fastidious, slow-growing organisms at 37° C and have not been found in human specimens.

Photorhabdus

This genus includes three species: *P. luminescens,* with subspecies *luminescens, akhurstii,* and *laumondii; P. asymbiotica;* and *P. temperate.* Their natural habitat is the lumen of entomopathogenic nematodes, but strains have occasionally been isolated from human specimens. They occur in two phases with the property of luminescence in phase 1 only. Most strains produce pink, red, orange, yellow or green pigmented colonies on nutrient agar and especially on nutrient-rich media, such as trypticase soy agar and egg yolk agar. They are also negative for nitrate reduction.

Pragia

Pragia fontium is the only species in this genus. It produces H$_2$S, a *Shigella*-like odor on nutrient agar, and a "pig sty–like" odor on Endo agar overlaid with a sloping surface of agar. Other key reactions include utilization of citrate and oxidation of gluconate. Most strains are positive for methyl red as well. There has been one isolate from the stool of a healthy human, but no indication of pathogenicity for humans or animals.

Rahnella

Rahnella aquatilis is the name given to a group of water bacteria that are psychrotolerant, growing at 4° C. These organisms have no single characteristic that distinguishes them from the other members of the Enterobacteriaceae. They resemble *Enterobacter agglomerans;* however, they can be distinguished by a weak phenylalanine deaminase reaction; the fact that they are negative for potassium cyanide (KCN), gelatin, lysine, ornithine, and motility; and their lack of yellow pigmentation. They have been occasionally isolated from human clinical specimens, including wound infections, bacteremias, feces from patients with acute gastroenteritis, and septicemia, especially from immunocompromised patients.

Tatumella

Tatumella ptyseos is the only species of the genus *Tatumella.* This organism is unusual for the family Enterobacteriaceae in several ways: stock cultures may be kept frozen in sheep red blood cells or freeze-dried, but they will die in a few weeks on agar slants; show more biochemical reactions at 25° C than at 35° C; are motile at 25° C but not at 35° C; and demonstrate large 15- to 36-mm zones of inhibition around penicillin disks. In addition, *Tatumella* isolates are slow-growing, produce tiny colonies, and are relatively nonreactive in laboratory media. These organisms have been isolated from human sources, especially sputum, and may be a rare cause of infection.

Trabulsiella

Trabulsiella guamensis is the only species in this genus, and although it is very rarely isolated, it is biochemically similar to *Salmonella.* The type strain was isolated from vacuum-cleaner contents on the island of Guam when environmental indoor dirt samples were being collected. It has been isolated from human feces as well.

Xenorhabdus

The genus *Xenorhabdus* is composed only of *X. nematophilus,* an organism that grows best at 25° C and does not reduce nitrate to nitrite. *X. nematophilus,* which has been isolated from nematodes, has not been found in human specimens.

Yokenella

Yokenella regensburgei was first thought to be another species of *Hafnia,* but DNA hybridization showed a 15% relatedness, which was not sufficient to include these organisms in that genus. They are biochemically similar to *Hafnia* but differ primarily by yielding negative Voges-Proskauer test results. *Yokenella* strains have been isolated from human specimens, but further study will be required to determine their significance in human disease.

LABORATORY DIAGNOSIS OF ENTEROBACTERIACEAE

Specimen Collection and Transport

Members of the family Enterobacteriaceae may be isolated from a wide variety of clinical samples. Most often these bacterial species are isolated with other organisms, including more fastidious pathogens. Therefore to ensure isolation of both opportunistic and fastidious pathogens, laboratories must provide appropriate transport media such as Cary-Blair, Amies, or Stuart media. Microbiology personnel must encourage immediate transport of clinical samples to the laboratory for processing, regardless of the source of the clinical sample.

Isolation and Identification

To determine the clinical significance of the isolate, the microbiologist must consider the site of origin. Generally enteric opportunistic organisms isolated from sites that are normally sterile are highly significant. However, careful examination is critical of organisms recovered from, for example, the respiratory tract, urogenital tract, stool, and wounds in open sites that are inhabited by other endogenous microbiota.

Members of the family Enterobacteriaceae are routinely isolated from stool cultures; therefore complete identification should be directed only toward true intestinal pathogens. On the other hand, sputum cultures from hospitalized patients may contain enteric organisms that may require complete identification.

Direct Microscopic Examination

Unlike the case with gram-positive bacteria, in which microscopic morphology may help provide a presumptive identification, the microscopic characteristics of enterics are indistinguishable from other gram-negative bacteria. However, smears prepared directly from CSF, blood, and other body fluids or exudates from an uncontaminated site can be examined microscopically for the presence of gram-negative bacteria. Although this examination is nonspecific for enteric organisms, this presumptive result may aid the clinician in the preliminary diagnosis of the infection, and appropriate therapy can be instituted immediately.

On the other hand, direct smears prepared from samples, such as sputum, that contain endogenous microbiota do not provide valuable information because their significance cannot be fully assessed unless the gram-negative bacteria are prevalent and endogenous inhabitants are absent. Direct smear examination of stool samples is not particularly helpful in identifying enteric pathogens but may reveal the presence of inflammatory cells. This information may be helpful in determining whether a GI disease is toxin-mediated or an invasive process.

Culture

Members of the family Enterobacteriaceae are facultatively anaerobic and most clinically significant species grow at an optimal temperature of 35° C to 37° C. Certain species can grow at low temperatures (1° to 5° C, such as *Serratia* and

TABLE 19-11 Stool Culture Screening for Enteric Pathogens Utilizing TSI and LIA in Combination

LIA Reactions	TSI Reactions							
	K/A H₂S	K/AG H₂S	K/AG	K/A	A/A H₂S	A/AG	A/A	K/K
R/A		P. vulgaris P. mirabilis	M. morganii Providencia	M. morganii Providencia	P. vulgaris P. mirabilis	—	Providencia	—
K/K H₂S	Salmonella* Edwardsiella	Salmonella* Edwardsiella*	Salmonella*	Salmonella*	—	—	—	—
K/K	Salmonella	—	Hafnia Klebsiella Serratia	Salmonella* Plesiomonas† Hafnia	—	Klebsiella Enterobacter E. coli	Serratia	Pseudomonas†
K/A H₂S	—	Salmonella*	—	Serratia	—	—	—	—
K/A	—	Citrobacter	Salmonella* Shigella Aeromonas† E. coli Enterobacter Citrobacter	Shigella* Yersinia Aeromonas† E. coli Enterobacter	Citrobacter	Aeromonas*† E. coli Citrobacter Enterobacter	Aeromonas*† Yersinia Citrobacter Enterobacter	—

Data from the Microbiology Laboratory, The Ohio State University Hospitals and Maureta Ott, Columbus, Ohio.
LIA, Lysine-iron agar; TSI, triple sugar iron; K, alkaline; A, acid; G, gas; R, deamination (red slant).
*Results of TSI and LIA reactions in this category indicate a potential pathogen; additional tests must be performed.
†Oxidase positive.

Yersinia) or tolerate high temperatures (45° to 50° C, such as E. coli). Colonies become visible on nonselective and differential media after 18 to 24 hours of incubation.

Most laboratories use a wide variety of nonselective media, such as SBA and CHOC agar, as well as selective media, such as MAC, to recover enteric organisms from wounds, respiratory tract secretions, urine, and sterile body fluids. On CHOC agar or SBA plates, enteric bacteria produce large, grayish, smooth colonies. On SBA, colonies may be β-hemolytic or nonhemolytic.

Screening Stool Cultures for Pathogens

Because of the mixed microbial biota of fecal specimens, efficient screening methods should be used for the recovery and identification of stool pathogens. Enteric pathogens include *Salmonella, Shigella, Yersinia, E. coli* O157:H7, *Aeromonas, Campylobacter, Vibrio,* and *Plesiomonas shigelloides.* All fecal specimens should be routinely screened for *Salmonella, Shigella,* and *Campylobacter* (see Chapter 20). In addition, many laboratories screen for *E. coli* O157:H7. Screening routinely for the remaining organisms may not be cost effective; therefore these organisms should be addressed on the basis of patient history (e.g., travel near coastal areas where certain organisms are endemic) and gross description of the specimen (bloody or watery).

Stool specimens contain enteric organisms as normal colon microbiota; therefore, in processing stool samples, laboratories may develop their own protocol for the maximum recovery of enteric pathogens. Fecal pathogens are generally nonlactose fermenters (NLFs). These organisms appear as clear or colorless and translucent colonies on MAC agar. However, many of the bacteria that compose common fecal microbiota also appear as NLFs, for example, *Proteus, Providencia,* and *Pseudomonas,* as well as the delayed lactose-fermenting organisms (*Serratia* and *Citrobacter*). For this reason,

it is necessary to set up screening tests to differentiate these organisms from stool pathogens. An easy approach is to take a well-isolated, NLF colony and perform a screening battery of tests consisting first of an oxidase test and the inoculation of lysine iron agar (LIA) and TSI agar slants (Table 19-11). If the screening battery identifies a group of organisms that are nonpathogens, the process is complete and the culture is discarded (after 48 hours of incubation).

Most clinical microbiologists inoculate stool samples on highly selective media, such as HE or XLD agars, in addition to regular MAC and SMAC agar for *E. coli* O157:H7. An enrichment broth has been traditionally inoculated to enhance recovery; however, this practice is slowly being eliminated. As previously mentioned, CIN agar can serve the dual purpose of screening for both *Y. enterocolitica* and most *Aeromonas* spp., but one must remember that *Yersinia* is oxidase negative, *Aeromonas* is oxidase positive, and testing for this trait must be done on SBA, not on selective or differential media.

On HE agar, lactose-fermenting species produce yellow colonies, whereas NLFs such as *Shigella* spp. produce green colonies (Figure 19-12). However, *Proteus* are NLFs and species that produce hydrogen sulfide will also appear green with black centers on HE agar. *Citrobacter freundii* usually produces yellow colonies with black centers. NLF species such as *Salmonella enterica,* which produces lysine decarboxylase, produce red colonies with black centers on XLD medium (Figure 19-13). Another selective and differential medium is SS (Salmonella-Shigella) agar, a light straw-colored medium where *Salmonella* colonies will appear as colorless with dark black centers from the production of hydrogen sulfide and *Shigella* colonies will appear as colorless colonies only. On CHROMagar Salmonella (CHROMagar Co., Paris, France), *Salmonella* isolates will produce mauve-colored colonies (Figure 19-14) due to the activity of an esterase on a patented substrate. Other members of the family Enterobacteriaceae produce blue or white colonies.

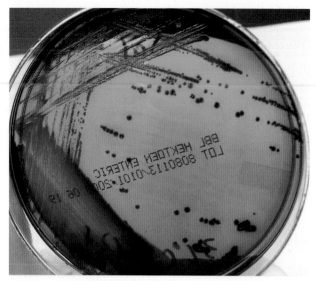

FIGURE 19-12 Clear, green colonies of *Shigella* growing on Hektoen enteric (HE) agar. (Courtesy R. Abe Baalness.)

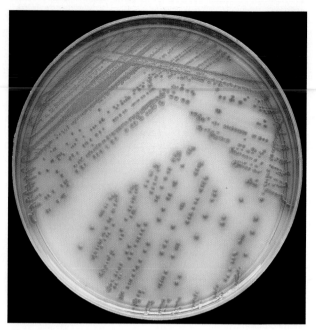

FIGURE 19-14 *Salmonella* growing on CHROMagar Salmonella differential agar. (Courtesy BD Diagnostic Systems, Sparks, Md.)

FIGURE 19-13 Hydrogen sulfide–producing colonies of salmonellae growing on xylose-lysine-desoxycholate agar. (Courtesy American Society for Clinical Laboratory Science, Education and Research Fund, Inc., 1982.)

Identification

The identification of members of the family Enterobacteriaceae can be done in several ways. Certain laboratories might prefer to use conventional biochemical tests in tubes, whereas others may prefer miniaturized or automated commercial identification systems. For a thorough description of the currently available rapid and automated commercial identification systems, consult Chapter 9. The use of conventional biochemical tests in tubes is cumbersome to test isolates with all the biochemical tests available. Therefore most clinical laboratories develop identification tables and protocols using a limited number of tests that suit their needs and capabilities. These tables are based on the key features necessary to iden-

tify each particular genus and clinically relevant species. Figure 19-15 shows an example of a schematic diagram for the identification of commonly isolated enterics using conventional biochemical tests. Table 19-12 shows the differentiating characteristics of the species, biogroups, and enteric groups of the Enterobacteriaceae.

To identify an isolate, the clinical microbiologist must first determine whether the isolate belongs to the family Enterobacteriaceae. All members of the family (1) are oxidase negative except for *Plesiomonas shigelloides* (see Chapter 20), (2) ferment glucose, and (3) reduce nitrate to nitrite (except *Photorhabdus* and *Xenorhabdus*). Gram-negative isolates, especially NLFs, should be tested for cytochrome oxidase production. The oxidase test should always be performed using young growth from an SBA plate. Testing colonies from highly selective media such as CIN may give a false-negative reaction, whereas MAC and EMB agars may give the appearance of a false-positive reaction from the pH indicators and dyes present in the media.

Regardless of the identification system used, the clinical microbiologist may presumptively determine utilization of carbohydrates by observing the colony morphology of the isolate on a differential or selective medium, such as MAC, SMAC, CIN, HE, or XLD. The traditional biochemical tests to perform for identification include the following:

- TSI agar or Kligler iron agar (KIA) to determine glucose and lactose or sucrose, utilization (sucrose in TSI only) and hydrogen sulfide production
- LIA to determine lysine decarboxylase activity
- Urease test to determine hydrolysis of urea
- Simmons citrate to determine the ability to use citrate as the sole carbon source
- Semisolid motility agar

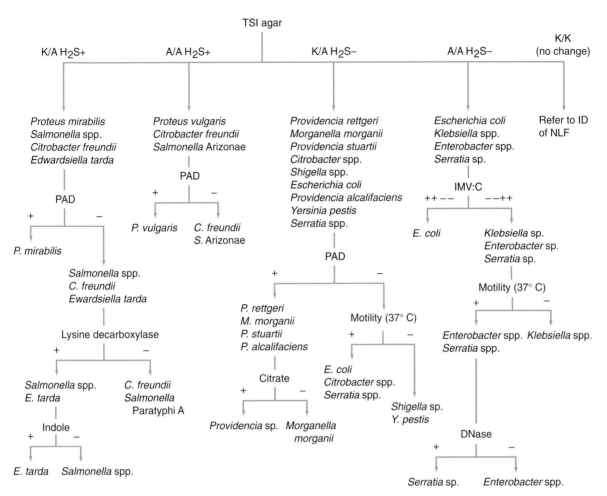

FIGURE 19-15 Flowchart for the presumptive identification of commonly encountered Enterobacteriaceae on triple sugar iron (TSI) agar. *K*, alkaline; *A*, acid; *PAD*, phenylalanine deaminase; *IMV:C*, indole, methyl red, Voges-Proskauer, citrate; *NLF*, nonlactose fermenter. (Data from Koneman E et al: *Color atlas in diagnostic microbiology,* ed 5, Philadelphia, 1997, Lippincott-Raven.)

- Sulfide, indole, motility (SIM) or motility, indole, and ornithine (MIO) media
- Carbohydrate fermentation

Serologic Grouping

Once an isolate is biochemically identified as *Salmonella* or *Shigella,* serologic grouping of the isolate for the O serogroups (somatic antigen) must be performed for confirmation. Serologic grouping is also important in the identification of the enterovirulent *E. coli.*

Salmonella

Based on the common O antigens, *Salmonella* may be placed into major groups designated by capital letters. Approximately 60 somatic O antigenic groups exist; however, 98% of *Salmonella* isolates from humans belong to serogroups A through G. Laboratories may report isolates as *Salmonella* groups (A-G) when specific serotyping is not available; isolates may be sent to a state or reference laboratory for serotyping. If an isolate is suspected of being one of these three serotypes, *Salmonella* Typhi, *Salmonella* Paratyphi, or *Salmo-*

nella Choleraesuis, because of its medical implications it must be biochemically identified and serologically confirmed. Their identification is very important in providing proper therapy for the patient and in limiting any possible complications that might develop.

It is imperative for any laboratory performing bacteriology to be able to identify serologically *S.* serotype Typhi particularly and other members of *Salmonella* in O groups A through G. Other isolates can be identified as "biochemically compatible with *Salmonella*" and submitted to a reference laboratory for further testing. To perform serologic grouping by slide technique, a suspension from a pure culture of the organism is prepared in sterile saline. Serologic typing is best performed on a colony taken from a pure culture growing on nonselective media, such as an SBA plate, although TSI or MAC can be used for presumptive serologic identification.

A slide with wells is easy to use for the agglutination test. A regular microscope slide may be used by marking separate circles with a wax pencil. The laboratory scientist places one drop of antisera on the appropriately labeled slide. One drop

Text continued on p. 460

TABLE 19-12 Biochemical Reactions of the Named Species and Unnamed Groups of the Family Enterobacteriaceae

Organism	Indole production	Methyl red	Voges-Proskauer	Citrate (Simmons)	Hydrogen sulfide (TSI)	Urea hydrolysis	Phenylalanine deaminase	Lysine decarboxylase	Arginine dihydrolase	Ornithine decarboxylase	Motility	Gelatin hydrolysis (22° C)	Growth in KCN	Malonate utilization	D-Glucose, acid	D-Glucose, gas	Lactose fermentation	Sucrose fermentation	D-Mannitol fermentation	Dulcitol fermentation	Salicin fermentation	Adonitol fermentation
Budvicia aquatica	0	93	0	0	80	33	0	0	0	0	27	0	0	0	100	53	87	0	60	0	0	0
Buttiauxella agrestis	0	100	0	100	0	0	0	0	0	100	100	0	80	60	100	100	100	0	100	0	100	0
Buttiauxella brennerae	0	100	0	0	0	0	0	0	0	33	100	0	100	100	100	100	67	0	100	0	100	67
Buttiauxella ferragutiae	0	100	0	0	0	0	0	100	0	80	60	0	40	0	100	100	0	0	100	0	100	0
Buttiauxella gaviniae	0	100	0	20	0	0	0	0	20	0	80	0	60	100	100	40	60	0	100	0	100	100
Buttiauxella izardii	0	100	0	0	0	0	0	0	0	100	100	0	67	100	100	100	100	0	100	0	100	0
Buttiauxella noackiae	33	100	0	33	0	0	100	0	67	0	100	0	100	100	100	100	0	0	100	0	100	0
Buttiauxella warmboldiae	0	100	0	33	0	0	100	0	0	0	100	0	33	100	100	100	0	0	100	0	100	0
Cedecea davisae	0	100	50	95	0	0	0	0	50	95	95	0	86	91	100	70	19	100	100	0	99	0
Cedecea lapagei	0	40	80	99	0	0	0	0	80	0	80	0	100	99	100	100	60	0	100	0	100	0
Cedecea neteri	0	100	50	100	0	0	0	0	100	0	100	0	65	100	100	100	35	100	100	0	100	0
Cedecea species 3	0	100	50	100	0	0	0	0	100	0	100	0	100	0	100	100	0	50	100	0	100	0
Cedecea species 5	0	100	50	100	0	0	0	0	50	50	100	0	100	0	100	100	0	100	100	0	100	0
Citrobacter amalonaticus	100	100	0	95	5	85	0	0	85	95	95	0	99	1	100	97	35	9	100	1	30	0
Citrobacter braakii	33	100	0	87	60	47	0	0	67	93	87	0	100	0	100	93	80	7	100	33	0	0
Citrobacter farmeri	100	100	0	10	0	59	0	0	85	100	97	0	93	0	100	96	15	100	100	2	9	0
Citrobacter freundii	33	100	0	78	78	44	0	0	67	0	89	0	89	11	100	89	78	89	100	11	0	0
Citrobacter gillenii	0	100	0	33	67	0	0	0	33	0	67	0	100	100	100	100	67	33	100	0	0	0
Citrobacter koseri (C. diversus)	99	100	0	99	0	75	0	0	80	99	95	0	0	95	100	98	50	40	99	40	15	99
Citrobacter murliniae	100	100	0	100	67	67	0	0	67	0	100	0	0	100	100	100	67	33	100	100	33	0
Citrobacter rodentium	0	100	0	0	0	100	0	0	0	100	0	0	0	100	100	100	100	0	100	0	0	0
Citrobacter sedlakii	83	100	0	83	0	100	0	0	100	100	100	0	100	100	100	100	100	0	100	100	17	0
Citrobacter werkmanii	0	100	0	100	100	100	0	0	100	0	100	0	100	100	100	100	17	0	100	0	0	0
Citrobacter youngae	15	100	0	75	65	80	0	0	50	5	95	0	95	5	100	75	25	20	100	85	10	0
Cronobacter sakazakii	11	5	100	99	0	1	50	0	99	91	96	0	99	18	100	98	99	100	100	5	99	0
Enteric Group 137 (5 strains)	100	100	0	0	0	70	0	0	20	100	100	0	100	0	100	0	100	100	100	0	100	0
Edwardsiella hoshinae	50	100	0	0	0	0	0	100	0	95	100	0	0	100	100	35	0	100	100	0	50	0
Edwardsiella ictaluri	0	0	0	0	0	0	0	100	0	65	0	0	0	0	100	50	0	0	0	0	0	0
Edwardsiella tarda	99	100	0	1	100	0	0	100	0	100	98	0	0	0	100	100	0	0	0	0	0	0
Edwardsiella tarda biogroup 1	100	100	0	0	0	0	0	100	0	100	100	0	0	0	100	50	0	100	100	0	0	0
Enterobacter aerogenes	0	5	98	95	0	2	0	98	0	98	97	0	98	95	100	100	95	100	100	5	100	98
Enterobacter amnigenus biogroup 1	0	7	100	70	0	0	0	0	9	55	92	0	100	91	100	100	70	100	100	0	91	0
Enterobacter amnigenus biogroup 2	0	65	100	100	0	0	0	0	35	100	100	0	100	100	100	100	35	0	100	0	100	0
Enterobacter asburiae	0	100	2	100	0	60	0	0	21	95	0	0	97	3	100	95	75	100	100	0	100	0

From the Centers for Disease Control and Prevention, Atlanta, Ga.

TSI, Triple sugar iron; *KCN*, potassium cyanide; *ONPG*, o-nitrophenyl-β-D-galactopyranoside.

*Each number is the percentage of positive reactions after 2 days of incubation at 36° C unless noted otherwise. Most of these positive reactions occur within 24 hours. Reactions that become positive after 2 days are not considered.

myo-Inositol fermentation	D-Sorbitol fermentation	L-Arabinose fermentation	Raffinose fermentation	L-Rhamnose fermentation	Maltose fermentation	D-Xylose fermentation	Trehalose fermentation	Cellobiose fermentation	Alpha-methyl-D-glucoside fermentation	Erythritol fermentation	Esculin hydrolysis	Melibiose fermentation	D-Arabitol fermentation	Gllycerol fermentation	Mucate fermentation	Tartrate, Jordan's	Acetate utilization	Lipase (corn oil)	DNase (25° C)	Nitrate nitrite	Oxidase, Kovacs	ONPG test	Yellow pigment	D-Mannose fermentation	Tyrosine utilization	D-Galactose	Citrate, Christensen's
0	0	80	0	100	0	93	0	0	0	0	0	0	27	0	20	27	0	0	0	100	0	93	0	0			
0	0	100	100	100	100	100	100	100	0	0	100	100	0	60	100	60	0	0	0	100	0	100	0	100			
0	0	100	100	33	100	100	100	100	0	0	100	100	67	67	67	0	0	0	0	100	0	100	0	100			
0	100	100	0	100	100	100	100	100	40	0	100	0	0	0	60	0	0	0	0	100	0	100	0	100			
0	0	100	0	100	60	100	100	100	0	0	100	0	80	0	80	40	0	0	0	100	0	100	0	100			
0	0	100	33	100	100	100	100	100	0	0	100	67	0	33	100	67	0	0	0	100	0	100	0	100			
0	0	100	0	100	100	100	100	100	33	0	100	0	0	0	100	100	0	0	0	100	0	100	0	100			
67	0	100	0	100	100	100	100	100	0	0	100	0	0	0	0	0	0	0	0	100	0	100	0	100			
0	0	0	10	0	100	100	100	100	5	0	45	0	100	0	0	0	0	91	0	100	0	90	0	100			
0	0	0	0	0	100	0	100	100	0	0	100	0	100	0	0	0	60	100	0	100	0	99	0	100			
0	100	0	0	0	100	100	100	100	0	0	100	0	100	0	0	0	0	100	0	100	0	100	0	100			
0	0	0	100	0	100	100	100	100	50	0	100	100	100	0	0	0	50	100	0	100	0	100	0	100			
0	100	0	100	0	100	100	100	100	0	0	100	100	100	0	0	0	50	50	0	100	0	100	0	100			
0	99	99	5	100	99	99	100	100	2	0	5	0	0	60	96	96	86	0	0	99	0	97	0	100			
0	100	100	7	100	100	100	100	73	33	0	0	80	0	87	100	93	53	0	0	100	0	80	0	100			
0	98	100	100	100	100	100	100	100	75	0	0	100	0	65	100	93	80	0	0	100	0	100	0	100			
0	100	100	44	100	100	89	100	44	11	0	0	100	0	100	100	100	44	0	0	100	0	89	0	100			
0	100	100	0	100	100	100	100	67	0	0	0	67	0	67	67	100	0	0	0	100	0	67	0	100			
0	99	99	0	99	100	100	100	99	40	0	1	0	98	99	95	90	75	0	0	100	0	99	0	100			
0	100	100	33	100	100	100	100	100	0	0	0	33	0	100	100	100	33	0	0	100	0	100	0	100			
0	100	100	0	100	100	100	100	100	0	0	0	0	0	0	100	100	0	0	0	100	0	100	0	100			
0	100	100	0	100	100	100	100	100	0	0	17	100	0	83	100	100	83	0	0	100	0	100	0	100			
0	100	100	0	100	100	100	100	0	0	0	0	0	0	100	100	100	100	0	0	100	0	100	0	100			
5	100	100	10	100	95	100	100	45	0	0	5	10	5	90	100	100	65	0	0	85	0	90	0	100			
75	0	100	99	100	100	100	100	100	96	0	100	100	0	15	1	1	96	0	0	99	0	100	98	100			
0	100	100	100	100	100	100	100	100	80	0	100	100	0	100	100	50	100	0	0	100	0	100	0	100	0	100	90
0	0	13	0	0	100	0	100	0	0	0	0	0	0	65	0	0	0	0	0	100	0	0	0	100			
0	0	0	0	0	100	0	0	0	0	0	0	0	0	0	0	0	0	0	0	100	0	0	0	100			
0	0	9	0	0	100	0	0	0	0	0	0	0	0	30	0	25	0	0	0	100	0	0	0	100			
0	0	100	0	0	100	0	0	0	0	0	0	0	0	0	0	0	0	0	0	100	0	0	0	100			
95	100	100	96	99	99	100	100	100	95	0	98	99	100	98	90	95	50	0	0	100	0	100	0	95			
0	9	100	100	100	100	100	100	100	55	0	91	100	0	0	35	9	0	0	0	100	0	91	0	100			
0	100	100	0	100	100	100	100	100	0	0	100	100	0	0	100	0	0	0	0	100	0	100	0	100			
0	100	100	70	5	100	97	100	100	95	0	95	0	0	11	21	30	87	0	0	100	0	100	0	100			

Continued

TABLE 19-12 Biochemical Reactions of the Named Species and Unnamed Groups of the Family Enterobacteriaceae—cont'd

Organism	Indole production	Methyl red	Voges-Proskauer	Citrate (Simmons)	Hydrogen sulfide (TSI)	Urea hydrolysis	Phenylalanine deaminase	Lysine decarboxylase	Arginine dihydrolase	Ornithine decarboxylase	Motility	Gelatin hydrolysis (22° C)	Growth in KCN	Malonate utilization	D-Glucose, acid	D-Glucose, gas	Lactose fermentation	Sucrose fermentation	D-Mannitol fermentation	Dulcitol fermentation	Salicin fermentation	Adonitol fermentation
Enterobacter cancerogenus (E. taylorae)	0	5	100	100	0	1	0	0	94	99	99	0	98	100	100	100	10	0	100	0	92	0
Enterobacter cloacae	0	5	100	100	0	65	0	0	97	96	95	0	98	75	100	100	93	97	100	15	75	25
Enterobacter dissolvens	0	0	100	100	0	100	0	0	100	100	0	0	100	100	100	100	0	100	100	0	100	0
Enterobacter gergoviae	0	5	100	99	0	93	0	90	0	100	90	0	0	96	100	98	55	98	99	0	99	0
Enterobacter hormaechei	0	57	100	96	0	87	4	0	78	91	52	0	100	100	100	83	9	100	100	87	44	0
Enterobacter intermedium	0	100	100	65	0	0	0	0	0	89	89	0	65	100	100	100	100	65	100	100	100	0
Enterobacter nimipressuralis	0	100	100	0	0	0	0	0	0	100	0	0	100	100	100	100	0	0	100	0	100	0
Enterobacter pyrinus	0	29	86	0	0	86	0	100	0	100	43	0	0	86	100	100	14	100	100	0	100	0
Escherichia albertii	0	0	0	0	0	0	0	100	0	100	0	0	0	0	100	100	0	0	100	0	0	0
Escherichia blattae	0	100	0	50	0	0	0	100	0	100	0	0	0	100	100	100	0	0	0	0	0	0
Escherichia coli	98	99	0	1	1	1	0	90	17	65	95	0	3	0	100	95	95	50	98	60	40	5
Escherichia coli, inactive	80	95	0	1	1	1	0	40	3	20	5	0	1	0	100	5	25	15	93	40	10	3
Escherichia fergusonii	98	100	0	17	0	0	0	95	5	100	93	0	0	35	100	95	0	0	98	60	65	98
Escherichia hermannii	99	100	0	1	0	0	0	6	0	100	99	0	94	0	100	97	45	45	100	19	40	0
Escherichia vulneris	0	100	0	0	0	0	0	85	30	0	100	0	15	85	100	97	15	8	100	0	30	0
Ewingella americana	0	84	95	95	0	0	0	0	0	0	60	0	5	0	100	0	70	0	100	0	80	0
Hafnia alvei	0	40	85	10	0	4	0	100	6	98	85	0	95	50	100	98	5	10	99	0	13	0
Hafnia alvei biogroup 1	0	85	70	0	0	0	0	100	0	45	0	0	0	45	100	0	0	0	55	0	55	0
Klebsiella oxytoca	99	20	95	95	0	90	1	99	0	0	0	0	97	98	100	97	100	100	99	55	100	99
Klebsiella ornithinolytica	100	96	70	100	0	100	0	100	0	100	0	0	100	100	100	100	100	100	100	10	100	100
Klebsiella planticola	20	100	98	100	0	98	0	100	0	0	0	0	100	100	100	100	100	100	100	15	100	100
Klebsiella pneumoniae subsp. ozaenae	0	98	0	30	0	10	0	40	6	3	0	0	88	3	100	50	30	20	100	2	97	97
Klebsiella pneumoniae subsp. pneumoniae	0	10	98	98	0	95	0	98	0	0	0	0	98	93	100	97	98	99	99	30	99	90
Klebsiella pneumoniae subsp. rhinoscleromatis	0	100	0	0	0	0	0	0	0	0	0	0	80	95	100	0	0	75	100	0	98	100
Klebsiella terrigena	0	60	100	40	0	0	0	100	0	20	0	0	100	100	100	80	100	100	100	20	100	100
Kluyvera ascorbata	92	100	0	96	0	0	0	97	0	100	98	0	92	96	100	93	98	98	100	25	100	0
Kluyvera cryocrescens	90	100	0	80	0	0	0	23	0	100	90	0	86	86	100	95	95	81	95	0	100	0
Kluyvera georgiana	100	100	0	100	0	0	0	100	0	100	100	0	83	50	100	17	83	100	100	33	100	0
Leclercia adecarboxylata	100	100	0	0	0	48	0	0	0	0	79	0	97	93	100	97	93	66	100	86	100	93
Leminorella grimontii	0	100	0	100	100	0	0	0	0	0	0	0	0	0	100	33	0	0	0	83	0	0
Leminorella richardii	0	0	0	0	100	0	0	0	0	0	0	0	0	0	100	0	0	0	0	0	0	0
Moellerella wisconsensis	0	100	0	80	0	0	0	0	0	0	0	0	70	0	100	0	100	100	60	0	0	100

From the Centers for Disease Control and Prevention, Atlanta, Ga.

TSI, Triple sugar iron; *KCN*, potassium cyanide; *ONPG*, o-nitrophenyl-β-D-galactopyranoside.

*Each number is the percentage of positive reactions after 2 days of incubation at 36° C unless noted otherwise. Most of these positive reactions occur within 24 hours. Reactions that become positive after 2 days are not considered.

myo-Inositol fermentation	D-Sorbitol fermentation	L-Arabinose fermentation	Raffinose fermentation	L-Rhamnose fermentation	Maltose fermentation	D-Xylose fermentation	Trehalose fermentation	Cellobiose fermentation	Alpha-methyl-D-glucoside fermentation	Erythritol fermentation	Esculin hydrolysis	Melibiose fermentation	D-Arabitol fermentation	Gllycerol fermentation	Mucate fermentation	Tartrate, Jordan's	Acetate utilization	Lipase (corn oil)	DNase (25° C)	Nitrate nitrite	Oxidase, Kovacs	ONPG test	Yellow pigment	D-Mannose fermentation	Tyrosine utilization	D-Galactose	Citrate, Christensen's
0	1	100	0	100	99	100	100	100	1	0	90	0	0	1	75	0	35	0	0	100	0	100	0	100			
15	95	100	97	92	100	99	100	99	85	0	30	90	15	40	75	30	75	0	0	99	0	99	0	100			
0	100	100	100	100	100	100	100	100	100	0	100	100	0	0	100	0	100	0	0	100	0	100	0	100			
0	0	99	97	99	100	99	100	99	2	0	97	97	97	100	2	97	93	0	0	99	0	97	0	100			
0	0	100	0	100	100	96	100	100	83	0	0	0	0	4	96	13	74	0	0	100	0	95	0	100			
0	100	100	100	100	100	100	100	100	100	0	100	100	0	100	100	100	0	0	0	100	0	100	0	100			
0	100	100	0	100	100	100	100	100	100	0	100	100	0	0	100	0	0	0	0	100	0	100	0	100			
100	0	100	0	100	100	0	100	100	0	0	100	0	0	0	0	0	0	0	0	100	0	100	0	100			
0	0	100	0	0	60	0	60	0	0	0	20	0	0	100	0		100	0	0	100	0	100	0	100			
0	0	100	0	100	100	100	75	0	0	0	0	0	0	100	50	50	0	0	0	100	0	0	0	100			
1	94	99	50	80	95	95	98	2	0	0	35	75	5	75	95	95	90	0	0	100	0	95	0	98			
1	75	85	15	65	80	70	90	2	0	0	5	40	5	65	30	85	40	0	0	98	0	45	0	97			
0	0	98	0	92	96	96	96	96	0	0	46	0	100	20	0	96	96	0	0	100	0	83	0	100			
0	0	100	40	97	100	100	100	97	0	0	40	0	8	3	97	35	78	0	0	100	0	98	98	100			
0	1	100	99	93	100	100	100	100	25	0	20	100	0	25	78	2	30	0	0	100	0	100	50	100			
0	0	0	0	23	16	13	99	10	0	0	50	0	99	24	0	35	10	0	0	97	0	85	0	99			
0	0	95	2	97	100	98	95	15	0	0	7	0	0	95	0	70	15	0	0	100	0	90	0	100			
0	0	0	0	0	0	0	70	0	0	0	0	0	0	0	0	30	0	0	0	100	0	30	0	100			
98	99	98	100	100	100	100	100	100	98	2	100	99	98	99	93	98	90	0	0	100	0	100	1	100			
95	100	100	100	100	100	100	100	100	100	0	100	100	100	100	96	100	95	0	0	100	0	100	0	100			
100	92	100	100	100	100	100	100	100	100	0	100	100	100	100	100	100	62	0	0	100	0	100	1	100			
55	65	98	90	55	95	95	98	92	70	0	80	97	95	65	25	50	2	0	0	80	0	80	0	100			
95	99	99	99	99	98	99	99	98	90	0	99	99	98	97	90	95	75	0	0	99	0	99	0	99			
95	100	100	90	96	100	100	100	100	0	0	30	100	100	50	0	50	0	0	0	100	0	0	0	100			
80	100	100	100	100	100	100	100	100	100	0	100	100	100	100	100	100	20	0	0	100	0	100	0	100			
0	40	100	98	100	100	99	100	100	98	0	99	99	0	40	90	35	50	0	0	100	0	100	0	100			
0	45	100	100	100	100	91	100	100	95	0	100	100	0	5	81	19	86	0	0	100	0	100	0	100			
0	0	100	100	83	100	100	100	100	100	0	100	100	0	33	83	50	83	0	0	100	0	100	0	100			
0	0	100	66	100	100	100	100	100	0	0	100	100	96	3	93	83	28	0	0	100	0	100	37	100			
0	0	100	0	0	0	83	0	0	0	0	0	0	0	17	100	100	0	0	0	100	0	0	0	0			
0	0	100	0	0	0	100	0	0	0	0	0	0	0	0	50	100	0	0	0	100	0	0	0	0			
0	0	0	100	0	30	0	0	0	0	0	0	0	100	75	10	0	30	10	0	90	0	90	0	100			

Continued

TABLE **19-12** **Biochemical Reactions of the Named Species and Unnamed Groups of the Family Enterobacteriaceae—cont'd**

Organism	Indole production	Methyl red	Voges-Proskauer	Citrate (Simmons)	Hydrogen sulfide (TSI)	Urea hydrolysis	Phenylalanine deaminase	Lysine decarboxylase	Arginine dihydrolase	Ornithine decarboxylase	Motility	Gelatin hydrolysis (22° C)	Growth in KCN	Malonate utilization	D-Glucose, acid	D-Glucose, gas	Lactose fermentation	Sucrose fermentation	D-Mannitol fermentation	Dulcitol fermentation	Salicin fermentation	Adonitol fermentation
Morganella morganii subsp. morganii	95	95	0	0	20	95	95	1	0	95	95	0	98	1	99	90	1	0	0	0	0	0
Morganella morganii subsp. sibonii	50	86	0	0	7	100	93	29	0	64	79	0	79	0	100	86	0	7	0	0	0	0
Morganella morganii biogroup 1	100	95	0	0	15	100	100	100	0	80	0	0	90	5	100	93	0	0	0	0	0	0
Obesumbacterium proteus biogroup 2	0	15	0	0	0	0	0	100	0	100	0	0	0	0	100	0	0	0	0	0	0	0
Pantoea agglomerans	20	50	70	50	0	20	20	0	0	0	85	2	35	65	100	20	40	75	100	15	65	7
Pantoea dispersa	0	82	64	100	0	0	9	0	0	0	100	0	82	9	100	0	0	1	100	0	0	0
Photorhabdus luminescens (all tests at 25° C)	50	0	0	50	0	25	0	0	0	0	100	50	0	0	75	0	0	0	0	0	0	0
Photorhabdus DNA hybridization group 5	0	0	0	20	0	60	0	0	0	0	100	80	20	0	100	0	0	0	0	0	0	0
Pragia fontium	0	100	0	89	89	0	22	0	0	0	100	0	0	0	100	0	0	0	0	0	78	0
Proteus mirabilis	2	97	50	65	98	98	98	0	0	99	95	90	98	2	100	96	2	15	0	0	0	0
Proteus myxofaciens	0	100	100	50	0	100	100	0	0	0	100	100	100	0	100	100	0	100	0	0	0	0
Proteus penneri	0	100	0	0	30	100	99	0	0	0	85	50	99	0	100	45	1	100	0	0	0	0
Proteus vulgaris	98	95	0	15	95	95	99	0	0	0	95	91	99	0	100	85	2	97	0	0	50	0
Providencia alcalifaciens	99	99	0	98	0	0	98	0	0	1	96	0	100	0	100	85	0	15	2	0	1	98
Providencia heimbachae	0	85	0	0	0	0	100	0	0	0	46	0	8	0	100	0	0	0	0	0	0	92
Providencia rettgeri	99	93	0	95	0	98	98	0	0	0	94	0	97	0	100	10	5	15	100	0	50	100
Providencia rustigianii	98	65	0	15	0	0	100	0	0	0	30	0	100	0	100	35	0	35	0	0	0	0
Providencia stuartii	98	100	0	93	0	30	95	0	0	0	85	0	100	0	100	0	2	50	10	0	2	5
Rahnella aquatilis	0	88	100	94	0	0	95	0	0	0	6	0	0	100	100	98	100	100	100	88	100	0
Salmonella bongori	0	100	0	94	100	0	0	100	94	100	100	0	100	0	100	94	0	0	100	94	0	0
Salmonella enterica subsp. arizonae	1	100	0	99	99	0	0	99	70	99	99	0	1	95	100	99	15	1	100	0	0	0
Salmonella enterica subsp. diarizonae	2	100	0	98	99	0	0	99	70	99	99	0	1	95	100	99	85	5	100	1	0	0
Salmonella enterica subsp. enterica	1	100	0	95	95	1	0	98	70	97	95	0	0	0	100	96	1	1	100	96	0	0
Salmonella enterica subsp. houtenae	0	100	0	98	100	2	0	100	70	100	98	0	95	0	100	100	0	0	98	0	60	5
Salmonella enterica subsp. indica	0	100	0	89	100	0	0	100	67	100	100	0	0	0	100	100	22	0	100	67	0	0
Salmonella enterica subsp. salamae	2	100	0	100	100	0	0	100	90	100	98	2	0	95	100	100	1	1	100	90	5	0
Salmonella serotype Choleraesuis	0	100	0	25	50	0	0	95	55	100	95	0	0	0	100	95	0	0	98	5	0	0
Salmonella serotype Gallinarum	0	100	0	0	100	0	0	90	10	1	0	0	0	0	100	0	0	0	100	90	0	0

From the Centers for Disease Control and Prevention, Atlanta, Ga.

TSI, Triple sugar iron; *KCN*, potassium cyanide; *ONPG*, o-nitrophenyl-β-D-galactopyranoside.

*Each number is the percentage of positive reactions after 2 days of incubation at 36° C unless noted otherwise. Most of these positive reactions occur within 24 hours. Reactions that become positive after 2 days are not considered.

myo-Inositol fermentation	D-Sorbitol fermentation	L-Arabinose fermentation	Raffinose fermentation	L-Rhamnose fermentation	Maltose fermentation	D-Xylose fermentation	Trehalose fermentation	Cellobiose fermentation	Alpha-methyl-D-glucoside fermentation	Erythritol fermentation	Esculin hydrolysis	Melibiose fermentation	D-Arabitol fermentation	Gllycerol fermentation	Mucate fermentation	Tartrate, Jordan's	Acetate utilization	Lipase (corn oil)	DNase (25° C)	Nitrate nitrite	Oxidase, Kovacs	ONPG test	Yellow pigment	D-Mannose fermentation	Tyrosine utilization	D-Galactose	Citrate, Christensen's
0	0	0	0	0	0	0	0	0	0	0	0	0	0	5	0	95	0	0	0	90	0	10	0	98			
0	0	0	0	0	0	0	100	0	0	0	0	0	0	7	7	100	0	0	0	100	0	0	0	100			
0	0	0	0	0	0	0	0	0	0	0	0	0	0	100	0	100	0	0	0	90	0	20	0	100			
0	0	0	0	15	50	15	85	0	0	0	0	0	0	0	0	15	0	0	0	100	0	0	0	85			
15	30	95	30	85	89	93	97	55	7	0	60	50	50	30	40	25	30	0	0	85	0	90	75	98			
0	0	100	0	91	82	100	100	55	0	0	0	0	100	27	0	9	100	0	0	91	0	91	27	100			
0	0	0	0	0	25	0	0	0	0	0	0	0	0	0	0	50	0	0	0	0	0	0	50	100			
0	0	0	0	0	0	0	0	0	0	0	0	0	0	0	0	60	20	0	0	0	0	0	60	100			
0	0	0	0	0	0	0	0	0	0	0	78	0	0	0	0	0	0	0	0	100	0	0	0	0			
0	0	0	1	1	0	98	98	1	0	0	0	0	0	70	0	87	20	92	50	95	0	0	0	0			
0	0	0	0	0	100	0	100	0	100	0	0	0	0	100	0	100	0	100	50	100	0	0	0	0			
0	0	0	1	0	100	100	55	0	80	0	0	0	0	55	0	85	5	45	40	90	0	1	0	0			
0	0	0	1	5	97	95	30	0	60	1	50	0	0	60	0	80	25	80	80	98	0	1	0	0			
1	1	1	1	0	1	1	2	0	0	0	0	0	0	15	0	90	40	0	0	100	0	1	0	100			
46	0	0	0	100	54	8	0	0	0	0	0	0	0	92	0	69	0	0	0	100	0	0	0	100			
90	1	0	5	70	2	10	0	3	2	75	35	5	100	60	0	95	60	0	0	100	0	5	0	100			
0	0	0	0	0	0	0	0	0	0	0	0	0	0	5	0	50	25	0	0	100	0	0	0	100			
95	1	1	7	0	1	7	98	5	0	0	0	0	0	50	0	90	75	0	10	100	0	10	0	100			
0	94	100	94	94	94	94	100	100	0	0	100	100	0	13	30	6	6	0	0	100	0	100	0	100			
0	100	94	0	88	100	100	100	0	0	0	0	94	0	0	88	0	100	0	0	100	0	94	0	100			
0	99	99	1	99	98	100	99	1	1	0	1	95	1	10	90	5	90	0	2	100	0	100	0	100			
0	99	99	1	99	98	100	99	1	1	0	1	95	1	10	30	20	75	0	2	100	0	92	0	100			
35	95	99	2	95	97	97	99	5	2	0	5	95	0	5	90	90	90	0	2	100	0	2	0	100			
0	100	100	0	98	100	100	100	50	0	0	0	100	5	0	0	65	70	0	0	100	0	0	0	100			
0	0	100	0	100	100	100	100	0	0	0	0	89	0	33	89	100	89	0	0	100	0	44	0	100			
5	100	100	0	100	100	100	100	0	8	0	15	8	0	25	96	50	95	0	0	100	0	15	0	95			
0	90	0	1	100	95	98	0	0	0	1	0	45	1	0	0	85	1	0	0	98	0	0	0	95			
0	1	80	10	10	90	70	50	10	0	1	0	0	0	0	0	50	100	0	0	10	100	0	0	100			

Continued

TABLE 19-12 Biochemical Reactions of the Named Species and Unnamed Groups of the Family Enterobacteriaceae—cont'd

Organism	Indole production	Methyl red	Voges-Proskauer	Citrate (Simmons)	Hydrogen sulfide (TSI)	Urea hydrolysis	Phenylalanine deaminase	Lysine decarboxylase	Arginine dihydrolase	Ornithine decarboxylase	Motility	Gelatin hydrolysis (22° C)	Growth in KCN	Malonate utilization	D-Glucose, acid	D-Glucose, gas	Lactose fermentation	Sucrose fermentation	D-Mannitol fermentation	Dulcitol fermentation	Salicin fermentation	Adonitol fermentation
Salmonella serotype Paratyphi A	0	100	0	0	10	0	0	0	15	95	95	0	0	0	100	99	0	0	100	90	0	0
Salmonella serotype Pullorum	0	90	0	0	90	0	0	100	10	95	0	0	0	0	100	90	0	0	100	0	0	0
Salmonella serotype Typhi	0	100	0	0	97	0	0	98	3	0	97	0	0	0	100	0	1	0	100	0	0	0
Serratia entomophila	0	20	100	100	0	0	0	0	0	0	100	100	100	0	100	0	0	100	100	0	100	0
Serratia ficaria	0	75	75	100	0	0	0	0	0	0	100	100	55	0	100	0	15	100	100	0	100	0
Serratia fonticola	0	100	9	91	0	13	0	100	0	97	91	0	70	88	100	79	97	21	100	91	100	100
Serratia liquefaciens	1	93	93	90	0	3	0	95	0	95	95	90	90	2	100	75	10	98	100	0	97	5
Serratia marcescens	1	20	98	98	0	15	0	99	0	99	97	90	95	3	100	55	2	99	99	0	95	40
Serratia marcescens biogroup 1	0	100	60	30	0	0	0	55	4	65	17	30	70	0	100	0	4	100	96	0	92	30
Serratia odorifera biogroup 1	60	100	50	100	0	5	0	100	0	100	100	95	60	0	100	0	70	100	100	0	98	50
Serratia odorifera biogroup 2	50	60	100	97	0	0	0	94	0	0	100	94	19	0	100	13	97	0	97	0	45	55
Serratia plymuthica	0	94	80	75	0	0	0	0	0	0	50	60	30	0	100	40	80	100	100	0	94	0
Serratia rubidaea	0	20	100	95	0	2	0	55	0	0	85	90	25	94	100	30	100	99	100	0	99	99
Shigella boydii	25	100	0	0	0	0	0	0	18	2	0	0	0	0	100	0	1	0	97	5	0	0
Shigella dysenteriae	45	99	0	0	0	0	0	0	2	0	0	0	0	0	0	0	0	1	100	0	0	0
Shigella flexneri	50	100	0	0	0	0	0	0	5	0	0	0	100	0	100	3	1	1	95	1	0	0
Shigella sonnei	0	100	0	0	0	0	0	0	2	98	0	0	0	0	100	0	2	1	99	0	0	0
Tatumella ptyseos	0	0	5	2	0	0	90	0	0	0	0	0	0	0	100	0	0	98	0	0	55	0
Trabulsiella guamensis	40	100	0	88	100	0	0	100	50	100	100	0	100	0	100	100	0	0	100	0	13	0
Xenorhabdus nematophilus	40	0	0	0	0	0	0	0	0	0	100	80	0	0	80	0	0	0	0	0	0	0
Yersinia aldovae	0	80	0	0	0	60	0	0	0	40	0	0	0	0	100	0	0	20	80	0	0	0
Yersinia bercovieri	0	100	0	0	0	60	0	0	0	80	0	0	0	0	100	0	20	100	100	0	20	0
Yersinia enterocolitica	50	97	2	0	0	75	0	0	0	95	2	0	2	0	100	5	5	95	98	0	20	0
Yersinia frederiksenii	100	100	0	15	0	70	0	0	0	95	5	0	0	0	100	40	40	100	100	0	92	0
Yersinia intermedia	100	100	5	5	0	80	0	0	0	100	5	0	10	5	100	18	35	100	100	0	100	0
Yersinia kristensenii	30	92	0	0	0	77	0	0	0	92	5	0	0	0	100	23	8	0	100	0	15	0
Yersinia mollaretii	0	100	0	0	0	20	0	0	0	80	0	0	0	0	100	0	40	100	100	0	20	0
Yersinia pestis	0	80	0	0	0	5	0	0	0	0	0	0	0	0	100	0	0	0	97	0	70	0
Yersinia pseudotuberculosis	0	100	0	0	0	95	0	0	0	0	0	0	0	0	100	0	0	0	100	0	25	0
Yerrsinia rohdei	0	62	0	0	0	62	0	0	0	25	0	0	0	0	100	0	0	100	100	0	0	0
Yersinia ruckeri	0	97	10	0	0	0	0	50	5	100	0	30	15	0	100	5	0	0	100	0	0	0
Yokenella regensburgei (Koserella trabulsii)	0	100	0	92	0	0	0	100	8	100	100	0	92	0	100	100	0	0	100	0	8	0
Enteric Group 58	0	100	0	85	0	70	0	100	0	85	100	0	100	85	100	85	30	0	100	85	100	
Enteric Group 59	10	100	0	100	0	0	30	0	60	0	100	0	80	90	100	100	80	0	100	0	100	
Enteric Group 60	0	100	0	0	0	50	0	0	0	100	75	0	100	100	100	0	0	50	0	0		
Enteric Group 68	0	100	50	0	0	0	0	0	0	0	0	0	100	0	100	0	0	100	100	0	50	
Enteric Group 69	0	0	100	100	0	0	0	0	100	100	100	0	100	100	100	100	100	25	100	100	100	0

From the Centers for Disease Control and Prevention, Atlanta, Ga.

TSI, Triple sugar iron; *KCN*, potassium cyanide; *ONPG*, o-nitrophenyl-β-D-galactopyranoside.

*Each number is the percentage of positive reactions after 2 days of incubation at 36° C unless noted otherwise. Most of these positive reactions occur within 24 hours. Reactions that become positive after 2 days are not considered.

myo-Inositol fermentation	D-Sorbitol fermentation	L-Arabinose fermentation	Raffinose fermentation	L-Rhamnose fermentation	Maltose fermentation	D-Xylose fermentation	Trehalose fermentation	Cellobiose fermentation	Alpha-methyl-D-glucoside fermentation	Erythritol fermentation	Esculin hydrolysis	Melibiose fermentation	D-Arabitol fermentation	Gllycerol fermentation	Mucate fermentation	Tartrate, Jordan's	Acetate utilization	Lipase (corn oil)	DNase (25° C)	Nitrate nitrite	Oxidase, Kovacs	ONPG test	Yellow pigment	D-Mannose fermentation	Tyrosine utilization	D-Galactose	Citrate, Christensen's
0	95	100	0	100	95	0	100	5	0	0	0	95	0	10	0	0	0	0	0	100	0	0	0	100			
0	10	100	1	100	5	90	90	5	0	0	0	0	0	0	0	0	0	0	0	100	0	0	0	100			
0	99	2	0	0	97	82	100	0	0	0	0	100	0	20	0	100	0	0	0	0	0	0	0	100			
0	0	0	0	0	100	40	100	0	0	0	100	0	60	0	0	100	80	20	100	100	0	100	0	100			
55	100	100	70	35	100	100	100	100	8	0	100	40	100	0	0	17	40	77	100	92	8	100	0	100			
30	100	100	100	76	97	85	100	6	91	0	100	98	100	88	0	58	15	0	0	100	0	100	0	100			
60	95	98	85	15	98	100	100	5	5	0	97	75	0	95	0	75	40	85	85	100	0	93	0	100			
75	99	0	2	0	96	7	99	5	0	1	95	0	0	95	0	75	50	98	98	98	0	95	0	99			
30	92	0	0	0	70	0	100	4	0	0	96	0	0	92	0	50	4	75	82	83	0	75	0	100			
100	100	100	100	95	100	100	100	100	0	0	95	100	0	40	5	100	60	35	100	100	0	100	0	100			
100	100	100	7	94	100	100	100	100	0	7	40	96	0	50	0	100	65	65	100	100	0	100	0	100			
50	65	100	94	0	94	94	100	88	70	0	81	93	0	50	0	100	55	70	100	100	0	70	0	100			
20	1	100	99	1	99	99	100	94	1	0	94	99	85	20	0	70	80	99	99	100	0	100	0	100			
0	43	94	0	1	20	11	85	0	0	0	15	0	50	0		50	0	0	0	100	0	10	0	100			
0	30	45	0	30	15	4	90	0	0	0	0	0	0	10	0	75	0	0	0	99	0	30	0	100			
0	29	60	40	5	30	2	65	0	0	0	0	55	1	10	0	30	8	0	0	99	0	1	0	100			
0	2	95	3	75	90	2	100	5	0	0	0	25	0	15	10	90	0	0	0	98	0	90	0	100			
0	0	0	11	0	0	9	93	0	0	0	0	25	0	7	0	0	0	0	0	98	0	0	0	100			
0	100	100	0	100	100	100	100	100	0	0	40	0	0	0		100	50	88	0	100	0	100	0	100			
0	0	0	0	0	0	0	0	0	0	0	0	0	0	0	0	60	0	0	20	20	0	0				60	80
0	60	60	0	0	0	40	80	0	0	0	0	0	0	0		100	0	0	0	100	0	0	0	100			
0	100	100	0	0	100	100	100	100	0	0	20	0	0	0	0	100	0	0	0	100	0	80	0	100			
30	99	98	5	1	75	70	98	75	0	0	25	1	40	90	0	85	15	55	5	98	0	95	0	100			
20	100	100	30	99	100	100	100	100	0	0	85	0	100	85	5	55	15	55	0	100	0	100	0	100			
15	100	100	45	100	100	100	100	96	77	0	100	80	45	60	6	88	18	12	0	94	0	90	0	100			
15	100	77	0	0	100	85	100	100	0	0	0	0	45	70	0	40	8	0	0	100	0	70	0	100			
0	100	100	0	0	60	60	100	100	0	0	0	0	0	20	0	100	0	0	0	100	0	20	0	100			
0	50	100	0	1	80	90	100	0	0	0	50	20	0	50	0	0	0	0	0	85	0	50	0	100			
0	0	50	15	70	95	100	100	0	0	0	95	70	0	50	0	50	0	0	0	95	0	70	0	100			
0	100	100	62	0	0	38	100	25	0	0	0	50	0	38	0	100	0	0	0	88	0	50	0	100			
0	50	5	5	0	95	0	95	5	0	0	0	0	0	30	0	30	0	30	0	75	0	50	0	100			
0	0	100	25	100	100	100	100	100	0	0	67	92	0	0	0	25	0	0	0	100	0	100	0	100			
0	100	100	0	100	100	100	100	100	55	0	0	0	0	30	0	60	45	0	0	100	0	100	0	100			
0	0	100	0	100	100	100	100	100	10	0	100	0	10	10	60	50	50	0	0	100	0	100	25	100			
0	0	25	0	75	0	0	100	0	0	0	0	0	0	75	0	75	0	0	0	100	0	100	0	100			
0	0	0	0	50	0	100	0	0	0	0	0	0	50	0		0	0	0	100	100	0	0		100			
0	100	100	100	100	100	100	100	100	100	0	100	100	0	0	100	0	25	0	0	100	0	100	0	100			

of bacterial suspension is added to each drop of antisera for a direct agglutination assay. Antisera kits usually consist of a polyvalent A through G, Vi, and individual antisera for serogroups A, B, C1, C2, D, E, and G. Latex agglutination kits offer improved visibility of agglutination reactions; this is an example of reverse passive agglutination.

In the event of a positive agglutination in the Vi antisera with no agglutination in the other groups, the suspension should be heated to 100° C for 10 minutes to inactivate the capsular Vi antigen. The suspension is then cooled and retested with antisera A to G. Larger laboratories usually maintain antisera to serotype salmonellae for all the somatic types. H antigen or flagella typing is usually performed in a state or reference laboratory that provides epidemiologic information in outbreaks.

Shigella

Similar serogrouping procedures may be used in the serologic testing for *Shigella*. Serologic grouping of *Shigella* is also based on the somatic O antigen. *Shigella* spp. may belong to one of the four serogroups: A *(S. dysenteriae)*, B *(S. flexneri)*, C *(S. boydii)*, and D *(S. sonnei)*. The O antisera used for serogrouping are polyvalent, containing several serotypes within each group (with the exception of group D, which contains only a single serotype). If agglutination fails, the suspension must be heated to remove the capsular antigen that may be present, and subsequently the agglutination test procedure is repeated.

BIBLIOGRAPHY

Abbott SL: *Klebsiella, Enterobacter, Citrobacter, Serratia, Plesiomonas,* and other Enterobacteriaceae. In Murray PR et al, editors: *Manual of clinical microbiology,* ed 9, Washington, DC, 2007, ASM Press.

Brenner DJ, Farmer III JJ: Enterobacteriaceae. In Brenner DJ et al, editors: *Bergey's manual of systematic bacteriology,* ed 2, vol 2, New York, 2005, Springer-Verlag, p. 587.

Centers for Disease Control and Prevention: Surveillance for foodborne outbreaks—United States, 1993-1997, *MMWR* 49(SS01):1, 2000. Available at: www.cdc.gov/mmwr/preview/mmwrhtml/ss4901a1.htm. Accessed September 30, 2008.

Centers for Disease Control and Prevention: Investigation update: outbreak of *Salmonella* Litchfield infections associated with a hotel—Atlantic City, New Jersey, 2007. Available at: www.cdc.gov/mmwr/preview/mmwrhtml/mm5728a4.htm. Accessed September 30, 2008.

Centers for Disease Control and Prevention: Multistate outbreak of *Salmonella* serotype Tennessee infections associated with peanut butter—United States, 2006-2007, *MMWR* 56:521, 2007. Available at: www.cdc.gov/mmwr/preview/mmwrhtml/mm5621a1.htm. Accessed September 30, 2008.

Centers for Disease Control and Prevention: Investigation of outbreak of infections caused by *Salmonella* Agona. Available at: www.cdc.gov/salmonella/agona. Accessed September 30, 2008.

Centers for Disease Control and Prevention: *Salmonella* Wandsworth outbreak investigation June-July 2007. Website: www.cdc.gov/salmonella/wandsworth.htm. Accessed September 30, 2008.

Centers for Disease Control and Prevention: Turtle-associated salmonellosis in humans—United States, 2006-2007, *MMWR* 56:649, 2007. Available at: www.cdc.gov/mmwr/preview/mmwrhtml/mm5626a1.htm. Accessed on July 1, 2008.

Centers for Disease Control and Prevention: Multi-state outbreaks of *Salmonella* infections associated with raw tomatoes eaten in restaurants—United States, 2005-2006, *MMWR* 56:909, 2007. Available at: www.cdc.gov/mmwr/preview/mmwrhtml/mm5635a3.htm Accessed on July 1, 2008.

Centers for Disease Control and Prevention: *Yersinia enterocolitica* gastroenteritis among infants exposed to chitterlings—Chicago, Illinois, 2002, *MMWR* 52:956, 2003. Available at: www.cdc.gov/mmwr/preview/mmwrhtml/mm5240a2.htm. Accessed July 1, 2008.

Centers for Disease Control and Prevention: Outbreaks of multi-drug-resistant *Shigella sonnei* gastroenteritis associated with day care centers—Kansas, Kentucky, and Missouri, 2005, *MMWR* 55:1068, 2006. Available at: www.cdc.gov/mmwr/preview/mmwrhtml/mm5539a3.htm. Accessed on July 1, 2008.

Centers for Disease Control and Prevention: Multistate outbreak of *E. coli* O157:H7 infection linked to eating raw, refrigerated prepackaged cookie dough (Website). www.cdc.gov/ecoli/2009/0807.html. Accessed September 4, 2009.

Centers for Disease Control and Prevention: Investigation update: outbreak of *Salmonella* Typhimurium infections, 2008-2009 (Website). www.cdc.gov/salmonella/typhimurium/update.html. Accessed September 4, 2009.

Ewing WH: *Edwards and Ewing's identification of Enterobacteriaceae,* ed 4, New York, 1986, Elsevier.

Farmer III JJ et al: Enterobacteriaceae: introduction and identification. In Murray PR et al, editors: *Manual of clinical microbiology,* ed 9, Washington, DC, 2007, ASM Press.

Iversen C et al: *Cronobacter* gen. nov., a new genus to accommodate the biogroups of *Enterobacter sakazakii,* and proposal of *Cronobacter sakazakii* gen. nov., comb. nov., *Cronobacter malonaticus* sp. nov., *Cronobacter turicensis* sp. nov., *Cronobacter muytjensii* sp. nov., *Cronobacter dublinensis* sp. nov., *Cronobacter* genomospecies 1, and of three subspecies, *Cronobacter dublinensis* subsp. *dublinensis* subsp. nov., *Cronobacter dublinensis* subsp. *lausannensis* subsp. nov. and *Cronobacter dublinensis* subsp. *lactaridi* subsp. nov, *Int J Syst Evol Microbiol* 58:1442, 2008.

Judicial Commission of the International Committee on Systematics of Prokaryotes: Opinion: the type species of the genus *Salmonella lignieres* 1900 is *Salmonella enterica* (ex Kauffmann and Edwards 1952) Le Minor and Popoff 1987, with the type strain LT22, and conservation of the epithet *enterica* in *Salmonella enterica* over all earlier epithets that may be applied to this species, *Opinion* 80:519, 2005.

Karolis DK et al: Cloning of the RDEC-1 locus of enterocyte effacement (LEE) and functional analysis of the phenotype on HEp-2 cells, *Adv Exp Med Biol* 412:241, 1997.

Kehl KS et al: Evaluation of the premier EHEC assay for detection of Shiga-toxin producing *Escherichia coli, J Clin Microbiol* 35:2051, 1997.

Levine M et al: *Escherichia coli* strains that cause diarrhea but do not produce heat-labile or heat-stable enterotoxins and are noninvasive, *Lancet* 1:1119, 1978.

Nataro JP et al: *Escherichia, Shigella,* and *Salmonella.* In Murray PR et al, editors: *Manual of clinical microbiology,* ed 9, Washington, DC, ASM Press, 2007.

Nowicki B et al: Family of *Escherichia coli* Dr adhesins: decay-accelerating factor receptor recognition and invasiveness, *J Infect Dis* 183:S24, 2001.

Popoff MY, Minor LE: Genus *Salmonella.* In Brenner DJ et al, editors: *Bergey's manual of systematic bacteriology,* ed 2, vol 2, New York, 2005, Springer-Verlag, pp 764.

Tindall BJ et al: Nomenclature and taxonomy of the genus *Salmonella, Int J Syst Evol Microbiol* 55:521, 2005.

Yanger A: *Yersinia.* In Murray PR et al, editors: *Manual of clinical microbiology,* ed 9, Washington, DC, 2007, ASM Press.

Yoh M et al: Importance of *Providencia* species as a major cause of travellers' diarrhoea, *J Med Microbiol* 54:1077, 2005.

Points to Remember

- Nearly any of the genera discussed in this chapter could conceivably be isolated from almost any clinical specimen, especially when dealing with immunocompromised patients.
- Whereas most isolates of *E. coli* are considered normal fecal microbiota, several strains are known to cause intestinal tract infections. *E. coli* is the most significant cause of urinary tract infections.
- *Salmonella* and *Shigella* are enteric pathogens and are not considered normal fecal biota.
- *Yersinia pestis,* one of the most virulent species in the family Enterobacteriaceae, causes the extraintestinal infection called plague.
- A good patient history, combined with the proper types of selective screening agar (e.g., Hektoen enteric [HE] agar, xylose-lysine-desoxycholate [XLD] agar, and MacConkey agar with sorbitol [SMAC], are available for the presumptive identification of enteric pathogens), can be very helpful in a timely and accurate identification of enteric pathogens associated with diarrheal disease.
- The use of an initial battery of selective agar media and key biochemical tests such as triple sugar iron, urea, and motility agars can usually result in a presumptive genus identification that can then be confirmed with either conventional biochemical test or with the use of one of several available multitest or rapid and automated identification systems.
- There are notable exceptions to the Enterobacteriaceae family "gold standard" definition of glucose fermenters that are able to reduce nitrate to nitrite and are oxidase negative.

Learning Assessment Questions

1. What are the three general characteristics a gram-negative bacillus must possess to belong to the family Enterobacteriaceae with three exceptions?

2. Match the *Shigella* spp. with the corresponding group antigen: A, B, C, and D.
   a. *S. sonnei*
   b. *S. boydii*
   c. *S. dysenteriae*
   d. *S. flexneri*

3. Which of the following test results is most helpful in categorizing an isolate as a member of the Tribe *Proteeae*?
   a. Positive Voges-Proskauer
   b. Positive urea
   c. Positive phenylalanine deaminase
   d. Positive lactose fermentation

4. The causative agent of plague is:
   a. *Yersinia pestis*
   b. *Klebsiella rhinoscleromatis*
   c. *Citrobacter freundii*
   d. *Serratia marcescens*

5. A patient who had just returned from Mexico was admitted to the hospital with a 3-day history of vomiting and diarrhea, without fever, and no fecal leukocytes were found in the stool. When he was admitted to the hospital, a stool culture grew an organism identified as *Escherichia coli.* Which of the following strains is the most likely cause of the infection?
   a. Enteropathogenic *E. coli* (EPEC)
   b. Enterotoxigenic *E. coli* (ETEC)
   c. Enterohemorrhagic *E. coli* (EHEC)
   d. Enteroinvasive *E. coli* (EIEC)

6. A gram-negative, oxidase-negative coccobacillus was isolated from the cerebrospinal fluid of an infant in the newborn nursery. The organism produced dark pink colonies on MacConkey agar and had the following biochemical results: triple sugar iron, acid over acid with gas; phenylalanine deaminase, negative; sulfide-indole-motility agar, hydrogen sulfide negative, indole positive, and motile; urease negative; and citrate negative. The most probable identity of this organism is:
   a. *Escherichia coli*
   b. *Enterobacter aerogenes*
   c. *Klebsiella pneumoniae*
   d. *Serratia marcescens*

7. An organism often associated with lobar pneumonia in elderly hospitalized patients:
   a. *Shigella* spp.
   b. *Proteus vulgaris*
   c. *Escherichia coli*
   d. *Klebsiella pneumoniae*

8. The most common cause of community-acquired urinary tract infections:
   a. *Klebsiella pneumoniae*
   b. *Escherichia coli*
   c. *Providencia stuartii*
   d. *Citrobacter freundii*

9. An opportunistic pathogen, this organism causes wound and urinary tract infections and may cause the production of kidney stones:
   a. *Yersinia enterocolitica*
   b. *Citrobacter freundii*
   c. *Proteus vulgaris*
   d. *Enterobacter cloacae*

10. Acquired by eating improperly cooked or preserved contaminated food, this enteric organism produces dysentery in affected individuals:
    a. *Proteus vulgaris*
    b. *Salmonella* Typhi
    c. *Serratia marcescens*
    d. *Shigella* spp.

Vibrio, Aeromonas, Plesiomonas, and Campylobacter Species

Amy J. Horneman, Deborah Ann Josko

OBJECTIVES

After reading and studying this chapter, you should be able to:

1. Describe the colony morphology and microscopic characteristics of each organism.

2. Discuss the habitat in which these organisms are found.

3. Discuss the appropriate specimen collection, transport, and processing for maximum recovery of each organism.

4. List the media of choice for each organism.

5. Identify key biochemical reactions that will help differentiate among the different genera and various species.

6. Compare the confirmatory tests commonly used to identify these isolates.

7. Discuss the criteria used to differentiate the bacterial species that cause gastrointestinal illnesses from other diarrheal agents.

8. Compare and contrast each group of organisms with respect to macroscopic and microscopic morphology, biochemical reactions, media, epidemiology, clinical infection, specimen collection, and specimen transport.

9. Describe the disease states associated with each group of organisms.

Case in Point

A 65-year-old Chinese man, in obvious shock, was examined in the emergency department for a painful swelling of the left hand. His medical history revealed bilateral knee joint pain and posthepatic cirrhosis. The day before admission, he had pricked his left index finger while selecting shrimp at a fish market. At first he noticed only a local reaction in his finger, but after 12 hours the left hand began to swell, accompanied by nausea, vomiting, and diarrhea. The patient was now clammy with a weak pulse, marked swelling, and bullous formation with gangrenous changes apparent on the left hand. A diagnosis of septic shock was made, and antimicrobial therapy was instituted. Blood and wound cultures subsequently grew an oxidase-positive, gram-negative rod that produced pink colonies on MacConkey agar and green colonies on thiosulfate citrate bile salt sucrose agar and required 3% to 6% NaCl for growth. No acceptable identification could be made with a rapid identification system for gram-negative bacilli, and final identification was made with conventional biochemicals supplemented with 1% NaCl. The patient suffered a cardiac arrest and died 11 hours after admission.

Issues to Consider

After reading the patient's case history, consider:

- Various pathogenic organisms associated with aquatic life that cause human infections
- Disease spectrum and states associated with these organisms
- Presentation of clinical signs and symptoms
- Media of choice to aid in a rapid diagnosis
- Key biochemical reactions to presumptively and definitively identify the organism responsible for this infection
- Treatment of choice

Key Terms

Cholera	Kanagawa phenomenon
Cholera toxin	Microaerophilic
Choleragen	Thiosulfate citrate bile salts
"Darting" motility	sucrose (TCBS) agar
El Tor	Type B gastritis
Halophilic	Urea breath test

This chapter discusses agents of diarrheal diseases and other infections caused by species of *Vibrio, Aeromonas, Plesiomonas, Campylobacter,* and *Helicobacter.* The microscopic and macroscopic characteristics as well as the epidemiology and clinical infection of each organism are discussed. Specimen collection, transport, growth requirements, and key biochemical reactions used for diagnosis are also included in this chapter. This group of organisms is important because some of them, the *Vibrio* spp. in particular, have been associated with large epidemics and pandemics. In addition, *Campylobacter* spp. infection may play a role in Guillain-Barré syndrome, and *Helicobacter pylori* can cause ulcers and has been linked to gastric carcinoma.

VIBRIO

The genus *Vibrio* resides in the family Vibrionaceae and encompasses more than 75 validly published species, although to date only 12 of these species have been found in human clinical specimens. However, the most recent ninth edition of the *Manual of Clinical Microbiology* supports the classification of *Vibrio hollisae* in the new genus *Grimontia* as *G. hollisae,* and reports on the proposal to possibly reclassify *Vibrio damsela* as *Photobacterium damsela.*

Vibrio spp. are commonly found in a wide variety of aquatic environments, including fresh water, brackish or estuarine water, and marine or salt water. They are temperature sensitive in that in temperate climates when water temperatures exceed 20° C, as in the summer months, vibrios can easily be isolated from water, suspended particulate matter, algae, plankton, fish, and shellfish. However, their numbers decline markedly in the winter months, and they are generally found only in the sediments. Therefore the risk of infection from all *Vibrio* spp. can be reduced by the avoidance of eating raw or undercooked shellfish, particularly in warmer summer months. This is especially pertinent to persons who are immunocompromised or have serious underlying liver disease. Additionally, those who are severely immunosuppressed should avoid exposure of wounds to fresh, estuarine, and marine water sources.

Pandemics (worldwide epidemics) of **cholera,** a devastating diarrheal disease caused by *V. cholerae,* have been documented since 1817. Recently a large epidemic of cholera occurred in Dhaka, the capital city of Bangladesh, with an estimated 30,000 cases. This outbreak was due to the resurgence of *V. cholerae* 0139, the newest serotype associated with the disease cholera that was initially recognized in Madras, India in 1992.

A general increase in the number of reported cases of *Vibrio* infections, both gastrointestinal and extraintestinal, caused by other species has been seen. Some of the various reasons for this significant rise in the clinical isolation of *Vibrio* include the following:
- Increased travel to either coastal or cholera endemic areas
- Increased consumption of seafood (particularly raw or undercooked)
- Increased use of recreational water facilities, which encourages aquatic exposure
- Larger populations of immunocompromised individuals
- Increased awareness of the existence and significance of these organisms in the clinical microbiology laboratory

General Characteristics

Clinical Manifestations

Vibrio spp. can be isolated from a number of clinical sources, and most species have been implicated in more than one disease process, ranging from mild gastroenteritis to cholera and from simple wound infections to fatal septicemia and necrotizing fasciitis. Table 20-1 lists the various clinical infections associated with *Vibrio* spp. The four *Vibrio* spp. most likely to be encountered in the clinical laboratory are *V. cholerae* (serogroups O1 and non-O1), *V. parahaemolyticus, V. vulnificus,* and *V. alginolyticus.*

Because most laboratories, except those in coastal areas, have a fairly low frequency of isolation of *Vibrio* spp., a good medical history is extremely important. Often the best indication of a possible *Vibrio* infection is the presence of certain recognized factors, such as the following:
- Recent consumption of raw seafood (especially oysters)
- Recent immigration or foreign travel
- Gastroenteritis with cholera-like or rice-water stools
- Accidental trauma incurred during contact with fresh, estuarine, or marine water or associated products (e.g., shellfish, oyster or clam shells, fishhooks)

Microscopic Morphology

Vibrio spp. are asporogenous, gram-negative rods that measure approximately 0.5 to 0.8 μm in diameter by 1.5 to 3.0 μm in length. These organisms possess polar, sheathed flagella when grown in broth, but they can produce peritrichous, unsheathed flagella when grown on solid media. They have been described classically as "curved" gram-negative rods, but this morphology is often seen only in the initial Gram stain of the clinical specimen (Figure 20-1). Vibrios usually appear as small, straight, gram-negative rods, but they can be highly pleomorphic, especially under suboptimal growth conditions.

Physiology

The vibrios are facultatively anaerobic, and all 12 clinically significant species are oxidase positive and able to reduce nitrate to nitrite, except for *V. metschnikovii*. Most species are generally susceptible to the vibriostatic compound O/129 (2,4-diamino-6,7-diisopropylpteridine), exhibiting a zone of inhibition to a 150-µg Vibriostat disk (Oxoid, Cambridge, United Kingdom) on either a Mueller-Hinton or trypticase soy agar (Figure 20-2). However, this test is not as valuable with isolates from India and Bangladesh, where resistance to O/129 is common in *V. cholerae* isolates.

Most vibrios, including *V. cholerae*, also exhibit a positive string test observed as a mucoid "stringing" reaction after emulsification of colonies in 0.5% sodium desoxycholate. All species, except for *V. cholerae* and *V. mimicus*, are **halophilic** or salt-loving and require the addition of Na⁺ for growth. Vibrios can be differentiated from the similar genera *Aeromonas* and *Plesiomonas* by means of key biochemical and growth requirement characteristics, as shown in Table 20-2.

TABLE 20-1   Clinical Infections Associated with *Vibrio* Species

Species	Clinical Infection	Frequency
V. cholerae O1	Cholera, gastroenteritis, wound infections, bacteremia	Common
V. cholerae O139	Cholera	Relatively common
V. cholerae non-O1	Gastroenteritis, septicemia, ear infections	Relatively common
Vibrio parahaemolyticus	Gastroenteritis, wound infections	Common
Vibrio vulnificus	Septicemia, wound infections	Common
Vibrio alginolyticus	Wound infections, ear infections, conjunctivitis, respiratory infections, bacteremia	Common
Vibrio mimicus	Gastroenteritis, ear infections	Uncommon
*Vibrio damsela**	Wound infections	Uncommon
Vibrio fluvialis	Gastroenteritis	Uncommon
Vibrio furnissii	Gastroenteritis	Uncommon
Vibrio cincinnatiensis	Meningitis	Rare
Vibrio metschnikovii	Septicemia, peritonitis	Rare
Vibrio harveyi (*Vibrio carchariae*)	Wound infections	Rare
Grimontia (*Vibrio*) *hollisae*†	Gastroenteritis	Uncommon

Abbott SL et al: *Vibrio* and related organisms. In Murray PR et al, editors: *Manual of clinical microbiology,* ed 9,Washington, DC, 2007, ASM Press.
*Proposed as *Photobacterium damsela.*
†Reclassified as *Grimontia hollisae.*

TABLE 20-2   Salient Features for the Identification of *Vibrio, Aeromonas,* and *Plesiomonas*

	Vibrio	Aeromonas	Plesiomonas
Gram-stain reaction	–	–	–
Oxidase activity	+	+	+
Resistance to 0/129*			
10 µg	+/–	+	+/–
150 µg	–	+	–
Growth in nutrient broth with:			
0% NaCl	–/+	+	+
6.5% NaCl	+	–	–
Acid from:			
Glucose	+	+	+
Inositol	–	–	+
Mannitol	+	+/–	–
Sucrose	+/–	+/–	–
Gelatin liquefaction	+	+	–

Carnahan AM: Update on *Aeromonas* identification, *Clin Microbiol Newsl* 13:169, 1991.
+, Most strains positive; –, most strains negative; +/– or –/+, predominant reaction first.
*Vibriostatic agent (2, 4-diamino-6, 7-diisopropylpteridine).

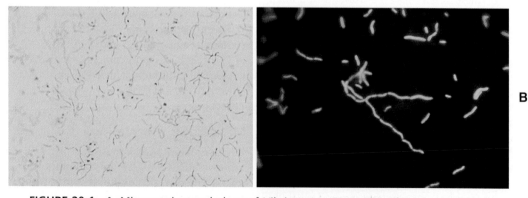

FIGURE 20-1   A, Microscopic morphology of *Vibrio* sp. on Gram-stained smear. **B,** Acridine orange stain of *Vibrio cholerae.* (**A,** Courtesy J. Michael Janda. **B,** Courtesy Rita R. Colwell.)

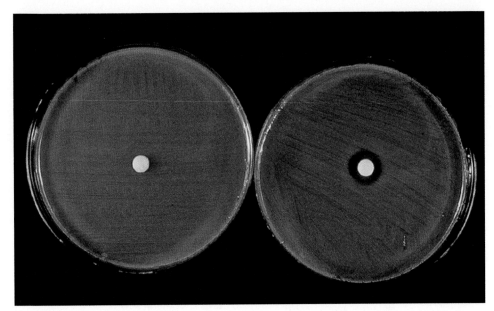

FIGURE 20-2   O/129 Susceptibility test for *Vibrio* sp. *Left,* Resistant; *right,* susceptible. (Courtesy J. Michael Janda.)

Antigenic Structure

Little is known about the antigenic structure of *Vibrio* except for *V. cholerae, V. parahaemolyticus,* and to a lesser degree *V. fluvialis* and *V. vulnificus.* The three major subgroups of *V. cholerae* are *V. cholerae* O1, *V. cholerae* O139, and *V. cholerae* non-O1, all of which share a common flagellar (H) antigen and somatic (O) antigen. Based on the composition of the O antigen, *V. cholerae* O1 organisms are divided into the following serotypes: Ogawa (A, B), Inaba (A, C), and Hikojima (A, B, C). Strains of *V. cholerae* O1 and *V. cholerae* O139 are associated with epidemic cholera. Strains that phenotypically resemble *V. cholerae* but fail to agglutinate in O1 antisera are referred to as *V. cholerae* non-O1. *V. parahaemolyticus* can also be serotyped by means of its O and K (capsule) antigens, but this generally is done only during epidemiologic studies conducted by reference laboratories.

Vibrio cholerae

Epidemiology

Vibrio cholerae O1 is the causative agent of cholera, also known as *Asiatic cholera* or *epidemic cholera.* It has been a disease of major public health significance for centuries. Most epidemics occur in developing countries, where it is endemic; in particular, cholera is prevalent in the Bengal region of India and Bangladesh. The seventh pandemic of cholera originated in Indonesia in 1961. The pandemic strain, *V. cholerae* O1, spread quickly throughout Asia and reached the African continent in 1970. Cholera returned to South America in 1991 for the first time in almost a century and has now advanced northward into South America, Central America, and even into Mexico. Cases of cholera are not commonly reported in the United States, and in most cases are considered "imported" cases.

Clinical Manifestations

Cholera is an acute diarrheal disease that is spread mainly through contaminated water. However, improperly preserved and handled foods including fish and seafood, milk, ice cream, and unpreserved meat, have been responsible for outbreaks. The disease manifests in acute cases as a severe gastroenteritis accompanied by vomiting followed by diarrhea. The stools produced by patients with cholera are described as "rice-water," and the number of stools, which are watery and contain numerous flecks of mucus, may be as many as 10 to 30 per day. If left untreated, cholera can result in a rapid fluid and electrolyte loss that leads to dehydration, hypovolemic shock, metabolic acidosis, and death in a matter of hours.

The devastating clinical scenario is the result of a powerful enterotoxin known as **cholera toxin,** or **choleragen.** Once ingested, the bacteria colonize the small intestine, where they multiply and produce choleragen. The toxin consists of two toxic A subunits and five binding B subunits. The toxin initially binds to the GM_1-ganglioside receptor on the cell membrane via the B subunits. Then the A2 subunit facilitates the entrance of the A1 subunit. Once inside the cell, the active A1 subunit stimulates the production of adenylate cyclase through inactivation of the G protein. This leads to an accumulation of cyclic adenosine monophosphate (cAMP) along the cell membrane, which stimulates hypersecretion of electrolytes (Na^+, K^+, HCO_3^-) and water out of the cell and into the lumen of the intestine, as shown in Figure 20-3. The net effect is that the gastrointestinal tract's absorptive ability is overwhelmed, resulting in the massive outpouring of watery stools.

Treatment and management of cholera are best accomplished by the administration of copious amounts of intravenous or oral fluids to replace fluids lost from the severe diarrhea. The administration of antimicrobial agents can shorten the duration of diarrhea and thereby reduce fluid

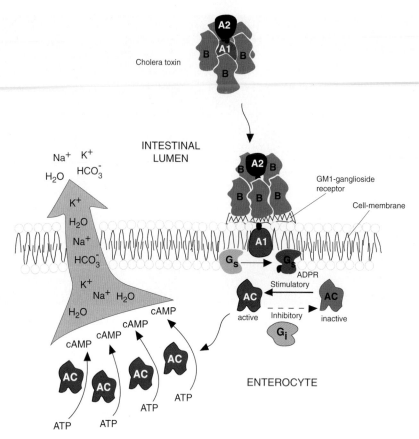

FIGURE 20-3 The action of cholera toxin. The complete toxin is shown binding to the GMI-ganglioside receptor on the cell membrane via the binding (B) subunits. The active portion (A1) of the A subunit catalyzes the adenosine diphosphate (ADP)–ribosylation of the Gs (stimulatory) regulatory protein, "locking" it in the active state. Because the G protein acts to return adenylate cyclase from its active to inactive form, the net effect is persistent activation of adenylate cyclase. The increased adenylate cyclase activity results in accumulation of cyclic adenosine 3' 5'-monophosphate (cAMP) along the cell membrane. The cAMP causes the active secretion of sodium (Na), chloride (Cl^-), potassium (K^+), bicarbonate (HCO_3^-), and water out of the cell into the intestinal lumen. (From Ryan KJ: *Vibrio* and *Campylobacter.* In Sherris J, editor: *Medical microbiology: an introduction to infectious diseases,* ed 4, New York, 2004, McGraw-Hill.)

losses. However, resistance to tetracycline and doxycycline has been reported. Therefore administration of additional antimicrobials may be necessary.

Epidemic *V. cholerae* O1 strains occur in two biogroups: classic and **El Tor.** El Tor has been the predominant biogroup in the last two pandemics. Recent studies in Bangladesh, however, indicate a rapidly occurring re-emergence of the classic biogroup. The El Tor biogroup differs from the classic in that El Tor is Voges-Proskauer positive, hemolyzes erythrocytes, is inhibited by polymyxin B (50 μg), and is able to agglutinate chicken red blood cells. The two biogroups also have different phage susceptibility patterns.

Numerous cases of *Vibrio* infections have been reported involving other serogroups, such as *V. cholerae* non-O1. Most of these strains are phenotypically similar to toxigenic *V. cholerae* O1, but most lack the cholera toxin gene and appear to cause a milder form of gastroenteritis or cholera-like disease. However, *V. cholerae* serogroup O141 appears to be associated with sporadic cholera-like diarrhea and bloodstream infections in the United States. Other non-O1 serogroup strains have been implicated in a variety of extraintestinal infections, including cholecystitis, ear infections, cellulitis, and septicemia.

The emergence of *V. cholerae* serogroup O139 has led to a widespread occurrence of cholera cases throughout India and Bangladesh. It is believed that resurgence of this strain may well be the beginning of what will heretofore be known as the "eighth pandemic" of cholera. Of interest is that some of these O139 strains share cross-reacting antigens with *Aeromonas trota,* a somewhat uncommon cause of diarrheal disease that is discussed later in this chapter.

Vibrio parahaemolyticus

Epidemiology

Vibrio parahaemolyticus is the second most common *Vibrio* species implicated in gastroenteritis. It was first recognized as a pathogen in Japan in 1950, when it was the cause of a large food-poisoning outbreak; even today it is the number-one cause of "summer diarrhea" in Japan. *V. parahaemolyticus* has also been isolated in Europe, the Baltic area, Australia, Africa, Canada, and nearly every coastal state in the United States. Most cases of *V. parahaemolyticus* reported before 1996 were associated with various serotypes; however, after 1996 a pandemic strain of *V. parahaemolyticus* serotype O3:K6 emerged and has since been implicated in numerous food-borne outbreaks in various parts of the world.

Like other vibrios, *V. parahaemolyticus* is found in aquatic environments, but it appears to be limited to coastal or estuarine areas, despite a halophilic requirement of 1% to 8% NaCl. *V. parahaemolyticus* has an association with at least 30 different marine animal species, including oysters, clams, crabs, lobsters, scallops, sardines, and shrimp. Hence most cases of gastroenteritis can be traced to recent consumption of raw, improperly cooked, or recontaminated seafood, particularly oysters.

Of note is a report of 177 cases of *V. parahaemolyticus* infection associated with consumption of raw shellfish in three different states (New York, Oregon, and Washington) between May 20 and July 31, 2006. In these outbreaks, 122 of the cases were associated with 17 specific clusters, and in two of the New York City clusters, vibriosis was associated with cooked seafood (e.g., lobster, scallops, crab, shrimp) that had been eaten in a restaurant. This suggests that the food may have been cross-contaminated by raw shellfish after cooking.

Clinical Manifestations

The gastrointestinal disease caused by *V. parahaemolyticus* is generally self-limited. Patients have watery diarrhea, moderate cramps or vomiting, and little if any fever. Symptoms begin about 24 to 48 hours after ingestion of contaminated seafood. *V. parahaemolyticus* has occasionally been isolated from extraintestinal sources such as wounds, ear and eye infections, and even in a case of pneumonia. Invariably the patient has a history of recent aquatic exposure or a water-associated traumatic injury to the infected site.

The pathogenesis of *V. parahaemolyticus* is not as well understood as *V. cholerae*. However, there is a possible association between hemolysin production and virulence, known as the **Kanagawa phenomenon.** It has been observed that most clinical *V. parahaemolyticus* strains produce a heat-stable hemolysin that is able to lyse human erythrocytes in a special high-salt mannitol medium (Wagatsuma agar). These strains are considered Kanagawa toxin positive, whereas most environmental isolates are Kanagawa toxin negative. There are exceptions to both these observations, however, and the exact role of this hemolysin in pathogenesis of the disease is still not understood. It is also important to note the recent emergence of atypical urease-positive *V. parahaemolyticus* strains from clinical sources along the Pacific coast of North America.

Vibrio vulnificus

Vibrio vulnificus can be found in marine environments on the Atlantic, Gulf, and Pacific coasts of North America. Until 1976 *V. vulnificus* was commonly referred to as the "lactose-positive" *Vibrio*. After cholera the second most serious type of *Vibrio*-associated infections are those caused by *V. vulnificus*. Infections caused by *V. vulnificus* generally fall into two categories: primary septicemia and wound infections. The former is surmised to occur through the gastrointestinal route after the consumption of shellfish, especially raw oysters. Patients with liver dysfunction and syndromes that result in increased serum levels of iron (e.g., hemochromatosis, cirrhosis, thalassemia major, hepatitis) are particularly predisposed to this scenario. Within hours, septicemia can develop, with a mortality rate of 40% to 60%. The Centers for Disease Control and Prevention recently made cases of *V. vulnificus* reportable to local and state public health departments, starting in 2007.

Patients with wound infections from *V. vulnificus* invariably have a history of some type of traumatic aquatic wound that often presents as a cellulitis, similar to that in the Case in Point. Such cases have also been documented as progressing to necrotizing fasciitis and/or multiple organ system failure. Although such infections can occur in healthy hosts, the most serious cases are in individuals who are immunocompromised and have experienced a mild to severe injury to the infected site. One such case involved a fatal episode of multiple organ dysfunction, only 7 days after a 58-year-old Canadian developed a septicemia with *V. vulnificus* after merely handling raw *Tilapia* species fish he had purchased for dinner.

Vibrio alginolyticus

Of the four major *Vibrio* spp. likely to be encountered in the clinical laboratory, *V. alginolyticus* is the least pathogenic for humans and is the one most infrequently isolated. It is a common inhabitant of marine environments and is a strict halophile, requiring at least 1% NaCl, and is able to tolerate up to 10% NaCl. Nearly all isolates originate from extraintestinal sources, such as eye and ear infections or wound and burn infections. The organism can be an occupational hazard for people in constant contact with seawater, such as fishermen or sailors.

Laboratory Diagnosis

Specimen Collection and Transport

Vibrios are not fastidious, and only a few special collection and processing procedures are necessary to ensure the recovery of vibrios from clinical material. Whenever possible, body fluids, pus, or tissues should be submitted, but swabs are acceptable if they are transported in an appropriate holding medium, such as Cary-Blair, to prevent desiccation. Buffered glycerol saline is not recommended as a transport or holding medium because the glycerol is toxic for vibrios. Even strips of blotting paper soaked in liquid stool and placed in airtight plastic bags are considered viable specimens for up to 5 weeks. Stool specimens should be collected as early as possible in the course of the illness, before the administration of any antimicrobial agents.

Culture Media

The salt concentration (0.5%) in most commonly used laboratory media, such as nutrient agar or sheep blood agar (SBA), is sufficient to support the growth of any vibrios present. On

SBA or chocolate (CHOC) agar, vibrios produce medium to large colonies that appear smooth, opaque, and iridescent with a greenish hue. The SBA plate should also be examined for the presence of α- or β-hemolysis. On MacConkey (MAC) agar, the pathogenic vibrios usually grow as nonlactose fermenters. However, lactose-fermenting species such as *V. vulnificus* may be overlooked and incorrectly considered to be members of the family Enterobacteriaceae, such as *Escherichia coli*. It therefore is imperative to determine the oxidase activity of any suspicious *Vibrio*-like colony. This can be accomplished by either directly testing colonies from SBA or CHOC agar plates with oxidase reagent or by subculturing any suspicious lactose-fermenting colonies on MAC to an SBA plate for next-day testing. This is necessary because lactose-positive colonies from selective-differential media such as MAC or cefsulodin-irgasin-novobiocin agar may give false-positive oxidase reactions.

If a selective medium is warranted, either because of the clinical history (exposure to seafood or seawater) or for geographic reasons (coastal area resident or recent foreign travel), **thiosulfate citrate bile salts sucrose (TCBS) agar** is recommended. It differentiates sucrose-fermenting (yellow) species (Figure 20-4) such as *V. cholerae, V. alginolyticus, V. fluvialis, V. furnissii, V. cincinnatiensis, V. metschnikovii,* and some *V. vulnificus* strains from the nonsucrose-fermenting (green) vibrios: *V. mimicus, V. parahaemolyticus, V. damsela,* and most *V. vulnificus* strains. About 50% of *V. harveyi* (formerly *V. carchariae*) isolates are sucrose positive. Although TCBS generally inhibits all other organisms, it should be monitored with stringent quality-control measures. There is great lot-to-lot variation in performance, and not all *Vibrio* spp. grow on TCBS, especially *Grimontia* (formerly *Vibrio*) *hollisae*. If an enrichment procedure is desired to enhance isolation of vibrios, alkaline peptone water with 1% NaCl (pH 8.5) can be inoculated (at least 20 mL) and incubated for 5 to 8 hours at 35° C before subculturing to TCBS.

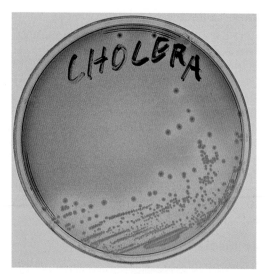

FIGURE 20-4 *Vibrio cholerae* on thiosulfate citrate bile salts sucrose agar. (Courtesy S.W. Joseph.)

Presumptive Identification

Several key tests can aid in the initial identification of a *Vibrio* isolate. Vibrios can be easily confused with other genera, including *Aeromonas, Plesiomonas,* Enterobacteriaceae, and even *Pseudomonas.* Their general susceptibility to the vibriostatic agent O/129 (150 µg) and positive "string test" distinguishes them from *Aeromonas.* Inability to ferment inositol (except for *V. cincinnatiensis* and some strains of *V. metschnikovii*) separates them from *Plesiomonas.* Their positive oxidase reaction (except for *V. metschnikovii*) separates them from the Enterobacteriaceae (excluding *Plesiomonas shigelloides*), and a fermentative metabolism separates them from the oxidative *Pseudomonas.*

Definitive Identification

Numerous useful biochemical tests aid in the definitive identification of most isolates to the species level. Table 20-3 outlines eight key differential tests to divide the 12 clinically significant *Vibrio* spp. into six groups as an initial identification step. Some of the additional tests necessary to identify eight clinical *Vibrio* spp. from Groups 1, 5, and 6 are summarized in Table 20-4. It is important to note that with the halophilic or salt-loving vibrios, it often is necessary to add at least 1% NaCl to most biochemical media to obtain reliable reaction results.

Rapid and Semiautomated Identification Systems. Although rapid and semiautomated identification systems contain databases of the more commonly encountered clinical vibrios, they generally are inadequate for accurate identification of these species, particularly the less commonly encountered species. In particular their inoculating suspensions should contain at least 0.85% NaCl, such as that found with the API-20E identification strips (bioMérieux Vitek, Hazelwood, Mo.). Even then the halophilic vibrios might grow poorly, if at all, and they often are confused with other genera, such as *Aeromonas.* Most authorities advocate identification with conventional biochemicals, supplemented with additional NaCl where warranted; alternatively the rapid-system identification should be confirmed at a reference laboratory or state public health department laboratory.

Serology. It generally is considered sufficient for most clinical laboratories below the level of reference laboratory simply to screen their presumptive *V. cholerae* isolates with commercially available polyvalent O1 antiserum. However, some non-O1 *V. cholerae* isolates misidentified as *V. cholerae* O1, and vice versa, have been reported. In any case, all isolates with a presumptive biochemical identification of *V. cholerae* should be promptly reported to the appropriate public health authorities, and the isolate should be forwarded to the health department or a reference laboratory for serotyping.

Antimicrobial Susceptibility

Both Mueller-Hinton agar and broth contain sufficient salt to support the growth of the *Vibrio* spp. most often isolated from clinical specimens. The recommended antimicrobial susceptibility testing methods are standardized disk diffusion (Kirby-Bauer) or dilution susceptibility testing methods. The Clinical and Laboratory Standards Institute (CLSI), formerly National

TABLE 20-3 Key Differential Tests for the Six Groups of 12 *Vibrio* Species That Occur in Clinical Specimens

| | Reactions of the Species in*: | | | | | | | | | | |
| | Group 1 | | Group 2 | Group 3 | Group 4 | Group 5 | | Group 6 | | | |
Test	*V. cholerae*	*V. mimicus*	*V. metschnikovii*	*V. cincinnatiensis*	*G. hollisae*	*V. damsela*	*V. fluvialis*†	*V. alginolyticus*	*V. parahaemolyticus*	*V. vulnificus*	*V. harveyi*
Growth in nutrient broth with:											
No NaCl added‡	+	+	−	−	−	−	−	−	−	−	−
1% NaCl added	+	+	+	+	+	+	+	+	+	+	+
Oxidase production	+	+	−	+	+	+	+	+	+	+	+
Nitrate reduced to nitrite	+	+	−	+	+	+	+	+	+	+	+
Myo-Inositol fermentation			V	+			−	−	−	−	−
Arginine dihydrolase					−/NG	+	+	−	−	−	−
Lysine decarboxylase					−/NG	V	−	+	+	+	+
Ornithine decarboxylase					−/NG						

Used with permission from Abbott SL et al: *Vibrio* and related organisms. In Murray PR et al: editors: *Manual of clinical microbiology,* ed 9, Washington, DC, 2007, ASM Press.
+, 90% to 100% positive; V, variable, 11% to 89% are positive; −, negative, 0% to 10% positive; NG, no growth, possibly because the NaCl concentration is too low, even when 1% NaCl is added. See Table 20-4 for the exact percentages.
*All data except those for oxidase production and nitrate reduction are for reactions that occur within 2 days at 35° to 37° C; oxidase production and nitrate reduction reactions are done only at day 1.
†Includes *V. furnissii,* which differs from *V. fluvialis* primarily by production of gas in D-glucose.
‡Species that require salt should have salt added to each biochemical tested.

TABLE 20-4 Key Differential Biochemicals to Separate Species within Groups 1, 5, and 6

| | % Positive for*: | | | | | | | |
| | Group 1 | | Group 5 | | Group 6 | | | |
Test	V. cholerae	V. mimicus	V. damsela	V. fluvialis*	V. alginolyticus	V. parahaemolyticus	V. vulnificus	V. harveyi
Voges-Proskauer (1% NaCl)	75	9	95	0	95	0	0	50
Motility	99	98	25	70-89	99	99	99	0
Acid production from:								
Sucrose	100	0	5	100	99	1	15	50
D-Mannitol	99	99	0	97	100	100	45	50
Cellobiose	8	0	0	30	3	5	99	50
Salicin	1	0	0	0	4	1	95	0

Used with permission from Abbott SL et al: *Vibrio* and related organisms. In Murray PR et al, editors: *Manual of clinical microbiology,* ed 9, Washington, DC, 2007, ASM Press.

*The numbers indicate the percentages of strains that are positive after 48 hours of incubation at 36° C (unless other conditions are indicated). Most of the positive reactions occur during the first 24 hours.

Committee for Clinical Laboratory Standards (NCCLS), has interpretive guidelines only for *V. cholerae* limited to ampicillin, tetracyclines, folate pathway inhibitors, and chloramphenicol. In general most strains of *V. cholerae* are susceptible to doxycycline or ciprofloxacin. Increased resistance from the acquisition of plasmids is relatively uncommon in the United States, but there are reports of multiple resistant strains from both Asia and Africa.

Because most vibrios grow rather rapidly and are similar to enteric bacteria in many ways, it is often useful for a first approximation to use the interpretive guidelines for the Enterobacteriaceae when testing *Vibrio* isolates other than *V. cholerae* for agents not currently covered by the most recent CLSI document. In general, fluoroquinolones alone or the synergistic combination of ciprofloxacin and cefotaxime displays excellent in vitro activity against *V. vulnificus* strains. Most vibrios are also susceptible to gentamicin, tetracyclines, chloramphenicol (except *V. damsela*), monobactams, carbapenems, and fluoroquinolones.

AEROMONAS

The genus *Aeromonas* consists of ubiquitous oxidase-positive, glucose-fermenting, gram-negative rods (Figure 20-5) that are widely distributed in freshwater, estuarine, and marine environments worldwide. They are frequently isolated from retail produce sources and animal meat products. Aeromonads are responsible for a diverse spectrum of disease syndromes among a variety of warm- and cold-blooded animals including fish, reptiles, amphibians, mammals, and humans.

Previously the genus *Aeromonas* resided in the family Vibrionaceae. However, phylogenetic evidence from molecular studies resulted in the proposal of a separate family Aeromonadaceae. With the publication of the second edition of *Bergey's Manual of Systematic Bacteriology,* this genus does indeed now reside in the family Aeromonadaceae. Currently more than 17 proposed species and eight subspecies are within the genus *Aeromonas.* However, to date only eight species, and

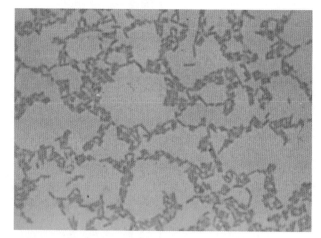

FIGURE 20-5 Gram stain of *Aeromonas.* (Courtesy J. Michael Janda.)

two biovars within *A. veronii,* have been isolated with any frequency from clinical specimens. Aeromonads have a seasonal pattern of increased isolation from May through October, reflecting their increased numbers in aquatic environments in the warmer months of the year in the United States.

General Characteristics

Aeromonads are straight rods (1.0 to 3.5 µm long by 0.3 to 1.0 µm wide), and most are motile by means of a single polar flagellum. Aeromonads are classified into one of two groups: the mesophilic group or the psychrophilic group. The mesophilic group consists of three different complexes or groups of species. One is the *A. hydrophila* complex which includes *A. hydrophila, A. bestiarum,* and certain motile strains of *A. salmonicida.* Another is the *A. veronii* complex, and this includes *A. veronii* biovar sobria (formerly misidentified as *A. sobria), A. veronii* biovar veronii, *A. jandaei, A. trota,* and *A. schubertii.* The last mesophilic complex is the *A. caviae* complex and this includes the species *A. caviae, A. media,* and *A. eucrenophila.* These organisms are considered mesophiles because they grow well at 37° C. They are all motile.

The psychrophilic group consists of only one species, *A. salmonicida,* which is a fish pathogen with several subspecies. This organism is nonmotile and is considered a psychrophile because it grows best at 22° to 25° C, and when such strains are found to be nonmotile, they are not considered human pathogens. All aeromonads, in general, can typically grow from 4° to 42° C.

Clinical Manifestations

Intestinal Infections

The aeromonads are recognized as enteric pathogens, albeit not in the same manner as the more common enteric pathogens like *Salmonella, Shigella,* or *V. cholerae.* The level and pattern of virulence is more like the multifactorial patterns of the various *E. coli* subgroups associated with enteric disease (e.g., enterotoxigenic *E. coli,* enterohemorrhagic *E. coli*). Therefore screening of stool specimens for the presence of these organisms, followed by further identification to the species level, is appropriate. This is especially true in cases of pediatric diarrhea or any type of immunocompromised individual.

The medical history of patients displaying diarrhea and harboring aeromonads often, but not always, involves aquatic exposure, such as an association with untreated groundwater or consumption of seafood, particularly raw oysters or clams. Infections have also been linked to fresh produce and dairy products. Five diarrheal presentations are observed in patients in whom an *Aeromonas* has been isolated from their stools:

1. An acute, secretory diarrhea often accompanied by vomiting
2. An acute, dysenteric form of diarrhea (similar to shigellosis) with blood and mucus
3. A chronic diarrhea usually lasting more than 10 days
4. A cholera-like disease including rice-water stools
5. The nebulous syndrome commonly referred to as "traveler's diarrhea" (similar to enterotoxigenic *E. coli*

Most cases are self-limiting, but in the pediatric, geriatric, and immunocompromised populations, supportive therapy and antimicrobials are often indicated.

A. caviae is the species most frequently associated with gastrointestinal infections, especially in neonate and pediatric populations, and has been associated with inflammatory bowel disease. Other species associated with diarrhea include *A. hydrophila* and *A. veronii* (biovars sobria and veronii). More serious complications, usually from infections with *A. hydrophila* and *A. veronii* biovar sobria, include hemolytic uremic syndrome or kidney disease that may require a kidney transplant. *A. veronii* biovar sobria has also been linked to cholera-like disease characterized by abdominal pain, fever, and nausea.

Extraintestinal Infections

Aeromonads are also responsible for extraintestinal infections; septicemia, meningitis, and wound infections are the most common. Aeromonads have also been implicated in cases of osteomyelitis, pelvic abscesses, otitis, cystitis, endocarditis, peritonitis, cholecystitis, keratitis associated with contact lens wear, and endophthalmitis in both healthy and immunocompromised individuals. Wound infection invariably involves a recent traumatic aquatic exposure such as a boating or fishing accident or even just playing mud football in Australia, and generally occurs on the extremities. The most common presentation is cellulitis, although there are a few instances of myonecrosis, necrotizing fasciitis, and even a rare case of ecthyma gangrenosum associated with sepsis.

Most aeromonad wound isolates are *A. hydrophila, A. veronii* biovar sobria, or *A. schubertii.* This last species has to date been isolated almost exclusively from aquatic wound infections and bloodstream infections. Elevated numbers of *Aeromonas* spp. were recorded in floodwater samples in New Orleans following Hurricane Katrina in 2005. Moreover, *Aeromonas* spp. were the most common cause of skin and soft tissue infections among the survivors of the 2004 tsunami in southern Thailand.

An interesting association between *A. veronii* biovar veronii and surgical wound infections involving the use of leeches for medicinal therapy following plastic surgery to relieve venous congestion has been noted. These patients can develop serious aeromonad wound infections. It appears that the leech *Hirudo medicinalis* has a symbiotic relationship with this particular aeromonad species within its gut, wherein the organisms aid in the enzymatic digestion of the blood ingested by the leech.

Aeromonad sepsis appears to be the most invasive type of *Aeromonas* infection and likewise has a strong association with the species *A. veronii* biovar sobria, *A. jandaei,* and *A. hydrophila.* Such patients are most likely to be immunocompromised and to have a history of liver disease or dysfunction, hematologic malignancies, hepatobiliary disorders, or traumatic injuries. Also at high risk are individuals with leukemia, lymphoma, or myeloma. Although the original source of infection has not been determined, it is surmised that it is the gastrointestinal tract, the biliary tract, or even more rarely the respiratory tract.

Laboratory Diagnosis

Culture Media

Aeromonads grow readily on most media used for both routine and stool cultures. After 24-hour incubation at 35° C, aeromonads appear as large round, raised, opaque colonies with an entire edge and a smooth, often mucoid surface. Frequently, an extremely strong odor is present, and pigmentation ranges from translucent and white to buff colored. Hemolysis is variable on SBA, but most major clinical species, such as *A. hydrophila, A. veronii* biovar sobria, and *A. jandaei,* display strong β-hemolysis (Figure 20-6). Oddly, the most commonly isolated species, *A. caviae,* is nearly always nonhemolytic or at best weakly α-hemolytic on SBA.

Although aeromonads grow on nearly all enteric media, they often are overlooked on MAC agar, especially in stool cultures because a number of aeromonads ferment lactose. This is of particular concern because the most commonly isolated species, especially in pediatric cases of diarrhea, is the

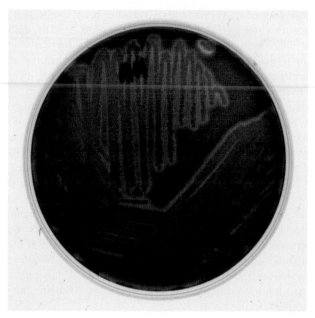

FIGURE 20-6 *Aeromonas hydrophila* exhibiting β-hemolysis on sheep blood agar. (Courtesy A.J. Horneman.)

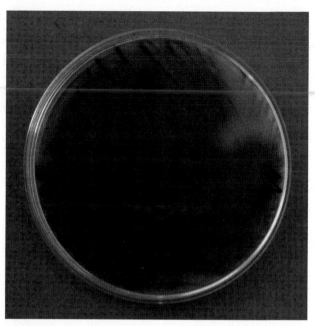

FIGURE 20-7 *Aeromonas caviae* exhibiting lactose fermentation on MAC agar. (Courtesy A.J. Horneman.)

lactose-fermenting *A. caviae*. This particular species is nearly always pink on MAC agar because of positive lactose fermentation and is therefore generally overlooked as "normal biota" *E. coli* (Figure 20-7).

The combined use of ampicillin sheep blood agar and a modified cefsulodin-irgasin-novobiocin (CIN II) plate (with only 4 μg of cefsulodin instead of 15 μg), might yield the highest recovery of aeromonads. However, the incorporation of ampicillin in the blood agar may inhibit some *A. caviae* as well as all *A. trota* strains because the hallmark feature of *A. trota* is its unusual universal susceptibility to ampicillin. Therefore SBA without ampicillin is preferred. On CIN medium (either the standard CIN formulation for enteric *Yersinia* or the modified CIN II), *Aeromonas* will form pink-centered colonies from the fermentation of mannitol, with an uneven, clear apron-resembling *Yersinia enterocolitica*. However, an oxidase test performed on SBA colonies will easily separate the oxidase-positive aeromonads from the oxidase-negative yersinias. The use of an enrichment broth generally is not considered necessary. However, if such a medium is warranted for detecting chronic cases or asymptomatic carriers, alkaline peptone water is recommended. This can be inoculated, incubated overnight at 35° C, and subsequently subcultured to appropriate plate media.

Presumptive Identification

An important screening procedure for aeromonads is to perform an oxidase test and a spot indole on suspicious colonies on SBA, especially β-hemolytic colonies. A positive oxidase distinguishes aeromonads from the family Enterobacteriaceae (except for *Plesiomonas shigelloides*), and most clinically relevant aeromonads are indole positive. The presence and type of hemolysis among multiple aeromonad-colony types in a single culture often are the only clues to an infection involving more than one species of *Aeromonas*.

Members of the genera *Aeromonas, Plesiomonas,* and *Vibrio* organisms have many similar characteristics. Table 20-2 lists key tests to help separate these three genera. The best tests to distinguish the aeromonads from *Vibrio* spp. are the string test (usually negative for aeromonads and positive for vibrios) and testing for sensitivity to O/129 (usually aeromonads and plesiomonads are resistant and most vibrios are susceptible; see Figure 20-2). An additional test to separate aeromonads and plesiomonads from most vibrios is that of determining the ability to grow in the presence of NaCl. Aeromonads and plesiomonads grow quite well in nutrient broth with 0% NaCl, but not in 6% NaCl. Conversely, most vibrios (specifically the halophilic species) cannot grow in 0% NaCl but thrive in 6% NaCl and even higher concentrations of NaCl (Figure 20-8). However, because both *V. cholerae* and *V. mimicus* are nonhalophilic and grow quite well without additional salt, any salt tolerance test must be used in conjunction with both the string test and the O/129 disk to distinguish aeromonads from this major pandemic cholera species and the less common sucrose-negative *V. mimicus*. For separation of aeromonads from plesiomonads, one can utilize the fermentation of inositol—where aeromonads are negative and plesiomonads are positive. Lastly, the ability to ferment glucose, with or without the production of gas, distinguishes *Aeromonas* from oxidase-positive nonfermenting *Pseudomonas* isolates.

Definitive Identification

Definitive identification of the aeromonads is accomplished with a small number of conventional and readily available biochemical tests and antimicrobial markers and the use of a

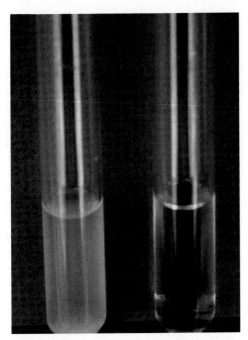

FIGURE 20-8 Both *Aeromonas* and *Plesiomonas* spp. will grow in nutrient broth with 0% NaCl *(left)*, whereas neither will grow in nutrient broth with 6% NaCl *(right)*. (Courtesy A.J. Horneman.)

simple dichotomous key, Aerokey II. When used in conjunction with the additional tests from Table 20-5, the clinical microbiologist should be able to easily identify nearly all *Aeromonas* isolates to the species level. However, it should be noted that the esculin hydrolysis test requires an agar-based medium (with or without bile), but never a standard broth or miniaturized cupule broth version. Furthermore, any antimicrobial resistance marker tests for Aerokey II, as well as all CLSI antimicrobial susceptibility studies for use in patient therapy, should always be determined by the standard Kirby-Bauer disk diffusion method. This is because of possible serious discrepancies in β-lactamase detection by rapid minimal inhibitory concentration methods that would directly impact the proper treatment of aeromonad infections.

Although a few rapid and semiautomated identification systems can identify an isolate as belonging to either the *A. caviae* complex or the *A. hydrophila* complex, most are currently inadequate for identification to the species level. This is due to a lack of sufficient discriminatory markers to detect interspecies differences and to poor correlation between conventional test results and rapid or miniaturized versions, specifically esculin hydrolysis, decarboxylase reactions, and sugar fermentation. A number of species-related disease syndromes (exist: *A. hydrophila* and *A. schubertii* from aquatic wounds, *A. veronii* biovar sobria from septicemia and meningitis, *A.*

TABLE 20-5 Differential Characteristics for Mesophilic Clinical *Aeromonas* Species

Characteristic	*Aeromonas hydrophila*	*Aeromonas veronii* biovar *sobria*	*Aeromonas veronii* biovar *veronii*	*Aeromonas caviae*	*Aeromonas schubertii*	*Aeromonas jandaei*	*Aeromonas trota*
Esculin hydrolysis	+	−	+	+	−	−	−
Voges-Proskauer	+	+	+	−	V+	−	
Pyrazinamidase activity	+	−	−	+	−	−	−
Arginine dihydrolase	+	+	−	V	+	+	+
Fermentation							
Arabinose	V	−	−	+	−	−	−
Cellobiose	−	−	+	V	−	−	+
Mannitol	+	+	+	+	−	+	+
Sucrose	+	+	+	+	−	−	−
Susceptibility							
Ampicillin	R	R	R	R	R	R	S
Carbenicillin	R	R	R	R	R	R	S
Cephalothin	R	S	S	R	S	R	R
Colistin*	V	S	S	S	S	R	S
Decarboxylase							
Lysine	+	+	+	−	+	+	+
Ornithine	−	−	+	−	−	−	−
Indole	+	+	+	V+	−	+	+
H₂S†	+	+	+	−	−	+	+
Glucose (gas)	+	+	+	−	−	+	+
Hemolysis (5% sheep RBCs)	+	+	+	V	+	+	V

Horneman AJ et al: *Aeromonas*. In Murray PR et al, editors: *Manual of clinical microbiology,* ed 9, Washington, DC, 2007, ASM Press.
+, Positive; −, negative; *V,* variable; *R,* resistant; *RBC,* red blood cells; *S,* susceptible.
*MIC single dilution 4 μg/mL.
†H₂S from gelatin-cysteine-thiosulphate media, not the conventional TSI media.

caviae from pediatric diarrhea, and *A. veronii* biovar sobria from medicinal leech therapy cases. The disease associations; coupled with differences in antimicrobial susceptibilities among the species, strongly suggest that conventional identification to the species level and antimicrobial susceptibilities using the Kirby-Bauer method should be performed on all clinical aeromonad isolates, if at all possible.

Antimicrobial Susceptibility

Although most cases of *Aeromonas*-associated gastroenteritis are self-limited, antimicrobial therapy is often indicated. It is always warranted in wound infections and septicemia. As a genus, aeromonads are nearly uniformly resistant to penicillin, ampicillin, and carbenicillin, except for the susceptibility of all *A. trota* isolates and a moderate number of *A. caviae* isolates to ampicillin. Aeromonads are variable with regards to ticarcillin or piperacillin as well as the cephalosporins. Thus far, *A. veronii* biovar veronii isolates still appear to be susceptible to cephalothin, but only *A. veronii* biovar veronii is 100% susceptible to cefoxitin. Otherwise aeromonads are generally susceptible to trimethoprim-sulfamethoxazole, aminoglycosides, and quinolones. However, there have been reports of a case of sepsis with an extended-spectrum β-lactamase (ESBL)–producing *A. hydrophila* and a case of necrotizing fasciitis with the probable in vivo transfer of a TEM-24 plasmid-borne ESBL gene from *Enterobacter aerogenes.*

PLESIOMONAS

Because of phenotypic characteristics, the genus *Plesiomonas* was formerly in the family Vibrionaceae. Like the vibrios and aeromonads, these organisms are oxidase-positive, glucose-fermenting, facultatively anaerobic, gram-negative bacilli that are motile by polar flagella. However, recent phylogenetic studies have presented evidence that *Plesiomonas* is actually closely related to members of the family Enterobacteriaceae. In the second edition of *Bergey's Manual of Systematic Bacteriology,* *Plesiomonas* has been moved to the family Enterobacteriaceae and is the only oxidase-positive member. *P. shigelloides* is still the only species in this genus.

Epidemiology

Plesiomonas shigelloides is found in both soil and aquatic environments, but because of intolerance to increased NaCl and a minimum growth temperature of 8° C, they are generally found only in the fresh and estuarine waters of tropical and subtropical climates. Like the genus *Aeromonas,* they are widely distributed among both warm- and cold-blooded animals, including dogs, cats, pigs, vultures, snakes, lizards, fish, newts, and shellfish. They have emerged as a potential cause of enteric disease in humans and have also been isolated from a number of extraintestinal infections. Cases are probably underreported because of the similarity to *E. coli* on most ordinary enteric media. However, increased laboratory awareness of the existence of *Plesiomonas,* coupled with the knowledge of previously outlined recreational, immunologic, and gastronomic risk factors, has resulted in a gradual but steady increase in the number of reported cases, mostly in adults.

Clinical Manifestations

Gastroenteritis

Unlike the genus *Aeromonas,* at least three well-documented outbreaks of diarrheal disease caused by *Plesiomonas* have occurred: two in Japan and one in Cameroon. The most common vehicle of transmission is the ingestion of contaminated water or food, particularly uncooked or undercooked seafood such as oysters, clams or shrimp. However, only a few possible virulence features have been defined to explain this organism's association with enteric disease. At least three major clinical types of gastroenteritis are caused by *Plesiomonas:*

- The more common watery or secretory diarrhea
- A subacute or chronic disease that lasts between 14 days and 2 to 3 months
- A more invasive, dysenteric form that resembles colitis

On average, 25% to 40% of all patients present with fever or vomiting or both, and the single most common clinical symptom for all such patients is abdominal pain. Most cases are self-limiting, but antimicrobial therapy is indicated in severe and prolonged cases.

Reports of *P. shigelloides* infection in patients with human immunodeficiency virus infections are increasing, as are associations with inflammatory bowel disease.

Extraintestinal Infection

Because of the organism's wide dissemination among animal populations and aquatic environments, it is apparent that occupational exposure can be a source of infections for veterinarians, zookeepers, aquaculturists, fish handlers, and athletes participating in water-related sports. More serious infections, such as bacteremia and meningitis, usually occur only in severely immunocompromised patients or neonates. Recent reports include cases of continuous ambulatory peritoneal dialysis-associated peritonitis. Furthermore, biliary tract disease has been identified as a possible risk factor for bacteremia with this organism.

General Characteristics

Plesiomonads are straight (0.8 to 1 μm by 3 μm), gram-negative bacilli that occur singly, in pairs, or in short chains or filamentous forms. They do not form spores or capsules and are motile by monotrichous or two to five lophotrichous flagella.

The genera *Plesiomonas* and *Shigella* share both biochemical and antigenic features, and plesiomonads often cross-agglutinate with *Shigella sonnei, S. dysenteriae,* and even *S. boydii*—hence the species name *shigelloides.* However, unlike *Shigella,* the organism *P. shigelloides* appears to possess a much lower virulence potential, with a low symptomatic carriage rate among humans, and is oxidase-positive. *Plesiomonas* can be serotyped by somatic O antigens (50 groups) and their flagellar H antigens (17 groups). Some of the 107 serovars are ubiquitous, and others are confined to certain regions only.

Laboratory Diagnosis

Culture Media

Plesiomonas spp. grow readily on most media routinely used in the clinical laboratory. After 18 to 24 hours incubation at 35° C, shiny, opaque, nonhemolytic colonies appear, with a slightly raised center and a smooth and entire edge. Because most strains ferment lactose, albeit as a "delayed" positive reaction, the easiest screening procedure is an oxidase test performed on colonies from nonselective media, such as SBA or CHOC agar. Although a specialized medium is not recommended for the detection of plesiomonads from stool specimens, and because certain strains are inhibited on eosin-methylene blue or MAC agars, the use of inositol brilliant green bile salts agar can enhance the isolation of plesiomonads. *Plesiomonas* colonies are white to pink on this medium, and most coliform colonies are either green or pink. *Plesiomonas* will not grow on TCBS agar but will grow quite well on CIN, a selective agar for *Yersinia* spp., as opaque (non-mannitol fermenting) colonies with an opaque apron. However, they must be distinguished from other oxidase-positive organisms, such as *Aeromonas* and *Pseudomonas,* that will also grow on CIN. Because plesiomonads are often susceptible to ampicillin, any agar used as a possible means of detecting plesiomonads in clinical samples should not contain this antibiotic.

Identification

Plesiomonas shigelloides can be presumptively differentiated from similar genera with several key tests (see Table 20-2). The positive oxidase activity separates it from the Enterobacteriaceae, sensitivity to the vibriostatic agent O/129 separates it from *Aeromonas,* and its ability to ferment inositol separates it from all *Aeromonas* and nearly all *Vibrio* spp. It can also be separated from the halophilic *Vibrio* spp. by its ability to grow in nutrient broth with 0% NaCl coupled with its inability to grow in nutrient broth with 6% NaCl (see Figure 20-8).

Most rapid identification systems include *P. shigelloides* in their databases and appear to be able to identify it with a fairly high degree of accuracy. This is in large part because of its unique "positive trio" profile of positive ornithine and lysine decarboxylases and arginine dihydrolase reactions, combined with the fermentation of inositol. Because of its association with the ingestion of raw or undercooked seafood, particularly clams and oysters, a quantitative polymerase chain reaction assay for *P. shigelloides* in foodstuff has been developed.

Antimicrobial Susceptibility

Although most cases of plesiomonad gastroenteritis are self-limiting, antimicrobial therapy is indicated in patients with severe or chronic gastroenteritis. Likewise, extraintestinal infections, particularly among neonates, often require antimicrobial therapy. Studies have shown a general resistance to the penicillin class of antibiotics, but penicillins combined with a β-lactamase inhibitor, as well as trimethoprim-sulfamethoxazole, are active. There are reports of resistance to more than one aminoglycoside (e.g., gentamicin, tobramycin, amikacin), but the quinolones, cephalosporins, and carbapenems appear to be an effective therapy.

CAMPYLOBACTER AND CAMPYLOBACTER-LIKE SPECIES

Campylobacter and *Campylobacter*-like species, which include *Helicobacter* and *Wolinella,* have recently undergone changes in taxonomy. Campylobacters were formerly classified with the vibrios because of their positive oxidase and characteristic microscopic morphology, but DNA homology studies have shown that *Campylobacter* spp. do not belong with the vibrios. In addition, unlike the vibrios, which are fermentative, most campylobacters are asacchrolytic.

Based on ribosomal RNA (rRNA) sequence studies, *Wolinella recta* and *Wolinella curva* have been found to be similar to the campylobacters. Therefore these two species have been transferred to the genus *Campylobacter* as *C. rectus* and *C. curvus.* Although they may appear to be strict anaerobes, they have been grown in a **microaerophilic** environment. Microaerophilic organisms require oxygen, but at a concentration less than that of room air; 5% is normally optimal. As a result of rRNA studies, a new genus, *Arcobacter,* and a new family, Campylobacteraceae, were proposed. Many of the current members comprising the family Campylobacteraceae and other *Campylobacter*-like organisms are listed in Box 20-1.

BOX 20-1   Members of the Family Campylobacteraceae and Other *Campylobacter*-Like Organisms

Campylobacter jejuni subsp. *jejuni*
Campylobacter jejuni subsp. *doylei*
Campylobacter coli
Campylobacter lari
Campylobacter fetus subsp. *fetus*
Campylobacter fetus subsp. *venerealis*
Campylobacter hyointestinalis
Campylobacter sputorum biovar sputorum
Campylobacter sputorum biovar paraureolyticus
Campylobacter sputorum biovar faecalis
Campylobacter upsaliensis
Campylobacter mucosalis
Campylobacter concisus
Campylobacter curvus
Campylobacter rectus
Campylobacter gracilis
Arcobacter cryaerophilus
Arcobacter nitrofigilis
Arcobacter butzleri
Arcobacter skirrowii
Helicobacter pylori
Helicobacter mustelae
Helicobacter felis
Helicobacter muridarum
Helicobacter fennelliae
Helicobacter cinaedi
Helicobacter canadensis

This box also includes *Campylobacter* spp. that are rarely isolated from human specimens.

Epidemiology

Campylobacter spp. have been known to cause abortion in domestic animals, such as cattle, sheep, and swine. Although these organisms were suspected of causing human infections earlier, campylobacters were not established as human pathogens until sensitive isolation procedures and media were developed. Today the most common cause of bacterial gastroenteritis worldwide is *Campylobacter jejuni*. The transmission of campylobacterioses has been attributed to direct contact by exposure to animals and handling infected pets, such as dogs, cats, and birds, and indirectly by the consumption of contaminated water and dairy products and improperly cooked poultry. Person to person transmission has been reported, and some *Campylobacter* spp. are also sexually transmitted.

Although the first reported cases of *Campylobacter* gastroenteritis in humans involved primarily children, later investigations showed that the diarrheal disease also occurs in adults. The population that most often manifests the disease includes children younger than 1 year of age and adults between 20 and 40 years of age. Besides *C. jejuni*, other *Campylobacter* spp. that cause gastrointestinal disease (enteric campylobacters) are *C. coli* and *C. lari*.

Campylobacter fetus subsp. *fetus* has been isolated most frequently from blood cultures and is rarely associated with gastrointestinal illness. Most infections occur in immunocompromised and elderly patients. Table 20-6 summarizes the clinical significance of *Campylobacter*, *Arcobacter*, and *Helicobacter* organisms. *Helicobacter pylori* has been strongly associated with gastric, peptic, and duodenal ulcers as well as with gastrointestinal carcinoma. *H. pylori* has been identified in as many as 80% of gastric ulcer patients. Although the organisms were previously found in human gastric tissue, it was difficult to assess their significance because the samples were taken at autopsy. It is estimated that half of the population worldwide is infected with *H. pylori*. In developing countries in Africa, Asia, and South America, the incidence is reported to be as high as 80% to 90%. This greater incidence is attributed to poor sanitary conditions, and it appears that infection occurs early in life. Some data suggest human-to-human transmission and the possibility of human reservoirs. Although it is not conclusively proven, fresh groundwater is the likely source of many infections.

Clinical Manifestations

Campylobacter

Several *Campylobacter* spp. have been implicated in human infection: *C. fetus, C. jejuni, C. coli, C. sputorum, C. concisus, C. curvus,* and *C. rectus. C. fetus* contains two subspecies: *C. fetus* subsp. *fetus* and *C. fetus* subsp. *venerealis*. Patients infected with *C. jejuni* present with a diarrheal disease that begins with mild abdominal pain within 2 to 10 days after ingestion of the organisms. Cramps and bloody diarrhea often follow the initial signs. Patients may experience fever and chills and, rarely, nausea and vomiting. In most patients,

TABLE 20-6 *Campylobacter* Species and Campylobacter-Like Organisms and Their Clinical Significance

Campylobacter Species	Clinical Significance
Arcobacter butzleri	Associated with diarrheal disease and bacteremia in humans and in children with recurring gastrointestinal illness (abdominal cramps)
Arcobacter cryaerophilus	Isolated from cases of human bacteremia and diarrhea
Arcobacter nitrofigilis	
Campylobacter fetus subsp. *venerealis*	Rarely involved in human infections
Campylobacter sputorum biovar faecalis	
Campylobacter concisus	Involved in periodontal disease; has also been recovered from individuals with gastrointestinal illness
Campylobacter fetus subsp. *fetus*	Bacteremia in immunocompromised patients
Campylobacter hyointestinalis	Enteric disease in swine; occasionally associated in human enteric illness
Campylobacter jejuni	Most common cause of bacterial diarrhea worldwide
Campylobacter lari	Enteritis very similar to that caused by *Campylobacter jejuni*
Campylobacter mucosalis	
Campylobacter sputorum biovar bubulus	
Campylobacter rectus	Associated with periodontal disease; has been recovered from patients with root canal infections and Crohn disease
Campylobacter upsaliensis	Potential pathogen in humans, causing gastrointestinal illness and bacteremia in both immunocompetent and immunocompromised patients
Helicobacter canadensis	Isolated in stool specimens from patients with diarrhea, pathogenesis unknown
Helicobacter cinaedi	Recovered from blood of homosexual males with or without AIDS and from blood and feces of children and adult females
Helicobacter felis	
Helicobacter fennelliae	Recovered from rectal swabs and blood of homosexual men with or without AIDS presenting with proctitis, proctocolitis, and enteritis
Helicobacter muridarum	
Helicobacter mustelae	
Helicobacter pylori	Common cause of duodenal ulcers and type B gastritis; possibly a risk factor in gastric carcinoma

AIDs, Acquired immunodeficiency syndrome.

the illness is self-limited and usually resolves in 2 to 6 days. Untreated patients can remain carriers for several months. Other enteric *Campylobacter* infections (i.e., those caused by *C. coli* and *C. lari*) have similar clinical manifestations.

Strong evidence suggests that *Campylobacter* infection plays a role in Guillain-Barré syndrome, an autoimmune disorder characterized by acute paralysis due to damage to the peripheral nervous system. Many patients with GBS test positive for antibodies to *Campylobacter.* It is believed that antibodies produced during a *Campylobacter* infection bind to gangliosides found on peripheral nerves. Cross-reactivity with these nerve cells in an autoimmune response may be responsible for this debilitating nerve disorder.

Helicobacter pylori

Helicobacter pylori has been primarily linked to gastric infections. Once acquired, *H. pylori* colonizes the stomach for a long time and can cause a low-grade inflammatory process, producing a chronic superficial gastritis. Although it does not invade the gastric epithelium, the infection is recognized by the host immune system, which initiates an antibody response. The antibodies produced are not protective, however.

H. pylori is also recognized as a major cause of **type B gastritis,** a chronic condition formerly associated primarily with stress and chemical irritants. In addition, based on recent data, the strong association between long-term *H. pylori* infection and gastric cancer has raised more questions regarding the clinical significance of this organism. There is speculation that long-term *H. pylori* infection resulting in chronic gastritis is an important risk factor for gastric carcinoma. Other species of helicobacters, including *H. cinaedi* and *H. fennelliae,* have been associated with human gastroenteritis, generally in immunocompromised patients. More recently gastroenteritis has also been linked to *H. canadensis, H. canis, H. pullorum,* and *H. winghamensis.* In addition, *H. cinaedi* has been isolated from blood of patients with bacteremia and patients with human immunodeficiency virus infection.

Laboratory Diagnosis

Specimen Collection and Transport

Campylobacter fetus subsp. *fetus* can be recovered in several routine blood culture media. *Campylobacter* spp. that cause enteric illness are isolated from stool samples and rectal swabs, the less-preferred specimen. If a delay in processing the stool specimen is anticipated, it can be placed in a transport medium such as Cary-Blair to maintain the viability of the organisms. A common stool transport medium, buffered glycerol-saline, is toxic to enteric campylobacters and should therefore be avoided.

H. pylori can be recovered from gastric biopsy materials. Samples must be transported quickly to the laboratory. Stuart medium can be used to maintain the viability of the organisms if a delay in processing is anticipated. Tissue samples may also be placed in cysteine-Brucella broth with 20% glycerol and frozen at −70° C.

Culture Media

An enriched selective agar, CAMPY-BAP (blood agar plate), is a commonly used medium to isolate *C. jejuni* and other enteric campylobacters. This commercially available medium contains Brucella agar base, 10% sheep red blood cells, and a combination of antimicrobials: vancomycin, trimethoprim, polymyxin B, amphotericin B, and cephalothin. Other selective media that have been successful in recovering *Campylobacter* spp. are Butzler medium and Skirrow's medium.

TABLE 20-7   Selective Media for the Cultivation of *Campylobacter* Species

Medium	Base	Antimicrobial Agent
CAMPY blood agar plate	Brucella agar 10% sheep red blood cells	Vancomycin Trimethoprim Polymyxin B Amphotericin B Cephalothin
Skirrow's	Oxoid blood agar base Lysed, defibrinated horse red blood cells	Vancomycin Trimethoprim Polymyxin B
Butzler	Thioglycolate fluid with agar added 10% sheep red blood cells	Bacitracin Novobiocin Actidione Colistin Cefazolin
CCDA	Nutrient agar Charcoal Sodium deoxycholate	Cefoperazone Amphotericin B

CCDA, Charcoal cefoperazone deoxycholate agar (Oxiod, Inc., Cambridge, United Kingdom.).

Table 20-7 shows the composition of each of these selective media.

Medium V, a modification of the original Butzler medium, contains cefoperazone, rifampin, colistin, and amphotericin B; it seems to inhibit normal colon microbiota better than the original formulation. CAMPY-CVA (cefoperazone-vancomycin-amphotericin B) medium has been reported to provide better suppression of fecal biota, even when this medium is incubated at 37° C. Incubation at 37° C allows the recovery of *Campylobacter* spp. that are inhibited at 42° C. *C. fetus* subsp. *fetus, C. rectus,* and *C. curvus* can be isolated using routine culture media. Charcoal-based blood-free media, such as charcoal cefoperazone deoxycholate agar, are also available. To recover *H. pylori,* a combination of a nonselective medium, such as CHOC agar or Brucella agar with 5% horse red blood cells, and a selective medium, such as Skirrow's agar, may be used. It is important that the inoculated medium be fresh and moist and that the culture be incubated in a microaerophilic environment with increased humidity.

Incubation

There is a double purpose for incubating stool cultures at 42° C to recover *C. jejuni.* First, *C. jejuni* and other enteric campylobacters grow optimally at 42° C. Second, growth of normal colon organisms is inhibited at this higher temperature. *C. fetus* subsp. *fetus,* on the other hand, is a rare stool isolate, and growth is suppressed at 42° C; therefore to isolate this organism, media should be incubated at 37° C.

Enteric *Campylobacter* and *Helicobacter* species require a microaerophilic and capnophilic environment. The ideal atmospheric environment for these organisms contains a gas mixture of 5% O_2, 10% CO_2, and 85% N_2 for *Campylobacter* spp. and 5% to 10% O_2 and 5% to 12% CO_2 for *Helicobacter* spp. Except for *C. rectus* and *C. curvus,* a strict anaerobic environment does not support the growth of most *Campylo-*

bacter spp. Several methods can be used to obtain the required environment for campylobacters. With the GasPak EZ Gas Generating Container System (BD Diagnostic Systems, Sparks, Md.), specimen plates along with a sachet are placed into a clear plastic incubation container, sealed, and incubated at the appropriate temperature. The sachet is activated upon exposure to air once the foil pouch is removed. The number of sachets needed per container depends on the container used. The GasPak EZ Gas Generating Pouch Systems (BD Diagnostic Systems) can hold up to four plates but requires at least two plates per resealable pouch. One sachet is added to each pouch and is activated upon exposure to air similar to the procedure above. For optimal results, a paper towel or moistened cotton ball with 5 ml of water should be placed inside the pouch. The pouch is sealed by closing the zipper part of the pouch and then incubated at the appropriate temperature.

An evacuation replacement system similar to that used to obtain a strict anaerobic condition may also be used. The anaerobic jar is evacuated to a pressure of 15 inches Hg at least twice and refilled each time with one of the following gas mixtures: 10% CO_2, 90% N_2; 5% CO_2, 10% H_2, 85% N_2; or 10% CO_2, 10% H_2, 80% N_2. A candle jar may be used if none of the aforementioned systems can be obtained. However, this method provides the least ideal environmental condition. The incubation time should be extended to 72 hours to isolate more efficiently enteric *Campylobacter* spp. This procedure allows facultative organisms present on the medium to reduce the O_2 tension created by the candle to a more suitable concentration for campylobacters.

Presumptive Identification

Microscopic Morphology. *Campylobacter* spp. are curved, non–spore-forming, gram-negative rods that measure approximately 0.2 to 0.9 μm × 0.5 to 5.0 μm (Figure 20-9). Enteric campylobacters may appear as long spirals, S shapes, or seagull-wing shapes. These organisms may appear as coccobacilli in smears prepared from older cultures. On Gram-

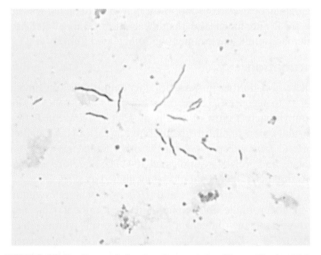

FIGURE 20-9 *Campylobacter* Gram stain. (From Marler LM et al: *Bacteriology Atlas CD-ROM,* Indiana Pathology Images, 2005.)

stained smears, these organisms stain poorly. For better visualization, carbolfuchsin is recommended as a counterstain; if safranin is used, counterstaining should be extended to 2 to 3 minutes. They exhibit a characteristic **"darting" motility** on hanging drop preparations or when visualized under phase-contrast microscopy.

Arcobacter spp. have a microscopic morphology similar to that of *Campylobacter* spp. *H. pylori* also appears similar to campylobacters, but one ultra structural study has shown that *Helicobacter* has multiple flagella at one pole, unlike the single polar flagellum of campylobacters.

Colony Morphology. The typical colony morphology of *C. jejuni* and other enteric campylobacters is moist, "runny looking," and spreading. Colonies are usually nonhemolytic; some are round and raised and others may be flat. *C. fetus* subsp. *fetus* produces smooth, convex, translucent colonies. A tan or slightly pink coloration is observed in some enteric campylobacter colonies. Other *Campylobacter* species produce colonies similar to those of *C. jejuni*. Although most do not produce pigment, *C. mucosalis* and *C. hyointestinalis* can produce a dirty yellow pigment.

Definitive Identification

Isolates from stool specimens and rectal swabs can be presumptively identified as *Campylobacter* spp. by being oxidase positive, observing the characteristic Gram-stained microscopic morphology, and the characteristic motility. The microscopic morphology is very important because it differentiates *Campylobacter* from other bacterial species (i.e., *Aeromonas, Pseudomonas* that are oxidase positive and can grow at 42° C in a microaerophilic environment. To observe the typical motility, organisms should be suspended in *Brucella* or tryptic soy broth. Distilled water and saline seem to inhibit motility. A positive hippurate hydrolysis is an important characteristic for the identification of *C. jejuni*. Table 20-8 lists the biochemical tests most useful in definitively identifying the most commonly encountered *Campylobacter, Helicobacter,* and *Arcobacter* species.

Helicobacter infections usually are identified by nonculture methods. *H. pylori* may be presumptively identified in a gastric biopsy specimen by testing for the presence of a rapid urease reaction (Figure 20-10). The collected tissue sample is placed onto Christensen's urea medium and incubated at 37° C for 2 hours. A rapid color change suggests the presence of *H. pylori*. Other rapid tests commercially available include the CLOtest Rapid Urease Test (Kimberly-Clark/Ballard Medical Products, Neenah, Wis.), Hp Fast Rapid Urea Test (GI Supply, Camp Hill, Pa.), and a paper strip test by PyloriTek (BARD, Murray Hill, N.J.).

Urease activity can also be detected by the **urea breath test,** which is reportedly both sensitive and specific and is recommended for monitoring therapy. In this test the patient is given [13]C- or ^{14}C-labeled urea orally. Urea degraded by the urease activity of *H. pylori* releases [13]CO_2 or [14]CO_2, which is absorbed into the bloodstream and detected in the exhaled breath by a scintillation counter. *H. pylori* infection can also be diagnosed by fecal antigen detection, microscopic examination of stained gastric tissue, and DNA amplification tests (i.e., polymerase chain reaction).

TABLE 20-8 Biochemical Tests to Differentiate *Campylobacter*, *Arcobacter*, and *Helicobacter* Species

Species	Catalase	Nitrate Reduction	Urease	H₂S Production (TSI)	Hippurate Hydrolysis	Indoxyl Acetate Hydrolysis	Growth at 15° C	25° C	42° C	Susceptibility to Nalidixic Acid (30 mcg)	Cephalothin (30 mcg)
Campylobacter jejuni subsp. *jejuni*	+	+	–	–	+	+	–	–	+	+	–
Campylobacter jejuni subsp. *doylei*	V	–	–	–	V	+	–	–	–	+	+
Campylobacter coli	+	+	–	V	–	+	–	–	+	+	–
Campylobacter lari	+	+	–	–	–	–	–	–	+	–	–
Campylobacter fetus subsp. *fetus*	+	+	–	–	–	–	–	+	–	–	+
Campylobacter hyointestinalis	+	+	–	+	–	–	–	+	+	–	+
Campylobacter upsaliensis	–	+	–	–	–	+	–	–	+	+	+
Campylobacter concisus	–	+	–	V	–	–	–	–	+	–	–
Campylobacter curvus	–	+	–	V	V	V	–	–	+	+	ND
Campylobacter rectus	V	+	–	–	V	V	–	–	W	+	ND
Arcobacter butzleri	–W	+	–	–	–	+	+	+	V	V	–
Helicobacter pylori	+	V	+	–	–	–	–	–	V	–	+
Helicobacter fennelliae	+	–	–	–	–	+	–	–	–	+	+
Helicobacter cinaedi	+	+	–	–	–	V	–	–	–	+	+

From Fitzgerald C, Nachamkin I: *Campylobacter* and *Arcobacter* and from Fox JG, Megraud F: *Helicobacter.* In Murray PR et al, editors: *Manual of clinical microbiology,* ed 9, Washington, DC, 2007, ASM Press.
TSI, Triple sugar iron agar slant; +, positive result; –, negative result; *W,* weak; *V,* variable result; *ND,* not determined; –*W,* mostly negative, some weak.

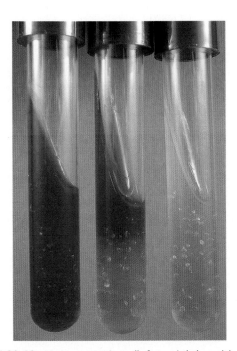

FIGURE 20-10 Urease reactions (left to right) positive, weak positive, and negative. (From Marler et al: *Bacteriology Atlas CD-ROM,* Indiana Pathology Images, 2005.)

Immunologic Assays

Latex agglutination tests are available for rapid identification of colonies of enteric campylobacters on primary isolation media. Two commercial kits are available in the United States for culture identification: INDX-Campy (JCL) (Hardy Diagnostics, Santa Maria, Calif. and Fisher Scientific, Hampton, N.H.) and Dry Spot campylobacter test kit (Remel, Lenexa, Kan). The kits can detect the presence of *C. jejuni*, *C. coli*, *C. upsaliensis*, *C. lari*, and sometimes *C. fetus* subsp. *fetus*. However, neither system differentiates among the *Campylobacter* spp. Commercial kits are also available for detecting *Campylobacter* antigen in fecal samples.

Specific antibodies in serum can be detected by enzyme-linked immunosorbent assay or by indirect immunofluorescent assay methods. These methods have been reported to be reasonably sensitive and specific indicators of *Campylobacter* and *H. pylori* infections. Serologic testing is useful for epidemiologic studies for *Campylobacter* but is not recommended for routine diagnosis. Serologic testing is an important screening method for diagnosis of *H. pylori* infection.

Antimicrobial Susceptibility

Antimicrobial susceptibility testing for *Campylobacter* spp. is not routinely performed in the clinical microbiology laboratory and is not standardized. The drug of choice for treating intestinal campylobacteriosis is erythromycin, although most patients recover without antimicrobial intervention. Ciprofloxacin as well as other quinolones can also be used. Gentamicin is used to treat systemic infections. Tetracycline, erythromycin, and chloramphenicol can be substituted for gentamicin.

The standard therapy for treating *H. pylori* infections consists of a macrolide, amoxicillin, and a proton pump inhibitor. An alternative regimen consisting of metronidazole, tetracycline, and bismuth salt can also be used. Treatment for *H. pylori* infections should be administered for 7 to 14 days to eradicate the infection.

BIBLIOGRAPHY

Abbott SL et al: *Klebsiella, Enterobacter, Citrobacter, Serratia, Plesiomonas,* and other Enterobacteriaceae. In Murray PR et al, editors: *Manual of clinical microbiology*, ed 9, Washington, DC, 2007, ASM Press.

Abbott SL et al: *Vibrio* and related organisms. In Murray PR et al, editors: *Manual of clinical microbiology*, ed 9, Washington, DC, 2007, ASM Press.

Abbott SL, Cheung WK, Janda JM: The genus *Aeromonas*: biochemical characteristics, atypical reactions, and phenotypic identification schemes, *J Clin Microbiol* 41:2348, 2003.

Centers for Disease Control and Prevention: *Vibrio parahaemolyticus* infections associated with consumption of raw shellfish—three states, 2006, *MMWR* 55:854, 2006. Available at: www.cdc.gov/mmwr/preview/mmwrhtml/mm5531a5.htm. Accessed October 21, 2008.

Clinical and Laboratory Standards Institute: *Performance standards for antimicrobial susceptibility testing, 18th Informational Supplement, CLSI document M100-S18*, Wayne, Pa, 2008, Clinical and Laboratory Standards Institute.

Crump JA et al: Toxigenic *Vibrio cholerae* serogroup O141-associated cholera-like diarrhea and bloodstream infection in the United States, *J Infect Dis* 187:866, 2003.

Dechet AM et al: Nonfoodborne *Vibrio* infections: an important cause of morbidity and mortality in the United States, 1997-2006, *Clin Infect Dis* 46:970, 2008.

Faruque SM et al: Reemergence of epidemic *Vibrio cholerae* O139, Bangladesh, *Emerg Infect Dis* 9:1116, 2003.

Fitzgerald C, Nachamkin I: *Campylobacter* and *Arcobacter*. In Murray PR et al, editors: *Manual of clinical microbiology*, ed 9, Washington, DC, 2007, ASM Press.

Fox JG, Megraud F: *Helicobacter*. In Murray PR et al, editors: *Manual of clinical microbiology*, ed 9, Washington, DC, 2007, ASM Press.

Gilbert DN et al: *The Sanford guide to antimicrobial therapy 2009*, Hyde Park, Vt, 2009, Antimicrobial Therapy, Inc.

Gu W, Levin RE: Quantitative detection of *Plesiomonas shigelloides* in clam and oyster tissue by PCR, *Int J Food Microbiol* 111:81, 2006.

Hiransuthikul N et al: Skin and soft-tissue infections among tsunami survivors in southern Thailand, *Clin Infect Dis* 41:e93, 2005.

Horneman AJ et al: *Aeromonas*. In Murray PR et al, editors: *Manual of clinical microbiology*, ed 9, Washington, DC, 2007, ASM Press.

Horneman AJ, Morris JG: *Aeromonas* infections. In *UpToDate, CD-ROM* for infectious diseases, version 16.2, Waltham, Mass, 2008.

Horneman AJ, Morris JG: *Plesiomonas shigelloides* infections. In *UpToDate, CD-ROM* for infectious diseases, version 16.2, Waltham, Mass, 2008.

Janda JM: Genus *Plesiomonas*. In Brenner DJ et al, volume editors: *Bergey's manual of systematic bacteriology: the proteobacteria*, vol 2, ed 2, New York, 2005, Springer, p 740.

Kim DM et al: In vitro efficacy of the combination of ciprofloxacin and cefotaxime against *Vibrio vulnificus, Antimicrob Agents Chemother* 49:3489, 2005.

Lee CH et al: Necrotizing fasciitis caused by *Vibrio vulnificus* in a man with cirrhosis, *Lancet Infect Dis* 8:399, 2008.

Martin-Carnahan AJ, Joseph SW: Genus *Aeromonas stanier* 1943, 213[AL]. In Brenner DJ et al, volume editors: *Bergey's manual of systematic bacteriology: the proteobacteria*, vol 2, ed 2, New York, 2005, Springer.

Morris JG: Infections due to "non-cholera" vibrios. In *UpToDate CD-ROM* for infectious diseases, version 16.2, Waltham, Mass, 2008.

On SLW et al: Genus *Helicobacter*. In Brenner DJ et al, volume editors: *Bergey's manual of systematic bacteriology*, vol 2, ed 2, New York, 2005, Springer.

Ouderkirk JP et al: *Aeromonas* meningitis complicating medicinal leech therapy, *Clin Infect Dis* 38:e36, 2004.

Pinna A et al: *Aeromonas caviae* keratitis associated with contact lens wear, *Ophthalmology* 111:348, 2004.

Presley SM et al: Assessment of pathogens and toxicants in New Orleans, LA following Hurricane Katrina, *Environ Sci Technol* 40:468, 2006.

Vally H et al: Outbreak of *Aeromonas hydrophila* wound infections associated with mud football, *Clin Infect Dis* 38:1084, 2004.

van der Gaag EJ, Roelofsen E, Tummers RF: *Aeromonas caviae* infection mimicking inflammatory bowel disease in a child, *Ned Tijdschr Geneeskd* 149:712, 2005.

Vandamme P et al: Genus *Arcobacter*. In Brenner DJ et al, volume editors: *Bergey's manual of systematic bacteriology*, vol 2, ed 2, New York, 2005, Springer.

Vandamme P et al: Genus *Campylobacter* Sebald and Véron 1963, 907,[AL] emmend. Vandamme, Falsen, Rossau, Hoste, Segars, Tytgat and De Ley 1991a, 98. In Brenner DJ et al, editors: *Bergey's manual of systematic bacteriology*, vol 2, ed 2, New York, 2005, Springer.

Vinh DC et al: *Vibrio vulnificus* septicemia after handling *Tilapia* species fish: a Canadian case report and review, *Can J Infect Dis Med Microbiol* 17:129, 2006.

Vila J et al: *Aeromonas* spp. and traveler's diarrhea: clinical features and antimicrobial resistance, *Emerg Infect Dis* 9:552, 2003.

Woo PC et al: Two cases of continuous peritoneal dialysis-associated peritonitis due to *Plesiomonas shigelloides, J Clin Microbiol* 42:933, 2004.

Woo PC, Lau SK, Yuen KY: Biliary tract disease as a risk factor for *Plesiomonas shigelloides* bacteraemia: a nine-year experience in a Hong Kong hospital and review of the literature, *New Microbiol* 28:45, 2005.

Points to Remember

- Most species in this chapter are found in fresh, estuarine, or marine water.
- Twelve species of *Vibrio* have been implicated in human infection and most are agents of diarrheal disease.
- *V. cholerae* produces a powerful enterotoxin and is responsible for large numbers of epidemics as well as pandemics.
- Other *Vibrio* spp. are common causes of diarrheal disease related to consumption of raw shellfish or related to aquatic wound infections with serious sequelae like septicemia and death.
- TCBS agar is the medium of choice to differentiate the *Vibrio* spp. This medium distinguishes sucrose-fermenting strains from nonsucrose fermenting strains.
- *Aeromonas* spp. can also cause several types of diarrhea and a variety of extraintestinal infections that can lead to septicemia, meningitis, hemolytic uremic syndrome, and death.

- *Plesiomonas shigelloides* phenotypically resembles the vibrios and aeromonads, but recent molecular analyses have moved this organism to the position of being the only "oxidase-positive" member of the family Enterobacteriaceae.
- Human *Campylobacter* spp. are generally responsible for enteritis, and *C. jejuni* is one of the most common causes of bacterial diarrhea worldwide.
- Patients suffering from Guillain-Barré syndrome (GBS) often test positive for *Campylobacter* antibodies. GBS is believed to be an autoimmune disorder resulting from cross-reactivity of *Campylobacter* antibodies with the nerve ganglia.
- *H. pylori* is strongly associated with gastric and duodenal ulcers and has been implicated in cases of gastric carcinoma.

Learning Assessment Questions

1. A gram-negative bacillus isolated from a stool specimen produces clear colonies on MacConkey agar and yellow colonies on thiosulfate citrate bile salts sucrose medium. The isolate is subcultured to a sheep blood agar plate with an O/129 disk. The isolate is sensitive to O/129 and is oxidase positive. You should suspect:
   a. *Vibrio parahaemolyticus*
   b. *Vibrio cholerae*
   c. *Plesiomonas*
   d. *Aeromonas*

2. Which of the following *Vibrio* spp. would you expect to be most likely isolated from a blood culture?
   a. *V. cholerae*
   b. *V. parahaemolyticus*
   c. *V. vulnificus*
   d. *V. alginolyticus*

3. Which of the following genera is typically microaerophilic?
   a. *Helicobacter*
   b. *Aeromonas*
   c. *Plesiomonas*
   d. *Vibrio*

4. *Campylobacter jejuni* is most noted for causing:
   a. Wounds
   b. Septicemia
   c. Gastric ulcers
   d. Gastroenteritis

5. Which of the following is a risk factor for acquiring *V. alginolyticus* infection?
   a. Farming
   b. Hunting
   c. Fishing or swimming in ocean water
   d. Drinking unpasteurized milk

6. An oxidase-positive, indole-positive, β-hemolytic, gram-negative bacillus that is resistant to O/129, cannot grow in 6% NaCl broth, and is a non-lactose fermenter on MacConkey agar is isolated from an adult stool culture. You should suspect:
   a. *Aeromonas hydrophila*
   b. *Aeromonas caviae*
   c. *Plesiomonas shigelloides*
   d. *Vibrio parahaemolyticus*

7. Darting motility is a characteristic of:
   a. *Aeromonas*
   b. *Campylobacter*
   c. *V. cholerae* O1
   d. *V. cholerae* non-O1

8. Which of the following tests is most helpful in differentiating *C. jejuni* from the other *Campylobacter* spp.?
   a. Nitrate reduction
   b. Urease activity
   c. Hippurate hydrolysis
   d. Susceptibility to nalidixic acid

9. When attempting to recover enteric *Campylobacter* spp., what specimen, media, and incubation conditions should be used?

10. What nonculture methods are used to diagnosis *Helicobacter pylori* infections?

Nonfermenting and Miscellaneous Gram-Negative Bacilli

Gerri S. Hall

OBJECTIVES

After reading and studying this chapter, you should be able to:

1. Describe the general characteristics of nonfermentative gram-negative bacilli.

2. Compare the metabolic pathways used by nonfermentative and fermentative organisms.

3. Discuss the natural habitat of the nonfermentative gram-negative bacilli.

4. Describe how nonfermentative organisms cause infections.

5. Recognize the initial clues to nonfermentative organisms isolated in clinical laboratories.

6. Describe the typical reactions and characteristic features of most of the commonly encountered nonfermentative organisms.

Case in Point

A 25-year-old woman who received a bone marrow transplant as treatment for aplastic anemia had the following presenting symptoms: fever, chills, and malaise of approximately 2 days' duration. Blood cultures were drawn according to standard procedure (i.e., two sets of 20 mL each). The patient was admitted, and approximately 5 hours later another two sets of blood cultures were collected because her fever persisted. At this point the patient was given a broad-spectrum antimicrobial agent; the plan was to give her antifungal agents if the fever persisted. About 12 hours after the first blood cultures were drawn, the clinician was called because both blood cultures tested positive for a gram-negative bacillus. In another 4 hours, the other two sets were also positive for a gram-negative bacillus. The next day the clinician was informed that the gram-negative bacillus was an oxidase-positive, non–lactose fermenter. The isolate would be identified and antimicrobial susceptibility testing would be performed.

Issues to Consider

After reading the patient's case history, consider:

■ The risk factors in this patient for infection with a nonfermenting gram-negative bacillus

■ The significance of the number of positive blood cultures for a similar organism

■ How you might rapidly identify this organism for better clinical care

Key Terms

Asaccharolytic	Nonfermentative
Dysgonic fermenter	Nonoxidizer
Eugonic fermenter (EF)	Oxidizer
Eugonic oxidizer	Pyocyanin
Fermentative	Pyoverdin

BOX 21-1 Risk Factors for Diseases Caused by Nonfermentative Gram-Negative Bacilli

Immunosuppression
Diabetes mellitus
Cancer
Steroids
Transplantation

Trauma
Gun shot, knife wounds, punctures
Surgery
Burns

Foreign Body Implantation
Catheters: urinary or blood stream
Prosthetic devices: joints, valves
Corneal implants or contact lenses

Infused Fluids
Dialysate
Saline irrigations

This chapter discusses miscellaneous nonfermentative gram-negative organisms that have become more clinically significant because of the increasing numbers of immunocompromised patients. These patients often have multiple risk factors for infection with these uncommon pathogens. The groups of organisms discussed in this chapter include the *Pseudomonas* spp., *Acinetobacter* spp., *Stenotrophomonas maltophilia* and other lactose-negative oxidizers, and asaccharolytic species of gram-negative bacilli. Aerobic gram-negative bacilli can be divided into at least two large groups: those that ferment carbohydrates, called **fermentative** or fermenters; and those that do not ferment carbohydrates, called **nonfermentative** or nonfermenters.

GENERAL CHARACTERISTICS OF NONFERMENTERS

Nonfermenting gram-negative bacilli are grouped together because they fail to acidify oxidative-fermentative (O-F) media when it is overlaid with mineral oil or fail to acidify triple sugar iron (TSI) agar. They prefer and grow much better in an aerobic environment; some do not grow in an anaerobic environment at all. Some group members oxidize carbohydrates to derive energy for their metabolism; they are referred to as **oxidizers.** Others do not break down carbohydrates at all and are inert or biochemically inactive; they are referred to as **nonoxidizers** or **asaccharolytic.** Additional characteristics can differentiate this group of nonfermenters from other gram-negative bacilli: motility, pigmentation, and their ability or lack of ability to grow on selective gram-negative media such as MacConkey (MAK) agar. Most nonfermentative gram-negative bacilli are oxidase positive, a feature that differentiates them from the Enterobacteriaceae (*Plesiomonas* sp. is the only oxidase-positive member of the family Enterobacteriaceae).

In general, nonfermentative gram-negative bacilli or coccobacilli are ubiquitous and found in most environments: in soil and water, on plants and decaying vegetation, and in many foodstuffs. They prefer moist environments, and in hospitals they can be isolated from nebulizers, dialysate fluids, saline, and catheters and other devices. Nonfermenters can withstand treatment with chlorhexidine and quaternary ammonium compounds. They are rarely, if ever, part of the normal host microbiota but can easily colonize hospitalized patients, especially those who are immunocompromised. Nonfermentative gram-negative bacilli tend to be resistant to multiple classes of antimicrobial agents.

Clinical Infections

Nonfermenters account for about 15% of all gram-negative bacilli isolated from clinical specimens. Although there are differences among the clinical diseases caused by each species, some common disease manifestations and risk factors can be found. Nonfermenters can be responsible for a number of infections, including septicemia, meningitis, osteomyelitis, and wound infections, usually following surgery or trauma. Common risk factors for development of these infections are listed in Box 21-1 and include immunosuppression, foreign body implantation, trauma, or the introduction of fluids via dialysates, catheters, or irrigations. Usually the individual who contracts infection with one of these organisms is hospitalized or has been recently discharged from the hospital.

Biochemical Characteristics and Identification

As mentioned, all the nonfermenters fail to ferment carbohydrates and thus will not yield acidic reactions in the anaerobic portion of media such as TSI or Kligler's iron agar (KIA). A fermenter (e.g., *Escherichia coli*) typically produces an acid (yellow) butt with an acid or alkaline (red) slant on TSI or KIA within 18 hours of incubation on either of these media. A nonfermenter (either an oxidizer or nonoxidizer) produces no change in the butt and slant or may produce an alkaline slant. The principles of the TSI reactions are explained in Chapter 9. In addition to these types of organisms, some "true" fermenters are fastidious (e.g., *Pasturella multocida*) and do not easily acidify the butt or slant of a TSI like other fermenters, but they do show reactions if more sensitive or nutritious media are used.

Some characteristics or initial clues can indicate the presence of a nonfermenter in the clinical laboratory:
- Thin, gram-negative bacilli or coccobacilli on Gram stain
- Oxidase-positive reaction, although reaction can be weak and variable
- Nonreactivity in 24 hours in commercial systems for the identification of Enterobacteriaceae

- No acid production in the slant or butt of TSI or KIA
- Resistance to a variety of classes of antimicrobial agents, such as aminoglycosides, third-generation cephalosporins, penicillins, and fluoroquinolones

Many classification systems have been devised for grouping the nonfermenters. One system uses the reactions of three common tests: (1) growth on MAK agar, (2) oxidase reaction, and (3) glucose oxidation/fermentation (O-F test). The eight possible combinations of results are then used to group the nonfermenters as shown in Figure 21-1. Included in this figure are some nonfermentative gram-negative bacilli not always considered with the more "typical" nonfermenters. Organisms such as *Brucella* spp. and *Bordetella* spp. are biochemically similar and are discussed in Chapter 18.

For the identification of nonfermentative gram-negative bacilli, conventional tube biochemical testing, multi-test systems, automated systems, or combinations of these can be used. Three genera of nonfermenters make up the majority of isolates routinely seen in clinical laboratories: *Pseudomonas aeruginosa, Acinetobacter* spp., and *Stenotrophomonas maltophilia*. Any of the aforementioned systems perform adequately to identify these three groups. For the remainder of the nonfermenters, for which there is great variability, depending on the system used, decisions need to be made about whether a full identification is needed based on the clinical situation and relevance of the isolate. As a result of nucleic acid studies, the nonfermentative gram-negative bacilli continually undergo taxonomic changes. Table 21-1. Box 21-2 summarizes characteristics common to some gram-negative nonfermenters.

TABLE 21-1 Taxonomic Changes of Some Gram-Negative Nonfermenters

New Name	Old Name
Achromobacter xylosoxidans	Achromobacter xylosoxidans var. xylosoxidans
Achromobacter denitrificans	Achromobacter xylosoxidans var. denitrificans
Bergeyella zoohelcum	Weeksella zoohelcum
Brevundimonas diminuta	Pseudomonas diminuta
Chryseobacterium gleum	Flavobacterium gleum
Chryseobacterium indologenes	Flavobacterium indologenes
Cupriavidus pauculus	Ralstonia paucula
Cupriavidus gilardii	Ralstonia gilardii
Delftia acidovorans	Comomonas acidovorans
Elizabethkingia meningosepticum	Chryseobacterium meningosepticum
Empedobacter brevis	Flavobacterium brevis
Methylobacterium mesophilicum	Pseudomonas mesophilica
Myroides odoratus	Flavobacterium odoratum
Ochrobactrum anthropi	Achromobacter biovar 1, 2, or Vd-1
Pandoraea spp.	CDC group WO-2
Paracoccus yeei	CDC EO-2
Pseudomonas luteola	Chryseomonas luteola
Pseudomonas oryzihabitans	Flavimonas oryzihabitans
Psychrobacter phenylpyruvicus	Moraxella phenylpyruvica
Ralstonia pickettii	Pseudomonas pickettii
Rhizobium radiobacter	Agrobacterium radiobacter
Sphingobacterium multivorum	Flavobacterium multivorum
Sphingobacterium spiritivorum	Flavobacterium spiritivorum
Sphingomonas paucimobilis	Pseudomonas paucimobilis

BOX 21-2 Characteristics Common to Groups of Nonfermenters

Pigmentation
Yellow
Chryseobacterium spp. and *Elizabethkingia* spp. (weak fermenters)
Pseudomonas (Chryseomonas) luteola
Pseudomonas oryzihabitans
Sphingobacterium spp.
Pseudomonas stutzeri (light yellow)

Pink
Methylobacterium spp.

Blue-green
Pseudomonas aeruginosa

Violet
Chromobacterium violaceum (fermenter)

Lavender to lavender-green (blood agar)
Stenotrophomonas maltophilia

Tan (occasionally)
P. stutzeri
Shewanella putrefaciens

Wrinkled Colonies
P. stutzeri
Burkholderia pseudomallei

Odors
Sweet
Alcaligenes faecalis
Myroides odoratus
P. aeruginosa (grapes)

Popcorn
EO-4
EF-4ab

Nonmotile
Acinetobacter sp.
Moraxella sp.
Chryseobacterium spp. and *Elizabethkingia* spp. (weak fermenters)
Sphingobacterium spp. (May "glide")
Oligella sp. (nonureolytica)

Oxidase Negative
Acinetobacter sp.
S. maltophilia
Chryseomonas spp.
Pseudomonas cepacia ±
Pseudomonas luteola
Pseudomonas oryzihabitans

H₂S Positive
Shewanella putrefaciens
Shewanella algae

Courtesy Anne Morrissey, George Manuselis, and Connie Mahon.

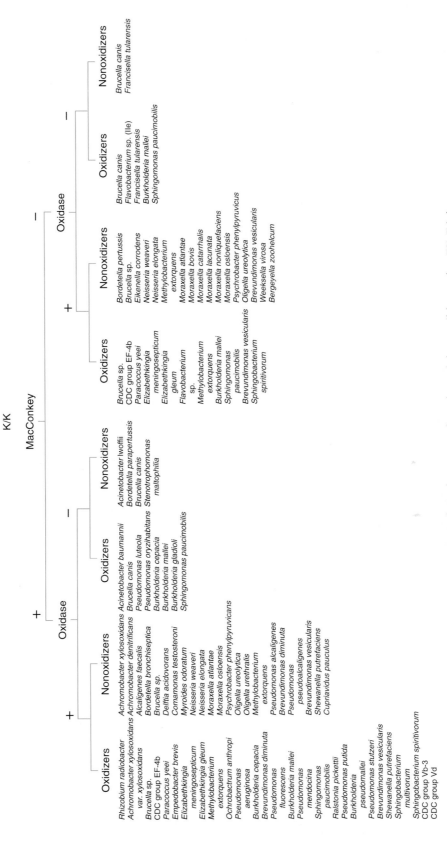

FIGURE 21-1 Grouping of nonfermenters based on eight possible results. *TSI*, Triple sugar iron; *K/K*, alkaline/alkaline. Some bacteria have variable results and belong to more than one group.

The decision to identify many of the nonfermenters is based on the site from which they have been isolated, that is, whether they have been isolated from a sterile site in pure culture or from a nonsterile site in which three or four other bacterial species are also present. In the former case, it may be decided that definitive identification and susceptibility testing are required. Use of a kit or automated system with or without conventional biochemicals should then be used. In the nonsterile site, a genus identification may be appropriate, and this can be achieved through use of a few biochemical tests (e.g., oxidase, growth on MAK agar, glucose utilization, indole, and motility). Alternatively, identification as a "nonfermenter, not *P. aeruginosa, Acinetobacter* sp., or *S. maltophilia,* may be all that is needed, especially when cultures are mixed with many other bacterial species.

Definitive identification of every nonfermenter is time consuming and can be costly. Figure 21-2 gives typical biochemical and morphologic characteristics for a large number of nonfermentative gram-negative bacilli. If definitive identification is considered necessary for epidemiologic purposes or for academic reasons, such as for publication of an unusual case report involving the organism, laboratory scientists should consider sending the isolate to a reference laboratory that is better equipped to achieve these identifications in a cost-effective manner. Today, many of these reference laboratories would probably use a DNA sequencing method of identification and not rely on biochemical or phenotypic identification.

In vitro susceptibility testing of the nonfermenters is not always necessary. For clinically significant isolates of *P. aeruginosa, S. maltophilia, Acinetobacter* spp., and *Burkholderia cepacia,* the Clinical and Laboratory Standards Institute (CLSI) recommends that a broth microdilution or Kirby-Bauer disk diffusion assay be performed. For other species, broth microdilution, not disk diffusion, is recommended if antimicrobial susceptibility testing is done at all.

CLINICALLY SIGNIFICANT NONFERMENTATIVE GRAM-NEGATIVE BACILLI

The genus *Pseudomonas* accounts for the largest percentage of all nonfermenters isolated from clinical specimens. Characteristics common to most of the pseudomonads, including members of the genus *Pseudomonas* and several *Pseudomonas*-like organisms include the following:

- Gram-negative bacillus or coccobacillus
- Motile with polar or polar tufts of flagella, except *Burkholderia mallei*
- Oxidase and catalase positive
- Usually growth on MAK agar
- Usually an oxidizer of carbohydrates, but some species are asaccharolytic

Fluorescent Pseudomonad Group

Pseudomonas aeruginosa

Pseudomonas aeruginosa is the most commonly isolated species of the genus in clinical specimens. It is an uncommon part of the normal bacterial biota and is isolated from fewer than 12% of normal stool specimens. It can, however, account for 5% to 15% of all nosocomial infections, especially pneumonia and bacteremia. *P. aeruginosa* is the leading cause of nosocomial respiratory tract infections. A large variety of clinical diseases have been documented as being caused by *P. aeruginosa*, including bacteremia, often presenting with ecthyma gangrenosum of the skin; wound infections; pulmonary disease, especially among individuals with cystic fibrosis (CF); nosocomial urinary tract infections (UTIs); endocarditis; infections following burns or trauma; and, in rare cases; central nervous system infections, including meningitis.

Pseudomonas aeruginosa has a propensity to invade vascular walls of blood vessels, which facilitates its spread in the body. *P. aeruginosa* accounts for up to 6% of all bacteremias and as many as 75% of nosocomial bacteremias, and it is the third most common cause of gram-negative bacillary bacteremia, after *E. coli* and *Klebsiella pneumoniae*. Poor prognostic factors associated with *P. aeruginosa* bacteremia include septic shock, granulocytopenia, inappropriate antimicrobial therapy, and the presence of septic metastatic lesions. In the Case in Point, *P. aeruginosa* was the organism identified from the blood cultures. Other less serious conditions associated with *P. aeruginosa* infection are otitis externa, particularly in swimmers or divers; a necrotizing skin rash, referred to as *Jacuzzi* or *hot tub syndrome,* that develops in users of these recreational facilities; and infections of the nail beds in people who wear artificial nails. Figure 21-3 illustrates the Gram stain of a bronchial specimen containing *P. aeruginosa*.

Virulence Factors. *Pseudomonas aeruginosa* can produce a variety of factors that lend to its pathogenicity, such as endotoxin (lipopolysaccharide), motility, pili, capsule, and several exotoxins: proteases, hemolysins, lecithinase, elastase, and DNase. The most important exotoxin is exotoxin A, which functions similarly to diphtheria toxin by blocking protein synthesis. In lower respiratory tract infections of patients with CF, most *P. aeruginosa* strains produce mucoid colonies because of the overproduction of alginate—a polysaccharide polymer (Figure 21-4). The production of mucoid colonies in strains isolated from patients with CF can be a helpful identifying characteristic. *P. aeruginosa* is also inherently resistant to a number of antimicrobial agents. Despite the vast array of virulence factors, *P. aeruginosa* is still considered an opportunistic pathogen.

Identifying Characteristics. Members of the fluorescent pseudomonad group, which includes *P. aeruginosa, P. fluorescens, P. putida, P. veronii, P. monteilii,* and *P. mosselii,* produce **pyoverdin,** a yellow-green or yellow-brown pigment. Pyoverdin is water soluble and fluoresces under short-wavelength ultraviolet light. Many strains of *P. aeruginosa* will also produce the blue, water-soluble pigment **pyocyanin.** When pyocyanin combines with pyoverdin, the green color characteristic of *P. aeruginosa* is produced (Figure 21-5). No other nonfermentative, gram-negative bacillus produces pyocyanin, so its presence specifically indicates *P. aeruginosa*. If needed, pyocyanin typing can be used to epidemiologically link strains of *P. aeruginosa*. About 4% of clinical strains of *P. aeruginosa*, however, do not produce pyocyanin. Other water-soluble pigments, (e.g., pyorubin [red] and pyomelanin [brown or black]), are occasionally produced.

	MOTILE, STRONGLY SACCHAROLYTIC NONFERMENTERS										MOTILE, WEAK, OR NONSACCHAROLYTIC NONFERMENTERS										
	Pseudomonas aeruginosa	*Pseudomonas fluorescens/putida*	*Burkholderia cepacia*	*Achromobacter xylosoxidans*	*Stenotrophomonas maltophilia*	*Burkholderia pseudomallei*	*Pseudomonas stutzeri*	*Sphingomonas paucimobilis*	*Pseudomonas mendocina*	*Ralstonia pickettii*	*Delftia acidovorans*	*Pseudomonas pseudoalcaligenes*	*Alcaligenes faecalis*	*Achromobacter denitricans*	*Oligella ureolytica*	*Bordetella bronchiseptica*	*Pseudomonas alcaligenes*	*Brevundimonas diminuta*	*Brevundimonas vesicularis*	*Comamonas testosteroni*	*Shewanella putrefaciens*
Oxidase	+	+	+	+	−	+	+	+	+	+	+	+	+	+	+	+	+	+	+	+	+
Pyocyanin	+/−	−	−	−	−	−	−	−	−	−	−	−	−	−	−	−	−	−	−	−	−
Fluorescein	+	−/+	−	−	−	−	−	−	−	−	−	−	−	−	−	−	−	−	−	−	−
Glucose	+	+	+	+/−	+/−	+	+	+/−	+	+	−	−/+	−	−	−	−	−	−	−	+	−
Xylose	+	+	+/−	+	−	+	−/+	+/−	+	+	−	−	−	−	−	−	−	−	−	−	−
Mannitol	+/−	+/−	+/−	−	−	+	−/+	−	−	−	+/−	−	−	−	−	−	−	−	−	−	−
Lactose	−	−	+/−	−	−	+	+/−	+/−	−	−	−	−	−	−	−	−	−	−	−	−	−
Maltose	−	−	+/−	−	−	+	+	+/−	+/−	−	−	−/+	−	−	−	−	−	−	+	−	−
42° C	+	−	+/−	+	+/−	+	+	−	+	+/−	−	+	+/−	−/+	−	+	+/−	−/+	+/−	+/−	+/−
Esculin	−	−	−/+	−	+	+/−	−	+	−	−	−	−	−	−	−	−	−	−	+	−	−
Urea	+	−/+	+/−	−	+/−	−/+	−/+	−/+	+/−	+	−	−	−/+	−	+	+	−/+	+/−	−	−	+/−
DNase	−	−	−	−	+	−	−	+	−	−	−	−	−	−	−	−	−	−	+	+	+
ONPG	−	−	+/−	−	+	−	−	+/−	−	−	−	−	−	−	−	−	−	−	−	−	−
Indole	−	−	−	−	−	−	−	−	−	−	−	−	−	−	−	−	−	−	−	−	−
Motility	+	+	+	+	+	+	+	−	+	+	+	+	+	+	+	+	+	+	+	+	+
Flagella	1	>1	>1	P	>1	>1	1	1	1	1	>1	1	P	P	P	P	1	1	1	>1	1
H₂S	−	−	−	−	−	−	−	−	−	−	−	−	−	−	−	−	−	−	−	−	+
N₂ gas	+/−	−	−	−	−	+	+	−	+	−/+	−	−	+	+/−	+	−	−	−	−	−	−
Pigment	B,F,G	F	Y	−	Y	−	B,Y	Y	−	−	−	−	−	−	−	−	−	−	B,Y	−	B
Growth on MacConkey	+	+	+	+	+	+	+	−	+	+	+	+	+	+	+	+	+	+	−/+	+/−	+

FIGURE 21-2 Biochemical and morphologic characteristics of selected nonfermentative gram-negative bacilli. *ONPG,* o-Nitrophenyl-β-ᴅ-galactopyranoside; +, most strains positive; −, most strains negative; *B,* brown; *F,* fluorescein; *G,* green; *Y,* yellow. (Data from the Ohio State University Hospital, Columbus, Ohio.)

| | NONMOTILE, PIGMENTED, INDOLE-POSITIVE NONFERMENTERS | | | | NONMOTILE COCCOBACILLI | | |
| | | | | | | Oxidase negative | |
	Elizabethkingia meningosepticum	*Myroides odoratus*	*Bergeyella zoohelcum*	*Weeksella virosa*	*Moraxella sp.*	*Acinetobacter lwoffii*	*Acinetobacter baumannii*
Oxidase	+	+	+	+	+	−	−
Pyocyanin	−	−	−	−	−	−	−
Fluorescein	−	−	−	−	−	−	−
Glucose	+/−	−	−	−	−	−	+
Xylose	−	−	−	−	−	−	+
Mannitol	−/+	−	−	−	−	−	−
Lactose	−	−	−	−	−	−	+
Maltose	−/+	−	−	−	−	+/−	−
42° C	+/−	−	−	−/+	−/+	−	+
Esculin	+	−	−	−	−	−	−
Urea	−/+	+	+	−/+	−	−/+	−/+
DNase	+	+	+	+	−	−	−/+
ONPG	+/−	−	−	−	−	−	−
Indole	+	−	−/+	+	−	−	−
Motility	−	−	−	−	−	−	−
Flagella	−	−	−	−	−	−	−
H₂S	−	−	−	−	−	−	−
N₂ gas	−	−/+	−	−	−	−	−
Pigment	Y	Y	B	B	−	−	−
Growth on MAC	+	+	−	−	+/−	+	+

Flagella

1, Polar monotrichous

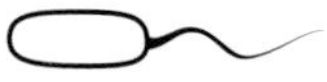

>1, Polar tuft (>1 flagellum)

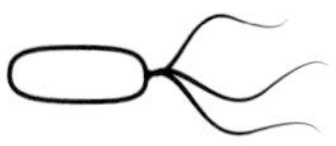

P, Peritrichous

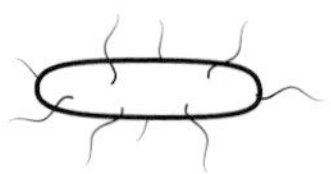

FIGURE 21-2, cont'd.

Most isolates of *P. aeruginosa* are β-hemolytic on sheep blood agar (SBA) and will produce flat spreading colonies with a characteristic metallic sheen. Many strains of *P. aeruginosa* produce a fruity, grapelike odor caused by the presence of 2-aminoacetophenone. Other key characteristics of *P. aeruginosa* include gluconate production from glucose via oxidation, arginine dihydrolase (ADH) positive, growth at 42° C, citrate positive, and acetamide utilization. Cetrimide agar is a selective and differential medium for the identification of *P. aeruginosa*. Cetrimide acts as a detergent and inhibits most bacteria; the medium also enhances the production of the two pigments produced by *P. aeruginosa*: pyoverdin and pyocyanin.

Treatment. *Pseudomonas aeruginosa* is innately resistant to many antimicrobial agents including penicillin, ampicillin, first- and second-generation cephalosporins, trimethoprim-sulfamethoxazole (SXT), and chloramphenicol, along with other agents to which most gram-negative bacilli are resistant. *P. aeruginosa* is usually susceptible to aminoglycosides; semisynthetic penicillins such as piperacillin and ticarcillin; the third- and fourth-generation cephalosporins, ceftazidime and cefepime, respectively; and carbapenems (except ertapenem);

and fluoroquinolones. Resistance to any of these agents may develop while a patient is on therapy; the incidence of resistance is much higher in nosocomial strains of *P. aeruginosa*. Treatment of severe *P. aeruginosa* infections usually requires combination therapy, often ceftazidime, piperacillin, or a carbapenem (imipenem or meropenem) with an aminoglycoside (tobramycin or amikacin).

Pseudomonas fluorescens and *Pseudomonas putida*

Both *P. fluorescens* and *P. putida* are of very low virulence, rarely causing clinical disease. They have been isolated from respiratory specimens, contaminated blood products, urine, cosmetics, hospital equipment, and fluids. *P. fluorescens* and *P. putida* have been documented, although rarely, as causes of UTIs, postsurgical abscesses, empyema, septic arthritis, and other wound infections. Both species can grow at 4° C and have been linked to transfusion-associated septicemia.

P. fluorescens and *P. putida* produce pyoverdin, but neither produces pyocyanin or grows at 42° C. Key characteristics of *P. aeruginosa*, *P. fluorescens*, and *P. putida* are that they cannot reduce nitrate to nitrogen gas, but they can produce acid from xylose, characteristics that separate them from the other fluorescent pseudomonads. Gelatin hydrolysis can be used to differentiate the two species: *P. putida* (negative) and *P. fluorescens* (positive). They are usually susceptible to the aminoglycosides, polymyxin, and piperacillin, but they are resistant to carbenicillin and SXT.

Acinetobacter

The genus *Acinetobacter*, a member of the family Moraxellaceae, consists of 25 DNA homology groups or genomospecies. Only 11 species have been officially named. The two species most commonly seen in clinical specimens are *A. baumannii*, a glucose-oxidizing nonhemolytic strain, and *A. lwoffii*, glucose negative nonhemolytic strain. Most hemolytic strains of *Acinetobacter* are *A. haemolyticus*.

Acinetobacter spp. are ubiquitous in the environment in soil, water, and foodstuffs; in the hospital environment, they

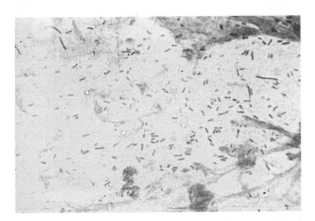

FIGURE 21-3 Gram stain of bronchial specimen positive for *Pseudomonas aeruginosa*.

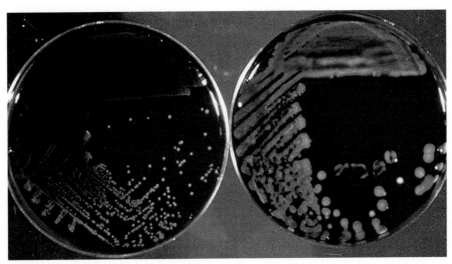

FIGURE 21-4 *Pseudomonas aeruginosa* on sheep blood agar. *Left:* Nonmucoid colonies. *Right:* Mucoid colonies. Note discoloration of media, especially on the left.

A

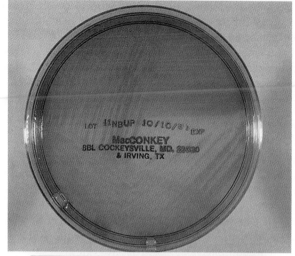

B

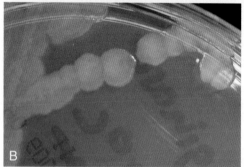

FIGURE 21-5 **A**, *Pseudomonas aeruginosa* on MacConkey agar and, **B**, Mueller-Hinton agar. Note the blue-green pigment.

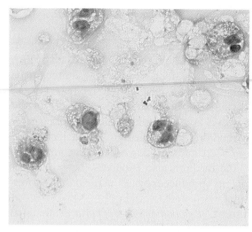

FIGURE 21-6 *Acinetobacter baumanii* on Gram stain. Note the coccoid nature of the cells as well as the pleomorphic forms.

have been associated with ventilators, humidifiers, catheters, and other devices. About 25% of adults carry the organisms on their skin, and about 7% carry the organism in their pharynx. If not harboring *Acinetobacter* spp. already, hospitalized patients may become easily colonized. As many as 45% of patients with a tracheotomy may be colonized. When *Acinetobacter* spp. are isolated from urine, feces, vaginal secretions, and many different types of respiratory specimens, they are often considered insignificant colonizers or contaminants. However, with the increased isolation of *Acinetobacter* spp. with resistance to most antimicrobial agents, their clinical significance when isolated from respiratory or urine specimens in a hospitalized immunocompromised patient cannot be dismissed routinely.

Clinical Infections

Acinetobacter spp. are opportunistic pathogens, accounting for 1% to 3% of all nosocomial infections; they are second only to *P. aeruginosa* in frequency of isolation of all nonfermenters in the clinical microbiology laboratory. Diseases with which they, in particular *A. baumanii*, have been associated include urinary tract infection (UTI); pneumonia, tracheobronchitis, or both; endocarditis, with up to a 22% mortality;

septicemia; meningitis (often as a complication of intrathecal chemotherapy for cancer); and cellulitis, most often as a result of contaminated indwelling catheters, trauma, burns, or introduction of a foreign body. More recently, *A. baumanii*, because of its increasing resistance to carbapenems and most other antimicrobial agents, has been involved in more clinically relevant situations and needs to be considered as a potential pathogen before being discarded as a colonizer or contaminant. The literature contains reports of eye infections caused by *A. baumanii*, including endophthalmitis, conjunctivitis, and corneal ulcerations. *A. lwoffii* is much less virulent and when isolated most often indicates contamination or colonization rather than infection.

Identifying Characteristics

All the *Acinetobacter* spp. are strictly aerobic, gram-negative coccobacilli (Figure 21-6) that are oxidase-negative, catalase-positive, and nonmotile. It should be noted that *Acinetobacter* organisms can appear as gram-positive cocci in smears made from blood culture bottles. They possess few growth requirements and thus are capable of growing on most laboratory media, including MAK agar. The purplish hue produced by some species on this medium may resemble a lactose-fermenting bacterium (Figure 21-7). Lower temperatures (30° to 35° C) and pH 5.5 to 6.0 are preferred. *A. baumannii* is saccharolytic, and *A. lwoffii* is asaccharolytic.

Isolates of *A. baumannii* are often resistant to many antimicrobials, including penicillins, first- and second-generation cephalosporins, and fluoroquinolones. Many strains have become resistant to carbapenems; carbapenemases have been reported in isolates throughout the United States. *A. baumannii* demonstrates variable susceptibility to the aminoglycosides and β-lactam plus β-lactamase inhibitor combinations (e.g., ampicillin/sulbactam or piperacillin/tazobactam). *A. lwoffii* is usually susceptible to almost all antimicrobial agents.

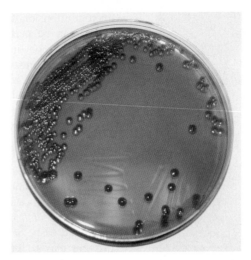

FIGURE 21-7   *Acinetobacter calcoaceticus* on MacConkey agar after 24 hours of incubation.

Stenotrophomonas maltophilia

Stenotrophomonas maltophilia is the third most common non-fermentative gram-negative bacillus isolated in the clinical laboratory. It was determined through DNA homology and sequencing analysis that it be classified as a member of the genus *Stenotrophomonas*, where it remains today. Isolates are ubiquitous in the environment, being found in water, sewage, and plant materials. *S. maltophilia* is common to the hospital environment, where they can be found contaminating blood-drawing equipment, disinfectants, transducers, and other equipment.

When *S. maltophilia* is isolated from clinical specimens, it is initially regarded as a saprophyte or colonizer. Although not considered part of the normal human microbiota, *S. maltophilia* can quickly colonize the respiratory tract of hospitalized patients, in particular those exposed to antimicrobial agents to which *S. maltophilia* may be inherently resistant. These antimicrobials include cephalosporins, penicillins, carbapenems, and aminoglycosides. With increased use of agents to which it is innately resistant, there have been more reports of disease attributed to this organism. Reported diseases include endocarditis, especially in a setting of prior intravenous drug abuse or heart surgery; wound infections, including cellulitis and ecthyma gangrenosum; bacteremia; and rarely, meningitis and UTI. With rare exceptions, infections have occurred in a nosocomial setting. *S. maltophilia* is rarely associated with lower respiratory tract infections, although it has been isolated from 6.4% to 10.2% of patients with CF. Pseudoinfections have also occurred as a result of contaminated collection tubes or cups (e.g., blood collection tubes). The single most important risk factor in affected individuals was the presence of a venous catheter. Most patients with bacteremia responded well to therapy unless they had concomitant pneumonia or shock.

S. maltophilia is an oxidase-negative, nonfermentative, gram-negative bacillus. In addition, it is positive for catalase, DNase, esculin and gelatin hydrolysis, and lysine decarboxylase (LDC). *S. maltophilia* is usually susceptible to SXT, and this is the drug of choice for most infections. Other agents to which it might demonstrate in vitro susceptibility include ticarcillin-clavulanate; the fluoroquinolone levofloxacin; and tetracyclines, including tigecycline. The CLSI recommends broth microdilution testing for *S. maltophilia;* in addition Etest (AB BIODISK, Solna, Sweden) or agar dilution can be performed. Interpretive criteria are provided for ticarcillin-clavulanic acid, ceftazidime, minocycline, levofloxacin, and SXT. Methods for disk diffusion are provided in the January 2008 CLSI supplements, but it is recommended that only minocycline, levofloxacin, and SXT results be reported for *S. maltophilia* if this method is used.

Burkholderia

Burkholderia cepacia

Burkholderia cepacia is a complex of nine distinct genomic species (genomovars) that has in the past been called *Pseudomonas cepacia, P. multivorans, P. kingii,* and CDC unnamed group EO-1. Clinically *B. cepacia* (this species will be used as representative of the complex*)* is a low-grade, nosocomial pathogen most often associated with pneumonia in patients with CF or chronic granulomatous disease. It has also been reported to cause endocarditis (specifically in drug addicts), pneumonitis, UTI, osteomyelitis, dermatitis, and other wound infections resulting from use of contaminated water. It has been isolated from irrigation fluids, anesthetics, nebulizers, detergents, and disinfectants. Research supports the association of *B. cepacia* and increased severity of disease and death in patients with CF and chronic granulomatous disease. In the United States, about 3% of the CF population are infected with *B. cepacia,* but rates up to 30% in some adult CF patient populations have been reported. Outside these populations, morbidity and mortality rates remain low, and consideration needs to be given to the

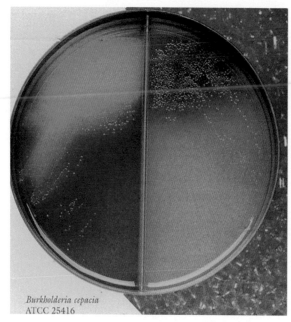

FIGURE 21-8 *Burkholderia cepacia* on selective/differential media. *Left:* Colonies of *B. cepacia* on oxidative-fermentative base, polymyxin B, bacitracin, lactose (OFPBL) agar are yellow. *Right:* Colonies of *B. cepacia* on *Burkholderia cepacia* selective agar.

possibility of contamination rather than infection when it is isolated in an individual without CF or chronic granulomatous disease.

The organism grows well on most laboratory media but might lose viability on SBA in 3 to 4 days without appropriate transfers. *B. cepacia* grows on MAK agar, but selective media containing antimicrobials to reduce the growth of *P. aeruginosa*, as well as other gram-negative bacilli, are available to increase the recovery of *B. cepacia* (Figure 21-8). These media include PC *(P. cepacia),* OFPBL (oxidative-fermentative base, polymyxin B, bacitracin, lactose), and BCSA (*B. cepacia* selective agar). Studies have suggested that BCSA is the most effective in reducing overgrowth while maintaining good recovery of *B. cepacia*.

B. cepacia complex often produces a weak, slow, positive oxidase reaction. Nearly all strains oxidize glucose, and many will oxidize maltose, lactose, and mannitol. Most strains are LDC and o-nitrophenyl-β-D-galactopyranoside (ONPG) positive, whereas most strains are ornithine decarboxylase (ODC) negative and fail to reduce nitrate to nitrite. Isolates are motile by means of polar tufts of flagella. They do not fluoresce like *P. aeruginosa*, but they can produce a nonfluorescing yellow or green pigment that may diffuse into the media. Colonies of *B. cepacia* are nonwrinkled, and this trait may be used to differentiate isolates from *P. stutzeri*, which also produces a yellow pigment.

B. cepacia is intrinsically resistant to aminoglycosides and polymyxins; in addition, many strains are resistant to β-lactam antibiotics. Isolates might be susceptible to chloramphenicol, ceftazidime, piperacillin, minocycline, some fluoroquinolones, and SXT. Susceptibility to the carbapenems is variable. Resistance can develop quite rapidly during treatment. A broth

microdilution or Etest minimal inhibitory concentration (MIC) can be performed, and CLSI provides interpretive criteria for reporting ticarcillin-clavulanic acid, ceftazidime, meropenem, minocycline, levofloxacin, chloramphenicol and SXT. The CLSI recommends that if disk diffusion is the method of susceptibility testing, strict criteria for reading the zones of inhibition should be followed and only ceftazidime, meropenem, minocycline, and SXT should be reported.

Burkholderia gladioli

Primarily a plant pathogen, *Burkholderia gladioli* resembles *B. cepacia* and is sometimes mistaken for it. Isolates have been found in patients with CF and chronic granulomatous disease. Rarely *B. gladioli* organisms have been recovered from the blood and tissue of immunocompromised patients. A yellow pigment may be produced. These organisms are motile by means of one or two polar flagella and are catalase and urease positive. *B. gladioli* oxidizes glucose, is mannitol positive and decarboxylase negative, grows on MAK agar, and is 100% resistant to polymyxin B. *B. gladioli* produces variable results with oxidase and nitrate reduction, but results are usually negative. Specific species identification of *B. gladioli* is difficult without the use of molecular tools for confirmation; however, *B. gladioli* isolates are more susceptible to antimicrobials than *B. cepacia*. *B. gladioli* is usually susceptible to aminoglycosides, carbapenems, ciprofloxacin, and SXT but resistant to aztreonam and the cephalosporins.

Burkholderia mallei

Burkholderia mallei causes glanders, a zoonosis primarily affecting livestock such as horses, mules, and donkeys. It is rare in humans but can produce severe local suppurative or acute pulmonary infections. The organism is considered by government agencies to be a potential bioterrorist agent. The only case of glanders in the United States in the last 50 years was due to a laboratory accident. *B. mallei* is a nonmotile gram-negative coccobacillus with nonpigmented colonies and no distinctive odor. Growth on MAK agar and oxidase production is variable; glucose is oxidized and nitrates are reduced to nitrites and isolates are ADH positive.

Burkholderia pseudomallei

Burkholderia pseudomallei causes melioidosis, an aggressive granulomatous pulmonary disease caused by ingestion, inhalation, or inoculation of the organisms with further metastatic abscess formation in lungs and other viscera. Overwhelming septicemia can occur. Local infections, including orbital cellulitis, dacryocystitis, and draining abscesses, might occur. Pneumonia is the most common presentation. The incubation period can be prolonged. The organisms are found in water and muddy soils in Southeast Asia (including Vietnam and Thailand), Northern Australia, and Mexico. Those who have traveled to endemic areas are at risk for infection with *B. pseudomallei*.

B. pseudomallei should be considered when a nonfermentative, wrinkled colony is isolated (Figure 21-9) that demonstrates bipolar staining on Gram-stained smears. *Pseudomonas stutzeri*, which may also appear as wrinkled colonies, does not utilize lactose, in contrast to *B. pseudomallei*. A selective medium, Ashdown, is supplemented with colistin; colonies on

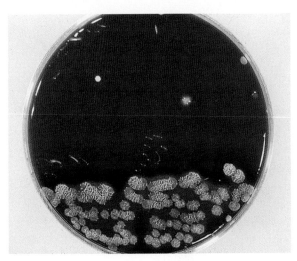

FIGURE 21-9 *Burkholderia pseudomallei* on sheep blood agar.

this agar are deep pink because of the absorption of neutral red in the medium. Colonies will also exhibit an "earthy" odor; however, work should be done in a biological safety cabinet when *B. pseudomallei* is suspected. As with all organisms, "sniffing" of plates should be discouraged.

B. pseudomallei has been placed on the list of organisms considered agents of bioterrorism (see Chapter 30). If *B. pseudomallei* is isolated from someone who never traveled to an endemic area, the occurrence should be reported to local or state public health departments. Although isolates may be susceptible in vitro to many antimicrobial agents, including SXT, chloramphenicol, tetracycline, semisynthetic penicillins, and ceftazidime, the clinical response to therapy is usually slow, and relapses are common. SXT and the fluoroquinolones do seem to work clinically. As with many of the nonfermenters, the CLSI does not recommend disk diffusion for testing, and specific breakpoints for resistance have not been determined.

Moraxella and Oligella

Members of the genus *Moraxella* are strongly oxidase positive, nonmotile, and coccobacillary to bacillary gram-negative bacilli. They are in general biochemically inert with regard to carbohydrate oxidation. They are strictly aerobic and most often susceptible to penicillin, an unusual characteristic for the nonfermenters. These isolates are opportunists that reside on the mucous membranes of humans and lower animals and can be isolated from the respiratory tract, urinary tract, and eyes; however, they rarely cause disease in humans. Members of the genus *Moraxella* that are commonly encountered include *M. catarrhalis, M. nonliquefaciens, M. lacunata, M. osloensis, M. lincolnii,* and *M. atlantae. M. phenylpyruvica* has been reclassified as *Psychrobacter phenylpyruvicus.*

Moraxella catarrhalis is frequently isolated from clinical specimens, especially from respiratory and ear specimens. This species resembles the *Neisseria* by exhibiting gram-negative coccal morphology, and at one time it was called *N. catarrhalis* and also *Branhamella catarrhalis. M. catarrhalis* is discussed in Chapter 17.

Moraxella nonliquefaciens is the second most commonly isolated member of the genus after *M. catarrhalis.* It often

resides as normal biota in the respiratory tract and rarely causes disease in humans. Rare cases of bacteremia, keratitis, and endophthalmitis caused by *M. nonliquefaciens* have been reported. The organism is gelatin hydrolysis negative and urease negative and does not usually grow on MAK agar. It is phenylalanine deaminase (PDA) negative as well.

Moraxella osloensis is similar morphologically and biochemically to *M. nonliquefaciens;* unlike the latter, however, it grows and produces an alkaline reaction in acetate medium and acidifies ethanol. *M. osloensis* is found as normal biota in the genitourinary tract. *P. phenylpyruvicus* has been isolated from urine, blood, cerebrospinal fluid (CSF), and the genitourinary tract. It is urease positive and also PDA positive. *M. atlantae,* similar to *P. phenylpyruvicus,* is more fastidious but will grow on MAK agar. It can also spread and pit the agar surfaces of the medium on which it grows. It is gelatin negative, PDA negative, and nitrate negative. *M. lacunata,* a common conjunctival isolate, is a small coccobacillus that is usually gelatin positive, urease negative, and unable to grow on MAK agar. It may be PDA positive.

The genus *Oligella* is related to the genus *Moraxella.* Members of the genus *Oligella* include *O. urethralis* and *O. ureolytica. Oligella* are small, paired, gram-negative bacilli or coccoid organisms, most often isolated from the urinary tract. There has been one report of a blood culture isolate from a patient with obstructive uropathy in which the isolate was believed to be significant. These organisms are nonoxidative, PDA positive, oxidase positive, nitrate and nitrite positive with nitrogen gas formation, and gelatinase and indole negative. Most strains of *O. ureolytica* are motile by means of peritrichous flagella—hence the relationship to *Alcaligenes* as well as to *Taylorella.* The positive PDA helps to differentiate them from *Alcaligenes* spp. *O. urethralis* is nonmotile. *Oligella* spp. usually do not grow on MAK agar and, unlike members of the genus *Moraxella,* they alkalinize citrate when the test is performed on an aerobic low-glucose peptone slant. *O. urethralis* is susceptible to most antimicrobials including penicillin. The susceptibility pattern of *O. ureolytica* to antimicrobial agents is variable and, if needed, should be performed on each isolate.

LESS COMMONLY ENCOUNTERED NONFERMENTATIVE GRAM-NEGATIVE BACILLI

Alcaligenes and Achromobacter

The medically important species of *Alcaligenes* and *Achromobacter* are divided into the asaccharolytic species (*Alcaligenes faecalis, Achromobacter piechaudii,* and *Achromobacter denitrificans*) and the sacchrolytic species (*Achromobacter xylosoxidans* and the unnamed *Achromobacter* groups B, E, and F). Isolates of these genera are found in water (e.g., swimming pools, tap water, dialysis fluids) and are resistant to disinfectants such as chlorhexidine and quaternary ammonium compounds. They are isolated in specimens from hospitalized patients such as urine, feces, sputum, and wounds.

The asaccharolytic members of this group are less likely isolated from clinical specimens than the saccharolytic species;

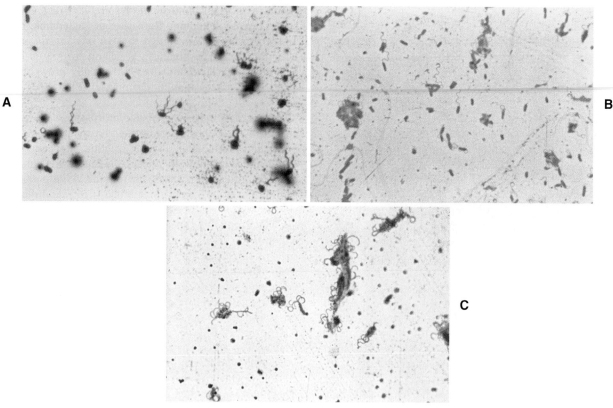

FIGURE 21-10 Flagella stains of gram-negative bacilli. **A,** Peritrichous flagella (e.g., *Alcaligenes* sp.) **B,** Polar, monotrichous (e.g., *Pseudomonas aeruginosa*.) **C,** Polar, multitrichous (e.g., *Comamonas* spp.)

among the former, *A. faecalis* is the species most often seen in clinical specimens and has been isolated from the blood of patients with and without septicemia. *A. piechaudii* has been isolated from the ear of a diabetic patient. Gram-stained smears of the exudate were positive for gram-negative bacilli and gram-positive cocci. Both coagulase-negative staphylococci and *A. piechaudii* were repeatedly isolated. The patient recovered once the diabetes was stabilized. *A. xylosoxidans* is the most commonly isolated member of the genera *Alcaligenes* and *Achromobacter;* it has been associated with cases of otitis media, meningitis, pneumonia, surgical wound infections, UTI, peritonitis, and bacteremia. *A. xylosoxidans* is a frequent colonizer in patients with CF.

Alcaligenes faecalis and the *Achromobacter* spp. possess peritrichous flagella (Figure 21-10), are oxidase positive, and are obligately aerobic gram-negative bacilli. These organisms usually grow well on most laboratory media, including Mac-Conkey agar. On SBA most species are nonpigmented (Figure 21-11). Some strains may produce a fruity odor and cause a green discoloration on SBA. In O-F medium, most isolates are nonoxidative and produce a deep blue color at the top, except for *A. xylosoxidans*, which produces an acid reaction in both glucose and xylose (hence the name). All species reduce nitrates to nitrites; *A. xylosoxidans* and *A. faecalis* can further reduce nitrites to nitrogen gas. Isolates are negative for indole production and esculin hydrolysis.

The asaccharolytic members of the group, *A. faecalis* and *A. piechaudii* are usually susceptible to SXT, piperacillin,

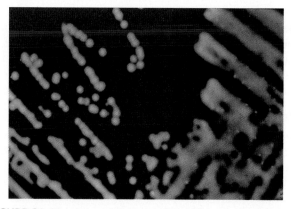

FIGURE 21-11 *Achromobacter xylosoxidans* on sheep blood agar.

ticarcillin, ceftazidime, and quinolones (although variability occurs). Resistance to aztreonam and the aminoglycosides is common. Some strains of *A. piechaudii* may be susceptible to amoxicillin. *A. xylosoxidans* is usually resistant to aminoglycosides, ampicillin, first- and second-generation cephalosporins, chloramphenicol, and fluoroquinolones, but usually are susceptible to piperacillin, third-generation cephalosporins, carbapenems, and SXT. Resistance to all of these antimicrobial agents has been increasing, however, especially in immunocompromised patients in which *A. xylosoxidans* is isolated.

A new genus *Advenella* containing one species, *A. incenata,* was described in 2005 as a novel member of the family Alcaligenaceae. Colonies are light brown in color and oxidase and catalase positive with variability demonstrated for motility and oxidation of glucose. They have been isolated from sputa, wounds, and blood, although their significance is unclear.

Two other genera of oxidase positive, indole negative, asaccharolytic nonfermenters closely associated to the Alcaligenaceae are *Aquaspirillum* and *Laribacter hongkongensis.* *Aquaspirillum* spp. produced pale yellow, buttery-like colonies that do not grow in the presence of 3% NaCl. Cells are helical on Gram stain. Species of *Aquaspirillum* have an aquatic habitat and have been isolated from laboratory distilled water tanks. Clinically, the Centers for Disease Control and Prevention (CDC) has reported isolates from blood cultures in at least three patients. Identification of this organism has been accomplished with molecular techniques. *L. hongkongensis* has yet to be isolated in North America, but it has been isolated in Asia from blood, pleural fluid, and diarrheic stool.

Balneatrix

The genus *Balneatrix* contains a single species, *B. alpaca,* a curved to straight rod that is motile by polar flagella. It was first isolated in 1987 during an outbreak of pneumonia and meningitis associated with persons attending a hot spring spa. Colonies of *B. alpaca* are pale yellow, becoming brown with age. No growth occurs on MAK agar. The isolates are positive for oxidase, indole, nitrate reduction, gelatin, and lecithinase. The organism oxidizes glucose, mannose, fructose, and other sugars. It is similar to *Elizabethkingia meningoseptica,* (formerly *Chryseomonas meningosepticum*) in appearance, but motility and nitrate reduction should help to differentiate *Balneatrix* from *Elizabethkingia.* Isolates are usually susceptible to all β-lactams, aminoglycosides, SXT, quinolones, nalidixic acid, and tetracycline. *Balneatrix* is resistant to clindamycin and vancomycin, unlike *E. meningoseptica.*

Brevundimonas

Brevundimonas spp. are infrequent isolates in clinical microbiology laboratories. *B. diminuta* has been found in blood, CSF, urine, and wounds; it is usually considered a contaminant. The isolates are motile and possess a short wavelength on their single polar flagellum. *B. diminuta* oxidizes glucose and is indole negative and oxidase positive; most colonies are white, but some isolates produce a brown, water-soluble pigment on heart infusion agar with tyrosine added. Most strains grow on MAK agar. In vitro, the organism demonstrates resistance to ampicillin, cefoxitin, and nalidixic acid; intrinsic resistance to fluoroquinolones has been detected.

Brevundimonas vesicularis has been reported as a cause of meningitis, infective endocarditis, and infections in a patient undergoing chronic peritoneal dialysis. It has also been isolated, with unknown significance, from urine and eye specimens. Like *B. diminuta,* *B. vesicularis* is a slender rod with short-wavelength polar flagella. Only about 25% of *B. vesicularis* strains will grow on MAK agar. Most strains of *B. vesicularis* produce an orange intracellular pigment. *B. vesicularis* is also oxidase positive and oxidizes glucose and maltose. Esculin hydrolysis is the best test to differentiate the two species; approximately 88% of *B. vesicularis* isolates are positive, whereas *B. diminuta* is rarely positive. *B. vesicularis* has been described as susceptible to fluoroquinolones and piperacillin/tazobactam but resistant to carbapenems, aztreonam, and the cephalosporins.

CDC Groups EO-3, EO-4, *Paracoccus,* and *Psychrobacter*

The taxonomy of CDC groups, EO-3, and EO-4, and *Paracoccus,* and *Psychrobacter* is unclear; EO refers to **eugonic oxidizer.** Isolates of *Paracoccus yeei* have been recovered from blood cultures and cutaneous bullae in a 67-year-old man. It was also found in at least one case of uveitis for which it was considered the potential pathogen. 16S rRNA sequencing of EO-3 strains has shown it to closely match *Fulvimarina pelagi;* however, it has not as yet been renamed. EO-3 has been reported in a case of chronic ambulatory peritoneal dialysis infection. Isolates of *P. yeei,* EO-3, and EO-4 have been obtained from urine, eye discharge, blood, pleural fluid, CSF, and from lung, throat, and genitourinary tract specimens in which their clinical significance remains unclear.

Isolates of *P. yeei,* EO-3, and EO-4 are oxidase positive, indole negative, nonmotile, saccharolytic coccobacilli that grow weakly if at all on MAK agar. They all oxidize glucose and xylose but differ in oxidation of lactose and mannitol. They are all negative for decarboxylases, esculin, and gelatin but may be positive for urease. EO-3 and many EO-4 isolates have a yellow nondiffusible pigment. *P. yeei* is further characterized by the production of characteristic coccoid or O-shaped cells on Gram stain, the latter of which results from the presence of vacuolated or peripherally stained cells. Susceptibility to antimicrobial agents is not well known.

Psychrobacter immobilis differs from the EO organisms by being psychrotrophic (optimal temperature for growth is 20° C). They have been isolated from fish, processed meat, and poultry. Clinically they have been isolated from the eye of a newborn, who had acquired the infection nosocomially via a water source. *P. immobilis* organisms were also reportedly isolated from the blood and CSF of a 2-day-old infant. *P. immobilis* is a nonmotile, oxidase positive, oxidative diplococcus. Isolates resemble *Moraxella* but are usually not penicillin susceptible. Isolates grow well at 5° to 25° C but rarely at 35° C. They are nitrate positive and can grow on Thayer-Martin medium. An odor of roses (resembling phenylethyl alcohol) has been reported.

Chromobacterium

Chromobacterium violaceum is the only species in the genus *Chromobacterium.* Reservoirs are soil and water; isolates are more commonly found in tropical and subtropical climates. *C. violaceum* is an opportunistic pathogen, attacking the immunocompromised patient with neutrophil deficits (including patients with chronic granulomatous disease), usually as a result of contamination of wounds with water or soil. It has been isolated from cases of osteomyelitis, abscesses and septicemia, as well as from urine and gastrointestinal infections. A skin lesion is the typical portal of entry.

C. violaceum is a fermentative gram-negative bacillus that can be oxidase positive, and hence it might be mistaken initially as a nonfermenter. It is motile with polar flagella and, as its name implies, produces a violet pigment (about 91% of the time). The pigment, violacein, is ethanol-soluble and water-insoluble. The presence of the pigment may hamper proper oxidase reactions. Isolates are usually indole negative, but nonpigmented strains may be indole positive. Isolates ferment glucose and, variably, sucrose; they grow on MacConkey agar and most enteric media, reduce nitrate, and grow at 42° C. On Gram stain, the organisms may appear as curved bacilli that might resemble vibrios, which are oxidase positive. Nonpigmented strains have been confused with *Aeromonas* spp. If the oxidase reaction is negative, *C. violaceum* can resemble members of the family Enterobacteriaceae.

C. violaceum isolates are sensitive to fluoroquinolones, tetracyclines, carbapenems, gentamicin and SXT. However, they are resistant to β-lactam antibiotics. A high mortality rate with *C. violaceum* has been recognized even with adequate therapy because of the underlying disease of the patients involved.

Comamonas

Comamonas spp. resemble vibrios or spirillum-like bacteria, produce alkalinity in O-F medium, are catalase and oxidase positive, are usually motile by multitrichous polar flagella, and accumulate hydroxybutyrate intracellularly. Ubiquitous in soil and water, *Comamonas* spp. are rarely isolated from clinical specimens but have been found in hospital equipment and fluids. Rare isolates have been reported to cause nosocomial bacteremia, corneal ulcerations, endocarditis in intravenous drug abusers, sepsis, and pyoarthrosis. It is phenotypically difficult to distinguish among the *Comamonas* spp.; therefore isolates are usually reported as *Comamonas* spp. *C. acidovorans*, which may be more resistant to antimicrobial agents, including aminoglycosides, than other members of the genus, has been renamed *Delftia acidovorans*. *D. acidovorans* can oxidize fructose and mannitol; some strains produce a fluorescent pigment and some a soluble yellow to tan hue.

Flavobacteriaceae

The genus *Flavobacterium* has undergone extensive revision. What once was a large diverse group of gram-negative, weak to nonfermentative bacilli belonging to a single genus has been separated into several new genera. *Flavobacterium, Chryseobacterium, Elizabethkingia, Empedobacter, Myroides, Weeksella, Bergeyella,* and several unnamed CDC groups belong to the family Flavobacteriaceae. The remaining *Flavobacterium* spp. are indole negative and are not found in human specimens. Members of the family Flavobacteriaceae are ubiquitous in soil and water and are not considered part of the normal human biota. Because isolates often contaminate hospital equipment, they can be important causes of nosocomial infections. Even though the organisms are weak fermenters, the reactions are usually delayed, and the isolates initially appear to be nonfermenters.

Chryseobacterium (Flavobacterium) indologenes is the most frequently isolated species, although it is rarely significant. It has been linked to nosocomial infections such as

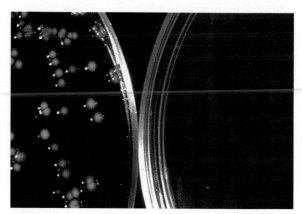

FIGURE 21-12 *Elizabethkingia (Chryseobacterium) meningosepticum.* Note the growth with yellow pigment on sheep blood agar *(left)* and absence of growth on MacConkey plate *(right).*

bacteremia. Most diseases produced by members of this group are due to *Elizabethkingia (Chryseobacterium) meningosepticum.* The disease typically presents as a meningitis or septicemia in a newborn, especially in conjunction with prematurity. In adults *E. meningosepticum* can cause pneumonia, endocarditis, bacteremia, and meningitis. Isolated cases of peritonitis and keratitis have been recently reported.

Members of the family Flavobacteriaceae are nonmotile and often possess a yellow intracellular pigment, which is especially prominent in species IIb (Figure 21-12). On media with blood, a lavender-green discoloration of the agar may occur because of the proteolytic activity of the organisms. Some species release a characteristic fruity odor. Most are DNase positive, oxidase positive, gelatin hydrolysis positive, and weakly indole positive (the more sensitive Ehrlich indole test is recommended over the Kovac test). All except *Myroides odoratus* and *Myroides odoratimimus* are indole positive, a distinctive characteristic. *M. odoratus* and *M. odoratimimus* are very difficult to separate and are rarely isolated in the clinical laboratory. Microscopically, *E. meningosepticum* and *C. indologenes* are long, thin bacilli, often with bulbous ends.

In vitro, most species are resistant to aminoglycosides and β-lactam antibiotics, but some species are susceptible to vancomycin and rifampin, which is an unusual characteristic for gram-negative bacilli, including the nonfermenters. However, one report of susceptibility testing of more than 50 isolates of *Chryseobacterium* spp. demonstrated reduced activity to vancomycin as compared to what had been previously reported by others. Activity to SXT, fluoroquinolones, and piperacillin/tazobactam was good. The response to other antimicrobial agents is variable, and an in vitro susceptibility test is needed if the isolate is considered clinically relevant.

The previously unnamed *Flavobacterium* spp., IIf and IIj, have been renamed as members of the genus *Weeksella*. These isolates are asaccharolytic, indole and oxidase positive, and fail to grow on MAK agar. *W. virosa* (formerly CDC group IIf) colonies may be mucoid or "slimy" and possess a yellow-green pigment. Isolates have been found from genitourinary specimens and will grow on Thayer-Martin or other media selective for *Neisseria gonorrhoeae*. *Bergeyella* (*Weeksella*) *zoohelicum* is nonmucoid, although its colonies may be sticky. It is urease positive and polymyxin B resistant but otherwise similar to *W. virosa*. *B. zoohelicum* has been isolated from many sources, in particular from dog and cat bite wounds. *Weeksella* and *Bergeyella* spp. are susceptible to penicillin and a variety of other antimicrobial agents.

Groups EF-4a and EF-4b

Eugonic fermenter (EF) is a group of nonfastidious fermenters distinguished from the unnamed **dysgonic fermenters,** which are fastidious fermenters. Dysgonic fermenters were placed into the genus *Capnocytophaga* and are discussed in Chapter 18. EF-4a and EF-4b both belong to the family Neisseriaceae and are part of the normal biota of dogs, cats, and rodents. They have been isolated from infected areas after dog and cat bites or contact with these animals.

Eugonic fermenter isolates are nonmotile, short rods to coccobacilli and are oxidase and catalase positive. EF-4a is a glucose fermenter. It can produce a yellow to tan pigment, reduces nitrate to gas, may grow on MAK agar, and may liquefy gelatin or grow at 42° C. EF-4a ferments only glucose and is negative for indole and urea and can be ADH positive. Colonies give off a characteristic popcorn like odor, a trait shared with EF-4b. EF-4b is an oxidizer of glucose, not a fermenter, and is ADH negative. In addition, EF-4b is gelatinase negative and does not reduce nitrates to gas. Both EF-4a and EF-4b are susceptible to most β-lactams, chloramphenicol, tetracycline, fluoroquinolones, and variably susceptible to penicillin, aminoglycosides and the macrolides.

Methylobacterium and *Roseomonas*

The genus *Methylobacterium* contains 20 named species plus additional unnamed biovars; isolates produce a characteristic pink to coral pigment and are able to utilize methanol as a sole source of carbon and energy. Epidemiologically the *Methylobacterium* are isolated from soil, vegetation, sewage, water, and hospital nebulizers. They have also been recovered from clinical specimens such as throat swabs, bronchial washes, and even blood specimens. Clinically these organisms have been reported to cause bacteremia (one case), peritonitis, synovitis, and skin ulcers. Contaminated tap water has been implicated as a cause of positive blood cultures in a patient receiving irrigations who had recently undergone a bone marrow transplant.

Methylobacterium mesophilicum (formerly *Pseudomonas mesophilica* and *P. extorquens*) and *M. zatmanii* are the species most often isolated in clinical specimens; they prefer a lower temperature (25 to 35° C), produce distinctive large vacuolated pleomorphic rods, are oxidase positive, and are motile with a polar flagellum. Oxidation of carbohydrates is weak; urea and starch are hydrolyzed. Isolates are slow growers, producing 1-mm sized dry colonies in 4 to 5 days. They are often first seen on fungal media, such as Sabouraud dextrose agar, and do not grow as well on blood, chocolate, Thayer-Martin, or buffered charcoal yeast extract agars. No growth on MAK agar is typical.

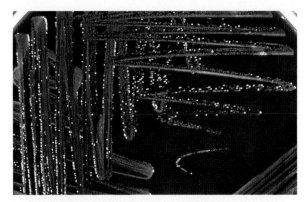

FIGURE 21-13 *Roseomonas* sp. on sheep blood agar; note the pink to red colonies.

The other pink-pigmented, nonfermentative bacilli are a group of bacteria now classified in the genus *Roseomonas*. These bacteria have been isolated from blood, CSF, sputum, abscesses, and wounds, as well as from the environment. One species, *R. gilardii* may have more pathogenic potential than other species in the genus, including the cause of catheter-related bacteremia. Distinguishing them from *Methylobacterium* spp. may be difficult. *Roseomonas* spp. are unable to oxidize methanol or assimilate acetamide. On Sabouraud dextrose agar, they produce pink, mucoid, almost "runny" colonies (Figure 21-13); however, they do not appear black under long-wavelength ultraviolet light as do the *Methylobacterium* spp. *Roseomonas* spp. are nonvacuolated, coccoid bacteria, forming pairs and short chains. They are variable in the oxidase reaction, often weak to negative, but are catalase and urease positive.

Methylobacterium spp. are usually susceptible to the aminoglycosides and SXT. Susceptibility to β-lactam antibiotics is variable. If needed, susceptibility tests should be incubated at 30° C for 48 hours. *Roseomonas* spp. are susceptible to the aminoglycosides, fluoroquinolones, and carbapenems. Susceptibility to β-lactams and SXT is variable.

Nonfluorescent Pseudomonad Group

Pseudomonas stutzeri

Pseudomonas stutzeri, although a rare isolate and even rarer pathogen in the clinical laboratory, is usually easily recognizable because of its characteristic macroscopic colony appearance—wrinkled, leathery, adherent colonies that can produce a light-yellow or brown pigment (Figure 21-14). In the immunocompromised host, *P. stutzeri* has been reported to be responsible for diseases that include septicemia, pneumonia (especially in patients with CF and immunocompromised patients), endocarditis, postsurgical wound infections, septic arthritis, conjunctivitis, and UTIs. Isolates are usually susceptible to the aminoglycosides, SXT, ampicillin and polymyxin, tetracyclines, fluoroquinolones, and third-generation cephalosporins (e.g., ceftazidime) but resistant to chloramphenicol and the first- and second-generation cephalosporins. Because of the adherent nature of colonies of *P. stutzeri*, in vitro susceptibility testing can be unreliable.

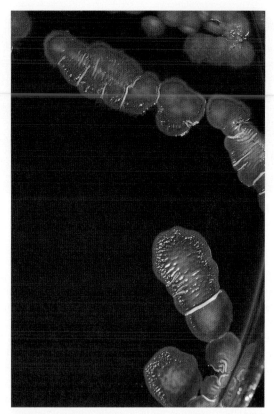

FIGURE 21-14 *Pseudomonas stutzeri* on sheep blood agar. Note the wrinkled appearance of the colonies.

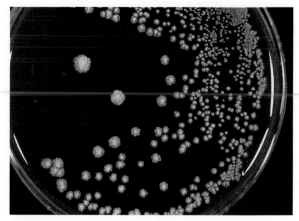

FIGURE 21-15 *Pseudomonas oryzihabitans* wrinkled yellow colonies on sheep blood agar plate at 48 hours.

Pseudomonas mendocina

Pseudomonas mendocina can be found in soil and water, but it is rarely isolated from human specimens; when it is, it is usually considered a contaminant. *P. mendocina* resembles a nonpigmented *P. aeruginosa* isolate, but it is acetamide and 2-ketogluconate negative. *P. mendocina* is motile by means of a single polar flagellum, it oxidizes glucose and xylose, is positive for oxidase and ADH, and is nonproteolytic.

Pseudomonas luteola and Pseudomonas oryzihabitans

The natural habitat of *Pseudomonas luteola* (formerly *Chryseomonas luteola*) and *P. oryzihabitans* (formerly *Flavimonas oryzihabitans*) is unknown, although members of both genera have been isolated from soil and water. *P. oryzihabitans* has been found in Japanese rice paddies and has been isolated from hospital drains and respiratory therapy equipment. These two pseudomonads are rarely recovered from humans, but they have been isolated from wounds, abscesses, blood cultures, peritoneal and chronic ambulatory peritoneal dialysis fluids, and other sources. They have also been implicated in cases of peritonitis and possibly meningitis, although many times in association with each other or with other bacteria. *P. luteola* has been recovered as the only isolate from a case of prosthetic valve endocarditis and subdiaphragmatic abscess.

P. oryzihabitans has been isolated in eye cultures and was described as the cause of "sticky eye" in one patient who responded to antimicrobial therapy. There appears to be higher risk for infection by these organisms in the presence of foreign materials (e.g., catheters), corticosteroid use, and immunocompromised states.

P. luteola and *P. oryzihabitans* are gram-negative, nonfermentative, oxidase-negative bacilli. They both are catalase positive and motile, oxidize glucose and other sugars, grow on MAK agar, and often produce an intracellular nondiffusible yellow pigment (Figure 21-15). Both species typically produce wrinkled or rough colonies at 48 hours. *P. luteola* can be differentiated from *P. oryzihabitans* by ONPG and esculin hydrolysis.

Both *P. luteola* and *P. oryzihabitans* are susceptible to aminoglycosides, third-generation cephalosporins, ureidopenicillins, and quinolones. *P. oryzihabitans* isolates are resistant to first- and second-generation cephalosporins but are usually susceptible to penicillin. *P. luteola* is usually sensitive to all β-lactams. Both demonstrate variable susceptibilities to tetracycline, chloramphenicol, and SXT.

Ralstonia and Cupriavidus

Ralstonia pickettii is the most common species of the genus *Ralstonia* isolated from humans. Isolates of *R. pickettii* can be found contaminating sterile hospital fluids and can be isolated from human specimens such as urine, nasopharynx, abscesses, wounds, and blood, usually as colonizers or contaminants. It has been isolated from respiratory specimens of patients with CF, but it has not been associated with any disease in this group. *R. pickettii* isolates are slow growers; it can take more than 72 hours on primary cultures before colonies are visible. *R. pickettii* is oxidase, catalase (although catalase negative strains exist), and urease positive; grows on MAK agar; reduces nitrate; oxidizes glucose and xylose, and is motile by means of a single polar flagellum. *R. pickettii* is susceptible to most agents, except for the aminoglycosides and polymyxin.

Cupriavidus pauculus, formerly *Ralstonia paucula,* has been isolated from a number of aquatic environments and was recently recognized as an opportunistic pathogen causing serious infections including septicemia, peritonitis, abscesses, and tenosynovitis, most notably in immunocompromised patients. *C. pauculus* is a motile (peritrichous flagella), oxidase-positive, catalase-positive, asaccharolytic, gram-negative bacillus. Isolates are urease positive but negative for gelatinase, esculin hydrolysis, and indole. Isolates cannot reduce nitrates to nitrites and are PDA negative. They usually grow on MAK agar. Isolates are resistant to aminoglycosides, ampicillin, and first- and second-generation cephalosporins. They are usually susceptible to quinolones, third-generation cephalosporins, piperacillin, and doxycycline, although not many isolates have been tested.

Shewanella

Shewanella putrefaciens and *S. algae,* although infrequent isolates, have been recovered from a variety of human specimens. These organisms are rarely pathogenic; isolates can be obtained from abscesses and traumatic ulcers, but they are usually present in mixed culture and probably represent colonization rather than infection. Environmental sources—such as stagnant water, natural gas, petroleum brine, and spoiled dairy products—can contain *S. putrefaciens. S. algae* is more frequently isolated from clinical specimens than *S. putrefaciens,* whereas *S. putrefaciens* is more frequently isolated from environmental sources.

Both species produce profuse H_2S in TSI agar, possibly resembling H_2S producers of the family Enterobacteriaceae. The oxidase test should differentiate *Shewanella* from the family Enterobacteriaceae. *S. putrefaciens* produces a tan to brown pigment that might cause a discoloration to the media. *S. algae* requires NaCl (halophilic) and is asaccharolytic, whereas *S. putrefaciens* is nonhalophilic and saccharolytic. The organisms are usually susceptible to ampicillin, tetracycline, chloramphenicol, erythromycin, and the aminoglycosides, but resistant to penicillin and first-generation cephalosporins.

Sphingobacterium

Members of the genus *Sphingobacterium* at one time were regarded as members of the genus *Flavobacterium.* Several species are currently placed in this genus; the two most frequently isolated species are *S. multivorum* and *S. spiritovorum.* Clinically *S. multivorum* has been isolated from the blood of patients with septicemia and from cases of peritonitis. *S. spiritovorum* has also been isolated from clinical specimens, primarily blood and urine, and from hospital environments. *S. mizutae,* formerly called *Flavobacterium mizutaii,* has been isolated from a case of meningitis in premature birth and suspected in a case of cellulitis.

These isolates are aflagellate but can produce gliding motility. They are oxidase, catalase, and esculin positive but indole negative. The presence of sphingophospholipids in the cell wall is unique to the group. They are truly fermenters and oxidize some carbohydrates. Growth on MAK agar is sparse to none, but these organisms will grow in the presence of 40%

bile. *S. spiritovorum* and *S. multivorum* are very similar biochemically, but *S. spiritovorum* produces acid from mannitol, ethanol, and rhamnose, and *S. multivorum* does not. Both species produce a yellow pigment similar to that of isolates of *Chryseobacterium, Weeksella,* and *Empedobacter* spp. Most isolates of *Sphingobacterium* spp. are sensitive to SXT and the fluoroquinolones and resistant to aminoglycosides, clindamycin, and polymyxin B. Susceptibility to β-lactam antibiotics is variable.

Sphingomonas

Sphingomonas paucimobilis can be isolated environmentally from water, including that in swimming pools, as well as from hospital equipment and laboratory supplies. The genus *Sphingomonas* contains at least 12 species, but only two are believed to be clinically significant: *S. paucimobilis* and *S. parapaucimobilis.* Documented *S. paucimobilis* infections include peritonitis associated with chronic ambulatory peritoneal dialysis, septicemia, meningitis, leg ulcer, empyema, and splenic and brain abscesses. *S. parapaucimobilis* has been isolated from sputum, urine, and vaginal specimens. Although isolates have been found to produce esterases, endotoxin, lipases, and phosphatases, inherent virulence is limited, and most isolates must be regarded as colonizers or contaminants.

The yellow-pigmented *S. paucimobilis* does not grow on MAK agar and requires more than 48 hours for growth on SBA (Figure 21-16). Isolates are weakly oxidase positive (some strains may be negative), motile at 18° to 22° C but not at 37° C, urease negative, indole negative, and oxidizers. *S. parapaucimobilis* resembles *S. paucimobilis* except that isolates of *S. parapaucimobilis* are H_2S positive by the lead acetate method, Simmon's citrate positive, and DNase negative. *S. paucimobilis* isolates demonstrate variable resistance to antimicrobial agents, although most are susceptible to the aminoglycosides, tetracyclines, chloramphenicol, and SXT; susceptibility to the third-generation cephalosporins (e.g., ceftazidime, ceftriaxone, ceftizoxime) and fluoroquinolones varies has been reported. They are susceptible to polymyxin B, which differentiates isolates from members of the genus *Sphingobacterium,* to which it is similar.

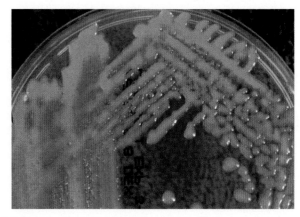

FIGURE 21-16 *Sphingomonas paucimobilis* on trypticase soy agar; note the yellow colonies.

BIBLIOGRAPHY

Aisenberg G et al: Bacteremia caused by *Achromobacter* and *Alcaligenes* species in 46 patients with cancer (1989-2003), *Cancer* 101:2134, 2004.

Arora U et al: *Ochrobactrum anthropi* septicaemia, *Indian J Med Microbiol* 26:81, 2008.

Blondel-Hill E et al: *Pseudomonas*. In Murray PR et al, editors: *Manual of clinical microbiology*, ed 9, Washington, DC, 2007, ASM Press.

Brisse S et al: Comparative evaluation of the BD Phoenix and VITEK 2 automated instruments for identification of isolates of *Burkholderia cepacia* complex, *J Clin Microbiol* 40:1743, 2002.

Casalta JP et al: Prosthetic valve endocarditis caused by *Pseudomonas luteola*, *BMC Infect Dis* 5:82, 2005.

Chihab W et al: *Chryseomonas luteola* identified as the source of serious infections in a Moroccan University Hospital, *J Clin Microbiol* 42:1837, 2004.

Christakis GB et al: *Chryseobacterium indologenes* non-catheter-related bacteremia in a patient with a solid tumor, *J Clin Microbiol* 43:2021, 2005.

Clinical and Laboratory Standards Institute: *Performance standards for antimicrobial susceptibility testing, eighteenth international supplement*, CLSI Document M100-S18, Wayne, Pa, 2008, CLSI.

Coenye T et al: Characterization of unusual bacteria isolated from respiratory secretions of cystic fibrosis patients and description of *Inquilinus limosus* gen. nov., sp. nov, *J Clin Microbiol* 40:2062, 2002.

Coeyne T et al: *Advenella incenata* gen. nov., sp. nov., a novel member of the *Alcaligenaceae*, isolated from various clinical specimens, *Int J Syst Evol Microbiol* 55:251, 2005.

Daneshvar MI et al: *Paracoccus yeei* sp. nov. (formerly CDC group EO-2), a novel bacterial species associated with human infection, *J Clin Microbiol* 41:1289, 2003.

Daneshvar MI et al: Assignment of CDC weak oxidizer group 2 (WO-2) to the genus *Pandoraea* and characterization of three new *Pandoraea* genomospecies, *J Clin Microbiol* 39:1819, 2001.

Davies J, Rubin BK: Emerging and unusual gram-negative infections in cystic fibrosis, *Semin Respir Crit Care Med* 28:312, 2007.

De I, Rolston KV, Han XY: Clinical significance of *Roseomonas* species isolated from catheter and blood samples: analysis of 36 cases in patients with cancer, *Clin Infect Dis* 38:1579, 2004.

Drancourt M et al: High prevalence of fastidious bacteria in 1520 cases of uveitis of unknown etiology, *Medicine (Baltimore)* 87:167, 2008.

Funke G, Funke-Kissling P: Evaluation of the new VITEK 2 card for identification of clinically relevant gram-negative rods, *J Clin Microbiol* 42:4067, 2004.

Funke G et al: First comprehensively documented case of *Paracoccus yeei* infection in a human, *J Clin Microbiol* 42:3366, 2004.

Gómez-Cerezo J et al: *Achromobacter xylosoxidans* bacteremia: a 10-year analysis of 54 cases, *Eur J Clin Microbiol Infect Dis* 22:360, 2003.

Hansen PS, Jensen TG, Gahrn-Hansen B: *Dysgonomonas capnocytophagoides* bacteraemia in a neutropenic patient treated for acute myeloid leukaemia, *APMIS* 113:229, 2005.

Hofstad T et al: *Dysgonomonas* gen. nov. to accommodate *Dysgonomonas gadei* sp. nov., an organism isolated from a human gall bladder, and *Dysgonomonas capnocytophagoides* (formerly CDC group DF-3), *Int J Syst Evol Microbiol* 50:2189, 2000.

Hoshino T et al: *Neisseria elongata* subsp. *nitroreducens* endocarditis in a seven-year-old boy, *Pediatr Infect Dis J* 24:391, 2005.

Janknecht P, Schneider CM, Ness T: Outbreak of *Empedobacter brevis* endophthalmitis after cataract extraction, *Graefes Arch Clin Exp Ophthalmol* 240:291, 2002.

Jitmuang A: Human *Chromobacterium violaceum* infection in Southeast Asia: case reports and literature review, *Southeast Asian J Trop Med Public Health* 39:452, 2008.

Lee CH, Tang YF, Liu JW: Underdiagnosis of urinary tract infection caused by *Methylobacterium* species with current standard processing of urine culture and its clinical implications, *J Med Microbiol* 53:755, 2004.

Lee SM et al: Experience of *Comamonas acidovorans* keratitis with delayed onset and treatment response in immunocompromised cornea, *Korean J Ophthalmol* 22:49, 2008.

Lin PY et al: Clinical and microbiological analysis of bloodstream infections caused by *Chryseobacterium meningosepticum* in non-neonatal patients, *J Clin Microbiol* 42:3353, 2004.

Lowe P, Engler C, Norton R: Comparison of automated and non-automated systems for identification of *Burkholderi pseudomallei*, *J Clin Microbiol* 40:4625, 2002.

Manjunath B: Fatal septicaemia due to *Chromobacterium violaceum*, *West Indian Med J* 56:380, 2007.

Marín M et al: Infection of Hickman catheter by *Pseudomonas* (formerly *Flavimonas*) *oryzihabitans* traced to a synthetic bath sponge, *J Clin Microbiol* 38:4577, 2000.

McLean TW et al: Catheter-related bacteremia due to *Roseomonas* species in children with cancer, *Pediatr Blood Cancer* 46:514, 2005.

Moissenet D et al: *Ralstonia paucula* (formerly CDC group IV c-2): unsuccessful strain differentiation with PCR-based methods, study of the 16s-23s spacer of the rRNA operon, and comparison with other *Ralstonia* species (*R. eutropha, R. pickettii, R. gilardii,* and *R. solanacearum*), *J Clin Microbiol* 39:381, 2001.

Mondello P, Ferrari L, Carnevale G: Nosocomial *Brevundimonas vesicularis* meningitis, *Infez Med* 14:235, 2006.

Nolan JS, Waites KB: Nosocomial ventriculitis due to *Roseomonas gilardii* complicating subarachnoid haemorrhage, *J Infect* 50:244, 2005.

O'Hara CM: Manual and automated instrumentation for identification of Enterobacteriaceae and other aerobic gram-negative bacilli, *Clin Microbiol Rev* 18:147, 2005.

O'Hara CM, Miller JM: Evaluation of the MicroScan rapid neg ID3 panel for identification of Enterobacteriaceae and some common gram-negative nonfermeters, *J Clin Microbiol* 38:3577, 2000.

O'Hara CM, Miller JM: Ability of the MicroScan rapid gram-negative ID-type3 panel to identify nonenteric glucose fermenting and nonfermenting gram-negative bacilli, *J Clin Microbiol* 40:3750, 2002.

O'Hara CM, Miller JM: Evaluation of the Vitek 2 ID-GNB assay for identification of members of the family Enterobacteriaceae and other nonenteric gram-negative bacilli and comparison with the Vitek GNI+ card, *J Clin Microbiol* 41:2096, 2003.

Rolston KV et al: Nonfermentative gram-negative bacilli in cancer patients: increasing frequency of infection and antimicrobial susceptibility of clinical isolates to fluoroquinolones, *Diagn Microbiol Infect Dis* 51:215, 2005.

Romero Gómez MP et al: Prosthetic mitral valve endocarditis due to *Ochrobactrum anthropi*: case report, *J Clin Microbiol* 42:3371, 2004.

Sahm DF et al: Evaluation of current activities of fluoroquinolones against gram-negative bacilli using centralized in vitro testing and electronic surveillance, *Antimicrob Agents Chemother* 45:267, 2001.

Saiman L et al: Synergistic activities of macrolide antibiotics against *Pseudomonas aeruginosa, Burkholderia cepacia, Stenotrophomonas maltophilia,* and *Alcaligenes xylosoxidans* isolated from patients with cystic fibrosis, *Antimicrob Agents Chemother* 46:1105, 2002.

Schreckenberger PC et al: *Acinetobacter, Achromobacter, Chryseobacterium, Moraxella,* and other nonfermentative gram-negative rods. In Murray PR et al, editors: *Manual of clinical microbiology*, ed 9, Washington, DC, 2007, ASM Press.

Shukla SK et al: Isolation of a fastidious *Bergeyella* species associated with cellulitis after a cat bite and a phylogenetic comparison with *Bergeyella zoohelcum* strains, *J Clin Microbiol* 42:290, 2004.

Subudhi CP et al: Fatal *Roseomonas gilardii* bacteremia in a patient with refractory blast crisis of chronic myeloid leukemia, *Clin Microbiol Infect* 7:573, 2001.

Tronel H et al: Bacteremia caused by a novel species of *Sphingobacterium*, *Clin Microbiol Infect* 9:1242, 2003.

Tsai CK, Liu CC, Kuo HK: Postoperative endophthalmitis by *Flavimonas oryzihabitans*, *Chang Gung Med J* 27:830, 2004.

Winn W et al, editors: *Koenman's color atlas and textbook of diagnostic microbiology*, ed 6, New York, 2006, Lippincott Williams & Wilkins.

Yang ML et al: Case report: infective endocarditis caused by *Brevundimonas vesicularis*, *BMC Infect Dis* 6:179, 2006.

Points to Remember

- Nonfermenters will not acidify the butt of triple sugar iron or Kligler's iron agar.
- Most nonfermenters are usually oxidase positive, a key test in differentiation from the Enterobacteriaceae.
- Nonfermenters are environmental isolates, which rarely cause disease in healthy humans.
- Nonfermenting gram-negative bacilli are found in a variety of hospital environments and can colonize inanimate objects and solutions, serving as a possible source of infection, especially in compromised hosts.
- Of the gram-negative bacilli isolated from clinical specimens, about 30% will be nonfermenters. The three most common nonfermentative gram-negative bacilli seen in clinical specimens are *Pseudomonas aeruginosa*, *Acinetobacter baumanii* complex, and *Stenotrophomonas maltophilia*.
- *P. aeruginosa* is the only nonfermentative gram-negative bacillus producing pyocyanin, which combines with pyoverdin to form a soluble green pigment.
- Nonfermenters may be more resistant to antimicrobial agents than members of the family Enterobacteriaceae.

Learning Assessment Questions

1. What is the difference between nonfermentative and fermentative organisms?
2. What is the typical natural habitat of most nonfermenters?
3. What types of infections do nonfermenters cause?
4. What risk factors are associated with infections caused by nonfermentative gram-negative bacilli?
5. What are the three most common nonfermentative gram-negative bacilli isolated in the clinical laboratory?
6. What are the susceptibility patterns of the most common nonfermenters?
7. What initial clues indicate that an isolate is a nonfermenter?
8. How would you differentiate *Pseudomonas aeruginosa* from other members of the fluorescent pseudomonad group?
9. What are the identifying characteristics of *Acinetobacter* spp.?
10. How would you differentiate *Burkholderia pseudomallei* from *Pseudomonas stutzeri*?

Anaerobes of Clinical Importance

*Robert C. Fader**

OBJECTIVES

After reading and studying this chapter, you should be able to:

1. Describe anaerobic bacteria including their sensitivity to oxygen and where they may be found in the environment and the human body.

2. Differentiate the various types of anaerobes with regard to atmospheric requirements (i.e., obligate anaerobes, facultative anaerobes, and aerotolerant anaerobes).

3. Describe how anaerobes, as part of endogenous microbiota, initiate and establish infection.

4. Name the endogenous anaerobes commonly involved in human infections.

5. Recognize specimens that are acceptable and unacceptable for anaerobic culture.

6. Describe each of the following as they relate to the culture and isolation of anaerobes:
   ◼ Atmospheric requirements
   ◼ Isolation media
   ◼ Identification systems

7. Given the clues (signs and manifestations) to an anaerobic infection, name the most probable etiologic agent of the following:
   ◼ Wound botulism
   ◼ Tetanus
   ◼ Gas gangrene
   ◼ Actinomycosis
   ◼ Pseudomembranous colitis
   ◼ Bacterial vaginosis

*This chapter builds on the chapter in previous editions written by Paul Engelkirk and Janet Duben-Engelkirk.

8. Compare the microscopic and colony morphology and the results of differentiating tests of anaerobic isolates.

9. Evaluate the laboratory diagnostic methods for *Clostridium difficile.*

10. Compare the pigments produced by various anaerobic bacteria.

11. Discuss antimicrobial susceptibility testing of anaerobes including acceptable susceptibility methods, when anaerobe susceptibility testing should be performed, β-lactamase testing, resistance patterns of anaerobes, and antimicrobial agents to be tested.

12. Describe the four major approaches to treat anaerobe-associated diseases: antimicrobial therapy, surgical therapy, hyperbaric oxygen, and administration of antitoxins.

Case in Point

A 45-year-old male farmer was admitted to the hospital for complications resulting from a tractor accident that caused traumatic injury to his left leg. The patient's leg was painful, bluish, and edematous. A radiograph revealed pockets of gas in the tissue. A complete blood count revealed a marked increase in neutrophils and a total white blood cell count of 33,000/mL. A Gram stain of the wound specimen revealed numerous large, rectangular-shaped, gram-positive bacilli with no spores and very few leukocytes. The patient was immediately scheduled for surgical debridement and was placed on a broad spectrum antimicrobial agent.

Issues to Consider

After reading the patient's case history, consider:
- The clinical significance of anaerobes in human infections
- Indications of an anaerobic infection
- The importance of proper selection, collection, transport, and processing of anaerobic specimens
- Various anaerobes that may be found in different types of specimens
- Extent of anaerobe identification
- When and how to perform susceptibility testing of anaerobes

Key Terms

Actinomycosis	Exogenous anaerobe
Aerotolerance test	Facultative anaerobe
Aerotolerant anaerobe	Hydroxyl radical
Anaerobe	Microaerophilic
Anaerobic chamber	Myonecrosis
Bacterial vaginosis (BV)	Obligate anaerobe
Botulism	Pseudomembranous colitis
Capnophilic	Superoxide anion
Catalase	Superoxide dismutase
Endogenous anaerobe	Tetanus
Enteritis necroticans	

Anaerobic bacteria are important in human and veterinary medicine because they play a role in serious, often fatal, infections and intoxications. They are involved in infectious processes in virtually any organ or tissue of the body and consequently can be recovered from most clinical specimens. This chapter discusses how anaerobes differ from aerobic bacteria, the importance of anaerobes as endogenous microbiota and their role as disease-causing agents, the proper techniques for the recovery and identification of anaerobes, susceptibility testing of anaerobic isolates, and treatment of anaerobic infections.

IMPORTANT CONCEPTS IN ANAEROBIC BACTERIOLOGY

Anaerobes Defined

An **anaerobe** is a bacterium able to replicate in the absence of oxygen. In order to recover all potential pathogens, the clinical microbiology laboratory must use a variety of atmospheric conditions for culturing bacteria (Table 22-1). Ambient air contains approximately 21% oxygen and 1% carbon dioxide. **Obligate,** or strict, **aerobes** require oxygen for metabolism, and they can grow well in an ambient air incubator. **Capnophilic** organisms, such as *Capnocytophaga,* grow best when the concentration of carbon dioxide is increased to 5% to 10% in a CO_2 incubator. This increase in CO_2 reduces the oxygen concentration to 15%, which is still sufficient to allow aerobic organisms to replicate. **Microaerophilic** organisms, such as *Campylobacter,* require the oxygen concentration to be reduced to 5% or less. **Facultative anaerobes,** such as *Escherichia coli* and *Staphylococcus aureus,* preferentially use oxygen if it is available but can grow well in the absence of oxygen. However, in order to grow anaerobes, the laboratory needs to use growth conditions free from oxygen. This can be accomplished by a variety of mechanisms described later in this chapter.

Anaerobes also vary in their response to the presence of oxygen. Some anaerobes are killed almost immediately in the presence of oxygen (e.g., *Clostridium novyi*). These are referred to as **obligate,** or **strict, anaerobes.** Other anaerobes can survive some oxygen exposure but will not be able to perform metabolic processes unless placed into an anaerobic environment. These organisms are referred to as **aerotolerant,** or moderate, **anaerobes.** Many of the pathogens encountered in the clinical microbiology laboratory fall into this group (e.g., *Bacteroides fragilis*).

Why Some Organisms Are Anaerobes

Molecular oxygen can be toxic to some anaerobes, but substances produced when oxygen becomes reduced through metabolic processes are even more toxic. During oxidation-reduction reactions that occur during normal

TABLE 22-1 Classification of Bacteria on the Basis of Their Relationship to Oxygen and Carbon Dioxide

Category	Requirement	Examples
Obligate aerobe	15%-21% O_2 (as found in a CO_2 incubator or air)	Mycobacteria, fungi
Microaerophile	5% O_2	*Campylobacter, Helicobacter* spp.
Facultative anaerobe	Multiplies equally well in the presence or absence of O_2	Enterobacteriaceae, most staphylococci some streptococci
Aerotolerant anaerobe	Reduced concentrations of O_2 (anaerobic system and a microaerophilic environment)	Most strains of *Propionibacterium, Lactobacillus*, some *Clostridium* spp.
Obligate anaerobe	Strict anaerobic environment (0% O_2)	Most *Bacteroides* spp., many *Clostridium, Eubacterium, Fusobacterium* spp., *Peptostreptococcus* spp., *Porphyromonas* spp.
Capnophile	5%-10% CO_2	Some anaerobes, *Neisseria, Haemophilus* spp.

Modified from Engelkirk PG et al: *Principles and practice of clinical anaerobic bacteriology*, Belmont, Calif, 1992, Star.

cellular metabolism, molecular oxygen is reduced to **superoxide anion** (O_2^-) and hydrogen peroxide (H_2O_2) in a stepwise manner by the addition of electrons, as shown in the following equations:

$$O_2 + e^- \rightarrow O_2^- \text{(superoxide anion)}$$

$$O_2^- + e^- + 2H^+ \rightarrow H_2O_2 \text{(hydrogen peroxide)}$$

Furthermore, one hypothesis of oxygen toxicity proposes that the superoxide anion reacts with hydrogen peroxide in the presence of iron (Fe^{3+}/Fe^{2+}) to generate the **hydroxyl radical** (OH^-). This short-lived molecule is the most potent biological oxidant known. Reaction between the hydroxyl radical and the superoxide anion forms singlet oxygen, which is also damaging to the cell. It becomes obvious that cells need a way to remove these harmful molecules if they are to survive in the presence of oxygen. Strict aerobic and facultative anaerobic bacteria that use oxygen have the enzymes **superoxide dismutase** and/or **catalase** to protect them from superoxide anions and their toxic derivatives, as shown in the following equations:

$$4O_2^- + 4H^+ \xrightarrow[\text{dismutase}]{\text{superoxide}} 2H_2O_2 + O_2$$

$$2H_2O_2 \xrightarrow{\text{catalase}} 2H_2O + O_2$$

Superoxide dismutase converts the superoxide anion to oxygen and hydrogen peroxide. Hydrogen peroxide can be toxic to cells but not to the degree of the superoxide anion or the hydroxyl radical. Hydrogen peroxide will diffuse out from the cell, but many organisms also possess the enzyme catalase that breaks hydrogen peroxide down to oxygen and water, thereby negating its toxic effect. Because the hydroxyl radical is a product of the further reduction of the superoxide anion, elimination of the superoxide anion by superoxide dismutase will inhibit the formation of the hydroxyl radical.

Anaerobes, on the other hand, are particularly susceptible to these toxic derivatives of oxygen because they lack the protective enzymes superoxide dismutase and/or catalase, or the enzymes are present in low concentrations. Extended exposure to oxygen results in cell death for strict anaerobes and cessation of growth for the more oxygen tolerant anaerobes. Strict anaerobes also may require an environment that has a low oxidation-reduction (redox) potential. This may be

in part because certain enzymes that are essential for bacterial growth require fully reduced sulfhydryl (–SH) groups to be active. Reducing agents such as thioglycollate, cysteine, and dithiothreitol often are added to microbiologic media to obtain a low redox potential. In vivo bacteria have a tendency to lower the redox potential at their site of growth. Consequently, anatomic sites colonized with mixtures of organisms, such as found on mucosal surfaces, frequently provide conditions favorable to the growth of obligate anaerobes.

Where Anaerobes Are Found

In a world where oxygen abounds, anaerobes are found only in specific ecologic niches. They can be found in soil, in freshwater and saltwater sediments, and as components of the **endogenous microbiota** of humans and other animals. Anaerobes that exist outside the bodies of animals are referred to as **exogenous anaerobes**, and the infections they cause are referred to as *exogenous infections*. Conversely, anaerobes that exist inside the bodies of animals (endogenous microflora) are referred to as *endogenous anaerobes* and are the source of endogenous infections.

Exogenous anaerobic infections are usually caused by gram-positive, spore-forming bacilli belonging to the genus *Clostridium*. Clostridia, or their toxins, initiate infection when spores are ingested by way of contaminated food or gain access to the body through open wounds contaminated with soil. However, the anaerobes most frequently isolated from infectious processes in humans are those of endogenous origin. Table 22-2 shows endogenous anaerobes commonly encountered in human infections. Endogenous anaerobes can contribute to an infectious disease in any anatomic site of the body if suitable conditions exist for colonization and penetration of the bacteria. Although many different species of anaerobes can be isolated from human clinical specimens, the number of species routinely isolated is relatively small. Table 22-3 lists the anaerobes most frequently recovered from clinical specimens at a university medical center and includes members of the *B. fragilis* group; *Porphyromonas* and *Prevotella* spp.; *Fusobacterium* spp.; *Clostridium* spp.; *Propionibacterium* spp.; and the anaerobic cocci. One of the most frequently encountered pathogenic anaerobes is *Clostridium difficile*, a cause of antibiotic-associated diarrhea, in which the diagnostic test is most often based on the detection of the

TABLE 22-2 Endogenous Anaerobes Commonly Involved in Human Infections

Infection	Anaerobe
Actinomycosis	*Actinomyces israelii,* other *Actinomyces* spp.
Antibiotic-associated diarrhea; Pseudomembranous colitis	*Clostridium difficile*
Bacteremia	*B. fragilis* group, fusobacteria, clostridia, peptostreptococci
Brain abscess	*Bacteroides* spp., *Prevotella* spp., *Porphyromonas* spp., *Fusobacterium* spp., *Clostridium* spp. (these infections are often polymicrobial)
Infections of female genitourinary tract	Peptostreptococci, *Bacteroides* spp., *Clostridium* spp.; *Prevotella bivia, P. disiens, Actinomyces israelii* (IUD associated)
Intra-abdominal infections, liver abscess, peritonitis, perineal and perirectal infections	*Bacteroides fragilis* group, other *Bacteroides* spp., *Fusobacterium* spp., *C. perfringens,* other *Clostridium* spp., peptostreptococci (frequently polymicrobial)
Myonecrosis	*Clostridium perfringens, C. novyi, C. septicum* (80% to 95% of the cases)
Oral, sinus, dental infections	Peptostreptococci, *Porphyromonas* spp., *Fusobacterium* spp. (often polymicrobial)
Aspiration pneumonia, pleuropulmonary infections	*Porphyromonas* spp., *F. nucleatum,* peptostreptococci, *B. fragilis* group, *Actinomyces* spp.

Modified from Engelkirk PG et al: *Principles and practice of clinical anaerobic bacteriology,* Belmont, Calif, 1992, Star.
IUD, Intrauterine device.

TABLE 22-3 Incidence of Anaerobes at a University Medical Center

Organism Group	Total	Blood Isolates
Bacteroides fragilis group	377	16
Fusobacterium	47	4
Prevotella/Porphyromonas group	244	6
Clostridium	40	13
Propionibacterium	148	60*
Peptostreptococci	155	6
Veillonella	7	0

Data provided by the author.
*Mostly considered contaminants.

toxins produced by the bacterium rather than by culturing the organism from feces.

Anaerobes at Specific Anatomic Sites

Anaerobes outnumber aerobes at mucosal surfaces, such as the linings of the oral cavity, gastrointestinal (GI) tract, and genitourinary (GU) tract. These heavily colonized surfaces are the usual portals of entry into the tissues and bloodstream

TABLE 22-4 Endogenous Anaerobes of Various Anatomical Sites

Site	Anaerobes
Skin	*Propionibacterium,* peptostreptococci
Upper respiratory tract	Peptostreptococci, *Actinomyces, Propionibacterium, Campylobacter, Fusobacterium, Prevotella, Veillonella*
Oral cavity	*Actinomyces, Eubacterium/Eggerthella,* peptostreptococci, *Campylobacter, Fusobacterium, Prevotella, Bifidobacterium, Porphyromonas, Veillonella*
Intestine	*Bifidobacterium, Eubacterium/Eggerthella, Clostridium,* peptostreptococci, *Bacteroides fragilis* group, *Bilophila, Campylobacter, Fusobacterium, Porphyromonas, Prevotella, Sutterella, Veillonella*
Genitourinary tract	Peptostreptococci, *Bifidobacterium, Fusobacterium, Lactobacillus, Mobiluncus, Prevotella, Veillonella*

From Jouseimies HR et al: *Wadsworth-KTL anaerobic bacteriology manual,* ed 6, Belmont, Calif, 2002, Star.

for endogenous anaerobes. Under ordinary circumstances, microorganisms that are members of the microbial biota do not cause disease. Indeed, many actually can be beneficial. However, when some of these organisms gain access to usually sterile body sites such as the bloodstream, brain, and lungs, they can cause serious or even fatal infections.

Knowledge of the composition of the microbiota at specific anatomic sites is useful for predicting the particular organisms most likely to be involved in infectious processes that arise at or adjacent to those sites. Table 22-4 summarizes the variety of endogenous anaerobes that may be found at specific body sites. Finding site-specific organisms at a distant and/or unusual site can serve as a clue to the underlying origin of an infectious process. For example, the isolation of oral anaerobes from a brain abscess may suggest invasion from the oral cavity, perhaps due to poor dentition. Some anaerobes have a fairly predictable antimicrobial susceptibility pattern; such knowledge may be of value to physicians considering empirical antimicrobial therapy.

Skin

Indigenous members of the skin microbiota include anaerobes that colonize the sebaceous glands and hair follicles. *Propionibacterium acnes* is frequently isolated from blood cultures, but its presence often represents contamination from the patient's skin resulting from poor site preparation during the phlebotomy procedure. Nevertheless, *P. acnes* is considered an opportunistic pathogen and has been associated with cases of endocarditis and surgical wound infections. Other anaerobes found on the skin include gram-positive cocci (e.g., *Peptostreptococcus*). Superficial wound or abscess specimens aspirated by needle and syringe are much better specimens for anaerobic bacteriology than material collected by swabs; the latter often are contaminated with anaerobes of the skin microflora.

Respiratory Tract

Of the bacteria present in saliva, nasal washings, and gingival and tooth scrapings, 90% are anaerobes. Gram-negative anaerobic bacilli *(Prevotella, Porphyromonas,* and *Fusobacterium)* and anaerobic cocci are the anaerobes occurring in the largest numbers. These particular anaerobes should be suspected as participants in any infectious process occurring in the oral cavity and in suspected cases of aspiration pneumonia. In addition, invasion through the oral mucosa should be suspected whenever oral anaerobes such as *F. nucleatum* and *Porphyromonas* are recovered from the bloodstream or from abscesses located far from the oral cavity.

Gastrointestinal Tract

Of the estimated 500 to 1000 species of bacteria that inhabit the human body, approximately 300 to 400 live in the colon. Microbiota studies have found that anaerobes outnumber facultative anaerobes by a factor of 1000:1. Although *Bacteroides fragilis* is the most common species of anaerobic bacteria isolated from soft tissue infections and bacteremia, it accounts for less than 1% of the human intestinal biota. Other members of the *B. fragilis* group, such as *B. vulgatus, B. thetaiotaomicron,* and B. *distasonis,* are among the most common species of bacteria isolated from human feces. Other species commonly inhabiting the GI tract include *Bifidobacterium, Clostridium, Eubacterium,* and the anaerobic gram-positive cocci. Any infection in the peritoneal cavity would likely be caused by organisms that have been able to escape from the GI tract.

Genitourinary Tract

Although anaerobic bacteria colonize the distal urethra, they are not considered to be a cause of uncomplicated urinary tract infections. Similarly, 50% of the bacteria in cervical and vaginal secretions are anaerobes. These include the anaerobic cocci, *Fusobacterium, Prevotella, Bacteroides,* and *Lactobacillus.* For this reason, GU tract swabs and voided or catheterized urine specimens are unacceptable for anaerobic bacteriology because recovery of these organisms would not distinguish whether they were present as pathogens or endogenous microbiota.

Factors That Predispose Patients to Anaerobic Infections

Factors that commonly predispose the human body to anaerobic infections include trauma to mucous membranes or the skin, vascular stasis, and decreased oxygenation of tissue leading to tissue necrosis and a decrease in the redox potential of tissue. The precise mechanisms by which anaerobic bacteria cause disease are not always known. Like other pathogenic bacteria, anaerobes can produce a variety of virulence factors. Toxins, enzymes that break down tissue, capsules that inhibit phagocytosis by macrophages, and adherence factors that aid in attachment to mucosal surfaces are thought to play a role in pathogenicity (Table 22-5).

Generally, infectious diseases involving anaerobic bacteria follow some type of trauma to protective barriers such as the skin and mucous membranes. Trauma at these sites allows anaerobes of the endogenous biota (or in some cases, soil anaerobes) to gain access to deeper tissues. Vascular stasis prevents oxygen from entering a particular site, which results in an environment conducive to growth and multiplication of any anaerobe that might be present at that site. Similar results might occur in the presence of tissue necrosis and when redox potential in tissue is decreased. Box 22-1 lists examples of conditions that may predispose a patient to anaerobic infections.

TABLE 22-5 Potential Virulence Factors of Anaerobic Bacteria

Potential Virulence Factor	Possible Role	Anaerobes Known or Thought to Possess
Polysaccharide capsules	Promotes abscess formation; antiphagocytic function	*Bacteroides fragilis, Porphyromonas gingivalis*
Adherence factors	Certain fimbriae, fibrils enable organisms to adhere to cell surfaces	*B. fragilis, P. gingivalis*
Clostridial toxins/exoenzymes		
Collagenases	Catalyzes the degradation of collagen	Certain *Clostridium* spp.
Cytotoxins	Toxic to specific types of cells	*C. difficile*
DNases	Destroy DNA	Certain *Clostridium* spp.
Enterotoxins	Toxic to cells of the intestinal mucosa	*C. difficile*
Hemolysins	Liberate hemoglobin from red blood cells by lysing the cells	Certain *Clostridium* spp.
Hyaluronidase	Catalyze the hydrolysis of hyaluronic acid, the cement substance of tissues	Certain *Clostridium* spp.
Lipases	Catalyze the hydrolysis of ester linkages between fatty acids and glycerol of triglycerides and phospholipids	Certain *Clostridium* spp.
Neurotoxins (e.g., botulinum toxin, tetanospasmin)	Destroy or disrupt nerve tissue	*C. botulinum, C. tetani*
Phospholipases	Catalyze the splitting of phospholipids (lecithinase)	Certain *Clostridium* spp.
Proteases	Splits proteins by hydrolysis of peptide bonds	Certain *Clostridium* spp.

Modified from Engelkirk PG et al: *Principles and practice of clinical anaerobic bacteriology,* Belmont, Calif, 1992, Star.

Indications of Anaerobe Involvement in Human Disease

Infectious processes involving anaerobes are usually purulent, with many polymorphonuclear leukocytes present. However, the absence of leukocytes does not rule out the possibility that anaerobes are contributing to the process because some anaerobes such as *Clostridium perfringens* produce enzymatic virulence factors that destroy neutrophils, macrophages, and other cells.

Box 22-2 contains a list of indications of anaerobe involvement in infectious processes. Although any of these indicators should alert the physician to the possible involvement of anaerobes, most are not specific for anaerobes. For example, large quantities of gas in the specimen might be due to gas-producing organisms such as *E. coli* or a mixture of enteric bacteria other than anaerobes. Similarly, the foul odor usually associated with specimens containing anaerobes could be absent. Many of the infectious processes involving anaerobes are polymicrobial, consisting of mixtures of obligate anaerobes or mixtures of obligate or aerotolerant anaerobes and facultative organisms. A symbiotic relationship between facultative anaerobes and obligate anaerobes frequently exists in polymicrobial infections, which can contribute to an infectious disease.

FREQUENTLY ENCOUNTERED ANAEROBES AND THEIR ASSOCIATED DISEASES

Taxonomically, anaerobic bacteria encountered in human clinical specimens may be divided into gram-negative and gram-positive genera. Gram-positive anaerobes can be further divided between those organisms capable of forming endospores (spore formers) and those unable to (non–spore formers). The presence or absence of spores, coupled with the Gram-stain reaction and cellular morphology, can be helpful in making the initial or presumptive identification of anaerobic bacteria and determining the appropriate identification tests to be performed.

As with other areas of clinical microbiology, the use of molecular methods rather than phenotypic characteristics to determine taxonomic placement of an organism has resulted in an explosion of taxonomic changes. It is beyond the scope of this chapter to list all the current names of rarely encountered anaerobes. Instead, this chapter will concentrate on the clinically important anaerobes most likely to be encountered in specimens submitted to the clinical microbiology laboratory.

Gram-Positive, Spore-Forming Anaerobic Bacilli

All spore-forming anaerobic bacilli are classified in the genus *Clostridium* and are collectively referred to as *clostridia*. Although all clostridia are capable of producing spores, some species do so readily, whereas others require extremely harsh conditions. Spores are often not observed in Gram-stained smears of clinical specimens containing clostridia or in smears of colonies from an agar plate unless the culture has been incubated for many days. It is sometimes necessary to use heat or alcohol shock to induce sporulation.

Clostridia may be grouped according to the location of the endospore within the cell. Spores are described as *terminal* when the spore is located at the end of the bacterial cell and *subterminal* when the spore is found at a location other than the end of the cell. Terminal spores typically cause swelling of the cell. Figure 22-1 shows a clostridial species that produces terminal spores and a clostridial species that produces subterminal spores. Spores located in the center of the cell are called *central spores*.

Clinical Infections

Clostridium spp. are frequently encountered in exogenous anaerobic infections or intoxications. Clostridia or their toxins usually gain access to the body through ingestion or open wounds that have become contaminated with soil. Clostridia cause classic diseases such as tetanus, gas gangrene (myonecrosis), **botulism,** and food poisoning (foodborne intoxication). In tetanus, gas gangrene, and wound botulism, clostridial spores enter through open wounds and germinate in vivo. The vegetative bacteria then multiply and produce toxins. In foodborne disease caused by *C. perfringens*, organisms are acquired through consumption of contaminated food that has been improperly stored. Almost any *Clostridium* spp. can cause wound or abscess infection, usually as part of mixed biota, and most can be isolated from the blood in cases of bacteremia. One clostridial infection that is of endogenous origin is antibiotic-associated pseudomembranous colitis caused by *C. difficile*.

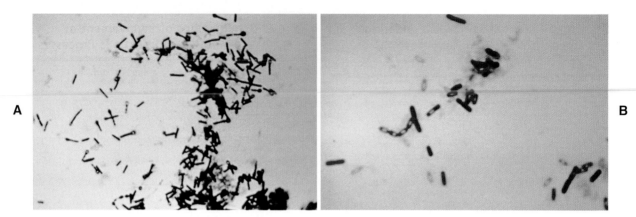

FIGURE 22-1 Classification of some clinically encountered clostridia by endospore location. **A,** Gram-stained appearance of terminal spores of *Clostridium tetani.* **B,** Gram-stained appearance of subterminal spores of *Clostridium sordellii.* (Courtesy Bartley SL, Howard JD, Simon R: Centers for Disease Control and Prevention, Atlanta, Ga.)

***Clostridium perfringens* Food Poisoning.** *Clostridium perfringens* is associated with two types of food poisoning: type A, a relatively mild and self-limited gastrointestinal illness, and type C, a more serious but rarely seen disease. *C. perfringens* foodborne disease usually follows ingestion of enterotoxin-producing strains in contaminated food. *C. perfringens* lacks the ability to produce a number of essential amino acids; therefore meats and gravies are commonly implicated in outbreaks. Foods are often heat-treated, which kills vegetative bacteria but allows the spore-forming clostridia to survive. Improperly stored food allows germination of the spores and growth of vegetative bacteria. Food poisoning due to *C. perfringens* type A is caused by a *C. perfringens* enterotoxin linked to sporulation. After an 8- to 12-hour incubation period, the patient experiences diarrhea and cramping abdominal pain for about 24 hours. Other than fluid replacement, therapy is usually unnecessary.

Clostridium perfringens type C food poisoning **(enteritis necroticans)** is associated with strains that produce β-toxin and less commonly α-toxin. After an incubation period of at least 5 to 6 hours, symptoms begin as an acute onset of severe abdominal pain and diarrhea, which is often bloody, and may be accompanied by vomiting. Early symptoms are followed by necrotic inflammation of the small intestines. Without treatment, the disease is often fatal; even with treatment the fatality rate is 15% to 25%. In general, the clinical microbiology laboratory, unless serving a public health function, usually does not have a role in recovering *C. perfringens* from food or feces during outbreaks.

Botulism. Foodborne **botulism** results from the ingestion of preformed botulinum toxin, produced in the food by *C. botulinum.* Although there are seven antigenically different botulinum toxins (A through G), only types A, B, and E are associated with human infections. Botulinum toxin is an extremely potent neurotoxin; it takes only a small amount to produce paralysis and death. Botulinum toxin attaches to the neuromuscular junction of nerves and prevents the release of acetylcholine, which results in a flaccid type of paralysis and death. Botulinum toxin type A is also used medically to treat strabismus ("wandering eye") and as a beauty enhancer by temporarily improving "frown lines."

Common food sources involved in botulism include home-canned vegetables, home-cured meat such as ham, fermented fish, and other preserved foods. Clinical manifestations develop as early as 2 hours or as late as 3 to 8 days following ingestion of food containing the botulinum toxin. The toxin is absorbed through the small intestine and enters the systemic circulation to reach the nervous system. Weakness and paralysis are the main features of botulism. Double or blurred vision, impaired speech, and difficulty in swallowing are also commonly seen. Respiratory paralysis may occur in severe cases. Treatment of foodborne botulism involves the use of antitoxin and supportive care. Infant botulism, unlike that in adults, follows ingestion of *C. botulinum* spores. Honey contaminated with the *C. botulinum* spores is the food most commonly associated with infant botulism. Once ingested, the spores germinate and the vegetative cells then colonize the colon and subsequently produce toxins.

Wound botulism is the result of contamination of wounds with spores of *C. botulinum,* which germinate, multiply, and produce toxins. Clinical manifestations of wound botulism are similar to those of foodborne intoxication. Botulism toxin and *C. botulinum* are considered potential agents of bioterrorism; laboratorians or physicians are required to notify state laboratories if *C. botulinum* is isolated or if a case of botulism is suspected. See Chapter 30 for a discussion of *C. botulinum* as an agent of bioterrorism. In 2007, the Centers for Disease Control and Prevention (CDC) reported 32 cases of foodborne botulism, 85 cases of infant botulism, and 27 cases of wound or other botulism infections.

Tetanus. The clinical manifestations of **tetanus** are attributed to the neurotoxin tetanospasmin produced by *Clostridium tetani.* Tetanospasmin acts on inhibitory neurons, preventing the release of neurotransmitters. This results in a spastic type of paralysis with continuous muscular spasms leading to trismus ("lockjaw"), risus sardonicus (distorted grin), and difficulty breathing.

Tetanus occurs when spores in the environment enter the skin through puncture wounds. The spores germinate into vegetative cells that produce tetanospasmin. Symptoms usually appear approximately 7 days after the injury, but the incubation period has been reported to range from 3 to 21 days. The length of incubation is related to the distance from the injury to the central nervous system. Clinical manifestations include muscular rigidity, usually in the jaw, neck, and lumbar region. Difficulty in swallowing results from muscular spasms in the pharyngeal area. Rigidity of the abdomen, chest, back, and limbs may also occur. As a result of the widespread use of the diphtheria-pertussis-tetanus (DPT) vaccine, tetanus is no longer a common disease in the United States; only 28 cases were reported to the CDC in 2007. Therapy for tetanus requires the injection of antitoxin, muscle relaxants, and intensive therapy. Although most treated patients completely recover, long-term disability and even death can occur. From 1998 to 2000, an 18% mortality was associated with tetanus infections in the United States.

Myonecrosis. **Myonecrosis,** or gas gangrene, usually occurs when organisms contaminate wounds, through either trauma or surgery. *C. perfringens, C. histolyticum, C. septicum, C. novyi,* and *C. bifermentans* have all been associated with myonecrosis. *C. perfringens,* however, is the most common cause. Under favorable conditions, the organisms are able to grow, multiply, and release potent exotoxins. In gas gangrene, exotoxins, such as α-toxin produced by *C. perfringens,* cause necrosis of the tissue and allow deeper penetration by the organisms.

α-Toxin is a lecithinase (phospholipase C) produced by all strains of *C. perfringens.* Clinical manifestations of myonecrosis include pain and swelling in the affected area. Bullae (fluid-filled blisters), serous discharge, discoloration, and tissue necrosis are observed. The onset and spread of myonecrosis can be rapid, and extensive surgical debridement of the necrotic tissue is often required. If treatment is delayed, amputation of the affected limb is not uncommon.

Bacteremia. Many of the clostridia have been recovered from blood cultures, but *C. perfringens* is by far the most common. When *C. septicum* is present in the bloodstream, it is often a marker organism for a malignancy in the GI tract. *C. bifermentans* and *C. tertium* have also been isolated from blood cultures from patients with serious underlying disease.

***Clostridium difficile*–Associated Diseases.** *Clostridium difficile* is the most common cause, but not the sole cause, of antibiotic-associated diarrhea and **pseudomembranous colitis.** This organism is found as part of the gastrointestinal biota in about 5% of individuals, although the colonization rate in patients associated with long-term care facilities such as nursing homes and rehabilitation facilities can reach 20% of the population. Following antimicrobial therapy, many bowel biota organisms other than *C. difficile* are killed, thus allowing *C. difficile* to multiply and produce two toxins: toxin A, an enterotoxin, and toxin B, a cytotoxin. Bloody diarrhea with associated necrosis of colonic mucosa is seen in patients with pseudomembranous colitis. *C. difficile* is a common cause of health care–associated (nosocomial) infection. The organism is frequently transmitted among hospitalized patients and is present occasionally on the hands of hospital personnel. Diarrhea caused by *C. difficile* is being seen with increasing frequency in outpatients who have received antimicrobial therapy. Recently, a strain of *C. difficile* associated with hyperproduction of toxins was recovered from patients with severe and sometimes fatal cases of pseudomembranous colitis leading to bowel perforation and sepsis.

Gram-Positive, Non–spore-forming Anaerobic Bacilli

Gram-positive, non–spore-forming anaerobic bacilli have undergone considerable taxonomic revision in recent years. In general, the group can be divided into two phyla: the Actinobacteria and the Firmicutes. Important clinical genera of the Actinobacteria include *Actinomyces, Bifidobacterium, Eggerthella, Mobiluncus,* and *Propionibacterium.* The Firmicutes include many genera, but *Lactobacillus* is the only member encountered on a routine basis in the clinical microbiology laboratory. All of these organisms are found as part of the endogenous microbiota of humans, and they are considered opportunistic pathogens. The microscopic morphology of these organisms varies, ranging from very short rods to long, branching filaments.

Clinical Infections

Actinomycosis. **Actinomycosis** is a chronic, granulomatous, infectious disease characterized by the development of sinus tracts and fistulae, which erupt to the surface and drain pus that may contain "sulfur granules" (dense clumps of bacteria that may be colored). Examinations of wet mounts and Gram-stained preparations of pus from draining sinuses are useful diagnostic procedures for demonstrating the non–spore forming, thin, gram-positive bacilli that frequently exhibit branching in clinical specimens (Figure 22-2). Since *Actinomyces* spp. are endogenous biota of the oral cavity, many cases of actinomycosis can be seen in the maxillary region with draining sinuses in the neck and thorax. Another common site of actinomycosis is the female genital tract where the infection is often associated with long-standing intrauterine devices. Although *Actinomyces israelii* is the most common cause of actinomycosis, other gram-positive anaerobes such as *Propionibacterium* and *Bifidobacterium* have also been noted to cause this type of infection.

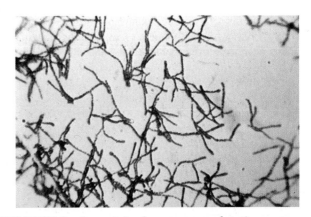

FIGURE 22-2 Gram-stained appearance of *Actinomyces israelii,* illustrating the term *Actinomyces-like.*

Bacterial Vaginosis. **Bacterial vaginosis (BV)** is thought to arise because of a shift in the ecology of the endogenous microbiota of the vagina. *Lactobacillus* spp. usually comprise the largest portion of the vaginal biota. In BV, a shift in the vaginal biota occurs resulting in the overgrowth of other endogenous anaerobes of the vagina such as *Mobiluncus* spp., *Bacteroides* spp., *Prevotella* spp., anaerobic gram-positive cocci, and the aerobic bacterium *Gardnerella vaginalis*. Clinical features of BV include a gray-white, homogenous, malodorous vaginal discharge with little or no discomfort and no inflammation. BV is most often diagnosed on clinical appearance and a Gram stain of the vaginal secretions that reveals a shift in the vaginal biota from predominantly the gram-positive lactobacilli to a mixture of *Gardnerella* spp. (gram-variable bacilli) and mixed gram-negative anaerobes. Because many of the anaerobic organisms associated with BV are members of the endogenous microbiota of the female genitourinary tract, culture of vaginal secretions is not performed as part of the diagnosis.

Lactobacillus. *Lactobacillus* spp. are gram-positive, highly pleomorphic bacilli, which may appear on Gram stain as a coccoid or spiral-shaped organism. There are over 100 species of *Lactobacillus*. They are considered aerotolerant anaerobes growing better under anaerobic conditions. Lactobacilli are widely distributed in nature and foods, as well as in normal biota in the human mouth, GI tract, and female genital tract.

Lactobacillus spp. play an important role in the health of the female vaginal tract, in that they help protect the host from urogenital infections. Lactobacilli produce lactic acid from glycogen, which lowers the vaginal pH and suppresses the overgrowth of organisms such as *Mobiluncus, Prevotella,* and *G. vaginalis*. BV may result if the delicate balance between lactobacilli and other bacteria representing the normal vaginal biota is disrupted. BV is associated with an increased risk of a woman acquiring human immunodeficiency virus infection, adverse outcomes in pregnancy, and possibly with the pathogenesis of pelvic inflammatory disease. *Lactobacillus acidophilus* complex constitutes the majority of the lactobacilli of the healthy vagina, but *L. fermentum, L. vaginalis, L. salivarius, L. plantarum,* and others have also been recovered.

Lactobacillus spp. can often be recovered from urine cultures and genital cultures where their role in the infectious process is doubtful. Systemic human infections are rare and are associated with the patient's endogenous organisms. Serious infections, primarily bacteremia and endocarditis, are known to occur in immunocompromised patients. Endocarditis is the most common clinical disease caused by lactobacilli and has a high mortality rate (23% to 27%). Other infections associated with lactobacilli include intra-abdominal abscesses, meningitis, oral infections, and conjunctivitis. Opportunistic infections such as endocarditis and polymicrobial abscesses caused by lactobacilli are sometimes seen in patients who previously received the antimicrobial vancomycin. Although vancomycin is normally effective in treating infections caused by almost all gram-positive bacteria, many lactobacilli are resistant to the agent and consequently will be able to overgrow other inhibited gram-positive organisms during vancomycin therapy.

Colony morphology of the lactobacilli varies greatly, with some species appearing as pinpoint α-hemolytic colonies on sheep blood agar (SBA). Others have been described as medium in size with a rough appearance and gray color. Lactobacilli are catalase negative and, unless a Gram stain is performed, differentiation from *Streptococcus* sp. viridans group is difficult. In addition to vancomycin, lactobacilli are frequently resistant to the cephalosporins. Once the organism is confirmed as clinically significant and not a contaminant, treatment is usually penicillin with an aminoglycoside.

Anaerobic Gram-Negative Bacilli

Gram-negative anaerobic bacilli are all non–spore forming and are often found as members of the endogenous microbiota. They can be found as part of the oral microbiota, as a major component of the GI flora, and as members of the biota of the GU tract. The genera most commonly encountered in clinical specimens include the *B. fragilis* group, *Porphyromonas, Prevotella,* and *Fusobacterium.*

Clinical Infections

Anaerobic gram-negative bacilli are frequently found in mixed infections such as abscesses occurring beneath mucosal surfaces. As predominant members of the GI biota, the organisms are often associated with peritoneal infections following disruption of the GI lining. Members of the *B. fragilis* group are the most commonly isolated anaerobes from blood cultures. Brain abscesses are frequently caused by anaerobic organisms such as *Prevotella, Porphyromonas,* and *Fusobacterium* that are found as endogenous microbiota of the oral cavity. The anaerobic gram-negative bacilli are often associated with mixed biota in diabetic foot ulcers and decubitus pressure sores. It is often difficult to determine whether the organisms recovered in culture from these specimens are pathogens or just colonizers.

Anaerobic Cocci

Most of the gram-positive anaerobic cocci were classified previously in the genus *Peptostreptococcus,* with the exception of *Peptococcus niger,* an infrequently isolated anaerobic coccus. However, the genus *Peptostreptococcus* has been reclassified recently into at least four different genera: *Peptostreptococcus, Anaerococcus, Finegoldia,* and *Peptoniphilus.* Taxonomy of this group is still in a state of flux, so this chapter will continue to use the term "peptostreptococci" or anaerobic gram-positive cocci when discussing these organisms as a group.

Although several genera of gram-negative anaerobic cocci are found in the endogenous microbiota, only *Veillonella* spp. are implicated as pathogens. *Veillonella* are very small (0.3 to 0.5 μm in diameter) and inhabit the oral cavity. They are most often seen as mixed flora in abscesses.

Clinical Infections

The anaerobic cocci are isolated from a wide variety of infections, including brain abscess, meningitis, aspiration pneumonia, lung abscess, and gingivitis and other periodontal diseases. They are most often associated with polymicrobial infections but can occasionally be recovered from blood cultures and can be a cause of infections following orthopedic surgery.

Finegoldia magna is the most pathogenic of the anaerobic cocci and the one most often isolated in pure culture.

SPECIMEN SELECTION, COLLECTION, TRANSPORT, AND PROCESSING

Specimen Quality

When physicians suspect an infection involving anaerobes, the specimen they collect must be from the actual site of the infection and not just a swab of a mucosal surface. It must also be collected in a manner that avoids prolonged exposure to oxygen and must be transported as quickly as possible to the laboratory under anaerobic conditions. The laboratory plays an important preanalytical role in specimen selection by providing guidelines for specimen collection and by ensuring that a suitable anaerobic transport system is available. As previously mentioned, most anaerobic infections are caused by members of the endogenous microbiota. An improperly collected specimen may result in the growth of many different anaerobes, but determining which, if any, are responsible for the infection may be impossible. The consequences of working up improper or incorrectly collected or transported specimens places a burden on the laboratory and may provide misleading results to the physician. Consequently, the laboratory, with the cooperation of the medical staff, must develop criteria for the rejection of inappropriate specimens. Specimens that are acceptable for anaerobic culture are listed in Table 22-6. Conversely, Box 22-3 provides a list of specimens not recommended for anaerobic culture. All of these specimens are likely to result in the growth of many different anaerobes that are colonizing the mucosal surface at the site of specimen collection, making it impossible to determine which, if any, are causing infection.

BOX 22-3 Unacceptable Specimens* for Anaerobic Bacteriology

Throat swabs, nasopharyngeal swabs; sputum obtained by nasotracheal or endotracheal suction; bronchial washings or other specimens obtained via a bronchoscope (unless a protected double-lumen catheter is used); expectorated sputum

Gingival swabs or any other intraoral surface swabs

Large bowel contents[†]; feces[†]; ileostomy and colostomy effluents; rectal swabs; gastric and small bowel contents

Voided or catheterized urine

Vaginal, cervical, or urethral swabs; female genital tract specimens collected via the vagina[‡]; swabs of a vaginal discharge

Surface swabs from decubitus ulcers, perirectal abscesses, foot ulcers, exposed wounds, eschars, pilonidal sinuses, and other sinus tracts

Any material adjacent to a mucous membrane that has not been adequately decontaminated

Modified from Engelkirk PG et al: *Principles and practice of clinical anaerobic bacteriology*, Belmont, Calif, 1992, Star.
*All would contain endogenous anaerobic microbiota.
[†]Except for *Clostridium difficile*, *Clostridium botulinum*, and other specific etiologic agents.
[‡]Except for suction curettings or other specimens collected via a double-lumen catheter.

Specimen Transport and Processing

Regardless of the type of specimen submitted for anaerobic bacteriology, it must be transported and processed as rapidly as possible and with minimum exposure to oxygen. Specimens usually are collected from a warm, moist environment that is low in oxygen. Thus it is important to avoid "shocking" the anaerobes by exposing them to oxygen or permitting them to dry out. In addition, the specimens should not be refrigerated and the amount of time they remain at room temperature should be minimized.

Aspirates

Abscess specimens collected by needle and syringe are better for anaerobic bacteriology than those collected by swab because they are less likely to be contaminated by endogenous microbiota present at the mucosal or skin surface. Following aspiration of the specimen, any air present in the syringe and needle should be expelled. To prevent a potentially infectious aerosol, an alcohol-soaked gauze pad can be placed over the needle while air is expelled. The aspirate should be injected into an oxygen-free transport tube or vial, preferably one containing a prereduced, anaerobically sterilized (PRAS) transport medium, such as the one shown in Figure 22-3. PRAS media (Anaerobe Systems; Morgan Hill, Calif.) are

---

TABLE 22-6 Acceptable Specimens for Anaerobic Bacteriology

Anatomic Source	Specimens and Recommended Methods of Collection
Central nervous system	Cerebrospinal fluid, aspirated abscess material, tissue from biopsy or autopsy
Dental/ENT specimens	Aspirated abscess material, biopsied tissue
Localized abscesses	Needle and syringe aspiration of closed abscesses
Decubitus ulcers	Aspirated pus
Sinus tracts or draining wounds	Aspirated material
Deep tissue or bone	Specimens obtained during surgery from depths of wound or underlying bone lesion
Pulmonary	Aspirate obtained by direct lung puncture; pleural fluid obtained by thoracentesis; open lung biopsy; "sulfur granules" from draining fistula
Intra-abdominal	Aspirate from abscess, ascites fluid, peritoneal fluid, tissue
Urinary tract	Suprapubic bladder aspiration
Female genital tract	Aspirate from loculated abscess; culdocentesis specimen
Other	Blood, bone marrow, synovial fluid, biopsied tissue from any normally sterile site

Modified from Engelkirk PG et al: *Principles and practice of clinical anaerobic bacteriology*, Belmont, Calif, 1992, Star.
ENT, Ear, nose, and throat.

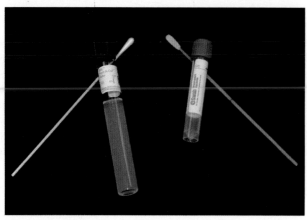

FIGURE 22-3 Anaerobic specimen collection and transport systems. *Left:* BBL Port-A-Cul with prereduced gel (BD Diagnostic Systems, Sparks, Md.). *Right:* ESwab with prereduced liquid Amies (Copan Diagnostics, Corona, Calif.).

prepared by boiling (to remove dissolved oxygen), autoclaving (to sterilize the mixture), and replacing any air with an oxygen-free gas mixture.

Once in the laboratory, aspirates in transport containers should be vortexed to ensure even distribution of the material, especially when the sample is grossly purulent. Using a sterile Pasteur pipette, one drop of purulent material or two to three drops of nonpurulent material should be added to each plate and streaked in such a manner as to obtain well-isolated colonies. A few drops of the specimen may also be inoculated into the bottom of a tube of enriched thioglycollate or cooked meat broth. Finally, one drop of material is spread evenly over an alcohol-cleaned glass slide for Gram staining.

Swabs

Swabs should be used only when aspiration of material is not possible and a biopsy specimen is not available. When swabs are deemed necessary, they should always be transported under anaerobic conditions. A number of swab transport systems suitable for anaerobes are commercially available. On arrival in the laboratory, the swab should be placed into a tube containing about 0.5 mL of sterile thioglycollate broth. The swab is then vortexed vigorously to remove the clinical material from the swab and then pressed firmly against the inner wall of the tube to remove as much liquid as possible. The remaining liquid suspension is used to inoculate media as previously described for an aspirate. Alternatively, a new transport system called the ESwab (see Figure 22-3; Copan Diagnostics, Corona, Calif.) contains a swab that is transported in 1 mL of a prereduced Amies liquid that can maintain both aerobic and anaerobic organisms for up to 48 hours at room temperature.

Tissue

Tissue specimens collected by biopsy or at autopsy from usually sterile sites are acceptable specimens for anaerobic culture. Small pieces of tissue can be placed in anaerobic transport tubes or vials containing PRAS medium to keep the tissue moist. When inserting either swabs or small pieces of tissue into an anaerobic transport container, care must be taken not to tip the container. This would cause the heavier-than-air, oxygen-free gas mixture to be displaced by room air, thus defeating the primary purpose of using such a transport medium.

Larger tissues of greater than 1 cm² can maintain a reduced atmosphere as long as the transport time to the laboratory is minimized. These specimens can be sent in a sterile container with wet gauze. If a delay in transport is expected, tissue may be transported in pouches containing an oxygen-free atmosphere. Such bags or pouches are available commercially from BD Diagnostic Systems (GasPak Pouches, Sparks, Md.), Mitsubishi Gas Chemical America (AnaeroPack System, New York, N.Y.), and other companies. These containers are described in more detail under Anaerobic Incubation of Inoculated Media later in this chapter. To process the tissue or bone fragments in the laboratory, 1 mL of sterile thioglycollate broth is added to a sterile tissue grinder. The piece of tissue or bone fragment is homogenized until a thick suspension is obtained. Ideally, this procedure can be performed within an **anaerobic chamber.** If a chamber is not available, the grinding must be accomplished as quickly as possible at the workbench. The suspension is used to inoculate media as described previously for an aspirate.

Blood

Blood must be cultured in such a manner as to recover any and all bacteria or yeasts that may be present. This usually requires aseptic inoculation of both an anaerobic and aerobic blood culture bottles. Once inoculated, bottles should be rapidly transported to the laboratory, where they are incubated at 35° to 37° C. Blood for culture must be carefully collected to minimize contamination with skin biota. This usually is accomplished by meticulous preparation of the venipuncture site with a bactericidal agent, such as tincture of iodine, an iodophor, or more recently, chlorhexidine gluconate in combination with 70% isopropyl alcohol.

Processing Clinical Samples for Recovery of Anaerobic Pathogens

To ensure that results of anaerobic cultures are clinically significant, only properly selected, collected, and transported specimens should be processed. Ideally, once a specimen arrives in the laboratory, it should be placed immediately into an anaerobic chamber to prevent further exposure to oxygen. Anaerobic chambers allow all steps in the processing of a specimen to be performed in an oxygen-free environment. In laboratories not equipped with anaerobic chambers, holding systems (described under Inoculation Procedures later in this chapter) may be used. To comply with mandatory infectious disease safety policies, laboratory scientists must follow appropriate safety precautions. Disposable gloves should be worn and a biosafety cabinet used when handling clinical specimens containing potentially infectious agents. The following procedures should be performed on clinical specimens for the recovery of anaerobic bacteria:
- Macroscopic examination of the specimen
- Preparation of Gram-stained smears for microscopic examination

TABLE 22-7 Characteristics to Note During the Macroscopic Examination of a Specimen

Questions to Ask	Comments
Is it an appropriate specimen?	Inappropriate specimens should be rejected
Was it submitted in an appropriate transport container or medium?	Improperly transported specimens should be rejected
Does the specimen have a foul odor?	Many anaerobes, especially *Fusobacterium* and *Porphyromonas,* have foul-smelling metabolic end products
Does the specimen fluoresce brick-red when exposed to long-wave (366 nm) ultraviolet light?	Pigmented species of *Porphyromonas* and *Prevotella* produce substances that fluoresce under long-wave, ultraviolet light prior to becoming darkly pigmented; although a brick-red fluorescence is presumptive evidence of these organisms, some members of this group fluoresce colors other than brick-red
Is the necrotic tissue or exudate black?	Such discoloration may be due to the pigment produced by pigmented species of *Porphyromonas* and *Prevotella*
Does the specimen contain sulfur granules?	Such granules are associated with actinomycosis, a condition caused by *Actinomyces, Propionibacterium propionicum,* and closely related organisms, such as *P. acnes*

Modified from Engelkirk PG et al: *Principles and practice of clinical anaerobic bacteriology,* Belmont, Calif, 1992, Star.

- Inoculation of appropriate plated and tubed media, including media specifically designed for culturing anaerobes
- Anaerobic incubation of inoculated media

Macroscopic Examination of Specimens

Each specimen received in the anaerobic bacteriology section should be examined macroscopically and pertinent observations recorded either in an electronic workcard or on a paper worksheet. Some of the characteristics to note during the macroscopic examination are listed in Table 22-7.

Direct Microscopic Examination of Specimens

Direct smears for Gram stain should be prepared on all specimens received for anaerobic culture for several reasons:

- The Gram stain reveals the various morphotypes and the relative number of microorganisms present in the specimen. The presence of multiple distinct morphologic forms suggests that a polymicrobic infectious process is present.
- Certain morphotypes may provide a presumptive identification of organisms and serve as a guide to media selection. For example, if large, gram-positive bacilli suggestive of clostridia are seen, the laboratory may want to inoculate an egg-yolk agar plate to detect lecithinase or lipase activity, in addition to the routine media normally inoculated. Thin, gram-negative bacilli with tapered ends are suggestive of *Fusobacterium nucleatum,* whereas extremely pleomorphic, gram-negative bacilli with bizarre shapes are suggestive of *Fusobacterium mortiferum* or *F. necrophorum.* Tiny, round to oval, gram-negative cocci with a tendency to stain gram-variable are suggestive of *Veillonella,* whereas gram-negative coccobacilli may be *Bacteroides, Porphyromonas,* or *Prevotella.*
- The Gram stain often reveals the presence of leukocytes indicating an inflammatory response at the site of the infection. However, certain anaerobes produce necrotizing toxins (leukocidins) that destroy leukocytes.

Thus the absence of leukocytes in a Gram-stained smear can never rule out the involvement of anaerobes.

- The Gram stain may also reveal the presence of squamous epithelial cells that would suggest mucosal surface contamination during specimen collection. Such a specimen would likely not provide useful information to the clinician. The laboratory should be cautious in processing such a specimen.
- Finally, the Gram stain can serve as a valuable quality control tool. Failure to isolate certain organisms observed in the Gram-stained smear might indicate problems exist with the anaerobic culture technique being used. In addition, failure to recover certain morphotypes could be the result of oxygen exposure during specimen collection and transport or perhaps be the result of the patient receiving antimicrobial agents that inhibited growth of the organisms on the plated media.

It is recommended that direct smears for Gram stain be methanol fixed rather than heat fixed. Methanol fixation preserves the morphology of leukocytes and bacteria better than heat fixation. Gram-negative anaerobes frequently stain a pale pink when safranin is used as the counterstain and thus may be overlooked in Gram-stained smears of clinical specimens and blood cultures. To enhance the red color of gram-negative anaerobes, use of 0.1% basic fuchsin as the counterstain or extending the counterstaining with safranin for 3 to 5 minutes is recommended.

Inoculation of Appropriate Plated and Tubed Media

The choice of media for use in the anaerobic bacteriology laboratory is an extremely important aspect of successful anaerobic bacteriology. Anaerobes have special nutritional requirements for vitamin K, hemin, and yeast extract, and all primary isolation media for anaerobes should contain these three ingredients. No one medium is likely to support the growth of all anaerobic bacteria; however, CDC agar provides the best recovery.

TABLE 22-8 Primary Setup Media Recommended for Recovery of Anaerobes

Medium	Organisms	Comments
Anaerobic blood agar (CDC)	Supports growth of virtually all obligate and facultative anaerobes, best for anaerobic gram-positive cocci	An enriched medium containing sheep blood for enrichment and detection of hemolysis, vitamin K (required by some *Porphyromonas* spp.), and yeast extract
Bacteroides bile esculin (BBE) agar	Supports growth of bile-tolerant *Bacteroides* spp., some strains of *Fusobacterium mortiferum*, *Klebsiella pneumoniae*, enterococci, and yeast may grow to a limited extent	A selective medium containing gentamicin (which inhibits most aerobic organisms), 20% bile (which inhibits most anaerobes), and esculin; used primarily for rapid isolation and presumptive identification of members of the *B. fragilis* group, which grow well on BBE (due to their bile-tolerance) and turn the originally light-yellow medium to brown (due to esculin hydrolysis)
Brucella blood agar (BRU/BA)	Supports growth of virtually all obligate and facultative anaerobes, best for gram-negative bacteria	An enriched medium containing sheep red blood cells for enrichment and detection of hemolysis, casein peptones, dextrose, yeast extract, vitamin K, and hemin
Kanamycin-vancomycin-laked blood (KVLB) agar	Supports growth of *Bacteroides* and *Prevotella* spp., yeasts and kanamycin-resistant, facultative, gram-negative bacilli will also grow	A selective medium containing kanamycin (which inhibits most facultative gram-negative bacilli), vancomycin (which inhibits most gram-positive organisms and vancomycin-sensitive strains of *Porphyromonas* spp.), and laked blood (which accelerates production of brown-black pigmented colonies by certain *Prevotella* spp.); used primarily for rapid isolation and presumptive identification of pigmented species of *Prevotella*
Phenylethyl alcohol (PEA) agar	Supports growth of virtually all obligate anaerobes (both gram-positive and gram-negative) and gram-positive, facultative anaerobes	A selective medium containing phenylethyl alcohol; used primarily to suppress the growth of any facultative, gram-negative bacilli (e.g., Enterobacteriaceae) that might be present in the clinical specimen, especially swarming *Proteus* spp.
Colistin nalidixic acid (CNA) blood agar plate	Supports growth of virtually all obligate anaerobes (both gram-positive and gram-negative) and gram-positive, facultative anaerobes	A selective medium containing sheep blood and the antimicrobials colistin and nalidixic acid; used primarily to suppress the growth of any facultative, gram-negative bacilli (e.g., Enterobacteriaceae) that might be present in the clinical specimen, especially swarming *Proteus* spp.
Anaerobic broth (e.g., thioglycollate [THIO] and chopped or cooked meat)	Supports growth of virtually all types of bacteria; in THIO, obligate aerobes and microaerophiles grow near the top, obligate anaerobes at the bottom, and facultative anaerobes throughout the broth	Because obligate anaerobes can be overgrown by more rapidly growing facultative organisms present in the specimen and killed by their toxic, metabolic by products, THIO serves only as a backup source of culture material (e.g., in the event that there is no growth on plated media due to a jar failure or the presence of antimicrobial agents in the specimen); chopped meat carbohydrate broth can be used in place of THIO; broth cultures should never be relied on exclusively for isolating anaerobes from clinical material

Modified from Engelkirk PG et al: *Principles and practice of clinical anaerobic bacteriology*, Belmont, Calif, 1992, Star.

Primary Plating Media for Anaerobic Cultures. Table 22-8 lists the primary media recommended for recovery of anaerobes. Although these media are designed for anaerobes, they also support the growth of most aerobes. No single medium exists that supports all common species of anaerobes while inhibiting all aerobes. At a minimum, specimens for anaerobic culture should be plated onto a nonselective blood agar (such as brucella or CDC blood agar), a biplate containing *Bacteroides* bile esculin (BBE) and kanamycin and vancomycin with laked sheep blood (KVLB) agars. Laked blood is blood lysed through a series of freeze/thaw cycles. Many laboratories also inoculate specimens onto a phenylethyl alcohol (PEA) or colistin nalidixic acid (CNA) blood agar plate. Either of these media will inhibit facultative anaerobic gram-negative bacteria that may overgrow anaerobes present in the specimen. Surgical specimens or sterile site specimens may also be inoculated into a broth medium such as thioglycollate or prereduced chopped meat to serve as a backup source of culture material.

The ideal media for use in the culture of anaerobes are those that have never been exposed to oxygen or have been exposed only briefly. Media should be at room temperature when inoculated. Media exposed to air for extended periods may contain toxic substances, produced as a result of the reduction of molecular oxygen. Such media may also have redox potentials above those required for anaerobes to initiate growth. To provide the best recovery of anaerobes, fresh, plated media should be stored within an anaerobic chamber or holding system until used. An alternative is to use commercial media, such as PRAS media, that have been prepared, packaged, shipped, and stored under anaerobic conditions. With PRAS media shown in Figure 22-4, growth is initiated

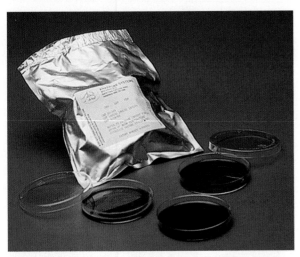

FIGURE 22-4   Prereduced, anaerobically sterilized (PRAS) plated media. PRAS plated media are manufactured, packaged, shipped, and stored under anaerobic conditions. (Courtesy Anaerobe Systems, Morgan Hill, Calif.)

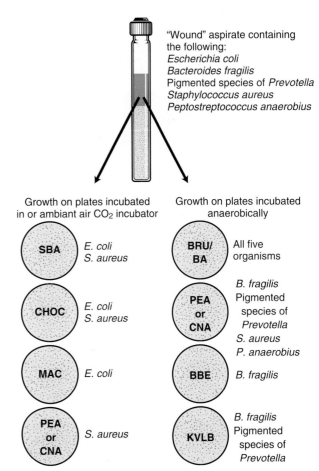

FIGURE 22-5   Culture results that might be obtained from the primary isolation setup of a hypothetical "wound" specimen. This diagram illustrates the media and atmospheric conditions that would support growth of various organisms contained in the specimen. *SBA,* Blood agar; *BBE,* Bacteroides bile-esculin agar; *BRU,* brucella blood agar; *CHOC,* chocolate agar; *KVLB,* kanamycin-vancomycin-laked blood agar; *MAC,* MacConkey agar; *PEA,* phenylethyl alcohol blood agar; *CNA,* Colistin nalidixic acid blood agar. (Modified from Engelkirk PG et al: *Principles and practice of anaerobic bacteriology,* Belmont, Calif, 1992, Star.)

quickly. Many anaerobes produce sufficient growth after only 24 hours of incubation. Studies have demonstrated that these media perform better than other commercially available media.

Media for Aerobic Incubation. In most instances, a request for anaerobic culture on a specimen is also accompanied by a request for aerobic culture. In addition to the battery of selective anaerobic media to be incubated anaerobically, a variety of plated media to be incubated aerobically (in a CO_2 incubator) is also inoculated. The specific media vary somewhat from one laboratory to another and will depend on the specimen type; nevertheless, 5% sheep blood, MacConkey, and chocolate agar plates are usually included. Some laboratories also routinely include a CNA blood agar plate to select for gram-positive bacteria. Figure 22-5 shows a typical plating protocol for a wound sample and the types of results that might be expected.

Inoculation Procedures. In laboratories not equipped with an anaerobic chamber, inoculation of appropriate plated and tubed media could be performed in an area with a suitable nitrogen gas holding system. Such a holding system, which may employ a jar, box, or other small chamber, allows plates that have not been inoculated to be held under anaerobic conditions until needed. Inoculated plates should be held under near-anaerobic conditions until placed into an anaerobic jar or bag. Care should be taken to ensure that inoculated plates do not remain in the holding jar at room temperature for extended periods (i.e., not longer than 1 hour). Also, so the holding jar can maintain as low an oxygen concentration as possible, care should be taken to minimize convection currents whenever freshly inoculated plates are added to the jar. A good quality control procedure to ensure that the agar is maintained under proper conditions is to inoculate an agar plate with *F. nucleatum* and place the plate in the holding jar. After all the specimens have been inoculated, the agar plate can be incubated anaerobically. Growth of *F. nucleatum* indicates that the agar was maintained under near anaerobic conditions.

Some microbiologists believe it is better to batch-process specimens than to process each specimen as it arrives in the laboratory. This relieves their concern that freshly inoculated plates will remain at room temperature in a holding system that may contain some oxygen. Batch processing is an acceptable alternative for aspirates and specimens received in proper transport containers (i.e., those kept moist under anaerobic conditions). It would be unacceptable, however, to batch-process improperly submitted specimens (e.g., dry swabs) or clinical specimens apt to contain rapidly growing bacteria. The delay would further expose anaerobes to molecular oxygen, increase the likelihood of specimens drying out, and decrease the probability of recovering anaerobes.

Anaerobic Incubation of Inoculated Media

After specimens are processed and inoculated onto the appropriate media, the inoculated plates must be incubated anaero-

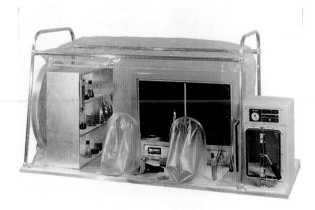

FIGURE 22-6 "Glove box" type of anaerobic chamber (Coy Laboratory Products, Grand Lake, Mich.). The flexible, clear vinyl chambers are available in three lengths (36, 59, and 78 inches), including one fitted with two pairs of gloves so that two microbiologists can use the chamber simultaneously. (Modified from Engelkirk PG et al: *Principles and practice of clinical anaerobic bacteriology*, Belmont, Calif, 1992, Star.)

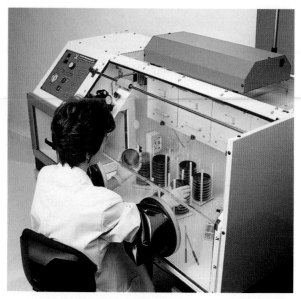

FIGURE 22-7 "Gloveless" type of anaerobic chamber with dissecting microscope attachment. This stainless steel and Plexiglas chamber is manufactured by Anaerobe Systems. (Courtesy Anaerobe Systems, Morgan Hill, Calif.; Sheldon Manufacturing, Inc., Cornelius, Ore.)

bically at 35° to 37° C. The most common and practical choices for anaerobic incubation systems for clinical laboratories are anaerobic chambers, anaerobic jars, and anaerobic bags or pouches. The choice of system is influenced by a number of factors including financial considerations, the number of anaerobic cultures performed, and space limitations.

Anaerobic Chambers. The ideal anaerobic incubation system is an anaerobic chamber, which provides an oxygen-free environment for inoculating media and incubating cultures. Identification and susceptibility tests also can be performed within the chamber. Anaerobic chambers are available as sealed glove boxes and gloveless chambers. Glove boxes are fitted with airtight rubber gloves (Figure 22-6). The microbiologist inserts his or her hands into the gloves and manipulates specimens, plates, and tubes inside the chamber. They have the disadvantage of trying to accommodate many different hand sizes into one pair of gloves. This cumbersome disadvantage has been overcome by the development of the gloveless anaerobic chamber (Figure 22-7). Airtight rubber sleeves that fit snugly against the user's bare forearms are used in place of gloves, enabling the microbiologist to work within an anaerobic environment with bare hands. However, to comply with mandatory infectious disease safety precautions, it is recommended that disposable gloves be worn if clinical specimens are being processed within gloveless chambers. Subsequent operations may be performed with bare hands, if preferred. Some gloveless models also have a dissecting microscope mounted on the front of the rigid Plexiglas chamber. This enables the user to observe colony morphology within the chamber, eliminating the need to remove the plates from the chamber resulting in exposure of the colonies to oxygen.

All anaerobic chambers contain a catalyst, a desiccant, an oxidation-reduction indicator, and anaerobic gas (5% hydrogen, 5% to 10% CO_2, and 85% to 90% nitrogen). The catalyst, usually palladium-coated alumina pellets, removes residual oxygen from the atmosphere within the chamber. With time, the catalyst pellets become inactivated by gaseous metabolic end products produced by the anaerobes. A product called Anatox (Don Whitley Scientific, Shipley, West Yorkshire, England) has been shown to absorb these metabolites and prolong catalyst life. Silica gel is used as a desiccant to absorb the water formed when hydrogen combines with free oxygen in the presence of the catalyst. The silica gel desiccant turns from blue to pink when saturated with water, and it needs to be heated daily to rejuvenate.

Carbon dioxide is required for the growth of many anaerobic organisms, and inert nitrogen gas is used as filler for the remaining percentage of the anaerobic atmosphere. The College of American Pathologists requires that laboratories performing anaerobic cultures verify on a daily basis that anaerobiasis is achieved. This requires the use of an oxygen reduction indicator, which can be either methylene blue or resazurin. Methylene blue remains white in the absence of oxygen (reduced) and turns blue in the presence of oxygen; resazurin goes from colorless in the absence of oxygen to pink in the presence of oxygen.

Anaerobic Jars. For small laboratories, where the volume of anaerobic cultures may not justify the purchase of anaerobic chambers, alternative systems are available. One such alternative is the GasPak jar (BD Diagnostic Systems; Figure 22-8). The jars have been used in clinical laboratories for many years, enabling even small laboratories to perform satisfactory anaerobic bacteriology. Newer models accommodate a larger number of plates as well as microtiter susceptibility trays and anaerobic identification strips or trays. Other anaerobic jars or containers are available from other companies. None of these systems provide all the features or advantages of anaer-

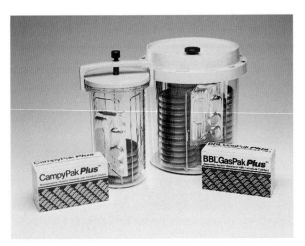

FIGURE 22-8   Anaerobic jars. This photograph depicts two of the many different types of anaerobic jars that are available commercially. As can be seen in this photograph, the jars can also be used to culture microaerophilic organisms. (Courtesy BD Diagnostic Systems, Sparks, Md.)

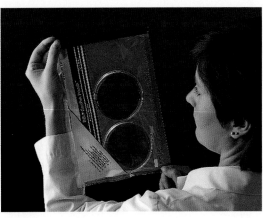

FIGURE 22-9   Anaerobic pouch. This photograph depicts the GasPak Pouch, one of the commercially available anaerobic bag or pouch systems. Identification and susceptibility testing systems requiring anaerobic incubation can be incubated within some of the bags or pouches. (Courtesy BD Diagnostic Systems, Sparks, Md.)

obic chambers, and cost analysis reveals that, over time, a chamber is actually more cost effective.

Anaerobic jar systems use an envelope gas generator. Numerous gas-generating systems are available and can be divided into newer systems that are waterless and the older systems that require water. When water is added to the GasPak envelope, two gases are generated: carbon dioxide and hydrogen. The two gases have a function similar to that in the anaerobic chamber. Hydrogen is explosive, and if the catalyst is not functioning properly, hydrogen gas will accumulate in the jar. An individual should never open the jar in the vicinity of an open flame. A methylene blue oxidation-reduction indicator strip is always added to the jar to verify that an anaerobic atmosphere has been achieved. It takes about 30 to 45 minutes to obtain an anaerobic environment. However, it may take several hours for the methylene blue indicator to change from blue to white. If the catalyst performs properly, water vapor will be present on the inside of the jar, and the indicator strip will be white. Some of the newer gas-generating packets contain a built-in indicator.

Failure to achieve anaerobic conditions could be the result of a "poisoned" catalyst or a crack in the jar, lid, or O-ring. A poisoned catalyst results from the gases, particularly H_2S, produced by anaerobes. The reusable catalyst pellets can be rejuvenated after every use by heating in a 160° C oven for a minimum of 2 hours. The newer waterless gas generating systems (AnaeroPack System; Mitsubishi Gas Chemical America, Inc.) are single-use disposable packets that are designed to produce anaerobic conditions without the use of water or catalyst. Once the packet is removed from its foil container, it must be rapidly (within 1 minute) placed in the anaerobe jar or bag. The atmospheric oxygen in the container is rapidly absorbed with the simultaneous generation of carbon dioxide. The reaction proceeds without the generation of hydrogen, so it eliminates the need for a catalyst. No water is produced in response to the anaerobic atmosphere generation, so plates in bags can be more easily viewed.

The major disadvantage of any anaerobic jar system is that the plates have to be removed from the jar to be examined and worked on. This exposes the bacteria to oxygen, which is especially harmful to the anaerobes during their first 48 hours of growth. For this reason, a suitable holding system ideally should be used in conjunction with anaerobic jars. Plates can be removed from the anaerobic jar, placed in an oxygen-free holding system, removed one by one for rapid microscopic examination of colonies, and then quickly returned to the holding system. Plates never should remain in room air on the open bench.

Anaerobic Bags. Another alternative to an anaerobic chamber or jars are anaerobic bags or pouches (Figure 22-9). Such products are available from BD Diagnostic Systems, Mitsubishi, Oxoid (Hampshire, England)/Inaria, Hardy Diagnostics (Santa Monica, Calif.), and other companies. One or two inoculated plates are placed into a bag, an oxygen-removal system is activated, and the bag is sealed and incubated. Theoretically, the plates can be examined for growth without removing the plates from the bags—thus without exposing the colonies to oxygen. However, with some of the products, a water vapor film on the inner surface of the bag or the lid of the plate can sometimes obscure vision. In such cases, the plates must be removed from the bag to observe for growth, and a new bag and oxygen-removal system must be used whenever additional incubation is required. As with the anaerobic jar, plates must be removed from the bags in order to work with the colonies at the bench. Thus an anaerobic holding system should be used in conjunction with any of the anaerobic bags.

Any of these bags are also useful transport devices. For example, a biopsy specimen can first be placed in a sterile screw-capped tube containing sterile saline, which is then placed in one of these bags. Once the oxygen-removal system is activated, the specimen is transported to the laboratory within the bag, thereby minimizing exposure to oxygen. This is especially important if delays in transport of the specimen are expected.

TABLE 22-9 Options Available for Identifying Anaerobic Bacteria

Identification Technique	Time to Obtain Results	Extent of Identification
Presumptive identification based on colony morphology, Gram-stain observations, and results of simple tests (e.g., disks, catalase, spot indole)	Same day that the PC/SC plate is available	Limited capability; many clinically encountered anaerobes cannot be identified
Definitive identification Commercially available, preexisting enzyme-based identification systems (e.g., ANIDENT, MicroScan, RapID ANA-II, BBL Crystal, Vitek ANI card)	Same day that the PC/SC plate is available (4-hr incubation)	Most commonly encountered, clinically significant anaerobes can be identified
Commercially available biochemical-based identification systems (e.g., API 20A, Minitek, Sceptor)	24-48 hours after PC/SC plate is available	Most commonly encountered saccharolytic anaerobes can be identified, but many asaccharolytic anaerobes cannot be
Cellular fatty acid analysis by high resolution GLC (e.g., MIDI Inc., Newark, Del. system)	24-48 hours after PC/SC plate is available	Most clinically encountered anaerobes can be identified
Conventional tubed biochemical tests and metabolic endproduct analysis by GLC	24-72 hours after PC/SC plate is available	Most clinically encountered anaerobes can be identified
16S rDNA sequencing	5 hours after PC/SC plate is available	Most clinically encountered anaerobes can be identified

PC/SC, Pure culture/subculture; *GLC,* gas-liquid chromatography.

PROCEDURES FOR IDENTIFYING ANAEROBIC ISOLATES

Various methods are available to clinical microbiologists for identifying anaerobic isolates; Table 22-9 lists several options. The method and level of identification usually depends on the size and capabilities of the laboratory and whether the organism is from a mixed infection or from a sterile site such as the blood or other sterile body fluid, for example, synovial, peritoneal, or pleural fluid. Presumptive identifications of microorganisms have become more popular in recent years due primarily to increased emphasis on speed and cost-reduction. Many anaerobic bacteria can be identified in the laboratory using presumptive identification criteria, thereby providing physicians with timely information concerning the presence of anaerobes in clinical specimens. The following sections on identification techniques will be based on progressively more complex procedures that ultimately can provide the genus/species of an anaerobic bacterium. However, keep in mind that often the most actionable information for the physician can be based on the presumptive identification procedures described below, and full identification may not be necessary. Communication with the physician is important to determine how far to go with an identification and whether susceptibility testing is required for proper patient management.

The Clinical Laboratory Standards Institute (CLSI) offers a document (M35-A2, *Abbreviated Identification of Bacteria and Yeast*) that provides guidelines for the rapid presumptive identification of many of the commonly encountered anaerobic bacteria. It is an individual laboratory decision whether such identification will suffice, or whether definitive identifications on some isolates are necessary. By using the guidelines in the CLSI document, an isolate can be identified with greater than 95% accuracy. Consequently, by combining readily observable colony and Gram-stain features with results of simple test procedures, even small laboratories are capable of making presumptive identification of many commonly isolated and clinically important anaerobes.

Preliminary Procedures

When to Examine Primary Plates

Recently the emphasis on anaerobic bacteriology has shifted from full identification of all isolates to rapid, presumptive identification of the most commonly isolated anaerobes. Because many anaerobic infections consist of a mixture of aerobic and anaerobic organisms, the most actionable information that can be provided to the physician is a rapid answer as to whether the specimen contains anaerobes or not. The physician can then select the most appropriate empirical antimicrobial agents to treat the infection.

Plates incubated in an anaerobic chamber can be examined at any time without exposing the colonies to oxygen. However, those incubated in anaerobic jars, bags, or pouches will be exposed to the potentially damaging effects of oxygen whenever the containers are opened. This may inhibit the growth of strict anaerobes due to the toxic effect of oxygen. If a holding system is available at the anaerobe workstation and is used in conjunction with jars, bags, or pouches, exposure to oxygen will be minimized, and plates can be removed and examined at 24 hours and then placed immediately into the holding system. As soon as all plates are examined, those requiring additional incubation are returned to an anaerobic system and incubated for an appropriate period before reexamination. If a holding system is not used, inoculated plates should be held until 48 hours before initial examination. This delays the time to detection, and is certainly not the optimal method, but may be necessary in small laboratories lacking resources. Anaerobic cultures are routinely held 5 to 7 days to allow growth of particularly slow-growing anaerobes and at least 10 days whenever *Actinomyces* is suspected.

Indications of the Presence of Anaerobes in Cultures

Several clues can alert the microbiologist that anaerobes may be present on the primary plates. These include:

- A foul odor upon opening an anaerobic jar or bag. Some anaerobes, especially *C. difficile, Fusobacterium,* and *Porphyromonas,* produce foul-smelling metabolic end products that are readily apparent when the jars, bags, or pouches are opened.
- Colonies present on the anaerobically incubated blood agar plates but not on the CO_2-incubated blood or chocolate agar plates.
- Good growth, more than 1 mm in diameter, of gray colonies on a BBE plate, characteristic of members of the *B. fragilis* group.
- Colonies on either KVLB or anaerobic blood agar plates that fluoresce brick-red under ultraviolet light, or are brown to black in ordinary light, characteristics of pigmented *Porphyromonas* and *Prevotella,* although most strains of *Porphyromonas* will not grow on KVLB because of their sensitivity to vancomycin.
- Double zone of hemolysis on sheep blood agar plate incubated anaerobically, suggestive of *C. perfringens.*

When anaerobes are suspected, the following steps must be performed and recorded for each colony morphotype present on the anaerobic blood agar plate to initiate presumptive identification of the isolates:

- Describe the colony morphology and note whether growth occurred on each of the selective (e.g., BBE, KVLB) and nonselective anaerobic blood agar plates.
- Describe the Gram-stain reaction and cell morphology.
- Set up an aerotolerance test.
- Inoculate pure subculture plate and add appropriate identification disks.

Colony Morphology and Gram-Stain Reaction. The use of a dissecting microscope to observe the fine details of each colony morphotype and to pick colonies for isolation is recommended. Figure 22-10 depicts the appearance of colo-

nies as seen through a dissection microscope. Growth of a particular morphotype can be semiquantitated using terms such as "light," "moderate," and "heavy" or by using a coding system (e.g., 1+, 2+, 3+, etc.). The Gram-stain reaction and morphologic appearance of the organism aid in the presumptive identification of isolates, as shown in a schematic diagram in Figure 22-11.

Aerotolerance Testing. The **aerotolerance test** determines whether a microorganism isolated under anaerobic conditions is a strict anaerobe or a facultative anaerobe. Incubating the suspected isolate in both aerobic and anaerobic environments determines the true atmospheric requirements of the organism. Suspected colonies should be inoculated with a short streak onto a chocolate agar plate for incubation in a CO_2 incubator and an anaerobic blood agar incubated anaerobically. By using this technique, many different organisms can be tested for aerotolerance on a single plate. Some laboratories also prefer to inoculate a sheep blood agar plate in the same manner to be incubated in an ambient air

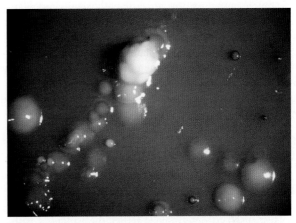

FIGURE 22-10 Anaerobic blood agar plate from an intrauterine device culture as seen through a dissection microscope. The heavy mixture of sizes and types of colonies makes the task of isolating and identifying colonies very difficult without the enhancement obtained with a dissection microscope.

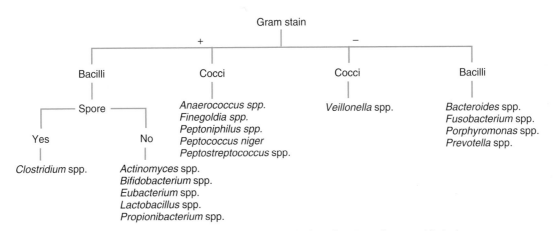

FIGURE 22-11 Schematic diagram for the initial identification of anaerobic isolates based on Gram-stain morphology. Not all *Clostridium* spp. readily sporulate in clinical specimens or in culture.

TABLE 22-10 Interpretation of Aerotolerance Test Results

	Aerobe	Capnophilic Aerobe	Facultative Anaerobe	Obligate Anaerobe
Blood agar plate incubated aerobically in a non-CO₂ incubator	+	−	+	−
Chocolate agar plate incubated aerobically in a CO₂ incubator	+	+	+	−
Blood agar plate incubated anaerobically	−	−*	+	+

Haemophilus influenzae will grow on an anaerobically incubated *Brucella* blood agar plate but can be differentiated from an anaerobe by its growth on the chocolate agar plate incubated in the CO₂ incubator.

incubator. This enables differentiation between aerobic and capnophilic organisms.

All aerotolerance test plates should be incubated at 35° C for up to 48 hours. Following incubation, the aerotolerance test plates are examined for growth. Theoretically, an anaerobe should grow only on the anaerobically incubated plates. However, some aerotolerant anaerobes (e.g., certain *Clostridium, Actinomyces, Propionibacterium,* and *Lactobacillus*) can grow on the CO₂-incubated chocolate agar, but they usually grow much better on the anaerobically incubated plate. A facultative, noncapnophilic organism will grow on all plates, but a capnophilic aerobe should grow only on the CO₂-incubated chocolate agar plate. *Haemophilus influenzae,* however, will grow on the anaerobic plate and the CO₂-incubated chocolate agar plate but not on the aerobically incubated sheep blood agar plate. Table 22-10 describes how the aerotolerance test is interpreted.

Presumptive Identification of Clinically Significant Anaerobes

A presumptive identification of a bacterium is derived from simple colony and Gram-stain observations and the results of several relatively rapid and inexpensive tests. The aerotolerance test, used to determine whether the isolate is truly an anaerobic organism, needs to be one of the first tests performed. The following section describes tests, some rapid (results in about 1 hour or less), that are of value in presumptively identifying many of the anaerobes commonly encountered in clinical specimens.

Rapid Tests

Fluorescence. Many strains of pigmented *Porphyromonas* and *Prevotella* fluoresce brick-red under long-wave (366 nm) ultraviolet (UV) light (Figure 22-12, *A*). However, some strains fluoresce colors other than brick-red (e.g., brilliant red, yellow, orange, and pink-orange). *F. nucleatum* and *C. difficile* fluoresce chartreuse (Figure 22-12, *B*). *Veillonella* spp. often fluoresce red, but the fluorescence is dependent on the culture medium. It is weaker than the fluorescence produced by pigmented species of *Porphyromonas* and *Prevotella* and fades completely if the colonies are exposed to air for 5 to 10 minutes. Table 22-11 lists the fluorescence characteristic of commonly isolated anaerobic bacteria.

Catalase Test. To perform a catalase test, a plastic, disposable inoculating loop or a wooden applicator stick is used to place some of the colony onto a small area of a glass microscope slide. A drop of 15% hydrogen peroxide is added, and the production of bubbles of oxygen gas is a positive

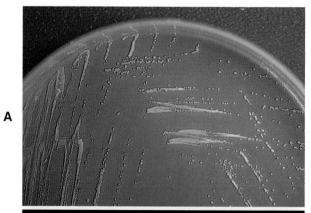

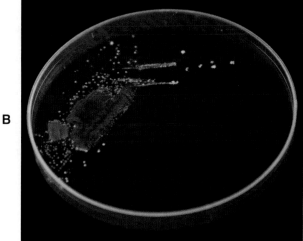

FIGURE 22-12 Examples of fluorescence observed with long-wave ultraviolet light. **A,** Brick-red fluorescence observed with *Porphyromonas asaccharolytica*. **B,** Chartreuse fluorescence of *Fusobacterium nucleatum*. (**A,** From Engelkirk PG et al: *Principles and practice of clinical anaerobic bacteriology*, Belmont, Calif, 1992, Star.)

result. Among other uses, the catalase test is valuable in differentiating aerotolerant strains of *Clostridium* (catalase-negative) from *Bacillus* (catalase-positive).

Spot Indole Test. The spot indole test uses a small piece of filter paper saturated with para-dimethylaminocinnamaldehyde. An inoculating loop or wooden applicator stick is used to transfer some growth from the culture plate onto the saturated filter paper. Rapid development of a blue or green color indicates a positive test (i.e., production of indole from the amino acid tryptophan), whereas a pink or orange color indicates a negative test. The spot indole test also can be performed directly on a pure culture plate. The spot indole test is useful in identifying *Propionibacterium acnes* (indole positive) from other *Propionibacterium* spp. (indole negative).

Urease Test. A rapid urease test can be accomplished by adding a Wee-Tab Urease Test Tablet (Key Scientific Products, Stamford, Tex.) into 1 mL of distilled water. The isolate is then heavily inoculated into the water and incubated at 37° C. A positive reaction can occur within 15 minutes, but the tube must be held for up to 6 hours before a true negative reaction is determined. Rapid urea broths are also available from various manufacturers. *C. sordellii* is the only *Clostridium* sp. urease positive.

Motility Test. Motility may be determined by wet mount using either very young (4 to 6 hours old) broth cultures or 24- to 48-hour-old colonies on agar. Using a wooden applicator stick, a small portion of a colony should be touched to a drop of saline on a microscope slide. A coverslip is carefully placed over the drop, and the slide is examined with a light microscope. A positive motility test is indicated when organisms exhibit purposeful movement and should not be confused with Brownian motion. Motile gram-negative anaerobes include some *Campylobacter* spp. (e.g., *Campylobacter concisus, C. curvus,* and *C. rectus*) and *Mobiluncus* spp., among many others.

Special-Potency Antimicrobial Disks. Although the Gram stain is helpful in the initial identification of an anaerobic isolate, certain species of *Clostridium* may stain pink and thus appear to be gram-negative bacilli. To determine the true Gram-stain reaction of the isolate, special-potency disks can be used. These disks—kanamycin (1000 μg), vancomycin (5 μg) and colistin (10 μg)—are used for identification purposes and are not meant to predict treatment options for the physician (Figure 22-13).

The disks are placed on the heavily inoculated area of the plate (usually the first quadrant of the subculture plate). Disks of the proper potency must be pressed firmly to the surface of the plate to ensure uniform diffusion of the agent into the medium. The disk results for *C. ramosum* are shown in Figure 22-14. Other disks may be used for identification purposes. Disk results are interpreted as listed in Table 22-12.

Sodium Polyanethol Sulfonate Disk. A sodium polyanethol sulfonate (SPS) disk aids in the identification of anaerobic gram-positive cocci. An SPS-sensitive, gram-positive anaerobic coccus can be presumptively identified as *Peptostreptococcus anaerobius,* whereas an SPS-resistant, spot indole–positive, gram-positive anaerobic coccus can be presumptively identified as *Peptoniphilus (Peptostreptococcus) asaccharolyticus.*

Nitrate Disk. The nitrate reduction disk test is a miniaturized version of the conventional nitrate reduction test. This determines an organism's ability to reduce nitrate to nitrite or nitrogen gas.

Bile Disk. This disk can be used to determine an organism's ability to grow in the presence of relatively high concentrations (20%) of bile; however, it is not necessary if BBE agar is used as a primary plating medium. The bile disk may be added to the anaerobic subculture plate whenever the Gram stain reveals the isolate to be a gram-negative bacillus. Good growth on a BBE plate or growth in 20% bile indicates bile tolerance. A bile-tolerant, gram-negative anaerobic bacillus indicates the isolate is likely a member of the *B. fragilis* group.

Lecithinase, Lipase, and Proteolytic Reactions. An egg-yolk agar (EYA) plate can be used to determine the activities of lecithinase, lipase, and proteolytic enzymes. These reac-

TABLE 22-11 Fluorescence Under Long-Wave Ultraviolet Light

Organism	Color of Fluorescence
Prevotella (pigmented)	Brick red
P. bivia, P. disiens	Light orange to pink (coral)
Porphyromonas	Brick red (some no fluorescence)
Fusobacterium	Chartreuse
Veillonella	Red but fades rapidly
Clostridium ramosum	Red
C. innocuum, C. difficile	Chartreuse
Eggerthella lenta	Red or no fluorescence

TABLE 22-12 Interpretation of Special-Potency Antimicrobial Disk Results

Vancomycin*	Kanamycin†	Colistin‡	Interpretation
S	V	R	Probably a pink-staining, gram-positive bacillus such as *Clostridium ramosum* or *C. clostridioforme;* however, if the kanamycin result is resistant, it could be a *Porphyromonas* sp.
S	R	R	*Porphyromonas* sp.
R	R	R	Probably a member of the *Bacteroides fragilis* group, but could be a *Prevotella* sp.
R	R	V	*Prevotella* sp.
R	R	S	Probably a *Prevotella* sp.
R	S	S	*Bacteroides ureolyticus, Bilophila wadsworthia,* or a *Fusobacterium* sp.; *Veillonella*

From Mangels JI: Anaerobic bacteriology. In Isenberg HD: *Essential procedures for clinical microbiology,* Washington, DC, 1998, American Society for Microbiology.
R, Resistant; *S,* susceptible (A zone of inhibition 10 mm or more is considered susceptible.); *V,* variable.
*Vancomycin, 5 μg.
†Kanamycin, 1000 μg.
‡Colistin, 10 μg.

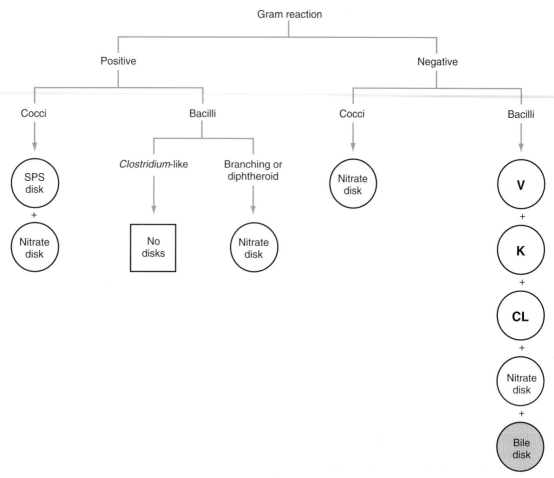

FIGURE 22-13 Disks to add to the pure culture/subculture plate. *SPS,* Sodium polyanethol sulfonate; *V,* vancomycin (5 μg); *K,* kanamycin (1000 μg); *CL,* colistin (10 μg). *Clostridium*-like organisms are large, unbranched, gram-positive rods, with or without spores. (Not all clostridia are large, and not all clostridia will stain as gram-positive rods.) (Modified from Engelkirk PG et al: *Principles and practice of clinical anaerobic bacteriology,* Belmont, Calif, 1992, Star.)

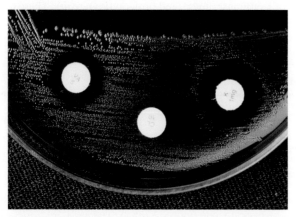

FIGURE 22-14 Typical special-potency antimicrobial disk results for *Clostridium ramosum*: susceptible to vancomycin *(left)* and kanamycin *(right)*, and resistant to colistin *(center disk)*. (Courtesy Anaerobe Systems, Morgan Hill, Calif.)

tions are of value in identifying many species of clostridia. Lecithinase cleaves lecithin found in egg yolk, releasing insoluble fat (diglyceride) that produces an opaque zone around the colony. This opacity is actually in the medium and is not a surface phenomenon. The appearance of the lecithinase reaction is shown in Figure 22-15. Lipases hydrolyze triglycerides and diglycerides to fatty acids and glycerol. Lipase-positive organisms produce a colony covered with an iridescent, multicolored sheen, sometimes described as resembling the appearance of gasoline on water or mother-of-pearl. This multicolored sheen also may appear on the surface of the agar in a narrow zone around the colony. In contrast to the lecithinase reaction, the lipase reaction is essentially a surface phenomenon. The appearance of the lipase reaction is depicted in Figure 22-16. Organisms that produce proteolytic enzymes (proteases) have a completely clear zone, often quite narrow, around their colonies. Proteolysis is best observed by holding the plate up to a strong light source. It is reminiscent of the complete clearing seen with β-hemolytic organisms on sheep blood agar plates.

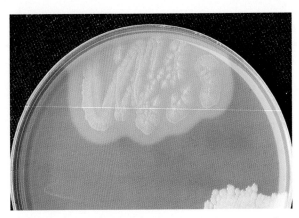

FIGURE 22-15 Positive lecithinase reaction on egg-yolk agar. The reaction occurs within the agar. *Clostridium perfringens* is shown here. (Courtesy Anaerobe Systems, Morgan Hill, Calif.)

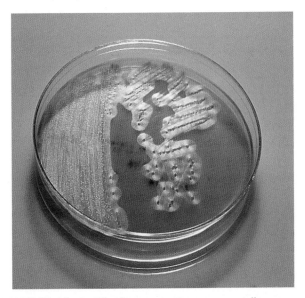

FIGURE 22-16 Positive lipase reaction on egg-yolk agar. The reaction occurs on the surface of colonies and the surrounding medium. A positive reaction by *Fusobacterium necrophorum* is shown here. (Courtesy Anaerobe Systems, Morgan Hill, Calif.)

Presumptive Identification of Gram-Positive Anaerobes

Many gram-positive anaerobes can also be presumptively identified with simple procedures (Table 22-13). None of these organisms will grow on BBE or LKVB media so identification is based on the colony appearance on nonselective anaerobic blood and egg-yolk agars.

- Large, irregular-shaped colonies on sheep blood agar demonstrating a double zone of beta-hemolysis can be identified as *C. perfringens* (Figure 22-17). These organisms will stain as large, boxcar-shaped bacilli.
- Large, flat colonies that produce a "barnyard" or "horse stable" odor and fluoresce chartreuse under long-wave UV light can be identified as *C. difficile*.
- A rapidly growing colony exhibiting smooth swarming (as opposed to the waves observed with *Proteus*) and staining as thin rods with subterminal spores is likely to be *C. septicum*. Colonies often show beta-hemolysis at 48 hours.
- Small, peaked, circular colonies appearing after 24 hours that stain as gram-positive cocci can be considered *Peptostreptococcus* spp. The CLSI M-35-A2 document suggests continued use of the terms *Peptostreptococcus* spp. or "anaerobic gram-positive cocci" as a presumptive

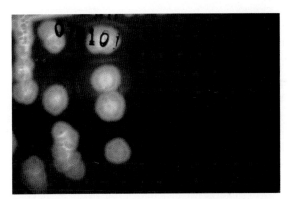

FIGURE 22-17 Double zone of hemolysis produced by *Clostridium perfringens*: inner zone of complete β-hemolysis and outer zone of partial β-hemolysis. (Courtesy Anaerobe Systems, Morgan Hill, Calif.)

TABLE 22-13   Presumptive Identification of Gram-Positive Anaerobes*

Identification	Colony Morphology on Blood Agar	Cellular Morphology	Spot Indole
Clostridium difficile	Large, flat colonies; barnyard odor, chartreuse fluorescence	Thin rods, rare spores	Negative
C. perfringens	Large, irregular-shaped, double zone of beta-hemolysis	Boxcar, large, square rods	Not done
C. septicum	Smoothly swarming	Thin rods, subterminal spores	Negative
C. sordellii	Very large, lobate, irregular, flat	Thin rods, subterminal spores	Positive
C. tetani	Smoothly swarming but slow growing	Swollen terminal spores	Positive
Peptostreptococci	Small, peaked, circular	Cocci, pairs and chains	Not done
Propionibacterium acnes	Small, opaque, enamel-white, circular (catalase positive)	Coryneform rods	Positive

*Additional information about presumptive identification of aerobes and facultative anaerobes can be found in *Abbreviated identification of bacteria and yeast: approved guidelines—second edition*, CLSI document M35-A2, vol. 28, no. 18, Wayne, Pa, 2008, Clinical Laboratory Standards Institute.

TABLE 22-14 Presumptive Identification of Gram-Negative Anaerobes*

Identification	Colony Morphology on Blood/KVLB Agar	Colony Morphology on BBE	Cellular Morphology	Spot Indole
B. fragilis group	Large (>1 mm)	Large, convex Black-gray	Regular	Not done
B. ureolyticus	Translucent, pitting (some)	No growth	Tiny rods or coccobacilli	Negative
Bilophila wadsworthia	Tiny, translucent	Translucent with black center at 72 hr	Regular to filamentous	Negative
Fusobacterium nucleatum	Ground-glass or breadcrumb	No growth	Fusiform, thin with pointed ends	Positive
Porphyromonas	Small, translucent or opaque, brick red fluorescence on blood agar, no growth on KVLB	No growth	Tiny coccobacilli	Positive
Prevotella intermedia	Small, translucent or opaque, brick red fluorescence on blood and KVLB agar	No growth	Tiny coccobacilli	Positive
Prevotella				Negative
Veillonella	Small, translucent or opaque, brick red fluorescence on blood agar, no growth on KVLB	No growth	Tiny diplococci	Negative

KVLB, Kanamycin and vancomycin with laked sheep blood; *BBE, Bacteroides* bile esculin.
*Additional information about presumptive identification of aerobes and facultative anaerobes can be found in *Abbreviated identification of bacteria and yeast: approved guidelines,* CLSI document M35-A2, vol. 22, no. 18, Wayne, Pa, 2002, Clinical Laboratory Standards Institute.

identification rather than identifying these organisms with the newer nomenclature.
- *Peptococcus niger* produces colonies that are initially black to olive-green and become light gray when exposed to air, but it is only rarely isolated from clinical specimens.
- Small, opaque colonies that are catalase and indole positive and stain as coryneform rods can be identified as *P. acnes.*

Presumptive Identification of Gram-Negative Anaerobes

Using Gram-stain results, growth characteristics on primary plating media (e.g., nonselective anaerobic blood, BBE, KVLB) and a few rapid tests, many gram-negative anaerobes can be presumptively identified, often within 24 hours of inoculation (Table 22-14).
- Growth of large (greater than 1 mm) gray-black colonies on BBE agar with growth on the KVLB agar after an overnight incubation is sufficient to identify an isolate as a member of the *B. fragilis* group (Figure 22-18).
- Translucent, pitting colonies observed on the anaerobic blood agar plate, with no growth observed on BBE or KVLB agars, are characteristic of *Bacteroides ureolyticus.*
- Translucent colonies with a black "bull's eye" center observed on BBE agar (usually at 48-72 hours) can be used to presumptively identify *Bilophila wadsworthia* (Figure 22-19).
- Ground-glass or breadcrumb like colonies of long, slender gram-negative rods with pointed ends are usually *Fusobacterium nucleatum* (Figure 22-20).
- Organisms that grow on anaerobic blood agar and KVLB but not BBE and fluoresce brick-red can be identified as *Prevotella.*
- Small, translucent or opaque colonies of tiny gram-negative cocci or diplococci can be identified as *Veillonella.*

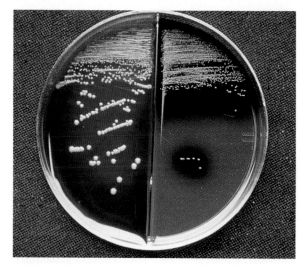

FIGURE 22-18 Appearance of *Bacteroides fragilis* on a kanamycin-vancomycin-laked blood agar *(left)* and *Bacteroides* bile-esculin (BBE) agar biplate *(right).* Browning of the BBE medium is the result of esculin hydrolysis. (Courtesy Anaerobe Systems, Morgan Hill, Calif.)

Definitive Identification of Anaerobic Isolates

For sterile site and some surgical isolates, it is important for the laboratory to provide full identification. A variety of techniques exist for making definitive identification (see Table 22-9):
- Biochemical-based and preexisting enzyme-based minisystems
- PRAS and non-PRAS tubed biochemical test media
- Gas-liquid chromatography (GLC) analysis of metabolic end products
- Cellular fatty acid analysis by GLC
- Sequencing of the 16S ribosomal gene

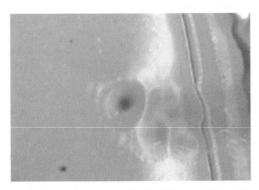

FIGURE 22-19 Appearance of *Bilophila wadsworthia* on BBE agar. Note the "fish-eye" appearance of the colonies.

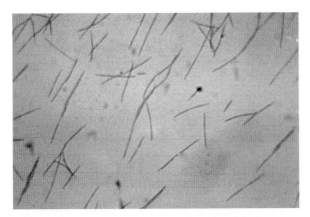

FIGURE 22-20 Gram-stained appearance of *Fusobacterium nucleatum* subsp. *nucleatum*, illustrating the fusiform morphology of this organism. (Courtesy Suzette L. Bartley, James D. Howard, and Ray Simon, Centers for Disease Control and Prevention, Atlanta, Ga.)

The majority of today's clinical microbiology laboratories use one of the commercially available biochemical-based or preexisting enzyme-based minisystems for making definitive identifications, but it is important to remember that none of these will identify all the anaerobes that could potentially be isolated from clinical specimens. Most are designed to identify those anaerobes that are most frequently encountered in clinical specimens. It is far more important for a system to identify such organisms than to identify obscure anaerobes that are only rarely isolated from clinical specimens or involved in infectious processes.

Biochemical-Based Multitest Systems

A commercially available alternative to conventional tubed media is the biochemical-based identification systems manufactured by Analytab Products (API; bioMérieux, Durham, N.C.). This system provide many of the same tests as the conventional systems but in the form of a small plastic strip or tray. The biochemical-based multitest system is easier and faster to inoculate than a conventional system of plates and tubes. Although they can be inoculated aerobically, they require anaerobic incubation. The larger model BBL anaerobic jars and some of the commercially available bags and pouches can be used to incubate biochemical-based trays and strips if an anaerobic chamber is not available. After 24 to 48 hours of incubation, test results are read, a code number is generated for each isolate, and the identification is determined from a compendium codebook. It is notable that the databases from which the codebooks are developed do not contain all the anaerobes that can potentially be isolated from clinical specimens.

Preformed Enzyme-Based Systems

Many of the newer commercial identification systems are based on the presence of preformed (preexisting) bacterial enzymes. Because these systems do not depend on enzyme induction, the results are available in about 4 hours. The small plastic panels or cards are easy to inoculate, can be inoculated at the bench, and do not require anaerobic incubation. Most of the systems generate code numbers, which are referenced in a manufacturer-supplied codebook. Like the biochemical-based multitest systems, these systems are primarily of value for identifying only the most commonly isolated anaerobes. One potential pitfall with these systems is that the codebook compendium is divided by Gram-staining characteristics of the organism. Hence, it is vital to have an accurate Gram stain in order to arrive at an accurate identification. Special potency disks to determine the true Gram stain of an organism can play a major role in the use of the preformed enzyme-based identification systems.

Examples of preexisting enzyme-based systems include the Vitek ANI Card (bioMérieux), the AN-IDENT (bioMérieux), the RapID-ANA II (Remel, Lenexa, Kans.), the MicroScan Rapid Anaerobe Identification Panel (Siemens Biomedical Diagnostics, Inc., Deerfield, Ill.) and the BBL Crystal Anaerobe ID System (BD Diagnostic Systems). The RapID-ANA II System is shown in Figure 22-21. In general, the systems use the same or similar substrates. They contain a number of nitrophenyl and naphthylamide compounds, which are colorless substances that produce yellow or red products, respectively, in the presence of appropriate enzymes. The results of some of these systems can be read via instrumentation.

Conventional Tubed Biochemical Identification Systems

In general, conventional or traditional systems for the identification of anaerobic isolates employ large test tubes containing a variety of PRAS or non-PRAS biochemical test media. Biochemical reactions are measured either by measuring the pH with a probe or by color changes based on a bromthymol blue indicator. Identification of anaerobes by conventional biochemicals is expensive and time consuming and has been replaced largely in clinical laboratories by the systems mentioned above.

Gas-Liquid Chromatography. Identification of anaerobes by GLC analysis of metabolic end products was pioneered at the Virginia Polytechnic Institute (VPI), and the VPI guidelines were modified by the CDC. The anaerobe to be

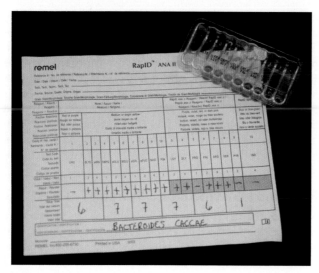

FIGURE 22-21 RapID ANA-II preformed enzyme system (Remel, Lenexa, Kans.). One of many systems available for rapid definitive identification of commonly isolated anaerobes.

tested is grown in a tube of peptone–yeast extract–glucose (PYG) medium. After incubation, the metabolic end products are extracted with chloroform and ether, injected into the chromatograph, volatilized, and carried as a gas through a packed column. Aliquots of the extraction solutions are used to analyze volatile (ether-extracted) and nonvolatile (chloroform-extracted) acids. The acids are separated and recovered in a specific order, based on their chemical and physical properties. The acids are identified based on their position on the chromatogram by their relative retention time as compared to a standard.

Short-chain volatile acids produced by anaerobes include formic, acetic, propionic, isobutyric, isovaleric, valeric, isocaproic, butyric, caproic, and heptanoic. Figure 22-22, *A* and *B*, shows chromatograms of a volatile acid standard and *Fusobacterium*, respectively. The chloroform extract recovers nonvolatile, low–molecular-weight aliphatic and aromatic acids. These include pyruvic, lactic, oxaloacetic, oxalic, malonic, fumaric, succinic, benzoic, phenylacetic, and hydrocinnamic acids. In Figure 22-22, *C* and *D*, chromatograms show the nonvolatile acid standard and *Actinomyces*, respectively. These procedures were used extensively in the early days of anaerobic bacteriology, but because of cost, safety, and time commitment they have been largely abandoned for more rapid identification procedures.

Cellular Fatty Acid Analysis by High-Resolution GLC

Cellular fatty acid analysis is another method of identifying anaerobes. The term *cellular fatty acid* refers to fatty acids and related compounds (aldehydes, hydrocarbons, and dimethylacetals) that are present within organisms as cellular components. Cellular fatty acids are coded for on bacterial chromosomes, as opposed to plasmids, and are not affected by simple mutations or plasmid loss. Thus the fatty acid composition of a particular organism is relatively stable when

grown under specific growth conditions (medium, incubation temperature, and time). Although fatty acid profiles can be identified manually, computerized, high-resolution GLC and specialized software programs are available to analyze cellular fatty acids of unknown bacteria and compare the results to patterns of known species.

The MIDI Sherlock Microbial Identification System (MIDI, Inc., Newark, Del.) is a fully automated gas chromatographic system that can be used to identify bacteria (including anaerobes) and yeasts. The organism is grown in pure culture in peptone–yeast extract–glucose (PYG) broth or another standardized medium. The bacterial cells are removed by centrifugation and then saponified to release the fatty acids from the bacterial lipids. After extraction, the methyl esters are analyzed by GLC. A chromatogram depicting the unknown organism's fatty acid composition and a comparison to a database of fatty acids of known anaerobes are generated as a computer printout or report. The report includes statistical values or "similarity indices," which are based on deviations in the unknown organism's fatty acid composition from the known profiles contained in the database. Because no subjective interpretations are required, the identifications are objective and highly reproducible.

16S Ribosomal RNA Gene Sequencing

Many of the techniques mentioned above have been replaced largely in research and reference laboratories by 16S ribosomal RNA gene sequencing. The 16S ribosomal RNA gene (rDNA) has highly conserved and highly variable regions that can be used for microbial identification. The rDNA is first extracted from the organism; the target segment of about 500 base pairs is amplified through polymerase chain reaction technology and then sequenced on an automated sequencer. The resulting nucleotide sequence is compared to known sequences in public databases such as GenBank, a repository of sequences maintained by the National Institutes of Health. The MicroSeq Microbial Identification System (Applied Biosystems, Foster City, Calif.) has kits and an electronic database that can be used for bacterial or fungal identification. The results can be obtained in approximately 5 hours.

Identification of *Clostridium* species

An identification algorithm for some *Clostridium* spp. is shown in Figure 22-23. Identification of clinically encountered clostridia using cultural and biochemical characteristics is summarized in Table 22-15. The clostridial cell wall structure is similar to that of other gram-positive bacteria. However, some species appear gram-variable, and some, such as *C. ramosum* and *C. clostridioforme*, routinely stain gram-negative. The vancomycin special-potency antimicrobial disk set up at the same time as the aerotolerance test is used to determine the true Gram-stain reaction of a pink-staining anaerobic bacillus. Gram-positive clostridia are always susceptible to vancomycin.

Certain cultural characteristics may be used to initially identify clostridial isolates. As previously mentioned, a boxcar-shaped, gram-positive anaerobic bacillus that produces a characteristic double zone of hemolysis on sheep blood agar can be presumptively identified as *C. perfringens*. Double zone

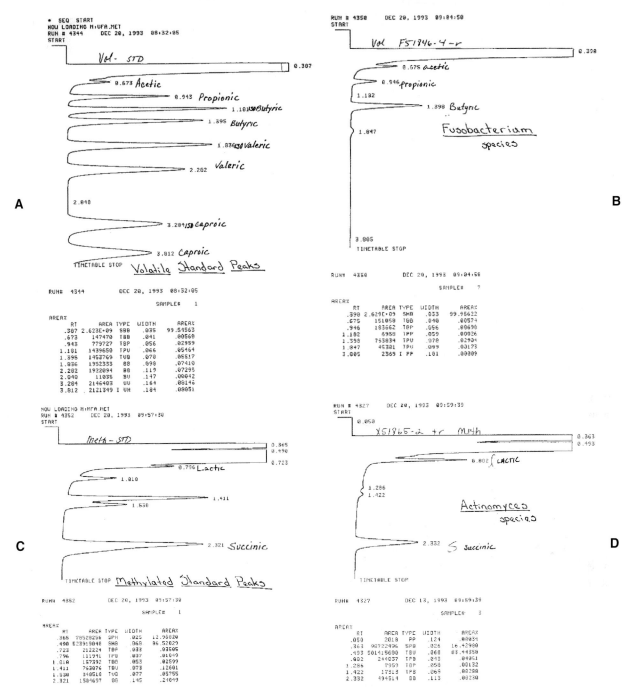

FIGURE 22-22 **A,** Volatile acid standard chromatogram. Elution times of known acids and their peaks are depicted in the extract of the standard solution. **B,** Volatile acid chromatogram of an unknown organism identified as *Fusobacterium* sp. after comparison of the retention times of the acids with those for the standard solution. Numbers located near the acid peaks are retention times. **C,** Methylated acid standard chromatogram. Elution times of known acids and their peaks are depicted in the extract of the standard solution. **D,** Methylated acid chromatogram of an unknown organism identified as *Actinomyces* sp. after comparison of the retention times of the acids with those of the standard solution. Numbers located near the acid peaks are retention times in minutes. *RT,* Retention time.

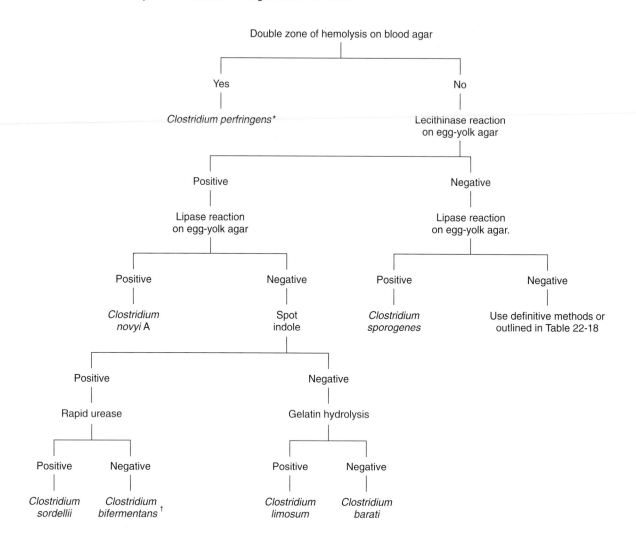

Double zone of hemolysis on blood agar

Yes → *Clostridium perfringens**

No → Lecithinase reaction on egg-yolk agar

Positive → Lipase reaction on egg-yolk agar

Negative → Lipase reaction on egg-yolk agar.

Positive → *Clostridium novyi* A

Negative → Spot indole

Positive → *Clostridium sporogenes*

Negative → Use definitive methods or outlined in Table 22-18

Positive → Rapid urease

Negative → Gelatin hydrolysis

Positive → *Clostridium sordellii*

Negative → *Clostridium bifermentans*†

Positive → *Clostridium limosum*

Negative → *Clostridium barati*

* Boxcar-shaped bacilli; lecithinase-positive; reverse CAMP (Christie, Atkins, and Munch-Petersen) test–positive; subterminal spores, but spores rarely observed
† Produces chalk-white colonies on egg-yolk agar

FIGURE 22-23 Identification of *Clostridium* spp. Use this chart for organisms fulfilling the following three criteria: (1) anaerobic, (2) gram-positive bacilli, and (3) spore formers. (Data from Mangels JI: Anaerobic bacteriology. In Isenberg HD: *Essential procedures for clinical microbiology*, Washington, DC, 1998, American Society for Microbiology.)

of hemolysis appears as an inner zone of complete β-hemolysis and an outer zone of partial β-hemolysis due to two different hemolysins (see Figure 22-17). A swarming, gram-positive, anaerobic bacillus with terminal spores is probably *C. tetani*, whereas one with subterminal spores is most likely *C. septicum*. Egg-yolk agar is useful for detecting lecithinase, lipase, and proteolytic enzymes produced by some clostridia. Lecithinase-positive clostridia include *C. bifermentans, C. sordellii, C. perfringens,* and *C. novyi type A.* Examples of lipase-positive clostridia are *C. botulinum, C. novyi* type A, and *C. sporogenes.*

C. sordellii is the only member of the clostridia to exhibit urease activity. *C. bifermentans* and *C. sordellii* are spot-indole positive. Finally, it is important to remember that *C. tertium* will grow minimally on the aerotolerance plate and can be mistaken for a facultative anaerobe. However, growth on the

anaerobic subculture plate will exhibit much heavier growth than on the aerotolerance test plate.

Clostridium difficile can be recovered from feces by inoculating a cycloserine-cefoxitin-fructose agar (CCFA) plate. CCFA is a selective and differential medium for the recovery and presumptive identification of *C. difficile.* On CCFA, *C. difficile* produces yellow "ground-glass" colonies, and the originally pink agar turns yellow in the vicinity of the colonies because of the fermentation of fructose. In reduced conditions the indicator, neutral red, turns yellow in the presence of an acid pH. Although other organisms may grow on CCFA, their colonies are smaller and do not resemble the characteristic colonies of *C. difficile.* In addition, *C. difficile* has a characteristic odor resembling a horse stable, and colonies on blood agar fluoresce chartreuse under UV light.

TABLE 22-15 Characteristics of Some Clinically Encountered *Clostridium* species

Clostridium species	Aerotolerant Growth	Swarming	Double-Zone β-Hemolysis	Chartreuse Fluorescence	Gram-Stain Reaction	Spore Position	Motility	Indole	Lecithinase	Lipase	Proteolysis in Milk	Gelatin Hydrolysis	Acid from Lactose	Urease
C. bifermentans	−	−	−	−	+	ST	+	+	+	−	+	−	−	−
C. clostridioforme	−	−	−	−	−	ST	−⁺	−	−	−	−	−	+	−
C. difficile	−	−	−	+	+	ST	+	−	−	−	−	−⁺	−	−
C. novyi type A	−	−	−	−	+	ST	+⁻	−	+	+	−	+	−	−
C. perfringens	−	−	+	−	+	−ˢᵀ	−	−	+	−	−	+	+	−
C. ramosum	−	−	−	−	−	(T)	−	−	−	−	−	−	+	−
C. septicum	−	+	−	−	+	ST	+	−	−	−	−	−	+	−
C. sordellii	−	−	−	−	+	ST	+	+	+	−	+	−	−	+
C. sporogenes	−	−	−	−	+	ST	+	−	−⁺	+	+	−⁺	−	−
C. tertium	+	−	−	−	+	T	+	−	−	−	−	−	+	−
C. tetani	−	+	−	−	+	T	+	−⁺	−	−	−	+	−	−

Modified from Engelkirk PG et al: *Principles and practice of clinical anaerobic bacteriology*, Belmont, Calif, 1992, Star.
ST, Subterminal; *T*, terminal; −ˢᵀ, usually not observed but subterminal when seen; *(T)*, variable but usually terminal; +⁻, most strains positive; −⁺, most strains negative.

Organisms that are isolated must be tested for toxin production because a small percentage of the human population can carry *C. difficile* as normal biota, and some isolates may not be toxin producers. Culture for *C. difficile* has largely been replaced by assays designed to detect the toxins produced by the organism. The cell culture cytotoxicity assay that detects toxin B in fecal samples by tissue culture is generally considered the gold standard. However, this assay is technically demanding and can take 2 to 3 days for results. A number of rapid detection tests are available that detect toxin A, toxin B, an enzyme called *glutamate dehydrogenase*, or a combination of toxins A and B. Many of the kits employ microwell or membrane enzyme immunoassay methodologies. Glutamate dehydrogenase is not a virulence factor, but it is an enzyme frequently associated with *C. difficile*. Detection of glutamate dehydrogenase requires confirmation that the organism produces toxins A and B, but a negative test can be used as rapid screening test to rule out *C. difficile*–associated disease. Because not all strains of *C. difficile* produce both toxin A and B, assays that detect both toxins are generally more sensitive. Molecular based assays that can detect the presence of toxin A and B genes in feces are currently under development.

Identification of Anaerobic Non–spore-forming Gram-Positive Bacilli

Identifying characteristics of clinically encountered non–spore-forming gram-positive bacilli are listed in Table 22-16. In general, non–spore-forming gram-positive bacilli are difficult to identify because the preformed enzyme system databases often do not contain many of the less commonly isolated species. GLC of volatile and nonvolatile fatty acids may be required to adequately place isolates within a genus. Sequencing of the 16S rDNA gene has been used most recently to redefine many of these organisms to new genera.

Actinomyces

Actinomyces spp. are straight to slightly curved bacilli of varying lengths, from short rods to long filaments. Short rods may have clubbed ends and may be seen in diphtheroid arrangements, short chains, or small clusters. Longer rods and filaments may be straight or wavy and branched. Although the *Actinomyces* are gram-positive, irregular staining may produce a beaded or banded appearance, much like that seen with *Nocardia* spp. The typical branching, filamentous, Gram-stained appearance of an *Actinomyces* sp., depicted in Figure 22-20, is referred to as "*Actinomyces*-like."

Investigators at the CDC Anaerobic Bacteria Branch found that members of the genus *Actinomyces* are seldom obligate anaerobes. However, some are quite fastidious, requiring special vitamins, amino acids, and hemin for adequate growth. Young *Actinomyces* colonies are frequently spider-like or wooly, whereas older colonies of *A. israelii* usually have a molar tooth appearance (Figure 22-24). Depending on the species, colonies may be red, pink, tan, yellow, white, or grayish.

Bifidobacterium

Bifidobacterium spp. are variable in shape, ranging from coccobacilli to long, branching rods. The ends of the cells may be pointed, bent, club-shaped, spatulated, or bifurcated (forked). Cells may appear singly or in chains and as starlike aggregates, V arrangements, or "palisade" clusters. Colonies of *Bifidobacterium* spp. are convex, entire, and cream to white, smooth, glistening, and soft.

TABLE 22-16 Characteristics of Some Clinically Encountered Gram-Positive Non–spore-forming Anaerobic Bacilli

	48-hr colony <1 mm	Red-pigment colony	β-hemolytic colony	Rough colony	Branched bacilli	Catalase	Indole	Major products in PYG by GLC	Comments
Actinomyces israelii	+	−	−	+	+	−	−	A,L,S	Molar tooth colony, slow growth
A. meyeri	−⁺	−	−	−	+	−	−	A,L,S	
A. naeslundii	−⁺	−	−	−⁺	+	−	−	A,L,S	
A. odontolyticus	−	+	−	−	+	−	−	A,L,S	
A. viscosus	−	−	−	−⁺	+	+	−	A,L,S	
Bifidobacterium spp.	−	−	−	−	−	−	−	A,L	Rods with forked ends
Eggerthella lenta	−	−	−	−	−	V	−	(A)	Nitrate positive
Eubacterium spp.	−	−	−	−	−	−	−	A,B	
Propionibacterium acnes	−	−	−	−	−	+	+	A,P,(L),(S)	
P. propionicum	+	−	−	+	+	−	−	A,P,L	

Modified from Engelkirk PG et al: *Principles and practice of clinical anaerobic bacteriology*, Belmont, Calif, 1992, Star.
PYG, Peptone–yeast extract–glucose medium; *GLC*, gas liquid chromatography; *A*, acetic acid; *P*, propionic acid; *L*, lactic acid; *S*, succinic acid; −⁺, most strains are negative; *V* or (), strains are variable.

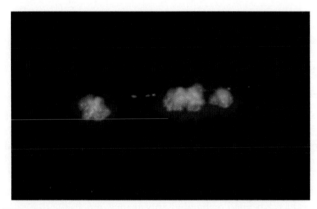

FIGURE 22-24 Appearance of *Actinomyces israelii* showing the "molar tooth" colonies typical for this anaerobe.

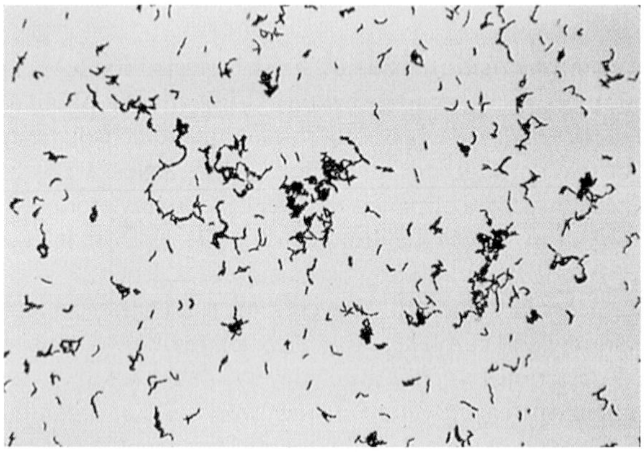

FIGURE 22-25 Gram-stained appearance of *Propionibacterium acnes*, illustrating the term "diphtheroid." (Courtesy Suzette L. Bartley, James D. Howard, and Ray Simon, Centers for Disease Control and Prevention, Atlanta, Ga.)

Eggerthella/Eubacterium

Eggerthella (previously classified as a *Eubacterium*) and *Eubacterium* spp. may be observed as either uniform or pleomorphic (variable in shape) gram-positive rods with no branching. They may be coccoid, diphtheroidal, or filamentous and range in width from thin to plump. *Eubacterium* colonies are usually small, circular, and convex, with an entire margin. An indole-negative, nitrate-positive, gram-positive anaerobic diphtheroid can be presumptively identified as *Eggerthella (Eubacterium) lenta*.

Propionibacterium

Propionibacterium spp. are pleomorphic rods with a diphtheroid appearance. The Gram-stained appearance of *P. acnes* is shown in Figure 22-25. Because *P. acnes* is a common member of the skin microbiota, it is frequently isolated from blood culture bottles as a contaminant. However, *P. acnes*, like coagulase-negative staphylococci, can cause subacute bacterial endocarditis and bacteremia and thus is not always a contaminant. A gram-positive anaerobic diphtheroid that is both catalase and spot-indole positive can be presumptively identified as *P. acnes*.

Propionibacterium propionicus can cause actinomycosis. This organism varies considerably in size and shape, ranging from coccoid and short diphtheroidal rods to long, branched filaments. Individual cells may be of uneven diameter and have distended or clubbed ends. As the genus implies, *Propionibacterium* spp. are characterized by having a major propionic acid peak by GLC.

TABLE 22-17 Phenotypic Characteristics of Anaerobic Gram-Negative Bacilli

	Vancomycin	Kanamycin	Colistin	Bile Resistant	Growth on KVLB	Esculin Hydrolysis	Red Fluorescence	Chartreuse Fluorescence	Indole	Oxidase	Catalase	Urease	Lipase	Nitrate	Pitting Colony	Formate/Fumarate*	Comment
***Bacteroides fragilis* Group**																	
B. fragilis	R	R	R	+	+	+	–	–	–	–	+	–	–	–	–		
B. caccae	R	R	R	+	+	+	–	–	–	–	–⁺	–	–	–	–		
B. distasonis	R	R	R	+	+	+	–	–	–	–	+	–	–	–	–		The genus name *Parabacteroides* recently proposed
B. ovatus	R	R	R	+	+	+	–	–	+	–	+	–	–	–	–		
B. thetaiotaomicron	R	R	R	+	+	+	–	–	+	–	+	–	–	–	–		
B. uniformis	R	R	R	+	+	–	–	–	+	–	V	–	–	–	–		
B. vulgatus	R	R	R	+	+	+	–	–	–	–	–⁺	–	–	–	–		
***Bacteroides ureolyticus* Group**																	
B. ureolyticus	R	S	S	–	–	–	–	–	–	+	±	+	–	+	±	+	Pitted and nonpitted
Campylobacter spp.	R	S	S	±	–	–	–	–	–	–	–	–	–	+	±	+	Pitted and nonpitted
Sutterella wadsworthensis	R	S	S	+	–	–	–	–	–	–	–	–	–	+	±	+	Pitted and nonpitted
Bilophila wadsworthia	R	S	S	+	+	+	–	–	–	–	+	±	–	+	–		"Fish-eye" on BBE
Prevotella																	
P. bivia	R	R	R	–	+	–	+	–	–	–	–	–	–	–	–		Delayed pigment
P. disiens	R	R	V	–	+	–	+	–	–	–	–	–	–	–	–		Delayed pigment
P. denticola	R	R	V	–	+	–	+	–	–	–	–	–	–	–	–		Brown colonies
P. intermedia	R	R	V	–	+	–	+	–	+	–	–	–	+	–	–		
P. loescheii	R	R	V	–	+	–	+	–	–	–	–	–	+	–	–		
P. melaninogenica	R	R	V	–	+	–	+	–	–	–	–	–	–	–	–		Brown colonies
Porphyromonas																	
P. asaccharolyticus	S	R	R	–	–	–	+	–	+	–	–	–	–	–	–		
P. endodontalis	S	R	R	–	–	–	+	–	+	–	–	–	–	–	–		
P. gingivalis	S	R	R	–	–	–	–	–	+	–	–	–	–	–	–		
Fusobacterium																	
F. nucleatum	R	S	S	–	–	–	–	+	+	–	–	–	–	–	–		Slender, pointed cells
F. mortiferum	R	S	S	+	+	–	–	+	–	–	–	–	–	–	–		Bizarre, round bodies
F. necrophorum	R	S	S	–⁺	+	–	–	+	+	–	–	–	+⁻	–	–		Large, pleomorphic cells
F. varium	R	S	S	+	–	–	–	+	+	–	–	–	–⁺	–	–		Large, rounded ends

Modified from Engelkirk PG et al: *Principles and practice of clinical anaerobic bacteriology*, Belmont, Calif, 1992, Star.

KVLB, Kanamycin and vancomycin with laked sheep blood; *R,* resistant; *S,* sensitive; *V,* strains are variable, +⁻, most strains are positive, –⁺, most strains are negative; *BBE, Bacteroides* bile esculin.

Identification of Anaerobic Gram-Negative Bacilli

Key tests for the identification of gram-negative anaerobic bacilli are listed in Table 22-17. Definitive identification of many of the commonly occurring gram-negative anaerobes can be accomplished by the preformed enzyme systems, so reliance on more extensive methods is usually not necessary.

Bacteroides

The genus *Bacteroides* was divided previously into bile-tolerant and bile-sensitive species. However, most of the bile sensitive species were transferred to the genera *Prevotella* and *Porphyromonas*. Bile tolerant species grow in the presence of 20% bile, so colonies will be present on BBE agar. They will exhibit robust growth on KVLB agar.

Bacteroides fragilis* Group and Other Bile-Resistant *Bacteroides. Bile-tolerant *Bacteroides* spp. include members of the *B. fragilis* group and the less frequently encountered *B. splanchnicus*. Members of the *B. fragilis* group, which contains about 13 related species, are especially pathogenic. *B. fragilis* is the most common species of anaerobic bacteria isolated from infectious processes of soft tissue and anaerobic bacteremia, and it is responsible for more than 60% of the infections caused by the *B. fragilis* group. *B. thetaiotaomicron* is the next most frequently encountered member of the *B. fragilis* group and often exhibits the highest degree of antimicrobial resistance. Gram-stained smears of *Bacteroides* spp. colonies reveal gram-negative coccobacilli or bacilli, but cells in broth cultures are frequently pleomorphic. The Gram-stained appearance of a typical *Bacteroides* species is shown in Figure 22-26.

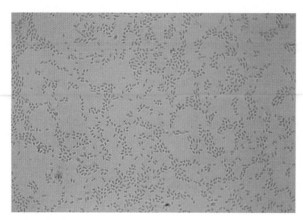

FIGURE 22-26 Gram-stained appearance of *Bacteroides thetaiotaomicron*, illustrating the typical appearance of *Bacteroides* spp. (Courtesy Suzette L. Bartley, James D. Howard, and Ray Simon, Centers for Disease Control and Prevention, Atlanta, Ga.)

Colonies of the *B. fragilis* group on BBE agar plate are gray and a minimum of 1 mm in diameter at 24 hours. The originally light-yellow medium turns brown to black in the area around the colonies. Good growth is the result of bile tolerance, and darkening of the medium is due to esculin hydrolysis. A dark precipitate (stippling) in the medium around the areas of heavy growth is suggestive of the species *B. fragilis*, although some strains of *Bacteroides ovatus* also cause stippling. The appearance of *B. fragilis* group organisms on a biplate of BBE and KVLB agar is shown in Figure 22-18. Caution must be taken, however, when interpreting results on BBE agar. *B. vulgatus*, a member of the *B. fragilis* group, often does not hydrolyze esculin and therefore may not produce a brown to black discoloration of the medium. Depending on the commercial source, age, and storage conditions of the medium, other organisms such as *F. mortiferum*, *Klebsiella pneumoniae*, *Enterococcus* spp., and some yeasts may also grow on BBE agar. Their colony size (which tends to be smaller), Gram-stain morphology, and aerotolerance will aid in the recognition of these other organisms.

Characteristics of the most commonly isolated members of the *B. fragilis* group can be found in Table 22-17. All members will be resistant to colistin, kanamycin, and vancomycin special potency disks. The members of the *B. fragilis* group can be divided into those that produce indole (*B. thetaiotaomicron*, *B. uniformis*, and *B. ovatus*) and those that do not (*B. fragilis*, *B. vulgatus*, *B. caccae*, and *B. distasonis*). Catalase activity can be found in *B. distasonis*, *B. fragilis*, *B. ovatus*, and *B. thetaiotaomicron*.

Bilophila

Bilophila wadsworthia is a bile resistant anaerobe that will grow on BBE agar with a characteristic "fish-eye" appearance (see Figure 22-19). Growth also occurs on KVLB agar. The organism is strongly catalase positive and will also be nitrate positive.

Prevotella

Prevotella spp. will grow on KVLB agar but not BBE agar. They are resistant to vancomycin and kanamycin but are variable in their susceptibility to the colistin special potency disk. Certain species of *Prevotella* produce protoporphyrin, a dark pigment that causes their colonies to become brown to black with age. Colony pigmentation may take 2 to 3 weeks of incubation before it becomes evident on routine *Brucella* blood agar (BRU/BA) plates, but it appears sooner on KVLB agar. Therefore, nonpigmented colonies on KVLB agar or BRU/BA should be subjected to long-wave UV light, such as a Wood's lamp, to detect the typical brick-red fluorescence of pigment-producing *Prevotella* spp. that appears before the brown pigment. The brick-red fluorescence under UV light is similar to that shown in Figure 22-12, *A*. Some species of pigmented *Prevotella* fluoresce colors other than brick-red, such as brilliant red, yellow, orange, and pink-orange, and some do not fluoresce at all. Only brick-red fluorescence allows presumptive identification of the pigmented *Prevotella* group. *P. intermedia* and *P. loescheii* produce lipase, and *P. intermedia* is spot-indole positive. In a Gram stain, *Prevotella* spp. appear as gram-negative coccobacilli or bacilli, very similar to *Bacteroides* spp.

Porphyromonas

Porphyromonas spp. will produce brick-red fluorescence under UV light, similar to *Prevotella*, but some species do not fluoresce. Because most *Porphyromonas* strains are susceptible to vancomycin, they will not grow on KVLB agar; but in contrast to *Prevotella*, they are resistant to colistin with the special potency disks. Most *Porphyromonas* spp. are spot-indole positive.

Bacteroides ureolyticus group

The *B. ureolyticus* group consists of bile-sensitive and bile-tolerant nonpigmented organisms (see Table 22-17). Recent reports have shown that the so-called pitting anaerobes of the *B. ureolyticus* group (which includes *B. ureolyticus*, *Campylobacter gracilis*, *C. curvus*, and *C. rectus*, and *Sutterella wadsworthensis*) are actually microaerophiles rather than obligate anaerobes. One useful identifying characteristic of this group is the colony appearance. Many of the organisms have colonies that appear to "pit" the agar. However, not all strains actually pit agar, and among those strains that do pit, not all colonies will appear to be pitting. Thus they may resemble a mixed culture. Growth in broth is enhanced by the addition of formate or fumarate, a characteristic unique to this group. The members of this group are positive in the nitrate test, whereas *B. ureolyticus* is able to hydrolyze urea and is spot-oxidase positive. *B. ureolyticus* is bile sensitive; *Sutterella* spp. are bile tolerant, whereas the campylobacters are variable in bile sensitivity.

Fusobacterium

Fusobacterium spp. are often described microscopically as long, thin, and tapered rods, a morphology characteristically referred to as *fusiform*. It is important to note, however, that only *F. nucleatum* has cells that are consistently fusiform in shape, and clinically encountered bacteria that are fusiform in shape are not necessarily *Fusobacterium*. The Gram-stained appearance of *F. nucleatum* is depicted in Figure 22-20. Other fusobacteria, such as *F. mortiferum*, appear pleomorphic, exhibiting globular forms, swellings, and other bizarre shapes. The pleomorphism of *F. mortiferum* is depicted in Figure 22-27. Organisms other than fusobacteria may also have fusiform-shaped cells; examples include *C. gracilis*, *Bacteroides forsythus*, and microaerophilic *Capnocytophaga*.

Fusobacteria are resistant to vancomycin but susceptible to colistin and kanamycin with the special potency disks. However, all except *F. nucleatum* will grow on the KVLB agar because the level of kanamycin is reduced from that of the special potency disk. With the exception of *F. mortiferum*, the fusobacteria are indole positive, and all will fluoresce chartreuse under long-wave UV light. In addition, *F. necrophorum* is positive for lipase when grown on egg-yolk agar.

Identification of Anaerobic Cocci

An algorithm depicting the presumptive identification of the anaerobic gram-positive cocci is shown in Figure 22-28. The Gram-stain appearance of a typical anaerobic coccus is seen

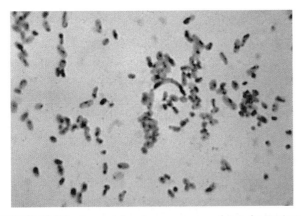

FIGURE 22-27 Gram-stained appearance of *Fusobacterium mortiferum*, illustrating pleomorphism. (Courtesy Suzette L. Bartley, James D. Howard, and Ray Simon, Centers for Disease Control and Prevention, Atlanta, Ga.)

in Figure 22-29. Other characteristics used to identify anaerobic cocci are listed in Table 22-18. As previously mentioned, presumptive identification of gram-positive anaerobic cocci can be reported as *Peptostreptococcus* spp. or "anaerobic gram-positive cocci." Full identification by preformed enzyme systems or other methods should be reported with the current terminology, with *Peptostreptococcus* inserted between the genus and species until these names become more familiar to physicians, for example, *Finegoldia (Peptostreptococcus) magna*. A black-pigmented anaerobic gram-positive coccus can be identified as *Peptococcus niger*. *Peptostreptococcus anaerobius* can be identified by a zone of inhibition around an SPS disk. Spot-indole positive isolates are often members of the genus *Peptoniphilus*, with *P. indolicus* identified by a positive nitrate test.

The only urease-positive anaerobic coccus is *Anaerococcus tetradius*. *Veillonella parvula* is the only commonly encountered gram-negative cocci and can be identified with Gram-stain, positive-catalase reaction, and red fluorescence under long-wave UV light. It is also positive for nitrate reduction.

ANTIMICROBIAL SUSCEPTIBILITY TESTING

Traditionally, the isolation, identification, and susceptibility testing of anaerobes have been quite slow when compared to aerobic bacteria isolated from the same specimen. As a result, when physicians suspect an anaerobic infection, they routinely select a broad-spectrum agent for empirical therapy that will cover most anaerobes, pending outcome of the culture. This practice was based on the fact that many antimicrobial agents could be relied upon to have good activity against the most commonly isolated anaerobes. However, resistance to antimicrobial agents has increased in recent years, and the susceptibility patterns of many anaerobes to certain antimicrobial agents can no longer be guaranteed. Antimicrobial resistance has mainly been observed in the *B. fragilis* group but has also been noted to a lesser extent in most of the clinically significant anaerobes.

The CLSI offers a document that provides guidelines for susceptibility testing of anaerobes, *Methods for Antimicrobial*

TABLE 22-18 Characteristics of Some Clinically Encountered Anaerobic Cocci

	Gram-Stain Reaction	Catalase	Indole	Urease	Nitrate Reduction	Red Fluorescence	Major Products in PYG by GLC	Comments
Peptostreptococcus anaerobius	+	−	−	−	−+	−	A, IB, IV, IC	Inhibited by SPS disk
Peptostreptococcus micros	+	−	−	−	−	−	A	
Peptoniphilus asaccharolyticus	+	−+	+	−	−	−	A, B	
Peptoniphilus indolicus	+	−	+	−	+	−	A, P, B	
Finegoldia magna	+	−+	−	−	−	−	A	
Anaerococcus prevotii	+	−+	−	−	−	−	A, P, B	
Anaerococcus tetradius	+	−	−	+	−	−	A, B, L	
Veillonella parvula	-	+	−	−	−+	+−	A, P	

Modified from Engelkirk PG et al: *Principles and practice of clinical anaerobic bacteriology*, Belmont, Calif, 1992, Star.
PYG, Peptone–yeast extract–glucose; *GLC*, gas liquid chromatography; *A*, acetic acid; *P*, propionic acid; *IB*, isobutyric acid; *B*, butyric acid; *IV* isovaleric acid; *IC*, isocaproic acid; *L*, lactic acid; +−, most strains positive; −+, most strains negative; *SPS*, sodium polyanethol sulfonate.

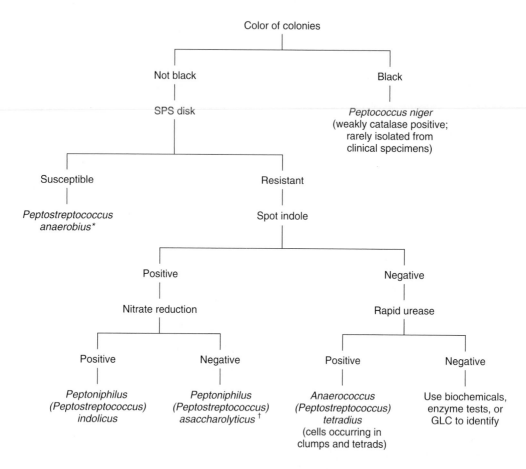

Color of colonies

Not black — SPS disk

Black — *Peptococcus niger* (weakly catalase positive; rarely isolated from clinical specimens)

SPS disk:
- Susceptible — *Peptostreptococcus anaerobius**
- Resistant — Spot indole
  - Positive — Nitrate reduction
    - Positive — *Peptoniphilus (Peptostreptococcus) indolicus*
    - Negative — *Peptoniphilus (Peptostreptococcus) asaccharolyticus* †
  - Negative — Rapid urease
    - Positive — *Anaerococcus (Peptostreptococcus) tetradius* (cells occurring in clumps and tetrads)
    - Negative — Use biochemicals, enzyme tests, or GLC to identify

* Some strains of *Peptostreptococcus micros* are susceptible to SPS, but they generally produce smaller zones of inhibition
† Anaerococcus (*Peptostreptococcus*) *hydrogenalis* is also indole-positive but unlike *P. asaccharolyticus* is alkaline phosphatase-positive.

FIGURE 22-28 Identification of anaerobic gram-positive cocci. Anaerobic gram-positive cocci (AGPC) are susceptible to metronidazole, whereas microaerophilic gram-positive cocci are not. An 80-μg metronidazole elution disk (BD Diagnostics Systems, Sparks, Md.) can be used to presumptively determine metronidazole susceptibility. Although metronidazole-resistant strains of AGPC have been reported, they appear to be rare. *GLC,* Gas-liquid chromatography; *SPS,* sodium polyanethol sulfonate. (Data from Mangels JI: Anaerobic bacteriology. In Isenberg HD: *Essential procedures for clinical microbiology,* Washington, DC, 1998, American Society for Microbiology.)

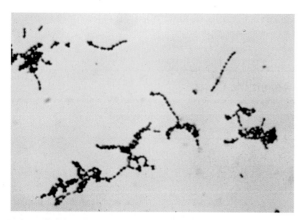

FIGURE 22-29 Gram-stained appearance of a *Peptostreptococcus* sp. illustrating the chain formation that occurs with some species of anaerobic gram-positive cocci. (Courtesy Suzette L. Bartley, James D. Howard, and Ray Simon, Centers for Disease Control and Prevention, Atlanta, Ga.)

Susceptibility Testing of Anaerobic Bacteria (Approved Standard, M11-A7). The document suggests that susceptibility testing should be performed when anaerobes are recovered from the following infections:

- Brain abscess
- Endocarditis
- Infection of a prosthetic device or vascular graft
- Joint infections
- Osteomyelitis
- Bacteremia

Because many anaerobe-associated infectious processes are polymicrobial, deciding which anaerobic isolates warrant susceptibility testing is frequently difficult. The CLSI suggests that the following anaerobes, recognized as highly virulent and/or commonly resistant to antimicrobial agents, should be considered for testing:

- *Bacteroides fragilis* group
- *Prevotella*

TABLE 22-19 Suggested Antimicrobial Susceptibility Testing for Anaerobic Bacteria from CLSI Document M11-A7

	B. fragilis Group, β-Lactamase Positive or β-Lactamase Unknown	Gram-Negative β-Lactamase-Negative	*Clostridium* spp. Other Than *C. perfringens*	*C. perfringens*, Gram-Positive Cocci, Other Gram-Positive Rods
Primary choices	Ampicillin-sulbactam *or* Piperacillin-tazobactam *or* Ticarcillin-clavulanic acid	Ampicillin *or* penicillin	Ampicillin *or* penicillin	Ampicillin *or* penicillin
	Clindamycin	Clindamycin	Ampicillin-sulbactam *or* Piperacillin-tazobactam *or* Ticarcillin-clavulanic acid	Clindamycin
	Ertapenem *or* Imipenem *or* Meropenem Metronidazole	Metronidazole	Cefotetan* *or* Cefoxitin	Metronidazole
			Clindamycin	
			Ertapenem *or* Imipenem *or* Meropenem Metronidazole	
Supplemental choices	Ceftizoxime Ceftriaxone	Cefotetan* Cefoxitin Ceftizoxime Ceftriaxone	Ceftizoxime Ceftriaxone	Cefotetan* Cefoxitin Ceftizoxime Ceftriaxone
	Cefotetan* Cefoxitin	Ampicillin-sulbactam *or* Piperacillin-tazobactam *or* Ticarcillin-clavulanic acid	Tetracycline	Ampicillin-sulbactam *or* Piperacillin-tazobactam *or* Ticarcillin-clavulanic acid
	Moxifloxacin	Moxifloxacin	Moxifloxacin	Tetracycline Moxifloxacin

Modified from Clinical Laboratory Standards Institute (CLSI): *Methods for antimicrobial susceptibility testing of anaerobic bacteria: approved standard,* ed 7, CLSI document M11-A7, Wayne, Pa, 2007, CLSI. Available from Clinical and Laboratory Standards Institute, 940 West Valley Road, Suite 140, Wayne, Pa 19087-1898, USA.
*As of 2008, cefotetan is currently no longer being manufactured.

- *Clostridium*
- *Fusobacterium*
- *Bilophila wadsworthia*
- *Sutterella wadsworthensis*

The CLSI working group suggests that larger laboratories periodically test several of the anaerobes listed above to determine whether the emergence of resistance to certain antimicrobial agents has occurred. Likewise, if a new antimicrobial agent has been added to the hospital formulary, testing should be performed to determine the agent's range of activity. The microbiology laboratory's decision as to which antimicrobial agents to test will be made following consultation with the hospital's infectious disease practitioners, pharmacists, and infection control committees. Table 22-19 lists the CLSI recommendations for the antimicrobial agents that should be considered for testing.

Problems in Susceptibility Testing of Anaerobic Isolates

One problem that has limited the routine susceptibility testing of anaerobes is a convenient and reproducible testing methodology. The difficulties include a lack of reproducibility, failure of some anaerobes to grow on or in particular media, difficulty in reading endpoints with certain methods, and a lack of comparability between methods. Cost and procedure complexity are other factors that inhibit laboratories from

performing susceptibility testing of anaerobes. Of far greater concern, however, are the accuracy of the methods and their correlation with the in vivo or clinical situation.

Susceptibility Testing Options

The CLSI document M11-A7 describes only two methods for susceptibility testing of anaerobes: agar dilution and broth microdilution. Although it is considered the gold standard method, agar dilution is labor intensive and is not a practical method for use in smaller clinical laboratories. It is used primarily in reference laboratories and institutions that test large numbers of isolates simultaneously. Broth microdilution panels are commercially available and can be stored frozen or lyophilized for extended periods of time. However, the CLSI M11-A7 document suggests that, at present, this method be used only for testing members of the *B. fragilis* group.

The Etest (AB BIODISK, Solna, Sweden) methodology, described in Chapter 13, is an alternative method for anaerobic susceptibility testing that has gained popularity in recent years. Testing can be performed on Mueller-Hinton agar supplemented with 5% sheep red blood cells, and plates can be incubated in anaerobe bags, jars, or chambers. Testing is limited to six antimicrobial agents on one agar plate, but that is usually sufficient for most clinical situations. One critical aspect of the Etest procedure is limiting exposure to oxygen during set up and quickly achieving anaerobiosis. This is because the commonly used antimicrobial agent metronidazole is very oxygen sensitive.

β-Lactamase Testing

β-Lactamases are enzymes that destroy the β-lactam ring of penicillins (penicillinases) and cephalosporins (cephalosporinases), thus rendering these antibiotics ineffective. The first anaerobes shown to produce β-lactamases were members of the *B. fragilis* group, but it is now known that many different anaerobes (e.g., *Prevotella, B. wadsworthia, Fusobacterium, Clostridium*) produce these enzymes. The ability of an anaerobe to produce β-lactamase enzymes can be determined using simple, commercially available methods (see Chapter 13).

β-Lactamase testing was used extensively when penicillin had reliable activity against a broad range of anaerobes. This is no longer the case, and with the development of β-lactam combination antibiotics that inactivate β-lactamases, the test has limited utility. Another limitation to β-lactamase testing is that a negative result does not necessarily mean that an organism will be susceptible to β-lactam antibiotics. Anaerobes can be resistant to such agents by mechanisms other than β-lactamase (e.g., by altering the number or type of penicillin-binding proteins or blocking penetration of the drug into the active site through alteration of the bacterial outer membrane pores). Anaerobes known to be resistant to β-lactam drugs by mechanisms other than production of β-lactamase include *C. gracilis, B. wadsworthia,* and some strains of *Bacteroides distasonis* and *B. fragilis.* Thus β-lactamase testing may be used as an adjunct to susceptibility testing but never as a replacement for it.

Many laboratories amend their anaerobic culture reports with statements suggesting empirical agents that continue to have broad anaerobic activity. These include the carbapenems (e.g., ertapenem, imipenem, and meropenem), metronidazole, and the β-lactam combination antibiotics (ampicillin/sulbactam, amoxicillin/clavulanic acid, piperacillin/tazobactam, and ticarcillin/clavulanic acid). This provides physicians with valuable information concerning empirical treatment of anaerobic infections.

TREATMENT OF ANAEROBE-ASSOCIATED DISEASES

There are essentially four approaches to the management of anaerobic infections.

1. **Surgical therapy.** Because most anaerobic infections are abscesses caused by mixtures of aerobic and anaerobic bacteria, the most important therapy is surgical drainage of the abscess. In less serious infections, this may be the only therapy required. Other surgical procedures include removing dead tissue (debridement), eliminating obstructions, decompressing tissues, releasing trapped gas, and improving circulation in and oxygenation of tissues.

2. **Hyperbaric oxygen.** The use of a hyperbaric oxygen chamber to force oxygen into necrotic tissue has been used as adjunct therapy for anaerobic infections for a number of years. Hyperbaric oxygen has also been suggested to be useful therapy in cases of osteomyelitis caused by anaerobes. However, the routine use of hyperbaric oxygen in the treatment of anaerobic infections remains controversial.

3. **Antimicrobial therapy.** The primary role of antimicrobial agents is to limit the local and systemic spread of the organisms. Selection of the correct antimicrobial agent depends on a number of factors including types of organisms involved, known resistance factors, the site of the infection, and the toxicity of the antimicrobial agent. Although antimicrobial resistance has been observed with virtually every agent known to have anaerobic coverage, the carbapenems, metronidazole, and the β-lactam combination antibiotics continue to have activity against most anaerobes and are used as empirical therapy.

4. **Antitoxins.** In cases of tetanus and botulism, antitoxins are used to neutralize the effect of neurotoxins produced by *Clostridium tetani* and *C. botulinum*, respectively.

BIBLIOGRAPHY

Allen SD et al: Anaerobic bacteriology. In Truant AL, editor: *Manual of commercial methods in microbiology*, Washington, DC, 2002, ASM Press.

Barenfanger J et al: Comparison of chlorhexidine and tincture of iodine for skin antisepsis in preparation for blood sample collection, *J Clin Microbiol* 42:2216, 2004.

Brook I: Management of anaerobic infection, *Expert Rev Anti-Infect Ther* 2:153, 2004.

Brynestad S, Granum PE: *Clostridium perfringens* and foodborne infections, *Int J Food Microbiol* 74:195, 2002.

Centers for Disease Control and Prevention: Summary of notifiable diseases—United States, 2007. Available at: www.cdc.gov/mmwr/PDF/wk/mm5653.pdf. Accessed September 8, 2009.

Citron DM et al: *Bacteroides, Porphyromonas, Prevotella, Fusobacterium,* and other anaerobic gram-negative rods. In Murray PR et al, editors: *Manual of clinical microbiology*, ed 9, Washington, DC, 2007, ASM Press.

Clinical Laboratory Standards Institute: *Methods for antimicrobial susceptibility testing of anaerobic bacteria: approved standard*, ed 7, CLSI document M11-A7, Wayne, Pa, 2007, CLSI.

Clinical Laboratory Standards Institute: *Abbreviated identification of bacteria and yeast: approved guideline*—second edition, CLSI Document M35-A2, Wayne, Penn. 2008, CLSI.

Englekirk PG et al: *Principles and practice of clinical anaerobic bacteriology*, Belmont, Calif, 1992, Star.

Fader RC et al: *CACMLE self-study course #117: Anaerobic bacteriology for today's clinical laboratory*, Denver, 2007, Colorado Association for Continuing Medical Laboratory Education.

Finegold SM et al: Taxonomy—general comments and update of clostridia and anaerobic cocci, *Anaerobe* 8:283, 2002.

Johnson EA et al: *Clostridium*. In Murray PR et al, editors: *Manual of clinical microbiology*, ed 9, Washington, DC, 2007, ASM Press.

Jousimies-Somer H, Summanen P: Recent taxomonic changes and terminology update of clinically significant anaerobic gram-negative bacteria (excluding spirochetes), *Clin Infect Dis* 35(Suppl 1):S17-S21; 2002.

Jouseimies-Somer HR et al: *Wadsworth-KTL anaerobic bacteriology manual*, ed 6, Belmont, Calif, 2002, Star.

Kõnõnen E, Wade W: *Propionibacterium, Lactobacillus, Actinomyces,* and other non–spore-forming anaerobic gram-positive rods. In Murray PR et al, editors: *Manual of clinical microbiology*, ed 9, Washington, DC, 2007, ASM Press.

Simmon KE et al: Genotypic diversity of anaerobic isolates from bloodstream infections, *J Clin Microbiol* 46:1596, 2008.

Song Y, Finegold SM: *Peptostreptococcus, Finegoldia, Anaerococcus, Peptoniphilus, Veillonella,* and other anaerobic cocci. In Murray PR et al, editors: *Manual of clinical microbiology,* ed 9, Washington, DC, 2007, ASM Press.

Points to Remember

- Anaerobes are organisms that do not require oxygen for life.
- Anaerobes are important in human and veterinary medicine because they play a role in serious, often fatal, infections and intoxications.
- Anaerobic infections of exogenous origin are usually caused by gram-positive, spore-forming bacilli belonging to the genus *Clostridium.*
- The anaerobes most frequently isolated from infectious processes in humans are those of endogenous origin.
- Factors that commonly predispose the human body to anaerobic infections include trauma of mucous membranes or skin, vascular stasis, tissue necrosis, and decrease in redox potential of tissue.
- Significant clinical infections caused by anaerobes include mixed microbiota abscesses, tetanus, botulism, myonecrosis, antibiotic-associated diarrhea, and actinomycosis.
- Many types of specimens are unacceptable for anaerobic bacteriology because they are likely to be contaminated with anaerobes of the endogenous microbiota.
- Proper selection, collection, and transport of specimens for anaerobic culture are critical for quality results and maximum recovery of pathogens.
- The anaerobes most commonly associated with infectious processes and those most often isolated from specimens include members of the *B. fragilis* group, certain *Clostridium* spp. (e.g., *C. perfringens, C. ramosum, C. clostridioforme, C. septicum, C. difficile*), *Fusobacterium nucleatum, F. necrophorum, Propionibacterium acnes, Actinomyces israelii, Porphyromonas, Prevotella,* and the anaerobic gram-positive cocci.
- Presumptive identifications are based upon Gram stain, colony appearance on different media, and the results of simple, inexpensive, rapid test procedures.
- Definitive identifications are made using preformed enzyme-based identification kits, analysis of metabolic end products or cellular fatty acids or by rDNA sequencing.
- Susceptibility testing of anaerobes is not recommended for all anaerobic isolates, but it is warranted in some clinical situations, for specific types of serious infections, and whenever especially virulent or drug-resistant anaerobes have been isolated.
- Practical methods for anaerobe susceptibility testing include microwell broth dilution panels and the Etest.
- Some anaerobes are capable of producing β-lactamases, enzymes that destroy the β-lactam ring of penicillins and cephalosporins, thereby rendering them ineffective.
- Anaerobe-associated diseases may be treated by surgery, hyperbaric oxygen, antitoxins, and antimicrobial therapy.

Learning Assessment Questions

1. Match the following infectious diseases with their associated causative organism:
   _____ Myonecrosis
   _____ Tetanus
   _____ Botulism
   _____ Pseudomembranous colitis
   _____ Actinomycosis
   A. *Clostridium difficile*
   B. *Clostridium perfringens*
   C. *Clostridium tetani*
   D. *Clostridium botulinum*
   E. *Actinomyces* spp.

2. An organism that can live and grow in reduced concentrations of oxygen but prefers an anaerobic environment is known as a(n):
   a. Capnophile
   b. Obligate anaerobe
   c. Facultative anaerobe
   d. Aerotolerant anaerobe

3. Some anaerobes are particularly susceptible to oxygen because they lack the enzyme:
   a. Amylase
   b. β-Lactamase
   c. Superoxide dismutase
   d. Glucose-6-phosphate dehydrogenase

4. Endogenous anaerobes least likely to be involved in cases of bacteremia are:
   a. *Bacteroides*
   b. *Eubacterium*
   c. *Fusobacterium*
   d. *Peptostreptococcus*

5. Which of the following specimens would be unacceptable for anaerobic culture?
   a. Aspirated pus
   b. Cerebrospinal fluid
   c. Tissue from biopsy
   d. Urethral swab

6. A gram-positive bacillus was isolated from a wound specimen and had the following characteristics: double zone of β-hemolysis, lecithinase positive, lipase negative, indole negative. What is the most likely identification of this organism?
   a. *Clostridium perfringens*
   b. *Clostridium ramosum*
   c. *Clostridium septicum*
   d. *Clostridium tetani*

7. An anaerobic, pleomorphic, gram-negative bacilli was recovered from a liver abscess. The special-potency antimicrobial disks demonstrated that the organism was vancomycin-resistant, and colistin- and kanamycin-sensitive. Other results were as follows: chartreuse fluorescence, spot-indole positive, and lipase positive.
   What is the most likely identification of the organism?
   a. *Fusobacterium mortiferum*
   b. *Fusobacterium necrophorum*
   c. *Fusobacterium nucleatum*
   d. *Fusobacterium varium*

Indicate whether the following statements are true or false.

_____ **8.** Exogenous anaerobes more commonly cause infectious diseases than do endogenous anaerobes.

_____ **9.** *Clostridium* spp. are especially easy to identify in Gram-stained smears of clinical specimens. because they always appear as gram-positive rods with terminal or subterminal spores.

_____ **10.** Failure to isolate fusiform gram-negative organisms that were observed on a Gram-stained smear of a clinical specimen could be an indication that a problem exists with either the primary media used for the isolation of anaerobes or the system being used for anaerobic incubation of primary plates.

_____ **11.** Large, dark colonies (greater than 1 mm) growing on a BBE plate at 24 hours can presumptively be called a member of the *Bacteroides fragilis* group.

_____ **12.** A pleomorphic gram-positive bacillus that is spot indole and catalase positive can be presumptively identified as *Propionibacterium acnes*.

The Spirochetes

A. Christian Whelen

■ **LEPTOSPIRES**
General Characteristics
Virulence Factors and Pathogenicity
Infections Caused by Leptospires
Epidemiology
Laboratory Diagnosis
Antimicrobial Susceptibility

■ **BORRELIAE**
General Characteristics
Clinically Significant Species

Borrelia recurrentis and Similar Borreliae
Borrelia burgdorferi

■ **TREPONEMES**
General Characteristics
Clinically Significant Species
Treponema pallidum subsp. *pallidum*
Other Treponemal Diseases

OBJECTIVES

After studying this chapter, you should be able to:

1. Describe the general characteristics of the *Leptospira*.

2. List the clinical infections caused by *Leptospira* spp.

3. State the general characteristics of the genus *Borrelia*.

4. Compare the etiologic agents and the arthropod vectors of relapsing fever and Lyme disease.

5. Describe the classic skin lesion, erythema chronicum migrans (ECM), of Lyme disease.

6. Compare the four human pathogens of the genus *Treponema*.

7. Discuss the primary, secondary, and tertiary clinical manifestations of syphilis.

8. Discuss the clinical manifestations of congenital syphilis.

9. Describe and evaluate the diagnostic tests used to identify *Treponema pallidum* in the clinical laboratory.

10. Describe the three nonvenereal treponemal diseases.

Case in Point

A 29-year-old male arrived at a local medical clinic in Los Angeles complaining of diarrhea, fever, chills, muscle aches, and headaches. He had returned two days earlier after competing in the "Eco-Challenge" in Malaysian Borneo. During the competition he had completed various events that included mountain biking, caving, climbing, jungle trekking, swimming, and kayaking in both fresh and salt water. He was still recovering from multiple abrasions from the jungle trekking and mountain biking. While kayaking the Segama River, his kayak capsized and he inadvertently swallowed several mouthfuls of river water. His two teammates were on doxycycline as malaria prophylaxis before and during the race. Neither of them became ill.

Issues to Consider

After reading the patient's case history, consider:
■ Risk factors for the patient
■ Etiologic agents that cause influenza-like illness (ILI) and methods to identify or rule out those agents

■ Effective prophylaxis, if available, for ILIs
■ Empirical therapy options

Key Terms

Chancre
Endemic relapsing fever
Endemic syphilis
Epidemic relapsing fever
Erythema chronicum migrans (ECM)
Gummas
Jarisch-Herxheimer reaction
Leptospirosis
Lyme borreliosis
Periplasmic flagella

Pinta
Rapid plasma reagin (RPR) test
Spirochetes
Syphilis
Venereal Disease Research Laboratory (VDRL) test
Weil disease
Yaws
Zoonoses

The order *Spirochaetales* contains two families: Leptospiraceae and Spirochaetaceae. The family Leptospiraceae contains the genus *Leptospira*, and the family Spirochaetaceae contains *Borrelia* and *Treponema*. These three genera include the causative agents of important human diseases such as **syphilis**, zoonoses (transmitted from animals to humans) such as **leptospirosis**, and vector-borne diseases such as Lyme disease and relapsing fever.

The **spirochetes** are slender, flexuous, helically shaped, unicellular bacteria ranging from 0.1 to 0.5 μm wide and from 5 to 20 μm long, with one or more complete turns in the helix. They differ from other bacteria in that they have a flexible cell wall around which several fibrils are wound. These fibrils, termed the **periplasmic flagella** (also known as axial fibrils, axial filaments, endoflagella, and periplasmic fibrils), are responsible for motility. A multilayered outer sheath similar to the outer membrane of gram-negative bacteria completely surrounds the protoplasmic cylinder (the cytoplasmic and nuclear regions enclosed by the cytoplasmic membrane–cell wall complex and periplasmic flagella). The spirochetes exhibit various types of motion in liquid media. They are free living, or survive in association with animal and human hosts as normal biota or pathogens. In addition, they are chemoheterotrophic and can utilize carbohydrates, amino acids, long-chain fatty acids, or long-chain fatty alcohols as carbon and energy sources. Metabolism can be anaerobic, facultatively anaerobic, or aerobic depending on the species. *Treponema* reproduce via transverse fission, whereas *Leptospira* and *Borrelia* divide by the more common binary fission.

LEPTOSPIRES

General Characteristics

Organisms of the genus *Leptospira* are tightly coiled, thin, flexible spirochetes, 0.1 μm wide and 5 to 15 μm long (Figure 23-1). In contrast to both *Treponema* and *Borrelia* organisms, the spirals are very close together, so the organism may appear to be a chain of cocci. One or both ends of the organism have hooks rather than tapering off. Their motion is rapid and rotational. Historically, pathogenic organisms were identified as *Leptospira interrogans* and saprophytes were categorized as *Leptospira biflexa*. More than 200 different serovars (serotypes) of *L. interrogans* sensu lato have been reported. Although genetic typing has established relatedness based on nucleic acid similarities and is taxonomically correct, serogroup-based nomenclature continues to be preferred among scientists and physicians.

Electron microscopy reveals a long axial filament covered by a very fine sheath, similar to treponemes and borreliae. All species have two periplasmic flagella. The organisms cannot be readily stained, but they can be impregnated with silver and visualized. Unstained cells are not visible by bright-field microscopy but are visible by dark-field, phase-contrast, and immunofluorescent microscopy. Leptospires are obligately aerobic and can be grown in artificial media such as Fletcher's semisolid, Stuart liquid, or Ellinghausen-McCullough-Johnson-Harris (EMJH) semisolid media.

FIGURE 23-1 Dark-field image of *Leptospira interrogans* serotype Sejroe Wolffi 3705 (1000× oil). The tight coils and bent ends are characteristic of this organism. (Courtesy of State Laboratories Division, Hawaii Department of Health.)

Virulence Factors and Pathogenicity

Leptospiral disease in the United States is caused by more than 20 different serovars, the most common of which are icterohaemorrhagiae, australis, and canicola. Some serovars of *L. interrogans* sensu lato and *L. biflexa* sensu lato are pathogenic for a wide range of wild and domestic animals and humans, but mechanisms of pathogenicity are not well understood. Factors that may play a role in pathogenicity include reduced phagocytosis in the host, a soluble hemolysin produced by some virulent strains, cell-mediated sensitivity to leptospiral antigen by the host, and small amounts of endotoxins produced by some strains. The clinical findings in animals with leptospirosis suggest the presence of endotoxemia.

Infections Caused by Leptospires

Leptospires are most likely to enter the human host through small breaks in the skin or intact mucosa. The initial sites of multiplication are unknown. Nonspecific host defenses do not stop multiplication of leptospires, and leptospiremia occurs during the acute illness. Late manifestations of the disease may be caused by the host's immunologic response to the infection.

The incubation period of leptospirosis is usually 10 to 12 days but ranges from 3 to 30 days. The onset of clinical illness is usually abrupt, with nonspecific, influenza-like constitutional symptoms such as fever, chills, headache, severe myalgia, and malaise. The subsequent course is protean, frequently biphasic, and often results in hepatic, renal, and central nervous system involvement. The major renal lesion is an interstitial nephritis with associated glomerular swelling and hyperplasia that does not affect the glomeruli. The most characteristic physical finding is conjunctival suffusion, but this is seen in less than half of the patients. Severe systemic disease

(Weil disease) includes renal failure, hepatic failure, and intravascular disease and can result in death. Duration of the illness varies from less than 1 week to 3 weeks. Late manifestations may be caused by the host immunologic response to the infection. In patients with a leptospiral bacteremia, immunoglobulin M (IgM) antibodies are detected within a week after onset of disease and may persist in high titers for many months. Immunoglobulin G (IgG) antibodies are usually detectable a month or more after infection. Convalescent serum contains protective antibodies.

Epidemiology

Leptospirosis is a zoonoses primarily associated with occupational or recreational exposure. Working with animals or in rat-infested surroundings poses hazards for veterinarians, dairy workers, swine handlers, slaughterhouse workers, miners, sewer workers, and fish and poultry processors. In the United States, the majority of leptospirosis disease results from recreational exposures. In California residents, 59% of the leptospirosis cases were acquired during freshwater recreation from 1982 to 2001; in the last 5 of those years, the rate was 85%. Leptospirosis ceased to become a nationally notifiable disease in 1995. Of the 38 cases reported in 1994, 22 were in Hawaii. Leptospirosis is still reportable in Hawaii, and from 2000 to 2004, Hawaii averaged 25 cases per year. Cases are surely unrecognized nationwide, and go unreported in Hawaii.

In the natural host, leptospires live in the lumen of renal tubules and are excreted in the urine. Dogs, rats, and other rodents are the principal animal reservoirs. Hosts acquire infections directly by contact with the urine of carriers or indirectly by contact with bodies of water contaminated with the urine of carriers. Leptospires can survive in neutral or slightly alkaline waters for months. Protective clothing (boots and gloves) should be worn in situations involving possible occupational exposure to leptospires. Control measures include rodent elimination and drainage of contaminated waters. Vaccination of dogs and livestock has been effective in preventing disease but not the initial infection and leptospiruria. Short-term prophylaxis consisting of weekly doxycycline may be appropriate in high-risk groups with expected occupational exposure.

Laboratory Diagnosis

Specimen Collection and Handling

During the acute phase (first week) of the disease, blood or cerebrospinal fluid (CSF) should be collected. Optimal recovery occurs if fresh specimens are inoculated directly into laboratory media. Urine can also be collected, but yield is much higher after the first week of illness, and shedding can occur intermittently for weeks.

Microscopic Examination

Although direct demonstration of leptospires in clinical specimens during the first week of the disease by special stains, dark-field, or phase-contrast microscopy is possible, it is not recommended. Direct demonstration is only successful in a small percentage of cases, and false-positive results may be reported because of the presence of artifacts, especially in urine.

Isolation and Identification

Isolation of leptospires is accomplished by direct inoculation of 1 to 2 drops of freshly drawn blood or CSF into laboratory media such as Fletcher's, Stuart, or EMJH, and incubating the media in the dark at room temperature. Urine can also be cultured and is most productive after the first week of illness. Several dilutions should be used (undiluted, 1:10, and 1:100) and/or filtered (0.45 µm) to minimize the effects of inhibitory substances. Tubes are examined weekly for evidence of growth such as turbidity, haze, or a ring of growth. A drop taken from a few millimeters below the surface is examined by dark-field microscopy for tightly coiled, rapidly motile spirochetes with hooked ends. Serotypes have historically been identified by microscopic agglutination testing (MAT) using sera of defined reactivity; however, other methods such as pulsed-field gel electrophoresis and 16s ribosome DNA sequencing are also being investigated.

Serologic Tests

In patients with a leptospiral bacteremia, IgM antibodies are detected within a week after onset of disease and may persist in high titers for many months. A month or more after the onset of illness, IgG antibodies can be detected in some patients. A U.S. Food and Drug Administration-approved, visually-read IgM ELISA (Pan Bio INDx, Baltimore, Md.) is available and has been shown to have high sensitivity (98%) and specificity (90.6%) in acute leptospirosis cases. A macroscopic slide agglutination test for rapid screening as well as a more sensitive MAT is available for detection of leptospiral antibodies, but both require the maintenance of defined serotypes in culture, so performance is typically limited to confirmatory laboratories.

Antimicrobial Susceptibility

Susceptibility testing of leptospires is not normally performed in the clinical laboratory; however, leptospires have been shown to be susceptible in vitro to streptomycin, tetracycline, doxycycline, and the macrolide antimicrobials in vitro. Although treatment data are too sparse to be definitive, penicillin is considered beneficial and alters the course of the disease if treatment is initiated before the fourth day of illness. Doxycycline appears to shorten the course of the illness in adults and reduce the incidence of convalescent leptospiruria.

BORRELIAE

General Characteristics

The genus *Borrelia* comprises several species of spirochetes that are morphologically similar but have different pathogenic properties and host ranges. Most species cause relapsing fever with the notable exception of Lyme disease (**Lyme borreliosis**), which is caused by several species in the *Borrelia burgdorferi* sensu lato complex. All pathogenic *Borrelia* are arthropod-borne.

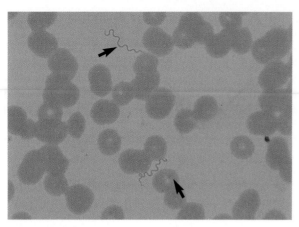

FIGURE 23-2 Appearance of *Borrelia recurrentis* in blood. Giemsa stain (850×).

The borreliae are highly flexible organisms varying in thickness from 0.2 to 0.5 μm and in length from 3 to 20 μm. The spirals vary in number from 3 to 10 per organism and are much less tightly coiled than those of the leptospires (Figure 23-2). Unlike the leptospires and treponemes, the borreliae stain easily and can be visualized by bright-field microscopy. Electron microscopy shows the same general features as are seen with the treponemes—long, periplasmic flagella (15 to 20 per cell) coated with sheaths of protoplasm and periplasm. The borreliae are typically cultivated in the clinical laboratory using Kelly medium.

Clinically Significant Species

A number of borreliae, including *Borrelia recurrentis* and *Borrelia duttonii*, cause relapsing fever. The complex *B. burgdorferi* sensu lato causes a spectrum of syndromes known as Lyme disease.

Borrelia recurrentis and Similar Borreliae

Virulence Factors

As the disease name suggests, relapsing fever is characterized by acute febrile episodes that subside spontaneously and tend to recur over a period of weeks. *Borrelia* species responsible for this disease first evade complement by acquiring and displaying suppressive complement regulators: C4b-binding protein and factor H. The relapses are potentiated by antigenic variation; the borreliae systematically change their surface antigens, thereby rendering specific antibody production ineffective in completely clearing the organisms.

Clinical Manifestations

After an incubation period of 2 to 15 days, a massive spirochetemia develops and remains at varying levels of severity during the entire course of relapsing fever. The infection is accompanied by sudden high temperature, rigors, severe headache, muscle pains, and weakness. The febrile period lasts about 3 to 7 days and ends abruptly with the development of an adequate immune response. The disease recurs several days to weeks later, following a less severe but similar course. The spirochetemia worsens during the febrile periods and wanes between recurrences.

Epidemiology

Relapsing fever can be either tickborne (**endemic relapsing fever**) or louse-borne (**epidemic relapsing fever**). The tickborne borreliae are transmitted by a large variety of soft ticks of the genus *Ornithodoros*. Species-specific borreliae often bear the same epithet as their vectors (e.g., *Ornithodoros hermsii* transmits *Borrelia hermsii*). Tickborne borreliae are widely distributed throughout the eastern and western hemispheres, and transmission to a vertebrate host takes place via infected saliva during tick attachment.

Louse-borne fever is transmitted via the body louse, *Pediculus humanus*, and humans are the only reservoir. The borreliae infect the hemolymph of the louse. Unlike tickborne disease, transmission of the louse-borne disease occurs when infected lice are crushed and scratched into the skin rather than through the bite of an infected arthropod. Relapsing fever is best prevented by control of exposure to the arthropod vectors. For tickborne relapsing fever, exposure control includes wearing protective clothing, rodent control, and the use of repellents. For louse-borne relapsing fever, control is best achieved by good personal and public hygiene, especially improvements in overcrowding and delousing.

Laboratory Diagnosis

Microscopic Examination. Diagnosis of borreliosis is readily made by observing Giemsa- or Wright-stained blood smears of blood taken during the febrile period. Relapsing fever is the only spirochetal disease in which the organisms are visible in blood with bright-field microscopy. The appearance of the spirochete among the red cells is characteristic (Figure 23-2).

Isolation and Identification. Borreliae can be recovered using Kelly medium or animal inoculation (involving suckling Swiss mice or suckling rats), but it is rarely attempted. *B. recurrentis*, *B. hermsii*, *Borrelia parkeri*, *Borrelia turicatae*, and *Borrelia hispanica* have been successfully cultivated. Antigenic variation in the spirochetes that cause relapsing fever makes the serodiagnosis of their diseases difficult and impractical.

Antimicrobial Susceptibility

Borreliae are susceptible to many antimicrobial agents; however, tetracyclines are the drugs of choice because they reduce the relapse rate and rid the central nervous system of spirochetes. Studies indicate that up to 39% of patients treated with antimicrobial agents experience fever, chills, headache, and myalgias believed to be caused by the sudden release of endotoxin from the spirochetes (**Jarisch-Herxheimer reaction**).

Borrelia burgdorferi

Virulence Factors

Bacterial spread may occur by the organism's ability to bind plasminogen and urokinase-type plasminogen activator to its surface. This binding could convert plasminogen to plasmin, which is a potent protease and could facilitate tissue invasion.

Binding factor H allows for complement evasion and immune system suppression might explain, in part, why IgM antibody does not peak for 3 to 6 weeks. In vitro, the organism can stimulate proinflammatory cytokines such as tumor necrosis factor and interferons, which can be important in controlling disease but may also contribute to inflammatory manifestations as untreated disease progresses.

Clinical Manifestations

Lyme borreliosis is a complex disease that can generally be divided into three stages. Early infection includes two stages, the first of which is localized (stage 1). About 60% of patients exhibit **erythema chronicum migrans (ECM),** the classic skin lesion that is normally found at the site of the tick bite. It begins as a red macule and expands to form large annular erythema with partial central clearing. A regional lymphadenopathy is common with minor constitutional symptoms. Stage 2 is early disseminated and produces widely variable symptoms that are not limited to secondary skin lesions, migratory joint and bone pain, alarming neurologic and cardiac pathology, splenomegaly, and severe malaise and fatigue. Late manifestations, or late persistent infections (stage 3), focus on the cardiac, musculoskeletal, and neurologic systems. Arthritis is the most common symptom, occurring weeks to years later.

Epidemiology

Lyme disease was first described after an outbreak among children in Lyme, Connecticut, in 1975. Organisms are transmitted via the bite of infected *Ixodes* ticks, so the majority of cases occur during June through September, when more people are involved in outdoor activities and ticks are more active. A total of 27,444 cases were reported in the United States in 2007.

At least three species of the *B. burgdorferi* sensu lato cause Lyme disease (Lyme borreliosis). *B. burgdorferi* sensu stricto occurs in North America. *B. garinii* and *B. afzelii* have been confirmed in Asia, and all three species have caused disease in Europe. Protective clothing and repellents should be worn in areas in which tick exposure is intense. Attached ticks should be removed immediately because pathogen transmission is associated with the length of attachment.

Laboratory Diagnosis

Specimen Collection and Handling. The most common and productive specimen collected for the laboratory diagnosis of *B. burgdorferi* sensu lato infection is serum for serology. Serology can also be used to detect antibodies in the CSF, which is indicative of neuroborreliosis. Direct examination of blood or skin specimens is rarely productive. Culture from skin biopsies (ECM margin) or joint fluid (in patients with arthritis) in Kelly medium permits definitive diagnosis but is labor intensive and not widely available.

Serologic Tests. Diagnosis is typically supported serologically, either by indirect fluorescent antibody or enzyme immunoassay (EIA). EIA is often used because of its superior sensitivity, specificity, and ease of use. False-positive results are unusual with current commercial kits, especially when initial results are confirmed with a Western blot for specific

B. burgdorferi antigens; however, a *Treponema pallidum* infection could produce a false-positive result. Consequently, a nontreponemal test, such as **rapid plasma reagin (RPR) test** for syphilis, should be performed on positive sera to exclude cross reactivity.

The specific IgM antibody response begins during the first 10 days after infection but does not peak until 3 to 6 weeks after the onset of the disease. Peak levels of IgG antibodies are not observed until 4 to 6 months after the illness onset, and they typically persist in untreated patients with late manifestations of Lyme borreliosis. Western blot confirmation of IgM antibody presence includes reactivity for two of the three following bands: 24, 39, and 41 kDa. Confirmation of IgG antibody presence is acceptable when five of the following bands are present: 18, 21, 28, 30, 39, 41, 45, 58, 66, and 93 kDa.

Antimicrobial Susceptibility

Early diagnosis and antimicrobial treatment are important for preventing neurologic, cardiac, and joint abnormalities that can occur late in the disease. Doxycycline and amoxicillin are equally effective in treating early stages of Lyme disease without complications. For refractile or late stages, prolonged treatment with ceftriaxone has been effective.

TREPONEMES

General Characteristics

Pathogenic treponemes are thin, spiral organisms about 0.1 to 0.2 μm in thickness and 6 to 20 μm in length. They are difficult to visualize with a bright-field microscope because they are so thin, but they can be seen very easily using dark-field microscopy. The spirals are regular and angular with 4 to 14 spirals per organism (Figure 23-3). Three periplasmic flagella are inserted into each end of the cell. The ends are pointed and covered with a sheath. The cells are motile, with graceful flexuous movements in liquid.

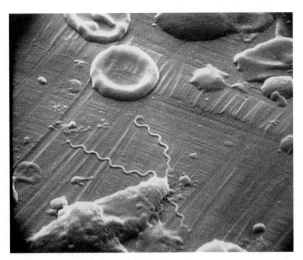

FIGURE 23-3 Scanning electron micrograph of *Treponema pallidum* (Nichols stain). Two treponemes are shown adjacent to an erythrocyte (2500×).

Clinically Significant Species

The genus *Treponema* comprises four microorganisms that are pathogenic for humans: *T. pallidum* subsp. *pallidum*, the causative agent of syphilis; *T. pallidum* subsp. *pertenue*, the causative agent of **yaws**; *T. pallidum* subsp. *endemicum*, the causative agent of **endemic syphilis;** and *Treponema carateum*, the causative agent of **pinta**. The four pathogenic strains exhibit a high degree of DNA homology and shared antigens. At least six nonpathogenic species have been identified in the normal biota, and they are particularly prominent in the oral cavity.

Treponema pallidum subsp. *pallidum*

Virulence Factors

Treponema pallidum subsp. *pallidum* has the ability to cross intact mucous membranes and the placenta, disseminate throughout the body, and infect virtually any organ system. It has also been postulated that antigenic variation of cell surface proteins contributes to the organism's ability to evade host immune response and establish persistent infection.

Clinical Manifestations

Treponema pallidum subsp. *pallidum* causes syphilis. The word *syphilis* comes from a poem written in 1530 that described a mythical shepherd named Syphilus who was afflicted with the disease as punishment for cursing the gods. The poem represented the compendium of knowledge at the time regarding the disease.

  Treponema pallidum subsp. *pallidum* transmission normally occurs during direct sexual contact with an individual who has an active primary or secondary syphilitic lesion. Consequently, the genital organs—the vagina and cervix in females, and the penis in males—are the usual sites of inoculation. Syphilis can also be acquired by nongenital contact with a lesion (e.g., on the lip) or transplacental transmission to a fetus, resulting in congenital syphilis. After bacterial invasion through a break in the epidermis or penetration through intact mucous membranes, the natural course of syphilis can be divided into primary, secondary, and tertiary stages based on the clinical manifestations. Coinfection with human immunodeficiency virus (HIV) can result in variation of the natural course of the disease. Furthermore, ulcers caused by syphilis may contribute to the efficiency of HIV transmission in populations with high rates of both infections. Syphilis has a wide variety of clinical manifestations, which gave rise to the name the "great imitator."

  Primary Stage of Syphilis. After inoculation, the spirochetes multiply rapidly and disseminate to local lymph nodes and other organs via the bloodstream. The primary lesion develops 10 to 90 days after infection and is a result of an inflammatory response to the infection at the site of the inoculation. The lesion, known as the **chancre**, is typically a single erythematous lesion that is nontender but firm with a clean surface and raised border. The lesion is teeming with treponemes and is extremely infectious. Because the chancre is commonly found on the cervix or vaginal wall, it may not be apparent in females. The lesion can also be found in the anal canal of either sex and remain undetected. No systemic signs or symptoms are evident in the primary stages of the disease.

  Secondary Stage of Syphilis. Approximately 2 to 12 weeks after development of the primary lesion, the patient may experience secondary disease, with clinical symptoms of fever, sore throat, generalized lymphadenopathy, headache, lesions of the mucous membranes, and rash. The rash can present as macular, papular, follicular, papulosquamous or pustular and is unusual in that it can also occur on the palms and soles. All secondary lesions of the skin and mucous membranes are highly infectious. The secondary stage can last for several weeks and may relapse. It might also be mild and go unnoticed by the patient.

  Tertiary Stage of Syphilis. After the secondary stage heals, individuals are not contagious; however, relapses of secondary syphilis occur in about 25% of untreated patients. Following the secondary stage, patients enter latent syphilis, when clinical manifestations are absent. Latency within 1 year of infection is referred to as early latent, whereas latency greater than 1 year is late latent syphilis. Approximately one third of untreated patients exhibit a biologic cure, losing serologic reactivity. Another one third remain latent for life but have reactive serology. The remaining one third ultimately develop tertiary or late syphilis, generally decades later. Symptoms of tertiary syphilis include the development of granulomatous lesions **(gummas)** in skin, bones, and liver (benign tertiary syphilis); degenerative changes in the central nervous system (neurosyphilis); and syphilitic cardiovascular lesions, particularly aortitis and aortic valve insufficiency. Patients in the tertiary stage are usually not infectious. In the United States, the tertiary stage of disease is not often seen because most patients are adequately treated with antimicrobial agents before the tertiary stage is reached.

  Congenital Syphilis. Treponemes can be transmitted from an infected mother to her fetus by crossing the placenta. Congenital syphilis affects many body systems and is therefore severe and mutilating. Early onset congenital syphilis, onset less than 2 years of age, is characterized by mucocutaneous lesions, osteochondritis, anemia, hepatosplenomegaly, and central nervous system involvement and occurs when mothers have early syphilis during pregnancy. Late onset congenital syphilis results following pregnancies when mothers have chronic, untreated infections. Symptoms of late onset congenital syphilis occur after 2 years of age but generally are not apparent until the second decade of life. Symptoms include interstitial keratitis, bone and tooth deformities, eighth nerve deafness, neurosyphilis, and other tertiary manifestations.

Epidemiology

Treponema pallidum subsp. *pallidum* is an exclusively human pathogen under natural conditions. Syphilis was first recognized in Europe at the end of the fifteenth century, when it reached epidemic proportions. Two theories have been proposed concerning the introduction of syphilis to Europe. The first theory suggests that Christopher Columbus's crew brought the disease from the West Indies back to Europe. The second theory suggests that the disease was endemic in Africa and transported to Europe via the migration of armies and civilians. The venereal transmission of syphilis was not recognized until the eighteenth century. The causative agent of syphilis was not discovered until 1905.

The rates of both primary and secondary syphilis in the United States had dropped through the 1990s, and the fewest cases (31,575) since reporting began in 1941 was reached in 2000. However, since 2000 there has been a steady increase through 2007 when 40,920 cases were reported. Overall increases in syphilis cases have been due to increases among white males; however, recent increases among all races, women, men who have sex with men, and congenitally acquired disease are also disturbing. High-risk sexual behavior and coinfection with HIV continue to complicate syphilis control efforts. Educating people about sexually transmitted diseases, including the proper use of barrier contraceptives; reporting each case of syphilis to the health authorities for contact investigation; and treating all sexual contacts of persons infected with syphilis are cornerstones of syphilis control efforts. Serologic screening of high-risk populations should be performed, and to avoid congenital syphilis, pregnant women should have serologic examinations early and late in the pregnancy.

Laboratory Diagnosis

Specimen Collection and Handling. Lesions of primary and secondary syphilis typically contain large numbers of spirochetes. The surface of primary or secondary lesions is cleaned with saline and gently abraded with dry, sterile gauze; bleeding should not be induced. Serous transudate is placed onto a slide, diluting with nonbacteriocidal saline if the preparation is too thick. A coverslip is added and the slide is transported immediately to a laboratory where dark-field microscopy is performed. Oral lesions should not be examined because numerous nonpathogenic spirochetes present in these specimens will lead to misinterpretation. Culture methods are not available and dark-field microscopy equipment and expertise is uncommon, so serology is the normal basis of diagnosis.

Microscopic Examination. Organisms are too thin to be observed by bright-field microscopy, so spirochetes are illuminated against a dark background. Dark-field microscopy requires considerable skill and experience; however, demonstration of motile treponemes in material from the chancre is diagnostic for primary syphilis.

Serologic Tests. Serology is the primary method used for the laboratory diagnosis of syphilis. Two major types of serologic tests exist: nontreponemal tests and treponemal tests. Both have lower sensitivities in the primary stage but have sensitivities of nearly 100% in the secondary stage of syphilis. The treponemal tests retain a very high sensitivity in the tertiary stage as well. A coinfection with HIV can result in false-negative serologic tests. Comparisons between CSF and serum antibody responses can be helpful in potential cases of neurosyphilis. With congenital syphilis, comparing antibody responses in mother and baby serum can aid diagnosis.

The nontreponemal tests detect reaginic antibodies that develop against lipids released from damaged cells. Although they are biologically nonspecific and known to react with organisms of other diseases and conditions (causing false-positive reactions), the nontreponemal tests are excellent screening tests. The antigen employed is a cardiolipin-lecithin complex made from bovine hearts.

The two nontreponemal tests widely used today are the **Venereal Disease Research Laboratory (VDRL)** and RPR tests. These tests are inexpensive to perform, demonstrate rising and falling reagin titers, and correlate with the clinical status of the patient. The VDRL test uses a cardiolipin antigen that is mixed with the patient's serum or CSF. Flocculation occurs in a positive reaction and is observed microscopically. RPR is the more common test used; it employs carbon particles and is read macroscopically. When mixed with a positive serum on a disposable card, the black charcoal particles clump together with the cardiolipin-antibody complexes. Flocculation is easily observed without a microscope. Reactive or weakly reactive sera should undergo titration and be tested with treponemal tests.

The treponemal tests detect antibodies specific for treponemal antigens. They are helpful in the detection of late-stage infections and the confirmation of positive nontreponemal test results. Treponemal test titers remain high and usually do not drop in response to therapy as the nontreponemal test results do. Thus, treponemal tests are not useful in following therapy or detecting reinfection. The antigens used are spirochetes derived from rabbit testicular lesions. Two commonly used treponemal test methods are the *Treponema pallidum*–particulate agglutination (TP-PA) Test (Fujirebio America, Fairfield, N.J.) and EIAs. The fluorescent treponemal antibody absorption (FTA-ABS) test is becoming less frequently used.

In the FTA-ABS test, the patient's serum is first absorbed with extracts of a cultivated, nonpathogenic Reiter treponeme, which is not *T. pallidum*, to remove nonspecific treponemal antibody. Then the absorbed serum is placed on a slide that has *T. pallidum* Nichols strain organisms affixed to it. After specific antibody from the patient is allowed to react with the organisms, unbound antibodies in the serum are removed by washing. The presence of anti–*T. pallidum* antibody is then detected by application of fluorescein-labeled, anti–human globulin and examination of the slide with an ultraviolet (UV) microscope. Positive results are indicated by fluorescence of the *T. pallidum* organisms. An FTA-ABS 19S-IgM test has also been developed for evaluation of congenital syphilis; however, the test is still considered provisional.

The TP-PA test uses gelatin particles sensitized with *T. pallidum* antigens. The TP-PA test is simpler to perform than the FTA-ABS test, does not require an absorption step or expensive UV microscope, and is more specific than the microhemagglutination-TP test. Several EIA kits are commercially available. EIA tests have sensitivities and specificities similar to other treponemal tests and are generally easier to perform.

Antimicrobial Susceptibility

Penicillin is the drug of choice for treating patients with syphilis. It is the only proven therapy that has been widely used for patients with neurosyphilis, congenital syphilis, and syphilis during pregnancy. Resistant strains have not developed. Long-acting penicillin such as benzathine penicillin is preferred. Alternative regimens for patients who are allergic to penicillin and not pregnant include doxycycline, tetracycline, and chloramphenicol. A typical Jarisch-Herxheimer reaction and exacerbation of cutaneous lesions may occur within hours following treatment. For further discussion on recommendations for appropriate therapy and interpretation of serologic tests, refer to the *Sexually Transmitted Diseases Treatment Guidelines* published by the Centers for Disease Control and Prevention.

Other Treponemal Diseases

Three nonvenereal treponemal diseases occur in different geographic locations. These treponematoses are found in developing countries where hygiene is poor, little clothing is worn, and direct skin contact is common because of overcrowding. All three diseases have primary and secondary stages, but tertiary manifestations are uncommon. All diseases respond well to penicillin or tetracycline. These infections are rarely transmitted by sexual contact, and congenital infections do not occur. The three nonvenereal treponemal diseases are yaws, pinta, and endemic syphilis.

Yaws

Yaws is a spirochetal disease caused by *T. pallidum* subsp. *pertenue*. It is endemic in the humid, tropical belt—the tropical regions of Africa; parts of South America, India, and Indonesia; and many of the Pacific Islands. It is not seen in the United States. The course of yaws resembles that of syphilis, but the early stage lesions are elevated, granulomatous nodules.

Endemic Syphilis

Endemic syphilis (bejel) is caused by *T. pallidum* subsp. *endemicum* and closely resembles yaws in clinical manifestations. It is found in the Middle East and the arid, hot areas of the world. The primary and secondary lesions are usually papules that often go unnoticed. They can progress to gummas of the skin, bones, and nasopharynx. Dark-field microscopy is not useful because of normal oral spirochetal biota. Poor hygienic conditions are important in perpetuating these infections. Bejel is transmitted by direct contact or sharing contaminated eating utensils.

Pinta

Pinta, which is caused by *T. carateum*, is found in the tropical regions of Central and South America. It is acquired by person-to-person contact and is rarely transmitted by sexual intercourse. Lesions begin as scaling, painless papules and are followed by an erythematous rash that becomes hypopigmented with time.

BIBLIOGRAPHY

Aguero-Rosenfeld ME et al: Diagnosis of Lyme borreliosis, *Clin Microbiol Rev* 18:484-509, 2005.

Centers for Disease Control and Prevention: *Sexually transmitted disease surveillance 2006*, Washington, DC, 2007, U.S. Department of Health and Human Services.

Centers for Disease Control and Prevention, Workowski KA, Berman SM: Sexually transmitted diseases treatment guidelines, 2006, *MMWR* 55(RR-11):1, 2006. Available at: www.cdc/gov/mmwr/preview/mmwrhtml/rr5511a1.htm. Accessed December 16, 2009.

Centers for Disease Control and Prevention: Summary of notifiable diseases—United States, 2007, *MMWR* 56, 2009. Available at: www.cdc.gov/mmwr/preview/mmwrhtml/mm5653a1.htm. Accessed December 16, 2009.

Dworkin MS et al: The epidemiology of tick-borne relapsing fever in the United States, *Am J Trop Med Hyg* 66:753, 2002.

Hawaii Department of Health Communicable Disease Division: Communicable Disease Report, September/October 2004. Personal communication for 2004 leptospirosis data.

Kassutto S, Doweiko JP: Syphilis in the HIV era, *Emerg Infect Dis* 10:1471, 2004.

Katz AR et al: Leptospirosis in Hawaii, 1974-1998: epidemiologic analysis of 353 laboratory-confirmed cases, *Am J Trop Med Hyg* 66:61-78, 2002.

Levett PN et al: Two methods for rapid serological diagnosis of acute leptospirosis, *Clin Diagn Lab Immunol* 8:349, 2001.

Levett PN: Leptospira. In Murray PR et al, editors: *Manual of clinical microbiology*, ed 9, Washington, DC, 2007, ASM Press.

Meri T et al: Relapsing fever spirochetes *Borrelia recurrentis* and *B. duttonii* acquire complement regulators C4b-binding protein and factor H, *Infect Immunity* 74:4157, 2006.

Pope V et al: *Treponema* and other human host-associated spirochetes. In Murray PR et al, editors: *Manual of clinical microbiology*, ed 9, Washington, DC, 2007, ASM Press.

Sejvar JB et al: Leptospirosis in "Eco-Challenge" athletes, Malaysian Borneo, 2000. *Emerg Infect Dis* 9:702, 2003.

Steere AC: *Borrelia burgdorferi* (Lyme disease, Lyme borreliosis). In Mandell GL et al, editors: *Mandell, Douglas, and Bennett's principles and practice of infectious diseases*, ed 5, New York, 2000, Churchill Livingstone.

Points to Remember

- Spirochetes are slender, flexuous, helically shaped, unicellular bacteria.
- Leptospires are most likely to enter the human host through small breaks in the skin or intact mucosa.
- The incubation period of leptospirosis is usually 10 to 12 days but ranges from 3 to 30 days after inoculation. The onset of clinical illness is usually abrupt, with nonspecific, influenza-like constitutional symptoms such as fever, chills, headache, severe myalgia, and malaise.
- The pathogenic borreliae commonly are arthropod-borne (by a tick or louse) and cause relapsing fever and Lyme disease.
- *Borrelia recurrentis* and similar species cause relapsing fever. The relapses are caused by immune evasion including antigenic variation. During the course of a single infection, borreliae systematically change their surface antigens.
- During the febrile period, diagnosis of relapsing fever is readily made by Giemsa or Wright staining of blood smears. Relapsing fever is the only spirochetal disease in which the organisms are visible in blood with bright-field microscopy.
- Diagnosis of Lyme borreliosis caused by *Borrelia burgdorferi* sensu lato is typically supported serologically. False-positive results are unusual with current commercial kits. However, a *Treponema pallidum* infection could produce a false-positive result. Consequently, a nontreponemal test (such as the rapid plasma reagin) for

syphilis should be performed on positive sera to exclude the factor of cross-reactivity.

- The rates of both primary and secondary syphilis in the United States dropped through the 1990s, and the lowest rate since reporting began in 1941 was reached in 2000. However, since 2000 there has been a steady increase in the incidence of syphilis.
- Treponemes can cross the placenta and be transmitted from an infected mother to her fetus. Congenital syphilis affects many body systems and is therefore severe and mutilating. All pregnant women should have serologic testing for syphilis early in pregnancy.

Learning Assessment Questions

1. Describe the general morphology of spirochetes.
2. What risk factors are associated with *Borrelia* spp. endemic relapsing fever infection?
3. Which tickborne species of *Borrelia* is associated with a skin rash or lesion?
4. What is the significance on infectious disease transmission of finding partially engorged ticks attached to the skin?
5. What is the test of choice for the laboratory diagnosis of relapsing fever borreliosis?
6. Where are most cases of leptospiroses contracted within the United States, and why is this important when considering the typical incubation period of the infection?
7. What are the stages of a *Treponema pallidum* subsp. *pallidum* infection? Is the final stage usually seen in the United States?
8. Name the four strains of the genus *Treponema* that are pathogenic for humans.
9. What is erythema chronicum migrans?
10. Compare the difference(s) between treponemal and nontreponemal tests for syphilis.

Chlamydia and Rickettsia

Donald C. Lehman, Connie R. Mahon*

■ **CHLAMYDIACEAE**
General Characteristics
Chlamydia trachomatis
Chlamydophila (Chlamydia) pneumoniae
Chlamydophila (Chlamydia) psittaci

■ **RICKETTSIACEAE AND SIMILAR ORGANISMS**
Rickettsia
Orientia
Anaplasmataceae
Coxiella

OBJECTIVES

After reading and studying this chapter, you should be able to:

1. List the members of the family Chlamydiaceae.
2. Discuss the unique growth cycle of *Chlamydia*, describing elementary and reticulate bodies.
3. Compare *Chlamydia* and *Rickettsia* and distinguish them from other bacteria and viruses.
4. Discuss the most important human diseases caused by the species of *Chlamydia*, *Chlamydophila*, *Rickettsia*, and similar microorganisms.
5. Describe the modes of transmission for each species of *Chlamydia*, *Chlamydophila*, *Rickettsia*, and similar microorganisms.
6. Define the appropriate cultures for detection of *Chlamydia trachomatis*.
7. Compare the available assays for the laboratory diagnosis of *C. trachomatis* and *Chlamydophila pneumoniae* infections.
8. Discuss the problems with serologic cross-reactivity among the rickettsial species.
9. For the following human rickettsial diseases, link the causative agent and compare the mode of transmission to humans:
   - Louse-borne typhus
   - Rocky Mountain spotted fever
   - Scrub typhus
10. Compare the characteristics of the *Rickettsia* and *Coxiella* and the diseases they cause.

Case in Point

A 7-day-old newborn girl was brought by her grandmother to the emergency department of a large city hospital. She had been discharged 3 days after birth, with the last nursing note indicating that the child was "fussy." The child presented to the emergency department with a fever of 39° C, loss of appetite, a profuse yellow discharge from the right eye, and general "irritability." Medical history revealed the mother to be a 17-year-old intravenous drug abuser with no prenatal care and who had a vaginal delivery in the parking lot of a local hospital. Eye discharge and cell scrapings were cultured. Routine bacterial cultures were negative; however, the cell cultures were diagnostic.

Issues to Consider

After reading the patient's case history, consider:
- The various organisms that can be recovered from exudative material from newborns
- The clinical infections and disease spectrum associated with these organisms
- How these organisms are transmitted and the risk factors associated with the diseases produced
- The appropriate methods of laboratory diagnosis

*This chapter was prepared by C.R. Mahon in her private capacity. No official support or endorsement by the FDA is intended or implied.

Key Terms

Brill-Zinsser disease

Bubo

Elementary body (EB)

Human granulocytic
anaplasmosis (HGA)

Human monocytic ehrlichiosis
(HME)

Lymphogranuloma venereum
(LGV)

Morulae

Pelvic inflammatory disease
(PID)

Reiter syndrome

Reticulate body (RB)

Trachoma

The genus *Chlamydia* is in the family Chlamydiaceae; members of the family share selected characteristics (Table 24-1) and have a unique life cycle. Within the genus *Chlamydia*, four species were recognized: *C. pecorum*, *C. pneumoniae*, *C. psittaci*, and *C. trachomatis*. All except *C. pecorum* have been associated with human disease. However, based on analysis of 16S and 23S rRNA gene sequences a new taxonomic classification has been accepted. The family Chlamydiaceae now consists of two genera: (1) *Chlamydia* to include *C. trachomatis* and (2) *Chlamydophila* to include *C. pneumoniae*, *C. psittaci*, and *C. pecorum*. The creation of a second genus was somewhat controversial and is still being

debated. Therefore, readers may find both taxonomic classifications in published literature.

The term *rickettsiae* can specifically refer to the genus *Rickettsia* or it can refer to a group of organisms included in the order Rickettsiales. There has been significant reorganization in the order Rickettsiales in recent years. The order includes the families Rickettsiaceae and Anaplasmataceae. The family Rickettsiaceae includes the genera *Rickettsia* and *Orientia*. The family Anaplasmataceae includes the genera *Ehrlichia*, *Anaplasma*, *Cowdria*, *Neorickettsia*, and *Wolbachia*. As a result of this reorganization, *Coxiella* has been removed from the family Rickettsiaceae.

CHLAMYDIACEAE

General Characteristics

As shown in Table 24-2, initial differentiation of the *Chlamydia* spp. was based on selected characteristics of the growth cycle, susceptibility to sulfa drugs, and DNA relatedness. Table 24-2 also lists additional properties of the Chlamydiaceae species that have helped further differentiate the three human species on the basis of natural host, major diseases, and number of antigenic variants (i.e., serovars).

Chlamydiae are deficient in energy metabolism and are therefore obligate intracellular parasites. Their unique growth

---

TABLE 24-1 Comparative Properties of Microorganisms

Characteristic	Organisms				
	Typical Bacteria	Chlamydiae	Rickettsiae	Mycoplasmas	Viruses
DNA and RNA	+	+	+	+	−
Obligate intracellular parasites	−	+	+	−	+
Peptidoglycan in cell wall	+	+	−	−	−
Growth on nonliving medium	+	−	−	+	−
Contain ribosomes	+	+	+	+	−
Sensitivity to antimicrobial agents	+	+	+	+	−
Sensitivity to interferon	−	+	−	−	+
Binary fission (replication)	+	+	+	+	−

+, Characteristic is present; −, characteristic is absent.

TABLE 24-2 Initial Differentiation of *Chlamydiaceae* Species

Properties	*Chlamydia trachomatis*	*Chlamydophila pneumoniae*	*Chlamydophila psittaci*
Inclusion morphology	Round, vacuolar	Round, dense	Variable shape, dense
Glycogen in inclusions	+	−	−
Elementary body morphology	Round	Pear-shaped	Round
Sulfa drug sensitivity	+	−	−
DNA relatedness (against *C. pneumoniae*)	10%	100%	10%
Natural hosts	Humans	Humans	Birds, lower animals
Major human diseases	Sexually transmitted diseases	Pneumonia	Pneumonia
	Trachoma	Pharyngitis	FUO
	Lymphogranuloma venereum	Bronchitis	
Number of serovars	20	1	10

FUO, Fever of unknown origin; +, characteristic is present; −, characteristic is absent.

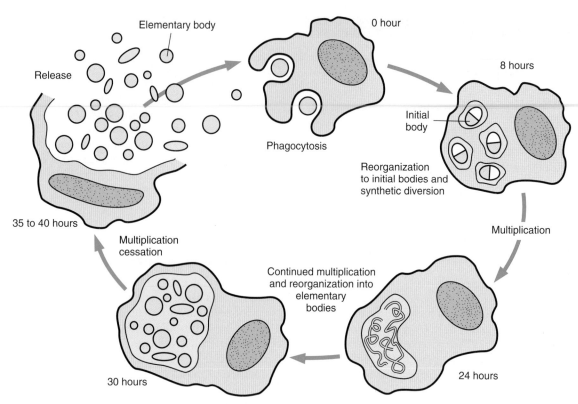

FIGURE 24-1 Life cycle of *Chlamydia*.

cycle involves two distinct forms of the organism: an **elementary body (EB),** which is infectious, and a **reticulate body (RB),** which is noninfectious. The growth cycle (Figure 24-1) begins when the small EB infects the host cell by inducing energy-requiring active phagocytosis. In vivo, host cells are primarily the nonciliated, columnar, or transitional epithelial cells that line the conjunctiva, respiratory tract, urogenital tract, and rectum. During the next 8 hours, they organize into larger, less dense RBs, which divert the host cell's synthesizing functions to their own metabolic needs and begin to multiply by binary fission. About 24 hours after infection, the dividing organisms begin reorganizing into infective EBs. At about 30 hours, multiplication ceases, and by 35 to 40 hours, the disrupted host cell dies, releasing new EBs (Figure 24-2) that can infect other host cells, continuing the cycle.

The EB has an outer membrane similar to that of many gram-negative bacteria. The most prominent component of this membrane is the major outer membrane protein (MOMP). The MOMP is a transmembrane protein that contains both species-specific and subspecies-specific epitopes that can be defined by monoclonal antibodies. The chlamydial outer membrane also contains lipopolysaccharide (LPS). This extractable LPS, with ketodeoxyoctonate, is shared by most members of the family and is the primary antigen detectable in genus-specific tests and serologic assays for the chlamydiae.

Chlamydia trachomatis

Chlamydia trachomatis has been divided into three biovars: trachoma, lymphogranuloma venereum, and mouse pneumo-

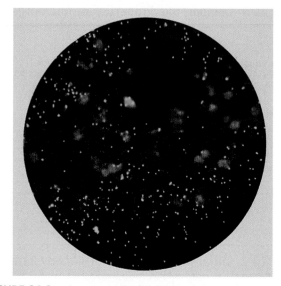

FIGURE 24-2 Elementary bodies and cells in *Chlamydia trachomatis*–positive direct specimen. (Courtesy Syva Microtrak, Palo Alto, Calif.)

nitis (renamed *C. muridarum*). In addition, characterization of an MOMP has separated *C. trachomatis* into 20 serovariants, or serovars (Table 24-3). The trachoma biovar includes serovars A through K. Serovars A, B, Ba, and C are associated with the severe eye infection **trachoma,** while serovars D through K, Da, Ia, and Ja are associated with inclusion conjunctivitis, a milder eye infection, and urogenital infections.

TABLE 24-3 Human Diseases Caused by Chlamydiaceae Species

Species	Serovars*	Disease	Host
Chlamydia trachomatis	A, B, Ba, C	Hyperendemic trachoma	Humans
	D, Da, E, F, G, H, I, Ia, J, Ja, K	Inclusion conjunctivitis (adult and newborn)	Humans
		Nongonococcal urethritis	
		Cervicitis	
		Salpingitis	
		Pelvic inflammatory disease	
		Endometritis	
		Acute urethral syndrome	
		Proctitis	
		Epididymitis	
		Pneumonia of newborns	
		Perihepatitis (Fitz-Hugh–Curtis syndrome)	
	L_1, L_2, L_{2a}, L_{2b}, L_3	Lymphogranuloma venereum	
Chlamydophila pneumoniae	1	Pneumonia, bronchitis	Humans
		Pharyngitis	
		Influenza-like febrile illness	
Chlamydophila psittaci	10 serotypes	Psittacosis	Birds
		Endocarditis	
		Abortion	

*Predominant serovars associated with disease.

Serovars L_1, L_2, L_{2a}, L_{2b}, and L_3 are associated with **lymphogranuloma venereum (LGV),** an invasive urogenital tract disease.

Chlamydia trachomatis is unique in that it carries 10 stable plasmids whose function is currently unknown. This unique characteristic is a major reason for the applications of nucleic acid amplification by polymerase chain reaction (PCR) and identification by hybridization.

Clinical Infections

Trachoma. Initially, *C. trachomatis* was linked to the chronic eye infection trachoma (Figure 24-3), the number one cause of preventable blindness in the world. Trachoma is associated with serotypes A, B, Ba, and C. These serovars are most frequently found near the equator and are seen in climates with high temperature and high humidity; they are not commonly seen in the United States. These serovars produce a chronic infection resulting in scarring and continual abrasion of the cornea as the eyelid turns downward toward the cornea and, if left untreated, infection generally ends in blindness in adults. Prevention includes either or both antimicrobial treatment and a simple surgical procedure on the eyelid.

Lymphogranuloma Venereum. *Chlamydia trachomatis* serovars L_1, L_2, L_{2a}, L_{2b}, and L_3 cause LGV, a sexually transmitted disease (STD); these serovars are more invasive than the others. In LGV, patients have inguinal and anorectal symptoms (Figure 24-4). The serovars causing LGV are able to survive inside mononuclear cells. The bacteria enter the lymph nodes near the genital tract and produce a strong inflammatory response that often results in **bubo** formation and subsequent rupture of the lymph node. LGV is uncommon in the United States and is usually seen in immigrants from and returning travelers to countries where the disease is endemic, typically the tropics and subtropics. The LGV

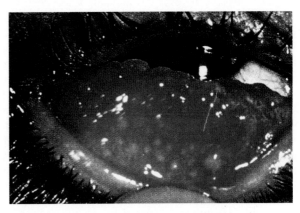

FIGURE 24-3 Conjunctival scarring and hyperendemic blindness caused by *Chlamydia trachomatis* in ocular infections.

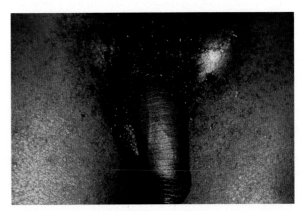

FIGURE 24-4 Inguinal swelling and lymphatic drainage due to *Chlamydia trachomatis* serovars L_1, L_{2a}, L_{2b}, or L_3, that is, lymphogranuloma venereum.

serovars have also been linked to Parinaud oculoglandular conjunctivitis.

Other Urogenital Diseases. *Chlamydia trachomatis* infections in adult men include nongonococcal urethritis (NGU), epididymitis, and prostatitis. Serovars D through K are associated with these clinical infections, which can be persistent and subclinical as well as acute and demonstrable. Between 45% and 68% of female partners of men with *Chlamydia*-positive NGU yield chlamydial isolates from the cervix. Approximately 50% of current male partners of women with a cervical chlamydial infection are also infected.

Infections in adult women include urethritis, follicular cervicitis (leukorrhea hypertrophic cervical erosion), endometritis, proctitis, salpingitis, **pelvic inflammatory disease (PID),** and perihepatitis. **Reiter syndrome** (urethritis, conjunctivitis, polyarthritis, and mucocutaneous lesions) in adults is believed to be caused by *C. trachomatis*. Salpingitis can lead to scarring and dysfunction of the oviductal transport system, resulting in infertility or ectopic pregnancy. In the United States, this is a major cause of sterility.

Chlamydia trachomatis is the most common sexually transmitted bacterial pathogen in the United States. In 2007, a total of 1,108,374 cases of genital infections were reported, but many infections are undiagnosed. The number of cases has been increasing by over 5% annually since 1997. Only genital warts caused by human papillomavirus is a more common sexually transmitted disease in the United States. *Neisseria gonorrhoeae* is a distant third, with 355,991 confirmed cases in 2007 and an estimated 600,000 new cases per year. The reported rate of chlamydial infections in women increased from 78.5 cases per 100,000 population in 1987 to 496.5 cases per 100,000 population in 2005. This rate is over three times that of males. The Centers for Disease Control and Prevention (CDC) attributed these increases in the reported national *C. trachomatis* infection rate to increased screening, increased use of nucleic acid amplification tests, better reporting, and ongoing high burden of disease.

Chlamydia Infection in the Newborn. Traveling through an infected birth canal, infants can be infected with *Chlamydia* spp. Chlamydial infection in an infant delivered by cesarean section is rare, and infection from seronegative mothers has not been reported. Infants suffering from chlamydial infection can experience conjunctivitis, nasopharyngeal infections, and pneumonia. Table 24-4 shows selected features associated with neonatal inclusion conjunctivitis. The portal of entry is ocular or aspiration, with colonization of the oropharynx being a necessary event before infection.

Between 20% and 25% of neonates born to *Chlamydia*—culture-positive mothers develop conjunctivitis, 15% to 20% develop nasopharyngeal infection, and 3% to 18% develop pneumonia. Otitis media is a less frequent infection. Infants born in the United States receive prophylactic eyedrops, generally erythromycin, to prevent eye infections by *C. trachomatis* and *N. gonorrhoeae*.

Clinically, it is believed that pneumonia in infants younger than 6 months of age is associated with *C. trachomatis*, unless proven otherwise. This pneumonia also can occur as a mixed infection with gonococcus, cytomegalovirus and other viruses, and *Pneumocystis*. The incubation period is variable, but symptoms generally appear 2 to 3 weeks after birth.

Laboratory Diagnosis

There are numerous methods for the laboratory diagnosis of *C. trachomatis* that vary in sensitivity, specificity, and positive predictive value. Table 24-5 identifies the situations in which the tests may be most applicable and identifies the population groups at greatest risk. Table 24-6 provides the predictive values for isolation, detection, and identification methods. The most appropriate tests or combinations of assays used depend on the following factors:

- Knowledge of the population at risk
- Capability and facilities available for testing
- Cost of assays
- Ability to batch specimen types
- Experience of laboratory scientist

Prevalence in the population to be tested is an important criterion in determining which method or combination of methods should be used. For any assay, the positive predictive value increases (assuming optimum technical conditions) when the prevalence of the disease in the population is high. The type of specimen selected for laboratory processing depends on the symptoms of the patient and the clinical presentation. Regardless of the source, however, the specimen should consist of infected epithelial cells and not exudate. Dacron, cotton, and calcium alginate swabs can be used, but it should be noted that toxicity has been associated with different lots of each. Furthermore, it is important to remember that swabs with plastic or metal shafts are superior to those with wooden shafts, which are toxic to cells. Table 24-7 lists the optimum specimens for detection of *Chlamydia* spp. in patients with a variety of clinical manifestations.

Direct Microscopic Examination. Direct specimen examination by cytologic methods primarily involves trachoma and inclusion conjunctivitis (Figure 24-5). Investigators have estimated this method as nearly 95% sensitive, but it is technically demanding and influenced by the quality of the specimen and expertise of the laboratory scientist. Although this method is difficult to use with large numbers of specimens, it does offer rapidity in selected cases, particularly in detecting ocular infection in newborns. When direct fluorescent antibody (DFA) testing is used for endocervical or urethral specimens, characteristic fluorescence of EBs is suggestive, but verification by alternative methods employing a different epitope is needed. Direct specimen examination offers one additional important advantage: it allows for immediate quality control of the specimen, revealing whether columnar epithelial cells are present. Figure 24-6 shows

---

TABLE 24-4 Inclusion Conjunctivitis in the Neonate Caused by *Chlamydia trachomatis*

Characteristic	Comments
Incubation period	4 to 5 days
Signs	Edematous eyelids
Discharge	Copious, yellow
Course	Untreated, weeks to months
Complications	Corneal panus formation, conjunctival scarring

TABLE 24-5 Appropriate *Chlamydia trachomatis* Assays for Selected Patient Population

| | Patient Population | | | | | | | |
| | Prenatal | | Newborn | | Clinics* | | Legal Applicability (Rape or Child Abuse?) | Test of Cure |
Assay	Low Risk	High Risk	Eye	Throat	Low Risk	High Risk		
Culture	A/B	A	B	A	A/B	B	Yes	Yes
Nonculture, nonamplified								
DFA	B	A	A	A	B	A	No	No
EIA	A/B	A	A	A	A/B	A	No	No
OIA	—	—	—	—	B	B	No	No
Nonculture, amplified								
Probe	B	B	IUO	IUO	B	A	No	No
PCR	A	A	IUO	IUO	A	A	IUO	IUO
Serology								
CF	B, LGV	B, LGV	NA	NA	B, LGV	B, LGV	No	No
EIA	B	B	A	A	B	B	NA	NA
Micro-IF	NA	B	A	A(IgM)	B	B	No	No

A, Most useful, stands alone; *B*, probable, but needs verification or complementary assay recognizing different *Chlamydia trachomatis* macromolecules, i.e., LPS (EIA) vs. MOMP; (DFA) or competition assay for DNA probes; *DFA*, direct fluorescent antibody; *EIA*, enzyme immunoassay; *OIA*, optical immunoassay; *IUO*, investigational use only; *PCR*, polymerase chain reaction; *CF*, complement fixation; *LGV*, lymphogranuloma venereum; *Micro-IF*, microimmunofluorescence; *NA*, not available; *MOMP*, major outer membrane proteins.
*A low-risk population is defined as one with a <5% incidence, such as in an obstetrics-gynecology or family practice patient group (e.g., birth control, annual gynecologic examination). A high-risk population is defined as one with a >10% incidence, such as those in sexually transmitted disease clinics, university or college student health centers, and emergency department patients.

TABLE 24-6 Detection Capabilities of Various Methods for *Chlamydia trachomatis*

| | | | | | Specimen Site | | | | | | |
	SENS* (%)	SPEC* (%)	PPV* (%)	NPV* (%)	Cervical-Urethral	Rectal	Urine	Eye	False +/−	Reported Cross-Reactivity	Comments
Culture	50 to 85	100	73 to 98	90 to 100	+	+	+	+	False −	None	Labor-intensive gold standard for specificity
Nonculture, nonamplified											
DFA	70 to 95	92 to 98	73 to 98	95 to 99	+	+	−	+	False −/+	Staphylococci	Screen only; experience in FA needed
EIA	72 to 95	90 to 99	45 to 92	95 to 99	+	−	LA	LA	False +/−	Streptococci, GC, *Acinetobacter*	Verify with complementary assay
Probe	60 to 90	92 to 98	85 to 99	98 to 99	+	−	−	−	False +/−	Selected bacteria	Screen and verify with complementary assay
Nonculture, amplified											
PCR, LCR, TMA	85 to 95	99 to 100	85 to 95	100	+	−	+	RUO	False −	None reported	No verification necessary

SENS, Sensitivity; *SPEC*, specificity; *PPV*, positive predictive value; *NPV*, negative predictive value; *DFA*, direct fluorescent antibody; *FA*, fluorescent antibody; *EIA*, enzyme immunoassay; *LA*, limited availability; *PCR*, polymerase chain reaction; *TMA*, transcription-mediated amplification; *RUO*, research use only.
*RANGE: Low to high prevalence as described in the text.

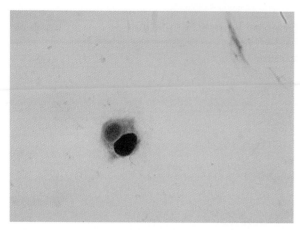

FIGURE 24-5 Giemsa stain showing inclusion body from ocular swab of a 7-day-old newborn who was discharged but then readmitted with fever, weight loss, lack of eating, and "fussiness." At 3 days after delivery, *Neisseria gonorrhoeae* was isolated from ocular discharge, although the patient had been given silver nitrate eye drops. Eye cultures confirmed the presence of *Chlamydia trachomatis*.

inclusion bodies demonstrated by direct examination of cytologic stains of endocervical smears.

Cell Culture. Until the development of PCR assays, chlamydial cell culture was considered the gold standard for detecting *C. trachomatis* infection; however, cell culture utility has been limited because of the inherent technical complexity, time and specimen handling requirements, expense, and labile nature of the organism. Even under the most stringent and optimal conditions, isolation of chlamydiae is only approximately 80% sensitive. Cell lines commonly used for the detection of chlamydiae include McCoy, HEp-2, HeLa, and buffalo green monkey kidney. The cell lines are grown on coverslips in 1-dram shell vials or on the surface of multiwell cell culture dishes containing cell culture media with cycloheximide. Because multiple blind passes are not necessary to maximize the isolation rate in a 1-dram vial, the shell vial technique (see Chapter 29) has been found to be more sensitive than the microwell method. The specimen is centrifuged onto the cell monolayer and incubated for 72 hours.

Fluorescein-labeled monoclonal antibodies can be used to detect the chlamydial inclusions. Alternatively, iodine or

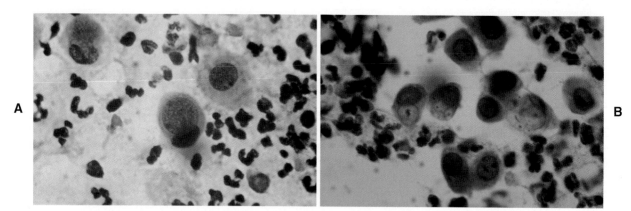

FIGURE 24-6 **A** and **B**, Cytologic examination of endocervical specimens demonstrating inclusion bodies consistent with *Chlamydia trachomatis*. Papanicolaou stain. (**B**, 600×).

TABLE 24-7 Appropriate Specimens for Detection of Chlamydial Infections

Clinical Manifestation/Site of Infection	Specimen Site/Type	Comments
Inclusion conjunctivitis and trachoma	Conjunctival swab, scraping with spatula or tears	Specimen collection in neonates is difficult
Urethritis	Urethral swab	In males, >4 cm and do not use discharge
Epididymitis	Epididymis aspirate	
Cervicitis	Endocervical swab	Remove exudate first
Salpingitis	Fallopian tube (lumen) or biopsy	
Lymphogranuloma venereum	Bubo or cervical lymph node aspirate	
Infant pneumonia	Throat swab, nasopharyngeal aspirate, or lung tissue	
Sexually transmitted disease, male sex partner	Urine	Noninvasive diagnostic procedure
		EIA antigen detection is 80% accurate; PCR, 98%
Psittacosis	Sputum, lung tissue	
Chlamydophila pneumoniae pneumonia or pharyngitis	Sputum, throat swab, or lung tissue	Tissue culture isolation and direct immunofluorescence are relatively new and need further evaluation
Sexually transmitted disease, result clarification	Rectal, vaginal swabs	May be used for supplemental information and in clarifying previous isolates or diagnostic dilemmas

EIA, Enzyme immunoassay; *PCR*, polymerase chain reaction.

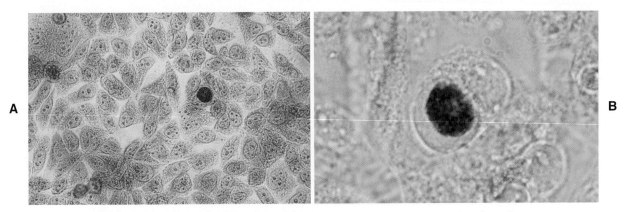

FIGURE 24-7 Iodine-stained inclusion bodies from *Chlamydia trachomatis*–infected McCoy cells. (**A**, 40×; **B**, 100×.) Note the size and half-moon shape of the inclusion.

Giemsa stain can be used, but these methods are less sensitive and specific (Figure 24-7). There are a number of commercially available fluorescent antibodies. Some researchers use species-specific monoclonal antibodies that bind to the MOMP, whereas others prefer the family-specific antibody, which binds to an LPS component. Monoclonal antibodies against the MOMP are reported to offer the brightest fluorescence with consistent bacterial morphology and less nonspecific staining than monoclonal antibodies against the LPS. Many studies determining the specificity, sensitivity, and positive and negative predictive values of the fluorescent monoclonal antibody method have been published. Studies reveal a sensitivity range of 70% to 95% and a specificity range of 92% to 99%.

Immunoassays. The most commonly employed rapid antigen assay for the detection of *C. trachomatis* is the enzyme immunoassay (EIA). Depending on the manufacturer, the EIA detects either the outer membrane LPS chlamydial antigen or the MOMP. Many commercial kits are available, all having similar advantages. These include the ability to screen large volumes of specimens; to obtain objective results; to have test results available in 3 to 5 hours; and to use various specimen types, including urine for males, which may be important when evaluating partner contact. A summary of the published sensitivity, specificity, and negative and positive predictive values as well as test specimens is listed in Table 24-6. However, none of them equals the sensitivity of culture, and most are significantly less sensitive. Discrepancies in sensitivity could be based on differences in sample size, disease prevalence, population characteristics, collection sampling techniques, and laboratory standards.

One additional caution must be observed when EIA is employed for chlamydial antigen detection. A positive result must be considered preliminary and should be verified, because antigen detection methods may give a false-positive result when used in low-prevalence (<5%) populations. Verification of a positive specimen can be made on the same specimen using a monoclonal blocking antibody and a repeated EIA test using DFA or, alternatively, competitive binding for probe assays. A modification of EIA is optical immunoassay. This membrane capture technology provides results in less than 30 minutes. It is approved for use in physicians' offices and focuses on a "near-to-patient" or point-of-care rapid tests approach.

Nucleic Acid Hybridization and Amplification Assays. The newest advances in *Chlamydia* spp. identification have dealt with detection of nucleic acids. Initially, only one probe was commercially available, a nonisotopically labeled DNA probe that detected *C. trachomatis* rRNA (PACE 2; Gen-Probe, Inc., San Diego, Calif.) in urogenital specimens. Although the sensitivity, specificity, and positive and negative predictive values have been in the same range or higher than those reported for EIA, this DNA probe assay has the added advantage of detecting two STDs—gonorrhea and *C. trachomatis* infection—in one sample.

More recently, nucleic acid amplification tests (NAATs) have become the preferred diagnostic method to detect *C. trachomatis* genital infections. NAATs amplify and detect organism-specific DNA or RNA sequences and have been reported to be significantly more sensitive than the first-generation nonculture methods. In-house PCR tests as well as U.S. Food and Drug Administration (FDA)–approved systems for detection of *C. trachomatis* in clinical specimens such as the PCR-based Roche Amplicor (Roche Molecular Systems, Indianapolis, Ind.), APTIMA (Gen-Probe, Inc., San Diego, Calif.), and the ProbeTec (BD Diagnostic Systems, Sparks, Md.) are commercially available. Although commercial tests differ in their amplification methods and target nucleic acid sequences, the increased sensitivity of NAATs is ascribed to their ability to produce positive signals from as little as a single copy of the target DNA or RNA. The ProbeTec uses strand displacement amplification to amplify *C. trachomatis* DNA sequences. The APTIMA Combo 2 (Gen-Probe, Inc., San Diego, Calif.) assay for *C. trachomatis* uses transcription-mediated amplification to detect a specific ribosomal RNA target. All three commercial systems offer the ability to simultaneously detect *N. gonorrhoeae* infection.

The commercial NAATs have been cleared by the FDA to detect *C. trachomatis* in endocervical swabs from women, urethral swabs from men, and urine from both men and women. The concomitant use of a rapid screen for white cells (leukocyte esterase test) in urogenital specimens, however, may heighten suspicion, demonstrate leukorrhea, and target specimens that would have the highest probability of detecting a true STD infectious agent. Conversely, there are significant selected clinical limitations for the use of rapid screening methods employing EIA, DFA, or nucleic acid hybridization. As established by the CDC, these assays cannot be used in rape or child abuse cases, nor should they be used in the measurement of treatment success. Because established appropriate antimicrobial agents have a predictable 95% cure rate, the false-positive rate (due to less than 5% potentially uncured) would obscure follow-up results and suggest treatment failure. The nonculture amplified assays may also be most useful in low-risk patient populations because they have essentially no false-positive result. In fact, these methods will most likely become the gold standard, often called "expanded gold standard," recognizing the problems with culture.

Antibody Detection. Serologic assays can be used in the detection of *C. trachomatis* infections. Historically, these were thought to be limited and problematic. Many individuals have chlamydial antibodies from previous infections, and because chlamydial infections tend to be localized, they do not cause the traditional fourfold rise in antibody titer between acute and convalescent specimens. Today, the interpretation and significance of serologic assays are being reevaluated, and serologic testing is growing as a complementary diagnostic tool in certain selected scenarios such as the following:

- With microimmunofluorescence (micro-IF), when a specific IgM response to a different serovar of *C. trachomatis* is observed, new infections can be diagnosed in patients who have had previous infections with other serovars.
- Ascending infections by *C. trachomatis* involving fallopian tubes and additional organs of the upper female genital tract are almost never detected by endocervical cultures. Hence, patients at risk for chronic infections would be missed with the standard screening methods employing a cervical swab. The best screening test for patients at risk, particularly as part of a prenatal workup, may be detecting antibodies to the serovars of *C. trachomatis*. Prenatal patient sera are often kept for approximately 1 year following initial serologic evaluations—for example, for hepatitis B virus, human

immunodeficiency virus, and the TORCH agents (*Toxoplasma gondii*, rubella virus, cytomegalovirus, and herpes simplex virus). This is a serum reservoir that needs to be recognized and used more effectively.

- Complement fixation (CF) detects family-reactive antibody, including elevated levels of antibody in systemic infections, such as LGV. Diagnosis of LGV is supported by CF titers of 1:64 or more (Table 24-8). It must be noted, however, that CF generally is not useful in nonsystemic chlamydial conjunctivitis or routine urogenital tract infections.

Micro-IF detects antibodies to chlamydial EBs; these antibodies are serovar-specific antibodies. Hence, high levels of chlamydial IgM by micro-IF are diagnostic of systemic *C. trachomatis* infection in infants. In fact, because same-day diagnosis is possible, IgM micro-IF is the method of choice for diagnosis of *C. trachomatis* pneumonia in infants, preferable even to culture. Furthermore, infants with inclusion conjunctivitis normally do not have detectable IgM antibodies unless they have a systemic infection. Chlamydial IgG is generally not useful in infants, because rising titers are seldom observed, and when high titers are detected they probably reflect maternal antibody.

Results Reporting

With such great latitude in current testing choices, it is important for each laboratory to clearly report and define results. Some key points in the development of an approach to ordering and reporting results of tests for *C. trachomatis* and related organisms in a patient specimen are as follows:

- Agreeing in advance with the obstetrics/gynecology and emergency departments on which organisms are associated with which clinical syndrome, then testing accordingly, using profiles
- Reporting which tests were and were not performed for each patient profile
- Reporting unusual observations. Pure isolates of *Pseudomonas*, *Haemophilus*, *Neisseria meningitidis*, and yeast are not normal, and the physician needs to be aware of their presence.

TABLE 24-8 Detection of *Chlamydia* Species by Various Serologic Methods

		Serologic Findings		
			Micro-IF	
	CF Total	IgM		IgG
Chlamydia trachomatis	≥256			
A-C (trachoma)	*	*		*
D-K		Newborn pneumonia ≥32		
L1-L3 (LGV)				≥128
Chlamydophila pneumoniae	≥256		Four fold rise (A/C) or	
		≥16		≥512
Chlamydophila psittaci	≥256		Four fold rise (A/C) or	
		≥16		≥512

CF, Complement fixation (using LPS common to all members of the Chlamydiaceae); *Micro-IF*, microimmunofluorescence; *A/C*, acute/convalescent sera.
*Serological techniques have limited diagnostic value for trachoma.

Chlamydophila (Chlamydia) pneumoniae

Chlamydophila pneumoniae was formerly known as *Chlamydia* sp., strain TWAR, and it was originally identified in 1965 from a conjunctival culture of a child (TW) enrolled in a Taiwan trachoma vaccine study. In 1983 at the University of Washington, a similar organism was isolated in HeLa cells from a pharyngeal specimen of a college student (AR). Today, *C. pneumoniae* is recognized as an important respiratory pathogen. It is known to be a cause of acute respiratory disease, pneumonia, and pharyngitis. It also has been isolated from patients with otitis media with effusion, pneumonia with pleural effusion, and aseptic pharyngitis. Infection with *C. pneumoniae* has been established as a risk factor for Guillain-Barré syndrome, an immunologically mediated neurologic disease. There also appears to be a relationship between sarcoidosis and *C. pneumoniae*, but considerable work needs to be done to establish the existence and degree of this relationship. To date, only a single *C. pneumoniae* serovar has been found.

Chlamydia pneumoniae has been implicated as a possible factor in asthma and cardiovascular disease. *C. pneumoniae* has been isolated from atherosclerotic tissue, but its possible pathogenic role remains under investigation. Association of this organism with other vascular diseases, such as abdominal aortic aneurysm, has also been considered. Because of the evidence implicating *C. pneumoniae* with the development or outcome of cardiovascular disease, antimicrobial therapy was recommended in treating vascular disease by up to 4% of physicians in the United States, according to a 1999 survey. Results from clinical studies, however, have not shown benefits of antimicrobial therapy in individuals with coronary heart disease. Furthermore, results suggest that conventional antimicrobial therapy may not eradicate the organism or reduce mortality in these patients, although *C. pneumoniae* remains a potential risk factor in cardiovascular disease.

Clinical Infections

Although probably 90% of infections are asymptomatic or mildly symptomatic, infection with *C. pneumoniae* is thought to be fairly common, with an estimated 200,000 to 300,000 cases annually in the United States. In adults, antibodies have been demonstrated in more than 50% of infections, but there is virtually no antibody detectable in children younger than 5 years of age. It is thought that the attack rate is highest between the ages of 6 and 20 years, with a particular emphasis in college-age students. Unlike viral respiratory diseases, there seems to be no seasonal incidence, although some Scandinavian data have indicated the possibility of epidemics every 4 to 6 years. Reinfection with *C. pneumoniae* appears to be common and can be either milder or more severe than the initial infection. The epidemiologic and clinical features of *C. pneumoniae* are listed in Table 24-9.

The clinical picture in college-age students, although it may be varied, is a biphasic clinical course. *C. pneumoniae* infection results in prolonged sore throat (5 to 7 days) and hoarseness, followed by flulike lower respiratory tract symptoms (8 to 15 days). Because of its striking clinical similarity

TABLE 24-9 Summary of Key Epidemiologic and Clinical Features of *Chlamydophila pneumoniae* Infections

Epidemiologic	Clinical
Virtually no antibody detectable before 5 years of age	Estimated to account for approximately 6% to 10% of outpatient and hospitalized pneumonia
Antibodies present in >50% of adults	90% of infections are asymptomatic or mildly symptomatic
Attack rate highest between the ages of 6 years and mid-20s, often focusing on college-age students	Biphasic illness: prolonged sore throat and crouplike hoarseness followed by lower respiratory (flulike) symptoms
No seasonal incidence; epidemics have been reported every 4 to 6 years	Pneumonia and bronchitis, rarely accompanied by sinusitis
Reinfection is common	Fever relatively uncommon
	Chest radiograph shows isolated pneumonitis
	1 in 9 infections results in pneumonia
	Sarcoidosis, cardiovascular relationships?

to bacterial pharyngitis, the result of a streptococcal antigen test often is thought to be falsely negative. The second phase of the biphasic illness often results in pneumonia (approximately 1 in 9 infections) and bronchitis but is rarely accompanied by sinusitis. Fever is relatively uncommon, and radiographs show isolated pneumonitis. *C. pneumoniae* is recognized as the third most common cause of infectious respiratory disease. It accounts for approximately 6% to 10% of outpatient and hospitalized cases of pneumonia. The mode of transmission, incubation period, and infectiousness of *C. pneumoniae* infections are still largely unknown. No animal reservoir or vector is known. Table 24-10 summarizes situations and/or populations at risk that would benefit from detection of *C. pneumoniae*, usually by serologic methods.

Laboratory Diagnosis

Chlamydia pneumoniae may be cultured on selected cell lines and visualized with fluorescein-conjugated monoclonal antibodies. Human lines (HL) and HEp-2 from the human respiratory tract are the most sensitive. Monoclonal antibodies specific for *C. pneumoniae* are used to identify inclusions in cell culture. It should be noted that a family-reactive monoclonal antibody can identify *C. pneumoniae* inclusions but cannot differentiate this organism from the other chlamydiae. Attempts to culture *C. pneumoniae*, if undertaken, should take into account the organism's lability. *C. pneumoniae* seems to be considerably more labile than *C. trachomatis*, although its viability is relatively stable at 4° C. Specimens used for detection of chlamydial infections are listed in Table 24-7. An indirect fluorescent antibody method has been reported for detecting *C. pneumoniae* in respiratory secretions; the antibody reacts with the MOMP (Figure 24-8). This same antibody can be used to identify infected cell culture monolayers.

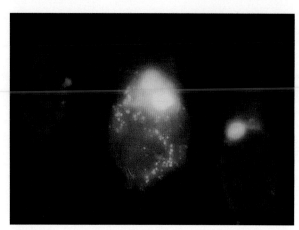

FIGURE 24-8 *Chlamydophila pneumoniae* detection from direct sputum smear using fluorescent-labeled monoclonal antibody, highlighting cytoplasmic inclusion (200×). (Courtesy DAKO Reagents, Carpinteria, Calif.)

TABLE 24-10 **Evaluating for** *Chlamydophila pneumoniae*

Population/Situation	Evaluation Methods	Comments
Pneumonias requiring hospitalization (age 6 to 20 years)	*C. pneumoniae*–specific IgM and IgG: acute and convalescent, use micro-IF IgM, single visit	12% antibody prevalence
Pharyngitis in college students		9% antibody prevalence
Retrospective, undiagnosed outbreaks in young adults, college or military	CF or micro-IF, IgG-specific	
Serious pneumonia, undiagnosed; clinically presents like *Mycoplasma pneumoniae*	*C. pneumoniae*–specific IgM and IgG by micro-IF	Rather than repeat cultures for similar respiratory pathogens (i.e., *Mycoplasma pneumoniae*), establish etiology and impact on diagnosis-related group reimbursement

IgM, Immunoglobin M; *IgG*, immunoglobin G; *CF*, complement fixation; *micro-IF*, microimmunofluorescence.

Given the difficulty of and lack of standardization for isolation of *C. pneumoniae*, serologic tests have been the method of choice for diagnosis. A CF test had been the traditional assay most often employed for *C. pneumoniae* detection, but it is rarely used today. The present method of choice is the micro-IF assay, which is more sensitive and specific than CF. Furthermore, it does not cross-react with *C. trachomatis*

and *C. psittaci*. Micro-IF also can distinguish an IgM from an IgG response. Single titer evaluations, although not diagnostic, may be suggestive. An IgM titer greater than 1:32 or an IgG single titer greater than 1:512 may suggest *C. pneumoniae* as a recent etiologic agent, warranting further evaluation. An IgG titer greater than or equal to 1:16 but less than 1:512 is evidence of past infection or exposure.

Two antibody response patterns have been identified for *C. pneumoniae* infections. In the primary response, most often seen in adolescents, university students, and military trainees, CF antibodies usually appear first. By micro-IF, *C. pneumoniae*–specific IgM does not appear until 3 weeks after onset of symptoms, and often *C. pneumoniae*–specific IgG does not reach diagnostic levels for 6 to 8 weeks. Therefore the traditional convalescent serum obtained approximately 14 to 21 days after onset does not contain micro-IF–detectable *C. pneumoniae* antibody. In contrast, during reinfection, a CF antibody change is not detected, but by micro-IF, an IgG titer of 1:512 or more can appear within 2 weeks. IgM levels may be detectable but are low. More recently, some partially automated enzyme-linked immunosorbent assays (ELISAs) have become commercially available. Studies have shown a concurrence between the ELISAs and micro-IF test results. The ELISAs have major advantages, namely being less time consuming, and the method does not rely on the quality of the fluorescent microscope used or the experience of the laboratory scientist.

Chlamydophila (Chlamydia) psittaci

Chlamydophila psittaci is the cause of psittacosis among psittacine birds, also known as ornithosis or parrot fever. The former mammalian *Chlamydophila psittaci* strains that cause feline conjunctiva, rhinitis, and respiratory infections among cats; guinea-pig conjunctivitis; and abortion among ruminants have been replaced in three new species, *C. felis*, *C. caviae,* and *C. abortus,* respectively. Diagnosis of psittacosis is usually based on a history of exposure to psittacines and a fourfold rise in antibody to the chlamydial group LPS antigen. In the United States, fewer than 50 cases of *C. psittaci* are reported annually. Retrospective serologic testing of sera from patients with acute respiratory disease have shown that many people previously thought to have *C. psittaci* infections due to "transient bird exposure" were, in fact, actually infected with *C. pneumoniae*. Hence, misdiagnosis of *C. psittaci* is a problem, and physicians need to know the tests that are most appropriate for differentiating these microorganisms.

Isolation of *C. psittaci* in culture, although diagnostic, is difficult, dangerous, and is not routinely employed or recommended. Therefore almost all diagnoses of *C. psittaci* are based on serologic evaluation. A single antibody titer greater than 1:32 is suggestive of acute illness in a symptomatic patient during an outbreak of psittacosis. The rise in antibodies is usually not demonstrable until the acute illness is over, however, and it often is weak or absent if appropriate antimicrobial therapy is given. This is most often a "rule-out" disease. If *C. pneumoniae* and *C. trachomatis*–specific IgG and IgM are not detected by micro-IF and a fourfold rise in chlamydiae antibodies is detected by CF, then *C. psittaci* should be strongly suspected. A good history is paramount in evaluating bird exposure, incubation time, and disease process.

RICKETTSIACEAE AND SIMILAR ORGANISMS

The genera *Rickettsia* and *Orientia* belong to the family Rickettsiaceae. Most of the members of the rickettsial group are arthropod-borne, obligately intracellular pathogens that can grow only in the cytoplasm of host cells. These bacteria have become extremely well adapted to their arthropod hosts. The primary hosts usually have minimal or no disease from their rickettsial infection. The arthropod host allows rickettsiae to persist in nature in two ways. First, rickettsiae are passed through new generations of arthropods by transovarial transmission. Because of this mechanism, arthropods are not only vectors for rickettsioses but also reservoirs. Second, arthropods directly inoculate new hosts with rickettsiae during feeding. An exception to this pattern occurs with *Rickettsia prowazekii*. In this case, the arthropod vector, the body louse, can die of the rickettsial infection, and humans act as a natural reservoir.

Rickettsia

Rickettsiae are short, nonmotile, gram-negative bacilli about 0.8 to 2.0 μm × 0.3 to 0.5 μm in size. The members of the genus *Rickettsia* have not been grown in cell-free media, but they have been grown in the yolk sacs of embryonated eggs and several monolayer cell lines. *Rickettsia* spp. are divided into groups according to the types of clinical infections they produce. The typhus group contains only two species: *R. prowazekii* and *R. typhi*. The spotted fever group includes a number of species generally recognized as human pathogens such as *R. rickettsii*, *R. akari*, *R. coronii*, and *R. africae*. Both *R. bellii* and *R. canadensis* are excluded from either group.

Spotted Fever Group

Rocky Mountain Spotted Fever. The most severe of the rickettsial infections, Rocky Mountain spotted fever (RMSF) is caused by *R. rickettsii*. It was first described in the western United States during the latter part of the nineteenth century. It was not until the early 1900s that researchers demonstrated the infectious nature of the disease, when they infected laboratory animals with the blood of infected patients. The nature of the agent was a mystery, because no bacteria were apparent on direct examination or on culture. However, researchers had to discount a viral etiology, because the agent was filterable. The organism was first seen using light microscopy in 1916.

Humans are accidental hosts and acquire the infection by tick bites. Ticks are the principal vector and reservoir for RMSF. The most common tick vectors are *Dermacentor variabilis* (Figure 24-9) in the southeastern United States and *D. andersoni* in the western part of the country. Other species of ticks, however, can be vectors. Ticks transmit the organism into humans via saliva, which is passed into the host during the tick's feeding. Once in the host tissue, the rickettsiae are phagocytosed into endothelial cells, where they replicate in

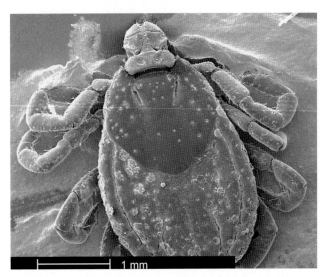

FIGURE 24-9 The dorsal view of *Dermacentor variabilis,* the American dog tick, a vector for Rocky Mountain spotted fever. (Photograph by Janice Carr; courtesy Centers for Disease Control and Prevention, Atlanta, Ga.)

the cytoplasm of the host cell. Replication in the nucleus also occurs. The rickettsiae pass directly through the plasma membranes of infected cells into adjacent cells without causing damage to the host cells. The rickettsiae are spread throughout the host hematogenously and induce vasculitis in internal organs, including the brain, heart, lungs, and kidneys.

Clinically, the patient experiences flulike symptoms for approximately 1 week, which follows an incubation period of approximately 7 days. The symptoms include fever, headache, myalgia, nausea, vomiting, and rash. The rash, which may be hard to distinguish in individuals of color, begins as erythematous patches on the ankles and wrists during the first week of symptoms. The rash can extend to the palms of the hands and soles of the feet but normally does not affect the face. The maculopapular patches eventually consolidate into larger areas of ecchymoses.

Once disseminated, the organisms cause vasculitis in the blood vessels of the lungs, brain, and heart, leading to pneumonitis, central nervous system manifestations, and myocarditis. The patient experiences symptoms secondary to vasculitis, including decreased blood volume, hypotension, and disseminated intravascular coagulation. The mortality rates for untreated or incorrectly treated patients can be as high as 20%, although correct antimicrobial therapy with tetracycline or chloramphenicol lowers the rates to 3% to 6%.

Rickettsialpox. Another cause of spotted fever is rickettsialpox, caused by *R. akari*. The reservoir is the common house mouse, and the vector is the mouse mite *Liponyssoides sanguineus*. Rickettsialpox occurs in Korea and the Ukraine as well as in the eastern United States, including the cities of New York, Boston, and Philadelphia. The infections occur in crowded urban areas where rodents and their mites exist.

Rickettsialpox has similarities to RMSF but is a milder infection. The rickettsial organism enters the human host following a mite (chigger) bite. The incubation period is about

10 days, after which a papule forms at the site of inoculation. The papule progresses to a pustule, then to an indurated eschar. The patient becomes febrile as the rickettsiae are disseminated throughout the body via the bloodstream. The patient also experiences headache, nausea, and chills. Unlike RMSF, the rash of rickettsialpox appears on the face, trunk, and extremities and does not involve the palms of the hands or soles of the feet. Rickettsialpox symptoms resolve without medical attention.

Boutonneuse Fever. Boutonneuse fever, also known as *Mediterranean spotted fever,* caused by *R. conorii,* occurs in France, Spain, and Italy. *R. conorii* also causes Kenya tick typhus, South African tick fever, and Indian tick typhus. Like the agent for RMSF, this rickettsia is tickborne, and its reservoirs include ticks and dogs.

Boutonneuse fever is also clinically similar to RMSF. The rash involves the palms of the hands and soles of the feet, just as in RMSF. The rash of boutonneuse fever, however, also involves the face. Also in contrast with RMSF, this disease is characterized by the presence of taches noires (black spots) at the primary site of infection. Taches noires are lesions caused by the introduction of *R. conorii* into the skin of a nonimmune person. As the organism spreads to the blood vessels in the dermis, damage occurs to the endothelium. Edema secondary to increased vascular permeability reduces blood flow to the area and results in local necrosis.

Typhus Group

The typhus group of rickettsiae includes the species *R. typhi* (endemic typhus, also referred to as murine typhus) and *R. prowazekii* (epidemic louse-borne typhus and **Brill-Zinsser disease**). Generally, the typhus rickettsiae differ from the other rickettsial groups in that they replicate in the cytoplasm of the host cell and cause cell lysis, thereby releasing the rickettsiae. The infection causes host cell lysis, thereby releasing the rickettsiae. Other rickettsiae pass directly through an uninjured cell.

Murine Typhus. The arthropod vector for *R. typhi* is the oriental rat flea *Xenopsylla cheopis,* and the rat *(Rattus exulans)* is the primary reservoir. Apparently, the cat flea, *Ctenocephalides felis,* can also harbor the organism. Because this flea infests a large number of domestic animals, it may be an important factor in the persistence of infection in urban areas.

The rickettsiae also survive in nature, to a lesser extent, by transovarial transmission. When a flea feeds on an infected host, the rickettsiae enter the flea's midgut, where they replicate in the epithelial cells. They are eventually released into the gut lumen. Humans become infected when fleas defecate on the surface of the skin while feeding. The human host then reacts to the bite by scratching the site, allowing direct inoculation of the infected feces into abrasions. *R. typhi* can also be transmitted to humans directly from the flea bite itself.

In the 1940s, approximately 5000 cases of murine typhus were reported annually in the United States. Rigid control measures have reduced that number to fewer than 100 cases annually. The disease essentially occurs only in southern Texas and southern California in this country but continues to be a problem in areas of the world where rats and their

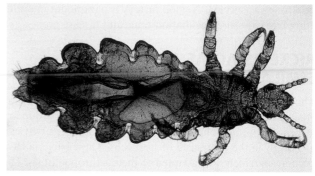

FIGURE 24-10 The female head louse, *Pediculus humanus,* which is a vector for *Rickettsia prowazekii,* the agent of epidemic typhus. (Photograph by Dr. Dennis D. Juranek; courtesy Centers for Disease Control and Prevention, Atlanta, Ga.)

fleas are present in urban settings. As is the case with RMSF, the clinical course of endemic typhus includes fever, headache, and rash. Unlike RMSF, endemic typhus does not always produce a rash; only about 50% infected will have a rash. When the rash is present, however, it usually occurs on the trunk and extremities. Rash on the palms of the hands occurs rarely. Complications are rare, and recovery usually occurs without incident.

Louse-Borne Typhus. Louse-borne (epidemic) typhus is caused by *R. prowazekii.* The vectors include the human louse (*Pediculus humanus;* Figure 24-10), the squirrel flea *(Orchopeas howardii),* and the squirrel louse *(Neohaematopinus sciuriopteri).* The reservoirs are primarily humans and flying squirrels located in the eastern United States. The louse often dies of its rickettsemia, unlike vectors of other rickettsiae.

Louse-borne typhus is still found commonly in areas of Africa and Central and South America where unsanitary conditions promote the presence of body lice. As seen during World War II, epidemic louse-borne typhus can recur even in developed countries when sanitation is disrupted. More than 20,000 cases were documented during the 1980s, with the vast majority originating in Africa. Louse-borne typhus is similar to the other rickettsioses.

Lice are infected with *R. prowazekii* when feeding on infected humans. The organisms invade the cells lining the gut of the louse. They actively divide and eventually lyse the host cells, spilling the organisms into the lumen of the gut. When the louse feeds on another human, it defecates, and the infected feces are scratched into the skin, just as in murine typhus. The disease progression is similar to that of RMSF, including involvement of the palms of the hands and soles of the feet with the rash. Unlike the case with RMSF, the face may also be affected by rash. The mortality rates for untreated patients can approach 40%, although mortality rates in treated patients are very low.

Brill-Zinsser disease, also called *recrudescent typhus,* is seen in patients who have previously had louse-borne typhus. *R. prowazekii* lies dormant in the lymph tissue of the human host until the infection is reactivated. Brill-Zinsser disease is a milder disease than louse-borne typhus, and death is rare. Patients with latent infections constitute an important reservoir for the organism.

Orientia

Scrub typhus is a disease that occurs in India, Burma, eastern Russia, Asia, and Australia. The causative agent is *Orientia* (formerly *Rickettsia*) *tsutsugamushi.* The vector is the chigger, *Leptotrombidium deliensis,* and the main reservoir is the rat. The bacteria are transmitted transovarially in the chiggers.

The transmission of *O. tsutsugamushi* to the human host is followed by an incubation period of approximately 2 weeks. A tache noire, similar to that of boutonneuse fever, forms at the site of inoculation. The normal rickettsial symptoms of fever, headache, and rash are also present. The rash starts on the trunk and spreads to the extremities. Unlike the case with RMSF, the rash does not involve the palms of the hands and soles of the feet, and the face is also not involved.

Laboratory Diagnosis of Rickettsial Diseases

Because of their infectious nature, isolation of the rickettsiae is not recommended and should only be attempted by biosafety level 3 laboratories. The immunohistochemical detection of rickettsiae is an established method for diagnosis of these infections. Monoclonal antibodies directed against either the spotted fever or typhus group have been used, but no antibody is commercially available. PCR assays have also been described, but they too are not readily available.

Typically, serologic assays are the only laboratory tests performed for the diagnosis of rickettsial diseases. Unfortunately, these methods are only able to confirm a diagnosis in convalescent specimens and offer little help in diagnosing acute infections that could guide antimicrobial therapy. The immunofluorescent antibody (IFA) test is considered the gold standard method for antibody detection. Because of cross-reactivity among members of the same groups (spotted fever and typhus), generally only group-specific antibody is available. Antibodies to certain rickettsial species are known to cross react with bacteria in the genus *Proteus.* This gave rise to the Weil-Felix agglutination test. Because the assay does not use rickettsial antigen, it is nonspecific and not used much in the United States. However, because of its low cost, it is used in some other countries. An agglutination test utilizing latex beads coated with rickettsial antigens is commercially available for the diagnosis of RMSF (Panbio, Inc., Baltimore, Md.).

Anaplasmataceae

Ehrlichia

Ehrlichiosis was first noted in France in the 1930s when dogs infected with brown dog ticks became ill and died. Postmortem examination revealed rickettsial-like inclusions in the monocytes of the dead animals. These newly described rickettsiae were named *Rickettsia canis.* They were obligately intracellular, arthropod-borne, gram-negative coccobacilli. They differ from the other members of the rickettsiae in that they multiply in the phagosomes of host leukocytes and not in the cytoplasm of endothelial cells.

Because these organisms grew within host cell vacuoles, they were reclassified into a new genus, *Ehrlichia,* in 1945. The ehrlichiae have a developmental cycle similar to that of the

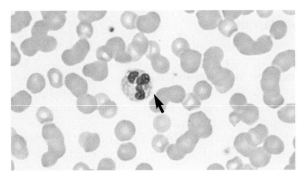

FIGURE 24-11   *Ehrlichia morula* in an infected white blood cell.

chlamydiae. The infective form of the organism is the EB, which replicates in the phagosome and prevents phagolysosome formation. These bodies give rise to inclusions with initial bodies inside. As the inclusions mature, they develop **morulae** (mulberry-like bodies; Figure 24-11). As the host cell ruptures, the morulae break into many individual EBs that continue the infective cycle.

Ehrlichia chaffeensis causes **human monocytic ehrlichiosis (HME),** which occurs in the United States, Europe, Africa, and South and Central America. In the United States, most cases are found in the southeastern and south central states, as well as in the mid-Atlantic states. Fewer than 2000 cases have been definitely or presumptively identified since its description in 1986, although cases may be underreported. Natural hosts of the organism include dogs and deer, as well as humans, with the lone star tick *(Amblyomma americanum)* being the primary vector.

Many patients with HME may experience asymptomatic infection. The organism has an incubation period of 5 to 10 days. Patients often experience high fever, headache, malaise, and myalgia. Nausea, vomiting, diarrhea, cough, joint pain, and confusion are rarely present. As many as 67% of the pediatric patients infected with *E. chaffeensis* have a rash; however, adults rarely experience a rash. Patients may also have evidence of leukopenia and neutropenia, thrombocytopenia, and elevated liver enzymes. Patients can experience severe complications including toxic shock–like syndrome, central nervous system involvement, and adult respiratory distress syndrome. Mortality rates are approximately 2% to 3%.

Direct staining (Giemsa or Wright) of peripheral blood smears or buffy coats for morulae can be used for diagnosing *E. chaffeensis* infections; however, this method is not very sensitive (29%). The bacteria are primarily found in monocytes. Antigen detection in tissues such as bone marrow, liver, and spleen has been described. Again the sensitivity is low (40%), and cross-reaction with other species has been noted. This leaves NAATs as the most frequently used method for direct detection of *E. chaffeensis.* The bacteria have also been isolated from peripheral blood in cell monolayers. Most cases of HME are diagnosed retrospectively by serologic testing; IFA is the most widely used method.

Anaplasma

Anaplasma phagocytophilum, formerly known as *Ehrlichia phagocytophilum*, causes a disease now referred to as **human granulocytic anaplasmosis (HGA)**. The disease is identical to that which *Ehrlichia equi* causes in horses and *Ehrlichia phagocytophilum* causes in ruminants. All three of these organisms are now classified as *A. phagocytophilum*. The incubation period for HGA is 5 to 11 days. The symptoms closely resemble HME; less than 11% of infected individuals have a rash.

Although HGA is probably underreported, there was an average yearly rate of 16 cases per 100,000 population in northern Wisconsin from 1990 to 1995. More than 2000 cases were reported nationwide between 1999 and 2004. Most cases are identified in the upper Midwest and Northeast United States. Natural hosts include deer, rodents, horses, cattle, and humans. Tick vectors include *Ixodes scapularus* and *I. pacificus*.

As with HME, staining of peripheral blood and buffy coats can be used to diagnose HGA. The morulae are found in granulocytes, and the sensitivity is about 60%. Diagnosis can also be made by direct antigen detection, NAATs, and isolation in cell cultures. IFA serologic kits are available for detection of antibodies to *A. phagocytophilum*.

Coxiella

Coxiella burnetii is the only species in the genus. This organism differs in several ways from many members of the families Rickettsiaceae and Anaplasmataceae. For example, although *C. burnetii* is an obligate intracellular parasite, it develops within the phagolysosome of infected cells. The acidic environment activates its metabolic enzymes. Spore formation by *C. burnetii* allows it to survive harsh environmental conditions. In addition, *C. burnetii* is generally not transmitted by arthropods, although it is known to infect more than 12 genera of ticks and other arthropods. The bacteria can infect fish, birds, rodents, livestock, and other mammals.

Coxiella burnetii is the causative agent of Q (query) fever. This is a disease found worldwide. Q fever is highly contagious and, as such, is considered a potential bioterror agent (see Chapter 30). Most infections are spread by inhalation of dried birthing fluids. The ingestion of unpasteurized milk is also a recognized risk factor. Acute Q fever generally has an abrupt onset of high fever that can be accompanied by headaches, myalgia, arthralgia, cough, and rarely a rash. Patients may present with elevated liver enzymes and erythrocytic sedimentation rate and thrombocytopenia.

The laboratory diagnosis of Q fever can be made by direct immunofluorescence assays of infected tissue. However, with the exception of heart tissue in cases of endocarditis, infected tissue contains low numbers of bacteria. NAATs, such as PCR, have also been successful in diagnosing infections. *C. burnetii* is highly contagious; isolation in cell cultures should be attempted only in biosafety level 3 facilities. Several serologic assays have been described for detecting antibodies in acute and chronic cases. IFA is the method of choice.

BIBLIOGRAPHY

Beninati T et al: First detection of spotted fever group rickettsiae in *Ixodes ricinus* from Italy, *Emerg Infect Dis* 8:983, 2002.

Bengis RG et al: The role of wildlife in emerging and re-emerging zoonoses, *Rev Sci Tech* 23:497, 2004.

Brouqui P et al: *Coxiella*. In Murray PR et al, editors: *Manual of clinical microbiology*, ed 9, Washington, DC, 2007, ASM Press.

Centers for Disease Control and Prevention: Screening tests to detect *Chlamydia trachomatis* and *Neisseria gonorrhoeae* infections–2002, *MMWR* 51(RR-15):1, 2002. Available at: www.cdc.gov/mmwr/PDF/rr/rr5115.pdf. Accessed December 5, 2008.

Centers for Disease Control and Prevention: Screening tests to detect *Chlamydia trachomatis* and *Neisseria gonorrhoeae* infections–2002, *MMWR* 51(RR-15):1, 2002. Available at: www.cdc.gov/mmwr/PDF/rr/rr5115.pdf. Accessed December 5, 2008.

Centers for Disease Control and Prevention: Summary of notifiable diseases—United States, 2007, *MMWR* 56:1, 2009. Available at: www.cdc.gov/mmwr/preview/mmwrhtml/mm5653a1.htm. Accessed December 17, 2009.

Danesk J et al: *C. pneumoniae* IgA titer and cardiovascular heart disease: prospective study and meta-analysis, *Eur Heart J* 23:371, 2002.

Dumler JS et al: Reorganization of the genera in the families Rickettsiaceae and Anaplasmataceae in the order Rickettsiales: unification of some species of *Ehrlichia* with *Anaplasma*, *Cowdria* with *Ehrlichia* and *Ehrlichia* with *Neorickettsia*, description of six new species combinations and designation of *Ehrlichia canis* and "HGE agent" as subjective synonyms of *Ehrlichia phagocytophila*, *Int J Syst Bacteriol* 51:2145, 2001.

Essig A: *Chlamydia* and *Chlamydophila*. In Murray PR et al, editors: *Manual of clinical microbiology*, ed 9, Washington, DC, 2007, ASM Press.

Gaydos C: Nucleic acid amplification tests for gonorrhea and *Chlamydia*: practice and applications, *Infect Dis Clin North Am* 19:367, 2005.

Gomes JP et al: Polymorphisms in the nine polymorphic membrane proteins of *Chlamydia trachomatis* across all serovars: evidence for serovar Da recombination and correlation with tissue tropism, *J Bacteriol* 188:275, 2006.

Hammerschlag MR: *Chlamydia trachomatis* and *Chlamydia pneumoniae* infections in children and adolescents, *Pediatr Rev* 25:43, 2004.

Hermann C et al: Comparison of quantitative and semiquantitative enzyme-linked immunosorbent assays for immunoglobulin G against *Chlamydophila pneumoniae* to a microimmunofluorescence test for use with patients with respiratory tract infections, *J Clin Microbiol* 42:276, 2004.

Kalayoglu MV: *Chlamydia pneumoniae* in cardiovascular disease: update on Chsp60 and other emerging virulence determinants, *Medicinal Chemistry Reviews—Online* 1:475, 2004. Available at: www.bentham.org/mcro/mcro1-4.htm. Accessed December 5, 2008.

Krusell A et al: Rickettsial pox in North Carolina: a case report, *Emerg Infect Dis* 8:727, 2002.

Olano JP, Aguero-Rosenfeld ME: *Ehrlichia, Anaplasma,* and related intracellular bacteria. In Murray PR et al, editors: *Manual of clinical microbiology*, ed 9, Washington, DC, 2007, ASM Press.

Verkooyen RP et al: Reliability of nucleic acid amplification methods for detection of *Chlamydia trachomatis* in urine: results of the first international collaborative quality control study among 96 laboratories, *J Clin Microbiol* 41:3013, 2003.

Walker DH, Bouyer DH: *Rickettsia* and *Orientia*. In Murray PR et al, editors: *Manual of clinical microbiology*, ed 9, Washington, DC, 2007, ASM Press.

Points to Remember

- Chlamydiae and rickettsiae are obligate intracellular organisms.
- *Chlamydia trachomatis* is the most common sexually transmitted bacterial pathogen, and certain serovars are associated with trachoma, which can result in blindness.
- Nucleic acid amplification tests are better assays for the diagnosis of *C. trachomatis* infections than cultures.
- *Chlamydophila pneumoniae* is a relatively common respiratory tract pathogen considered responsible for many cases of community-acquired pneumonia. It has also been linked to chronic illnesses such as atherosclerosis, coronary heart disease, and stroke.
- *Chlamydophila psittaci* is the cause of psittacosis, also known as parrot fever or ornithosis. This bacterium produces lower respiratory tract infections in humans.
- The *Rickettsia* spp. are important human pathogens responsible for a number of diseases including Rocky Mountain spotted fever, rickettsialpox, and typhus.
- The *Rickettsia, Orientia, Ehrlichia*, and *Anaplasma* are typically transmitted to humans by the bites of arthropods.
- *Ehrlichia* and *Anaplasma* are intracellular parasites of white blood cells: mononuclear cells and granulocytes, respectively.
- *Coxiella burnetii* is the causative agent of Q fever. Infection is most often transmitted by inhalation of dried birthing fluids. The ingestion of unpasteurized milk is also a risk factor.

Learning Assessment

1. What organisms should be considered as possible causes of neonatal conjunctivitis?
2. What stains should be performed on the discharge or conjunctival scraping for microscopic examination?
3. For the infant described in the Case in Point, what other clinical conditions could be due to the causative organisms?
4. What sexually transmitted disease (STD) is caused by *Chlamydia trachomatis* serotypes L_1, L_2, L_{2a}, L_{2b}, and L_3?
5. How does lymphogranuloma venereum differ from other STDs caused by *C. trachomatis*?
6. With what types of infections are *Chlamydophila pneumoniae* associated?
7. What is psittacosis or ornithosis?
8. What is the most common laboratory method used to diagnose rickettsial diseases? Explain.
9. What cells do the *Ehrlichia* and *Anaplasma* species typically infect in humans?
10. How does *Coxiella burnetii* differ from the *Rickettsia* spp.?

Mycoplasma and Ureaplasma

Donald C. Lehman, Connie R. Mahon*

- ■ GENERAL CHARACTERISTICS
- ■ CLINICAL INFECTIONS
  Mycoplasma pneumoniae
  Mycoplasma hominis and *Ureaplasma* Species
  Other *Mycoplasma* Species
- ■ LABORATORY DIAGNOSIS
  Specimen Collection and Transport
  Direct Examination

Culture
Serologic Diagnosis
- ■ ANTIMICROBIAL SUSCEPTIBILITY
- ■ INTERPRETATION OF LABORATORY RESULTS

OBJECTIVES

After reading and studying this chapter, you should be able to:

1. Describe the general characteristics of the *Mycoplasma* spp. and how they differ from other bacterial species.
2. Compare the clinical diseases caused by *Mycoplasma pneumoniae*, *Mycoplasma hominis*, and *Ureaplasma urealyticum*.
3. Identify the preferred stain for demonstration of the mycoplasmas.
4. Discuss the possible roles of *M. hominis* and *U. urealyticum* in infections of low-birthweight and high-risk neonates.
5. Discuss the clinical manifestations of other *Mycoplasma* spp. in immunocompromised patients.
6. Analyze the diagnostic methods appropriate for detection of mycoplasmal and ureaplasmal infections.
7. Discuss the use of serologic assays for diagnosing *M. pneumoniae* infections.
8. Name two selective media for detection of the mycoplasmas.
9. Explain the effects of antimicrobial therapy on mycoplasmal infections.
10. Provide recommendations for the proper interpretation and reporting for *Mycoplasma* and *Ureaplasma*.

Case in Point

A premature male infant in the neonatal intensive care unit, who weighed 1.5 lb at birth (low birthweight), developed signs of meningitis, and a lumbar puncture was performed. Results of a white blood cell count of the cerebrospinal fluid were negative, the Gram stain was reported as "no organisms seen," and routine culture at 3 days was "no growth." The infant was still symptomatic at this time, and the pediatric infectious disease physician, after consultation with the microbiology laboratory, performed another spinal tap and ordered additional cultures. An organism was recovered by the laboratory.

Issues to Consider

After reading the patient's case history, consider:

- ■ The etiology of meningeal infections in the given patient population
- ■ Supporting laboratory findings and how they help establish the diagnosis
- ■ Methods for recovery of the suspected etiologic agent

Key Terms

Cell-wall deficient
L-forms
Pleuropneumonia-like
  organism (PPLO)

Primary atypical
  pneumonia
T-strain mycoplasma

This chapter discusses a group of organisms once thought to be viruses because of their size. Mycoplasmas are the smallest self-replicating organisms in nature. This group of bacteria belongs within the class Mollicutes. *Mycoplasma* and *Ureaplasma* are the two genera in the family Mycoplasmataceae. At least 16 species of mollicutes have been repeatedly isolated from humans. Although there are numerous species of *Mycoplasma* and *Ureaplasma* identified in plants and animals, the following species are the most significant human pathogens (Table 25-1):

- • *Mycoplasma pneumoniae*, which causes respiratory disease
- • *Mycoplasma hominis*, associated with urogenital tract disease

*This chapter was prepared by C.R. Mahon in her private capacity. No official support or endorsement by the FDA is intended or implied.

TABLE 25-1 Divergent Ecosystems Inhabited by Genera of the Class Mollicutes

Ecosystem	Mycoplasma	Ureaplasma	Acholeplasma	Spiroplasma	Thermoplasma	Anaeroplasma
Soil and grasses	–	–	–	+	–	–
Crops and plants	–	–	–	+	–	–
Mown hay	–	–	–	–	+	–
Water	–	–	+	–	–	–
Deciduous trees	–	–	–	+	–	–
Humans	+	+	–	–	–	+
Cattle	+	+	–	–	–	+

+, Present in ecosystem; –, rarely associated with ecosystem.

TABLE 25-2 Pathogens in the Class Mollicutes

Feature	Mycoplasma	Ureaplasma	Acholeplasma
Cell-wall deficient	+	+	+
Gram stain	–	–	–
Penicillin susceptible	–	–	–
Urease activity	–	+	–
Induced in hypertonic solution and penicillin, lysozyme, or salts	–	–	–
Derivation: exists in nature as free-living organism	+	+	+
Contains cell wall components but lacks true cell wall	+	+	+
Reverts to parental form (or reestablishes cell wall) when induction is eliminated	–	–	–
Pleomorphic shape	+	+	–
Other shared characteristics	+	+	+
	Smaller than bacteria—close in size to myxoviruses		
	Limited metabolic activity (i.e., fastidious)		
	Lower guanidine/cytosine (GC) ratio than most bacteria		
	Many mollicutes contain DNase		
	Smaller genome than bacteria		

+, Feature present; –, feature absent.

• *Ureaplasma urealyticum,* associated with urogenital tract disease

GENERAL CHARACTERISTICS

Mycoplasmas are pleomorphic organisms that do not possess a cell wall, a characteristic that makes them resistant to cell-wall–active antibiotics such as the penicillins and cephalosporins. Because of the permanent absence of a cell wall, they were originally grouped under the general term **cell-wall deficient** bacteria. They are not, however, classified as **L-forms,** which are bacteria that have temporarily lost their cell wall as a result of environmental conditions. The mollicutes range in size for coccoid forms from approximately 0.2 to 0.3 μm in diameter to tapered rods of approximately 1 to 2 μm in length and 0.2 to 0.3 μm in diameter. Table 25-2 compares features of three genera known to be pathogenic for humans.

Mollicutes are generally slow-growing, highly fastidious, facultative anaerobes requiring complex media containing cholesterol and fatty acids for growth; important exceptions include aerobic *M. pneumoniae* and the more rapidly growing *M. hominis.* The mollicutes produce small colonies ranging in size from about 15 μm to over 300 μm in diameter. *Mycoplasma* spp. often grow embedded beneath the surface of solid

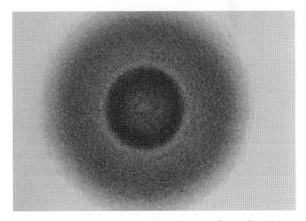

FIGURE 25-1 Typical large *Mycoplasma* colony showing "fried egg" appearance. (Courtesy Bionique Testing Laboratories, Saranac Lake, N.Y.)

media; therefore transferring colonies with a loop is ineffective. On solid media, some species (e.g., *M. hominis*) form colonies with slightly raised centers giving the classic "fried egg" appearance (Figure 25-1). In the laboratory, mycoplasmas are common and hard-to-detect contaminants of cell cultures.

TABLE 25-3 *Mycoplasma* Species Indigenous to Humans

Mycoplasma Species	Usual Habitat	Reported Frequency	Colony Morphology*
M. salivarium	Oropharynx	Very common	Large, fried egg
M. orale	Oropharynx	Common	Small, spherical
M. buccale	Oropharynx	Uncommon	Large, fried egg
M. faucium	Oropharynx	Uncommon	Large, fried egg
M. lipophilum	Oropharynx	Rare	Large, fried egg
M. pneumoniae	Oropharynx	Common (with disease)	Small, spherical, granular
M. fermentans	Oropharynx	Rare	Small, fried egg, spherical
	Urogenital tract	Uncommon	
M. hominis	Oropharynx	Uncommon	Large, fried egg, vesiculated peripheral zone
	Urogenital tract	Common (9% to 50% women)	
M. genitalium	Urogenital tract	Common?	
Ureaplasma urealyticum	Urogenital tract	Very common (81% women; 30% to 50% men)	Tiny, spherical, fried egg, granular

*Relative sizes: large >100 nm; small = 50 to 100 nm; tiny <50 nm.

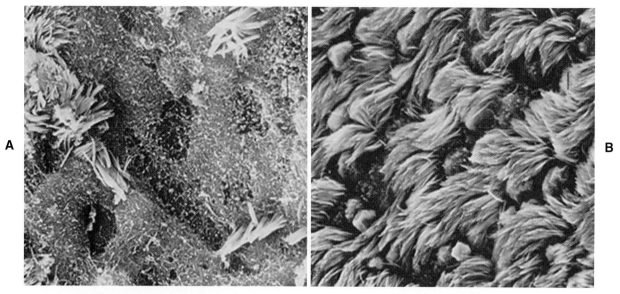

FIGURE 25-2   Electron micrographs showing effect of *Mycoplasma pneumoniae* on ciliated tracheal cells. **A,** Infected animal model. **B,** Uninfected animal model.

The first *Mycoplasma* was isolated in the late 1800s from a cow with pleuropneumonia. Later, a mycoplasma was isolated from humans and was referred to as **pleuropneumonia-like organism (PPLO)** and the Eaton agent, after the researcher who first isolated it from humans. This human isolate became known as *M. pneumoniae.* The mycoplasmas adhere to the epithelium of mucosal surfaces in the respiratory and urogenital tracts and are not eliminated by mucous secretions or urine flow. Figure 25-2 depicts electron micrographs of ciliated tracheal epithelial cells before and after *M. pneumoniae* adherence. Figure 25-3 is an electron micrograph demonstrating the shape of *M. pneumoniae* and its orientation of attachment. *Mycoplasma* spp. indigenous to humans are listed in Table 25-3. The human mycoplasmas are susceptible to adverse environmental conditions such as heat and drying. Transmission of mycoplasmas and ureaplasmas in humans may occur via direct sexual contact, from mother to child

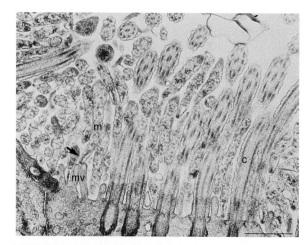

FIGURE 25-3   Electron micrograph of *Mycoplasma pneumoniae* attaching by specific attachment features to ciliated trachea. *mv,* Microvilli; *m,* mycoplasma; *c,* cilia.

during delivery or in utero, and by respiratory secretions or fomites in cases of *M. pneumoniae* infections.

CLINICAL INFECTIONS

Mycoplasma pneumoniae

Mycoplasma pneumoniae may cause bronchitis, pharyngitis, or a relatively common respiratory infection known as **primary atypical pneumonia** or walking pneumonia. The clinical manifestations resemble those due to *Chlamydophila pneumoniae*. The disease differs from the typical pneumonia caused by *Streptococcus pneumoniae* in that it is milder, has a higher incidence in young adults, and is not seasonal. *M. pneumoniae* does not occur as a normal commensal; therefore its isolation is always significant and pathognomonic. *M. pneumoniae* causes approximately 20% of reported pneumonias in the general population and up to 50% in confined populations such as military settings. School-age children and young adults are especially susceptible to infection. Clinical disease is uncommon in very young children and older adults. Other groups at risk include closed-in populations such as prisoners, college students, and military personnel. Epidemics are known to occur in these populations. Infection is not considered seasonal, but many cases occur in autumn and early winter. Outbreaks also have been noted when adolescents return to school in the fall. Transmission is probably through aerosol droplet spray produced while coughing.

Many infections are completely asymptomatic or very mild; however, about one third of infected patients demonstrate clinically apparent pneumonia (Figure 25-4). The incubation period is usually 2 to 3 weeks, and early symptoms are nonspecific, consisting of headache, low-grade fever, malaise, and anorexia. Sore throat, dry cough, and earache are accompanying symptoms. Extrapulmonary complications, including

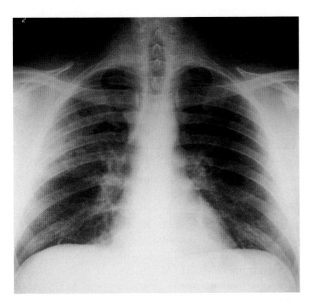

FIGURE 25-4 Typical chest radiograph of a patient with a 3-week course of atypical pneumonia. Note nonspecific interstitial pneumonia and patchy infiltrate delineated by feathery outline.

cardiovascular, central nervous system, dermatologic, and gastrointestinal problems, are rare occurrences. *M. pneumoniae* is not associated with infections of the urogenital tract. It has, however, been implicated as a co-infection or cofactor in epidemic group A meningococcal meningitis and infant pneumonitis.

Mycoplasma hominis and *Ureaplasma* Species

Although the mollicutes do not cause vaginitis, both *M. hominis* and *U. urealyticum* are associated with infections of the urogenital tract. They are, however, frequently isolated from asymptomatic individuals, making interpretation of a positive culture difficult. Because they are opportunistic pathogens, the immune status of the host is an important factor in the occurrence and severity of disease. In addition, it has been reported that among sexually active individuals, the rate of colonization is directly related to the number of sexual partners. Higher rates of colonization have been noted in adults of lower socioeconomic status. The organisms do not persist in infants colonized at birth, but they can be found in the lower genital tract in many sexually active individuals. Table 25-4 summarizes the known association of genital mollicutes with urogenital and newborn diseases.

Mycoplasma hominis is found in the lower genitourinary tracts of approximately 50% of healthy adults and has not been reported as a cause of nongonococcal urethritis (NGU). The organism may, however, invade the upper genitourinary tract and cause salpingitis, pyelonephritis, pelvic inflammatory disease (PID), or postpartum fevers. *Ureaplasma parvum* and *U. urealyticum* do not cause disease in the female lower genital tract but have been associated with approximately 10% of cases of NGU in men, as well as with upper female genitourinary tract disorders. *U. urealyticum* has been recovered from more than 60% of normal sexually active females, and it has been associated with reproduction disorders, chorioamnionitis, congenital pneumonia, and the development of chronic lung disease in premature infants. Although it is not a primary cause of chronic lung disease, *U. urealyticum* is a common organism isolated from tracheal aspirates of low-birthweight infants with respiratory disease. Fourteen percent of infections were in newborns delivered by cesarean section, thus indicating that infection occurred in utero and not during passage through the birth canal.

Mycoplasma hominis and *Ureaplasma* spp. can be transmitted to the fetus at delivery and have been recovered from the cerebrospinal fluid (CSF) of certain high-risk newborns, including preterm and low-birthweight babies. In particular, *U. parvum* has been linked to respiratory distress in premature infants. It has been recommended that culture for these organisms be attempted when the CSF specimen from a newborn with evidence of meningitis is negative for both Gram stain and routine bacteriology culture (Table 25-5).

In immunocompromised individuals, bacteremia and invasive disease of the joints and respiratory tract caused by mycoplasmal species has occurred. *U. urealyticum* has been reported to cause chronic inflammatory diseases such as arthritis and cystitis in hypogammaglobulinemic patients. *Mycoplasma* isolates have been intermittently associated with

TABLE 25-4 Summary of the Association of Genital Mollicutes with Urogenital and Newborn Diseases

Disease	Mycoplasma hominis	Ureaplasma urealyticum	Comments
Nongonococcal urethritis	None	Strong	Ureaplasmas cause some cases, but the proportion is unknown
Prostatitis	Weak	None	An association with a few cases of chronic disease has been reported; a causal relation is unproven
Epididymitis	None	None	Mycoplasmas are not an important cause
Reiter disease	None	None	The role of ureaplasmas should be studied
Bartholin gland abscess	Weak	None	*M. hominis* may cause some disease but is not an important cause
Vaginitis and cervicitis	None	None	*M. hominis* often associated with disease, but a causal relation is unproven
Pelvic inflammatory disease	Strong	Weak	*M. hominis* causes some cases, but the proportion is unknown
Postabortal fever	Strong	None	*M. hominis* is responsible for some cases, but the proportion is unknown
Postpartum fever	Strong	None	Recent work indicates *M. hominis* may be a major cause
Urinary calculi	None	Weak	Ureaplasmas cause calculi in male rats, but no convincing evidence exists that they cause natural human disease
Pyelonephritis	Strong	None	*M. hominis* causes some cases
Involuntary infertility	None	Weak	Ureaplasmas are associated with altered motility of sperm
Repeated spontaneous abortion and stillbirth	None	Weak	Maternal and fetal infections have been associated with spontaneous abortion, but a causal relation is unproven
Chorioamnionitis	None	Strong	An association exists, but a causal relation is unproven
Low birthweight	None	Strong	An association exists, but a causal relation is unproven
Neonatal infections, including sepsis, pneumonia, meningitis	Strong	Strong	Further clarification is needed, but importance is growing in a selected prenatal population

TABLE 25-5 Summary of the Association of Genital Mycoplasmas with Neonatal Disease

Condition/Target Population	Isolates		Comments
	Mycoplasma hominis	Ureaplasma urealyticum	
Neonatal period, including preterm delivery, very low birthweight.			These findings need further clarification because most neonatal infections resolve without therapy, but in low socioeconomic groups, "diagnostic workup" of newborns should now include CSF and blood cultures for detection of mycoplasmas. This includes low–birthweight and preterm newborns, in whom traditional CSF cell counts and cultures would be negative.
Clinical signs compatible with			
Meningitis (CSF)	+	+	
Pneumonia (trachea)	+	+	
Sepsis (blood)	+	+	

CSF, cerebrospinal fluid.

patients with endocarditis, sternal wound infections, and arthritis.

Other *Mycoplasma* Species

Mycoplasma genitalium, first isolated in 1980, has been associated with NGU, cervicitis, endometriosis, and PID. There is evidence linking *M. genitalium* to some cases of tubal sterility. Its prevalence is not known, but it may be primarily a resident of the gastrointestinal tract that occurs secondarily in the genitourinary or respiratory tracts. Using polymerase chain reaction (PCR) assays, *M. genitalium* has been found more frequently in urethral samples taken from men with acute NGU than in those from men without urethritis.

Mycoplasma fermentans has been noted as a likely opportunistic respiratory pathogen. It is not known how often *M. fermentans* occurs in the respiratory tracts of healthy children, but it has been detected in throats of patients with lower respiratory tract infection, in some of whom a specific etiologic agent was not identified. Other groups of patients from whom *M. fermentans* has been recovered include adult patients with respiratory illness and those with acquired immunodeficiency syndrome (AIDS). *M. fermentans* has been isolated from tissue in patients both with and without AIDS who died of systemic infection. *M. fermentans* has also been isolated from synovial fluid of patients with rheumatoid arthritis. *M. penetrans* has been demonstrated in urine of homosexual males with human immunodeficiency virus-associated disease.

TABLE 25-6 Major Clinical and Corresponding Diagnostic Manifestation of *Mycoplasma pneumoniae*

Manifestation	Days after Onset						
	5	10	15	20	25	35	40
Headache and malaise	+1	+3	+3	+2	+1		
Dry cough	+2	+4	+4	+1			
Chest soreness	+3	+3	+1				
Fever							
104° F							
102° F							
100° F							
Chest radiograph	+2	+3	+2	+2	+1		
Mycoplasma culture with or without antibiotic treatment	+	+	+	+	+	+	
Complement fixation (titer)	≤8	8	32	64	256	256	128
Mycoplasma-specific Ig							
IgM	–	+	+	+	+	+	+
IgG	–	–	+	+	+	+/–	–

+4, Most severe; +1, least severe; +, present or positive; –, absent or negative; ▌, patient treated without appropriate antibiotic; ▌, patient treated with optimum antibiotic therapy, dose, and duration; *IgM*, immunoglobin M; *IgG*, immunoglobin G.

M. salivarium has been recovered from culture or detected by PCR in synovial fluid from patients with rheumatoid arthritis; however, the significance of this organism in this disease condition is unclear.

LABORATORY DIAGNOSIS

Because recovery from culture is difficult (sensitivity is approximately 40%), isolation of *M. pneumoniae* from respiratory sites is infrequently attempted. Growth may take several weeks, and technical expertise is necessary. *M. hominis* and *Ureaplasma* spp. are less stringent in their growth requirements but require cholesterol for synthesis of plasma membranes. *M. hominis* is the only species that will grow on sheep blood and chocolate agars. Diagnosis of *M. pneumoniae* infection is usually established serologically, traditionally with acute and convalescent sera collected 2 to 3 weeks apart to demonstrate a fourfold rise in titer. A schematic representation of classic clinical and corresponding diagnostic manifestations of *M. pneumoniae* is shown in Table 25-6. As noted previously, many of the early symptoms are nonspecific, and a thorough understanding of the disease process is necessary for interpretation of both serum and culture results.

Specimen Collection and Transport

Specimens for mycoplasmal culture include body fluids such as blood, sputum, synovial fluid, CSF, amniotic fluid, and urine, as well as wound aspirates, and nasopharyngeal, cervical, and vaginal swabs. Tissue samples may also be submitted for culture. Owing to the lack of a cell wall, all mycoplasmas are extremely sensitive to drying and heat. Ideally, specimens should be inoculated at bedside. If this is not possible, specimens should be delivered immediately to the laboratory in a transport medium. Cotton-tipped swabs and wooden shafts should be avoided because of possible inhibitory effects. Most references recommend swabs made of Dacron polyester or calcium alginate with aluminum or plastic shafts and that swabs be removed when the sample is placed in a transport medium. Trypticase soy broth with 0.5% albumin and 400 units/mL of penicillin or SP4 medium (sucrose phosphate buffer, *Mycoplasma* base, horse serum [20%], and neutral red) can be used. On arrival in the laboratory, the specimens should be frozen at −70° C if immediate plating is not possible within 24 hours.

Direct Examination

Because they lack a cell wall, the mollicutes will not be visible by Gram staining. A DNA fluorescent stain (e.g., acridine orange) can be used, but this is not specific for the mollicutes. Antigen detection assays have been used, but they are generally low in sensitivity and are not recommended. The PCR has been described for the detection of many mollicutes with varied results. Patients with *M. pneumoniae* infections can persistently harbor the organism for varied lengths of time after the acute infection. Therefore it is difficult to interpret a positive PCR result. No commercial kits are currently available.

Culture

Media

Several media have been developed for the recovery of mollicutes, and no single medium is suitable for all species isolated from humans. Penicillin can be added to minimize bacterial contamination. SP4 broth and agar are ideal for *M. pneumoniae* and *M. hominis*. *M. pneumoniae* and *M. genitalium* require glucose (their major energy source), *M. hominis* requires arginine, and *Ureaplasma* spp. require urea. *Ureaplasma* spp. also require media to have a pH near 6.0 (Shepherd's 10B arginine broth). It is difficult to maintain *Ureaplasma* spp. in culture, because death occurs rapidly when the urea is depleted, and the bacteria are sensitive to changes in pH because of urea utilization. Because mycoplasmas do not produce turbidity in broth media, a pH indicator such as phenol red should be added to detect growth. A8 agar can be used as a solid medium to recover both *M. hominis* and *Ureaplasma* spp.

Recovery of mycoplasma from blood can be performed by collecting uncoagulated blood and placing the sample into mycoplasmal broth media. A ratio of 1:10 (blood:broth) and 10 mL of blood for adults is recommended. Sodium polyanethol sulfonate (SPS), an additive often found in commercial blood culture media, is inhibitory to mycoplasma. The addition of 1% (wt/vol) of gelatin may help overcome the inhibitory effect of SPS; nevertheless, the use of commercial blood culture media, whether or not used in automated instruments, is not recommended. Figure 25-5 presents a schematic representation of media and methods used in the traditional isolation and identification of *Mycoplasma* spp.

Fluids should be centrifuged and the pellet resuspended in a small volume of liquid for media inoculation. It is important that specimens be diluted in broth up to 10^{-3} before plating each dilution. This helps to minimize the inhibitory effects of antimicrobial agents, antibodies, and other inhibitors that may be present in the specimen.

Commercial culture media and kits for detection and recovery of mycoplasmal organisms have been developed and are available in Europe but not in the United States. Such products may detect, quantify, identify, and determine antimicrobial susceptibility of genital mycoplasmas from urogenital specimens and *M. pneumoniae* from respiratory secretions.

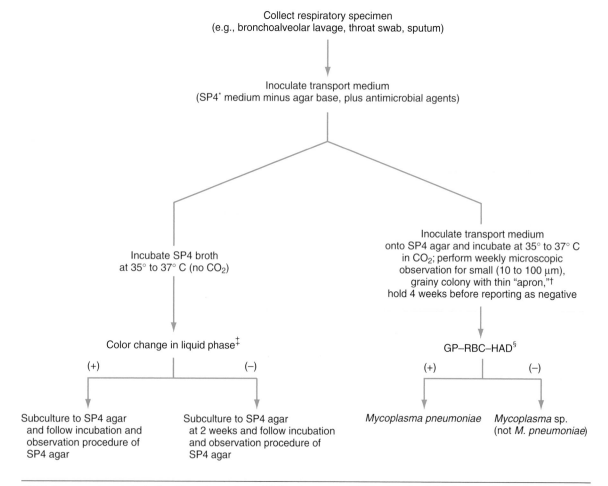

*SP4, Sucrose phosphate buffer, Mycoplasma base, fetal bovine serum (20%), phenol red. Medium stabilizes and decontaminates specimen. Storage at −70° C for repeat testing is recommended.

†Thin colony periphery. Examine with Stereomicroscope using 20× to 60× magnification.

‡Color change: positive, yellow color with no gross turbidity; negative, red color.

§GP–RBC–HAD = Guinea pig red blood cell hemadsorption. b-Hemolysis test for presumptive identification of Mycoplasma pneumoniae may be used in lieu of GP–RBC–HAD.

NOTE: Methylene blue on Dienes stain can be used for detection of Mycoplasma spp. on SP4 agar; plate immunofluorescence using labeled antibody can be used for identification.

FIGURE 25-5 Flow diagram for *Mycoplasma* spp. isolation using classic methods.

Isolation and Identification

Once inoculated, broth media should be placed at 37° C under atmospheric conditions, whereas solid agar media may be incubated in an environment of room air enhanced with 5% to 10% CO_2, or in an anaerobic atmosphere of 95% N_2 with 5% CO_2. Incubation in a candle jar is adequate.

Mycoplasma hominis and *Ureaplasma* spp. colonies may appear within 2 to 4 days, while *M. pneumoniae* may take 21 days or more. Because the organisms do not stain with the Gram stain, mycoplasma-like colonies are stained with the Dienes or methylene blue stains. Staining is performed by placing a small block of the agar on a glass slide, covering the colony with the stain, adding a coverslip, and examining the agar microscopically under low power. *M. hominis* has a typical "fried-egg" appearance, with the periphery staining a light blue and the center dark blue (Figure 25-6). *Mycoplasma* spp. almost universally show a mixed colony presentation on primary isolation when examined with a stereomicroscope (Figure 25-7).

Identification is often made by typing methods employing immunofluorescence and observation of plate media using a stereomicroscope. A direct plate immunofluorescent method also can be used. Fluorescent-labeled anti–*M. pneumoniae*

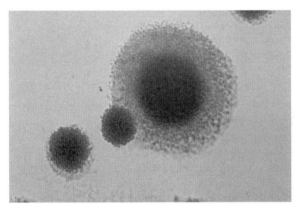

FIGURE 25-6 Dienes stain of *Mycoplasma* spp. colonies demonstrating typical "fried-egg" appearance.

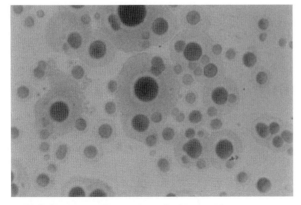

FIGURE 25-7 Typical mixed sizes of *Mycoplasma* spp. on primary isolation media: *Mycoplasma salivarium*. (Courtesy Bionique Testing Laboratories, Saranac Lake, N.Y.)

antibody is flooded on colonies on the plate; the plate is then washed and examined for immunofluorescence. The Chen assay is a fluorochrome method used to identify *Mycoplasma*-infected cell cultures. It uses a DNA fluorochrome stain (Hoechst 33258), which highlights *Mycoplasma* spp. as small ovoid bodies distributed throughout the glacial acetic acid–fixed cell culture. Figure 25-8 shows Vero cells (a monkey kidney cell line) artificially infected with *Mycoplasma orale* (Figure 25-8, *A*) and *M. salivarium* (Figure 25-8, *C*). Note the differences in morphotypes and distribution. Vero cell nuclei, which are rich in DNA, fluoresce with Hoechst 33258 stain in the negative control (Figure 25-8, *B*) as well as in the infected cell cultures. This method offers a unique way for diagnostic and clinical virology laboratories to perform quality control on their continuous cell cultures. The characteristic of guinea pig red blood cells (0.4% in saline) adhering to colonies of *M. pneumoniae* and not *M. hominis* is another standard assay that helps distinguish the two species. Furthermore, guinea pig cells do not adhere to large-colony mycoplasma, which are common inhabitants of the upper respiratory tract.

Ureaplasma spp., once called **T-strain mycoplasma** (*T* for "tiny"), form extremely small colonies that are difficult to see with the naked eye; hence, mycoplasmal cultures on solid media should always be examined with a stereomicroscope. Figure 25-9 shows both *M. hominis* and *U. urealyticum* grown on New York City (NYC) agar. Urease activity of ureaplasma may be detected on solid agar containing urea and manganese chloride (U9B urease color test medium). Urease-positive colonies are a dark golden-brown color due to the deposition of manganese dioxide.

Both *M. hominis* and *U. urealyticum* require cholesterol for synthesis of plasma membranes and other undetermined growth factors; fetal calf serum (20% v/v) is the traditional nutrient source. Although uncommon, extragenital *M. hominis* infections are emerging, and this organism should be considered whenever many polymorphonuclear cells are seen on Gram stain but there is no growth on routine bacterial culture. *M. hominis* grows well anaerobically and will appear as pinpoint (0.05 mm), clear, glistening, raised colonies on Columbia colistin–nalidixic acid agar or anaerobic blood agar (Centers for Disease Control and Prevention formula) in 48 hours. Under these anaerobic conditions, the colonies do not display the "fried egg" morphology characteristic of some mycoplasma. The anaerobic plate should be examined using oblique light. Those colonies that do not Gram stain should be subcultured to A7 medium, on which they demonstrate typical "fried egg" growth and stain positive with Dienes or methylene blue stains, if they are mycoplasmas.

Serologic Diagnosis

Because of the inherent difficulties of cultures and interpretations of a positive PCR assay, *M. pneumoniae* has historically been diagnosed by serologic methods. Optimally, serum samples for serologic testing should be collected at the onset of symptoms and 2 to 3 weeks later for acute and convalescent measurements; however, this often is not practical. With newer methods, single serum samples collected during the disease may rule out the infection or suggest additional evaluations. The cold agglutinin antibody titer had been used for

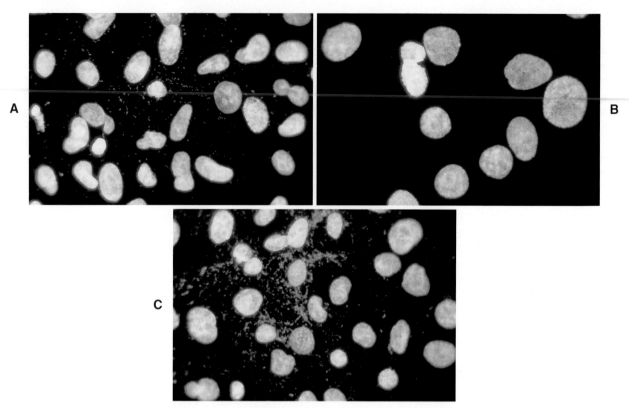

FIGURE 25-8 Identification of *Mycoplasma*-infected cell culture employing DNA-fluorochrome stain (Hoechst no. 33258 stain). **A,** *Mycoplasma orale.* **B,** Uninfected Vero cell culture highlighting the DNA-rich nucleus. **C,** *Mycoplasma salivarium.* The mycoplasma appear as small pinpoint fluorescent bodies throughout the background. (Courtesy Bionique Testing Laboratories, Saranac Lake, N.Y.)

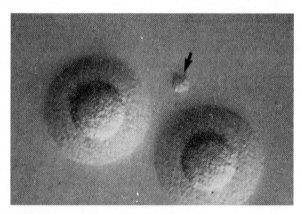

FIGURE 25-9 Mixed isolation of *Mycoplasma hominis* and *Ureaplasma urealyticum* showing why *U. urealyticum* was originally called "T" for "tiny-strain" *(arrow).*

Previously, the most commonly used technique for demonstration of *M. pneumoniae* specific antibodies was the micro-method complement fixation assay, which was time consuming and had inherent technical problems. Several commercially available enzyme immunoassays and microimmunofluorescence assays are now available for detection of serum antibodies and in some cases detect either IgM or IgG. Table 25-7 highlights selected features of these immunologic assays and other methods. Detection methods were added for comparative analysis and completeness. It is important to remember that demonstration of a significant rise in antibody titer in conjunction with culture isolation is preferable for definitive diagnosis. Serologic methods are available for *M. hominis* and *U. urealyticum*, but they are generally performed only by reference laboratories.

ANTIMICROBIAL SUSCEPTIBILITY

Because they lack a cell wall, the mollicutes are inherently resistant to the β-lactams: penicillins and cephalosporins. *M. pneumoniae* has remained susceptible to the tetracyclines, newer fluoroquinolones, and the macrolides (e.g., erythromycin). Because of side effects, tetracycline is used only for treatment of adults. *M. hominis*, which is more resistant than *M. pneumoniae*, is usually resistant to erythromycin but susceptible to clindamycin and lincomycin, whereas *U. urealyticum*

many years as an indicator of primary atypical pneumonia, but it is both insensitive and nonspecific for *M. pneumoniae*. Approximately 50% of patients with primary atypical pneumonia produce a detectable cold agglutinin antibody titer. This assay is no longer recommended for the diagnosis of *M. pneumoniae* infection.

TABLE 25-7 Comparative Features of Various Laboratory Methods Used in the Detection of *Mycoplasma pneumoniae*, *Mycoplasma hominis*, and *Ureaplasma urealyticum*

Detection Method	M. pneumoniae	M. hominis	U. urealyticum
Nonserologic			
Culture	Traditionally difficult	Method of choice, but must differentiate infection from colonization	Method of choice using urease detection, but must differentiate infection from colonization
Indirect immunofluorescence	Respiratory antigen for early-stage infection Research use only but is promising		
Polymerase chain reaction	Assays are being evaluated	Assays are being evaluated	Assays are being evaluated
Serologic			
Complement fixation	Traditional assay but <50% seroconvert; need fourfold rise between acute and convalescent sera >32 single titer may be suggestive		
Immunofluorescent antibody	Measures IgG and IgM separately	Measures IgG and IgM separately; not recommended	
Latex agglutination	IgM/IgG	IgG only	
Enzyme immunoassay	Method of choice M. pneumoniae reactive IgM, IgG, and IgA, but IgM may remain elevated for 1 yr		

IgM, Immunoglobin M; *IgG*, immunoglobin G.

is generally resistant to clindamycin and lincomycin and sensitive to erythromycin. Both organisms are often sensitive to tetracycline, but high-level resistance is emerging.

Standard methods have not been developed for susceptibility testing of mycoplasma, and protocols have varied considerably among laboratories. The agar dilution has been regarded as the reference method; however, because of the high degree of technical expertise required and the few mycoplasmal isolates, this assay is not offered by most hospital laboratories. The broth microdilution is the most commonly used method to determine minimal inhibitory concentrations. With reported antimicrobial resistance increasing, availability of newer, broad-spectrum antimicrobials, and the emergence of more infections due to the mycoplasma, antimicrobial susceptibility testing methods are being reevaluated. Because of the variable susceptibility pattern of *M. hominis*, antimicrobial susceptibility testing is usually recommended for clinically significant isolates; these isolates should be forwarded to a reference laboratory. *M. pneumoniae* has a more predictable sensitivity pattern; therefore antimicrobial susceptibility testing is not often warranted.

INTERPRETATION OF LABORATORY RESULTS

Mycoplasma pneumoniae detected by any method from pulmonary or nonpulmonary specimens should be considered significant and a pathogen. Interpretation of *M. hominis* isolation is not as obvious; differentiation from colonization and infection requires detailed clinical analysis and potentially repeat cultures. *U. urealyticum* is the most difficult to assess. In urogenital specimens, it has been reported to colonize up to 70% of men and 45% of women with no apparent infection. Its isolation is not indicative of pathogenicity, and it is incumbent on the laboratory to educate the physician, usually including a statement with culture results suggesting its potential for colonization versus pathogenicity. In nonurogenital specimens, particularly CSF isolates, it is reasonable to evaluate cautiously the clinical significance of ureaplasma.

Respiratory specimens received in the laboratory often provide limited clinical information. Specimens are processed and inoculated onto the appropriate media given the most likely candidate for the disease, clinical presentation, age of patient, and seasonability, recognizing that there is a certain predictability with selected pathogens. Table 25-8 presents laboratory methods used to diagnose infections caused by several pathogens—*Mycoplasma*, *Chlamydia*, *Legionella*, mycobacteria, fungi, and viruses—in various age groups. All respiratory specimens should be stored at −70° C. Acute sera should also be stored frozen for subsequent antibody titer testing.

TABLE 25-8 Laboratory Detection of Frequent Respiratory Pathogens

	Epidemiologic Factors				Laboratory Methods			
Age	Age/Organism Frequently Involved	Disease	Season	Specimen Source	Stains	Culture	Nonculture
Newborn	1, 3, 4	Pneumonia, aseptic workup		Tracheal suction	Gram	Traditional, plus mycoplasmal	
Grade school	2, 4	Atypical pneumonia	Fall	Sputum	Gram, acid-fast bacillus	Traditional, plus mycoplasmal	EIA, mycoplasmal, IgM
College student	1, 2	Biphasic disease with pharyngitis and, later, bronchitis	Spring?	Sputum	DFA	Cell culture, mycoplasmal	EIA, micoplasmal IgM
Adult	2, 4, 5, 6	Pneumonia or immunocompromised		Sputum Bronchoalveolar lavage specimen	DFA, acid-fast bacillus Gomori methenamine silver, toluidine blue, and/or calcofluor white	Cell culture Traditional plus fungal, acid-fast bacillus	IgG, mycoplasmal

1, Chlamydophila pneumoniae; 2, Mycoplasma pneumoniae (outbreak); *3, Mycoplasma hominis; 4,* viral (outbreak) adenovirus/respiratory virus/influenza (seasonal); *5,* other: acid-fast bacilli, fungus, *Legionella,* or *Pneumocystis* pneumonia; *6, Streptococcus pneumoniae. EIA,* Enzyme immunoassay; *DFA,* direct fluorescent antibody; *IgM,* immunoglobin M; *IgG,* immunoglobin G.

BIBLIOGRAPHY

Cuccuru MA et al: PCR analysis of *Mycoplasma fermentans* and *M. penetrans* in classic Kaposi's sarcoma, *Acta Derm Venereol* 85:459, 2005.

Cultrera R et al: Molecular evidence of *Ureaplasma urealyticum* and *Ureaplasma parvum* colonization in preterm infants during respiratory distress syndrome, *BMC Infect Dis* 6:166, 2006.

Dhawan B et al: Evaluation of the diagnostic efficacy of PCR for *Ureaplasma urealyticum* infection in Indian adults with symptoms of genital discharge, *Japn J Infect Dis* 59:57, 2006.

Shyh-Ching Lo et al: *Mycoplasma penetrans* infections and seroconversion in patients with AIDS: identification of major mycoplasmal antigens targeted by host antibody response, *Immunol Med Microbiol* 44:277, 2005.

Waites KB, Taylor-Robinson D: *Mycoplasma* and *Urealyticum.* In Murray PR et al, editors: *Manual of clinical microbiology,* ed 9, Washington, DC, 2007, ASM Press.

Points to Remember

- *Mycoplasma* spp. are minute organisms characterized by the lack of a cell wall.
- The most significant species of Mycoplasmataceae include *M. pneumoniae, M. hominis,* and *Ureaplasma* spp., although others are beginning to be recognized as opportunistic pathogens.
- *M. pneumoniae* is an important cause of community-acquired pneumonia.
- *M. hominis* and *Ureaplasma* spp. are genital mycoplasma commonly diagnosed by culture, although polymerase chain reaction technology is also available.

Learning Assessment Questions

1. From what source did the infant described in the Case in Point likely acquire the infection?
2. Would routine prenatal culture of the mother have yielded this organism?
3. Why was the Gram stain negative?
4. How does primary atypical pneumonia differ from pneumonia caused by *Streptococcus pneumoniae?*
5. Name the four common species of mollicutes associated with the genitourinary tracts of humans.
6. What special stain is used on suspected colonies of *Mycoplasma?*
7. What culture media are used to isolate *Mycoplasma pneumoniae, M. hominis,* and *Ureaplasma urealyticum?*
8. Why is cold agglutinin titer not a useful diagnostic tool for *M. pneumoniae?*
9. What current serologic assays are available to demonstrate *M. pneumoniae* antibodies?
10. Why are the mollicutes universally resistant to penicillin?

Mycobacterium tuberculosis and Other Nontuberculous Mycobacteria

Olarae Giger

- ■ GENERAL CHARACTERISTICS
- ■ CLINICAL SIGNIFICANCE OF THE *MYCOBACTERIUM TUBERCULOSIS* COMPLEX
  Mycobacterium tuberculosis
  Mycobacterium bovis
- ■ CLINICAL SIGNIFICANCE OF NONTUBERCULOUS MYCOBACTERIA
  Slowly Growing Species
  Rapidly Growing Species
- ■ *MYCOBACTERIUM LEPRAE*
- ■ ISOLATION AND IDENTIFICATION OF MYCOBACTERIA
  Laboratory Safety Considerations

Specimen Collection
Digestion and Decontamination of Specimens
Concentration Procedures
Staining for Acid-Fast Bacilli
Culture Media and Isolation Methods
Laboratory Identification
- ■ SUSCEPTIBILITY TESTING OF *MYCOBACTERIUM TUBERCULOSIS*
- ■ IMMUNODIAGNOSIS OF *MYCOBACTERIUM TUBERCULOSIS*
  Skin Testing
  Serology

OBJECTIVES

After studying this chapter, you should be able to:

1. Describe the general characteristics of mycobacteria and compare them with other groups of microorganisms.

2. Discuss the safety precautions to be followed while working in a mycobacteriology laboratory.

3. Describe the appropriate specimen collection and processing procedures to recover mycobacteria from clinical samples.

4. Explain why clinical samples for mycobacterial isolation sometimes require digestion and decontamination procedures.

5. Describe the principles and procedures for the stains used to demonstrate mycobacteria in clinical samples and isolates.

6. Compare the different culture media used for the isolation of mycobacteria.

7. Discuss the different tests used to identify mycobacteria.

8. Compare the new methods of detecting mycobacterial species in clinical samples.

9. Discuss the clinical disease caused by *Mycobacterium tuberculosis*.

10. Describe the use of the tuberculin skin test.

11. Discuss the clinical significance of nontuberculous mycobacteria.

Case in Point

A 56-year-old white male came to the emergency department complaining of fatigue and mild weight loss (10 lb) over the past 12 months. During questioning the patient also complained of a cough for 3 months that produced sputum with red streaks. The patient indicated a history of night fever and chills but denied dyspnea or chest pain. The patient also had a family history of pulmonary tuberculosis from his original home in Mexico. He reported that his last purified protein derivative (PPD) skin test, approximately 5 years ago, was negative. Vital signs included temperature of 36.5° C (97.7° F), pulse of 63 beats per minute, respirations 15 per minute, and blood pressure of 96/56 mm Hg. The patient's chest radiograph revealed an infiltrate in the right upper lobe. A computed tomography scan of the chest showed nodular patchy opacity in the right upper lobe. The patient was admitted for further evaluation. A PPD skin test showed a 10 × 7-mm induration. Three sputum samples were obtained over a 3-day period for acid-fast bacilli (AFB) smears and culture. Direct smears on all three samples were reported as no organisms seen. Processed samples were inoculated onto Löwenstein-Jensen medium and into BACTEC 12B bottles. After 12 to 14 days of incubation the BACTEC bottles from all three specimens yielded positive results. Smears of the bottles revealed

AFB by Kinyoun stain. Polymerase chain reaction DNA amplification for *Mycobacterium tuberculosis* of the BACTEC medium was positive. A four-drug antituberculosis regimen of isoniazid, rifampin, pyrazinamide, and ethambutol was recommended.

Issues to Consider

After reading the patient's case history, consider the following:

- What might be significant about this patient's family history?
- What are the characteristic symptoms of tuberculosis?
- What is the typical length of time for a culture to yield pathogenic *Mycobacterium*?

Key Terms

Acid fastness

Auramine/auramine-rhodamine fluorochrome stains

Kinyoun stain

Löwenstein-Jensen (LJ) medium

Middlebrook 7H10 medium

Middlebrook 7H11 medium

Mycobacterium avium complex (MAC)

Mycobacterium tuberculosis complex

Nonchromogenic

Nontuberculosis mycobacteria (NTM)

Photochromogenic

Pott disease

Purified protein derivative (PPD)

Scotochromogenic

Ziehl-Neelsen stain

The genus *Mycobacterium* is composed of approximately 100 recognized and proposed species. The most familiar of the species are *Mycobacterium tuberculosis* (MTB) and *Mycobacterium leprae*, the causative agents of tuberculosis (TB) and Hansen disease (leprosy), respectively. Both diseases have long been associated with chronic illness and social stigma. Tuberculosis remains a major cause of morbidity and mortality in the world today. Additionally, the growing number of immunocompromised patients worldwide has led to a resurgence of tuberculosis as well as diseases caused by **nontuberculosis mycobacteria (NTM).**

In addition to TB and Hansen disease, *Mycobacterium* spp. produce a spectrum of infections in humans and animals. A large group of mycobacteria, excluding the *M. tuberculosis* complex and *M. leprae*, normally inhabit the environment and can cause disease that often resembles tuberculosis in humans. These organisms are sometimes referred to as atypical mycobacteria or mycobacteria other than the tubercle bacillus (MOTT). The term *nontuberculous mycobacteria* is used here. Box 26-1 shows the usual clinical significance of *Mycobacterium* spp. isolates.

Epidemiologic changes have led to challenges within the mycobacteriology laboratory, including rapid identification of all clinically significant mycobacteria and antimicrobial susceptibility testing of *Mycobacterium* spp. Fortunately new developments in the field of clinical mycobacteriology are helping to meet these challenges. Rapid methods may eliminate the need for lengthy culturing for isolation and protracted biochemical methods of identification. Future developments

BOX 26-1 Usual Clinical Significance of *Mycobacterium* Species Isolates

Pathogen
Mycobacterium tuberculosis
Mycobacterium bovis
Mycobacterium ulcerans

Often Pathogen, Potential Pathogen
Mycobacterium avium complex
Mycobacterium kansasii
Mycobacterium marinum
Mycobacterium haemophilum
Mycobacterium xenopi
Mycobacterium genavense

Potential Pathogen
Mycobacterium abscessus
Mycobacterium chelonae
Mycobacterium fortuitum
Mycobacterium malmoense
Mycobacterium scrofulaceum
Mycobacterium simiae
Mycobacterium szulgai

Usual Saprophyte, Rare Pathogen
Mycobacterium gordonae
Mycobacterium flavescens
Mycobacterium gastri
Mycobacterium nonchromogenicum
Mycobacterium terrae
Mycobacterium phlei
Mycobacterium smegmatis
Mycobacterium vaccae
Mycobacterium thermoresistibile

in the application of molecular biology to mycobacteriology may further diminish the time required for identification, increase accuracy and reproducibility, ease performance, and reduce cost. This chapter discusses the following:

- The clinical significance of the *Mycobacterium* spp.
- The general characteristics of mycobacteria
- Safety precautions that must be observed in the mycobacteriology laboratory
- Appropriate specimen collection and handling
- Laboratory procedures for isolation and identification of mycobacterial isolates

GENERAL CHARACTERISTICS

Mycobacteria are slender, slightly curved or straight, rod-shaped organisms 0.2 to 0.6 μm × 1 to 10 μm in size. They are nonmotile and do not form spores. The cell wall has extremely high lipid content; thus mycobacterial cells resist staining with commonly used basic aniline dyes at room temperature. Mycobacteria do take up dye with increased staining time or application of heat; however, they resist decolorization with acid-ethanol. This characteristic is referred to as **acid fastness**—hence the term acid-fast bacilli (AFB)—and is a basic characteristic in distinguishing mycobacteria from most other genera and species.

Mycobacteria are strictly aerobic, but increased carbon dioxide (CO_2) will enhance the growth of some species. The mycobacteria grow more slowly than most bacteria pathogenic for humans. The most rapidly growing species generally grow on simple media in 2 to 3 days at temperatures of 20° to 40° C. Most mycobacteria associated with disease require 2 to 6 weeks of incubation on complex media at specific optimum temperatures. One of the mycobacteria pathogenic for humans, *M. leprae*, fails to grow in vitro.

CLINICAL SIGNIFICANCE OF THE *MYCOBACTERIUM TUBERCULOSIS* COMPLEX

The *Mycobacterium tuberculosis* **complex** consists of *M. tuberculosis, M. bovis* (including the vaccination strain bacillus Calmette-Guérin), *M. africanum, M. canettii,* and *M. microti. M. africanum* has been associated with human cases of TB in tropical Africa, and *M. microti* has been linked to TB in both immunocompetent and immunocompromised individuals. The latter three species are rarely encountered in the United States.

Mycobacterium tuberculosis

Mycobacterium tuberculosis was first described by Robert Koch in 1882; however, TB is one of the oldest documented communicable diseases. Today there are more than 1 billion cases of TB infection worldwide, with 8 to 10 million new cases of disease and 3 million deaths attributed to TB per year. A person is infected with *M. tuberculosis* when exposed to the organism. Whether or not a person develops TB is determined by the person's cellular immune response, the amount of exposure, and the virulence of the strain.

In the United States before 1985, the actual number of TB cases was continually declining at a rate of about 5% per year. In 1985 this decline ended, and the number of documented TB cases per year in the United States increased until the early 1990s. The increase in the 1980s could be attributed to several factors, including the acquired immunodeficiency syndrome (AIDS) epidemic (which increases a person's risk for TB), increased use of intravenous drugs, and greater spread among inhabitants of closed environments, such as nursing homes, correctional facilities, and shelters for the homeless. In the 1990s, the Centers for Disease Control and Prevention (CDC) allocated additional funds for public laboratories to improve identification and susceptibility testing of mycobacteria. As a result, the incidence of TB in the United States steadily declined from a high of 26,673 in 1992 to 13,299 in 2007. Currently, in the United States more cases are associated with foreign-born individuals from endemic areas than with U.S.–born persons.

Primary Tuberculosis

Clinically, TB is usually a disease of the respiratory tract. Tubercle bacilli are acquired from persons with active disease who are excreting viable bacilli by means of coughing, sneezing, or talking. Airborne droplet nuclei containing bacteria, 1 to 5 μm, enter the respiratory tract of an exposed individual and are deposited in the lung alveoli. *M. tuberculosis* cells are phagocytized by alveolar macrophages and are capable of intracellular multiplication. In a person with adequate cellular immunity, T cells arrive within 4 to 6 weeks with macrophage-activating polypeptides called *lymphokines*. This enables the macrophage in the area of infection to destroy the intracellular mycobacteria. There is then a regression and healing of the primary lesion and any disseminated foci of infection by the *M. tuberculosis* organisms.

In many exposed individuals, the immune system does not eliminate the bacteria. The pathologic features of TB are the result of a hypersensitivity reaction to mycobacterial antigen. If there is little antigen and a great deal of hypersensitivity reaction, a hard tubercle or granuloma may be formed. The granuloma is an organization of lymphocytes, macrophages, giant cells, fibroblasts, and capillaries. With granuloma formation, healing occurs, along with fibrosis, encapsulation, and scar formation as a reminder of the past infection. If the antigen load and hypersensitivity reaction are both high, tissue necrosis from enzymes of degenerating macrophages may occur; the tissue response is less organized, and no granuloma is formed. Without granuloma or necrosis, lesions may heal without obvious pathology. With necrosis a caseous material may be present at the site of the primary lesion as a result of solid or semisolid amorphous material laid down at the site of necrosis. After healing of first-degree infection, the bacilli are not totally eradicated but can remain viable in granulomas for months or years. In infected individuals, there is a potential for reactivation of TB.

Clinical diagnosis of primary TB is usually limited to signs and symptoms and a positive **purified protein derivative (PPD)** skin test. Children may demonstrate a nonproductive cough and fever with or without shortness of breath; these symptoms are unusual in adults. Chest radiographs are usually normal, although rarely there may be infiltrates without cavitation in the anterior segment of the upper, middle, or lower lobe with hilar or paratracheal lymphadenopathy. Along with these limited clinical findings there is a paucity of bacteriologic findings. If sputum or bronchial washings are cultured during the primary infection, the yield is only 25% to 30% positive. A small percentage of individuals who are infected with TB develop progressive (active) pulmonary disease, most often from a failed cellular immune response and hence a failure to stop multiplication of the bacilli. In young children or older adults who are primarily infected and in people with an underlying immunodeficiency, massive lymphohematogenous dissemination may occur and lead to meningeal or miliary (disseminated) TB. In addition, 10% of young adults may progress to active disease from their primary infection. This will resemble reactivation TB in older adults, and the only way to differentiate it is by finding a positive PPD in a previously negative individual.

Reactivation Tuberculosis

The risk of reactivation of TB is about 3.3% during the first year after a positive tuberculin (i.e., PPD) skin test and a total of 5% to 15% thereafter in the person's lifetime. Progression from infection to active disease varies with age and the intensity and duration of exposure. Malnutrition, with or without other factors such as alcoholism, homelessness, incarceration, immunosuppression, and acquired immunodeficiency syndrome (AIDS), can contribute greatly to the progression to active TB.

Reactivation TB occurs when there is an alteration or a suppression of the cellular immune system in the infected host that favors replication of the bacilli and progression to disease. The symptoms of disease are slow in developing and consist of fever, shortness of breath, night sweats and chills, fatigue, anorexia, and weight loss. About 20% of individuals may have no symptoms, but most patients eventually have cough, chest pain, and productive sputum. Hemoptysis occurs in 25% of cases. The radiographs of patients with reactivation TB reveal a patchy or confluent consolidation with increased linear densities extending to the hilum; thick-walled cavities without air-fluid levels usually are found in apical or posterior segments of the upper lobe or superior segment of the middle lobe of the lung. If there is bronchogenic spread of the bacilli, multiple alveolar densities will be seen; rarely is there enlargement of the lymph nodes.

If the disease has been chronic, fibrosis, loss of lung volume, and calcifications will be demonstrated. The PPD skin test may be negative in up to 25% of these cases; diagnosis is confirmed by smear and culture of sputum, gastric aspirates, or bronchoscopy specimens. Fiberoptic bronchoscopy has been found to yield a 95% recovery; postbronchoscopic sputa are usually positive as well. In any case of pulmonary TB disease, there may be complications if diagnosis and treatment are delayed. These include empyema, pleural fibrosis, massive hemoptysis, adrenal insufficiency (rare), and hypercalcemia (up to 25% of cases). In patients with AIDS and TB with drug-resistant bacilli, the risk of progression to disease from infection is quite high, although the clinical findings may vary from those in the non-AIDS patient with reactivation TB. The diagnosis is usually made by smears and culture, with a rate of sensitivity similar to that in the non-AIDS patient.

Extrapulmonary Tuberculosis

Extrapulmonary TB occurred much less commonly than pulmonary tuberculosis (<15%) before the AIDS epidemic; however, as cases of pulmonary TB in the United States declined, the number of cases of extrapulmonary TB remained constant. Cases of extrapulmonary disease have increased since 1988 because it is a common presentation in individuals with human immunodeficiency virus (HIV) infection, although it is most often in association with pulmonary disease.

Miliary TB refers to the seeding of many organs outside the pulmonary tree with AFB through hematogenous spread. This usually occurs shortly after primary pulmonary disease but can take place anywhere in the course of acute or chronic TB. The most common sites of spread of *M. tuberculosis* are the spleen, liver, lungs, bone marrow, kidney, adrenal gland, and eyes, usually in that order of occurrence. Other forms of extrapulmonary TB include pleural, lymphadenitis, gastrointestinal, skeletal, meningeal, peritoneal, and genitourinary infections. Virtually any organ of the body can be infected by *M. tuberculosis*; additional uncommon manifestations include gastrointestinal infection, peritonitis, cutaneous TB, laryngitis, otitis, and involvement of the adrenal glands, eyes, and breast infections.

Overall, children account for most cases of miliary TB, but it is also a common form of TB disease in HIV-infected individuals. The mortality is 20% or higher in most studies; the finding of meningitis is an extremely poor prognostic indicator. Up to 70% of HIV-infected patients may have extrapulmonary TB alone or, most often, in combination with pulmonary disease. The most common extrapulmonary sites in this population are lymph nodes (especially mediastinal), genitourinary tract, and the abdominal cavity. Bacteremia is not uncommon.

Pleurisy, an unexplained pleural effusion with mononuclear pleurocytosis, manifests as cough, fever, and chest pain, resembling the presentation of bacterial pneumonia; it occurs in about 5% of all cases of TB. In endemic areas, pleurisy is a presentation in young individuals; in the United States, middle-aged to older persons are most affected. Resolution is common. AFB are rarely seen in pleural fluid, but cultures may be positive in 20% to 50% of cases; pleural biopsies offer a higher yield of microbiologic diagnosis.

Lymphadenitis is usually a disease of children, appearing as painless head or neck swellings. Lymph node involvement, particularly mediastinal, has been a common extrapulmonary manifestation in patients with AIDS. Genitourinary TB can involve the kidneys and genital organs. Renal TB accounts for 2% of all cases of TB and manifests as typical urinary tract symptoms and sterile pyuria. Cultures may be positive in up to 80% of cases. Male genital TB usually appears as a scrotal mass and occurs most often along with renal TB. In men and women, hematogenous spread is usually the source of genitourinary TB. Skeletal TB of the spine is referred to as **Pott disease**. Back pain is the most common characteristic. Cultures of bone and tissue are needed to confirm the diagnosis. Peripheral skeletal bones and joints also may be involved, with the hip and knee being the most common sites.

Meningitis due to *M. tuberculosis* is usually the result of a rupture of a tubercle into the subarachnoid space and not usually hematogenous spread. In childhood it occurs rarely after primary pulmonary infection. Most infections occur at the base of the brain, and patients may develop very thick, gelatinous, masslike lesions there. With more chronic disease, a fibrous mass may surround cranial nerves. Involvement of arteries can cause infarctions. Cerebrospinal fluid (CSF) examination usually reveals elevated protein, decreased glucose, and predominance of lymphocytes.

Identification of *Mycobacterium tuberculosis*

Colonies of this slowly growing species are typically raised with a dry, rough appearance. The colonies are nonpigmented and classically described as being buff colored (Figure 26-1). Elaboration of cord factor can result in characteristic cord formation. Optimum growth occurs at 35° to 37° C.

Biochemically, *M. tuberculosis* is characteristically positive for niacin accumulation, reduction of nitrate to nitrite, and production of catalase, which is destroyed after heating (heat-stable catalase negative). Isoniazid-resistant strains may not produce catalase at all. *M. tuberculosis* is inhibited by nitroimidazopyran or p-nitroacetylamino-β-hydroxyproplophenone (NAP). This species can be distinguished from *M. bovis* by the inhibition of *M. bovis* by thiophene-2-carboxylie acid hydrazide (T2H) and pyrazinamidase activity.

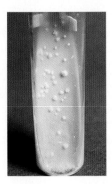

FIGURE 26-1 *Mycobacterium tuberculosis* growing on Löwenstein-Jensen medium.

Treatment

The treatment of TB involves the use of more than one anti-mycobacterial agent. For pulmonary TB, treatment usually involves a 9-month course of therapy with isoniazid and rifampin, usually once per day the first month and twice a week thereafter. Many regimens also include a 2- to 8-week initial course of streptomycin or ethambutol. Most individuals clear their sputum of AFB within the first 2 months. Pyrazinamide (PZA) may be added to the regimen if there is a suspicion of lowered cellular immunity and a need to obtain bactericidal levels of antituberculous activity intracellularly in macrophages. PZA is usually recommended for a shorter course, initially along with isoniazid and rifampin.

Multidrug-Resistant *Mycobacterium tuberculosis*

The incidence of multidrug-resistant (MDR) TB in the United States decreased from 2.5% of isolates in 1993 to 1.1% in 2007. Since 1997, the percentage of United States-born patients with MDR-TB has remained low, less than or equal to 1.0%. However, of the total number of reported MDR-TB cases, the proportion occurring in foreign-born persons increased from 25.5% in 1993 to 80% in 2007.

Within any population of *M. tuberculosis*, resistance to a single agent can develop at a fairly well-defined rate. For example, with isoniazid and streptomycin the chance that a resistant isolate will develop is approximately 1 in 10^6. The rate of spontaneous mutation of resistance to both drugs in one cell is the product of the rates of resistance to the individual drugs or 1 in 10^{12}. In a patient with pulmonary tuberculosis, the pulmonary cavity may contain 10^7 to 10^9 bacterial cells. Random drug resistance has a good likelihood of developing when only one antimycobacterial agent is used or if the patient is on multidrug therapy and fails to complete the course of medication. Therefore the use of combination therapy (i.e., three or more drugs) to treat mycobacterial infections is common.

Risk factors for drug resistance may include previous treatment for TB, residence in an area endemic for drug resistance, or close contact with an individual who is infected with MDR-TB. Drug resistance is usually acquired by spontaneous mutations as a result of the inappropriate use of antimicrobial agents to treat *M. tuberculosis* and the lack of patient compliance. If compliance is an issue, directly observed therapy is recommended to ensure proper medication. Otherwise resistance may be assumed and tested for in vitro.

Primary MDR-TB is defined as no previous history of TB disease and resistance to at least isoniazid and rifampin, drugs recognized as the primary treatments for drug susceptible *M. tuberculosis*. Extensively drug resistant tuberculosis (XDR-TB) is defined as resistance to isoniazid and rifampin plus resistance to any fluoroquinolone and at least one of three injectable second-line anti-TB drugs (i.e., the aminoglycosides amikacin, kanamycin, or capreomycin). In the United States, two cases of XDR-TB were reported in 2007; however, clusters of XDR-TB have been reported in other areas of the world. Because of the threat of MDR-TB and XDR-TB it is important for laboratories to identify *Mycobacterium* spp. rapidly and to perform antimicrobial susceptibility testing so that appropriate therapy can be administered as quickly as possible.

MDR-TB requires an extended treatment period compared with drug-susceptible isolates. For cases of resistance to isoniazid or rifampin, second-line antituberculosis drugs may include aminoglycosides and fluoroquinolones. In communities where at least 4% of the isolates are drug resistant, a regimen of four drugs is usually recommended. With the numbers of cases of MDR-*M. tuberculosis* increasing, newer agents are being tested in vitro to determine their efficacy.

Mycobacterium bovis

Mycobacterium bovis produces TB primarily in cattle but also in other ruminants, as well as dogs, cats, swine, parrots, and humans. The disease in humans closely resembles that caused by *M. tuberculosis* and is treated similarly. In some areas of the world, a significant percentage of cases of TB are due to *M. bovis*, but in the United States the number of isolates of this organism is very low.

Mycobacterium bovis is closely related taxonomically to *M. tuberculosis* and belongs to the *M. tuberculosis* complex. It grows very slowly on egg-based media, producing small, granular, rounded, white colonies with irregular margins after 21 days of incubation at 37° C. Growth is nonpigmented. On **Middlebrook 7H10 medium,** colonies are similar to those of *M. tuberculosis* but slower to mature. Most strains of *M. bovis* are niacin negative, do not reduce nitrate, and do not grow in the presence of T2H, characteristics that distinguish the species from most strains of *M. tuberculosis*.

CLINICAL SIGNIFICANCE OF NONTUBERCULOUS MYCOBACTERIA

Most NTM are found in soil and water. They have been commonly implicated as opportunistic pathogens in patients with underlying lung disease, immunosuppression, or percutaneous trauma. AIDS has contributed greatly to the incidence and awareness of NTM disease. Chronic pulmonary disease resembling TB is the usual clinical presentation associated with these organisms, although a few species are more often associated with cutaneous infections. Infections caused by the NTM are not considered transmissible from person to person. Regional differences in the incidence of NTM disease are quite striking.

Slowly Growing Species

Mycobacterium avium Complex

Epidemiology. *Mycobacterium avium* and *M. intracellulare* are part of the **M. avium complex (MAC).** These organisms are common environment saprophytes and have been recovered from soil, water, house dust, and other environmental sources. Certain areas, such as coastal marshes, have higher concentrations of the organism. *M. avium* is a cause of disease in poultry and swine, but animal-to-human transmission has not been shown to be an important factor in human disease. Environmental sources, especially natural waters, seem to be the reservoir for most human infections. Moreover there appears to be a close association between many of the organisms that cause disease in humans and those commonly found in animals, suggesting that some infections may qualify as a zoonosis. A large increase in MAC infections has occurred in the past decade, primarily owing to the number of infections in patients with AIDS. MAC is now the most common NTM causing tuberculosis in the United States.

Clinical Infections. Pulmonary disease resulting from MAC infection presents a clinical picture similar to that of TB: cough, fatigue, weight loss, low-grade fever, and night sweats. Radiologic examination demonstrates cavitary disease in most patients, whereas solitary nodules or diffuse infiltrates may be observed in others. Disseminated disease has become more common, usually occurring in immunocompromised patients or patients with hematologic abnormalities. MAC infections are the most common systemic bacterial infection in patients with AIDS. The loss of CD4+ T cells reduces the capability of the macrophage to become activated to kill MAC.

The clinical outcome of MAC lung disease is unpredictable; thus the management of affected patients can be difficult. Observation, therapy for underlying pulmonary disease (e.g., bronchodilators, broad-spectrum antimicrobials, smoking cessation), and periodic sputum cultures may be all that is required for most patients. For patients with significant symptoms and advanced or progressive radiographic disease, multidrug therapy is indicated. For children with cervical lymphadenitis from MAC, excisional surgery without chemotherapy is usually successful. A combination of surgical excision and chemotherapy is the usual treatment for adults with localized, nonpulmonary disease. Most cases of disseminated disease in immunosuppressed patients without AIDS respond to multidrug regimens. Multidrug therapy consisting of ethambutol, rifampin (or rifabutin), clofazimine, and an aminoglycoside has resulted in symptomatic and clinical improvement in most (but not all) patients with AIDS. Physicians experienced in pulmonary or mycobacterial disease may best direct the treatment of MAC disease.

Laboratory Diagnosis. Because the two species within the MAC are so similar, most laboratories do not distinguish between them but report isolates of both species as MAC. On primary isolation media, these organisms grow slowly, producing thin, transparent or opaque, homogeneous, smooth colonies. A small proportion of strains may exhibit rough colonies. Usually the colonies are nonpigmented, but they may become yellow with age. Rarely are the colonies pigmented from the onset of detectable growth. Optimum growth temperature is 37° C.

On microscopic examination, the cells are short and coccobacillary and uniformly stained without beading or banding. Long, thin, beaded bacilli resembling *Nocardia* spp. may be seen in stains of very young cultures or under certain other conditions. MAC species are inactive in most physiologic tests used to identify the mycobacteria. Exceptions are the production of a heat-stable catalase and the ability to grow on media containing 2 μg/mL of T2H. Nonisotopic nucleic acid probes are available for the identification of MAC as well as the two individual species.

Susceptibility Testing. In laboratory tests members of the MAC are generally resistant to the relatively low concentrations of anti-TB drugs currently used for testing *M. tuberculosis*. Treatment recommendations have been based largely on empiric data rather than in vitro susceptibility testing. For this reason, routine agar dilution susceptibility testing with the anti-TB agents, as currently performed for testing *M. tuberculosis*, is not recommended for MAC isolates. Currently the usefulness of testing at higher drug concentrations than used for *M. tuberculosis* or determination of minimun inhibitory concentration (MIC) is being evaluated. In vitro susceptibility studies using combinations of drugs have shown significant synergism between drugs. The significance of in vitro tests in predicting clinical response and recommendations for testing individual isolates have yet to be determined.

Mycobacterium avium subsp. *paratuberculosis*

Mycobacterium avium subsp. *paratuberculosis* is the causative agent of Johne disease, an intestinal infection occurring as a chronic diarrhea in cattle, sheep, goats, and other ruminants. A *Mycobacterium* sp. that closely resembles *M. avium* subsp. *paratuberculosis* was isolated from samples taken from resected terminal ileum of three patients with Crohn disease, although other studies have not found a link between Crohn disease and *M. avium* subsp. *paratuberculosis* or *M. avium* subsp. *silvaticum*. *M. avium* subsp. *paratuberculosis* is difficult to cultivate because of its very slow growth rate (3 to 4 months) and its need for a mycobactin-supplemented medium for primary isolation. Mycobactin is an iron-binding hydroxamate compound produced by other mycobacterial species.

Mycobacterium kansasii

Epidemiology. *Mycobacterium kansasii* is second to MAC as the cause of NTM lung disease. In the United States, most cases of *M. kansasii* infections have been reported from the southern states of Texas, Louisiana, and Florida; from Illinois and Missouri in the Midwest; and from California. *M. kansasii* strains have been isolated from water, but the natural source of human infection is not clear. As with other NTM, infections are not normally considered contagious from person to person.

Clinical Infections. The most common manifestation is chronic pulmonary disease involving the upper lobes, usually with evidence of cavitation and scarring. Extrapulmonary infections, including lymphadenitis, skin and soft tissue infections, and joint infection, have been reported occasionally. Disseminated *M. kansasii* infection rarely occurs in immunocompetent individuals but has been reported in severely immunocompromised patients, particularly those with AIDS.

When tested in vitro using the current drug concentrations recommended for *M. tuberculosis*, most strains of *M. kansasii* are susceptible to rifampin and ethambutol, partially resistant to isoniazid and streptomycin, and resistant to pyrazinamide. For treatment of pulmonary disease caused by *M. kansasii*, a multidrug regimen of isoniazid, rifampin, and ethambutol is currently recommended.

Laboratory Diagnosis. *Mycobacterium kansasii* is a slowly growing organism that appears as long rods with distinct cross-banding. *M. kansasii* has an optimal growth temperature of 37° C, and colonies appear smooth to rough with characteristic wavy edges and dark centers when grown on Middlebrook 7H10 agar. Some cording can usually be seen with low-power magnification. Colonies are **photochromogenic** (Figure 26-2); with prolonged exposure to light, most strains form dark red crystals of 10-β-carotene on the surface of and inside the colony. Photoreactivity is discussed later in this chapter. **Scotochromogenic** and **nonchromogenic** strains are rarely isolated. Most strains are strongly catalase positive (greater than 45 mm); less commonly isolated are strains that are low catalase producers (less than 45 mm).

Characteristics that distinguish this species are a growth rate similar to that of *M. tuberculosis* at 37° C, strong photochromogenic properties, ability to hydrolyze Tween 80 in 3 days, strong nitrate reduction, catalase production, and pyrazinamidase production. A nonisotopic nucleic acid probe for the identification of *M. kansasii* isolates is available commercially.

Mycobacterium asiaticum

Mycobacterium asiaticum is a normally saprophytic and rarely causes human infection. The cells are acid-fast coccoid rods. Growth on inspissated egg medium after 15 to 21 days at 37° C is dysgonic and smooth. Members of this species are usually photochromogenic. Occasional strains fail to develop pigment after exposure to light. *M. asiaticum* fails to reduce nitrate and produces a high level of heat-stable catalase. No accumulation of niacin and the hydrolysis of Tween 80 are useful characteristics in differentiating this organism from *M. simiae*.

Mycobacterium celatum

Mycobacterium celatum is a slowly growing, nonphotochromogenic organism that is very similar in biochemical characteristics to the MAC and *M. malmoense*. Mycolic acid patterns of this species, as determined by high-performance liquid chromatography (HPLC), are most similar to those of *M. xenopi* but are distinct from other described species. In contrast to *M. xenopi*, *M. celatum* grows best at 35° C and poorly at 42° C, produces large colonies on Middlebrook 7H10 agar, and is usually resistant to rifabutin. *M. celatum* is most frequently isolated from respiratory specimens but has also been recovered from stool and blood samples of both immunocompromised and immunocompetent individuals.

Mycobacterium genavense

Mycobacterium genavense has been reported as a cause of disseminated infections in patients with AIDS. It has also been associated with enteritis and genital and soft tissue infections in HIV-positive and HIV-negative immunocompro-

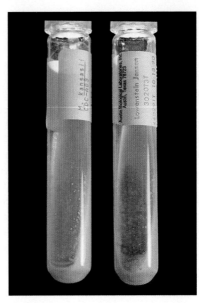

FIGURE 26-2 *Mycobacterium kansasii* growing on Löwenstein-Jensen medium showing photoreactivity. *Left,* Before exposure to light; *right,* after exposure to light.

mised patients. This slowly growing, fastidious mycobacterium has been recovered in BACTEC (BD Diagnostic Systems, Sparks, Md.) culture systems, but it failed to grow on subculture to routine solid media. Dysgonic growth was obtained when subculture medium Middlebrook 7H11 agar was supplemented with mycobactin. Isolates yield positive test results for semiquantitative and heat-stable catalase, pyrazinamidase, and urease.

Mycobacterium gordonae

Mycobacterium gordonae is commonly found in water taps and soil and is generally referred to as the "tap-water bacillus." This organism is frequently found in clinical specimens as a casual resident, but it is rarely implicated in disease. Infections reported in the literature have been isolated cases of meningitis secondary to ventriculoatrial shunts, hepatoperitoneal disease, endocarditis in a prosthetic aortic valve, synovitis, cutaneous lesions of the hand, and possible cases of pulmonary disease. In laboratory antituberculosis drug-resistance tests, *M. gordonae* is resistant to isoniazid, streptomycin, and p-aminosalicylic acid but susceptible to rifampin and ethambutol.

Growth of *M. gordonae* appears on egg-based medium after 10 to 14 days as smooth, yellow-orange colonies pigmented with both absence of and exposure to light. Optimum growth temperature range is 22° to 37° C. Differential characteristics are negative nitrate reduction, ability to hydrolyze Tween 80, and the production of heat-stable catalase. Isolates of *M. gordonae* can be rapidly identified with the use of a commercially available nucleic acid probe specific to the species.

Mycobacterium haemophilum

The rare infections associated with *M. haemophilum* occur primarily in patients who are immunocompromised. Cases have been reported in patients with Hodgkin disease and

AIDS. Submandibular lymphadenitis, subcutaneous nodules, painful swellings, ulcers progressing to abscesses, and draining fistulas are often the clinical manifestations.

A unique characteristic of this organism is its requirement for hemoglobin or hemin for growth. Isolation of this species is accomplished on media supplying the needed growth supplement, such as chocolate (CHOC) agar, Mueller-Hinton agar with 5% Fildes enrichment, and LJ medium containing 2% ferric ammonium citrate. Successful isolation on Middlebrook 7H10 agar with an X-factor disk planted in the inoculated area has been reported. Optimum growth temperature is 28° to 32° C; little or no growth occurs at 37° C. Colonies are rough to smooth and nonpigmented. Microscopically the cells are strongly acid-fast, short, occasionally curved bacilli without banding or beading and arranged in tight clusters or cords.

Mycobacterium malmoense

Pulmonary disease associated with *M. malmoense* has been reported more commonly outside the United States in Sweden, England, Wales, and Scotland. Reports of cases of chronic pulmonary disease and cervical lymphadenitis in the United States have appeared, however. In laboratory studies using conventional antituberculosis drug-resistance testing, *M. malmoense* is resistant to isoniazid, streptomycin, p-aminosalicylic acid, and rifampin and is susceptible to ethambutol and cycloserine.

Mycobacterium malmoense appears as a short coccobacillus without cross-bands on acid-fast–stained smears. Colonies are smooth (Figure 26-3), glistening, and opaque with dense centers. Color is nonpigmented to buff; exposure to light does not induce pigment production. Growth rate is slow; optimum growth temperature is 37° C. Growth at 22° C may require as much as 7 weeks of incubation. Some strains may require longer incubation (up to 12 weeks) before colonies become visible. For this reason some investigators suspect that *M. malmoense* may be underreported in the United States because most laboratories incubate cultures for 6 weeks, 2 to 6 weeks less than the incubation period needed for some strains of this organism. The increase in the isolation of *M. malmoense* may be attributed to the implementation of radiometric culture techniques in larger laboratories. Differential characteristics of *M. malmoense* are no accumulation of niacin, absence of nitrate reduction, ability to hydrolyze Tween 80, and the production of a heat-stable catalase. *M. malmoense* can be differentiated from biochemically similar *M. gastri* on the basis of the urease-negative and pyrazinamidase-positive reactions of *M. malmoense*.

Mycobacterium marinum

Mycobacterium marinum has been implicated in diseases of fish and isolated from aquariums. Cutaneous infections in humans have occurred when traumatized skin came in contact with inadequately chlorinated freshwater or with saltwater. Outbreaks of cutaneous lesions in lifeguards have been reported. The typical presentation of a tender red or blue-red subcutaneous nodule, or "swimming pool granuloma," usually occurs on the elbow, knee, toe, or finger. In some cases an abscess develops at the primary site of inoculation, with sec-

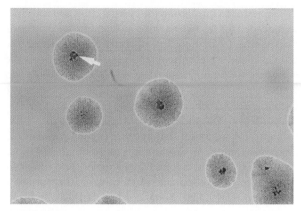

FIGURE 26-3 *Mycobacterium malmoense* on Middlebrook 7H10 medium.

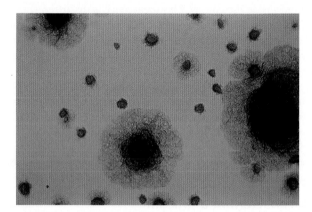

FIGURE 26-4 *Mycobacterium marinum* on Middlebrook 7H10 medium producing rough colonies.

ondary ascending spread along the lymphatics. Treatment modalities include simple observation of minor lesions, surgical excision, anti-TB drug therapy, and the use of single antimicrobial agents. In standard in vitro susceptibility testing currently used to test *M. tuberculosis*, *M. marinum* is susceptible to rifampin and ethambutol, resistant to isoniazid and pyrazinamide, and partially resistant or intermediate to streptomycin.

Cells of *M. marinum* are moderately long to long rods with cross-barring. Colonies of this slowly growing organism are smooth to rough (Figure 26-4) and wrinkled on inspissated egg medium but may be smooth when grown on Middlebrook 7H10 or 7H11 agar. *M. marinum* is photochromogenic; young colonies grown in the dark may be nonpigmented or buff, whereas colonies grown in or exposed to light develop a deep yellow color. Growth is optimum at incubation temperatures of 28° to 32° C. These preferences for growth at the lower incubation temperatures, along with photochromogenicity, are clues to the identification of *M. marinum*. Some strains of *M. marinum* produce niacin; however, none reduces nitrate or produces heat-stable catalase. The organisms hydrolyze Tween 80 and produce urease and pyrazinamidase.

Mycobacterium scrofulaceum

The most common form of disease associated with *M. scrofulaceum* is cervical lymphadenitis in children. The infection manifests in one or more enlarged nodes, often adjacent to the mandible and high in the neck, with little or no pain. Patients are usually treated by surgical incision and drainage; anti-TB drugs usually are not necessary. Pulmonary infections caused by *M. scrofulaceum* have been reported. Before being replaced by the MAC, *M. scrofulaceum* was the most common cause of cervical lymphadenitis in children. *M. scrofulaceum* is resistant to isoniazid, streptomycin, ethambutol, and p-aminosalicylic acid when tested in vitro using the current procedure for testing *M. tuberculosis*.

On microscopic examination, *M. scrofulaceum* is a uniformly stained, acid-fast, medium to long rod. The organism grows slowly (4 to 6 weeks) at incubation temperatures ranging from 25° to 37° C. Colonies are smooth with dense centers and pigmentation from light yellow to deep orange. The organism is scotochromogenic (Figure 26-5). Members of this species do not hydrolyze Tween 80 or reduce nitrate, but they do produce urease and are high (greater than 45 mm) catalase producers. These characteristics aid in differentiating this organism from other slowly growing scotochromogens, including certain strains of MAC, *M. gordonae*, and *M. szulgai*.

Mycobacterium simiae

The original strains of *M. simiae* were isolated from the lymph nodes of monkeys. Although the organism has been recovered from tap water, there seems to be significant geographic variation in the incidence. For example, *M. simiae* is rarely isolated in most parts of the United States, but in parts of Texas, it is a relatively common isolate. Infrequent cases of human infection from *M. simiae* have been reported and are most often pulmonary disease in patients with preexisting lung damage. Many isolates are resistant to most anti-TB drugs.

Cells of *M. simiae* appear as short coccobacilli. When they are grown on inspissated egg medium at 37° C, smooth colonies appear in 10 to 21 days. Colonies on Middlebrook 7H10 agar are thin, transparent or tiny, and filamentous. The species is usually photochromogenic. Development of the yellow pigment may require prolonged incubation, whereas some strains may fail to produce pigment on exposure to light. Differential biochemical characteristics are the accumulation of niacin, negative nitrate reduction, and high-level (greater than 45 mm) heat-stable catalase. *M. simiae* is one of the very few NTM that produces niacin, making it possible to confuse the identification with *M. tuberculosis* if pigment production under light is not performed.

Mycobacterium szulgai

Of the reported infections with *M. szulgai*, the most common manifestation is pulmonary disease similar to TB. Extrapulmonary infections, including lymphadenitis and bursitis, also have been reported. This organism is much more susceptible than MAC to the conventional anti-TB drugs.

On microscopic examination of an acid fast–stained smear, cells of *M. szulgai* are medium to long rods with some cross-barring. When the organism is cultured on egg-based medium at 37° C, smooth and rough colonies are observed. At 37° C, yellow to orange pigment develops in the absence of light and intensifies with exposure to light (scotochromogenic). Colo-

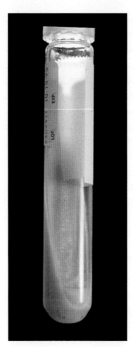

FIGURE 26-5 *Mycobacterium scrofulaceum* on Löwenstein-Jensen medium.

nies grown at 22° C are nonpigmented or buff in the absence of light and develop yellow to orange pigment with light exposure (photochromogenic). Based on 16s rRNA sequences, *M. szulgai* most closely resembles *M. malmoense*. Characteristics that differentiate *M. szulgai* from other slowly growing mycobacteria are slow hydrolysis of Tween 80, positive nitrate reduction, and inability to grow in the presence of 5% sodium chloride.

Mycobacterium terrae Complex

The *M. terrae* complex includes three species: *M. terrae, M. nonchromogenicum*, and *M. triviale*. A few cases of human infection associated with the *M. terrae* complex have been reported: septic arthritis, synovitis, osteomyelitis, respiratory infection, and tenosynovitis of the fingers, hands, and wrists. Isolates from the sputum and gastric lavage of humans are not uncommon and often are considered casual residents. Primary lung disease due to *M. nonchromogenicum* has been reported.

Microscopically members of the *M. terrae* complex appear as acid-fast, short to medium coccobacilli. The species grows slowly at an optimum temperature of 37° C and is nonphotochromogenic. Colonies of *M. triviale* on egg-based medium are rough, dry, and heaped, whereas the colonies of *M. terrae* tend to be smoother. Colonies of *M. nonchromogenicum* are smooth to rough and white to buff. Characteristics that differentiate the complex from other mycobacteria are hydrolysis of Tween 80, reduction of nitrate, and the presence of a heat-stable catalase. Members of the complex can only be differentiated by molecular techniques.

Mycobacterium ulcerans

Mycobacterium ulcerans is a rare cause of mycobacteriosis, also referred to as Buruli ulcer, in the United States but may be underreported as a result of difficulty in isolation. Worldwide *M. ulcerans* is the third most common *Mycobacterium* sp., behind *M. tuberculosis* and *M. leprae*. The disease manifests as a painless nodule under the skin after previous trauma. A shallow ulcer develops that may be quite severe. Patients rarely develop fever or systemic symptoms.

The acid-fast cells of *M. ulcerans* are moderately long without beading or cross-banding. Optimal growth temperature is 30° to 33° C with little growth at 25° C and usually none at 37° C. The organism grows slowly, often requiring 6 to 12 weeks of incubation before colonies are evident. Colonies are smooth and rough and nonpigmented or lightly buff, and they do not develop pigment with exposure to light. *M. ulcerans* produces a heat-stable catalase but is inert in most other conventional biochemical tests.

Mycobacterium xenopi

Mycobacterium xenopi has been recovered from hot- and cold-water taps (including water storage tanks of hospitals) and birds. The organism was first isolated from an African toad and was considered nonpathogenic for humans until 1965. Isolation of *M. xenopi* is relatively uncommon in the United States, yet it has been reported as one of the most commonly found NTM in southeast England. The reported human cases of *M. xenopi* infection are mostly slowly progressive pulmonary infections in individuals with predisposing conditions. Preexistent lung disease, alcoholism, malignancy, and diabetes mellitus are some of the conditions associated with reported *M. xenopi* infections. The pulmonary infections presented clinical pictures similar to those seen in patients with *M. tuberculosis, M. kansasii,* or MAC infection. Disseminated and extrapulmonary infections have been reported. Strains of *M. xenopi* are susceptible to the quinolones (ciprofloxacin and ofloxacin); some isolates are susceptible to vancomycin, erythromycin, or cefuroxime. In vitro susceptibility to anti-TB drugs is variable, with resistance to ethambutol only being the most common pattern.

On acid-fast–stained smears, *M. xenopi* are long, filamentous rods. Colonies of this slowly growing mycobacterium on Middlebrook 7H10 agar are small with dense centers and filamentous edges. Microscopic observation (low-power magnification) of colonies growing on cornmeal-glycerol agar reveals distinctive round colonies with branching and filamentous extensions; aerial hyphae are usually seen in rough colonies. Furthermore, young colonies grown on cornmeal agar show a "bird's nest" appearance with characteristic sticklike projections. Optimal growth temperature is 42° C; the organism grows more rapidly at this temperature than at 37° C and fails to grow at 25° C. *M. xenopi* has been classified with the nonphotochromogenic group; however, colonies are frequently bright yellow on primary isolation when incubated in the absence of light and when exposed to light. Distinctive characteristics, in addition to optimum growth at 42° C and yellow scotochromogenic pigment, are negative reactions for niacin accumulation, nitrate reduction, and positive reactions for the production of heat-stable catalase, arylsulfatase, and pyrazinamidase.

Rapidly Growing Species

Mycobacterium chelonae–Mycobacterium abscessus Group

The three most important rapidly growing mycobacteria causing human infections are *M. chelonae, M. abscessus,* and *M. fortuitum. M. chelonae* is found in the environment and associated with many of the same opportunistic infections as *M. fortuitum. M. chelonae* is the species of rapidly growing mycobacteria most likely isolated from disseminated cutaneous infections in immunocompromised patients. Both *M. fortuitum* and *M. chelonae* have been associated with a variety of infections of the skin, lungs, bone, central nervous system, and prosthetic heart valves. However, the two species vary in their susceptibility to antimicrobial agents. For this reason, determination of species of clinically significant isolates may be warranted. *M. chelonae* exhibits more resistance to antimicrobial agents than *M. fortuitum* does but sometimes is susceptible to amikacin and a sulfonamide.

Mycobacterium chelonae is closely related to *M. abscessus,* formerly designated as *M. chelonae* subsp. *abscessus. M. abscessus* is a commonly isolated rapidly growing mycobacterium that has been associated with chronic lung disease, otitis media following tympanostomy tube insertion, and disseminated cutaneous infections. In fact, 80% of cases of pulmonary disease due to rapidly growing mycobacteria are caused by *M. abscessus.* Infections by this organism have also been seen in patients with cystic fibrosis. Unlike with *M. chelonae,* tap water is an important reservoir for *M. abscessus.* Microscopically, young cultures of *M. chelonae* are strongly acid fast, with pleomorphism ranging from long, tapered to short, thick rods. This rapidly growing mycobacterium produces rough or smooth, nonpigmented to buff colonies within 3 to 5 days of incubation at 37° C. A positive 3-day arylsulfatase test, no reduction of nitrate, and growth on MacConkey agar without crystal violet are characteristics that help differentiate *M. chelonae* and *M. abscessus* from other nonchromogenic rapidly growing mycobacteria.

Mycobacterium fortuitum Group

Historically, the *M. fortuitum* group contained the species *M. fortuitum, M. peregrinum,* and an unnamed third species. However, in the past several years, seven new species have been added. Common in the environment, *M. fortuitum* has been isolated from water, soil, and dust. The organism has been implicated frequently in infections of the skin and soft tissues, including localized infections and abscesses at the site of puncture wounds. The *M. fortuitum* group is the most common rapidly growing mycobacteria associated with localized cutaneous infections. Infections associated with long-term use of intravenous and peritoneal catheters, injection sites, and surgical wounds following mammoplasty and cardiac bypass procedures have been reported. A variety of other infections have been associated with *M. fortuitum.* Differences in susceptibility to antimicrobial agents occur among the species; thus in vitro susceptibility testing is often recommended for clinically significant isolates. A test method using a broth microdilution MIC determination has been studied for the rapidly growing mycobacteria.

After 3 to 5 days of incubation at 37° C, colonies of *M. fortuitum* appear rough or smooth and either nonpigmented, creamy white, or buff. Microscopic examination of growth on cornmeal-glycerol and Middlebrook 7H11 agars after 1 to 2 days of incubation reveals colonies with branching, filamentous extensions and rough colonies with short aerial hyphae. On microscopic examination, cells are pleomorphic, ranging from long and tapered to short, thick rods. Cells from most cultures, especially older ones, tend to decolorize and appear partially acid-fast on any of the acid-fast staining techniques. Additional characteristics that distinguish *M. fortuitum* from other rapidly growing mycobacteria are the positive 3-day arylsulfatase test and the reduction of nitrate.

Mycobacterium smegmatis Group

The *M. smegmatis* group contains the three species *M. smegmatis* sensu stricto, *M. goodii,* and *M. wolinskyi.* However, recent studies based on DNA sequencing indicate that *M. wolinskyi* should be placed into a different group. Commonly considered saprophytic, *M. smegmatis* has been implicated in rare cases of pulmonary, skin, soft tissue, and bone infections.

Microscopically, on acid-fast stain, cells are long and tapered or short rods with irregular acid fastness. Occasionally rods are curved with branching or Y-shaped forms; swollen with deeper staining, beaded, or ovoid forms are sometimes seen. Colonies appearing on egg medium after 2 to 4 days are usually rough, wrinkled, or coarsely folded; smooth, glistening, butyrous colonies may also be seen. Colonies on Middlebrook 7H10 agar are heaped and smooth or rough with dense centers. Pigmentation is rare or late; colonies appear nonpigmented, creamy white, or buff to pink in older cultures. In addition to the rapid growth rate and the nonpigmented, rough colonies, characteristics valuable in the identification of this organism are its negative arylsulfatase reaction, positive iron uptake, ability to reduce nitrate, and growth in the presence of 5% NaCl and on MacConkey agar without crystal violet.

MYCOBACTERIUM LEPRAE

Mycobacterium leprae is the causative agent of Hansen disease (leprosy), an infection of the skin, mucous membranes, and peripheral nerves. The disease is rare in the United States and other Western countries, yet it remains a major problem in other parts of the world. At one time, the World Health Organization (WHO) estimated that 11 million people had Hansen disease. However, the WHO launched an eradication program, and since 1985, the incidence of Hansen disease has been reduced by about 90%. Since 1995, WHO has provided treatment free of charge to all patients with Hansen disease. The annual incidence of new cases has steadily declined since 2001 to about 254,000 cases in 2007. In the United States, generally fewer than 100 cases are reported annually; cases are generally acquired abroad.

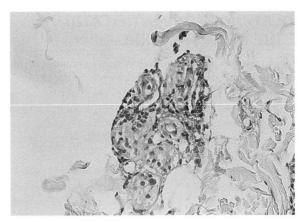

FIGURE 26-6 *Mycobacterium leprae* from a skin biopsy from a patient with lepromatous leprosy (acid-fast smear stained with Ziehl-Neelsen stain).

Despite its reputation, Hansen disease is not considered a highly contagious disease. Two major forms of the disease exist: tuberculoid leprosy and lepromatous leprosy. Symptoms of tuberculoid leprosy include skin lesions and nerve involvement that can produce areas with loss of sensation. Patients eventually exhibit an effective cell-mediated immune (CMI) response. The optimal growth temperature for *M. leprae* is approximately 30° C, and because the patient mounts an adequate immune response, the bacteria tend to remain in the extremities. Spontaneous recovery often occurs with tuberculoid leprosy.

Conversely, patients with lepromatous leprosy do not produce an effective CMI response. The disease is slowly progressive, malignant, and if untreated, life threatening. It is characterized by skin lesions and progressive, symmetric nerve damage. Lesions of the mucous membranes of the nose may lead to destruction of the cartilaginous septum, resulting in nasal and facial deformities. Current therapy usually consists of a combination of diaminodiphenylsulfone (dapsone), clofazimine, and rifampin. Laboratory diagnosis of Hansen disease depends on the microscopic demonstration of AFB that cannot be cultured from skin biopsy specimens. *M. leprae* has not been grown on artificial media.

In patients with tuberculoid leprosy, organisms are extremely rare and may not be detected in skin scrapings or biopsy specimens. However, AFB are usually abundant in samples from patients with lepromatous leprosy (Figure 26-6). *M. leprae* is a rod-shaped bacterium, usually 1 to 7 μm long and 0.3 to 0.5 μm wide. After examination of the entire smear, the number of organisms present per oil immersion field (1000×) is reported as the bacteriologic index (BI). The number of solid-staining cells per 100 total bacilli examined is reported as the morphologic index (MI). Solid-staining cells are those with dense, uniform staining of the entire bacillus with even sides and rounded ends in which the length of the bacillus is at least five times the width of the bacillus. The BI and MI aid the clinician in determining the progress of the disease. The definitive laboratory diagnosis is the development of disease in laboratory mice following inoculation of patient biopsy material to the mouse footpad.

ISOLATION AND IDENTIFICATION OF THE MYCOBACTERIA

Rate of growth, colony morphology, pigmentation, nutritional requirements, optimum incubation temperature, and biochemical test results are traditional characteristics used to differentiate species within the genus *Mycobacterium* (Table 26-1). More rapid techniques include broth-based culture systems, including some that monitor cultures continuously during the incubation period. A limited number of species-specific nucleic acid probes offer rapid identification of culture isolates. Researchers have developed polymerase chain reaction (PCR) assays, which increase the sensitivity of nucleic acid probes. Other techniques, such as HPLC, have been used to distinguish mycobacterial species. The application of PCR and chromatography methods has moved out of the research and larger reference mycobacteriology laboratories to routine laboratories, and these methods are being increasingly adopted by clinical laboratories.

Laboratory Safety Considerations

The serious nature of tuberculosis disease and the usual airborne route of infection require that special safety precautions be used by anyone handling mycobacterial specimens. The incidence of tuberculosis infection (i.e., skin test positivity) in those who work in the mycobacteriology laboratory is at least three times higher than that among other laboratory personnel in a given institution. The hazard of working in a mycobacteriology laboratory is minimal, however, when the laboratory is well designed, appropriate equipment is available, and precautions are followed closely.

Personnel Safety

The administration of the microbiology laboratory must ensure that each employee is (1) provided with adequate safety equipment, (2) trained in safe laboratory procedures, (3) informed of the hazards associated with the procedures, (4) prepared for action following an unexpected accident, and (5) monitored regularly by medical personnel. Laboratory personnel must be responsible for using appropriate safety equipment and following established procedures. A skin test (Mantoux) with PPD should be administered the first day of employment and thereafter regularly to persons previously skin test negative (nonreactors). Individuals known to be previously skin test positive (reactors) should be counseled regularly and referred for medical evaluation if their health status changes.

Ventilation

Laboratory design and ventilation play important roles in mycobacteriology laboratory safety. Ideally the mycobacteriology laboratory should be separate from the remainder of the laboratory and have a nonrecirculating ventilation system. The area in which specimens and cultures are processed should have negative air pressure in relation to other areas; that is, the airflow should be from clean areas, such as corridors, into less clean areas (mycobacteriology laboratory). Six to 12 room-air changes per hour effectively remove 99% or more of airborne particles within 30 to 45 minutes. A much higher number of room-air changes per hour can cause problems of air turbulence within the biologic safety cabinets.

Biological Safety Cabinet

Because the route of infection by mycobacteria is primarily through inhalation, it is essential that the dispersal of organisms into the air be minimized and that inhalation of airborne bacilli be avoided. The biological safety cabinet is the single most important piece of equipment in a mycobacteriology laboratory. Various types of safety cabinets are available, including class I negative-pressure cabinets and class II vertical-laminar flow cabinets. Proper installation, maintenance, and testing are essential to their performance. Each safety cabinet should be tested and recertified at least yearly by trained personnel with special monitoring equipment. Processing clinical specimens or transferring viable cultures outside a safety cabinet should not be permitted.

To prevent the dispersal of infectious aerosols into the laboratory area, all potentially infectious materials should be tightly covered when they are outside the biological safety cabinet. Specimens should be centrifuged in aerosol-free safety carriers, and the tubes should be removed from the safety carriers only inside the biological safety cabinet. Specimens taken out of the safety cabinet for transport to a decontamination area must be covered. After the safety cabinet work area has been cleaned with disinfectant, the ultraviolet (UV) light (which kills microorganisms) inside the cabinet should be used to eliminate further any contamination of surfaces and airborne bacteria. Because of the hazards to skin and eyes associated with excess UV light, the UV light should be turned on only when the safety cabinet is not in use.

Use of Proper Disinfectant

Covering the work surface with a towel or absorbent pad soaked in a disinfectant reduces the accidental creation of infectious aerosols. In the selection of a disinfectant for the mycobacteriology laboratory, the product brochure should be consulted to ensure that the disinfectant is bactericidal for mycobacteria (tuberculocidal). The following types of disinfectants are suitable for cleaning work areas, but some have limitations on their use.

- *Sodium hypochlorite* is effective at a concentration of 0.1% to 0.5% (e.g., a 1:50 to 1:10 dilution of most household bleaches). The solution should be made fresh daily, and contact time should be 10 to 30 minutes. Sodium hypochlorite loses effectiveness in the presence of a large amount of protein material.
- *Phenol*, 5%, with a contact time of 10 to 30 minutes is adequate. Phenol is irritating to the skin and hazardous to the eyes.
- *Phenol-soap mixtures* containing orthophenol or other phenolic derivatives are effective with contact periods of 10 to 30 minutes.
- *Formaldehyde*, 3% to 8%, or alkaline glutaraldehyde, 2%, is effective. Contact time should be at least 30 minutes.

Other Precautions

For sterilizing a wire-inoculating loop, an electric incinerator should be used within the biological safety cabinet. An

TABLE 26-1   Identification of Clinically Important Mycobacteria*

Descriptive term	Species (Subspecies)	Colony Morphology	Temp. Growth Range (°C)	Growth Rate (R=Rapid, S=Slow)	Pigment (Photo, Scoto, Nonphoto)	Arylsulfatase 3 Days	Arylsulfatase 2 Weeks	Carbon: Sodium Citrate	Carbon: Inositol	Carbon: Mannitol	Catalase Semi-Quant >45	Catalase Heat Stable (68°C)	Iron Uptake	Growth on MacConkey	Niacin	Nitrate Reduction	Pyrazinamidase†	Growth on 5% NaCl	Tellurite Reduction	Growth on T2H	Tween Hydrolysis +10 Day	Tween Opacity (1 Week)	Urease‡
Rapid growers	M. fortuitum biovar fortuitum	Smooth, Rough (13) (87)	22-40	R	N (99)	+(97)	+(99)	−(99)	−(99)	−(99)	(98)	+(94)	+(99)	+(96)	−(99)	+(99)		+(75)	+(97)	+(99)	+−(50)	+(91)	+(93)
	M. fortuitum biovar peregrinum	Smooth	22-37				+(98)	−(99)	−(99)	+(99)													
	M. fortuitum‖ third biovariant complex	Smooth	22-37	R(97)	N (99)			−(99)	+(99)	+(99)													
	M. chelonae subsp. chelonae	Smooth, Rough 60/40	22-35	R(97)	N (99)	+(96)	+(98)	+(99)	−(99)	−(99)	(97)	+/−(53/47)	−(98)	+(96)	−(92)	−(99)		−(99)	+(85)	+(98)	+/−(93/47)		+(99)
	M. chelonae subsp. abscessus		22-40					−(99)	−(99)	−(99)			+−Tan(99)					+(90)					
	M. chelonae (turtlelike)	Rough	22-30	R(30°)				+(99)	−(99)	−(99)		−(74)	−(99)	−(99)	−(99)	+(99)		−(99)	+(99)	+(99)	+(99)		+(96)
	M. fallax§ (looks like M. tb.)	Rough	30-37	S(37°)	N = 99%	−(99)		−(99)	−(99)	−(99)				−(99)	−(99)	+(99)		−(99)	+(87)	+(99)	+(75)		+(66)
	Other rapid growers	Smooth or Rough	17-52		P = 4%, S = 38%, N = 58%	−(72)	+(75)	−(70)	+(59)	+(60)	+(66)	+(63)	−(56)	+(52)	−(95)	−(51)		−(52)		+(99)		V	
	M. ulcerans	Smooth, Rough	25-33	S	N	−					−	+			−			−		+			−
TB complex	M. tuberculosis	Rough, Cords	33-39	S	N = 99%	−(99)	−(93)				−(99)	−(99)		−(99)	+(98)	+(99)	+(98)	−(99)	−(70)	+(92)	+(68)	−(83)	+(98)
	M. africanum	Rough	35-38	S	N	−(99)	−				−	−(99)		−(99)	−(95)	−(99)		−(99)	−(99)	Var.	−	Var.	+(99)
	M. bovis	1710 = R, LJ = S	35-38	S	N = 99%	−(99)	−(87)				−(97)	−(92)		−(99)	−(95)	−(94)	−(98)	−(99)	−(55)	−(94)	−(84)	−(75)	+(99)

Modified from Kent PT, Kubica GP: *Public health mycobacteriology: a guide for the level III laboratory,* Atlanta, 1985, Centers for Disease Control and Prevention.

*Test reactions listed as "+" or "−" followed by percentage of strains reacting as indicated. If no percentage is given or space is blank, insufficient data were available or test is of no apparent value.

†Pyrazinamidase data (Wayne Method) from both Wayne and Hawkins. Unless indicated, results are those at 4 days. Strains of *M. tuberculosis* resistant to PZA are often pyrazinamidase-negative. Within *M. terrae* complex, *M. nonchromogenicum* usually "+" and *M. terrae* usually "−".

‡Urease data (Murphy-Hawkins Disk Method) primarily from Dr. Jean E. Hawkins. Reference Laboratory for Tuberculosis and Other Mycobacterial Diseases, Veterans Administration Medical Center, West Haven, Conn., and Department of Laboratory Medicine, Yale University School of Medicine, New Haven, Conn.

§Data on *M. fallax* from Levy-Frebault et al (IJSB 33:336, 1983).

‖Several strains in this complex have varied in carbon sources as follows: "+" sodium citrate, "+" mannitol, "−" inositol.

Continued

TABLE 26-1 Identification of Clinically Important Mycobacteria—cont'd

Descriptive term	Species (Subspecies)	Colony Morphology	Temp. Growth Range (°C)	Growth Rate (R = Rapid, S = Slow)	Pigment (Photo, Scoto, Nonphoto)	Arylsulfatase 3 Days	Arylsulfatase 2 Weeks	Sodium Citrate	Inositol	Mannitol	Semi-Quant >45	Catalase Heat Stable (68°C)	Iron Uptake	Growth on MacConkey	Niacin	Nitrate Reduction	Pyrazinamidase†	Growth on 5% NaCl	Tellurite Reduction	Growth on T2H	Tween Hydrolysis +10 Day	Tween Opacity (1 Week)	Urease†
Nonphotochromogens	M. avium complex	Smooth / Rough / Trans. (99)	22-45	S = 99%	N = 85%, S = 12%, P = 3%	-(99)	+(51)				-(99)	+(76)		-(68)	-(99)	-(92)	+(86) 4d	-(99)	+(82)	+(99)	-(98)	-(99)	+(99)
	M. xenopi	Smooth	35-45	S	N = 80%, S = 20%	+(76)	+(99)				+(99)	+(83)		-(99)	-(99)	-(94)	+(51)	-(99)	-(59)	+(99)	-(99)	-(99)	-(99)
	M. shimoidei	Rough	30-45	S	N	-	-				-	+		-	-	-	+	-	+	+	+		-
	M. gastri	Smooth	25-40	S = 80%, R = 20%	N = 99%	-(96)	+(99)				-(99)	-(99)		-(84)	-(99)	-(99)	+(99) 4d	-(99)	-(74)	+(99)	+(99)	-(99)	+(79)
	M. terrae complex	(Smooth few / Rough)	22-37	S = 77%, R = 23%	N = 95%, S = 4%	-(99)	-(51)				+(99)	+(96)		-(77)	-(99)	+(72)	+(63) 4d, +(86) 7d	-(94)	-(75)	+(99)	+(99)	-(93)	-(91)
	M. triviale	Rough	22-37	S	N = 99%	-(66)	+(99)				+(93)	+(99)		-(99)	-(97)	+(99)	+(60) 4d, +(90) 7d	+(99)	-(99)	+(99)	+(99)		-(86)
	M. malmoense	Smooth	22-37	S	N = 90%, S = 10%	-(99)	-(89)				-(99)	+(69)		-(99)	-(99)	-(99)	+ 4d	-(99)	+(71)	+(99)	+(97)		-(67)
	M. haemophilum (Needs hemin)	Rough	22-35	S	N	-(99)	-				-	-	-		-	-	+		-	+	-		
Photochromes	M. simiae	Smooth	22-37	S	P = 91%, N = 9%	-	-(84)				+(99)	+(95)	-(99)	-(99)	+(85)	-(85)	+	-(99)	+(85)	+(99)	-(85)	-(64)	+(64)
	M. kansasii	Smooth / Rough	25-40	S = 98%, R = 2%	N = 99%, S = <1%, P = <1%	-(99)	+(55)				+(99)	+(95)		-(99)	-(99)	+(99)	+(99) 4d, +(69) 7d	-(99)	-(84)	+(99)	+(99)	-(97)	+(97)
	M. marinum	Smooth	25-35	R = 61%, S = 39%	P = 99%	-(66)	+(99)				-(79)	-(58)	-(99)	-(99)	-(80)	-(96)	+(99)	-(97)	-(79)	+(99)	+(99)		+(99)
	M. asiaticum	Smooth	33-37	S = 95%	P = 99%	-(99)	-(67)				+(91)	+(91)		-(99)	-(99)	-(99)	+(99)	-(99)	-(70)	+(99)	+(91)		-(99)
Scotochromogens	M. scrofulaceum	Smooth	22-37	S = 5%	S = 97%, P = 3%	-(99)	-(64)				+(93)	+(96)		-(99)	-(99)	-(85)	+(60) 4d, +(99) 7d	-(99)	-(57)	+(99)	-(98)	-(99)	+(99)
	M. szulgai	(Smooth / Rough)	22-37	S = 99%	S P (99), 37° 25°	-(99)	-(62)				+(99)	+(81)		-(99)	-(99)	+(99)	+ 4d	-(99)	+(56)	+(99)	±(50)	-(99)	+(94)
	M. scrofulaceum	(Smooth / Rough)	22-37	R = 1%, S = 99%	S = 99%	-(99)	+(57)				+(92)	+(97)		-(99)	-(99)	-(95)	-(67) 4d, +(78) 7d	-(99)	-(77)	+(98)	+(99)	-(99)	-(85)
	M. flavescens	Smooth	25-42	R = 59%, S = 41%	S = 99%	-(84)	+(78)				+(85)	+(99)		-(99)	-(99)	+(96)	+(99)	+(71)	-(67)	+(99)	+(97)	+(99)	+(71)

alcohol-sand flask can also be used to clean the waxy culture material from the wire before flaming in a Bunsen burner. Disposable sterile applicator sticks or plastic transfer loops are convenient and efficient for making smears and transfers. Splash-proof discard containers must be used to prevent aerosol formation and possible cross-contamination of samples.

Personal protective equipment provides extra safety for staff working in the mycobacteriology laboratory. All manipulations with cultures or specimens should be done with gloves and laboratory coats or gowns. In addition, respiratory protection must be used when performing procedures outside of the biological safety cabinet when aerosolization could result. The minimum level of respiratory protection is a respirator that contains a National Institute for Occupational Safety and Health–certified N series filter with 95% efficiency rating (N-95). In addition to being trained to use the respirator, laboratory staff must be fit-tested. Some laboratory directors believe that caps and shoe covers should also be worn.

Specimen Collection

Mycobacteria may be recovered from a variety of clinical specimens, including respiratory specimens, urine, feces, blood, CSF, tissue biopsies, and aspirations of any tissue or organ. Thus successful isolation of mycobacteria from clinical specimens begins with properly collected and handled specimens. Whenever possible, diagnostic specimens should be collected before the initiation of therapy. All specimens should be transported to the laboratory immediately after collection. If immediate transport is not possible, the specimen may be refrigerated overnight. Ideally, laboratories should process specimens for mycobacteria daily as delays in processing may lead to false-negative cultures and increased bacterial contamination.

Each specimen should be confined to a single collection in an individual collection container recommended by the laboratory providing the requested diagnostic service. The most commonly recommended container is a sterile, wide-mouth cup with a tightly fitted lid. Also, special sterile receptacles containing a 50-mL centrifuge tube for sputum collection are available commercially. Because of small sample volume, the use of swabs for clinical specimens is discouraged. As with all specimens for microbiologic examination, aseptic collection is important. The spectrum of illness caused by *Mycobacterium* spp. is so broad that almost any site can yield an acceptable specimen. Each specimen type, even when properly collected, transported, and processed, may have an intrinsic maximal yield. This can be the result of tubercle burden at the collection site or of environmental effects, such as pH, that can affect recovery. Emphasis should be placed on collecting the number and types of specimens that, when transported and processed correctly, maximize the diagnostic yield. Box 26-2 lists the types of clinical samples acceptable for mycobacteriologic culture.

Sputum and Other Respiratory Secretions

Although a variety of clinical specimens may be submitted to the laboratory to recover MTB and NTM, respiratory secretions such as sputum and bronchial aspirates are the most

---

BOX 26-2   Acceptable Specimens for Processing

Respiratory Specimens
Spontaneously expectorated sputum
Normal saline–nebulized, induced sputum
Transtracheal aspirate
Bronchoalveolar lavage
Bronchoalveolar brushing
Laryngeal swab
Nasopharyngeal swab

Body Fluids
Pleural fluid
Pericardial fluid
Joint aspirate
Gastric aspirate
Peritoneal fluid
Cerebrospinal fluid
Stool
Urine
Pus

Body Tissues
Blood
Bone marrow biopsy/aspirate
Solid organ
Lymph node
Bone
Skin

---

common. An early-morning specimen should be collected on three consecutive days. Pooled specimens are unacceptable because of increased contamination. The number of specimens necessary to obtain culture confirmation and perform susceptibility testing is related to the frequency of smear positivity. If at least two of the first three sputum direct smears are positive, then three specimens are often sufficient to confirm a diagnosis. However, when none, or only one, of the first three sputum smears is positive, additional specimens are needed for culture confirmation. Smear positivity and culture yield vary with the extent of the disease (i.e., whether there is cavitary or noncavitary pulmonary disease or endobronchial or laryngeal disease).

A volume of 5 to 10 mL of sputum produced by a deep cough of expectorated sputum or induced by inhalation of an aerosol of hypertonic saline should be used. When sputum is not obtainable, bronchoscopy may be performed, at which time samples such as bronchial washing, bronchoalveolar lavage (BAL), or transbronchial biopsy specimens are obtained. Brushings appear to be more commonly diagnostic than washing or biopsy, possibly because of an inhibitory effect on the mycobacteria by lidocaine used in adults during bronchoscopy or of dilution of the specimen with saline. Often patients are able to produce sputum for several days after bronchoscopy; these samples should be collected and examined.

Gastric Aspirates and Washings

Gastric aspirates are used to recover mycobacteria that may have been swallowed during the night. Use of this type of specimen should be only for patients who do not produce sputum by aerosol induction, for children under 3 years of age, and for nonambulatory individuals. Children with primary pulmonary tuberculosis typically have closed caseous lesions with relatively small numbers of organisms, resulting in a low yield from sputum analysis. Gastric lavage has been reported better than BAL for the detection of mycobacteria in children. When BAL was compared with three morning gastric lavage specimens, diagnosis of childhood pulmonary TB could be made in 10% versus 50% of children, respectively. This has not appeared to be the case in adults. Gastric lavage may offer a diagnostic alternative only in those unable to expectorate sputum and in whom BAL might be contraindicated. Gastric aspirates should be obtained in the morning after an overnight fast. Three specimens should be collected within 3 days. Sterile water, 30 to 60 mL, is instilled either orally or via nasogastric tube aspiration. Prolonged exposure to gastric acid kills mycobacteria and diminishes culture yield. Specimen processing should be done expeditiously, or the specimen should be neutralized with sodium carbonate or another buffer to pH 7.0 as soon as possible after specimen collection.

Urine

For examination of urine, a first morning midstream specimen is preferred. The entire volume of voided urine, or a minimum of 15 mL, is collected in a sterile container. A specimen may be collected through an indwelling catheter with a sterile needle and syringe. Urine specimens should be refrigerated during the interval between collection and processing; specimens should be processed promptly. As a general rule, pooled specimens collected over 12 to 24 hours are not recommended. Such specimens are more subject to contamination and may contain fewer viable tubercle bacilli.

Stool

Examination of stool specimens for the presence of AFB can be useful in identifying patients, such as individuals with AIDS, who may be at risk for developing disseminated mycobacterial disease resulting from the MAC. Frequently the number of organisms found in the bowel in these patients is quite high, although it has been reported that 68% of MAC culture-positive stool specimens are acid-fast–smear negative. Stool specimens should be collected in clean containers without any preservative and sent directly to the laboratory for processing. If processing within a few hours is not possible, the specimen should be frozen at −20° C until processed. Culture of feces for mycobacteria from patients other than those with or at risk for AIDS is usually not warranted.

Blood

Mycobacteremia, once considered rare, is now often seen in patients with AIDS but is seen less frequently in other immunocompromised hosts. Most infections are caused by MAC. Recovery of the organism from blood is associated with clinical disease. The Isolator lysis-centrifugation system (Wampole Laboratories, Cranbury, N.J.) or direct inoculation of blood into BACTEC 13A medium is effective for the collection and culture of blood samples. The two collection systems have been considered equivalent, although the Isolator system

allows for quantitative analysis, which may be used to monitor therapy and evaluate prognosis.

Tissue and Other Body Fluids

At times tissue and other body fluids may be needed for microscopic examination and culture. Whenever possible, CSF specimens should be from large-volume spinal taps to increase diagnostic yield. Diagnosis of tuberculous meningitis is extremely difficult. Peritoneal (ascitic fluid) smears are also rarely positive for AFB. Culture of large volumes and inoculation of the specimen into mycobacterial liquid media might help maximize yield in dilute specimens.

When noninvasive techniques have failed to provide a diagnosis, surgical procedures may need to be considered. Specimens obtained from the lung, pericardium, lymph nodes, bones, joints, bowel, or liver may be appropriate. The tissue or fluid should be collected aseptically and placed in a sterile container. If the tissue is not processed immediately, a small amount (10 to 15 mL) of sterile saline should be added to prevent dehydration. It may be necessary to collect fluid containing fibrinogen (e.g., pleural, pericardial, peritoneal) into a container with an anticoagulant. The amount of fluids recommended for culture varies: 2 mL for CSF, 3 to 5 mL for exudates and pericardial and synovial fluids, and 10 to 15 mL for abdominal and chest fluids. Immediate processing of these samples is important. When tissue is collected, histologic evaluation may reveal caseating or noncaseating granuloma formation with the presence of multinucleated giant cells. These histologic changes are consistent with but not specific for mycobacterial disease.

Digestion and Decontamination of Specimens

To ensure optimal recovery of mycobacteria from clinical specimens, many specimens must be processed before inoculation onto culture media. Each step must be carried out with precision. Specimens from sterile body sites can simply be concentrated by centrifugation (if a large volume) and inoculated. However, specimens that may contain commensal bacteria should be decontaminated and then concentrated.

Most clinical specimens, such as sputum, contain mucin or organic debris that surrounds the bacteria within the sample. An abundance of nonmycobacterial organisms, as well as possible mycobacteria, make up the microbiota of these specimens. When placed onto culture medium, the abundant nonmycobacterial organisms can quickly overgrow the more slowly growing mycobacteria. The purposes of the digestion-decontamination process are (1) to liquefy the sample through digestion of the proteinaceous material and (2) to allow the chemical decontaminating agent to contact and kill the nonmycobacterial organisms. The high lipid content in the cell wall of mycobacteria makes them somewhat less susceptible to the killing action of various chemicals. With liquefaction of the specimen, the surviving mycobacteria can be concentrated with centrifugation. Additionally, liquefying the mucin enables the mycobacteria to contact and use the nutrients of the medium to which they are subsequently inoculated. Specimens that contain mucus and require both digestion and decontamination are sputum, gastric washing, BAL, bronchial washing, and transtracheal aspirate. Voided urine, autopsy tissue, abdominal fluid, and any contaminated fluid require decontamination. Specimens from normally sterile sites, such as blood, CSF, synovial fluid, and biopsy tissue from deep organs, do not require decontamination. Sterility should be strictly maintained in collection and transport. Stool decontamination is especially difficult and may require repeated attempts.

Decontamination and Digestion Agents

Each laboratory should maintain a proper balance between rate of recovery of mycobacteria and the suppression of contaminating growth. Failure to isolate mycobacteria from patients with signs and symptoms of classic mycobacterial disease may indicate that the decontamination is too harsh. On the other hand, if more than 5% of all specimens cultured are contaminated, the decontamination procedure may be inadequate. In general a range that is considered acceptable in this delicate balance is between 2% and 5% of bacterially contaminated mycobacterial cultures. The bactericidal action of a decontaminating agent is influenced by the concentration of the chemical agent, exposure time, and temperature; therefore alterations in any of these factors can affect the bactericidal effect. The optimal decontamination procedure requires an agent that is mild and yields growth of mycobacteria while controlling contaminants. The use of selective media may diminish the need for harsh decontamination procedures.

Sodium Hydroxide. Sodium hydroxide (NaOH)—usual concentration 2%, 3%, or 4%—serves as both a digestant and a decontaminating agent. It must be used with caution because it is only slightly less harmful to the mycobacteria than to the contaminating organisms.

N-Acetyl-L-cysteine. A combination of a liquefying agent, such as N-acetyl-L-cysteine (NALC) or dithiothreitol, and NaOH is commonly used. The liquefying agent has no inhibitory effect on bacterial cells; however, liquefaction of the sample allows the decontaminating chemical to come into uniform contact with the contaminating bacteria more readily. When contamination can be controlled with a lower concentration of NaOH, the recovery of mycobacteria is indirectly improved using the milder procedure because fewer mycobacteria are lost in the process. See Appendix D for the NALC-NaOH digestion and decontamination procedure.

Benzalkonium Chloride. Another digestant-decontamination procedure uses benzalkonium chloride (Zephiran) combined with trisodium phosphate (Z-TSP). TSP liquefies sputum rapidly but requires a long exposure time to decontaminate the specimen. Benzalkonium chloride shortens the exposure time and effectively destroys many contaminants with little bactericidal effect on the tubercle bacilli. The addition of phosphate buffer to digested specimens results in greater isolation of mycobacteria. Zephiran is bacteriostatic for tubercle bacilli, necessitating either neutralization before plating or use of egg-based media to exploit its inherent neutralizing capacity.

Oxalic Acid. Oxalic acid, 5%, is used to decontaminate specimens contaminated with *Pseudomonas aeruginosa*, such as sputum specimens from patients with cystic fibrosis. This method is reported to be better than other alkali decontamination procedures when *P. aeruginosa* and certain other contaminants are present. Oxalic acid–treated specimens can be used with the broth-based culture systems.

Concentration Procedures

The specific gravity of the tubercle bacilli ranges from 0.79 to 1.07. Because of the low specific gravity of the AFB, a low centrifugal force has a buoyant rather than a sedimenting effect. Excess mucus will compound this phenomenon. Treatment with mucolytic agents such as NALC splits mucoprotein, allowing greater sedimentation. Therefore concentration centrifugation speeds must be at least $3000 \times g$ to maximize recovery.

Lower g force necessitates longer centrifuge time. The consequences of longer centrifuge time are prolonged exposure to the toxic effects of both the digestion-decontamination agents used and the higher temperatures generated by unrefrigerated centrifuges. Alternatives to high-speed centrifugation concentration have been explored. In summary, the digestion-decontamination agent used, its concentration, the length of exposure of the agent to the specimen, and the centrifugation speed and temperature all affect the recovery of *Mycobacterium* spp.

Staining for Acid-Fast Bacilli

When Gram-stained, *Mycobacterium* spp. stain faintly or not at all, giving a beaded appearance because of irregular uptake of the stain due to the increased lipid content of the cell wall. Acid-fast smears are prepared directly from clinical specimens and from digested, decontaminated, and concentrated specimens.

The conventional acid-fast staining methods, **Ziehl-Neelsen** and **Kinyoun stains**, use carbolfuchsin as the primary stain, acid-alcohol as a decolorizing agent, and a methylene blue counterstain. The Ziehl-Neelsen staining procedure involves the application of heat with the carbolfuchsin stain, whereas the Kinyoun acid-fast stain is a cold stain. Because of the potential cross-contamination of AFB from one smear to another, careful attention should be paid to the staining technique. Staining jars should not be used. Smears should not come in contact with one another. Slides are examined using a 100× oil immersion objective on a light microscope for 15 minutes, viewing a minimum of 300 fields before a slide is called negative.

The **auramine** or **auramine-rhodamine fluorochrome stains** are more sensitive than the carbolfuchsin stains. About 18% of all culture-positive specimens have smears that are positive on auramine-rhodamine stain but negative on Kinyoun or Ziehl-Neelsen stain. In addition, smears may be screened at a lower magnification (250× to 400×), thus allowing for more fields to be examined in a shorter time. A fluorescence microscope equipped with an appropriate filter system is needed for the examination of a fluorochrome-stained smear. The smear is examined under a mercury vapor lamp with a strong blue-filtered light. Positive stains reveal bright, yellow-orange bacilli against a dark background. Smears being examined for AFB should be carefully examined with a minimum of 300

Carbolfuchsin stain: # acid-fast bacilli seen (1000×)	Fluorochrome stain: # acid-fast bacilli seen (450×)	Quantitative report
0	0	No acid-fast bacilli seen
1-2/300 fields	1-2/70 fields	Doubtful acid-fast bacilli seen; resubmit another specimen for examination
1-9/100 fields	1-2/70 fields	1+
1-9/10 fields	2-18/50 fields	2+
1-9/fields	4-36/fields	3+
>9/fields	>36/fields	4+

Modified from Kent PT, Kubica GP: *Public health mycobacteriology: a guide for the level III laboratory*, Atlanta, 1985, U.S. Department of Health and Human Service, Public Health Service, Centers for Disease Control.

fields, and three horizontal sweeps of a smear that is 2 cm long and 1 cm wide should be performed. Less than 10% of the rapidly growing mycobacteria may be acid fast, and they may not stain at all with fluorochrome stains. If rapidly growing mycobacteria are suspected, smears should be stained with carbolfuchsin and a weaker decolorizing process used.

Individuals with extensive disease shed large numbers of organisms. However, many individuals have subtle infections in which fewer organisms will be shed. Thus the overall sensitivity of the acid-fast smear varies from 20% to 80%, depending on the extent of the infection. Even with concentration techniques, the number of organisms observed on a smear will be considerably less than organisms seen on a smear from an individual with bacterial pneumonia. The United States Department of Health and Human Services has made recommendations regarding the interpretation and reporting of acid-fast smears (Box 26-3). In the interpretation of a smear as positive for AFB, laboratory scientists must realize that organisms other than *Mycobacterium* might stain at least partially acid fast. *Nocardia* spp., *Legionella micdadei*, and *Rhodococcus* spp. may all appear acid fast.

Culture Media and Isolation Methods

Mycobacteria are strictly aerobic and grow more slowly than most bacteria pathogenic for humans. The generation time of mycobacteria is more than 12 hours; *M. tuberculosis* has the longest replication time at 20 to 22 hours. The rapidly growing species generally form colonies in 2 to 3 days, whereas most pathogenic mycobacteria require 2 to 6 weeks of incubation. The growth of *M. tuberculosis* is enhanced by an atmosphere of 5% to 10% CO_2. Mycobacteria require a pH between 6.5 and 6.8 for the growth medium and grow better at higher humidity. One of the mycobacteria pathogenic for humans, *M. genavense*, does not grow on media used routinely to isolate mycobacteria and requires extended incubation (6 to 8 weeks), whereas another, *M. leprae*, fails to grow on artificial media.

The many different media available for the recovery of mycobacteria from a clinical specimen are variations of three general types (Table 26-2): egg-based media, serum albumin agar media, and liquid media. Within each general type, there are nonselective formulations and formulations that have been made selective by the addition of antimicrobial agents. Because some isolates do not grow on a particular agar and each type of culture medium offers certain advantages, a combination of culture media is generally recommended for primary isolation. The use of a solid-based medium, such as **Löwenstein-Jensen (LJ) medium**, in combination with a liquid-based medium is recommended for routine culturing of specimens for the recovery of AFB.

Egg-Based Media

The basic ingredients in an inspissated egg medium, such as LJ, Petragnani, and American Thoracic Society (ATS) media, are fresh whole eggs, potato flour, and glycerol, with slight variations in defined salts, milk, and potato flour. Each contains malachite green to suppress the growth of gram-positive bacteria. Löwenstein-Jensen medium is most commonly used in clinical laboratories. Selective media that contain antimicrobial agents, such as Gruft modification of LJ and Mycobactosel (BD Diagnostic Systems, Sparks, Md.), are sometimes used in combination with nonselective media to increase isolation of mycobacteria from contaminated specimens. The nonselective egg-based media have a long shelf life of 1 year, but distinguishing early growth from debris is sometimes difficult.

Agar-Based Media

Serum albumin agar media, such as Middlebrook 7H10 and 7H11 agars, are prepared from a basal medium of defined salts, vitamins, cofactors, glycerol, malachite green, and agar combined with an enrichment consisting of oleic acid, bovine albumin, glucose (dextrose), and beef catalase (Middlebrook OADC enrichment). **Middlebrook 7H11 medium** also contains 0.1% casein hydrolysate, which improves recovery of isoniazid-resistant strains of *M. tuberculosis*. The addition of antimicrobial agents to either 7H10 or 7H11 makes the media more selective by suppressing the growth of contaminating bacteria. Mitchison's selective 7H11 contains polymyxin B, amphotericin B, carbenicillin, and trimethoprim lactate.

In contrast to opaque egg-based media, clear agar-based media can be examined using a dissecting microscope for early detection of growth and colony morphology. Drug susceptibility tests may be performed on agar-based media without altering drug concentrations, which occurs with egg-based media. When specimens are inoculated to Middlebrook 7H10 and 7H11 media and incubated in an atmosphere of 10% CO_2 and 90% air, 99% of the positive cultures are detected in 3 to 4 weeks, earlier than for those detected on egg-based media. Certain precautions should be followed in the preparation, storage, and incubation of Middlebrook media. Both excess heat and exposure of the prepared media to light can result in the release of formaldehyde, which is toxic to mycobacterial growth.

Liquid Media

Mycobacterium spp. grow more rapidly in liquid media. Middlebrook 7H9 broth is a nonselective liquid medium used for subculturing stock strains, picking single colonies, and preparing inoculum for in vitro testing. The BACTEC 460TB

TABLE 26-2 Mycobacterial Culture Media

Medium	Composition	Inhibitory Agents
American Thoracic Society	Fresh whole eggs, potato flour, glycerol	Malachite green (0.02%)
Löwenstein-Jensen (LJ)	Fresh whole eggs, defined salts, glycerol, potato four	Malachite green (0.025%)
Petragnani	Fresh whole eggs, egg yolks, whole milk, potato, potato flour, glycerol	Malachite green (0.052%)
Middlebrook 7H10	Defined salts, vitamins, cofactors, oleic acid, albumin, catalase, glycerol, glucose	Malachite green (0.00025%)
Middlebrook 7H11	Defined salts, vitamins, cofactors, oleic acid, albumin, catalase, glycerol, 0.1% casein hydrolysate	Malachite green (0.0001%)
Middlebrook 7H9, 7H12 (BACTEC 12B)	Broth base, casein hydrolysate, bovine serum albumin, catalase, C-14–labeled palmitic acid, deionized water	Polymyxin B Amphotericin B Nalidixic acid Trimethoprim Azlocillin
Middlebrook 7H9, 7H13 (BACTEC 13A)	Broth base, casein hydrolysate, bovine serum albumin, catalase, C-14–labeled palmitic acid, SPS, polysorbate 80	Polymyxin B Amphotericin B Nalidixic acid Trimethoprim Azlocillin
Gruft (modification of LJ)	Fresh whole eggs, defined salts, glycerol, potato flour, RNA	Malachite green Penicillin Nalidixic acid
Mycobactosel (BBL, BD Diagnostic Systems, Sparks, Md.) LJ	Fresh whole eggs, defined salts, glycerol, potato flour	Malachite green Cycloheximide Lincomycin Nalidixic acid
Middlebrook 7H10 (selective)	Defined salts, vitamins, cofactors, oleic acid, albumin, catalase, glycerol, glucose	Malachite green Cycloheximide Lincomycin Nalidixic acid
Mitchison's selective 7H11	Defined salts, vitamins, cofactors, oleic acid, albumin, catalase, glycerol, glucose, casein, hydrolysate	Carbenicillin Amphotericin B Polymyxin B Trimethoprim lactate

SPS, Sodium polyanethol sulfonate; *RNA*, ribonucleic acid.

system is an automated radiometric method using Middlebrook 7H12 and 7H13 (BACTEC 12B and 13B) containing a ^{14}C-labeled substrate (palmitic acid) that is metabolized by mycobacteria, liberating radioactive CO_2 ($^{14}CO_2$) into the headspace of a glass vial. The amount of $^{14}CO_2$ liberated is detected by the BACTEC 460TB instrument and interpreted as a "growth index." It is assumed that the release of CO_2 denotes growth of the organism. The recommended inoculum for the BACTEC 12B 4 mL vial is 0.5 mL of decontaminated concentrated specimen. Antimicrobial agents supplied by the manufacturer—polymyxin B, amphotericin B, nalidixic acid, trimethoprim, and azlocillin (PANTA) reconstituted into polyoxyethylene stearate, a growth-enhancing agent—are added to each vial at the time of inoculation.

The Middlebrook 7H13 medium (BACTEC 13B) was introduced for culturing larger volumes of blood or bone marrow. Its components are similar to those of the BACTEC 12B vial except that an anticoagulant, sodium polyanethol sulfonate (SPS), and polysorbate 80 have been added. Five milliliters of blood may be added directly to this 30-mL vial. Numerous studies have shown that the radiometric BACTEC isolation method significantly improves the isolation rate of mycobacteria and reduces the recovery time compared with conventional isolation media. The BACTEC vials should be read within 4 days of inoculation. Negative vials should be retested every 3 to 4 days for the first 2 weeks and then once weekly for the remaining 6 weeks.

With the BACTEC method, mycobacteria may be detected in clinical specimens in less than 2 weeks. *M. tuberculosis* is detected on average in 9 to 14 days, and the NTM are detected in less than 7 days. In general the time required for isolation and identification of *M. tuberculosis* is reduced from 6 weeks to 3 weeks. The time in which the radiometric system will detect growth reflects the quantity of viable *Mycobacterium* organism in the submitted sample, which is indirectly reflected by smear positivity. In smear-positive samples, *M. tuberculosis* may be detected as early as 7 to 8 days and *M. avium* as early as 5 to 8 days. In smear-negative samples, *M. tuberculosis* and NTM are usually detected in 14 to 28 days and 8 to 12 days, respectively, by the BACTEC 460 system. These detection times are an obvious improvement in the recovery time from conventional media. In conventional agar cultures, recovery from smear-positive TB specimens may require 16 days, and from smear-negative specimens, 26 days. By the end of the fourth week, 96.8% of all effectual positives will have been detected by the BACTEC system, and by the end of the fifth week, 98.8%. The greater sensitivity of the BACTEC system has resulted in a higher yield from smear-negative specimens.

The disadvantage of the BACTEC system is that when the BACTEC vial is positive before a companion agar or egg-medium culture, no colony morphology or pigmentation is available to suggest that the growth is of a mycobacterial species. The BACTEC system also may not be as good in recovery of all species of *Mycobacterium*, specifically *M. fortuitum* and MAC. False-positive results from cross-contamination have been reported. The BACTEC system can also be used for the antimicrobial susceptibility testing of *M. tuberculosis*. Currently it is not recommended for sensitivity testing of NTM.

Automated, nonradiometric microbial detection systems designed for the recovery of mycobacteria from clinical specimens are also available. The MGIT 960 system (BD Diagnostic Systems) uses a modified Middlebrook 7H9 broth in conjunction with a fluorescence quenching-based oxygen sensor to detect growth of mycobacteria. The MB/BacT Alert 3D System (bioMérieux, Durham, N.C.) employs a colorimetric carbon dioxide sensor in each bottle to detect the growth. The VersaTrek Culture System (Trek Diagnostics, Cleveland, Ohio) is based on the detection of pressure changes in the headspace above the broth medium in a sealed culture bottle resulting from gas production or consumption during the growth of microorganisms. Each manufacturer provides a mixture of antimicrobial agents to be added to each culture vial at the time of inoculation. These continuous monitoring systems have similar performance and operational characteristics. All share the advantage over the radiometric broth system of using no radioisotopes and elimination of the potential for cross-contamination. Because these systems are monitored continuously, bottles are incubated in the instrument for the entire monitoring period. Options for electronic data management are also available. A limitation of the continuous monitoring systems is that cultures with mycobacteria with a lower optimum temperature, such as *M. haemophilum*, *M. marinum*, and *M. ulcerans*, may not be detected.

Other Culture Media for Recovery of Mycobacteria

A CHOC agar plate should be included in the primary isolation media for skin and other body surface specimens for the recovery of *M. haemophilum*, which requires ferric ammonium citrate or hemin for growth. The plate should be incubated at 30° C, the optimum temperature for recovery of this organism and for *M. marinum*. Alternatively, hemin (X) strips or disks used for the identification of *Haemophilus* spp. can be placed on Middlebrook agar plates.

A biphasic media system for the detection and isolation of mycobacteria, Septi-Chek AFB (Figure 26-7), is available commercially (BBL Septi-Chek AFB, BD Diagnostic Systems). The system consists of a bottle containing Middlebrook 7H9 broth with an atmosphere of 5% to 8% CO_2, an enrichment consisting of growth-enhancing factors and antimicrobial agents, and a paddle with agar media. One side of the paddle is covered with nonselective Middlebrook 7H11 agar. One of the two sections on the reverse side of the paddle contains a modified egg-based medium for differentiating *M. tuberculosis* from other mycobacteria, and the other contains CHOC agar for the detection of contaminating bacteria. The biphasic media system provides for rapid growth and identification and drug susceptibility testing without the need for

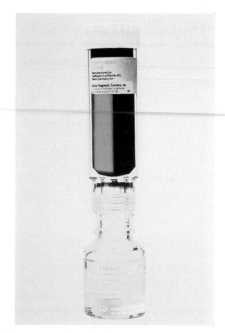

FIGURE 26-7 Septi-Chek biphasic media system for acid-fast bacilli.

routine subculturing. The biphasic media system is sensitive and does not require use of radioactivity and a CO_2 incubator. Detection times are shorter than with conventional agar but significantly longer than with the BACTEC system.

Isolator Lysis–Centrifugation System

Isolator (Wampole Laboratories, Cranbury, N.J.) is a blood collection system that contains saponin to liberate intracellular organisms. After treatment with the saponin, the sample is inoculated onto mycobacteria media plates or tubes. The system allows for higher yields and shorter recovery times for mycobacteria than conventional blood culture methods. It offers the advantage of yielding isolated colonies and the ability to quantify mycobacteremia, which may be useful in monitoring the effectiveness of therapy in disseminated MAC infection. For maximal recovery of mycobacteria, many laboratories use a battery of media that includes an egg-based medium, one agar medium, and the radiometric broth method for primary isolation. A selective medium is often reserved for specimens in which heavy contamination is anticipated.

Laboratory Identification

Laboratory Levels or Extents of Service

A change in the distribution of mycobacterial laboratory testing led to development of levels of service by the ATS and extents of service by the College of American Pathologists to maintain quality of service. Laboratories must decide which level of mycobacterial services to offer: level 1, specimen collection only; level 2, perform microscopy and isolate and identify and sometimes perform susceptibility tests for *M. tuberculosis*; or level 3, perform microscopy, isolation, identification, and susceptibility testing for all species of *Mycobacterium* (Box 26-4). A facility's selection of a level of service depends on the volume of specimens submitted, the patient populations served, the ability to perform the requested tests according to comfort and training in performance of each requested test, as well as the time, effort, and funds allocated for the service.

The CDC has developed separate training courses designed for each level of service as well as manuals for reference. Procedures available within a particular mycobacteriology laboratory vary with the level of service of that laboratory. In addition, the methodology within laboratories varies. The CDC, in collaboration with the Association of State and Territorial Public Health Laboratory Directors, surveyed mycobacterial laboratories for their practices in isolation, identification, and susceptibility testing of MTB. Those laboratories that used conventional mycobacteriologic methods for culturing and identification were not able to report results as quickly as those that have already incorporated newer methodologies, the amount of time needed being 43 versus 22 days, respectively.

Preliminary Identification of Mycobacteria

Once an isolate has been recovered in the mycobacteriology laboratory, certain characteristics may be used to classify the isolate before performing biochemical tests. The first step is to confirm that the isolate recovered in broth or on solid media is an acid-fast organism by performing an acid-fast stain. Then, once the organisms are growing on solid media, phenotypic characteristics such as colony morphology, growth rate, optimum growth temperature, and photoreactivity help to speciate mycobacteria. These characteristics do not allow for definitive identification but are presumptive and help in the selection of other, more definitive tests. Figures 26-8 and 26-9 show schematic diagrams for the identification of slowly growing and rapidly growing *Mycobacterium* spp., respec-

tively. See Table 26-1 for a summary of the identification characteristics of clinically important mycobacteria.

Colony Morphology. Colonies of mycobacteria are generally distinguished as having either a smooth and soft or a rough and friable appearance. Colonies of *M. tuberculosis* that are rough often also exhibit a prominent patterned texture referred to as cording (curved strands of bacilli); this texture is the result of tight cohesion of the bacilli. Colonies of MAC have a variable appearance: glossy, whitish colonies often occurring with smaller translucent colonies.

Growth Rate. Growth rate and recovery time depend on the species of mycobacteria but are also influenced by media, the incubation temperature, and the initial inoculum size. The range in recovery time is wide, from 3 to 60 days. Mycobacteria are generally categorized as rapid growers, having visible growth in fewer than 7 days, or slow growers, producing colonies in more than 7 days. Determination of growth rate should be evaluated from the time of subculture, not the time of detection from clinical sample. The inoculum should be sufficiently small to produce isolated colonies. Microscopic examination of agar for microcolonies allows earlier detection of growth.

Temperature. The optimum temperature and range at which a mycobacterial species can grow may be extremely narrow, especially at the time of initial incubation. *M. marinum, M. ulcerans,* and *M. haemophilum* grow best at 30° to 32° C and poorly, if at all, at 35° to 37° C. At the other extreme, *M. xenopi* grows best at 42° C.

Photoreactivity. *Mycobacterium* spp. have traditionally been categorized into three groups according to their photoreactive characteristics (Box 26-5). Species that produce carotene pigment upon exposure to light are photochromogens. Color ranges from pale yellow to orange. Species that produce pigment in the light or the dark are scotochromogens. Growth temperature may influence the photoreactive characteristics of a species. Other species, such as *M. tuberculosis,* are nonchromogenic or nonphotochromogenic. These colonies are a buff (i.e., tan) color and are nonphotoreactive; exposure to light does not induce pigment formation.

Biochemical Identification

A panel of biochemical tests can identify most mycobacteria isolates, but because growth of *Mycobacterium* spp. is so slow, accomplishing this may take several weeks. Progress in molecular technology has diminished the frequency with which biochemical tests are routinely performed in the identification of mycobacteria. Because mycobacterial species may show only quantitative differences in enzymes used in biochemical identification, no single biochemical test should be relied on for the identification of a species. For expediency, all necessary biochemical tests should be set up at one time. The biochemical tests are based on the enzymes the organisms possess, the substances that their metabolism produce, and the inhibition of growth on exposure to selected biochemicals. Appropriate positive and negative controls should be included for each biochemical test.

Niacin Accumulation. Most mycobacteria possess the enzyme that converts free niacin to niacin ribonucleotide. However, 95% of *M. tuberculosis* isolates produce free niacin (nicotinic acid) because the species lacks the niacin-connect-

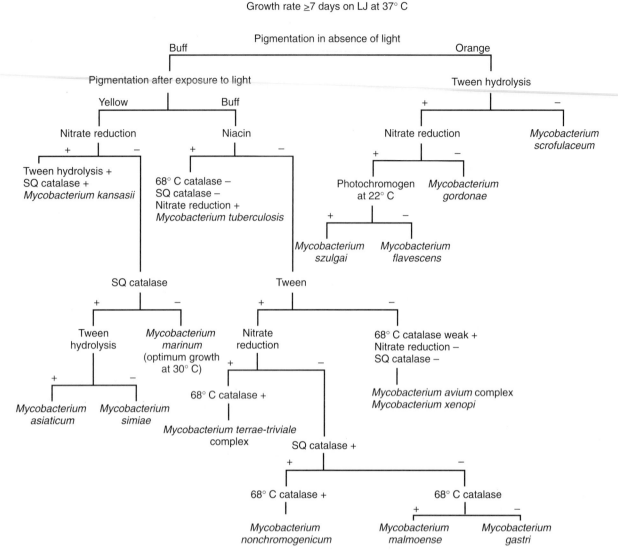

FIGURE 26-8 Schematic diagram for the identification of slowly growing *Mycobacterium* spp. Exceptional reactions occur. Organisms should be subjected to a battery of morphologic and physiologic tests before final identification is made. *SQ,* Semiquantitative; *LJ,* Löwenstein-Jensen.

ing enzyme. Accumulation of niacin, detected as nicotinic acid, is the most commonly used biochemical test for the identification of MTB. Nicotinic acid reacts with cyanogen bromide in the presence of an amine to form a yellow-pigmented compound (Figure 26-10). Reagent-impregnated strips have eliminated the need to handle and dispose of cyanogen bromide, which is both caustic and toxic. Cyanogen bromide must be alkalinized with NaOH before disposal.

The niacin test may be negative when performed on young cultures with few colonies. It is recommended that the test be done on egg agar cultures 3 to 4 weeks old and with at least 50 colonies. Tests that yield negative results may need to be repeated in several weeks. The test should not be performed on scotochromogenic or rapidly growing species because *M. simiae,* bacillus of Calmette-Guérin (BCG) strain of *M. bovis, M. africanum, M. marinum, M. chelonae,* and *M. bovis* may be positive, although this occurs rarely. Results are most consistent when the test is performed on egg-based media.

Nitrate Reduction. The production of nitroreductase, which catalyzes the reduction of nitrate to nitrite, is relatively uncommon among *Mycobacterium* spp., but a positive result may be seen in *M. kansasii, M. szulgai, M. fortuitum,* and *M. tuberculosis.* Bacteria are incubated in 2 mL of sodium nitrate at 37° C for 2 hours. Hydrochloric acid (50 mL HCL in 50 mL of water), sulfanilamide, and N-naphthylenediamine dihydrochloride are then added; if the bacteria reduced the nitrate to nitrite, a red color forms (Figure 26-11). When no color change develops, however, either no reaction has occurred or the reaction has gone beyond nitrite. The addition of zinc detects nitrate and results in a pink color change in a true-negative reaction. Commercially available strips have simplified the assay. The nitrate reduction test differentiates *M. tuberculosis* from the scotochromogens and MAC.

Catalase. Catalase is an enzyme that can split hydrogen peroxide into water and oxygen. Mycobacteria are catalase positive. However, not all strains produce a positive reaction

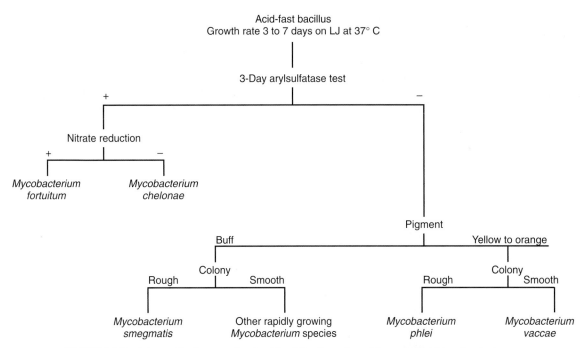

Acid-fast bacillus
Growth rate 3 to 7 days on LJ at 37° C

3-Day arylsulfatase test

+   −

Nitrate reduction

+   −

Mycobacterium fortuitum   *Mycobacterium chelonae*

Pigment

Buff   Yellow to orange

Colony

Rough   Smooth

Colony

Rough   Smooth

Mycobacterium smegmatis   Other rapidly growing *Mycobacterium* species   *Mycobacterium phlei*   *Mycobacterium vaccae*

FIGURE 26-9 Schematic diagram for the identification of rapidly growing *Mycobacterium* species. Exceptional reactions occur. Organisms should be subjected to a battery of morphologic and physiologic tests before final identification is made. *LJ,* Löwenstein-Jensen.

BOX 26-5 Photoreactivity of Clinically Important Mycobacteria

Nonchromogens
Slow Growers
M. tuberculosis
M. avium-intracellulare*
M. bovis
M. celatum
M. gastri
M. genavense
M. haemophilum
M. malmoense
M. terrae complex
M. ulcerans

Rapid Growers
M. chelonae
M. fortuitum group

Photochromogens
Slow Growers
M. asiaticum
M. kansasii
M. marinum
M. simiae

Scotochromogens
Slow Growers
M. gordonae
M. szulgai†
M. scrofulaceum
M. xenopi‡

Rapid Growers
M. phlei
M. smegmatis group

---

*Some *M. avium-intracellulare isolates* are scotochromogens.
†Some *M. szulgai* isolates are photochromogens.
‡Young cultures may be nonchromogenic.

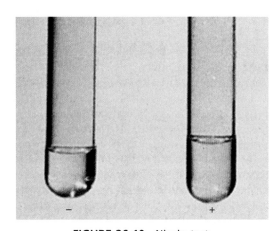

FIGURE 26-10 Niacin test.

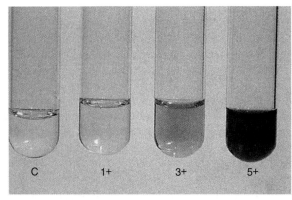

FIGURE 26-11 Nitrate reduction test.

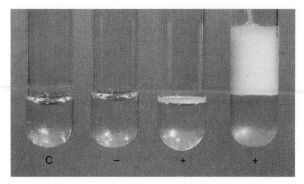

FIGURE 26-12 Catalase test.

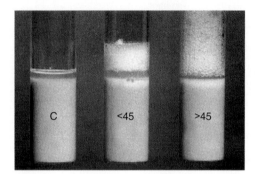

FIGURE 26-13 Semiquantitative catalase test.

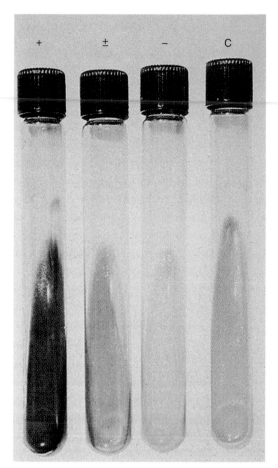

FIGURE 26-14 Iron uptake.

after the culture is heated to 68° C for 20 minutes. Isolates that are catalase positive after heating have a heat-stable catalase (Figure 26-12). Most *M. tuberculosis* complex organisms do not produce heat-stable catalase; exceptions are certain strains resistant to isoniazid. Other heat-stable catalase negative species include *M. gastri, M. haemophilum,* and *M. marinum.* Semiquantitation of catalase production uses the addition of Tween 80 (a detergent) and hydrogen peroxide to a 2-week-old culture grown in an agar deep. The reaction is read after 5 minutes, and the resulting column of bubbles is measured (Figure 26-13). The column size is recorded as either greater than or less than 45 mm.

Hydrolysis of Tween 80. Some mycobacteria possess a lipase that can split the detergent Tween 80 into oleic acid and polyoxyethylated sorbitol. The pH indicator, neutral red, is initially bound to Tween 80 and has an amber color. After hydrolysis of Tween 80, neutral red can no longer bind, and it is released, causing a pink color to form. The time required for the hydrolysis is variable. Results are recorded as positive after 24 hours, 5 days, or 10 days. This test is helpful in distinguishing scotochromogenic and nonphotochromogenic mycobacteria.

Iron Uptake. Some mycobacteria are able to convert ferric ammonium citrate to an iron oxide. After growth of the isolate appears on an egg-based medium slant, rusty brown colonies appear in a positive reaction upon the addition of 20% aqueous solution of ferric ammonium citrate; color formation is the result of iron uptake (Figure 26-14). The test is most useful in distinguishing *M. chelonae,* which is generally negative, from other rapid growers, which are positive.

Arylsulfatase. Most members of the genus *Mycobacterium* possess the enzyme arylsulfatase. This enzyme hydrolyzes the bond between the sulfate group and the aromatic ring structure in compounds with the formula $R—OSO_3H$. Tripotassium phenolphthalein sulfate is such a molecule, from which phenolphthalein is liberated with exposure to arylsulfatase. The liberation of phenolphthalein causes a pH change in the presence of sodium bicarbonate, indicated by formation of a pink color change. The *M. fortuitum* complex, *M. chelonae, M. xenopi,* and *M. triviale* have rapid arylsulfatase activity that can be detected in 3 days. *M. marinum* and *M. szulgai* exhibit activity with 14 days of incubation.

Pyrazinamidase. Pyrazinamidase hydrolyzes pyrazinamide to pyrazinoic acid and ammonia in 4 days. Ferrous ammonium sulfate combines with pyrazinoic acid, producing a red pigment (Figure 26-15). This reaction occurs in about 4 days and may be useful in distinguishing *M. marinum* from *M. kansasii* and *M. bovis* from *M. tuberculosis.*

Tellurite Reduction. Reduction of colorless potassium tellurite to black metallic tellurium in 3 to 4 days is a characteristic of MAC (Figure 26-16) and thus is useful in distinguishing MAC from other nonchromogenic species. In addition, all rapid growers are able to reduce tellurite in 3 days.

Urease. Detection of urease activity can be used to distinguish *M. scrofulaceum,* urease positive, from *M. gordonae,*

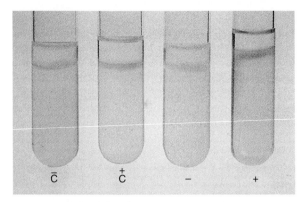

FIGURE 26-15   Pyrazinamidase test.

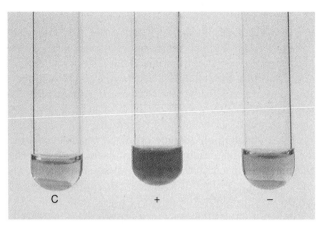

FIGURE 26-17   Urease test.

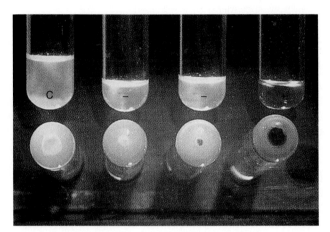

FIGURE 26-16   Test for tellurite reduction.

urease negative (Figure 26-17). A loopful of test organism is grown in 4 mL of urea broth at 37° C for 3 days. A pink to red color is indicative of a positive reaction.

Inhibitory Tests

NAP. NAP (p-nitroacetylamino-β-hydroxypropiophenone) is a precursor in the synthesis of chloramphenicol. NAP selectively inhibits the *M. tuberculosis* complex. A radiometric application was the first assay developed to detect the selective inhibition. Performance of the test either with isolated colonies or with broth from a BACTEC medium with a growth index of 50 to 100 or more is recommended. An aliquot of the original BACTEC medium is transferred to the BACTEC-NAP vial, which contains 5 mg of NAP. Growth is then closely monitored and compared with the original BACTEC vial, which serves as a growth control. A 20% increase in growth index is considered significant and rules out *M. tuberculosis* complex. About 4 to 6 additional days are required for identification if such indirect NAP testing is performed. Testing should be done with positive and negative controls. Direct specimen BACTEC-NAP testing, eliminating prior isolation, has been reported to identify *M. tuberculosis* in an average of 7.8 days but with diminished sensitivity.

T2H. T2H (thiophene-2-carboxylic acid hydrazide) distinguishes *M. bovis* from *M. tuberculosis*. *M. bovis* is susceptible to lower levels of T2H than MTB. Variability in inhibition

exists, depending on the concentration of the inhibitory agent and the temperature of incubation. This selective inhibitory agent has also been applied to radiometric systems.

Sodium Chloride Tolerance. High salt concentration (5% NaCl) in egg-based media (i.e., LJ) inhibits the growth of most mycobacteria. *M. flavescens, M. triviale*, and most rapidly growing *Mycobacterium* spp. are exceptions that do grow in the presence of 5% NaCl.

Growth on MacConkey Agar. *Mycobacterium fortuitum-chelonae* complex can grow on MacConkey agar without crystal violet, whereas most other mycobacteria cannot. This is not the same formulation of MacConkey agar typically used for the isolation of enteric bacilli.

Chromatography

The cell walls of *Mycobacterium* spp. contain long-chain fatty acids called mycolic acids, which may be detected chromatographically. The type and quality of mycolic acids are species specific. Identification of *Mycobacterium* spp. by chromatographic methods has been of long-standing interest, and assays have changed as technology evolved. Earlier methods, such as column chromatography and thin-layer chromatography, have been replaced by gas-liquid chromatography and, most recently, HPLC. Current methods allow sufficient amount of mycolic acid to be easily extracted from small quantities of bacterial cultures. A basic saponification followed by acidification and chloroform extraction allows accurate identification of most mycobacterial species using chromatograms and colony characteristics. Species identifications made with HPLC have been shown to agree well with biochemical and nucleic acid probe identifications. Many state health departments and the CDC use this method for identification of mycobacterial isolates. Chromatography is rapid and highly reproducible, but the initial cost of equipment is high.

Hybridization and Nucleic Acid Amplification Tests for *Mycobacterium tuberculosis*

The use of nucleic acid hybridization techniques allows rapid identification of certain common mycobacterial species. Commercially available nucleic acid probes (AccuProbe; Gen-Probe Inc., San Diego, Calif.) are available for the *M.*

tuberculosis complex, the MAC, *M. avium, M. intracellulare, M. kansasii,* and *M. gordonae.* These tests use nonisotopically labeled (e.g., an acridine ester–labeled nucleic acid) probes specific to mycobacterial ribosomal RNA (rRNA). The rRNA is released from the cell after sonication. The DNA probe is allowed to react with the test solution. If specific rRNA is present, a stable DNA-RNA complex, or hybrid, is formed. Unbound probe is chemically degraded. The complex is detected by adding an alkaline hydrogen peroxide solution. The hybrid-bound acridine ester is available to cause a chemiluminescent reaction, resulting in the emission of light. The amount of light emitted is related to the amount of hybridized probe.

The sensitivity of the assay varies between 95% and 100%, depending on the species and species complexes. The amount of organism required for testing in the case of MTB is a single colony of at least 1 mm in diameter or in the case of MAC a barely visible film of growth on the surface of the medium. Most positive results are well above the cutoff value of 10% hybridization. When a probe is used on a contaminated specimen, the resulting hybridization percentage may incorrectly fall below accepted cutoff hybridization levels, leading to a false negative result. DNA hybridization identification can be applied to growth on conventional agar as well as to growth in liquid media. The combination of broth based growth for detection and DNA hybridization identification using the probe technology allows rapid recovery and identification.

In addition to hybridization assays, many laboratories are using PCR tests to identify the mycobacteria. The INNO-LiPA Mycobacteria test (Innogenetics, Ghent, Belgium) is a PCR assay which targets the 16S-23S rRNA spacer region of mycobacteria species and has been used to directly detect and identify *M. tuberculosis* complex, *M. avium* complex, *M. kansasii, M. xenopi, M. gordonae,* and *M. chelonae.* The Geno-Type *Mycobacterium* (Hain Lifescience GmbH, Nehrin, Germany) uses a similar format and has additional probes for *M. celatum, M. malmoense, M. peregrinum,* and *M. fortuitum.*

Restriction enzyme analysis, or restriction fragment length polymorphism, has also been used to identify mycobacteria. In this approach, a highly conserved gene such as *hsp*65 is amplified by PCR. Following restriction enzyme digestion, the digested products are separated by gel electrophoresis with subsequent sizing of the resulting fragments. The restriction fragment patterns are species-specific and can be used to differentiate many species of the nontuberculous mycobacteria.

Automated DNA sequencing is also used by some laboratories for identification of mycobacterial isolates. The target that has been most commonly used is the gene coding for 16S rRNA. This gene is present in all bacteria and contains both conserved and variable regions. Identification is accomplished by PCR amplification of DNA followed by sequencing of the amplicons (i.e., amplified products). The organism is identified by comparison of the nucleotide sequence with reference sequences. Although this method holds great promise, sequences in some reference databases are not accurate and procedures are not yet standardized. As more molecular biology methods become available commercially and increasingly automated, identification and detection of mycobacteria will become faster, less costly, and more specific.

Direct Nucleic Acid Amplification Tests. Nucleic acid amplification assays designed to detect *M. tuberculosis* complex bacilli directly from patient specimens can be performed in as few 6 to 8 hours on processed specimens and offer the promise of same-day reporting of results for detection and identification of *M. tuberculosis.* The amplified *Mycobacterium tuberculosis* direct test (AMTD, Gen-Probe, Inc.) consists of transcription-mediated amplification of a specific 16S rRNA target performed at a constant temperature for the detection of *M. tuberculosis* complex rRNA in smear-positive and negative respiratory specimens. The Amplicor *Mycobacterium tuberculosis* PCR assay (Roche Molecular Systems, Branchburg, N.J.) consists of PCR amplification of the 584-bp region of the 16S rRNA gene sequence. The Amplicor assay is approved for use with smear-positive respiratory specimens.

SUSCEPTIBILITY TESTING OF *MYCOBACTERIUM TUBERCULOSIS*

Along with increased incidence of mycobacterial disease, the development of MDR strains of mycobacteria is being observed. So that patients can be placed on appropriate therapy, the CDC currently recommends that, when isolated, *M. tuberculosis* be tested for susceptibility to isoniazid, rifampin, ethambutol, and streptomycin. Pyrazinamide is to be considered as well. Likewise, testing should be repeated if the patient's cultures for *M. tuberculosis* remain positive after 3 months of therapy. Susceptibility testing of *M. tuberculosis* requires meticulous technique and experienced personnel in interpreting results. Therefore laboratories that isolate few *M. tuberculosis* isolates should consider sending isolates to a reference laboratory for susceptibility testing. Currently four methods are used for determining susceptibility of *M. tuberculosis*: absolute concentration, resistance ratio, and proportional and broth-based methods.

The absolute concentration method determines the minimum inhibitory concentration (MIC). For each drug tested, a standardized inoculum is added to control (drug-free) media and media containing several dilutions of the drug. Resistance is expressed as the lowest concentration of drug that inhibits all or almost all of the growth, that is, the MIC. The resistance ratio method compares the resistance of the test organism with that of a standard laboratory strain. Both strains are tested in parallel by adding a standardized inoculum to media containing twofold serial dilutions of the drug. Resistance is expressed as the ratio of the MIC of the test strain divided by the MIC of the standard strain for each strain.

Historically, the proportion method has been the most commonly used assay in the United States. In clinical correlations with in vitro data, if 1% of a patient's bacilli are resistant to a particular drug, treatment fails. Laboratory tests then must demonstrate the rate of resistant organisms. To do so, the inoculum of bacilli used is adjusted to enable this 1%—usually 100 to 300 colony-forming units (CFU) per milliliter—to be determined. The test is often referred to as the *proportion method* because it allows one to predict the probability that 1% of the cells are resistant or not. For each drug tested, drug-containing agar is prepared and dispensed in quadrant Petri dishes. An inoculum of mycobacteria is prepared to yield about 100 to 300 CFU/mL, which appears as a barely turbid broth. The broth is then diluted 10^2-fold and 10^4-fold. The two dilutions provide a set of plates that should be countable (i.e., 100 to 300 CFU on the control plate). A control plate is set up in each test of drugs so that the numbers of colonies on the test quadrants can be counted and compared with the number on the control quadrant. If the test growth is less than 1% of the control growth, the organism is susceptible, and if greater, it is resistant. By this method, results can be obtained in 2 to 3 weeks, depending on the growth rate of the organism. Plates are incubated at 37° C.

Currently four commercial methods are approved by the FDA to determine susceptibility of *M. tuberculosis* to antimycobacterial agents: BACTEC 460TB, BACTEC MGIT 960, ESPII Culture System (Trek Diagnostic Systems), and MB/Bac T Alert 3D (bioMérieux). Employing the principles of the agar proportion method, these methods use liquid media. Growth is indicated by the amount of ^{14}C-labeled-CO_2 release, as measured by the BACTEC 460 instrument, or the amount of fluorescence or gas measured by the BACTEC MGIT 960, the MB/BacT Alert 3D, or the ESPII, respectively. For each drug tested, a standardized inoculum is added into a drug-free and a drug-containing vial. The rate and amount of CO_2 produced in the absence or presence of drug is then compared. Broth-based susceptibility results are usually available in 5 to 7 days because one does not wait to visually detect growth.

Table 26-3 lists drugs and their concentrations to be used in susceptibility tests. The susceptibility test is performed on a pure culture, identified as *M. tuberculosis*. A direct susceptibility test may be performed, however, using clinical specimens that are positive on smear, provided appropriate dilutions are made on the basis of numbers of AFB seen. The advantage of this direct assay is a quicker susceptibility report, that is, within 2 to 3 weeks of culture, rather than 5 to 7 weeks or longer. If, however, cultures are not thoroughly decontami-

nated, overgrowth is a problem. Likewise, the mycobacteria isolated may be other than *M. tuberculosis*. Researchers are looking for more rapid methods involving nucleic acid amplification and the detection of resistance genes. The INNO-LiPA Rif TB (Innogenetics) is a reverse hybridization-based probe assay for rapid detection of rifampin mutations leading to rifampin resistance in *M. tuberculosis*.

Susceptibility testing of most NTM is not performed routinely. Correlations between clinical outcome and in vitro test results have not been shown. In addition, no standardized method currently exists for performing these tests. The one exception is the rapidly growing mycobacteria. Broth microdilution and agar disc diffusion may be used. The Etest (AB BIODISK, Solna, Sweden) is being used with increasing frequency for performing susceptibility testing on the rapid growers.

IMMUNODIAGNOSIS OF MYCOBACTERIUM TUBERCULOSIS INFECTION

Skin Testing

The tuberculin skin test has been used for many years to determine an individual's exposure to *M. tuberculosis*. Protein extracted and purified from the cell wall of culture-grown *M. tuberculosis* is used as the antigen, that is, PPD. A standardized amount of antigen is injected intradermally into the patient's forearm. Reactivity is read at 48 hours; in immunocompetent individuals the presence of a raised firm area (induration) 10 mm or larger is considered reactive. A reactive tuberculin skin test indicates past exposure to *M. tuberculosis*; other *Mycobacterium* spp. generally result in induration less than 10 mm. Immunocompromised patients with previous *M. tuberculosis* infection may also produce induration less than 10 mm. The skin test detects a patient's cell-mediated immune response to the bacterial antigens in a type IV hypersensitivity reaction.

Serology

Clinical, radiologic, and microbiologic tests are currently used for the diagnosis of *M. tuberculosis* infection. In December 2004 a new diagnostic test kit for *M. tuberculosis* infection was approved for the use in the United States. The Quantiferon-TB Gold assay (Cellestis Limited, Carnegie, Victoria, Australia) measures the cell-mediated immune response in whole blood samples to mycobacterial antigens. Quantiferon-TB Gold is a patented technology for the measurement of interferon-gamma production by cells that have been stimulated by two secretory, low–molecular-weight mycobacterial peptides: early secreted antigenic target 6 (ESAT-6) and culture filtrate protein 10 (CFP-10). Quantiferon-TB Gold is analogous to the tuberculin skin test used to detect latent tubercular infection and is less affected by BCG vaccination and cross-reactivity with antigens derived from other mycobacterial species. It has the potential to distinguish between responses caused by nontuberculous mycobacteria and avoids the inconsistency and bias that may be associated with the tuberculin skin test used for diagnosis and screening of *M. tuberculosis* infection.

TABLE 26-3 Antituberculosis Drugs and Their Recommended Concentrations

Drug	Concentration (μg/mL)*
Primary	
Isoniazid	0.2
Isoniazid	1.0
Streptomycin	2.0
Streptomycin	10.0
Rifampin	1.0
Ethambutol	5.0
Secondary[†]	
Ethionamide	5.0
Capreomycin	10.0
Cycloserine	20.0
Kanamycin	5.0
Pyrazinamide (at pH 5.5)	25.0

*In 7H10 Medium.
[†]Modified from National Committee for Clinical Laboratory Standards: *Antimycobacterial susceptibility testing: Proposed Standard Document M24-P*, vol 10, Villanova, Pa, 1990, NCCLS.

BIBLIOGRAPHY

Bothamley GH: Immunological tests in tuberculosis and leprosy. In Detrick B et al, editors: *Manual of molecular and clinical laboratory immunology*, ed 7, Washington, DC, 2006, American Society for Microbiology.

Brown-Elliott BA, Wallace RJ: *Mycobacterium*: clinical and laboratory characteristics of rapidly growing mycobacteria. In Murray PR et al, editors: *Manual of clinical microbiology*, ed 9, Washington, DC, 2007, ASM Press.

Centers for Disease Control and Prevention: Emergence of *Mycobacterium tuberculosis* with extensive resistance to second-line drugs—worldwide, 2000-2004, *MMWR* 55:301, 2006. Available at: www.cdc.gov/mmwr/preview/mmwrhtml/mm5511a2.htm. Accessed December 18, 2008.

Centers for Disease Control and Prevention: Extensively drug-resistant tuberculosis—United States, 1993-2006, *MMWR* 56:250, 2007. Available at: www.cdc.gov/mmwr/preview/mmwrhtml/mm5611a3.htm. Accessed December 18, 2008.

Centers for Disease Control and Prevention: Reported tuberculosis in the United States, 2007. Available at: www.cdc.gov/tb/surv/2007/default.htm. Accessed December 18, 2008.

Centers for Disease Control and Prevention: Trends in tuberculosis, 2007 – United States. Available at: www.cdc.gov/tb/pubs/tbfactsheets/TBTrends.htm. Accessed December 18, 2008.

Clinical and Laboratory Standards Institute: *Susceptibility testing of mycobacteria, nocardiae, and other actinomcyes; approved standards*, M24-A, Wayne, Penn, 2008.

Della-Latta, P et al: Mycobacteriology and antimycobacterial susceptibility testing. In Isenberg HD, editor: *Clinical microbiology procedures handbook*, ed 2, Washington, DC, 2004, ASM Press.

Di Perri G, Bonora S: Which agents should we use for the treatment of multidrug-resistant *Mycobacterium tuberculosis*? *J Antimicrob Chem* 54:593-602, 2004.

Pfyffer GE: *Mycobacterium*: general characteristics, isolation, and staining procedures. In Murray PR et al, editors: *Manual of clinical microbiology*, ed 9, Washington, DC, 2007, ASM Press.

Sharma SK, Mohan A: Multidrug-resistant tuberculosis, *Indian J Med Res* 120:354-376, 2004.

Thorel MF et al: *Mycobacterium avium* and *Mycobacterium intracellulare* infection in mammals, *Rev Sci Tech* 20:204-218, 2001.

Vincent V, Gutiérrez MC: *Mycobacterium*: Laboratory characteristics of slowly growing mycobacteria. In Murray PR et al, editors: *Manual of clinical microbiology*, ed 9, Washington, DC, 2007, ASM Press.

World Health Organization: Report of the global forum on the elimination of leprosy as a public health problem: Geneva, Switzerland, 26 May 2006. Available at: www.whqlibdoc.who.int/hq/2006/WHO_CDS_NTD_2006.4_eng.pdf. Accessed December 19, 2008.

Points to Remember

- The mycobacteria are important causes of human diseases such as tuberculosis and Hansen disease.
- The mycobacteria have a unique cell wall and require special stains to visualize the microorganisms.
- Many *Mycobacterium* spp. are environmental isolates infrequently isolated from clinical specimens.
- Isolation of mycobacteria requires specific safety precautions, including laboratories with negative air pressure, biological safety cabinets, the use of respirators and other personal protective equipment, and electric incinerators instead of flame incinerators.
- Most pathogenic mycobacteria are slow growers, taking up to several weeks for isolation on artificial media.

- Some *Mycobacterium* spp. produce a pigment, which can be a helpful characteristic in the identification scheme of the mycobacteria.
- Other key tests for the identification of mycobacteria include rate of growth, nitrate reduction, niacin production, presence of heat stable catalase, and sensitivity to T2H.

Learning Assessment Questions

1. Describe the current recommendations for the identification of *Mycobacterium tuberculosis* in the clinical laboratory.

2. Describe the reason mycobacterial infections have to be treated for 6 months or longer, and explain the need to use multiple drugs when treating *M. tuberculosis* infections.

3. Compare and contrast the different levels of mycobacterial laboratory testing, and cite the reasons why smaller-volume laboratories should consider not performing full identification and susceptibility testing on mycobacterial isolates.

4. Discuss the methods used to process clinical specimens for mycobacterial culture and the reasons specimens need to be decontaminated and digested before culture.

5. With respect to laboratory technique in the isolation and identification of mycobacteria, discuss some causes of false-negative and false-positive results.

6. Describe important safety considerations for laboratories attempting mycobacterial isolation and identification.

7. Which of the following is/are fluorescent stain(s) used in the detection of the mycobacteria?
   a. Auramine/rhodamine
   b. Kinyoun's
   c. Ziehl-Neelsen
   d. Both b and c

8. A nonpigmented mycobacterium is isolated that reduces nitrate to nitrite and is niacin positive. You should suspect:
   a. *M. kansasii*
   b. *M. xenopi*
   c. *M. tuberculosis*
   d. *M. avium* complex

9. The causative agent of Hansen disease:
   a. Is highly contagious
   b. Readily grows on most mycobacterial media
   c. Grows best at core body temperature (37° C)
   d. None of the above

10. The skin test for tuberculosis:
    a. Detects antibodies to mycobacterial antigens
    b. Detects a cell-mediated immune response to mycobacterial antigens
    c. Uses the bacillus of Calmette-Guérin strain as the antigen source
    d. Both a and b

Medically Significant Fungi

Annette W. Fothergill

OBJECTIVES

After reading and studying this chapter, you should be able to:

1. Describe the general characteristics of fungi.

2. Describe the structures associated with fungi.

3. Compare asexual and sexual reproduction of fungi.

4. List the four divisions of fungi.

5. Describe diseases caused by fungi.

6. Identify the major causes of fungal infections.

7. List the common opportunistic saprobes associated with infections in immunocompromised hosts.

8. Characterize the following different types of mycoses, defining the tissues they affect:

   a. Superficial

   b. Cutaneous

   c. Subcutaneous

   d. Systemic

   e. Opportunistic saprobic

9. Analyze the appropriate specimen collection procedures, staining methods, and culture techniques used in the mycology laboratory.

10. Compare and contrast the methods used to identify fungi.

Case in Point

A 32-year-old woman developed a fever 12 days after a bone marrow transplant. Broad-spectrum antimicrobial therapy was initiated, but the fever persisted. On day 17 the patient developed skin lesions across her body and lower extremities; a biopsy was obtained. Microscopic evaluation of the tissue revealed hyphal elements. That same day, after 5 days of incubation, the patient's blood cultures were positive with a yeastlike colony. Although antifungal therapy was initiated, the patient died on day 22.

Issues to Consider

After reading the patient's case history, consider:

- Which fungi are most likely to be implicated in this patient's infection.
- How the laboratory will resolve the discrepancy between what is seen in the tissue slides and what grows from the blood culture.
- The steps necessary to arrive at a final identification of this agent of disease.

Key Terms

Anamorph	Mycelia
Arthroconidium	Mycoses
Ascospore	Onychomycosis
Ascus	Polymorphic fungi
Blastoconidium	Pseudogerm tube
Conidium	Pseudohyphae
Dermatophyte	Rhizoids
Dimorphic fungi	Saprobe
Eumycotic mycetoma	Sporangiophores
Germ tube	Sporangiospores
Hyphae	Synanamorph
Macroconidium	Teleomorph
Microconidium	Yeast
Mould	

Fungi constitute an extremely diverse group of organisms and are generally classified as either **moulds** or **yeasts.** Some have been recognized as classic pathogens, whereas others are recognized only as environmental **saprobes.** Fungi can cause mild infections, trigger allergic reactions including asthma, and produce serious life-threatening disease. With the advent of chemotherapy, radiation therapy, and diseases such as acquired immunodeficiency syndrome (AIDS) that affect the immune system, the line between pathogen and saprobe has been blurred. The isolation of all organisms, especially in the immunocompromised patient, must initially be considered a significant finding and evaluated in light of the patient history and physical examination results.

GENERAL CHARACTERISTICS

The characteristics of the fungi differ from those of plants or bacteria. Fungi are eukaryotic; that is, they possess a true nucleus with a nuclear membrane and mitochondria. Bacteria are prokaryotic, lacking these structures. Unlike plants, fungi lack chlorophyll and must absorb nutrients from the environment. In addition, fungal cell walls are made of chitin, whereas those of plants contain cellulose. Most fungi are obligate aerobes that grow best at a neutral pH, although they tolerate a wide pH range. Moisture is necessary for growth, but spores and conidia survive in dry conditions.

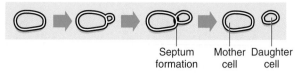

FIGURE 27-1 Formation of blastoconidia in yeast.

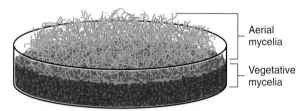

Aerial mycelia

Vegetative mycelia

FIGURE 27-2 Aerial mycelia give mould the "woolly" appearance. Vegetative mycelia are responsible for absorbing nutrients from the medium.

Yeasts versus Moulds

Yeasts are single vegetative cells that typically form a smooth, creamy, bacterial-like colony without aerial hyphae. Because both their macroscopic and microscopic morphologies are similar, identification of yeasts is based primarily on biochemical testing. Yeasts reproduce by budding, with subsequent production of a **blastoconidium** (daughter cell), as shown in Figure 27-1. This process involves lysis of the yeast cell wall so that a blastoconidium can form. As this structure enlarges, the nucleus of the parent cell undergoes mitosis. Once the new nucleus is passed into the daughter cell, a septum forms and the daughter cell breaks free.

Most moulds have a "fuzzy" or woolly appearance because of the formation of **mycelia** (Figure 27-2). The mycelia are made up of many long strands of tubelike structures called **hyphae,** which are either aerial or vegetative. Aerial mycelia extend above the surface of the colony and are responsible for the fuzzy appearance. In addition, mycelia can support the reproductive structures that produce conidia. Conidia can be used to identify the different fungal genera. The vegetative mycelia extend downward into the medium to absorb nutrients.

The microscopic appearance often aids in the identification of moulds. In some species, antler, racquet, or spiral hyphae are formed (Figure 27-3, *A*). Antler hyphae have swollen, branching tips that resemble moose antlers. Racquet hyphae contain enlarged, club-shaped areas. Spiral hyphae are tightly coiled. Rhizoids (Figure 27-3, *B*), rootlike structures, might be seen in some of the Zygomycetes, and their presence and placement can assist with identification. Frequently, when fungal hyphae are being described, they are referred to as *septate* or *sparsely septate*. Septate hyphae (Figure 27-4, *A*) show frequent cross-walls occurring perpendicularly to the outer walls of the hyphae, whereas sparsely septate hyphae (Figure 27-4, *B*) have few cross-walls at irregular intervals. The term *aseptate,* meaning the absence of septations, has historically been used to describe the hyphae of the Zygomycetes. Microscopic examination of hyphae associated with the

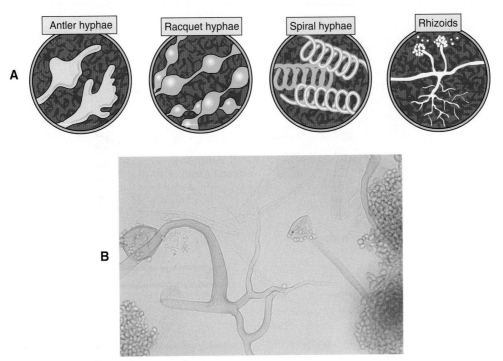

FIGURE 27-3 **A,** Specialized structures that are formed in vegetative mycelia by certain fungal species. **B,** *Rhizopus* spp. showing rhizoids.

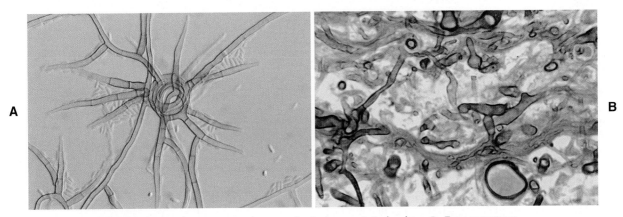

FIGURE 27-4 **A,** *Phaeoacremonium* sp. displaying septate hyphae. **B,** *Zygomycetous* hyphae in tissue appears sparsely septate.

Zygomycetes often reveals occasional septations; therefore these hyphae are more correctly termed *sparsely septate* as opposed to *aseptate*.

Hyaline versus Dematiaceous

Another characteristic useful in identification is pigmentation. Hyaline (moniliaceous) hyphae are either nonpigmented or lightly pigmented, whereas dematiaceous hyphae are darkly pigmented (Figure 27-5) because of the presence of melanin in the cell wall. Depending on the amount of melanin present, the hyphae will appear pale to dark brown or nearly black. Note that the dark hyphae seen in the tissue section in Figure 27-4, *B,* is dark-colored because of stains that enable better visualization of fungal elements in tissue and not because of

melanin. All fungal elements appear black when Gomori methylene stain is used. Another stain that is often used to determine hyphal pigmentation in tissue is the Fontana-Masson stain. This stain specifically stains melanin causing dematiaceous hyphae to appear brown whereas hyaline hyphae remain pink to red.

Dimorphism and Polymorphism

Dimorphism refers to the ability of some fungi to exist in two forms, depending on growth conditions. These **dimorphic fungi** include a mould phase and either a yeast or spherule phase. The yeast or tissue state is seen in vivo or when the organism is grown at 37° C with increased CO_2. The mould phase is seen when the organism is grown at room tempera-

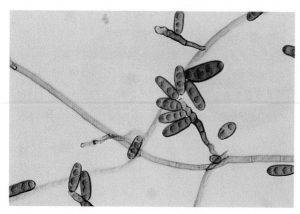

FIGURE 27-5 *Bipolaris* sp. is an example of a dematiaceous fungus. Note the dark pigmentation, which is due to the presence of melanin in the cell wall.

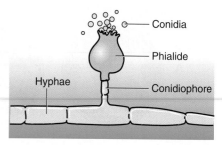

FIGURE 27-6 An example of asexual reproduction is the production of phialoconidia. Conidia are formed from conidiogenous cells like phialide (a vaselike structure). Phialoconidia are "blown out" of the phialide.

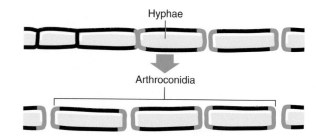

FIGURE 27-7 Arthroconidia, another form of asexual reproduction, are formed by fragmentation of fertile hyphae.

ture (22° to 25° C) in ambient air conditions. Thermally dimorphic fungal species associated with human disease include *Blastomyces dermatitidis, Coccidioides immitis, Histoplasma capsulatum* var. *capsulatum, Paracoccidioides brasiliensis, Sporothrix schenckii,* and *Penicillium marneffei.* Several other fungi also possess this ability but have not been described as agents of human **mycoses** (infections due to fungi). **Polymorphic fungi** have both yeast and mould forms in the same culture. This characteristic occurs despite growth conditions and is best observed in *Exophiala* spp., where the yeast phase is typically observed initially followed by the mould phase as the colony ages.

Reproduction

Fungi can reproduce either asexually (imperfect) or sexually (perfect). Asexual reproduction results in the formation of conidia (singular: **conidium**) following mitosis. Asexual reproduction is carried out by specialized fruiting structures known as *conidiogenous cells.* These structures form conidia, which contain all the genetic material necessary to create a new fungal colony. Two common conidiogenous cells are the phialide, vaselike structures that produce phialoconidia (Figure 27-6), and the annellide, ringed structures that produce annelloconidia. Both form their conidia blastically (budding) like many yeasts; the parent cell enlarges and a septum forms to separate the conidial cell. Another type of conidia is the arthroconidia (singular, **arthroconidium**). These conidia are formed by fragmentation of fertile hyphae (Figure 27-7).

In the clinical laboratory, most mould identifications are based on the structures formed as a result of asexual reproduction. Sexual reproduction requires the joining of two compatible nuclei, followed by meiosis (Figure 27-8). A fungus that reproduces sexually is known as a **teleomorph.** Occasionally a teleomorph will also reproduce asexually. When this occurs, the asexual form is termed the **anamorph.** If more than one anamorph is present for the same teleomorph, the anamorphs are termed **synanamorphs.** The best example of the phenomenon is the teleomorph *Pseudallescheria boydii,* which has two anamorphs: *Scedosporium apiospermum* and *Graphium* sp. These two anamorphs are synanamorphs to each other.

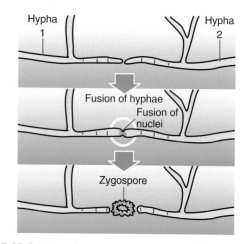

FIGURE 27-8 Sexual reproduction occurs by the fusion of compatible nuclei and subsequent production of a zygospore.

TAXONOMY

Most of the etiologic agents of clinical infections are found in four groups of fungi. They consist of the divisions Zygomycota, Ascomycota, Basidiomycota, and the form-division Fungi Imperfecti (Deuteromycota).

Zygomycota

Members of the class Zygomycetes are rapidly growing organisms normally found in the soil. They are often opportunistic

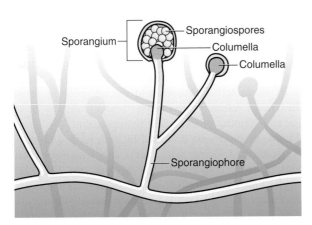

FIGURE 27-9 Asexual reproduction by Zygomycetes is characterized by the production of spores (sporangiospores) from within a sporangium.

pathogens in immunocompromised hosts. Zygomycetes generally produce profuse, gray to white, aerial mycelium characterized by the presence of sparsely septate hyphae. Asexual reproduction of Zygomycetes is characterized by the presence of **sporangiophores** and **sporangiospores.** The asexual spores (sporangiospores) are produced in a structure known as a *sporangium*, which develops from a sporangio-phore (Figure 27-9). Although some Zygomycetes are capable of sexual reproduction resulting in the production of zygo-spores, these structures are not routinely seen in clinical labo-ratories. Common Zygomycetes include *Mucor, Rhizopus,* and *Absidia.*

Ascomycota

Fungi associated with the class Ascomycetes are characterized by the production of sexual spores known as **ascospores.** Ascospores are formed within a saclike structure known as an **ascus.** It is important to note, however, that they are usually identified on the basis of characteristic asexual structures. Representative organisms include *Microsporum* spp., *Tricho-phyton* spp., and *Pseudallescheria boydii.*

Basidiomycota

Clinically significant basidiomycetes are few. The only known major pathogen is *Filobasidiella neoformans,* the perfect form of *Cryptococcus neoformans* var. *neoformans.* When basidio-mycetous moulds are recovered in the laboratory, they typi-cally remain sterile, complicating the identification process. One clue that a mould is a basidiomycete is the presence of clamp connections. Clamp connections occur at the septa-tions in the vegetative hyphae and are easily visible with light microscopy. A portion of the hypha on one side of the septation grows out and connects to the hypha on the other side of the septation, thereby bypassing the septation. Basid-iomycetous moulds are being recovered in increasing numbers in the laboratory, but their role in infectious disease is not readily understood. Close communication between the physi-cian and the laboratory may assist with determining whether the isolate is an environmental contaminant or an agent of disease.

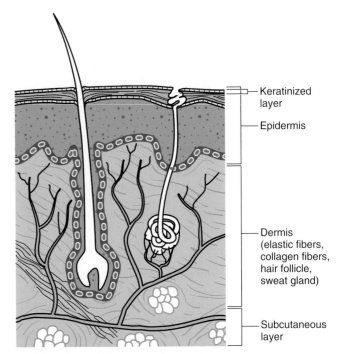

FIGURE 27-10 Diagram of the layers of skin and tissues in which fungal infections can occur.

Fungi Imperfecti

The form-division Fungi Imperfecti contains the largest number of organisms that are etiologic agents of mycoses, including cutaneous, subcutaneous, and systemic disease. Organisms are placed within this group when no mode of sexual reproduction has been identified. Therefore they are identified on the basis of characteristic asexual reproductive structures.

MYCOSES

Mycoses (singular: mycosis) are diseases caused by fungi. Fungal disease is frequently categorized based on the site of the infection. These categories include superficial, cutaneous, subcutaneous, and systemic mycoses. Figure 27-10 shows the different layers of tissues where fungal infections may occur. Following this diagram, it becomes easier to classify infec-tions of the skin, depending on where the infection occurs. Infections not involving the skin or deeper tissues just under the skin are termed *systemic.*

Superficial Mycoses

Superficial mycoses are infections confined to the outermost layer of skin or hair. Because infections of the skin, hair, and nails were at one time believed to be the result of burrowing worms that formed ring-shaped patterns in the skin, the term *tinea* was applied to each disease, along with a Latin term for the body site. An example of nondermatophytic tinea is the disease *tinea versicolor* (pityriasis versicolor). This disease is characterized by discoloration or depigmentation and scaling of the skin and is caused by the yeast identified as *Malassezia*

TABLE 27-1 Various Forms of Dermatophytoses and the Respective Affective Sites

Type of Ringworm	Site Affected
Tinea capitis	Head
Tinea favosa	Head (distinctive pathology)
Tinea barbae	Beard
Tinea corporis	Body (glabrous skin)
Tinea manuum	Hand
Tinea unguium	Nails
Tinea cruris	Groin
Tinea pedis	Feet
Tinea imbricata	Body (distinctive lesion)

furfur complex. The disease becomes apparent in individuals with dark complexions or in those that fail to tan normally.

Another nondermatophytic superficial infection is tinea nigra. This disease is almost always caused by *Phaeoannellomyces werneckii* and is characterized by brown or black macular patches primarily on the palms. Biopsy and culture of the site is important to distinguish this infection from a much more serious disease, melanoma. Finally, piedra is another superficial infection that is confined to the hair shaft and is characterized by nodules composed of hyphae and a cementlike substance that attaches it to the hair shaft. Black piedra is caused by *Piedraia hortae*, and white piedra is caused by *Trichophyton ovoides* and *T. inkin*.

Cutaneous Mycoses

Dermatomycoses are defined as fungal diseases of the keratinized tissues of humans and other animals. Although nondermatophyte species are capable of causing similar infections, this syndrome is most often a result of infection with a dermatophyte, thus the term *dermatophytosis*. Note that this term should not be used until the etiologic agent has been identified to be a dermatophyte. Genera in this group include *Trichophyton*, *Microsporum*, and *Epidermophyton*. Dermatophytic infections usually involve a restricted region of the host; traditionally these diseases are named with respect to the portion of the body affected. We continue to describe the various forms of "ringworm" in these terms, as shown in Table 27-1.

Each ringworm lesion is the result of a local inoculation of the skin with the etiologic agent. Lesions enlarge with time, usually with most inflammation occurring at the advancing edge of the lesion. Some cases of ringworm are subclinical, exhibiting only a dry, scaly lesion without inflammation. Symptoms of cutaneous mycoses include itching, scaling, or ringlike patches of the skin; brittle, broken hairs; and thick, discolored nails.

Subcutaneous Mycoses

Subcutaneous mycoses involve the deeper skin layers, including muscle, connective tissue, and bone. Except in certain patient populations, dissemination through the blood to major organs does not occur. Characteristic clinical features include progressive, nonhealing ulcers and the presence of draining sinus tracts. In tropical areas, agents such as *Phialophora* spp. and *Cladosporium* spp. cause chromoblastomycosis, characterized as verrucous nodules that often become ulcerated and crusted. This disease is diagnosed by the presence of characteristic lesions and the microscopic sclerotic bodies, often referred to as *copper pennies* because of their shape and staining properties in tissue sections.

Eumycotic mycetoma is caused by both fungi and bacteria and results in draining sinus tracts and tissue destruction. Grains (granules), tightly bound hyphae, can be collected from the fluids that drain from the sinus tracks. *Sporothrix schenckii* commonly presents as a progressive lymphocutaneous infection beginning with a single lesion and progressing along the limbs via the lymph system. Dissemination of this species causing systemic sporotrichosis is much more common.

Systemic Mycoses

Systemic, or disseminated, mycoses are infections that affect internal organs or deep tissues of the body. Frequently the initial site of infection is the lung, from which the organism disseminates hematogenously to other organs or the skin. Generalized symptoms include fever and fatigue. Chronic cough and chest pain might also accompany these infections. Historically the term *systemic mycoses* has been used to describe diseases caused by thermally dimorphic fungi, including *Histoplasma*, *Coccidioides*, and *Blastomyces* species. Other fungal agents are capable of causing systemic disease and include *Aspergillus*, *Fusarium*, and *Bipolaris* species as well as some monomorphic yeast: *Candida albicans* and *Cryptococcus neoformans*. It is important to note that any fungus is capable of disseminating from the primary site of infection in the immunocompromised host.

CLINICALLY SIGNIFICANT SPECIES

Agents of Superficial Mycoses

Superficial mycoses are fungal diseases that affect only the cornified layers (stratum corneum) of the epidermis. Patients who suffer from superficial fungal infections do not show any overt symptoms because the fungal agents do not activate any tissue response or inflammatory reaction. Patients usually seek medical attention to address cosmetic rather than medical concerns caused by these fungi.

Malassezia furfur

Clinical Manifestations. The *M. furfur* complex causes tinea versicolor, a disease characterized by patchy lesions or scaling of varying pigmentation. It is also thought to be a cause of dandruff. Lesions associated with tinea versicolor typically appear as pale patches in individuals with darkly pigmented skin, but they can also be described as "fawn-colored liver spots" in individuals with fair complexions. Lesions become especially evident in warm months where sun exposure is more likely. Tinea versicolor may involve any area of the body, but the most prevalent sites include the face, chest, trunk, or abdomen. Antifungal therapy is not typically indicated, but the appearance of lesions may be diminished by treatment with antidandruff shampoos. Interestingly, *M. furfur* complex has also been implicated in disseminated infections in patients receiving high-dose lipid replacement therapy, particularly in infants. Removal of indwelling feeding lines is usually sufficient to clear infections without the use of antifungal therapy.

M. furfur is a common endogenous skin colonizer. Although reasons for overgrowth by *M. furfur* resulting in clinical manifestation are still unknown, it appears to be related to squamous cell turnover rates. This is evidenced by the higher incidence of tinea versicolor among persons receiving corticosteroid therapy, which decreases the rate of squamous epithelial cell turnover. Some investigators have identified genetic influence, poor nourishment, and excessive sweating as other factors that contribute to the overgrowth of the organism on the skin. This organism is found worldwide, with the greatest prevalence in hot, humid, and tropical locations. *M. furfur* requires lipids and will not grow on routine fungal media.

Laboratory Diagnosis. *M. furfur* can be identified by visualizing skin scrapings from characteristic lesions in a potassium hydroxide (KOH) preparation or by observing yellow fluorescence with a Wood's lamp on examination of the infected body site. Microscopic examination of the direct smear in KOH preparations reveals budding yeasts, approximately 4 to 8 μm, along with septate, sometimes branched, hyphal elements. This microscopic appearance has gained *M. furfur* the term "the spaghetti and meatballs" fungus (Figure 27-11).

Because of the special nutritional requirements of this organism, routine fungal cultures are negative for growth. Typical yeastlike colonies may be observed only after the

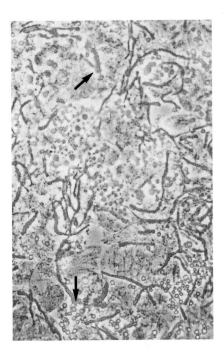

FIGURE 27-11 Diagram of the typical "spaghetti and meatballs" appearance of *Malassezia furfur* in a potassium hydroxide preparation.

culture medium is overlaid with olive oil. Colonies are cream colored, moist, and smooth.

Piedraia hortae

Clinical Manifestations. *Piedraia hortae* is the causative agent of black piedra, an infection that occurs on the hairs of the scalp. The infecting organism produces hard, dark brown to black gritty nodules that are firmly attached to the hair shaft. These nodules consist of asci (sacklike structures) containing eight ascospores. The disease is endemic in tropical areas of Africa, Asia, and Latin America.

Laboratory Diagnosis. When infected hair shafts are removed and placed in 10% to 20% KOH, the nodules may be crushed open to reveal the asci. Thick-walled rhomboid cells containing ascospores are seen. *P. hortae* grows slowly on Sabouraud dextrose agar at room temperature. It forms brown, restricted colonies that remain sterile.

Trichosporon spp.

Clinical Manifestations. *Trichosporon beigelii* has been described in the literature as an extremely variable human pathogen. Examination of the genome of members of the genus has revealed that *T. beigelii* is no longer a valid species but rather a complex of at least 17 distinct species. *T. ovoides, T. asteroides, T. cutaneum,* and *T. inkin* have been implicated in superficial mycoses. The most important species in this genus is *T. asahaii,* which is implicated in severe and frequently fatal disease in immunocompromised hosts.

Trichosporon spp. are occasionally found as part of the normal skin biota. White piedra occurs on the hair shaft and is characterized by a soft mycelial mat surrounding hair of the scalp, face and pubic region. Members of this genus have also been recognized as opportunistic systemic pathogens. Although rare, systemic disease caused by these fungi are frequently fatal and occurs most often in the immunocompromised host, commonly people who have hematologic disorders or malignancies or are undergoing chemotherapy. Infections in immunocompromised patients include infections of the blood, cerebrospinal fluid (CSF), and organs. Widely distributed in nature, white piedra is endemic in tropical areas of South America, the Far East, and the Pacific.

Laboratory Diagnosis. *Trichosporon* spp. produce both arthroconidia and blastoconidia (Figure 27-12) and grow rapidly on primary fungal media. The colonies are cream-colored and yeastlike. Colonies remain smooth or may eventually become wrinkled as they mature. Identification of species is confirmed by biochemical reactions, including the absence of carbohydrate fermentation or utilization of potassium nitrate and the assimilation of many sugars; they are also urease positive.

Hortaea werneckii

Clinical Manifestations. Tinea nigra, characterized by brown to black nonscaly macules that occur most often on the palms of the hands and soles of the feet, is caused by *H. werneckii.* Synonyms for *H. werneckii* include *Phaeoannellomyces werneckii, Exophiala werneckii,* and *Cladosporium werneckii.* Disease involves no inflammatory or other tissue reaction to the infecting fungus. However, the clinical presen-

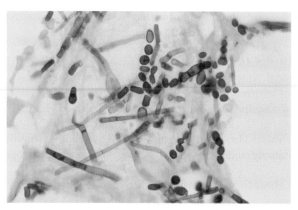

FIGURE 27-12 Microscopic appearance of *Trichosporon* species on lactophenol cotton blue preparation showing the presence of both blastoconidia and arthroconidia.

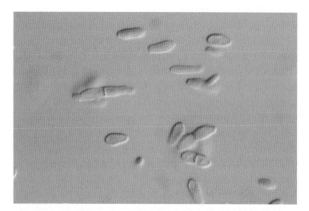

FIGURE 27-13 Microscopic structures of *Phaeoannellomyces werneckii*, showing characteristic budding annelloconidia. *P. werneckii* causes tinea nigra.

tation is so similar to other conditions that misdiagnosis could occur, resulting in unnecessary surgical procedures, especially when confused with malignant melanoma. The disease is endemic in the tropical areas of Central and South America, Africa, and Asia.

Laboratory Diagnosis. Diagnosis of tinea nigra can be made by direct examination of skin scrapings placed in 10% to 20% KOH. Microscopic examination shows septate hyphal elements and budding cells (Figure 27-13). Younger cultures are primarily composed of budding blastoconidia, whereas the older mycelial portion of the colony shows hyphae with blastoconidia in clusters. *Annelloconidia* are seen in older hyphal colonies. *P. werneckii* produces shiny, moist, yeastlike colonies that start with a brownish coloration that eventually turns olive to greenish black.

Agents of Cutaneous Mycoses

General Characteristics

Three genera of fungi, *Trichophyton*, *Microsporum*, and *Epidermophyton*, are etiologic agents of dermatophytoses. Species within these genera are keratinophilic; that is, they are adapted to grow on hair, nails, and cutaneous layers of skin that contain the scleroprotein keratin. Infection of deep tissue by these fungi is rare, but occasionally extensive inflammation and nail-bed involvement or disseminated disease may result.

By way of a single developmental process, dermatophytes typically form two sizes of reproductive cells, termed a **macroconidium** or a **microconidium**. Both of these are anamorphic or asexual conidia, and their distinctive size, shape, and surface features make them valuable structures for species identification. Some dermatophytes are known to also have teleomorphic stages, in which ascospores are the reproductive cells. Teleomorphs in this group of organisms are not observed in routine laboratory studies of patient isolates because dermatophytes are heterothallic—requiring the combination of two distinct mating types. Although a few reference laboratories perform mating tests with known "tester strains," this is not a procedure regularly used in clinical laboratories.

Most of the agents of dermatophytoses live freely in the environment, but a few have adapted almost exclusively to living on human host tissues, and they are rarely recovered from any other source. Distribution of these species, referred to as **dermatophytes,** is generally worldwide, although a few are found only in restricted geographic regions. Approximately 43 species of dermatophytes and dermatophyte-like fungi have been described, and just over two dozen of these have been documented to cause human infection.

Dermatophytes that primarily inhabit the soil are termed *geophilic*. Most geophilic fungi produce large numbers of conidia and therefore are among the most readily identified species. Zoophilic dermatophytes are typically adapted to live on animals and are not commonly found living freely in soil or on dead organic substrates. They often cause infections in animal hosts and may be spread as agents of disease in humans. Fewer conidia are produced by zoophilic fungi than by geophilic species. A few dermatophytes have become adapted exclusively to human hosts and are termed *anthropophilic*. Although they are encountered almost always as agents of human disease, the infections are seldom inflammatory. Species identification may be quite difficult because most anthropophilic species produce few conidia.

Not only are diverse sites on the host involved in infections but also certain species cause distinctive lesions. The notable example is tinea imbricata, caused by *Trichophyton concentricum*. Over time, involved portions of the trunk develop diagnostically distinctive concentric rings of scaling tissue. In some forms of ringworm, a persistent allergic reaction, dermatophytid, is manifested in the formation of sterile, itching lesions on body sites distant from the point of infection. Symptoms of dermatophyte infections vary from slight to moderate and occasionally severe.

Infections Involving Hair

Different body sites manifest different symptoms. Infections in the scalp, where hair follicles are the initiation sites, can be among the most severe and disfiguring forms of the disease. Tinea favosa, or favus, begins as an infection of the hair follicle by *Trichophyton schoenleinii* and progresses to a crusty lesion made up of dead epithelial cells and fungal mycelia.

Crusty, cup-shaped flakes called *scutula* are formed. Hair loss and scar tissue formation commonly follow.

Two distinct forms of tinea capitis, gray-patch ringworm and black-dot ringworm, are caused by different species of dermatophytes. Gray-patch ringworm is a common childhood disease that is easily spread among children. The fungus colonizes primarily the outer portion of hair shafts, the so-called ectothrix hair involvement. The lesions are seldom inflamed, but luster and color of the hair shaft may be lost. *Microsporum audouinii* and *M. ferrugineum* are agents of this disease. Black-dot ringworm consists of endothrix hair involvement. The hair follicle is the initial site of infection, and fungal growth continues within the hair shaft, causing it to weaken. The brittle, infected hair shafts break off at the scalp, leaving the "black-dot" stubs. *Trichophyton tonsurans* and *T. violaceum* are the most common fungi implicated in this form of dermatophytosis.

Infections Involving the Nails

Onychomycosis, infections of the nails, is most often caused by dermatophytes but also may be the result of infection by other fungi. These nail and nail-bed infections may be among the most difficult dermatomycoses to treat. Long-term, costly therapy with terbinafine or itraconazole is considered the best treatments, but results are often unsatisfactory. There is a direct association between dermatophytic infections of the feet or hands and infections of the nails. It is unlikely that anyone suffering from tinea pedis will escape onychomycosis to some extent. Subungual is the most common form of onychomycosis, which is described as lateral, distal, or proximal. Either of the ends of the nail is first infected with spread continuing to the nail plate. Nails become thick, discolored and flakey. Some common agents that infect the nails are *Trichophyton rubrum, T. mentagrophytes,* and *T. tonsurans,* as well as *Epidermophyton floccosum.*

Tinea Pedis

Among the shoe-wearing human population, tinea pedis (athlete's foot) is a common disease. Infection arises from contact with infected skin scales coming into contact with exposed skin in carpet, showers, and other environments. It is believed that individuals have a genetic predisposition to developing the disease because not everyone coming into contact with infected skin scale becomes infected. Infections within a family are common. Various sites on the foot may be involved, but most often tinea pedis affects the soles of the feet and toe webs. In more severe cases, the sole of the foot may develop extensive scaling with fissuring and erythema. The disease may progress around the sides of the foot from the sole, giving rise to use of the term "moccasin foot," descriptive of the appearance of the infected area. Infections of the glabrous skin range from mild with only minimal scaling and erythema to severely inflamed lesions.

Systemic Dermatophyte Infections

Immunocompromised persons may suffer systemic dermatophyte infections. Disseminated disease appears in different forms. In some patients, it manifests as granulomas whereas in others it develops into nodules ranging from pea to walnut size. Biopsy of these nodules reveals fungal elements that are easily recovered in culture. This phenomenon has been seen primarily in kidney transplant patients and is thought to have spread from athlete's foot or onychomycosis.

Epidermophyton floccosum

Despite the fact that *Epidermophyton floccosum* produces only one size of conidia, these conidia are described as macroconidia because of their size. The smooth, thin-walled macroconidia are produced in clusters or singly. The distal end of the conidium is broad, or spatulate, and reminiscent of a beaver's tail. Occasionally conidia may be single celled, but usually they are separated into two to five cells by perpendicular cross-walls.

Colonies of *E. floccosum* are yellow to yellow-tan, flat with feathered edges, and remain small in diameter. Epidermophyton isolates are notorious for developing pleomorphic tufts of sterile hyphae in older cultures. Epidermophyton is distributed worldwide.

Microsporum canis

Macroconidia from *Microsporum canis* are spindle shaped with echinulate, thick walls; they measure 12 to 25 μm × 35 to 110 μm and have 3 to 15 cells (Figure 27-14). The tapering, sometimes elongated, spiny distal ends of the macroconidia are key features that distinguish this species. Microconidia are abundantly formed by most isolates, and these may be the only conidia maintained in cultures that have been serially transferred. Colonies are fluffy and white, with the reverse side of the colony usually developing a lemon-yellow pigment, especially on potato dextrose agar. This fungus has a worldwide distribution.

Microsporum gypseum

The fusiform, moderately thick-walled conidia (Figure 27-15) typical of *Microsporum gypseum* measure 8 to 15 μm × 25 to 60 μm and can have as many as six cells. In some isolates, the distal end of the macroconidium might bear a thin, filamentous tail. Abundant macroconidia and microconidia produced by most isolates of this species result in a powdery,

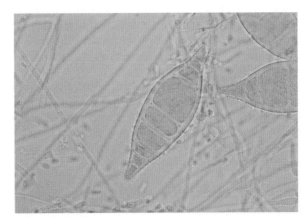

FIGURE 27-14 *Microsporum canis* showing spindle-shaped, echinulate macroconidia with thick walls and tapered ends, which are key features in identification of this species.

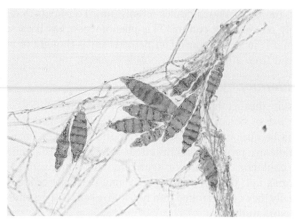

FIGURE 27-15 *Microsporum gypseum* showing fusiform, moderately thick-walled macroconidia containing several cells.

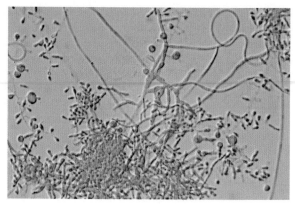

FIGURE 27-16 *Trichophyton mentagrophytes* showing globose, teardrop-shaped microconidia. (Nomarski optics, 1250×).

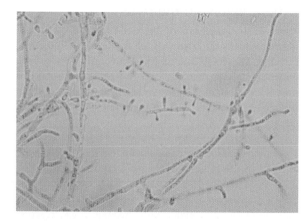

FIGURE 27-17 *Trichophyton rubrum* showing clavate- or peg-shaped microconidia.

granular appearance on colony surfaces. Colonies that form tan to buff conidial masses are typical of fresh isolates, but this species tends to develop pleomorphic tufts of white, sterile hyphae in aging cultures and after serial transfers. Abundant brown to red pigment can form beneath some strains, but others remain colorless. *M. gypseum* is a rapidly growing geophilic species found in soils worldwide.

Microsporum audouinii

A slow-growing anthropomorphic dermatophyte, *Microsporum audouinii* was responsible for most of the gray-patch tinea capitis of children until a few decades ago, when *T. tonsurans* replaced it as the leading cause of scalp infection. In culture, conidia are only rarely produced. Some isolates form chlamydoconidium-like swellings terminally on hyphae. Colonies of *M. audouinii* appear cottony white and generally form little or no pigment on the reverse.

Trichophyton mentagrophytes

Trichophyton mentagrophytes makes both microconidia and macroconidia. Microconidia (Figure 27-16) are primarily globose but may appear tear-shaped and measure 2.5 to 4 μm in diameter. Microconidia are found primarily in clusters described as grapelike or "engrape." Macroconidia are thin walled, smooth, and cigar shaped, with four to five cells separated by parallel cross-walls. These conidia measure about 7 μm × 20 to 50 μm and are produced singly on undifferentiated hyphae.

Colony morphology varies with the extent of conidia production. Granular colonies are noted when abundant microconidia are formed. In the downy form, conidia are less abundant. Compared with other dermatophytes, *T. mentagrophytes* is a relatively rapidly growing fungus. This species is distributed worldwide.

Trichophyton rubrum

Although *Trichophyton rubrum* is known to produce three- to eight-celled cylindrical macroconidia measuring somewhat smaller than those of *T. mentagrophytes,* these are seldom seen in clinical isolates. A typical microscopic picture of *T.*

rubrum contains clavate- or peg-shaped microconidia (Figure 27-17) formed along undifferentiated hyphae, and even these may be sparse. Colonies usually remain white on the surface but may be yellow to red. Most strains develop a red to deep burgundy wine-colored pigment on the reverse that diffuses into the agar. This species has a worldwide distribution.

Trichophyton tonsurans

Trichophyton tonsurans possess microconidia that are extremely variable in shape, ranging from round to peg shapes. When grown on Sabouraud dextrose agar, colonies usually form a rust-colored pigment on the colony's reverse. *T. tonsurans*, which infects skin, hair, and nails, has become the leading cause of tinea capitis in children in many parts of the world, including the United States.

Agents of Subcutaneous Mycoses

Subcutaneous mycoses are fungal diseases that affect subcutaneous tissue. These mycoses are usually the result of the traumatic implantation of foreign objects into the deep layers of the skin, permitting the fungus to gain entry into the host. The etiologic agents responsible are organisms commonly found in soil or on decaying vegetation; therefore, agricultural workers are most often affected. Organisms causing subcutaneous mycoses belong to a variety of genera in the form-class Hyphomycetes. Although some are moniliaceous (hyaline or light colored), many are dematiaceous, producing darkly pigmented colonies and containing melanin in their cell walls. The infections are commonly chronic and usually incite the development of lesions at the site of trauma. Subcutaneous fungal infections may be grouped together by the disease processes they cause or by the etiologic agents involved.

Chromoblastomycosis

Also known as *verrucous dermatitidis* and *chromomycosis,* chromoblastomycosis occurs worldwide but is most common in tropical and subtropical regions of the Americas and Africa. In the United States, most cases have occurred in Texas and Louisiana. Several organisms are responsible for the disease, and certain organisms appear to reside in specific areas of endemicity throughout the world. Chromoblastomycosis is caused by several infectious agents, namely *Fonsecaea compacta, F. pedrosoi, Phialophora verrucosa, Cladophialophora carrionii,* and *Rhinocladiella aquaspersa.*

Clinical Manifestations. Chromoblastomycosis is a chronic mycosis of the skin and subcutaneous tissue that develops over a period of months or, more commonly, years. It is mostly asymptomatic in the absence of secondary complications, such as bacterial infections, carcinomatous degeneration, and elephantiasis. Lesions are usually confined to the extremities, often the feet and lower legs, and are a result of trauma to these areas. Lesions of chromoblastomycosis frequently appear as verrucous nodules that may become ulcerated and crusted. Longstanding lesions have a cauliflower-like surface. Brown, round sclerotic bodies, which are nonbudding structures occurring singly or in clusters, are seen in tissues. These sclerotic bodies reproduce by dividing in various planes, resulting in multicellular forms. Occasionally short hyphal elements are also seen. The presence of sclerotic bodies is diagnostic for this disease.

Laboratory Diagnosis. The microscopic morphology of each of the agents is described in Table 27-2. *P. verrucosa* and *C. carrionii* are shown in Figure 27-18. Etiologic agents are

identified on the basis of characteristic structures, such as arrangement of conidia and the manner in which conidia are borne. Organisms causing chromoblastomycosis are darkly pigmented or dematiaceous moulds. Growth is moderate to slow, and colonies are velvety to woolly and gray-brown to olivaceous black. Species are not differentiated by colony morphologies because they all produce similar characteristics.

Eumycotic Mycetomas

Mycetoma is an infection of the subcutaneous tissues that arises at the site of inoculation. The disease is characterized

---

TABLE 27-2 Microscopic Morphology of Fungi Causing Chromoblastomycosis

Organism	Microscopic Morphology
Phialophora verrucosa	Conidiogenous cells dematiaceous, flask-shaped phialides with collarettes
	Conidia oval, one-celled, occur in balls at tips of phialides
Fonsecaea pedrosoi	Primary one-celled conidia formed on sympodial conidiophores
	Primary conidia function as conidiogenous cells to form secondary one-celled conidia
	Some conidia similar to those seen in *Cladosporium* organisms, some like those in *Rhinocladiella* organisms, and others like those in *Phialophora* sp.
Fonsecaea compactum	Similar to *F. pedrosoi* but with more compact conidial heads
	Conidia are subglobose rather than ovoid
Cladophialophora carrionii	Erect conidiophores bearing branched chains of one-celled, brown blastoconidia
	Conidium close to tip of conidiophore termed "shield cell"
	Fragile chains
Rhinocladiella aquaspersa	Conidiophores erect, dark, bearing conidia only on upper portion near the tip
	Conidia elliptical, one-celled, produced sympodially

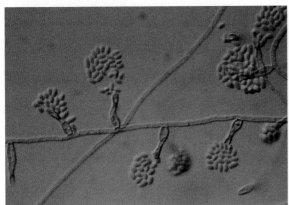
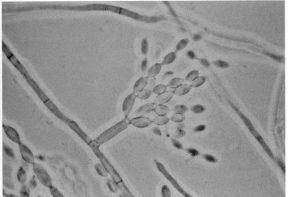

FIGURE 27-18 **A,** Conidia of *Phialophora verrucosa* at the tips of phialides with collarettes (Nomarski optics, 1250×). **B,** Conidial arrangement of *Cladophialophora carrionii.* (Courtesy Dr. Michael McGinnis.)

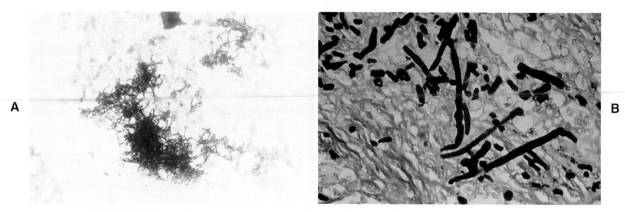

FIGURE 27-19 *Actinomycotic mycetoma* showing fine-branching, filamentous rods in tissue sample **(A)**, compared with the hyphal elements **(B)** seen in eumycotic infections (1250×).

TABLE 27-3 Description of Granules Seen in Eumycotic Mycetomas

Fungus	Color	Size (mm)	Texture
Pseudallescheria boydii	White	0.5-1.0	Soft
Acremonium falciforme	White	0.2-0.5	Soft
Madurella mycetomatis	Black	0.5-5.0	Hard
Madurella grisea	Black	0.3-0.6	Soft
Exophiala jeanselmei	Black	0.2-0.3	Soft

by swelling with characteristic exudate draining to the skin surface through sinus tracts. Mycetomas may be caused by either fungi or bacteria. Those caused by bacteria are referred to as *actinomycotic mycetomas,* and those caused by fungal agents are referred to as *eumycotic mycetomas.* Although clinical manifestations are similar for both types, the etiology must be determined before appropriate therapy is begun.

Mycetomas occur in tropical and subtropical areas but are also seen in temperate zones. The disease is endemic in India, Africa, and South America. Although mycetoma is an uncommon mycosis in the United States, the following species (in order of occurrence) are the most commonly incriminated agents: *Pseudallescheria boydii, Acremonium falciforme, Madurella mycetomatis, M. grisea,* and *Exophiala jeanselmei.* Direct microscopic examination of the granules collected from the draining lesion immediately differentiates eumycotic from actinomycotic mycetomas (Table 27-3). Figure 27-19, *A,* shows the branching filamentous rods of actinomycetes in contrast to the hyphal elements (Figure 27-19, *B*) seen in eumycotic infections.

Pseudallescheria boydii. The anamorphic form of *Pseudallescheria boydii* is the septate filamentous fungus *Scedosporium apiospermum.* Opinions differ regarding this fungus in relation to it being hyaline or dematiaceous. It produces oval conidia singly at the tips of conidiogenous cells (cells that make conidia) known as *annellides* (Figure 27-20). The teleomorph is noted by the formation of cleistothecia containing ascospores (Figure 27-21). This phenomenon occurs in fungi that are homothallic (ability of a single organism to undergo

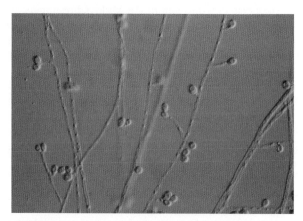

FIGURE 27-20 The *Scedosporium apiospermum* anamorph of *Pseudallescheria boydii.* (Nomarski optics, 625×).

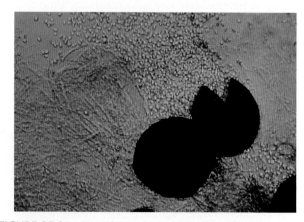

FIGURE 27-21 Sexual structures (cleistothecia containing ascospores) of *Pseudallescheria boydii.* (Nomarski optics, 325×).

sexual reproduction without a mate). This isolate grows rapidly and produces white to dark gray colonies on potato dextrose agar at both 22° and 35° C.

Acremonium falciforme. *Acremonium falciforme* produces mucoid clusters of single or two-celled, slightly curved conidia borne from phialides at the tips of long, unbranched, multiseptate conidiophores. Conidia are held together in mucoid clusters at the apices of the phialides. This isolate is a hyaline, septate, filamentous mould. Colonies grow slowly and are grayish brown, becoming grayish violet.

Madurella. *Madurella* spp. are dematiaceous, septate fungi. Approximately half of the isolates of *M. mycetomatis* produce conidia from the tips of phialides, but many remain sterile. This species grows very slowly but is initially white, and becomes yellow, olivaceous, or brown with a characteristic diffusible brown pigment with age. It grows best at 37° C and with slower growth at 40° C.

In colonies of *M. grisea,* only sterile hyphae are observed. This isolate grows slowly, produces olive brown to black colonies, and may produce a reddish brown pigment. Optimum growth temperature is 30° C.

Subcutaneous Phaeohyphomycosis

Phaeohyphomycosis is a mycotic disease caused by darkly pigmented fungi or fungi that have melanin in their cell walls. This term was coined to separate several clinical infections caused by dematiaceous fungi from those distinct clinical entities known as chromoblastomycosis. In tissue, these fungi may form yeastlike cells that are solitary or in short chains or hyphae that are septate, branched, or unbranched and often swollen to toruloid (irregular or beaded). Agents responsible for these mycoses are organisms commonly found in nature, encompassing many genera of Hyphomycetes, Coelomycetes, and Ascomycetes. Fungi that appear to be regularly associated with this condition include *Exophiala* spp. such as *E. dermatitidis*. A more complete list of genera associated with subcutaneous phaeohyphomycosis is found in Box 27-1.

With most *Exophiala* spp., conidia are borne from annellides, with conidia aggregating in masses at the tips of the conidiophore, as seen in Figure 27-22. *E. dermatidis*, however, forms conidia at the tips of phialides (Figure 27-23). This group of fungi produces olivaceous to black colonies that are initially yeastlike but become velvety at maturity.

Sporothrix schenckii

Clinical Manifestations. The most commonly seen presentation of *S. schenckii* infection is lymphocutaneous sporotrichosis. This chronic infection is characterized by nodular and ulcerative lesions along the lymph channels that drain the primary site of inoculation. Less commonly seen disease states include fixed cutaneous sporotrichosis, in which the infection is confined to the site of inoculation and mucocutaneous sporotrichosis, a relatively rare condition. Primary and secondary pulmonary sporotrichosis as well as extracutaneous and disseminated forms of the disease may also occur.

Sporothrix schenckii is commonly recovered from the soil and is associated with decaying vegetation. It is distributed worldwide but especially in warm, arid areas such as Mexico and also in moist, humid regions such as Brazil, Uruguay, and South Africa. In temperate countries such as France, Canada, and the United States, most cases of sporotrichosis are associated with gardening, particularly with exposure to rose thorns (rose-handler's disease) and sphagnum moss.

Laboratory Diagnosis. Direct examination of tissue might reveal *S. schenckii* as small, cigar-shaped yeast (Figure 27-24, *A*). Although the organism is occasionally seen in a Gram-stained smear, wet-mounts of material are often unrewarding because of the small numbers of organisms present. Microscopic examination from culture reveals thin, delicate hyphae bearing conidia developing in a "rosette" pattern at the ends of delicate conidiophores. Dark-walled conidia are also produced along the sides of the hyphae and may be more readily viewable than the rosettes in mature cultures (Figure 27-24, *B*).

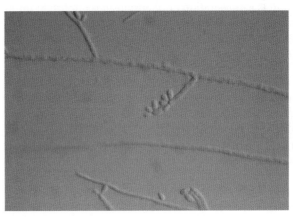

FIGURE 27-22 Conidia of *Exophiala* sp. borne at the tips of annellides. (Nomarski optics, 1250×).

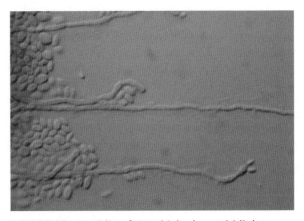

FIGURE 27-23 Conidia of *Exophiala dermatitidis* borne at the tips of phialides as well as the black yeast synanamorph. (Nomarski optics, 1250×).

BOX 27-1 Dematiaceous Genera Inciting Subcutaneous Phaeohyphomycosis*

Alternaria	Mycocentrospora
Bipolaris	Ochronosis
Chaetomium	Oidiodendron
Cladosporium	Phaeosclera
Curvularia	Phialophora
Dactylaria	Phoma
Exophiala	Ulocladium
Fonsecaea	Xylohypha

*This list is not all-inclusive.

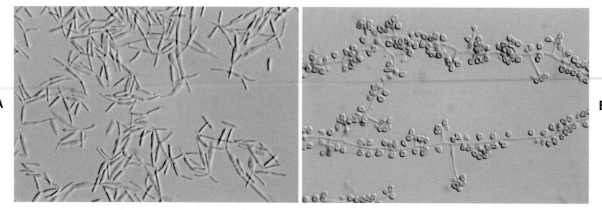

FIGURE 27-24 A, Yeast phase of *Sporothrix schenckii* showing cigar-shaped yeast cells typical of the species. **B,** Mould phase of *S. schenckii* revealing hyaline conidia borne at the ends of conidiophore in "rosettes" as well as dematiaceous conidia along the sides of the hyphae. (Nomarski optics, 625×).

Because *S. schenckii* is dimorphic, cultures are examined at 22° and 37° C. This fungus grows well on most culture media, including those containing cycloheximide. The colony morphology of *S. schenckii* at 22° C can be quite variable. At room temperature, colonies are often initially white, glabrous, and yeastlike, turning darker and more mycelial as they mature. Demonstration of dimorphism is important for identification of *S. schenckii*. To induce mycelia to yeast conversion, the fungus is inoculated onto brain heart infusion agar supplemented with sheep red blood cells and incubated at 37° C, in a CO_2 incubator. The formation of yeast colonies may require several subcultures. Complete conversion seldom occurs, but a portion of the colony will develop yeastlike cells.

Agents of Systemic Mycoses

Organisms that cause classic systemic fungal diseases have historically been categorized together because they share several characteristics, such as mode of transmission, dimorphism, and systemic dissemination. Although the term systemic generally refers to the organisms described here, it must be understood that any fungus, given an immunocompromised host, has the potential to become invasive and to disseminate to sites far removed from the portal of entry.

The term dimorphic, refers to the ability to grow as the mould form in the natural environment or in the laboratory at 22° to 30° C as shown in Table 27-4 or in the yeast or spherule form when incubated at 35° to 37° C on enriched media (Table 27-5). Each agent has a fairly well-defined area of endemicity, and the diseases they cause are contracted by the inhalation of infectious conidia. Table 27-6 provides a summary of systemic mycoses, their agents, and their characteristics. All laboratory procedures to recover and identify these agents must be performed in a biological safety cabinet.

Blastomyces dermatitidis

Clinical Manifestations. Blastomycosis is most prevalent in middle-aged men, as are other systemic mycoses, presumably owing to men's greater occupational and recreational exposure to the soil. Although patients with primary infection may exhibit flulike symptoms, most are asymptomatic and cannot

TABLE 27-4 Morphology of Systemic Fungi at 22° C

Fungus	Macroscopic Morphology	Macroscopic Morphology
Blastomyces dermatitidis	Slow to moderate growth White to dark tan Young colonies tenacious, older colonies glabrous to woolly	Oval, pyriform, to globose smooth conidia borne on short, lateral hyphalike conidiophores
Histoplasma capsulatum	Slow growth White to dark tan with age Woolly, cottony, or granular	Microconidia small, one-celled, round, smooth (2-5 μm) Tuberculated macroconidia large, round (7-12 μm) Hyphalike conidiophores
Coccidioides immitis/ Coccidioides posadasii	Rapid growth White to tan to dark gray Young colonies tenacious, older colonies cottony Tend to grow in concentric rings	Alternating one-celled, "barrel-shaped" arthroconidia with disjunctor cells
Paracoccidioides brasiliensis	Slow growth White to beige Colony glabrous, leathery, flat to wrinkled, folded or velvety	Colonies frequently only produce sterile hyphae Fresh isolates may produce conidia similar to those of *B. dermatitidis*

accurately define the time of onset. When the primary disease fails to resolve, pulmonary disease may ensue, with cough, weight loss, chest pain, and fever. Progressive pulmonary or invasive disease may follow, resulting in ulcerative lesions of the skin and bone. In the immunodeficient patient, multiple organ systems may be involved, and the course may be rapidly fatal.

Blastomycosis is also known as *Gilchrist disease, North American blastomycosis,* and *Chicago disease.* It occurs primarily in North America and parts of Africa. In the United States it is endemic in the Mississippi and Ohio River basins. Sporadic point-source outbreaks have also occurred in the St. Lawrence River basin. The natural reservoir has not been unequivocally established, although the organism has been recovered from the soil and from some natural environments. Apparently, only a very narrow range of conditions supports its growth. In areas where the organism appears endemic, natural disease occurs in dogs and horses, with the disease process mimicking that seen in human infections.

The teleomorph or sexual form of *B. dermatitidis* was described in 1967 and named *Ajellomyces dermatitidis*. It occurs only in rigidly controlled environments by mating of isolates with tester strains to produce gymnothecia containing ascospores. This teleomorph does not occur in the routine laboratory because the species is heterothallic—requiring two mating strains to produce the sexual form.

Laboratory Diagnosis. Examination of tissue or purulent material in cutaneous skin lesions may reveal large, spherical, refractile yeast cells, 8 to 15 µm in diameter, with a double-contoured wall and buds connected by a broad base (Figure 27-25). KOH (10%) or calcofluor white may be used to aid examination for the presence of the yeast cells. In the mould phase, conidia are borne on short lateral branches that are ovoid to dumbbell shaped and vary in diameter from 2 to 10 µm. Because they resemble a variety of other fungi, the microconidia are not diagnostic (Figure 27-26).

In culture at 22° C, the organism can produce a variety of colony morphologies. Colonies may be white, tan, or brown and may be fluffy to glabrous. Frequently, raised areas termed *spicules* are seen in the centers of the colonies. When grown

TABLE 27-5 Mould to Yeast Conversion of Thermally Dimorphic Fungi*

Fungus	Culture Media and Temperature	Yeast Form
Blastomyces dermatitidis	Blood agar, 37° C	Large yeast (8-12 µm) Blastoconidia attached by broad base
Histoplasma capsulatum	Pines medium, glucose-cysteine blood, or BHI-blood, 37° C	Small, oval yeast (2-5 µm)
Paracoccidioides brasiliensis	BHI-blood, 37° C	Multiple blastoconidia budding from single, large yeast (15-30 µm)

Coccidioides immitis can be converted to the spherule phase in a modified Converse medium at 40° C in 5%-10% CO_2. Exoantigen testing is preferred to this procedure in the routine clinical laboratory.
BHI, Brain heart infusion.

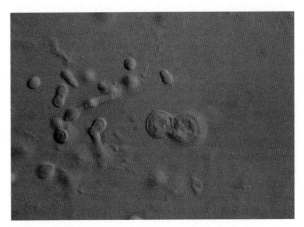

FIGURE 27-25 Conversion of the mould phase of *Blastomyces dermatitidis* to the "broad-based bud" yeast form. (Nomarski optics, 1250×).

TABLE 27-6 Summary of Systemic Mycoses

Fungus	Ecology	Clinical Disease	Tissue Form
Blastomyces dermatitidis	Mississippi and Ohio River valleys	Primary lung Chronic skin/bone Systemic, multiorgan	Large yeast (8-12 µm) Broad-based bud
*Histoplasma capsulatum**	Ohio, Missouri, and Mississippi River valleys Bird and bat guano Alkaline soil	Primary lung Asymptomatic Immunodeficient hosts prone to disseminated disease	Small, oval yeast (2-5 µm) in histiocytes, phagocytes
Coccidioides immitis/ Coccidioides posadasii	Semiarid regions: southwest United States, Mexico, Central and South America In soil	Primary lung Asymptomatic Secondary cavitary Progressive pulmonary Multisystem	Spherules (30-60 µm) containing endospores
Paracoccidioides brasiliensis	Central and South America In soil	Primary lung Granulomatous Ulcerative nasal and buccal lesions Lymph node involvement Adrenals	Thick-walled yeasts (15-30 µm) Multiple buds "Mariner's wheel

Histoplasma capsulatum var. *capsulatum* (teleomorph *Ajellomyces capsulatus*). *Histoplasma capsulatum* var. *duboisii is* endemic in Central Africa and is not discussed in this chapter.

at 37° C on suitable media, *B. dermatitidis* produces characteristic broad-based budding yeast cells.

The mycelial phase of the systemic dimorphic fungi, *B. dermatitidis, C. immitis, H. capsulatum,* and *P. brasiliensis,* require confirmatory identification. A simple and relatively rapid confirmatory test is detection of cell-free antigens, known as exoantigens. These exoantigens are detected by using a double-diffusion immunoassay. The principle of the double-diffusion immunoassay is discussed in Chapter 10. Control antigen and reference antisera to several antigens are commercially available. The exoantigens from mycelial cultures are extracted and placed into wells cut into an agarose plate. Wells are arranged in a circular fashion, and extracted antigens are placed in wells along with control antigen. One of

the reference antisera is added to the center well approximately 1 hour previously (Figure 27-27). The agar plate is incubated for 24 hours at room temperature. The plates are examined with indirect light for lines of identity; any line of identity to control antigen-antibody is considered significant.

Coccidioides immitis

Clinical Manifestations. *Coccidioides* spp. are probably the most virulent of all human mycotic agents. Two very similar species that infect humans are *C. immitis* and *C. posadasii.* The inhalation of only a few arthroconidia produces primary coccidioidomycosis. Clinical infections include asymptomatic pulmonary disease and allergic manifestations. Allergic manifestations can manifest as toxic erythema, erythema nodosum (desert bumps), erythema multiforme (valley fever), and arthritis (desert rheumatism). Primary disease usually resolves without therapy and confers a strong, specific immunity to reinfection, which is detected by the coccidioidin skin test.

In symptomatic patients fever, respiratory distress, cough, anorexia, headache, malaise, and myalgias can manifest for 6 weeks or longer. The disease might then progress to secondary coccidioidomycosis, which can include nodules, cavitary lung disease, or progressive pulmonary disease. Single or multisystem dissemination follows in about 1% of this population. Filipinos and Blacks run the highest risk of dissemination with meningeal involvement being a common result of disseminated disease. The sex distribution ratio for clinically apparent disease is approximately 9:1 (male:female). The exception is in pregnant women, in whom the dissemination rate equals or exceeds that for men.

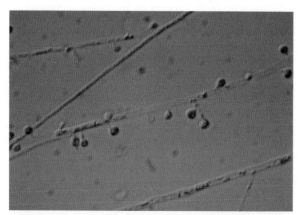

FIGURE 27-26 Mould phase of *Blastomyces dermatitidis* grown on potato flakes agar. (Nomarski optics, 1250×).

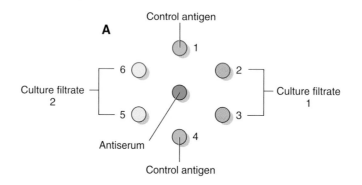

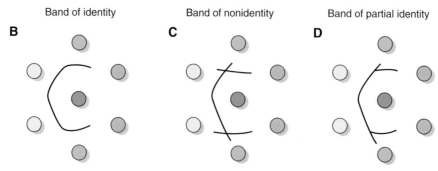

FIGURE 27-27 The exoantigen immunodiffusion test **(A)**; a band of identity between culture filtrate 2 and control antigen **(B)**; a band of nonidentity **(C)**; and a band of partial identity **(D)**.

Coccidioides spp. reside in a narrow ecologic niche known as the Lower Sonoran Life Zone, characterized by low rainfall and semiarid conditions. Highly endemic areas include the San Joaquin Valley of California, the Maricopa and Pima counties of Arizona, and southwestern Texas. Outside the United States, areas of high endemicity are found in northern Mexico, Guatemala, Honduras, Venezuela, Paraguay, Argentina, and Columbia. Because they are morphologically identical, molecular evaluation is required to differentiate *C. immitis* from *C. posadasii*. It appears that the species can be traced to specific geographic locations. *C. immitis* is encountered in the San Joaquin Valley region of California, whereas *C. posadasii* is found in the desert southwest of the United States, Mexico, and South America.

Laboratory Diagnosis. After inhalation, the barrel-shaped arthroconidia, which measure 2.5 to 4 µm × 3 to 6 µm, round up as they convert to spherules. At maturity the spherules (30 to 60 µm) produce endospores by a process known as progressive cleavage; rupture of the spherule wall releases the endospores into the bloodstream and surrounding tissues. These endospores, in turn, form new spherules (Figure 27-28). Direct smear examination of secretions may reveal the spherules containing the endospores. Caution must be exercised when diagnosis is made by histopathologic means only. Small, empty spherules may resemble the yeast cells of *B. dermatitidis*, and the endospores can be confused with the cells of *C. neoformans*, *H. capsulatum*, and *P. brasiliensis*.

Microscopic examination of the culture shows fertile hyphae arising at right angles to the vegetative hyphae, producing alternating (separated by a disjunctor cell), hyaline arthroconidia (Figure 27-29). When released, conidia have an annular frill at both ends. As the culture ages, the vegetative hyphae also fragment into arthroconidia. Although *Coccidioides* spp. do not readily convert to the spherule stage at 37° C in the laboratory, they produce a variety of mould morphologies at 22° C. Initial growth, which occurs within 3 to 4 days, is white to gray, moist, and glabrous. Colonies rapidly develop abundant aerial mycelium, and the colony appears to enlarge in a circular "bloom." Mature colonies usually become tan to brown to lavender.

Histoplasma capsulatum

Clinical Manifestations. Histoplasmosis is acquired by the inhalation of the microconidia of *Histoplasma capsulatum* var. *capsulatum*. The microconidia are phagocytized by macrophages in the pulmonary parenchyma. In the host with intact immune defenses, the infection is limited and is usually asymptomatic, with the only sequelae being areas of calcification in the lungs, liver, and spleen. With heavy exposure, however, acute pulmonary disease may occur. In the mild form of the disease, viable organisms remain in the host, quiescent for years, which are the presumed source of reactivation in individuals with abrogated immune systems. In immunocompromised individuals, *H. capsulatum* may cause a progressive and potentially fatal disseminated disease. Chronic pulmonary histoplasmosis in patients with chronic obstructive pulmonary disease may also occur. Other various manifestations of the disease are mediastinitis, pericarditis, and mucocutaneous lesions.

Histoplasma capsulatum var. *capsulatum* causes histoplasmosis, also known as reticuloendothelial cytomycosis, cave disease, spelunker's disease, and Darling disease. Histoplasmosis occurs worldwide. The highest endemicity in the United States occurs in the Ohio, Missouri, and Mississippi river deltas. This organism resides in soil containing high nitrogen content, particularly in areas heavily contaminated with bat and bird guano. Skin testing of long-term residents in endemic areas indicates that about 80% of the population has been infected. *H. capsulatum* var. *duboisii*, endemic in Central Africa, causes a clinically distinct form of disease primarily involving the skin and bones. Another variant, *H. capsulatum* var. *farciminosum*, causes epizootic lymphangitis in horses and mules. *H. capsulatum*, like *B. dermatitidis*, is also a heterothallic ascomycete that produces the teleomorphic state, *A. capsulatus*, when mated with appropriate tester strains.

Laboratory Diagnosis. Careful examination of direct smear preparations of specimens for histoplasmosis frequently reveals the small yeast cells of *H. capsulatum*, particularly in infections seen in immunodeficient hosts. The yeast cells measure 2 to 3 µm × 4 to 5 µm. When smears are stained with Giemsa or Wright stains, the yeast cells are commonly

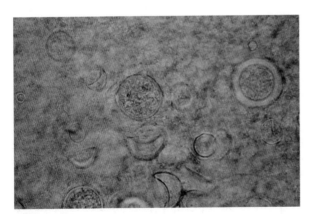

FIGURE 27-28 Spherules of *Coccidioides immitis* in tissue (300×).

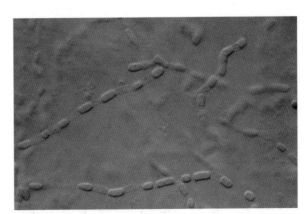

FIGURE 27-29 Mould phase of *Coccidioides immitis*, 25° C. (Nomarski optics, 1250×).

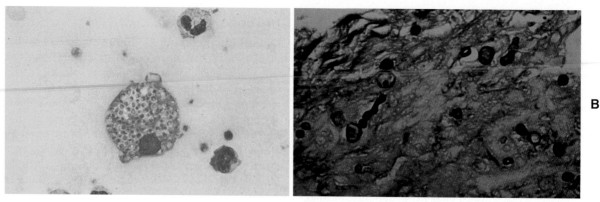

FIGURE 27-30 **A,** Bone marrow aspirate stained with Giemsa showing the yeast cells of *Histoplasma capsulatum* var. *capsulatum* inside the monocytes (1200×). **B,** Tissue phase of *H. capsulatum* var. *capsulatum*. (Gomori methylene stain, 1200×).

seen within monocytes and macrophages occurring in significant numbers, as shown in Figure 27-30, *A.* The small cells, when found in tissue (Figure 27-30, *B*), resemble the blastoconidia of *Candida glabrata,* but they can be differentiated by fluorescent antibody (FA) techniques or culture.

Although microconidia may resemble *Chrysosporium* spp. and the macroconidia resembles *Sepedonium* spp., neither saprobe produce two types of conidia in a single culture, nor are they dimorphic. Conversion of the mould form to the yeast form, utilizing brain-heart infusion agar incubated at 37° C, is confirmatory for *H. capsulatum.* Although complete conversion is seldom noted, a combination of both mycelial and yeast forms is sufficient for identification. *H. capsulatum* grows as a white to brownish mould. Early growth of the mycelial culture produces round to pyriform microconidia measuring 2 to 5 μm. As the colony matures, large echinulate or tuberculate macroconidia characteristic for the species are formed (Figure 27-31).

Serologic procedures for the diagnosis of histoplasmosis might be an adjunct to culture methods. Tests that may be employed include skin tests; complement fixation, immunodiffusion, and latex agglutination to detect circulating antibody; and FA microscopy to detect either viable or nonviable fungal elements in tissue sections. Currently the most useful serologic application for the diagnosis of histoplasmosis appears to be the combination of complement fixation and immunodiffusion tests, in which rising titers in serial dilutions are considered significant. The exoantigen test can also be used for culture identification.

Paracoccidioides brasiliensis

Clinical Manifestations. Although the primary route of infection for *Paracoccidioides brasiliensis* is pulmonary and infection is usually unapparent and asymptomatic, subsequent dissemination leads to the formation of ulcerative granulomatous lesions of the buccal, nasal, and occasionally gastrointestinal mucosa. A concomitant striking lymph node involvement is also evident. Although *P. brasiliensis* has a rather narrow range of temperature tolerance, as evidenced by its predilection for growth in cooler areas of the body (nasal and oropharyngeal), dissemination to other organs,

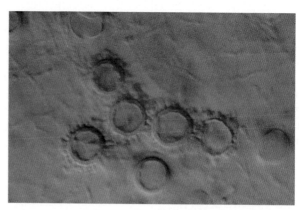

FIGURE 27-31 Large tuberculate macroconidia of *Histoplasma capsulatum* var. *capsulatum* (Nomarski optics, 1250×).

particularly the adrenals, occurs with diminished host defenses.

P. brasiliensis is the causative agent of paracoccidioidomycosis (South American blastomycosis, Brazilian blastomycosis, Lutz-Splendore-Almeida disease, paracoccidioidal granuloma), a chronic, progressive fungal disease that is endemic to Central and South America. Geographic areas of highest incidence are typically humid, high-rainfall areas with acidic soil conditions.

Laboratory Diagnosis. Direct microscopic examination of cutaneous and mucosal lesions demonstrates the characteristic yeast cells. The typical budding yeast measures 15 to 30 μm in diameter with multipolar budding at the periphery, resembling a mariner's wheel (Figure 27-32). These "daughter" cells (2 to 5 μm) are connected by a narrow base, unlike the broad-based attachment in *B. dermatitidis.* Many buds of various sizes may occur, or there may be only a few buds, giving the appearance of a "Mickey Mouse cap" to the yeast cell.

P. brasiliensis produces a variety of mould morphologies when grown at 22° C. Flat colonies are glabrous to leathery, wrinkled to folded, floccose to velvety, pink to beige to brown with a yellowish brown reverse, resembling those of *B. derma-*

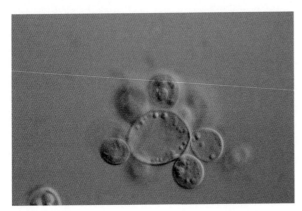

FIGURE 27-32 Yeast phase ("mariner's wheel") of *Paracoccidioides brasiliensis* with multipolar budding. (Nomarski optics, 1250×).

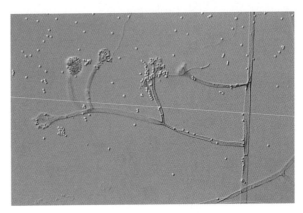

FIGURE 27-33 *Absidia* sp.

titidis. Microscopically, the mould form produces small (2 to 10 μm in diameter), one-celled conidia, generally indistinguishable from those observed with the mould phase of *B. dermatitidis* or the microconidia of *H. capsulatum*. On brain-heart infusion (BHI)–blood agar at 37° C, the mycelial phase rapidly converts to yeast phase.

Penicillium marneffei

Clinical Manifestations. *Penicillium marneffei* is unique among the *Penicillium* species being dimorphic. It is the only true pathogen in the genus. *P. marneffei* is a common cause of systemic infection in immunocompromised patients who have visited the endemic region of Southeast Asia. This includes patients with AIDS or hematological malignancies. Infections are usually disseminated with multiple organ involvement. The fungus can be isolated from cutaneous lesions, which are frequently present in infected patients. Disseminated disease is typically fatal.

Laboratory Diagnosis. The yeastlike cells of *P. marneffei* can be detected in Wright-stained smears from skin lesions or biopsy specimens. The cells of *P. marneffei* resemble those of *H. capsulatum*—oval to cylindrical measuring 3 to 6 μm long and may have a cross-wall. The mould form is described as having sparse green aerial and reddish brown vegetative hyphae and production of a red diffusible pigment. Exoantigen and polymerase chain reaction tests have been described for identification confirmation.

Agents of Opportunistic Mycoses

Saprobe and saprophyte have been used to describe free-living microorganisms in the environment that are not typically of concern in human disease. The line between saprobic and parasitic or pathogenic organisms is increasingly blurred. The major reason for this development is the growing number of persons with defects in their immune systems. For several decades medical science has made advances in life-sustaining and life-lengthening treatments. A serious side effect of procedures, such as organ transplants and cancer chemotherapy, is the short- or long-term insult to the host defenses. Magnifying the problem greatly during the last two decades has been the spread of AIDS. All these persons constitute the prime targets for infection by a wide variety of microorganisms, including the recognized pathogenic fungi and a growing list of fungi heretofore regarded as harmless.

The types of disease caused by these fungi are as varied as the species, sometimes more so, because a given fungus may cause multiple disease forms. Surgical wounds are ideal points of inoculation, allowing these saprobes to become opportunistic agents of disease. Skin and nail-bed infections as well as severe respiratory infections may be caused by a variety of fungi in patients with AIDS. Following is a discussion of the most common saprobes that have been associated with opportunistic infections. Characteristic morphologic features of each fungal species are described. These fungi are found worldwide in the environment, often associated with decaying vegetation.

Zygomycetes

Absidia. The Zygomycetes are aseptate or sparsely septate hyaline fungi. *Absidia* spp. have a predilection for vascular invasion causing thrombosis and necrosis of the tissues. This agent, along with other fungi in the class Zygomycetes, is most frequently found in diabetic patients suffering from ketoacidosis. In this patient population, the infection usually begins in the sinuses where conidia are inhaled and take up residence. From the sinuses, infection rapidly spreads to the orbits, face, palate, and brain. This presentation is known as rhinocerebral zygomycosis. Other sites of infection have been noted in cancer patients to include cutaneous, subcutaneous, and systemic disease. *Absidia* spp. are found worldwide and are often associated with soil or decomposing organic matter.

Absidia hyphae are broad and ribbonlike with few septations (Figure 27-33). Erect sporangiophores either solitary or in groups terminate in an apophysis surrounded by a sporangium. Sporangiospores are smooth and ovoid. Internodal **rhizoids** are present. Colonies are wooly and grow rapidly, completely covering the culture medium. Colony color is initially white, becoming gray to gray-brown with age.

Cunninghamella. *Cunninghamella* spp. can be recovered from the sinuses or other organs from disseminate disease. Found worldwide, this isolate is common in the environment. Sporangiophores are erect, branching into several vesicles that bear sporangioles (Figure 27-34) and can be covered with

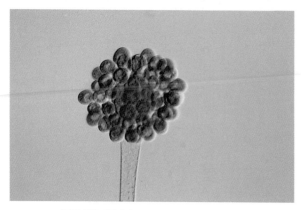

FIGURE 27-34   *Cunninghamella* sp.

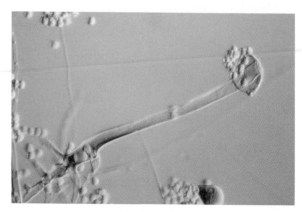

FIGURE 27-36   *Rhizopus* sp.

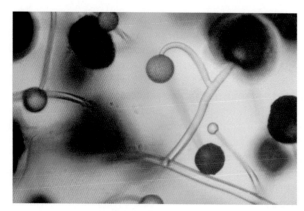

FIGURE 27-35   *Mucor* sp.

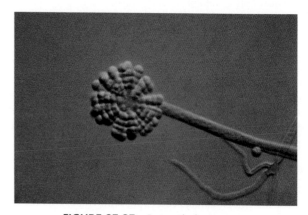

FIGURE 27-37   *Syncephalastrum* sp.

long, fine spines. These organisms are rapidly growing Zygomycetes that form a cottony colony that is initially white but becomes gray with age.

Mucor. As with other Zygomycetes, *Mucor* spp. have been implicated in rhinocerebral zygomycosis in addition to disseminated disease. *Mucor* spp. are commonly isolated from the environment worldwide. Sporangiospores are formed in sporangia on erect sporangiophores (Figure 27-35). Rhizoids, typical of some Zygomycetes, are not found in *Mucor* spp. The sporangia frequently remain intact, as opposed to *Rhizopus* spp. where the sporangia typically collapse. *Mucor* spp. are rapidly growing Zygomycetes that form cottony, dirty white colonies that become mousy-brown to gray with age.

Rhizopus. *Rhizopus* sp. is the most common zygomycete that causes human disease. It is classically involved in diabetic patients with ketoacidosis, presenting as rhinocerebral zygomycosis. *Rhizopus* sp. is extremely refractory to treatment and may be recovered from virtually any source. With worldwide distribution, this isolate is easily recovered from the environment in decaying vegetation.

Rhizopus sp. has erect sporangiophores terminated by dark sporangia and sporangiospores (Figure 27-36). At the base of the sporangiophores are brown rhizoids. Separate clusters of sporangiophores are joined by stolons—arching filaments that terminate at the rhizoids. The sporangia are typically fragile and are not easily retained when making slide culture preparations, resulting in an umbrella-shaped structure at the

end of the conidiophores. *Rhizopus* spp. produce rapidly growing, woolly colonies that cover the entire surface of the culture medium. Colonies are initially white but become gray to brown with age.

Syncephalastrum. *Syncephalastrum* is rarely implicated in human disease, but it has been documented in cutaneous infections. This fungus is found in the soil and decaying vegetation. Microscopically, erect sporangiophores are noted. Each sporangiophore has a large columella on which merosporangia, containing stacks of sporangiospores, are formed (Figure 27-37). Care should be taken when reviewing this isolate, as it is sometimes confused with *Aspergillus* on initial examination. Colonies are initially white and become gray with age. The growth rate is rapid, as with other Zygomycetes, with colonies covering the entire surface of the agar.

Septate and Hyaline Saprophytes

Aspergillus. *Aspergillus* spp. are the second most isolated fungus after *Candida* spp. *A. fumigatus* is the species most commonly isolated; other pathogenic species include *A. flavus*, *A. terreus*, and *A. niger*. Mortality from infections caused by the aspergilli remains extremely high, frequently above 90% in the immunocompromised host.

Neutropenia is the single most predictive factor for developing aspergillosis. *Aspergillus* spp. are the most frequent cause of disease in the bone marrow transplant recipient in addition to other cancer and transplant patients. Infection is initiated following inhalation of fungal conidia. In the lung air spaces, conidia begin to germinate and invade the tissue. Within a few days the patient develops a severe fever that fails to respond to antifungal therapy. Although not all patients suffer from chest pain, it is not uncommon for pneumonia-like symptoms to appear. The infection easily spreads hematogenously, and it is not uncommon to find in multiple organ system involvement, including the brain, liver, heart, and bone. Allergic reactions to *Aspergillus* spp. are a problem to those with sensitivities to moulds. Another frequent presentation is "fungus balls" in the lungs of agricultural workers who routinely are in contact with fungal conidia from environmental sources.

The conidia are readily found in the environment and may be recovered in air-settling plates. Many species of aspergilli have been implicated in human disease. Although some are easily distinguished from others, some aspergilli require extensive testing to determine a definitive identification at the species level.

Aspergilli may be either uniseriate or biseriate. Uniseriate species are those whose phialides attach directly to the vesicle at the end of the conidiophore. Biseriate species possess a supporting structure called a *metula*. Metulae attach directly to the vesicle, and attached to each of the metula are phialides (Figure 27-38). Conidia are produced from the phialides. Other characteristics include an erect conidiophore arising from a "foot cell" within the vegetative hyphae and whether or not phialoconidia remain in long chains or are easily disturbed. Chains of conidia can be aligned in very straight, parallel columns or in a radiating pattern around the vesicle, and the conidia can be either rough or smooth.

The color of *Aspergillus* spp. colonies is derived from the conidia. Colors range from black to white and include yellow, brown, green, gray, pink, beige, and tan. Some species also form diffusible subsurface pigments on a variety of media. Granular texture is seen in species with abundant conidial formation. Most known pathogens in this group form green-to tan-colored colonies.

Beauveria. *Beauveria bassiana* is a rare human isolate, uncommonly associated with keratitis. This fungus is a known insect pathogen and is found worldwide on vegetation and in the soil. Abundant, single-celled, tear-shaped sympoduloconidia are formed on sympodulae, which taper extremely from a rather swollen base (Figure 27-39). Conidiophores may cluster in some isolates to form radial tufts. Colonies are hyaline, moderately rapidly growing, fluffy colonies, sometimes developing a powdery surface reminiscent of *T. mentagrophytes*.

Chrysosporium. A rare cause of disease, *Chrysosporium* spp. have been recovered from nails and skin lesions. They are found in the environment worldwide. Microscopically simple, wide-based, single-celled conidia are produced on nonspecialized cells (Figure 27-40). The conidiogenous cell disintegrates or breaks to release the conidia. Both arthroconidia and aleurioconidia may be seen. Colonies are hyaline with a moderate growth rate that, with age, can develop light shades of pink, gray, or tan pigment.

Fusarium. *Fusarium* spp. are frequently seen in mycotic keratitis. In fact, a multistate outbreak involving more than 100 individuals wearing soft contact lenses was reported in 2006. The outbreak was associated with a particular brand of contact lens solution. In bone marrow transplant patients, mortality from infections caused by the fusaria approaches 100%. Unless a patient regains some cell-mediated immunity, mortality is certain because of the ability of these fungi to grow and continue to invade despite antifungal therapy. Patients present with high fever, possibly disseminated skin lesions and, in some patients, fungemia. *Fusarium* spp. are easily recovered in blood culture systems. Care should be

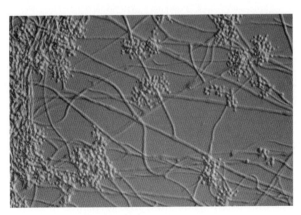

FIGURE 27-39 *Beauveria* sp.

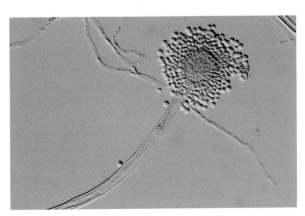

FIGURE 27-38 *Aspergillus* sp.

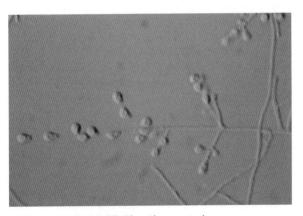

FIGURE 27-40 *Chrysosporium* sp.

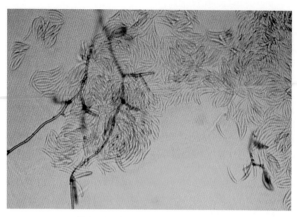

FIGURE 27-41 *Fusarium* sp.

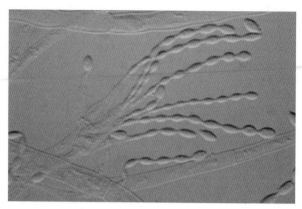

FIGURE 27-43 *Paecilomyces* sp.

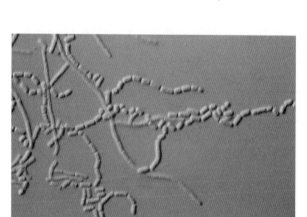

FIGURE 27-42 *Geotrichum* sp.

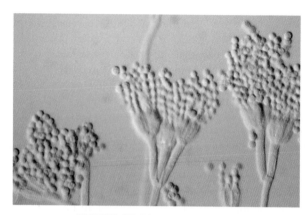

FIGURE 27-44 *Penicillium* sp.

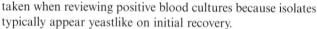

taken when reviewing positive blood cultures because isolates typically appear yeastlike on initial recovery.

Normally, abundant macroconidia with fewer microconidia are produced on vegetative hyphae (Figure 27-41). Macroconidia are banana or canoe shaped and are formed singly, in small clusters, or clustered together in mats termed *sporodochia*. Macroconidia typically are multicelled. *Fusarium* is a rapidly growing hyaline fungus that can develop various colors with age, ranging from rose to mauve to purple to yellow.

Geotrichum. *Geotrichum* has been implicated in pulmonary disease in immunocompromised patients. Microscopic evaluation reveals abundant arthroconidia formed from the vegetative hypha that occurs either singly or may be branched (Figure 27-42). Colonies are white to cream, yeastlike and can be confused with *Trichosporon* spp. Occasionally, aerial mycelium form, producing colonies that resemble *C. immitis*.

Paecilomyces. *Paecilomyces lilacinus* is extremely refractory to treatment and has been recovered in a hospital outbreak with high associated mortality. Microscopically, care must be taken to avoid confusion between *Paecilomyces* and *Penicillium* spp. Phialides of *Paecilomyces* are generally longer and more obviously tapered, and they may be singly formed or arranged in a verticillate pattern, on which long chains of spindle-shaped or somewhat cylindrical conidia are formed (Figure 27-43).

Paecilomyces spp. grow rapidly and usually form flat, granular to velvety colonies in shades of tan, brownish gold, or mauve. Green or blue-green colors are not seen. Infections with *Paecilomyces* spp. are potentially serious and difficult to treat; care should be taken when encountering fungi that are mauve.

Penicillium. *Penicillium* spp. rarely cause infections; most reports of disease involve chronic fungal sinusitis. Ubiquitous in nature, these fungi may be recovered from any location worldwide. Conidiophores are erect, sometimes branched with metulae bearing one or several phialides on which oval to ovoid conidia are produced in long, loose chains (Figure 27-44). This commonly seen fungus is a rapid grower with colonies most often in shades of green or blue-green.

Scopulariopsis. *Scopulariopsis* spp. are not uncommonly isolated from nail specimens and have been implicated in pulmonary disease in immunocompromised patients. This isolate is recovered from the environment worldwide. Conidiophores are formed singularly or can be in clusters (Figure 27-45). Conidia are formed from annellides, which increase in length as conidia are formed. The truncate-based conidia tend to remain in chains on the annellides. *Scopulariopsis* grows moderately rapidly and forms colonies covered by tan to buff conidia. Some species are dematiaceous.

Trichoderma. *Trichoderma* sp. is an emerging pathogen in the immunocompromised host that can cause a range of

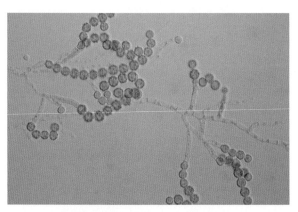

FIGURE 27-45 *Scopulariopsis* sp.

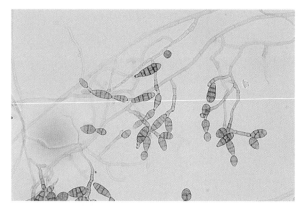

FIGURE 27-47 *Alternaria* sp.

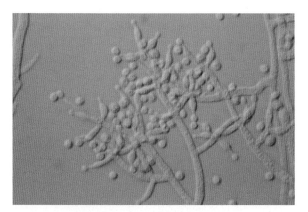

FIGURE 27-46 *Trichoderma* sp.

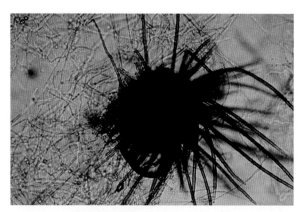

FIGURE 27-48 *Chaetomium* sp.

infections, including pulmonary and skin. This isolate is readily recovered from the environment worldwide. *Trichoderma* sp. is rapidly growing and forms hyaline hyphae that give rise to yellow-green to green patches of conidia formed on clusters of tapering phialides (Figure 27-46). Conidia may remain clustered in balls at the phialide tips. Colonies are intensely green and granular with an abundance of conidia.

Septate and Dematiaceous Saprophytes

Alternaria. Although *Alternaria* spp. isolates may be recovered from virtually any source, they are primarily implicated in chronic fungal sinusitis. Patients are often misdiagnosed and treated for an extended time for bacterial sinusitis. This type of infection rarely travels outside the sinuses in the immunocompetent host but can be found systemically in those suffering from immune suppression. *Alternaria* spp. are found worldwide on grasses and leaves. They have been implicated in tomato rot and are readily recovered from the environment in air-settling plates.

Microscopic evaluation reveals short conidiophores bearing conidia in chains that lengthen in an acropetal fashion (Figure 27-47). Multicelled conidia have angular cross-walls and taper toward the distal end. *Alternaria* spp. are dematiaceous, rapidly growing fungi with colonies ranging from shades of gray, to brown, to black.

Aureobasidium. Infections by *Aureobasidium* spp. are rare but can be traced to contaminated dialysis lines and other similar devices. This organism may be recovered from blood, tissues, and abscesses. It is recovered worldwide primarily in wet conditions, such as shower tiles and water lines.

Microscopic evaluation reveals hyaline hyphae giving rise to hyaline conidia directly from the vegetative hyphae. With age, dematiaceous hyphae develop and break up into arthroconidia, which do not bear hyaline conidia. These arthroconidia are responsible for the darkening colony morphology. *Aureobasidium* spp. grow moderately to rapidly and have a yeasty consistency. Young cultures are off-white to pink, but with age they become black with the production of darkly pigmented arthroconidia.

Chaetomium. Infections by *Chaetomium* organisms have been reported in the brains of patients with central nervous system disease. Several of these patients have been identified as intravenous drug abusers. These fungi are found in the environment and have a predilection for cellulose products. They have been known to devastate printed literature and library holdings and have been associated with indoor air-quality problems.

Microscopically, numerous perithecia are typically seen (Figure 27-48). These perithecia are pineapple shaped and are ornamented with straight or curled "hairs" or setae. The asci contained within the perithecia are evanescent, so at maturity the pigmented, lemon-shaped ascospores are released within the perithecium. Colonies are moderately to rapidly growing and begin dirty gray, becoming dematiaceous with age. Some

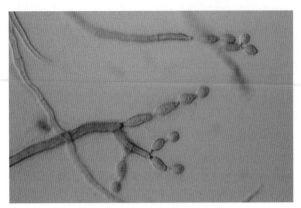

FIGURE 27-49 *Cladosporium* sp.

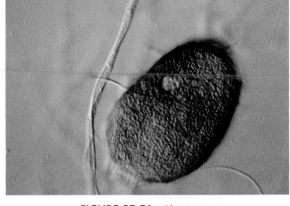

FIGURE 27-51 *Phoma* sp.

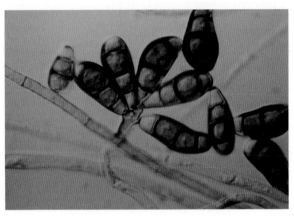

FIGURE 27-50 *Curvularia* sp.

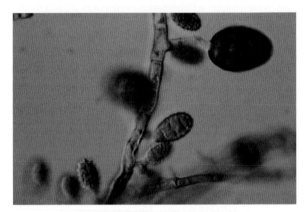

FIGURE 27-52 *Pithomyces* sp.

species produce a diffusible pigment that turns the agar completely red.

Cladosporium. An infrequent cause of disease, *Cladosporium* sp. are primarily recovered as laboratory contaminants. Infections are typically confined to the sinuses or following traumatic inoculation. Ubiquitous in nature, this isolate can be recovered from nearly any location in the world. *Cladosporium* sp. forms brown to olive to black hyphae and conidia (Figure 27-49). Conidiophores are erect and may branch into several conidiogenous cells. Spherical to ovoid conidia form blastically on the end of each previously formed conidium. Branched conidium-bearing cells may dislodge, and the three scars on each of these cells give them the appearance of a shield. Generally, conidial chains of the saprophytic species break up easily, whereas those of pathogenic species remain connected. These organisms are slowly to moderately growing dematiaceous fungus with granular velvety to fluffy colonies, ranging in color from olive to brown or black.

Curvularia. *Curvularia* spp. isolates are most often implicated in chronic sinusitis in immunocompetent patients. Found worldwide, this fungus is frequently recovered from grass, leaves, and decaying vegetations. Multicelled conidia are produced on sympodial conidiophores (Figure 27-50). This genus is among the easiest to identify because of the frequently crescent-shaped conidia with three to five cells of unequal size and an enlarged central cell. These fungi form a

rapidly growing dematiaceous colony that is cottony and dirty gray to black.

Phoma. Disease caused by the *Phoma* spp. is usually secondary to traumatic inoculation. *Phoma* spp. produce pycnidia, which appear as black fruiting bodies that are globose and lined inside with short conidiophores (Figure 27-51). Large numbers of hyaline conidia are generated in the pycnidium and flow out a small apical pore. *Phoma* spp. produce a moderately rapid growing gray to brown colony.

Pithomyces. Disease caused by *Pithomyces* spp. is usually secondary to traumatic inoculation. Conidia are somewhat barrel-shaped, formed singly on simple short conidiophores (Figure 27-52). Conidia have both transverse and longitudinal cross-walls and are often echinulate. *Pithomyces* spp. produce rapidly growing dematiaceous colonies.

Ulocladium. *Ulocladium* spp. are sometimes implicated in subcutaneous infections, usually following traumatic inoculation. Conidiophores bear dark, multicelled conidia on sympodial conidiophores (Figure 27-53). Conidia have angular cross-walls and, in some species, echinulate surfaces. *Ulocladium* spp. are rapidly growing dematiaceous fungi, forming colonies ranging from brown to olivaceous to black.

Agents of Yeast Infections

The escalating incidence of yeast and yeastlike fungi isolated from patient specimens has increased the importance of iden-

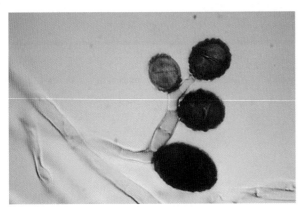

FIGURE 27-53 *Ulocladium* sp.

tifying yeast isolates to the species level. With greater immunosuppression, the variety of organisms implicated in disease also expands. *Candida albicans* has become the fourth most common cause of blood-borne infection in the United States today. Isolation of other yeasts from clinical samples, including *Candida glabrata, C. parapsilosis,* and *C. tropicalis,* is also increasing. Infections caused by these yeasts are extremely aggressive and difficult to treat.

Yeast fungi can be classified into one of two groups: yeasts and yeastlike fungi. Isolates that reproduce sexually, either by forming ascospores or basidiospores, are truly yeasts. Most isolates that are not capable of sexual reproduction or whose sexual state has not yet been discovered are correctly called *yeastlike fungi.* For ease of discussion, all isolates are referred to here as yeasts.

General Characteristics

Moulds and yeasts are very different morphologically, but some of the macroscopic characteristics used as aids in identifying moulds can also be used to identify yeasts. Macroscopic characteristics include color and colony texture. The color of a yeast colony ranges from white to cream or tan, with a few species forming pink to salmon colonies. Some yeast isolates, referred to as *dematiaceous yeasts,* are darkly pigmented because of melanin in their cell walls. Dematiaceous yeasts are associated with several species of the polymorphic fungi and are discussed elsewhere in this chapter.

The texture of the yeast colonies also varies. For example, *Cryptococcus* spp. tend to be mucoid and can flow across the plate, a trait shared by some bacterial isolates, such as *Klebsiella* spp. Some yeasts are butterlike, and others range in texture from velvety to wrinkled. Strain-to-strain variation in texture may be noted within a species.

Candida

Candida spp. are commonly present as normal biota of the mucosa, skin, and digestive tract, and they are also the most notorious agents of yeast infection. Clinical disease ranges from superficial skin infections to disseminated disease. *C. albicans* currently reigns as the premier cause of yeast infection in the world. It is recovered as normal biota from a variety of sites, including skin, oral mucosa, and vagina.

When host conditions are altered, however, this isolate is capable of causing disease in virtually any site. In individuals with an intact immune system, infections are localized and limited. One of the most widely recognized manifestations of *C. albicans* infection is thrush, an infection of the oral mucosa. Thrush is also recognized as an indicator of immunosuppression. Among individuals infected with human immunodeficiency virus (HIV), as well as those receiving prolonged antimicrobial therapy or other chemotherapeutic agents, thrush manifests as a serious infection capable of dissemination.

Candida glabrata is probably the second most common *Candida* species to cause disease and may account for 21% of all urinary yeast isolates. Infections associated with *C. glabrata* tend to be aggressive and difficult to treat with traditional antifungal therapy. This organism has different sugar assimilation patterns, notably rapid assimilation of trehalose, from those of *C. albicans* and therefore can easily be differentiated.

Other notable species of *Candida* are *C. krusei* and *C. tropicalis.* In addition, *C. parapsilosis* has become a major cause of outbreaks of nosocomial infections. These isolates are identified by the differences in their carbohydrate assimilation patterns and other secondary testing procedures. Table 27-7 shows important differentiating characteristics among *Candida* spp. and other yeasts.

Cryptococcus

Cryptococcus spp. are important causes of meningitis, pulmonary disease, and septicemia. *C. neoformans,* the most notable pathogen in this genus, has become a major cause of opportunistic infection in patients with AIDS. The organism is commonly found in soil contaminated with pigeon droppings and is most likely acquired by inhalation.

Cryptococcus spp. are surrounded by a capsule that produces the characteristic mucoid colony appearance. The capsule can be detected surrounding the budding yeast in spinal fluid with the aid of India ink (Figure 27-54). The background fluid is black, and clear halos are seen around individual yeast cells. The use of India ink preparation is being replaced by the latex agglutination test for cryptococcal antigen because of the former's low sensitivity. The latex agglutination test is recommended for routine use in most clinical microbiology laboratories.

Cryptococcus spp. are noted for producing blastoconidia only, without producing true hyphae or **pseudohyphae** on cornmeal agar. Although all species of the genus are urease positive, nitrate reaction varies. Production of phenol oxidase is a feature differentiating *C. neoformans* from other *Cryptococcus* spp. Sugar assimilations also vary for each species. *C. neoformans* can be differentiated by using the characteristics described in Table 27-7.

Rhodotorula

Rhodotorula spp. are noted for their bright salmon-pink color. They are closely related to the cryptococci because they bear a capsule and are urease positive. Some species are also nitrate positive. They are not common agents of disease, but have been known to cause opportunistic infection.

TABLE 27-7 Differentiating Characteristics of Yeasts

	Temperature Growth at			Cornmeal Agar					
	37° C	42° C	45° C	Pseudohyphae	True Hyphae	Arthroconidia	Cycloheximide	Urea	Nitrate
Candida									
C. albicans	+	+	+	+	+	–	R	–	–
C. dubliensis	+	–	–	+	+	–	R	–	–
C. glabrata	+	+	+	–	–	–	S	–	–
C. guilliermondii	+	+	–	+	–	–	R	–	–
C. krusei	+	+	–	+	–	–	S	V	–
C. lusitaniae	+	+	+	+	–	–	V	–	–
C. parapsilosis	+	–	–	+	–	–	S	–	–
C. stellatoidea	+	+	+	+	+	–	S	–	–
C. tropicalis	+	+	+	+	–	–	V	–	–
Cryptococcus									
C. albidus	–	–	–	–	–	–	S	+	+
C. neoformans	+	–	–	–	–	–	S	+	–
Trichosporon spp.	+	V	–	+	+	+	R	+	–

+, Positive; –, negative; *R*, resistant; *S*, sensitive; *V*, variable.

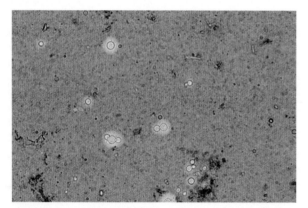

FIGURE 27-54 India ink preparation is used primarily to examine cerebrospinal fluid for the presence of the encapsulated yeast *Cryptococcus neoformans*. This is an India ink preparation from an exudate containing encapsulated budding yeasts.

Pneumocystis

Pneumocystis spp. can inhabit the lungs of many mammals. *P. carinii* was originally classified with the protozoa, but nucleic acid sequencing showed conclusively that the organism was a fungus. It is now apparent from nucleic acid studies that *P. carinii* is not a single species. *P. carinii* is the species most commonly found in rats, and *P. jiroveci* is the species most often recovered from humans. Future studies will likely lead to the naming of many other species.

Clinical Manifestations

Pneumocystis spp. infection is acquired early in life; serologic studies have shown that most humans have antibodies or antigens by 2 to 4 years of age. In immunocompetent individuals, infection is asymptomatic; however, in immunocompromised patients, serious life-threatening pneumonia can develop. *Pneumocystis* sp. initially was identified as the etiologic agent in interstitial plasma cell pneumonia seen in mal-

nourished or premature infants. Since the early 1980s, it has remained one of the primary opportunistic infections found in patients with AIDS. A high incidence of disease also results from the use of immunosuppressive drugs in patients with malignancies or organ transplants. Underlying defects in cellular immunity apparently make patients susceptible to clinical infection with the organism.

Patients infected with *Pneumocystis* sp. may have fever, nonproductive cough, difficulty breathing, and a low-grade fever. Chest radiographs can be normal or show a diffuse interstitial infiltrate. The immune response to the organism after it attaches to and destroys alveolar cells is partly responsible for this radiographic pattern. When the infiltrate is examined, it is found to contain cells from the alveoli and plasma cells.

Life Cycle

Pneumocystis sp. is a nonfilamentous fungus. Terminology referring to the various life cycle forms, however, is reflected in the fact that it was first considered a protozoan. The life cycle of *Pneumocystis* sp. has three stages: the trophozoite, which is 1 to 5 μm in size and is irregularly shaped; the precyst, 5 to 8 μm; and the cyst, which is a thick-walled sphere of about 8 μm containing up to eight intracystic bodies.

Transmission of the organism is known to occur through the respiratory route, with the cyst being the infective stage. The spores or intracystic bodies are released from the cyst in the lung, and these trophic forms multiply asexually by binary fission on the surface of the epithelial cells (pneumocyte) lining the lung. Sexual reproduction by trophozoites also occurs, first producing a precyst and then the cyst containing spores or intracystic bodies.

Laboratory Diagnosis

Traditionally, diagnosis was made by finding the cyst or trophozoite in tissue obtained through open lung biopsy. Specimens now used include bronchoalveolar lavage, transbronchial biopsy, tracheal aspirate, pleural fluid, and induced sputum.

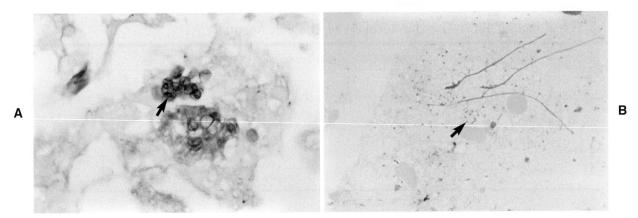

FIGURE 27-55 **A,** *Pneumocystis jiroveci* cysts (silver stain). **B,** *P. jiroveci* (Giemsa stain). Notice the circular arrangement of intracystic bodies within a faint outline of cyst wall in center of field.

Sputum, however, is the least productive specimen. Lavage and sputum specimens are often prepared using a cytocentrifuge.

Histologic stains such as Giemsa and Gomori methenamine silver are used. With the methenamine silver stain, the cyst wall stains black. Cysts often have a punched-out "ping-pong ball" appearance. With the Giemsa stain, the organism appears round, and the cyst wall is barely visible. Intracystic bodies are seen around the interior of the organism. Figure 27-55, *A,* shows the characteristic black-staining cyst of *P. jiroveci* with methenamine silver stain. Figure 27-55, *B,* shows the cyst stained with Giemsa stain. The cyst wall does not pick up the stain, but the nuclei of all forms stain pink, and the intracystic bodies can be demonstrated as a circular arrangement within the cyst.

Calcofluor white can be used to screen specimens for *Pneumocystis* and other fungi. This stain detects any organism that contains chitin in its cell wall. Fungi, yeast, and *Pneumocystis* spp. will fluoresce with a blue-white color when stained and viewed under ultraviolet light. Immunofluorescent monoclonal antibody stains are commercially available and have gained wide use.

Treatment includes trimethoprim-sulfamethoxazole or pentamidine isethionate. Some patients with AIDS have been given aerosolized pentamidine as a prophylactic treatment. However, disseminated *Pneumocystis* spp. infection in such patients has been reported. *Pneumocystis* spp. infections do not respond to most antifungal and antiprotozoan agents.

LABORATORY DIAGNOSIS OF FUNGI

Safety Issues

Standard safety precautions apply to the mycology laboratory. Because of the additional hazard of airborne conidia, a class II biological safety cabinet should be used to reduce personnel exposure to fungal elements. Specimen processing and plating must be performed in a properly maintained and operating safety cabinet. The use of an enclosed electric incinerator is recommended to eliminate the hazards of open gas flames and to contain particles emitted when loops or needles are incinerated. The cabinet should be checked daily to see that none of the airflow inlets or outlets is blocked by supplies, incinerators, or waste disposal jars.

Use of Petri dishes in the mycology laboratory is hazardous; screw-top tubes are recommended instead. The chance for the release of airborne conidia is less likely with tubed media. Screw-capped tubes also tend to show less media dehydration than Petri dishes and are more easily handled and stored. On the other hand, Petri dishes have a greater surface area for colony isolation and are easier to manipulate when making preparations for microscopic examination.

Specimen Collection, Handling, and Transport

Collection of appropriate specimens is the primary criterion for accurate diagnosis of mycotic infections. All specimens for mycology should be transported and processed as soon as possible. Because many pathogenic fungi grow slowly, any delay in processing compromises specimen quality and decreases the probability of isolating the causative agent as a result of overgrowth by contaminants. In addition, all laboratories should maintain a protocol for rejection of unsatisfactory or improperly labeled specimens.

Although almost any tissue or body fluid can be submitted for fungal culture, the most common specimens are respiratory secretions, hair, skin, nails, tissue, blood or bone marrow, and CSF. Table 27-8 presents the predominant culture sites for recovery of etiologic agents of fungal diseases. Figure 27-56 presents a schematic guideline to assist in how to proceed to make a diagnosis of a mycosis.

Hair, skin, or nails submitted for dermatophyte culture are generally contaminated with bacteria or rapidly growing fungi or both. With these types of specimens, primary isolation medium should contain antimicrobial agents. The following procedures are recommended for collecting and processing clinical samples submitted for fungal studies.

Hair

A Wood's lamp can be useful in identifying infected hairs. Hairs infected with fungi such as *Microsporum audouinii* fluo-

TABLE 27-8 Predominant Culture Sites for Recovery of Etiologic Agents*

Infection	Respiratory	Blood	Bone Marrow	Tissue	Skin	Mucus	Bone
Blastomycosis	+				+	+	+
Histoplasmosis	+	+	+				
Coccidioidomycosis	+				+	+	
Paracoccidioidomycosis	+				+	+	
Sporotrichosis	+			+	+	+	
Chromoblastomycosis				+	+		
Eumycotic mycetoma				+	+		
Phaeohyphomycosis				+	+		

*Organisms may be recovered from multiple sites in disseminated infections.

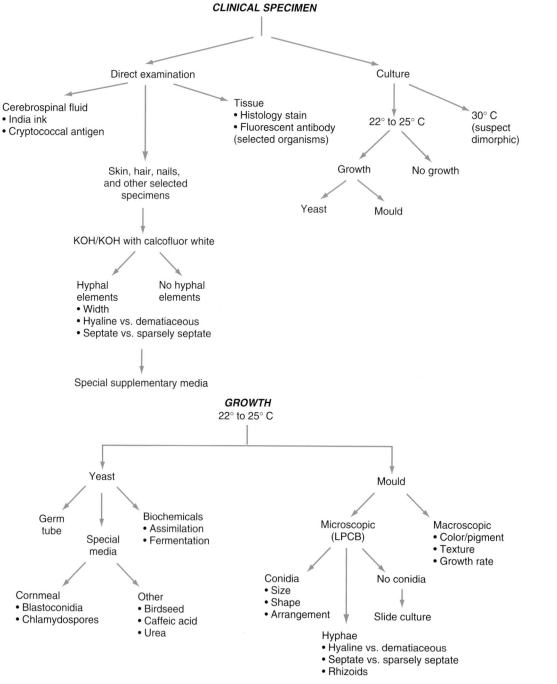

FIGURE 27-56 Guideline for the identification of fungal isolates. *LPCB,* lactophenol cotton blue.

resce when a Wood's lamp is shone on the scalp. Sterile forceps should be used to pull affected hair. A less useful method involves cutting the hairs close to the scalp with sterile scissors. Hairs are placed directly into a sterile Petri dish. A few pieces of hair are inoculated onto fungal medium and incubated at 22° to 30° C.

Skin

Skin samples are scraped from the outer edge of a surface lesion. Skin must be cleaned with 70% isopropyl alcohol before sampling. A KOH wet mount is prepared with some of the scrapings; the KOH breaks down tissue and allows fungal hyphae to be seen. The remaining material is inoculated directly onto the agar.

Nails

Nail specimens may be submitted as either scrapings or cuttings and occasionally as a complete nail. Nails are cleaned with 70% isopropyl alcohol before the surface is scraped. Deeper scrapings are necessary to prepare a KOH preparation and inoculate media. Sterile scissors are used to cut complete nails into small thin strips, which are used to inoculate media.

Blood and Bone Marrow

Blood from septicemic patients can harbor both known pathogenic and opportunistic fungi. The lysis centrifugation system, the Isolator tube (Wampole, Cranbury, N.J.), is the most sensitive method for the recovery of some fungi. The lysis of white blood cells and red blood cells releases microorganisms, which are then concentrated into sediment during centrifugation. The sediment is inoculated onto culture media. A biphasic system (broth and agar), such as the Septi-Chek (BD Diagnostic Systems Sparks, Md.), can also be used. Heparinized bone marrow specimens should be plated directly onto media at bedside; blood culture bottles are not recommended.

Cerebrospinal Fluid

CSF and other sterile body fluids should be concentrated by centrifugation before inoculation. One drop of the concentrate is used for India ink preparation or latex agglutination for *Cryptococcus*, and the remainder is inoculated onto media. If more than 5 mL is submitted, the CSF may be filtered through a membrane filter, and portions of the filter placed on media. Use of media with antimicrobial agents should not be needed because CSF is normally sterile.

Abscess Fluid, Wound Exudates, and Tissue

Using a dissecting microscope, one can examine abscess fluid and exudate from wounds for the presence of granules. If no granules are present, the material may be plated directly onto the media. Tissue should be gently minced before inoculation. Grinding of tissue has been recommended, but this process might destroy fragile fungal elements and prevent recovery of etiologic agents, particularly if a zygomycete is present. Although grinding of tissue may be necessary for KOH and calcofluor white preparations, it should not be done unless sufficient tissue is present for both mincing and grinding.

When large sections of tissue are submitted, suspicious areas, such as purulent or discolored sections, are selected for both mincing and grinding prior to subsequent culture.

Respiratory Specimens

Because many fungal infections have a primary focus in the lungs, lower respiratory tract secretions (sputum, transtracheal aspirates) and pleural lavage fluids are commonly submitted. Patients should obtain sputa from a deep cough shortly after arising in the morning. If the patient cannot produce sputum, a nebulizer may be used to induce sputum. All sputum specimens should be collected into a sterile, screw-top container.

If the material is not too viscous, the specimens can be inoculated onto media with a sterile pipette. With viscous materials such as a thick tracheal aspirate, either a cotton swab may be used to inoculate the material onto the media, or the specimen can be digested with the mucolytic agent N-acetyl-l-cysteine and concentrated before inoculation. In addition to nonselective media, a medium with antimicrobial agents should be used to prevent bacterial overgrowth. A KOH preparation should also be made.

Oropharyngeal candidiasis is easily diagnosed by direct smear and culture. Routine fungal media can be used, but the selective chromogenic agars such as CHROMagar *Candida* (CHROMagar, Paris, France) and *Candida* ID (bioMérieux, Hazelwood, Mo.) provide a rapid preliminary identification. Nasal sinus specimens obtained surgically can be plated directly to media containing antimicrobial agents except for cycloheximide, which can inhibit some fungi.

Urogenital and Fecal Specimens

Laboratory scientists often receive specimens such as urine, feces, and vaginal secretions for bacteriologic culture; on occasion these specimens grow yeast that requires identification. Urine submitted specifically for fungal culture should be centrifuged and the sediment used to inoculate media. A first-voided morning urine specimen is preferred.

Direct Microscopic Examination of Specimens

Direct examination of clinical material for fungal elements serves several purposes. First, it provides a rapid report to the physician, which may in turn result in the early initiation of treatment. Second, in some cases specific morphologic characteristics provide a clue to the genus of the organism. In turn any special media indicated for species identification can be inoculated immediately. Third, direct examination might provide evidence of infection despite negative cultures. Such a situation can occur with specimens from patients who are on antifungal therapy, which may inhibit growth in vitro even though the infection may still be present in the patient.

Although the Gram stain performed in the routine microbiology laboratory often gives the first evidence of infections with bacteria and yeast, other direct stains give more specific information about mould infections. The types of direct examination used in identification of fungal infections include wet preparations such as KOH, India ink, and calcofluor white. Histologic stains for tissue may also be useful.

KOH Preparation

A 10% to 20% solution of KOH is useful for detecting fungal elements embedded within skin, hair, nails, and tissue. In this procedure, a drop of the KOH preparation is added to a slide. Nail scrapings, hair, skin scales, or thin slices of tissue are added to the drop, and a coverslip is added. The slide is then gently heated and allowed to cool for approximately 15 minutes. The KOH breaks down the keratin and skin layers to see more easily any fungi present in the specimen. Interpreting KOH slides remains difficult, and fungal elements may evade detection.

Modifications of the KOH test can provide easier and more reliable results. These preparations incorporate dimethyl sulfoxide (DMSO) and a stain into the KOH solution. The DMSO facilitates more rapid breakdown of cellular debris without requiring heat while the stain is taken up by fungal elements, making them readily visible upon microscopic examination of the slide preparation.

KOH with Calcofluor White

A drop of calcofluor white (a fluorescent dye) can be added to the KOH preparation before adding a cover slip. Calcofluor white binds to polysaccharides present in the chitin of the fungus or to cellulose. Fungal elements fluoresce apple green or blue-white, depending on the combination of filters used on the microscope; therefore any element with a polysaccharide skeleton fluoresces. The actual fungal structure must be seen before a positive preparation is reported. Care must be taken when using this process because much variability exists between manufacturers and even from lot to lot of the stain prepared by the same manufacturer.

India Ink

India ink preparations can be used to examine CSF for the presence of the encapsulated yeast *Cryptococcus neoformans*. A drop of India ink is mixed with a drop of sediment from a centrifuged CSF specimen, and the preparation is examined on high magnification (400×). With this negative stain, budding yeast surrounded by a large clear area against a black background is presumptive evidence of *C. neoformans* (see Figure 27-54). White blood cells and other artifacts may resemble encapsulated organisms; therefore careful examination is necessary. Many laboratories, however, now use the latex agglutination test for cryptococcal antigen in place of the India ink examination.

Tissue Stains

Common tissue stains used in the histology department for detection of fungal elements are the periodic acid–Schiff (PAS), Gomori methenamine–silver nitrate, hematoxylin and eosin, Giemsa, and the Fontana-Masson stains. The Giemsa stain is used primarily to detect *Histoplasma capsulatum* in blood or bone marrow (Figure 27-57). PAS attaches to polysaccharides in the fungal wall and stains fungi pink. The Fontana-Masson method stains melanin in the cell wall and identifies the presence of dematiaceous fungi. Table 27-9 lists the characteristic fungal reactions seen with selected stains.

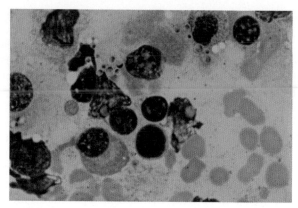

FIGURE 27-57 Bone marrow stained with Giemsa stain showing the yeast phase of *Histoplasma capsulatum* var. *capsulatum*.

TABLE 27-9 Staining Characteristics of Fungi

Stain	Color of Fungal Element	Background Color
Periodic acid–Schiff	Magenta	Pink or green
Gomori methenamine silver	Black	Green
Giemsa	Purple-blue yeast with clear halo (Capsule)	Pink-purple
India ink	Yeast with clear halo	Black
KOH	Refractile	Clear
KOH-calcofluor white	Fluorescent	Dark
Masson-Fontana	Brown	Pink-purple

KOH, Potassium hydroxide.

Isolation Methods

Culture Media

In general fungi do not share the broad range of nutritional and environmental needs that characterize bacteria; and therefore relatively few types of standard media are needed for primary isolation. These media include Sabouraud dextrose agar (SDA), SDA with antimicrobial agents, potato dextrose agar (PDA) or the slightly modified potato flakes agar, and BHI agar enriched with blood and antimicrobial agents. Gentamicin or chloramphenicol and cycloheximide are the antimicrobials usually included in fungal media. Gentamicin and chloramphenicol inhibit bacterial growth, whereas cycloheximide inhibits both bacteria and many of the environmental fungi typically considered contaminants. The pH of the Emmons modification of SDA is close to neutral and is a more efficient medium for primary isolation than the original formulation. Table 27-10 shows the expected growth results with some of the standard fungal media.

Fungal media can be poured into Petri dishes or large test tubes. Petri dishes have the advantage of a larger surface area, but they are more prone to dehydration because of prolonged incubation necessary for the recovery of some fungi. Petri dishes must be poured thicker than a standard medium for bacterial growth. The plates can be sealed with tape or para-

TABLE 27-10 Summary of Primary Fungal Culture Media

Medium	Expected Growth Results
At 22° C	
SDA	Initial isolation of pathogens and saprobes
	Dimorphic fungi may exhibit their mycelial phase
SDA with antibiotics*	Saprobes are generally inhibited on this medium
	Dermatophytes and most of the fungi considered primary pathogens grow
BHI	Initial isolation of pathogens and saprobes
BHI with antibiotics	Recovery of pathogenic fungi
	Dermatophytes not usually recovered
Inhibitory mould agar	Initial isolation of pathogens except dermatophytes
Cycloheximide	Primary recovery of dermatophytes
At 37° C	
SDA	The yeast form of dimorphic fungi and other organisms grow
	Dermatophytes grow poorly
BHI with blood	Yeasts such as *Cryptococcus* grow well
	The yeast form of *Histoplasma capsulatum* takes up some of the heme pigment in the medium and becomes light tan with a grainy, wrinkled texture

SDA, Sabouraud dextrose agar; *BHI,* brain-heart infusion agar.
*Antibiotics generally used are cycloheximide and chlorophenical.

film or sealed in semipermeable bags to minimize dehydration and to prevent the spread of fungal spores. Tubed media have the advantage of being safer to handle and less susceptible to drying. Fungal plates and tubes should be opened only in a biological safety cabinet.

Incubation

Most laboratories routinely incubate fungal cultures at room temperature or at 30° C. Fungi grow optimally at these temperatures, whereas bacteria have a slower growth rate. If the etiologic agent suspected is a dimorphic fungus, cultures should also be incubated at 37° C. Cultures are generally maintained for 4 to 6 weeks and should be examined twice weekly for growth. Zygomycetes, such as *Mucor* and *Rhizopus* spp., grow rapidly and may fill the tube with aerial mycelium within a few days, whereas more slowly growing organisms such as *Fonsecaea* or *Phialophora* spp. might require 2 weeks or more before growth is seen.

Information that should be recorded about an isolate includes the number of days until first visible growth and the number of days required to see fruiting structures, whether mould or yeast forms are recovered, media on which the fungus is isolated, temperature at which growth occurs, and the morphology of the colonies.

Identification of Fungi

Although the number of fungal species described exceeds 100,000, the number known to cause human disease is a fraction of this number, and although the number of species that are routinely seen causing infection is quite low, new species are continually being implicated. Most diseases are caused by

a handful of species making identification, at least to the genus level, easier. The traditional starting place is to decide whether the isolate is a yeast or a mould.

None of the following tests alone is sufficient for proper identification, but when they are used together, accurate identification is often easily accomplished. Armed with these test procedures, the laboratory scientist should be able to identify the most commonly encountered fungal isolates.

Macroscopic Examination of Cultures

Once an organism has grown, colonies must be examined for macroscopic characteristics. Gross morphologic traits, such as color, texture, and growth rate, are initial observations that should be made. Rapidly growing organisms such as the Zygomycetes usually appear within 1 to 3 days, whereas intermediate growers may take 5 to 9 days, and slow growers up to 2 weeks. Pigment on the reverse side of the colony or in the aerial mycelium can be noted but is not always helpful, especially with the dematiaceous fungi.

Microscopic Examination

The most common procedure for microscopic examination is a direct mount of the fungal isolate. This is achieved by preparing a tease mount or cellophane tape mount. Many fungi routinely recovered can be identified by either of these two methods. Because of the risk of airborne conidia, these slide preparations must be performed in a biological safety cabinet. When fungi are atypical or are a species not routinely recovered, a slide culture should be prepared. Whereas tease and tape mounts typically disturb conidia, preventing viewing of how they are formed, slide cultures provide a more intact specimen. Fruiting structures, as well as conidial arrangement, are better observed by this method. Microscopic characteristics that should be observed are the following:
- Septate versus sparsely septate hyphae
- Hyaline or dematiaceous hyphae
- Fruiting structures
- The types, size, shape, and arrangement of conidia

Tease Mount. For the tease mount, two teasing needles are used to remove a portion of the mycelium from the middle third of the colony. The mycelium is placed in a drop of lactophenol cotton blue (LPCB) on a slide and is gently teased apart using the needles. A modification of this procedure is more practical and permits retention of more of the fruiting structure. Instead of using two teasing needles, a portion of the colony may be removed by either one teasing needle or by a sterile applicator stick. The mycelium is then placed into a drop of LPCB on a slide, a cover slip is added and the slide is examined microscopically at both low (100×) and high magnification.

LPCB is used to fix and stain tease or tape mounts from cultures. The combination of lactic acid, phenol, and the blue dye kills, preserves, and stains the organism. The hyphae take up the LPCB, but the stain does not work well with the dematiaceous fungi because they retain their dark color. The major disadvantage of this procedure is the disruption of conidia during the teasing process.

Cellophane Tape Preparation. Cellophane tape preparations involve gently touching a piece of clear tape, sticky side down, to the surface of the colony and then removing it. The tape should not be pressed into the colony but rather just permitted to touch the surface. Note that frosted tape does not work because the fungi are not visible through this type of tape. The tape is placed onto a drop of LPCB on a slide and examined. An advantage of this procedure is that the conidial arrangement is retained. A major disadvantage is the potential contamination of the colony and the temporary nature of this preparation. Tape preparations should be read within 30 minutes and then discarded. A cover slip is not needed if the cellophane tape technique is used because the tape serves as a cover slip.

Slide Culture. Slide cultures are useful for demonstrating the natural morphology of fungal structures and for encouraging conidiation in some poorly fruiting fungi. Several methods have been devised for constructing slide cultures (see Appendix D). Another advantage to this type of slide is that it can be preserved indefinitely. This is particularly useful when the slide culture from a known isolate is stored in a collection for future comparison against isolates awaiting identification.

Miscellaneous Tests for the Identification of Moulds

Hair Perforation Test. In the hair perforation tests, sterile 5- to 10-mm hair fragments are floated on sterile water supplemented with a few drops of sterile 10% yeast extract. Conidia or hyphae from the dermatophyte in question are inoculated onto the water surface. Hair shafts are removed and microscopically examined in LPCB at weekly intervals for up to 1 month. *T. rubrum*, which may be morphologically similar to *T. mentagrophytes*, usually causes only surface erosion of hair shafts in this test, whereas *T. mentagrophytes* typically forms perpendicular penetration pegs in the hair shafts (Figure 27-58). Some laboratories also use this test to distinguish penetration-capable *Microsporum canis* from *M. equinum*, which does not penetrate hair.

Urease Test. Another test used to help differentiate *T. mentagrophytes* from *T. rubrum* is the 5-day urease test. Tubes

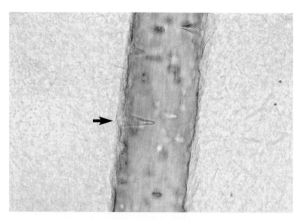

FIGURE 27-58 A positive hair perforation test shows penetration of the fungal agent in the hair shaft. This is the typical reaction by *Trichophyton mentagrophytes*, whereas *Trichophyton rubrum* causes only surface erosion of hair shaft.

of Christensen urea agar are very lightly inoculated with the dermatophyte and held for 5 days at room temperature. Most isolates of *T. mentagrophytes* demonstrate urease production, resulting in a color change of the medium from peach to bright fuchsia within that time, whereas most *T. rubrum* isolates are negative or require more than 5 days to give a positive reaction. This test is also useful for other moulds, fungi, and yeast.

Thiamine Requirement. Some dermatophytes cannot synthesize certain vitamins and therefore do not grow on vitamin-free media. Although several vitamin deficiencies are recognized in fungi, the test for thiamine requirement is perhaps the single most useful nutritional test for dermatophytes. Tubes of media with and without the vitamin are inoculated with a tiny, medium-free portion of the colony and observed for growth after 10 to 14 days. Great care must be exercised to avoid transfer of culture medium with the inoculum because even minuscule amounts of vitamin carried over can adequately supply the requirement and thereby mask an otherwise negative reaction.

Trichophyton Agars. Seven different Trichophyton agars, numbered 1 through 7, are used to determine the nutritional requirements of the *Trichophyton* spp. Each of the media has different nutritional ingredients; after inoculation and incubation growth is scored on a scale of 1 to 4. Based on the growth pattern, identification is made.

Growth on Rice Grains. Poorly sporulating isolates of *M. canis* can be difficult to differentiate from *M. audouinii*, a species that typically forms few spores. Sterile, nonfortified rice is inoculated lightly with a portion of a colony. After 10 days of incubation at room temperature, the medium is observed for growth. *M. canis* and virtually all other dermatophytes grow well and usually form many conidia, whereas *M. audouinii* does not grow but rather turns the rice grains brown.

Miscellaneous Tests for the Identification of Yeasts

Germ-Tube Production. The **germ-tube** test is probably the most important and easiest test to perform for identification of yeasts. Figure 27-59 shows a schematic diagram of how the germ-tube test can be used presumptively to identify yeast species. Both *Candida albicans* and *C. dubliniensis* are identified by germ-tube production (Figure 27-60). The standard procedure, (see Appendix D), requires the use of serum or plasma such as fetal bovine serum. Expired fresh-frozen plasma from the blood bank is useful in this test and can be stored at 4° C almost indefinitely. Many other liquid media (e.g., BHI, trypticase soy broth, or nutrient broth) have been used successfully as alternative media. The substrate is inoculated then incubated at 37° C for 3 hours. Care must be taken not to incubate the test beyond 3 hours because other species are capable of forming germ tubes with extended incubation.

A presumptive identification of either *C. albicans* or *C. dubliniensis* can be made when true germ tubes are present. This test provides only a presumptive identification because not all strains of *C. albicans* will be positive, and other species can provide false-positive results. True germ tubes lack con-

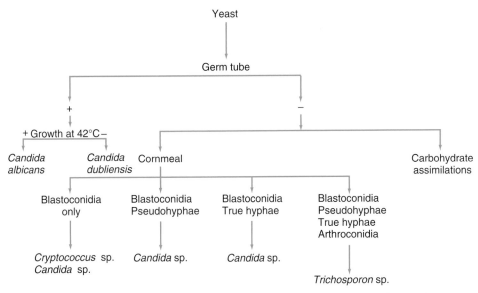

FIGURE 27-59 Schematic diagram showing how the germ-tube test can be used to presumptively identify yeasts.

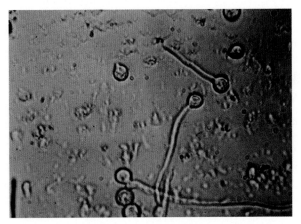

FIGURE 27-60 Germ-tube production by *Candida albicans*. A positive germ tube has no constriction at its base.

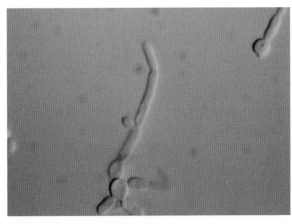

FIGURE 27-61 *Candida tropicalis* shows constriction at the base of the germ tube, called a *pseudogerm* tube.

striction at their bases, where they attach to the mother cell. If a constriction is present at the base of a germ tube, the yeast is not either species. Such constricted germ tubes, called **pseudogerm tubes,** are more characteristic of *C. tropicalis* (Figure 27-61). *C. dubliniensis* is differentiated from *C. albicans* by its inability to grow at 42° C.

Carbohydrate Assimilation. Sugar fermentation tests, although valuable, are time and labor intensive, making them impractical for the routine microbiology laboratory. Carbohydrate assimilation tests, however, can be readily performed as part of the routine procedures. Assimilation tests identify which carbohydrates a yeast can utilize as a sole source of carbon aerobically. Assimilation patterns can be determined from methods as sophisticated as an automated identification system or as simple as the various manual procedures and commercial kits. The individual laboratory should adopt the method that can be practically implemented into its particular working environment.

Although many such kits are available for yeast identification, the API 20C (bioMérieux) yeast identification system is probably the most commonly used. In this method a series of freeze-dried sugars are placed into wells on a plastic strip. Yeast isolates are suspended in an agar basal medium, pipetted into the wells, and incubated at 30° C for 72 hours. As sugars are assimilated, the wells become turbid with growth. Wells remain clear when the sugar is not assimilated. A code is derived from the assimilation patterns and matched against a computerized database. Identifications are accompanied by a percentage, which indicates the probability that the identification is correct. Although this test is reliable, other auxiliary testing should accompany assimilation results before a final identification is made. Automated systems are also available for yeast identification. Many of these systems use enzyme reactions as well as assimilation reactions to aid in yeast identification.

Chromogenic Substrates. A number of media containing chromogenic substrates are available for the presumptive identification of yeasts. CHROMagar *Candida* presumptively identifies *C. albicans, C. tropicalis,* and *C. krusei.* Identification is based on different colony colors, depending on the breakdown of chromogenic substrates by the different species.

Cornmeal Agar. Yeast morphology on cornmeal agar is second in importance to sugar assimilations in determining yeast identification (see Appendix D). Recognition of four different types of morphology is an important clue to yeast identification: blastoconidia, chlamydoconidia, pseudohyphae, and arthroconidia.

Blastoconidia are the characteristic budding yeast forms most often seen on direct mounts. *C. albicans* produces chlamydoconidia along with hyphae, as shown in Figure 27-62. Pseudohyphae (Figure 27-63) occur when the blastoconidia germinate to form a filamentous mat. The cross-walls help determine whether the structures are true hyphae or pseudohyphae. Cross-walls of pseudohyphae are constricted and not true septations, whereas true hyphae remain parallel at cross-

walls with no indentation. Arthroconidia begin as true hyphae but break apart at the cross-walls with maturity. Rectangular fragments of hyphae should be accompanied by blastoconidia for an isolate to be considered a yeast.

Potassium Nitrate Assimilation. Potassium nitrate (KNO_3) assimilation patterns provide valuable information for separating the clinically significant yeasts. Use of the modified KNO_3 agar is a fairly rapid, easy, and accurate method to determine the ability of yeast to use nitrate as the sole source of nitrogen. A positive KNO_3 assimilation result turns the medium blue, and a negative result turns the medium yellow. Control organisms that may be used are *Cryptococcus albidus* (positive) and *C. albicans* (negative).

Temperature Studies. Temperature studies offer information for yeast identification. *Cryptococcus* spp. have weak growth at 35° C and no growth at 42° C. The optimal temperature for growth is about 25° C. Several *Candida* spp. have the ability to grow well at temperatures as high as 45° C. *C. albicans* grows at 45° C, whereas *C. dubliniensis* is negative.

Urease. Yeast isolates producing the enzyme urease can be detected easily with urea agar. The slants are inoculated and incubated at room temperature for 48 hours. Positive test results turn the medium bright fuchsia pink, whereas negative results cause little if any change. Nearly all clinically encountered *Candida* spp. are urease negative, whereas all *Cryptococcus* and *Rhodotorula* organisms are urease positive. Most strains of *Trichosporon* spp. are urease positive.

IMMUNODIAGNOSIS OF FUNGAL INFECTIONS

Immunodiagnostic assays to aid in the identification of fungal isolates and the diagnosis of infections have been available for several years. Antisera reacting against cell-wall antigens are commercially available for a number of *Candida* spp. and *Cryptococcus neoformans.* The Pastorex *Candida* (Bio-Rad, Hercules, Calif.) and Cand-Tec (Ramco Laboratories, Houston, Tex.) are latex agglutination assays that detect *Candida*-specific mannan. However, these assays tend to have low sensitivity, possibly from transient mannan antigenemia. In addition, *C. albicans* cannot be differentiated from *C. dubliniensis* by this method. An enzyme immunoassay for mannan, Platelia *Candida* (Bio-Rad), is available. Latex agglutination assays are also available for detecting *C. neoformans* polysaccharide antigen.

Detecting *Aspergillus*-specific galactomannan by enzyme-linked immunosorbent assay (ELISA) in patient samples has demonstrated high sensitivity and specificity. The ELISA method seems to be more accurate than previously used latex agglutination assays. The concentration of circulating *Aspergillus* antigen correlates with fungal tissue burden in neutropenic animal models. In addition, antigen titer corresponds to clinical outcomes; therefore, this assay could be used to monitor patient response to treatment.

The Fungitec (Seikagaku Corp., Tokyo, Japan) is an assay method for glucan, a cell-wall component found in most fungi except the zygomycetes. The assay is based on the sensitivity of factor G in the horseshoe crab to glucan. Activation of factor G by glucan produces coagulation. This assay can

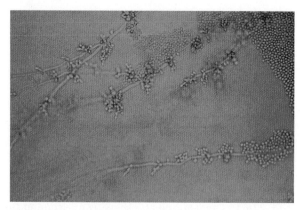

FIGURE 27-62 *Candida albicans* on cornmeal agar showing typical chlamydospores.

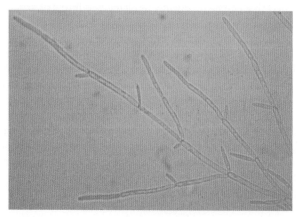

FIGURE 27-63 Pseudohyphae occur when the blastoconidia germinate and form a filamentous mat.

determine the concentration of glucan in patient serum. Normal individuals typically have glucan concentrations less than 10 pg/mL, whereas concentrations greater than 20 pg/mL correlate with fungal infections.

Skin test reactivity to fungal antigens is sometimes used in the diagnosis of fungal allergies and infections. For example, *Aspergillus* spp. antigen extract is used for suspected allergic bronchopulmonary aspergillosis, atopic dermatitis, or allergic asthma. Although few are commercially available, assays to detect antibodies to fungi have also been used to help diagnose infection. Results depend on the antigen chosen and its quality. Cross-reactivity among related fungi has been reported. Double-immunodiffusion is probably the most commonly used method. Interlaboratory discrepancies have been reported. One problem with serologic assays is the ubiquitous nature of many of the opportunistic fungi. Individuals can have detectable antibodies but not an active infection. It has also been shown that some individuals with *Aspergillus* spp. infections do not have detectable levels of antibody.

ANTIFUNGAL SUSCEPTIBITY

Antifungal Agents

In the last 25 years, fungal infections have steadily increased in incidence, with *C. albicans* now ranked as the fourth leading cause of nosocomial infection. This increase can be attributed to advances in medicine that have permitted prolonged life expectancy. Advances in the area of transplant medicine and chemotherapy, combined with immunosuppression from HIV infection, have created new patient populations susceptible to fungal infections.

Physicians have far fewer options for treating fungal infection than for bacterial counterparts. Current options for treating fungal infection include drugs from three classes: the polyenes, azoles, and candins. The primary antifungal agent is amphotericin B (AMB), a polyene. This antifungal drug is the only agent known to kill most fungi. Not only is this agent lethal for fungi, but it is toxic for patients as well. Patients being treated with AMB may suffer from many side effects, including fever, rigors, renal impairment, and possibly shock. Frequently the physician must decide between treating the fungal infection and risk damaging the patient's kidneys. Despite these problems, AMB remains the drug of choice for most life-threatening fungal disease. Unfortunately resistance to AMB has been documented with *P. boydii, P. lilacinus,* and in about 6% of *Candida lusitaniae* isolates.

The class that has provided the largest number of agents is the azoles. The most noteworthy compounds in this class include fluconazole (FLU), itraconazole (ITRA), and voriconazole (VORI). The azoles are important because they exhibit reasonable activity against the fungi while maintaining fewer side effects. Fluconazole is the leading agent for treating yeast infections but has limited to no activity against moulds. It is widely used by many practitioners for all types of infection, including vaginitis and thrush. Unfortunately its overuse or misuse has resulted in the development of resistance, most notably with *C. glabrata.* For patients who have been on long-term antifungal therapy, it is extremely important to deter-

mine the susceptibility pattern for a specific isolate prior to prescribing FLU for severe infections.

Three other azoles, ITRA, VORI, and posaconazole (POSA) are more frequently prescribed for mould infections. Itraconazole was released about the time of FLU and is especially useful for the aspergilli and dematiaceous fungi. POSA is the newest azole and has perhaps the best activity against most fungal species. VORI has shown improved activity against the aspergilli in addition to several emerging pathogens. Although prophylaxis with VORI is effective in decreasing infections by *Aspergillus* spp., it is also feared that an increase in zygomycete infections might be attributed to this same agent.

The first agent to be released in the candins group was caspofungin (CAS). This agent is lethal for yeast and, although effective against the aspergilli, is not generally lethal. This class targets cell-wall synthesis, which makes it an attractive option for treating fungi that have developed resistance to other agents. Two newer candins have been released: anidulafungin and micafungin. These two antifungals tend to have lower minimum inhibitory concentrations (MICs) than CAS and may be options when MICs to CAS are above desired limits.

Antifungal Susceptibility Testing

Until the last several years, many laboratories used methods that had been developed in-house to determine susceptibility patterns for the fungi. The CLSI (Clinical Laboratory Standards Institute), formerly the NCCLS (National Committee of Clinical Laboratory Standards), has released three methods for fungal testing. These methods include M27-A3 for yeast testing, M38-A2 for mould testing, and M44-A for disk diffusion testing for yeasts. The most recent method, M44-A, was developed as a cost-effective method that could easily be incorporated into busy microbiology laboratories that routinely perform this type of antimicrobial testing for bacteria. As with bacterial testing, Mueller-Hinton agar is used, alleviating the necessity of multiple media to perform antimicrobial susceptibility testing. Work is underway to release M51-P for disk diffusion testing of moulds. This should give microbiology laboratories options that make antifungal susceptibility testing a more viable option for in-house testing.

Although much debate exists regarding antifungal susceptibility testing, it is gaining popularity with more laboratories. The Food and Drug Administration has approved a microtiter method provided by Trek Diagnostic Systems (Cleveland, Ohio) and a diffusion method developed by **AB BIODISK** (Etest, Solna, Sweden). Before this product was developed, only laboratories that could prepare their own reagents performed testing. The largest barrier to widespread antifungal testing is the lack of established breakpoints for most of the agents. Currently only seven agents have established breakpoints; 5-fluorocytosine, an agent used only in combination with other antifungals, primarily AMB, shares categorical designations with bacteria. These categories are S (susceptible), I (intermediate), and R (resistant). The azoles FLU, ITRA, and VORI are categorized as S, SDD (susceptible-dose-dependent), and R. The SDD category indicates isolates that may be considered susceptible when high-dose therapy, as opposed to standard therapy, is used. The candins are the newest agents to have breakpoints and all three share two categories S and NS (non-susceptible). Until other drugs are studied and breakpoints are established, the utility of antifungal susceptibility testing will most likely remain limited.

BIBLIOGRAPHY

Brandt ME, Warnock DW: *Histoplasmosis, Blastomyces, Coccidioides,* and other dimorphic fungi causing systemic mycoses. In Murray PR et al, editors: *Manual of clinical microbiology,* ed 9, Washington, DC, 2007, ASM Press.

Cushion MT: *Pneumocystis.* In Murray PR et al, editors: *Manual of clinical microbiology,* ed 9, Washington, DC, 2007, ASM Press.

de Hoog GS et al: Fungi causing eumycotic mycetoma. In Murray PR et al, editors: *Manual of clinical microbiology,* ed 9, Washington, DC, 2007, ASM Press.

de Hoog GS, Vitale RG: *Bipolaris, Exophiala, Scedosporium, Sporothrix,* and other dematiaceous fungi. In Murray PR et al, editors: *Manual of clinical microbiology,* ed 9, Washington, DC, 2007, ASM Press.

Erjavec Z, Verweij PE: Recent progress in the diagnosis of fungal infections in the immunocompromised host, *Drug Resist Updates* 5:3, 2002.

Hazen KC, Howell SA: *Candida, Cryptococcus,* and other yeasts of medical importance. In Murray PR et al, editors: *Manual of clinical microbiology,* ed 9, Washington, DC, 2007, ASM Press.

Larone DH: *Medically important fungi: a guide to identification,* ed 4, Washington, DC, 2002, ASM Press.

Richardson MD et al: *Rhizopus, Rhizomucor, Absidia,* and other agents of systemic and subcutaneous zygomycoses. In Murray PR et al, editors: *Manual of clinical microbiology,* ed 9, Washington, DC, 2007, ASM Press.

Stevens DA: Diagnosis of fungal infections: current status, *J Antimicrob Chemother* 49(Suppl S1):11, 2002.

Summerbell RC et al: *Trichophyton, Microsporum, Epidermophyton,* and agents of superficial mycoses. In Murray PR et al, editors: *Manual of clinical microbiology,* Washington, DC, 2007, ASM Press.

Verweij PE, Brandt ME: *Aspergillus, Fusarium,* and other opportunistic moniliaceous fungi. In Murray PR et al, editors: *Manual of clinical microbiology,* ed 9, Washington, DC, 2007, ASM Press.

Points to Remember

- Yeasts typically reproduce by budding whereas moulds often reproduce by forming spores.
- The fungi provide a fascinating array of isolates that cause human disease.
- Fungi can be isolated from nearly any type of clinical specimen.
- Fungal identification is based on a variety of characteristics, including macroscopic appearance, microscopic appearance, ability to grow at various temperatures, and biochemical reactions.
- Dematiaceous fungi produce dark pigments.
- Dermatophytoses are caused by *Trichophyton, Microsporum,* and *Epidermophyton* species.

- The thermally dimorphic fungi are often associated with systemic mycoses.
- Clinically important Zygomycetes include *Rhizopus, Mucor, Absidia, Cunninghamella,* and *Syncephalastrum.*
- Because of its microscopic morphology, *Geotrichum* is a mould that is often initially mistaken for a yeast.
- Saprobic fungi are most problematic in the immunocompromised host.
- *C. albicans* is the most commonly isolated yeast.
- *Pneumocystis* sp. is an important pathogen of patients with AIDS.
- Extreme care should be taken when working with dimorphic fungi in the laboratory.
- The identification of fungi is based primarily on colony and microscopic morphologies.
- Antifungal therapy is frequently ineffective when diagnosis is delayed.

Learning Assessment Questions

1. For each of the following dimorphic fungi, describe the characteristic microscopic appearance at 37° C or and when grown at 22° C:
   a. *Blastomyces dermatitidis*
   b. *Coccidioides immitis*
   c. *Histoplasma capsulatum* var. *capsulatum*
   d. *Sporothrix schenckii*

2. Describe the microscopic morphology for each of the following organisms:
   a. *Microsporum gypseum*
   b. *Microsporum canis*
   c. *Trichophyton rubrum*
   d. *Trichophyton mentagrophytes*

3. Compare the results of the urease test and the hair perforation test for *T. rubrum* and *T. mentagrophytes.*

4. Describe the significance of isolating a saprobe from an infection in an immunocompromised patient.

5. Compare the macroscopic and microscopic morphology of the following saprobes: *Penicillium* spp., *Aspergillus fumigatus, Fusarium* spp., and *Curvularia* spp.

6. Describe the difference between chromoblastomycosis and eumycotic mycetoma.

7. Discuss the differences between bacteria and fungi.

8. Discuss the difference between hyaline and dematiaceous.

9. Define teleomorph, anamorph, and synanamorph.

10. You suspect that a yeast isolated from the oral cavity of a patient with HIV infection is *Candida albicans.* Describe the results of the germ tube test. What morphology would you see if you inoculated the colony onto cornmeal agar?

Diagnostic Parasitology

Linda A. Smith

- ■ **GENERAL CONCEPTS IN PARASITOLOGY LABORATORY METHODS**
  Fecal Specimens
  Other Specimens Examined for Intestinal and Urogenital
     Parasites
  Examination of Specimens for Blood and Tissue
     Parasites

Immunologic Diagnosis
Quality Assurance in the Parasitology Laboratory
- ■ **MEDICALLY IMPORTANT PARASITIC AGENTS**
  Protozoa
  Apicomplexa
  Microsporidia
  Helminths

OBJECTIVES

After reading and studying this chapter, you should be able to:

1. List the major considerations in the collection and handling of specimens for identification of intestinal and blood and tissue parasites.

2. Describe the general procedures for performing the direct wet mount, fecal concentration, and permanent stained smears.

3. Describe procedures such as the preparation of blood films, wet mounts, concentration methods, and staining methods for blood and tissue parasites.

4. List the stages of parasites found during microscopic examination of fecal material with each of the following: direct wet mount, fecal concentration, and permanent stained smears.

5. Compare the procedure and uses of thick and thin blood smears for the identification of blood parasites.

6. Compare the general characteristics of the major phyla of human parasites.

7. Compare the morphology and clinical infections of *Naegleria fowleri* and *Acanthamoeba*.

8. For the major human pathogens, describe the mechanism of pathogenesis, clinical symptoms, treatment, and prevention.

9. Develop protocols for sample collection, handling, and transport of specimens for blood and tissue parasites.

10. For each organism presented, describe the morphology, the life cycle, including the infective stage and the diagnostic stage, and the usual procedure for identification.

Case in Point

A 4-year-old boy was seen in the public health clinic because of intermittent bouts of diarrhea lasting almost 4 weeks. The mother did not note any bright-red blood in the stool. The child was pale, listless, and had a protuberant abdomen. He had a number of small erythematous vesicles on his feet. His mother said that he sometimes ate dirt but otherwise always had a good appetite. The family lived in a rural part of Georgia and had a well from which they got their drinking water. This part of the county had only recently been connected into the local city's sanitation system. The physician initially ordered a complete blood count. The white blood cell count was 10,200 cell/mL, and the differential showed 14% eosinophils. The hemoglobin was 6.2 g/dL and the reticulocyte count was 8%. The red blood cell morphology was described as microcytic and hypochromic. The physician ordered a stool culture for bacterial pathogens and an ova and parasite (O & P) examination. The bacterial culture was negative for enteric pathogens, but the O & P examination revealed parasitic organisms and the presence of Charcot-Leyden crystals.

Issues to Consider

After reading the patient's case history, consider:
- ■ What features about the patient's history are significant.
- ■ What intestinal parasites should be considered part of the patient's differential diagnosis.
- ■ What additional laboratory tests could aid the diagnosis.

Key Terms

Amastigote	Metacercaria
Asexual reproduction	Microfilariae
Blackwater fever	Peripheral chromatin
Bradyzoites	Polyvinyl alcohol (PVA)
Cercaria	Proglottids
Chromatoidal bars	Rhabditiform larva
Cysts	Schizogony
Cysticercus	Schizont
Definitive hosts	Schüffner's stippling
Erythrocytic phase	Scolex
Exoerythrocytic phase	Sexual reproduction
Filariform larvae	Sporoblast
Gametes	Sporocysts
Gametocytes	Sporogony
Hexacanth embryo (oncosphere)	Sporozoites
Intermediate hosts	Tachyzoites
Karyosomes	Trophozoites
Kinetoplast	Trypomastigote
Merozoites	Vectors
	Ziemann's dots

Parasites are an important cause of human morbidity and mortality. In the United States and other developed countries, they are seldom regarded as major causes of disease. Health care professionals, however, have become increasingly aware that parasites must be considered as possible etiologic agents in a patient's clinical condition. Factors that have led to this greater awareness include the rising number of immunocompromised patients who are susceptible to infections caused by known pathogens and opportunistic organisms, the increasing number of people who travel to countries that have less than ideal sanitation and a large number of endemic parasites, and the growing population of immigrants from areas with endemic parasites.

When a primary care provider is confronted with an infection that may be due to a parasite, the patient's symptoms and clinical history, including travel history, are significant data to be gathered and shared with the laboratory scientist. The clinician and laboratory scientists should collaborate to make sure that the appropriate specimen is properly collected, handled, and examined. Knowledge of common pathogens and of nonpathogens that exist in specific geographic regions and for a given body site is necessary to ensure identification and, if necessary, therapy. Parasitic infections can be difficult to diagnose, however, because patients often have nonspecific clinical symptoms that can be attributed to a number of disease agents. Detection and identification of a parasite depend not only on the adequacy of the submitted specimen but also on the procedures established by the clinical laboratory, including the criteria for specimen collection, handling, and transport, and for the laboratory methods used. This chapter discusses the major medically important parasites, their epidemiology and life cycle, and the clinical infections

they cause. In addition, the diagnostic features that characterize these agents are presented. Readers are referred to standard parasitology references for detailed procedures, reagent preparation, and a comprehensive description of parasites that have been implicated in human disease.

GENERAL CONCEPTS IN PARASITOLOGY LABORATORY METHODS

Fecal Specimens

Collection, Handling, and Transport

The collection and handling of a stool specimen prior to laboratory examination may have an effect on whether or not organisms will be identified. The stool should be delivered to the laboratory as soon as possible after collection or a portion placed immediately in a preservative. **Trophozoites** of some amebae or eggs of some helminths may disintegrate if not examined or preserved within a short time. Because many intestinal organisms are shed into the stool irregularly, a single stool specimen may be insufficient to detect an intestinal parasite. Traditionally for optimal detection of intestinal parasites, a series of three stool specimens spaced a day or two apart collected within a 10-day period has been recommended. This procedure of examining each specimen submitted is time consuming and labor intensive. Published articles suggest that in some circumstances, pooling of the three formalin-preserved specimens gives a parasite recovery rate comparable to that of individual examination of formalin-preserved stools. Although this method saves time, there is a risk that if organisms are present in small numbers, they may be missed on microscopic examination of wet mounts due to a dilution effect (i.e., reduced sensitivity). Most studies have shown increased sensitivity when multiple specimens are examined. Many laboratories establish an algorithm that takes into account the types of parasitology examinations routinely performed (e.g., concentration and permanent stained smear), the patient population, and specific criteria (travel, symptoms, immune status, in- or outpatient classification) to determine if a single specimen or multiple stool specimens should be examined.

It has been recommended that permanent stained smears be made and examined for each specimen individually. In addition, whether the cases are inpatient or outpatient, the presence of symptoms should dictate whether three specimens are needed. For example, although inpatients frequently acquire nosocomial bacterial infections, it is highly unlikely that an inpatient would acquire a nosocomial parasitic infection. In addition to routine testing, an immunoassay for *Giardia lamblia* or *Cryptosporidium parvum* may be requested on specimens from immunocompromised patients with diarrhea or children in daycare settings who are symptomatic.

The appropriate collection container for feces is clean, dry, sealed tightly, and waterproof (e.g., a plastic container with lid). Commercial systems that incorporate collection container and preservatives are also available. Stool specimens should never be collected from bedpans or toilet bowls; such a practice might contaminate the specimen with urine or water, resulting in the destruction of trophozoites or introduction of free-living protozoa. As an alternative, the specimen could be collected on a clean piece of waxed paper or newspaper and transferred to the container. Another alternative is to use a disposable collection containers that can be fitted under the toilet bowl rim. The specimen should be submitted as soon as possible after passage. Information on the container should include the patient's name and the date and time the stool was collected. The laboratory requisition should include the same information and any additional pertinent clinical data, such as the suspected diagnosis.

Stool specimens for parasites should be collected before a barium enema or before the start of antimicrobial therapy. Antimicrobials can reduce the number of organisms present. If the patient has undergone a barium enema, stool examination should be delayed for 7 to 10 days, because barium obscures organisms when specimens are examined microscopically even after concentration procedures. If a purged specimen is to be collected, it is recommended that a saline or phosphosoda purgative be used, because mineral oil droplets interfere with identification of parasites, especially protozoan **cysts.** The second or third specimen after the purge is more likely to contain trophozoites that inhabit the cecum.

Preservation

Several methods are available for stool preservation if the specimen will not be delivered immediately to the laboratory. The preservative to be used is determined by the procedure to be performed on the fecal sample. Regardless of the preservative used, the ratio of three parts preservative to one part feces should be maintained for optimal fixation. Table 28-1 presents some of the more common preservatives and their appropriate use. The time that the stool was passed and the time that it was placed in the fixative should be noted on the laboratory requisition and the container. A commercially available two-vial system using **polyvinyl alcohol (PVA)** in one vial and 10% formalin in the other vial is commonly used. The system comes with patient instructions and a self-sealing plastic bag for transport. PVA fixative, which consists of mercuric chloride (for fixation) and PVA (a resin to increase adhesion of the stool to the slide), is used when a permanently stained smear will be made.

TABLE 28-1 Preservatives Commonly Used for Fecal Samples

Preservative	Laboratory Examination Method
Polyvinyl alcohol (PVA)	Permanently stained smear DNA-PCR
10% Formalin	Formalin–ethyl acetate concentration, direct wet mount, and immunoassays
Sodium acetate–acetic acid–formalin (SAF)	Permanently stained smears and concentration
Merthiolate-iodine-formalin (MIF)	Concentration and direct wet mount
Single-vial systems	Concentration, direct wet mount, permanently stained smears, and immunoassays

PCR, Polymerase chain reaction.

Concern about disposal of hazardous mercury compounds has led to development and evaluation of a number of alternative nontoxic fixatives. Ecofix (Meridian Diagnostics, Inc., Cincinnati, Ohio), Parasafe (Scientific Device Laboratory, Des Plaines, Ill.), and Prot-fix (Alpha-Tec, Vancouver, Wash.) are single-vial fixatives for wet mounts and permanent stained slides that do not use formaldehyde or mercury compounds. Evaluation of stains made from stools preserved with these compounds showed varying quality of the stained preparations. In some cases the background quality was poor, and in others a less sharp morphology of the organism was observed. Overall, however, most provided a satisfactory substitute for the standard PVA containing mercuric chloride. The alternative compounds do not contain PVA, so the smears dry faster. Formalin can be used when either a wet mount or concentration procedure (either sedimentation or flotation) will be performed. The fixative sodium acetate–acetic acid–formalin (SAF) can be used for the preservation of fecal specimens when both concentration procedures and permanent stains will be used. Vials of merthiolate-iodine-formalin (MIF) can also be used to preserve trophozoites, cysts, larvae, and helminth eggs for wet mount or concentration procedures. This preservative, however, is not routinely used for permanently stained smears.

Macroscopic Examination

The examination of an unpreserved stool specimen should include macroscopic (gross) and microscopic procedures. The initial laboratory procedure is the macroscopic examination. During gross examination, intact worms or **proglottids** (tapeworm segments) may be identified on the surface of the stool. Gross examination of the specimen also reveals the consistency (liquid, soft, formed) of the stool sample. Consistency may help determine the type of preservation to be used, can indicate the forms of parasites expected to be present, or may dictate the immediacy of examination. Figure 28-1 shows the relationship between stool consistency and protozoan stage. For example, a soft or liquid stool specimen or a purged specimen primarily contains motile protozoan trophozoites; hence purged specimens should be examined immediately after passage. Soft or liquid specimens should be examined within one-half hour of passage to ensure motility of the organisms. If examination will be delayed, a portion should also be placed in a fixative such as PVA, so that permanent stained smears for definitive identification can be made.

During the gross examination, the color of the stool specimen is noted. A normal stool sample usually appears brown. Stool that appears black may indicate bleeding in the upper gastrointestinal tract, whereas the presence of fresh blood may indicate bleeding in the lower portion of the intestinal tract. Any portion of the stool that contains blood or blood-tinged mucus should be selected for wet mount preparations and be placed in preservative. A formed stool specimen should be examined within 2 to 3 hours of passage if held at room temperature; however, examination may be delayed up to 24 hours after passage if the specimen is placed in the refrigerator. A portion of the formed stool should be placed in formalin for concentration procedures and another portion placed in PVA for permanently stained smears. The specimen should

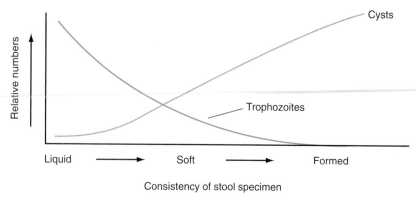

FIGURE 28-1 Relationship of stool consistency to protozoan stage.

not be placed in a 37° C incubator, which increases the rate of disintegration of organisms present and enhances overgrowth by bacteria.

Microscopic Examination

Several diagnostic methods can be used in the microscopic examination of a fecal specimen:

- Direct wet mount examination (stained and unstained) of fresh stool specimens
- Concentration procedures with wet mount examination of the concentrate
- Preparation of permanently stained smears

In general, the concentration and permanent staining procedures should be performed on all specimens.

Wet Mount Preparations. The direct wet mount of unpreserved fecal material is primarily used to detect the presence of motile protozoan trophozoites in a fresh liquid stool or from sigmoidoscopy material. Because of the low diagnostic yield and labor-intensiveness, a wet mount should not be performed on formed stool. Wet mounts are also made from the fecal specimen following a concentration procedure. This procedure detects protozoan cysts, helminth eggs, and helminth larvae.

The wet mount procedure uses a glass slide on which a drop of physiologic saline (0.85%) has been placed at one end and a drop of iodine (Dobell and O'Connor, D'Antoni, or a 1:5 dilution of Lugol solution) at the other end. A small amount (2 mg) of feces is added to each drop and mixed well. Each preparation should be covered with a No. 1, 22-mm square coverslip. The preparation should be thin enough so that newsprint can be read through it and should not overflow beyond the edges of the coverslip. The edges of the coverslip can be sealed with either clear nail polish or vaspar (50:50 mixture of petroleum jelly and paraffin). Sealing the preparation prevents rapid drying and allows further examination. Because the PVA becomes cloudy when exposed to air, PVA-preserved specimens are not acceptable for wet mounts.

If the specimen has been preserved in 10% formalin, the drop of saline may be omitted from the unstained preparation. In unfixed stool specimens, the saline preparation is useful for detection of helminth eggs or larvae, motile trophozoites, and refractile protozoan cysts. Iodine emphasizes nuclear detail and glycogen masses but kills trophozoites.

Stains such as buffered methylene blue have been used to enhance nuclear morphology in trophozoites but may inhibit motility and cause the organisms to round up. Reading the wet mount involves thorough examination of each coverslipped preparation at low power, starting at one corner and following a systematic vertical or horizontal pattern until the entire preparation has been examined. A high-power objective is used to identify any suspicious structures. Oil immersion should not be used on a wet preparation unless the preparation has been sealed with either clear nail polish or vaspar.

Concentration Techniques. Concentration techniques are designed to concentrate the parasites present into a small volume of fluid and remove as much debris as possible. Either fresh or formalin-preserved stool specimens may be used. The concentrate may then be examined either unstained or stained with iodine. Protozoan trophozoites do not survive the procedure; protozoan cysts, helminth larvae, and helminth eggs are usually detected using this method.

Sedimentation and flotation methods, both of which are based on the difference in specific gravity between the parasites and the concentrating solution, are used to concentrate parasites into a small volume for easier detection. In sedimentation methods, the organisms are concentrated in sediment at the bottom of the centrifuge tube. In flotation methods, the organisms are suspended at the top of a high-density fluid. Overall, sedimentation methods concentrate a greater diversity of organisms, including cysts, larvae, and eggs. The formalin–ethyl acetate sedimentation (FES) method was the standard sedimentation method. A number of manufacturers now market self-contained fecal concentration kits that do not use ethyl acetate. One example is the Para-Pak SpinCon system (Meridian Diagnostics, Inc.), which uses a centrifuge tube with a prefilter and two metal filters. A solvent is not needed; specimens fixed in 10% formalin, SAF, or Ecofix can be concentrated. The pellet is used for wet mounts and permanent stained slides. Although these kits offer easier disposability and a cleaner preparation owing to the filtration method used, studies indicate that their use is more expensive than the traditional FES method.

The zinc sulfate method is the usual flotation procedure. Although the zinc sulfate method yields less fecal debris in the finished preparation than the FES method, the zinc sulfate causes operculated eggs to open or collapse. It also tends to distort protozoan cysts. Infertile *Ascaris lumbricoides* eggs and *Schistosoma* spp. eggs may be missed if this procedure is used. Because of their high density, these eggs sink to the bottom of the tube. Most organisms tend to settle after about 30 minutes. Therefore, the examination should be made as soon as possible after the procedure has been completed to ensure optimum recovery of organisms. Special flotation procedures, such as the Sheather sugar flotation method, have been used in detection of specific organisms such as *Cryptosporidium* spp. Although oocysts of *Cryptosporidium* spp. can be detected with either the FES or the zinc sulfate method, Sheather flotation allows for better visibility of the oocysts because of the greater refractivity of the oocyst against the background solution. Fresh or formalin-fixed feces can be used in this procedure. A newer concentration method that involves laying sediment from an FES concentration procedure over saturated sodium chloride has been described. This method increases separation of oocysts from fecal debris and enhances detection. It has particular application for oocysts of organisms such as *Cryptosporidium* spp.

Permanently Stained Smears. Permanently stained smear preparations of all stool specimens should be made to detect and identify protozoan trophozoites and cysts. Characteristics needed for identification of the protozoa, including nuclear detail, size, and internal structures, are visible in a well-made and properly stained smear. Permanent stains commonly used include iron hematoxylin and trichrome (Wheatley modification of the Gomori stain). The stain of choice in most laboratories is the trichrome stain, because results are somewhat less dependent on technique and the procedure is less time consuming. Although some laboratories prepare the stain in-house, manufacturers provide prepared stains and reagents for this procedure. A trichrome stain can be performed on a smear made from a fresh stool specimen fixed in Schaudinn fixative or from one that has been preserved in PVA. Specimens preserved in SAF do not stain well with trichrome and should be stained with iron hematoxylin.

To prepare a trichrome-stained smear on a fresh specimen, applicator sticks are used to smear a thin film of stool across a 1- by 3-inch slide. The smear is placed immediately in Schaudinn fixative; it must not be allowed to dry before fixation. For PVA-fixed specimens, several drops of specimen are placed on a paper towel to drain excess fluid; the material on the paper towel is collected to prepare the smear in the same way as for a fresh specimen. This specimen is allowed to air-dry thoroughly before staining.

In a well-stained trichrome smear, the cytoplasm of protozoan cysts and trophozoites stains a blue-green, although *Entamoeba coli* often stains purple. Nuclear chromatin, **karyosomes, chromatoidal bars,** and red blood cells (RBCs) stain a dark red-purple. Eggs and larvae stain red; background debris and yeasts stain green. In an iron hematoxylin stain, the organisms stain gray-black, nuclear material stains black, and background material is light blue-gray. With either stain, poor fixation of fecal material results in poorly staining or nonstaining organisms. A number of modifications of the trichrome staining procedure have been developed to allow detection of microsporidia. Stained smears should be examined by first scanning for thick and thin areas using lower power magnification (10× or 40× objective). Thin areas should be selected and examined under oil immersion (100× objective) for identification of organisms. It should take approximately 10 to 15 minutes to adequately examine selected areas. Organisms that stain lightly and may be difficult to identify are *Entamoeba hartmanni, Dientamoeba fragilis, Endolimax nana, Chilomastix mesnili,* and *Giardia lamblia.*

Modified Acid-Fast Stain. Use of a Kinyoun modified acid-fast stain enhances detection of oocysts of *Cryptosporidium, Isospora belli,* and *Cyclospora cayetanensis.* With this procedure, the oocysts appear as magenta-stained organisms against a blue background. The use of a stain combining iron hematoxylin with carbol fuchsin for simultaneous staining of *Isospora, Cryptosporidium,* and protozoa has been reported.

Other Specimens Examined for Intestinal and Urogenital Parasites

Cellophane Tape Preparation for Pinworm

The life cycle of the pinworm *(Enterobius vermicularis)* includes migration of the female from the anus at night to lay eggs in the perianal area. Therefore a fecal specimen is not the optimal specimen for diagnosis of infection with this organism. Instead, the cellophane tape preparation is routinely used for detection of suspected pinworm infections. This procedure involves swabbing the child's perianal area with a tongue blade covered with cellophane tape (sticky side out). The collection should take place first thing in the morning, before the child uses the bathroom or is bathed. After the sample has been taken, the sticky side of the tape is placed on a microscope slide and scanned at low- and high-power magnification for the characteristically shaped eggs. An adaptation of this procedure using paddles with a sticky surface is commercially available (Starplex Scientific, Inc., Etobicoke, Canada).

Duodenal Aspirates

Material obtained from duodenal aspirates or from the duodenal capsule Enterotest (HDC Corp., San Jose, Calif.) may be submitted in cases of suspected giardiasis or strongyloidiasis when clinical symptoms are suggestive of infection but routine stool examination results are negative. In the Enterotest, the patient swallows a gelatin capsule containing a weighted string. One end of the string has been taped to the side of the patient's mouth; the weighted end is carried into the upper small intestine. After about 4 hours, the string is brought up, and part of the mucus adhering to the surface is stripped off and examined on a wet mount for motile trophozoites. The remainder of the specimen is placed in a fixative for a permanently stained smear. Eggs of *Fasciola hepatica* or *Clonorchis sinensis,* as well as oocysts of *Cryptosporidium* or *Isospora belli,* may also occasionally be recovered.

Sigmoidoscopy Specimens

Scrapings or aspirates obtained by sigmoidoscopy may be used to diagnose amebiasis or cryptosporidiosis. These specimens are examined immediately for motile trophozoites, and a portion of the sample is placed in PVA fixative so that permanently stained smears can be prepared for examination.

Urine, Vaginal, and Urethral Specimens

Eggs of *Schistosoma haematobium* and *E. vermicularis* and trophozoites of *Trichomonas vaginalis* can be detected in the sediment of a urine specimen. *T. vaginalis* can also be detected in a wet mount of vaginal or urethral discharge. Envelope culture methods for *T. vaginalis*, such as the InPouch TV (BioMed Diagnostics, San Jose, Calif.), are also available. The specimen is added to the medium and incubated. Growth of the organism can be observed through the pouch within 3 days.

Sputum

In cases of *Strongyloides stercoralis* hyperinfection, the **filariform larvae** may be seen in a direct wet mount of sputum. Eggs of the lung fluke *Paragonimus westermani* can also be identified in a sputum wet mount. If the patient is suspected of having a pulmonary abscess caused by *Entamoeba histolytica*, the sputum specimen should be examined as a permanently stained smear.

Examination of Specimens for Blood and Tissue Parasites

Blood Smears

Examination of a blood smear stained with Giemsa or Wright stain is the most common method of detecting malaria, *Babesia*, *Trypanosoma*, and some species of microfilaria. Although motile organisms such as *Trypanosoma* and **microfilariae** can be detected on a wet preparation of a fresh blood specimen under low- and high-power magnification, identification is made on the basis of characteristics seen on a permanently stained smear. Concentration methods using membrane filters can be used to detect *Trypanosoma* spp. or microfilariae, but these methods are rarely performed in the clinical laboratory. Tissue parasites such as *Trichinella spiralis*, *Leishmania* spp., and *Toxoplasma gondii* can be identified by examination of tissue biopsy or by serologic methods.

Collection and Preparation. Blood taken directly from a fingerstick is the ideal specimen for a malarial smear because it tends to give the best staining characteristics. Blood collected in ethylenediaminetetraacetic acid (EDTA) gives adequate staining if processed within 1 hour. Distortion of the organism may occur if time to preparation of the slide is greater than1 hour, and organisms may be lost if the time exceeds 4 hours. For example, the **gametocytes** of *Plasmodium falciparum* may lose their characteristic banana shape and round up. With Giemsa stain, the cytoplasm of the parasite stains bluish, and the chromatin stains red to purple-red. If malarial stippling is present, it appears as discrete pink-red dots. Giemsa staining gives the best morphologic detail but is a time-consuming procedure. Wright stain has a shorter staining period, but the color intensity for differentiation of parasites is not as good as that with Giemsa stain.

Identification Procedure. For suspected cases of blood parasites, both a thick film and a thin film should be made. Both preparations can be made on the same slide or on separate slides. Because the two preparations are treated differently before staining, however, use of two slides may be more

efficient. Giemsa stain provides the best staining of the organisms and should be used on both thick and thin films. Thin smears must first be fixed in methanol before staining with the Giemsa stain. RBCs in the unfixed thick smear will lyse during the staining procedure. Unless the RBCs on the slide are first lysed in distilled water, Wright stain cannot be used for a thick film because the stain contains methanol, which will fix RBCs.

A thick film is best for detection of parasites (high sensitivity), because of the larger volume of blood and the fact that organisms are concentrated in a relatively small area. The thick film is made by pooling several drops of blood on the slide and then spreading it into a 1.5-cm area. A film that is too thick peels from the slide; thickness is optimal when newsprint is barely visible through the drop of blood before it dries. The blood should be allowed to dry for at least 6 hours before staining. It should not be fixed with methanol before staining; fixing prevents lysis of the RBCs. Giemsa stain lakes hemoglobin (releases hemoglobin by lysing RBCs) from unfixed red cells. Initial scanning of the stained smear at 10× detects microfilariae. At least 100 oil immersion fields should be examined before a negative result is reported. In the thick film, the RBCs are destroyed so that only white cells, platelets, and parasites are visible. In a thick film, the organisms may be difficult to identify, and there is no way to compare size of infected and noninfected erythrocytes. Therefore, species identification should be made from a thin film because the characteristics of the parasite and the RBCs can be seen.

The thin film is made in the same way as that for a differential cell count. It should be fixed in methanol for 1 minute and air dried before staining with Giemsa stain. The entire smear should be scanned at 100× for detection of large organisms such as microfilariae; then at least 100 oil immersion fields (1000×) must be examined for the presence of organisms such as *Trypanosoma* or for intracellular organisms such as *Plasmodium* or *Babesia*. For a symptomatic patient, several blood smears from samples collected at approximately 6-hour intervals over 36 to 48 hours should be examined before a final negative diagnosis is made.

Biopsy Specimens

Biopsy specimens are usually needed to diagnose infections with *Leishmania* spp. because the organisms are intracellular. Depending on the species present, the **amastigote** stage can be detected in tissues such as skin, liver, spleen, and bone marrow. Cutaneous lesions should be sampled below the edges of the ulcer; surface samples do not yield infected cells.

Cerebrospinal Fluid

Viable organisms in suspected cases of amebic meningitis or sleeping sickness can occasionally be seen in a cerebrospinal fluid (CSF) specimen. The **trypomastigote** is readily visible because of the motion of the flagellum and undulating membrane. It requires a skillful microscopist, however, to discern amebic motility in a field of neutrophils. If amebic meningoencephalitis caused by *Naegleria fowleri* is suspected, the CSF can be cultured. Non-nutrient agar is seeded with an *Escherichia coli* overlay, and the spinal fluid sediment is inoculated onto the medium. The specimen is sealed and incubated at 35° C. The medium is examined daily for thin tracks in the bacterial growth, which indicate that amebae have been feeding on the bacteria.

Immunologic Diagnosis

The parameters that should be considered by a laboratory in selecting methods to be used include not only cost but also diagnostic yield, patient population, relative incidence of the parasite in the area, and number of specimens to be processed. Classically, methods such as hemagglutination or complement fixation were used, especially in the detection of antibodies to parasitic organisms. Some tests may use fluorescent or enzyme immunoassay (EIA) techniques. Immunoassay tests for antibodies to *T. gondii* or *E. histolytica* (extraintestinal infections) are available for use in clinical laboratories.

Enzyme Immunoassays

Problems with using EIA methods for the detection of antibody to intestinal parasites include difficulty in obtaining a parasite antigen that is appropriate for detection, cross-reactivity of antibodies, and poor sensitivity and specificity of tests. Parasites that invade tissue are the primary organisms that stimulate antibody production. Many serologic tests are useful if invasive methods cannot be used for identification. In most cases, however, tests for antibody serve only as epidemiologic markers, especially in endemic areas. Detection of IgM class antibody can be useful in identifying infection during the acute phase, but this class of antibody generally declines to nondetectable levels as the infection begins to resolve. Detection of IgG class antibody does not distinguish between relatively recent or past infection, because this class of antibody may persist for years. In some cases, however, detection of antibody is useful. For example, a patient who lives in a nonendemic area for a parasite has recently traveled to an endemic area and now shows symptoms, but the organism has not been detected in a clinical specimen. A positive test for antibody would help confirm a diagnosis. Another disadvantage of antibody tests is that they can have a large number of cross reactions, which limit their diagnostic usefulness. In addition, many serologic tests used by reference laboratories such as the Centers for Disease Control and Prevention (CDC) are not commercially available.

The major use of EIA has been to detect parasite antigens in clinical specimens. These tests, in contrast to antibody tests, provide information about current infection. A number of EIAs are available to detect the presence of *Giardia lamblia*, *Cryptosporidium* spp., and *E. histolytica/Entamoeba dispar*. Some are able to detect more than one parasite in the specimen by detecting antigens of the organism in the stool using organism-specific antibodies immobilized on a membrane. Rapid EIA kits that can be used with fresh or preserved fecal specimens and kits using monoclonal antibody to detect both *Giardia* and *Cryptosporidium* organisms are also available. Not all kits detecting *E. histolytica*, however, can differentiate between *E. histolytica* and *E. dispar*.

Another growing area of EIA application testing is the field diagnosis of malaria. Although most of these tests are used in endemic areas, one has been approved by the Food and Drug Administration for use in the United States. These tests, based on the principle of immunochromatographic antigen capture, are likened to dipstick tests and use whole blood to detect malarial proteins. Patient's blood is reacted with monoclonal antibody labeled with dye or gold particles. The antigen-antibody complex moves up the reaction strip until it attaches to a bound antibody. Color changes reflect the binding of the antigen-antibody complex with bound antibody. Some tests are relatively nonspecies-specific and detect a protein such as parasite lactate dehydrogenase (pLDH) or aldolase that is common to all four human *Plasmodium* spp. Other tests may detect a species-specific protein such as histidine rich protein (HDT-2) which is associated with *P. falciparum*. Some tests combine both types of protein on the dipstick to provide a more complete picture of the possible infective agent.

Fluorescent Antibody Techniques

Direct fluorescent antibody (DFA) techniques using monoclonal antibodies have been developed to detect *Cryptosporidium* oocysts in fecal specimens. These methods are more expensive than the modified acid-fast procedure but demonstrate greater sensitivity, especially when only rare oocysts are present. A DFA combination reagent for *G. lamblia* and *Cryptosporidium* antigens is also available. The monoclonal antibodies eliminate false-positive and false-negative results. Such procedures are useful in screening large numbers of specimens during epidemiologic studies. A fluorescent method Quantitative Buffy Coat (QBC; Becton-Dickinson, Sparks, Md.) that stains nuclear material using acridine orange is available for detecting malarial organisms in blood.

Quality Assurance in the Parasitology Laboratory

Quality assurance procedures in the parasitology laboratory are similar to those in other sections of the laboratory. An updated procedures manual, controls for staining procedures, records of centrifuge calibration, ocular micrometer calibration, and refrigerator and incubator temperatures should be available. Reagents and solutions must be properly labeled. In addition, the parasitology laboratory should have the following:

- A reference book collection including texts and atlases
- A set of 2 × 2 Kodachrome slides or digital images of common parasites
- A set of clinical reference specimens, including permanently stained smears and formalin-preserved feces

The department should also be enrolled in an external proficiency testing program. An ongoing internal proficiency testing program should be used to enhance identification skills of the laboratory scientists, especially if a full-time parasitologist is not employed. It has been shown that approximately twice as many parasites are detected when a single laboratory scientist staffs the parasitology department compared to departments that rotate personnel through the department. Internal proficiency programs are important. One type of program might assess the reproducibility of results in the examination of fecal specimens. Preserved specimens that have been reported are reexamined as part of this program to see if the initial results (organism identification and quantification) are duplicated.

Size is an important diagnostic criterion for parasites, and use of a properly calibrated ocular micrometer ensures accurate measurement of organisms. The micrometer should be calibrated for each objective on the microscope. Calibration requires two parts: the stage micrometer, a 0.1-mm line that is ruled in 0.01-mm units, and the ocular micrometer, which is ruled in 100 units but has no value assigned to the units. Values for each ocular unit can be calculated by using the stage micrometer according to procedure found in Appendix D.

MEDICALLY IMPORTANT PARASITIC AGENTS

Medically important parasites can be found in phyla representing single-celled organisms such as the protozoa and complex, multicelled organisms such as tapeworms and roundworms. Table 28-2 lists the characteristics of the classes in which most medically important human parasites are found; they are described in the remainder of this chapter.

Protozoa

Intestinal Amebae

In general, amebae present the most difficult challenge in regard to identification. Their average size range is smaller than that of most other parasitic organisms, and they must be distinguished from artifacts and cells that appear in the clinical specimen. Species identification, whether in the cyst or trophozoite stage, often rests on the following characteristics: size, number of nuclei, nuclear structure, and presence of specific internal structures. In a wet preparation, the motility of the trophozoite may aid in presumptive identification. Overall, however, the permanently stained smear is the best preparation for identification of the amebae.

Entamoeba histolytica is recognized as a true pathogen, and *Blastocystis hominis* is an opportunistic pathogen; the remainder of the amebae are considered nonpathogens. All the organisms discussed here live in the large intestine. All of the amebae possess a trophozoite and cyst stage. *B. hominis* has additional morphologic stages. The trophozoite is the motile, feeding stage that reproduces by binary fission. The cyst is a resistant stage that is infective for humans. Multiplication of nuclei in the cyst stage also serves a reproductive function.

Life Cycle

The life cycle of the amebae is relatively simple, with direct fecal-oral transmission in food or water via the cyst stage and no **intermediate hosts.** Humans ingest the infective cysts, which excyst in the intestinal tract and multiply by binary fission. Trophozoites colonize the cecal area. Figure 28-2 illustrates a generalized life cycle for amebae, as well as the extraintestinal phase of *E. histolytica*.

Treatment. Treatment is given only for *E. histolytica* infections; treatment for nonpathogens is not indicated.

TABLE 28-2 Characteristics of Phyla of Medically Important Parasites

Organisms	Characteristics
Phylum: Sarcomastigophora	
-Subphylum: Sarcodina (ameba)	Single celled Move by pseudopodia Trophozoite and cyst stages Asexual reproduction
-Subphylum: Mastigophora (flagellates)	Single celled Most move by action of flagella Trophozoite and cyst stages for intestinal organisms, except for *Dientamoeba fragilis* Asexual reproduction Some blood flagellates
Phylum: Ciliaphora (ciliates)	Single celled Move by action of cilia Trophozoite and cyst stages Asexual reproduction
Phylum: Apicomplexa (sporozoa)	Single celled Usually inhabit tissue and blood cells Insects and other mammals are involved as part of life cycle May have both sexual and asexual life cycles
Phylum: Platyhelminthes (flatworms)	
-Class: Trematoda (flukes)	Multicelled and bilaterally symmetric Most are hermaphroditic Egg, miracidium, cercaria, and adult are life cycle stages Fish, snails, crabs are involved as intermediate hosts in life cycle
-Class: Cestoda (tapeworms)	Multicellular, ribbonlike body Hermaphroditic Egg, larva, and adult worm are life cycle stages Mammals and insects are involved as intermediate hosts in life cycle
Phylum: Aschelminthes	
-Class: Nematoda (roundworms)	Adults of both sexes Egg, larva, and adult worm are life cycle stages May have free-living form or may require intermediate host

Luminal amebicides such as metronidazole are given to carriers in nonendemic areas to prevent the invasive phase and to reduce the risk of transmission. In endemic areas with a high risk of reinfection, treatment may not be indicated. Patients with invasive amebiases are treated with systemic drugs as well as luminal amebicides. In cases of *B. hominis* infection, treatment may be indicated if the patient is symptomatic.

Entamoeba histolytica and Entamoeba dispar. *Entamoeba histolytica* and *E. dispar* are morphologically identical organisms that differ in their effects on the host. Historically, studies demonstrated a large number of people were infected with an organism identified as *E. histolytica*. However, only about 10% of these individuals developed clinical symptoms or invasive disease. It was thought that perhaps two strains of

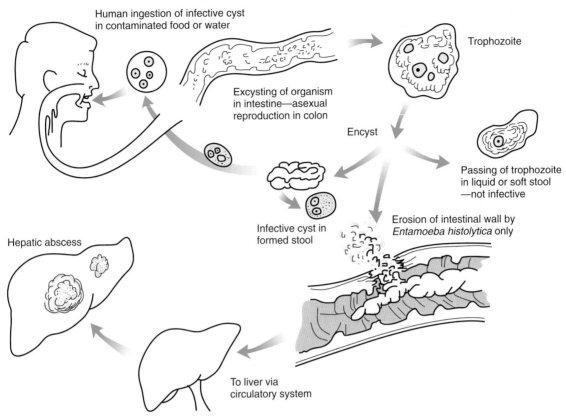

FIGURE 28-2 Generalized life cycle of intestinal ameba.

the organism existed: one pathogenic and one nonpathogenic. For many years this hypothesis was unproven—there was no way to differentiate the strains morphologically.

Clinical studies that took place after the emergence of the human immunodeficiency virus (HIV) provided the impetus to explain the discrepancy. Research studies using electrophoresis identified differing isoenzyme (zymodeme) patterns between organisms that caused clinical symptoms and those found in asymptomatic persons. The studies showed that most strains in asymptomatic cyst passers and in most men who have sex with men were nonpathogenic, whereas several strains from areas with high rates of endemic disease were pathogenic. Further immunologic and DNA probe studies supplied additional evidence, such as differences in epitopes of the galactose-specific binding lectin and differences in surface antigens as well as differences in gene expression. Based on this evidence, the noninvasive organism, formerly referred to as nonpathogenic *E. histolytica*, was named *E. dispar*. The pathogenic organism remained *E. histolytica*.

The organisms are morphologically identical and must be distinguished based on identification of surface antigens. However, the presence of ingested erythrocytes in the trophozoite stage will distinguish *E. histolytica*. *E. histolytica* is found worldwide but especially in the tropics and subtropics. It is a major protozoan pathogen for humans, causing an estimated 40 to 50 million cases of colitis and hepatic abscesses per year. It ranks third behind malaria and schistosomiasis as a cause of death due to parasitic infection, accounting for an estimated 40,000 to 100,000 deaths annually. Prevalence of infection varies according to socioeconomic levels and sanitary practices; infection is more common in poorly developed countries. Travelers to those areas are at increased risk of acquiring infection. The organism has also been identified as a sexually transmitted agent among men who have sex with men.

Clinical Infection. The pathogenicity of *E. histolytica* is reflected in its ability to cause invasive intestinal amebiasis and extraintestinal amebic infections. The organism adheres to the mucous layer of the intestine, invades and disrupts the mucosal barrier, produces contact-dependent killing, and induces apoptosis of the intestinal cells. The organism in turn lyses and phagocytizes the cell. Invasion of the deeper layers of the intestinal wall is medicated by cysteine proteases that destroy collagen and fibronectin. The host secretes proinflammatory cytokines leading to an acute inflammatory response and migration of neutrophils and macrophages into the tissue. The organism demonstrates resistance to host immune defense mechanisms. Although *E. histolytica* can activate the alternative and mannose binding lectin complement pathways, it is relatively resistant to destruction by C5b-9 (membrane attack complex). This may be mediated by the Gal/GalNAc lectin, which inhibits C8 and C9 assembly into the membrane attack complex. In addition, enzymes from the parasite can degrade C3a and C5a (anaphylotoxins) and immunoglobulin molecules. The organism can also secrete chemoattractants for neutrophils. It kills these cells by contact-dependent lysis, and the subsequent release of lysozymes, superoxides, and collagenases from the neutrophil granules produces additional damage to the intestinal mucosa.

The host has innate and acquired immune responses that come into play to attempt to prevent colonization. Mucin in the intestinal mucus competes for attachment to the lectin and protects epithelial cells from attack. The host may have intestinal IgA that helps prevent colonization and repeated infection, and antigen-specific T cells secrete cytokines that have direct cytotoxicity for the trophozoites.

Entamoeba histolytica infection presents in several ways: asymptomatic colonization, amebic dysentery (colitis), and extraintestinal amebiasis. Individuals who have colonization but remain asymptomatic pose a great risk to others because they are "cyst passers" and therefore infective. Symptomatic clinical infection may appear as an acute or chronic form. In acute infections, the patient may experience vague abdominal symptoms such as tenderness and cramping, fever, and up to 20 diarrheic stools per day that contain the trophozoite form, blood, and mucus. In severe cases, the patient may shed pieces of intestinal mucosa. Some patients with *E. histolytica* infection develop an ameboma (amebic granuloma), a tumor like lesion that forms in the submucosa of the intestine. This represents an area of chronic lysis and infiltration with neutrophils, lymphocytes, and eosinophils. In chronic infections, on the other hand, the patient may alternate between periods in which there are no symptoms and diarrheal episodes.

The characteristic lesion in the intestinal mucosa, referred to as "flask-shaped" ulcer, is a result of lysis of the intestinal mucosa. The lesion shows a pinpoint ulceration on the mucosal surface and a gradual widening in the submucosal areas as the parasites invades the tissue. The organisms may completely erode the intestinal mucosa and enter the circulation. When this occurs, the organ most commonly colonized is the right lobe of the liver, because organisms are trapped in the venules of the liver. Patients with hepatic abscesses may have symptoms such as fever and pain in the upper right quadrant or may be asymptomatic. Weight loss, increased white blood cell counts, or elevated liver enzymes may be present. Lung abscesses may be seen as the result of penetration of the diaphragm by amebae from hepatic abscesses or from hematogenous spread. Invasion of the lung may cause

the patient to have chest pain, dyspnea, and a productive cough. Other sites, such as the perianal area or bladder, also may be colonized, with resulting tissue destruction.

Laboratory Diagnosis. Patients with diarrhea are most likely to have trophozoites in the stool, which may be seen in direct wet mounts or trichrome-stained smears. Sigmoid biopsies may be used to demonstrate the characteristic morphology of the intestinal ulcers or to identify trophozoites in tissue when none can be isolated from the stool specimen. Table 28-3 summarizes the characteristics of *E. histolytica* trophozoites and cysts and compares *E. histolytica* to other amebae. In a direct saline wet mount of a diarrheic stool, the trophozoite of *E. histolytica* may exhibit a progressive, directional motility by extending long, thin pseudopods. The size of the organism ranges from 10 to 50 μm, averaging 15 to 25 μm. The organism is refractile, and the characteristic "bull's-eye" nucleus, consisting of a small central karyosome and even, fine **peripheral chromatin,** may be only slightly visible.

In a trichrome-stained smear, the cytoplasm of the organism appears clean and free of ingested bacteria and vacuoles. Finely granular nuclear chromatin, which is evenly distributed on the nuclear membrane, and the small central karyosome stain a dark purple-red. Ingested RBCs are diagnostic for *E. histolytica* trophozoites but usually are not seen. If there are no ingested RBCs, the organism must be reported as *E. histolytica/E. dispar.* Immunoassays are necessary to differentiate these two species. Figure 28-3 shows trichrome-stained trophozoites of *E. histolytica.* The trophozoite in Figure 28-3, *B,* contains an ingested RBC. The average size of the cyst is 10 to 20 μm (Figure 28-4).

Cysts of *E. histolytica* may have one to four nuclei, each with a small central karyosome and fine, evenly distributed peripheral chromatin. The cytoplasm may contain chromatoidal bars composed of ribonucleic acid. The chromatoidal bars are cigar-shaped with rounded ends. In young cysts there are often multiple bars, and mature cysts may show only one. In an iodine wet mount, the nuclei appear as yellowish refractile bodies within the cyst; chromatoidal bars do not take up stain and appear as colorless areas. With trichrome stain, the cyst

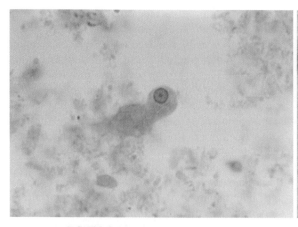
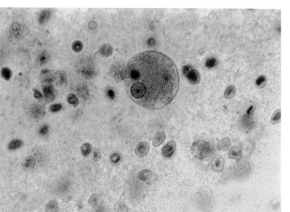

A

B

FIGURE 28-3 **A,** *Entamoeba histolytica* trophozoite (trichrome stain). **B,** *E. histolytica* trophozoite. Notice darkly staining, ingested red blood cell near the nucleus (trichrome stain).

TABLE 28-3 Comparisons of Amebae

| Organism | Trophozoite | | | | Cyst | | | |
	Size (μm)	Motility	Cytoplasm	Trophozoite and Cyst Nuclear Structure	Size (μm) and Shape	Number of Nuclei in Mature Cyst	Chromatoidal Bars	Glycogen Vacuole
Entamoeba histolytica	15-25	Progressive, directional	Finely granular May contain ingested red blood cells	Small, central karyosome Fine, evenly distributed peripheral chromatin	10-20, round	4	Rounded Elongated Usually seen	Not usually seen Diffuse in young cyst
Entamoeba coli	15-50	Nondirectional	Vacuolated Ingested bacteria	Large, eccentric karyosomes Coarse, uneven peripheral chromatin	15-25, round	8	Elongated Splintered ends Not always seen	Not seen
Entamoeba hartmanni	4-12	Nondirectional	Finely granular	Small, central karyosomes Fine, evenly distributed peripheral chromatin	5-10, round	4	Rounded ends Elongated Not always present	Not seen
Endolimax nana	5-12	Nondirectional	Vacuolated May contain ingested bacteria	Large, irregularly shaped karyosome No peripheral chromatin	5-12, oval	4	Not present	Not seen
Iodamoeba bütschlii	6-20	Nondirectional	Vacuolated May contain ingested bacteria	Large karyosome surrounded by achromatic granules No peripheral chromatin	6-15, oval or irregular	1	Not present	Single, defined

is light green-gray; nuclear material and chromatoidal bars stain a dark purple-red. Young cysts may show discrete glycogen masses that stain light brown in an iodine wet mount, but in the more mature cyst, the glycogen is diffuse. Cysts can persist 2 to 4 weeks in a moist environment but may be killed by drying, temperatures over 55° C, superchlorination, or addition of iodine to drinking water.

Amebic ulcers of the liver often are detected by ultrasonographic or radiographic tests. Subsequent aspiration of the abscess may yield motile trophozoites and necrotic material composed of lysed cells. Serologic methods of detecting antibody to *E. histolytica* are available, and the results are positive in more than 90% of patients with extraintestinal disease. These antibody levels rise after tissue invasion but are not protective. Tests for antibody, however, are not particularly useful in distinguishing between past and current infection, because antibodies may persist for years after an infection has resolved. In addition, these tests provide limited information in patients from endemic areas.

Tests that detect *E. histolytica* antigen in stool provide evidence of current infection. These tests involve EIA methodology using monoclonal antibodies to proteins or adhesion lectins. A number of kits detect *E. histolytica* antigens without excluding *E. dispar*; currently, only one differentiates *E. histolytica* from *E. dispar*. Point-of-care tests using immunochromatographic techniques are being developed to assist with

rapid diagnosis of *E. histolytica* infection. Some are designed to detect antigen in the stool and others to detect antibodies in the serum.

Entamoeba hartmanni. *Entamoeba hartmanni*, once known as "small race" *Entamoeba histolytica*, is a nonpathogen. It generally resembles *E. histolytica* in a trichrome-stained smear but is more likely to have an eccentric karyosome or uneven peripheral chromatin resembling that of *Entamoeba coli*. Size is a major determinant in differentiating *E. histolytica* and *E. hartmanni*. The average size of the trophozoites of *E. hartmanni* is 4 to 12 μm; trophozoites with an average size measuring greater than 12 μm are identified as *E. histolytica* or *E. dispar*. *E. hartmanni* cysts measure 5 to 10 μm; those of 10 μm or more are identified as *E. histolytica* or *E. dispar*. Figure 28-5, *A* shows the trichrome-stained trophozoite, and Figure 28-5, *B* is an enlarged view of *E. hartmanni* to demonstrate the irregular peripheral chromatin. Figure 28-6 shows the cyst of *E. hartmanni* with three nuclei visible and at least one chromatoidal bar.

Entamoeba coli. *Entamoeba coli* is a commonly found intestinal commensal transmitted by ingestion of cysts in fecally contaminated food or water. The average size of the trophozoite is 15 to 50 μm with most measuring 25 μm (Figure 28-7, *A*). The nuclear structure is characterized by a large, eccentric karyosome and coarse, uneven peripheral chromatin on the nuclear membrane. Figure 28-7, *B* is an enlargement of the organism to demonstrate the characteristic nuclear morphology. The motility of the trophozoite in a wet preparation is sluggish and nondirectional. In a permanently stained preparation, the cytoplasm of the trophozoite may stain a dark purplish gray and contains vacuoles and ingested materials.

The mature cyst has eight nuclei; the immature cyst may have one or two large nuclei with a large glycogen vacuole. Cysts often stain darkly and unevenly, giving an irregular appearance to the cyst. The large eccentric karyosome is visible, but peripheral chromatin may be difficult to see surrounding all of the nuclei. Chromatoidal bars, when present, have a pointed, splintered appearance. The average size of the cyst is 15 to 25 μm. Figure 28-8, *A* shows an MIF wet mount of a cyst of *E. coli*, and Figure 28-8, *B* shows a trichrome-stained cyst.

Endolimax nana. The trophozoite of *E. nana* has a large karyosome with no peripheral chromatin on the nuclear mem-

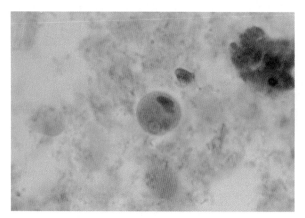

FIGURE 28-4 *Entamoeba histolytica* cyst with round-end chromatoidal bars. Two nuclei are visible (trichrome stain).

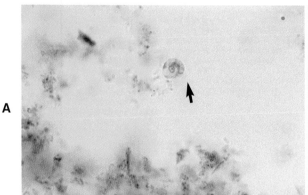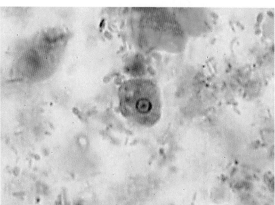

FIGURE 28-5 **A,** *Entamoeba hartmanni* (trichrome stain). **B,** Enlarged view of *E. hartmanni.*

brane. The trophozoite ranges in size from 5 to 12 µm with the average being less than 10 µm (Figure 28-9). The cytoplasm is granular and vacuolated. In a wet preparation, the motility is sluggish. In a wet mount it may be difficult to distinguish the large karyosome of *E. nana* from the karyosome of *E. hartmanni*, and the organisms may be misidentified. The cyst of *E. nana* is oval or spherical, 5 to 12 µm, and has up to four large karyosomes (Figure 28-10, *A*). Figure

28-10, *B* shows an enlargement of the cyst with three of the characteristic large "buttonhole" nuclei easily visible. A fourth is partially visible. At least one of the nuclei shows evidence of the thin nuclear membrane.

Iodamoeba bütschlii. *Iodamoeba bütschlii* is less commonly encountered than *E. coli* or *E. nana*. The nucleus is composed of a single, irregularly shaped karyosome surrounded by achromatic granules and a thin nuclear membrane with no peripheral chromatin. The trophozoites of *I. bütschlii*, which are 6 to 20 µm, show a vacuolated cytoplasm in a permanently stained smear (Figure 28-11). The oval cyst is 6 to 15 µm (average 9 to 10 µm) and contains a single large karyosome and a large, well-defined glycogen vacuole. The vacuole stains dark brown in an iodine wet mount and appears empty in a permanently stained smear. Figure 28-12 demonstrates a trichrome-stained cyst of *I. bütschlii*.

Blastocystis hominis. *Blastocystis hominis* is one of the most common intestinal protozoa and has a prevalence of greater than 50% in developing countries, and infection occurs in both immunocompetent and immunocompromised individuals. *B. hominis* has come to prominence as a possible cause of diarrhea in humans, although controversy concerning its pathogenicity still exists because of the conflicting outcomes of numerous studies. Although not considered a

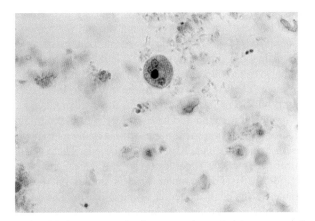

FIGURE 28-6 **Entamoeba hartmanni** cyst (trichrome stain).

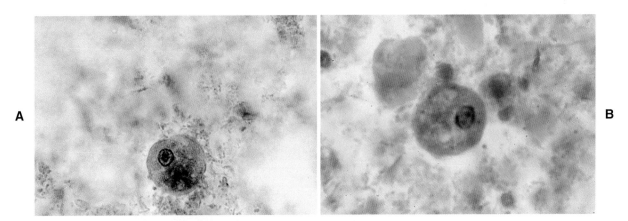

FIGURE 28-7 **A,** *Entamoeba coli* trophozoite. Notice dark staining, highly vacuolated cytoplasm (trichrome stain). **B,** Enlarged view of *E. coli* trophozoite to demonstrate peripheral chromatin (trichrome stain).

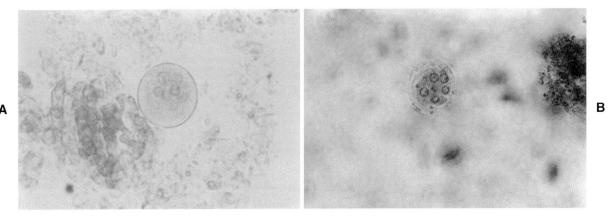

FIGURE 28-8 **A,** *Entamoeba coli* cyst (merthiolate-iodine-formalin) wet mount. **B,** *E. coli* cyst with five nuclei visible (trichrome stain).

common cause of diarrheal disease, this organism neverthe-less has been found in patients with abdominal pain and diarrhea who have no other intestinal pathogens present. These patients often have a history of travel abroad and of consuming untreated water. There have also been some studies that link presence of *B. hominis* to colitis and irritable bowel syndrome. Other authors suggest that *B. hominis* has no role as a pathogen. Several strains may exist, which could explain the differences in clinical presentation. Patients infected with

B. hominis may present with diarrhea, abdominal pain, anorexia, and flatulence. Laboratories often report the pres-ence of the organism quantitatively, with the presence of more than five organisms per high-power field and no other known enteric pathogens in symptomatic patients considered to be evidence of *B. hominis* as the cause of gastrointestinal symptoms.

The taxonomy of *B. hominis* is also unresolved. Originally classified as a yeast, it is currently regarded as an ameba. However, ribosomal RNA (rRNA) analysis indicates it is related to the stramenopiles (brown algae and water moulds). *B. hominis* is a polymorphic organism that exists in four forms: ameboid, granular, vacuolar, and cyst. The vacuolar form, also called the central body form, is the most commonly identified. The average size for the vacuolar form is 5 to 15 μm, but up to 20% of organisms are smaller than 5 μm. The organism is round and has a ring of cytoplasm lining the inside of the plasma membrane with as many as four nuclei present, which are usually pushed to the side. There is a large central vacuole that occupies up to 90% of the cell volume (Figure 28-13). The granular form is similar but possesses granules in the central vacuole and cytoplasm. The ameboid form, which may be seen in diarrheic stools, is 3 to 8 μm and often lacks a vacuole but possesses several pseudopods. In an iodine mount, the cytoplasm and the central area of the vacu-

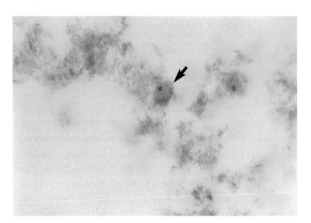

FIGURE 28-9   *Endolimax nana* trophozoite (trichrome stain).

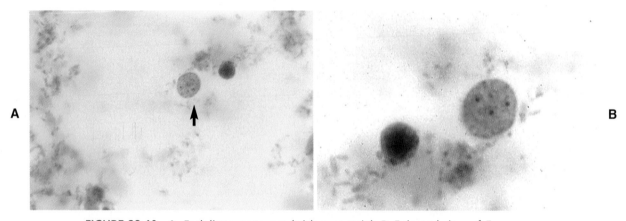

FIGURE 28-10   A, *Endolimax nana* cyst (trichrome stain). **B,** Enlarged view of *E. nana* cyst (trichrome stain).

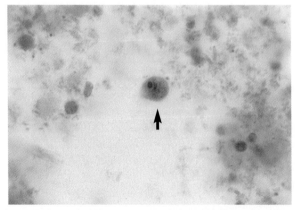

FIGURE 28-11   *Iodamoeba bütschlii* trophozoite (trichrome stain).

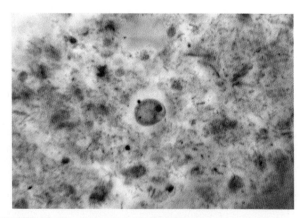

FIGURE 28-12   *Iodamoeba bütschlii* cyst with prominent glycogen vacuole (iron hematoxylin stain).

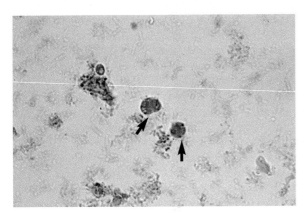

FIGURE 28-13 *Blastocystis hominis* vacuolar form (trichrome stain).

olar form stain brown. With the trichrome stain, the cytoplasm stains dark green and the central area may stain pale to intensely green with the nuclei a dark purple-black. The cyst form, which was identified in the 1990s, can be found in stool and in culture. The cyst stage is small (3 to 5 μm), oval to round, and possesses one to four nuclei and multiple vacuoles. Because of its small size, it may resemble fecal debris. It is resistant to the usual chlorine levels in drinking water, and water has been implicated in transmission of the organism.

Tissue Amebae

Free-living, thermotolerant amebae found in soil and water (freshwater sources, domestic water supplies, and swimming pools) usually feed on bacteria in the environment but are known to be capable of causing human disease. They are able to gain access to the central nervous system (CNS) either by inhalation into the upper respiratory tract, which allows them to travel along the olfactory nerve to the brain, or by hematogenous spread from the lungs or skin lesions. While the number of infections caused by these organisms is low compared to those caused by intestinal protozoans, they are very difficult to diagnose and treat and are associated with a high mortality rate. *Naegleria fowleri* and *Acanthamoeba* spp. have been recognized for many years as the amebae most commonly associated with CNS invasion in humans. In recent years *Balamuthia mandrillaris* has been identified as another agent of CNS infection in humans.

The ameboflagellate *N. fowleri* is the etiologic agent of primary amebic meningoencephalitis (PAM), a rapidly fatal condition involving the CNS. *Acanthamoeba* spp. have been associated with a more chronic condition, granulomatous amebic encephalitis (GAE), especially in individuals with impaired cell mediated immunity. In addition, *Acanthamoeba* spp. have been linked with amebic keratitis in soft contact lens wearers and with cutaneous infections in patients with acquired immunodeficiency syndrome (AIDS). *B. mandrillaris* is primarily associated with GAE and cutaneous lesions in humans. A comparison of the CNS infections caused by *N. fowleri* and *Acanthamoeba* spp. is given in Table 28-4.

Naegleria fowleri. PAM has been reported from countries worldwide. It is a relatively rare infection; however, many studies have shown the presence of antibodies directed against *N. fowleri* in healthy individuals. In the United States, PAM

TABLE 28-4 Comparison of Central Nervous System Infections Caused by Amebae

	Primary Amebic Meningoencephalitis	Granulomatous Amebic Encephalitis
Etiologic agent	*Naegleria fowleri*	*Acanthamoeba* spp.
Stages in		
Cerebrospinal fluid	Trophozoite	Trophozoite
Brain biopsy	Trophozoite	Trophozoite and cyst
Characteristics	Trophozoite 10-12 μm	Trophozoite 10-45 μm
	Large karyosome	Spinelike pseudopod
	Broad pseudopods	Cyst
		15-20 μm
		Wrinkled double wall
Entry	Nasal passage olfactory nerve to CNS	Lungs and skin with hematogenous spread to CNS
Clinical course	Fulminant (death within 1 week of onset)	Slow and chronic
Population at risk	Children to young adults, healthy (history of water activities in stagnant, warm water)	Immunocompromised

CNS, Central nervous system.

is most frequently reported in Texas, Florida, Virginia, and California. It occurs in healthy, immunocompetent children and young adults with no predisposing condition. A common factor in infection is the report of recent swimming or other water-related activities in warm, artificial lakes or brackish or muddy water. The life cycle of *N. fowleri* is relatively simple, consisting of three stages: a free-living amebic trophozoite, a transient flagellate form that appears when there is a scarcity of nutrients, and an environmentally resistant cyst.

The organism enters the nasal cavity through inhalation of contaminated water or soil. The amebic form colonizes the nasal cavity, invades the nasal mucosa, attaches to olfactory nerves, penetrates the cribriform plate, moves along the olfactory nerve to the olfactory bulb, and moves into the arachnoid space. From there, it is free to disseminate throughout the CNS. Infections are thought to be related to inhalation of a large number of organisms or forceful entry of water into the nose (microtrauma) and to the virulence of the strain.

Clinical Infection. Clinically, the disease cannot be distinguished from bacterial meningitis. The incubation period is usually 2 to 3 days but may range up to 2 weeks. Initial symptoms include severe bifrontal headache, fever (38° to 41° C), stiff neck, and nausea and vomiting. The organism multiplies within brain tissue, and within 2 to 4 days, the patient may suffer drowsiness, confusion, and seizures, and progress into a coma. The disease usually is fatal within 1 week of the appearance of clinical symptoms. At autopsy, there will be evidence of trophozoites along with a purulent exudate, edema, and hemorrhagic and necrotic areas of infection in the brain. *N. fowleri* is capable of ingesting erythrocytes and other cells including nerve cells. The invasive

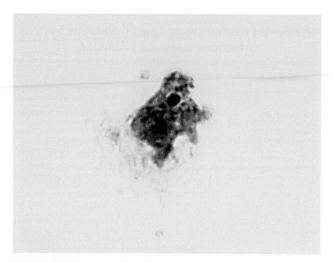

FIGURE 28-14 *Naegleria fowleri* trophozoite. Note prominent karyosome (iron hematoxylin stain).

properties of the organism are related to its ability to counteract the host immune response in a number of ways. The organism produces a CD59-like protein that inhibits the complement cascade, can 'shed' the C5b-C9 (membrane attack) complex, and is able to inhibit insertion of the complex into the cell membrane. Macrophages and neutrophils are the primary host defense against the organism as the trophozoites are relatively resistant to actions of host cytokines. Infection with *N. fowleri* has greater than 95% mortality. Because the symptoms resemble bacterial meningitis, specific treatment may be delayed. Yet the possibility of cure depends on early diagnosis. Aggressive therapy with intravenous and intrathecal amphotericin B has been used. Rifampin, miconazole, and tetracycline have been used in addition to amphotericin B.

Laboratory Diagnosis. Diagnosis can be made by finding motile amebic trophozoites in the CSF. The trophozoite ranges in size from 10 to 30 μm and moves by explosively extending large, broad pseudopods (lobopodia). The nucleus contains a large central karyosome that is surrounded by a halo. Figure 28-14 shows a trophozoite of *N. fowleri* as it appears in a CSF specimen stained with iron hematoxylin. The CSF in PAM contains many segmented neutrophils and RBCs and demonstrates elevated protein and decreased glucose values, which are characteristic of bacterial meningitis.

Naegleria fowleri does not stain well with the Gram stain, but motile trophozoites can be seen in a wet mount of the CSF. The ameba can be converted to the flagellate stage by adding one drop of CSF sediment to 1 mL of distilled water and incubating it at 37° C. Conversion to the flagellate form occurs in 2 to 20 hours. The organisms can be cultured by overlaying nonnutrient agar with *Escherichia coli* and inoculating the agar with a drop of the CSF sediment. Clearing of the agar in thin tracks is evidence of the organism feeding on the bacteria. Cysts, which are approximately 10 μm in diameter and have a round, smooth double wall and a single pore, are not seen in clinical specimens. Immunofluorescent staining of CSF with monoclonal antibody is available in some reference laboratories for detection of the trophozoite. Molecular methods are used to identify strains.

Acanthamoeba. *Acanthamoeba* spp., which are also soil and water organisms, have been linked to several clinical conditions, including GAE, cutaneous infections, and amebic keratitis. Cutaneous acanthamebiasis has been associated primarily with patients with AIDS whose CD4 count is less than 250/mL. The condition is characterized by chronic, nonhealing lesions, especially on the extremities and face. Lesions may develop at the site of inoculation or may occur as a result of hematogenous dissemination from the lungs. Trophozoites and cysts can be seen in biopsy preparations of the lesion. Unlike PAM, GAE is characterized by hematogenous spread to the CNS from a primary inoculation site in either the lungs or the skin. The infection is subacute, and incubation time is unknown but may range from months to years. Symptoms include drowsiness, seizures, hemiparesis, headache, stiff neck, and personality disorders. The trophozoite is uncommonly seen in CSF, and diagnosis is typically made by brain biopsy demonstrating either or both cysts and trophozoites. Histologic preparations of the brain at autopsy show inflammatory lesions containing many segmented neutrophils, eosinophils, and trophozoites. A specific therapeutic regimen has not been established because most infections have been diagnosed at autopsy. However, disseminated *Acanthamoeba* infections have been treated with pentamidine isethionate, fluconazole, ketoconazole, and cotrimoxazole (trimethoprim-sulfamethoxazole).

Amebic keratitis, associated with *Acanthamoeba* spp., has been identified since the 1980s. The primary group at risk for developing this condition is individuals who wear contact lenses, especially the soft and extended-wear types. Factors in these infections include the preparation of homemade saline solution using tap water, a history of corneal trauma, or wearing contact lenses during swimming—all of which may cause corneal trauma and subsequent colonization by the organism. The organism binds to corneal epithelium and produces a protein that causes cell lysis. Patients experience photophobia, blurred vision, inflammation, ring infiltrates, and pain. Because of the similarity in tissue damage, the infection may initially be confused with bacterial or herpes simplex viral infection and treatment is delayed. Phase contrast microscopy of direct wet mount preparations of corneal scrapings may reveal the trophozoite or cyst. The use of calcofluor white increases detection of the organisms. Permanent stains such as trichrome and Giemsa may also demonstrate the trophozoite in clinical specimens.

Isolation of *Acanthamoeba* may be performed in a manner similar to that for *N. fowleri*. *Acanthamoeba* spp. have only two stages, the resistant cyst and the motile trophozoite. The trophozoite ranges from 20 to 45 μm in diameter and has a single nucleus with a central prominent endosome. Blunt pseudopods and characteristic spinelike projections of the cytoplasm (acanthopodia) may also be seen on a wet mount. The cyst is approximately 15 to 20 μm, spherical, and double walled, with the walls having a wrinkled appearance. Topical applications of chlorhexidine gluconate and ketoconazole have been used to treat cutaneous infections. Corticosteroids are used to reduce inflammation. Despite treatment, systemic infections have a poor prognosis, and many patients with keratitis lose the sight in the affected eye.

Balamuthia mandrillaris

Balamuthia mandrillaris is an emerging opportunistic pathogen that has been identified as a cause of skin lesions and GAE. Since 1990 when it was first linked to human illness, this free-living ameba has caused more than 150 cases with a mortality of greater than 95%. Over 50% of the cases reported occurred in individuals of Hispanic origin. It is not known if there is a genetic predisposition or if the type of work the individuals engage in increases exposure risk. Unlike infections with *Acanthamoeba* spp., which occur primarily in immunocompromised hosts, infection with *B. mandrillaris* can occur in both immunocompetent and immunocompromised hosts. Humans become infected by inhaling airborne cysts of the organism or by direct inoculation through skin lesions.

Skin infections present as a relatively painless nodule. Once the organism has entered through the lungs or through the skin it spreads hematogenously. Only rarely will it invade nasally and spread along nerve fibers to the olfactory bulb. Once the organism reaches the blood-brain barrier, it is able to bind to microvascular endothelial cells through receptor molecules. The organism produces proteolytic enzymes such as collagenases and metalloproteases that facilitate tissue damage, and the host's inflammatory response helps increase the permeability of the barrier. In the CNS, the organism multiplies by binary fission and causes a necrotizing hemorrhagic infection similar to that of *Acanthamoeba* spp. The onset is insidious, with fever, headache, stiff neck, vomiting, and photophobia, and progresses to personality changes and seizures. Onset of symptoms may occur weeks to months after infection, but once the brain has been invaded, the time to death is short. Treatment involves multiple antimicrobial regimen including fluconazole, clarithromycin, and sulfadiazine.

In the majority of cases, infection is identified at autopsy by finding trophozoites and cysts in the tissue. The trophozoite is 30 to 60 µm, with broad pseudopods and a large single nucleus with multiple nucleoli. The cyst is round, 10 to 30 µm in diameter, and has a single nucleus. There is a wrinkled outer wall and smooth inner wall. The CSF will usually exhibit increased protein, normal or decreased glucose, and increased lymphocytes. Serum antibodies can be detected by indirect fluorescent antibody methods using ameba-coated slides. The methods for culture using nonnutrient agar seeded with *E. coli* does not work because this organism will not feed on gram-negative bacteria.

Ciliates

Only one ciliate, *Balantidium coli,* is considered pathogenic for humans. Pigs are the natural host for this organism, and humans serve as accidental hosts. The organism lives in the large intestine, where it may cause mucosal lesions but not extraintestinal infections. Most people with this infection are asymptomatic, but the organism may cause a self-limiting diarrhea with nausea, vomiting, and abdominal tenderness.

The life cycle is similar to that of the amebae, with the cyst being the infective stage. The organism is quite large and covered with short cilia. The oval trophozoite (Figure 28-15, *A*) demonstrates two size ranges: 45 to 60 µm × 30 to 40 µm and 90 to 120 µm × 60 to 80 µm. The cilia-lined cytostome is located at the slightly pointed anterior end. The cytoplasm contains food vacuoles. A small opening at the posterior, the cytopyge, is used to expel the contents of food vacuoles. In a wet mount, the cilia are seen propelling the organism with a rotary motion. The rounded, thick-walled cyst (Figure 28-15, *B*) averages 45 to 75 µm. Cilia may be seen retracted within the cyst wall. Both stages are characterized by the presence of two nuclei: a kidney bean–shaped macronucleus and a small, round micronucleus that usually is situated in the small curvature of the macronucleus. The micronucleus is rarely visible in routinely stained smears.

Pathogenic Intestinal and Urogenital Flagellates

The flagellates constitute another major group of parasites that may inhabit the intestinal tract. The life cycle is relatively simple, resembling that of the amebae (Figure 28-16). Most flagellates have both cyst and trophozoite stages. *Dientamoeba fragilis, T. vaginalis,* and *Trichomonas hominis* lack a cyst stage, however, and the trophozoite of these organisms serves as the infective stage.

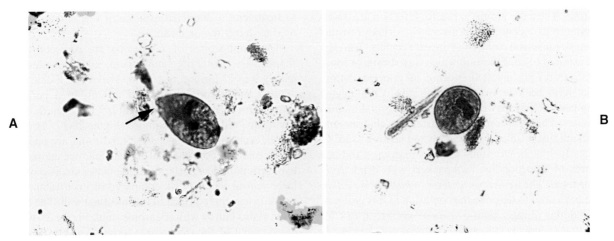

FIGURE 28-15 **A,** *Balantidium coli* trophozoite. Arrow denotes the cytostome (trichrome stain). **B,** *B. coli* cyst (trichrome stain).

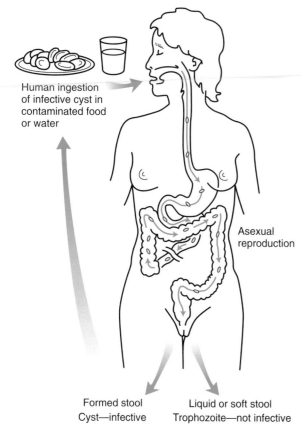

Human ingestion
of infective cyst in
contaminated food
or water

Asexual
reproduction

Formed stool
Cyst—infective

Liquid or soft stool
Trophozoite—not infective

FIGURE 28-16 Generalized life cycle for intestinal flagellates.

Giardia lamblia, also known as *G. intestinalis* or *Giardia duodenalis,* originally was considered the only pathogenic intestinal flagellate. However, *D. fragilis* is now recognized as a pathogen. *T. vaginalis,* a pathogen of the genitourinary tract in both men and women, is also discussed in this section. Table 28-5 shows the characteristics of the trophozoite and cyst stages of the intestinal and genitourinary flagellates.

Giardia lamblia. *Giardia lamblia* has a worldwide distribution and has frequently been identified as the etiologic agent of outbreaks of gastroenteritis and traveler's diarrhea. It is the most commonly reported intestinal protozoan in the United States. The main groups at risk for infection are travelers returning from endemic areas, hikers who drink untreated water from streams, and children in daycare centers. Travelers are often exposed to conditions in which waterborne or foodborne cysts (rare) are ingested because of poor sanitation. Outbreaks have been reported from focally contaminated swimming pools. Cysts may remain viable for several months in cold water. They are somewhat resistant to chlorine and iodine, but are susceptible to desiccation and heating to 50° C.

Animals such as beavers may serve as reservoirs and can be a source of infection for backpackers who drink from streams or rivers. The names *beaver fever* or *backpacker's diarrhea* have been used to describe the condition in this group of people. Children younger than 5 years of age are at risk for infection, and *G. lamblia* has caused outbreaks of diarrhea in nurseries and daycare centers as a result of person-to-person

contact. Along with *E. histolytica, G. lamblia* has been identified as a sexually transmitted pathogen among those who practice oral-anal sex.

Clinical Infection. A low number of cysts, often as few as 10 to 100, can initiate infection with *G. lamblia.* Once the cysts are ingested, the organism reacts to the pH in the stomach and begins to excyst. The organism then responds to the slightly alkaline pH in the small intestine and completes the process in the duodenal area, where the presence of carbohydrates and bile stimulates trophozoite growth. Although it does not invade the mucosal surface, it does attach to the surface of columnar epithelial cells. Adherence to the intestinal mucosa is achieved by the ventral sucking disk and possibly binding by a mannose binding lectin (similar to the mechanism of *E. histolytica*). Pathologic mechanisms associated with *G. lamblia* include irritation and damage to the mucosa, as well as interference with absorption of nutrients, fats, and fat-soluble vitamins. Damage to the mucosal surface results in atrophy of the microvilli. Bacterial overgrowth may contribute to symptoms. The intestinal mucus layer, the presence of secretory IgA and influx of mast cells that produce interleukins such as IL-6 help prevent colonization by the organism.

In most patients, the acute infection manifests as a self-limiting diarrhea with malaise, cramps, nausea, and abdominal tenderness after an incubation period of 12 to 14 days. Explosive, foul-smelling, nonbloody diarrhea is present. Symptoms last 1 to 4 weeks, and the patient may lose a significant amount of weight. Patients with secretory IgA deficiency or achlorhydria seem not only to be more apt to acquire the infection but also to develop chronic disease. In chronic giardiasis, there may be a malabsorption-like syndrome with up to 20% weight loss, fatigue, anorexia, and steatorrhea with large amounts of gas. Fats and vitamin B_{12} are two of the substances that may be incompletely absorbed in chronic infection. Metronidazole (Flagyl), which has been the drug of choice for treating giardiasis, may be prescribed. Albendazole is another drug that may be used.

Laboratory Diagnosis. Feces serve as the usual diagnostic specimen, but shedding of the cysts is irregular, and multiple stool specimens are often required for diagnosis. When clinical symptoms persist and the organism cannot be demonstrated in the feces, or when the patient does not respond to treatment, a duodenal aspirate or the Enterotest may be used to detect the organism.

The trophozoites of *G. lamblia* are pear- or teardrop-shaped, are bilaterally symmetrical, and measure approximately 9 to 21 μm × 5 to 15 μm. They show a characteristic "falling leaf" motility in a wet mount. In a permanently stained smear, the binucleate organism has been described as having an "old man" appearance (Figure 28-17, *A*). Two oval nuclei, each with a large central karyosome, are on each side of the midline. Four pairs of flagella, midline axonemes, and two median bodies posterior to the nuclei are also present. A large ventral sucking disk composed of microtubules is used by the organism to attach to the intestinal wall. The organism often stains faintly with trichrome stain. Figure 28-17, *B* is an enlargement of the trophozoite to reveal several of the morphologic features. Table 28-5 summarizes the characteristics

TABLE 28-5 Comparison of Intestinal and Urogenital Flagellates

Organism	Trophozoite			Cyst		
	Size (μm)	Motility	Number of Nuclei	Other Features	Size (μm) and Shape	Number of Nuclei	Other Features
Giardia lamblia	9-21 × 5-15	"Falling leaf"	2	Sucking disk, ventral surface Parabasal bodies and axonemes	8-12, oval	4	Cytoplasm retracted from cyst wall Fibrils and flagella inside cyst
Chilomastix mesnili	10-20 × 3-10	Rotary	1	Spiral groove Cytostome	6-10, lemon-shaped	1	Anterior of cyst has nipplelike protrusion
Trichomonas hominis	6-14	Jerky	1	Undulating membrane the entire length of the organism Axostyle through body			No cyst stage
Dientamoeba fragilis	5-12	Nondirectional	2 (20% have 1)	Nucleus made of 4 to 8 clustered granules Resembles ameba			No cyst stage
Trichomonas vaginalis	7-23 × 5-12; average, 15-18	Jerky, nondirectional	1	Undulating membrane half the length of the body Found in urine			No cyst stage

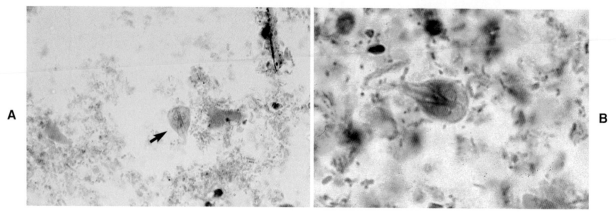

FIGURE 28-17 **A,** *Giardia lamblia* trophozoite (trichrome stain). **B,** Enlarged view of *G. lamblia* trophozoite (trichrome stain).

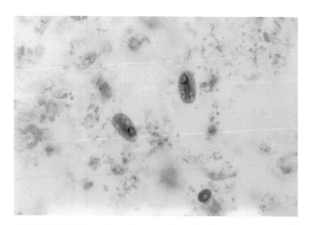

FIGURE 28-18 *Giardia lamblia* cysts (trichrome stain).

of *G. lamblia* and compares them with those of other flagellates. Cysts of *G. lamblia* are oval and measure approximately 8 to 12 μm × 7 to 10 μm. There are up to four nuclei, and the cytoplasm is often pulled away from the cyst wall. On a permanently stained smear, the retracted flagella and other internal structures give the cyst a cluttered appearance (Figure 28-18).

EIAs using monoclonal antibodies to detect soluble antigens of *G. lamblia* in stool are available. Direct fluorescent antibody tests are frequently used to identify the cyst of *Giardia* in a stool specimen. Several of these tests also contain a monoclonal antibody that identifies *Cryptosporidium*. Some patients who remain symptomatic but show no evidence of the organism after repeated stool tests may require a duodenal aspirate or use of Enterotest to demonstrate the trophozoite in the small intestine.

Dientamoeba fragilis. For many years there have been questions about the pathogenicity of *D. fragilis*. The organism was isolated from the stools of patients who were asymptomatic as well as from those who had gastrointestinal symptoms such as abdominal pain or tenderness, or diarrhea. Although it is circumstantial, evidence now suggests that the organism has a role as a pathogen. Case reports show that treatment with a drug such as metronidazole results in the clearance of

the organism and alleviation of symptoms. Molecular methods show that there are at least two genetic types, but the significance of these is unknown. The organism lacks a cyst stage and the life span of the trophozoite outside the body is very short, so direct transmission is unlikely. Some studies suggest that the trophozoite may be transmitted to humans by ingestion in a helminth egg, especially that of *Enterobius vermicularis* because co-infection of *D. fragilis* and *E. vermicularis* is more common than coinfection of *D. fragilis* with other organisms. Molecular studies, however, have provided no evidence of coinfection.

The morphology of *D. fragilis* closely resembles that of the amebae, but electron microscopy studies of ultrastructure demonstrate the presence of a flagellum, indicating that it belongs to the subphylum Mastigophora. The lack of a cyst stage and analysis of small-subunit rRNA show its relationship to the trichomonads. The organism is characteristically binucleate, with 50% to 80% of the organisms demonstrating this characteristic. The delicate nuclear membrane has no peripheral chromatin, and the karyosome consists of four to eight discrete granules, one of which is often larger than the others. The size of the trophozoite ranges from 5 to 12 μm, and the cytoplasm contains many food vacuoles and bacteria (Figure 28-19). This organism degenerates within hours after excretion, and rapid preservation of the stool is important. The organism can be difficult to see on a trichrome-stained smear because its outline often is indistinct and blends into the background.

Trichomonas vaginalis. *Trichomonas vaginalis*, a pathogen of the urogenital tract in men and women, causes trichomoniasis, one of the most common nonviral sexually transmitted diseases with an estimate of 180 million cases worldwide. Approximately 3 million to 5 million new cases are reported in the United States each year with up to two thirds of these in women 15 to 24 years of age. Humans are the only host, and presence of infection with the organism is associated with other sexually transmitted diseases, especially gonorrhea. Trichomoniasis has been associated with increased adverse pregnancy outcomes including transmission of the organism to the newborn, in addition to cervical neoplasia and pelvic inflammatory disease. The most significant com-

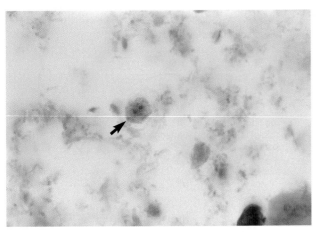

FIGURE 28-19   *Dientamoeba fragilis* binucleate trophozoite (trichrome stain).

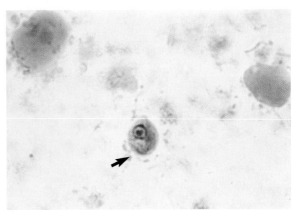

FIGURE 28-20   *Chilomastix mesnili* cyst (trichrome stain).

plication is increased risk of HIV transmission due primarily to the inflammatory response that compromises the mucosal barriers to HIV. *T. vaginalis* lacks a cyst stage, and the trophozoite stage is infective through sexual contact. The organism is susceptible to rapid drying in the environment; but a few cases of nonsexual transmission have been reported.

In women, the infection is primarily localized to the vagina, resulting in itching and the production of a frothy, creamy, mucopurulent vaginal discharge as well as dysuria. About one third of infected women, however, are asymptomatic. A chronic state can develop with mild symptoms of pruritus and scanty discharge. Women with this form of infection are often a major source of transmission to sexual partners. Men infected with *T. vaginalis* are usually asymptomatic and serve as carriers, although they may develop nonspecific urethritis with a milky discharge that lasts up to 4 weeks. *T. vaginalis* is now considered an important cause of nongonococcal urethritis.

Infections in either sex are usually treated with metronidazole. Treatment of sexual partners is suggested to obtain optimum cure and prevent reinfection. Long-term immunity is not developed after an acute infection, and reinfection can occur. In women, the diagnosis was classically made by finding the trophozoite in vaginal discharge or occasionally in urine; in men the trophozoite is seen in urine or prostatic secretions. The organism is 5 to 18 µm in diameter, has four anterior flagella, and an undulating membrane that extends half the length of the body. In a wet mount, the trophozoite has a characteristic jerky motility, and the motion of the flagella and undulating membrane may be seen. The preparation should be examined immediately as the organism loses viability quickly. In a Giemsa-stained preparation, the pear-shaped organism shows the presence of an axostyle extending the length of the organism, a single nucleus near the anterior end, and chromatic granules extending the length of the axostyle. Fluorescent staining of exudates using acridine orange will demonstrate a typical fluorescent morphology with a yellow-green nucleus. Although most clinicians rely on wet mount preparations, the method has relatively low sensitivity (30% to 70%).

Until the advent of molecular methods, culture of the organism from exudate was considered the most sensitive and specific method of detection, although an inoculum of 300 to 500 organisms is necessary. Commercial systems using a plastic pouch containing culture medium are available for microscopic detection of the organisms. The specimen should be inoculated into the pouch within 30 minutes of collection to ensure optimal organism viability. Culture specimens should be held for up to 5 days. Polymerase chain reaction (PCR) methods and antigen detection assays are also available commercially. The rapid antigen detection tests are based on immunochromatographic enzyme immunoassay procedures using monoclonal antibodies. These tests have relatively high sensitivity when compared to examination of a wet preparation. PCR tests are especially useful in detecting infection in asymptomatic males.

Nonpathogenic Intestinal Flagellates

Chilomastix mesnili and *Trichomonas hominis* are intestinal nonpathogens that must be differentiated from pathogenic flagellates. *C. mesnili* trophozoites are pear shaped and approximately 10 to 20 µm long × 3 to 10 µm wide. The cytostome and nucleus are prominent in the anterior of the organism, and a spiral groove encircles the body of the organism. The nucleus has a small central karyosome and is surrounded by fibrils that curl around the cytostome to give a "shepherd's crook" appearance. The cytostome is elongate and rounded at the anterior and posterior. The cyst of *C. mesnili*, which measures 6 to 10 µm, is lemon shaped with an anterior nipple. The nucleus, cytostome, and curved fibrils are visible in a stained smear (Figure 28-20).

Trichomonas hominis is a small organism not usually identified in the stool. The trophozoite is 6 to 14 µm long with a prominent axostyle extending through the posterior of the organism, four anterior flagella, and an oval nucleus with a small karyosome. The undulating membrane extends the length of the organism and is joined to the body along the costa.

Blood and Tissue Flagellates

The hemoflagellates in the genera *Leishmania* and *Trypanosoma* differ in several ways from the intestinal flagellates.

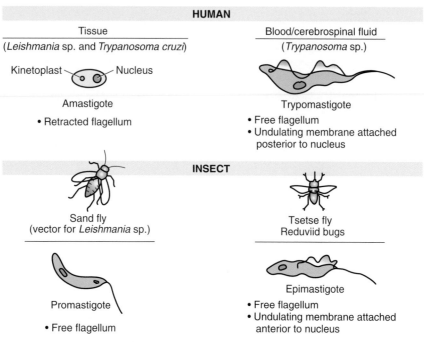

FIGURE 28-21 Life cycle stages of the blood and tissue flagellates.

First, they are transmitted by insect **vectors,** which are necessary for completion of the life cycle. Second, these organisms have different life cycle stages for diagnosis. Figure 28-21 shows the four life cycle stages of the hemoflagellates. The trypomastigote and the amastigote (Leishman-Donovan body) are the diagnostic stages found in humans. The amastigote is an obligate intracellular organism, 2 to 5 μm in diameter, found within macrophages, liver or spleen cells, or bone marrow cells in diseases caused by the *Leishmania* spp. In addition, the amastigote stage may be seen in cells of patients infected with *Trypanosoma cruzi*. The trypomastigote, a flagellated form measuring 15 to 20 μm, is found in the blood, lymphatic fluid, and CSF of patients infected with *Trypanosoma* spp. The epimastigote and promastigote stages are seen in the insect vectors.

Leishmania. The genus *Leishmania* contains several complexes of at least 20 species that cause disease in humans: *Leishmania tropica* complex, *Leishmania mexicana* complex, *Leishmania braziliensis* complex, and *Leishmania donovani* complex. Leishmaniasis is a zoonotic infection in which dogs and rodents serve as the primary reservoir hosts for all species and humans serves as an accidental host. The insect vectors are sand flies of the genera *Phlebotomus* and *Lutzomyia*.

Clinical Infections. Clinical infections range from single, self-healing skin ulcers to visceral disease affecting multiple organs. *Leishmania tropica* complex, the cause of cutaneous leishmaniasis or Oriental sore, is found primarily in the Orient and North-Central Africa. *L. mexicana* complex, the cause of New World cutaneous leishmaniasis, is found in South and Central America. The condition is characterized by the presence of a crusted circular lesion on any of the exposed body surfaces, especially the face and extremities. The lesion begins as a small, red papule at the site of the insect bite and progresses to a lesion with an elevated, indurated margin that may reach 8 cm. The lesion resolves in several months and provides some level of immunity (incomplete) against future infection. Another form of the disease, chiclero ulcer—often associated with *L. mexicana* complex—is characterized by lesions on the ear. The infection is self-limiting and does not invade mucosal surfaces, but secondary bacterial infection can occur.

Leishmania braziliensis complex is the causative agent of mucocutaneous leishmaniasis or espundia. This infection manifests as an initial lesion that may increase in size, invading and destroying the mucosal surfaces of the nose and mouth. It may also destroy cartilage, leaving the patient with significant disfigurement. *L. braziliensis* complex is primarily found in Mexico and Central and South America. The most severe infection, visceral leishmaniasis or kala-azar, is endemic in parts of South America, Africa, Southern Europe, and Asia. The etiologic agents are organisms of the *L. donovani* complex. In this disease, organisms spread through the lymphatics and invade organs of the reticuloendothelial system, including the liver, spleen, lymph nodes, and bone marrow. Patients with kala-azar exhibit malaise, anorexia, weight loss, headache, and fever. In addition, they may show splenomegaly and hepatomegaly with elevated liver enzymes, hypogammaglobulinemia and hypoproteinemia. *Leishmania*-containing macrophages invade the bone marrow. The kidneys and heart may also be affected. If untreated, visceral leishmaniasis is often fatal within 2 years. Cases of cutaneous leishmaniasis and visceral leishmaniasis have been seen in a number of military personnel serving in Mideast countries such as Iraq and Afghanistan. Standard therapy for all leishmanial infections is pentavalent antimony compounds.

Life Cycle. Figure 28-22 shows the generalized life cycle for *Leishmania* spp. When the female insect takes a blood meal, she ingests the amastigote stage. The parasite develops as a promastigote in the gut of the insect and migrates to the salivary glands when mature. The promastigote is transmitted to humans through the salivary glands of the insect when it

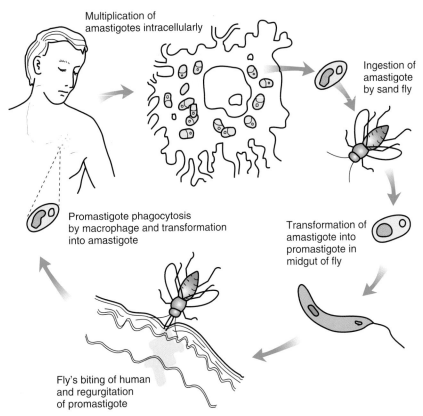

Multiplication of
amastigotes intracellularly

Ingestion of
amastigote
by sand fly

Promastigote phagocytosis
by macrophage and transformation
into amastigote

Transformation of
amastigote into
promastigote in
midgut of fly

Fly's biting of human
and regurgitation
of promastigote

FIGURE 28-22 Life cycle of *Leishmania* spp.

takes a blood meal. The promastigote is taken up via receptor-mediated phagocytosis by a macrophage. In addition, uptake is enhanced because the organism can be coated with C3b, which binds to specific macrophage receptors. Within the macrophage it converts to the amastigote stage and multiplies within the cell. When the cell ruptures, amastigotes are released and invade other macrophages.

Laboratory Diagnosis. The amastigote is the diagnostic stage in humans. It is a small intracellular stage found in macrophages or histiocytes around the periphery of the skin lesions (*L. tropica* or *L. braziliensis*) or within cells of a bone marrow aspirate or liver or spleen biopsy specimens (*L. donovani*). Wright stain reveals an oval organism 2 to 5 μm in diameter, with pale blue cytoplasm, a large red nucleus, and a rodlike **kinetoplast** within the cytoplasm (Figure 28-23). The amastigote has also been reported extracellularly in cases of cutaneous leishmaniasis. The same authors reported finding promastigotes (the insect form of the parasite) in 76% of 42 patient samples; 52% of the time the promastigote was the only form found. Serologic tests such as direct agglutination and indirect fluorescent assays can be used in individuals from nonendemic areas. A dipstick test for detecting infection is under development.

Trypanosoma. Trypanosomes are blood and CSF flagellates that require an insect vector, the tsetse fly (genus *Glossina*) for transmission. *Trypanosoma brucei rhodesiense* and *Trypanosoma brucei gambiense* are the causative agents of sleeping sickness, which is seen primarily in central Africa. West African sleeping sickness, caused by *T. brucei gambiense*,

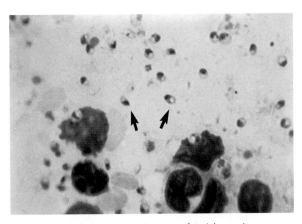

FIGURE 28-23 Amastigotes of *Leishmania* spp.

is the milder and more chronic of the two diseases. A long asymptomatic stage is followed by death years later. East African sleeping sickness, caused by *T. brucei rhodesiense,* is characterized by a rapid course often resulting in death within 6 months after the onset of symptoms. Both infections are zoonoses, and game animals serve as important reservoir hosts of *T. rhodesiense. T. cruzi,* the agent of American trypanosomiasis or Chagas disease, is discussed in the next section.

Clinical Infections. Initial symptoms of African sleeping sickness include a local inflammatory reaction to the parasites at the site of the insect bite. This occurs within 2 to 3 days and may last up to 4 weeks. During this time the organisms

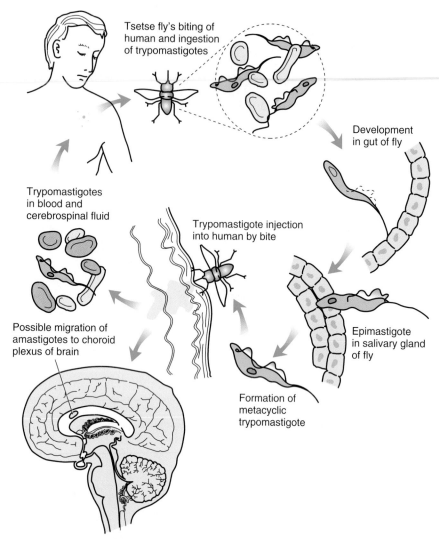

FIGURE 28-24 Life cycle of the agents of sleeping sickness (*Trypanosoma brucei gambiense* and *Trypanosoma brucei* rhodesiense).

are reproducing and beginning to enter the bloodstream. About 1 to 3 weeks after the metacyclic trypomastigotes enter the blood and lymphatics, the patient experiences generalized symptoms including fever, headache, joint and muscle pain, weakness, and lymphadenopathy. Enlargement in the postero-lateral triangle of the neck is known as Winterbottom's sign. Edema in the legs and arms and around the eyes is possible. While circulating, the organisms are able to resist antibody-mediated destruction by continuous antigenic variation. A protective glycoprotein layer helps the organism resist direct lysis by complement. As the trypomastigotes invade the CNS, the patient develops severe headaches, mental dullness, and apathy and may experience coordination problems, altered reflexes, and paralysis. Eventually, the patient has convulsions, lapses into a coma, and dies.

Life Cycle. The tsetse fly (genus *Glossina*) is the biologic vector for agents of sleeping sickness. Figure 28-24 shows a generalized life cycle for these agents. The fly ingests the try-pomastigote stage when it takes a blood meal from a human. The organisms migrate to the insect gut and develop into

epimastigotes, which, when mature, migrate to the salivary gland. There they develop into infective metacyclic trypomas-tigotes, which are transmitted to humans in saliva when the fly bites. The trypomastigote form first circulates in the blood and lymphatic system, ultimately invading the central nervous system.

Laboratory Diagnosis. The diagnostic stage in humans is the trypomastigote, which is usually seen in a Wright-stained blood smear, although wet films may be used to detect the motile trypomastigote. The organism can also be detected in lymphatic fluid and CSF. The CSF in infected individuals will often show increased lymphocytes and elevated protein levels. The trypomastigote is 15 to 20 μm long with a single large nucleus and a posterior kinetoplast to which is attached the flagellum of the undulating membrane (Figure 28-25). The anterior flagellum is not visible in this organism. *Try-panosoma* spp. cannot be differentiated on a blood smear; therefore the organism is reported as *Trypanosoma* sp. Final determination of species may be made based on clinical symptoms as well as the geographic area.

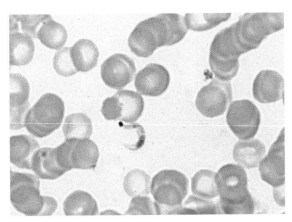

FIGURE 28-25 *Trypanosoma* trypomastigote in a blood smear.

The QBC method, which has been used in the detection of malarial parasites, has also been adapted for detection of trypomastigotes. Field diagnosis of infection is important in endemic areas, and a serologic method using a card agglutination test (CATT) and a micro-CATT have been developed. The test uses lyophilized *T. gambiense* antigen to detect antibodies in the blood. The test cannot distinguish current from past infection; therefore microscopy should be used to confirm the presence of organisms in the blood. Molecular dipstick methods are under development.

Trypanosoma cruzi. Chagas disease is a zoonotic infection found primarily in rural areas of Mexico and Central and South America. There are estimates that up to 20 million people in these countries may have the disease. It is caused by the hemoflagellate *T. cruzi*, which is transmitted by the triatomid bug, also known as the reduviid or kissing bug (*Triatoma* sp. or *Panstrongylus* sp.). These insects live within mud or thatch walls of a dwelling during the day and come out at night to take a blood meal from the human inhabitants. Animals such as armadillos and opossums may also be infected with the organism and serve as a reservoir for infection. Although insect transmission is most common, the organism has been transmitted by blood transfusion, transplanted organs, and congenital infection. In endemic areas of the world, transmission by transfusion is relatively common, and in North America, several cases of transfusion-transmitted Chagas disease have been reported. Donors in these cases were asymptomatic and in the latent or chronic state of the disease. There are estimates that 50,000 to 100,000 immigrants to the United States are chronically infected and could be capable of causing transfusion- or transplant-transmitted Chagas disease. Screening of blood donors for antibodies to *T. cruzi* in some countries of Central and South America has decreased the rate of transfusion transmission. Screening tests for blood donors in the United States have been developed.

Clinical Infections. The infection is divided into three phases, acute, intermediate (latent), and chronic. After the insect bites, there is an incubation period that ranges from 2 to 4 weeks. As the organisms enter the blood, the acute phase begins. Individuals in the acute phase may be asymptomatic or have local symptoms including the presence of a chagoma (ulcerative skin lesion at the site of the insect bite) or a uni-

lateral edema around the eye (Romaña sign) if the bite is on the ocular conjunctiva. Systemic manifestations include fever, lymphadenitis, hepatosplenomegaly, malaise, muscular pains, and diarrhea and vomiting. Whereas adults often have a milder form of the disease, the most severe form of acute infection usually occurs in children. This may manifest as myocarditis or meningoencephalitis.

The latent period develops as the trypomastigotes disappear from the circulation and invade the cells of the cardiac or gastrointestinal system. The latent phase may last 10 to 40 years after infection, but only about 30% to 40% of patients develop the chronic form of Chagas disease. Chronic myocarditis develops in many cases and may progress to tachycardia and eventually congestive heart failure. In some patients the chronic form may manifest as megacolon, megastomach, or megaesophagus that results in difficulty in swallowing and disturbances to intestinal motility. Once the patient enters the chronic stage of the disease, there are periods of intermittent parasitemia of trypomastigotes during which time the organism may be transmitted.

Life Cycle. Transmission of the organism to humans occurs when the insect vector defecates in the area surrounding its bite site. Metacyclic trypomastigotes in the feces are scratched into the bite site and invade the bloodstream as. The trypomastigotes circulate in the blood and eventually enter a cell, where they transform into an amastigote. Cells of the cardiac muscle and skeletal muscle are most commonly infected. Within the cell the amastigote multiplies and causes the cell to rupture. Free amastigotes then invade other cells. A few of the released amastigotes will transform back into trypomastigotes in the bloodstream, which can be taken in by the insect to continue the life cycle and transmission. Figure 28-26 shows the life cycle of *T. cruzi*.

Laboratory Diagnosis. The primary diagnostic stage in the blood is the trypomastigote. It is an elongated structure 15 to 20 μm long that often appears in a C or U shape. Like the other trypomastigotes, it shows a single large nucleus midbody, a single anterior flagellum, and a posterior kinetoplast to which is attached the undulating membrane. In most Wright's stained smears, the nucleus and kinetoplast and parts of the undulating membrane are well stained, but only the suggestion of a flagellum can be seen at the anterior end. In a cardiac or other tissue biopsy specimen, the organism can be seen in the amastigote stage. The morphology of all trypomastigotes is similar (see Figure 28-25); therefore a complete patient history is necessary to determine the species present. Serologic tests for detecting IgG antibodies to *T. cruzi* include complement fixation, immunofluorescence, and EIA.

Xenodiagnosis is used in Central and South America as a diagnostic method. A laboratory-raised triatomid bug is allowed to feed on patients suspected of having *T. cruzi* infection. When the insect is returned to the laboratory, its feces are examined on a regular basis for the presence of the parasite. Presence of the parasite in the insect's feces indicates that the patient was infected. This method is most helpful for diagnosing infections in the chronic stage when fewer parasites are present. Rapid diagnostic tests using whole blood are under evaluation for testing individuals in remote areas.

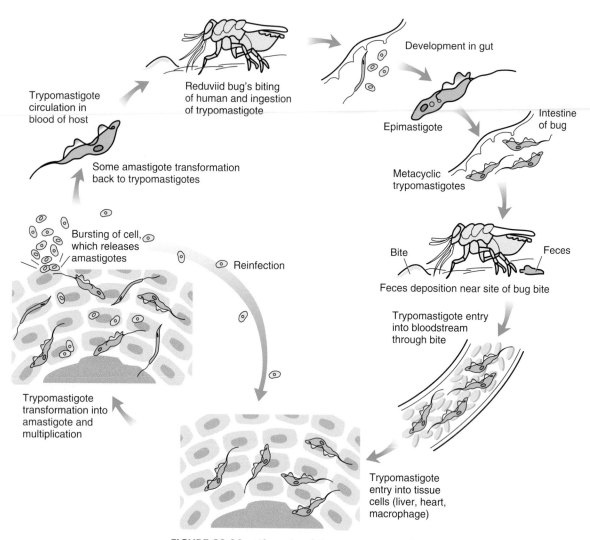

FIGURE 28-26 Life cycle of *Trypanosoma cruzi.*

Apicomplexa

The phylum Apicomplexa includes blood and tissue parasites that represent both age-old pathogens and newly recognized agents of opportunistic infection. This group of organisms shows a diversity of morphology and transmission methods and can infect many different body sites. Life cycles are complex and are characterized by sexual and **asexual reproduction** phases. In addition, some may require an insect vector or intermediate host for completion of the life cycle. Humans can serve as **definitive hosts** when **sexual reproduction** takes place in human tissues and as intermediate hosts when asexual reproduction occurs.

Plasmodium

Plasmodium spp., which cause malaria, remain endemic throughout the world in tropical and subtropical countries with an estimated 300 million to 500 million cases annually. *Plasmodium vivax, Plasmodium ovale, Plasmodium malariae,* and *Plasmodium falciparum* are the etiologic agents of human malaria. Along with schistosomiasis and amebiasis, malaria is a major cause of mortality in people in underdeveloped countries. Between 1 and 2 million deaths worldwide are caused by malaria each year, primarily due to infection with *P. falciparum.* Mortality in children who have malaria is also significantly associated with infection by *P. falciparum.* In the United States, approximately 1000 cases are reported annually, with *P. falciparum* being the etiologic agent in more than 50% of the cases. Most of these cases are in travelers to endemic areas.

Plasmodium vivax has the widest geographic distribution and is the one most likely to be found in temperate climates. *P. vivax* and *P. falciparum* cause the majority of infections. *P. ovale* is confined to Africa; *P. falciparum* and *P. malariae* have similar distributions throughout Africa and tropical countries. In general, infections caused by *P. vivax, P. ovale,* and *P. malariae* are less severe than those caused by *P. falciparum.*

Clinical Infections. Although malaria is transmitted most commonly through the bite of an anopheline mosquito, transmission through blood transfusion and infected needles has been reported. Transplacental infection also has been documented. In these cases, the organism is sequestered in the placenta and can compromise fetal development because it affects transplacental transport. The malarial paroxysm, which begins 10 to 15 days after the bite of an infected mosquito, is the primary symptom associated with the erythrocytic cycle. It is linked to rupture of RBCs and release of **merozoites,** malarial metabolites, and endotoxin-like substances into the bloodstream.

The prodromal phase of the paroxysm involves headache, bone pain, nausea, or flulike symptoms. A shaking chill (the cold stage) of 15 to 60 minutes initiates the paroxysm and is followed by a fever (hot stage) with headache, myalgia, and nausea, and a temperature of up to 40° C. This stage lasts about 2 to 4 hours, after which the fever finally breaks. The patient begins to sweat profusely and is left exhausted and sleepy. This cycle repeats itself at regular intervals, depending on the species of malarial organism present. Long-term infection with any malarial organism may result in damage to the liver and spleen caused by deposits of malarial pigment (hemozoin). In small children and in heavy infections, severe anemia can develop.

Plasmodium vivax and *P. ovale* infections generally do not have the range of complications seen with other species. However, the persistence of hypnozoites that remain dormant in the liver can lead to relapses within 3 years of initial exposure. *P. malariae* infections may lead to nephrotic syndrome, which arises from deposition of circulating immune complexes of malarial antigen and antibody on the basement membrane of the glomeruli, causing an autoimmune reaction. This organism has the most chronic course, and recrudescence occurs even decades after the initial infection.

The most severe form of malaria is caused by *P. falciparum*, with the primary complication being the development of cerebral malaria. Between 20% and 50% of deaths caused by *P. falciparum* are the result of CNS complications. The parasite-infected RBCs demonstrate sticky "knobs" that mediate adhesion to the endothelial cells of the capillary walls. The parasite protein *P. falciparum* erythrocyte membrane protein 1 (PfMP1) is involved in mediating this attachment. Blood flow is slowed in the microcirculation, reducing oxygen delivery to the tissues, with resultant tissue anoxia. In addition, proinflammatory cytokines mediate damage to tissue. The patient has severe headaches, may be confused, and ultimately lapses into a coma.

A second but less common complication of infection with *P. falciparum* is **blackwater fever.** It usually develops in patients with repeated infections and those undergoing quinine therapies. Blackwater fever may be mediated by an antigen-antibody reaction caused by the development of an autoantibody to the RBCs. The black appearance of the urine is the result of massive intravascular hemolysis and resulting hemoglobinuria. In addition, the high parasitemia that often accompanies *P. falciparum* infection may lead to anemia and deposits of malarial pigment in organs such as the spleen. Renal complications such as nephrotic syndrome or even renal failure can occur with *P. falciparum* infection as a result of tubular necrosis brought about by tissue anoxia.

Although complete immunity to malaria does not exist, individuals in endemic areas develop antibodies against asexual stages, which help reduce the parasite load and the severity of illness. In addition, reports of antibodies directed against **sporozoites** and **gametes** indicate that these also may help reduce the rate of infection and the severity of illness. Patients with hemoglobinopathies, such as sickle cell disease, hemoglobin C, and glucose-6-phosphate dehydrogenase deficiency, are somewhat protected against severe malaria because the parasite cannot replicate or in some cases exist in these RBCs.

Treatment. Chloroquine remains the primary drug for prophylaxis and treatment of malaria. It is effective against all asexual stages of malarial organisms and all gametocytes except those of *P. falciparum*. Many strains of *P. falciparum* have become resistant to the drug. Recent reports indicate that strains of *P. vivax* in Southeast Asia and Papua New Guinea show diminished response to treatment with chloroquine as well.

Plasmodium falciparum has also demonstrated resistance to sulfadoxine-pyrimethamine (Fansidar) and mefloquine (Lariam) in parts of South America, Southeast Asia, and Africa. Doxycycline, Malarone, or quinine use has been reestablished in some cases of multidrug-resistant *P. falciparum*. Chloroquine-resistant *P. vivax* may be treated with mefloquine or quinine sulfate with doxycycline. Primaquine phosphate, which is effective against hypnozoites that persist in the liver, is used to treat individuals infected with *P. vivax* and *P. ovale* to prevent relapses of these infections. There is also evidence that some strains of *P. vivax* in the geographic areas of chloroquine resistance may be refractory to primaquine. Recently artemisinin-based drugs have been used in combination with classic drugs in areas with emergence of highly resistant strains of *P. falciparum*.

Life Cycle. The life cycle of *Plasmodium* involves both sexual reproduction **(sporogony)** and asexual reproduction **(schizogony),** as shown in Figure 28-27. The female *Anopheles* mosquito serves as biologic vector and definitive host. Asexual reproduction, which occurs in humans, has an **exoerythrocytic phase** that takes place in the liver and an **erythrocytic phase** that takes place in RBCs.

In human infections, the earliest stage is the ring-form trophozoite (Figure 28-28) in which the organism has a prominent, red-purple chromatin dot and a small, blue ring of cytoplasm surrounding a vacuole. The growing trophozoite is characterized by an increase in cytoplasm, the disappearance of the vacuole, and the appearance of malarial pigment in the organism's cytoplasm. The immature **schizont** is characterized by a splitting of the chromatin mass. The mature schizont contains merozoites, which are individual chromatin masses, each surrounded by cytoplasm. Microgametocytes (male) have pale blue cytoplasm and a diffuse chromatin mass that stains pale pink-purple. The chromatin may be surrounded by a clear halo. Macrogametocytes (female) show a well-defined, compact chromatin mass that stains dark pink, and the cytoplasm stains a darker blue than in microgametocytes. The chromatin mass often is set eccentrically in the organism. Pigment is distributed throughout the cytoplasm except in *P. falciparum,* in which it often is clumped near the chromatin mass.

Exoerythrocytic Phase. Humans serve as intermediate host and acquire the infection when the female mosquito takes a blood meal and injects the infective sporozoites with salivary secretions. The sporozoites enter the human circula-

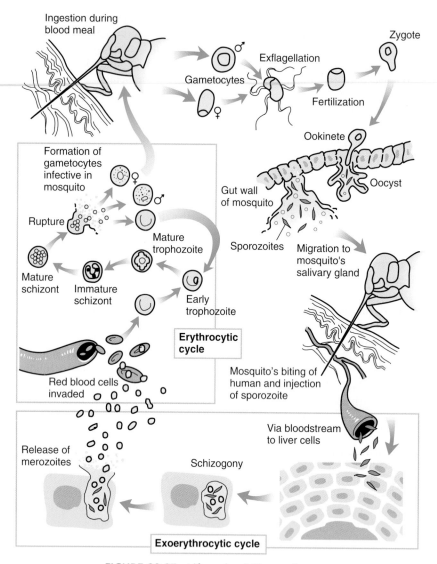

FIGURE 28-27 Life cycle of *Plasmodium* spp.

tion and take approximately 30 to 60 minutes to reach the liver, where they begin the exoerythrocytic phase by penetrating parenchymal cells. Maturation through the trophozoite and schizont phases results in production of merozoites. Each schizont produces a large number of merozoites. Release of mature merozoites from liver cells and invasion of RBCs signal the beginning of the erythrocytic phase. Generally, only one cycle of merozoite production occurs in the liver before RBCs are invaded. *P. vivax* and *P. ovale*, however, may persist in the liver in a dormant stage known as hypnozoites, which accounts for the relapse (recurrence) of the disease within 1 to 3 years after the primary infection. Neither *P. malariae* nor *P. falciparum* has a persistent liver phase, although recrudescence in untreated individuals with either of these organisms may be the result of a continued subclinical erythrocytic infection.

Erythrocytic Phase. Merozoites have structures and proteins (such as erythrocyte binding antigen) that selectively adhere to receptors on the RBC membrane. *P. vivax* uses antigens of the Duffy blood group as receptors, whereas *P.* *falciparum* may simply attach to receptors that are integral parts of the red cell membrane itself. Once merozoites have attached, endocytic invagination of the red cell membrane allows the organism to enter the red cell within a vacuole.

Once inside the RBC, the organism feeds on hemoglobin and initiates the erythrocytic phase. Malarial pigment, which is composed of iron deposits, is formed in the growing trophozoite as a result of incomplete metabolism of the hemoglobin. Once the organism has reached the mature trophozoite stage, the chromatin begins to divide (schizont). When the chromatin split has been completed, each chromatin mass is surrounded by its own bit of malarial cytoplasm (merozoite). Each malarial species has a typical number of merozoites, which may be used as an identifying characteristic. When the RBC ruptures, merozoites are released to invade other RBCs. At this point, two outcomes are possible: one is that the merozoite enters a cell and repeats development into a schizont; the other is that it enters a cell and develops into one of the sexual stages—either the microgametocyte or the macrogametocyte.

Sexual Phase. Sporogony, which takes place in the mosquito, results in production of sporozoites infective for humans. Both microgametocyte and macrogametocyte are infective for the female mosquito when she takes a blood meal. In the insect's stomach, exflagellation by the male and subsequent fertilization of the female result in formation of an ookinete that migrates through the gut wall and forms an oocyst on the exterior gut wall. Sporozoites are produced within the oocyst. Mature sporozoites are released into the body cavity of the mosquito and migrate to the salivary glands. The female then injects sporozoites into a human as she takes her blood meal.

Laboratory Diagnosis. History of travel to an endemic area and the presence of classic clinical symptoms, including the malarial paroxysm of fever and chills, should alert a clinician to request Giemsa-stained thick and thin smears for malaria. Examination of these blood smears remains the classic method of diagnosing malaria. Laboratory identification of malarial species involves examination of both the morphology of infected RBCs and the characteristic morphology of the parasite. The thick smear is used to detect malarial parasites; however, distortions of parasite morphology and the lack of intact RBCs require that a thin smear be examined to identify the species. Trophozoites, schizonts, and gametocytes may be seen in the blood smear. Table 28-6 gives the general characteristics of trophozoites and schizonts of the malarial species.

The QBC system uses a microhematocrit tube coated with acridine orange for the detection and identification of malarial species. This method demonstrates the presence of parasites, but a thin smear must still be made for definitive identification. DNA probes have been proposed as another method for diagnosing malaria. However, the extended time and costly equipment required do not make the procedure cost effective or efficient, especially for field work. Several different immunoassays, collectively referred to as rapid diagnostic tests, use malarial antibody impregnated dipsticks to detect *P. falciparum* infection. These use an antigen capture immunochromatographic principle to detect soluble proteins from malarial organisms in the blood. Some may detect an antigen specific to *P. falciparum*, while others detect a protein common to all species. One brand is available for use in the United States. Serologic tests for antibody to malaria are not useful in an endemic area but may be useful for diagnosis in individuals who have traveled to an endemic area and who have clinical symptoms of malaria.

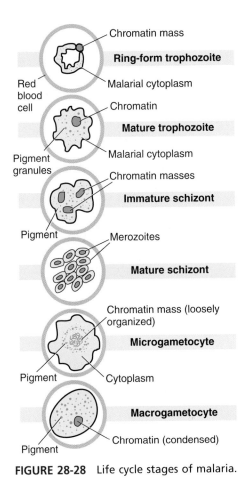

FIGURE 28-28   Life cycle stages of malaria.

TABLE 28-6 Comparisons of Malarial Species

Plasmodium Species	Red Blood Cell Morphology	Trophozoite	Number of Merozoites in Schizont	Reproductive Cycle (Hours)	Other Characteristics
P. vivax	Enlarged (1½ to 2×) Schüffner's dots	Ameboid Large vacuoles Golden-brown pigment	12-24 Average: 16	48	Wide range of stages in peripheral blood
P. malariae	Normal size May have dark hue Ziemann's dots (rare)	Compact May assume "band form" across cell Coarse, dark brown pigment	6-12 Average: 8 with daisy petal–like arrangement around clumped pigment	72	Wide range of stages in peripheral blood
P. ovale	Enlarged, oval Fringed edge Schüffner's dots	Compact Golden-brown pigment (resembles *P. vivax*)	6-16 Average: 8	48	Wide range of stages in peripheral blood
P. falciparum	Normal size Multiple infections	Small, delicate Double chromatin dots Appliqué forms Dark pigment	12-36 Average: 20-24	Irregular, 36-48	Crescent-shaped gametocyte Ring and gametocyte stages only in peripheral blood

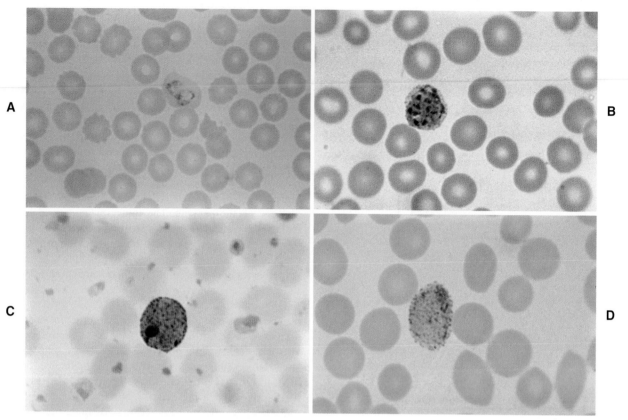

FIGURE 28-29 **A,** *Plasmodium vivax* trophozoite. **B,** *P. vivax* mature schizont. **C,** *P. vivax* macrogametocyte. **D,** *P. vivax* microgametocyte.

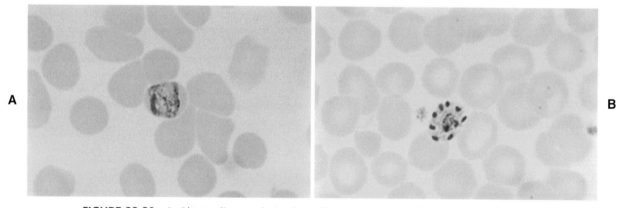

FIGURE 28-30 **A,** *Plasmodium malariae* band form trophozoite. **B,** *P. malariae* schizont.

Plasmodium vivax. *Plasmodium vivax* has a tertian life-cycle pattern—that is, it takes approximately 48 hours for the life cycle to be completed. The invasion of a new group of RBCs begins on the third day. *P. vivax* usually invades young RBCs (reticulocytes) and therefore is characterized by enlarged infected RBCs, often 1½ to 2 times normal size. A fine pink stippling known as **Schüffner's stippling** (or dots) may be present in the cell. The young trophozoite is characterized by its ameboid appearance; by maturity, it usually fills the RBC, and golden brown malarial pigment is present. The mature schizont contains 12 to 24 merozoites, with an average of 16. Gametocytes are rounded and fill the cell. Macrogame-

tocytes are often difficult to differentiate from mature trophozoites. Figure 28-29 shows several stages of *P. vivax.*

Plasmodium malariae. *Plasmodium malariae* usually invades older RBCs, perhaps accounting for the occasional darker appearance of the invaded RBC. The life cycle is characterized as quartan, with reproduction occurring every 72 hours and invasion of new RBCs every fourth day. The trophozoite is compact and may assume a characteristic "band" appearance, in which it stretches across the diameter of the RBCs (Figure 28-30, *A*). Notice the presence of dark, coarse, brown-black pigment in the band form. Occasionally, a few pink cytoplasmic dots, called **Ziemann's dots**, may be seen.

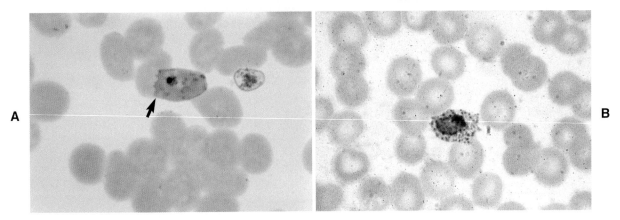

FIGURE 28-31 **A,** *Plasmodium ovale* trophozoite. **B,** Schüffner's stippling of *P. ovale* clearly visible.

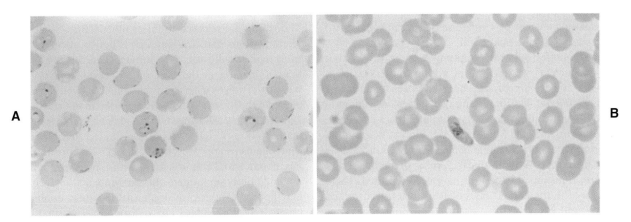

FIGURE 28-32 **A,** *Plasmodium falciparum* ring-form trophozoites. **B,** *P. falciparum* gametocyte.

The mature schizont contains 6 to 12 merozoites (Figure 28-30, *B*), with an average of 8. Merozoites may be arranged in a characteristic loose "daisy petal" arrangement around the clumped pigment; however, they may also be randomly arranged.

Plasmodium ovale. *Plasmodium ovale,* the least commonly seen species, resembles *P. vivax.* In *P. ovale* infections, the RBC is enlarged and may assume an oval shape with fimbriated or fringelike edges. Schüffner's dots are less commonly seen than with *P. vivax.* The parasite remains compact, has golden-brown pigment, and has a range of 6 to 12 merozoites in the mature schizont. It also exhibits a tertian life cycle. Figure 28-31, *A,* shows trophozoites of *P. ovale.* The Schüffner's stippling in Figure 28-31, *B,* has stained almost a bluish pink, but the compact organism and fimbriated cell are characteristic.

Plasmodium falciparum. Although identified as having a tertian life cycle, *P. falciparum* often demonstrates an asynchronous life cycle with rupture of the RBCs taking place at irregular intervals ranging from 36 to 48 hours. The life cycle stages seen in peripheral blood are usually limited to the ring-form trophozoite and the gametocyte. Other stages mature in the venules and capillaries of the major organs. *P. falciparum* invades RBCs of any age and, for this reason, often exhibits

the highest parasitemia—reaching 50% in some cases. The ring forms of *P. falciparum* (Figure 28-32, *A*) are more delicate than those of other species and often have two chromatin dots. Appliqué forms, parasites at the edge of the RBC, and multiple ring forms in a single RBC are common. In this figure, the appliqué form is seen in the lower left and upper right of the photograph. The mature trophozoite is small and compact and may have dark-brown pigment. The schizont has 8 to 36 merozoites, with an average of 20 to 24. Gametocytes have a characteristic banana or crescent shape (Figure 28-32, *B*).

Babesia microti

Babesia microti is an intraerythrocytic, zoonotic parasite causing infections in humans. *Babesia* spp. had been known to infect cattle and other animals, but the first cases reported in humans occurred in the 1950s. These initial cases were limited to patients who had undergone splenectomy, but since then, cases of babesiosis have been reported in patients who are not asplenic. The first documented cases in the United States were in the Martha's Vineyard and Nantucket Island area, where a hard tick (*Ixodes* spp.) served as the vector and the white-tailed deer as the host. White-footed mice are the usual reservoir host. There also have been reports indicating

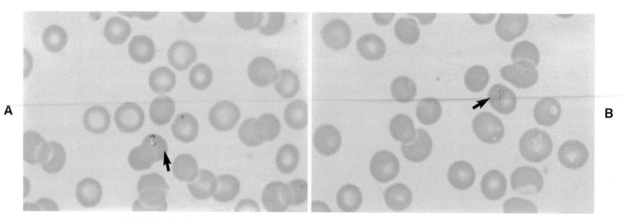

FIGURE 28-33 **A,** *Babesia microti* trophozoite. **B,** *B. microti* tetrad form.

simultaneous transmission of *B. microti* and *Borrelia burgdorferi* (the causative agent of Lyme disease) because these two organisms use the same tick vector.

Patients manifest clinical symptoms of one disease but show a concurrent rise and fall in antibody titers to both *Babesia* spp. and *B. burgdorferi*. There have been a number of cases of *B. microti*–like organisms isolated in Washington state (WA1) and California (CA1). Recently there have been reports of an organism in Missouri (MO1) and in Washington state that more closely resemble *Babesia divergens*, a parasite of cattle in Europe. As with malaria, cases of perinatal and transfusion-transmitted babesiosis have been reported. There are reports of more than 50 cases of transfusion-transmitted babesiosis, and many of these occurred in immunocompromised recipients. Efforts to develop methods to inactivate pathogens such as malaria and babesia have shown promise and are used in some European countries.

Clinical Infections. Most infections occur from May to September when outdoor activities peak and exposure to ticks is highest. Infection is often asymptomatic, but the very young, elderly, and immunosuppressed patients are likely to exhibit symptoms. Symptoms are related to the asexual reproductive cycle, lysis of RBCs, and the level of parasitemia. The time from infection to development of symptoms is 1 to 6 weeks. Patients with babesiosis may have malaria-like symptoms such as malaise, fever, chills, sweating, and myalgia; however, many cases are asymptomatic. The fever does not exhibit the cyclic nature seen in malaria. Anemia may develop if hemolysis is severe or prolonged. The clinical course tends to be more severe if the patient has undergone splenectomy, is immunosuppressed, or is elderly. Complications may include respiratory, liver, or renal failure or disseminated intravascular coagulation. Treatment with quinine sulfate and clindamycin is effective in eliminating the infection. Recently the use of azithromycin and atovaquone has been recommended.

Life Cycle. As with *Plasmodium* spp., the life cycle of *Babesia* spp. have alternating sexual and asexual reproduction stages. Production of the infective stage (sexual reproduction) takes place in the tick. The zygote migrates to the salivary glands of the tick where sporozoites are formed. These sporozoites enter mammals during a blood meal, infect RBCs,

become trophozoites, and divide by asexual reproduction. Merozoites are released to infect other RBCs. Some will differentiate into gametes, but this is not an identifiable stage from the asexual form. One difference in this life cycle from that of malaria is the lack of an exoerythrocytic cycle in humans. Transovarian transmission can occur in the tick, allowing the life cycle to persist without an intermediate host.

Laboratory Diagnosis. The diagnosis of babesiosis is made from a Wright- or Giemsa-stained thin blood smear. The organisms appear as small, delicate, ring-form trophozoites, about 1 to 2 µm in length, with a prominent chromatin dot and faintly staining cytoplasm. More mature trophozoites may appear as pyriform organisms in single, double, or the classic tetrad (Maltese cross) formation within the RBC. Figure 28-33, *A,* shows the small, compact, ringlike trophozoites of *B. microti*; Figure 28-33, *B,* demonstrates the tetrad formation characteristic of the organism. The morphology initially may be confused with that of *P. falciparum*. Lack of pigment, the presence of extraerythrocytic organisms, and absence of other life cycle stages serve as keys to differentiate *Babesia* from *P. falciparum*. Although they are characteristic for babesiosis, the tetrad forms are not always seen.

Serologic studies such as immunofluorescence assays can be used to detect circulating antibody. Titers greater than 1:64 are generally considered diagnostic. Although transfusion-transmitted babesiosis has been reported, there is no screening test for blood donors. Molecular methods to detect parasite DNA have been developed and may be used when there is a high suspicion of babesiosis but the smears remain negative.

Toxoplasma gondii

Toxoplasma gondii is an obligate intracellular parasite found in mammals worldwide. Serologic studies indicate that the rate of infection often varies from country to country. In the United States, more than 20% of the population shows serologic evidence of infection, but in parts of Europe the figures may be as high as 80%. Toxoplasmosis can present with a wide range of clinical symptoms and complications that are often related to the immunologic status of the patient. Whereas most immunocompetent individuals do not have serious infection, the most serious forms of the infection are found

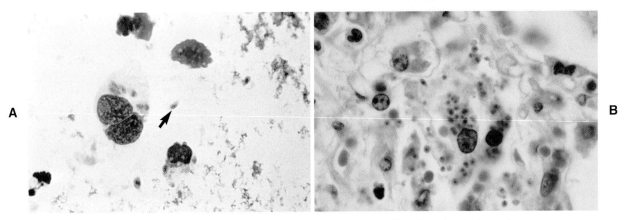

FIGURE 28-34 **A,** *Toxoplasma gondii* tachyzoites. **B,** *T. gondii* tachyzoites in lung tissue.

in HIV patients and in transplant patients. In addition, infants may contract the disease in utero and present with varying degrees of congenital problems.

Clinical Infections. The clinical presentation of toxoplasmosis varies based on the immunologic status of the individual. Immunocompetent patients with acute infections may be asymptomatic or may have mild flulike or mononucleosis-like symptoms, including low-grade fever, lymphadenopathy, malaise, and muscle pain. Once the acute infection has resolved, the organism enters a relatively inactive stage in which tissue cysts containing a large number of slowly growing forms of the organism are found.

The organism may also be transmitted congenitally due to a transient parasitemia in pregnant women who have a primary infection. Congenital transmission occurs when **tachyzoites** in the maternal circulation cross the placenta and enter the fetal circulation and tissues. Children who acquire *T. gondii* in this way may have a range of serious complications, including mental retardation, microcephaly, seizures, hydrocephalus, retinochoroiditis, and blindness. If the fetus is exposed to the infection early in the pregnancy, more severe complications are likely to result. Infections acquired later in pregnancy may result in the child being asymptomatic at birth but developing complications, especially ocular problems, later in childhood.

Immunosuppressed patients, particularly those with leukemia or lymphoma and those undergoing chemotherapy, may suffer from a serious primary infection or reactivation of a latent infection that may manifest as a fulminating encephalitis and result in rapid death. There are also a number of reports that up to 10% of the deaths of patients with AIDS are caused by reactivation of latent toxoplasmosis, resulting in encephalitis. Computed tomographic (CT) scans may demonstrate lesions in the brain that represent *Toxoplasma* spp. cysts. Pulmonary toxoplasmosis may be present in conjunction with the CNS infections or may be the presenting condition; however, the organism is capable of disseminating to any organ of the body. The organism can also be transmitted via organ transplantation. In this case, the organ may contain the tissue cysts with **bradyzoites** that reactivate in the immunocompromised recipient. This frequently occurs when the organ recipient is seronegative for *T. gondii* (lacks antibodies

to *T. gondii*) and the organ donor is seropositive. In these patients the infection usually occurs within the first 3 months after transplant and may disseminate to multiple organs. In the case of a seropositive organ transplant recipient, immunosuppressive treatment to prevent organ rejection may reactivate a latent infection in the transplant recipient.

In general toxoplasmosis in the immunocompetent host is not treated. When treatment is necessary, combinations of antimicrobials such as trimethoprim and sulfamethoxazole are used for the tachyzoite stage. The drugs are not effective against bradyzoites in cysts located in muscle and brain.

Life Cycle. *Toxoplasma gondii* has two life-cycle stages in human: the tachyzoite and the bradyzoite. Tachyzoites are capable of invading any nucleated cell and are the actively motile and reproducing forms. They are crescent shaped, 4 to 6 µm long, and have a prominent nucleus (Figure 28-34, *A*). Figure 28-34, *B* shows lung tissue containing free tachyzoites as well as a number of intracellular forms. Bradyzoites are the slowly growing and reproducing forms found within a cystlike structure during the dormant phase of the infection.

As shown in the life cycle illustrated in Figure 28-35, humans can acquire infection with *T. gondii* several ways: ingestion or inhalation of the oocyst from soil or water, ingestion of undercooked meat containing the cystlike structure containing bradyzoites, and congenital transmission. Primary risk factors for acquiring the infection include cleaning a cat litter box, gardening without gloves, and eating raw or undercooked meat or unwashed vegetables and fruit. The household cat and other members of the family Felidae serve as definitive hosts for the organism. Sexual and asexual reproduction occur in the intestine of the cat, whereas only asexual reproduction occurs in humans and other intermediate hosts. The result of sexual reproduction is the production of an oocyst, which is passed in cat feces. The oocyst requires 2 to 5 days in the environment to mature and become infective.

When a human ingests the infective oocyst, sporozoites in the oocyst are liberated in the intestine, penetrate the intestinal wall, gain access to the circulation, and migrate to the organs. These tachyzoites, as they are now called, are responsible for tissue destruction. They invade cells, multiply, cause cells to rupture, and release tachyzoites to invade other cells. The immune system, in particular T cells, responds strongly

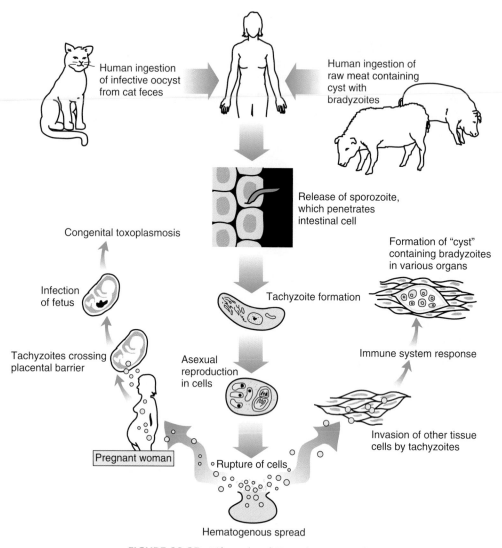

Human ingestion of infective oocyst from cat feces

Human ingestion of raw meat containing cyst with bradyzoites

Release of sporozoite, which penetrates intestinal cell

Congenital toxoplasmosis

Formation of "cyst" containing bradyzoites in various organs

Infection of fetus

Tachyzoite formation

Tachyzoites crossing placental barrier

Asexual reproduction in cells

Immune system response

Pregnant woman

Rupture of cells

Invasion of other tissue cells by tachyzoites

Hematogenous spread

FIGURE 28-35 Life cycle of *Toxoplasma gondii.*

when tachyzoites invade the tissues. This immune response results in formation of a large cystlike structure. As a result of this immune response, the tachyzoites convert to bradyzoites, and eventually the cystlike structure contains hundreds to thousands of the slowly growing and reproducing bradyzoites. At this point, the infection generally remains dormant for the life of the host unless the immune system is compromised. In the immunocompromised patient, the bradyzoites are released from the cyst and become active tachyzoites that invade multiple organs, resulting in disseminated infection.

If a human ingests raw or undercooked meat containing the tissue cysts, the cyst wall is dissolved and bradyzoites are liberated. Studies show that these organisms are resistant to digestive tract enzymes for about 6 hours, during which time they convert to tachyzoites and invade the intestinal wall. They then gain access to the circulation and subsequently invade various organs. All types of meat, including lamb, pork, beef, and game animals such as deer and bear, have been implicated in this mechanism.

Laboratory Diagnosis. Identification of the tachyzoite or pseudocysts with bradyzoites in tissue is very difficult,

because no single organ is invaded. Finding free tachyzoites in CSF, bronchoalveolar lavage specimens, or other sites such as lymph nodes is unusual unless the infection is disseminated. Antibodies to the organism show a rapid rise during infection, and tests for antibodies are most commonly used for diagnosis. The Sabin-Feldman dye test was the first antibody test developed but is not used in clinical laboratories because it requires live organisms. Indirect fluorescent antibody tests and EIAs using *T. gondii* organisms as antigen are routinely used for diagnosis.

Because most people have developed an antibody titer to the organism, interpretation of the titer must be linked to clinical symptoms and the patient's history. A significant rise in titer (fourfold) between acute and convalescent specimens may indicate acute infection. An IgM-specific test may also be used to diagnose acute infections and can be useful in the diagnosis of toxoplasmosis in pregnant women suspected of having been exposed to the organism or in neonates in whom congenital infection is suspected. IgM titers usually peak within the first month of infection. Antibody titers may be unreliable in immunocompromised patients, because these patients lack the ability to produce sufficient antibody to cause a significant rise in titer. In disseminated toxoplasmosis, histologic stains of biopsy materials may demonstrate the cyst with bradyzoites, or, in some cases, the tachyzoites. Noninvasive technology, such as magnetic resonance imaging (MRI) and CT scans, may be used in the diagnosis of patients suspected of having disseminated toxoplasmosis. PCR assays to detect *T. gondii* DNA may be used for CSF or amniotic fluid and are useful in detecting congenital infection in utero. Molecular methods are also being used in bone marrow transplant patients to detect infection.

Opportunistic Intestinal Apicomplexa

Cryptosporidium parvum and *Isospora belli* have been recognized as organisms that cause self-limiting gastrointestinal infection in the immunocompetent host. Both organisms, however, have also been identified as opportunistic pathogens in immunocompromised hosts, particularly those with AIDS. *Cyclospora cayetanensis* was initially seen in immunocompetent hosts with a history of travel to specific areas in which the organism is endemic. Recently, prolonged and more severe infections have been seen in individuals who are immunocompromised. All of these organisms are transmitted by the fecal-oral route, and sexual and asexual reproduction occurs in the human intestinal tract.

Cryptosporidium parvum. *Cryptosporidium* spp. are recognized animal parasites that were initially identified as zoonotic infections in veterinarians and other animal handlers. Along with *Giardia* these organisms account for the majority of outbreaks caused by waterborne parasites. Outbreaks in daycare centers and from environmental contamination of municipal water supplies have been reported. *Cryptosporidium* spp. are obligate intracellular parasites transmitted by ingestion of the infective oocyst. In the 1980s, cryptosporidiosis was identified as a major opportunistic infection in patients with AIDS. The primary organism associated with human outbreaks is *C. parvum*. The oocysts are infective at a low dose (as few as 10 oocysts) and are resistant to common chlorine- and ammonia-based disinfectants.

Clinical Infections. In immunocompetent patients, *C. parvum* causes a transient profuse, watery diarrhea along with mild to severe nausea and vomiting, headache, and cramps. The mucosa is inflamed, and there is an influx of segmented neutrophils, macrophages, and lymphocytes. The onset is rapid (within 3 to 7 days after ingestion of the oocyst), but the infection is self-limiting. Symptoms resolve in several weeks, although infections can last up to a month. Infection begins in the small intestine but may spread to the large intestine. Antibodies (IgG, IgA, and IgM) are produced, but it is not clear how much of a role they play in control. In addition, the host mounts a cell-mediated immune response that includes production of several cytokines. The organism alters osmotic pressure in the gut, with a resulting influx of fluid. The diarrhea is cholera-like, with bits of mucus and little fecal material. Fluid loss has been reported to range from 3 to 6 L/day to as much as 17 L/day. In addition to weight loss, patients show signs of dehydration and electrolyte imbalance. In patients with AIDS whose cell-mediated immunity is compromised and whose CD4 count is less than 50 cells/mL, the

infection is more likely to become fulminant or life threatening or disseminate to extraintestinal sites.

In chronic cases, the intestinal villi may show signs of atrophy due to inflammation, and the brush border of the cells is disrupted due to invasion by the organism. This damage alters intestinal permeability and can result in decreased uptake of fluids, electrolytes, and nutrients. Malabsorption syndrome may occur. No antimicrobial is completely effective against this infection. Paromomycin and azithromycin, which can suppress the infection, have been used with mixed results. Nitazoxanide, which is a relatively new agent, has been used for *Giardia* and *Cryptosporidium* infection in children and may also be effective in adults.

Life Cycle. The sexual and asexual life cycles of *C. parvum* occur in the same host. Life cycle stages, as shown in Figure 28-36, develop under the brush border of the intestinal mucosal epithelial cells. Oocysts are infective when passed and may be ingested in contaminated water or food or passed by person-to-person contact. Ingestion of the infective oocyst initiates the asexual cycle (sporogony) with release of sporozoites. These attach to receptors on the intestinal mucosal border, penetrate cells, and mature into trophozoites. Once trophozoites have matured, the development of meronts with merozoites begins. The nucleus and cytoplasm divide to form individual organisms known as merozoites. When the meront ruptures, merozoites are released and penetrate other cells, either to continue asexual reproduction or to transform into a gamete, either a microgamete or a macrogamete. Fertilization of the macrogamete results in formation of the oocyst, which contains four sporozoites. Two types of oocysts may be formed—the thin-walled oocyst, which ruptures within the intestine and results in autoinfection, and the thick-walled oocyst, which is infective when passed in the stool. Key factors in the life cycle of this organism that contribute to its pathogenicity include the following:

- The oocysts are infective when passed.
- Rupture of thin-walled oocysts in the intestine creates the potential for continual autoinfection.
- Patients may remain infective and continue to shed oocysts for a time after the diarrhea ceases.

Laboratory Diagnosis. The small size (4 to 6 μm), refractile appearance, and round shape of the oocyst make detection difficult with routine concentration procedures because the organism may resemble a yeast or RBC. More oocysts are seen in a liquid stool than in a formed stool. The Sheather sugar flotation method improved detection of *C. parvum*, but other intestinal parasites are not easily identified using this method. In addition, one study showed that concentration of a stool by the FES method may lead to a significant decrease in the number of oocysts seen. Another concentration method involving use of the traditional FES method and subsequent overlay of sediment with saturated sodium chloride has been described. This method improves the recovery rate of oocysts.

Trichrome and iron hematoxylin stains are not useful permanent stains for identification of *Cryptosporidium* spp. The recommended detection methods when *Cryptosporidium* infection is suspected are the modified acid-fast stain and a direct fluorescent antibody test using a monoclonal antibody directed against *Cryptosporidium* spp. With the acid-fast

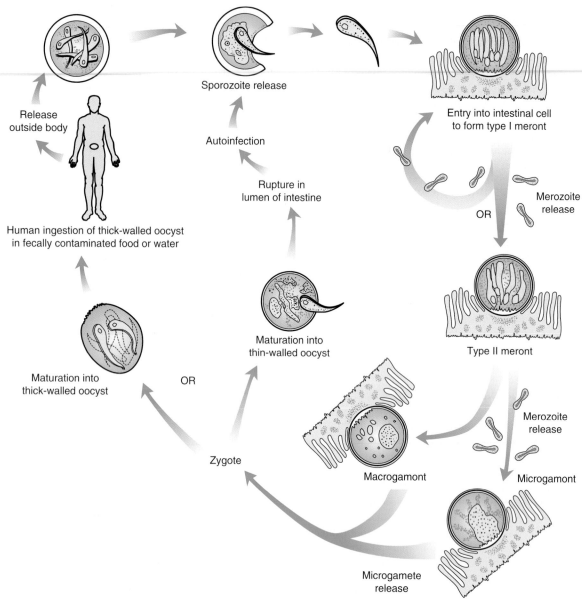

FIGURE 28-36 Life cycle of *Cryptosporidium* sp.

stain, the organism stains as a bright red sphere, which distinguishes it from yeasts, which stain green. Figure 28-37 shows an acid-fast stain of *Cryptosporidium* spp. Studies indicate that the monoclonal antibody test demonstrates greater sensitivity and specificity than the modified acid-fast stain. EIA methods can also be used but are less sensitive than fluorescent antibody methods. Methods such as flow cytometry are being investigated as a means to detect low number of oocysts in a stool specimen. Although biopsy specimens initially were required to identify life cycle stages, they are not routinely used for laboratory diagnosis.

Isospora belli. *Isospora belli* is an opportunistic organism seen less frequently than *C. parvum*. Acute infections with *I. belli* are usually clinically indistinguishable from those with *Cryptosporidium* spp. Most patients infected with *I. belli* are asymptomatic, but symptoms such as low-grade fever, headache, diarrhea, and colicky abdominal pain may be present.

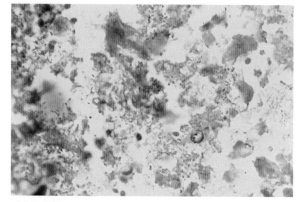

FIGURE 28-37 *Cryptosporidium* oocysts (modified acid-fast stain).

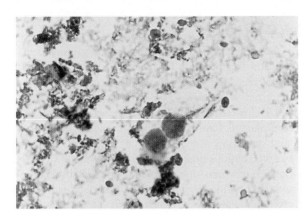

FIGURE 28-38 *Isospora belli* oocysts (modified acid-fast stain).

The infection is self-limiting and usually resolves in several weeks in an immunocompetent host. The infection is often more serious in immunocompromised patients including those with AIDS as well as those with conditions such as Hodgkin disease, lymphoproliferative disorders, or lymphoblastic leukemia. These patients may have watery diarrhea and concurrent weight loss or develop a chronic infection. Treatment with trimethoprim-sulfamethoxazole has been effective in eliminating diarrhea, but patients often show recurrence of infection when therapy is discontinued.

The life cycle of *I. belli* is similar to that of *Cryptosporidium* spp. but occurs within the cytoplasm of epithelial cells of the small intestine. The oocyst of this organism is not infective when passed in the feces and requires 24 to 48 hours outside the body before it is infective. There is no thin-walled oocyst to cause continued autoinfection. The mature oocyst of *I. belli* is oval, 20 to 33 μm by 10 to 19 μm, with a hyaline cell wall. The immature oocyst usually shows a single **sporoblast;** the mature oocyst has two **sporocysts,** with four elongated sporozoites within each. Both may be seen in wet mounts.

The modified acid-fast stain has been used to detect *I. belli.* The oocyst wall does not stain but often shows a faint outline owing to precipitated stain, and the sporoblasts or sporocysts stain dark red. Like oocysts of *Cyclospora cayetanensis,* the oocysts of *I. belli* will autofluoresce a bluish color at 365 nm and a bright green at 405 nm. Size and shape of the oocyst serve as the identification characteristics in this examination. Figure 28-38 shows the characteristic appearance of an acid-fast stain of the oocyst of *I. belli.*

Cyclospora cayetanensis. *Cyclospora cayetanensis* is another food-borne and waterborne organism implicated as a cause of endemic and epidemic diarrheal disease. Humans are the only known host for this organism, but other *Cyclospora* spp. are found in animals. The organism was first linked to human disease in the 1990s when it was found in human stool specimens. It was originally thought to be a *Cyanobacterium*-like body, blue-green algae, or large *C. parvum.*

Cyclospora cayetanensis is endemic in Nepal, Peru, and Haiti, but outbreaks have been reported in many countries, including those in Central and South America, parts of the Caribbean, India, and Europe. The usual mode of transmission is ingestion of fecally contaminated water or food. Most outbreaks in endemic areas occur during the rainy season. Persons living in these areas may acquire some level of immunity that increases resistance to future infection. Individuals who travel to endemic areas are susceptible to "traveler's diarrhea" caused by *C. cayetanensis.* The organism has also been linked to several large food-borne outbreaks in North America. Most of the outbreaks were associated with the consumption of contaminated fresh fruit, especially raspberries and strawberries imported from endemic areas of Central America. Subsequently, there have been isolated outbreaks associated with imported vegetables such as basil and snow peas. The infective dose is not known.

Although the organism is most commonly encountered in immunocompetent patients, it may be considered an opportunistic infection in patients with AIDS. Symptoms of infection with *C. cayetanensis* may vary based on age, infective dose, and host immune status. The incubation period is approximately 1 week. The organism infects cells in the upper portion of the small intestine and causes frequent, watery, but nonbloody stools that may alternate with bouts of constipation. Symptoms, which may mimic those of cryptosporidiosis or isosporiasis, include anorexia, weight loss, abdominal cramping and bloating, vomiting, low-grade fever, and nausea. Patients often report a flulike syndrome before the onset of diarrhea. In immunocompetent hosts, the symptoms are self-limiting and persist for several weeks, but may occur in a relapsing pattern for up to 2 months. Immunocompromised patients suffer a prolonged course and may be symptomatic for as long as 4 months. Some cases of malabsorption due to inflammation and damage to the intestinal villi and a few cases of extraintestinal infection have occurred in immunocompromised patients. Trimethoprim-sulfamethoxazole is used to treat the infection, and once treatment is started, symptoms usually abate within several days. In endemic areas, individuals may acquire a low level of immunity that increases resistance to infection.

The organism shares the general life cycle characteristics of other intestinal Apicomplexa. Once the mature oocyst has been ingested, the presence of bile and trypsin in the small intestine helps trigger release of sporozoites which invade the intestinal cells. Two types of meronts develop: type I, which produce merozoites that infect other intestinal cells (asexual cycle), and type II merozoites, which develop into sexual stages. Once fertilization occurs, a zygote forms and develops into an immature oocyst that is passed in the stool. Unlike *C. parvum,* however, immediate person-to-person transmission is unusual because these oocysts require about 1 to 2 weeks outside the body to mature and become infective.

The oocyst is similar to that of *C. parvum* but larger, with an average size of 8 to 10 μm. In wet mounts the oocyst appears nonrefractile, spherical, and unsporulated with multiple internal globules or granules. Sporulation occurs after several days, resulting in the production of two sporocysts with two sporozoites each. The organism does not stain with traditional trichrome or iron hematoxylin stains. The modified acid-fast stain demonstrates variably staining organisms, from dark pink to almost colorless, with no visible internal structures. One distinguishing characteristic of *C. cayetanen-*

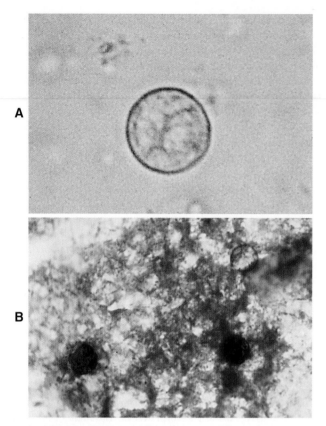

FIGURE 28-39 *Cyclospora cayetanensis* oocyst. **A,** Wet mount. **B,** Modified acid-fast stain.

sis is its autofluorescence. *C. cayetanensis* shows a bright blue fluorescence (365 nm) or mint green (450 to 490 nm) under ultraviolet light. Flow cytometry methods to screen large numbers of specimens are being developed. Figure 28-39, *A* shows an oocyst of *C. cayetanensis* in a wet mount, and Figure 28-39, *B* is an acid-fast stain.

Microsporidia

In the mid-1980s, a group of organisms in the phylum Microspora were linked to infections in patients who were infected with HIV. These organisms, collectively referred to as microsporidia, are obligate intracellular parasites common to invertebrates and other animals. Originally considered protists, based on the chitin present in the spore wall and rRNA sequencing they have been reclassified as fungi or to a kingdom related to the fungi. Only seven (*Nosema, Vittiforma, Encephalitozoon, Pleistophora, Brachiola, Trachipleistophora,* and *Enterocytozoon*) of the more than 150 genera have been implicated in human infections. While infection with the organisms is often linked to HIV infection, microsporidia have been identified in organ transplant patients, the elderly, and patients with traveler's diarrhea. The organisms are capable of infecting a wide variety of human organs including eyes, muscles, liver, kidneys, and the CNS. Intestinal infections are most often caused by *Enterocytozoon bieneusi* or *Encephalitozoon intestinalis*. Disseminated infections have also been reported. Unclassified organisms usually are referred to with the encompassing term microsporidia.

Clinical Infections

Symptoms vary with the species and organ infected. *E. bieneusi* and *E. intestinalis* both commonly infect the gastrointestinal tract, and infection in immunocompetent hosts is characterized by diarrhea, cramps, loss of appetite, and fatigue. Dehydration and weight loss are sometimes seen. Infected patients have four to eight liquid or loose stools a day, and symptoms may persist up to 8 months with spontaneous exacerbations and remissions. In patients with AIDS, the diarrhea may persist several years with malabsorption and cachexia as additional complications. Risk factors in patients with AIDS include sexual transmission, a CD4 count of less than 100 cells/μL, exposure to water by swimming, and contact with animals. Dissemination of *E. intestinalis* especially to the urinary tract, gallbladder, or respiratory tract has been seen. Dissemination to muscles may result in weakness and pain. Patients with AIDS may develop encephalitis, nephritis, or keratoconjunctivitis. Albendazole has been used to treat infections with *Encephalitozoon* spp., but most other microsporidial organisms are resistant to this and other drugs. Metronidazole may provide some relief, but the symptoms recur once the drug is discontinued.

Life Cycle

The infective stage for humans is the environmentally resistant spore. Once the infective spore is ingested, it gains access to host cells by inserting a coiled tube (polar tube or polar filament) through the cell membrane. The contents of the spore (sporoplasm) are then transferred into the cell. Within the cell, the sporoplasm divides and develops into meronts (proliferating forms). These structures subsequently develop into sporoblasts that differentiate into sporonts. As these structures mature into spores, they develop a thick membrane and the polar tube. The host cell ruptures, and spores are released to penetrate other host cells to repeat the reproductive cycle or to be passed out of the body. In the case of intestinal infection, spores are passed in the feces; in infection of the urinary tract they can be detected in urine. There is evidence that the spore might also gain access to the host cell by endocytosis and then discharge contents into the cell through the polar filament.

Laboratory Diagnosis

Initially, identification methods were limited to finding the small spores in Giemsa-stained tissue sections or in electron microscopic examination of biopsy specimens. Electron microscopy must be used to identify the species of the organism. Speciation is based on the number of coils in the polar tubule, septations in the spore, and size. Routine ova and parasite examination will not detect the spores in a fecal specimen. However, staining of formalin-preserved feces using the Weber modification of the trichrome stain and the Ryan trichrome blue stain can be used to detect microsporidial spores. The small size of the spores, however, makes them easy to overlook in clinical specimens. A thin smear of feces must be used so that debris does not obscure the small, faintly staining spores. Figure 28-40 shows the small spores (1.5 to 4.0 μm) in a chromotrope stain of a fecal specimen. Spores stain pink-

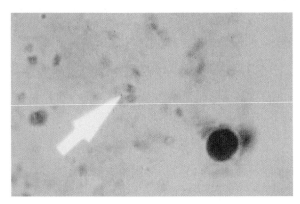

FIGURE 28-40 Microsporidia spores (chromotrope stain). (Courtesy Texas Department of Health.)

red and may have a diagonal or equatorial band that helps distinguish them from bacteria or yeast. Background staining in Weber stain is pale green, whereas in Ryan stain it is blue. A Gram-chromotrope stain will produce spores that are dark violet and demonstrate an equatorial band.

Calcofluor white, a fluorescent stain used for detection of fungi, can also be used to screen for microsporidia spores. The stain is a chemofluorescent agent, such as calcofluor white M2R (American Cyanamid Corp., Princeton, N.J.) or Fungi-Fluor (Polysciences, Inc., Washington, Pa.). The stain is nonspecific and binds to the chitin in the spore wall. Therefore, the presence of spores should be confirmed using one of the modified trichrome stains. Species-specific indirect fluorescent antibody staining is useful to identify spores in fluids such as urine or in biopsy specimens. There are also species-specific PCR assays for identification.

Helminths

Helminth infections in humans are caused by flukes, tapeworms, or roundworms. Humans may become infected by directly ingesting the egg, by ingesting larvae in an intermediate host, or through direct larval penetration of skin. Adult forms do not multiply in the human body; therefore the number of adult worms present is related to the number of eggs or larvae ingested. The pathologic consequences and severity of infection are related to the number of adults present, commonly referred to as the worm burden. Patients with only a few adult worms are usually asymptomatic, whereas a patient with a large number of adults shows clinical symptoms. Most of the parasites inhabit the intestinal tract, but species also infect the liver, lungs, lymphatics, and blood vessels.

Flukes

Flukes (trematodes) are members of the phylum Platyhelminthes, or flatworms. Most infections are seen in people from East Asia, Africa, South America, and some areas of the Caribbean. Adults can range in size from several millimeters to almost 8 cm. With the exception of the blood flukes, adult flukes are dorsoventrally flattened and have an oral sucker at the anterior end and a ventral sucker located midline,

posterior to the anterior sucker. Also, except for the blood flukes, flukes are hermaphroditic.

Figure 28-41 shows a generalized life cycle of the liver, lung, and intestinal flukes. In all species eggs must reach water to mature, and all have a snail species as the first intermediate host. The miracidium (first-stage larva) is ingested by a snail while within the egg or is released from eggs and penetrates the snail. Within the snail, a complex development of germinal tissue occurs, resulting first in sporocysts, which contain undifferentiated germinal structures, and then in rediae, which contain partially differentiated germinal material. The **cercaria** (second-stage larva) develops within the redia and is released into the water. The cercaria then attaches to aquatic vegetation or invades the flesh of aquatic organisms. At this stage the organism is referred to as a **metacercaria** and is infective for humans. With the exception of the schistosomes, which infect humans by direct cercarial penetration, infection occurs when an individual ingests the metacercaria in raw or undercooked aquatic animals or on water vegetation. Prevention includes adequate cooking of water vegetation, fish, and crustaceans. In the case of the blood flukes, individuals should wear clothing and shoes to prevent cercarial penetration.

The egg is the primary diagnostic stage. It is best detected on a wet mount of a concentrated specimen. Routine concentration procedures for feces, such as FES, may be used. The zinc sulfate method is not satisfactory, however, because all eggs except those of schistosomes are operculated. With the zinc sulfate method, the operculum may open and release the contents or cause the egg to sink. Table 28-7 shows a comparison of the characteristics of the fluke eggs.

Intestinal Flukes. *Fasciolopsis buski,* known as the giant intestinal fluke, is found in the Far East, including China, Vietnam, and India. Dogs and pigs may serve as reservoir hosts. Humans acquire the infection by ingesting metacercaria on freshwater vegetation such as bamboo shoots and water chestnuts. Adults of *F. buski* live in the duodenum, where they cause mechanical and toxic damage. Inflammation and ulceration of the mucosa may be present. Heavy infections may result in persistent diarrhea, anorexia, edema, ascites, nausea and vomiting, or intestinal obstruction.

Finding the adult or egg is diagnostic, although the egg is more commonly seen. The adult is flattened, is 2 to 7 cm long, and lacks the cephalic cone seen in *Fasciola hepatica*. Adults are usually not seen in a stool sample unless it is a purged specimen. Eggs are yellow-brown, average 130 to 140 μm by 80 to 85 μm, and have a small, relatively inconspicuous operculum. They are unembryonated when passed (Figure 28-42). These eggs are identical to those of *F. hepatica* and when seen should be reported as *F. buski/F. hepatica* eggs.

Metagonimus yokogawai and *Heterophyes heterophyes* are two small flukes found in the Far East and Mideast. Humans acquire infection with these organisms by ingesting the metacercaria in undercooked or raw fish. Adults live in the small intestine and produce few symptoms. A patient with a heavy worm burden may have diarrhea, colic, and stools with a large amount of mucus. Adults of both species are small (1 to 2 mm) and delicate. Eggs serve as the primary diagnostic stage. They are 28 to 30 μm long and have a vase or flask shape. They are embryonated and operculated with incon-

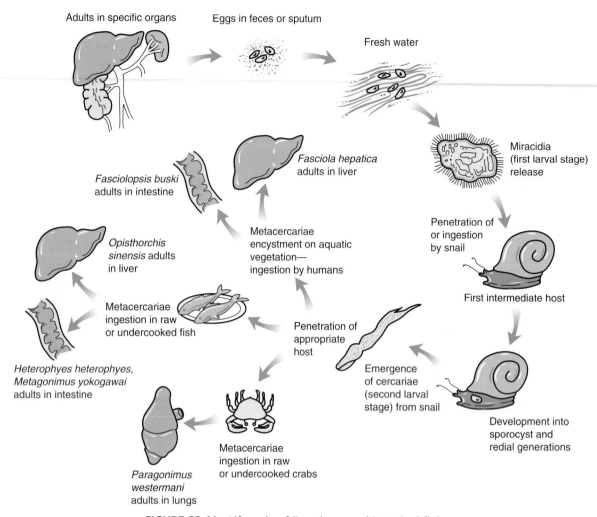

Adults in specific organs

Eggs in feces or sputum

Fresh water

Fasciola hepatica
adults in liver

Fasciolopsis buski
adults in intestine

Miracidia
(first larval stage)
release

Metacercariae
encystment on aquatic
vegetation—
ingestion by humans

*Opisthorchis
sinensis* adults
in liver

Penetration of
or ingestion
by snail

First intermediate host

Metacercariae
ingestion in raw
or undercooked fish

Penetration of
appropriate
host

Emergence
of cercariae
(second larval
stage) from snail

*Heterophyes heterophyes,
Metagonimus yokogawai*
adults in intestine

Development into
sporocyst and
redial generations

Metacercariae
ingestion in raw
or undercooked crabs

*Paragonimus
westermani*
adults in lungs

FIGURE 28-41 Life cycle of liver, lung, and intestinal flukes.

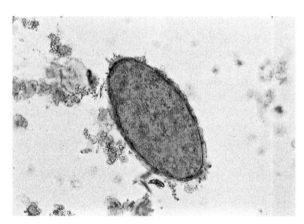

FIGURE 28-42 *Fasciola hepatica/Fasciolopsis buski* egg.

spicuous shoulders at the operculum. Eggs of these species resemble each other as well as those of *Clonorchis sinensis*.

Liver Flukes. *Fasciola hepatica,* the sheep liver fluke, is seen in the major sheep-raising areas of the world, including parts of the southwestern United States. In addition, the organism is found in some cattle-raising areas. In sheep, the organism causes a disease known as liver rot, which is char-

acterized by destruction of the liver. Humans acquire the infection by ingesting metacercaria on raw water vegetation, especially watercress. The larvae reach the liver by migrating through the intestinal wall and peritoneal cavity. Adults live in the biliary passages and gallbladder and rarely cause overt symptoms because infections are light. Tissue damage during migration through the liver may result in eosinophilia, an inflammatory reaction, secondary infection, and fibrosis in the biliary ducts. Heavy infections may induce diarrhea, upper right quadrant abdominal pain, hepatomegaly, cirrhosis, and liver obstruction, with resulting jaundice. Chronic infections are usually asymptomatic.

Adults are approximately 3 cm long and have a prominent cephalic cone. The unembryonated and operculated eggs are carried in the bile to the intestinal tract and are passed in the feces. The size range is 130 to 150 μm × 60 to 90 μm. They are virtually indistinguishable from eggs of *F. buski* (see Figure 28-42). As mentioned previously, eggs that have these characteristics should be reported as "*F. buski/F. hepatica* eggs seen."

The Chinese liver fluke, *Clonorchis* (also known as *Opisthorchis*) *sinensis*, is geographically limited to the Far East, where dogs and cats serve as reservoir hosts. The adults live

TABLE 28-7 Comparisons of Fluke Eggs

Organism	Average Size (μm) and Shape	Other Identifying Features
Fasciola hepatica	130 × 60-90 Ellipsoidal	Small, indistinct operculum Yellow-brown color Unembryonated when passed
Fasciolopsis buski	130 × 80-85 Ellipsoidal	Cannot be distinguished from *F. hepatica* Unembryonated when passed
Paragonimus westermani	80-118 × 48-60 Oval	Brown, thick shell Slightly flattened operculum Shoulders at operculum Unembryonated when passed
Clonorchis sinensis	29-35 × 12-19 Vase shaped	Domed operculum Prominent shoulders Knob at end opposite operculum Embryonated when passed
Heterophyes heterophyes and *Metagonimus yokogawai* Note: These two species, and *C. sinesis*, are virtually indistinguishable.	28-30 × 15-17 Vase shaped	Operculated Shoulders not distinct Small knob Embryonated Similar to *C. sinensis*
Schistosoma mansoni	115-175 × 45-75 Oval	Lateral spine No operculum Embryonated when passed
Schistosoma haematobium	110-170 × 40-70 Oval	Rounded anterior Terminal spine Embryonated when passed
Schistosoma japonicum	60-95 × 40-60 Round to slightly oval	Small, inconspicuous, hooked lateral spine Embryonated when passed

in the distal bile ducts. As with *F. hepatica*, light infections produce few or no symptoms. Repeated or heavy infections may cause inflammation due to mechanical irritation, fever, diarrhea, pain, fibrotic changes, or obstruction of the bile duct. Humans acquire the infection by ingesting the metacercaria in raw, undercooked, or pickled fish. The diagnosis is made by finding the egg in a stool specimen or, occasionally, in duodenal aspirates. Adults are thin, tapered at both ends, and 1 to 2.5 cm long. The egg is 29 to 35 μm long, embryonated when passed, flask shaped, and operculated with promi-

nent shoulders at the operculum and a knob at the opposite end (Figure 28-43).

Lung Flukes. Organisms of the genus *Paragonimus* usually infect tigers, leopards, dogs, and foxes. *P. westermani*, the lung fluke, is found primarily in Southeast Asia and in focal areas of Latin America and Africa. Humans acquire the infection by ingesting metacercariae in raw, pickled, wine-soaked, or undercooked freshwater crabs or crayfish. The metacercaria excysts in the small intestine and burrows through the duodenal wall into the peritoneal cavity. It even-

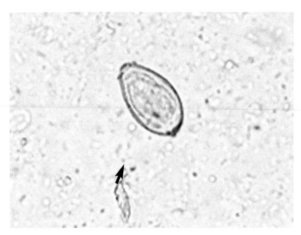

FIGURE 28-43 *Clonorchis sinensis* egg.

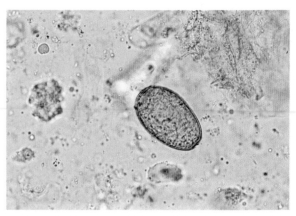

FIGURE 28-44 *Paragonimus westermani* egg.

tually penetrates the diaphragm and enters the lung. The host shows few symptoms during this migration but may exhibit intermittent coughing and chest pain. Within the lung the parasite induces an inflammatory response characterized by the presence of neutrophils and eosinophils. Major symptoms associated with lung habitation are nonspecific and may include persistent cough, chest pain, and hemoptysis. Adults, which are reddish brown and approximately 1 cm long, live within capsules in the bronchioles.

Sputum is the primary diagnostic specimen. Eggs are expelled from the capsule into the bronchioles and carried upward in the sputum. Eggs may be found in the feces if they have been coughed up and subsequently swallowed. Eggs are broadly oval, 80 to 118 μm × 48 to 60 μm, with a flattened operculum and slight shoulders. They are unembryonated when passed. The shell thickens at the end opposite the operculum (Figure 28-44). These eggs can appear similar to those of *Diphyllobothrium latum* and must be carefully examined when seen in the feces. A wet mount of sputum demonstrates the egg in some patients.

Blood Flukes. The blood flukes, *Schistosoma* spp., differ from other flukes:

- There is both a male and a female form; the female lives in an involuted chamber, the gynecophoral canal, which extends the length of the male.
- The eggs are unoperculated.
- Humans are infected by direct cercarial penetration of the skin.
- They have a cylindrical shape rather than being dorsoventrally flattened.

The three primary species of schistosomes pathogenic to humans are *Schistosoma mansoni, Schistosoma haematobium,* and *Schistosoma japonicum.* Adults of the schistosomes measure 7 to 20 mm for males and 7 to 26 mm for females. *S. mansoni,* which is most commonly found in Africa, parts of South America, the West Indies, and Puerto Rico, lives in venules of the mesentery and large intestines. *S. japonicum,* which is commonly found in the Far East, including Japan, China, and the Philippines, lives in venules of the small intestine. This species, unlike the other two, has many mammalian reservoir hosts. *S. haematobium,* which is primarily found in the Nile Valley, the Mideast, and East Africa, lives in the veins

surrounding the bladder. Two additional species pathogenic for humans are *S. intercalatum* and *S. mekongi.*

Clinical Infections. Schistosomiasis (bilharziasis) affects approximately 200 million people worldwide and, after malaria, is the second most prevalent tropical disease. The term is used to describe symptoms caused by any of the schistosomes. Symptoms are related to the phases of the fluke's life cycle. Cercarial penetration may cause a self-limiting local dermatitis, including irritation, redness, and rash, that persists for approximately 3 days. Larval migration through the body causes generalized symptoms such as urticaria, fever, and malaise, which may last up to 4 weeks. The presence of the migrating larva and the adults causes little inflammatory damage because they acquire host human leukocyte antigens and ABO blood group antigens on their surface that diminish the host's immune response.

Egg production and egg migration through the tissues are responsible for most of the acute damage, as the eggs are highly immunogenic. After the adult female dilates the vein to lay eggs, the vein contracts, and aided by secretion of enzymes, the eggs begin to penetrate vessel walls and tissue. Eggs subsequently find their way into the lumen of the intestines or bladder. The egg spines cause trauma to the tissues and walls of the vessels during the early stage of acute infections and may result in hematuria *(S. haematobium)* or diarrhea *(S. mansoni* and *S. japonicum).* In some individuals, especially those heavily infected with *S. japonicum,* an acute serum-sickness–like illness (Katayama fever) occurs during the initial egg laying period. This is induced by antigenic response to the egg and is characterized by increased circulating immune complexes and eosinophils.

In chronic infections, the eggs remaining in the tissue induce an immune response resulting in granuloma formation, which leads to thickening and fibrotic changes. Scarring of the veins, development of ascites, pain, anemia, hypertension, hepatomegaly, and splenomegaly are also seen. In urinary schistosomiasis, microscopic bleeding into the urine is present during the acute phase. In chronic stages, dysuria, urine retention, and urinary tract infections are present.

Penetration of humans by cercariae of the flukes of birds and other mammals cause schistosomal dermatitis, commonly referred to as "swimmer's itch." Foreign proteins from

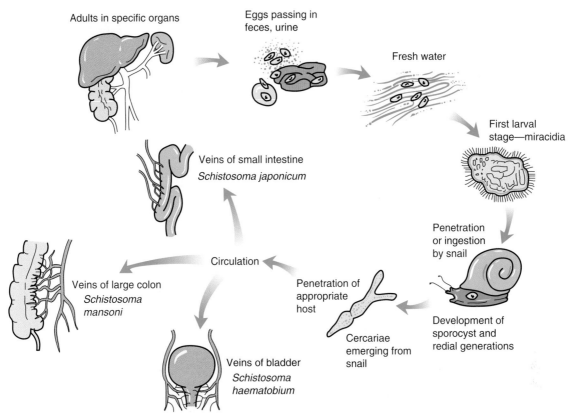

FIGURE 28-45 Life cycle of blood flukes (*Schistosoma* spp.).

these cercariae elicit a tissue reaction characterized by small papules 3 to 5 mm in diameter, edema, erythema, and intense itching. Symptoms last about a week and disappear as cercariae die and degenerate.

Life Cycle. The life cycles of all three schistosomes are identical (Figure 28-45). The eggs are embryonated when passed, and the miracidium is released when the egg reaches water. After the miracidium penetrates the snail (the first intermediate host), sporocysts and then cercariae are produced during a 6-week period. Cercariae migrate from the snail into water. Cercariae attach by oral and ventral suckers and, with the help of enzymes, are able to penetrate intact human skin. Once in the vasculature they shed their forked tails and are referred to as schistosomula. They circulate until they reach the lungs or enter the liver, where maturation and pairing of female and male is completed. The paired adult flukes use the portal system to reach veins of the intestine or bladder.

Laboratory Diagnosis. Diagnosis is made by finding embryonated eggs in the feces (*S. mansoni* and *S. japonicum*) or in the urine (*S. haematobium*). The egg of *S. mansoni* (Figure 28-46, *A*) is yellowish, elongated, and 115 to 175 μm × 45 to 75 μm and has a prominent lateral spine. *S. haematobium* eggs (Figure 28-46, *B*) are elongated and 110 to 170 μm × 40 to 70 μm and have a terminal spine. *S. japonicum* eggs (Figure 28-46, *C*), which resemble *S. mekongi* eggs, are round and 60 to 95 μm × 40 to 60 μm and have a small, curved, rudimentary spine. The best time to collect eggs in urinary schistosomiasis is during peak excretion time in early after-

noon (noon to 2 PM). Biopsies may also be used in the diagnosis of schistosomiasis. Serodiagnosis may be useful to diagnose infection in patients from nonendemic countries who develop symptoms after visiting endemic areas.

Tapeworms

Tapeworms (cestodes) are another group of human parasites in the phylum Platyhelminthes. They show a wide range of sizes, from 3 mm to 10 m, generally require intermediate hosts in their life cycle, and are hermaphroditic. They are ribbonlike organisms whose method of growth involves the addition of segments, called *proglottids.* Each proglottid, when mature, produces eggs that are infective for the intermediate host. Figure 28-47 shows a general diagram of the tapeworm. The **scolex** has suckers and, in some species, hooklets as a means of attachment to the intestinal mucosa. The neck is directly behind the scolex. Treatment is targeted at detaching the scolex from the mucosa, because the neck area is the origin of proglottid production. Gravid proglottids at the distal end of the organism contain eggs to be discharged into the feces.

Eggs of most of the tapeworms contain a **hexacanth embryo (oncosphere)** that is infective for the intermediate host. Transmission to humans involves ingestion either of a larval stage, called the **cysticercus,** cysticercoid, or plerocercoid larva (depending on the genus involved in infection) in raw or undercooked meat or fish or of insects harboring the larval stage. This larval stage contains an invaginated scolex of the tapeworm inside a protective membrane. The diagnosis of tapeworm infection is usually made by finding the eggs in

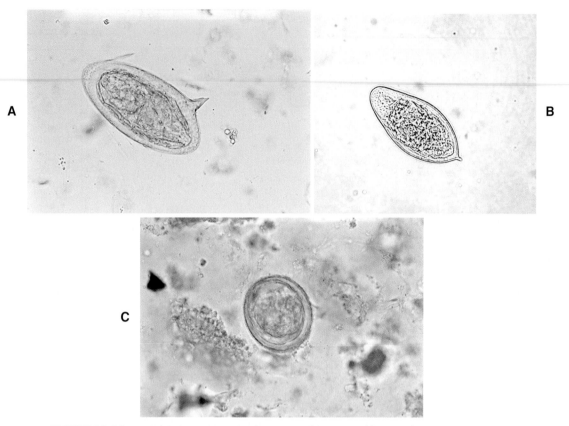

FIGURE 28-46   **A,** *Schistosoma mansoni* egg. **B,** *Schistosoma haematobium* egg. **C,** *Schistosoma japonicum* egg, unstained wet mounts.

feces, although proglottids can be used if passed intact. Table 28-8 presents a comparison of the characteristics of tapeworm eggs.

Diphyllobothrium latum. *Diphyllobothrium latum,* the fish tapeworm, is found worldwide in areas where the population eats pickled or raw freshwater fish. In the United States, it is primarily seen in the areas around the Great Lakes. Fish-eating mammals in endemic areas may also be infected. Humans usually harbor only a single worm, which attaches in the jejunum and may reach a length of up to 10 m. Most infected individuals demonstrate no clinical symptoms; others have vague gastrointestinal symptoms, including nausea and vomiting and intestinal irritation. The organism may cause a vitamin B_{12} deficiency, especially in persons of northern European descent, and long-term infection may lead to a megaloblastic anemia.

The life cycle of *D. latum* is somewhat of a hybrid between that of the flukes and that of the tapeworms. Figure 28-48 shows the life cycle of *D. latum.* The operculated, unembryonated egg, passed in human feces, must reach water to mature. The first larval stage (coracidium) is ingested by a copepod and develops into a procercoid larva within the copepod. When the infected copepod is ingested by a fish, the larva leaves the fish's intestine and invades the flesh, where it develops into a plerocercoid larva, which consists of a scolex with a thin, ribbon like portion of tissue. Humans ingest the plerocercoid larvae by eating raw or undercooked fish. The scolex is released in the intestine, where it develops into an adult worm.

The scolex, proglottid, and egg are diagnostic structures that can be found in a fecal specimen. The egg, however, is most commonly detected. The egg is unembryonated when passed, operculated, and yellow-brown (Figure 28-49). It is about 58 to 76 μm × 40 to 50 μm and has a small, knoblike protuberance at the end opposite the operculum. The knob may not be seen on all eggs, so size and lack of shoulders must be used to distinguish the egg from that of *Paragonimus westermani.* The proglottid is wider than it is long, with a characteristic rosette-shaped or coiled uterus. The scolex, which is 2 to 3 mm long, is elongated and has two sucking grooves, one located on the dorsal surface and the other on the ventral surface.

Taenia. Two *Taenia* spp. infect humans: *Taenia saginata,* the beef tapeworm, which is found primarily in beef-eating countries of the world, and *Taenia solium,* the pork tapeworm, which is found in areas of the world with a high consumption of pork, such as Latin America. Both organisms attach to the intestinal mucosa of the small intestine. Adults of *T. saginata* may reach a length of 10 m, whereas those of *T. solium* may reach only 7 m. Infection with the adult tapeworm of either species usually causes few clinical symptoms, although vague abdominal pain, indigestion, and loss of appetite may be present. The major complication of infection with *T. solium* is cysticercosis, in which the infected individual becomes the intermediate host and harbors the larvae in tissues. This infection is discussed in the section on tissue infections.

specimen. The egg is spherical to oval, measures 30 to 47 μm, and has a grayish color. The hexacanth embryo is contained within an inner membrane, and the area between the inner membrane and egg wall contains two polar thickenings from which four to eight polar filaments extend (Figure 28-53). Infection with *H. diminuta* is acquired by ingesting fleas that contain the infective cysticercoid. The adult tapeworm is 20 to 60 cm long. The egg, which must be distinguished from that of *H. nana*, is 50 to 75 μm, gray or straw colored, and oval. An inner membrane with inconspicuous polar thicken-

ings but no polar filaments surrounds the oncosphere (Figure 28-54).

Dipylidium caninum. Humans serve as accidental hosts for *Dipylidium caninum,* the dog tapeworm. Children are most often infected by ingesting fleas containing the larval stage. The resulting infections are usually asymptomatic. The proglottid may be seen in human feces and is characterized by its pumpkin seed shape, twin genitalia, and the presence of two genital pores, one on each side of the proglottid. The eggs are characteristically seen in packets of 15 to 25 eggs. Individual eggs are 20 to 40 μm and may resemble those of *Taenia* spp. (Figure 28-55).

Tissue Infections with Cestodes

Cysticercosis, sparganosis, and hydatid cyst disease are the major diseases caused by the tissue stage of tapeworms. They originate when a human accidentally becomes the intermediate host for the parasite.

Cysticercosis. Cysticercosis results when a human ingests the infective eggs of *T. solium,* the pork tapeworm thus becoming an intermediate host. The disease is endemic in areas of rural Latin America, Asia, and Africa. Contributing factors for infection include poor hygiene and sanitary habits that result in ingestion of food containing an infective egg, as well as residence in rural areas and hog raising. Once the egg is ingested, the hexacanth embryo is released into the intes-

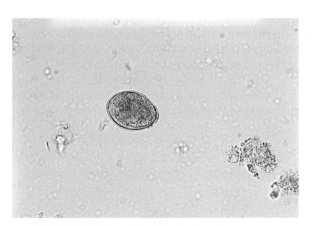

FIGURE 28-49 *Diphyllobothrium latum* egg.

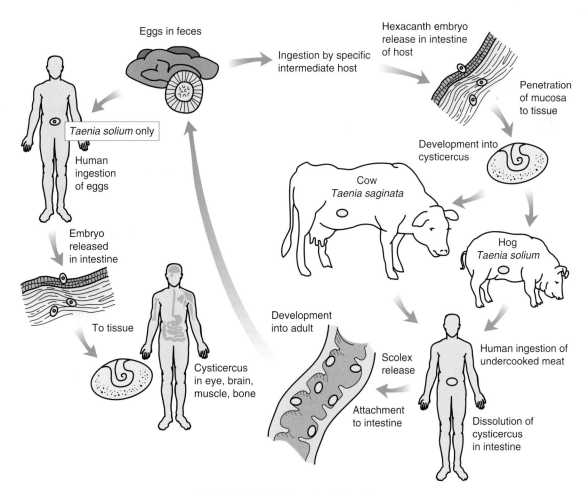

FIGURE 28-50 Life cycle of *Taenia* spp.

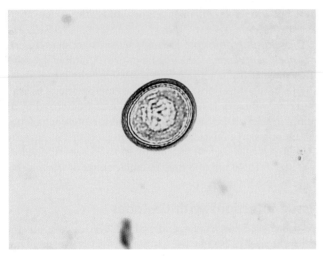

FIGURE 28-51 *Taenia* sp. ovum, unstained wet mount.

tines, penetrates the intestinal wall, and enters the circulation to develop as a cysticercus in any tissue or organ. The larva can live up to 7 years and elicits a host-tissue reaction, resulting in production of a fibrous capsule. However, once the organism dies and releases larval antigens, there is an intense host inflammatory reaction which leads to tissue damage in the area. Eventual calcification of the cysticercus will occur. The most commonly infected sites are striated muscle, the eye, and the brain.

Light infections usually cause no clinical symptoms. When present, symptoms depend on the organ affected and the size and number of cysticerci present. Muscular pain, weakness, and cramps characterize infections of the striated muscle. In the eye, a cysticercus forms in the vitreous or subretinal space. Retinal detachment, intraorbital pain, flashes of light, and blurred vision may occur. Neurocysticercosis which is the most serious manifestation, is the causative agent for up to 10% of neurologic problems seen in developing countries. In the United States, the condition is often seen in Hispanic

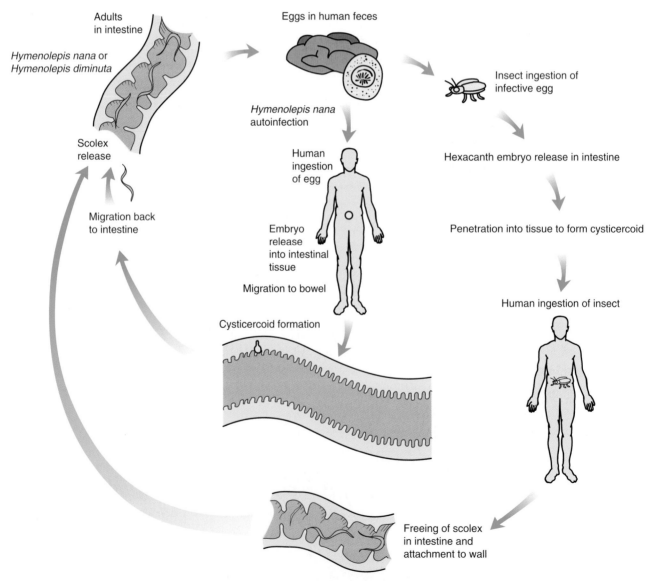

FIGURE 28-52 Life cycle of *Hymenolepis* spp.

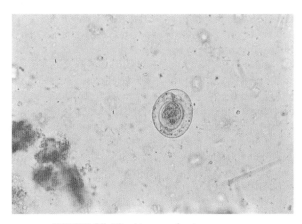

FIGURE 28-53 *Hymenolepis nana* egg.

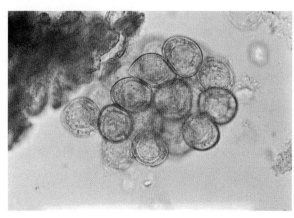

FIGURE 28-55 *Dipylidium caninum* egg packet.

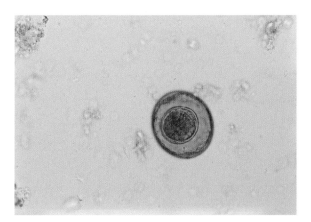

FIGURE 28-54 *Hymenolepis diminuta* egg.

immigrants from endemic areas. Infection may be manifested by headaches, symptoms resembling those seen with meningitis or a brain tumor, convulsions, or a variety of motor and sensory problems.

The cysticercus is oval, translucent, and about 5 to 18 mm in size. It contains an invaginated scolex containing four suckers and a circle of hooklets on the rostellum. Diagnosis of the infection may be made by a variety of methods, including radiography to detect calcified cysts, examination of the eye with an ophthalmoscope to detect cysticerci, imaging techniques (CT scan and MRI) to locate larvae in the brain, and biopsy and histologic staining of tissue. Serologic tests are sensitive when multiple lesions are present.

Sparganosis. Human infection with the plerocercoid larva (sparganum) of a dog or cat tapeworm can result in sparganosis. Humans acquire the infection by ingesting a copepod containing the procercoid larva; by ingesting reptiles, amphibians, or other animals containing the plerocercoid larva; or through invasion by the plerocercoid larva when the raw tissue from the second intermediate host is used as a poultice. The disease is most common in Southeast Asia. An infection is often seen in the eye after a poultice has been applied to relieve an infection. The organism may also cause migratory subcutaneous nodules, itching, and pain. The diagnosis of sparganosis is made by finding a small, white, ribbon-like organism with a rudimentary scolex. Size varies from

a few millimeters to 40 cm. The organism may be removed surgically.

Echinococcosis. Echinococcosis (hydatid cyst disease) is an infection by *Echinococcus granulosus* that normally involves the dog or other member of the family Canidae as the definitive host. Sheep and other herbivores are the usual host of the larval stage (hydatid cyst). The disease is primarily seen in sheep-raising areas of the world, including Australia, southern South America, and parts of the southwestern United States.

The adult worm is approximately 5 mm long and contains only three proglottids. The eggs are found in the feces of dogs or other definitive hosts and resemble those of *Taenia* spp. A human becomes an intermediate host by accidentally ingesting the eggs of *E. granulosus* containing the hexacanth embryo. The oncosphere is liberated in the intestine, penetrates the mucosa, enters the circulation, and usually lodges in the liver. The embryo develops a central cavity-like structure lined with a germinal membrane, from which brood capsules and protoscolices (hydatid sand) develop. The hydatid cyst's size is limited by the organ in which it develops. In bone, a limiting membrane never develops, so the cyst fills the marrow and eventually erodes the bone. Symptoms vary according to the organ infected. Pressure from the increasing size of a cyst may cause necrosis of surrounding tissue. Rupture of the cyst liberates large amounts of foreign protein that may elicit an anaphylactic response. In addition, freed germinal epithelium may serve as a source of new infection. The diagnosis may be made by radiologic examination, ultrasound, or other imaging techniques. Aspiration of the cyst contents usually reveals the presence of protoscolices.

Roundworms

Human roundworms include those that infect the intestinal tract and blood and tissue. These organisms, found worldwide, may be transmitted by ingestion of the embryonated egg or by direct penetration of the skin by larvae in the soil, or they may require an insect vector. Intestinal roundworms are the most common of all the helminths that infect humans in the United States. Infected individuals are found in highest numbers in the warm, moist area of the Southeast and in areas with poor sanitation.

Roundworms are characterized by the presence of two sexes and a life cycle that may involve larval migration throughout the body. The adults obtain nourishment by absorbing nutrients from partly digested intestinal contents or by sucking blood. Patients may be asymptomatic or symptomatic, and the severity of the symptoms is related to the worm burden, the host's nutritional status and age, and the duration of infection. Most roundworm infections can be treated with oral albendazole or mebendazole. Table 28-9 gives a comparison of diagnostic characteristics of the eggs and larvae of intestinal roundworms.

Enterobius vermicularis. *Enterobius vermicularis,* often called the *pinworm,* is a worldwide parasite commonly detected in children, especially those 5 to 10 years old. It is estimated that 20 million to 40 million individuals are infected in the United States alone. Enterobiasis is frequently found in families or in crowded conditions where the eggs may be easily transmitted. The eggs are resistant to drying and are easily spread in the environment. Adult worms live in the large intestine (cecum), although they have occasionally been found in the appendix or vagina. Ectopic infections have also caused endometritis, urethritis, and salpingitis. There is evidence that

TABLE 28-9 Comparisons of Intestinal Roundworm Eggs and Larvae

Organism	Average Size (μm) and Shape	Other Identifying Features
Ascaris lumbricoides Fertile 	45-75 × 35-50 Oval	Bile-stained shell Bumpy, mammillated In one-cell stage when passed Some eggs may be decorticated (lack mammillated coat)
Infertile 	85-95 × 43-47 Oval (some bizarrely shaped)	Mammillated Thin shell Undifferentiated internal granules
Enterobius vermicularis 	50-60 × 20-30 Oval, flattened on one side	Colorless shell Usually embryonated with C-shaped larva
Trichuris trichiura 	50-55 × 22-23 Barrel shaped	Bile-stained, thick shell Hyaline polar plugs Unembryonated when passed
Hookworm Egg 	50-60 × 35-40 Broadly oval	Thin shell, colorless In four- to eight-cell stage when passed
Rhabditiform larva 	250-300	Long buccal capsule Inconspicuous genital primordium
Filariform larva 	500	Pointed tail Esophageal-intestinal ratio 1:4
Strongyloides stercoralis Rhabditiform larva 	Egg rarely seen—resembles that of hookworm 200-250	Short buccal capsule Prominent genital primordium
Filariform larva 	500	Notched tail Esophageal-intestinal ratio 1:1

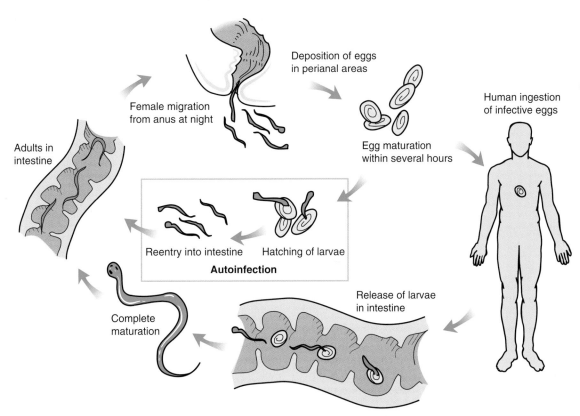

Deposition of eggs
in perianal areas

Human ingestion
of infective eggs

Female migration
from anus at night

Egg maturation
within several hours

Adults in
intestine

Reentry into intestine   Hatching of larvae
Autoinfection

Release of larvae
in intestine

Complete
maturation

FIGURE 28-56   Life cycle of *Enterobius vermicularis.*

the organism may also be associated with urinary tract infections in young girls.

Although infection with *E. vermicularis* is often asymptomatic, the patient may experience loss of appetite, abdominal pain, loss of sleep, and nausea and vomiting. Anal pruritus is caused by migration of the female to the perianal area. Treatment with mebendazole may need to be repeated in several weeks to eliminate organisms that matured as a result of ingestion of eggs remaining in the environment. The life cycle of this organism (Figure 28-56) is characterized by migration of the female out the anus during the night to lay eggs in the perianal area. The eggs are infective with a third-stage larva within several hours of being laid. Typically, transmission involves inhalation or ingestion of the infective egg. Direct anal-oral transmission because of poor handwashing or fingernail biting can occur in children. Autoinfection, in which the hatched larva reenters the intestine to mature into an adult, may also occur.

Because eggs are laid outside the body in the perianal area and are rarely present in the stool, a fecal specimen is unsatisfactory for diagnosis. The cellophane tape preparation or commercially available sticky paddle is considered the diagnostic method of choice. The procedure must be done as soon as the child arises in the morning. The perianal area is touched with the sticky side of the tape or paddle. The adult female occasionally can be seen in this preparation. Because the gravid female can migrate into the vagina, eggs can also be seen in vaginal specimens.

The adult female measures 8 to 13 mm long and has a long, pointed tail and three cuticle lips with alae at the anterior end.

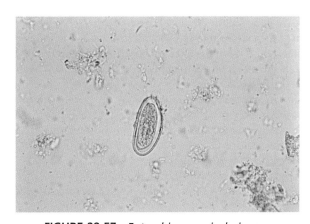

FIGURE 28-57   *Enterobius vermicularis* egg.

The less commonly seen male is 2 to 5 mm long with a curved posterior. The egg is oval, colorless, and slightly flattened on one side. It measures approximately 50 to 60 µm × 20 to 30 µm. The egg is usually seen embryonated with a C-shaped larva (Figure 28-57).

Trichuris trichiura. *Ascaris lumbricoides, Trichuris trichiura,* and the two genera of hookworms are the most common soil-transmitted helminths. The organisms have a worldwide distribution and are major causes of morbidity rather than mortality in developing areas of the world. Estimates indicate that a quarter of the world's population is infected with one or more of these organisms. Chronic infection due to these helminths, especially hookworm, can adversely affect both physical and mental development in children. A heavy worm burden

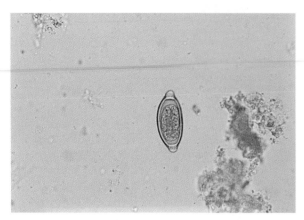

FIGURE 28-58 *Trichuris trichiura* egg.

is more likely to result in complications. Some of the risk factors for infection include sanitation (personal and community), poverty, occupation, and climate (necessary for maturation and survival of the eggs in the soil). *Strongyloides stercoralis* is also a soil-transmitted helminth but does not have the broad geographic distribution of the other organisms.

Trichuris trichiura, commonly referred to as the "whipworm," is found worldwide, especially in areas with a moist, warm climate. It occurs in the southeastern United States, often as a coinfection with *A. lumbricoides*. Light infections with *T. trichiura* rarely cause symptoms; heavy infections result in intestinal bleeding, weight loss, abdominal pain, nausea and vomiting, and chronic diarrhea. As the adults thread themselves through the intestinal mucosa, inflammation develops. Prolonged, heavy infection may result in colitis or diarrhea with blood-tinged stools. Rectal prolapse can be seen as the result of repeated heavy infections in undernourished children. Hypochromic anemia may occur with inadequate iron and protein intake in the presence of constant, low-level bleeding in chronic infection. Although treatment is not always necessary, albendazole has been reported as effective, especially in undernourished children.

Eggs are passed in the feces and require at least 14 days in warm, moist soil for embryonation to occur. Humans acquire infection by ingesting the infective egg. The larva is released in the small intestine and undergoes several molts before maturing into an adult worm in the cecum. The egg and occasionally the adult of *T. trichiura* may be seen in fecal specimens. The adult male measures 30 to 45 mm and has a thin anterior and a thick, coiled posterior. The female is 30 to 50 mm long with a thin anterior and thick, straight posterior. The brown barrel-shaped egg is unembryonated when passed, 50 to 55 μm × 22 to 23 μm, and has a thick wall and hyaline polar plugs at each end (Figure 28-58).

Ascaris lumbricoides. More than 1 billion people worldwide are infected with *A. lumbricoides*. The organism can be found in tropical as well as temperate areas, and children are most commonly infected. In the United States, the organism is most frequently seen in rural parts of the Southeast. Transmission is primarily fecal-oral, and clinical symptoms may be related to the different phases of the life cycle. The organism is often found concurrently with whipworm.

Abdominal discomfort, loss of appetite, and colicky pains are caused by the presence of adults in the intestine. There is evidence that heavy infections may contribute to lactose intolerance and malabsorption of some vitamins. In children large numbers of adult worms may cause intestinal obstruction. Because the worms feed on liquid intestinal contents, chronic infection with *A. lumbricoides* in children may hamper growth and development. Larvae migrating through the lungs may cause an immune response in the host characterized by asthma, edema, pneumonitis, and eosinophilic infiltration. Rarely, larvae are seen in the sputum in heavy infections. On some occasions, fever or other disease conditions may cause the adults to migrate from the intestine and invade other organs, resulting in peritonitis, liver abscess, or secondary infection in the lungs. Adults may also exit through the mouth, tear duct, or nose and have been reported to enter and block catheters. Eosinophilia may be present.

Eggs that are deposited in warm, moist soil become infective within about 2 weeks. After the egg is ingested, larvae hatch in the duodenum, penetrate the intestinal wall, and gain access to the hepatic portal circulation. They break out from capillaries into the lungs, travel up the bronchial tree and trachea and over the epiglottis, and are swallowed. Maturation is completed in the intestine. The life cycle (Figure 28-59) takes about 50 days after infection until adults are mature. The usual diagnostic stage is the egg. Fertile *Ascaris* eggs are oval, measure 45 to 75 μm × 35 to 50 μm, and have a thick hyaline wall surrounding a one-cell-stage embryo. Most eggs have a brown, bile-stained, mammillated outer layer (Figure 28-60). Some eggs, referred to as *decorticated,* lack the mammillated outer coat. Infertile eggs, whose size can range up to 90 μm, are often elongated and contain a mass of highly refractile granules. Adults, measuring 15 to 35 cm long and about the diameter of a lead pencil, may be seen in stool samples. The female has a straight posterior, and the male has a curved posterior. Both have three anterior lips with small, toothlike projections.

Hookworms. Two species of hookworm, *Necator americanus* (New World) and *Ancylostoma duodenale* (Old World), infect humans. *A. duodenale* is seen in southern Europe and northern Africa along the Mediterranean, as well as in parts of Southeast Asia and South America. *N. americanus* has a geographic distribution in Africa, Southeast Asia, and South and Central America and is endemic in rural areas of southeastern United States. There seems to be a racial distribution, with infections more prevalent in whites than in African Americans. Infection worldwide is estimated at close to 1 billion, and in the United States, hookworm is the second most commonly reported helminth infection. Unlike other helminths in which infection peaks in childhood and adolescence, hookworm burden often increases with age.

Adults of the two species can be differentiated by the morphology of the buccal capsule or, in the male, the copulatory bursa. The eggs, however, are identical. These worms live in the small intestine and attach to the mucosa by means of teeth *(A. duodenale)* or cutting plates *(N. americanus)*. They digest the tissue plug and pierce capillaries. Once attached, they continue to ingest blood as a source of nourishment by secreting anticoagulants, platelet inhibitors, and substances

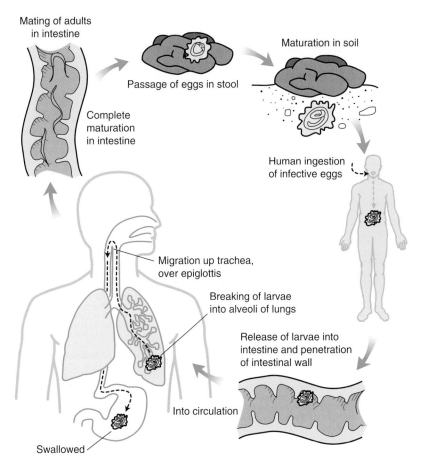

FIGURE 28-59 Life cycle of *Ascaris lumbricoides.*

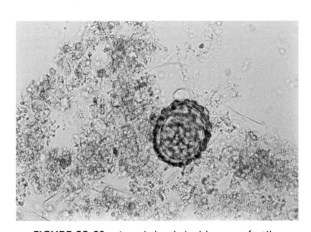

FIGURE 28-60 *Ascaris lumbricoides* egg, fertile.

that interfere with the VIIa-tissue factor complex. The organisms also secrete substances that interfere with the action of digestive enzymes and inhibit host absorption of nutrients.

Clinical symptoms vary according to the phase of the life cycle and worm burden. A small, red, itchy papule, referred to as *ground itch,* develops at the site of larval penetration. If large numbers of larvae are present during the lung phase of migration, the patient may have bronchitis, but unlike with *Ascaris* spp. larvae, no host sensitization occurs. The most severe symptoms are associated with the adult, including non-

specific symptoms such as diarrhea, fever, and nausea and vomiting. A few patients may experience pica and then ingest dirt (geophagia). Blood loss, ranging from 0.03 to 0.2 mL per worm per day, is primarily the result of the ingestion of blood by the adult worm. Hemorrhages at the site of attachment, however, also contribute to total blood loss. Chronic heavy infection with hookworm may lead to microcytic hypochromic anemia, especially in children whose diet is inadequate in iron and protein. The mental and physical development of a child may be affected by chronic heavy infections because of the complications of anemia and malnutrition.

Infection is usually treated with albendazole or mebendazole, which blocks glucose uptake by the organism. Supportive therapy, including iron and protein supplements, may be needed in severe cases, especially if the child shows evidence of anemia or if the infection is in a pregnant woman. Vaccine development using hookworm antigens is being targeted as a way to help control infections.

Once the eggs have been deposited in warm, moist soil, the first-stage **rhabditiform larva** develops within 1 to 2 days and feeds on bacteria in the soil. A nonfeeding, infective, filariform larva develops within a week. Humans are infected when the filariform larvae penetrate their skin. The organisms enter the circulation and break out of the capillaries into the lung, then migrate up the bronchial tree, over the epiglottis, and into the digestive tract. After additional larval molts, the worms attach to the mucosa in the small intestine. Eggs are produced within

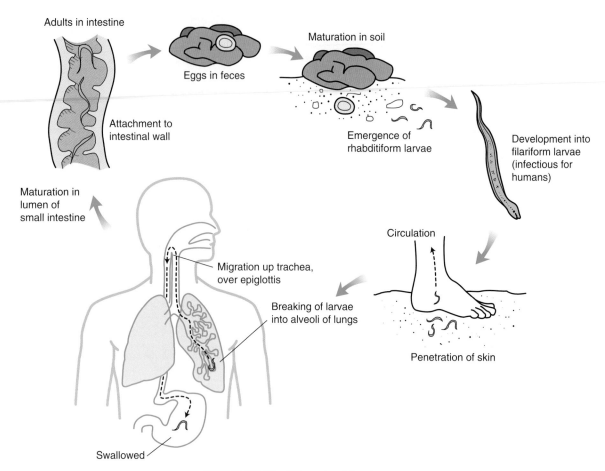

Adults in intestine

Eggs in feces

Maturation in soil

Attachment to intestinal wall

Emergence of rhabditiform larvae

Development into filariform larvae (infectious for humans)

Maturation in lumen of small intestine

Circulation

Migration up trachea, over epiglottis

Breaking of larvae into alveoli of lungs

Penetration of skin

Swallowed

FIGURE 28-61 Life cycle of hookworm.

6 to 8 weeks after skin penetration by the filariform larva. Figure 28-61 shows the life cycle of the hookworm.

Adult hookworms are rarely seen in stool specimens; the egg and the rhabditiform larva are the usual diagnostic stages. The eggs and rhabditiform larvae of the two species are indistinguishable; therefore the laboratory can report only "hookworm" when a characteristic egg or larva is found in a stool specimen. The egg is oval, colorless, thin-shelled, and 50 to 60 µm long and usually contains an embryo in the four- to eight-cell stage of cleavage (Figure 28-62). The rhabditiform larva must be differentiated from that of *S. stercoralis* because treatment is different. The hookworm rhabditiform larva is 250 to 300 µm long and has a small, inconspicuous genital primordium (Figure 28-63, *A*), and a long buccal capsule (Figure 28-63, *B*). The filariform larva also must be distinguished from that of *S. stercoralis*. Hookworm filariform larvae are about 500 µm, with a pointed tail and an esophageal-intestinal ratio of 1:4.

Strongyloides stercoralis. *Strongyloides stercoralis*, known as the *threadworm*, inhabits the small intestine but is also capable of existing as a free-living worm. It is endemic in the tropics and subtropics including Southeast Asia, Latin American, and sub-Saharan Africa. It is estimated that 100 million to 200 million people are infected worldwide. *S. stercoralis* has been identified in a number of United States military veterans who served in Vietnam and other Southeast

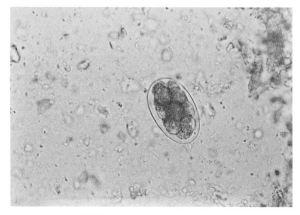

FIGURE 28-62 Hookworm egg.

Asian countries. In the United States, the prevalence rate ranges from 0.4% to 4%, with most cases found in people living in Appalachia or in rural areas of the Southeast or in immigrants from endemic areas.

Although many people with *S. stercoralis* infection are asymptomatic, patients may exhibit fever, nausea and vomiting, and sharp, stabbing pains that resemble those of an ulcer. Chronic mild diarrhea may be present. The eosinophil count may be elevated. Unlike hookworms, *S. stercoralis* larval penetration of the skin does not cause a prominent papule, and

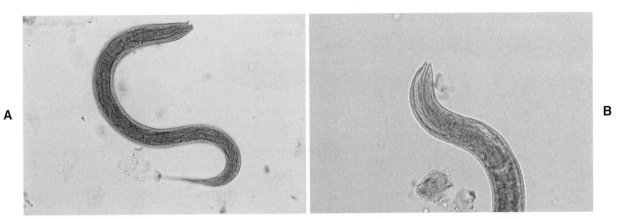

FIGURE 28-63 **A,** Hookworm rhabditiform larva. Notice long buccal capsule and lack of prominent genital primordium. **B,** Hookworm rhabditiform larva, buccal capsule.

migration through the lungs rarely elicits pneumonitis, but the patient may have wheezing and a mild cough. In contrast to the mild symptoms in an immunocompetent host, patients with a drug-induced immunocompromised state, lymphoma, malignancy, or other condition that causes T-cell depletion can develop severe infections, referred to as disseminated strongyloidiasis or hyperinfection. In this population, large numbers of the filariform larvae develop in the intestine in an autoinfective cycle and migrate from the intestine into the lungs and other organs, such as the liver, heart, and central nervous system, causing a fulminating, often fatal infection. Most cases in organ transplant patients are due to reactivation of latent or chronic infection. Secondary bacterial infections, which occur as a result of massive larval migration, may be seen in up to 40% of patients with disseminated strongyloidiasis. The mortality rate in immunocompromised patients is over 80%, and the usual causes of death are complications resulting in respiratory failure. Disseminated strongyloidiasis, however, is not common in patients with advanced AIDS despite their immunocompromised status. Research into this seeming contradiction has shown that individuals with severe immunosuppression may harbor larval stages that are more likely to develop into free-living females or males rather than into filariform larvae.

The life cycle of *S. stercoralis* can take one of three phases: direct, which is similar to that of hookworm; indirect, which involves a free-living phase; or autoinfection (Figure 28-64). In the direct life cycle, the fertile egg hatches in the intestine and develops into the rhabditiform larva (noninfective form), which is passed in the stool. In the soil, the rhabditiform larvae develop into filariform larvae, which are infective for humans by direct penetration. Once the larva has penetrated the skin, it enters the circulation, breaks out from capillaries in the lung, migrates up the bronchial tree and over the epiglottis, and enters the digestive tract, where it matures into the adult worm.

In the indirect life cycle, the rhabditiform larvae in the soil develop into free-living males and females that produce eggs. At any point, the free-living cycle may revert and result in production of infective filariform larvae. In most individuals, rhabditiform larvae develop into the filariform larvae in the intestine. These filariform larvae then penetrate the mucosa, enter the circulation, and return to the intestine to develop into adults. This part of the life cycle, called *autoinfection*, may allow an initial infection to persist at low levels for years.

The parasitic female threadworm is small (2.5 mm) and rarely seen in a stool specimen. No male has been identified in intestinal infections. The primary diagnostic stage in humans is the rhabditiform larva. It is 200 to 250 µm long with a short buccal capsule (Figure 28-65, *A*), a large bulb in the esophagus, and a prominent genital primordium located in its posterior half to posterior third (Figure 28-65, *B*). The egg, which is rarely seen except in cases of severe diarrhea, resembles that of a hookworm. It is thin shelled, measures 54 by 32 µm, and often is segmented. The filariform larva has a notched tail, is 500 µm long, and has an esophageal-intestinal ratio of 1 : 1. Filariform larvae may be identified in the sputum of patients with hyperinfection. If clinical symptoms suggest *Strongyloides* infection but multiple stool specimens test negative for the larvae, a duodenal aspirate, or the Enterotest may be used for diagnosis because the organism lives in the upper small intestine. Albendazole can be used to treat both intestinal and disseminated *Strongyloides* infection.

Blood and Tissue Roundworm Infections

Trichinella spiralis. Trichinosis is the infection of muscle tissue with the larval form of *T. spiralis*, a helminth whose adult stages live in the human intestine. Humans acquire the infection by eating undercooked meat, particularly pork that contains the larval forms. In recent years ingestion of wild game has led to infection by other species of *Trichinella*. The larvae are released from the tissue capsule in the intestine and mature into adults. The female produces liveborn larvae that penetrate the intestinal wall, enter the circulation, and are carried throughout the body. Once the larvae enter the striated muscle, they begin a maturation cycle that is completed in about 1 month. The larvae coil and become encapsulated. Although larvae may remain viable for many years, eventually the capsules calcify and the larvae die.

During the intestinal phase, infected individuals have few symptoms, although diarrhea and abdominal discomfort may be present. Most symptoms occur during the migration and

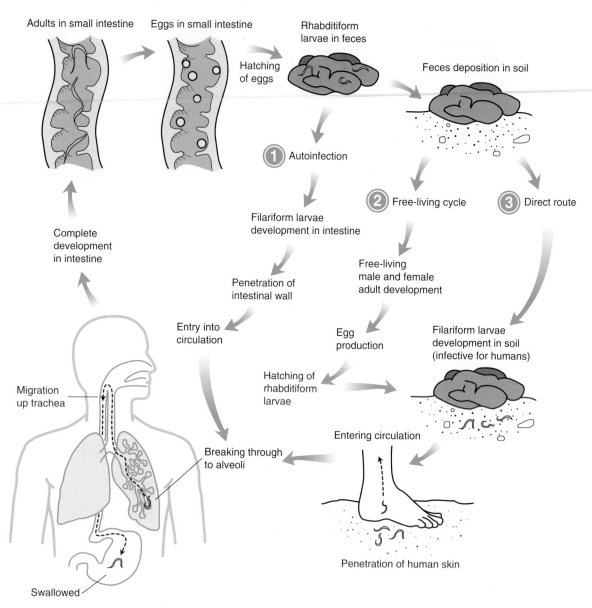

Adults in small intestine

Eggs in small intestine

Rhabditiform larvae in feces

Hatching of eggs

Feces deposition in soil

① Autoinfection

② Free-living cycle

③ Direct route

Filariform larvae development in intestine

Complete development in intestine

Penetration of intestinal wall

Free-living male and female adult development

Entry into circulation

Egg production

Filariform larvae development in soil (infective for humans)

Migration up trachea

Hatching of rhabditiform larvae

Breaking through to alveoli

Entering circulation

Swallowed

Penetration of human skin

FIGURE 28-64 Life cycle of *Strongyloides stercoralis.*

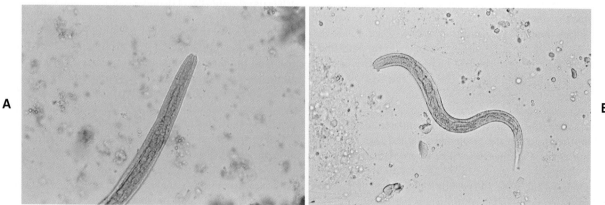

FIGURE 28-65 **A,** *Strongyloides stercoralis* rhabditiform larva, buccal capsule. **B,** *S. stercoralis* rhabditiform larva. Notice short buccal capsule and prominent genital primordium.

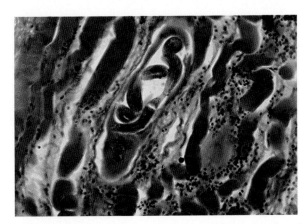

FIGURE 28-66 *Trichinella spiralis* larva (biopsy specimen).

encapsulation period, and the severity of the symptoms depends on the number of parasites, the tissues invaded, and the person's general health. Symptoms that occur during the larval phase are the result of an intense inflammatory response by the host. Common symptoms include periorbital edema, fever, muscular pain or tenderness, headache, and general weakness. Muscle enzyme levels may be elevated. Splinter hemorrhages beneath the nails can be seen in many patients. Eosinophilia of 40% to 80% is common. Patients with symptoms should be treated with analgesics and general supportive measures. Steroids are given only in rare cases.

Because it is difficult to recover adults or larvae in a stool specimen, the diagnosis often is based on clinical symptoms and the patient's history. Biopsy of muscle tissue and identification of the encapsulated, coiled larva is the definitive diagnostic method. Figure 28-66 shows a biopsy specimen of a muscle containing the larvae of *T. spiralis*. Specimens from large muscles, such as the deltoid and gastrocnemius, should be stained for histologic examination. The presence of calcified larvae on a radiographic film indicates infection, and numerous serologic tests are available.

Larva Migrans. Two forms of larva migrans exist in humans: cutaneous (creeping eruption) and visceral. In both cases humans are the accidental host of infection with nonhuman nematode larvae that are unable to complete their life cycle in humans. In the United States cutaneous larva migrans occurs primarily in the southwest, mid-Atlantic, and Gulf coast areas and is most commonly caused by the filariform larva of the dog or cat hookworm (*Ancylostoma braziliense*). The larva penetrates the human skin through a hair follicle or break in the skin, or through unbroken skin. Once inside the body, it does not enter the circulation but wanders through the subcutaneous tissue, creating long, winding tunnels. Secretions from the larva creates a severe allergic reaction with intensely itchy skin lesions that are vesicular and erythematous. Secondary bacterial infections may result from scratching. The infection resolves within several weeks when the larva dies. The diagnosis is based primarily on history and clinical symptoms.

In visceral larva migrans, a human accidentally ingests the eggs of the dog roundworm *(Toxocara canis)* or cat roundworm *(Toxocara cati)*. The larvae hatch in the intestine, pen-

etrate the intestinal mucosa, wander through the abdominal cavity, and may enter the lungs, eye, liver, or brain. The infection is seen primarily in children 1 to 4 years old. Clinical symptoms include malaise, fever, pneumonitis, and hepatomegaly. Eosinophilia ranging from 30% to 50%, and as high as 85%, has been reported. CNS complications may develop. When the eye is invaded it is referred to as *ocular larva migrans,* and in these cases, eosinophilia is usually absent. The diagnosis of these infections is made on the basis of clinical findings and the results of serologic tests using *Toxocara*-specific antigens.

Filarial Worms. Filarial worms are roundworms of blood and tissue that are found primarily in tropical areas of the world. A number of species infect humans. Those considered most pathogenic are *Brugia malayi, Wuchereria bancrofti, Onchocerca volvulus,* and *Loa loa.* Lymphatic filariasis (caused by *W. bancrofti* and *B. malayi*) is the second most common mosquito-borne disease after malaria. In addition, the nonpathogens *Mansonella ozzardi, Mansonella (Dipetalonema) perstans,* and *Mansonella (Dipetalonema) streptocerca* may be seen in clinical specimens. These roundworms give birth to liveborn larvae referred to as microfilariae. Identification of the various species depends on the morphology of the microfilaria, its periodicity, and its location in the host. Important morphologic characteristics include the presence or absence of a sheath (the remnant of the egg from which the larva hatched) and the presence and arrangement of nuclei in the tail. Table 28-10 presents a comparison of the species of microfilariae commonly found in humans.

Adults, which may range in size from 2 to 50 cm, live in human lymphatics, muscles, or connective tissues. Mature females produce liveborn microfilariae that are the infective stage for the insect during the insect's blood meal. Once ingested, microfilariae penetrate the insect's gut wall and develop into infective third-stage (filariform) larvae. These larvae enter the insect proboscis and are introduced into human circulation when the insect feeds. Figure 28-67 shows a generalized life cycle for microfilariae.

Wuchereria bancrofti. The causative agent of Bancroftian filariasis and elephantiasis, *W. bancrofti* is primarily limited to the tropical and subtropical regions. The insect vector is a mosquito, either *Culex* or *Aedes* sp. The adult filarial worm lives in the lymphatics and lymph nodes, especially those in the lower extremities. Presence of the adults initiates an immunologic response consisting of cellular reactions, edema, and hyperplasia. A strong granulomatous reaction with production of fibrous tissue around dead worms ensues. The end result of the reaction is that small lymphatics may be narrowed or closed, resulting in increased hydrostatic pressure with subsequent leakage of fluid into the surrounding tissue. During this period, the patient may experience generalized symptoms such as fever, headache, and chills as well as localized swelling, redness, and lymphangitis, primarily at sites in the male and female genitalia and the extremities.

Elephantiasis, a debilitating and deforming complication, occurs in less than 10% of infections, usually after many years of continual filarial infection. Chronic obstruction to the lymphatic flow results in lymphatic varices, fibrosis, and prolifera-

TABLE 28-10　Comparisons of Microfilariae

Organism	Arthropod Vector	Periodicity	Location of Adult/ Microfilaria	Tail Morphology	
Wuchereria bancrofti	Mosquito (*Culex, Aedes, Anopheles* spp.)	Nocturnal	Lymphatics, blood	Sheathed Nuclei do not extend to tip of tail	
Brugia malayi	Mosquito (*Aedes* sp.)	Nocturnal	Lymphatics, blood	Sheathed Terminal nuclei separated	
Loa loa	Fly (*Chrysops* sp.)	Diurnal	Subcutaneous tissue, blood	Sheathed Nuclei extend to tip of tail	
Onchocerca volvulus	Fly (*Simulium* sp.)	Nonperiodic	Subcutaneous nodule, subcutaneous tissue	Unsheathed Nuclei do not extend to tip of tail	
Mansonella ozzardi	Midge (*Culicoides* sp.)	Nonperiodic	Body cavity, blood, skin	Unsheathed Nuclei do not extend to tip of tail	
Mansonella perstans	Midge (*Culicoides* sp.)	Nonperiodic	Mesentery, blood	Unsheathed Nuclei extend to blunt tip of tail	
Mansonella streptocerca	Midge (*Culicoides* sp.)	Nonperiodic	Subcutaneous, skin	Unsheathed Nuclei extend to tip of hooked tail	

tion of dermal and connective tissue. The enlarged areas eventually develop a hard, leathery appearance. Diagnosis of *W. bancrofti* should include the examination of a blood specimen obtained at night (10 PM to 2 AM) for the presence of microfilariae. The blood may be examined immediately for live microfilariae or may be pooled on a slide and stained. Filtration of up to 5 mL of blood through a 5-µm Nuclepore filter (Nuclepore Corp., Pleasanton, Calif.) can detect light infections. The microfilariae of *W. bancrofti* are sheathed, and the nuclei do not extend to the tip of the tail (Figure 28-68). New immunochromatographic tests have limited applications for identification of *W. bancrofti* antigens in blood.

Brugia malayi. *Brugia malayi*, another nocturnal microfilarial species, is limited to the Far East, including Korea, China, and the Philippines. Mosquitoes of the genera *Mansonia, Anopheles*, and *Aedes* have been shown to transmit the organism. The pathology of the disease and the clinical symptoms are the same as those seen with *W. bancrofti* infections. The distinguishing characteristics of the microfilariae are the presence of a sheath and the arrangement of tail nuclei—the nuclei extend to the tip, but a space separates the two terminal nuclei.

Loa loa. Infection with *Loa loa,* the eye worm, is limited to the African equatorial rain forest, where the fly vector (*Chrysops* spp.) breeds. Adults migrate through the subcutaneous tissue, causing temporary inflammatory reactions, called Calabar swellings. These characteristic swellings may cause pain and pruritus that last about a week before disap-

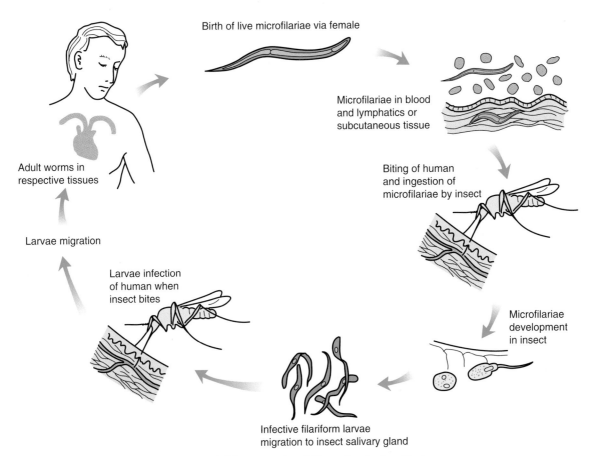

Birth of live microfilariae via female

Microfilariae in blood and lymphatics or subcutaneous tissue

Adult worms in respective tissues

Biting of human and ingestion of microfilariae by insect

Larvae migration

Larvae infection of human when insect bites

Microfilariae development in insect

Infective filariform larvae migration to insect salivary gland

FIGURE 28-67   Generalized life cycle of microfilaria.

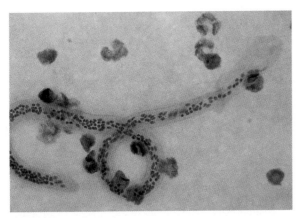

FIGURE 28-68   *Wuchereria bancrofti* microfilaria. Notice faintly staining sheath extending from both ends of organism.

pearing, only to reappear in another part of the body. The adult worm can often be seen as it migrates across the surface of the eye. Diagnosis can be based on the presence of Calabar swellings or of the adult worm in the conjunctiva of the eye. Microfilariae may be seen in a blood specimen if it is taken during the day, especially around noon, when migration peaks. The microfilaria is sheathed, and nuclei extend to the tip of the tail.

Onchocerca volvulus. Infection with *O. volvulus* is referred to as onchocercosis or river blindness. The organism can be found in Africa and South and Central America; transmission occurs by the bite of the black fly (*Simulium* spp.). Adults are encapsulated in fibrous tumors in human subcutaneous tissues. Microfilariae can be isolated from the subcutaneous tissue, skin, and the nodule itself but are rarely found in blood or lymphatic fluid.

The nodules in which adults live may measure up to 25 mm and can be found on most parts of the body. They are the result of an inflammatory and granulomatous reaction around the adult worms. Figure 28-69 shows a cross section of tissue containing these organisms. Blindness, the most serious complication, results when microfilariae collect in the cornea and iris, causing hemorrhages, keratitis, and atrophy of the iris. The presence of endosymbiotic bacteria of the genus *Wolbachia* have been linked to stimulation of the host immune response and may contribute to the inflammatory tissue reaction.

Diagnosis involves clinical symptoms, such as the presence of nodules, and microscopic identification of microfilariae. The diagnostic method used is the skin snip, in which a small slice of skin is obtained and placed on a saline mount. Microfilariae with no sheath and with nuclei that do not extend into the tip of the tail are characteristic of this organism. Because the skin snip is painful and poses a risk of infection, research-

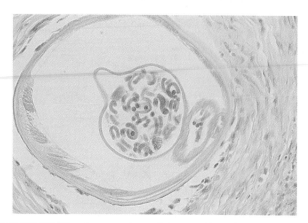

FIGURE 28-69 Cross-section of tissue infected with *Onchocerca volvulus.*

ers are developing immunochromatographic tests for parasite specific antigens in body fluids such as urine and tears.

Mansonella species. *Mansonella ozzardi, Mansonella streptocerca,* and *Mansonella perstans* are filarial worms not usually associated with serious infections. They are transmitted by midges belonging to the genus *Culicoides.* The microfilariae of *M. streptocerca* are found in the skin. They are unsheathed and have nuclei that extend to the end of the "shepherd's crook" tail. Microfilariae of *M. ozzardi* and *M. perstans* are found in the blood as unsheathed organisms. *M. ozzardi* microfilariae have tails with nuclei that do not extend to the tips, whereas the nuclei in the tail of an *M. perstans* microfilaria extend to the tip.

Dracunculus medinensis. *Dracunculus medinensis* (guinea worm, fiery serpent of the Israelites) causes serious infections in the Middle East, parts of Africa, and India. It is often found in areas in which "step-down" wells are used. In the 1990s, several health agencies, including the World Health Organization and the United Nations Children's Fund, launched an eradication program. In 1986, an estimated 3.5 million people were infected annually; in 2008, only about 4600 cases were reported.

Adult worms mature in the deep connective tissue, and the gravid females migrate to the subcutaneous tissue. Initially a painful, blisterlike, inflammatory papule appears on the leg in the area of the gravid female. The papule ulcerates, and when the person's body comes in contact with water, the female worm exposes her uterus through the ulceration and releases larvae into the water. Patients may have nausea and vomiting, urticaria, and dyspnea before the rupture of the worm's uterus. If the worm is broken during an attempt to remove it, the patient may experience a severe inflammatory reaction and secondary bacterial infection.

Humans acquire the infection by ingesting a copepod (*Cyclops* spp.) that contains an infective larva. The larva is released in the intestine, penetrates the intestinal wall, and migrates to the body cavity, where males and females mature. When mature and gravid, the female migrates through the subcutaneous tissues to the arm or leg to release liveborn larvae into the water. The rhabditiform larvae are then ingested by the copepod.

The diagnosis is made from the typical appearance of the lesion. Metronidazole is given to treat the infection. The ancient method of removal by rolling the worm a few inches at a time onto a stick is still practiced in some areas of the world.

BIBLIOGRAPHY

Ackers JP, Mirelman D: Progress in research on *Entamoeba histolytica* pathogenesis, *Curr Opin Microbiol* 9:367, 2006.

Al-Hasan MN et al: Invasive enteric infections in hospitalized patients with underlying strongyloidiasis, *Am J Clin Pathol* 128:622, 2007.

Ali SA, Hill DR: *Giardia intestinalis, Curr Opin Infect Dis* 16:453, 2003.

Amin O: Seasonal prevalence of intestinal parasites in the United States during 2000, *Am J Trop Med Hyg* 66:2002, 2002.

Arauco R et al: Human fascioliasis: a case of hyperinfection and an update for clinicians, *Foodborne Pathog Dis* 4:305, 2007.

Barbosa JM et al: A flow cytometric protocol for detection of *Cryptosporidium* spp. *Cytometry A:J Int Soc Analyt Cytology* 73:44, 2008.

Behera B et al: Parasites in patients with malabsorption syndrome: a clinical study in children and adults, *Dig Dis Sci* 53:672, 2008.

Bell D et al: Ensuring quality and access for malaria diagnosis: how can it be achieved? *Nat Rev Microbiol* 4:682, 2006

Bern C et al: Chagas disease and the U.S. blood supply, *Curr Opin Infect Dis* 21:476, 2008.

Bethany J et al: Soil-transmitted helminth infections: ascariasis, trichuriasis, and hookworm, *Lancet* 367:1521, 2006.

Bialek R et al: Comparison of autofluorescence and iodine staining for detection of *Isospora belli* in feces, *Am J Trop Med Hyg* 67:304, 2002.

Blevins SM et al: Blood smear analysis in babesiosis, ehrlichiosis, relapsing fever, malaria, and Chagas disease, *Cleve Clin J Med* 75:7, 2008.

Borowski H et al: Active invasion and/or encapsulation? A reappraisal of host-cell parasitism by *Cryptosporidium, Trends Parasitol* 24:509, 2008.

Branda JA et al: A rational approach to the stool ova and parasite examination, *Clin Infect Dis* 42:972, 2006.

Brown HL et al: Clinical evaluation of Affirm VPlll in the detection and identification of *Trichomonas vaginalis, Gardnerella vaginalis,* and *Candida* species in vaginitis/vaginosis, *Infect Dis Obstet Gynecol* 12:17, 2004.

Brun R, Balmer O: New developments in human African trypanosomiasis, *Curr Opin Infect Dis* 19:415, 2006.

Bungiro R, Cappello M: Hookworm infection: new developments and prospects for control, *Curr Opin Infect Dis* 17:421, 2004.

Burkhart CN, Burkhart CG: Assessment of frequency, transmission, and genitourinary complications of enterobiasis (pinworms), *Int J Dermatol* 44:837, 2005.

Buzoni-Gatel D, Werts C: *Toxoplasma gondii* and subversion of the immune system, *Trends Parasitol* 22:448, 2006.

Cable RG, Leiby DA: Risk and prevention of transfusion-transmitted babesiosis and other tick-borne diseases, *Curr Opin Hematol* 10:405, 2003.

Campbell AL et al: First case of toxoplasmosis following small bowel transplantation and systematic review of tissue-invasive toxoplasmosis following noncardiac solid organ transplant, *Transplantation* 81:408, 2006.

Campbell L et al: Evaluation of the OSOM *Trichomonas* rapid test versus wet preparation examination for detection of *Trichomonas vaginalis* vaginitis in specimens from women with a low prevalence of infection, *J Clin Microbiol* 46:3467, 2008.

Centers for Disease Control and Prevention: Two cases of visceral leishmaniasis in U.S. military personnel—Afghanistan, 2002-2004, *MMWR Morb Mortal Wkly Rep* 53:265, 2004. Available at: www.cdc.gov/mmwr/preview/mmwrhtml/mm5312a.htm. Accessed February 13, 2009.

Centers for Disease Control and Prevention: Update: Cutaneous leishmaniasis in U.S. military personnel—Southwest/Central Asia, 2002-2004, *MMWR Morb Mortal Wkly Rep* 53:264, 2004. Available at: www.cdc.gov/mmwr/preview/mmwrhtml/mm5312a4.htm. Accessed February 13, 2009.

Chappuis F et al: Options for field diagnosis of human African trypanosomiasis, *Clin Microbiol Rev* 18:133, 2005.

Chilton D et al: Use of rapid diagnostic tests for diagnosis of malaria in the UK, *J Clin Pathol* 59:862, 2006.

Daboul MW: Is the amastigote form of *Leishmania* the only form found in humans infected with cutaneous leishmaniasis? *Lab Med* 39:38, 2008.

Dacombe RJ et al: Time delays between patient and laboratory selectively affect accuracy of helminth diagnosis, *Trans R Soc Trop Med Hyg* 101:140, 2007.

deSilva MR et al: Soil-transmitted helminth infections: updating the global picture, *Trends Parasitol* 19:547, 2003.

Desjeux P: The increase in risk factors for leishmaniasis worldwide, *Trans R Soc Trop Med Hyg* 95:239, 2001.

Didier ES: Microsporidiosis: an emerging and opportunistic infection in humans and animals, *Acta Tropica* 94:61, 2005.

Didier ES, Weiss LM: Microsporidiosis: current status, *Curr Opin Infect Dis* 19:485, 2006.

Didier ES et al: Epidemiology of microsporidiosis: sources and modes of transmission, *Vet Parasitol* 126:145, 2004.

Dixon BR et al: Detection of *Cyclospora cayetanensis* oocysts in human fecal specimens by flow cytometry, *J Clin Microbiol* 43:2375, 2005.

Doel ID et al: Encephalitis due to a free-living amoeba (*Balamuthia mandrillaris*): case report with literature review, *Surg Neurol* 53:611, 2000.

Döller PC et al: Cyclosporiasis outbreak in Germany associated with the consumption of salad, *Emerg Infect Dis* 8:992, 2002.

Eckmann L: Mucosal defenses against *Giardia*, *Parasite Immunol* 25:259, 2003.

Foulks GN: *Acanthamoeba* keratitis and contact lens wear: static or increasing problem, *Eye Contact Lens* 33:412, 2007.

Fox LM et al: Neonatal babesiosis: case report and review of the literature, *Pediat Infect Dis J* 25:169, 2006.

Franzen C: Microsporidia: how can they invade other cells? *Trends Parasitol* 20:275, 2004.

Fritzinger AE et al: identification of a *Naegleria fowleri* membrane protein reactive with anti-human CD59 antibody, *Infect Immun* 74:1189, 2006.

Gascon J: Epidemiology, etiology, and pathophysiology of traveler's diarrhea, *Digestion* 73(Suppl 1):102, 2006.

Girginkardesler N et al: Transmission of *Dientamoeba fragilis*: evaluation of the role of *Enterobius vermicularis*, *Parasitol Int* 57:72, 2008.

Gurtler RE et al: Congenital transmission of *Trypanosoma cruzi* infection in Argentina, *Emerg Infect Dis* 9:29, 2003.

Hanscheid T et al: Screening of auramine-stained smears of all fecal samples is a rapid and inexpensive way to increase the detection of coccidial infections, *Int J Infect Dis* 12:47, 2008.

Herwaldt BL et al: Transmission of *Babesia microti* in Minnesota through four blood donations from the same donor over a 6-month period, *Transfusion* 42:1154, 2002.

Herwaldt BL et al: *Babesia divergens*-like infection, Washington state, *Emerg Infect Dis* 10:622, 2004.

Heukelbach J, Feldmeier H: Epidemiological and clinical characteristics of hookworm-related cutaneous larva migrans, *Lancet Infect Dis* 8:302, 2008.

Hill D, Dubey JP: *Toxoplasma gondii*: transmission, diagnosis and prevention, *Clin Microbiol Infect* 8:634, 2002.

Ho AY et al: Outbreak of cyclosporiasis associated with imported raspberries, Philadelphia, Pennsylvania, 2000, *Emerg Infect Dis* 8:783, 2002.

Hobbs MM et al: Methods for detection of *Trichomonas vaginalis* in the male partners of infected women: implications for control of trichomoniasis, *J Clin Microbiol* 44:3994, 2006.

Homer MJ et al: Babesiosis, *Clin Microbiol Rev* 13:451, 2000.

Hong DK et al: Severe cryptosporidiosis in a seven-year-old renal transplant recipient—case report and review of the literature, *Pediatr Transplant* 11:94, 2007.

Hopkins H et al: Comparison of HRP2- and pLDH-based rapid diagnostic tests for malaria with longitudinal follow-up in Kampala, Uganda, *Am J Trop Med Hyg* 76:1092, 2007.

Hotez PJ et al: Hookworm infection, *N Engl J Med* 351:799, 2004.

Huston CD: Parasite and host contributions to the pathogenesis of amebic colitis, *Trends Parasitol* 20:23, 2004.

Jensen B et al: Comparison of polyvinyl alcohol fixative with three less hazardous fixatives for detection and identification of intestinal parasites, *J Clin Microbiol* 38:1592, 2000.

Johnson EH et al: Emerging from obscurity: biological, clinical, and diagnostic aspects of *Dientamoeba fragilis*, *Clin Microbiol Rev* 17:553, 2004.

Johnston VJ, Mabey DC: Global epidemiology and control of *Trichomonas vaginalis*, *Curr Opin Infect Dis* 21:56, 2008.

Karanis P et al: Waterborne transmission of protozoan parasites: a worldwide review of outbreaks and lessons learnt, *J Water Health* 5:1, 2007.

Katanik MT et al: Evaluation of ColorPAC *Giardia/Cryptosporidium* rapid assay and ProSPect *Giardia/Cryptosporidium* microplate assay for detection of *Giardia* and *Cryptosporidium* in fecal specimens, *J Clin Microbiol* 29:4523, 2001.

Khan NA: *Acanthamoeba* and the blood-brain barrier: the breakthrough, *J Med Microbiol* 57:1051, 2008.

Kiderlen AF, Laube U: *Balamuthia mandrillaris*, an opportunistic agent of granulomatous amebic encephalitis, infects the brain via the olfactory nerve pathway, *Parasitol Res* 94:49, 2004.

Kiderlen AF et al: Cytopathogenicity of *Balamuthia mandrillaris*, an opportunistic causative agent of granulomatous amebic encephalitis, *J Eukaryot Microbiol* 53:456, 2006.

Kimura K et al: Comparison of three microscopic techniques for diagnosis of *Cyclospora cayetanensis*, *FEMS Micro Letters* 238:263, 2004.

Krause PJ: Babesiosis, *Med Clin North Am* 86:361, 2002.

Kravetz JD, Federman DG: Toxoplasmosis in pregnancy, *Am J Med* 118:212, 2005.

Kucik CJ et al: Common intestinal parasites, *Am Fam Physician* 69:1161, 2004.

Lagace-Wiens PR et al: *Dientamoeba fragilis*: an emerging role in intestinal disease, *CMAJ* 175:468, 2006.

Lam CS et al: Disseminated strongyloidiasis: a retrospective study of clinical course and outcome, *Eur J Clin Microbiol Infect Dis* 25:14, 2006.

Leder K et al: No correlation between clinical symptoms and *Blastocystis hominis* in immunocompetent individuals, *J Gastroenterol Hepatol* 20:1390, 2005.

Leiby DA: Threats to blood safety posed by emerging protozoan pathogens, *Vox Sang* 87(Suppl 2):S120, 2004.

Leiby DA: Babesiosis and blood transfusion: flying under the radar, *Vox Sang* 90:157, 2006.

Lejon V, Buscher P: Cerebrospinal fluid in human African trypanosomiasis: a key to diagnosis, therapeutic decision and post-treatment follow-up, *Trop Med Int Health* 10:395, 2005.

Leo M et al: Evaluation of *Entamoeba histolytica* antigen and antibody point-of-care tests for rapid diagnosis of amebiasis, *J Clin Microbiol* 44:4569, 2006.

Lewthwaite P et al: Gastrointestinal parasites in the immunocompromised, *Curr Opin Infect Dis* 18:427, 2005.

Libman MD et al: Detection of pathogenic protozoa in the diagnostic laboratory: result of reproducibility, specimen pooling, and competency assessment, *J Clin Microbiol* 46:2200, 2008.

Luquetti AO et al: Chagas' disease diagnosis: a multicentric evaluation of Chagas Stat-Pak, a rapid immunochromatographic assay with recombinant proteins of *Trypanosoma cruzi, Diagn Microblol, Infect Dis* 46:265, 2003.

Mansfield LS, Gajadhar AA: *Cyclospora cayetanensis*, a food- and waterborne coccidian parasite, *Vet Parasitol* 126:73, 2004.

Marciano-Cabral F, Cabral G: *Acanthamoeba* spp. as agents of disease in human, *Clin Microbiol Rev* 16:273, 2003.

Marciano-Cabral F, Cabral GA: The immune response to *Naegleria fowleri* amebae and pathogenesis of infection, *FEMS Immunol Med Microbiol* 51:243, 2007.

Matin A et al: Increasing importance of *Balamuthia mandrillaris*, *Clin Microbiol Rev* 21:435, 2008.

Matlashewski G: *Leishmania* infection and virulence, *Med Microbiol Immunobiol* 190:37, 2001.

McAuley JB: Toxoplasmosis in children, *Pediatr Infect Dis* 27:161, 2008.

Meamar AR et al: *Strongyloides stercoralis* hyper-infection syndrome in HIV/AIDS patients in Iran, *Parasitol Res* 101:663, 2007.

Mir A et al: Eosinophil-selective mediators in human strongyloidiasis, *Parasite Immunol* 28:397, 2006.

Montoya JG: Laboratory diagnosis of *Toxoplasma gondii* infection and toxoplasmosis, *J Infect Dis* 185(Suppl 1):573, 2002.

Montoya JG, Liesenfeld O: Toxoplasmosis, *Lancet* 363:1865, 2004.

Moody A: Rapid diagnostic tests for malaria parasites, *Clin Microbiol Rev* 15:66, 2002.

Nowicki MJ et al: Prevalence of antibodies to *Trypanosoma cruzi* among solid organ donors in Southern California: a population at risk, *Transplantation* 81:477, 2006.

Padgett JJ, Jacobsen KH: Loiasis: African eye worm, *Trans R Soc Trop Med Hyg* 102:983, 2008.

Pantenburg B et al: Intestinal immune response to human *Cryptosporidium* sp. infections, *Infect Immun* 76:23, 2008.

Patel G et al: *Strongyloides* hyperinfection syndrome after intestinal transplantation, *Transpl Infect Dis* 10:137, 2008.

Petro M et al: Unusual endoscopic and microscopic view of *Enterobius vermicularis*: a case report with a review of the literature, *South Med J* 98:926, 2005.

Ponce C et al: Validation of a rapid and reliable test for diagnosis of Chagas disease by detection of *Trypanosoma cruzi*–specific antibodies in blood of donors and patients in Central America, *J Clin Microbiol* 43:5065, 2005.

Price RN et al: *Vivax* malaria: neglected and not benign, *Am J Trop Med Hyg* 77(Suppl 6):79, 2007.

Riles JA et al: Point prevalence of *Cryptosporidium, Cyclospora,* and *Isospora* infections in patients being evaluated for diarrhea, *Am J Clin Pathol* 122:28, 2004.

Roberts LJ et al: Leishmaniasis, *BMJ* 321:801, 2000.

Roddy P et al: Field evaluation of a rapid immunochromatographic assay for detection of *Trypanosoma cruzi* infection by use of whole blood, *J Clin Microbiol* 46:2022, 2008.

Roxstrom-Lindquist K et al: Giardia immunity—an update, *Trends Parasitol* 22:26, 2006.

Schuster FL, Visvesvara GS: Amebae and ciliated protozoa as causal agents of waterborne zoonotic disease, *Vet Parasitol* 126:91, 2004.

Schwebke JR, Burgess D: Trichomoniasis, *Clin Microbiol Rev* 17:794, 2004.

Sena AC et al: *Trichomonas vaginalis* infection in male sexual partners: implications for diagnosis, treatment, and prevention, *Clin Infect Dis* 44:13, 2007.

Shafri SC, Sorvillo FJ: Viability of *Trichomonas vaginalis* in urine: epidemiologic and clinical implications, *J Clin Microbiol* 44:3787, 2006.

Sharp SE et al: Evaluation of the Triage Micro Parasite Panel for detection of *Giardia lamblia, Entamoeba histolytica/Entamoeba dispar,* and *Cryptosporidium parvum* in patient stool specimens, *J Clin Microbiol* 39:332, 2001.

Shields JM, Olson BH: *Cyclospora cayetanensis*: a review of an emerging parasitic coccidian, *Int J Parasitol* 33:371, 2003.

Siddiqui R, Khan NA: *Balamuthia* amoebic encephalitis: an emerging disease with fatal consequences, *Microb Pathog* 44:89, 2008.

Simon MW, Simon NP: Cutaneous larva migrans, *Pediatr Emerg Care* 19:350, 2003.

Sorvillo FJ et al: Deaths from cysticercosis, United States, *Emerg Infect Dis* 13:230, 2007.

Stanley SL: Pathophysiology of amoebiasis, *Trends Parasitol* 17:280, 2001.

Stark D et al: *Dientamoeba fragilis* as a cause of travelers' diarrhea: report of seven cases, *J Travel Med* 14:1195, 2007.

Stark DJ et al: Dientamoebiasis: clinical importance and recent advances, *Trends Parasitol* 22:92, 2006.

Stark D et al: Irritable bowel syndrome: a review on the role of intestinal protozoa and the importance of their detection and diagnosis, *Int J Parasitol* 37:11, 2007.

Stauffer W, Ravdin JI: *Entamoeba histolytica*: an update, *Curr Opin Infect Dis* 16:479, 2003.

Sternberg JM: Human African trypanosomiasis: clinical presentation and immune response, *Parasite Immunol* 26:469, 2004.

Suresh K, Smith H: Comparison of methods for detecting *Blastocystis hominis, Eur J Clin Microbiol Infect Dis* 23:509, 2004.

Sutton M et al: The prevalence of *Trichomonas vaginalis* infection among reproductive-age women in the United States, 2001-2004, *Clin Infect Dis* 45:1319, 2007.

Tan KSW et al: Recent advances in *Blastocystis hominis* research: hot spots in terra incognita, *Int J Parasitol* 32:789, 2002.

Torno MS et al: Cutaneous acanthamoebiasis in AIDS, *J Am Acad Dermatol* 42:351, 2000.

Tzipori S, Ward H: Cryptosporidiosis: biology, pathogenesis and disease, *Microbes Infect* 4:1047, 2002.

Utzinger J et al: FLOTAC: a new sensitive technique for the diagnosis of hookworm infections in humans, *Trans R Soc Trop Med Hygiene* 102:84, 2008.

van Doorn HR et al: Use of enzyme-linked immunosorbent assay and dipstick assay for detection of *Strongyloides stercoralis* infection in humans, *J Clin Microbiol* 45:438, 2007.

van Doorn HR et al: Use of rapid dipstick and latex agglutination tests and enzyme-linked immunosorbent assay for serodiagnosis of amebic liver abscess, amebic colitis, and *Entamoeba histolytica* cyst passage, *J Clin Microbiol* 4:4801, 2005.

Vannier E et al: Human babesiosis, *Infect Dis Clin N Am* 22:469, 2008.

Vega-Lopez F: Diagnosis of cutaneous leishmaniasis, *Curr Opin Infect Dis* 16:97, 2003.

Vijayan, VK: How to diagnose and manage common parasitic pneumonias, *Curr Opin Pulmonary Med* 13:218, 2007.

Viney ME et al: Why does HIV infection not lead to disseminated strongyloidiasis? *J Infect Dis* 190:2175, 2004.

Wasson K, Peper RL: Mammalian microsporidiosis, *Vet Pathol* 37:113, 2000.

Welburn SC, Odiit M: Recent developments in human African trypanosomiasis, *Curr Opin Infect Dis* 15:477, 2002.

Wendel KA et al: *Trichomonas vaginalis* polymerase chain reaction compared with standard diagnostic and therapeutic protocols for detection and treatment of vaginal trichomoniasis, *Clin Infect Dis* 35:576, 2002.

Wichro E et al: Microsporidiosis in travel-associated chronic diarrhea in immune-competent patients, *Am J Trop Med Hyg* 73:285, 2005.

Williams TN: Red blood cell defects and malaria, *Mol Biochem Parasitol* 149:121, 2006.

World Health Organization: dracunculiasis eradication, Available at: www.who.int/dracunculiasis/en/. Accessed August 25, 2009.

Yakoob J et al: Irritable bowel syndrome: in search of an etiology: role of *Blastocystis hominis, Am J Trop Med Hyg* 79:383, 2004.

Young C et al: Transfusion-acquired *Trypanosoma cruzi* infection, *Transfusion* 47:540, 2007.

Zhang X et al: Morphology and reproductive mode of *Blastocystis hominis* in diarrhea and in vitro, *Parasitol Res* 101:43, 2007.

Points to Remember

- Protozoan cysts, helminth eggs, and helminth larvae can be identified on a wet mount preparation of a fecal concentrate. The identification of protozoan trophozoites and cysts is confirmed on a permanently stained smear.

- Fecal-oral transmission is the route of infection for enteric protozoa. The cyst is the infective stage, and the trophozoite is the stage that causes tissue damage.

- The major intestinal protozoan pathogens include *E. histolytica* and *G. lamblia*. *D. fragilis* and *B. hominis* cause symptomatic infections in some patients.

- *E. histolytica* and *E. dispar* are morphologically identical, and specific immunoassay techniques must be performed to differentiate the pathogenic *E. histolytica* from the nonpathogenic *E. dispar*. However, if ingested RBCs are present in the trophozoite, then the organism can be reported as *E. histolytica*.

- *N. fowleri* and *Acanthamoeba* spp. are free-living amebae that can infect humans. *N. fowleri* causes an acute condition called primary amebic meningoencephalitis that is rapidly fatal. *Acanthamoeba* spp. cause keratitis or granulomatous amebic encephalitis.

- The genera *Leishmania* and *Trypanosoma* are blood flagellates of humans and are transmitted by insects.

- Human malaria may be caused by four different *Plasmodium* spp.: *P. vivax, P. ovale, P. malariae,* and *P. falciparum*.

- The life cycle of malaria is complicated, with asexual reproduction taking place in RBCs of humans and sexual reproduction in the gut of the mosquito.

- Identification of the *Plasmodium* spp. is made by observing characteristics of the infected RBC and the malarial organism on a Wright- or Giemsa-stained peripheral blood smear.

- *B. microti*, an intraerythrocytic parasite, morphologically resembles *P. falciparum* on blood smears.

- The intestinal Apicomplexa include *C. parvum, I. belli,* and *C. cayetanensis*, and the infective stage for humans is the acid-fast–positive oocyst.

- *T. gondii* causes a tissue infection that is usually asymptomatic in the immunocompetent host. In patients with AIDS, a latent infection may reactivate and cause encephalitis or pneumonia. Congenital transmission can result in serious complications.

- For most flukes, diagnosis is made by finding the egg in a fecal specimen. For the lung fluke (*P. westermani*), the egg may be found in sputum; for *S. haematobium*, the egg is found in urine.

- Humans are the definitive host and animals or insects serve as the intermediate host for most tapeworms infecting humans.

- Eggs of the beef tapeworm, *T. saginata*, and the eggs of the pork tapeworm, *T. solium*, are identical and must be reported as *Taenia* sp.

- The diagnostic stage for a roundworm may be an egg or a larval form, depending on the species.

- Pinworm, *E. vermicularis*, infection is common in children and is diagnosed by finding eggs on a cellophane tape preparation. Eggs are laid on the perianal area when the female migrates out the anus at night.

- Human hookworm infection may be caused by *N. americanus* and *A. duodenale*. The eggs are identical and are reported as "hookworm eggs."

- Eggs of *S. stercoralis* are not usually present in the stool; the typical diagnostic stage is the rhabditiform larva.

- *T. spiralis* is acquired when humans ingest raw or undercooked pork containing the larval form.

- Diagnosis of trichinosis is made through biopsy of tissue to identify the coiled larval stage.

- Diagnosis of filarial worm infection is made by observing the microfilariae in blood or tissue specimens. Larval characteristics include the presence or absence of a sheath, and the location and arrangement of nuclei in the tail of the microfilariae.

Learning Assessment Questions

1. A trichrome-stained smear of a patient's fecal specimen shows the presence of cysts that are oval, approximately 11 μm in size, have four nuclei characterized by large karyosomes with no peripheral chromatin, and a "cluttered" appearance in the cytoplasm. What is the most likely identification of the organism? Is the organism considered a pathogen?

2. A patient with a history of travel to Africa has fever and chills. The physician suspects malaria and orders a blood smear for examination. Why should you do both a thin film and a thick film? Why would final species identification be made from the thin smear?

3. Give the major characteristics (including size) that you would use to identify eggs of the following organisms: *Taenia* spp., *Ascaris lumbricoides*, *Trichuris trichiura*, and hookworm.

4. Describe the diagnostic method you would use to detect *Enterobius vermicularis* eggs that would not be used with the other types of eggs of intestinal helminths. Explain why.

5. Describe the microscopic characteristics you would use to differentiate the oocysts of *Cyclospora cayetanensis* and *Cryptosporidium parvum*. Include size, appearance on routine wet mount or trichrome, and appearance with special stains.

6. You identify a trophozoite on a trichrome stained smear of a stool sample that is approximately 22 μm in diameter. There is a single nucleus that shows even peripheral chromatin and a small central karyosome. The cytoplasm is relatively "clean" but ingested red blood cells are seen. What is the most likely identification of the organism? Is the organism considered a pathogen? If yes, describe the typical patient symptoms and possible complications.

7. For both *Cryptosporidium parvum* and *Strongyloides stercoralis*, explain the mechanism of autoinfection in the life cycle and why this phase contributes to increased severity of infection.

8. You are examining a blood smear and find an extracellular structure that is approximately 18 μm long. It is tapered at both ends and has an anterior flagellum. An undulating membrane extends the length of the body. What is the genus of this organism? What is the morphologic stage of this organism? With what two diseases do you see this stage in the blood?

9. Compare primary amebic meningoencephalitis and granulomatous amebic encephalitis. Include the following in your discussion: causative organism, population usually infected, route of infection, clinical symptoms, and method of diagnosis.

10. For the following three organisms, *Toxoplasma gondii*, *C. parvum*, and *S. stercoralis*, compare the clinical presentation in the immunocompetent host and in the immunocompromised host.

Clinical Virology

Brian J. Robinson, Sarah L.L. Pierson

OBJECTIVES

After reading and studying this chapter, you should be able to:

1. Describe the characteristics of viruses and differentiate them from bacteria.

2. Describe how viruses multiply.

3. Describe the proper procedures for collection and transport of viral specimens.

4. Name the appropriate specimen for maximum recovery of the suspected viral agent.

5. Compare the different methods used in the diagnosis of viral infections.

6. Explain the advantages and limitations of conventional cell cultures for diagnosing viral infections.

7. Explain the advantages and limitations of rapid viral antigen detection methods.

8. Discuss the indications and limitations of serologic assays in the diagnosis of viral infections.

9. Define cytopathic effect and describe how it is used to presumptively identify viral agents.

10. Create an algorithm for the serologic diagnosis of human immunodeficiency virus infection.

11. Compare the genomes and mode of transmission of the human hepatitis viruses.

12. Develop an algorithm for the serologic diagnosis of viral hepatitis.

13. For each of the viral agents presented in this chapter, discuss how the virus is transmitted or acquired, the infection the virus produces, and the most effective method of laboratory diagnosis.

Case in Point

A 36-year-old man was admitted to the hospital after going to the emergency department and stating that for 7 months he had been experiencing numbness and weakness in his right leg. He had lost 25 lb, was experiencing bowel incontinence, and had been unable to urinate for 3 days. Two years previously the patient had been diagnosed with human immunodeficiency virus infection. A physical examination demonstrated bilateral lower extremity weakness, and his reflexes were slowed throughout his body. Kaposi sarcoma lesions were noted, especially on the lower extremities. Thrush and herpes lesions in the perianal region were also observed. The patient was afebrile. A magnetic resonance imaging (MRI) examination ruled out spinal cord compression. The patient had a history of intravenous drug abuse, chronic diarrhea for 1½ years, Kaposi sarcoma for 2 years, and pancytopenia for several weeks. The patient had large right arachnoid cysts of congenital origin. No previous laboratory reports indicated infectious agents in the cerebrospinal fluid (CSF). Meningitis was suspected, and the patient was admitted with a diagnosis of polyradiculopathy secondary to acquired immunodeficiency syndrome. Blood and CSF were collected. Although numerous white blood cells were found, the CSF produced no growth on routine bacteriologic culture. The blood cultures were also negative. Acyclovir was administered after culture results were received.

Issues to Consider

After reading the patient's history, consider the following:

- In what ways the patient's history could relate to the current complaint
- What information is obtained from the laboratory and MRI results
- How the information presented helps to determine the most likely cause of the patient's complaint

Key Terms

Antigenic drift	Heteroploid
Antigenic shift	Koplik spots
Arboviruses	Nucleocapsid
Capsid	Obligate intracellular parasites
Cell cultures	Primary cell cultures
Continuous cell cultures	Prions
Cytopathic effect	Syncytia
Diploid	Tissue culture
Envelope	Vaccinia virus
Hemagglutinin	Virion

Clinical virology is one of the most exciting fields of clinical microbiology. The "older" views of virology as clinically irrelevant have fallen as new rapid diagnostic tests have been developed, allowing rapid laboratory-directed diagnosis in some cases. Rapid laboratory results without appropriate medical interventions would be only half a service, but antiviral therapy is keeping pace with the progress in rapid diagnostic assays. In the recent past new viral threats have literally leapt into our lives: the introduction of West Nile virus into North America; the explosion, spread, mortality, and then withdrawal of severe acute respiratory syndrome (SARS); the increase of highly pathogenic avian viruses in Asia, and the jump of the virus directly into human hosts with high mortality rates, the unexpected transfer of monkeypox from Africa to the midwestern United States, and most recently the worldwide spread of the novel influenza A (H1N1), or "swine flu."

Virology has puzzles that defy management. Human immunodeficiency virus (HIV) continues to ravage entire continents, effectively reducing large portions of generations. Mosquitoes continue to spread dengue virus throughout the world. Despite reliable vaccines and dependable antiviral medications, more than 30,000 U.S. citizens die each year of influenza. This chapter discusses the advances and the challenges of clinical virology. The virology practiced in clinical laboratories today is different from the services provided 5 years ago, and the clinical virology practiced 5 years from now will likely be different from what is done today. The challenges demand better services and better tools for diagnosis.

CHARACTERISTICS OF VIRUSES

Structure

At a minimum, viruses contain a viral genome of either RNA or DNA and a protein coat—the **capsid**. The genome can be either double stranded (ds) or single stranded (ss). The genome and its protein coat together are referred to as a **nucleocapsid.** The entire virus particle is called a **virion.** Some viruses also have a phospholipid **envelope** surrounding the virion. Enveloped viruses are often more susceptible to inactivation by high temperature, extreme pH, and chemicals than nonenveloped (naked) viruses. The envelopes are of host origin, but they contain virus-encoded proteins. The viruses acquire the lipid membrane as they bud from host cells.

The morphology of virions is helical, icosahedral (a geometric shape with 20 triangular sides), or complex. The envelope masks the shape of the virion, so most enveloped viruses are pleomorphic, or variably shaped. The poxviruses are the largest viruses (250 × 350 nm), and the smallest human virus is the poliovirus, which is 25 nm in diameter.

Taxonomy

Originally viruses were classified by their host range and the type of diseases they caused. Now viruses are classified in orders, families, genera, and species based on genome type (RNA or DNA), the number of strands in the genome (ds or ss), morphology, and presence or absence of an envelope. Nucleotide sequencing of the genome is also a valuable tool for taxonomic placement of viruses. A summary of the clinically significant viruses is shown in Table 29-1.

Viral Replication

Viruses are **obligate intracellular parasites,** meaning they must be inside a living cell in order to replicate. For infection of a cell to occur, virions must absorb or attach to the cell surface. Absorption is specific for certain cell receptors. Most host cell receptors are glycoproteins, some of which include the immune globulin superfamily molecules (for poliovirus), acetylcholine (for rabies virus), sialic acid (for influenza virus), CD4 (for HIV), and complement receptor C3d (for Epstein-Barr virus [EBV]). The virus attaches to specific receptors on the surface of a susceptible cell by means of specialized structures on its surface, called *adhesion molecules.*

The next step in viral replication is penetration. Viruses can penetrate the cell by several different mechanisms, depend-

TABLE 29-1 List of Viruses Causing Human Disease, Based on Nucleic Acid Characteristics and Taxonomy

Genome Strand	Family (Subfamily)	Genus	Species
dsDNA	Adenoviridae	*Mastadenovirus*	Human adenovirus C
	Herpesviridae		
	Alphaherpesvirinae	*Simplexvirus*	Human herpesvirus 1, 2
		Varicellovirus	Human herpesvirus 3
	Betaherpesvirinae	*Cytomegalovirus*	Human herpesvirus 5
		Roseolovirus	Human herpesvirus 6
			Human herpesvirus 7
	Gammaherpesvirinae	*Lymphocryptovirus*	Human herpesvirus 4
		Rhadinovirus	Human herpesvirus 8
	Papillomaviridae	*Papillomavirus*	Human papillomavirus
	Poxviridae	*Orthopoxvirus*	Variola virus, vaccinia virus
ds/ssDNA	Hepadnaviridae	*Orthohepadnavirus*	Hepatitis B virus
ssDNA	Parvoviridae	*Erythrovirus*	Parvovirus B-19
		Bocavirus	Human *Bocavirus*
dsRNA	Reoviridae	*Rotavirus*	Rotavirus A
		Coltivirus	Colorado tick fever virus
ssRNA	Arenaviridae	*Arenavirus*	Lymphocytic choriomeningitis virus, Lassa virus
	Astroviridae	*Mamastrovirus*	Human astrovirus 1
	Bunyaviridae	*Orthobunyavirus*	California encephalitis virus
		Hantavirus	Hantaan virus, Sin Nombre
		Nairovirus	Crimean-Congo hemorrhagic fever virus
		Phlebovirus	Rift Valley fever virus
	Caliciviridae	*Norovirus*	Norwalk virus
		Sapovirus	Sapporo virus
	Coronaviridae	*Coronavirus*	SARS-coronavirus
	Filoviridae	*Marburgvirus*	Lake Victoria marburgvirus
		Ebolavirus	Zaire ebolavirus
	Flaviviridae	*Flavivirus*	Yellow fever virus
		Japanese encephalitis complex	West Nile virus
	Hepeviridae	*Hepacivirus*	Hepatitis C virus
		Hepevirus (was "Hepatitis E-like viruses")	Hepatitis E virus
	Orthomyxoviridae	*Influenzavirus A*	Influenza A virus
		Influenzavirus B	Influenza B virus
		Influenzavirus C	Influenza C virus
	Paramyxoviridae		
	Paramyxovirinae	*Respirovirus*	Sendai virus
		Morbillivirus	Measles virus
		Rubulavirus	Mumps virus
		Henipavirus	Hendra virus
	Pneumovirinae	*Pneumovirus*	Human respiratory syncytial virus
		Metapneumovirus	Human metapneumovirus
	Picornaviridae	*Enterovirus*	Poliovirus
		Rhinovirus	Human rhinovirus A
		Hepatovirus	Hepatitis A virus
	Rhabdoviridae	*Lyssavirus*	Rabies virus
	Retroviridae	*Lentivirus*	Human immunodeficiency virus 1, human immunodeficiency virus 2
	Togaviridae	*Alphavirus*	Venezuelan equine encephalitis, eastern equine encephalitis, western equine encephalitis
		Rubivirus	Rubella virus

ing on the virus. Naked virions can directly penetrate the cell membrane. Enveloped viruses may enter the cell by fusion with the cell membrane, and a third method of penetration is *endocytosis,* whereby the enveloped virus enters the cell in a cytoplasmic vacuole. Once inside the cell, the virus loses its protein coat, releasing the genome. This process is called *uncoating.* RNA viruses usually release the genome into the cytoplasm, whereas most DNA viruses release their genome into the host nucleus. The viral genome then directs the host cell to make viral proteins and replicate the viral genome. Depending on the virus, the metabolism of the host cell may be completely stopped (as with polioviruses), or it may continue on a restricted scale (as with influenza viruses).

The next step is the assembly or maturation of the virus particles. The capsid protein subunits aggregate to form capsomers, and the capsomers combine to form the capsid. The capsid and genome associate to form the nucleocapsid. The new virions are then released by lysis of the cell, if infected with a naked virus, or by budding through the cell, plasma membrane if infected by enveloped viruses. During budding, part of the plasma membrane surrounds the viral capsid and becomes the viral envelope.

LABORATORY DIAGNOSIS OF VIRAL INFECTIONS

Laboratories can provide different levels of services, based on mission, financial resources, and need. Full-service virology laboratories provide viral culture and identification using different mammalian **cell cultures** to support the growth of viruses from clinical specimens. Although not all medical treatment facilities provide full virology services, these laboratories can still provide information about viral infections using a variety of rapid tests that detect specific viruses in clinical specimens. These rapid tests can involve the detection of viral antigens by a number of methods such as immuno-fluorescence (IF) or enzyme immunoassay (EIA). Some tests are Clinical Laboratory Improvement Act (CLIA) waived, bringing viral identification services into physicians' offices and clinics. Other laboratories limit their virology services to viral serology—determining the patient's immune response to viruses—rather than detecting the viruses directly.

Specimen Collection and Transport

Because viral shedding is usually greatest during the early stages of infection, the best specimens are those collected as early as possible. The sensitivity of viral culture may decrease rapidly 3 days after acute onset of symptoms. Specimens should be collected aseptically. Aspirated secretions are often preferable, but swabs are easier to use for collection. Swabs must be made of Dacron or rayon. Calcium alginate swabs inhibit the replication of some viruses and can interfere with nucleic acid amplification tests. Tissue samples must be kept moist. Viral transport medium, saline, or trypticase soy broth can be added to sterile containers to keep tissues from drying out.

Several viral transport systems are commercially available. Most transport media consist of a buffered isotonic solution with some type of protein, such as albumin, gelatin, or serum, to protect less stable viruses. Antibacterial and antifungal agents are added in some transport systems to inhibit contaminating bacterial and fungal biota. Samples that can be collected with viral transport media are respiratory, swab, and tissue samples. Samples that should be collected without viral transport media include blood, bone marrow, cerebrospinal fluid (CSF), amniotic fluid, urine, pericardial fluid, and pleural fluid. It is also important for the transport container to be unbreakable and able to withstand freezing and thawing.

It is optimal to process viral specimens for culture immediately. Some viruses, such as respiratory syncytial virus (RSV), become more difficult to recover even a few hours after collection. If specimens cannot be processed immediately after collection, however, they should be stored at 4° C. Specimens should not be frozen unless a significant delay, more than 4 days, in processing is anticipated. In that case,

specimens should be frozen and held at –70° C. Specimens should not be stored at –20° C. This temperature facilitates the formation of ice crystals, which disrupts the host cells and results in significant loss of viral viability.

Appropriate Specimens for Maximum Recovery

Logically, specimens for viral isolation should be collected from the affected site. For example, secretions from the respiratory mucosa are most appropriate for viral diagnosis of respiratory infections. Aspirates, or surface swabs, are usually appropriate for lesions. If the intestinal mucosa is involved, a stool specimen is most appropriate. However, if systemic, congenital, or generalized disease is involved, specimens from multiple sites, including blood (buffy coat), CSF, and the portals of entry (oral or respiratory tract) or exit (urine or stool), are appropriate. Enteroviruses can cause respiratory infections and may be recovered from the stool after the respiratory shedding has ceased. In addition, enteroviruses are a major cause of aseptic meningitis and can be isolated from urine specimens. Table 29-2 lists suggested specimens to be collected for viral diagnosis according to the affected body site.

Methods in Diagnostic Virology

The laboratory uses four major methods to diagnose viral infections:
- Direct detection of the virus in clinical specimens
- Nucleic acid–based detection
- Isolation of viruses in cell cultures
- Serologic assays to detect antiviral antibodies

Each laboratory must decide which of these methods to offer based on the spectrum of infections encountered, the population of patients served, and the financial resources. In most circumstances, a combination of these methods is used.

Direct Detection

Direct-detection methods are generally not as sensitive as culture methods, but they can offer valuable assistance to the laboratory scientist. Many of these tests can be performed in a few minutes. Viral detection allows clinicians to make relevant decisions about therapy and hospitalization. In some situations, virology results might be available before routine bacteriology culture results.

Microscopy. Except for the poxviruses, individual virus particles are too small to be seen by bright-field microscopy. Electron microscopy has a greater magnification and can be used to detect virions. However, electron microscopy is expensive, labor intensive, and not a very sensitive method of detecting viruses. For these reasons electron microscopy is rarely used in clinical laboratories, although it can detect noncultivatable viruses, such as the Norwalk viruses in stool filtrates.

Many viruses produce characteristic visual changes in infected cells, referred to as **cytopathic effect** (CPE). The CPE can be detected in cell scrapings from infected sites. For instance, a Tzanck smear can detect Cowdry type A bodies from herpes simplex virus (HSV) and varicella-zoster virus (VZV) lesions, and Papanicolaou (Pap) smears can reveal human papillomavirus (HPV)–associated koilocytosis—squamous cells with an enlarged nucleus surrounded by a non-

TABLE 29-2 Tests Available for Common Viral Pathogens and Specimens for Culture

Body System Affected	Antigen Detection	Virus Isolation	Serology	Culture Specimens
Respiratory tract	Adenovirus, herpes simplex virus (HSV), cytomegalovirus (CMV), influenza virus types A and B, parainfluenza virus, respiratory syncytial virus (RSV)	Adenovirus, coxsackie A, coxsackie B, echovirus, HSV, CMV, influenza virus types A and B, parainfluenza virus, RSV, reovirus, rhinovirus	Adenovirus, coxsackie A virus, coxsackie B virus, Echovirus, HSV, CMV, influenza virus types A and B, parainfluenza virus, RSV	Nasal aspirate, nasopharynx (NP) or throat swabs, bronchoalveolar lavage, lung biopsy
Gastrointestinal	Adenoviruses 40 and 41, rotavirus	Adenovirus 40 and 41, coxsackie A, reovirus	Adenoviruses 40 and 41, coxsackie A	Stool, rectal swab
Hepatitis			Hepatitis A virus (HAV), hepatitis B virus (HBV), hepatitis C virus (HCV), hepatitis D virus (HDV), hepatitis E virus (HEV), Epstein-Barr virus (EBV)	
Cutaneous	HSV, adenovirus, varicella-zoster virus (VZV)	HSV, adenovirus, coxsackie group A virus, coxsackie group B virus, echovirus, enterovirus, measles virus, VZV, reovirus, rubella virus, vaccinia virus	HSV, adenovirus, coxsackie group B virus, dengue virus, echovirus, human herpes virus 6 (HHV-6), measles virus, VZV, parvovirus B19, rubella virus, vaccinia virus	Vesicle aspirate, NP aspirate and stool, lesion swab
Central nervous system	HSV, mumps virus	Coxsackie group A virus, Coxsackie group B virus, echovirus, enterovirus, poliovirus, HSV, mumps virus	Coxsackie group A virus, coxsackie group B virus, echovirus, poliovirus, HSV, HHV-6, mumps virus	Cerebrospinal fluid, brain biopsy, NP swabs, stool
Ocular	Adenovirus, HSV	Adenovirus, HSV, coxsackie group A, Enterovirus	HSV, coxsackie group A virus	Corneal swabs, conjunctival scrapings
Genital	HSV	HSV	HSV	Vesicle aspirate, vesicle swab

staining halo. Rabies is sometimes diagnosed by detecting Negri bodies, which are eosinophilic cytoplasmic inclusions, in neurons.

Immunofluorescence can be a flexible tool to detect various viral agents directly in clinical specimens. In direct fluorescent antibody (DFA) tests, cells from a patient are fixed to a microscope slide and fluorescence-labeled antibodies are added. If viral antigens are present, the labeled antibody will bind and fluorescence will be seen microscopically (see Chapter 10 for a more detailed description). DFA assays are available for numerous viruses, including adenovirus, influenza viruses A and B, measles, parainfluenza viruses 1 through 4, and RSV from respiratory specimens; HSV-1 and HSV-2 and VZV from cutaneous lesion material; and cytomegalovirus (CMV) from blood.

Enzyme Immunoassays. Many EIA tests for viral detection are commercially available; most are packaged as microtiter plate assays. These tests can be used to detect RSV and influenza A from respiratory specimens, hepatitis B virus (HBV) and HIV-1 from serum or plasma, the enteric adenoviruses from stool, and HSV from cutaneous lesions and conjunctival swabs. Other tests are packaged in single-test platforms, with positive specimens being detected either by colorimetric changes or optical density changes on membrane

or silicon surfaces (Figure 29-1). These tests can be used to detect RSV, influenza viruses A and B from respiratory specimens, rotavirus and enteric adenovirus from rectal swabs, and West Nile virus from serum. EIA tests are often less sensitive than cell cultures or IF tests, so negative results are confirmed with IF tests, cell culture, or gene amplification.

Nucleic Acid–Based Detection

An increasing interest in nucleic acid–based detection assays compared with traditional cell culture methods has shifted the focus of clinical virology. Although cell culture–based virology is still important to confirm the presence of viruses in clinical samples, not only can rapid analysis determine the presence or absence of a virus but, depending on the assay utilized, a quantitative result can also be generated. The use of these assays has led to a better understanding of viruses as well as insights into better patient therapies.

Nucleic acid–based detection assays in the virology laboratory provide both advantages and disadvantages. Advantages include quicker turnaround times, better sensitivity than cell culture and DFA, assays that can be quantitative and can detect viruses unculturable by cell culture (i.e., norovirus, hepatitis viruses), and the ability to detect multiple viruses simultaneously (multiplex) and potentially characterize the

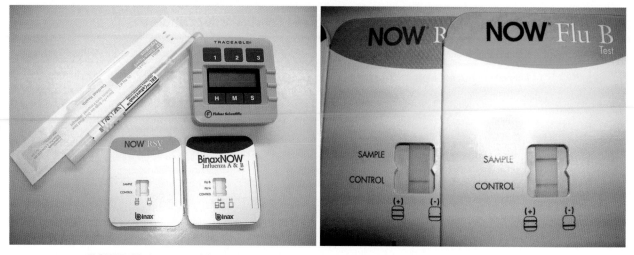

FIGURE 29-1 A, Card format rapid immunochromatographic membrane assay, BinaxNow (Scarborough, Me.), for three common respiratory viruses: influenza A and B and respiratory syncytial viruses. **B,** Examples of positive and negative results.

virus genetically (i.e., genotype). Disadvantages include detection of both active and inactivated virus, increased cost, need for specialized training and facilities, and lack of Food and Drug Administration (FDA)-cleared assays. The use of nucleic acid–based detection assays in the virology laboratory is at the discretion of the individual laboratory and is determined by available resources, populations served, and requests for tests by clinicians.

Techniques involved in providing rapid more detailed results are polymerase chain reaction (PCR), including both traditional and real-time PCR; branched DNA; nucleic acid sequence-based amplification; or a combination of PCR and flow cytometry, such as the Luminex System (Luminex Corporation, Austin, Tex.) for multiplex detection. Zitterkopf et al. demonstrated the detection of influenza A virus by PCR was not only more sensitive than the traditional cell culture and shell vial methods, but allowed earlier administering of antiviral treatment for patients and better overall management of patients. Lodes et al. established a microarray assay to rapidly subtype influenza A virus isolates, stating that this technology would be valuable in the event of an outbreak or pandemic. Mahony et al. developed a Luminex assay to detect and type/subtype 20 different viral pathogens within 5 hours. This flow cytometry–based technology should help the public health community by rapidly identifying viral pathogens and improve management of patients if an outbreak occurs.

Nucleic acid hybridization tests can detect viruses from various clinical specimens. Assays are available to detect a number of viruses, including the HPV from endocervical specimens, and to classify them into high-risk and low-risk HPV types for cancer. Other hybridization tests can detect CMV from blood and HBV from plasma and serum. Numerous gene amplification techniques are available for the amplification and detection of viral genomes, primarily the blood-borne pathogens such as HIV-1, HBV, hepatitis C virus (HCV), and West Nile virus (WNV).

Viral Isolation

In clinical virology, isolating viruses is still the gold standard against which all other methods are compared. Traditionally three methods are used for isolation of viruses in diagnostic virology: cell culture, animal inoculation, and embryonated eggs. Of these three methods, the most commonly used by clinical virology laboratories is cell culture. Animal inoculation is extremely costly and is used only as a special resource and in reference or research laboratories. For example, certain coxsackie A viruses require suckling mice for isolation of the virus. Embryonated eggs are rarely used; isolation of influenza viruses is enhanced in embryonated eggs, but this is generally much more easily accomplished in cell culture.

Establishing at least a limited clinical virus isolation capability in routine laboratories is amply justified. Most of the clinical workload focuses on the detection of HSV in genital specimens and respiratory viruses. A significant percentage of common clinical viruses can often be identified within 48 hours of inoculation, including HSV, influenza A and B viruses, parainfluenza viruses 1 through 4, RSV, adenovirus, and many enteroviruses.

Cell Culture. The term *cell culture* is technically used to indicate culture of cells in vitro; the cells are not organized into a tissue. The term **tissue culture** or *organ culture* is used to denote growth of tissues or an organ in a way that preserves the architecture or function of the tissue or organ. However, many clinical virologists use these terms interchangeably.

Cell cultures can be divided into three categories: primary, low passage (or finite), and continuous. **Primary cell cultures** are obtained from tissue removed from an animal. The tissue is finely minced and then treated with an enzyme such as trypsin to disperse individual cells further. The cells are then seeded onto a surface to form a monolayer, such as in a flask or test tube. With primary cell lines, only minimal cell division occurs. To maintain cell viability, they must periodically be removed from the surface, diluted, and placed into a new container. This process is referred to as *splitting* or *passaging*. Primary cell lines can only be passaged a few times. An example of a commonly used primary cell culture is primary monkey kidney (PMK) cells.

Finite cell cultures can divide, but passage is limited to about 50 generations. Finite cell lines, like primary cell lines, are **diploid,** meaning they contain two copies of each chromosome. Diploid is the normal genetic make up for eukaryotic cells. With increasing passage, these cells become more insensitive to viral infection. Human neonatal lung (HNL) is an example of a standard finite cell culture used in diagnostic virology.

Continuous cell cultures are capable of infinite passage and are **heteroploid,** meaning they have an abnormal and variable number of chromosomes that is not a multiple of the normal haploid number. HEp2 (derived from a human laryngeal epithelial carcinoma), A549 (derived from a human lung carcinoma), and Vero (derived from monkey kidney) are examples of continuous cell lines used in diagnostic virology. Each laboratory must decide which cell lines to use based on the spectrum of viral sensitivity, availability, and cost. Optimally several different cell lines will be used for a single specimen to recover a variety of different viruses that might be present, much like the use of artificial media for the recovery of bacteria. Table 29-3 lists some cell culture lines commonly used in clinical virology.

Mixed or engineered cell cultures are lines of cells that contain a mixture of two different cell types or are made up of cells genetically modified to make identification of viral infection easier. Mixed cell lines have been developed by combining two cell lines that are susceptible to certain types of viruses such as respiratory or enteric viruses. The mixed line can then give greater sensitivity to a wider range of viruses.

Cytopathic Effect on Cell Cultures. Some viruses produce characteristic CPE, which can provide a presumptive identification of a virus isolated from a clinical specimen. For example, HSV grows rapidly on many different cell lines and frequently produces CPE within 24 hours. A predominantly cell-associated virus, HSV produces a focal CPE (in which adjacent cells become infected) and *plaques*, or clusters of infected cells. The combination of rapid growth, plaque formation, and growth on many different cell types, such as MRC-5, human fibroblasts, Vero, HEp-2, mink lung, and PMK, is presumptive evidence for the identification of HSV. HSV is one of the few viruses that can grow on rabbit kidney cells (Figure 29-2); therefore it is a useful cell line for HSV detection.

CMV produces HSV-like CPE (Figure 29-3), but it grows much more slowly and only on diploid fibroblasts. VZV grows on several types of cells, including diploid fibroblasts, A549, and Vero cells. Enteroviruses characteristically produce rather

TABLE 29-3 Cell Cultures Commonly Used in the Clinical Virology Laboratory

Virus	PMK	HDF	HEp2	RK	A549	CPE
Herpes simplex virus	−	+ + +	+ + +	+ + +	+ + +	Large, rounded cells
Cytomegalovirus	−	+ + +	−	−	−	Large, rounded cells
Varicella-zoster virus	−	+ + +	−	−	+/−	Foci or rounded cells; possible syncytia
Enterovirus	+	+	+ +	−	+	Refractile, round cells in clusters
Adenovirus	+	+ +	+ + +	−	+ +	Large, rounded cells in clusters
Respiratory syncytial virus	+/−	+	+ + +	−	+ +	Syncytia
Influenza/parainfluenza	+ + +	+/−	−	−	−	Variable—none to granular appearance

Modified from Costello MJ et al: Guidelines for specimen collection, transportation, and test selection, *Lab Med* 24:19, 1993.
PMK, Primary monkey kidney; *HDF*, human diploid fibroblasts; *HEp2*, human laryngeal carcinoma cell line; *RK*, rabbit kidney; *A549*, human lung carcinoma cell line; *CPE*, cytopathic effect.

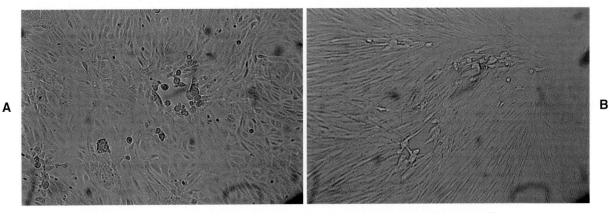

FIGURE 29-2 A, Herpes simplex virus (HSV) from the skin, showing cytopathic effect (CPE) in less than 1 day on rabbit kidney cells. **B,** HSV showing CPE in less than 1 day on HeLa cells.

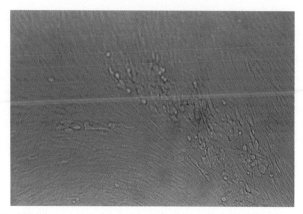

FIGURE 29-3 Cytomegalovirus from cerebrospinal fluid forming cytopathic effect on diploid fibroblast cells.

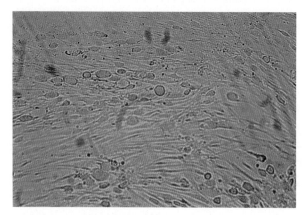

FIGURE 29-4 Cytopathic effect of adenovirus on HeLa cells.

small, round infected cells that spread diffusely on PMK, diploid fibroblasts, human embryonal rhabdomyosarcoma (RD) cells, and A549 cells. Adenoviruses also produce cell rounding (Figure 29-4), usually larger than that caused by enteroviruses, on a number of cell types, including diploid fibroblasts, HEp-2, A549, and PMK. The rounding may be diffuse or focal, appearing like a cluster of grapes.

The respiratory viruses may not produce characteristic CPE. RSV can produce classic syncytial formation in HEp2 or even MKC cells. **Syncytia** are giant multinucleated cells formed from cell fusion as a result of virus infection. Parainfluenza type 2, and to a lesser extent parainfluenza type 3, viruses can also produce syncytia. Influenza virus commonly does not exhibit a well-defined CPE. Specimens submitted for influenza virus cultures are usually inoculated onto PMK, LLC-MK2 (a continuous line derived from rhesus monkey kidney), or MDCK (canine kidney) cells. Because influenza viruses typically do not produce CPE, a hemagglutination or hemadsorption test is done to detect these viruses. Cells infected with influenza virus express a viral **hemagglutinin** (H) protein on their surface that binds red blood cells. In the hemadsorption test, a suspension of red blood cells is added to the infected cell monolayer. If influenza virus is present, the red blood cells will "stick" or adsorb to the infected cells.

In the hemagglutination assay, supernatant from the infected monolayer containing influenza virus is mixed with a suspension of red blood cells. Influenza viruses also have on their surface the H protein; therefore the red blood cells will agglutinate. Fluorescent antibody stains that detect viral antigen, like those used directly on clinical specimens, can also be used to screen cell cultures before a final negative result is reported. Besides IF, EIA and nucleic acid amplification assays can be applied to detecting and identifying viruses in cell cultures.

Centrifugation-Enhanced Shell Vial Culture. The shell vial culture technique is a simple method that more rapidly identifies viruses than does the traditional cell culture method. Cells are grown on a round coverslip in a shell vial. A shell vial is a small, round, flat-bottom tube, generally with a screw cap. The shell vial is inoculated with the clinical sample and then centrifuged to promote viral absorption. The shell vial is incubated for 24 to 48 hours, after which the coverslip is removed and the IF technique performed. Based on the type of clinical specimen and suspected viruses, a variety of fluorescent-labeled antibodies can be used. A modification of this procedure is to use flat-bottom microtiter plates.

Serologic Assays

Viral serology provides limited information, and certain problems are inherent in the methods. First, serologic assays measure host response rather than directly detecting the virus. Second, the antibody-producing capabilities of human hosts vary widely. Third, the antibody level does not necessarily correlate with the acuteness or activity level of the infection.

With few exceptions, paired sera (acute and convalescent) demonstrating seroconversion or a fourfold rise in titer are required to establish a diagnosis of recent infection. Therefore serologic studies are usually retrospective. Some assays are able to distinguish between immunoglobulin M (IgM) and immunoglobulin G (IgG); the presence of IgM indicates an acute infection. Cross-reactions with nonspecific antibodies can occur, which makes interpretation of results difficult. Interpretation is also difficult because of passive transfer of antibodies, such as in transplacental or transfusion transmission. The following are indications for serologic testing:

- Diagnosis of infections with nonculturable agents such as hepatitis viruses
- Determination of immune status in regard to rubella, measles, VZV, HAV, and HBV
- Monitoring of patients who have immunosuppression or have had transplants
- Epidemiologic or prevalence studies

DOUBLE-STRANDED DNA VIRUSES

Viruses are discussed herein in groups based on nucleic acid types: dsDNA, ssDNA, dsRNA, and ssRNA viruses. As an exception, the hepatitis viruses will be discussed as one group, despite the fact that they do not all have the same type of nucleic acid. This exception is primarily to accommodate the fact that these viruses are so closely associated in a clinical laboratory because of their common tissue tropism.

Adenoviridae

Human adenoviruses belong to the genus *Mastadenovirus*. Adenoviruses are naked icosahedral viruses with dsDNA (Figure 29-5). Adenovirus has 49 distinct serotypes (six subgenera: A through F), and the different serotypes are associated with numerous clinical manifestations. The most common serotypes are 1 to 8, 11, 21, 35, 37, and 40. Although half of all adenovirus infections are asymptomatic, the virus causes about 10% of all pneumonia and 5% to 15% of all gastroenteritis in children. The viruses cause upper respiratory tract infections, acute respiratory distress, epidemic keratoconjunctivitis, acute hemorrhagic cystitis, and pharyngoconjunctival fever. Adenovirus infections occur throughout the year and strike every age group. Adenovirus serotype 14 is rarely reported but causes severe and sometimes fatal acute respiratory disease (ARD) in patients of all ages. An outbreak of adenovirus 14 was reported in four states from 2006 to 2007. The outbreak included one infant in New York and 140 additional cases from Oregon, Texas, and Washington. Although no link could be found between the New York case and the other cases, all isolates were identical by hexon and fiber gene sequencing.

Adenovirus is shed in secretions from the eyes and respiratory tract. Viral shedding in stool and urine can occur for days after the disease has disappeared. The viruses are spread by aerosols, fomites, the oral-fecal route, and personal contact. Most infections are mild and require no specific treatment. Until the sole manufacturer ceased production, oral vaccination was available from 1971 to 1999 for types 4 and 7 and was used only for preventing ARD among military recruits. A new vaccine is in development. Good infection control measures, including adequate chlorination of swimming pools, prevent adenovirus infection, such as adenovirus-associated conjunctivitis.

Adenoviruses type 40 and 41 are called *enteric* adenoviruses because they cause epidemics of gastroenteritis in young children. Diarrhea is a prominent feature of the illness, but less vomiting and fever occur than with rotavirus infections. Enteric adenoviruses have a worldwide, endemic distribution, and numbers of cases increase during the warmer months. These adenoviruses can be identified but not serotyped by EIA. Commercial antigen detection kits are available. Adenoviruses are quite stable and can be isolated in human embryonic kidney and many continuous epithelial cell lines. They produce characteristic CPE, with swollen cells in grapelike clusters. Isolates can be identified by FA and EIA methods. Serotyping is accomplished by serum neutralization or hemagglutination inhibition.

Herpesviridae

The herpesviruses belong to the family Herpesviridae. The herpesviruses have a genome of linear dsDNA, an icosahedral capsid, an amorphous integument surrounding the capsid, and an outer envelope. In addition, all herpesviruses share the property of being able to achieve latency and lifelong persistence in their hosts. The virus is latent between active infections. Certain stimuli, including stress, caffeine, and sunlight, can activate the virus. Activation can cause lesions to reappear.

Eight species of human herpesviruses (HHV) are currently known:

- Herpes simplex virus type 1 (HSV-1), also known as *human herpes virus type 1 (HHV-1)*
- Herpes simplex virus type 2 (HSV-2), also known as *HHV-2*
- Varicella-zoster virus (VZV), also known as *HHV-3*
- Epstein-Barr virus (EBV), also known as *HHV-4*
- Cytomegalovirus (CMV), also known as *HHV-5*
- Human herpesvirus 6 (HHV-6)
- Human herpesvirus 7 (HHV-7)
- Human herpesvirus 8 (HHV-8), also known as *Kaposi sarcoma herpes virus*

Additional herpes viruses infect only primates, except for herpes B virus, which has produced fatal infections in researchers and others handling primates.

Herpes Simplex Viruses

HSV-1 and HSV-2 belong to the genus *Simplexvirus*. HSV infections are very common. By adulthood, about 80% of Americans have been infected with HSV-1. Approximately 20% of Americans have HSV-2 infections. Most infections with HSV are asymptomatic. Disease caused by HSV infection is classically divided into two categories: *primary* (first or initial infection) and *recurrent* (reactivation of the latent virus).

Infections are generally spread by contact with contaminated secretions. Lesions usually occur on mucous membranes after an incubation period of 2 to 11 days. Infected individuals are most infectious during the early days of a primary infection. Virus-infected cells are usually found at the edge and in the base of lesions; however, the virus can be transmitted from older lesions and asymptomatic patients. HSV infections can cause a wide spectrum of clinical manifestations, including the following:

- *Oral herpes.* Oral herpes infections are usually but not exclusively caused by HSV-1. The incubation period varies from 2 days to 2 weeks. Primary infections are usually asymptomatic, but when apparent, they commonly manifest as intraoral mucosal vesicles (which

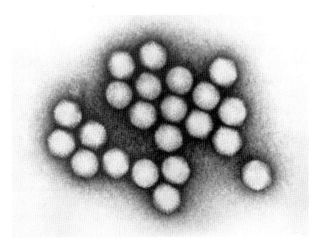

FIGURE 29-5 Transmission electron micrograph of adenovirus. (Courtesy Centers for Disease Control and Prevention, Dr. G. William Gary, Jr.)

are rarely seen) or ulcerations that may be quite widespread and involve the buccal mucosa, posterior pharynx, and gingival and palatal mucosae. In young adults, a primary herpes simplex infection may involve the posterior pharynx and appear as acute pharyngitis. Recurrent, or reactivation, HSV infection usually occurs on the border of the lips at the junction of the oral mucosa and skin. A prodrome of burning or pain followed by vesicles, ulcers, and crusted lesions is the typical pattern.

- *Genital herpes.* Genital herpes infections are usually caused by HSV-2, although HSV-1 virus can cause as many as one third of the infections. Many individuals with antibodies to HSV-2 have not been diagnosed with genital herpes. When the infection manifests, it appears in females as vesicles on the mucosa of the labia, vagina, or both. Cervical and vulvar involvement is not uncommon. In males, the shaft, glans, and prepuce of the penis are the commonly affected sites. The urethra is commonly involved in both sexes. Recurrent herpes infections involve the same sites as primary infections, but the urethra is less commonly involved. The symptoms are usually less severe in recurrent disease. Genital herpes infections can as much as double the risk of sexual transmission of HIV.

- *Neonatal herpes.* Transmission of HSV from infected mothers to neonates is less common than might be expected. However, mortality associated with disseminated neonatal disease is about 60% in treated patients. Infection may be acquired in utero, intrapartum (during birth), or postnatally (after birth). The infection is most commonly transmitted during a vaginal delivery and is more severe when HSV-2 is involved. Transmission is about 50% for a mother who has a primary infection. Most newborns are infected by mothers who are asymptomatically shedding the virus during a primary infection. The risk of transmission is very low when the mother has recurrent herpes. Cesarean section or suppressive antiviral therapy at delivery significantly reduces the risk of transmission.

- *HSV encephalitis.* HSV encephalitis is a rare but devastating disease, with a mortality of about 70%. In fact, HSV is the leading cause of fatal sporadic encephalitis in the United States. Encephalitis is usually caused by HSV-2 in neonates and HSV-1 in older children and adults. HSV encephalitis is also associated with immunocompromised patients. Survival rates and clinical outcomes are greatly improved with intravenous (IV) antiviral treatment.

- *Ocular herpes.* A herpes simplex infection of the conjunctiva can manifest as swelling of the eyelids associated with vesicles. Corneal involvement may result in destructive ulceration and even perforation of the cornea. HSV is the most common cause of corneal infection in the United States. Fortunately most infections involve only the superficial epithelial layer and heal completely with treatment.

Diagnosis of HSV infections is best made by antigen detection or viral isolation. The best specimens for culture are

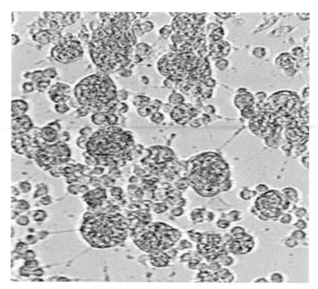

FIGURE 29-6 Advanced cytopathic effect in an A549 cell line due to herpes simplex virus infection. (Courtesy Sarah Pierson.)

aspirates from vesicles, open lesions, or host cells collected from infected sites. Culture of CSF is usually not productive. To get a culture-confirmed diagnosis of encephalitis, brain-biopsy material is required. Alternatively CSF can be assayed by PCR for detection of HSV. In some studies, gene amplification for HSV in CSF approaches 100% sensitivity.

In culture HSV replicates rapidly, and CPE can be seen within 24 hours (see Figure 29-2 and Figure 29-6). Therefore diagnosis and appropriate therapy can be readily accomplished. HSV can be isolated in numerous cell lines including human embryonic lung, rabbit kidney, HEp-2, and A549. HSV is one of the most frequently isolated viruses in the clinical virology laboratory. Once isolated, monoclonal antibodies can be used to type the virus. Typing genital lesion isolates can be prognostic in that HSV-2 reactivation occurs more readily than HSV-1. In addition, typing genital lesions from children might provide medicolegal evidence supporting potential sexual abuse.

Commercially available engineered cell lines improve the ease of detection of HSV. In the ELVIS (enzyme-linked virus inducible system) test, a gene for the enzyme β-galactosidase linked to a virus-induced promoter has been inserted into baby hamster kidney cells. If HSV-1 is present in the cell line, a viral protein will activate the promoter, resulting in β-galactosidase expression. Detection is accomplished by addition of a reagent, which is cleaved by the enzyme produced in virus infected cells, resulting in a color change. The color change is detectable with use of a light microscope.

Previously, serology provided only limited information to aid in the diagnosis of HSV infections. Reagents that could distinguish between antibodies to HSV-1 and to HSV-2 were not previously available. This was problematic because most adult patients have antibodies to HSV-1. Now, however, several FDA-approved type-specific assays are available that differentiate antibody response to HSV. The tests come in a variety of formats including EIA, strip immunoblot, and even simple membrane-based point-of-care assays. The difference between the newer tests and the previous generation lies in the antigens used. The newer tests use recombinant or affinity-purified type-specific glycoprotein G1 or G2, giving the tests the ability to distinguish between HSV-1 and HSV-2. Older-generation tests used crude antigen preparations from lysed cell culture of the virus and have been shown to have cross-reactivity rates of as much as 82% in positive specimens.

Cytomegalovirus

Cytomegalovirus is in the genus *Cytomegalovirus*. It is a typical herpesvirus but replicates only in human cells and much more slowly than HSV or VZV. CMV is spread by close contact with an infected person. Most adults demonstrate antibody against the virus, and those who live in overcrowded living conditions may acquire CMV at an early age. The virus is shed in saliva, tears, urine, stool, and breast milk. CMV infection can also be transmitted sexually via semen and cervical and vaginal secretions and through blood and blood products. CMV produces the most common congenital infection in the United States.

The vast majority of CMV infections are asymptomatic. Occasionally in immunocompetent patients the infection may manifest as a self-limiting, infectious mononucleosis-like illness with fever and hepatitis. In immunocompromised hosts, such as transplant recipients and HIV-infected patients, a CMV infection can become a life-threatening disseminated disease involving almost any organ including the lungs, liver, intestinal tract, retina, and central nervous system (CNS).

Congenital infections and infections in immunocompromised patients are often symptomatic and can be serious. A congenital infection is unlikely to occur if the mother was seropositive at the time of conception. Serious clinical manifestations may develop if the mother acquires the primary infection during pregnancy. Symptomatic congenital infection is characterized by petechiae, hepatosplenomegaly, microcephaly, and chorioretinitis. Other manifestations are low birth weight, CNS involvement, mental retardation, deafness, and death. CMV is one of the leading causes of mental retardation, deafness, and intellectual impairment.

The diagnosis of CMV infection is best confirmed by isolation of the virus from normally sterile body fluids, such as the buffy coat of blood or other internal fluids, or tissues. The virus can also be cultured from urine or respiratory secretions, but because shedding of CMV from these sites is common in normal hosts, isolation from such sources must be interpreted cautiously. More recently, a viral antigenemia test has gained widespread use among clinical virology laboratories. The antigenemia assay is specific, sensitive, rapid, and relatively easy to perform. The test is based on the immunocytochemical detection of the 65-kDa lower-matrix phosphoprotein (p65) in the nuclei of infected peripheral white blood cells. The antigenemia test may prove helpful in assessing the efficacy of antiviral therapy. CMV produces characteristic CPE that can sometimes be seen in clinical specimens (Figure 29-7).

Molecular-based testing is also widely used to detect virus particles in clinical samples. PCR, branched DNA, and hybridization assays are all used for blood donor screening

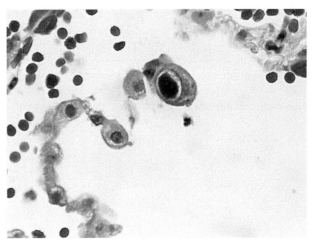

FIGURE 29-7 Active cytomegalovirus infection of lung in patient with acquired immune deficiency syndrome. Histopathology of lung shows cytomegalic pneumocyte containing characteristic intranuclear inclusion. (Courtesy Centers for Disease Control and Prevention, Edwin P. Ewing, Jr.)

and diagnostic applications. A congenital infection is best confirmed by isolation of CMV from the infant within the first 2 weeks of life. Isolation after the first 2 weeks of life does not confirm congenital infection. Urine is the most common source.

As with HSV, serology is not as helpful in diagnosing the infection as a culture. CMV can be isolated in cell culture only by using human diploid fibroblast cell lines, such as human embryonic lung or human foreskin fibroblasts (see Figure 29-3). The virus replicates slowly, so it may take up to 3 weeks for CPE to appear in culture. However, the use of shell vials can reduce the time of detection to as little as 1 day.

Epstein-Barr Virus

Epstein-Barr virus, in the genus *Lymphocryptovirus*, causes infectious mononucleosis (Figure 29-8). Signs and symptoms include sore throat, fever, lymphadenopathy, hepatomegaly, splenomegaly, and general malaise. The signs and symptoms usually resolve within a few weeks, although malaise may be prolonged. Complications of EBV infections are splenic hemorrhage and rupture, hepatitis, thrombocytopenia purpura with hemolytic anemia, Reye syndrome, encephalitis, and other neurologic syndromes. EBV can be recovered from the oropharynx of symptomatic and healthy persons, who can transmit the virus to susceptible persons via infected saliva.

The incubation period for EBV varies from 2 weeks to 2 months. As with the other herpes group viruses, infection is very common, and most adults demonstrate antibody against the virus. Infection in young children is almost always asymptomatic. As age at time of infection increases to young adulthood, a corresponding increase occurs in the ratio of symptomatic to asymptomatic infections. Some cancers also have been associated with EBV including Burkitt lymphoma, Hodgkin disease, and nasopharyngeal carcinoma (NPC). Burkitt lymphoma is a malignant disease of the lymphoid tissue and is seen most commonly in African children. The virus is also increasingly recognized as an important infectious agent in transplant recipients. The most significant clinical effect of EBV infection in these patients is the development of a B-cell lymphoproliferative disorder or lymphoma.

A viral culture for EBV requires human B lymphocytes, which is beyond the capabilities of most clinical virology laboratories. Therefore laboratory diagnosis of EBV is often

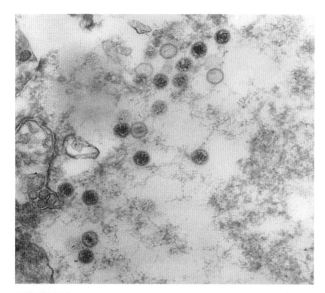

FIGURE 29-8 Negatively stained transmission electron micrograph revealing the presence of numerous Epstein-Barr virus virions. (Courtesy Centers for Disease Control and Prevention, Fred Murphy.)

accomplished with serologic tests. EBV infects circulating B lymphocytes and stimulates them to produce multiple (heterophile) antibodies, including antibodies to sheep and horse red blood cells and to *Proteus* OX19. The Paul-Bunnell heterophile antibody test is an excellent screen for these antibodies, although some false-positive reactions occur. A large number of rapid test kits, generally based on EIA or latex agglutination, are commercially available for detecting heterophile antibodies. These tests are 80% to 85% effective. Some false-positive tests represent patients who have had infectious mononucleosis and still have low levels of antibody. Young children can have false-negative results with the heterophile test; performing an EBV-specific antibody test on these individuals is appropriate. EBV-specific serologic tests (Table 29-4; Figure 29-9) measure the presence or absence of the following:

- *Anti-VCA* (antibodies against the viral capsid antigen): IgM to the VCA occurs early in the infection and disappears in about 4 weeks, so its presence indicates current infection. IgG often appears in the acute stage and will persist for life at lower titers.
- *Anti-EA IgG* (IgG antibody to early antigen): IgG to EA may appear in the acute phase, and its presence indicates either current or recent infection. The antibody usually cannot be detected after 6 months.
- *Anti-EA/D* (antibody to early antigen, diffuse): Antibodies to EA/D appear in the acute phase, and their presence indicates either current or recent infection. The antibodies usually cannot be detected after 6 months. Patients with NPC often have elevated IgG and IgA anti-EA/D antibodies.

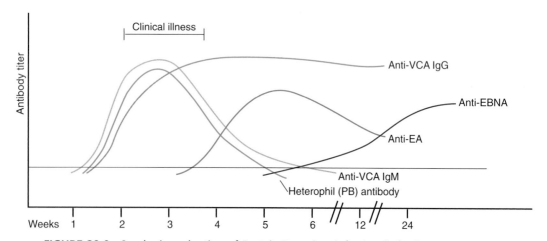

FIGURE 29-9 Serologic evaluation of Epstein-Barr virus infection (infectious mononucleosis) showing the rise and fall of detectable antibodies. *PB*, Paul-Bunnell.

TABLE 29-4 Interpretation of Epstein-Barr Virus Serologic Markers

PB	Anti–VCA-IgM	Anti–VCA-IgG	Anti-EA-IgG	Anti-EBNA	Interpretation
−	−	−	−	−	No previous exposure to Epstein-Barr virus
+	+	+	+/−	−	Acute infectious mononucleosis
+/−	+/−	+	+/−	+	Recent infection
−	−	+	−	+	Past infection

PB, Paul Bunnell antibody; *anti–VCA-IgM*, IgM antibodies against the viral capsid antigen; *anti–VCA-IgG*, IgG antibodies against the viral capsid antigen; *anti–EA-IgG*, antibody to early antigen; *anti-EBNA*, antibodies to the nuclear antigen.

- *Anti-EA/R* (antibody to early antigen, restricted): Antibodies to EA/R appear in the acute phase and disappear soon after anti-EA/D, but they can persist for up to 2 years and for life in some patients. Anti-EA/R IgG antibody is elevated in patients with Burkitt lymphoma.
- *Anti-EBNA* (antibody to the EBV nuclear antigen): Antibodies appear about 1 month after infection, with titers peaking in 6 to 12 months.

Varicella-Zoster Virus

Varicella-Zoster Virus, in the genus *Varicellovirus*, spreads by droplet inhalation or direct contact with infectious lesions. The virus causes two different clinical manifestations: varicella (chickenpox) and zoster (shingles). More than 90% of adults have antibody to VZV. Varicella is the primary infection and is highly contagious (Figure 29-10). In contrast to infections with the other herpes viruses, which are usually asymptomatic, varicella is usually clinically apparent. It commonly appears in childhood and includes symptoms such as a mild febrile illness, rash, and vesicular lesions. Usually the lesions appear first on the head and trunk and then spread to the limbs. The lesions dry, crust over, and heal in 1 to 2 weeks. Painful oral mucosal lesions may develop, particularly in adults.

Herpes zoster is the clinical manifestation due to reactivation of VZV and usually occurs in adults. Approximately one in three adults will develop herpes zoster in their lifetime. It is thought that the virus remains latent in the dorsal root or cranial nerve ganglia after primary infection. In a small proportion of patients the virus becomes reactivated, travels down the nerve, and causes zoster. The most common presentation is rash, followed by vesicular lesions in a unilateral dermatome pattern. These lesions may be associated with prolonged disabling pain that can remain for months, long after the vesicular lesions disappear.

VZV infection is usually diagnosed on the basis of characteristic clinical findings. In atypical cases, such as in immunosuppressed patients, the diagnosis may be more difficult or questionable. In such patients, culture of fresh lesions (vesicles) or use of fluorescent-labeled monoclonal antibodies against VZV confirms the diagnosis. VZV can be cultured on human embryonic lung or Vero cells. Cytopathic changes may not be evident for 3 to 7 days.

An attenuated vaccine to prevent chickenpox was licensed for use in the United States in 1995. Before routine use of the vaccine in children, an estimated 4 million cases occurred annually. The vaccine is expected to give lifelong immunity. In 2006, a single dose attenuated vaccine for shingles, Zostavax® (Merck & Co., Inc., Whitehouse Station, NJ), was approved. The vaccine is recommended for individuals 60 years of age and older.

Human Herpesvirus 6

Human herpesvirus 6 is in the genus *Roseolovirus.* The two variants, A and B, of the virus are indistinguishable serologically, but variant B appears to be the cause of disease. HHV-6 is a common pathogen; about 95% of young adults are seropositive. Studies have shown that the virus persists in the salivary glands and has been isolated from stool specimens, but most evidence indicates that saliva is the most likely route of transmission. Inhalation of respiratory droplets from and close contact with infected individuals are the most likely means of transmission.

In immunocompetent individuals, most infections are mild or subclinical. HHV-6 has been associated with the childhood disease roseola (which is also called *roseola infantum, exanthem subitum,* and *sixth disease,* reflecting its role as the sixth childhood rash). Children are protected by maternal antibodies until approximately age 6 months. Seroconversion occurs in 90% of children between the age of 6 months and 2 years. The disease is acute, febrile, and mild. A maculopapular rash appears as the fever resolves. About 30% to 40% of infected children with symptoms experience seizures. As with all members of the family Herpesviridae, reactivation of latent infections can become a clinical problem in immunocompromised individuals. HHV-6 has also been proposed as having some involvement in the development of both progressive multifocal leukoencephalopathy and multiple sclerosis.

The diagnosis of HHV-6 infection is usually made clinically. Isolation of the virus is most sensitive with lymphocyte cell culture, which is not practical for routine diagnosis. Serology may not be helpful unless paired sera are available. Patients do not usually have a positive IgM until about 5 days after infection; IgG appears several days later. PCR and viral load testing might offer sensitive and specific means of diagnosing primary HHV-6 infection.

Human Herpesvirus 7

First isolated from peripheral blood monocytes of infected patients in 1989, HHV-7 is classified in the genus *Roseolovirus*

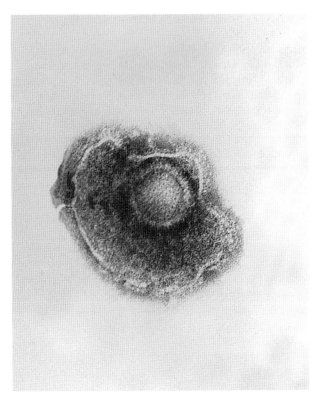

FIGURE 29-10 Electron micrograph of a varicella virus. (Courtesy Centers for Disease Control and Prevention, Erskine Palmer, B.G. Partin.)

with HHV-6. The CD4 molecule serves as a receptor for HHV-7 to infect T lymphocytes. It uses other receptors as well and has a broad range of host cells. Like HHV-6, HHV-7 is extremely common and is shed in the saliva of 75% of adults. The virus causes roseola that is clinically identical to that of HHV-6. HHV-7 causes latent infections in T lymphocytes. Despite the similarities between HHV-6 and HHV-7, their antigenic diversity is such that antibodies to one virus do not protect against infection from the other. In addition, exposure to HHV-7 seems to occur later in life than with HHV-6. Most 2 year olds are seronegative for HHV-7, but most children are seropositive by the age of 6 years.

HHV-7 can be isolated in culture in peripheral blood lymphocytes or in cord blood lymphocytes. Although the virus can be isolated from the saliva of healthy individuals, it is rarely isolated from peripheral blood mononuclear cells. PCR can detect the virus, but the ubiquitous nature of the virus can lead to difficulties in interpreting the results. Serologic results can be confusing because of cross-reactions, but patients with rising antibody levels to HHV-7 but not to HHV-6 may have an active HHV-7 infection.

Human Herpesvirus 8

Human herpesvirus 8, in the genus *Rhadinovirus,* can be detected in all forms of Kaposi sarcoma, including AIDS-related, Mediterranean, HIV-1–negative endemic to Africa, and posttransplantation Kaposi sarcoma. This association has earned it the more common name *Kaposi sarcoma–associated herpesvirus.* It has also been shown to play a role in the development of primary effusion lymphomas and multicentric Castleman disease.

In North America and much of Europe, HHV-8 appears to be transmitted primarily through sexual contact, but studies in Africa and some Mediterranean populations suggest transmission by more casual means. The pattern of infection is similar to that of HSV-2, although men who have sex with men seem to be more susceptible than heterosexuals. Prevalence ranges from close to zero in a study of Japanese blood donors to greater than 50% in parts of Africa. In HIV-positive persons, the seroprevalence can be as much as 20% to 50% higher than that of the surrounding healthy population. In the United States, as many as 20% of normal adults have antibodies to HHV-8, as do 27% of patients with HIV-1 who do not have Kaposi sarcoma and 60% of patients with HIV and Kaposi sarcoma.

Currently, the virus cannot be recovered in cell culture. PCR, although considered very sensitive, has been shown to be less so than some immunologic assays in detecting HHV-8 but has been used to detect the virus in various specimens, including tissue, blood, bone marrow, saliva, and semen. HHV-8 DNA or antigens are rarely detected in immunocompetent individuals, even if they are seropositive. In situ hybridization can detect HHV-8 affected tissue. The availability of commercially prepared monoclonal antibodies has made the identification of HHV-8 infected cells in various types of lesions by immunohistochemistry more common. Serologic tests are being evaluated.

Papillomaviridae

Papillomas, or warts, are caused by HPVs, which belong to the genus *Papillomavirus* within the family Papillomaviridae. Although associated with the common wart, some HPV types are linked to cancer including cervical cancer. More than 100 types of these small dsDNA viruses exist; more than 40 types are transmitted sexually, known as the *genital types.* HPV 1, 2, 3, and 4 are thought to infect universally all children or young adults with no significant consequences. Different HPV types exhibit different tissue tropism based on the type of epithelial cell the viruses preferentially infect: cutaneous or mucosal types. The genital HPVs are further categorized as low, intermediate, or high risk, based on their association with genital tract cancers. Table 29-5 lists some of the HPV types and their clinical significance.

Cervical HPV lesions typically consist of flat areas of dysplasia and are often difficult to see. Rinsing the area with 5% acetic acid, which turns the lesion white, makes the lesions more visible; however, this method is highly insensitive for diagnosis. Some types of HPV will result in genital wart for-

---

TABLE 29-5 Human Papillomaviruses and Their Clinical Significance

Human Papillomavirus Type	Clinical Manifestation	Association with Malignancy
Cutaneous		
1	Plantar warts	None
2-4	Common warts	None
5, 8, 9, 12, 14, 15, 17, 19-25, 36-38	Flat and macular warts	More than 30% of patients with epidermodysplasia verruciformis (a rare autosomal disease) with types 5, 8, 14, 17, and 20 develop malignancy
26-29, 34	Common and flat warts	Frequent, especially in immunosuppressed patients
Mucosal		
6, 11	Papillomatosis, primarily laryngeal, also upper respiratory tract and condylomata acuminate (genital warts)	Low risk
42, 43, 44	Condylomata acuminate	Low risk
31, 33, 35, 51, 52	Condylomata acuminate	Intermediate risk
16, 18, 45, 56, 58, 59, 68	Condylomata acuminate	High risk

Adapted from Patterson BK: Human papillomavirus. In Murray PR et al, editors: *Manual of clinical microbiology,* ed 9, Washington, DC, 2007, American Society for Microbiolgoy.

mation (condylomata acuminate), which can easily be identified by the physician. Lesions can be removed by surgery, cryotherapy, or laser.

The HPVs cannot be grown in cell cultures; therefore laboratory diagnosis of HPV infection often involves cytology sections. Cytotechnologists and cytopathologists read Pap smears and look for *koilocytes;* that is, cells with perinuclear clearing with an increase in density of the surrounding rim of cytoplasm, which are indicative of HPV infection. In addition, nucleic acid probe tests can detect HPV DNA in endocervical cells and identify the HPV type. PCR techniques are more sensitive and have shown that HPV is present in 90% or more of invasive cervical cancers, but the presence of the virus alone is not the sole factor in cancer development. As many as one third of all college-age women are infected with HPV, and most never develop anything beyond subclinical infections. Because finding HPV in cervical tissue is not the sole predictor of invasive disease, some doubt surrounds whether it is useful to look for the virus in cervical specimens routinely. A quadrivalent vaccine against HPV types 6, 11, 16, and 18 to prevent cervical cancer was approved by the FDA in 2006 for females ages 9 to 26 years.

Poxviridae

Poxviruses are among the largest of all the viruses, measuring in length from about 225 to 450 nm and width from about 140 to 260 nm. They have a characteristic brick shape and contain a dsDNA genome. Variola virus belongs to the genus *Orthopoxvirus*. Other members of the genus include vaccinia virus (the smallpox vaccine strain), monkeypox, cowpox, and various other poxviruses.

Variola Virus

Variola virus causes smallpox, a disease commonly occurring throughout early history (Figure 29-11). Edward Jenner demonstrated the efficacy of vaccination to smallpox in 1796, which ultimately led to control of the disease. The last reported case of smallpox in the United States occurred in 1949. The

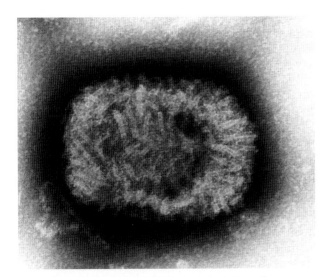

FIGURE 29-11 Negatively stained transmission electron micrograph of the smallpox (variola) virus. (Courtesy Centers for Disease Control and Prevention, J. Nakano.)

last case of smallpox on earth was in Somalia in 1977. The World Health Organization (WHO), after decades of aggressive eradication and vaccination, officially declared the world free of smallpox in May 1980. Although extinct in nature, at least two cultures are known to be maintained. One culture is kept in the United States at the Centers for Disease Control and Prevention (CDC), and one remains in Russia. These cultures remain under strict security and their very existence remains a point of contention between scientists who advocate their destruction and those who wish to continue their study.

Typically smallpox disease is characterized as producing a synchronous progressive rash with fever. The incubation period is approximately 10 to 17 days. The patient becomes febrile, and oral lesions may appear. At this point the patient is infectious. Within 24 to 48 hours, a faint macular rash appears on the body. The rash appears on all parts of the body, but lesions are present in greater concentration on the head and limbs *(centrifugal distribution),* including palms and soles. The macular rash progresses into papules, then vesicles, and finally, pustules that resemble lesions from chickenpox. Pustules are deeply embedded into tissues. All lesions change at the same time—thus the term *synchronous.* The average mortality rate for smallpox was 30%. Other forms of smallpox, including flat and hemorrhagic smallpox, occurred rarely but were almost always fatal.

Routine vaccination against smallpox in the United States ended in 1972, and other countries also have stopped their vaccination programs. Although smallpox was eradicated with the use of a relatively safe vaccine, the vast majority of today's population is now susceptible to infection because vaccination is thought to offer protection for up to 10 years. Because most humans are now susceptible to variola virus, it remains a threat as a weapon of bioterror. If an outbreak of smallpox did occur, there is sufficient smallpox vaccine to mount an effective vaccination program. An antiviral compound, cidofovir, may be effective in combating disease in humans. More information on smallpox as an agent of bioterror can be found in Chapter 30.

Monkeypox Virus

Monkeypox was first described in primates in 1958. The first case of human monkeypox was reported in 1970. In 2003 an unusual outbreak of monkeypox occurred in the United States. The virus was introduced into the country by rodents bought from Africa. Human monkeypox infection occurs primarily in central and western Africa. Human infections are rare but result in a vesicular, pustular febrile illness, similar to smallpox. Monkeypox infections are less severe in humans than smallpox, and mortality rates are significantly lower.

SINGLE-STRANDED DNA VIRUSES

Parvoviridae

The Parvoviridae are naked ssDNA viruses that are the smallest of the DNA viruses, measuring about 22 to 26 nm in diameter. Parvovirus B19 is the principal pathogen within the family, and it is classified in the genus *Erythrovirus*. Parvovirus

B19 was named after the serum sample (number 19 of panel B) in which the initial viral isolate was observed by electron microscopy.

Infections range from asymptomatic to potentially fatal. The most commonly recognized syndrome is erythema infectiosum (EI), or fifth disease. Patients with erythema infectiosum experience a prodrome of fever, headache, malaise, and myalgia with respiratory and gastrointestinal symptoms (nausea and vomiting). The prodromal phase lasts a few days, after which a rash often appears. The rash gives a "slapped-cheek" appearance and then spreads to the trunk and limbs. The rash occurs more commonly in children than in adults, lasts as long as 2 weeks, and can recur after heat and sunlight exposure. Adults may also experience arthralgia, arthritis, or both. In some cases this connective tissue manifestation occurs without the prodrome or rash stage. Most infections occur in children and adolescents, and 50% of adults are seropositive by the age of 50 years.

Parvovirus B19 viremia can cause transient aplastic crisis, a self-limited erythropoietic arrest. Erythroid precursor cells contain a receptor for the virus, allowing viral infection and replication. The disease is characterized by a decrease in red blood cell production in the bone marrow. In normal patients this decrease results in a short-lived anemia. The disease can be severe; complications include viremia, thrombocytopenia, granulocytopenia, pancytopenia, flu-like symptoms, and congestive heart failure. Within about a week, reticulocytosis occurs and the patient recovers.

The viremia of parvovirus B19 creates a risk for blood donors and fetuses. In utero infection can cause hydrops fetalis, resulting from anemia. Although the most vulnerable period for the fetus is the third trimester, most women exposed to the virus do not develop an acute disease, and few infections result in loss of the fetus. The infection usually does not require therapy, other than relief of symptoms, such as anti-inflammatory agents for painful joints.

A novel parvovirus was described in 2005 by Allander et al. This virus was named the human bocavirus (HBoV) and causes a variety of upper and lower respiratory tract illnesses. HBoV is closely related to the bovine parvovirus and canine minute virus, both members of the genus *Bocavirus* of the family Parvoviridae. Clinical symptoms of HBoV include cough, rhinorrhea, fever, difficulty breathing, diarrhea, conjunctivitis, and rash. HBoV has been increasingly present as a co-infection with respiratory syncytial virus and human metapneumovirus. Some studies have indicated a potential link to HBoV respiratory illness and gastroenteritis; however, researchers concluded that HBoV is indeed shed in high quantities in stool, but its link in gastroenteritis has not been demonstrated.

HBoV infection is highest during the winter months and has been detected worldwide in 5% to 10% of children 7 to 18 months in age with upper and lower respiratory tract infections. Since its first description, HBoV has been described in at least 19 countries on five continents. Detection of HBoV has improved with the development of sensitive and specific real-time PCR assays. HBoV was detected less frequently than common respiratory agents (influenza, parainfluenza, adenovirus, RSV) in South African children.

DOUBLE-STRANDED RNA VIRUSES

Reoviridae

Rotaviruses

Rotaviruses are naked viruses about 75 nm in diameter with two protein layers surrounding the capsid. They are classified in the genus *Rotavirus*. Rotaviruses are the most common cause of viral gastroenteritis in infants and children. Gastroenteritis is a major cause of infant mortality and the failure of young children to thrive. Rotaviruses have a worldwide distribution and cause an estimated 611,000 deaths each year. Outbreaks occur primarily in the winter months in the temperate zones and year-round in the tropics.

Rotaviruses are spread by the oral-fecal route and have an incubation period of 1 to 4 days. The sudden onset of symptoms includes vomiting, diarrhea, fever, and in some cases abdominal pain and respiratory symptoms. The vomiting and diarrhea can cause fatal dehydration. The rotavirus replicates in the epithelial cells in the tips of the microvilli of the small intestine. The microvilli are stunted and adsorption is reduced. The virus is shed in large quantities in the stool and can cause nosocomial outbreaks in the absence of good hygiene. Although the rotavirus is present in large numbers in stools, it can be isolated only with special procedures. Enzyme-linked immunosorbent assay (ELISA) and latex agglutination tests detect the viral antigens in fecal material. Rapid membrane-bound colorimetric tests are also available. Electron microscopy examination of stool samples can be used; however, this method is not very sensitive.

With the introduction in 2006 of a human-bovine rotavirus vaccine (RotaTeq, Merck & Co., Inc.) a delay in the onset of rotavirus season from mid-November to late February was seen. Additionally, the magnitude of the season based on laboratory reports of testing decreased by 37% and the number of positive tests by 78.5%. Although data are preliminary, and more must be collected before a definitive analysis can be made, the availability of this vaccine appears to have lowered infection rates in the United States. A second vaccine, Rotarix (GlaxoSmithKline, Middlesex, United Kingdom), was approved in June 2008.

Colorado Tick Fever Virus

The genus *Coltivirus* contains the Colorado tick fever virus, which causes a dengue-like infection in the western United States and Canada. It is an 80-nm spherical particle with two outer shells containing 12 RNA segments. Because Colorado tick fever is not a reportable infection, actual numbers of cases are unknown. However, it may be one of the most common diseases transmitted by ticks in the United States. Viruses that are transmitted by arthropods, such as ticks and mosquitoes, are referred to as **arboviruses.** The vector for the infection is *Dermacentor andersoni,* which has many hosts in nature, including deer, squirrels, and rabbits. Infected patients develop fever, photophobia, myalgia, arthralgia, and chills. Similar to dengue, patients can also have a biphasic fever with a rash, and children may experience hemorrhagic fever. No commercially produced laboratory tests are available, but recombinant immunoassays have been developed to detect Colorado tick fever IgG.

SINGLE-STRANDED RNA VIRUSES

Arenaviridae

The arenaviruses get their name from the Latin term *arena,* meaning "sand." Under an electron microscope, arenaviruses appear sandy and granular. More than 20 arenaviruses have been named, and the family includes many species that cause hemorrhagic fever. Arenaviruses are commonly split into two groups: the Old World and New World viruses. New World arenaviruses are the more extensive group and include Tacaribe, Guanarito, Junin, and Machupo. The Old World arenavirus group includes the lymphocytic choriomeningitis virus and Lassa virus.

The first arenavirus to be described was the lymphocytic choriomeningitis (LCM) virus in 1933. The Tacaribe virus was discovered in 1956, and since then several arenaviruses have been detected each decade. The first of the arenaviruses found to cause hemorrhagic fever was the Junin virus, which causes Argentine hemorrhagic fever. The Machupo virus, another hemorrhagic fever virus, was isolated from an outbreak in Bolivia in 1963. In 1969 the Lassa virus was isolated in Africa, which triggered a novel entitled *Fever,* written by John Fuller. The book details the emergence of Lassa fever, which in retrospect is eerily similar to the emergence of other hemorrhagic fevers that would be discovered later in Africa, including that of the Ebola virus.

The arenaviruses infect rodents, and humans are then exposed to the disease by zoonotic transmission. The rodents are infected for long periods and typically do not become ill from the viruses, which they shed in urine, feces, and saliva. In some parts of the United States, as many as 20% of the *Mus musculus* mice carry the LCM virus. Pet hamsters are also reservoirs. Humans become infected when they inhale the aerosolized virus or come in contact with fomites. The LCM virus causes an influenza-like illness; about 25% of infected patients develop meningitis.

Lassa virus is the most well known of the arenaviruses. Most exposed individuals develop an asymptomatic infection, but some patients experience fever, headache, pharyngitis, myalgia, diarrhea, and vomiting. Some patients develop pleural effusions, hypotension, and hemorrhaging. CNS involvement includes seizures and encephalopathy. The mortality rate is about 15% for patients ill enough to require hospitalization. West African nations suffer from more than 200,000 cases and approximately 3000 deaths per year.

Incidents of accidental importation of the disease from Africa by commercial air travelers underscore the vulnerability of large populations and have prompted vaccine development efforts with some promising early results. Most cases of Lassa fever are community acquired primarily by contact with excretions from the multimammate rat *Mastomys natalensis,* which sheds the virus throughout its life once infected. Humans either inhale the aerosolized virus or contract the virus directly through breaks in the skin. Lassa virus is present in throat secretions and can also be transmitted from person to person. It can also be transmitted through sexual contact and nosocomially. If therapy begins within the first 6 days of exposure, Lassa virus can be effectively treated with ribavirin.

Bunyaviridae

The family Bunyaviridae includes the genera *Orthobunyavirus, Phlebovirus,* and *Nairovirus,* which are classified as arboviruses. These viruses replicate initially in the gut of the arthropod vector and eventually appear in the saliva. The arthropod transmits the virus by feeding on the blood of vertebrate hosts, including humans. After a few days the infected host usually develops an asymptomatic viremia. Less commonly, the host becomes febrile. Some of the viruses in this family cause diseases that reflect damage to target organs. For instance, Rift Valley fever virus targets the brain and liver to cause encephalitis and hepatitis. LaCrosse (LACV) and California encephalitis viruses target the brain, causing encephalitis, and the Crimean-Congo hemorrhagic fever (CCHF) virus targets the vascular endothelium and liver. The hantaviruses, which also belong to this family, do not infect arthropod hosts. They are rodent-borne viruses.

Most members of the family Bunyaviridae cause a febrile illness, hemorrhagic fever, or encephalitis. CCHF virus causes a high mortality infection in humans. Infection begins with fever, myalgia, arthralgia, and photophobia. Patients develop mental status changes, ranging from confusion and agitation to depression and drowsiness. Petechiae and ecchymoses can form on mucosal surfaces and on skin. The patient may bleed from the bowel, nose, and gums. About 30% of the patients die. Others begin recovering after about 10 days of illness. Nosocomial transmission of CCHF has been reported. In the United States, LACV virus infects as many as an estimated 300,000 persons each year, of which about 100 result in severe disease of the CNS. The incidence is probably underestimated because the disease manifests as a nonspecific fever, headache, nausea, vomiting, and lethargy. The disease is commonly found in children and most often develops in the summer, frequently referred to as the "summer flu" or "summer cold." Because serology tests for LAC virus are not offered in most laboratories and because this disease has very low mortality (about 1%), definitive diagnosis does not occur often.

The genus *Hantavirus* includes Hantaan virus, Seoul virus, Puumala virus, and Dobrava virus. These viruses cause a disease referred to as *hemorrhagic fever with renal syndrome* (HFRS). These viruses occur in Asia and Europe, with the exception of the Seoul virus, which is found worldwide. Hantaviruses endemic to Europe and Asia are called *Old World hantaviruses.* The Puumala hantavirus is the most common member of this genus in Europe and causes a mild form of HFRS, called *nephropathia epidemica.* Viruses causing HFRS target the kidney. Patients develop a febrile prodrome and enter a phase of fever and shock accompanied by oliguria. The kidneys gradually regain function as the patient recovers. The mortality rate for HFRS is 1% to 15%.

In 1993 two adults from the same household in New Mexico died of an unusual respiratory illness. Serologic testing indicated these patients had been exposed to an unknown agent that was antigenically related to one of the

TABLE 29-6 Hantaviruses That Cause Hantavirus Pulmonary Syndrome

Hantavirus	Host	Location
Sin Nombre	*Peromyscus maniculatis* (deer mouse)	United States, western Canada
Black Creek Canal	*Sigmodon hispidus* (cotton rat)	United States, South America
Bayou	*Oryzomys palustris* (rice rat)	Southeastern United States
Monongahela	*Peromyscus maniculatis* (deer mouse)	Eastern United States
New York	*Peromyscus leucopus* (white-foot deer mouse)	New York
Oran	*Oligoryzomys longicaudatus*	Argentina
Andes	*Oligoryzomys longicaudatus*	Argentina, Chile
Lechiguanas	*Oligoryzomys flavescens*	Argentina
Laguna Negra	*Calomys laucha*	Paraguay, Bolivia

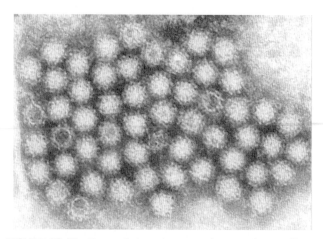

FIGURE 29-12 Transmission electron micrograph revealing the ultrastructure morphology of norovirus virions. (Courtesy Centers for Disease Control and Prevention, Charles D. Humphrey.)

Asian hantaviruses, despite the different clinical presentation. Serosurveys also determined that 30% of the tested deer mice in the New Mexico area were seropositive for the same unknown virus. The virus that occurred in mice that had infected the couple was ultimately characterized as a new hantavirus, and it was named *Sin Nombre* ("no name") virus (SNV). The disease caused by this virus is now known as *hantavirus pulmonary syndrome* (HPS). Molecular techniques subsequently were developed to detect many new hantaviruses in the Americas (Table 29-6), sometimes called the *New World hantaviruses*.

Sin Nombre virus is transmitted by inhaling aerosolized mouse urine, saliva, and feces. Generally person-to-person transmission does not occur with hantavirus. Patients with HPS have a 3- to 5-day febrile prodrome, with fever, chills, and myalgia. Patients then enter a phase of hypotensive shock and pulmonary edema. The patient develops tachycardia, hypoxia, and hypotension. In severe cases the patient may develop disseminated intravascular coagulation. The mortality rate for HPS is about 50%. Treatment for HPS is primarily supportive. No FDA-approved laboratory tests are available for the identification of a hantavirus infection. Some state health laboratories and the CDC perform EIAs to detect anti-SNV IgM and IgG. Immunohistochemistry is a sensitive method that is used to detect hantavirus antigens in capillary endothelium; an increased concentration of antigens is found in capillary tissue from the lung.

Caliciviridae

The family Caliciviridae contains four genera (*Sapovirus, Norovirus, Lagovirus,* and *Vesivirus*), which include Sapporo virus, Norwalk virus, rabbit hemorrhagic disease virus, and feline calicivirus, respectively. Sapoviruses (SaVs) and noroviruses (NoVs) are etiologic agents of human gastroenteritis.

The noroviruses (Figure 29-12) are the most common cause of infectious gastroenteritis in the United States, accounting for as many as 23 million cases annually. These small, ssRNA, round viruses of 27 to 30 nm in diameter were, until recently, called the *Norwalk-like viruses, caliciviruses,* and *small round structured viruses* (Figure 29-13). These viruses are currently placed in the genus *Norovirus,* family Caliciviridae. Noroviruses cause outbreaks of acute gastroenteritis in schools, colleges, nursing homes, and families, as well as on cruise ships. These viruses have been found in drinking water, swimming areas, and contaminated food. Transmission is most commonly food-borne, although waterborne and person-to-person transmission can be significant.

The incubation period is 24 to 48 hours, and the onset of severe nausea, vomiting, diarrhea, and low-grade fever is abrupt. The infection rate can be as high as 50%. The illness usually subsides within 72 hours. Immunity may be short-lived, leading to the potential for multiple infections throughout life.

The viruses cannot be grown in culture, so diagnosis is usually accomplished by examination of fecal material by electron microscopy. Immune electron microscopy and, more commonly, reverse transcriptase (RT)-PCR are also used to detect the virus in feces. In fact, it was the use of RT-PCR that led to the discovery of the high incidence of norovirus infections. Improved surveillance of outbreaks, development of rapid identification technology, such as PCR, and access to norovirus strain sequencing databases have led to a better understanding of norovirus and the morbidity and mortality associated with the virus.

Sapoviruses are small (30 to 35 nm in diameter) diarrhea-genic viruses distinguished by a cup-shaped morphology. They usually cause diarrhea and vomiting in infants, young children, and elderly patients. Originally discovered in Sapporo, Japan in 1977, these viruses must be detected by electron microscopy, molecular methods (e.g., RT-PCR or real-time RT-PCR), and/or immunologic methods (e.g., ELISA).

Coronaviridae

The coronaviruses, in the family Coronaviridae and the genus *Coronavirus*, are enveloped helical viruses with ssRNA. They have distinctive club-shaped projections on their surfaces (Figure 29-13). Coronaviruses may be responsible for 15% of cold-like infections in adults, but higher seroconversion rates are seen in children. Some coronaviruses are also responsible for a small percentage of pediatric diarrhea cases. The illness lasts for about a week, and blood may appear in the stool. Coronaviruses are extremely fragile and difficult to culture, but it is possible to test specimens directly by IF and EIA methods.

A novel coronavirus was the causative agent of a pandemic of respiratory disease that emerged from Hong Kong in late 2002. During a 6-month period, the infection spread rapidly to 26 countries in Asia, Europe, South America, and North America. The virus infected at least 8000 people and had a mortality rate of approximately 10%. The disease was characterized by high fever, pneumonia, and in some patients, acute respiratory distress syndrome. The disease was ultimately named *severe acute respiratory syndrome* (SARS), and the causative agent was designated as the SARS-associated coronavirus (SARS-CoV). No vaccine or antiviral agent was available to fight the pandemic, which ultimately ended with intense public health intervention, including massive screening programs, voluntary quarantine, and travel restrictions. This human infection apparently started as a coronavirus that jumped from its normal animal host, possibly a civet cat, into a human. SARS-CoV does highlight the public health risk that can occur when animal viruses suddenly appear in a susceptible human population.

The 2002 SARS outbreak created much interest in understanding the epidemiology, reservoir-host relationship, and vaccination possibilities associated with this human coronavirus. In 2007, SARS-CoV antibodies were detected in 47 (6.7%) of 705 South African and Democratic Republic of the Congo (DRC) bat sera sampled from 1986 to 1999. Researches in the United States tested bats from the Rocky Mountain region in 2006, detecting coronavirus RNA in two species of bats: *Eptesicus fuscus* and *Myotis occultus*. Animals such as civets may acquire infections with SARS-like CoV from contact with infected bats. Current data indicate that bats, primarily the horseshoe bat, are the most likely reservoir for the SARS-CoV, although the bat coronaviruses are species-specific. More than 10 mammalian species have been identified as susceptible to the SARS-CoV, by either natural or experimental infection. Infections of these secondary hosts may give rise to strains that could potentially infect humans.

The SARS-CoV targets the epithelial cells of the gastrointestinal tract, being transmitted person to person by direct contact, droplet, or airborne routes. Other organ systems are affected by SARS infection including spleen, lymph nodes, digestive tract, urogenital tract, central nervous system, bone marrow, heart, and others. Virus can also be isolated from urine and feces, suggesting other potential routes of transmission. Certain individuals may be genetically more susceptible to SARS than others.

Detection methods include electron microscopy, ELISA (EUROIMMUN AG, Lübeck, Germany), and RT-PCR. Antibody can be detected by Western blot. Although there is no current SARS vaccine, trials with an intranasal immunization and a UV/formalin inactivated vaccine have shown potential. The benefit of antivirals (e.g., ribavirin) during SARS infection is uncertain. Treatment is mostly supportive and precautions are made to quarantine infected individuals.

Filoviridae

The family Filoviridae includes two genera: *Marburgvirus* and *Ebolavirus*. The Lake Victoria marburgvirus (formerly Marburgvirus) is in the former genus, and the Ebola virus Zaire strain (EBO-Z), Ebola virus Sudan strain (EBO-S), Ebola virus Reston strain (EBO-R), and Ebola virus Tai Forest strain all belong to the latter. These viruses have some striking similarities: they rarely cause human infections; they cause infections with high mortality rates; and they have unknown reservoirs in nature, although human infections may result from contact with infected monkeys.

Lake Victoria Marburg virus hemorrhagic fever was named after the location of one of the first outbreaks, Marburg, Germany. In 1967, 32 people from Marburg and Frankfurt, Germany, and Belgrade, Yugoslavia, contracted an unknown

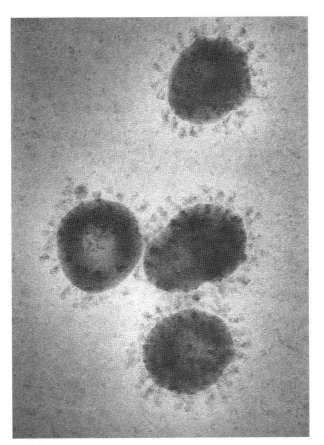

FIGURE 29-13 Electron micrograph of the coronavirus. This virus derives its name from the fact that under electron microscopy the virion is surrounded by a "corona" or halo. (Courtesy Centers for Disease Control and Prevention, Fred Murphy, Sylvia Whitfield.)

infection. Seven people died. Epidemiologists noted that the deceased individuals all worked in vaccine-producing facilities and had contact with monkeys that had recently arrived from Uganda. The virus had been transmitted to 24 other people through nosocomial transmission, casual contact, and sexual contact. Patients with secondary infection had a milder illness, and all survived the infection.

Outbreaks of Lake Victoria Marburg virus are noticeably rare, but some outbreaks have been fierce. In 1998 in the DRC, formerly Zaire, a large outbreak associated with gold miners resulted in 149 cases with a fatality rate of almost 83%. Another outbreak began in northern Angola in late 2004; by mid-2005, when reports of new cases began to decline, more than 350 people had died. Recent outbreaks have occurred in Angola (2005), Uganda (2007), and the Netherlands by Ugandan importation (2008).

Lake Victoria Marburg virus hemorrhagic fever begins with a febrile prodrome. The fever can last 12 to 22 days. At the end of the first week of infection, a maculopapular rash appears on the trunk and extremities, usually followed by the development of worsening nausea, vomiting, and diarrhea. Patients begin bleeding from the nose, gums, and gastrointestinal tract during the latter part of the first week. Liver hemorrhaging, myocarditis, kidney damage, and mental status changes occur, often followed by death. The infection can be diagnosed using PCR, immunohistochemistry, and IgM-capture ELISA. Treatment of infected patients is primarily supportive and includes replacement of blood and clotting factors.

The Ebola viruses are named after the Ebola River in the DRC, where the infection first emerged in 1976 (Figure 29-14). The virus emerged almost simultaneously in Sudan. In Zaire a patient treated at a village hospital for a bloody nose probably introduced the virus into the hospital, where it was then transmitted both nosocomially and via contact with infected individuals at home. Nuns in the hospital routinely reused syringes without sterilizing them. Therefore the hospital amplified the number of cases. Infections were also passed to

the victim's families, often during a process in which intestines of infected deceased males were cleaned to prepare the bodies for funerals.

Even though the two outbreaks of Ebola fever occurred simultaneously, they were caused by two different species, EBO-Z and EBO-S. EBO-Z is the more virulent species. In the initial outbreak, 318 patients in Zaire were infected; the mortality rate was 88%. In the Sudan outbreak, 284 people were infected and a mortality rate of 53% was reported. After the initial two large outbreaks, smaller outbreaks occurred. In Sudan 34 cases occurred in 1979, and 65% of the 34 patients died. The virus seemed to retreat back into the jungles for the next 15 years. However, an unusual sequence of events occurred in 1989, when monkeys imported to Reston, Virginia, from the Philippines experienced an epidemic of what eventually became the third type of Ebola virus, EBO-R. Four workers in the animal facility developed antibodies to EBO-R but did not develop disease. EBO-R was isolated from the bloodstream of one of the workers. Another outbreak of EBO-R occurred in monkeys at a Texas quarantine facility in 1996. Through 2004 Ebola Zaire continued to emerge periodically in the DRC. Additional outbreaks have occurred in DRC (2003 and 2007), Southern Sudan (2004), and Uganda (2007).

Symptoms of Ebola hemorrhagic fever include fever, chills, myalgia, and anorexia 4 to 16 days after infection. Patients develop a sore throat, abdominal pain, diarrhea, and vomiting and also start to bleed from injection sites and the gastrointestinal tract. Hemorrhaging in the skin and internal organs may occur as well. Diagnosis of the infection can be made using PCR, IF, or viral culture methods. Sometimes electron microscopy of clinical samples will yield the characteristic virions.

Flaviviridae

The family Flaviviridae contains a number of important human pathogens, many of which are zoonotic arboviruses, including Japanese encephalitis virus, dengue virus, yellow fever, St. Louis encephalitis virus, and West Nile virus. Japanese encephalitis (JE) virus is a major cause of encephalitis in Asia and is the most common cause of arboviral encephalitis in the world. Because it is being reported in regions previously free of JE, including Australia, JE virus is considered an emerging pathogen. Currently 30,000 to 50,000 cases of JE are reported each year. Most infections are asymptomatic. Disease ranges from influenza-like illness to acute encephalitis. Children assume the major burden of this infection, with a mortality as high as 30%; mortality in adults is much lower.

Another important member of the family Flaviviridae is dengue virus, which causes two distinct diseases: classic dengue fever (DF) and dengue hemorrhagic fever (DHF). Worldwide, tens of millions of cases of DF and approximately 500,000 cases of the more serious DHF occur. The average mortality associated with DHF is 5%, accounting for 24,000 deaths each year. Most deaths occur in children younger than 15 years. The virus is transmitted by *Aedes* mosquitoes, including *A. aegypti* and *A. albopictus*. These mosquitoes infest more than 100 countries and bring the risk of DF to 2.5 billion people.

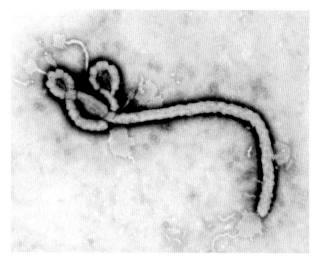

FIGURE 29-14 Transmission electron micrograph of the Ebola virus. (Courtesy Centers for Disease Control and Prevention, Fred A. Murphy.)

Dengue virus has four serotypes: 1 through 4. DF, which is a relatively mild infection, occurs when patients are bitten by mosquitoes carrying the virus. Patients with DF develop fever, headache, myalgia, and bone pain (resulting in the nickname "break-bone fever"). Some patients also develop a rash. The disease is self-limiting and often resolves in 1 to 2 weeks. Although classic DF is a mild disease, DHF is not. Patients develop DHF after they have already been exposed to one serotype of dengue virus and are then exposed to one of the other three serotypes. Exposure to two different serotypes of dengue virus appears necessary for developing DHF. Patients with DHF develop the symptoms of classic DF, along with thrombocytopenia, hemorrhage and shock, and sometimes death.

Yellow fever, caused by the yellow fever virus, is also considered an emerging infection. Although a safe vaccine has been available for decades, about 200,000 cases of yellow fever and 30,000 resulting deaths are reported annually worldwide. Actual incidence may greatly exceed these numbers. The emergence results from increased spread of the mosquito vectors, deforestation of Africa and South America, and increased travel by people into the endemic regions. The vaccine has greatly reduced or eliminated the transmission of yellow fever in some countries. However, yellow fever is still an epidemic in parts of Africa and South America, where about 80% of the population must be vaccinated to reduce the impact of the disease.

Patients bitten by mosquitoes carrying the yellow fever virus may develop an asymptomatic infection or an acute infection involving fever, myalgia, backache, headache, anorexia, nausea, and vomiting. Most patients experiencing acute disease recover after about 4 days. However, about 15% enter a systemic toxic phase in which fever reappears. The patient develops jaundice (thus the name "yellow" fever) and bleeding from the mouth, eyes, nose, or stomach or other areas. The kidneys may fail, and about 50% of the patients in the toxic phase die. The other 50% recover without serious sequelae. The three different transmission cycles for the yellow fever virus are the sylvatic, urban, and intermediate cycles. In the *sylvatic cycle,* yellow fever is maintained in monkey populations and transmitted by mosquitoes. Monkeys become sufficiently viremic to pass the virus to other mosquitoes as the mosquitoes feed on the monkeys, thus keeping the transmission cycle active. Humans are not the usual hosts when they enter jungle areas in which the sylvatic cycle exists.

The *urban cycle* occurs in larger towns and cities when infected *A. aegypti* mosquitoes transmit the infection to people. Because infected humans can continue the transmission when bitten by uninfected mosquitoes, large outbreaks can occur from a single case of yellow fever. The *intermediate transmission cycle* of yellow fever occurs in smaller villages in Africa. In the intermediate cycle, humans and monkeys are reservoirs and mosquitoes are reservoirs and the vectors for the high-morbidity, low-mortality outbreaks. In the intermediate cycle, mosquitoes can transmit the yellow fever virus from monkeys to humans and vice versa. If patients who develop yellow fever from the intermediate cycle travel to larger cities and if they are bitten by mosquitoes, they can trigger an outbreak of urban yellow fever.

In the United States the most common flavivirus infection is St. Louis encephalitis (SLE). During the past 35 years, an average of 193 cases has been reported annually in the United States. Epidemics are more likely to occur in midwestern or southeastern states, but cases have been reported in all of the lower 48 states. Patients with SLE are most likely to have an asymptomatic infection. Symptomatic patients may develop a fever only, whereas some patients develop meningoencephalitis. The mortality rate of symptomatic patients is 3% to 20%. Unlike many of the arboviral infections, SLE is milder in children than in adults; elderly patients have the greatest risk of serious illness and death. SLE is transmitted to humans by the bird-biting *Culex* mosquitoes. Most infections occur in the summer months.

First isolated and identified in 1937 from a febrile patient in the West Nile district of Uganda, WNV is a single-stranded RNA virus and a member of the Japanese encephalitis antigenic complex, similar to SLE. The virus is transmitted by a mosquito vector between birds and humans. The virus replicates actively inside the avian host; however, the virus does not replicate well in humans, making humans a dead-end host of infection. The incidence of WNV in the United States increased during the mid-1990s, prompting the development of a national surveillance system in 1999. In 2002 the CDC documented 4156 human cases of WNV in 44 states. More than 70% of these cases involved the CNS, in which 10% of those were fatal. The primary risk factor for serisus disease is age over 50 years. By 2008 the incidence of human WNV infections had dropped to 1356 with 44 deaths. Most individuals (approximately 80%) who become infected with WNV are asymptomatic. The remaining 20% display symptoms of what is termed "classic WNV infection" including fever, headache, fatigue, and occasional skin rash on the trunk, swollen lymph glands, and/or eye pain.

Laboratory tests approved for detection of WNV are IgG and IgM ELISA, including a rapid WNV ELISA assay, and indirect immunofluorescent assay to screen for flavivirus antibodies. WNV ELISA assays can cross-react with other flaviviruses and should be confirmed by antibody neutralization. WNV can be present in tissues, blood, serum, and CSF of infected humans or animals. A number of RT-PCR, Taqman, and nucleic acid sequence-based amplification assays have been used for successful confirmation of WNV. There is no specific treatment for WNV; however, in severe cases requiring hospitalization, supportive care including IV fluids, respiratory support, and prevention of secondary infection may be warranted.

Orthomyxoviridae

The influenza viruses types A (genus *Influenzavirus* A), B (genus *Influenzavirus* B), and C (genus *Influenzavirus* C) belong to the family Orthomyxoviridae. Influenza viruses have a worldwide distribution and originate as zoonotic infections, being carried by a number of different species of birds and mammals. Influenza season in the southern hemisphere is from May to October and in the northern hemisphere from November to April.

Influenza A virus remains one of the most crucial health problems worldwide. In the pandemic of 1918 and 1919, influenza is estimated to have killed between 20 and 50 million people, more than 500,000 of whom were Americans. Yet in the past 80 years, the world has been able only to react to the threat of influenza rather than to vanquish it. In six different years from 1972 to 1995, influenza deaths in the United States exceeded 40,000. A typical influenza season in the United States hospitalizes almost 200,000 and kills nearly 36,000.

Influenza viruses are enveloped, and types A and B have eight segments of ssRNA. Their major surface antigens are hemagglutinin (H) and neuraminidase (N). The H antigen is used to bind to host cells, and neuraminidase cleaves budding viruses from infected cells. There are 16 H antigens (H1 through H16), although human infections usually only occur with H1, H2, and H3. There are a total of 9 N antigens (N1 through N9); human infections usually occur with N1 and N2.

The Key to the persistence of the influenza virus is its antigenic variation. Each year **antigenic drifts** occur, caused by RNA replication errors of the virus. A *drift* is a minor change in antigenic structure as mutations accumulate. Antigenic drifts occur with all three types of influenza: A, B, and C. Sometimes the surface antigens can change drastically, causing an **antigenic shift,** resulting in a new H or N antigen. There are two mechanisms of antigenic shift. The first is *genetic reassortment* of the eight ssRNA strands of two separate influenza strains. Pigs have receptors for both avian and human influenza viruses, as well as swine influenza viruses, and can be co-infected with all three types of viruses. A reassortment occurs when the genome of both influenza viruses become mixed into a single virion, resulting in a new strain of influenza virus. The second mechanism is an *adaptive mutation,* in which a novel virus slowly adjusts and becomes transmissible from a mammalian (including human) host. Shifts result in novel strains of the influenza virus, so the human population is likely to have little or no historic exposure or resistance to the new strain, which greatly increases the risk of pandemics. Antigenic shift is only associated with influenza A.

Three major shifts occurred during the twentieth century; influenza A (H1N1) appeared in 1918 to 1919 (the "Spanish flu"). The H1N1 was the predominant strain until a shift to influenza A (H2N2) occurred in 1957 to 1958. That shift resulted in pandemic influenza, the "Asian flu." In 1968 another shift occurred, and a pandemic strain of influenza A (H3N2), the "Hong Kong flu," was the result. The dominant strains of influenza A since 1977 have been influenza A (H1N1) and influenza A (H3N2).

In early 1998 an outbreak of influenza A (H5N1), the "avian flu," appeared in poultry in Hong Kong. At least 18 humans acquired the disease via contact with the birds, and six deaths were reported. H5N1 is a highly pathogenic avian influenza (HPAI) virus, and historically HPAI has not been transmitted directly from birds to humans. The H5N1 influenza virus appeared in flocks in parts of Asia in 2004 and again in 2005, resulting in large poultry losses in Japan, Cambodia, China, Vietnam, and nearby countries. Some humans were infected during these poultry outbreaks; again the incidence of human disease was low, but the mortality rate was high, although it is possible that some mild cases have gone undiagnosed.

Recent studies documented wide dissemination of influenza A (H5N1) throughout Asia as a result of migrating birds. By early 2006, influenza A (H5N1) had been isolated from birds in the countries of Turkey, Greece, Italy, Germany, Iran, Iraq, Nigeria, and many others. The potential for the virus to adapt to the human host, through either genetic reassortment or adaptive mutation, remains an important concern for future influenza seasons. As of September 24, 2009, the WHO had recorded 442 human cases of influenza A (H5N1) infections and 262 deaths in 15 countries.

In spring of 2009, a highly infectious novel form of influenza (H1N1), swine flu, emerged. It was first reported throughout the country of Mexico and forced the closings of schools and cancellation of sporting events. As of October 9, 2009, the WHO received reports of more than 375,000 human cases and 4525 deaths. Because many countries stopped counting individual cases, the actual number is much larger. The outbreak quickly reached phase 6, a WHO definition of a pandemic. This was the first influenza pandemic in 40 years. Novel influenza A (H1N1) was found to contain RNA from bird, human, and swine strains of virus. Infection spreads in the same way as typical seasonal influenza viruses, mainly through coughing and sneezing of infected individuals. Infection may also be spread by handling fomites. Novel H1N1 infection causes a wide range of flu-like symptoms, including fever, cough, sore throat, body aches, headache, chills and fatigue. In addition, many people have reported nausea, vomiting, and/or diarrhea.

The first case of novel influenza H1N1 was reported in the United States on April 15, 2009, and by June 19, all 50 states, the District of Columbia, Puerto Rico, and the U.S. Virgin Islands had reported novel H1N1 infection. From April 15, 2009, to July 24, 2009, the CDC reported a total of 43,771 confirmed and probable cases of novel influenza A (H1N1) infection. Of the reported cases, 5,011 people were hospitalized, and 302 deaths occurred. Preliminary data for fall 2009 indicate that novel H1N1 has a much greater incidence than the seasonal flu strains. In September 2009, the United States FDA gave four manufacturers approval to use a monovalent swine flu vaccine; all four contain A/California/7/2009(H1N1)pdm, and none use an adjuvant. This vaccine was administered in addition to the regular seasonal flu vaccine.

Because the H and N antigens of the influenza A virus change continuously, the CDC and WHO make recommendations regarding the composition of the trivalent influenza vaccine several months before the influenza season begins. The vaccine usually contains two different strains of influenza A virus and a single strain of influenza B virus. Influenza B virus infections, which also can occur seasonally, are usually less common that influenza A virus infections, although epidemics of influenza B virus can occur every few years.

Influenza C is capable of causing mild upper respiratory illness in humans. The virus is enveloped, and its genome consists of only seven ssRNA segments, lacking the gene that codes for neuraminidase as in influenza A and B viruses. Studies have shown it to be more stable genetically than influenza A, and although reassortment does occur, it is less prone to major changes in infectivity.

Influenza viruses are spread by aerosols. The viruses attack the ciliated epithelial cells lining the respiratory tract, causing necrosis and sloughing of the cells. The incubation period is 1 to 4 days. Although asymptomatic infections can occur, infections are usually characterized by rapid onset of malaise, fever, myalgia, and often a nonproductive cough. Fever can be as high as 41° C. Infected patients are ill for as long as 7 days and convalescence may require more than 2 weeks. Influenza can also cause a fatal viral pneumonia. Complications include secondary bacterial pneumonia.

Nasopharyngeal swabs, washes, or aspirates collected early in the course of the disease are the best specimens. Flocked swabs (Copan Diagnostics, Corona, Calif.) are reported to collect significantly more epithelial cells than rayon swabs from the nasopharnyx. Specimens should never be frozen. A number of commercial rapid kits are available for diagnosis of influenza in about 30 minutes. Some of these kits are low-complexity and CLIA-waved. A kit can either (1) detect and distinguish between influenza A and B viruses, (2) detect both influenza A and B but not distinguish between them, or (3) detect only influenza A viruses. Influenza virus can be identified in respiratory secretions by DFA, EIA, and optical immunoassays. Influenza viruses grow in the amniotic cavity of embryonated chicken eggs and various mammalian cell culture lines, such as PMK and MDCK cells. As explained previously, influenza-infected culture cells adsorb red blood cells, a trait that can be used to detect positive cell cultures. Rapid culture assays can be performed using IF staining of infected monolayers grown in shell vials or flat-bottom wells of a microtiter plates.

The antiviral drugs amantadine and rimantadine can prevent infection or reduce the severity of symptoms if administered within 48 hours of onset. These antiviral drugs are effective only against influenza A. A newer class of antivirals, referred to as the *neuraminidase inhibitors,* is available. These agents, such as zanamivir (Relenza) and oseltamivir (Tamiflu), are more expensive than amantadine but provide coverage against influenza A and B infections. In the 2007-2008 flu season reports of oseltamivir resistant influenza A (H1N1) increased from about 1% of isolates to 15% globally.

Paramyxoviridae

Parainfluenza Viruses

Several genera belong to the family Paramyxoviridae, including *Morbillivirus, Paramyxovirus, Pneumovirus,* and *Rubulavirus.* Four types (1 through 4) of parainfluenza viruses (PIVs) can cause disease in humans. Human PIVs 1 and 3 belong to the genus *Paramyxovirus;* PIVs 2 and 4 belong to the genus *Rubulavirus.* The PIVs are enveloped helical RNA viruses with two surface antigens: hemagglutinin-neuraminidase (HN) antigen and the fusion (F) antigen. The HN antigen is the viral adhesion molecule, and the F antigen is responsible for the fusion of the virus to the cell and of one infected cell to another infected cell.

PIVs are a major cause of respiratory disease in young children. PIVs-1 and -2 cause the most serious illnesses in children between 2 and 4 years of age. PIV-1 is the primary cause of croup *(laryngotracheobronchitis)* in children. PIV-3 causes bronchiolitis and pneumonia in infants and is second in importance only to respiratory syncytial virus. PIV-4 generally causes mild upper respiratory tract infections. The viruses are spread through respiratory secretions, aerosols, and direct contact. Infection of the cells in the respiratory tract leads to cell death and an inflammatory reaction in the upper and lower respiratory tract. Rhinitis, pharyngitis, laryngotracheitis, tracheobronchitis, bronchiolitis, and pneumonia may result.

The best specimens for viral culture are aspirated secretions and nasopharyngeal washes. Specimens for viral isolation should be taken as early in the illness as possible, kept cold, and inoculated into PMK cells or LLC-MK2 cells. The viruses can be identified by hemadsorption, IF, or EIA techniques. Direct examination of nasopharyngeal secretions by IF can give rapid results. Serologic assays are more valuable for epidemiology studies than for diagnostic purposes. Aerosolized ribavirin can be used to treat infection. No vaccines are available, and infection control measures similar to those for RSV are employed to prevent spread in health care facilities.

Mumps Virus

Mumps virus is related to the PIVs and is classified in the genus *Rubulavirus.* It is an enveloped ssRNA virus with HN and F surface antigens. Mumps virus is spread by droplets of infected saliva and has a worldwide distribution. It causes an acute illness producing unilateral or bilateral swelling of the parotid glands, although other glands such as the testes, ovaries, and pancreas can be infected. The virus infects primarily children and adolescents and usually confers long-lasting immunity. The primary infection of the ductal epithelial cells in the glands results in cell death and inflammation.

A vaccine is available that has been effective in controlling the disease. From 2000 to 2003, roughly 250 cases of mumps were reported in the United States annually. However, from January to October 2006 a large multistate outbreak of almost 6000 cases of mumps was documented. The majority of the cases were reported in midwestern states among previously vaccinated persons 18 to 25 years of age. The reason for the outbreak is unknown. The mumps strain, genotype G, is the same one that has been circulating in the United Kingdom since 2004, where more than 70,000 cases have been reported. Most cases in the United Kingdom have occurred in unvaccinated individuals.

The mumps virus can be isolated from infected saliva and swabs rubbed over the Stensen's duct from 9 days before onset of symptoms until 8 days after parotitis appears. The virus can also be recovered from the urine and CSF. The mumps virus is relatively fragile. Specimens may be examined directly by IF and EIA methods. Studies have shown viral isolation using shell vial cultures of Vero or LLC-MK2 cells to be more successful than with either HEp2 or HeLa cell lines. Isolates can be identified by hemadsorption inhibition, IF, and EIA tests.

Paired sera can be tested for mumps antibody by EIA, IF, and hemagglutination inhibition tests. Paired sera taken as little as 4 to 5 days apart can demonstrate diagnostic or four-fold rise in titer. Cross-reactions between soluble and viral antigens can confuse interpretation of serologic results. Virus isolation is preferable, although physicians rarely have trouble recognizing mumps clinically.

Measles Virus

The measles virus is an enveloped virus classified in the genus *Morbillivirus*. It is found worldwide; in the temperate zones, epidemics occur during the winter and spring. At one time measles (rubeola) was the most common viral disease in children in the United States. An average of 500,000 cases of measles was reported annually in the 1950s, with an average mortality of 500. Immunization programs began in the United States in 1963, and the reported number of cases dropped to fewer than 1500 by 1983. A reemergence of measles occurred in 1989 through 1991. A decision to administer a second dose of vaccine to school-age children has drastically reduced the incidence of measles in the United States. On average, 63 cases per year were reported from 2001 to 2007. A spike of 131 cases in the first half of 2008 has been blamed on the rapid spread of the virus from a few imported cases mostly to unvaccinated school-age children. The WHO estimates that more than 30 million cases occur annually, with approximately 500,000 deaths in Africa alone.

Measles is highly contagious and spreads by aerosol. Initial replication takes place in the mucosal cells of the respiratory tract; measles virus then replicates in the local lymph nodes and spreads systemically. The virus circulates in the T and B cells and monocytes until eventually the lungs, gut, bile duct, bladder, skin, and lymphatic organs are all involved. After an incubation period of 7 to 10 days, there is an abrupt onset, with symptoms of sneezing, a runny nose and cough, red eyes, and rapidly rising fever. About 2 to 3 days later, a maculopapular rash appears on the head and trunk. **Koplik's spots,** lesions on the oral mucosa consisting of irregular red spots with a bluish-white speck in the center (Figure 29-15), generally appear 2 to 3 days before the rash and are diagnostic.

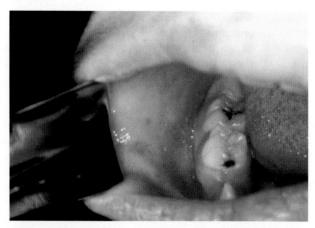

FIGURE 29-15 Patient presenting on the third pre-eruptive day with Koplik's spots indicative of the onset of measles. (Courtesy Centers for Disease Control and Prevention.)

Complications such as otitis, pneumonia, and encephalitis may occur. A progressive, highly fatal form of encephalitis may occur, but it is rare. In developing countries with malnutrition and poor hygiene, measles can have a high fatality rate. Infection confers lifelong immunity. An effective attenuated vaccine is available and recommended for all children.

Measles is easily diagnosed clinically, so few requests for laboratory identification are made. The virus is fragile and must be handled carefully. The specimens of choice are from the nasopharynx and urine, but the virus can only be recovered from these sources in the early stages of infection. The virus grows on PMK cells, causing formation of distinctive spindle-shape or multinucleated cells. The virus isolates can be identified using serum neutralization, EIA, or IF tests. Serologic diagnosis of measles is accomplished by demonstrating measles-specific IgM in the specimens collected during the acute phase of the disease.

Respiratory Syncytial Virus

Respiratory syncytial virus (RSV) is a member of the genus *Pneumovirus*. RSV is the most common virus isolated from infants with lower respiratory tract infections and causes croup, bronchitis, bronchiolitis, or interstitial pneumonia. Almost half of all infants are infected with RSV during their first year of life, and by the age of 2 years, almost all have been exposed to RSV. Because infection does not confer complete immunity, multiple infections can occur throughout life and can be severe in the elderly, the immunocompromised, and those with cardiac and respiratory problems. As many as 24 of 1000 children with RSV infection require hospitalization. For that reason health care–associated RSV is a problem in many medical treatment facilities. Testing hospital personnel and infants with upper respiratory tract infections for RSV, isolating RSV-infected infants, following good handwashing and personal protective equipment practices, limiting visitation, and organizing patients and staff members into cohorts are recommended to reduce the risk of nosocomial spread.

RSV can be a significant cause of morbidity and mortality in elderly patients as well. Unlike the bronchiolitis caused in children, adults often develop pneumonia. The virus spreads mostly through large-particle droplets and contact with fomites rather than through inhalation of small particle aerosols. The virus may be carried in the nares of asymptomatic adults. RSV occurs in yearly outbreaks that last 2 to 5 months and usually appears during the winter or early spring in the temperate zones.

RSV can be identified in specimens from nasopharyngeal swabs and washes by DFA or EIA. Because the virus is extremely fragile, recovering it from cultures is a significant problem. Specimens must be kept cold but cannot be frozen. RSV grows readily in continuous epithelial cell lines, such as HEp2, forming syncytia. It also grows in PMK and human diploid fetal cells. Once CPE is detected, RSV can be identified using IF, EIA, and serum neutralization tests. Rapid antigen detection kits are also available for RSV. The antiviral compound ribavirin is approved as a treatment for patients with RSV. Recently some controversy has developed regarding the efficacy of ribavirin therapy. In 1996 RSV immune globulin was released for pre-exposure prophylaxis of susceptible patients, but recommendation for its use is unresolved. No vaccine is available for RSV.

Human Metapneumovirus

The human metapneumovirus (hMPV) was first described in children with previously virus-negative cultures. Infected children display many clinical symptoms similar to infections caused by the respiratory syncytial virus, influenza virus, and parainfluenza virus. Clinical disease varies from mild upper respiratory tract to acute lower respiratory infection and includes fever, a nonproductive cough, sore throat, wheezing, congestion, shortness of breath, and lethargy. hMPV infections usually occur in the winter months, although outbreaks have been documented during the summer. Treatment for hMPV illness is mostly supportive.

Sequencing of the hMPV genome and database searches reveal a high degree of homology with other human respiratory pathogens in the family Paramyxoviridae as well as with the only member of a new genus, *Metapneumovirus,* the avian metapneumovirus. Serologic and RNA sequence research have shown that the virus is found virtually worldwide and that in some areas most children have been exposed by the time they reach 5 years of age.

hMPV will grow slowly but successfully in standard cell culture lines such as tertiary monkey kidney and A549 cell lines. Specimens can be collected from the nostrils using a swab and placed in transport media and transported on ice to the laboratory for culture or molecular analysis. Real-time RT-PCR and fluorescent monoclonal antibodies are currently being used for identification. The respiratory viral panel assay from Luminex Molecular Diagnostics, FDA-cleared in January 2008, claims 100% sensitivity and 98.2% specificity for hMPV in clinical specimens.

hMPV infections most often occur in children. A study in Finland surveyed 1338 children less than 13 years of age and found that 47 (3.5%) with respiratory illness were positive for hMPV. The highest concentration of illness (7.6%) was within children less than 2 years of age. Co-infections with another virus, including enterovirus, rhinovirus, influenza virus, and parainfluenza virus, were detected in 8 (17%) of the infected children. hMPV has also been documented causing outbreaks in some long-term care facilities. An outbreak of hMPV in the summer of 2006 affected 26 residents and 13 staff of a 171-bed California long-term care facility. All of the resident cases had an underlying medical condition; two were hospitalized, but none died. Analysis of respiratory samples by cell culture and PCR revealed hMPV as the causative agent, indicating a year-round risk of infection to institutionalized elderly patients. No other respiratory pathogens were detected in the confirmed cases.

Picornaviridae

The Picornaviridae is one of the largest families of viruses, with more than 230 members. It contains many important human and animal pathogens. Four genera with human clinical significance belong to the family Picornaviridae: *Enterovirus, Rhinovirus, Hepatovirus,* and *Parechovirus.* The genus *Hepatovirus* includes the hepatitis A virus. This virus is discussed in the hepatitis viruses section of this chapter.

Enteroviruses

The enteroviruses found in the genus *Enterovirus* include the following:

- Polioviruses 1 through 3
- Coxsackieviruses A1 through 23
- Coxsackieviruses B1 through 6
- Enteroviruses 68 through 72
- Echoviruses 1 through 32
- Parechovirus 1-4

These small, naked viruses cause various conditions including fever of unknown origin, aseptic meningitis, paralysis, sepsis-like illness, myopericarditis, pleurodynia, conjunctivitis, exanthemas, pharyngitis, and pneumonia. Enteroviruses have also been implicated in early onset diabetes, cardiomyopathy, and fetal malformations.

Most serotypes of the enteroviruses are distributed worldwide. In temperate zones, enterovirus epidemics occur in the summer and early fall. Enterovirus infections are more prevalent in areas with poverty, overcrowding, poor hygiene, and poor sanitation. Viruses are spread via aerosol, the fecal-oral route, and fomites. The portal of entry is the alimentary canal via the mouth. The viruses replicate initially in the lymphoid tissue of the pharynx and gut. Viremia can result in the virus spreading to the spinal cord, heart, and skin. Enterovirus infections often cause mild nausea and diarrhea except in neonates, in whom disease may be more severe because of the immaturity of the immune system.

The polioviruses tend to infect the nervous system and can cause paralysis in a small percentage of infected patients. The viruses destroy their host cells. In the intestines, damage is temporary because the cells lining the gut are rapidly replaced. In contrast, neurons are not replaced, so neuron death can result in permanent paralysis.

No vaccines are available for enteroviruses other than poliovirus; good personal and nosocomial hygiene and good sanitation can reduce the incidence of enterovirus infections. Excellent poliovirus vaccines of either attenuated or inactivated viruses are available. Since 1988 the polio vaccine has been crucial to the WHO's effort to eradicate polio worldwide. Countries with rates of polio considered to be endemic have decreased steadily since the program began. In 1988, 125 countries reported endemic rates; by 1999 that number had decreased to 30 and to only 6 by 2003. Unfortunately, interruptions in vaccine programs since 2003 have resulted in a re-emergence of polio in western Africa. The disease has since returned to four countries endemic for polio and 12 due to importations.

Enteroviruses can be cultured from the pharynx immediately before the onset of symptoms and for 1 to 2 weeks afterward; they can be isolated from the feces for as long as 6 weeks afterward. However, obtaining specimens early in the infection is ideal. Specimens from the throat, feces, rectum, CSF, and conjunctiva are recommended.

Polioviruses, type B coxsackieviruses, and echoviruses grow readily in a number of cell lines including PMK, continuous human and primate, and human fetal diploid fibroblast lines. The high-numbered enteroviruses (68 to 71) require special handling. The CPE appears quickly and is readily identifiable. Enteroviruses have no group antigen, so they must be identified individually by a serum neutralization test. The WHO distributes pools of enterovirus antisera that allow identification by neutralization patterns in the antisera. The CPE and resistance to detergent, acid, and solvents constitute a presumptive diagnosis of enterovirus infection.

Hand, foot, and mouth disease (HFMD) is caused primarily by coxsackievirus types A5, 10, and 16 and occasionally enterovirus type 71. HFMD is generally a disease that occurs in young children. It is spread by fomites or the oral-fecal route. A mild prodromal phase may develop, with malaise, headache, and abdominal pains. Small painful sores suddenly appear on the tongue, buccal mucosa, and soft palate. Simultaneously, a maculopapular rash appears on the hands, feet, and buttocks, followed by bullae on the soles of the feet and palms of the hands. The lesions regress in about a week. If a rash develops it is transient. The virus can be isolated from specimens from swabs of the mouth and bullae. Coxsackievirus A16 grows in PMK and human diploid fibroblast cells and can be identified by serum neutralization tests.

Rhinoviruses

Rhinoviruses, found in the genus *Rhinovirus,* are small, naked viruses closely related to the enteroviruses. Rhinoviruses are resistant to detergents, lipid solvents, and temperature extremes but are sensitive to a pH of less than 6. More than 100 serotypes exist. Rhinoviruses are the major cause of the common cold. Most people experience 2 to 5 colds each year, and about half of these colds are caused by the rhinoviruses. Rhinovirus infections occur throughout the year, but incidences increase in the winter and spring. Transmission is primarily via aerosols, but contact with secretions and fomites can also cause infection.

Rhinoviruses infect the nasal epithelial cells and activate inflammatory mediators. Symptoms include a profuse watery discharge, nasal congestion, sneezing, headache, sore throat, and cough. In severe cases, bronchitis and asthma may result. Unfortunately no cure has been found for the common cold. Treatment with interferon does block rhinovirus infection but has undesirable side effects such as nosebleeds.

Rhinoviruses grow best on human diploid fibroblast cells producing enterovirus-like CPE. They can be differentiated from enteroviruses by exposing the clinical isolate to an acidic buffer. Rhinoviruses are acid labile, whereas enteroviruses are acid stable.

Retroviridae

The family Retroviridae contains several subfamilies, including Oncovirinae and Lentivirinae. The retroviruses have a unique mode of replication; they require an RNA-dependent DNA polymerase (reverse transcriptase) to synthesize DNA from the RNA genome. The human T-lymphotropic viruses, HTLV-1, HTLV-2, and HTLV-5, belong to the subfamily Oncovirinae. These viruses are not cytolytic, but they are associated with a number of leukemias, sarcomas, and lymphomas.

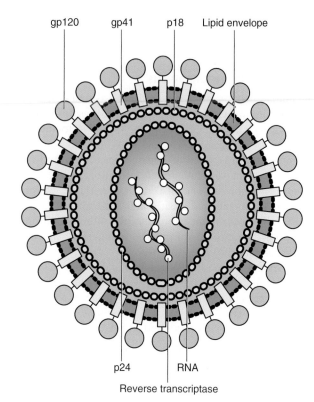

FIGURE 29-16 Human immunodeficiency virus (HIV).

HIV belongs to the subfamily Lentivirinae. Although pockets of individuals, mostly in West Africa, are infected with HIV-2, it is the impact of HIV-1 that continues to be felt around the world. HIV causes acquired immune deficiency syndrome (AIDS). HIV is a spherical virus with a three-layer structure (Figure 29-16). In the center are two identical copies of ssRNA and reverse transcriptase (RT) surrounded by an icosahedral capsid. The nucleocapsid is enclosed by a matrix shell to which an envelope of host cell origin is attached. Inserted into the viral envelop are viral glycoprotein (gp) trimers or spikes. The diagnostically important HIV antigens are the structural proteins p24, gp4l, gpl20, and gpl60.

More than 900,000 cases of HIV/AIDS have been reported in the United States since 1981, resulting in more than half a million HIV/AIDS-related deaths. It is estimated that 551,932 persons in the United States were living with HIV/AIDS at the end of 2007. In 2007, 73% of those infected were male; most adults and adolescents (64%) were infected by male-male sexual contact. Approximately 56,300 new cases of HIV infections occur in the United States each year. Globally in 2007, 33.2 million people were estimated living with HIV/AIDS, with 6800 new cases each day, demonstrating that the number of individuals living with HIV has leveled off and the number of people newly infected with HIV has decreased.

Approximately 2.1 million HIV/AIDS deaths occurred in 2007, and about 2.5 million new cases were diagnosed. The region most severely affected by HIV/AIDS is sub-Saharan Africa, which has approximately 22.5 million HIV-infected patients, accounting for 68% of the global total. Children share this burden; in 2007, approximately 2.5 million children under the age of 15 years had HIV/AIDS; 330,000 deaths in children and about 420,000 newly infected children during that same year were reported.

The virus is transmitted by blood and exchange of other body fluids. HIV is cell associated, so fewer viruses are found in cell-free plasma than in whole blood, and even less virus is found in saliva, tears, urine, or milk. HIV is not highly contagious, and normal, social, nonsexual contact poses no threat. Individuals at risk for contracting the virus are those having unprotected sex with multiple sex partners, IV drug users, blood and blood-product recipients, and children of infected mothers. Individuals with ulcerative sexually transmitted infections (e.g., syphilis, genital herpes, chancroid) are at the greatest risk. Today all donor blood and blood products are screened for HIV. As of 2006, new cases of HIV in the United States were associated with the following:

- Heterosexual contact (33%)
- Men who have sex with men (50%)
- IV drug use (13%)
- Heterosexual contact and IV drug use (3%)
- Transfusions or mother-to-infant transmission (1%)

Once HIV enters the body, the target cells are the CD4+ T cells, monocytes, and macrophages. Acute infections are generally mild and can resemble infectious mononucleosis. The individual will enter a period of clinical latency; even though the virus is replicating rapidly in lymphoid tissue, virus is not detectable in the bloodstream, and the patient remains asymptomatic. Eventually lymphopenia results, with the greatest losses in the CD4+ T-cell population. Lymph nodes become enlarged and hyperplastic. The virus destroys the cells (T-helper cells) that are critical in the immune response to infectious agents. The patient begins experiencing a number of chronic and recurrent infections such as those listed in Box 29-1. As the disease progresses, the CD4+ cell counts continue to decline and the opportunistic infections become more severe; the patient can also develop virus-induced cancers such as Kaposi sarcoma. Death usually

occurs from the resulting opportunistic infections, although HIV-1 itself can directly cause encephalitis and dementia.

For adults living in developed countries, the average length of time from HIV infection to development of AIDS is about 10 years. About 20% develop AIDS within 5 years, and fewer than 5% have an asymptomatic HIV infection for periods longer than 10 years. The rate at which the virus multiplies in the host is related to the development of AIDS. This rate can be measured with an HIV viral load assay, a quantitative gene amplification technique that measures the amount of HIV-1 RNA in the plasma of the patient.

Laboratory diagnosis of HIV infection is generally based on demonstration of anti-HIV antibodies and in some cases detection of viral antigens and RNA. HIV antibodies are normally produced within a few weeks after infection. A number of assays are commercially available as screening tests using different methodologies including EIA and IF. The early diagnostic kits, referred to as *first-generation* screening tests, used purified viral lysate as antigens. The second-generation tests used recombinant viral proteins, thus improving performance.

The third-generation tests rely on the double-antigen sandwich assay. In this procedure, viral antigen attached to a solid phase binds antibody to HIV from patient's serum. Then labeled HIV antigen is added and captured by the patient's antibody and measured. Fourth-generation kits detect both antibody and antigen.

A number of rapid assays can screen for HIV infection using serum, plasma, and even saliva. As of June 2008, the FDA had approved four rapid tests for the diagnosis of HIV infection: OraQuick Advance Rapid HIV-1/2 Antibody Test (Orasure, Bethlehem, Pa.), Uni-Gold Recombigen HIV test (Trinity Biotech, plc, Wicklow, Ireland), Reveal G2 Rapid HIV-1 Antibody Test (MedMira, Halifax, Nova Scotia), and Multispot HIV-1/2 Rapid Test (Bio-Rad Laboratories, Hercules, Calif.). OraQuick for whole blood and oral fluid specimens and Uni-Gold for whole blood samples are CLIA-waived. Currently the FDA has approved one home collection kit, Home Access HIV-1 Test System (Home Access Health Corporation, Maria Stein, Ohio).

Any reactive result on a screening test, usually an EIA, is retested in duplicate. If either of the tests is reactive, the specimen is reported as repeatedly reactive and is submitted for confirmation testing. Confirmation testing is usually performed by Western blot or IF. The Western blot test for HIV was developed in 1984 and has remained relatively unchanged. It is less sensitive than the screening tests, and it is prone to cross reactivity. Despite these flaws, the Western blot assay has remained the principal confirmatory assay for HIV antibody detection. The Western blot assay detects antibodies specific to viral antigens such as p24, p31, gp41, and gp120/gp160 (Figure 29-17). If the confirmatory test is reactive, the HIV test should be considered positive and the patient has an HIV infection. The presence of HIV antibodies is diagnostic, but a negative result simply means that no antibody was detected. It may take 6 weeks after infection before antibodies appear, and they disappear as immune complexes form in the late stages of the disease. Some other immunologic markers of HIV infection are listed in Box 29-2.

BOX 29-1 Opportunistic Infections and Cancers Commonly Seen in Patients with AIDS

- Candidiasis of the respiratory tract
- Coccidiomycosis
- Cryptococcal meningitis
- Cryptosporidiosis with persistent diarrhea
- Cytomegalovirus infections of organs other than the liver, spleen, or lymph nodes
- Histoplasmosis
- Persistent herpes simplex virus infections
- Kaposi sarcoma or lymphoma of the brain in patients younger than 60 years
- Oral hairy leukoplakia
- Lymphoid interstitial pneumonia, pulmonary lymphoid hyperplasia, or both in children younger than 13 years
- *Mycobacterium avium* complex, *Mycobacterium kansasii*, or *Pneumocystis jiroveci* pneumonia
- Progressive multifocal leukoencephalopathy
- Recurrent pneumonia
- Toxoplasmosis of the brain in infants older than 1 month
- Wasting disease

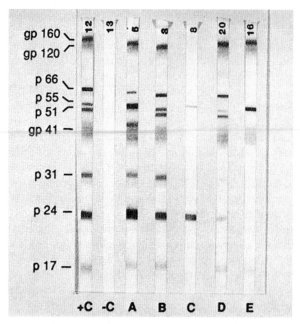

FIGURE 29-17 Human immunodeficiency immunoblot. Reactive protein (p) bands appear as purplish lines across the strip. Proteins with higher molecular weights appear at the top of the strip. Structural and nonstructural proteins are given RNA structural genome codes: *GAG,* group-specific antigens; *POL,* polymerase; and *ENV,* envelope. ENC codes for glycoprotein precursors (gp)—gp160, gp120, and gp41 through gp43. POL codes for p65, p51, and p31. GAG codes for p55, p24, and p17. Results are negative, indeterminate, or positive based on the pattern on the strip. *Positive:* Reactivity with a score of + or greater to GAG p24 or ENV gp120/gp160 or gp41. *Indeterminate:* The appearance of one or more bands in a pattern that does not satisfy the positive criteria. *Negative:* The absence of any band on the strips. (Courtesy Patricia A. Cruse.)

BOX 29-2   Important Immunologic Markers for AIDS

- Steady decline in number of CD4+ T cells
- Depression of the CD4+: CD8+ cell ration to less than 0.9 (reference value ≥1.5)
- Functional impairment of monocytes and macrophages
- Decreased natural killer cell activity
- Anergy to recall antigens in skin tests

Once HIV infection is diagnosed, therapeutic decisions are usually based on CD4+ T-cell counts and viral loads. Healthy individuals have CD4+ counts of at least 1000/mL, whereas HIV/AIDS patients can have counts fewer than 200/mL. Because these viruses readily develop resistance to drugs, HIV infections are often treated by combination therapy. Highly active antiretroviral therapy (HAART) involves aggressive combination therapy soon after HIV diagnosis is made.

Several classes of antiviral drugs are approved for treatment. Nucleoside analog reverse transcriptase inhibitors were the first class of retroviral drugs developed and are incorporated into viral DNA; examples include azidothymidine, dideoxyinosine, d4T (stavudine), 3TC (lamivudine), and tenofovir. Nucleotide analog RT inhibitors inhibit conversion of nucleoside analogs in the body to nucleotide analogs; examples include tenofovir and adefovir. Non-nucleoside analog RT inhibitors attach to the enzyme RT, preventing conversion of RNA to DNA; examples include delavirdine, nevirapine, and efavirenz. Other classes of antiviral drugs include protease inhibitors (ritonavir, saquinavir, indinavir, and amprenavir) and fusion inhibitors (T-20; enfuvirtide). HAART includes combinations such as two nucleoside analog RT inhibitors combined with a protease inhibitor.

HIV viral load assays can predict therapy efficacy. In different studies, suppression of HIV RNA levels to less than 5000 copies of RNA/mL for up to 2 years was correlated with an increase in CD4+ cell counts up to 90 cells/mL. In contrast, patients with HIV RNA loads of more than 5000 copies of RNA/mL generally showed declines in CD4+ cell counts.

Rhabdoviridae

Rabies is caused by several strains of viruses belonging to the genus *Lyssavirus.* The fear associated with the rabies virus is well deserved. Estimates of annual worldwide human deaths from rabies vary from 30,000 to 100,000. In the United States, human rabies is rare, with approximately two cases per year. However, rabies is an emerging infection in animals. Forty years ago, most rabies infections occurred in dogs, with some infections also occurring in cats, foxes, and skunks. Programs to vaccinate domestic animals reduced the number of rabid dogs and cats. However, rabies still occurs in raccoons, skunks, bats, foxes and coyotes.

Currently in the United States, rabid raccoons are found in the eastern part of the country, from Georgia to New England. Rabid skunks are found in California, the central United States, and New England. Rabid bats are found in all states except Alaska and Hawaii. Foxes and coyotes infected with rabies are found in an area that stretches from Arizona to Texas. Rabid coyotes may have been shipped accidentally from Texas to Florida, resulting in rabies outbreaks in dogs and cats.

Humans usually acquire the rabies virus when they are bitten or scratched by rabid animals. With the number of endemic areas increasing for wildlife, the risk of human exposure to rabies increases because of the increased likelihood of encountering a rabid animal or a domestic animal that has contracted rabies from wildlife. Humans infected with the rabies virus experience a brief prodromal period of pain in the exposure site and have vague, flulike symptoms. Mental status changes, such as anxiety, irritability, and depression, may also become evident. After the prodromal period, patients suffer additional CNS changes, including hallucinations, paralysis, excessive salivation, hydrophobia, bouts of terror, seizures, respiratory and cardiac abnormalities, and hypertension. These symptoms are followed ultimately by coma and death. In 2004, a Texas hospital encountered five cases of rabies when organs and tissues from what was later discovered to be a bat-bite victim were transplanted into four patients, all of whom subsequently died of the disease. It is likely the spread was due to the nerve tissue accompanying the new organs as rabies is not considered a blood-borne pathogen.

Laboratory diagnosis of rabies involves determining whether an animal that has bitten a human has rabies. The animal is killed, and its head is removed and sent to a reference laboratory. The fastest and most sensitive method of identifying rabies viruses in a specimen is by using direct IF techniques. Impression smears should be made from various areas of the brain, primarily the hippocampus, pons, cerebella, and medulla oblongata. In living patients suspected of having rabies, biopsies of skin (especially at the hairline) and impressions of the cornea can be made. The presence of rabies virus in such specimens is diagnostic, but its absence merely means that no virus is present in those particular specimens, not that the patient does not have rabies. Rabies viruses can be grown in suckling or young adult mice, murine neuroblastoma, or related cell lines. EIAs are currently the most sensitive assays to use for serologic tests.

Rabies cannot be successfully treated once symptoms appear. However, postexposure prophylaxis is 100% effective in preventing the disease if the patient is treated sufficiently early. Postexposure prophylaxis includes vigorously cleaning the wound site, providing human rabies immune globulin, and administering a three-injection series of the rabies vaccine. Two approved human vaccine preparations are available in the United States and can be given to persons who might be exposed to rabies, such as veterinarians, laboratory personnel, people who explore caves, and people visiting high-risk countries for more than 30 days. Only one unvaccinated person with rabies has ever survived. A female teenager in Wisconsin developed rabies about a month after being bitten by a rabid bat. She was put into a coma and treated with several antiviral compounds. The reason for her survival is not completely understood.

Togaviridae

The family Togaviridae contains the genera *Alphavirus, Rubivirus,* and *Arterivirus.* No member of the genus *Arterivirus* is known to infect humans. Many of the viruses in the genus *Alphavirus* are mosquito-borne and cause encephalitis. Eastern equine encephalitis (EEE) occurs primarily in the eastern half of the United States. About 220 cases have been reported since 1964, but infections have a significant mortality rate of about 36%. Infections can cause a range of effects, from very mild influenza-like symptoms to encephalitis. As many as half of those who survive the infection suffer permanent CNS damage. Birds are the natural reservoir of the virus, and it is spread to humans and horses via the bite of mosquitoes. Because horses and humans are dead-end hosts, equine EEE disease can be a predictor of human EEE cases.

The western equine encephalitis (WEE) virus also causes disease in humans and horses. WEE virus causes a milder disease than EEE virus, and patients develop either an asymptomatic or mild infection consisting of fever, headache, nausea, and mental status changes. As many as 30% of infected young children and infants will suffer permanent CNS damage. Mortality is about 3%. Since 1964 there have been 639 cases in the United States.

Venezuelan equine encephalitis (VEE) has caused large outbreaks of human and equine encephalitis in the Americas. During an outbreak that lasted from 1969 to 1971, 200,000 horses died of VEE. In 1995 VEE caused encephalitis in an estimated 75,000 to 100,000 people in Venezuela and Colombia. Mortality is much less common in patients with VEE infection than with WEE or EEE. Infected adults often develop an influenza-like illness, whereas encephalitis is more commonly seen in VEE-infected children.

Rubella virus is an enveloped virus belonging to the genus *Rubivirus.* It causes the disease rubella or German measles, a mild febrile illness accompanied by an erythematous, maculopapular, discrete rash with postauricular and suboccipital lymphadenopathy. Like measles, rubella occurs in the winter and spring. The diseases are so similar that as many as 50% of suspected measles cases are determined to be rubella. The rubella virus is transmitted by droplets. The virus is present in nasopharyngeal specimens or any secretion or tissue of infected infants, who shed the virus in large amounts for long periods. A rash starts on the face and spreads to the trunk and limbs. No rash appears on the palms and soles. As many as 50% of individuals with rubella are asymptomatic. Transient polyarthralgia and polyarthritis can occur in children and are common in adults.

Rubella would be of little concern if it did not cross the placenta of pregnant women and disseminate to fetal tissues, a condition referred to as *congenital rubella syndrome.* The results range from the birth of a normal infant to the birth of a severely impaired infant to fetal death and spontaneous abortion. The impact on the embryo is worse when the infection develops in the earliest stages of pregnancy, because the rubella virus halts or slows the growth of the cells it infects.

An effective attenuated vaccine is available and should be administered to all children and young women before they become sexually active. The incidence of rubella in the United States has dropped dramatically, from 364 cases in 1998 to approximately 10 cases annually since 2003. Rubella was declared no longer endemic in the United States in 2004. Direct examination of specimens by IF or EIA is recommended because isolation procedures are cumbersome. Serologic procedures are effective because any rubella antibody is presumed to be protective. The most sensitive serologic assays are the solid-phase and passive hemagglutination tests. Latex agglutination and antigen-coated red blood cell tests are useful but less sensitive.

HEPATITIS VIRUSES

The hepatitis viruses are grouped together, not because of structural or genetic similarities, but because they share a tissue tropism—the liver. Before the 1960s and 1970s, patients with hepatitis were classified as having either infectious hepatitis or serum hepatitis. Infectious hepatitis was transmitted from person to person via the fecal-oral route, and serum hepatitis resulted from transfusion of infected blood and blood products. During the past 30 years, at least eight different hepatitis viruses (Table 29-7) have been recognized: hepatitis A (HAV), hepatitis B (HBV), hepatitis C (HCV), delta hepatitis (or hepatitis D virus; HDV), hepatitis E (HEV),

TABLE 29-7 Clinical and Epidemiologic Differences of HAV, HBV, HDV, and HCV

Clinical Features	Hepatitis A (HAV)	Hepatitis B (HBV)	Hepatitis D (HDV)	Hepatitis C (HCV)
Incubation (days)	15-45	30-120	21-90	40-50
Type of onset	Acute	Insidious	Usually acute	Insidious
Mode of transmission				
Fecal/oral	Usual	Infrequent	Infrequent	
Parenteral	Increasing	Usual	Usual	Likely
Other	Food-borne, waterborne	Intimate contact, transmucosal transfer	Intimate contact, less efficient than for HBV	Vertical transmission Intranasal cocaine use
Sequelae				
Carrier	No	5%-10%	Yes	Yes
Chronic hepatitis	No	Yes	Yes	Yes
Mortality (%)	0.1-0.2	0.5-2.0	30 (chronic form)	0.2-0.3

hepatitis G (HGV), SEN, and transfusion transmitted virus (TTV). HAV and HEV are transmitted by the fecal-oral route, and HBV, HCV, HDV, HGV, SEN virus, and TTV are transmitted by infected blood and blood products. HBV, TT, and SEN have DNA genomes, whereas the others have an RNA genome.

The hepatitis viruses are unrelated and biologically and morphologically disparate. Many of the clinical symptoms caused by the different hepatitis viruses are similar, so differentiation on the basis of clinical findings is not reliable. Common symptoms are fatigue, headache, anorexia, nausea, vomiting, abdominal pain (right upper quadrant or diffuse), and jaundice and dark urine, which are the most characteristic symptoms.

Hepatitis A Virus

Hepatitis A virus is a small, icosahedral, naked ssRNA virus, the sole member of the genus *Hepatovirus* in the family Picornaviridae. HAV infects people of all ages. In the United States, children between the ages of 5 and 14 have the highest rate of infection. Nearly 30% of all cases occur in children under the age of 15 years. In the United States, reported cases have declined from an average of 25,000 per year in the 1990s to an average of 3,000 per year since 2006. Epidemics occur about every 10 to 15 years; the last two peaks in cases occurred in 1989 and 1995.

HAV is almost always transmitted by the fecal-oral route. Risk factors for HAV infection include sexual or household contact with an infected person, daycare contacts, food-borne or waterborne outbreaks, IV drug use, and international travel. However, almost half the cases in the United States have no established risk factor. The virus is shed in large amounts in the feces during the incubation period and early prodromal stage, and food and water contamination can result. The incubation for HAV is approximately 1 month. After individuals are infected with HAV, they experience a transient viremia, after which the virus reaches the liver and replicates in hepatocytes. The virus passes into the intestine, and viral shedding begins and can persist for months.

Infections in more than 90% of children aged younger than 5 years are asymptomatic. In adults, symptoms can range from mild to severe prolonged hepatitis. The onset is abrupt and patients experience fever, chills, fatigue, malaise, aches, pains, and in some cases jaundice. The infection is self-limiting, with convalescence possibly lasting weeks. Complete recovery can take months. HAV has a low mortality and no persistence, and it does not cause chronic liver damage.

The best method for laboratory diagnosis of HAV is to demonstrate IgM to HAV (Figure 29-18). Isolation of HAV is not practical because it is difficult to grow in culture and tends to mutate drastically when it does. Safe, effective vaccines for HAV are available. Vaccination of children in particular has the potential to reduce the incidence of HAV. Other vaccination target groups include people who travel to countries with endemic HAV, sexually active males, drug abusers, and patients with chronic liver disease. Persons who have not been vaccinated and have been exposed to HAV can receive immune globulin, which is 80% to 90% effective in preventing infection when administered in a timely fashion. Immune globulin can also be used as pre-exposure prophylaxis.

Hepatitis B Virus

Hepatitis B virus is a partially dsDNA virus. It is enveloped and belongs to the family Hepadnaviridae. The virus contains a surface antigen referred to as hepatitis B surface antigen (HBsAg) that circulates in the bloodstream as 22-nm particles. Complete viruses have a diameter of about 45 nm. The virion also contains a core antigen (HBcAg) and the hepatitis Be antigen (HBeAg). Eight genotypes of HBV have been identified (A-H), and some studies have shown a difference in clinical outcome based on the infecting genotype.

Almost half of the world's population lives in areas with endemic HBV, and more than 8% of the population is positive for HbsAg. Worldwide about 350 million people are chronic carriers, and in the United States there are more than a million chronic carriers of the virus. However, the incidence of acute hepatitis has declined over 81% in the United States since the mid-1980s, mostly as a result of aggressive screening and vaccination programs.

HBV is primarily a blood-borne pathogen. Infected patients can have as many as 1 million infectious particles per milliliter of blood. Lower concentrations of virus appear in semen, vaginal fluid, and saliva. Many other body fluids (e.g.,

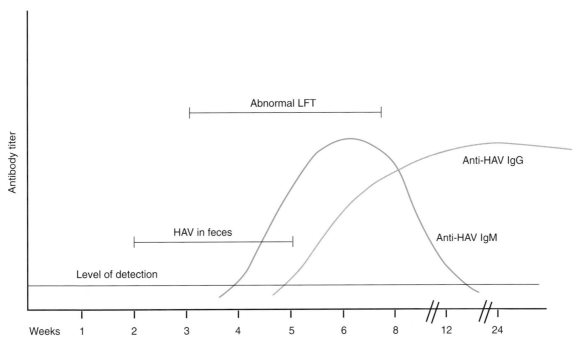

FIGURE 29-18 Serologic evaluation of hepatitis A virus infection showing the rise and fall of detectable antibodies. *LFT,* Liver function test.

tears, urine, sweat, breast milk) contain HbsAg but do not seem to be infective. The main modes of transmission are through sexual, perinatal, and parenteral routes. In the United States, heterosexual and homosexual sexual contact is the most common transmission routes. High-risk groups include IV drug abusers, men who have sex with men, individuals from endemic areas, persons who have household or sexual contacts with HBV carriers, health care personnel, people who have tattoos or body piercing, and infants born to HBV-positive mothers. Almost one third of the patients who become infected, however, have no known risk factor.

The human cost of the infection is high. As many as 1 million deaths per year are HBV related. Once HBV enters the host, it travels from the blood to the liver, and cytotoxic T cells attack the HBV-infected hepatocytes. The incubation period for HBV infection varies from 2 to 6 months, with an insidious onset that includes symptoms of fever, anorexia, and hepatic tenderness. Jaundice occurs in only about 10% of children who are younger than 5 years and is more common in older children and adults (30% to 50%).

As the immune response is activated, the virus is slowly cleared from the system, and most patients become noninfectious. About 5% to 70% of infections are asymptomatic; another 20% to 30% of the patients exhibit clinical jaundice but have a benign resolution of the infection. Therefore about 90% of infections do not cause serious sequelae. Nevertheless about 10% of infected individuals are chronic carriers for more than 6 months. Many of these individuals develop a chronic infection and have a higher risk of liver disease, such as cirrhosis or hepatic carcinoma. There is a safe and effective recombinant vaccine for preventing HBV infection.

Diagnosis of HBV infection is based on clinical presentation and demonstration of specific serologic markers for HBV

BOX 29-3 Serologic Markers for the Diagnosis of Hepatitis B Virus Infection

- HBsAg: Hepatitis B surface antigen, the envelope protein consisting of three polypeptides
- Anti-HBs: Antibody to hepatitis B surface antigen
- Anti-HBc: Antibody to hepatitis B core antigen
- HBeAg: Antigen associated with the nucleocapsid, also found as soluble protein in serum
- Anti-HBe: Antibody to hepatitis Be antigen

(Box 29-3). Serum aminotransferase levels also increase in infected patients. The presence of HBsAg in a patient's serum indicates that the patient has an active HBV infection, is a chronic carrier, or is in an incubation period. IgM anti-HBc appears early in the course of the disease and indicates an acute infection. In cases in which HBsAg is not detected and anti-HBs has not yet appeared, detection of IgM anti-HBc confirms the diagnosis of acute HBV infection. The time period between the inability to detect the HBsAg and the detection of Anti-HBs antibodies is often referred to as the core "window period" of immunity. The detection of anti-HBs in the serum indicates a convalescent or immune status.

When the infection resolves, IgG anti-HBc and anti-HBs become detectable in the patient's serum. The presence of HBsAg after 6 months of acute infection is a strong indication that the patient is a chronic carrier; the appearance of HBeAg in this case is indicative of a chronic infection and high infectivity. Table 29-8 shows the interpretation of HBV serologic markers. Figure 29-19 shows the rise and fall of detectable antibodies during acute HBV infection and resolution and of chronic HBV infection.

TABLE 29-8 Interpretation of Hepatitis B Serologic Markers

HBsAg	HBeAg	Anti-HBc	Anti-HBc IgM	Anti-HBs	Anti-HBe	Interpretation
−	NA	−		−	NA	No previous infection with HBV or early incubation
−	NA	+	−	+/−	NA	Convalescent or past infection
−	NA	−	−	±	NA	Immunization to HBsAg
+	−	−	+/−	−	−	Acute infection
+	+	+/−	+	−	−	Acute infection, high infectivity
+	−	+/−	+	−	+	Acute infection, low infectivity
+	+	+		−		Chronic infection, high infectivity
+	−	+	−	−	+	Chronic infection, low infectivity

−, Negative; +, positive; +/− positive or negative; *NA*, not applicable.

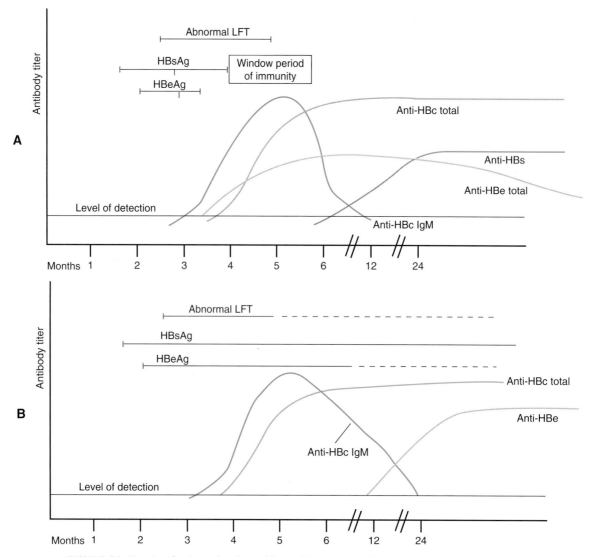

FIGURE 29-19 Serologic evaluation of hepatitis B virus infection showing the rise and fall of detectable antibodies. **A,** Serologic presentation in acute hepatitis infection with resolution. **B,** Serologic presentation in chronic hepatitis infection with late seroconversion. *LFT,* Liver function test.

TABLE 29-9 Interpretation of Hepatitis D Infection Serologic Markers

Clinical Variant	Serologic Markers			
	Anti-HBc IgM	HBsAg	Anti-HDV	Anti-HDV IgM
Co-infection	+	+	+	+
Superinfection	−	+	+	NA

NA, Not applicable.

Hepatitis D Virus

Hepatitis D virus, also known as the *delta hepatitis virus,* is a defective 1.7-kb ssRNA virus that requires HBV for replication. HDV requires the HBV HBsAg for its envelope. HDV is the sole member of the genus *Deltavirus.* The genus is not currently assigned to a family. HDV is transmitted primarily by parenteral means, although transmission by mucosal contact has been implicated in epidemics in endemic areas. At-risk groups in the United States are primarily IV drug users, although limited numbers of men who have sex with men in certain parts of the country are also at risk. Because of overlaps in the clinical presentation, a presumed low incidence of infection, and lack of an effective surveillance mechanism, the current epidemiology of delta hepatitis is minimal.

HDV infection is rare but usually severe and results in either acute disease with a fatality rate of 5% or chronic symptoms progressing to cirrhosis in two thirds of those infected. The viral infection can occur in one of two clinical forms: co-infection or superinfection. In a co-infection, the patient is simultaneously infected by HBV and HDV. In a superinfection, a chronic HBV carrier is infected with HDV; that is, an HDV infection develops in a patient with a chronic HBV infection. Patients with a co-infection suffer a more severe acute infection and have a higher risk of fulminant hepatitis than patients with a superinfection. However, chronic carriers of HBV who become superinfected with HDV also develop chronic HDV, which increases their chance of developing cirrhosis.

Diagnosis of HDV infection requires serologic testing for specific HDV antibody markers. Commercial tests are available for HDV IgG. Reference laboratories may offer IgM and HDV Ag testing as well as PCR for HDV. Table 29-9 shows interpretation of HDV serologic markers, and Figure 29-20 shows serologic presentations of HDV co-infection and superinfection.

Hepatitis C Virus

After methods for diagnosing HAV and HBV became available, it was apparent that they were not responsible for all hepatitis cases, in particular those related to blood transfusions. The resulting disease was merely called *non-A, non-B hepatitis* (NANB). The diagnosis of NANB hepatitis was primarily one of exclusion. In 1974, without any direct evidence, scientists predicted that a "hepatitis virus type C" must exist. Fifteen years later, with the aid of cloning techniques, the genomic sequence of HCV was determined before the virus was ever seen with an electron microscope.

HCV is an ssRNA virus in the genus *Hepacivirus,* family Flaviviridae, and accounts for about 90% of all previous cases of NANB hepatitis. Currently, fewer than 1000 new cases occur annually in the United States, However, because of the long incubation period, it is estimated that approximately 19,000 acute infections occur each year. Throughout the 1980s, the estimated number of infections hovered around 200,000 per year. A combination of factors, such as safer use of needles by IV drug abusers and reduction of posttransfusion infections because of better testing, has dropped the incidence dramatically in the United States. Worldwide, as many as 170 million new cases may develop each year. Although perinatal and sexual transmission of infection do occur, and parenteral transmission has been identified as a major route for infection, HCV antibody has been detected in patients in whom the routes of transmission are poorly understood or who have no evidence of identifiable risk factors.

Symptoms may be subtle and take time to become apparent. About 50% of HCV-positive patients become chronic carriers, and about 20% to 30% of patients with chronic infections develop cirrhosis. Cirrhosis is a major risk factor for hepatocellular carcinoma. About 3.5 million people are chronic carriers of HCV in the United States.

Gene amplification tests prove that HCV RNA appears in newly infected patients in as little as 2 weeks. However, most virus detection is accomplished by serologic testing, not by gene amplification. HCV is less immunogenic than HBV. Antibodies to HCV appear in about 6 weeks in 80% of patients and within 12 weeks in 90% of patients. HCV infection does not produce persistent, lifelong levels of antibody; rather, persistence of anti-HCV is linked to the presence of replicating HCV.

EIAs that detect serum antibodies to HCV proteins are available as screening tests; however, these assays have a high false-positive rate. Second-generation immunoblot assays use recombinant and or synthetic proteins to detect anti-HCV antibodies. A recombinant immunoblot assay (RIBA), manufactured by Chiron Corporation (St. Emeryville, Calif.), can be performed to confirm reactive results obtained with a screening test. The "blot" or "strip" contains separate bands of proteins 5-1-1, cl00, c33, and c22 to detect antibodies to these proteins by ELISA. Figure 29-21 shows a representation of the immunologic profile of HCV infection. Patients with a chronic HCV infection can be treated with interferon with or without ribavirin. Some laboratories offer HCV viral loads to help monitor efficacy of treatment in patients.

Hepatitis E Virus

Hepatitis E virus is a small (32 to 34 nm), naked, ssRNA virus classified in the genus *Hepevirus,* family Hepeviridae. Along with HCV, HEV is the other historic NANB hepatitis virus. Unlike HCV, HEV is a waterborne enteric agent transmitted by fecally contaminated drinking water. HEV has been identified as a cause of epidemics of enterically transmitted hepatitis in developing countries in Asia, Africa, and Central America. Although the virus has not been associated with outbreaks in the United States, it has been linked to sporadic cases in travelers returning from endemic areas.

HEV causes an acute, self-limiting disease with clinical symptoms that are similar to those of HAV. The incubation

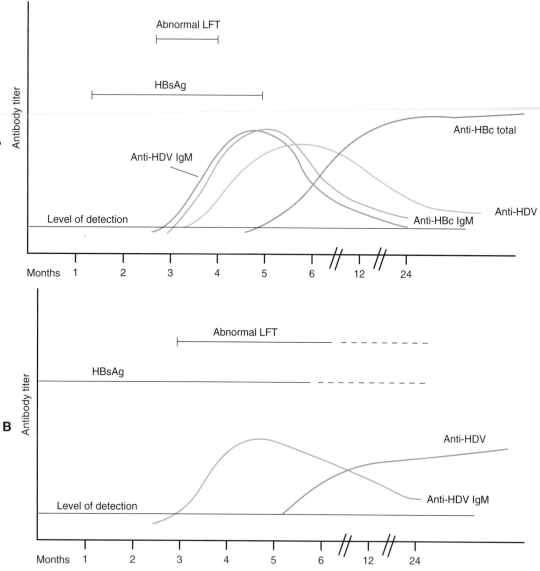

FIGURE 29-20 Serologic evaluation of hepatitis D virus (HDV) infection showing persistence of detectable antibodies indicating the presence of replicating HDV. *LFT,* Liver function test.

period is 2 to 9 weeks. Signs and symptoms of HEV infection include fever, malaise, nausea, vomiting, jaundice, and dark urine. Viral shedding in the feces has been shown to persist for several weeks. The mortality rate is 1% to 3% overall, with a higher likelihood of death in pregnant women (15% to 25%). Epidemics affect primarily young to middle-age adults. An ELISA test has been developed to detect IgG and IgM antibodies to HEV, although HEV testing is not currently performed in diagnostic laboratories in the United States.

Other Hepatitis Viruses

Evidence for HGV was derived originally from a patient with NANB hepatitis. This newly described RNA virus is a member of the family Flaviviridae and is genetically and antigenically similar to the virus GBV-C. Eventually sequencing data determined that they were actually different isolates of the same virus. In several studies HGV viremia has been demonstrated worldwide in 0.6% to 14% of blood donors, depending on geographic location. HGV viremia does not seem to be a common occurrence in the United States. The clinical significance of the virus is being studied. Experimental RT-PCR tests can be done to detect the virus, but routine testing is not yet recommended.

The most recently identified hepatitis viruses are SEN virus and TTV. SEN virus has a circular DNA genome. It is blood-borne and, although originally suspected to be a cause of hepatitis, it has not been definitively linked to any human disease. Transmission does appear to be linked to blood transfusions. About 30% of patients with HIV infection have antibodies to SEN. TTV was first identified in the serum of a Japanese patient in 1997. It is a single-stranded DNA virus related to the animal circoviruses. The role of TTV in human disease is unknown but may be associated with some cases of posttransfusion hepatitis.

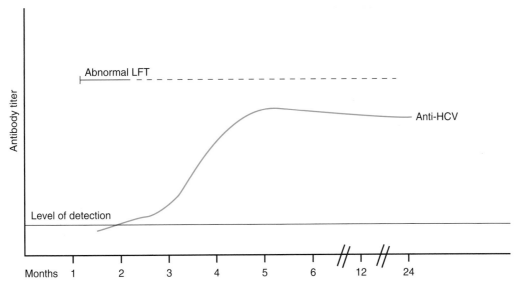

FIGURE 29-21 Serologic evaluation of hepatitis C virus (HCV) infection showing persistence of deectable antibodies, indicating the presence of replication HCV. *LFT,* Liver function test.

PRIONS

Prions are proteinaceous infectious particles that cause a group of diseases in mammals called *transmissible spongiform encephalopathies* (TSEs). The name *prion* was coined by Stanley B. Prusiner in 1982. Examples of TSEs include Kuru and Creutzfeldt-Jakob disease (CJD) in humans, scrapie in sheep, bovine spongiform encephalopathy (BSE) in cattle, and chronic wasting disease in deer and elk. BSE, also referred to as "mad cow disease," has been responsible for the loss of hundreds of thousands of cattle in the United Kingdom, most notably during the 1980s.

An increase in a variant form of CJD (vCJD) in the United Kingdom was noted about the same time as the surge of BSE. It appears that the agent of scrapie crossed species and infected cows and that it is the causative agent of BSE-infected humans causing vCJD. Three confirmed cases of BSE have been reported in the United States; the first case was discovered in 2003 in Washington state. Subsequent cases were reported in 2004 from Texas and 2006 in Alabama. Twelve cases of BSE have been reported in Canada. TSEs are known to be transmitted by ingestion. Sheep offal put into cattle feed was the likely cause of the prion moving from sheep to cattle.

The TSEs are characterized by progressive relentless degeneration of the CNS that is ultimately fatal. Typical histopathology is neuronal vacuolation and eventual loss of neurons, which is accompanied by proliferation and hypertrophy of fibrous astrocytes. The prion protein (PrP) found in animals with TSE is often referred to as PrP^{Sc}, named after the prion found in sheep with scrapie. Animals, including humans, have a similar but normal protein found on cells of the CNS referred to as PrP^{C}. Ingested PrP^{Sc} is absorbed into the bloodstream and makes its way into the CNS. PrP^{Sc} in some way converts PrP^{C} into PrP^{Sc}, which is released by neu-

ronal cells. PrP^{Sc} accumulates in the CNS, producing amyloid plaques and the characteristic histopathology.

The diagnosis of TSE is often based on clinical findings. Routine analysis of CSF is nonrevealing. Many patients with CJD will have 14-3-3 proteins in the CSF; however, these proteins are not specific for CJD. The presence of these proteins in CSF is a marker for rapid neuronal cell death, present not only in CJD but conditions such as hemorrhages and encephalitis. Histopathology stains and immunostaining of PrP^{Sc} remain the most specific diagnostic methods. Other detection methods include antigen detection, serologic testing, and nucleic acid sequencing. Recent findings have suggested the excretion of TSEs in urine.

The risk of infection to laboratory personnel is low, but material suspected of containing these agents must be handled carefully. Prion proteins are extremely resistant to inactivation; even 2 hours in a steam autoclave might not inactivate all prions in a specimen. Exposure to household bleach greater than 20,000 ppm available chlorine or 1 M sodium hydroxide is recommended.

ANTIVIRAL THERAPY

Some viral infections are treatable, especially if a laboratory can rapidly identify the pathogen. Antiviral compounds must target an essential viral replicative mechanism without destroying or damaging uninfected host cells. Several antiviral agents resemble nucleosides used in viral replication. The viruses insert these "counterfeit" nucleoside analogs into their own nucleic acid, resulting in a disruption of viral replication. Other antiviral compounds inhibit viral replication by targeting key viral proteins. For instance, phosphonoformic acid (foscarnet) is an analog of pyrophosphate that acts directly as a DNA polymerase inhibitor. Examples of some of the

TABLE 29-10 Examples of Antiviral Compounds

Antiviral	Inhibits	Active Against
Acyclovir	DNA polymerase	HSV, VZV
Cidofovir	DNA polymerase	CMV (retinitis)
Famciclovir	DNA polymerase	HSV-2
Ganciclovir	DNA polymerase	CMV (retinitis)
Valacyclovir	DNA polymerase	HSV-2
Idoxuridine, trifluridine	DNA synthesis (DNA base analog)	HSV (keratitis)
Amantadine, rimantadine	Uncoating	Influenza A (treatment and prophylaxis)
Inferferon-alpha	Viral replication (multiple mechanisms)	HPV (genital warts); chronic HCV, Kaposi sarcoma
Ribavirin	Viral replication (multiple mechanisms)	RSV; CCHF
ddI	Reverse transcriptase	HIV
3TC	Reverse transcriptase	HIV
d4T	Reverse transcriptase	HIV
ddC	Reverse transcriptase	HIV
ZDV	Reverse transcriptase	HIV
Indinavir	Proteases	HIV
Nelfinavir, ritonavir	Proteases	HIV
Saquinavir	Proteases	HIV
Lamivudine		Chronic HBV
Adefovir		Chronic HBV

HSV, Herpes simplex virus; *VZV*, Varicella-zoster virus; *CMV*, cytomegalovirus; *HPV*, human papillomavirus; *HCV*, hepatitis C virus; *RSV*, respiratory syncytial virus; *CCHF*, Crimean-Congo hemorrhagic fever; *HIV*, human immunodeficiency virus.

more commonly used antiviral agents are listed in Table 29-10.

Just as antibacterial agent use increases the risk of drug resistance in bacteria, the use of antiviral agents can result in viruses that are resistant to therapy. As more antiviral agents become available, antiviral susceptibility testing will become increasingly important. For example, foscarnet is being used to treat infections caused by HSV strains that are resistant to acyclovir and to treat CMV strains that are resistant to ganciclovir.

BIBLIOGRAPHY

Ablashi D et al: Spectrum of Kaposi's sarcoma-associated herpesvirus, or human herpesvirus 8, diseases, *Clin Micro Rev* 15:439, 2002.

Aguzzi AM et al: Transmissible spongiform encephalopathies. In Murray PR et al, editors: *Manual of clinical microbiology*, ed 9, Washington, DC, 2007, ASM Press.

Akiba J et al: SEN virus: epidemiology and characteristics of a transfusion-transmitted virus, *Transfusion* 45:1084, 2005.

Allander T et al: Cloning of a human parvovirus by molecular screening of respiratory tract samples, *PNAS* 102:12891, 2005.

Ashley R: Sorting out the new HSV type specific antibody tests, *Sex Transm Infect* 77:232, 2001.

Belay ED et al: Creutzfeldt-Jakob disease surveillance and diagnosis, *Clin Inf Dis* 41:834, 2005.

Canadian Food Inspection Agency: BSE completed investigations. Available at: www.inspection.gc.ca/english/anima/heasan/disemala/bseesb/comenqe.shtml. Accessed November 3, 2008.

Centers for Disease Control and Prevention: Brief report: update mumps activity—United States, January 1-October 7, 2006, *MMWR* 55:1152, 2006. Available at: www.cdc.gov/mmwr/preview/mmwrhtml/mm5542a3.htm. Accessed November 3, 2008.

Centers for Disease Control and Prevention: Update: measles—United States, January-July 2008, *MMWR* 57:893, 2008. Available at: www.cdc.gov/mmwr/preview/mmwrhtml/mm5733a1.htm. Accessed November 3, 2008.

Centers for Disease Control and Prevention: Acute respiratory disease associated with adenovirus serotype 14—four states, 2006-2007, *MMWR* 56:1181, 2007. Available at: www.cdc.gov/mmwr/preview/mmwrhtml/mm5645a1.htm. Accessed November 3, 2008.

Centers for Disease Control and Prevention: Statistics and surveillance, disease burden from hepatitis A, B, and C in the United States. Available at: www.cdc.gov/hepatitis/Statistics.htm#section3. Accessed November 3, 2008.

Centers for Disease Control and Prevention: Delayed onset and diminished magnitude of rotavirus activity—United States, November 2007-May 2008, *MMWR* 57:697, 2008. Available at: www.cdc.gov/mmwr/preview/mmwrhtml/mm5725a6.htm. Accessed November 3, 2008.

Centers for Disease Control and Prevention: Known cases and outbreaks of Marburg hemorrhagic fever, in chronological order. Available at: www.dcd.gov/ncidod/dvrd/spb/mnpages/dispages/marburg/marburgtable.htm. Accessed November 3, 2008.

Centers for Disease Control and Prevention: West Nile virus website. Available at: www.cdc.gov/ncidod/dvbid/westnile. Accessed November 3, 2008.

Centers for Disease Control and Prevention: HIV/AIDS in the United States. Available at: www.cdc.gov/hiv/topics/suveilance/resources/reports/2007report/pdf/2007SurveillanceReport.pdf. Accessed October 15, 2009.

Centers for Disease Control and Prevention: Human rabies prevention—United States, 2008. Recommendations of the Advisory Committee on Immunization Practices (ACIP), *MMWR* 57(RR03):1-26, 2008. Available at: www.cdc.gov/mmwr/preview/mmwrhtml/rr5703a1.htm. Accessed November 3, 2008.

Centers for Disease Control and Prevention: Progress toward interruption in wild poliovirus transmission—worldwide, January 2006-March 2007. *MMWR* 56:682, 2007. Available at: www.cdc.gov/mmwr/preview/mmwrhtml/mm5627a3.htm. Accessed November 3, 2008.

Centers for Disease Control and Prevention: Global polio eradication, Available at: www.cdc.gov/ncird/progbriefs/downloads/global-polio-eradic.pdf. Accessed November 3, 2008.

Centers for Disease Control and Prevention: Investigation of rabies infections in organ donor and transplant recipients—Alabama, Arkansas, Oklahoma, and Texas, 2004, *MMWR* 53:586, 2004. Available at: www.cdc.gov/mmwr/preview/mmwrhtml/mm5327a5.htm. Accessed November 3, 2008.

Centers for Disease Control and Prevention: Elimination of rubella and congenital rubella syndrome—the Americas, 2003-2008, *MMWR* 57: 1176, 2008. Available at: www.cdc.gov/mmwr/preview/mmwrhtml/mm5743a4.htm. Accessed November 3, 2008.

Centers for Disease Control and Prevention: Surveillance for acute viral hepatitis—United States, 2006, *MMWR* 57(SS-02): 1-24, 2008. Available at: www.cdc.gov/mmwr/preview/mmwrhtml/ss5702a1.htm. Accessed November 3, 2008.

Centers for Disease Control and Prevention: Brief report: respiratory syncytial virus activity—United States, 2004-2005, *MMWR* 54: 1259, 2005. Available at: www.cdc.gov/mmwr/preview/mmwrhtml/mm5449a3.htm. Accessed November 3, 2008.

Centers for Disease Control and Prevention: Prevention of herpes zoster: recommendations of the Advisory Committee on Immunization Practices, *MMWR* 57 (early release) 1, 2008. Available at: www.cdc.gov/mmwr/preview/mmwrhtml/rr57e0515a1.htm. Accessed October 14, 2009.

Daley P et al: Comparison of flocked and rayon swabs for collection of respiratory epithelial cells from uninfected volunteers and symptomatic patients, *J Clinic Microbiol* 44:2265, 2006.

Dowdle WR et al: Preventing polio from becoming a reemerging disease, *Emerg Inf Dis* 7:549, 2001.

Forman MS, Valsamakis A: Specimen collection, transport, and processing: Virology. In Murray PR et al, editors: *Manual of clinical microbiology*, ed 9, Washington, DC, 2007, ASM.

Gregori L et al: Excretion of transmissible spongiform encephalopathy infectivity in urine, *Emerg Inf Dis* 14:1406, 2008.

Gu J, Korteweg C: Pathology and pathogenesis of severe acute respiratory syndrome, *Am J Path* 170:1136, 2007.

Hall CB et al: Congenital infections with human herpesvirus 6 (HHV6) and human herpesvirus 7 (HHV7), *J Pediatrics* 145:472, 2004.

Heikkinen T et al: Human metapneumovirus infections in children, *Emerg Inf Dis* 14:101, 2008.

Horvat RT, Tegtmeier GE: Hepatitis B and D viruses. In Murray PR et al, editors: *Manual of clinical microbiology*, ed 9, Washington, DC, 2007, ASM.

Johnson NP, Mueller J: Updating the accounts: global mortality of the 1918-1920 "Spanish" influenza pandemic, *Bull Hist Med* 76:105, 2002.

Lodes M et al: Use of semiconductor-based oligonucleotide microarrays for influenza A virus subtype identification and sequencing, *J Clin Microbiol* 44:1209, 2006.

Louie JK et al: A summer outbreak of human metapneumovirus infection in a long-term-care facility, *J Inf Dis* 196:705, 2008.

Mahony J et al: Development of a respiratory virus panel test for detection of twenty human respiratory viruses by use of multiplex PCR and a fluid microbead-based assay, *J Clin Microbiol* 45:2965, 2007.

Matsuzaki Y et al: Frequent reassortment among influenza C viruses, *J Virol* 77, 2003.

Nolte F et al: MultiCode-PLx System for multiplexed detection of seventeen respiratory viruses, *J Clin Microbiol* 45:2779, 2007.

Parashar U et al: Rotavirus and severe childhood diarrhea, *Emerg Infect Dis* 12:304, 2006.

Parisi S et al: Both human immunodeficiency virus cellular DNA sequencing and plasma RNA sequencing are useful for detection of drug resistance mutations in blood samples from antiretroviral-drug-naive patients, *J Clin Microbiol* 45:1783, 2007.

Pellett PE, Tipples G: Human herpesviruses 6, 7, and 8. In Murray PR et al, editors: *Manual of clinical microbiology*, ed 9, Washington, DC, 2007, ASM.

Robinson C, Echavarria M: Adenoviruses. In Murray PR et al, editors: *Manual of clinical microbiology*, ed 9, Washington, DC, 2007, ASM.

Sauerbrei A, Wutzler P: Herpes simplex and varicella-zoster virus infections during pregnancy: current concepts of prevention, diagnosis and therapy. Part 1: herpes simplex virus infections, *Med Microbiol Immunol* 196:89, 2007.

Smuts H et al: Role of human metapneumovirus, human coronavirus NL63 and human bocavirus in infants and young children with acute wheezing, *J Med Virol* 80:906, 2008.

Stapleton JT et al: GB virus type C: a beneficial infection? *J Clin Microbiol* 42, 2004.

Tang YW, Crowe JE: Respiratory syncytial virus and human metapneumovirus. In Murray PR et al, editors: *Manual of clinical microbiology*, ed 9, 2007, ASM.

Taubenberger JK, Morens DM: The pathology of influenza virus infection, *Ann Rev Pathol* 3:499, 2008.

Thompson WW et al: Mortality associated with influenza and respiratory syncytial virus in the United States, *JAMA* 289:179, 2003.

Tsunetsugu-Yokota Y et al: Formalin-treated UV-inactivated SARS coronavirus vaccine retains its immunogenicity and promotes Th2-type immune responses, *Jpn J Infect Dis* 60:106, 2007.

van den Hoogen BG et al: A newly discovered human pneumovirus isolated from young children with respiratory tract disease, *Nature Med* 7:719, 2001.

World Health Organization: Hepatitis E fact sheet No. 280. Available at: www.who.int/mediacentre/factsheets/fs280/en/. Accessed November 3, 2008.

World Health Organization: *Fact sheet: measles*. Available at: www.who.int/mediacentre/factsheets/fs286/en/. Accessed November 3, 2008.

World Health Organization: *Cumulative number of confirmed human cases of avian influenza A(H5N1) reported to WHO*. Available at: www.who.int/csr/disease/avian_influenza/country/cases_table_2009_09_24/en/index.html. Accessed October 16, 2009.

World Health Organization: AIDS epidemic update, 2007. Available at: www.whqlibdoc.who.int. Accessed November 3, 2008.

World Health Organization: AIDS epidemic update, 2007. Available at: www.whqlibdoc.who.int. Accessed November 3, 2008.

World Health Organization: Pandemic (H1N1)—update 69. Available at: www.who.int/csr/don/2009_10_09/en/index.html. Accessed October 15, 2009.

Xu F et al: Trends in herpes simplex virus type 1 and type 2 seroprevalence in the United States, *JAMA* 296:964, 2006.

Zitterkopf N et al: Relevance of influenza A virus detection by PCR, shell vial assay, and tube cell culture to rapid reporting procedures, *J Clin Microbiol* 44:3366, 2006.

Points to Remember

- Clinical virology is an important component of clinical microbiology.
- Clinical virology services can consist of simple and rapid antigen or antibody detection kits, or they can be more sophisticated with cell culture capability and a variety of methods for identification of viral isolates.
- Clinically significant viruses can be isolated from patients with signs and symptoms that are commonly thought to be associated with bacterial infections, including pneumonia, gastrointestinal disease, cutaneous lesions, sexually transmitted infections, and sepsis, among others.
- Some viruses mutate rapidly, resulting in new strains which can be challenging to contain or treat.

- Antiviral compounds provide medical intervention for numerous viral infections.
- Many emerging infections are caused by viral agents that are unexpectedly transplanted into a susceptible human population.
- The hepatitis viruses are a diverse collection of viruses grouped together because they all infect primarily the liver.

Learning Assessment Questions

1. Which opportunistic infections or conditions are used as indicators of acquired immunodeficiency syndrome?

2. Which immunologic markers are used to diagnose a human immunodeficiency virus infection?

3. What disease does Epstein-Barr virus (EBV) produce? What complications may result from EBV infections?

4. How is an acute hepatitis B viral infection differentiated from a chronic infection? Which markers indicate resolution of the infection?

5. What are the differences between classic dengue fever and dengue hemorrhagic fever?

6. What are the methods commonly used to diagnosis rabies?

7. What is fifth disease? What is the cause of this disease?

8. Which viruses comprise the enteroviruses?

9. What are arenaviruses?

10. Which types of infections do human papillomaviruses produce?

11. Which viruses have the potential for latency?

12. Why are vaccines for influenza not always effective?

Agents of Bioterror

Wade Aldous, William F. Nauschuetz

- BIOSAFETY LEVELS
- GENERAL CHARACTERISTICS OF BIOTERROR AGENTS
- HISTORY OF CRIMINAL USE OF MICROBIAL AGENTS
- THE LABORATORY RESPONSE NETWORK
- AGENTS OF BIOTERROR
  Bacillus anthracis
  Yersinia pestis

Francisella tularensis
Brucella Species
Burkholderia Species
Coxiella burnetii
Variola Virus
Viral Hemorrhagic Fevers
Clostridium botulinum Toxin
Staphylococcal Enterotoxins
Ricin

OBJECTIVES

After reading this chapter, you should be able to:

1. Discuss the general characteristics of bioterror agents.

2. List the category A agents of bioterror that can be grown in cultures.

3. Compare the pathogenesis of the bioterror agents discussed in this chapter.

4. Compare the characteristics seen on initial culture of
   - *Bacillus anthracis*
   - *Yersinia pestis*
   - *Francisella tularensis*
   - *Brucella* spp.
   - *Burkholderia* spp.

5. Compare the roles of the three levels of Laboratory Response Network laboratories: sentinel, reference, and national.

Case in Point

On October 16, 2001, a 56-year-old African American man experienced fever, chills, headache, sore throat, and malaise. Symptoms progressed to difficulty in breathing, night sweats, nausea, and vomiting. He went to the hospital on October 19. At admission he was afebrile, and his heart rate was 100 beats per minute. Physical examination found decreased breath sounds and rhonchi. His complete blood count was unremarkable, and serum chemistries and renal functions were normal. Arterial blood gas did not show hypoxia. A chest radiograph showed a widened mediastinum, and a computed tomography scan showed mediastinal edema. Blood cultures were collected, and gram-positive bacilli presumptively identified as *Bacillus anthracis* grew within 11 hours. The patient was started on ciprofloxacin, rifampin, and clindamycin. On October 21, the patient developed respiratory distress, and he was treated with diuretics, corticosteroids, and thoracentesis. The patient eventually recovered.

Issues to Consider

After reading the patient's case history, consider:

- What signs and symptoms are characteristic of respiratory anthrax
- What key tests are used for the diagnosis of anthrax
- What tests should a sentinel laboratory perform to rule out *Bacillus anthracis*

Key Terms

Biosafety levels (BSLs)
Black death
Buboes
Bubonic plague
Category A agents
Eschar
Glanders
Inhalation anthrax
Laboratory Response Network (LRN)

Mediastinitis
Melioidosis
Pneumonic plague
Q fever
Tularemia
Vaccinia
Variola major
Variola minor

Bioterrorism is the intentional use of bacteria, viruses, fungi, or toxins to injure people, animals, or crops to cause civil and economic unrest. Bioterrorism can be classified as either overt or covert. In overt bioterrorism the impact will be immediate and there will be early recognition of the event, generally by emergency response personnel. Additionally, a group or society will often claim responsibility for the event. Covert events pose more of a challenge; clinical microbiologists and physicians will most likely be the first to suspect the attack. During covert bioterrorism the recognition, as well as the response, will be delayed. Biologic warfare is the deliberate use of bacteria, viruses, fungi, or toxins to injure people, animals, or crops to gain a military advantage.

The modern era of biologic weapons began during World War I, when Germany was believed to have used *Vibrio cholerae* and *Yersinia pestis* against humans and *Bacillus anthracis* and *Burkholderia mallei* against animals. Despite a Geneva Protocol prohibiting the use of biological agents during war signed by many nations, a number of countries began biological warfare research programs in the 1920s. This chapter discusses the pathogenesis of potential bioterror agents and their laboratory identification and summarizes the testing done at sentinel laboratories to rule out the presence of bioterror agents.

BIOSAFETY LEVELS

Microorganisms can be placed into one of four **biosafety levels (BSLs)** based on their disease potential. A BSL is a combination of standard procedures and techniques, safety equipment, and facilities designed to minimize the exposure of workers and the environment to infectious agents. BSL levels increase according to the nature of the organism(s) that is (are) studied or tested. Some organisms can fall under more than one category based upon the extent of culture studies. As an example, *B. anthracis* identified in a clinical laboratory is considered a BSL-2 agent, but if it is grown in larger quantities then it would be considered a BSL-3 organism. Additionally, *Mycobacterium tuberculosis* is a BSL-2 microorganism in clinical laboratories that perform only direct examination of clinical specimens. Laboratories that manipulate cultures and create an aerosolization risk should have a BSL-3 containment facility. It is important to remember that each higher level includes additional safety equipment, precautions, engineering, and work controls over the previous level.

BSL-1 organisms are those that do not ordinarily cause human disease and require minimal safety procedures and equipment. Examples of BSL-1 facilities would be a municipal water testing facility or a high school or community college teaching laboratory. *Bacillus subtilis* is an example of a BSL-1 microorganism. BSL-2 organisms, such as hepatitis B virus and salmonellae, are known to cause human disease but are not readily transmitted among hosts. Many bacteria recovered in a clinical laboratory setting are considered BSL-2. Class II biological safety cabinets are recommended for BSL-2 facilities.

TABLE 30-1 Examples of Categories A, B, and C Biothreat Agents

Category A Agents	Category B Agents	Category C Agents
Bacillus anthracis	*Brucella* spp.	Multiple drug–resistant *Mycobacterium tuberculosis*
Francisella tularensis	*Burkholderia mallei*	Hantavirus
Yersinia pestis	*Coxiella burnetii*	Yellow fever virus
Botulinum toxin	*Salmonella*	Tickborne hemorrhagic fever virus
Variola major	*Escherichia coli* O157:H7	
Hemorrhagic fever viruses	Eastern equine encephalitis virus	
	Staphylococcal enterotoxin B	
	Ricin	

BSL-3 organisms are typically indigenous or exotic agents that can be transmitted by the respiratory route and can produce serious disease. *Brucella melitensis* is an example of a BSL-3 agent. BSL-3 facilities typically have restricted access with a separate air ventilation system for containment. BSL-4 organisms can also be transmitted by the respiratory route, have a very high risk of serious disease, and no available treatment or vaccines. Examples of BSL-4 include Ebola and Congo-Crimean hemorrhagic fever viruses. BSL-4 facilities require even more strict precautions, including containment suits.

In 1999 academic infectious disease experts, national public health experts, Department of Health and Human Services agency representatives, civilian and military intelligence experts, and law enforcement officials met to comment on the threat potential of infectious agents to civilian populations. As a result of these meetings, agents were placed into one of three categories—A, B, or C—for initial public health preparedness efforts. The agents of bioterrorism are defined and categorized based on the impact an attack with that agent would have on the public health in this country. An abbreviated list can be found in Table 30-1. **Category A agents** (or biothreat level A) would have the greatest impact, whereas categories B and C would have less impact. Although *B. anthracis* is considered a BSL-2 in clinical laboratories, it is a category A agent in regard to a bioterror threat.

GENERAL CHARACTERISTICS OF BIOTERROR AGENTS

Because of the low cost and the lack of need for sophisticated equipment and supplies, bioterror agents cost less than conventional and other weapons, and cultivating bacteria does not require a lot of training or expertise. In addition small, mobile laboratories could be housed in large vans or semitrailers. In a covert attack, bioterrorists could produce large amounts of a biologic weapon in a small laboratory, release the agent, and move on before the attack was noticed.

Biologic weapons can enter the host via the respiratory tract, gastrointestinal tract, and also through the skin and mucous membranes. Dispensing bioterror agents in food or water may not be very efficient because dilution of the agents would occur. Even the highly toxic botulism toxin would be diluted to nontoxic levels in a large water supply. Also, usual water treatments such as chlorination, ozone treatment, and filtration would inactivate or remove many potential infectious agents. A potential risk is contamination of water near the end user (e.g., bottled water), which would likely involve a smaller volume of water.

The most efficient biologic weapons are probably those transmitted by aerosols; these agents would be expected to be more contagious than those dispersed by other deployment methods. A concern about aerosolized agents is person-to-person spread, which would enhance the effect of the attack. For example, person-to-person spread would be expected with smallpox virus and **pneumonic plague.** Agents dispersed as aerosols could be inactivated by extreme temperatures and ultraviolet (UV) light from the sun. Because bacterial spores, such as those of *B. anthracis,* are resistant to environmental stress (e.g., extreme temperatures, UV light, drying), spores are particularly attractive as bioterror agents. Other problems with aerosolized agents are that wind currents can carry the infectious particles far from the target site and sudden rainfall could cause the agent to fall to the ground. One of the greatest drawbacks to aerosolized weapons is producing particles small enough to enter the alveolar air sacs. The size limit is about 5 μm. Bacterial cells tend to clump, producing particles larger than 5 μm.

HISTORY OF CRIMINAL USE OF MICROBIAL AGENTS

Biocrime and *biothreat* are terms used to define situations in which a single person or group targets a specific individual or group. In the United States, agents of biocrime have been recently deployed. In 1984 the followers of Bhagwan Shree Rajneesh used *Salmonella* as a weapon to help influence election results in The Dalles, Oregon. By spraying liquid-based *Salmonella* culture into salad bars in restaurants, 750 persons developed culture-positive salmonellosis. Food- and water-borne pathogens, including *Salmonella,* are listed as category B biothreat agents.

Weaponized anthrax spores were used in Florida and New York in 2001. Anthrax-contaminated letters caused infection in 22 people, killing 5. Investigations recently attributed these attacks to an American scientist working at the United States Army Medical Research Institute of Infectious Disease (USAMRIID) in Fort Detrick, Maryland. Ricin, a toxin from castor beans, has been sent through the mail as well, and U.S. citizens have been arrested for producing ricin with the intent to use it as a weapon.

Previously, many of the bacteria and viruses associated with bioterror could be purchased easily through commercial laboratory suppliers. This availability led to possession of agents for potentially illegal purposes. In the 1990s, men were arrested in both Ohio and Nevada while carrying *Y. pestis* and anthrax spores in their car. Ironically, ordering and possessing these potential weapons did not necessarily constitute a crime. These cases identified gaps in the law and helped to define the need for stricter laws, such as the Public Health Security and Bioterrorism Preparedness and Response Act of 2002 and 42 CFR 73, Possession, Use and Transfer of Select Agents and Toxins; Final Rule (March 2005). As part of 42 CFR 73, rules were established for the possession, use, and transfer of select agents and toxins. The Centers for Disease Control and Prevention (CDC) and the U.S. Department of Agriculture developed a list of more than 80 select agents that potentially threaten public health and safety or animal and plant health. Any facility or individual possessing these agents must register them with either the CDC or the Animal and Plant Health Inspection Service.

Internationally, recent incidents highlight the availability and impact of bioweapon deployment. The cult Aum Shinrikyo successfully deployed sarin gas in the subways of Tokyo in 1995, killing 12 and injuring almost 5000 people; however, the Aum also had obtained and experimented with botulinum toxin, *B. anthracis, V. cholerae,* and *Coxiella burnetii* and had attempted to obtain Ebola virus from Zaire. From 1990 to 1995, the Aum tried several times to deploy botulinum toxin and anthrax spores, all unsuccessfully.

In the United States, it is illegal to threaten the release of biologic agents. In the late 1990's domestic hoaxes or threats to use biologic agents as weapons rose from 112 in 1998 to 187 in 1999 and then declined to 115 in 2000. Before the use of anthrax as a weapon in September 2001, there had been 67 threatened attacks. Hoaxes are assumed to be real until proven otherwise, thereby disrupting the affected area; specimen collection and testing during hoaxes occupy laboratory resources. Before 2001 the primary laboratories with capabilities to respond to agents of bioterror were the CDC in Atlanta, Georgia, and the USAMRIID in Fort Detrick, Maryland, and even capabilities at those laboratories to respond to large events were limited.

THE LABORATORY RESPONSE NETWORK

In an effort to increase responsiveness and to create a nation-wide ability to rapidly detect the covert or overt deployment of biologic weapons in the United States and its territories, the CDC, the Association of Public Health Laboratories, the Federal Bureau of Investigation (FBI), and USAMRIID established the **Laboratory Response Network (LRN)** in 1999; later that year, most states and territories were implementing training for the detection of biologic attacks using standardized LRN protocols. The goal of the LRN was to decentralize testing capabilities and to link state and local laboratories with advanced-capacity clinical, military, veterinary, agricultural, water, and food testing laboratories. There is also a chemical component of the LRN for chemical terror.

As defined by the LRN, community hospitals with microbiology capabilities are designated as sentinel (formerly level A) LRN laboratories. Sentinel laboratories must have a BSL-2 facility and utilize the laboratory protocols published on the CDC and American Society for Microbiology Web sites to

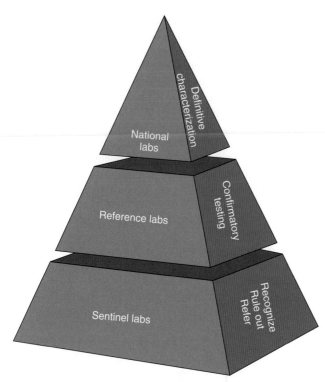

FIGURE 30-1 The structure of the Laboratory Response Network.

rule out the presence of biologic agents. Sentinel laboratory protocols are currently available for anthrax, avian influenza *Brucella,* botulinum toxin, *B. mallei* and *B. pseudomallei, C. burnetii,* plague, staphylococcal enterotoxin B, **tularemia,** and unknown viruses. A readiness plan guide is available to help laboratories develop their own readiness plan in case a bioterror event is encountered. When any of these agents cannot be ruled out, sentinel laboratories complete a chain of custody and refer the cultures to the nearest LRN Reference laboratory. The role of a sentinel laboratory is to rule out or refer suspicious isolates, not to identify. Because sentinel laboratories will refer isolates to a regional reference laboratory, laboratory scientists must be aware of the strict requirements for shipping and transporting infectious agents.

The LRN Reference laboratories have standardized confirmatory tests for several biothreat agents. Although the Reference laboratories do perform gene amplification and antigen detection, they rely heavily on culture identification and characterization when practical. LRN Reference laboratories are most often state public health laboratories and Department of Defense medical center laboratories. The LRN also includes national laboratories, which are the most technically capable laboratories. These laboratories can fulfill duties of the LRN Reference laboratories but also have the capabilities to perform complex forensic studies and definitive characterization of biothreat agents. The LRN National laboratories are the CDC, USAMRIID, and the Naval Medical Research Center. Both the CDC and USAMRIID have BSL-4 laboratories to handle the most dangerous agents (Figure 30-1). In the event of a bioterror event, clinical microbiologists would likely play a key role. Detection of a possible bioterror event requires active microbial surveillance programs; laboratory

scientists trained to recognize potential bioterror agents; and communication with clinicians, emergency response personnel, and infectious disease specialists. To help first responders, USAMRIID issued key indicators of a possible bioterrorism or biocrime event (Box 30-1).

AGENTS OF BIOTERROR

Bacillus anthracis

Bacillus anthracis is an aerobic gram-positive rod that produces endospores. Anthrax, the disease caused by *B. anthracis,* is primarily a disease of herbivores. Natural infections in humans usually occur as a result of interactions with animals or contaminated animal products. Evidence indicates that humans are somewhat resistant to anthrax infections, even when spores are inhaled. Anthrax infections in humans have been uncommon in this country for at least the past century. Most cases that were reported were cutaneous. A total of 224 cases of cutaneous anthrax were reported from 1944 until 1994 and only one case from 1992 to 1999. Until the anthrax attacks in 2001, the last reported case of **inhalation anthrax** was in 1978.

Because of the rarity of any form of human anthrax in the United States, especially inhalation anthrax, the diagnosis of inhalation anthrax in a 63-year-old man in Florida on October 4, 2001, attracted immediate national attention and action. The next month was historic, as letters with anthrax-containing powders had been sent to Florida; Washington, D.C.; and New York, resulting in 22 cases of anthrax: 11 cutaneous and 11 inhalation. Five of the patients with inhalation anthrax died. During the next 3 months, about 122,000 specimens were submitted to LRN laboratories for detection of anthrax and other bioterror agents. Civilian public health laboratories received and processed about 84,000 specimens, and the U.S. Army LRN National Laboratory and LRN Reference and Sentinel laboratories processed approximately 30,000 specimens. The vast majority of the specimens submitted for testing were environmental in nature, not clinical. Many specimens were submitted to trace the origin of the weaponized envelopes as they passed through various post offices. Recently, a senior scientist from USAMRIID who had been studying anthrax spores for many years was implicated by the FBI and the Department of Justice as the sole individual responsible for the attacks.

Clinical Manifestations

Once inside the host, *B. anthracis* spores undergo phagocytosis by macrophages. Spores can germinate into vegetative cells, which are capable of producing toxins. The virulence factors of *B. anthracis* include a glutamic acid capsule, which inhibits phagocytosis; lethal factor (LF); and edema factor (EF). For LF and EF to become biologically active toxins, they must first combine with *B. anthracis* protective antigen (PA).

Humans can present with three forms of anthrax: cutaneous, gastrointestinal, and inhalational. Worldwide, cutaneous anthrax is by far the most common form of the disease, accounting for about 95% of the cases. The disease occurs after spores are introduced into cuts or abrasions of human skin. After 1 to 5 days, a papule appears and then progresses to a 1- to 2-cm vesicle within the next 48 hours. The vesicle ruptures, resulting in a necrotic lesion that continues to grow into the characteristic black **eschar** (Figure 30-2). The lesion can be edematous, but the lesion itself is usually painless. The patient may or may not have systemic symptoms. The lesion usually heals without incident. Mortality is usually less than 1% with antimicrobial therapy but may be as high as 20% without treatment.

Gastrointestinal anthrax occurs when anthrax spores are introduced into the tissues of the gastrointestinal tract, often by eating meat containing anthrax spores. After an incubation period of 2 to 5 days, the patient experiences nausea and vomiting, which rapidly progress to bloody diarrhea, ascites, and often sepsis. Mortality of this form of anthrax is higher than that in cutaneous anthrax, with death resulting in about 50% of the patients.

Inhalation anthrax occurs when a patient inhales *B. anthracis;* it usually takes at least 8000 spores to initiate this form of the disease. Inhalation anthrax is the form of anthrax most likely to be seen in a bioterror event. Spore-containing particles 1 to 5 µm in size reach the alveoli of the lung. To weaponize *B. anthracis* spores, the spores cannot form aggregates larger than 5 µm. Macrophages ingest the spores, which are transported to the mediastinal lymph node. Spores germinate into vegetative cells, which then produce and release toxins. After an incubation period of 1 to 6 days, patients develop flulike symptoms with fever, malaise, and fatigue as vegetative *B. anthracis* invades the bloodstream from the lymph nodes. Respiratory symptoms become much more severe within the next few days as the patient experiences acute respiratory distress.

The differential diagnosis includes other causes, but the chest radiograph shows **mediastinitis** (Figure 30-3). Pneumonia is not usually supported by clinical findings. Data from the accidental spore release in Sverdlosk, Russia, in 1976 suggest a mortality rate of almost 100%; however, the mortality rate of patients with inhalation anthrax in the United States in 2001 was only 45% (5 of 11).

Specimen Collection and Preparation

The specimen of choice for cutaneous anthrax is vesicular fluid from fresh vesicles. Also, swabs can be used to collect material from under the edge of the crust of the eschar. The specimen of choice for patients with gastrointestinal anthrax is blood, particularly a few days after exposure. Although

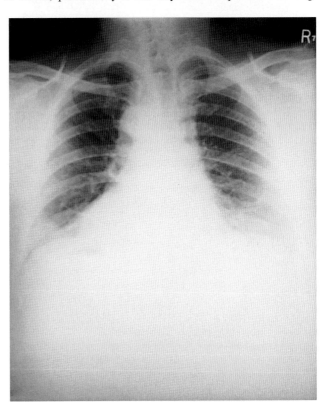

FIGURE 30-3 Chest radiograph of a patient who worked in a goat-hair processing mill. Note the widened mediastinum, often seen with inhalation anthrax. (Photograph by Arthur E. Keye, courtesy the Centers for Disease Control and Prevention.)

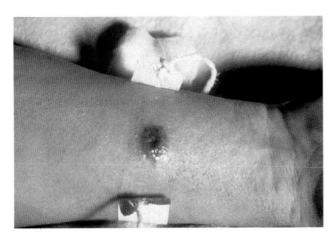

FIGURE 30-2 A cutaneous anthrax lesion on the right forearm. (Courtesy the Centers for Disease Control and Prevention.)

stool and rectal swabs can also be cultured, these specimens might not always yield positive results. The specimen of choice for patients with inhalation anthrax is also blood. Because inhalation anthrax usually does not result in pneumonia, and vegetative bacteria are not likely to be found in the lungs, the utility of sputa specimens is less than that of blood.

Direct Examination and Initial Culture

Smears from lesion fluid, eschars, blood, cerebrospinal fluid (CSF), or tissues may show large gram-positive bacilli. There may be evidence of a capsule around the cells. Spores most likely will not be evident in direct smears from clinical specimens, because spores form only in the presence of oxygen.

In aerobic culture, *B. anthracis* will yield large (2 to 5 mm) nonhemolytic colonies on 5% sheep blood agar (SBA). Colony

growth can be quite rapid: in as little as 8 hours. Mature colonies have a ground-glass appearance. The colony margins often have feathery projections coming from the margin, referred to as "Medusa-head" colonies (Figure 30-4). Colonies also have a tenacious consistency that when teased with a loop will stand up like an eggwhite (Figure 30-5). Cells are characteristically large gram-positive bacilli, possibly showing endospore formation (Figures 30-6 and 30-7). The spores are central or subterminal and do not cause the bacterial cell to swell.

Tests for Presumptive Identification

According to CDC protocols, a presumptive identification of *B. anthracis* can be made if an isolate has the following characteristics: aerobic growth; nonhemolytic colonies 2 to 5 mm in diameter; and catalase-positive, nonmotile, large gram-positive bacilli recovered from lesions, blood, CSF, or lymph nodes. Oval central to subterminal spores may be present.

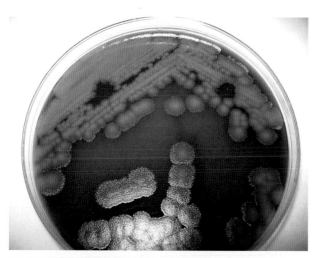

FIGURE 30-4 "Medusa-head" appearance of *Bacillus anthracis* nonhemolytic colonies with feathery projections from the edges at 24 hours. (Photograph by Edward F. Keen; courtesy Brooke Army Medical Center).

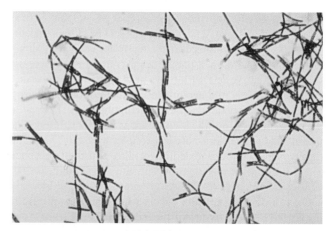

FIGURE 30-6 Gram stain of *Bacillus anthracis* from culture. (Courtesy the Centers for Disease Control and Prevention.)

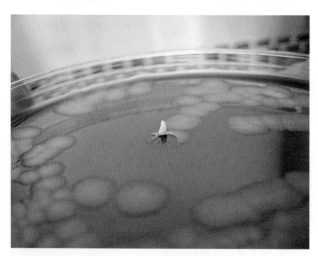

FIGURE 30-5 Tenacious consistency (stiff eggwhite appearance) of *Bacillus anthracis* colonies on sheep blood agar plate at 24 hours. (Photograph by Edward F. Keen; courtesy Brooke Army Medical Center).

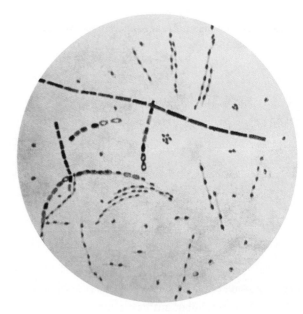

FIGURE 30-7 Spore stain of *Bacillus anthracis* culture. (Courtesy the Centers for Disease Control and Prevention.)

Some other bacilli, such as *B. cereus* var. *mycoides,* can also have this profile. Organisms with a presumptive identification of *B. anthracis* must be sent to an LRN Reference laboratory for confirmatory identification. The recovery of *B. anthracis* is a sentinel event in the United States.

Yersinia pestis

Throughout history, plague pandemics have demonstrated the efficacy of *Y. pestis* as a weapon against humankind. The first recorded pandemic of plague began in Egypt in AD 541 and lasted approximately 150 years. The pandemic may have reduced the population by as much as 60% throughout North Africa, Europe, and parts of Asia.

The second pandemic of plague started in Asia in 1330 and spread into Europe in 1347. The spread of plague into and throughout Europe was probably facilitated by the battle at Kaffa (at the site of the current city of Feodosiya, Ukraine) in 1346. Muslim Tartar soldiers laid siege on the walled city in an effort to defeat the Genoese Christians. The infection, commonly referred to as the **black death,** was decimating the Muslims, and in an effort to spread the disease to the Genoese in Kaffa, Tartar soldiers who had died of the black death were catapulted into the walled city. History tells us that the Genoese soldiers did start to contract the plague and ultimately evacuated the city, sailing back to Europe. However, this is really not a good example of biowarfare in that cold corpses do not transmit plague. In all likelihood, the disease was started as rats infested with fleas containing *Y. pestis* crawled into the walled city, spreading the infection via vectors. The Genoese carried infested rats on their ships and transplanted them to other ports throughout Europe, extending the spread of this disease. During the next 4 years, the plague killed as many as 20 to 30 million Europeans, with perhaps another 20 million victims over the next 50 years. Localized outbreaks and smaller epidemics occurred into the seventeenth century.

In 1894, Alexandre Yersin was the first person to describe the plague bacillus and to fulfill Koch's postulates linking this organism with **bubonic plague.** The major vector for the plague bacilli is the oriental rat flea, *Xenopsylla cheopis,* although many other fleas can transmit *Y. pestis.* More than 200 mammals can be involved in the transmission of the plague. *Rattus rattus,* the black rat, is the mammal most responsible for urban outbreaks of plague. In the United States, sylvatic plague still occurs in the desert Southwest. The reservoirs include deer mice, ground squirrels, prairie dogs, and other mammals. The most common vector in the United States is the flea, *Diamanus montanus.*

Clinical Manifestations

Yersinia pestis causes bubonic plague, septicemic plague, and pneumonic plague. These infections can occur as a result of being bitten by an infected flea, handling contaminated materials, or inhaling aerosolized plague bacteria. Natural infections rarely occur in the United States. Sixty-six cases of plague were reported in this country from 1996 to 2006, most of which occurred in the western part of the country, from New Mexico and Arizona north to Montana and Wyoming, although New Mexico accounted for almost 50% of the reported cases.

Bubonic plague, the most common form of disease, results from the bite of a flea and is characterized by fever, chills, headache, and malaise. The plague bacteria are transported to the local lymph nodes, most commonly the femoral, inguinal, or cervical. As the bacteria multiply, the lymph node becomes inflamed and painful, forming the characteristic *bubo* with evident erythema (Figure 30-8). **Buboes** are inflamed swollen lymph nodes that can be several centimeters in diameter. In some patients the lymph nodes are damaged, allowing hematogenous dissemination of the organism, causing secondary septicemic plague. This leads to disseminated intravascular coagulation (DIC) with petechiae and gangrene, often in the fingers and nose (Figure 30-9). These necrotic changes are the origin of the term *black death.*

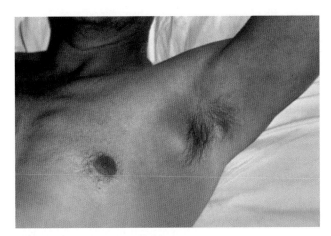

FIGURE 30-8 This patient has an axillary bubo and edema as a result of bubonic plague. (Photograph by Margaret Parsons and Dr. Karl F. Meyer; courtesy the Centers for Disease Control and Prevention.)

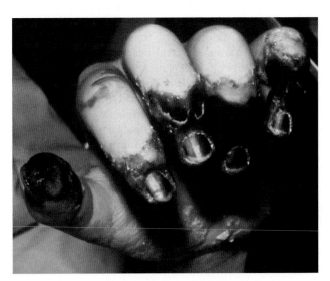

FIGURE 30-9 The patient presented with symptoms of plague that included gangrene of the right hand. (Photograph by Dr. Jack Pollard; courtesy the Centers for Disease Control and Prevention.)

Patients can also develop primary septicemic plague without the formation of buboes after being bitten by a plague-infected flea. Patients with primary septicemic plague have symptoms similar to those with bubonic plague, with the exception of the bubo. Rarely the bloodstream can carry the plague organisms to the lungs and cause secondary pneumonic plague, resulting in pneumonia, dyspnea, and hemoptysis. In the event of an attack with weaponized *Y. pestis*, it is likely that most patients would develop primary pneumonic plague as a result of inhaling aerosolized plague bacteria. Person-to-person transmission, with the potential of high mortality rates, could be expected in such an occurrence.

Specimen Collection and Preparation

Like anthrax, plague can manifest in numerous ways. If the patient has respiratory symptoms, lower respiratory secretions, such as sputum, bronchial wash, or transtracheal aspirate, are the specimens of choice. Patients who appear septic and have a fever should have blood drawn for cultures. It is recommended that if *Y. pestis* infection is suspected, one set of blood cultures be held at room temperature because this organism grows faster at 22° to 28° C.

The specimens of choice for patients with buboes would be either aspirated lesion fluid from the bubo or a biopsy of the lesion. Aspirates may be fairly nonproductive for culture purposes, so a saline wash injected into the bubo and then withdrawn might help recovery of the organism. Care must be taken to avoid aerosol generation to minimize risk of transmission during specimen collection.

Direct Examination and Initial Culture

Gram-stained preparations of respiratory secretions, aspirates, and tissues infected with *Y. pestis* will reveal plump, gram-negative rods, approximately 1 to 2 by 0.5 µm. They may appear as single cells or in short chains; longer chains can form in liquid media. This organism often shows bipolar staining characteristics; that is, the ends are darker than the middle of the cell, resulting in what is described as a "safety-pin" appearance (Figure 30-10). This appearance is not specific for *Y. pestis*, and the Gram stain may not always be the best choice of stains to reveal the bipolar nature. Smears stained with Wright stain may show more of the bipolar staining trait. Some literature describes staining with the Wayson stain, but this is not a common clinical laboratory stain.

Colonies of *Y. pestis* on SBA plates may grow slowly, and cultures may have to be held for as long as 48 hours for good colony growth. Colonies are nonhemolytic and can have a "fried egg" appearance (Figure 30-11). If specimens are plated into either a protein-based or thioglycolate broth, the organism may appear similar to stalagmites, connected to the tube and growing into the broth. As these formations break, cotton-like fragments accumulate at the bottom of the tube. Because the organism is fairly biochemically inert, it is worth noting that commercial identification systems might not correctly identify the isolate as *Y. pestis*.

Tests for Presumptive Identification

The LRN Sentinel protocols define a suspicious *Y. pestis* isolate as a bipolar staining, gram-negative rod that forms

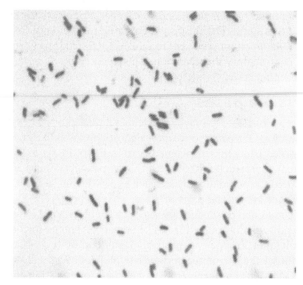

FIGURE 30-10 Gram stain of *Yersinia pestis*. Note the lighter staining intensity in the central portions of some cells, resulting in the "safety-pin" appearance. (Courtesy the Centers for Disease Control and Prevention.)

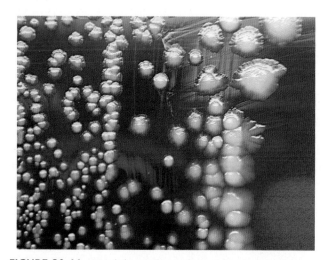

FIGURE 30-11 *Yersinia pestis* on sheep blood agar, 72 hours. Colonies are gray-white to slightly yellow opaque, raised, irregular "fried egg" morphology; alternatively, colonies may have a "hammered copper" shiny surface. (Photograph by Larry Stauffer, Oregon State Public Health Laboratory; courtesy the Centers for Disease Control and Prevention, Public Health Image Library, image 1921, phil.cdcgov/phil.).

very small colonies after 24 hours' incubation at 37° C, although colonies grown at room temperature can be larger. On media selective for gram-negative bacilli, such as MacConkey (MAC) agar, the organism will grow as small nonlactose fermenting colonies. *Y. pestis* is also positive for catalase but negative for oxidase and urease. Bacteria isolated from blood, respiratory specimens, or lesion aspirates with these characteristics should be submitted to an LRN Reference laboratory for definitive identification.

Francisella tularensis

Tularemia, like anthrax and plague, is a zoonotic disease. *Francisella tularensis* was first isolated and described in 1911, when it was found to be the cause of an outbreak in ground squirrels in Tulare County, California. Natural infections of *F. tularensis* do occur. From 2003 to 2007, 649 cases were in the United States; more than a third were in Arkansas and Missouri. Tularemia was not a national reportable disease between 1995 and 1999.

Infections in humans are almost always by accidental contact with the organism, which is found in water, soil, plants, and mammals. Hunters can get the infection after contact with infected carcasses and animals. Many infections are also transmitted by vectors including ticks, mosquitoes, and flies. In light of the numerous ways this infection can be transmitted, it has numerous nicknames to match, including deer-fly fever, rabbit fever, Ohara disease, market-men's disease, and water-trapper's disease. The most common reservoirs in the United States are several species of ticks, as well as numerous other arthropods. The most common mammal associated with tularemia in the United States is the rabbit.

Japan, the former Soviet Union, and the United States all recognize *F. tularensis* as a potential bioweapon. The infectious dose for the organism in humans is as low as 10 bacteria. The potential of this organism as a weapon was demonstrated during natural outbreaks of tularemia in Europe and in the Soviet Union during the 1930s and 1940s. Natural infections resulting from aerosolized *F. tularensis* have occurred in the past, often from handling infected vegetation. This high degree of infectivity increased interest in it as a potential biologic weapon. The World Health Organization (WHO) estimates that 50 kg of organism could infect 125,000 people in a city of five million people and could cause up to 19,000 deaths.

Clinical Manifestations

Depending on the source and route of infection, tularemia can have a number of different clinical manifestations. The most common is ulceroglandular tularemia, which results from the inoculation of the organism into the dermis of the patient (Figure 30-12). Inoculation occurs either via the bite of a tularemia-infested insect or from handling infectious materials. The latter is common among outdoor sportsmen. Ulceroglandular tularemia has an incubation period of about 3 to 10 days, after which patients become febrile with chills, headaches, cough, and chest pain. Patients develop lesions at the site of entry, and these lesions can persist for weeks to months. Organisms can be transported to the lymph nodes, and bubonic plague–like buboes can form. Hematogenous dissemination can occur, resulting in multiple-organ seeding. Even without antimicrobial therapy, patients who progress to this point rarely die of this form of the disease. Symptoms do resolve, but resolution may occur over a period of months as the patient experiences malaise and weight loss. Patients with all these symptoms, with the exception of the lesion, have the glandular form of the disease.

Less commonly patients develop oculoglandular, oropharyngeal, gastrointestinal (ingesting contaminated materials),

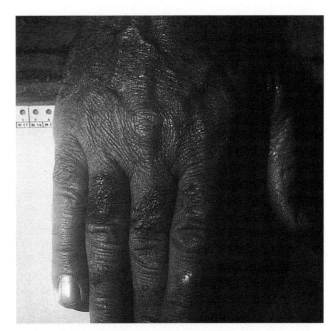

FIGURE 30-12 Cutaneous lesions of tularemia on the hand of a Vermont muskrat hunter. (Photograph by Roger Feldman; courtesy the Centers for Disease Control and Prevention.)

or inhalational disease. In the event of inhaling weaponized *F. tularensis,* patients would most likely develop pneumonic or inhalational tularemia. Patients would have fever and symptoms of a lower respiratory tract infection, similar to an influenza-like illness, which would progress to dyspnea, hemoptysis, sepsis, and shock. Chest radiographs will reveal a widened mediastinum, similar to that seen with inhalation anthrax. Natural cases of inhalational tularemia do occur, most commonly in rural areas. Mortality rates of untreated inhalational tularemia can be 30% to 60%. In the United States tularemia has an overall mortality of about 2%.

Direct Examination and Initial Culture

Although tularemia can manifest as a benign lesion at the site of entry, this form of tularemia usually merits medical care. The most usual clinical presentation involves ulceroglandular disease, during which the organism is transported to the local lymph nodes and disseminated throughout the bloodstream. Blood cultures are collected from patients with fever. If lesions are present, biopsies or cultures from the leading margin of the lesion can be collected and submitted for culture and direct examination. If clinical presentation or patient history is consistent with tularemia, the laboratory must be notified when specimens are submitted. *F. tularensis* is a BSL-3 isolate, and laboratory transmission of this organism can, and does, occur readily.

Tests for Presumptive Identification

Tiny pleomorphic gram-negative coccobacilli will be seen on Gram staining of positive blood culture bottles (Figure 30-13). *Francisella* is cysteine dependent and not easily isolated by culture. The organism will grow well on chocolate

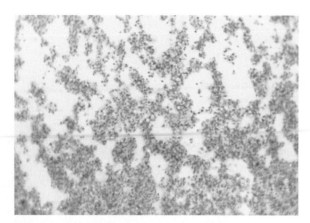

FIGURE 30-13 A microphotograph of *Francisella tularensis*. (Photograph by P.B. Smith; courtesy the Centers for Disease Control and Prevention.)

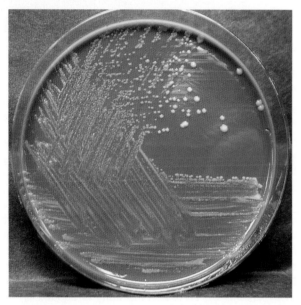

FIGURE 30-14 Colonies of *Francisella tularensis* growing on chocolate agar. (Photograph by Larry Stauffer, Oregon Public Health Laboratory; courtesy the Centers for Disease Control and Prevention.)

(CHOC) agar (Figure 30-14), Thayer-Martin medium, cysteine heart agar, and buffered charcoal yeast-extract agar. These media are supplemented with cysteine. *F. tularensis* does not grow rapidly, and colonies may not be visible on solid media until 36 to 48 hours. *F. tularensis* will not grow at all on MAC.

Pleomorphic, poorly staining, gram-negative coccobacilli from blood cultures that do not grow well, if at all, on SBA should lead the laboratory scientist to consider *F. tularensis*. As a safety precaution, laboratory procedures must be done inside a biological safety cabinet until *F. tularensis* has been ruled out. Catalase and β-lactamase tests are positive for *F. tularensis*, whereas requirements for X and V factors, urease, and oxidase are negative. Isolates with these reactions are presumptively identified as *F. tularensis* and must be sent to an LRN Reference laboratory for confirmation.

Brucella Species

The brucellae are small, gram-negative pleomorphic aerobic coccobacilli that can cause disease in a variety of animals, including humans. The species that are pathogenic to humans (followed by their normal hosts) include *Brucella melitensis* (sheep and goats), *B. suis* (swine), and *B. abortus* (cattle). Additional species are not associated with human disease: *B. ovis* (sheep), *B. neotomae* (desert wood rat), and *B. canis* (dogs). Synonyms for brucellosis include Malta fever, undulant fever, Mediterranean fever, Gibraltar fever, goat fever, Bang disease, and Cyprus fever, among others.

Brucellosis is endemic to many parts of the world, but its incidence has declined in the United States, where *B. abortus* has almost been eliminated from cattle, reducing the risk for occupational exposure. Food-borne transmission of *B. abortus* and *B. melitensis* is still a risk, primarily with unpasteurized milk products. Laboratory transmission of the organism does occur, and laboratorians are at risk unless BSL-3 containment is used when working with known cultures of brucellae.

Clinical Manifestations

Brucellosis can be transmitted through breaks in the skin, ingestion of contaminated food products, or inhalation. Hematogenous dissemination results in seeding of multiple organs, including the lung, liver, spleen, central nervous system (CNS), and bone marrow. The incubation period varies, generally from 5 to 35 days. The symptoms of brucellosis reflect the dissemination and infected sites. Symptoms may include malaise, night sweats, relapsing fever, chills, and myalgia. Brucellosis can persist for months, although patients ultimately recover even in the absence of antimicrobial therapy; however, even with treatment, relapse can occur.

Because many infections with the brucellae have historically occurred via the respiratory tract and occupational exposure, it has potential as an aerosolized weapon. The long incubation period and the nonspecific clinical findings might delay any association as a deployed weapon, features of a more affective bioterror weapon. The United States did study the use of *B. suis* as a biologic weapon more than 60 years ago. Before dismantling of the biologic weapons program in this country in 1972, the United States had weaponized the organism and tested the efficacy of the weapon in bombs. The brucellae have been weaponized, so their use in the future cannot be removed from all consideration.

Specimen Collection and Preparation

If a patient is suspected of having brucellosis, all work with specimens and cultures should be done in a biological safety cabinet while wearing appropriate personal protective equipment. Appropriate specimens to detect *Brucella* spp. include blood, bone marrow, tissues and fluids from affected organs, and abscess material. Fluids, tissues, and abscess material can be examined by direct Gram stain. If present, *Brucella* spp. will appear as tiny gram-negative coccobacilli (Figure 30-15). Because *Brucella* can grow more slowly than many other clinical isolates, it is prudent to hold all inoculated culture media as long as 7 days in a carbon dioxide

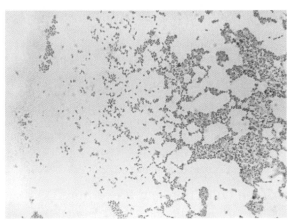

FIGURE 30-15 Gram stain of *Brucella melitensis*. (Courtesy the Centers for Disease Control and Prevention.)

(CO_2) incubator and to retain blood culture bottles for up to 10 days.

Tests for Presumptive Identification

Brucella spp. grow aerobically on SBA and CHOC within 48 to 72 hours. Only about 50% of the strains will grow on MAC, although there might be some breakthrough growth on these plates if held for 7 days. *Brucella* spp. colonies are small, circular, smooth, convex, nonpigmented, and nonhemolytic. On Gram stain, brucellae reveal tiny gram-negative coccobacilli. Results for a presumptive identification of *Brucella* spp. include the culture characteristics mentioned previously for an organism isolated from an appropriate specimen, along with catalase, oxidase, nitrate reduction, urease positivity, and lack of motility. The state public health laboratory must be notified of a presumptive identification of *Brucella,* and the specimen must be referred to them for confirmatory identification.

Burkholderia Species

The genus *Burkholderia* contains two species considered potential agents of bioterrorism: *B. mallei* and *B. pseudomallei*. *B. mallei* causes **glanders,** and *B. pseudomallei* is the causative agent of **melioidosis.**

Clinical Manifestations

Burkholderia mallei is an environmental isolate found in soil and water. The organism typically infects equids (horses, mules, and donkeys). Although the disease is endemic in livestock in Africa, Asia, the Middle East, and Central and South America, it is rare in the United States and Western Europe as a result of a campaign to eradicate seropositive animals. Infection in humans is usually initiated by direct contact with infected animals, and it is an occupational hazard for veterinarians and others working around animals. Although such cases are not well documented, the disease can be transmitted human to human. Two cases may have involved transmission via sexual and direct contact.

The incubation period varies, ranging from 1 day to 2 weeks. Disease in humans depends on the route of transmission. Symptoms of infection include fever, myalgia, headache,

and chest pain. Infection can result in localized cutaneous lesions, septicemia, and pneumonia. Bloodstream infections are often fatal. Although a human laboratory-acquired infection with *B. mallei* was documented in Maryland in 2000, no naturally acquired cases of human infection with *B. mallei* have been recorded in this country since 1945.

B. mallei was used by German agents during World War I as they tried to infect horses and mules in Allied countries. The livestock were due to be shipped to the European war front, where they were used as primary means of transportation. *B. mallei* is considered a potential agent of bioterror partly because of the apparently low dose required for infection. Melioidosis is similar to glanders, but it is found in different parts of the world. *B. pseudomallei* is endemic to Southeast Asia, the South Pacific, Africa, India, and the Middle East. Although not as common, the organism can also be isolated from patients in Mexico, Panama, Peru, and Haiti. The organism has also been recovered from human patients in Hawaii and Georgia. As many as five cases occur in the United States each year and are primarily travel related. This organism is also found commonly in soil and water.

Transmission is usually related to animal or human contact with soil and water, direct contact with infected animals, or inhalation. Rare documented cases of human-to-human transmission, primarily through blood and body fluids, have been reported. Clinical infection is similar to human cases of glanders. If the patient is infected through direct contact and entry through broken skin or mucous membranes, the clinical presentation is a localized nodule. Bloodstream dissemination can occur, resulting in acute sepsis; this occurs primarily in patients with underlying disease. Bloodstream dissemination of the organism can also result in chronic melioidosis, with lesions forming at multiple internal organs. If the organism was obtained by inhalation, the clinical presentation can vary from mild bronchitis to severe lower respiratory infections.

Specimen Collection and Preparation

Because laboratory transmission is a risk with these organisms, physicians suspecting infections with *B. mallei* and *B. pseudomallei* should notify the clinical microbiologists. Specimens appropriate for submission to detect either of these isolates are blood, bone marrow, sputum, bronchial alveolar lavage, abscess material, urine, and serum.

Direct Examination and Initial Culture

Direct Gram stain examination of aspirates and respiratory secretions will reveal gram-negative coccobacilli for *B. mallei* and small gram-negative bacilli, if positive for *B. pseudomallei*. These organisms will also be seen on direct examination of positive blood cultures from these patients.

Specimens are incubated at 35° C in 5% CO_2. If *B. mallei* or *B. pseudomallei* is suspected, cultures need to be incubated for a period of up to 5 days. *B. mallei* grows as a small, circular, butyrous colony after 24 to 48 hours' incubation on SBA. If held longer, the colonies will gradually convert to a dry, wrinkly appearance, resembling those of *Pseudomonas stutzeri*. *B. mallei* and *B. pseudomallei* typically grow on MAC. *B. pseudomallei* colonies are very similar to the colonies described already for *B. mallei*. *B. pseudomallei* may produce a smell similar to that of soil; however, smelling bacterial colonies with the plate open is hazardous and should never be done.

Tests for Presumptive Identification

Gram-negative coccobacilli or small gram-negative bacilli with poor growth at 24 hours, forming larger nonpigmented gray colonies at 48 hours that are indole negative, nonmotile, catalase positive, and resistant to polymyxin B discs or colistin discs are presumptively identified as *B. mallei* and must be submitted to the state public health laboratory or an LRN Reference laboratory. Gram-negative coccobacilli or small gram-negative bacilli with poor growth at 24 hours, forming larger nonpigmented gray colonies at 48 hours, that begin to wrinkle after 48 hours, grow on MAC, are oxidase positive and indole negative, and are resistant to polymyxin B or colistin discs cannot be ruled out as a *B. pseudomallei*. An isolate with these characteristics should be referred to an LRN Reference laboratory for identification. The Analytical Profile Index (API; bioMérieux, Hazelwood, Mo.) 20E, 20NE, and Vitek 1 (bioMérieux) are reliable in the identification of *B. pseudomallei*. Identification of this isolate by these systems should also be followed by referral to the closest LRN Reference laboratory.

Coxiella burnetii

Coxiella burnetii is a gram-negative coccobacillus that is an obligate intracellular pathogen. The microorganism has a complex developmental cycle. The tiny vegetative form of the bacterium transforms into a smaller spore-like body, called the *small-cell variant,* which has a spore-like resistance, allowing the organism to survive in the environment for longer than a month. The small-cell variant is the infective stage. Infection starts when a host cell, likely a macrophage, ingests the small-cell variant. The intracellular environment of the macrophage allows development of the vegetative cell, which is referred to as the *large-cell variant.*

Clinical Manifestations

Coxiella burnetii is the causative agent for the oddly named **Q fever.** The name of the disease was derived after an outbreak among slaughterhouse workers in Australia in 1935. The disease was called *query fever* because no cause was found. There are many natural reservoirs for *C. burnetii* including cattle, sheep, goats, dogs, cats, deer, fowl, and humans. The organism causes asymptomatic infection in most animals. Humans at risk for contracting Q fever are those with an occupational exposure, such as veterinarians and others who work closely with animals. Animals excrete the organism in urine, milk, and feces. The tissues and fluids expelled during birth can also be very infective. The organism can be transmitted by direct contact, ingestion, or inhalation, the last of which is the most common route of transmission to humans.

Approximately half of the infections in humans are symptomatic. Patients with acute Q fever develop an influenza-like illness with prolonged fever, headaches, cough, myalgia, and arthralgia. Some patients with acute Q fever develop pneumonia or hepatitis. The mortality rate of acute Q fever is about 2%. Some patients, such as those with heart valve damage or cancer, may develop the chronic form of the disease anywhere from 1 to 20 years after acute infection. The mortality rate of chronic Q fever can be as high as 65%. Several characteristics make *C. burnetii* a potentially attractive biologic weapon. It is resistant to environmental factors and extraordinarily infectious, with an infectious dose as low as one organism. It has a long incubation period, as long as 2 to 3 weeks, and the clinical course of the disease can be prolonged. In addition, it is hard to distinguish Q fever from more common causes of influenza-like illness.

Specimen Collection and Preparation

The laboratory should be notified if a physician suspects Q fever in a patient. Appropriate specimens include serum, blood, tissue, and body fluids. Because of the potentially high infectivity associated with specimens from patients with Q fever, most laboratories should send patient specimens to a state public health laboratory.

Direct Examination and Initial Culture

Because *C. burnetii* is an obligate intracellular parasite, it will not grow on any plated media. However, if laboratories process specimens for viral culture, *C. burnetii* may grow in the cell monolayers, thus presenting a potential hazard to unsuspecting laboratorians handling the cell monolayer culture fluids. In cultured monolayers, *C. burnetii* will result in cytoplasmic inclusions.

Infection can be diagnosed by serologic testing. Antibodies to phase I and phase II antigens can be measured. Patients with acute Q fever typically produce higher titers to phase II antigens, whereas patients with chronic Q fever have higher levels of anti-phase I antibodies. Polymerase chain reaction amplification assays have been developed, but are not yet approved for clinical use.

Variola Virus

Variola virus is the causative agent of smallpox. The virus belongs to the family Poxviridae, genus *Orthopoxvirus*. These brick-shaped, double-stranded DNA viruses are among the largest of all viruses, measuring approximately 200 nm in diameter.

Clinical Manifestations

Smallpox was a commonly occurring disease throughout history. The two major forms of the disease were **variola major** and **variola minor.** Until the late 1800s, variola major predominated. The mortality rate of variola major was about 30% in unvaccinated patients but only about 3% in vaccinated patients. Vaccinated patients can sometimes develop modified smallpox, which is not a serious infection. Variola minor was first described in the late nineteenth century in Africa and the United States. This form of smallpox spread throughout North America and eventually reached Europe. Although antigenically indistinguishable, variola minor caused a much less severe disease than variola major, having a mortality rate of about 1%.

Smallpox is normally transmitted through respiratory droplets or by direct contact. Fomite transmission also may have occurred. The dose required to initiate infection is quite low. Initially the virus replicates within cells of the oropharynx or respiratory mucosa. Later the virus spreads to the regional lymph nodes and multiplies. The patient undergoes a transient asymptomatic viremia resulting in the hematogenous dissemination of the virus. About 8 to 10 days after exposure, the patient develops fever and malaise, presenting with an influenza-like syndrome. Variola virions are present in white blood cells, which are transported to small blood vessels under the dermis and oral mucosa. Patients may then develop oral lesions; at this point, the patients are infectious via oral droplets.

The patient also develops a light macular rash, starting on the head and arms and then spreading to the trunk and legs. The macular rash then starts a progression to a vesicular rash after 1 to 2 days. One of the most characteristic signs of smallpox, differentiating it from other viral fever and rashes such as chicken pox, is the synchronous progression of the lesions; all lesions have nearly the same appearance. Also, lesions are more heavily concentrated on the extremities, as the virus prefers cooler body temperatures found in these locations. Another significant feature of smallpox infection is that the palms and soles are not spared as they are with varicella. Vesicles continue to progress into pustules (Figure 30-16). The pustules are unique in that they penetrate deeply into the tissue of the patient and are extremely turgid. It is at this stage, approximately 1 week after the start of the rash, when the patient is most likely to die. After about day 14 of rash, the pustules start to scab and heal, leaving significant scarring. The scab material is still highly infectious. The surviving patient will likely be resistant to future infections by

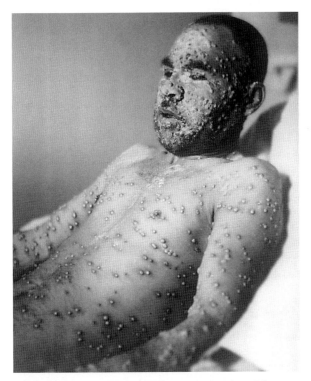

FIGURE 30-16 Smallpox pustules on an Iranian citizen. (Photograph by Dr. Don Millar; courtesy the Centers for Disease Control and Prevention.)

the virus. Variola minor disease is characterized by a less severe disease with a less dense rash.

Edward Jenner showed in 1796 that inoculation with the benign cowpox virus conferred resistance to smallpox. During the nineteenth century, vaccination programs began using **vaccinia** virus instead of cowpox. In 1967 the WHO began a smallpox eradication program based on detection and vaccination, which ultimately saw the end to smallpox infections. The last case of smallpox in the United States was in 1949, and the last documented case of natural smallpox on earth was in Somalia in 1977. The world was declared smallpox free in 1980. All known stocks of variola were destroyed except for two. One of the stocks remains at the CDC, and the second is maintained at the Institute of Virus Preparations in Moscow. It is possible that other undocumented stocks of smallpox virus are maintained by other countries. After the *B. anthracis* bioterror attack in the United States in 2001, several countries began stockpiling smallpox vaccine. In the United States, about 95 million doses of calf lymph vaccine prepared in 1978 by Wyeth (Madison, N.J.) and Aventis Pasteur (Lyon Cedex, France) are available. In addition, 200 million doses of vaccine produced in Vero cells by Acambis (Cambridge, Mass.) and Baxter (Deerfield, Ill.) were prepared.

History of Variola Virus as a Bioterror Agent

Variola virus has been used in warfare and terror several times throughout history. Sir Jeffrey Amherst, the commander of British troops in North America during the French and Indian War, wrote a letter to Colonel Henry Bouquet, suggesting the use of smallpox-contaminated materials to kill Native Americans sympathetic to the French. In 1763 Captain Simon Ecuyer, stationed at Fort Pitt, Pennsylvania, collected blankets and a handkerchief used by a soldier at Fort Pitt who had recently died of smallpox. These contaminated items were presented to the Delaware Native American tribe. An outbreak of smallpox did occur in the Native Americans, and the British were able to claim a military victory against a French military post, possibly as a result of the Native American deaths. It might be a stretch, however, to claim that the blankets led to the smallpox outbreak. The infections may very well have been transmitted through respiratory transmission as opposed to the contaminated blankets.

During the American Revolution, the British used smallpox against the Continental Army. Troops protected themselves against smallpox using variolation, the process of inoculating themselves with smallpox lesion fluid. This would often initiate a mild, localized infection that resulted in immunity. British troops forced variolation on citizens of Boston and Quebec, hoping the citizens would then become ill and spread the infection to the Continental Army. The strategy failed in Boston. However, Continental troops in Quebec did have an outbreak of smallpox as a result of the action, hastening a retreat of Continental forces from the region. The Japanese experimented with weaponization of smallpox during World War II as a part of operations at Unit 731 in Mongolia. Ken Alibek, a U.S. Defense Contractor and formerly a high-ranking officer in the Soviet bioweapon efforts, reported that the Soviets had extensive offensive capabilities with variola.

TABLE 30-2 Classification of Patients for Risk for Smallpox

Risk Level for Smallpox	Presentation	Minor and Major Criteria
Low	No fever prodrome, *or* Febrile prodrome and less than four of the minor criteria	Minor: Centrifugal rash; rash first in oral cavity, face, or forearms; lesions on palms and soles; patient appears toxic; slow evolution of rash
Moderate	Fever prodrome and one other major criterion *or* Febrile prodrome and more than four of the minor criteria	
High	Febrile prodrome *and* classic smallpox lesion *and* synchronous rash progression	Major: Febrile prodrome; classic smallpox lesions; synchronous rash progression

Because the technology does exist, and this virus was a component of an aggressive biowarfare program, it is considered a potential agent of bioterror.

Diagnosis of Smallpox

Detection and identification of smallpox virus are based on the patient's signs and symptoms as defined by the CDC: "Acute, Generalized Vesicular or Pustular Rash Protocol." Following this algorithm, patients seen by medical staff can be classified as being at low, moderate, or high risk for smallpox (Table 30-2). Specimens are collected from high-risk patients and are transmitted to either the CDC for laboratory confirmation or another LRN laboratory with special testing for variola virus identification. Positive variola virus test results by LRN laboratories are considered presumptive until confirmed by the CDC.

Viral Hemorrhagic Fevers

The hemorrhagic fever viruses include, but are not limited to, Ebola and Marburg viruses (family Filoviridae); Lassa fever virus (family Arenaviridae); Crimean-Congo hemorrhagic fever virus, Rift Valley fever virus, and several hantaviruses (family Bunyaviridae); and dengue, yellow fever, and Omsk hemorrhagic fever viruses (family Flaviviridae). All these viruses are small (40 to 130 nm), single-stranded RNA viruses. Generally these viruses persist in nature in arthropod vectors or animals, many in Africa. Not all reservoirs of these viruses have been discovered. In many cases human-to-human transmission occurs in nature. Exceptions are Rift Valley fever virus and the members of the Flaviviridae. As a group, these viruses tend to be relatively stable and can be very infectious if inhaled as an aerosol. Therefore they are considered a biothreat level A.

The viruses with the greatest name recognition of this group are likely to be the filoviruses: Marburg and Ebola. The first description of Marburg hemorrhagic fever was in 1967. Ebola virus was first recognized when epidemics occurred in both Sudan and the Democratic Republic of the Congo (formerly Zaire) in 1976. The latter epidemic resulted in 318 cases and 280 deaths; the former had 284 cases and 117 deaths. Since the first outbreak through January 2008, about 2200 cases have been reported with an overall fatality rate of 67%. The natural reservoirs of these viruses have not been determined. Contact with nonhuman primates appears instrumental in Ebola outbreaks, but the primates are not the natural reservoir. Some evidence points to a role for bats in the persistence of Ebola in the environment. Airborne or droplet transmission is not considered a common natural source of transmission with the filoviruses. Generally, effective use of personal protective equipment and contact precautions stops the transmission chain.

Although it was not described until 1969, Lassa fever is now endemic in West Africa. Seropositivity in various West African countries is as high as 50% in some groups. Lassa fever is commonly transmitted through contact with or ingestion of rats that harbor the virus. Some of the arenaviruses, including Lassa fever virus, can be found in semen and urine several months after infection, and transmission to spouses has been described in some of the arenaviruses, although transmission rates via sexual intercourse have not been clearly defined.

Clinical Manifestations

Clinical manifestations of these infections vary, depending on several factors. The incubation period for most of these infections is 2 to 3 weeks, after which the patient may experience fever, rash, myalgia and arthralgia, nausea, conjunctivitis, diarrhea, and CNS symptoms. Not all the viruses in this group cause hemorrhagic fevers as a common manifestation. Infections may include a varying degree of bleeding disorders, ranging from DIC, petechiae, and hemorrhage of the mucous membranes to blood in urine and vomitus.

Because of the lack of clinical experience with these infections, diagnosis as a result of a criminal release might not readily occur. Generally patients infected with filoviruses would be febrile and have a maculopapular rash, bleeding, and DIC. Patients with Lassa fever may exhibit a wider range of symptoms including fever, abdominal pain, and upper respiratory symptoms progressing to severe swelling in the head and neck area. Bleeding may not occur as commonly as in patients with filovirus infection.

Medical intervention for these infections varies. The antiviral compound ribavirin can be administered to patients with Lassa fever and other arenaviruses and Rift Valley fever. Care for patients with Ebola fever, Marburg fever, yellow fever, and Omsk hemorrhagic fever is generally supportive. Highest mortality rates are seen in the filovirus infections, as high as 90% with Ebola fever and as high as 70% in Marburg fever patients. Mortality rates for most other viral hemorrhagic fevers are less than 20%.

Specimen Collection and Preparation

Specimens should not be collected or processed from patients with suspected viral hemorrhagic fever until after consultation with state health officials. Specimens appropriate for the diagnosis of patients with symptoms compatible with viral hemorrhagic fever include serum, heparinized plasma, whole blood, respiratory aspirates, tissue, and urine.

Clostridium botulinum Toxin

Clinical Manifestations

Botulinum toxin (often referred to as *botox*) is a neurotoxin primarily produced by *Clostridium botulinum*, although other clostridia, including *C. butyricum* and *C. baratii,* can also produce the toxin. Seven different serotypes of toxin, designated A through G, have been identified. The serotypes implicated in human disease are A, B, and E, and rarely F.

C. botulinum spores can be recovered from soil specimens throughout the world. Although rare in the United States, naturally occurring botulism cases do occur. Approximately 150 cases of botulism are reported annually in the United States, with over half the cases occurring in California. Botulism can occur either by ingestion or by production of toxin by *C. botulinum* in either wounds or gut tissue. Food-borne botulism is associated with a variety of foods including potatoes, corn, beans, carrots, yogurt, cream cheese, and others. Most food-borne cases involve ingestion of preformed toxin, referred to as an intoxication.

The incubation period and symptoms vary, depending on the dose ingested. The incubation period varies from 2 hours to 8 days after ingestion. Because this is an intoxication and not an infection, fever is likely to be absent. Patients often develop trouble speaking, swallowing, and seeing. These effects are the result of a descending flaccid paralysis caused by the toxin. Paralysis of the respiratory muscles can result in death. Medical intervention, including mechanical ventilation or intubation, can reduce the rate of mortality to less than 15%. Respiratory support may be required for 2 to 8 weeks, although in some severe cases, support is needed for as long as 7 months. Other medical interventions include use of antitoxin and toxoid vaccine. Antitoxin is most beneficial when used before symptoms appear.

Botulinum toxin is the most lethal of all biologic compounds known. Theoretically, based on its lethal dose, 8 ounces would be enough to kill every human on earth. In reality, though, that degree of lethality is difficult to achieve. It might take as much as 8 kg of toxin to kill 50% of the people within a 100-km^2 area. Weaponizing the toxin entails producing an aerosol with particles between 1 and 5 μm in diameter to allow access to the lower respiratory tract and deploying the weapon in such a way that heat, acid, and UV light do not degrade the activity of the toxin. Wound-associated cases are not likely to be associated with a terrorist attack. It is more likely that inhalation of the toxin or food-borne ingestion would be associated with a criminal release.

The difficulty in deploying the weapon, once obtained, was seen in Japan in the early 1990s. The cult Aum Shinrikyo tried several times to deploy aerosols of botulinum toxin without success. Both the United States and the former Soviet Union included botulinum toxin in their arsenals, and yet it ultimately lost favor. Iraq, on the other hand, apparently considered botulinum toxin a bioweapon of choice. Iraq reportedly produced 19,000 L of botulinum toxin and had loaded 10,000 L into missiles, bombs, and other delivery systems. Still, many think that botulinum toxin is more of a threat in smaller attacks at the hands of terrorists than as a major weapon in a country's arsenal.

Specimen Collection and Diagnosis

Diagnosis of botulinum toxin ingestion or inhalation is likely to be based on symptoms as opposed to laboratory data. However, treatment should begin before laboratory confirmation. The LRN stresses that botulism is a public health emergency and that local and state public health officials should be notified as soon as the patient seeks medical consultation. Many local hospitals are not equipped to process specimens for the detection of botulinum toxin; therefore specimens should be submitted to the nearest LRN Reference laboratory. Specimens appropriate for referral include feces, gastric aspirate or vomitus, serum, tissues or exudates, and food specimens. Environmental specimens should always be submitted directly to the LRN Reference laboratory. Diagnosis of botulism can be confirmed by detection of botulinum toxin. The traditional method is a mouse toxicity assay that confirms botulinum toxin and identifies the serotype. Some enzyme immunoassay tests are sensitive enough to detect minute amounts of residual toxin found in the respiratory tract of affected patients.

Staphylococcal Enterotoxins

Staphylococcal enterotoxins are small-molecular-weight polypeptides belonging to the bacterial superantigen family. These toxins work by nonspecifically stimulating T cells, resulting in the release of proinflammatory cytokines such as tumor necrosis factor α, interleukin 2, and interferon-γ. Symptoms of mild exposure resemble a cell-mediated immune memory response, similar to a Mantoux skin test for tuberculosis.

Approximately 18 different staphylococcal enterotoxins have been identified. The symptoms depend on the enterotoxin and the route of entry. Staphylococcal enterotoxins are relatively stable and can be transmitted by aerosols or ingestions. Staphylococcal enterotoxin B (SEB) is classified as a category B bioterror agent. After inhalation of SEB, clinical features include fever, respiratory complaints (cough, dyspnea, and chest pain), and gastrointestinal symptoms. Severe intoxication results in pulmonary edema, respiratory distress syndrome, shock, and possibly death. SEB may cause food poisoning within 1 to 6 hours of ingestion, manifesting as acute salivation, nausea, and vomiting, followed by abdominal cramps and diarrhea. Because ingesting SEB does not usually result in pulmonary symptoms, gastrointestinal symptoms observed from inhalation intoxication likely result from secondary oral ingestion of SEB concomitant with the inhalation exposure.

Ricin

Ricin, from castor beans *(Ricinus communis),* is a potent biologic toxin that inhibits protein synthesis. Clinical manifestations depend on the route of exposure. Ingestion of ricin typically leads to profuse vomiting and diarrhea followed by multisystem organ failure and possibly death within 36 to 72 hours of exposure. Inhalation of ricin usually leads to respiratory distress, fever, and cough followed by the development of pulmonary edema, hypotension, respiratory failure, and possibly death within 36 to 72 hours.

Ricin toxin is a category B bioterror agent. It could be produced as a mist or powder to be inhaled. It could also be added to food or dissolved in water. If injected, a 500-µg dose would be lethal. In 1978 Georgi Markov, a Bulgarian writer and journalist living in London, died after he was injected with a poison ricin pellet by an umbrella containing an injection device. Like other toxins, ricin is not contagious and is not spread from person to person. In 2003 in South Carolina, an envelope with a threatening note and a sealed container was processed at a mail processing and distribution facility. The note threatened to poison water supplies if demands were not met. During the investigation the CDC confirmed that ricin was present in the container, although no evidence of environmental contamination and no cases of ricin-associated illness were found.

BIBLIOGRAPHY

American Society for Microbiology: *Sentinel guidelines for suspected agents of bioterrorism:* Brucella *species* (Web site). Available at: www.asm.org/ASM/files/LeftMarginHeaderList/DOWNLOADFILENAME/000000000523/Brucella101504.pdf. Accessed December 9, 2008.

American Society for Microbiology: *Sentinel laboratory guidelines for suspected agents of bioterrorism: botulinum toxin* (Web site). Available at: www.asm.org/ASM/files/LeftMarginHeaderList/DOWNLOADFILENAME/000000000522/Botulism.pdf. Accessed December 9, 2008.

American Society for Microbiology: *Sentinel laboratory guidelines for suspected agents of bioterrorism:* Burkholderia mallei *and* B. pseudomallei (Web site). Available at: www.asm.org/ASM/files/LeftMarginHeaderList/DOWNLOADFILENAME/000000002739/BpseudomalleiBmalleiRevision2008.pdf. Accessed December 9, 2008.

American Society for Microbiology: *Sentinel laboratory guidelines for suspected agents of bioterrorism:* Coxiella burnetii (Web site). Available at: www.asm.org/ASM/files/LeftMarginHeaderList/DOWNLOADFILENAME/000000001088/CoxiellaBurnetti.pdf. Accessed December 9, 2008.

American Society for Microbiology: *Sentinel laboratory guidelines for suspected agents of bioterrorism:* Staphylococcal enterotoxin B (Web site). Available at: www.asm.org/ASM/files/LEFTMARGINHEADERLIST/DOWNLOADFILENAME/0000001222/SEBrevised.pdf. Accessed December 9, 2008.

American Society for Microbiology: *Sentinel laboratory guidelines for suspected agents of bioterrorism: Unknown viruses* (Web site). Available at: www.asm.org/ASM/files/LEFTMARGINHEADERLIST/DOWNLOADFILENAME/0000001160/ukvirusesgl.pdf. Accessed December 9, 2008.

American Society for Microbiology: *Sentinel level clinical microbiology laboratory guidelines* (Web site). Available at: www.asm.org/Policy/index.asp?bid=6342. Accessed December 9, 2008.

American Society for Microbiology Centers for Disease Control and Prevention: *Basic diagnostic testing protocols for level A laboratories for the presumptive identification of* Bacillus anthracis (Web site). Available at: www.asm.org/ASM/files/LEFTMARGINHEADERLIST/DOWNLOADFILENAME/0000000521/bacillusanthracisprotocol[1].pdf. Accessed December 9, 2008.

American Society for Microbiology Centers for Disease Control and Prevention: *Basic protocols for level A laboratories: for the presumptive identification of* Francisella tularensis (Web site). Available at: www.asm.org/ASM/files/LEFTMARGINHEADER

LIST/DOWNLOADFILENAME/0000000525/tularemiaprotocol[1].pdf. Accessed December 9, 2008.

American Society for Microbiology Centers for Disease Control and Prevention: *Sentinel laboratory guidelines for suspected agents of bioterrorism:* Yersinia pestis (Web site). Available at: www.asm.org/ASM/files/LeftMarginHeaderList/DOWNLOADFILENAME/000000000524/Ypestis81505.pdf. Accessed December 9, 2008.

Arnon SS et al: Botulinum toxin as a biological weapon: medical and public health management, *JAMA* 285:1059, 2001.

Breman JG, Henderson DA: Diagnosis and management of smallpox, *N Engl J Med* 346:1300, 2002.

Burgess TH et al: Clinicopatholgic features of viral agents of potential use by bioterrorists, *Clin Lab Med* 21:475, 2001.

Centers for Disease Control and Prevention: Biological and chemical terrorism: strategic plan for preparedness and response. Recommendations of the CDC strategic planning workgroup, *MMWR* 49(RR-4): 2000. Available at: www.cdc.gov/mmwr/preview/mmwrhtml/rr4904a1.htm. Accessed December 9, 2008.

Centers for Disease Control and Prevention: Investigation of a ricin-containing envelope at a postal facility—South Carolina, 2003, *MMWR* 52:1129, 2003.Available at: www.cdc.gov/mmwr/preview/mmwrhtml/mm5246a5.htm. Accessed December 9, 2008.

Centers for Disease Control and Prevention: Laboratory exposure to *Burkholderia pseudomallei*—Los Angeles, California, 2003, *MMWR* 53:988, 2004. Available at: www.cdc.gov/mmwr/preview/mmwrhtml/mm5342a3.htm. Accessed December 9, 2008.

Centers for Disease Control and Prevention: Laboratory-acquired human glanders—Maryland, May 2000, *MMWR* 49:532, 2000. Available at: www.cdc.gov/mmwr/preview/mmwrhtml/mm4924a3.htm. Accessed December 9, 2008.

Centers for Disease Control and Prevention: Update: investigation of anthrax associated with intentional exposure and interim public health guidelines, October 2001, *MMWR* 50:889, 2001. Available at: www.cdc.gov/mmwr/preview/mmwrhtml/mm5041a1.htm. Accessed December 9, 2008.

Centers for Disease Control and Prevention: *Known cases and outbreaks of Ebola hemorrhagic fever, in chronological order* (website). Available at: www.cdc.gov/ncidod/dvrd/spb/mnpages/dispages/ebola/ebolatable.htm. Accessed December 9, 2008.

Centers for Disease Control and Prevention: Responding to detection of aerosolized *Bacillus anthracis* by autonomous detection systems in the workplace, *MMWR* 53(RR-7):1, 2004. Available at: Available at: www.cdc.gov/mmwr/preview/mmwrhtml/rr5307a1.htm. Accessed December 9, 2008.

Cheng AC, Currie BJ: Melioidosis: epidemiology, pathophysiology, and management, *Clin Microbiol Rev* 18:383, 2005.

Dembek ZF et al: Botulism: cause, effects, diagnosis, clinical and laboratory identification, and treatment modalities, *Disaster Med Public Health Prep* 1:122, 2007.

Dennis DT et al: Tularemia as a biological weapon: medical and public health management, *JAMA* 285:2763, 2001.

Department of Health and Human Services: *Possession, use, and transfer of select agents and toxins;* (Web site). Available at: www.selectagents.gov/resources/Biennial%20Review_CDC_20081016.pdf. Accessed October 20, 2009.

Drevets DA et al: Invasion of the central nervous system by intracellular bacteria, *Clin Microbiol Rev* 17:323, 2004.

Franz DA et al: Clinical recognition and management of patients exposed to biological warfare agents, *Clin Lab Med* 21:435, 2001.

Humes R, Snyder JW: Laboratory detection of potential agents of bioterrorism. In Murray PR et al, editors: *Manual of clinical microbiology*, ed 9, Washington, DC, 2007, ASM Press.

Inglesby TV et al: Plague as a biological weapon: medical and public health management, *JAMA* 283:2281, 2000.

Jernigan DB et al: Investigation of bioterrorism-related anthrax, United States, 2001: epidemiologic findings, *Emerg Infect Dis* 8:1019, 2002.

Jernigan JA et al: Bioterrorism-related inhalation anthrax: the first 10 cases reported in the United States, *Emerg Infect Dis* 7:933, 2001.

Klietmann WF, Ruoff KL: Bioterrorism: implications for the clinical microbiologist, *Clin Microbiol Rev* 14:364, 2001.

Lindström M, Korkeala H: Laboratory diagnostics of botulism, *Clin Microbiol Rev* 19:298, 2006.

Martin GJ, Marty AM: Clinicopathologic aspects of bacterial agents, *Clin Lab Med* 21:513, 2001.

Marty AM, Conran RM, Kortepeter MG: Recent challenges in infectious diseases: biological pathogens as weapons and emerging endemic threats, *Clin Lab Med* 21:411, 2001.

Marty AM: History of the development and use of biological weapons, *Clin Lab Med* 21:421, 2001.

Moran GJ, Talan DA, Abrahamian FM: Biological terrorism, *Infect Dis Clin North Am* 22:145, 2008.

Nigrovic LE, Wingerter SL: Tularemia, *Infect Dis Clin North Am* 22:489, 2008.

Reynolds KA, Mena KD, Gerba CP: Risk of waterborne illness via drinking water in the United States, *Rev Environ Contam Toxicol* 192:117, 2008.

Sinclair R et al: Persistence of category A select agents in the environment, *Appl Environ Microbiol* 74:555, 2008.

Points to Remember

- Bioterrorism is the use (or threatened use) of biologic agents to harm humans, animals, or crops to cause civil unrest. Biologic warfare is the use of biologic weapons to gain a military advantage.
- Many of the biothreat bacterial and viral agents are zoonotic.
- Most biothreat agents can also be isolated from patients with naturally occurring infections.
- Clinical microbiologists in all hospital laboratories should be able to recognize the basic colony and Gram stain characteristics of the bacterial biothreat agents included in this chapter.

- Laboratory Response Network (LRN) Sentinel laboratories have a crucial role in the rapid detection and reporting of potential biothreat isolates.
- The CDC provides information on minimal tests for the identification of potential bioterror agents for sentinel laboratories to use.
- Clinical microbiologists in LRN Sentinel laboratories should notify their state public health laboratories when a potential biothreat agent cannot be ruled out and receive instructions and guidance on chain of custody and shipping.

Learning Assessment Questions

1. What is the most typical clinical presentation for a patient who was a target of a criminal release of anthrax spores?

2. What clinical specimens are most appropriate to detect *Coxiella burnetii* from potentially exposed patients?

3. What is the most typical clinical presentation for a patient who was a target of a criminal release of *Yersinia pestis*?

4. What is the most toxic biologic compound known?

5. List five biothreat Level A agents.

6. List two characteristics of *Bacillus anthracis* leading to a presumptive identification of anthrax.

7. List the levels of the Laboratory Response Network for bioterrorism and compare the respective roles of each.

8. What is mediastinitis, and which bioterror agent is most closely associated with this syndrome?

9. What is modified smallpox?

10. What is the major clinical manifestation of a patient with botulinum toxin exposure?

Biofilms: Architects of Disease

Donald C. Lehman, Frederic J. Marsik

OBJECTIVES

After reading and studying this chapter, you should be able to:

1. Describe the proposed origin of biofilms, in a historical perspective, as a means of microbial survival.
2. Define *biofilm*.
3. Compare and contrast the planktonic phenotype to sessile phenotype.
4. Describe the interaction of multiple cells in a community.
5. Compare the five stages of biofilm formation.
6. Discuss the architecture of biofilms.
7. Describe the potential virulence mechanisms of biofilms.
8. Discuss the role of biofilm formation on periodontal disease.
9. Describe the role of indwelling medical devices and the pathogenicity associated with biofilms.
10. Discuss the consequence of biofilms for the clinical laboratory, particularly false-negative cultures, viable but nonculturable bacteria, low colony counts, inappropriate specimen collection, and loss of susceptibility.
11. Evaluate the limitations of biofilm interventions.
12. Analyze laboratory methods that may be used to study biofilms.

Case in Point

An 83-year-old woman was admitted to the hospital after developing a fever and having a hypotensive episode while in residence at a nursing home. The patient had a clinical history of rheumatoid arthritis, hypertension, atrioventricular block, gastroesophageal reflux disease, deep vein thrombosis with pulmonary embolism, and depression. The patient also had a history of recurrent prosthetic left knee joint infections subsequent to total knee arthroplasty 2 years earlier. Vancomycin-resistant enterococci (VRE), *Enterococcus faecium,* was the predominant organism isolated from synovial fluid taken from her knee. The patient was placed on multiple antimicrobial regimens with numerous revisions. The course of her illness was complicated by pancytopenia, most likely caused by injury to the bone marrow, possibly from a drug reaction. At this admission, blood and synovial fluid cultures were collected. The patient was given antimicrobial

therapy and supportive care, but her condition worsened and thereafter "comfort measures only" were instituted. When the patient died, an autopsy was requested by the family. The final pathologic diagnoses were as follows:

■ Nonhealing chronic wound infection (due to VRE) associated with prosthetic left knee joint and clinical history of sepsis
■ Pulmonary edema and pleural and peritoneal effusions
■ Pulmonary vascular calcifications and cardiomegaly

Issues to Consider

After reading the patient's case history, consider:

■ The role and significance of biofilms in infectious diseases
■ The difficulty of successfully treating infections due to biofilms

- Consequences of untreated biofilm diseases
- Whether laboratory standard practices should be altered to meet the challenges presented by biofilm-associated infections

Key Terms

Biofilm	Pheromone
Biofouling	Planktonic
Exopolysaccharide (EPS)	Quorum sensing (QS)
Persister cell	Sessile

Biofilms are communities of microorganisms attached to a solid surface; the surface can be either abiotic (nonliving) or living tissue. The organisms in a biofilm are specialized and have a great deal of genetic energy. Given the selected pressures of certain environments, notably aquatic systems, biofilms are the preferred method of growth. Their unique structure, which evolves over time, allows for a cohesive, robust community of cells with interspecies communication driven by the principle of survival. Microorganisms, be they prokaryotic or eukaryotic, have the potential to live in one of two phenotypes: *sessile* or *planktonic*. The **sessile** phenotype results from attachment and usually develops into a multispecies biofilm that has unique characteristics, making it similar in many ways to hydrated polymers. **Planktonic** forms are free-floating microorganisms.

Biofilms can be simple monospecies or complex co-biofilms. Co-biofilms, or multispecies biofilms, predominate in most environmental sites (Figure 31-1). Biofilms are known to form on a variety of surfaces such as ships' hulls and rocks in rivers and streams. Biofilms can also form inside pipes that carry drinking water, thereby making the water unsafe to drink, a process referred to as **biofouling.** Co-biofilms of bacteria and fungi have been found in ventilator systems of airplanes, in ice machines in restaurants and bars, and in mines,

where unique configurations have been found that result from the leeching process creating stress on the inanimate surface. Biofilms also have had an impact on agriculture involving mastitis in farm animals and on the wine industry by forming in barrels and causing wine to spoil. Co-biofilms of *Pseudomonas aeruginosa* and *Burkholderia cepacia* are associated with serious lung infections in patients with cystic fibrosis. Monospecies biofilms are associated with a variety of infections. Medically important biofilms are produced by bacteria such as *Pseudomonas fluorescens, Staphylococcus aureus,* and *Staphylococcus epidermidis.*

As patients live longer, in a state of more debilitated health, and undergo invasive procedures, they are more prone to infections by opportunistic pathogens and the development of biofilms. It is important for clinical microbiologists to become familiar with the role biofilms play in human disease. Until recently, the challenges that biofilms presented to the clinical microbiology laboratory had not been recognized. These challenges include significant problems in susceptibility testing, recovery of viable but nonculturable organisms in a mixed species biofilm, and the recognition that biofilms transform from gram-positive to gram-negative in an environment that is difficult to duplicate. This chapter presents an overview of biofilm properties and composition and discusses the consequences and challenges associated with biofilms that the clinical laboratorian has to confront. Diseases associated with biofilms are presented and potential interventions are introduced.

MICROBIAL BIOFILMS DEFINED

There are a number of definitions for *biofilm*. These definitions have evolved over time as our understanding of the forces and features of biofilms has emerged. However, the definition in Box 31-1 seems to "stand the test of time" and puts into perspective the concept of developmental biology and the uniqueness and cooperation required among members within the biofilm. A biofilm definition by Donlan and Costerton recognizes the components and imperative ingredients that characterize this multiorganism cooperative population. According to the definition, microbially derived sessile communities are characterized by cells irreversibly attached to a substratum, or interfaced to each other, embedded in a matrix of extracellular polymeric substance, that produce and exhibit an altered phenotype with respect to growth rate and gene transcription.

Microbial biofilms (phenotype biofilm [PBF]) are as common as planktonic microorganisms (phenotype planktonic; PPL). Virtually any liquid environment where organ-

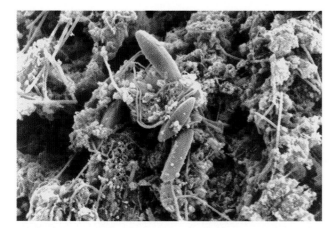

FIGURE 31-1 Natural biofilm on a metal surface. Scanning electron micrograph of a native biofilm that developed on a mild steel surface in an 8-week period in an industrial water system. (Courtesy Rodney Donlan and Donald Gibbon, by permission from ASM MicrobeLibrary.)

BOX 31-1 Biofilm Definition

A primitive type of developmental biology in which spatial organization of the cells within the matrix optimizes the utilization of the nutritional resources available, forming an immobilized enzyme system in which the milieu and the enzyme activities are constantly changing and evolving to appropriate steady state. The steady state can be radically altered by applying physical factors such as high shear force.

isms are subject to (1) shear forces and (2) nutrition alteration select for upregulation (i.e., increased expression of genes consistent with PBF) to the biofilm phenotype. PPL and PBF cells can have the same genetic potential but express a different phenotype. Given the environmental selective pressures, a significant number of bacteria will preferentially develop a biofilm phenotype. It is important to recognize that the two phenotypes are not mutually exclusive, but that the ratio of the PPL to the PFB may be a predictor of associated disease. Biofilms are a universal strategy for survival, horizontal gene transfer, and growth, as well as a probable ancestor of the planktonic free-floating organisms. The planktonic phenotype is genetically expensive, with sophisticated chemotactic and mobility mechanisms that may have developed post-biofilm. The primary purpose of the PPL is dissemination and colonization of new habitats.

There is growing evidence that the biofilm was the origin of survival and necessary for communication among microbes. Approximately 3.4 billion years ago, biofilms allowed microbes to survive, grow, and adapt to a hostile environment, including extreme pH and temperature and lack of water. As the Earth cooled and moved toward a multispecies adaptation with less environmental pressure, organisms were able to develop the ability to transfer to different ecologic niches and live outside of communities. Hence, the post-biofilm planktonic phenotype evolved, which had a reduced need for communities for survival.

Biofilms: Community of Cells

Although certain constituents are common to all biofilms, the contribution of the host relative to the microorganisms, such as immunologic components and the physical locations, has an impact on this structure. Several key environmental and cultural characteristics affect the selection of multispecies biofilm inhabitants (Figure 31-2). These features include (1) species attachment efficiency, (2) genotypic factors, (3) cyclic stage of biofilm, (4) substrata, (5) nutritional resources, (6)

mechanical factors and shear forces, (7) physicochemical environment, and (8) anti-infective hostile pressures forces.

Of these characteristics, the four most important are organism attachment efficiency, nutritional resources, substrata, and environmental shear stress or force. The shear stress, probably the most important characteristic, affects the physical morphology and dynamic behavior of the biofilm. The steady-state kinetics of the organisms within the biofilm can be radically altered by physical factors such as high shear, and the shear rate will determine the rate of erosion of cells and of the matrix from the biofilm. As a biofilm forms, "streamers" of cells extend from the surface. These cells can break off and establish new biofilms downstream. Not all microorganisms change with a high efficiency of upregulation between the planktonic and the biofilm phenotypes. It is no coincidence that coagulase-negative staphylococci, *P. aeruginosa,* and *Candida albicans* are some of the most efficient microbes prone to upregulation when selective pressures magnify the need for survival in a biofilm community. These microorganisms are also important human pathogens. Both prokaryotes and eukaryotes are important in biofilm-associated diseases. In particular, a co-biofilm of *Candida* and pseudomonad species is very difficult to eliminate because of its drug resistance. A co-biofilm increases in robustness and stability with maturity and numbers of organisms within the community.

Stages in Biofilm Formation

With biofilms it is possible to recognize a series of discrete and well-regulated steps that include attachment of cells to a substrate, the growth and aggregation of cells into microcolonies, and the maturation and maintenance of architecture, all of which are hallmarks of a developmental process in which many species of microorganisms progress through multiple developmental stages. There is a five-stage universal growth cycle of a biofilm with common characteristics independent of the phenotype of the organism.

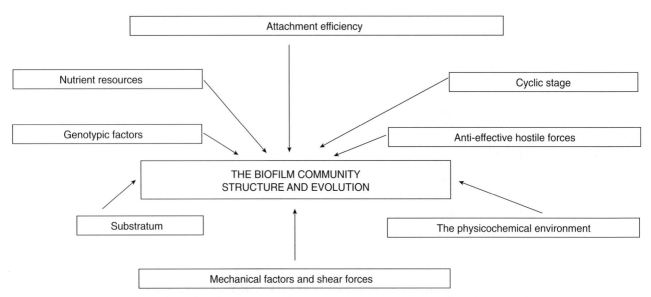

FIGURE 31-2 Environmental and cultural factors that affect biofilm development.

TABLE 31-1 Variables Important in Cell Attachment and Biofilm Formation

Properties of Substratum	Properties of Surrounding Fluid	Properties of the Cell
Texture or roughness	Flow velocity	Cell surface hydrophobicity
Hydrophobicity	pH	Fimbriae
Conditioning film	Temperature	Flagella
	Cations	Adhesion molecules

Stage I is the attachment phase that can take only seconds to initiate and is likely induced by environmental signals. These signals vary by organism, but they include changes in nutrients and nutrient concentrations, pH, temperature, oxygen and iron concentration, and osmolality. Even though biofilms can form on any surface, rough surfaces are more susceptible to biofilm formation. This is likely due to reduction of shear forces and increased surface area. Studies indicate that biofilms also tend to form more readily on hydrophobic material such as Teflon and other plastics (polymers) than on glass and metals. Table 31-1 lists some key factors in biofilm formation. The initial binding in stage I is reversible as some cells detach from the substratum. Binding to a surface is mediated by a number of adhesion molecules and pili. One example is *polysaccharide intercellular adhesion,* which is produced by enzymes encoded by the *ica* gene locus. In *Escherichia coli* there are genes that encode a similar polymer associated with adhesion designated *pga,* and they share sequence similarity with the staphylococcal *ica* genes.

Following attachment, the cells undergo changes in gene expression that lead to existence on a solid surface. It has been shown with *C. albicans* that a switch from yeast forms to hyphal growth is important in biofilm development. During stage I, bacterial cells exhibit a logarithmic growth rate. Stage II is characterized as irreversible binding and begins minutes after stage I. During stage II, cell aggregates are formed and motility is decreased. Toward the end of this stage, **exopolysaccharide (EPS)** is produced, which is able to trap nutrients and planktonic bacteria. In staphylococci and enterococci, iron deprivation and osmotic stress induce the expression of genes encoding proteins that synthesize EPS. It has been shown that alginate, an EPS, is increased threefold to fivefold in *P. aeruginosa* following attachment to a solid surface compared to planktonic cells.

When cell aggregates become progressively layered, with a thickness greater than 10 μm, the biofilm is in stage III. This stage is also referred to as *maturation-1.* When biofilms reach their ultimate thickness, generally greater than 100 μm, this is referred to as stage IV or *maturation-2.* It takes a biofilm several days to reach this stage. Some of the cell aggregates are displaced from the substratum but remain trapped in the biofilm EPS. During stage V, cell dispersion is noted. Some of the bacteria develop the planktonic phenotype and leave the biofilm. Stage V begins several days after stage IV.

Cycling of stages I to V is based on the organism pool and the timing of the growth characterization of the individual members. The formation of a biofilm has been compared to cell differentiation of a multicellular organism. One reason for this comparison is that microorganisms in a biofilm express great variability in metabolic activities. A biofilm is a dynamic system containing many species of bacteria with different characteristics. It is also recognized that there is a constant assessment of the need to remain within the cycle, attached or free-floating and, again, neither is mutually exclusive. Certain organisms, however, have evolved a much more efficient means of maintaining one phenotype or the other.

The organization of biofilms may take several forms, but it is important to recognize that a nonuniform spatial pattern and nonuniform susceptibility with physiologic heterogeneity equals survival in a harsh environment, such as one containing antimicrobial agents. **Persister cells,** essentially metabolically inert microorganisms analogous to bacterial spores, are present in all biofilms and bacterial populations. Persister cells are hypothesized to have disabled programmed cell death, or apoptosis. These cells have the greatest potential for maintenance of the gene pool and resistance to environmental stress, including antimicrobial agents.

Much of the development and structural integrity of the biofilm depends upon **quorum sensing (QS).** QS is the ability to use extracellular molecules, **pheromones,** to allow enhanced communication among bacteria. The most striking element of QS in gram-negative organisms is the highly conserved set of three-component regulatory networks used by these organisms to efficiently regulate a wide variety of bacterial density–dependent activates such as metabolism, virulence, chemotaxis and, notably, biofilm production and maturation. The viability of the biofilm community depends upon stress response genes and cell signaling from the cells via QS through biochemicals. QS is essential for biofilm formation, triggering expression of some genes and downregulation (i.e., silencing or reducing expression) of others. Pheromones are different for gram-positive and gram-negative bacteria. Gram-negative bacteria use low–molecular-weight homoserine molecules, such as N-acylhomoserine lactone, whereas gram-positive bacteria employ oligopeptides or proteins. The role QS plays for different organisms mechanistically in a biofilm community remains to be understood. Some challenges in the study of biofilms are (1) what parameters of a biofilm community influence the onset of QS and subsequent patterns of gene expression, (2) what are the functional challenges of QS, (3) does induction of QS influence the pathogenic potential of biofilm communities, (4) does induction of QS alter the antimicrobial tolerance of a biofilm community, (5) are there organisms in a biofilm community that eliminate or reduce signal transfer among organisms, and (6) does interspecies signaling occur in mixed species systems and what triggers this signaling? Physical contact, or cell aggregation, can also provide signals that are important in biofilm formation.

ARCHITECTURE OF BIOFILMS

It is important to recognize the interplay of biofilm and planktonic phenotypes and the three-dimensional architecture of the biofilm as universal, whether the biofilms are in

TABLE 31-2 Components of Biofilms

Component	Percent of Matrix
Water	Up to 97%
Microbial cells	2% to 5%, many species
Exopolysaccharide	1% to 2%
Proteins	Less than 1% to 2%
DNA and RNA	Less than 1% to 2%

animals, agricultural environments, or industrial settings. Biofilms are composed of stalks of mushroom-shaped microcolonies attached to the substratum surrounded by EPS. The biofilm matrix contains EPS, proteins, and DNA; EPS constitutes 50% to 90% of the organic carbon in the matrix. Biofilms are hydrated with fluid-filled channels running throughout the biofilm. The fluid-filled channels facilitate the exchange of nutrients and carry away waste products. In addition, motile microorganisms can be found swimming in the aqueous portion of a biofilm. Table 31-2 lists some commonly found constituents of biofilms.

The three-dimensional architecture of the mature biofilm often has three layers. The outermost layer of a biofilm is exposed to the highest concentration of nutrients and oxygen. It contains the most active organisms that primarily resemble the structure and activity of their planktonic counterparts. These organisms are generally closely aligned with selective pressures. Even though they are also part of the EPS, the organisms may slough off and initiate biofilm formation downstream. The second layer of the architecture is an intermediate level. Organisms in the second layer downregulate somewhat their metabolic activity, but they clearly have the capacity to utilize nutrients, exchange genes, and have the potential for multiple drug resistance. This spatial arrangement, physiologic heterogeneity, and non-uniformity are based on the proximity of microorganisms aligning next to one another. They benefit from that alignment, and it is not happenstance. The innermost layer of cells is attached to the substratum and represents the earliest part of the biofilm. These microorganisms also downregulate very efficiently and are the least metabolically active. This is where most persister cells are located. Generally, the innermost layer provides inheritance for future populations that transfer laterally.

BIOFILM PROPERTIES

As the understanding of biofilms increased, it became apparent that biofilm phenotypes cannot be defined by traditional principles of microbiology. Cell behavior in response to stress is much more than a group of microbes attached to a surface. In fact, the properties of a biofilm are similar to the properties of organic polymers. This explains why much of the early information about biofilms was defined by engineers. Engineers recognized early on that biofilms had key characteristics that could be quantified and mathematical formulas derived from the movement of hydrated polymers could be applied to biofilms.

Two key properties of a biofilm are attributable to their hydrated polymer gel-like material. First, biofilms exhibit viscoelasticity; that is, materials that have both elastic and viscous properties. The consequence of this viscoelastic property is magnified in the time-dependent response of biofilms. In short time periods, biofilms absorb increased shear by behaving elastically. In contrast, for long periods, shear is dissipated through viscous flow by a streamlining of the structure to reduce drag. This viscoelastic property can be measured by using principles of rheology, meaning that everything flows. The Greek philosopher Heraclitus (540-480 BC) of Ephesus said, "Everything flows and nothing abides; everything gives way and nothing stays fixed." In a more practical sense, will it flow or will it fracture? The outcome is determined by the applied forces. This also explains the phenomenon of "creeping," or rolling, which allows for a multispecies biofilm to literally move like lava flow when attached to an inanimate or abiotic surface. There is no detachment but rather the movement of a protective community down a surface as defined by viscoelastic properties of a material-like substance. This is of major concern when addressing movements of biofilms within the lumen of an endotracheal tube or of a central catheter line, for example.

Not only do biofilms share properties of organic polymers, they also have many properties common to neoplasia, another community of cells. Certainly, a neoplasia is a eukaryotic irreversible genotype. In contrast, members of a biofilm have "reversible phenotypes" and are more often prokaryotes. However, given those differences, several features are shared to some degree by neoplasia and a biofilm. Common to both are cycling or staging, metastasis, loss of contact inhibition, and cell-to-cell signaling. Similarities can also be observed in the three-dimensional architecture, heterogeneity, and virulence phenotype. The sharing of characteristics between neoplasia and a biofilm highlights the fact that biofilms are different from their free-floating counterparts.

MECHANISMS OF PATHOGENICITY

A great deal has been learned about the structure, function, and properties of biofilms. The mechanisms of pathogenicity, on the other hand, are a different matter. Do biofilms contribute to infectious disease? If so, what are the mechanisms of pathogenicity? Are some biofilms more pathogenic than others? Some observations appear to provide evidence of the significance of biofilms in the mechanisms of disease. Box 31-2 lists several potential pathogenic mechanisms concerning biofilms and disease.

Transitioning from acute to chronic infections is frequently associated with biofilm formation. In the environment and in patients, biofilms are the most advantageous method of growth by most microorganisms. Biofilms originate because of selective pressures in an environment where survival can be difficult, such as the presence of host defenses and antimicrobial agents.

Role of Biofilms in Attachment

Colonization is often a critical first step in development of an infectious disease, and biofilms may be an important mecha-

BOX 31-2 Biofilm Pathogenicity and Disease

- Allows attachment to a solid surface
- "Division of labor" increases metabolic efficiency of the community
- Evades host defenses such as phagocytosis
- Obtains a high density of microorganisms
- Exchanges genes that can result in more virulent strains of microorganisms
- Produces a large concentration of toxins
- Protects from antimicrobial agents
- Detachment of microbial aggregates transmits microorganisms to other body sites

nism of attachment to host tissue and indwelling medical devices (IMDs). Initial colonization involves bacterial adhesions such as surface proteins (e.g., teichoic acid, lipoteichoic acid) and pili. Motility is also important for initial colonization. However, after bacteria adhere to a surface and biofilm construction begins, changes in gene expression result in suppression of flagella and increased expression of adhesion molecules. This suggests that once a biofilm is established, other adhesion mechanisms are no longer needed.

Benefit of Biofilms on Metabolism

Biofilms allow members of the microbial community to withstand the shear forces of blood and urine flow, presumably keeping the microorganisms in a nutrient-rich environment. It has been shown with certain organisms, such as the pseudomonads, *E. coli*, *Vibrio cholerae*, and others, that the presence of an abundant usable carbon source (e.g., glucose) stimulates the production of EPS. The EPS can trap more microorganisms and may serve as a glucose storage mechanism at times when carbohydrates are plentiful. As nutrients in the surrounding environment become scarce, gene expression changes and some bacteria in the biofilm detach and become planktonic.

Because of the extreme variability in available nutrients, pH, and oxygen concentration in a large complex biofilm, there is great heterogeneity in the metabolic activity of microorganisms in the community. Even in monospecies biofilms, metabolic requirements and activities vary. This variability may be responsible in a "division of labor" whereby the metabolic efficiency of the microbial population is increased. Sharing of metabolic by-products is the basis of a beneficial symbiotic relationship. It has been proposed that bacteria living in a biofilm can exhibit mutually beneficial behavior. Evidence indicates that bacteria can undergo programmed cell death. Death of some cells in the community could relieve the metabolic load and release nutrients for nearby cells. This would help the biofilm survive. One of the major benefits of the biofilm configuration is the ability to produce a large number of organisms per unit mass. Generally in broth cultures, it is difficult to obtain greater than 10^8 cells/mL, but with configuration and upregulation of a biofilm phenotype, microorganisms are able to reach concentrations equal to or greater than 10^{12} cells/mL.

Biofilms as a Defense Mechanism

Biofilms can afford protection from host defenses including oxygen-reactive molecules, antimicrobial proteins, antimicrobial drugs, and phagocytosis. In addition, biofilms protect against pH changes and nutrient deprivation. A major benefit of the biofilm to microorganisms is its interference with immune function, particularly the activity of white blood cells. Phagocytic cells, such as polymorphonuclear cells (PMNs), generally are unable to penetrate the biofilm and phagocytize bacteria. When confronting a biofilm, PMNs will degranulate and cause damage to nearby host tissue. In periodontal disease, the consequence of interrupted white blood cell function is production of large quantities of collagenase of human origin that causes deterioration of support bone. In addition, biofilms can hide microbial antigens, preventing an immune response by blocking interaction with antibody.

How biofilms provide protection to its members is not completely known. Possibly, "sticky" EPS provides a physical barrier to penetration by phagocytic cells and antimicrobial molecules. Also, the heterogeneity of microbial metabolic activity may play a role. It is known that slow-growing organisms are more resistant to antimicrobial agents. This seems counterintuitive because one argument for forming a biofilm is the presence of a nutrient-rich environment; however, those microorganisms living near the substratum exist in a nutrient-poor environment and therefore grow slowly. The upregulation of the biofilm phenotype by microorganisms has the potential to out-compete normal biota. This is also particularly appropriate as bacteria transition from acute infections to chronic infections, more likely associated with the biofilm phenotype and the coaggregates of multispecies biofilms. The early bacterial population during an acute infection will be exceeded later in disease when the organisms reach a biofilm configuration. The microbial population is also often susceptible to antimicrobial agents early in the infections, as determined by genotyping, but become much more resistant as the population shifts to a biofilm phenotype. Removal of the selected pressure is critical in shifting the ratio of biofilm phenotype back to the planktonic phenotype in the nondisease state.

Biofilms afford a mechanism by which bacteria can be protected from antimicrobials. Several hypotheses may explain biofilm resistance to antimicrobial agents. However, it is critical to remember that the classic mechanisms of genetically encoded bacterial resistance can also operate in bacterial biofilms. Multidrug efflux pumps, antibiotic-modifying enzymes, and bacterial modifications are all viable modes of resistance for biofilms. However, these classic resistance mechanisms do not explain the resistance observed even in bacteria, which do not possess known antibiotic resistance genes. To explain this phenomenon, several biofilm specific alternative mechanisms of resistance have been proposed: (1) inability of an antimicrobial compound to penetrate all areas of the biofilm; (2) altered areas of metabolic activity of the bacteria or reduced growth rate, rendering antibiotics such as penicillin, which can only inhibit the growth of actively growing bacteria ineffective; and (3) differential gene expression within the biofilm community, which may allow certain bacteria to protect other bacteria by producing needed nutrients, compounds that inactivate antimicrobials (e.g., penicillinase), or other necessary compounds that regulate physiology of the biofilm community. Persister cells, which are phenotypic variants of the wild type, will neither grow nor die in the presence of a drug. When the antimicrobial agent is removed, the persister cells can give rise then to normal growing cells. These cells may be responsible for recurrent infections.

Gene Transfer and Expression

A biofilm is an optimal environment for the horizontal transfer of genetic material; that is, DNA. The microorganisms live in close proximity, which facilitates the uptake of DNA by transformation and conjugation. Plasmids, for example, are expensive for cells to maintain unless they offer a selective advantage. If a plasmid is lost by one cell, a nearby cell may take it up, a process called *transformation.* The horizontal transfer of genes may lead to the spread of antimicrobial resistance.

Upregulation to the biofilm phenotype has been associated with clustering of genes associated with virulence. In fact, some studies have indicated that the biofilm is a virulence factor and should be regarded as a means by which a disease process is enhanced. Endotoxin and the production of extracellular enzymes by the community are controversial, but there is no question that enzymatic activity for certain cohabitants is increased and that there is not universal growth of the biofilm on an inanimate surface.

Disaggregation

Disaggregation or detachment of aggregates clearly has the potential of transmitting already upregulated resistant aggregates of microorganisms to other body sites. Similar to cancer metastasis, this is most significant when aggregates spread via the bloodstream. This provides the microorganisms an opportunity to reach almost any body site. Important to disaggregation is the resulting ratio of PPL to PBF. As the ratio increases, the risk of the microorganisms spreading increases, leading to increased risk of more serious disease. There is some evidence, particularly in ventilator-associated pneumonia, that this ratio is a direct reflection of the disease process.

DISEASES ASSOCIATED WITH BIOFILMS

Medically, the primary location of biofilms is on IMDs, but they do exist in human tissue as well. Biofilms allow bacteria to grow to a density higher than normally established for planktonic forms, and biofilms may be one of the leading causes for a shift from acute phase diseases to chronic diseases. Hence, as we transition into an older population with more chronic infections and IMDs, it is important that the clinical laboratorian consider this population and associated biofilm diseases.

The list of human diseases associated with biofilms has grown significantly in the last several years and involves at least 30 bacteria and yeasts. Table 31-3 lists several medical or dental biofilm–associated conditions. These conditions include dental caries, periodontitis, otitis media, native valve endocarditis, pneumonia in patients with cystic fibrosis, colo-

TABLE 31-3 Partial List of Human Infections Involving Biofilms

Infection or Disease	Common Bacterial Species
Necrotizing fasciitis	Group A streptococci
Musculoskeletal infections	Gram-positive cocci
Osteomyelitis	Various species
Biliary tract infections	Enteric bacteria
Infectious kidney stones	Gram-negative bacilli
Periodontal disease	Various species
Infections Associated with Foreign Body Material	
Contact lenses	*Pseudomonas aeruginosa,* gram-positive cocci
Sutures	Staphylococci
Artificial heart valves	Staphylococci
Vascular grafts	Gram-positive cocci
Arteriovenous shunts	Gram-positive cocci
Endovascular catheter infections	Staphylococci
Peritoneal dialysis peritonitis	Various species
Urinary catheter infections	*Escherichia coli*, gram-negative bacilli
Intrauterine devices	*Actinomyces israelii* and other species
Penile prostheses	Staphylococci
Orthopedic prostheses	Staphylococci

nization of IMDs, kidney stones, and prostatitis. Newer diseases associated with biofilms are rhinosinusitis and soft tissue disease, particularly that of dystrophic epidermolysis bullosa. In nearly all cases, the biofilm plays a key role in helping the microorganisms survive or spread within the host.

Dental Biofilms

Dental biofilms, more commonly called *plaque,* are probably the most well-studied natural biofilm in humans. The microorganisms making up a dental biofilm are considered normal biota of the oral cavity. Plaque can lead to caries (dental cavities); gingivitis, a mild and irreversible form of periodontal disease; and periodontitis, inflammation of deep tissue below the gum surface that can result in tooth loss. In addition, poor oral hygiene and gum disease can allow normal oral microbiota to reach the bloodstream and contribute to cardiovascular disease.

Development of dental biofilms follows a sequence of events and involves hundreds of bacterial species. After a good dental cleaning at the dentist's office, tooth enamel becomes coated with a variety of proteins and glycoproteins of host origin. This coating develops almost immediately and is referred to as the *acquired pellicle.* After pellicle formation, the primary colonizers, first streptococci (particularly the sanguis streptococci) and later actinomycetes, colonize the surface of the teeth. Typical bacterial adhesion molecules and pili play a role in attachment to the pellicle. The bacteria are able to remain attached despite shearing forces of saliva and tongue movement.

The bacteria on the pellicle form cell-to-cell interactions (aggregates or coadhesions), both with the same species and with different species. The sessile organisms undergo cell-to-cell communication via QS. This initiates changes in gene expression. Notably, a number of streptococci, including *Streptococcus mutans* and related organisms, begin to synthesize insoluble glucan polymers used in the production of a glycolyx, an EPS. Bacteria from a number of species can bind to glucan via glucan-binding-proteins. Bridge bacteria, including members of the genus *Fusobacterium*, form aggregates with the primary colonizers. The bridge bacteria cannot bind to the pellicle, but they are able to bind to the primary colonizers. The primary colonizers cannot form aggregates with the late colonizers directly. The late colonizers forming aggregates with the fusobacteria include *Streptococcus salivarius*, propionibacteria, prevotellae, veillonellae, and *Selenomonas flueggei*. At this point in time, the biofilm consists primarily of nonpathogens. However, in the presence of dietary sucrose and other carbohydrates, acids are produced via fermentation. The production of organic acids on the tooth surface can result in demineralization of the tooth enamel and, over time, caries.

At the base of the tooth is a crevice, called a *sulcus*, between the tooth and the gingiva (gums). The plaque can extend into this space and is referred to as *subgingival plaque*. In immunocompetent individuals with good oral hygiene, the plaque remains composed primarily of gram-positive bacteria. This condition is not generally associated with disease because of a balance between host defenses and bacterial growth. If the plaque is allowed to remain undisturbed on the teeth for several days, the microbiota continues to change and becomes composed mainly of anaerobic and facultative anaerobic, gram-negative bacilli and spirochetes.

The last colonizers of the biofilm are considered pathogenic because of their role in periodontal disease. The most important pathogens include *Porphyromonas gingivalis*, *Bacteroides forsythus* (*Tannerella forsythensis*), *Aggregatibacter* (*Actinobacillus*) *actinomycetemcomitans*, and the spirochete *Treponema denticola*. These organisms require the presence of late colonizers in order to attach to the biofilm. The pathogens produce a number of virulence mechanisms allowing them to adhere to the epithelium lining the gums and invade the tissue, triggering an inflammatory response. PMNs arrive and degranulate; the contents of their granules enhance inflammation. Cell-mediated and humoral-mediated immune responses also contribute to the destruction of host tissue.

Initially the inflammation, called *gingivitis*, is reversible and relatively mild. If the disease is allowed to progress as a result of poor oral hygiene and lack of medical intervention, the inflammation can extend to the periodontal support structures (ligaments, cementum, and alveolar bone) resulting in periodontitis. If the disease continues to progress, it can result in destruction of the ligaments and alveolar bone that hold teeth in place, causing loosening of the teeth, pain, difficulty chewing, and eventually tooth loss. Gingivitis and mild periodontitis are considered relatively common in human populations. Periodontitis follows gingivitis, but it is not inevitable that periodontitis will develop following gingivitis.

Microbiology Changing Paradigm

In the industrialized world, chronic infections caused by organisms growing as biofilms (e.g., *S. epidermidis*) have become more important. The role of IMDs cannot be under-

TABLE 31-4 Microorganisms Commonly Associated with Biofilms on Indwelling Medical Devices

Microorganism	Indwelling Medical Device
Candida albicans	Artifical voice prosthesis
	Central venous catheter
	Intrauterine device
Coagulase-negative staphylococci	Artificial hip prosthesis
	Artificial voice prosthesis
	Central venous catheter
	Intrauterine device
	Prosthetic heart valve
	Urinary catheter
Enterococcus spp.	Artificial hip prosthesis
	Central venous catheter
	Intrauterine device
	Prosthetic heart valve
	Urinary catheter
Klebsiella pneumoniae	Central venous catheter
	Urinary catheter
Pseudomonas aeruginosa	Artificial hip prosthesis
	Central venous catheter
	Urinary catheter
Staphylococcus aureus	Artificial hip prosthesis
	Central venous catheter
	Intrauterine device
	Prosthetic heart valve

TABLE 31-5 Indwelling Medical Device–Risk Related Infections in the United States

Device	Usage	Infection Risk (%)
Bladder catheter	Tens of millions	10-30
Cardiac assisted devices	700	50-100
Cardiac pacemakers	400,000	1-5
Central venous catheters	5 million	5-8
Dental implants	1 million	5-10
Fracture fixators	2 million	5-10
Joint prostheses	600,000	1-3
Penile implants	15,000	2-10
Prosthetic heart valves	85,000	1-3
Vascular grafts	450,000	2-10

estimated in infections. IMDs are abiotic surfaces to which there is a natural aggregation of those organisms that have a predilection for biofilm upregulation and the phenotypes associated with multispecies aggregates. Table 31-4 lists the microorganisms associated with biofilms on IMDs. Table 31-5 lists the usage and infection risk associated with IMDs in the United States. The list is quite long and is expected to grow. In the area of dentistry alone, the use of implants and the growing recognition of the management of patients without teeth will have a significant impact on the number of biofilm-associated dental infections beyond caries and periodontitis.

Ventilator-associated pneumonia, a condition that consumes more resources in the intensive care unit than any single infectious disease, is another example where biofilms are an important disease-contributing factor. Ventilator-associated pneumonia is one of the most frequent nosocomial infections. The stress and shape of the endotracheal tube affect the cellular aggregation and fitness of the luminal biofilm, whether it is in the region closest to the ventilator, in the mid-section (where the greatest turbulent stress is found), or in the section closest to the lung–endotracheal interface.

There are both "good" and "bad" biofilms. In the human ecosystem, there are more than 10^{14} bacteria, more than all human cells. The Ecologic Hypothesis states that ecologic pressure is necessary for low numbers of pathogens to outcompete normal microbiota and achieve numerical dominance associated with diseases. Biofilms of stable normal biota represent a baseline organization. Biofilms of pathogenic organisms that overgrow normal biota and less virulent organisms because of selective pressures—that is, antimicrobial agents—are often associated with mismanagement. Microorganisms that are outcompeted often have low affinity for biofilm production or upregulation to the biofilm phenotype. It is also important to remember that biofilm composition is reflective of the normal biota and the location of IMDs placed close to the four reservoirs of normal biota: gastrointestinal tract, genitourinary tract, oral cavity, and skin.

LABORATORY CONSEQUENCES ASSOCIATED WITH BIOFILMS

Historically, laboratory protocols focused on the idea that free-floating microorganisms were the most clinically significant. Clinical laboratories have maximized techniques that support the growth of planktonic organisms. However, broth cultures will not always facilitate recovery of biofilm phenotypes given that environmental conditions are required to convert from a sessile to a planktonic phenotype. A broth culture incubated at 35° C with complex nutrients may not select for upregulation of an organism community. With greater understanding of biofilms, better practices in the clinical microbiology laboratory must also evolve.

With the emergence of biofilm-associated diseases, considerable diagnostic problems exist for the clinical laboratory. In general, these problems can be classified into five categories: false-negative cultures, viable but nonculturable organisms, underestimated or low colony count, inappropriate specimen, and loss of or decreased antimicrobial susceptibility. Biofilms are resilient, adherent, and with the EPS, quite resistant to culturing by swabs. False-negative culture results can occur because of improper sample collection. Studies have shown that cultures detect less than 10% of molecularly detectable methicillin-resistant staphylococci from vaginal specimens of biofilm communities. Some persister cells found in biofilms are viable but nonculturable bacteria for reasons not fully understood. Organisms upregulated to the biofilm phenotype may have significantly altered biochemical profiles. These organisms will not grow under normal laboratory conditions. They may be visible on Gram stain but might not be recovered in culture media.

Biofilms, by nature, are aggregates of cells surrounded by a matrix. When bacteria are recovered from a biofilm, often aggregates representing 10^5 cells/mL or greater can be recognized as a single colony on a bacteriologic plate. Hence, the colony count may be significantly falsely reduced. Ignoring the presence of a biofilm can result in collection of inappropriate specimens. Until the true nature of biofilms was understood and the importance of stress realized, most organisms could be considered attached (as in arterial line sepsis) on the outside of the inserted line. It is now apparent that bacteria preferentially select a luminal environment, often devoid of immunologic components. The only technique that has been associated with the recovery of organisms from extraluminal sources has been the rolling (Maki) technique. Today, it is recognized that line sepsis is often intraluminal and that methods need to address recovery of luminal organisms attached as biofilms.

Microbiology laboratories historically have performed antimicrobial susceptibility testing on organisms in the planktonic phenotype in pure culture. This is associated with expressed gene markers and detection of drug resistance of an organism. In contrast, a community of cells loses its susceptibility as a phenotypic expression of that community. It is now well established that a minimum inhibitory concentration against a free-floating planktonic isolate will increase 10- to 1000-fold when measured in the biofilm community. Drug resistance is even more amplified when multispecies are present, particularly with the accommodation of prokaryotic and eukaryotic cells. Consequently, bacterial isolates that appear sensitive in vitro will not respond to therapy or may relapse several months later because of the existence of biofilms in vivo. Biofilm colonization of IMDs often requires removal of the device for a successful outcome.

DETECTION OF BIOFILMS

The direct detection of biofilms on biopsied tissue such as on the middle ear mucosa in humans with chronic otitis media and on tissue or implants removed from diseased areas of the body is now possible. This detection is based on the use of combined methods such as polymerase chain reaction and pathogen-specific probes along with special microscopic methods such as confocal laser scanning microscopic (CLSM) imaging. Although not done routinely in clinical microbiology laboratories, these techniques provide valuable information about the role biofilms play in the disease process and what interventions may be possible to eliminate or prevent biofilms.

Techniques for the evaluation of biofilm formation potential by bacteria have become more available in the last decade. These techniques add to our knowledge about the organisms that form biofilms and allow us to study how to eliminate such organisms or prevent them from initiating biofilm formation. Such methods are observations by microscopic techniques (epifluorescence, CLSM, transmission electron, and scanning electron) or enumeration of sessile bacteria after detachment from the surface by scraping, vortexing, sonication, or the use of beads. These methods allow us to get detailed information, but they are laborious and time consuming and thus do not lend themselves to large-scale screening assays. Therefore more rapid and less laborious methods have been devised to evaluate the potential for bacteria to form biofilms in tubes or microtiter wells.

One such rapid method is a colorimetric assay in which a suspension of bacteria is prepared in a culture medium that is then placed in the wells of a microtiter plate or tubes. After incubation for 24 to 48 hours, the medium is removed from the wells and each well is rinsed several times to remove any bacteria not adhering to the sides. After rinsing, a stain, such as crystal violet or safranin, is added. After a specified time, the wells are rinsed several times, and then the wells are evaluated for the presence of stain with a spectrophotometer. The ability of the bacteria to form biofilms is determined by the degree of stain adhering to the bacteria in the wells or tubes after rinsing. Techniques such as this allow for studying the effects an antimicrobial agent might have on the formation of or inhibiting the growth of a biofilm. In a similar method, bacteria are incubated in the presence of silicone disks, and the ability of the bacteria to adhere to the disks is determined by a colorimetric method. The main problem with assays for the detection of biofilms or the potential of bacteria to form biofilms is that the methods have not been standardized; therefore analysis of data from these studies needs to include a critical assessment of the methods used.

POTENTIAL INTERVENTIONS

Because of the physical and chemical properties of biofilms, traditional antimicrobial therapy based on planktonic susceptibility profiles will have limited impact on resilient multispecies biofilms. Therapeutic modalities are refocusing on multiple interventions, recognizing that properties of biofilms are similar to organic polymers, not planktonic microbes.

Establishing biofilms in 96-well plates has allowed for a quantitative measurement of biofilms called *minimal biofilm elimination concentration*. This assay quickly screens biofilms for drug resistance. In theory, disk diffusion antimicrobial testing should be related to antimicrobial resistance testing, and biofilm testing or colonization resistance can be associated with antimicrobial susceptibility testing.

Disruption of the biofilm and its aggregates could have clinical consequences deleterious to the patient. Disaggregation of upregulated phenotypes could be associated with metastasis. Therefore the focus on reducing the bioburden and preventing attachment in the first place should continue. In addressing biofilm eradication, combinations of strategies have been used: (1) mechanical disruption/removal (sonication), (2) immune modulation, and (3) antimicrobial agents (silver and tobramycin). Other recognized schemes are presently employed to address biofilm-associated diseases, although success has been limited.

The effects that a variety of antimicrobials have on the elimination or reduction in the number of organisms in a biofilm or the prevention of biofilms have been studied. Such evaluations have found differences in the results for various antimicrobials when antimicrobials are used alone or in combination. For instance, a comparative analysis of the activities of daptomycin, linezolid, minocycline, tigecycline, and vancomycin used alone and in combination with rifampin against catheter-related methicillin-resistant *Staphylococcus aureus*

(MRSA) bacteremic isolates embedded in biofilm was performed. The study found that when used alone, minocycline, daptomycin, and tigecycline were more efficacious in inhibiting the MRSA in the biofilm than linezolid, vancomycin, and the negative control. Daptomycin by itself was found to be the fastest in eradicating the MRSA biofilm. Rifampin alone was not effective in eliminating the MRSA biofilm; however, when it was used in combination with other antimicrobials it enhanced the performance compared to when the antimicrobials were used alone. This study illustrates the effects antimicrobials may have on a biofilm formed by one specific organism. No generalization can be made at this time, however, about the effect of any one antimicrobial on biofilms formed by different bacteria or co-biofilms.

Another approach to eliminating biofilms uses bacteriophage genetically engineered to express a biofilm-degrading enzyme called *dispersion B* (DspB) to simultaneously attack the bacterial cells in the biofilm and the biofilm matrix (i.e., EPS). Initial studies showed that the engineered phage achieved a 99.9% removal of a biofilm produced by *E. coli* on plastic pegs. This approach removes the need to express, purify, and deliver large doses of enzyme to specific sites of infection, all of which can be difficult. The ultimate evaluation of such a method will be testing in animals and humans to determine its efficacy in elimination of biofilms. This approach is an example of synthetic biology, which over the years has enabled the development of many engineered biologic devices. Synthetic biology is distinguished from traditional genetic engineering through the use of modularity, abstraction, and standardization to allow generalized principles and designs to be applied to different scenarios. This is a true example of applied microbiology.

BIBLIOGRAPHY

Carmen J et al: Treatment of biofilm infections on implants with low-frequency ultrasound and antibiotics, *Am J Infect Control* 33:78, 2005.

Costerton W et al: The application of biofilm science to the study and control of chronic bacterial infections, *J Clin Invest* 112:1466, 2003.

Dave S et al: Resolution of inflammation in periodontitis, *Sci Med* 9:162, 2003.

Donlan RM: Biofilm formation: a clinically relevant microbiological process, *Clin Infect Dis* 33:1387, 2001.

Donlan RM: Biofilms and device-associated infections, *Emerg Infect Dis* 7:277, 2001.

Donlan RM: Biofilms: microbial life on surfaces, *Emerg Infect Dis* 8:881, 2002.

Donlan RM, Costerton JW: Biofilms: survival mechanisms of clinically relevant microorganisms, *Clin Microbiol Rev* 15:167, 2002.

El-Solh AA et al: Colonization of dental plaques: a reservoir of respiratory pathogens for hospital-acquired pneumonia in institutionalized elders, *Chest* 126:1575, 2004.

Foster JS et al: Effects of antimicrobial agents on oral biofilms in a saliva-conditional flowcell, *Biofilms* 1:5, 2004.

Fux CA et al: Bacterial biofilms: a diagnostic and therapeutic challenge, *Expert Rev Anti Infect Ther* 1:667, 2003.

Goeres DM et al: Statistical assessment of a laboratory method for growing biofilms, *Microbiology* 151:757, 2005.

Hall-Stoodley L et al: Bacterial biofilms: from the natural environment to infectious diseases, *Nat Rev Microbiol* 2:95, 2004.

Hall-Stoodley L et al: Direct detection of bacterial biofilms on the middle-ear mucosa of children with chronic otitis media, *JAMA* 296:202, 2006.

Hanna HA et al: Antibiotic-impregnated catheters associated with significant decrease in nosocomial and multidrug-resistant bacteremias in critically ill patients, *Chest* 124:1030, 2003.

Harrison JJ et al: Biofilms: a new understanding of these microbial communities is driving a revolution that may transform the science of microbiology, *Am Scientist* 93:508, 2005.

Jefferson KK: What drives bacteria to produce a biofilm? *FEMS Microbiol Lett* 236:163, 2004.

Kuhn DM et al: Comparison of biofilms formed by *Candida albicans* and *Candida parapsilosis* on bioprosthetic surfaces, *Infect Immun* 70:878, 2002.

Lu TK, Collins JJ: Dispersing biofilms with engineered enzymatic bacteriophage, *Proc Natl Acad Sci U S A* 104:11197, 2007.

Marsh PD: Are dental diseases examples of ecological catastrophes? *Microbiology* 149:279, 2003.

Mermel LA et al: Guidelines for the management of intravascular catheter-related infections, *Clin Infect Dis* 32:1249, 2001.

Murga R et al: Biofilm formation by gram-negative bacteria on central venous catheter connectors: effect of conditioning films in a laboratory model, *J Clin Microbiol* 39:2294, 2001.

Nadell CD et al: The evolution of quorum sensing in bacterial biofilms, *PLoS Biol* 6(1):e14, 2008.

O'Grady NP et al: Guidelines for the prevention of intravascular catheter-related infections, *Infect Control Hosp Epidemiol* 23:759, 2002.

O'Grady NP et al: Guidelines for the prevention of intravascular catheter-related infections, *Clin Infect Dis* 35:1281, 2002.

Raad I et al: Comparative activities of daptomycin, linezolid, and tigecycline against catheter-related methicillin-resistant *Staphylococcus aureus* bacteremic isolates embedded in biofilm, *Antimicrob Agents Chemother* 51:1656, 2007.

Ramage G et al: Inhibition of *Candida albicans* biofilm formation by farnesol, a quorum-sensing molecule, *Appl Environ Microbiol* 68:5459, 2002.

Roberts M, Stewart PS: Modeling protection from antimicrobial agents in biofilms through formation of persister cells, *Microbiology* 151:75, 2005.

Ryder M: The role of biofilm in vascular catheter-related infections, *N Dev Vasc Dis* 2:15, 2001.

Sauer K et al: *Pseudomonas aeruginosa* displays multiple phenotypes during development as a biofilm, *J Bacteriol* 184:1140, 2002.

Saye DE: Recurring and antimicrobial-resistant infections: considering the potential role of biofilms in clinical practice, *Ostomy Wound Manage* 53:46, 2007.

Wilson LS et al: The direct cost and incidence of systemic fungal infections, *Value Health* 5:26, 2002.

Points to Remember

- All microorganisms, including prokaryotes and eukaryotes, have the ability to exist in two phenotypes: planktonic and sessile.
- Biofilms likely evolved as a means of increasing microbial survival.
- Biofilms have unique properties, which are described and quantified by physical and chemical measurements including rheology and viscoelasticity.
- Pathogenicity associated with biofilms is not a total of the individual phenotypes but rather a concert of the entire community of cells. Expression of disease is particularly associated with immunologic cascade and resultant tissue injury with limited microbial injury.
- Staging of biofilms is critical in disease progression, and the ratio of biofilm to planktonic phenotypes is a predictor of virulence or pathogenicity.
- Biofilms are innately more resistant to antimicrobial agents than their individual planktonic counterparts.
- The presence of indwelling medical devices increases the risk for biofilm formation and subsequent infection.
- Many infections in animals follow either monospecies or multispecies biofilm formation.
- Biofilms are not recovered or recognized by standard laboratory protocols, and routine susceptibility testing does not accurately predict the success of antimicrobial therapy for biofilm phenotypes.

Learning Assessment Questions

1. How does the planktonic phenotype differ from the sessile phenotype?
2. Describe the five cycles of biofilm formation.
3. How do biofilms aid microbial attachment to solid surfaces?
4. Describe the structure of a typical mature multispecies biofilm.
5. How do biofilms increase microbial resistance to antimicrobial therapy?
6. List three virulence mechanisms of biofilms.
7. What is the acquired pellicle and what role does it play in dental disease?
8. What is the primary cause of inflammation in gingivitis?
9. Why do indwelling medical devices increase the risk of bacterial infection?
10. List three areas that are of concern for clinical microbiologists when dealing with biofilm-associated microorganisms.
11. Discuss three methods that can be used to study biofilm formation in vitro.
12. Explain why the disruption of a biofilm can have serious consequences to a patient.

PART III

Laboratory Diagnosis of Infectious Diseases: An Organ System Approach to Diagnostic Microbiology

Upper and Lower Respiratory Tract Infections

Preeti Kaur, James L. Cook

OBJECTIVES

After reading and studying this chapter, you should be able to:

1. Describe the basic anatomy of the respiratory tract and explain the mechanical defenses of each anatomic site and how alterations to these defenses may lead to infectious diseases.

2. Define the importance of normal biota in the respiratory tract and explain how alterations in the normal biota may lead to infectious diseases.

3. Discuss the basic pathogenic mechanisms of infectious diseases of the respiratory tract and the virulence factors of the organisms that cause disease.

4. Describe the most common organisms causing various upper and lower respiratory tract infections.

5. Describe the pathogenesis, risk factors, and complications associated with respiratory tract infections as well as the types of specimens collected for diagnosis.

6. Determine the risk factors in immunocompromised hosts that predispose to infections and provide examples of respiratory tract diseases in different types of immunocompromised hosts.

7. Describe the principles and methods of proper specimen collection and transport of respiratory secretions.

8. Discuss the importance of visual examination and proper culturing of respiratory samples.

9. Have an increased awareness of newer and emerging infections.

10. Have a general understanding of agents of bioterrorism as related to respiratory tract infections.

11. Be able to appraise the important aspects of diagnosis of infections of the respiratory tract through case studies.

Case in Point

A 52-year-old woman came to the Emergency Department complaining of right-sided chest pain with each breath, a cough that produced rust-colored sputum, and fever. She reported that her symptoms had begun abruptly the day before with the onset of shaking chills. Examination revealed that the patient had a fever of 102° F (38.8° C) and coarse breath sounds in the right anterior chest. The chest radiograph (see Figure 32-6) showed a right upper lobe infiltrate; the laboratory analysis included an elevated white blood cell count.

Issues to Consider

After reading the patient case history, consider:

- How mechanical and functional changes in the upper and lower compartments of the respiratory tract can lead to infection
- The importance of the normal biota of the respiratory tract in preventing colonization by potential pathogens and how alterations in the normal biota as well as colonization of normally sterile areas may lead to infection
- How microorganism virulence factors relate to the establishment and progression of infection
- Clinical manifestations of upper and lower respiratory tract infections including the pathogenesis, risk factors, and complications of specific disease states
- Infections in normal hosts and how presentations of these infections differ in immunocompromised patients

Key Terms

Acute sinusitis	Epiglottitis
Aspiration pneumonia	Normal biota
Bioterrorism	Nosocomial infection
Bronchiolitis	Opportunistic infection
Bronchitis	Otitis media
Colonization	Pathogenic microorganism
Emerging infections	Pertussis
Empirical antimicrobial	Pharyngitis
therapy	Pneumonia
Empyema	Virulence

This chapter describes respiratory tract infections from the perspective of the clinical microbiologist working with the clinician who must make the differential diagnosis of these infections. General concepts of infectious diseases of the respiratory tract are discussed, including the role of normal microbial biota in preventing infection and the importance of the host immune status in determining the pathogens likely to cause disease. The anatomy of the respiratory tract is outlined, with consideration given to natural barriers of infection. The chapter proceeds with a discussion of specific respiratory tract infections organized according to anatomic site. The etiology, epidemiology, clinical manifestations, pathogenesis, and complications of specific diagnoses are discussed, and emphasis is placed on appropriate methods of laboratory diagnosis. There is a discussion of respiratory tract infections in immunocompromised hosts, including patients who are immunosuppressed as a result of human immunodeficiency virus (HIV) infection. The chapter ends with consideration of respiratory tract infections caused by agents considered to be the most likely to be used in acts of bioterrorism.

GENERAL CONCEPTS OF INFECTIOUS DISEASES OF THE RESPIRATORY TRACT

Anatomy of the Respiratory Tract

The function of the respiratory tract is not only to perform respiration (i.e., the exchange of oxygen and carbon dioxide) but also to deliver air from the outside of the body to the alveoli where gas exchange occurs. Consideration of the anatomy of the respiratory tract (Figure 32-1) must include the entire course that air must travel: from the mouth and nose past the sinuses, into the pharynx, past the epiglottis, through the larynx, into the trachea and bronchi, and eventually into the alveoli. In addition to a role in air transport, each of these areas also plays an important role in defending the respiratory tract from infection.

Barriers to Infection

The respiratory tract has many natural barriers to infection that inhaled organisms must penetrate before they can cause disease. Among the elements of the respiratory tract and its functions that help prevent infection are nasal hair, mucociliary cells that line mucosal surfaces, coughing, **normal biota,** secretory immunoglobulin, defensins, and phagocytic inflammatory cells.

In the nasopharynx and oropharynx, turbulent airflow causes large particles to impact on mucosal surfaces. Nasal hairs filter air as it passes through the nasal passages. Humidification of the air causes hygroscopic particles to increase in size, making it more likely for them to be cleared by mechanical mechanisms of the upper respiratory tract. The normal biota of the nasopharynx and oropharynx helps protect the host by preventing **colonization** by pathogenic organisms. The mucociliary blanket of the sinuses, middle ear, and tracheobronchial tree clears particulate matter and contains immunoglobulin and other antimicrobial substances. In addition, coughing aids in the clearance and expulsion of particulate matter. If particles reach the alveoli, resident macrophages ingest organisms; polymorphonuclear leukocytes and monocytes are recruited once the lung becomes inflamed. Alterations in these barriers may lead to infection. For example, cigarette smoking impairs the ability of the ciliated respiratory epithelium to clear particulate matter and interferes with phagocytic cell activity. Structural abnormalities of the bronchial tree such as bronchiectasis or extrinsic compression of the bronchus by a malignancy can alter clearance of mucus that may contain infectious agents.

The Role of Normal Biota

The normal microbial biota (formerly referred to as *flora*) protects the host from infection with **pathogenic microorgan-**

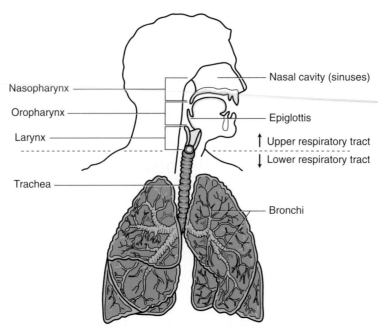

FIGURE 32-1   Anatomy of the respiratory tract.

isms. The normal biota can prevent proliferation and invasion of pathogenic organisms through competition for the same nutrients and the same receptor sites on host cells. In addition, these organisms produce bacteriocins, bacterial products that are toxic to potential pathogens. The presence of these organisms keeps the immune system primed for a rapid response to invading organisms and stimulates cross-protective immune factors known as *natural antibodies*. Under normal conditions, a balance of organisms is maintained that limits the quantity or dominance of any one type of organism.

Although a standard list of organisms can be routinely cultured from the upper respiratory tract (Box 32-1), it is interesting that the consensus concerning what is considered "normal biota" can change with time, as new associations between organisms and disease states are recognized. For example, in past years, *Moraxella catarrhalis* was considered part of the upper respiratory tract biota that was only rarely associated with serious infections. However, since the early 1970s, it has become clear that these organisms can cause respiratory tract infections in children and adults with chronic lung diseases. This indicates the importance of periodic reevaluation of the pathogenicity of all organisms.

Familiarity with the normal biota of respiratory tract compartments is important in determining the clinical relevance of an isolate. For example, isolation of α-hemolytic colonies from a pharyngeal culture from a patient with pharyngitis arouses little clinical interest, because α-hemolytic streptococci are normal biota in the oropharynx. In contrast, isolation of α-hemolytic colonies from a properly collected sputum specimen or bronchial aspirate in the clinical setting of lobar pneumonia should prompt full identification of the organism and perhaps initiation of empirical therapy for possible pneumococcal infection.

BOX 32-1   Common Nasopharyngeal and Oropharyngeal Organisms Isolated in the Normal Host

Bacteria
Usually present
Streptococcus mitis and other α-hemolytic streptococci
Non–group A β-hemolytic streptococci
Streptococcus pneumoniae
Streptococcus pyogenes
Streptococcus salivarius
Veillonella spp.
Bacteroides spp.
Fusobacterium spp.
Prevotella spp.
Porphyromonas spp.
Coagulase-negative staphylococci
Neisseria spp.
Nonhemolytic streptococci
Diphtheroids
Micrococcus spp.
Eikenella spp.
Capnocytophaga spp.

Occasionally present
Haemophilus influenzae
Haemophilus parainfluenzae
Peptostreptococcus
Actinomycetes
Staphylococcus aureus
Mycoplasma

Fungus
Candida spp.

Virus
Herpes simplex

Discriminating Among Normal Biota and Colonizing, and Pathogenic Microorganisms

The upper respiratory tract flora in an asymptomatic patient may change depending on the clinical setting. Patients who have previously received broad-spectrum antibiotics, have been hospitalized recently, or have chronic illnesses may have different pharyngeal biota. Gram-negative bacilli are commonly isolated from the pharynx in such patients in the absence of clinical signs of infection. Therefore it is important to distinguish between a positive culture for an organism that is a potential pathogen that is colonizing the respiratory tract and a clinical disease state caused by that pathogen. Box 32-2 lists organisms that are considered primary pathogens. Also shown are a number of organisms that may or may not be pathogens, depending on the clinical setting (i.e., possible pathogens). In this case, as in many others, proper communication between the clinical microbiologist and the clinician is essential.

Proper respiratory specimen collection improves the sensitivity and specificity of culture results. A high-quality sputum sample that minimizes contamination by oral biota and that is collected before initiation of antibiotic therapy can improve the clinical value of the culture results. Interpretation of the result must be based on several factors. Characteristics of the specimen, such as the presence of white blood cells and the number of organisms in the specimen, can help distinguish between colonization and infection. Most important, a compatible clinical syndrome should be present to determine whether the presence of a potential pathogen is clinically relevant. For example, the isolation of a few colonies of *Staphylococcus aureus* from a sputum specimen with many epithelial cells does not represent *S. aureus* pneumonia, but is more likely to be contamination with an organism that is part of the normal biota of the patient. In contrast, heavy growth of the same organism from a respiratory specimen with many white blood cells from an elderly man with post-influenza pneumonia is highly suggestive of *S. aureus* pneumonia, especially if the sputum culture is accompanied by a positive culture from a normally sterile site such as blood or pleural fluid.

Other organisms are potentially pathogenic and cause disease only when some interruption occurs in the pulmonary defense mechanisms. *Streptococcus pneumoniae* has been isolated from 5% to 70% of the normal adult population, yet only a very small proportion of these carriers will develop pneumococcal pneumonia. Pneumonia may also result from aspiration of upper respiratory tract secretions in patients with impaired pulmonary defenses, such as those with alcoholism or congestive heart failure. Other organisms are always considered pathogenic when isolated, even in small numbers. Isolation of *Mycobacterium tuberculosis* in any amount is significant because of the virulence of the organism and the risk for infection transmission from the infected patient to others.

HOST RISK FACTORS

Immune Status of the Host

The defenses of the host with a suspected infection must be evaluated when determining whether the identification of a specific microorganism is likely to be significant in causing disease. When considering the likelihood that a microorganism will cause infection in a given host, the laboratory professional must consider both the virulence of the organism and the defenses available to the host to counteract establishment and progression of infection. For these purposes, a normal host is considered to be one with mature immunologic defenses who may or may not have specific immunity against the microorganism in question. Examples of microorganisms that cause respiratory tract infections in normal hosts are the common respiratory viruses of childhood. In normal children, these viral infections occur at a high incidence but are relatively benign. The clinical outcomes of these and other respiratory tract infections in normal hosts depend on both the injurious effects of the microorganism and its products at the site of infection and the host immune response to infection.

Previous exposure of a normal host to pathogens such as the respiratory tract viruses is one example in which the host usually develops immunity to reinfection with the same organism. Immune responses may prevent or alter the course of subsequent infection. For example, adults previously infected with a given viral serotype as children usually do not manifest the same severity of infection when re-exposed to the same pathogen. Evidence of infection may not be present, or clinical signs and symptoms of infection are greatly reduced. In

---

BOX 32-2   Selected Nonviral Pathogens in the Respiratory Tract

Primary Pathogens

Streptococcus pneumoniae
Group A β-hemolytic streptococci
Neisseria meningitidis
Neisseria gonorrhoeae
Bordetella pertussis
Mycobacterium kansasii
Mycobacterium tuberculosis
Legionella pneumophila
Toxin-producing *Corynebacterium diphtheriae*
Mycoplasma pneumoniae
Chlamydia trachomatis
Chlamydophila pneumoniae
Pneumocystis jiroveci (carinii)

Possible Pathogens

Acinetobacter spp.
Enterics and other gram-negative bacilli
Fungi
Nocardia spp.
Staphylococcus aureus
Haemophilus influenzae
β-Hemolytic streptococci, non–group A
Moraxella catarrhalis
Anaerobes
Mycobacterium spp.
Actinomycetes

an immunocompromised host, however, microorganisms that are usually not pathogens in a normal host may cause serious infection. This type of infection is referred to as an **opportunistic infection** to indicate a combination of a reduced host response and a pathogen of low virulence that results in the establishment of infection. Of course, organisms exhibiting high levels of virulence also cause disease in immunocompromised hosts. Because the host response is diminished, infections with virulent pathogens are usually more severe and more rapidly progressive than in the normal host.

Age as a Risk Factor

Immunocompromise by reason of age is a form of functional immunodeficiency. Infants and the elderly are more susceptible to certain respiratory tract infections and are more likely to develop complications of these infections. For example, respiratory tract infections with *Haemophilus influenzae* are more commonly complicated by meningitis in infants than in older children or adults. Similarly, in the elderly, complications of common respiratory tract infections occur more frequently than in the younger adult population. One hallmark of seasonal outbreaks of influenza virus infection of the respiratory tract is the increased incidence of death from complicating bacterial pneumonias in the elderly.

It is apparent from these observations that one cannot determine the significance of a respiratory tract microbial isolate without considering the source of the specimen, the age and immunologic status of the host, and the clinical setting of the patient. The isolation of an organism that has potential to cause disease may represent either simple colonization of the upper respiratory tract or life-threatening disease. In contrast, isolation of a nonpathogenic organism that may be part of the normal biota of the upper respiratory tract may be an indication of disease if it is found in an unusual location or in a host with decreased defenses against infection. Availability of proper clinical data facilitates proper evaluation of the respiratory tract specimen by the clinical microbiologist.

Reduced Clearance of Secretions

In addition to the compromising factor of age, reduced clearance of secretions or obstruction of an area in either the upper or the lower respiratory tract predispose one to infection and can, on occasion, seriously compromise respiratory tract function. Mechanical clearance is important in limiting the numbers of potential pathogens and in the associated inflammatory response. Decreased clearance of respiratory secretions may result from the following:
- Immature anatomic development (e.g., eustachian tube anatomy in young children)
- Transient reduction in function of the mucociliary mechanism (e.g., after viral infection, as a result of cigarette smoking)
- Obstruction by a foreign body (e.g., aspirated food or foreign object)
- Previous disease that alters the normal respiratory tract anatomy (e.g., bronchiectasis; obstructing lymph node or tumor)
- Alterations in the viscosity of mucus (e.g., cystic fibrosis)

Infection-Induced Airway Obstruction

Another way in which respiratory tract obstruction can be a factor in infectious disease involves compromise of respiration. In these cases, the obstruction may be a consequence of infection, rather than the factor that precipitates infection. The anatomy of the area, rather than the type of pathogen, dictates the urgency with which treatment is initiated. An example of this type of respiratory tract infection is acute epiglottitis (see below) caused by infection of a nonimmune patient with *H. influenzae*. This inflammatory response to bacterial infection can cause life-threatening upper airway obstruction and is considered a medical emergency. In contrast, other infections caused by the same pathogen, such as sinusitis, can be treated more deliberately.

Seasonal and Community Trends in Infections

Awareness of the patterns of respiratory tract infections at different times of the year within the community in which the patient resides is important for the efficient use of diagnostic microbiology resources. Certain types of respiratory tract infections have peak seasonal incidences and may occur in epidemics in the community. Viral respiratory tract infections, for example, are more common in the fall and winter months. Therefore if influenza virus infection is epidemic in the community and a patient presents with symptoms and signs compatible with this viral illness, the likelihood is high that influenza is the cause of the infection. In such cases, performing extensive bacterial cultures to define the cause of the respiratory tract infection may be a wasteful use of resources.

In contrast, diseases associated with *Mycoplasma pneumoniae* typically occur throughout the year, without marked seasonal variability. The incidence of viral infections and secondary bacterial pneumonias is reduced during the summer months; therefore *M. pneumoniae* may cause as many as 50% of all pneumonias in the summer months. Communication among clinical microbiologists, physicians interested in infectious diseases, and state health department personnel with the purpose of sharing information on community trends in the pathogens causing respiratory tract infections helps focus diagnostic and therapeutic efforts.

Empirical Antimicrobial Therapy

To properly position the diagnostic microbiology laboratory in the scheme of the patient's care plan, it is important to understand the role of **empirical antimicrobial therapy** in the care of patients with respiratory tract infections. Although basing antimicrobial therapy on the results of diagnostic microbiologic studies is desirable, certain circumstances dictate that therapy be initiated before obtaining these results or even without submitting specimens for culture. For example, antimicrobial therapy should be initiated before obtaining microbial identification and susceptibility testing results in patients who are seriously ill with pneumonia. In some types of respiratory tract infections, it is standard to initiate antimicrobial therapy without obtaining any specimens for culture. This is the procedure in the case of a child who has a bacterial middle ear infection (otitis media). It can be predicted that the pathogen will usually be *S. pneumoniae, H. influenzae,* or *M. catarrhalis.* Considering the difficulty of obtaining cultures directly from the middle ear and the knowledge of the likely pathogens, treatment without obtaining cultures is reasonable. If treatment fails, then it may be necessary to do an invasive procedure to obtain specimens to test for antibiotic-resistant or unexpected pathogens. This same rationale applies to other respiratory tract sites that are difficult to culture directly, such as the sinuses.

When empirical antimicrobial therapy is necessary, it is important to have a working knowledge of the organisms most likely to cause the type of infection observed and of the antibiotics that are most likely to be effective. The microbiology laboratory can provide preliminary data on the possible identity of the pathogen, based upon Gram staining results and preliminary biochemical studies (e.g., lactose fermentation). If the infection is hospital-acquired (so-called **nosocomial infection**), it is important to know whether the antimicrobial susceptibility patterns of the infectious agent in question differ from those found in the community. Periodic reviews of bacterial antibiotic susceptibility patterns are published by clinical microbiology services to facilitate this type of decision-making process. These are called "antibiograms" for the specific institution. Empirical use of antibiotics and adjustment of therapy based on the results of subsequent microbiologic data represent other important interactions between the clinician and the clinical microbiologist.

VIRULENCE FACTORS OF PATHOGENIC ORGANISMS

The disease-producing capability of an organism is the clinical manifestation of its **virulence.** Microorganisms cause infection by entering the host, interacting with specific target tissues, evading the host's defenses, proliferating, damaging the host, and disseminating or elaborating products that cause systemic disease. Virulence factors involved in disease-producing mechanisms, such as adherence, toxin elaboration, and host evasion, enable the microorganism to complete this process.

Adherence

Attachment of the microorganism to the host tissue is a primary step in the pathogenic process of infection. Attachment is made possible by adhesins or other microbial surface molecules or organelles that bind the organism to a host surface. Specific bacterial adhesins interact with specific cellular receptors. Streptococci, for example, possess fimbriae, which are fine, irregular structures composed of M protein and lipoteichoic acid that bind to epithelial cells. Enterobacteriaceae such as *Escherichia coli* also use fimbriae to adhere to host cells.

Toxin Elaboration

Microorganisms may elaborate toxins that produce different pathogenic effects, depending on the activity of the toxin and the target cell it interacts with in the host. For example, *Corynebacterium diphtheriae* produces an ADP-ribosylating toxin that interferes with protein synthesis. Locally, the toxin induces necrosis, resulting in a "pseudomembrane" composed of necrotic respiratory epithelial cells, leukocytes, and organisms. This pseudomembrane can cause airway obstruction. Systemically, the toxin preferentially adheres to myocardial, nerve, and kidney tissue, causing myocarditis, neuritis, and renal tubular necrosis. The mechanism of action of *Pseudomonas* exotoxin A is similar to that of diphtheria toxin, but it has a different pathogenic effect because of the different target tissue and the involvement of other virulence factors. Another example of the role of toxins is provided by those produced by *Bordetella pertussis.* One is an adenylate cyclase toxin that enters target cells and increases intracellular cAMP levels, causing cell damage or cell death. Another is the pertussis toxin, which interrupts the transduction of signals from cell surface receptors to intracellular systems. During the paroxysmal phase of the illness when patients develop the characteristic whooping cough, the clinical signs and symptoms are attributed to toxin elaborated by the organism.

Evasion of Host Defenses

Evasion of host defenses enables microorganisms to proliferate and cause damage to the host. Certain respiratory pathogens, such as *S. pneumoniae, H. influenzae,* and mucoid *Pseudomonas aeruginosa,* evade host defenses by expressing polysaccharide capsules that prevent phagocytosis by host leukocytes. *Chlamydiae* are obligate intracellular parasites that are taken up by host cells, where they are protected from the host immune system. *M. tuberculosis,* another intracellular pathogen, survives by inhibiting phagosome-lysosome fusion. Other respiratory pathogens are able to cleave host secretory antibody by producing immunoglobulin A (IgA)–specific proteases.

BODY SITE INFECTIONS

UPPER RESPIRATORY TRACT INFECTIONS

Pharyngitis

> **Case Study**
>
> An 8-year-old girl was brought to an Emergency Department by her mother because the child was complaining of a sore throat and a low-grade fever. The mother stated that the girl had had a runny nose and cough for the last few days. On examination, the patient had a temperature of 99° F (37.2° C). Her pharynx was red, and her tonsils were slightly swollen, but no exudates were present. A neck examination revealed no tender lymph nodes.

Etiology

Table 32-1 summarizes the clinical syndromes encountered in the upper respiratory tract and the associated etiologic agents. The most commonly encountered etiologic agent of bacterial **pharyngitis** is group A streptococci. Identified in 15% to 30% of microbial isolates in school-aged children who present with pharyngitis, group A streptococci are isolated much less frequently in adults with a similar presentation (less than 10%

TABLE 32-1 Upper Respiratory Tract Infections

Clinical Syndrome	Causative Agents	Specimen Collection	Other
Pharyngitis	Group A streptococci (children), viral (adults)	Swab tonsils and posterior pharynx, and place in transport media; do not allow to dry; viral cultures not necessary	Culture for *Neisseria gonorrhoeae* or *Corynebacterium diphtheriae* if clinically indicated
Sinusitis	Most common: Rhinovirus Parainfluenza virus Influenza virus Less common: *Streptococcus pneumoniae* *Haemophilus influenzae*	Direct sinus sampling	Direct sampling indicated for patients who fail empirical therapy or who are severely ill or immunocompromised, or if unusual pathogen is suspected
Otitis media	Most common: *S. pneumoniae* *H. influenzae* Less common: *Streptococcus pyogenes* *Moraxella catarrhalis* *Staphylococcus aureus*	Direct culture by tympanocentesis	Direct culture indicated for patients who are severely ill or immunocompromised, or if unusual pathogen is suspected
Epiglottitis	Most common: *H. influenzae* type B Less common: *H. influenzae* type A and nontypable strains *Haemophilus parainfluenzae* Streptococci Staphylococci	Direct swab of epiglottis, blood cultures	Direct swab should be performed only if airway is secure
Pertussis	Most common: *Bordetella pertussis* *Bordetella parapertussis* Less common: *Bordetella bronchiseptica* Adenovirus	Nasopharyngeal swab: a. Plate directly onto Bordet-Gengou medium b. Direct fluorescent antibody stain c. Adenovirus shell vial culture for antigen detection	—

of microbial isolates). Most cases of pharyngitis are viral in origin and occur as part of the symptom complex of a common cold or an early case of influenza. The presence of exudates in the pharynx, fever, and painful adenopathy, or the lack of a cough, would suggest pharyngitis caused by *Streptococcus pyogenes*. This can be diagnosed by throat culture or rapid antigen tests. In certain cases of presumed viral pharyngitis, a specific pathogen can be isolated. However, many cases of pharyngitis do not have an identifiable pathogen. Cases of pharyngitis caused by unusual pathogens such as *Neisseria gonorrhoeae*, *Corynebacterium diphtheriae*, or other bacterial pathogens are suspected in patients with suggestive histories or in cases of pharyngitis refractory to conventional therapy.

Epidemiology

Most pharyngeal infections occur during the winter and early spring. The increase in person-to-person contact during these seasons favors transmission of the causative pathogens. The pathogens are usually inoculated by contamination of the hands and then gain entrance into the upper respiratory tract.

Clinical Manifestations

Clinically, differentiation between viral and streptococcal pharyngitis is difficult. With most cases of viral pharyngitis, symptoms of a common cold, including rhinorrhea, are

present, which is uncommon with streptococcal pharyngitis. Pharyngitis associated with influenza virus infection is accompanied by more numerous and more severe systemic symptoms, including fever, myalgias, and more profound fatigue. In contrast, other forms of viral pharyngitis that are associated with infectious mononucleosis are more commonly accompanied by cervical and generalized lymphadenopathy and enlargement of the spleen.

Streptococcal pharyngitis is associated with marked pharyngeal pain and difficulty in swallowing. Fever is more commonly a major component of the illness with streptococcal than with viral infection. In typical cases, a thick exudate covers the tonsils and posterior pharynx, which is uncommon in viral pharyngitis. It is important to realize, however, that documented streptococcal pharyngitis may also present in a manner that is indistinguishable from that of viral pharyngitis. Another uncommon form of pharyngitis is that seen in diphtheria caused by infection with *C. diphtheriae*. This is a highly contagious and potentially fatal form of bacterial pharyngitis transmitted through close contact with the infected patient or with bioaerosols from infected patients. It is classically associated with the presence of a tightly adherent pharyngeal membrane ("pseudomembrane") that attaches to the respiratory surfaces. Diphtheria is now uncommon in the United States and most of the developed world because of the widespread use of diphtheria-pertussis-tetanus (DPT) vaccination. This infection should be suspected in patient populations that have not received DPT vaccination; for example, in patients from developing countries and underserved U.S. populations, where vaccination rates are low.

Pathogenesis

The reasons for the symptom complex in patients with viral or streptococcal pharyngitis are incompletely understood. Some viruses (e.g., adenoviruses) that infect the pharyngeal mucosa cause cellular destruction (cytopathology) and all such agents elicit inflammatory cell responses. The combination of these events is responsible for the pharyngeal pain and swelling experienced by patients with pharyngitis. However, in other cases, the viral pathogens (e.g., rhinoviruses) cause symptoms of pharyngitis with little mucosal cell destruction. In some cases, these noncytopathic viruses have been shown to elicit production of inflammatory mediators that can reproduce the symptoms of pharyngitis.

The pathogenesis of streptococcal pharyngitis may be caused mainly by the inflammatory effects of a variety of extracellular products elaborated by the streptococci. These products exhibit a variety of activities, including toxicity to a variety of cells, pyrogenicity, and enhancement of the spread of streptococci through infected tissues.

Complications

Other than the infrequent problem of upper airway obstruction associated with severe, soft tissue swelling, few complications can be attributed directly to either bacterial or viral pharyngitis. The occasional complications of viral infections associated with pharyngitis usually are due to systemic manifestations of the infections or to secondary bacterial infections such as sinusitis, otitis media, or pneumonia. Displacement of either or both of the tonsils or asymmetric swelling of the soft tissues of the pharynx following pharyngitis should raise suspicion of peritonsillar or pharyngeal abscess. Although group A streptococci have often been associated with these soft-tissue infections, oral anaerobic bacteria should also be considered in the differential diagnosis.

Laboratory Diagnosis

Specimen Collection. The primary goal of obtaining cultures in most cases of acute pharyngitis is to differentiate streptococcal pharyngitis from more common cases of viral pharyngitis. A secondary goal is to be able to detect the uncommon causes of bacterial pharyngitis (e.g., diphtheria, gonorrhea) in cases in which the clinical history is suggestive or symptoms are persistent.

In collecting pharyngeal specimens for streptococcal cultures (Figure 32-2), it is important to vigorously swab the tonsillar areas and the posterior pharynx. The tongue and other oral structures should be avoided with the swab to minimize contamination with oral biota and dilution of the specimen. If any tonsillar exudate is seen, specific efforts should be made to directly swab the areas in which it is present. After collecting the specimen, swabs may be placed in transport medium.

Direct Microscopic Examination. Direct microscopic examination of pharyngeal secretions is not useful for clinical

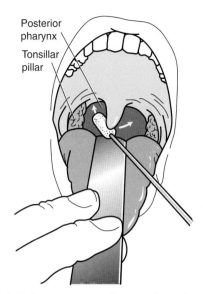

FIGURE 32-2 Specimen collection from the throat.

or laboratory diagnosis. Because respiratory exudates contain a wide variety of organisms, a direct Gram stain will not differentiate suspected pathogens from normal microbial biota.

Culture. Culture of the pharyngeal area will isolate bacterial pathogens such as β-hemolytic group A streptococci. A nonselective medium such as sheep blood agar (SBA) is commonly used. The addition of a selective medium containing an antimicrobial agent, such as sulfamethoxazole trimethoprim, may enhance the isolation of β-hemolytic streptococci.

Other Methods. Latex agglutination, coagglutination tests, and enzyme immunoassays have been introduced into clinical practice to rapidly detect group A streptococci directly from throat swabs. Currently available rapid antigen detection testing methods (RADTs) are highly specific (greater than 95% compared with conventional culture). False-positive test results are unusual; therefore therapeutic decisions can be made with confidence on the basis of a positive test result. Unfortunately, the sensitivity of RADTs is low—80% to 90% or lower. Negative results of specimens obtained from children and adolescents should generally be followed up by a conventional culture unless the laboratory is able to confirm that the RADT it uses has demonstrated sensitivity similar to that of throat culture. On the other hand, because of the low incidence of streptococcal infection in adults, negative RADT results on specimens obtained from adults need not be followed up with further culture testing.

Treatment. The goals of antibiotic treatment of streptococcal pharyngitis include amelioration of the symptoms, limitation of transmission of the infection to contacts (especially in school-aged children), and prevention of the serious complications of acute rheumatic fever and acute glomerulonephritis. Antibiotics such as penicillin or cephalosporins are commonly used and are highly effective. Other antibiotics that are effective and can be used in patients allergic to penicillin are macrolides, such as erythromycin, clarithromycin, and azithromycin. Ancillary treatment such as analgesics, saline gargles, and lozenges can provide symptomatic relief. With the exception of disease caused by influenza (for which there is specific antiviral therapy), viral pharyngitis, which is much more common than streptococcal pharyngitis, can currently be treated only with supportive management, pending development of effective antiviral agents.

Sinusitis

> ### Case Study
>
> A 40-year-old woman went to the doctor's office complaining of fever and nasal drainage. She stated that she had developed cold symptoms 1 week earlier and had been treating herself with over-the-counter medicines with little improvement. In fact, she had gotten worse over the last 48 hours with increasing headache and left face pain. The physical examination was notable for low-grade fever and tenderness over the left maxillary sinus as well as purulent drainage in the left side of the nose. Sinus radiographs showed an air-fluid level in the left maxillary sinus.

Etiology

A viral infection associated with the common cold is the most frequent etiology of **acute sinusitis,** a disease that results from the infection of one or more of the paranasal sinuses. Only a small percentage (up to 2%) of viral sinusitis is complicated by acute bacterial infection. Common viruses causing acute sinusitis include rhinovirus, parainfluenza, and influenza viruses. *S. pneumoniae* and *H. influenzae* are the bacterial pathogens identified historically as the most common causes of community-acquired infections in both adults and children. Introduction of *H. influenzae* type B vaccine has essentially eliminated this pathogen as a public health problem in children. *S. pyogenes, M. catarrhalis,* and *S. aureus* account for most of the other pathogens commonly associated with sinusitis. In hospital-acquired infections, *S. aureus* and gram-negative bacilli are recovered more frequently. The incidence of *M. catarrhalis* as a pathogen in acute sinusitis is much higher in children than in adults.

Acute fungal sinusitis is uncommon in normal patients; it occurs predominantly in immunosuppressed hosts treated with cytotoxic or immunosuppressive drugs or in patients with severe underlying illnesses such as uncontrolled diabetes mellitus. In contrast, chronic fungal colonization or sinusitis usually occurs in immunocompetent hosts in the clinical setting of other forms of chronic sinusitis (e.g., allergic sinusitis).

Epidemiology

The incidence of acute sinusitis follows that of other upper respiratory tract infections, occurring predominantly in the winter and spring months. The clinical diagnosis of acute sinusitis is less common in children than in adults, in part because of the incomplete development of most of the paranasal sinuses until adolescence.

Clinical Manifestations

The presentation of acute sinusitis in older children and adults is often that of a prolonged respiratory tract infection that involves a set of symptoms that are subtly different from those present early in the course of the illness. The most constant features include purulent nasal discharge and pain in the face. When the maxillary sinus is involved, facial pain is worse when leaning forward or when a jarring force is experienced, such as walking down stairs. Patients with maxillary sinusitis may also experience headache and pain that is perceived to come from the upper teeth. Fever is present in only about half the patients with acute sinusitis. In hospitalized patients, sinusitis can result from obstruction of the sinus openings (ostia) by indwelling nasal tubes.

In young children, the only symptoms observed may be persistent rhinorrhea and cough either directly after a viral upper respiratory tract infection or following a brief period of clinical improvement after such an infection. Ear examination is frequently abnormal in these children, with either middle ear infection or sterile fluid behind the tympanic membrane (serous otitis media). This involvement of the middle ear in young patients with sinusitis probably reflects the common problem of drainage obstruction in these two anatomic areas. In young children with signs and symptoms of persistent sinusitis, foreign bodies in the nose must always be considered. The most sensitive test for the routine diagnosis of acute and chronic sinusitis in adult patients is computed tomography (Figure 32-3). Computed tomography (CT) and magnetic resonance imaging (MRI) are clearly superior to plain radiographs for detailed analysis of the anatomy of the paranasal sinuses and are especially useful for studies of the ethmoid and sphenoid sinuses, which are difficult to image using plain films.

Pathogenesis

Acute sinusitis is usually a complication of common colds or other viral infections of the upper respiratory tract. Respiratory allergies also predispose individuals to acute sinusitis. When recurrent infectious sinusitis is associated with recurrent pulmonary infection over prolonged periods, it should suggest the possibility of cystic fibrosis, hypogammaglobulinemia, or ciliary dysfunction.

Obstruction is another predisposing factor in sinusitis. The sinuses normally undergo a continuous cleansing process through the action of ciliated epithelial cells. These ciliated epithelial cells move the mucous layer lining these areas toward the sinus ostia. This process normally clears the sinuses of bacteria from the adjacent nasopharynx. During acute rhinosinusitis, whether of viral or allergic origin, mucosal swelling may cause partial or complete obstruction of these sinus ostia, interrupting the flow of secretions and predisposing to bacterial overgrowth behind the obstruction. The function of the normal ciliated epithelial cells (altered by viral infection and bacterial toxins) and the viscosity of the mucous layer (which may be increased by the exudation and inflammation associated with infection or allergic reactions) may also be altered so that the clearance of sinus secretions is less efficient. Other processes that may limit normal drainage from the sinuses include foreign bodies, tumors, and congenital structural abnormalities of the nasopharynx. Nasotracheal tubes in hospitalized patients in respiratory failure and packing materials used during surgical procedures provide other forms of obstruction to normal sinus drainage that predispose to infection. Falling oxygen concentration has also been implicated in the pathogenesis of infectious sinus-

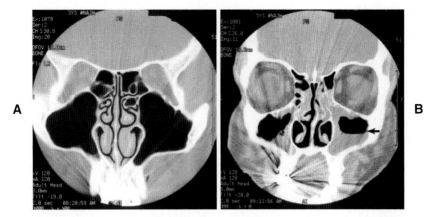

FIGURE 32-3 Computed tomography of the paranasal sinuses in a patient with normal maxillary sinuses **(A)** and in a patient with bilateral maxillary sinusitis **(B)**. **A,** The large (black) cavities on either side of the nasopharynx are the normal maxillary sinuses. Of note is the absence of thickening of the lining and the absence of any opacity within the cavity of the maxillary sinuses. **B,** The difference in the maxillary sinuses compared with image **A** is the presence of opacification in both maxillary sinuses. This opacification represents pus within the sinuses. The maxillary sinus on the right side of the figure also demonstrates an air-fluid level (the relatively straight, horizontal line between the air-filled black space above and the gray, fluid-filled space below *[arrow]*) that is characteristic of acute, purulent sinusitis.

itis. With obstruction of the sinus ostium, the partial pressure of oxygen in the sinus cavity falls, impairing the function of inflammatory cells and facilitating the growth of facultative and true anaerobic bacteria. After repeated bouts of acute sinusitis, the ciliated epithelium may be replaced by squamous epithelium, compromising the normal movement of the sinus mucous layer. This usually results in colonization of the chronically inflamed sinus with aerobic and anaerobic bacteria that are not present in the healthy sinus. The importance of this colonization in chronic sinusitis remains uncertain. It is generally believed that the presence of this colonization does not warrant treatment and that acute flare-ups of chronic sinusitis should be managed essentially the same as acute sinusitis in patients without chronic disease.

Complications

Complications of acute sinusitis result from extension of the infection to adjacent areas or structures. These complications include orbital cellulitis, osteomyelitis, meningitis, brain abscess, and cavernous sinus thrombosis.

Orbital cellulitis or retroorbital abscess can result from direct extension of infection from adjacent sinuses to the area around and behind the eye. Protrusion of the eye (proptosis) or limitation of ocular movements should suggest the possibility of extension of the infection to the retroorbital space. This is a serious complication that requires aggressive diagnosis and emergency management. Extension of frontal sinusitis can cause cellulitis in the area of the forehead overlying these sinuses. Osteomyelitis (infection of the bone) of the frontal bone, referred to as *Pott's puffy tumor,* also may develop. Further extension of frontal sinusitis may cause an abscess of the frontal lobes of the brain, a serious complication that is difficult to diagnose. Extension of infection from other sinuses (e.g., ethmoid, sphenoid) to the central nervous system (CNS) in the form of meningitis, brain abscess, or

cavernous sinus thrombosis is difficult to diagnose because of the deep location of these sinuses. Suspicion of such severe complications must remain high in patients who appear to have refractory sinusitis in the setting of altered mental status. In cases in which the adjacent bone is involved as in osteomyelitis, active sinusitis can complicate the interpretation of diagnostic radiologic studies. These complications can make the diagnosis difficult. It is usually necessary to follow serial studies of bone inflammation and integrity during therapy of sinusitis to establish the diagnosis of this complication.

Laboratory Diagnosis

Specimen Collection. The gold standard for making a microbial diagnosis of sinus infection is direct sinus puncture and aspiration. This invasive and potentially painful procedure is not appropriate for use in routine medical practice. Sinus aspirate culture should, however, be considered if there is a suspicion of intracranial extension of the infection, if patients have failed empirical antimicrobial therapy, or if the patient is severely ill or immunocompromised. Cultures of nasal secretions or of nasal swabs are unreliable indicators of the pathogen causing acute infection within the sinus, and most professionals agree that randomly collected cultures from the nasopharynx of either adult or pediatric patients are of no value in defining the bacterial cause of this disease.

Direct Microscopic Examination. Gram stain preparations are useful only for sinus specimens obtained by direct aspiration from the sinus ostia or from sinus puncture. In these cases, finding a predominant bacterial type can be of diagnostic and therapeutic value.

Culture. As mentioned previously, culture of sinus aspirations is useful only when performed on specimens obtained by sinus puncture or by direct aspiration of purulent secretions from sinus ostia. In these cases, samples are inoculated on culture media such as sheep blood (SBA), chocolate (CHOC), and MacConkey (MAC) agar, which are routinely used to isolate respiratory tract pathogens.

Treatment. Most symptoms of sinusitis resolve spontaneously in 1 to 2 weeks, especially if caused by infection with a nonbacterial pathogen, and there is no problem of sinus obstruction. However, antibiotics may need to be considered if the symptoms persist for more than 2 weeks and patients become symptomatic with facial swelling, facial pain, fever, and purulent discharge. Antibiotic choices may include amoxicillin, cephalosporins, macrolides, or fluoroquinolones, depending upon the clinical setting and history of previous antibiotic therapy or hospitalization. Supportive medications include nasal/oral decongestants and nasal saline sprays. In cases of empiric treatment failure, endoscopic or transantral specimen collection may be needed for Gram stain and culture to help guide antibiotic choice.

Otitis Media

Etiology

Otitis media is an infection of the middle ear that is an important cause of upper airway infection in the pediatric population. As in the case of acute sinusitis, the microbial etiology of the average case of acute otitis media has been clearly defined by cultures of infected middle ear specimens obtained by direct aspiration from the area. Considering the similarities in their pathogenesis, it is not surprising that the same group of pathogens is involved in both acute otitis media and acute sinusitis. *S. pneumoniae* and *H. influenzae* account for more than 50% of the isolates from cases of acute otitis media. *S. pyogenes, M. catarrhalis,* and *S. aureus* have also been implicated in this disease. In patients who have received multiple courses of broad-spectrum antibiotics for acute otitis media (or other infections), those who have tympanic membrane perforations or those with severe underlying disease, acute otitis media is more likely to be caused by gram-negative pathogens.

The analogy with the etiology of acute sinusitis also extends to the role of viruses in acute otitis media. Because most cases of acute otitis media occur on the heels of a viral infection of the upper respiratory tract, it is not surprising that viruses can be isolated from cultures from the middle ears of these patients. The most frequently isolated viruses are respiratory syncytial virus (RSV), rhinovirus, influenza viruses, and adenoviruses. Other possible causes of acute otitis media should be considered in unusual cases or circumstances. Theoretically, other pathogens that infect the upper and lower respiratory tract, such as *Mycoplasma pneumoniae* and *Chlamydia trachomatis,* can cause acute otitis media. However, the association between these potential pathogens and the average case of middle ear infection is not clear. In newborns, group B streptococci and gram-negative bacilli can be added to *S. pneumoniae* and *H. influenzae* as causes of occasional cases of acute otitis media. Acute otitis media occurs less often than acute sinusitis in the presence of nasal tubes in hospitalized patients with eustachian tube obstruction. Gram-negative bacillary pathogens are isolated more often in the hospital setting than in community-acquired acute otitis media.

Epidemiology

Otitis media is the most common localized infection of the upper respiratory tract in preschool-age patients. One study showed that almost one third of all visits by preschool children to pediatricians involved diseases of the middle ear. The increased incidence of these infections in preschoolers has been attributed to the crowding of susceptible hosts in daycare centers. In older children and adults, the syndrome of middle ear infection, although less common, is still a major precipitant of outpatient office visits during the winter and spring seasons, when viral respiratory infections are common.

Clinical Manifestations

Early signs and symptoms of acute otitis media may be nonlocalized, especially in young children. In these cases, fever and irritability may be the only signs of illness. In older children, tugging at the involved ear may be noticed during or at the end of the course of an upper respiratory tract infection. Other symptoms include ear pain, changes in hearing, and late in the course of the infection, drainage of purulent secretions from the ear canal, associated with perforation of the tympanic membrane. On direct examination of the tympanic membrane, the presence of acute otitis media may be indicated by a red, bulging membrane. However, the changes in the membrane are often more subtle. In these cases, it is important to perform pneumatic otoscopy to identify any evidence of fluid or pus behind the tympanic membrane, as evidenced by its reduced or absent movement in response to changes in air pressure in the canal.

Pathogenesis

The eustachian tube, which is the canal that links the middle ear to the nasopharynx, is shorter and travels a more direct course from the nasopharynx to the middle ear in young children than in older children and adults. This anatomic immaturity appears to predispose young patients to easier contamination of the middle ear with nasopharyngeal bacteria. This factor, coupled with the greater incidence of viral respiratory tract infections in preschool-age children, may explain the greater incidence of acute otitis media in this population.

Both the eustachian tube and the middle ear are lined with ciliated epithelium and mucus-secreting cells. This creates a situation similar to that seen in the paranasal sinuses, where a mucous layer clearance mechanism can defend against invasion and overgrowth of nasopharyngeal organisms. When this function is altered or impaired, infection may develop. Suppurative otitis media may result from relative or absolute obstruction of this drainage mechanism as a consequence of obstruction of the eustachian tube. Edema of the eustachian tube mucosa resulting from viral infections is much like the swelling that is induced around the ostia of the sinuses. Similarly, viral infections can cause impairment of the cleansing function of the ciliated epithelium of the eustachian tube–middle ear complex. In a manner similar to that associated with viral infection, the eustachian tube edema associated with allergic nasopharyngitis can cause obstruction and predispose to postobstructive infection of the middle ear. Infection behind the obstruction, regardless of the nature of the precipitating cause, can cause tissue damage that may affect hearing and can, if therapy is inadequate, lead to progressive infection of adjacent structures.

Complications

Progression of acute otitis media may lead to damage of the tympanic membrane and other associated problems that follow this destructive process. Tympanic membrane damage with subsequent hearing loss can have devastating effects on the speech development and education of young children, but it may be of less consequence in adults. A membrane perforation may heal without long-term effects on hearing or may become chronic, depending on the size of the perforation and the frequency of reinfection. If the perforation destroys crucial areas in the membrane, surgical correction may be necessary to close the perforation and restore membrane function. The necessity of such a procedure depends on multiple factors, the most important of which is the age of the patient. Unfortunately, most such complications occur in children who do not obtain adequate early medical care. Similar considerations apply to the approach to chronic adhesive changes in the repeatedly infected, but intact, tympanic membrane and chronic middle ear effusions (serous otitis media).

Acute mastoiditis is an uncommon complication of acute otitis media in the antibiotic era. As a result, surgical treatment (mastoidectomy) to prevent progressive disease and extension to the CNS is a rare procedure in modern practice. All the considerations discussed under acute sinusitis concerning the spread of infection to adjacent areas also apply to acute otitis media that goes untreated. Local extension of infection and spread to the CNS are potential problems. These problems are encountered less commonly in the antibiotic era in most clinical settings. However, in situations in which access to health care is limited for any reason, such severe late complications of middle ear infection must be considered.

Laboratory Diagnosis

Because the predominant pathogens for acute otitis media are known, obtaining specimens for culture before initiating therapy is unnecessary in the average case. If the patient is seriously ill or immunocompromised and likely to have rapidly progressive disease or if an unusual or drug-resistant organism is suspected, direct culture by tympanocentesis is indicated. As with acute sinusitis, probably no value exists in culturing the nasopharynx as an indicator of the type of pathogen that may be present in the middle ear.

Treatment

Antibiotic treatment is considered to be more important in children less than 2 years of age than for older children or adults, in which case observation maybe an option if disease is not severe. The initial drug of choice is high-dose amoxicillin. Failure to respond to this regimen may indicate a resistant organism as the possible pathogen, such as penicillin-resistant

pneumococci or β-lactamase-producing *Haemophilus* or *Moraxella*. Alternative antibiotics that may be indicated in such situations include amoxicillin-clavulanic acid, cephalosporins, macrolides, or fluoroquinolones (although the latter drug class is not generally approved for use in children). Ancillary therapy, including measures to relieve eustachian tube obstruction and treatment of associated symptoms should also be considered.

Epiglottitis

Case Study

A 4-year-old boy who immigrated recently with his parents from Mexico and who had not received his routine childhood vaccinations was brought to the pediatrician's office with a 6-hour history of fever and trouble swallowing. Inspiratory stridor was noted by the pediatrician. The patient was immediately taken to the Emergency Department, where the epiglottis was visualized, after assurance of airway protection, and noted to be red and edematous.

The epiglottis is a cartilaginous structure positioned at the anterior aspect of the opening of the trachea. It normally protects the airway from aspiration of secretions and food during swallowing. Acute **epiglottitis** is a rapidly progressive infection of this structure and the adjacent soft tissues in the upper airway that can result in partial airway obstruction, which can progress to a life-threatening emergency.

Etiology

Haemophilus influenzae type B was the most common bacterium associated with epiglottitis prior to the common use of vaccination against this organism. This organism was isolated from pharyngeal cultures in most children with this syndrome and from one fourth of adult cases. Positive blood cultures for *H. influenzae* were common in both children and adults with acute epiglottitis. Routine infant vaccination with *H. influenzae* type B protein-polysaccharide (Hib) conjugate vaccines has resulted in a dramatically decreased incidence and a shift of the microbial etiology of epiglottitis. Association of this syndrome with other bacteria such as *H. influenzae* type A and nontypable strains, staphylococci, and streptococci has been reported in the (Hib) vaccine era. Herpes simplex virus type 1, parainfluenza virus type 3, and influenza B viruses have all been implicated as rare viral causes of epiglottitis.

Epidemiology

Most cases of epiglottitis occur in preschool-age children. Although an uncommon occurrence in the average clinical practice, the fact that it is a potentially life-threatening infection because of the risk of airway obstruction warrants familiarity with the syndrome.

Clinical Manifestations

The presence of severe symptoms of pharyngitis and pain on swallowing in the absence of signs of pharyngitis on physical examination should suggest the diagnosis of epiglottitis. Patients are often noted to have stridor, which is a high-pitched sound noted during breathing that indicates the possibility of upper airway obstruction. The presence of stridor is a medical emergency. Visualization of the epiglottis is the most important step in the diagnosis of acute epiglottitis. However, this must be done in a setting where intubation or tracheostomy can be performed immediately because of the risk of airway obstruction during manipulation of the pharynx and the associated edema of epiglottitis. Generally, an endotracheal tube is inserted at the time of diagnosis to secure the airway until the inflammation and infection subside with treatment. Blood cultures and cultures of the epiglottis should be obtained, and intravenous antimicrobial therapy should be initiated immediately. The associated edema of the epiglottis can also cause the sudden onset of upper airway obstruction and respiratory arrest.

Early manifestations of epiglottitis include fever associated with severe sore throat and difficulty swallowing. Patients often prefer to lean forward and drool rather than to swallow their secretions, because of the extreme pain experienced. A rapid downhill course is more likely in children than in adults with epiglottitis. However, caution is warranted in the diagnostic approach to any patient suspected of having this disease. In small children, signs of upper airway obstruction should always prompt consideration of a foreign body lodged in the upper airway in the differential diagnosis of epiglottitis. The syndrome of croup associated with viral respiratory tract infections is the main condition to differentiate from epiglottitis in children. The viral illness that precedes and accompanies croup syndrome is not observed in patients with epiglottitis, and the cough typical of croup syndrome is not common in epiglottitis. In contrast, patients with epiglottitis usually have a relatively short history of illness. Patients with croup typically have predominant inflammation and airway narrowing below the epiglottis. As discussed in the section on the complications of pharyngitis, other soft tissue infections of the upper respiratory tract are associated with narrowing of the upper airway, such as retropharyngeal abscess. However, these processes usually do not exhibit the same symptom complex and fulminant course seen with *H. influenzae*–induced epiglottitis. In distinction from bacterial pharyngitis (e.g., streptococcal or, rarely, diphtheria pharyngitis), patients with epiglottitis usually do not have tonsillar or pharyngeal exudates.

Pathogenesis

The soft tissues of the epiglottis and the surrounding structures appear to be susceptible to significant accumulation of edema fluid during the inflammatory process incited by infection. Combined with the critical location of the epiglottis at the opening of the trachea, this creates the danger of partial or complete airway obstruction as the disease progresses.

Complications

The main complication is respiratory compromise associated with the sudden onset of airway obstruction. Some patients with epiglottitis have simultaneous pneumonia. However, the clinical significance of the lower respiratory tract involvement is relatively minor compared with the potential problems with upper airway obstruction early in the course of this infection.

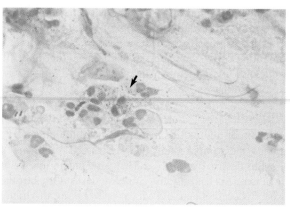

FIGURE 32-4 Gram-stained smear of sputum/exudate with *Haemophilus* organisms *(arrow)*.

Laboratory Diagnosis

Specimen Collection. Direct swab cultures from the area of the epiglottis are useful in establishing the etiologic diagnosis, but they should be taken only when the airway is secure. Blood cultures should also be performed in all patients in whom epiglottitis is suspected.

Direct Microscopic Examination. A direct smear of exudates for microscopic examination is a rapid method for early diagnosis. Exudates taken from the epiglottal area may reveal numerous white blood cells and pleomorphic, gramnegative bacilli characteristic of *H. influenzae* (Figure 32-4) or other bacterial pathogens.

Culture. *H. influenzae* are isolated from blood cultures and from exudates. An enriched medium such as CHOC is required to recover this organism. An environment with an enhanced concentration of carbon dioxide (5% to 10%) is also required for recovery. The organism is identified by determining the X and V factor requirements, porphyrin test, and hemolysis on Casman blood agar.

Treatment. Epiglottitis is a serious medical condition that requires hospitalization and administration of IV antibiotics, such as third-generation cephalosporin antibiotics (e.g., cefotaxime, ceftriaxone) or ampicillin-sulbactam. Patients should be monitored closely for signs and symptoms of respiratory distress that might require urgent intubation or tracheostomy. IV corticosteroids may help reduce inflammation and swelling of the airway.

Pertussis

Pertussis starts as mild respiratory illness that can progress to a paroxysmal cough syndrome.

Etiology

Bordetella pertussis and *Bordetella parapertussis* are most frequently associated with the pertussis syndrome. *Bordetella bronchiseptica* has also been associated with a similar clinical syndrome. Low-serotype adenoviruses (types 1, 2, 3, and 5) have been isolated from patients with an illness that can be indistinguishable from pertussis. The recent availability of rapid viral diagnostic tests makes it feasible to distinguish adenovirus infection based on culture data from *B. pertussis* during the acute illness. Formerly, this distinction between pertussis and viral illness required serologic studies that were useful only in retrospect.

Epidemiology

Pertussis is a highly transmissible respiratory illness in susceptible patient populations that occurs with little seasonal variation. The infection occurs more commonly in infants and young children, and serious complications are seen more often in this age group. In recent years, the incidence of this illness has increased in the teenage and adult population. Adolescents and adults with unusual (and often milder) manifestations of the illness may be undiagnosed because of a low clinical index of suspicion and can serve as reservoirs for transmission of the infection to susceptible children and others.

Clinical Manifestations

In the early phase of the illness, the symptom complex of pertussis is similar to that of a viral upper respiratory tract infection, and the differential diagnosis is difficult. Fever is uncommon throughout the course of the illness, unless a secondary bacterial infection has occurred. Following the early phase of the illness, the patient may experience exhausting paroxysms of coughing, often with multiple coughs during one expiratory cycle, which are typically worse at night. The cycle classically ends with an episode of vomiting resulting from the extreme nature of the cough. The "whooping" sound associated with the forceful inspiration through a narrowed airway after a prolonged episode of coughing is the source of the term "whooping cough," which has been used in common reference to B. pertussis infection. The whooping characteristic of the inspiratory cycle is not uniformly present during pertussis infection, however. Therefore it should not be used as a diagnostic criterion.

A major public health problem associated with the diagnosis of this infection in a child is limiting its spread within susceptible close contacts. Careful vaccination histories from contacts will allow the formulation of a plan for their protection by active immunization and antibiotic prophylaxis.

Pathogenesis

Although the pathogenesis of pertussis is incompletely understood, numerous studies suggest a significant role for pertussis toxin in the clinical presentation of this infection. Factors produced by these organisms have been implicated in several stages in the disease process, including damage to tracheal epithelial cells, impairment of host immunity, and induction of systemic symptoms of pertussis. It is apparent that pertussis is not a disease that is caused by the effects of a single toxin, as is the case in some other bacterial infections. Rather, it appears that the clinical syndrome may be a manifestation of the sum of several toxins produced by the pathogen and the host response that is elicited.

Complications

The most common complication of pertussis is the pneumonia that occurs in young children. These lower respiratory tract infections are commonly caused by secondary infections with other bacteria, although B. pertussis itself may cause pneumonia. Other secondary bacterial infections such as otitis media also occur.

Many of the complications associated with pertussis are a consequence of the severe and forceful coughing episodes that occur during this illness. Alveolar rupture may induce interstitial and subcutaneous emphysema. Forceful coughing has also been associated with subconjunctival (and other superficial) hemorrhages, epistaxis (nosebleed), rupture of the diaphragm, umbilical and inguinal hernias, and rectal prolapse. Among the most serious complications of pertussis are those that affect the CNS. These problems are most dangerous in infants with pertussis. Seizures during pertussis have been related to fever, cerebral hypoxia, and toxic encephalopathy. This infection has been implicated as a cause of bronchiectasis later in life.

Laboratory Diagnosis

Specimen Collection. Recovery of B. pertussis depends to a large extent on proper specimen collection and processing. Specimens should be plated directly onto selective media such as Bordet-Gengou or Regan-Lowe (RL). If delay is expected, a transport medium such as RL transport medium should be used.

Direct Microscopic Examination. Complementary data may be obtained by performing direct fluorescent antibody (DFA) staining of secretions from such swabs. Although DFA has limitations regarding false-negative and false-positive results, it can provide a rapid indicator that may be useful in initiating empirical therapy.

Culture. Isolation of B. pertussis from nasopharyngeal secretions remains the gold standard for diagnosis of pertussis. In addition to immunofluorescence studies, polymerase chain reaction (PCR) testing methods have been developed for rapid diagnosis. These techniques should not be used in place of culture data. At the same time that nasopharyngeal cultures are being collected for B. pertussis culture, specimens should be submitted for adenovirus culture using a rapid diagnostic assay such as the shell vial culture/antigen detection method. Specimens for viral culture are either inoculated directly or placed in a viral carrier medium containing antibiotics to suppress bacterial contamination.

Treatment. The macrolide antibiotics—erythromycin estolate, clarithromycin and azithromycin—are the antibiotics of choice. These help reduce the severity of paroxysms of cough if given during the catarrhal stage or early in the infection. Otherwise they are used to reduce the transmission of infection to others. These agents are also recommended as chemoprophylaxis of people exposed to an index case within 2 to 3 weeks of the onset of cough. Hospitalized patients should be kept in respiratory isolation for 5 days after initiation of antibiotic therapy.

Vaccination is the best form of prevention of this illness. Acellular pertussis vaccine is given in combination with diphtheria and tetanus toxoids (DTaP vaccine). Childhood vaccination does not, however, confer lasting immunity against pertussis. Therefore adults form a large reservoir for this infection. Consequently, an acellular pertussis vaccine in combination with diphtheria toxin (Tdap) is now recommended in adolescents and susceptible adults.

LOWER RESPIRATORY TRACT INFECTIONS

Infections in the lower respiratory tract usually occur when infecting organisms reach the lower airways or pulmonary parenchyma by bypassing the mechanical and other non-specific barriers of the upper respiratory tract. Infections may result from inhalation of infectious aerosols, aspiration of oral or gastric contents, or by hematogenous spread.

A series of host defenses must be overcome before a potential pathogen can establish infection in the lower respiratory tract. The sequence of events is somewhat different for respiratory viruses than for bacterial pathogens. The progression of viral pathogens from the upper to the lower respiratory tract is a process that involves both spread among adjacent cells and distant inoculation of susceptible cells by aspiration of infectious secretions and, to a lesser extent, by hematogenous transmission of the virus. Lung infections by bacterial pathogens usually occur via direct inoculation of organisms through aspiration from the upper respiratory tract. The ways in which mechanical host defenses are bypassed or suppressed, leading to lower respiratory tract infection, have been considered previously. Table 32-2 summarizes clinical syndromes encountered in the lower respiratory tract and the associated etiologic agents.

Bronchitis and Bronchiolitis

Etiology

Any of the respiratory viruses that cause upper respiratory tract infection can cause cough as a manifestation of acute **bronchitis** (infection and inflammation of the bronchi). The severity of the bronchial involvement varies with the different viral respiratory tract pathogens and, to some extent, with the patient population being studied. For example, during seasons when influenza is epidemic in the community, this viral respiratory pathogen is the most common cause of acute bronchitis and bronchiolitis in the general population. Respiratory syncytial virus also causes community-wide, seasonal outbreaks of **bronchiolitis** in infants. During nonepidemic periods, other respiratory viral pathogens such as rhinovirus, coronavirus, and parainfluenza virus are more likely to be isolated. In populations of young military recruits, adenovirus infections were the primary cause of acute bronchitis prior to the use of adenovirus vaccine. During the summer months, patients with enterovirus infection may exhibit acute bronchitis as part of the clinical syndrome, although this is not a major part of the illness in most cases.

Nonviral respiratory tract pathogens including *Mycoplasma pneumoniae*, *Chlamydia pneumoniae*, and *B. pertussis* can also induce the syndrome of acute bronchitis. Therefore the clinical presentation of these infections may be indistinguishable from cases of acute bronchitis caused by viral pathogens.

Epidemiology

Acute bronchitis can be viewed as the lower respiratory tract extension of many of the same viral infections that cause seasonal upper respiratory tract infections. The peak season for acute bronchitis is the winter months, which matches the period of peak incidence of these viral respiratory tract infections. It is somewhat artificial to separate the clinical syndromes of viral upper respiratory tract infections and acute bronchitis, because in many instances these represent a continuum of the same infection. The difference in the clinical presentations of these two conditions is often simply one of degree.

Clinical Manifestations

Patients with acute bronchitis often begin their illnesses with a syndrome typical of a nonbacterial upper respiratory tract infection. The course of the illness may exhibit a fairly rapid progression to lower respiratory tract involvement or, after several days of an upper respiratory tract syndrome, may evolve to symptoms of bronchitis. The typical patient with acute bronchitis has cough and fever as the primary manifestations of the illness. The amount of sputum produced with coughing varies with the individual, with the pathogen causing the illness, with the stage of the illness (the cough usually becomes more productive later in the course), and with the incidence of secondary bacterial infections that may follow nonbacterial acute bronchitis. Systemic symptoms such as diffuse myalgias and fatigue associated with viremic illnesses may also be seen early in the course of infection.

Acute Versus Chronic Bronchitis. The distinction between acute and chronic bronchitis is one of both definition and pathogenesis. For purposes of definition, chronic bronchitis is evidenced by the presence of a cough productive of sputum on most days for at least 3 months of the year for a minimum of 2 years in succession. Whereas acute bronchitis is usually of infectious etiology, chronic bronchitis is usually caused by long-term cigarette smoking and occasionally by other toxic exposures. From the perspective of infectious diseases of the respiratory tract, the main point to remember is that acute exacerbations of chronic bronchitis are usually initiated by the same pathogens that cause acute bronchitis in patients of the same age without underlying chronic respiratory tract disease. The difference is that patients with chronic bronchitis who experience an acute exacerbation of their illness resulting from intercurrent infection are more likely to have a severe primary illness or a prolonged illness associated with secondary bacterial infection than are otherwise healthy patients with acute bronchitis.

Acute Bronchiolitis. *Acute bronchiolitis* is a term reserved for an infectious disease of infants that is associated with a typical clinical picture. This syndrome is usually caused by respiratory syncytial virus infection, although other respiratory viruses (e.g., parainfluenza virus) can cause the same clinical picture. In addition to signs of a febrile upper respiratory tract infection, these patients present with signs of lower respiratory tract airway obstruction such as wheezing, respiratory distress, and air trapping. Chest radiographs do not usually show typical signs of pneumonia and can vary in presentation from a normal chest radiograph to one showing peribronchial thickening, hyperinflation, or patchy consolidation.

Pathogenesis

As previously mentioned, evidence almost always exists of antecedent or coexistent upper respiratory tract infection in

TABLE 32-2 Lower Respiratory Tract Infections

Clinical Syndrome	Causative Agents	Specimen Collection	Other	Special Comments
Bronchitis, bronchiolitis	**Most common:** Respiratory viruses **Less common:** *Mycoplasma pneumoniae* *Chlamydophila pneumoniae* *Bordetella pertussis*	Nasopharyngeal or lower respiratory culture if Influenza type A or Respiratory Syncytial Virus infection of the lower respiratory tract is suspected	Diagnostic cultures not indicated in uncomplicated cases	NP swabs, aspirates, and washings Requires special media for transport and culture Direct fluorescent antibody test (DFA) PCR Serology Viral culture (antigen assays) Viral PCR Other tests available include *S. pneumoniae* urinary antigen
Community-acquired pneumonia	**Children:** **Most common:** Respiratory Syncytial Virus Influenza A, B Parainfluenza 1, 2, 3 Adenovirus *M. pneumoniae* **Less common:** *Streptococcus pneumoniae* *Staphylococcus aureus* *Haemophilus influenzae* Group B Streptococcus (neonates) **Adults:** **Most common:** *S. pneumoniae* **Less common:** *M. pneumoniae* *H. influenzae* *Chlamydia pneumoniae* Respiratory viruses (e.g., Influenza)	"Deep" expectorated sputum	Avoid contamination with oropharyngeal flora; specimen collection via fiberoptic bronchoscopy or open lung biopsy may be indicated in some circumstances	
Nosocomial pneumonia	Gram-negative bacilli *Staphylococcus aureus* *Streptococcus pneumoniae* *Haemophilus influenzae* *Legionella* spp.	"Deep" expectorated sputum	Avoid contamination with oropharyngeal flora; specimen collection via fiberoptic bronchoscopy or open lung biopsy may be indicated in some circumstances	{*Legionella*} Cultures on selective media BCYE Urinary antigen test detects *Legionella pneumophila* serogroup 1
Aspiration pneumonia	Mixed anaerobes and aerobes	Expectorated sputum is of little value; bronchoscopic techniques required for specific diagnosis	Pleural fluid cultures may be useful with anaerobic empyema	
Chronic pneumonia	Mycobacteria *Mycobacterium tuberculosis* Non-tuberculous mycobacterium (especially *M. avium-intracellulare*) Fungi *Blastomyces* *Histoplasma* *Aspergillus* *Zygomyces* *Coccidioides* *Cryptococcus* Pneumocystis	Early morning "deep" expectorated sputum; bronchoscopy or open lung biopsy may be required to identify pathogen	—	Acid-fast bacillus stain Mycobacterial culture Nucleic acid amplification assays (for TB in sputum, especially when AFB smear positive) Fungal stains such as Gomori methenamine silver (GMS), calcofluor white, and periodic acid-Schiff (PAS) Cultures from tissue (lung), aspirate, or lavage fluid (Cross-reactive) antigen test on urine, blood, and respiratory secretions Histopathology Galactomannan assay Histopathology Serology Serum antigen assay Gomori methenamine silver (GMS) stain Fluorescent antibody (DFA) stain
Empyema	**Community acquired:** *S. aureus* *S. pneumoniae* *Streptococcus pyogenes* *Streptococcus anginosus* Anaerobes **Nosocomial:** Gram-negative bacilli Anaerobes	Pleural fluid should be aspirated directly into a sterile syringe with excess air removed from syringe immediately	Aliquots of specimen should be distributed to hematology and chemistry laboratories for other studies	

NP, Nasopharyngeal; *PCR,* polymerase chain reaction.

patients with acute bronchitis. The spread of these upper respiratory tract infections to the lower airways, manifested as acute bronchitis, represents infection and damage of respiratory epithelial cells by the same (usually viral) pathogens. The extent of destruction of the respiratory epithelium varies with the pathogen causing the illness. Viruses such as influenza and adenovirus are highly cytopathic and cause significant epithelial cell destruction; other viral infections such as rhinovirus cause epithelial cell dysfunction without inducing much cytopathology.

The inflammatory response, necrotic debris from epithelial cell destruction, and edema of the lower respiratory tract also contribute to the airway abnormalities and symptoms in these infections. In probably no clinical syndrome is this potential for airway obstruction more important than in bronchiolitis in infants. The resulting obliteration of the lumen of small airways appears to be the primary pathogenic mechanism in this infection. Indirect effects of viral infection on airway function are probably also important in the pathogenesis of some forms of acute bronchitis. The results of several studies suggest that alterations in airway β-adrenergic receptors and the production of inflammatory mediators during viral infections of the respiratory tract may be involved in many of the signs and symptoms associated with these infections.

Complications

A complication that is apparent in some patients with acute viral bronchitis is the development of secondary bacterial infection. Secondary infection can present in several ways. Some patients experience persistent or increasing symptoms of bronchitis, with an increase in the volume and purulence of the sputum produced. This usually occurs at a time in the course of the illness when most cases of acute bronchitis would be resolving. A further extension of this scenario is secondary bacterial infection presenting as acute or evolving pneumonia after an episode of acute bronchitis. These secondary bacterial infections of the lower respiratory tract are usually the common pathogens found in community-acquired pneumonia (e.g., *S. pneumoniae, H. influenzae*), although other bacterial pathogens (e.g., *M. catarrhalis,* gram-negative bacilli) may be involved in selected patient populations (e.g., patients with underlying respiratory diseases, hospitalized patients).

The long-term consequences of acute bronchitis continue to be debated. Several epidemiologic studies suggest an association between acute viral infections of the lower respiratory tract and subsequent asthma. Whether the infectious agents that caused acute bronchitis in these patients actually induced a permanent change in their airways that resulted in future airway hyperreactivity, or whether these infections occurred in patients who would have eventually developed asthma regardless of intercurrent episodes of acute bronchitis, remains an interesting puzzle. Speculation also exists that certain viruses that cause acute bronchitis can cause bronchiectasis. This is an abnormality in which inadequate drainage of respiratory secretions results from airway wall destruction, dilatation, and scarring that are associated with recurrent lower respiratory tract infections. Considering the cytopathic nature of some viral (e.g., influenza, adenovirus) infections

that can cause acute bronchitis, the suggested association between these pathogens and long-term development of bronchiectasis seems reasonable.

Laboratory Diagnosis

The collection of specimens for culture in cases of acute bronchitis largely follows the procedures outlined in the section on viral pharyngitis. Because acute bronchitis is an extension of a syndrome of nonbacterial upper respiratory tract infection, diagnostic cultures are not indicated in uncomplicated cases that follow the expected, self-limited course, unless there is some epidemiological reason for cultures (e.g., a suspected influenza outbreak. If, however, patients develop signs of secondary bacterial bronchitis or pneumonia, culture data may be useful in guiding therapy. When cultures are used to guide the treatment plan, it is important to attempt to obtain lower respiratory tract secretions that are minimally contaminated with oral biota.

In practice, collection of an adequate specimen is usually not difficult in patients with secondary bacterial bronchitis, because of the production of copious amounts of purulent sputum. The proper collection of lower respiratory tract secretions for the diagnosis of pneumonia is covered in the section on pneumonia. Other situations in which cultures might be indicated in cases of acute bronchitis or acute bronchiolitis are those in which effective antiviral agents are available against the viral pathogens suspected. For example, in cases of suspected influenza or respiratory syncytial virus infection of the lower respiratory tract, identification of these agents in respiratory tract secretions may be useful in guiding early antiviral therapy.

Treatment

Acute bronchitis and bronchiolitis are caused by viral infections in more than 95% of cases and therefore should not usually be treated with antibiotic therapy. Anti-influenza therapy must be started within 48 hours of the onset of symptoms to have a significant effect on clinical outcome. Symptom control and the additional use of inhaled bronchodilator medications and supplemental oxygen therapy may be required for patients with underlying pulmonary conditions that are made worse by viral lower respiratory tract infection. In a few such patients and in patients at the extremes of age (very young and very old), secondary bacterial bronchitis and/or pneumonia may follow viral bronchitis or bronchiolitis and may then require antibiotic therapy. In those cases, antibiotic treatment regimens can be designed using the same approach used for acute bacterial pneumonia (see later discussion).

Influenza

Respiratory tract infection with systemic symptoms of fever, myalgias, and fatigue is the most common manifestation of influenza, an acute illness caused by influenza A or B viruses. Influenza infections are usually first detected in the late fall and early winter. Influenza A viruses are categorized into subtypes on the basis of two surface antigens: hemagglutinin and neuraminidase. Influenza A is responsible for annual outbreaks or epidemics of varying intensity, whereas influenza B causes outbreaks every 2 to 4 years. Human influenza subtypes continuously undergo a process of antigenic drift, whereby amino acid substitutions allow the virus to evade preexisting host immunity. This antigenic drift is responsible for annual worldwide outbreaks. During the winter season, young children, elderly, and patients with underlying heart and lung disease, diabetes, renal disease, or immunosuppression are at increased risk for developing primary influenza pneumonia. Additionally, influenza infection predisposes patients to develop secondary bacterial pneumonias. Bacterial pathogens commonly seen in this setting include *S. pneumoniae, S. aureus,* and *H. influenzae.*

In the setting of an influenza outbreak, acute febrile respiratory illnesses can be diagnosed as influenza with a relatively high degree of certainty by clinical criteria. However, individual or sporadic cases cannot be reliably differentiated from infections caused by other respiratory viruses on clinical grounds. In this setting, specific laboratory tests may be helpful. Laboratory diagnosis is accomplished by the detection of virus viral antigen or viral nucleic acid in throat swabs, nasal washes, and sputum or bronchoalveolar lavage specimens. Isolation of the virus in tissue culture usually can be accomplished within 72 hours of inoculation. Rapid viral diagnostic tests employing immunologic and molecular techniques are increasingly available. Immunofluorescence assays, enzyme immunoassays, and PCR-based testing are all options. PCR tests are more sensitive than culture or immunological tests and are specific for both seasonal influenza A and B and for emerging influenza A variants (e.g., H5N1 and H1N1). Additionally, the diagnosis can be established retrospectively by serologic methods. A fourfold or greater rise in antibody titers between serum specimens obtained during acute illness and convalescent specimens obtained 10 to 14 days later is considered diagnostic.

Periodically, two strains of influenza will combine genetic material and result in the generation of a new reassorted virus to which there is little population immunity. This process of genetic reassortment is called *antigenic shift.* If the new virus contains virulence factors that include efficient person-to-person transmission, a pandemic influenza outbreak can occur with the potential for millions of worldwide deaths. The influenza pandemics in 1957 and in 1968 were caused by genetic reassortment between human influenza viruses and influenza viruses in birds. The influenza pandemic in 2009 was caused by reassortment of genetic elements of human, swine, and avian strains.

Prevention and Treatment

The best way to prevent influenza infection is by annual vaccination starting in the fall of each year. Vaccines are manufactured annually based upon global virus surveillance data, to allow inclusion in the vaccine of strains of both influenza A and influenza B that are most representative of those strains circulating worldwide. Other strategies that attempt to reduce influenza transmission, especially in health care and other institutional settings, include hand hygiene and respiratory protection. However, these methods are only ancillary measures that are markedly inferior to immunization of populations at risk. Antiviral drugs (e.g., osteltamivir [Tamiflu]) are available for chemoprophylaxis and treatment of influenza.

These drugs should not be substituted for vaccination as a means of disease prevention in immunocompetent persons but may have a role in protecting immunocompromised patients (who might not respond to vaccination) during local epidemics of influenza. Practical use of anti-influenza agents for treatment of infection is limited to the setting of community outbreaks of influenza. In this case, the diagnosis can be made on clinical grounds without waiting for confirmatory laboratory studies because of the high prevalence of such infections in the outbreak setting. This rapid clinical diagnosis is important, because antiviral therapy must be started within 48 hours of the onset of symptoms to have a significant beneficial effect on clinical outcome.

Emerging Viral Respiratory Tract Infections

Avian Influenza—H5N1

Between 2005 and 2007, attention was turned to the H5N1 strain of influenza A, a strain that is endemic in poultry across much of Southeast Asia, the Middle East, and Europe. This virus is but one of the **emerging infections** being studied. The first association of H5N1 influenza with clinical disease in humans was recognized during a poultry outbreak in live-bird markets in Hong Kong in 1997. In that outbreak, 18 people were infected with the H5N1 virus, and 6 died. Subsequent outbreaks of highly lethal illness among poultry were reported in at least eight Asian countries. Epidemiologic evidence suggested the virus was capable of person-to-person transmission in rare cases, and it is feared that further genetic alterations could result in a worldwide pandemic. However, no evidence has yet been found for such mutations or sustained, person-to-person transmission that would be required for a pandemic. Currently available methods used for diagnosis of influenza A have limited value for diagnosis of H5N1 influenza, because the commonly used testing kits are unable to distinguish influenza A subtypes.

Novel H1N1 Influenza

In the spring of 2009, an epidemic of H1N1 influenza A was first recognized in patients either living in or traveling to Mexico. Over the next several months, disease casused by this viral strain was recognized in the U.S. and throughout much of the world, and an influenza pandemic was declared by the World Health Organization in June of 2009. This novel viral strain has genetic elements derived from swine, avian, and human influenza strains previously recognized on multiple continents, but its epidemiologic history prior to the initial clinical outbreak in 2009 is still being resolved. Children appear to have no immunological memory of this novel virus, whereas adults, especially those who are 60 years of age or older, appear to have some level of pre-existing immunity, either because of previous experience with antigenically similar influenza infections or some degree of cross reactivity with H1N1 strains represented in previous vaccines. Perhaps as a result of this age-related difference in immunity, infections with novel H1N1 have been more of a problem in younger patients than older patients. Therefore, the immunization effort against H1N1 has been focused on younger patient populations, in addition to others at increased risk for negative outsomes, such as pregnant women and those with underlying medical conditions. Because of the increased global preparation for a possible H5N1 pandemic, there was a rapid response to the novel H1N1 problem. The most effective diagnostic method has been PCR-based testing of respiratory secretions for influenza A, followed by specific molecular testing for novel swine H1 sequences using real time PCR. As observed with previous influenza studies, molecular diagnostic testing has been more sensitive than rapid antigen detection assays. The molecular diagnostic studies have been useful for a variety of applications, including clinical decision making and epidemiological studies. However, use of these methods should be discussed and coordinated between clinicians, epidemiologists, and laboratory personnel to properly focus the effort and avoid creation of unnecessary burdens on the laboratory that can be caused by indiscriminate testing.

Severe Acute Respiratory Syndrome (SARS)

Severe acute respiratory syndrome (SARS) is the term used to describe outbreaks of viral pneumonia caused by a novel SARS-associated coronavirus (SARS-CoV) that was first recognized in southern China in late 2002. This virus was believed to be of animal origin. The Centers for Disease Control and Prevention (CDC) estimates 774 deaths were attributed to this outbreak until it was contained in China in 2004. Direct contact with respiratory secretions and spread via respiratory droplets were presumed to be the most important modes of transmission. A characteristic clinical picture is associated with SARS. After an incubation period of approximately 2 to 10 days, the most characteristic symptom was fever, with or without cough, or dyspnea and radiographic evidence of lung infiltrates consistent with pneumonia or respiratory distress syndrome. In most cases, symptoms resolved spontaneously after the first week; however, in more than 20% of patients, symptoms progressed to the more severe respiratory distress syndrome, and the patients required intensive care and respiratory support. Recommended viral diagnostic studies include viral culture, serological tests such as ELISA (enzyme-linked immunosorbent assay) or IFA (immunofluorescence assay; requires acute and 4-week follow-up sera) or detection of SARS coronavirus by nucleic acid amplification (e.g., reverse transcriptase polymerase chain reaction [RT-PCR] assay) using two different clinical specimens such as nasopharyngeal swab and stool specimen. Thorough diagnostic testing to rule out other etiologies, including influenza, should also be conducted. Respiratory specimens and blood, serum, and stool samples should be saved for additional testing until a specific diagnosis can be made. Strong clinical suspicion and early diagnosis is essential for early treatment and transmission prevention. Although the last reported symptomatic case was in 2004, global surveillance continues for recurrence of an outbreak.

Adenovirus Infections—Re-emergence in the Military

Since the discovery of adenoviruses in the 1950s, 51 serotypes have been described. Adenovirus infections have usually been associated with mild, febrile, respiratory tract illnesses in young children. Infections with certain adenovirus serotypes have been reported to cause outbreaks of pharyngoconjunctival fever in summer camps and public swimming pools and can also cause severe, disseminated disease in immunocompromised patients. Following recognition of infection with adenovirus (especially serotypes 4 and 7) as the cause of severe acute respiratory disease in military recruits in the 1950s, an effective military vaccination program was established. After the end of adenovirus vaccine production in 1995 and suspension of the military vaccination program in the late 1990s, adenovirus-related outbreaks were once again observed in military training facilities. This resulted in resumption of adenoviral vaccine production and plans for reinstitution of the military vaccine program. In addition to recurrence of problems with adenovirus serotypes 4 and 7 after discontinuation of vaccination, there emerged several adenovirus group B serotypes (including group B1 serotypes 3, 7, and 21 and group B2 serotype 14) that became a new problem in military training facilities. In some cases, these adenoviral infections were associated with severe cases of pneumonia and so-called acute respiratory distress syndroms (ARDS).

Metapneumovirus

Human metapneumovirus (hMPV) was first identified in 2001 in respiratory samples from children and adults with acute respiratory tract infection. hMPV is a new member of the family Paramyxoviridae that was first identified in the Netherlands by retrospectively examining respiratory samples of children with unidentified viral respiratory illness. hMPV can cause symptoms involving both the upper and lower respiratory tracts. It mostly affects the pediatric population, although it may cause severe disease in the elderly and immunocompromised adults. In children, it produces a clinical picture similar to that observed with other causes of viral bronchiolitis, with cough, rhinorrhea, and fever. In healthy adults, it presents with mild clinical symptoms, including mild cough, fatigue, and sore throat. Diagnosis can be made by testing cultures of respiratory secretions with indirect IFA and RT-PCR.

Human Bocavirus

Because an infectious etiology cannot be determined in many respiratory tract illnesses that present as viral syndromes, an ongoing search for new viral pathogens continues. In addition to hMPV, several other new viruses have been identified in recent years that are associated with these syndromes. Human bocaviruses are another example. The DNA sequences of human bocavirus closely resemble those of viruses in the Parvoviridae family. Bocavirus has been detected by PCR analysis of respiratory specimens, mostly from children less than 5 years of age, and can also be detected in stool and serum specimens. Because of the high co-infection rate with other potential viral pathogens and the lack of a clear bocavirus-related syndrome, the causal role of bocavirus infection in respiratory and other syndromes remains a challenge for future investigation. These agents likely represent the "tip of the iceberg" of undiscovered viral pathogens that will require new diagnostic methods and clinical studies before a proper perspective about their role in human disease can be determined.

Acute Pneumonia

The distinction between acute bronchitis and acute pneumonia may be subtle. Both are lower respiratory tract infections. The distinction depends on the degree and extent of involvement of the lower respiratory tract with the infectious process. By definition, patients who have bronchitis do not exhibit the physical, radiographic, and pathologic findings of pulmonary parenchymal involvement outside of the airways. Such lung tissue involvement with the infectious process defines **pneumonia.**

Pneumonia can be subdivided into diagnostic categories based upon the clinical setting, presentation of the illness, exposure to specific pathogens, and age and type of host infected. The importance of using such a strategy to make a presumptive determination of the infectious etiology of pneumonia is evident when one considers the long list of possible pathogens that can cause this type of infection. Table 32-3 lists the most common etiologic agents of lower respiratory tract infections and the usually affected patient populations. It is important to focus the clinical diagnosis on a subgroup of likely pathogens to allow the initiation of reasonable empirical therapy while awaiting a specific etiologic diagnosis and to make optimal use of the diagnostic microbiology laboratory in planning the diagnostic approach. The process of determining an etiologic diagnosis requires consideration of both the clinical setting and the age of the host affected. The highest incidence of both community-acquired and nosocomial pneumonias occurs in very young and very old patients. However, the types of etiologic agents that are most likely to cause pulmonary infections in these two groups are different. In infants and children, respiratory viruses cause the majority of pneumonias; in elderly adults, bacterial pathogens are more likely to be implicated.

Community-Acquired Pneumonia

Etiology. Respiratory syncytial virus is the most commonly identified cause of viral pneumonias in children, especially in infants, in most communities. This pathogen has also been recognized in infections among the elderly, those being cared for in nursing homes, and those who are immunosuppressed. Parainfluenza is the second-most commonly recognized viral pathogen to cause childhood pneumonias. Both respiratory syncytial virus and parainfluenza virus belong to the Paramyxoviridae family. Human metapneumovirus, the newly recognized member of this family, generally causes mild, self-limited upper respiratory infections in children and adults. Less frequently, it can cause severe pneumonia. Other less common etiologic agents to consider in pneumonias in this age group are low-serotype adenoviruses and mycoplasma.

Although much less common than viral pneumonias, bacterial pneumonias also occur in children and must be considered in the differential diagnosis. *S. pneumoniae* and *H. influenzae* type B were the most common pathogens isolated in childhood bacterial pneumonias prior to the routine use of *H. influenza* type B (Hib) conjugate vaccine for children. *H. influenza* type B is still a major bacterial cause of pneumonia in older infants and young children in underdeveloped countries or other areas where this vaccine is not available or implemented. Other bacterial pathogens must also be considered, depending on the clinical situation. For example, group B streptococci are more likely to be associated with pneumonia in neonates than in older children. In adults, *S. pneumoniae* remains the most common cause of community-acquired bacterial pneumonia in the general population. In addition, depending on the severity of the illness, the season of the year, and whether the community is experiencing an epidemic respiratory infection such as influenza, other pathogens such as respiratory viruses and *M. pneumoniae* are seen in community-acquired pneumonias (CAPs) in adolescents and adults and are responsible for the atypical pneumonia syndrome.

It is "atypical" in that the usual signs and symptoms of bacterial pneumonias that are more common in these age groups are absent or less impressive. The type of patient involved may also help determine which bacterial pathogens are more likely causes of CAP. For example, in adult patients with chronic lung disease, *H. influenzae* and *S. pneumoniae* are frequent colonizers. *H. influenzae* pneumonia is seen more frequently in these patients than in the general population. Patients with alcoholism and patients who have recently been hospitalized or treated with broad-spectrum antibiotics have an increased risk of being colonized with gram-negative bacillary pathogens that may cause pneumonia. Patients with recent influenza virus infection are at increased risk of developing pneumonia caused by *S. aureus* and by *S. pneumoniae*. These types of associations provide general guidelines that are useful for initiating empirical antibiotic therapy and for focusing diagnostic efforts.

Although *S. aureus* accounts for only 1% to 9% of cases of CAP, such infections deserve special attention because of a mortality rate of up to 30%. Most patients with *S. aureus* pneumonia are elderly and have serious underlying disorders such as cardiovascular disease, chronic pulmonary disease, diabetes, or cancer. Necrotizing pneumonia with pulmonary hemorrhage has been associated with *S. aureus* isolates that

---

TABLE 32-3 Most Common Pathogens of Lower Respiratory Infections by Age

Age	Etiology
Neonates	*Chlamydia trachomatis*
Children	
Infants	Respiratory syncytial virus
	Influenza virus
5 to 18 months	*Streptococcus pneumoniae*
	Haemophilus influenzae
3 months to teens	Viruses
	Staphylococcus aureus
	Mycoplasma pneumoniae
Young adults (18 to 45 years)	*M. pneumoniae*
Older adults	*S. pneumoniae*
	Legionella spp.
Institutionalized adults	Gram-negative rods
	S. pneumoniae
	S. aureus

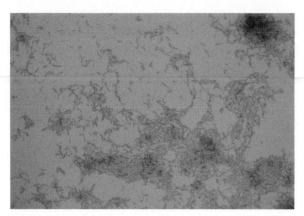

FIGURE 32-5 Gram-stained smear of *Legionella* species taken from culture.

produce Panton-Valentine leukocidin. Methicillin-resistant *Staphylococcus aureus* (MRSA) isolates were initially primarily associated with nosocomial infection. However, increasingly they have become a source of community-associated infection. Recent studies suggest that as many as 12% to 29% of adult and 35% to 50% of pediatric community-associated *S. aureus* infections are caused by MRSA, and the percentages continue to increase.

Another group of pathogens that has emerged in recent years as a cause of both atypical pneumonia and typical bacterial pneumonia is *Legionella pneumophila*. These cases can be difficult to diagnose because extraordinary laboratory efforts are required to identify the organism in the sputum or bronchial aspirate specimen. *Legionella* spp. do not stain well with Gram stain (Figure 32-5) and are often missed during culture of sputum or other types of respiratory secretions. The urinary antigen assay for *L. pneumophila* serogroup 1 reliably and rapidly detects as many as 80% to 90% of community-acquired cases of Legionnaire disease, but it is substantially less sensitive for nosocomial cases because of frequent involvement of serogroups other than serogroup 1. It is usually not possible to distinguish *Legionella* pneumonia from other forms of bacterial pneumonia without specific diagnostic studies. Of primary importance is the consideration of this diagnosis in atypical cases of pneumonia in which the pathogen is not defined early in the course of investigation, so that specific diagnostic studies can be planned to address the possibility of *Legionella* infection.

Epidemiology. Community-acquired pneumonias (CAPs) in children are usually attributable to viral pathogens that cause respiratory tract infections in the community during the winter months. It is useful, during such epidemic periods, to contact the local city and state health department virology laboratories to inquire about the prevalent viral pathogen(s) in the community, because seasonal viral respiratory infections often pass through the community in waves.

Unlike those seen in children, the majority of CAPs in adults are caused by bacterial infections. Although patients with no other known medical problems can present with acute bacterial pneumonia, the typical adult patient with CAP either is elderly or has an underlying disease, such as chronic lung disease, cardiovascular disease, diabetes mellitus, or alcohol-

ism, all of which predispose to lower respiratory tract bacterial infections. These patients may either present with a primary pneumonia or develop pneumonia as a secondary infection complicating a primary viral infection. This predisposition to bacterial pneumonias is the reason that the elderly and patients with underlying chronic illnesses are the major targets for influenza and pneumococcal vaccination programs. In the community, the major cause of death in patients with influenza virus infection is secondary bacterial pneumonia. Based on this observation, it has been reasoned that prevention of influenza by vaccination of these high-risk patients will also prevent the serious bacterial pneumonias that may follow.

Clinical Manifestations. The usual onset of nonbacterial pneumonia in children is indistinguishable from an average viral upper respiratory tract infection. However, instead of resolving in the time expected, the clinical course proceeds toward increasing severity of illness, with signs of respiratory distress. Few other signs may be seen in young children with viral pneumonia.

In older children and adolescents, the typical signs of systemic viral infection include general fatigue and myalgias associated with early signs of upper respiratory tract infection, including cough. Early in the course of the illness, the cough usually does not produce sputum. Low-grade fever is common. The findings on physical examination are variable, and the chest radiograph may show diffuse interstitial changes, patchy infiltrates, or lobar consolidation (dense localized changes restricted to one lobe of the lung; Figure 32-6). Lobar consolidation should always prompt evaluation for a bacterial pathogen, because this radiographic presentation is atypical for viral pneumonia but common with bacterial infection. Routine laboratory studies are rarely helpful in making the clinical diagnosis of viral pneumonia in either children or adults, although demonstration of a virus in the upper airway by DFA staining or culture in the clinical setting of pneumonia is usually considered diagnostic.

In adolescents and adults, the atypical pneumonia syndrome, represented by *M. pneumoniae*, has a symptom complex and clinical presentation that are not dramatically different from those of other nonbacterial pneumonias. Its onset is like that of other nonbacterial upper respiratory tract infections but progresses to produce symptoms and signs of lower tract involvement. Chest radiograph abnormalities are classically more dramatic than would be expected based on the physical examination. The time of the year during which the infection is seen may be helpful in narrowing the list of choices for the etiologic diagnosis. During the winter months, a nonbacterial pneumonia syndrome is often caused by a viral pathogen that is prevalent in the community; for example, influenza. During the summer months, however, when pneumonia caused by most other nonbacterial respiratory pathogens is uncommon, the likelihood that an atypical pneumonia will be caused by *M. pneumoniae* may approach 50%.

The clinical presentation of CAP in adults varies with the age and immunological status of the host. Most patients with bacterial pneumonia note a relatively sudden onset of fever associated with chills. In fact, they are often able to report the exact time their illness started. Cough productive of purulent sputum that may be blood-tinged is typical of this type of

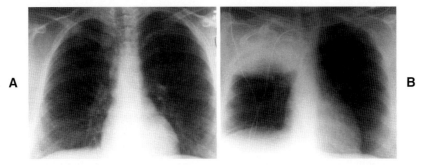

FIGURE 32-6   Chest radiographs before **(A)** and after **(B)** development of an acute, community-acquired, pneumococcal pneumonia. The patient is facing toward the reader. **B,** Consolidation of the right upper lobe of the lung is evidenced by the dense, whitish opacification of this lobe, which contrasts with the normal air (black) density of the remainder of the lung.

infection. Chest examination and radiographs typically show a localized area of lung involvement, described as lobar consolidation (see Figure 32-6). This abnormality in the lung parenchyma may be associated with reduced oxygenation, as measured by arterial blood gas monitoring, depending on the extent of lung involvement and the existence of underlying lung disease. Routine laboratory studies will usually show a neutrophilic leukocytosis with an increased percentage of immature forms of granulocytes in the differential white blood cell count (referred to as *left shift*).

Such is the presentation of the patient described in the case-in-point. This presentation is classic for pneumococcal (*S. pneumoniae*) pneumonia. Sputum Gram stain should show gram-positive lancet-shaped diplococci (see Chapter 7 for additional figures differentiating purulent sputums from oral contamination). Sputum culture should also grow *S. pneumoniae* if significant overgrowth from oral contaminants does not exist. These bacteria characteristically produce α-hemolytic colonies on blood agar. However, similar hemolysis can be produced by other streptococci, such as *S. viridans*, which are normal commensals in the upper respiratory tract. Biochemical tests, such as bile solubility and optochin sensitivity can distinguish *S. pneumoniae* from other streptococci. In approximately 25% of cases of pneumococcal pneumonia, patients demonstrate positive blood cultures for this organism (Figure 32-7). In adults, the pneumococcal urinary antigen assay is an acceptable test to augment the standard diagnostic methods of blood culture and sputum Gram stain and culture. This antigen assay is not likely to be useful for distinguishing children with pneumococcal pneumonia from those who are only colonized. The differential diagnosis should include other common causes of CAP such as *H. influenzae, M. catarrhalis,* or *Legionella* organisms. *Staphylococcus aureus* must be considered if a recent history of influenza exists. In cases of atypical pneumonia, patients have more constitutional symptoms and less sputum production. The chest radiograph is more likely to show patchy infiltrates rather than lobar consolidation. *Mycoplasma* spp., *Chlamydia* spp., *Legionella* spp., and viruses are potential causes of atypical pneumonia. In elderly or immunocompromised patients, the clinical presentation may be less impressive than in patients who are able to mount a normal immune response to pulmo-

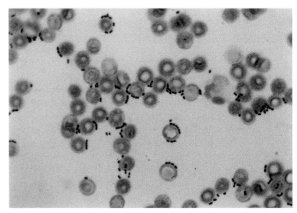

FIGURE 32-7   Gram-stained smear of *Streptococcus pneumoniae* isolated from the blood culture of a patient with pneumococcal pneumonia.

nary bacterial infection. These immunologically compromised patients may have few respiratory tract complaints and little or no fever. Nonspecific symptoms such as weakness, loss of appetite, and a minor cough may be the only manifestations of a progressive pneumonia. It is important to maintain a high index of suspicion in these patients and to routinely pursue changes in patterns of behavior with complete evaluations to avoid missing the diagnosis of pneumonia. These patients are also at increased risk for developing pneumonia after influenza infections. Therefore during influenza epidemics in the community, clinicians should have a heightened awareness of changes in respiratory symptoms that could be compatible with pneumonia in the elderly patient population.

Treatment. An initial decision regarding management of CAP is whether the patient should be hospitalized or can be treated as an outpatient. Several clinical parameters, such as age and presentation with ominous signs that predict increased mortality (e.g., hypotension, confusion, low oxygenation) can be used to make this decision. Increasing problems with antibiotic resistance must be considered during decisions about antibiotic treatment of CAP caused by infections with *S. pneumoniae* and MRSA. Antibiotic susceptibilities should be performed on all bacterial isolates obtained from critical sites (e.g., blood, empyema fluid). In 2008, the Clinical and Laboratory Standards Institute (CLSI) increased breakpoints for β-lactam antibiotics for treating extrameningeal *S. pneumoniae* infections, because of the increasing resistance of these bacteria to different groups of antibiotics. In sensitive *S. pneumoniae* infections, penicillin antibiotics are drugs of choice for inpatients, although they should be used in combination with a macrolide antibiotic to provide coverage for atypical pneumonias (e.g., those caused by *M. pneumoniae* or *Legionella*). Respiratory fluoroquinolones (e.g., levofloxacin) can be added for empiric treatment of patients with co-morbid conditions (e.g., alcoholism, cystic fibrosis). For patients in whom the severity of the CAP requires admission to the ICU, additional consideration should be given to adding antibiotic coverage for gram-negative pathogens, including *P. aeruginosa,* pending culture identification of the etiologic agent.

Nosocomial Pneumonia

Case Study

A 60-year-old man with a history of emphysema and chronic bronchitis was admitted to the hospital to have his gallbladder removed. He was given perioperative antibiotic prophylaxis with cefoxitin. Because of his underlying lung disease, there was difficulty weaning him from the ventilator postoperatively. His antibiotics were continued for a few more days. Seven days after surgery, he developed a high temperature, increased secretions from his endotracheal tube, and a new infiltrate in the right lower lung, as detected on his chest radiograph.

Nosocomial pneumonias include the spectrum of health care–associated pneumonia (HCAP) and ventilator-associated pneumonia (VAP). Hospital-acquired pneumonia (HAP) is defined as pneumonia that is acquired 48 hours or more after hospital admission, whereas VAP is defined as a HAP that is diagnosed 48 to 72 hours after airway intubation and initiation of mechanical ventilation. HCAP includes any patient who was hospitalized in an acute care hospital for 2 or more days within 90 days of infection; resided in a nursing home or a long-term care facility; received recent intravenous antibiotics, chemotherapy, or wound care within the past 30 days of the current infection or attended a hospital or hemodialysis clinic.

Etiology. The spectrum of pathogens associated with nosocomial pneumonia differs from that of CAP. Because microaspiration of upper airway secretions is the most common route of pathogen entry into the lower respiratory tract, the etiology of nosocomial pneumonia depends largely on the type of organisms colonizing the oropharynx. Patients with nosocomial pneumonia are at greater risk for colonization and infection with a wider spectrum of multidrug-resistant (MDR) bacterial pathogens, such as *P. aeruginosa,* extended-spectrum β-lactamase (ESBL+) *Klebsiella pneumoniae, Acinetobacter baumannii,* and MRSA. Mixed infections are common, although anaerobic infections are seen infrequently. Rates of hospital-acquired *L. pneumophila* vary

considerably among hospitals. More than 50% of nosocomial pneumonias caused by *S. aureus* are caused by MRSA strains. Methicillin resistance is mediated by the *mecA* gene, which encodes a penicillin-binding protein with reduced affinity for β-lactam antibiotics. MRSA isolates are resistant to all β-lactam agents, and most hospital-acquired strains are resistant to many other antistaphylococcal drugs. Because special infection control precautions are recommended for patients with MRSA infections, the role of the clinical microbiology laboratory in the differentiation of MRSA from susceptible strains of *S. aureus* is important.

Epidemiology. The causative agent of VAP may vary by time of onset (after intubation) and risk factors for colonization and infection with MDR isolates. Early-onset VAP, occurring within 5 days of intubation, generally has a better prognosis and is more likely to be caused by aspiration of antibiotic-sensitive bacteria. Late-onset VAP, occurring more than 5 days after intubation, tends to be caused by MDR, hospital-acquired pathogens and is associated with greater morbidity and mortality. Crude mortality rates for VAP range from 10% to 65%.

The spectrum of MDR pathogens is dynamic and may vary by geographic area, by hospital, or by specific intensive care unit within the hospital. Risk factors for the development of MDR pathogens include previous hospitalization, residence in a chronic care facility, late-onset disease relative to hospitalization, and previous exposure to antibiotics. The availability of current, local epidemiologic data on endemic MDR pathogens is essential in choosing appropriate empirical antibiotic therapy and for targeting infection-control strategies. It is best to collect specimens for culture before antibiotics are initiated or as soon thereafter as possible. However, specimen collection should not delay administration of empiric antibiotic therapy, because of the high mortality rate of such infections.

Pathogenesis. The pathogenesis of nosocomial pneumonia is related to upper respiratory tract colonization, the numbers and virulence of organisms entering the lower airway, and the response of the host's defenses to this invasion. Increased patient age, more severe illness, previous treatment with antibiotics, and manipulations that increase the gastric pH are all associated with increased oropharyngeal colonization with gram-negative bacilli (Figure 32-8). Such pathogens may be acquired from the patient's own gastrointestinal tract, but exposure of patients to the microbial biota encountered during hospitalization provides an exogenous source of colonization that can also be involved in subsequent nosocomial pneumonia. Hospitalized patients with altered levels of consciousness aspirate pharyngeal contents into the lung more often than normal volunteers (70% versus 45%). In addition, intubation of the lower airway greatly increases the risk of developing nosocomial pneumonia by bypassing the normal mechanical defenses provided by the glottis and cough reflex. Nasogastric intubation also increases the risk of aspiration resulting from interference with glottic function and increased reflux of gastric secretions into the oropharynx.

Complications. Patients with extensive viral or bacterial pneumonias may have insufficient ventilation to the involved

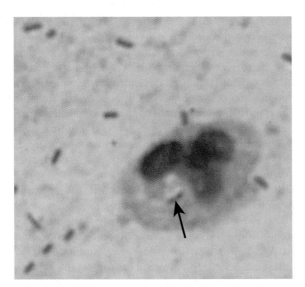

FIGURE 32-8 Gram stain of gram-negative bacilli in tracheal aspirate (*arrow* indicates intracellular gram-negative bacillus). They are common pathogens in nosocomial pneumonia. (Courtesy William M. Janda, PhD.)

lung to adequately support respiration. In rapidly progressive, multilobar pneumonias, ventilatory support may be needed as a result of overwhelming infection or an injury response of the lung termed *respiratory distress syndrome*. In these cases, mechanical support of ventilation and other supportive measures are used to provide time for antimicrobial therapy to control the pneumonia and to allow recovery of lung function. An example of tissue destruction caused by pneumonia is the development of a lung abscess. In this case, the pulmonary infection, usually an anaerobic infection of the lung, results in destruction of the lung parenchyma in the area of a necrotizing bacterial infection. These infections usually can be treated with antibiotic therapy alone. If the abscess is large and refractory to therapy, surgery may be required.

Extension of the infection beyond the chest occurs most commonly when bacterial invasion of the bloodstream occurs (bacteremia). The same type of spread is possible with viral pneumonias (viremia), although the consequences of viremia are usually much less severe than those of bacteremia. Patients with bacteremia as a complication of pneumonia have an increased mortality compared with patients with pneumonia without bacteremia. In some cases, this may simply be a reflection of the bacterial burden and the difficulty in controlling the infection. In other cases, such as gram-negative bacillary bacteremia, the presence of bacteria and their constituents (e.g., endotoxin) may be associated with severe shock, further complicating the care of the patient and increasing the likelihood of a fatal outcome. In addition to the direct consequences of bacteremia, in some instances an infection originally established in the lung may spread via the bloodstream to other sites, such as the CNS—a so-called metastatic infection.

Treatment. Broad-spectrum antibiotic therapy should be started initially and then modified and focused based upon culture data and clinical response. A shorter duration of 5 to 7 days of antibiotic therapy may be prescribed for uncomplicated pneumonia. However, pneumonia caused by infections with gram-negative bacilli requires longer duration of therapy. Empiric antibiotic therapy, pending culture results in nosocomial pneumonia, should be directed against virulent and drug-resistant strains such as *Enterobacter*, *Pseudomonas*, and *Acinetobacter*. These require therapy with extended spectrum β-lactams, carbapenems, or combinations of an antipseudomonal penicillin or antipseudomonal cephalosporin with a fluoroquinolone or aminoglycoside antibiotic. Vancomycin and linezolid are drugs of choice for treatment of MRSA pneumonia. In cases where *Legionella* is suspected as the etiology, a macrolide antibiotic should be added. In addition to empiric and culture-based tailored antibiotic therapy, ancillary measures that include chest physical therapy to aid with secretion clearance and elevation of the head of the patient's bed to reduce the likelihood of ongoing aspiration of upper respiratory and gastrointestinal secretions into the lungs may be needed.

Aspiration Pneumonia

Case Study (Aspiration Pneumonia)

A 63-year-old man who was a nursing home resident was admitted to the hospital for treatment of repeated urinary tract infections. He had several episodes of vomiting while he was an inpatient. A nurse found him to be somnolent, and pulse oximetry revealed oxygen desaturation. A chest X-ray done by the bedside showed a new infiltrate in the right middle lobe. He was transferred to the ICU for management of acute respiratory distress.

Etiology. **Aspiration pneumonia,** which occurs in both children and adults, follows the abnormal entry of fluid, particulate substances, or upper airway secretions into the lower respiratory tract. Three syndromes seen clinically, as a consequence of aspiration, are chemical pneumonitis, airway obstruction, and bacterial infection. Chemical pneumonitis refers to the aspiration of substances that are toxic, such as acidic gastric contents, into the lower respiratory tract in the absence of bacterial infection. Aspiration of food or other particulate matter may cause lower airway obstruction. In addition to associated problems with gas exchange, such lower airway obstruction can result in post-obstructive lung collapse (so-called "atelectasis") and associated infection, as a result of blocked clearance of secretions contaminated with bacteria from the upper airway or gastrointestinal tract. Even in the absence of airway obstruction, aspiration of upper airway bacteria may result in bacterial pneumonia after aspiration.

Epidemiology. Aspiration of oropharyngeal secretions is common in the general population and is more common in hospitalized patients or those who have reduced consciousness for a variety of reasons (e.g., alcohol or sedative use). The likelihood of developing infectious pneumonia after aspiration depends on the frequency of aspiration, quality and quantity of material aspirated, and host defenses. Patients with nosocomial aspiration pneumonia are more likely to have aerobic pathogens (predominantly gram-negative bacilli) than are patients with community-acquired aspiration pneumonia. Seriously ill, hospitalized patients have an increased risk of lower respiratory tract infection with aerobic gram-negative bacilli because of increased colonization with these organisms as a result of hospitalization and bacterial selection resulting from prior antibiotic therapy. Patients who are immunosuppressed by underlying disease and/or chemotherapy and patients with altered lung defenses (e.g., cigarette smoking, chronic lung disease, advanced age) are at increased risk for the development of infection after aspiration of a bacterial inoculum. In community-acquired aspiration pneumonia, the presence of periodontal disease, associated with an increased burden of oral anaerobic bacteria, increases the risk for the establishment of lung infection after aspiration.

Clinical Manifestations. The typical clinical presentation of patients with aspiration pneumonia and its complications may vary from an acute pneumonitis to a chronic, indolent respiratory condition presenting as chronic productive cough. If treatment fails, aspiration pneumonia may progress to a necrotizing pneumonia and lung abscess.

Patients with anaerobic lung abscess usually have a longer history of illness (weeks) with a more subtle onset of symptoms than patients with common acute bacterial pneumonia. Patients with lung abscess are also more likely to have putrid sputum and to complain of halitosis resulting from the involvement of anaerobic bacteria in the lung infection. On chest radiographs, areas of necrotizing pneumonia and lung abscess resulting from aspiration are more likely to involve parts of the lung that are dependent in the supine position (superior segments of the lower lobes and posterior segments of the upper lobes), because this is the most common position in which aspiration into the lung occurs. Right-sided lung involvement is twice as common as left-sided involvement, because the right mainstem bronchus has a more direct course into the lower lobe of the lung than the left mainstem bronchus.

Treatment. Treatment for acute aspiration involves respiratory support as needed based upon parameters of gas exchange and may require nasogastric tube placement, if aspiration is secondary to uncontrolled emesis. Empiric therapy of aspiration pneumonia should include broad-spectrum antibiotics that provide coverage for both anaerobic and aerobic bacteria and then should be tailored to fit specific pathogens, if they are identified during culture analysis. Depending on the clinical setting and microbiological data available (e.g., common pathogens in an intensive care setting), broad-spectrum antibiotics such as piperacillin-tazobactam or a third-generation cephalosporin plus metronidazole can be used for initial therapy. Evaluation by speech therapists may be indicated to assess impairment of swallowing mechanisms and silent aspiration.

Laboratory Diagnosis of Acute Pneumonias

Specimen Collection. Studies of expectorated sputum, when compared with other procedures, involves no risk to the patient. However, care must be taken to avoid contamination of the specimen with oropharyngeal biota. Patients should be instructed to rinse their mouths and collect "deep" sputum specimen, with the goal of sampling lower, and not upper,

respiratory tract secretions. Patients should remove dentures during specimen collection.

The expectorated sputum specimen should be examined for its character, which provides a preliminary indication about the type of pneumonia. A patient with typical bacterial pneumonia (e.g., pneumococcal pneumonia) will usually produce purulent sputum that may be streaked with small amounts of blood or be rusty in color. In contrast, patients with atypical pneumonia (e.g., mycoplasma pneumonia) may produce no sputum or small amounts of sputum that is less purulent.

Other Specimen Collection Methods. In some cases of pneumonia, expectorated sputum specimens may be either unavailable or of unsatisfactory quality for analysis. Specimen collection using a flexible, fiberoptic bronchoscope is useful when direct specimens from the lower respiratory tract or specific lung areas are required. Proper use of a protected brush extended from the end of the bronchoscope to collect specimens from the area of pneumonia may be useful for diagnosing both aerobic and anaerobic infections.

The same general approach used to process expectorated sputum specimens is used to process specimens collected using bronchoscopy. Bronchoalveolar lavage adds an extra dimension that may increase diagnostic yield. The segment of the lung suspected of being involved in a pneumonic process is lavaged with sterile saline; after aspiration through the bronchoscope, this fluid can be concentrated before processing. Quantitative cultures can help determine whether the potential pathogen is the cause of pneumonia or a contaminant from the upper respiratory tract. Detection of greater than 10^3 colony-forming units of bacteria has become a standard threshold for a positive culture. When bronchoscopy procedures are unsuccessful in establishing an etiologic diagnosis and an infectious pneumonia is suspected, it may be necessary to proceed to a lung biopsy to obtain tissue for culture, staining, and histologic study. Transbronchial biopsy can be performed through the flexible bronchoscope. The tissue specimen collected by this technique is small and may be insufficient for diagnosis. Video-assisted thoracoscopic surgery (VATS) for lung biopsy has been introduced as a means of sampling peripheral lung lesions located near the pleura. VATS provides a means to do a more directed biopsy under direct visualization of the area of involved lung. As a final option, an open lung biopsy performed during a surgical procedure may be necessary to obtain a larger tissue specimen for microbiologic and histologic study, when empiric therapy fails and a specific diagnosis becomes essential for therapeutic decision making.

Direct Microscopic Examination. The quality of the sputum specimen is determined by a direct Gram-stained smear. The goal is to eliminate specimens that are contaminated with oropharyngeal contents by evaluating the relative numbers of neutrophils and epithelial cells under low-power magnification. As a general guideline, samples with greater than 25 neutrophils and fewer than 10 epithelial cells per microscopic field are considered to be relatively free of contamination (Figure 32-9); samples containing more than 25 squamous epithelial cells per field (Figure 32-10, *A*) should not be cultured. Gram stain of samples collected by invasive procedures can produce more meaningful results, because there is a reduced likelihood of contamination of the specimens with upper respiratory biota. In addition to the presence or absence of microorganisms and inflammatory cells, the microscopic morphology of the organisms present may lead to a presumptive microbiologic diagnosis (Figure 32-10, *B*).

Culture. Only high-quality specimens should be processed for culture. The protocol should include culture media such as SBA, MAC, and CHOC plates to recover all likely bacterial agents. Samples collected by invasive procedures are unlikely to be contaminated with upper respiratory biota and, when properly collected, can be processed for anaerobic as well as aerobic culture, particularly if the patient is suspected of having aspiration pneumonia, lung abscess, or empyema.

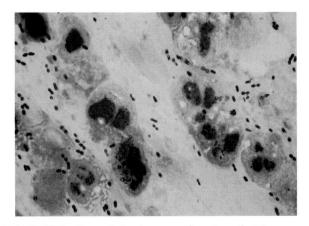

FIGURE 32-9 Gram-stained smear of sputum that is acceptable for culture, with white blood cells and gram-positive diplococci.

Empyema

Case Study

A 50-year-old hospitalized man with a history of community-acquired pneumonia continued to spike a low-grade fever despite a prolonged course of antibiotics. Chest X-ray showed left-sided pleural effusion. A CT scan of the chest showed that the effusion was loculated (i.e., was not free flowing but rather was trapped in multiple subcompartments because of fibrous reaction to an infection-induced purulent reaction).

Empyema is defined as a collection of purulent fluid in an existing body cavity, especially the pleural space between the lung and the chest wall. Empyema is distinguished from lung abscess, which is a collection of purulent fluid/material in a newly formed cavity in the lung. Although the accumulation of pleural fluid is fairly common in association with acute bacterial pneumonia, most such accumulations are sterile, and only a small percentage qualify as empyemas. The distinction between a sterile pleural effusion and empyema depends on the presence of a bacterial pathogen and an inflammatory response and is made using pleural fluid cell counts, chemistries, and cultures.

Etiology

In patients with community-acquired pneumonia, *S. aureus*, *S. pneumoniae*, and *S. pyogenes* are the most common causes of empyema. Empyema among hospitalized patients is caused primarily by aerobic gram-negative bacilli. Anaerobic bacteria are variably isolated from approximately one third to three fourths of empyemas. Empyemas, particularly if they are

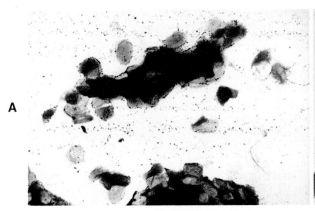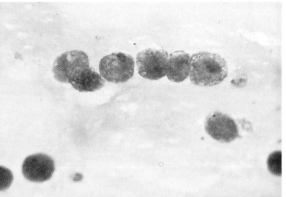

FIGURE 32-10 **A,** Expectorated sputum: smear and Gram stain visualized with light microscopy under low-power view (LPV). There is no presence of pus cells. It shows heavy presence of contaminating bacteria and epithelial cells. The sample is saliva, not sputum. There could be several reasons for submission of this sample to the laboratory. The patient could have been poorly directed and simply "spit" into the collection container, or the patient's cough may not be productive of sputum. **B,** Aspirated sputum: smear and Gram stain visualized with light microscopy under high-power view (HPV). There is no presence of pus cells or organisms. However, it shows specialized cells and mucus (pink-stained background) that are the local materials from the surface of the tracheobronchial tree. This smear confirms that sputum was sampled and that there is no suspicion for infection and no evidence of significant contamination (e.g., large numbers of epithelial cells, commonly found in the mouth). Routine bacterial culture of this specimen might still grow insignificant oral flora or pathogens.

mutiloculated (divided into multiple pleural spaces), may harbor multiple bacterial species. In patients with chronic pneumonias, such as those caused by *M. tuberculosis*, empyema may occur as a result of rupture of an underlying cavity into the pleural space.

Clinical Manifestations

The clinical presentation of a patient with empyema is usually an extension of the illness of the underlying lung (e.g., bacterial pneumonia, lung abscess). Patients may have chest pain on the affected side, fever, chills, and night sweats. If the empyema is large, it may be detected during the physical examination as an area of absent or reduced breath sounds. If empyema is not suspected based upon the physical findings, it is usually detected as an abnormality on the chest radiograph. Computed tomography of the chest may be necessary to differentiate empyema from underlying lung abscess or lung consolidation.

Pathogenesis

Empyema is usually a consequence of extension of infection directly from the underlying lung to the pleural space. Empyema may also complicate chest surgery or chest trauma, both of which provide a direct route of infection to the pleural space. Less commonly, empyema results from contamination of the pleural space as a result of peritoneal or gastrointestinal disease. Infection may extend to the pleural space from a pyogenic process beneath the diaphragm. Rarely, empyema results from infection of the pleural (and mediastinal) space after esophageal rupture.

Once organisms gain access to the pleural space, the resulting inflammatory response to this infection, along with the pleural response to the underlying process that seeded the pleural space, stimulates the exudation of fluid into this area. Typically, accumulation of large numbers of neutrophilic leukocytes occurs, resulting in the purulent appearance of most empyemas. Toward the later (or organizing) stages of an empyema, fibroblast infiltration into the area is associated with organization of the contents of the pleural space into a thick capsule that adheres to the lung and chest wall surfaces. Characteristics of the empyema fluid create an environment in which elimination of the offending pathogen is compromised. Opsonins and complement activity, which are necessary for the proper phagocytosis of bacteria by infiltrating granulocytes, are present in reduced concentrations in empyema fluid. In addition to this limitation of the host response, the usefulness of antibiotics in treating empyema is limited by the minimal blood supply to the area, resulting in reduced drug delivery, and by the low pH of empyema fluid, which can reduce the antimicrobial activity of antibiotics.

Complications

The complications associated with empyema depend primarily on the nature of the underlying disease. The main consequence of empyema is persistence of infection. If the empyema is not drained and treated with appropriate antibiotics, the infection causing the empyema may be difficult to eliminate. Persistent, poorly controlled infection may lead to the multiple complications associated with unresolved sepsis. A long-term complication of empyema is encasement of the lung in a thick capsule, which may alter lung function. This complication may necessitate removal of the thickened pleural lining (pleural decortication), which may or may not restore the function of the underlying lung, depending on the duration of the dysfunction.

Laboratory Diagnosis

Pleural fluid specimens for culture should be aspirated directly into an evacuated, sterile syringe. If the volume of the pleural fluid is relatively large, this procedure can usually be performed at the patient's bedside. If the volume is smaller or if the space is loculated, pleural fluid aspiration may have to be done in the radiology suite guided by ultrasound or CT scan. Because the volume of pleural fluid needed for diagnostic studies is small (a few milliliters), it is not necessary to remove the majority of the effusion for this purpose. Any excess air in the syringe should be expelled promptly to improve the yield of anaerobic bacteria.

The syringe containing the fluid should be transported immediately to the diagnostic microbiology laboratory so that Gram stain and processing for anaerobic and other bacteria can be performed promptly. The character (e.g., purulence, odor, presence of blood) of the fluid should be recorded. Aliquots of the fluid should be distributed to the hematology and chemistry laboratories for studies of cell count and differential count, total protein, lactic dehydrogenase concentration, and pH. These measurements provide parameters that are useful in differentiating an empyema from a transudative effusion.

An aliquot of the pleural fluid should be saved in case special studies are required to detect capsular polysaccharide antigens of pathogenic bacteria such as *S. pneumoniae* or *H. influenzae*. If malignancy is in the differential diagnosis, a fluid specimen should also be submitted for cytology. Because it is usually desirable to submit a large specimen for cytology when a malignant pleural effusion is suspected, a larger sample should be collected specifically for this purpose. If the diagnosis of tuberculous pleural effusion is suspected, it is useful to obtain a pleural biopsy to complement the pleural fluid sample for mycobacterial culture and, if available, for polymerase chain reaction (PCR) study for tuberculosis (TB). The combined data from such studies of two pleural biopsy specimens can be diagnostic in approximately 85% of cases, whereas culture of pleural fluid alone is positive in less than 25% of confirmed cases of tuberculous empyema.

Treatment

The mainstay of therapy of empyema is chest tube drainage. Other surgical management, such as decortication, may be needed in selected cases. If a pathogen is identified for an underlying pneumonia that is associated with empyema, it is appropriate to complement chest tube drainage with treatment using an antibiotic or antibiotics that are effective against the pathogen causing the pneumonia. This general principle of basing the choice of antibiotic therapy on the associated infectious lung pathology also applies to other conditions. Thus empyema associated with lung abscess should be treated with the same types of antibiotics that would be appropriate for the abscess. Because pleural fluid does not present the same problem of contamination with other respiratory biota as happens with sputum specimens and because

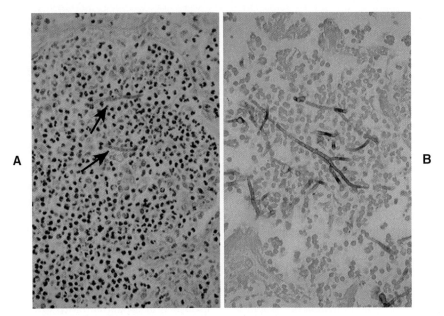

FIGURE 32-11   Lung exudate from a patient with hematologic disorder showing alveoli containing branching fungal elements. **A,** Hematoxylin and eosin stain; **B,** Gomori methylene silver (GMS) stain. (Courtesy Shirlyn B. McKenzie, PhD.)

pleural fluid should be sterile, a positive pleural fluid culture for a single pathogen (e.g., *S. pneumoniae*) can provide the definitive microbiologic diagnosis of the cause of a pneumonia (as is the case for positive blood cultures).

Tuberculosis and Other Chronic Pneumonias

Bacterial pneumonias usually resolve completely over a period of weeks. On occasion, however, resolution of pneumonia is delayed, with radiographic lung abnormalities that persist beyond improvement of clinical symptoms. Some bacteria that typically cause acute pneumonias induce necrotizing processes in the lung that can be slow to resolve despite clinical cure. Examples include anaerobic lung infections, gram-negative bacillary pneumonias, and pneumonias caused by *S. aureus*. Some pneumonias are inherently slow in progression and chronic in nature; the most common of these are mycobacterial and fungal infections of the lung.

Case Study

A 60-year-old man came to an Emergency Department complaining of cough and fever lasting several weeks. He reported night sweats and weight loss over the last few months. He admitted to drinking alcohol heavily on weekends and to staying in a shelter for the homeless most of the previous winter. The patient had a fever and appeared very thin. He coughed frequently during the examination. His chest radiograph revealed a right upper lobe infiltrate with a small area of cavitation.

Etiology

Mycobacteria are the most common pathogens that cause chronic pneumonias in immunocompetent hosts. Tuberculosis (TB) continues to be the most important cause of chronic

pneumonia globally and in certain regions of the United States. More than 50% of TB cases have been diagnosed in recent immigrants to the United States, and this percentage is steadily increasing. The remainder of cases tends to occur among socially disadvantaged, elderly, and immunocompromised patients (e.g., those with acquired immunedeficiency syndrome [AIDS]). Infections with nontuberculous mycobacteria (NTM) (e.g., *Mycobacterium avium* complex, *Mycobacterium kansasii,* and *Mycobacterium chelonae/abscessus*) can present with cavitary lung disease that is indistinguishable from TB, but more commonly present as nodular or patchy lung infiltrates superimposed on underlying lung disease (e.g., bronchiectasis, emphysema, pulmonary fibrosis, cystic fibrosis).

Opportunistic fungal pathogens, such as *Aspergillus* (Figure 32-11, *A* and *B*) and *Cryptococcus*, can cause acute and chronic pneumonia in immunosuppressed patients but rarely do so in immunocompetent patients. In contrast, the endemic fungal pathogens, *Histoplasma capsulatum, Blastomyces dermatitidis,* and *Coccidioides immitis* can cause chronic pneumonia in immunocompetent hosts.

Clinical Manifestations

The symptoms seen in the setting of acute pneumonia (e.g., fever, chills, productive cough) may also be observed in patients with chronic pneumonias, but these and other symptoms may be less intense and dramatic in onset. This may result in a greater delay between symptom onset and diagnosis. Because of the prolonged period of illness associated with chronic pneumonias, the patient may also exhibit signs that are not seen with acute infections, such as weight loss and slowly increasing debility.

Mycobacterial or fungal infections may be severe in immunocompromised patients, with local or disseminated infection causing life-threatening complications. For example, *Aspergil-*

lus spp. may cause overwhelming pneumonia in neutropenic patients, and cryptococcal pneumonia can cause fatal dissemination to the CNS in patients who are immunosuppressed after receiving chemotherapy or as a result of AIDS. Physical examination of patients with chronic pneumonia may show few signs, other than those associated with general debilitation. Routine laboratory studies are rarely helpful in making a specific diagnosis. In addition to the history, a chest radiograph and CT of the chest are the most important initial diagnostic studies in establishing a presumptive diagnosis of chronic pneumonia. For example, upper lobe cavitary lung disease is suggestive of TB or other mycobacterial disease. However, because many infections that cause chronic pneumonia present with similar radiographic abnormalities, further studies must be planned for a specific diagnosis.

Pathogenesis

Chronic pneumonias caused by mycobacterial or fungal pathogens typically elicit a granulomatous response in the lung that is distinct from the acute inflammatory response seen with acute bacterial pneumonias. Both humoral (specific antibody) and cellular (delayed type hypersensitivity) responses are elicited by these pathogens. The cellular immune response to chronic lung infections is involved in both protective and tissue-destructive aspects of these illnesses.

Complications

The complications of chronic infectious pneumonias depend on the extent of the local and systemic spread of the infection, the duration of the illness, and the immunologic status of the host. Patients who develop extensive lung involvement with a chronic infection, as a result of late or inadequate medical intervention or failed therapy, may eventually suffer from progressive debility and respiratory insufficiency. Infection dissemination beyond the lung in immunocompromised patients may result in infection of other vital organs, such as the CNS with *Cryptococcus* infection and multiple organ involvement in disseminated *Mycobacterium avium* complex infection in AIDS patients.

Laboratory Diagnosis

TB is usually the easiest to diagnose, among the chronic pneumonias. The presence of *M. tuberculosis* in expectorated sputum is diagnostic of disease that must be treated and that poses a public health risk. Because NTM can colonize the respiratory tract in the absence of invasive lung disease, repeated sputum specimens in the context of a progressive pulmonary process and in the absence of another pathogen may be needed to establish an association between the NTM infection and the illness. Therefore isolation of an organism (e.g., *M. avium* complex) from a single sputum specimen may be insufficient to establish an etiologic diagnosis.

Because of the public health implications of TB, any positive mycobacterial stain or culture should be reported, and proper respiratory isolation should be established until the organism is speciated. With chronic pneumonias of fungal etiology, it is difficult to isolate the pathogen from expectorated sputum. Therefore tissue specimens obtained by transbronchial biopsy at bronchoscopy, VATS lung biopsy, or open

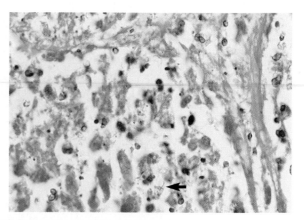

FIGURE 32-12 Acid-fast bacillus stain of sputum containing mycobacteria (red-stained organisms) *(arrow).*

lung biopsy are often required to identify the pathogen. Depending on the severity of the clinical illness, empirical therapy is often started based upon a presumptive diagnosis from the clinical presentation and the results of histopathology studies and special stains, while awaiting culture confirmation from the diagnostic microbiology laboratory.

Direct Microscopic Examination. Smears of concentrated sputum samples prepared for mycobacterial culture should be stained with acid-fast stains (Figure 32-12), such as Kinyoun, Ziehl-Neelsen, or with any of the fluorochrome stains—commonly referred to collectively as the *AFB (acid-fast bacillus) stain* of sputum. Direct microscopic examination of respiratory secretions should also include preparations to detect fungal agents. Potassium hydroxide and calcofluor white are commonly used to detect yeast cells and hyphal elements.

Rapid Diagnostic Tests for Tuberculosis. To complement the AFB stain of sputum specimens for rapid diagnosis, nucleic acid amplification (NAA) tests are available for *M. tuberculosis* infections of the lung. NAA tests use polymerase chain reaction and other methods to amplify and detect TB DNA and RNA in sputum, thus providing highly sensitive and specific methods to detect the presence of *M. tuberculosis* days to weeks before culture positivity. The sensitivity of these tests is greater for AFB smear-positive (more than 90%) than for smear-negative (approximately 70%) sputums. Nucleic acid amplification testing is recommended for all sputum specimens that contain AFB on direct sputum smears and for AFB-negative sputums when the clinical suspicion of TB is high. There is less experience with the use of NAA for TB diagnosis at other sites of infection; however, reports suggest that NAA methods are also useful for rapid diagnosis using spinal, pleural, and pericardial fluid specimens. These rapid assays require skilled personnel and are more costly per assay than conventional diagnostic methods. However, the increased speed of diagnosis can result in large overall savings, when considering the total costs of patient care.

Antigen Assays for Fungal Infections. Fungal pneumonias share with TB the problem of delays in culture-based diagnoses. Serum and urine fungal antigen testing can be a useful adjunct to microscopic studies for diagnosis of fungal infections, pending culture confirmation. Serum and urine antigen testing are increasingly available and useful as a complement to histology and culture studies—e.g., for *Histoplasma capsulatum* and *Blastomyces dermatitidis*. The value for diagnosis of other fungal antigen studies is under investigation.

Culture and Rapid Identification. Culture studies in patients with chronic pneumonias require close communication between the clinician and the clinical microbiologist. It is necessary to use special techniques to process respiratory secretions and lung tissue specimens for identification of mycobacterial and fungal pathogens. Furthermore, in some cases (e.g., TB, coccidioidomycosis), isolation of the pathogen creates a biohazard in the diagnostic laboratory. Therefore laboratory personnel must use special precautions when culturing these specimens.

Culture diagnosis of TB and NTM infections is commonly combined with early growth detection using new automated methods and molecular diagnostic probes. These assays speed detection of culture positivity and mycobacterial species identification, compared with what is possible using conventional bacterial colony detection on agar plates and biochemical studies on bacterial subcultures.

Treatment

The current standard for treatment of pulmonary TB is 6 months of therapy with multiple antibiotics if the *M. tuberculosis* isolate is susceptible to all first-line TB drugs. Patients with pansusceptible TB are started on a four-drug regimen of isoniazid (INH), rifampin, pyrazinamide, and ethambutol for an initial 2 months, followed by isoniazid and rifampin for an additional 4 months. Ideally, this therapy is delivered using what is termed "directly observed therapy" (DOT), because of the problems associated with failure of patients to adhere to the prolonged treatment. These problems include both treatment failure and emergence of TB drug resistance as a result of inadequate therapy and resulting bacterial selection. Because of these problems, there are ongoing studies of new anti-TB regimens to try to shorten the duration of therapy required for cure. Treatment duration must be prolonged (usually for 18 to 24 months) for MDR TB, which is defined as resistance of the *M. tuberculosis* isolate to at least INH and rifampin. In these cases, therapy should always be based upon antibiotic susceptibility testing results and done after consultation with an expert in TB therapy.

Chronic pneumonia caused by fungal infection also requires prolonged therapy. In cases of severe illness, therapy may be initiated with an intravenous amphotericin B preparation and then followed with an oral agent for prolonged treatment (12 to 24 months), whereas oral therapy may be used as initial treatment for patients with moderately severe illness. The oral antifungal agents of choice depend on the fungal pathogen being treated and should be selected with input from a specialist with expertise in treating chronic fungal pneumonias. For example, ketoconazole is often useful for treatment of infections with endemic mycoses, but the triazole drug, voriconazole, has replaced ketoconazole as the oral agent of choice for invasive *Aspergillus* infection. Extensive lung destruction resulting from fungal pneumonia may require a combined medical/surgical approach to treatment.

RESPIRATORY TRACT INFECTIONS IN THE IMMUNOCOMPROMISED HOST

Case Study

A 29-year-old man with a history of chronic myelogenous leukemia treated with bone marrow transplantation presented to the Oncology Clinic with a 3-day history of worsening fatigue and cough with yellowish, greenish sputum but no fever. A chest CT scan showed pulmonary micronodules and focal consolidation with necrosis and abscess formation within the areas of consolidation. The consolidation had worsened compared with a previous CT done a month ago. He had been on immunosuppressive medications for bone marrow transplant with tacrolimus and prednisone.

Opportunistic pathogens are so termed because they generally do not cause disease in normal hosts but require the "opportunity" of an impairment of host defense mechanisms to cause disease. Patients who are susceptible to opportunistic infections are called *immunocompromised hosts*. The expanded use of chemotherapeutic regimens for malignancy, the increased use of solid organ and hematopoietic transplantation for a variety of conditions, the prolonged survival of patients with congenital immune deficits and autoimmune disorders, and the HIV/AIDS epidemic have all contributed to increased numbers of immunocompromised hosts. Pulmonary infection is the most common form of documented infection in these individuals, because of exposure to potential pathogens through the respiratory route. Because early diagnosis and specific therapies are the cornerstones of successful treatment of infection in immunocompromised patients, the clinical microbiology laboratory plays an important role in their management.

Opportunistic Respiratory Tract Infections in Patients with HIV/AIDS

Case Study

An 18-year-old man with no significant past medical history presented to the Emergency Department with a history of cough, whitish sputum production, and shortness of breath, along with subjective fevers, chills, and rigors. The chest X-ray showed bilateral infiltrates in a diffuse "butterfly" pattern involving both central lung fields. The patient reported having unprotected sexual encounters with multiple other men and a history of IV drug use.

The occurrence of opportunistic disease in patients with HIV infection is a combined function of the extent of underlying host immunodeficiency and pathogen virulence. The absolute CD4 cell count remains the best surrogate marker for assessing the risk of HIV-associated, infectious complications. With CD4 cell counts greater than $500/mm^3$, it is more likely that infections will be caused by more virulent organisms that are capable of causing disease in immunocompetent hosts, such as *S. pneumoniae* or *M. tuberculosis*. When the CD4 cell count

TABLE 32-4 Common Respiratory Pathogens in HIV Infection in Relation to CD4 Count

Pathogen	CD4 Count
Bacteria	
Mycobacterium tuberculosis	Any
Mycobacterium avium complex	<100
Streptococcus pneumoniae	Any
Haemophilus influenzae	Any
Staphylococcus aureus	<500
Pseudomonas aeruginosa	<50
Rhodococcus equi	<100
Nocardia spp.	<100
Protozoa	
Toxoplasma gondii	<100
Fungi	
Pneumocystis jiroveci (carinii)	<200
Coccidioides immitis	<200
Histoplasma capsulatum	<100
Aspergillus spp.	<100
Viruses	
Influenza	Any
Cytomegalovirus	<50

HIV, Human immunodeficiency virus.

falls below 200/mm^3, the risk increases for infection with opportunistic pathogens that rarely cause disease in normal hosts, such as *Pneumocystis jiroveci* or *M. avium* complex (Table 32-4).

Epidemiology

The epidemiology of HIV-associated opportunistic infections has changed, along with the advent of highly active antiretroviral therapy (HAART) and the widespread use of improved preventive therapy. Nevertheless, pulmonary diseases remain a common complication of infection with HIV. *P. jiroveci (carinii)* pneumonia (PJP or PCP) remains the most common AIDS-associated opportunistic infection, although its incidence has decreased. Bacterial pneumonia is common and has increased as a proportion of diagnosed pulmonary infections despite an overall decrease in the number of cases. Tuberculosis is one of the most common AIDS-related opportunistic infections worldwide. Because patients with HIV infection have an elevated risk of progression of recent TB infection to active disease and of reactivation of latent TB infection, the diagnosis of TB remains an important consideration, even in areas of the world with low TB prevalence. The endemic fungi, *Histoplasma capsulatum* and *Coccidioides immitis,* cause pulmonary disease with increased incidence in patients with advanced HIV infection. Another important cause of fungal pneumonia in such patients is *Cryptococcus neoformans,* an encapsulated fungus that is widespread in the environment.

Although bacterial pneumonias can occur throughout the course of HIV infection, they tend to develop more frequently in individuals with advanced immunosuppression. *S. pneumoniae, H. influenzae,* and *S. aureus* are the most common etiologic agents. In addition, *P. aeruginosa* has been reported with increased frequency as a cause of recurrent community-acquired pneumonia in patients with advanced HIV infection. Nosocomial pneumonia in HIV-infected patients is most commonly caused by *S. aureus* and gram-negative organisms, including *P. aeruginosa, K. pneumonia,* and *Enterobacter* spp.

Cytomegalovirus (CMV) is a common isolate from respiratory specimens but a rare cause of clinical pneumonia in persons with advanced HIV infection. Influenza is a common cause of upper respiratory tract infections and bronchitis. Cases of influenza pneumonia may be complicated by bacterial superinfection with *S. pneumoniae, S. aureus,* and *H. influenzae.* Kaposi's sarcoma (KS) and non-Hodgkin lymphoma (NHL) are two common HIV-associated malignancies with strong viral associations and that frequently develop pulmonary involvement. KS is associated with human herpes virus 8 (HHV8). HHV8 DNA has been detected in sarcoma tissue and in the bronchoalveolar lavage fluid of patients with pulmonary KS. NHL is associated with Epstein-Barr virus. NHL usually develops at an advanced stage of HIV disease with extensive involvement at extranodal sites. Evidence of lung involvement may include pulmonary masses or nodules, parenchymal infiltrates, and pleural effusions.

Laboratory Diagnosis

Gram stain and bacterial cultures and AFB stain and mycobacterial cultures are appropriate for AIDS patients with expectorated sputum. In addition, blood cultures should be obtained. *S. pneumoniae* can be isolated in blood cultures in as many as 60% of HIV-infected patients with pneumococcal pneumonia. Sputum induction can increase the diagnostic yield of organisms such as *P. jiroveci* in patients who cannot produce sputum. If a specific diagnosis is not established, bronchoalveolar lavage can be used to identify HIV-related pathogens in secretions from the lower respiratory tract.

The diagnostic yield of sputum smear for *M. tuberculosis* is comparable to that found in HIV-negative patients. In more advanced stages of HIV disease, the sensitivity of sputum studies for AFB is lower, probably because of reduced sputum production associated with the reduced inflammatory response to infection. Sputum culture has a yield of approximately 90% in active TB. Bronchoalveolar lavage may increase the sensitivity of smear and culture. *P. jiroveci* was classified previously as a protozoan based on its morphologic appearance and response to antiprotozoal drugs. Genetic analysis, however, suggests *P. jiroveci (carinii)* is a fungus. *P. jiroveci (carinii)* cannot be cultured using fungal or other media. Diagnosis depends on cytopathology or immunologic detection of organisms in specimens of induced sputum or bronchoalveolar lavage. Induced sputum is stained with Giemsa or methenamine silver stain and examined for the presence of pneumocystic cysts. Monoclonal antibodies are available for direct and indirect immunofluorescence studies. In experienced laboratories, the diagnostic sensitivity of induced sputum approaches 90%, eliminating the need for more invasive diagnostic procedures in most cases (Figure 32-13). The serum cryptococcal antigen is less likely to be positive in localized cryptococcal pneumonia compared with disseminated cryptococcosis. However, its presence is useful in confirming the diagnosis, because the assay has excellent specificity. Histoplasma polysaccharide antigen (HPA) can be detected in the urine of 90% of patients with disseminated infection and 75%

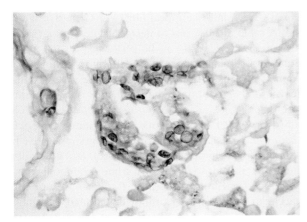

FIGURE 32-13 Gomori methylene silver (GMS) stain of bronchoalveolar lavage with *P. jiroveci (carinii)* cysts.

of those with diffuse acute pulmonary histoplasmosis. A recently developed *Blastomyces* urinary antigen has demonstrated similarly high sensitivity. Because the antigen assays for histoplasmosis and blastomycosis demonstrate considerable cross-reactivity, definitive diagnosis might require organism identification by characteristic histopathology or culture isolation.

Treatment

Starting antiretroviral therapy (ART), when indicated for advancing HIV disease, is the most important strategy for preventing opportunistic infections. One goal of ART is to maintain the host immune response—evidenced by the CD4 count—at a level that reduces susceptibility to these secondary infections. It is generally recommended to use preventive antimicrobial therapy, for patients with CD4 counts below 200/mm^3, to reduce the incidence of opportunistic infections. For example, weekly treatment with high-dose azithromycin is used to prevent infections with *M. avium*, and daily trimethoprim-sulfamethoxazole or dapsone treatment is used to prevent *Pneumocystis* and *Toxoplasma* disease.

Treatment of active disease caused by these opportunistic pathogens or by endemic fungal pathogens, TB, or *Mycobacterium avium intracellulare* infection (MAI), is done using the same antimicrobials agents used to treat immunocompetent patients, with a few exceptions.

Respiratory Tract Infections in Patients with Other Immunocompromised States

Severe granulocytopenia is defined as a reduction of the absolute granulocyte count to 500/mm^3 or less. This state is usually observed in patients with leukemia or those who have been treated with a variety of chemotherapeutic agents. In addition to causing granulocytopenia, chemotherapeutic agents can damage the mucosal membranes of the mouth and pharynx. This breakdown of normal barriers predisposes the patient to stomatitis and pharyngitis and to damage of the tracheal mucosa and cilia, increasing the risk of both upper respiratory tract infection and pneumonia. In these circumstances, respiratory pathogens colonize the oropharynx and nasopharynx of these patients before the development of pneumo-

nia. Patients who are immunosuppressed as a result of bone marrow or organ transplantation are also at increased risk for serious pneumonias. During the initial period of severe neutropenia after bone marrow transplantation, the same types of infections seen in other neutropenic states may be observed. Less commonly, congenital defects in antibody production (hypogammaglobulinemia), complement synthesis (classic and alternative complement pathway defects) and cellular components of the host immune response (functional neutrophil and lymphocyte defects) are observed and can predispose to opportunistic respiratory tract infections.

Epidemiology

Because neutropenic and transplant patients are immunocompromised, organisms that constitute part of the normal biota and that are not pathogenic in normal hosts may also become invasive pathogens. Furthermore, exposure of these patients to prolonged hospitalization and to repeated courses of broad-spectrum antibiotics often results in increased colonization with virulent and drug-resistant microorganisms. Antibiotic-resistant Enterobacteriaceae, staphylococci, and *Pseudomonas* are common pathogens that cause both bacteremia and pneumonia, often in association with skin and gastrointestinal lesions.

In bone marrow transplant patients being treated for chronic graft-versus-host disease, the incidence of *S. pneumoniae* infection is unusually high. Patients receiving solid organ transplants are particularly vulnerable to infection with *S. aureus* and *Legionella* species. Pneumonia with these organisms or with gram-negative bacilli can have a 60% mortality rate in solid organ transplant recipients.

Common causes of fungal pulmonary infection include *P. jiroveci (carinii)*, *Aspergillus* spp., and *Cryptococcus neoformans*. Chronic immune suppression that includes corticosteroids is most often associated with pneumocystosis. Invasive aspergillosis may present as a primary, nosocomial infection or as an invader of tissues (including sinuses and lung parenchyma) already damaged by prior illness. Fungal galactomannan assays may be used as an adjunct to culture-based techniques of isolating *Aspergillus*. The major importance of cryptococcal pulmonary infection is that the lung is the portal of entry for disseminated infection, which frequently involves the CNS. *Cytomegalovirus* is among the most important causes of viral pneumonia in transplant patients. The occurrence of *Pneumocystis* infection is highly associated with CMV infection; PCP and CMV are the two most common infections to coexist in transplant patients. CMV antigen or PCR assays, in addition to viral culture, can be used to establish the diagnosis.

The parasitic organism *Strongyloides stercoralis* can cause life-threatening infection in immunocompromised hosts. Once acquired, *Strongyloides* can remain dormant in the gastrointestinal tract for decades. In patients receiving steroids and in transplant recipients, larvae can penetrate the bowel wall, and invade surrounding tissues, causing a hemorrhagic enterocolitis and pneumonitis. Dissemination of the larvae is frequently accompanied by bloodstream invasion of gram-negative enteric bacteria.

Immunocompromised patients are also at increased risk for pneumonia with community-acquired respiratory viruses, including influenza, respiratory syncytial virus, and adenoviruses. Pulmonary involvement with herpes simplex virus (HSV) and varicella-zoster virus (VZV) in the immunocompromised host should be considered a life-threatening emergency. Nasal, oropharyngeal, or esophageal HSV and VZV infections may spread directly to the lungs with development of vesicular lesions in the trachea, or may cause viral pneumonitis as a result of viremia secondary to cutaneous reactivation. As with other types of immunodeficiency disease, most defective humoral immune responses are acquired as a result of specific immunosuppressive therapy or underlying disease states (e.g., multiple myeloma, chronic lymphocytic leukemia).

Pneumonias in patients with hypogammaglobulinemia are usually caused by encapsulated bacteria (e.g., *S. pneumoniae, H. influenzae*) resulting from the lack of specific opsonizing antibodies to enhance phagocytosis of these organisms by granulocytes. In addition to problems with other encapsulated bacteria, patients with complement defects may have serious infections with *N. meningitidis*.

Laboratory Diagnosis

The approach to diagnosis of opportunistic respiratory tract infections in this patient population is similar to that used for patients with AIDS. The same general principle also applies regarding the reduced ability to rely on parameters of host immune response (i.e., antibody production, inflammatory reactions) and the increased emphasis on histopathology and culture identification for diagnosis.

BIOTERRORISM AND RESPIRATORY INFECTIONS

Since the anthrax attack in the United States in 2001, the threat of biologic agents as weapons to cause mass mortality has become an important security and public health issue. The Centers for Disease Control and Prevention (CDC) has labeled anthrax, plague, Q fever, and tularemia as bacterial agents that constitute the highest level of threat (Category A). All of these organisms can be aerosolized for delivery to the respiratory tract. The initial clinical presentation of these pulmonary illnesses is similar to that observed with common bacterial respiratory pathogens but can be fulminant and rapidly fatal. Therefore the greatest diagnostic challenge is clinical suspicion of these unusual pathogens in the differential diagnosis of pneumonia and the related use of appropriate diagnostic studies or resources, when such infections are almost never seen in the general clinical setting.

Inhalational anthrax caused by *Bacillus anthracis* is most likely to be diagnosed in the clinical setting of pneumonia, with blood cultures positive for gram-positive bacilli that are nonhemolytic, nonmotile, and catalase positive. Such isolates are referred to reference laboratories in the Laboratory Response Network where identification can be confirmed by direct fluorescent antibody (DFA) and molecular diagnostic testing (polymerase chain reaction [PCR]).

Pneumonic plague is caused by *Yersinia pestis*. Sputum, tissue, and blood cultures from affected individuals may show plump, gram-negative bacilli that can exhibit bipolar staining ("closed safety-pin"–like appearance) with Giemsa or Wright's stains. A rapid dipstick test to detect plague capsular antigen has been developed that can be performed on the patient's sputum and serum. Confirmatory laboratory testing should be done through the Laboratory Response Network under strict biosafety conditions because of the risk of laboratory transmission.

Q (query) fever is a zoonotic illness caused by *Coxiella burnetii*, which is an obligate intracellular gram-negative bacterium that forms spores. It usually presents as a flulike illness that may be difficult to distinguish from a common, community-acquired pneumonia. Because *C. burnetii* is an obligate intracellular organism that cannot be cultured on routinely used bacteriologic media, the laboratory diagnosis is usually based on serologic testing. Laboratory precautions and biocontainment should still be used in cases where Q fever is in the differential diagnosis, because this organism is highly infectious and can be accidentally isolated in cell culture systems used for viral diagnosis. For this reason, it is recommended that specimens should not be handled in routine microbiology laboratories but should instead be referred directly to a higher-level Laboratory Response Network facility.

Tularemia is another zoonotic illness that is caused by an aerobic gram-negative coccobacillus called *Francisella tularensis*. Pulmonary tularemia is the clinical presentation that has a high mortality rate. As with plague, the microbiology laboratory should be notified if tularemia is suspected in the differential diagnosis of pneumonia. These organisms require stringent growth conditions and are therefore difficult to isolate in culture. This is another circumstance where the level of biocontainment must be considered during diagnostic studies because of the relatively high-level infectiousness of this agent in culture. Specimens should be referred to a Laboratory Response Network facility, where presumptive diagnosis may be made using direct fluorescent antibody, PCR, and culture.

BIBLIOGRAPHY

American Thoracic Society: Guidelines for the management of adults with hospital-acquired, ventilator-associated, and healthcare-associated pneumonia, *Am J Respir Crit Care Med* 171:388, 2005.

Bartlett JG et al: Practice guidelines for the management of community-acquired pneumonia in adults, *Clin Infect Dis* 31:347, 2000.

Baselski V: Microbiologic diagnosis of ventilator-associated pneumonia, *Infect Dis Clin North Am* 7:331, 1993.

Bennedsen J et al: Utility of PCR in diagnosing pulmonary tuberculosis, *J Clin Microbiol* 34:1407, 1996.

Bisno AL: Acute pharyngitis, *N Engl J Med* 344:205, 2001.

Bisno AL et al: Practice guidelines for the diagnosis and management of group A streptococcal pharyngitis, *Clin Infect Dis* 35:113, 2002.

Black S: Epidemiology of pertussis, *Pediatr Infect Dis J* 16:S85, 1997.

Boivin G et al: Virologic features and clinical manifestations associated with human metapneumovirus: a new paramyxovirus responsible for acute respiratory-tract infections in all age groups, *J Infect Dis* 186:1330, 2002.

Boldy DA, Skidmore SJ, Ayres JG: Acute bronchitis in the community: clinical features, infective factors, changes in pulmonary function and bronchial reactivity to histamine, *Respir Med* 84:377, 1990.

Boussaud V et al: Life-threatening hemoptysis in adults with community-acquired pneumonia due to Panton-Valentine leukocidin-secreting *Staphylococcus aureus*, *Intensive Care Med* 29:1840, 2003.

Brien JH, Bass JW: Streptococcal pharyngitis: optimal site for throat culture, *J Pediatr* 106:781, 1985.

Brook I, Frazier EH: Aerobic and anaerobic microbiology of empyema: a retrospective review in two military hospitals, *Chest* 103:1502, 1993.

Broughton WA et al: Bronchoscopic protected specimen brush and bronchoalveolar lavage in the diagnosis of bacterial pneumonia, *Infect Dis Clin North Am* 5:437, 1991.

Brubaker RR: Mechanisms of bacterial virulence, *Annu Rev Microbiol* 39:21, 1985.

Chapman SJ, Davies RJ: Recent advances in parapneumonic effusion and empyema, *Curr Opin Pulm Med* 10:299, 2004.

Chapman SW, Wilson JP: Nocardiosis in transplant recipients, *Semin Respir Infect* 5:74, 1990.

Chastre J, Fagon JY: Ventilator-associated pneumonia, *Am J Respir Crit Care Med* 165:867, 2002.

Cherry JD: Epiglottitis (supraglottitis). In Feigin RD, Cherry JD, editors: *Textbook of pediatric infectious diseases*, ed 4, Philadelphia, 1998, Elsevier.

Cherry JD: Epidemiological, clinical, and laboratory aspects of pertussis in adults, *Clin Infect Dis* 28(Suppl 2):S112, 1999.

Chotpitayasunondh T et al: Human disease from influenza A (H5N1), Thailand, 2004, *Emerg Infect Dis* 11:201, 2005.

Colice GL et al: Medical and surgical treatment of parapneumonic effusions: an evidence-based guideline, *Chest* 118:1158, 2000.

Committee on Infectious Diseases: Group A streptococcal infection. In Pickering LK, editor: *2000 Red book*, Elk Grove Village, Ill, 2001, American Academy of Pediatrics.

Corbett EL et al: The growing burden of tuberculosis: global trends and interactions with the HIV epidemic, *Arch Intern Med* 163:1009, 2003.

Craven DE, Palladino R, McQuillen DP: Healthcare-associated pneumonia in adults: management principles to improve outcomes, *Infect Dis Clin North Am* 18:939, 2004.

Cunha BA: Pneumonias in the compromised host, *Infect Dis Clin North Am* 15:591, 2001.

Daly KA, Giebink GS: Clinical epidemiology of otitis media, *Pediatr Infect Dis J* 19:S31, 2000.

DePaso WJ: Aspiration pneumonia, *Clin Chest Med* 12:269, 1991.

El-Solh AA et al: Microbiology of severe aspiration pneumonia in institutionalized elderly, *Am J Respir Crit Care Med* 167:1650, 2003.

Enright MC et al: The evolutionary history of methicillin-resistant *Staphylococcus aureus* (MRSA), *Proc Natl Acad Sci U S A* 99:7687, 2002.

Ettinger NA, Trulock EP: Pulmonary considerations of organ transplantation: parts I-III, *Am Rev Respir Dis* 143:1386, 1991.

Finegold SM: Aspiration pneumonia, *Rev Infect Dis* 13(Suppl 9):S737, 1991.

Fishman JA, Rubin RH: Infection in organ transplant recipients, *N Engl J Med* 338:1741, 1998.

Fauci AS et al, editors. *Harrison's principles of internal medicine*, ed 17, New York, 2008, McGraw-Hill.

Fridkin SK: Increasing prevalence of antimicrobial resistance in intensive care units, *Crit Care Med* 29(Suppl 4):N64, 2001.

Garner D, Weston V: Effectiveness of vaccination for *Haemophilus influenzae* type b, *Lancet* 361:395, 2003.

Gaston B: Pneumonia, *Pediatr Rev* 23:132, 2002.

George DL et al: Nosocomial sinusitis in patients in the intensive care unit: a prospective epidemiological study, *Clin Infect Dis* 27:463, 1998.

Good JT Jr et al: The diagnostic value of pleural fluid pH, *Chest* 78:55, 1980.

Gonzalez R et al: Principles of appropriate antibiotic use for treatment of uncomplicated acute bronchitis: background, *Ann Intern Med* 134:521, 2001.

Gwalty JM Jr: Acute community-acquired sinusitis, *Clin Infect Dis* 23:1209, 1996.

Gwalty JM Jr: Sinusitis. In Mandell GL et al, editors: *Principles and practice of infectious diseases*, ed 5, New York, 2000, Churchill Livingstone.

Hallander HO: Microbiological and serological diagnosis of pertussis, *Clin Infect Dis* 28(Suppl 2):S99, 1999.

Halm EA, Teirstein AS: Management of community-acquired pneumonia, *N Engl J Med* 347:2039, 2002.

Heikkinen T, Thint M, Chonmaitree T: Prevalence of various respiratory viruses in the middle ear during acute otitis media, *N Engl J Med* 340:260, 1999.

Hirschtick R et al: Bacterial pneumonia in persons infected with the human immunodeficiency virus, *N Engl J Med* 333:845, 1995.

Hsieh Y et al: Quarantine for SARS, Taiwan, *Emerg Infect Dis* 11:278, 2005.

Johnston RB Jr: Current concepts: immunology. Monocytes and macrophages, *N Engl J Med* 318:747, 1988.

Jonsson JS et al: Acute bronchitis in adults. How close do we come to its aetiology in general practice? *Scand J Prim Health Care* 15:156, 1997.

Kerr JR, Mathews RC: Bordetella pertussis infection: pathogenesis, diagnosis, management, and the role of protective immunity, *Eur J Clin Morcrobiol Infect Dis* 19:77, 2000.

Klein JO: Review of consensus reports on the management of acute otitis media, *Pediatr Infect Dis J* 18:1152, 1999.

Klein JO: Otitis externa, otitis media, mastoiditis. In Mandell GL, Bennett JE, Dolin R, editors: *Principles and practice of infectious diseases*, ed 6, New York, 2005, Churchill Livingstone.

Lien NT, Lim W: Lack of H5N1 avian influenza transmission to hospital employees, Hanoi, 2004, *Emerg Infect Dis* 11:210, 2005.

Longtin J et al: Human bocavirus infections in hospitalized children and adults, *Emerg Infect Dis* 14:217, 2008.

Mackowiak PA: The normal microbial flora, *N Engl J Med* 307:83, 1982.

Mandel LA et al: Update of practice guidelines for the management of community-acquired pneumonia in immunocompetent adults, *Clin Infect Dis* 37:1405, 2003.

McIntosh K: Community-acquired pneumonia in children, *N Engl J Med* 346:429, 2002.

McPhee SJ, Papadakis MA, Tierney LM Jr, editors: *Current medical diagnosis & treatment*, ed 47, New York, 2008, McGraw-Hill.

Mermel LA, Maki DG: Bacterial pneumonia in solid organ transplantation, *Semin Respir Infect* 5:10, 1990.

Michelow IC et al: Epidemiology and clinical characteristics of community-acquired pneumonia in hospitalized children, *Pediatrics* 113:701, 2004.

Müller FM, Hoppe JE, Wirsing von König CH: Laboratory diagnosis of pertussis: state of the art in 1997, *J Clin Microbiol* 35:2435, 1997.

Niederman MS et al: Guidelines for the management of adults with community-acquired pneumonia. Diagnosis, assessment of severity, antimicrobial therapy, and prevention, *Am J Respir Crit Care Med* 163:1730, 2001.

Okuma K et al: Dissemination of new methicillin-resistant *Staphylococcus aureus* clones in the community, *J Clin Microbiol* 40:4289, 2002.

Piccirillo JF: Clinical practice: acute bacterial sinusitis, *N Engl J Med* 351:902, 2004.

Reimer LG, Carroll KC: Role of the microbiology laboratory in the diagnosis of lower respiratory tract infections, *Clin Infect Dis* 26:742, 1998.

Richards MJ et al: Nosocomial infections in medical ICUs in the United States: National Nosocomial Infections Surveillance System, *Crit Care Med* 27:887, 1999.

Shah RK et al: Epiglottitis in the *Haemophilus influenzae* type b vaccine era: changing trends, *Laryngoscope* 114:557, 2004.

Shultz KD et al: The changing face of pleural empyemas in children; epidemiology and management, *Pediatrics* 113:1735, 2004.

Sinnott JT 4th, Emmanuel PJ: Mycobacterial infections in the transplant patient, *Semin Respir Infect* 5:65, 1990.

Stockton J et al: Human metapneumovirus as a cause of community-acquired respiratory illness, *Emerg Infect Dis* 8:897, 2002.

Stone WJ, Schaffner W: Strongyloides infections in transplant recipients, *Semin Respir Infect* 5:58, 1990.

Tablan OC et al: Guidelines for preventing healthcare-associated pneumonia, 2003 recommendations of CDC and the Healthcare Infection Control Practices Advisory Committee, *MMWR Morb Mortal Wkly Rep* 53(RR-3):1, 2004.

Takala A, Eskola J, van Alphen L, et al: Spectrum of invasive *Haemophilus influenzae* type b disease in adults, *Arch Intern Med* 150:2573, 1990.

Tanner K, Fitzsimmons G, Carrol ED, et al: Haemophilus influenzae type b epiglottitis as a cause of acute upper airways obstruction in children, *BMJ* 325:1099, 2002.

Teele DW et al: Middle ear disease and the practice of pediatrics: burden during the first five years of life, *JAMA* 249:1026, 1983.

Treanor JJ: Influenza virus. In Mandell GL, Bennett JE, Dolin R, editors: *Principles and practice of infectious diseases*, ed 5, New York, 2000, Churchill Livingstone, p 1823.

Turner D, Schwartz Y, Yust I: Induced sputum for diagnosing *Pneumocystis carinii* pneumonia in HIV patients: new data, new issues, *Eur Respir J* 21:204, 2003.

Wald ER et al: Clinical practice guideline: management of sinusitis, *Pediatrics* 108:798, 2001.

Wagner KR, Chaisson RE: Pulmonary complications of HIV infection. In Wormser GP, editor: *AIDS and other manifestations of HIV infection*, ed 4, Boston, 2004, Elsevier.

Wolff AJ, O'Donnell AE: Pulmonary manifestations of HIV in the era of highly active antiretroviral therapy, *Chest* 120:1888, 2001.

Wells RG, Sty JR, Landers AD: Radiological evaluation of Pott puffy tumor, *JAMA* 255:1331, 1986.

Wheat LJ et al: Pulmonary histoplasmosis syndromes: recognition, diagnosis, and management, *Semin Respir Crit Care Med* 25:129, 2004.

Wubbel L et al: Etiology and treatment of community-acquired pneumonia in ambulatory children, *Pediatr Infect Dis J* 18:98, 1999.

Points to Remember

- The method and site of collection, the quality of the clinical specimen, and the clinical context are all important factors to consider when distinguishing between colonization and infection.
- The age and immune status of the host will help determine likely infectious pathogens.
- The normal microbiologic biota and specific anatomic structures both play a role in defending the host from respiratory tract infection.
- Virulence factors of disease-producing organisms enable them to evade host defense mechanisms and cause clinical infection.
- The prevalence of differ ent viral respiratory pathogens varies according to seasonal changes in epidemiology.
- Newer pathogens such as novel ("swine") H1N1, H5N1 avian influenza, and the SARS coronavirus can cause fatal illness, and it is important to be aware of their existence and clinical significance.

- Nosocomial pathogens are likely to be resistant to multiple antimicrobial agents, and it is important to have a working knowledge of local antibiotic resistance patterns.
- The occurrence of opportunistic disease in patients with HIV infection is a function of both underlying host immunodeficiency and pathogen virulence.
- Immunocompromised patients, including those who have had bone marrow or organ transplants, are at increased risk for serious pneumonias caused by a broader spectrum of pathogens (opportunistic agents) than is observed with immunocompetent patients.
- The reader must be aware of potential agents of bioterrorism, as listed by the Centers for Disease Control and Prevention (CDC). It is important to retain these uncommon pathogens on the list of possible agents in the differential diagnosis.

Learning Assessment Questions

1. Why is it important to distinguish between normal microbial biota and pathogenic microorganisms?

2. Why is it important to assess the immune status of the host when determining the importance of a microorganism detected in the diagnostic microbiology laboratory? What is meant by opportunistic pathogens?

3. Why should the microbiologist maintain awareness of seasonal trends in respiratory tract infections? Give examples of infectious agents in which these trends are noted?

4. What are examples of *emerging viral respiratory pathogens*?

5. What are common pathogens that cause community-acquired pneumonia? What is meant by the term *atypical pneumonia* in the context of community-acquired pneumonia?

6. What is the epidemiologic importance of the distinction between antigenic drift and antigenic shift for influenza virus infections?

7. What is the difference between community-acquired and nosocomial pneumonia, as related to the likely bacterial pathogens? Why is there a different spectrum of pathogens for these two clinical circumstances?

8. What is the significance of the absolute CD4 cell count in determining the susceptibility to infection and the likely pathogens in a patient with HIV/AIDS?

9. What diagnosis should be suspected in a patient with a chronic pneumonia who is homeless and presents with a history of increasing fatigue, weight loss, and night sweats for several weeks to months?

10. What are the bacterial pathogens that have been designated as the highest threat level (Category A) by the CDC as potential agents of bioterrorism? What is the difference in laboratory protocol for diagnostic studies that should be considered for all agents of bioterrorism?

Skin and Soft Tissue Infections

Suzanne Templer, Nina M. Clark

■ **ANATOMY OF THE SKIN**
Skin Flora

■ **LOCALIZED BACTERIAL AND FUNGAL SKIN INFECTIONS**
Dermatitis
Pyoderma
Other Soft Tissue Infections
Nodular Lymphangitis

■ **DERMATOLOGIC MANIFESTATIONS OF SYSTEMIC BACTERIAL AND FUNGAL INFECTIONS**
Bacteria
Fungi

■ **VIRAL INFECTIONS**
Rubeola
Rubella
Parvovirus B19
Enteroviruses

Herpesviridae
Molluscum Contagiosum
Orf and Milker's Nodule
Human Papillomavirus
Hemorrhagic Fever Viruses

■ **PARASITIC INFECTIONS**
Helminths
Leishmania
Ectoparasites

■ **IMMUNE- OR TOXIN-MEDIATED DERMATOLOGIC MANIFESTATIONS OF INFECTIOUS AGENTS**
Immune-Mediated Cutaneous Disease
Toxin-Mediated Cutaneous Disease

■ **LABORATORY DIAGNOSIS**

OBJECTIVES

After reading and studying this chapter, you should be able to:

1. Describe the function of the skin as a host defense mechanism.

2. List the organisms that comprise normal skin flora.

3. Discuss the role of the microbial skin biota.

4. Name the manifestations and causative agents of each of the following types of skin infections:
■ Dermatitis
■ Various forms of pyoderma including folliculitis, furuncle, carbuncle, impetigo, erysipelas, and cellulitis
■ Diabetic foot infections
■ Infectious gangrene
■ Mycetoma
■ Nodular lymphangitis

5. Name some of the systemic bacterial and fungal infections that cause dermatologic manifestations and describe these manifestations.

6. Name the causes and manifestations of the common childhood viral exanthems.

7. Describe how herpesviruses can affect the skin.

8. Name some of the important parasitic causes of cutaneous infection.

9. Describe the characteristics and name causative agents of each of these manifestations of systemic infections:
■ Disseminated intravascular coagulation
■ Vasculitis
■ Toxic shock syndrome
■ Scarlet fever
■ Immune complex and embolic disease

10. Discuss the basic methods for making a laboratory diagnosis of the skin infections noted above.

Case in Point

A 55-year-old Caucasian man with type 2 diabetes presented to the hospital with high fever, chills, and severe pain and swelling in his right leg. He was unable to walk because of these symptoms. Two days prior to admission he was in his yard and noted a stinging sensation in his leg that he thought was an insect bite. This area became red, swollen, and progressively more painful over 48 hours. On physical examination, the patient was febrile to 39.5° C, his blood pressure was low at 90/50 mmHg, and the right leg was red, swollen, and markedly tender, with several purple bullae starting to develop. A white blood cell count was elevated at 22,000 cells/mm³. Blood cultures were obtained and intravenous antibiotics started. A computed tomography scan of the leg showed gas formation in the subcutaneous tissues. The patient was taken to surgery and found to have necrosis of the subcutaneous tissues down to the fascia with purulent material present. The area was extensively debrided, and tissue and pus were sent to the laboratory for Gram stain and culture. These specimens grew multiple organisms including *Escherichia coli*, *Bacteroides*, and *Peptostreptococcus*. The blood cultures also grew *E. coli*. After several additional debridements, a long hospitalization, and skin grafting, the patient fully recovered.

Issues to Consider

After reading the patient's case history, consider the following:

- The clinical clues (e.g., patient characteristics, information obtained from the history and physical exam) used by the clinician to diagnosis the patient's illness
- The type of specimen collection procedures appropriate to maximize recovery of the infectious agents
- The type of sample processing that should occur once the specimen arrives in the laboratory
- The types of organisms likely to be recovered on culture

Key Terms

Bullae
Carbuncle
Cellulitis
Chromoblastomycosis
Dermatophytosis
Ecthyma gangrenosum
Ectoparasite
Entomophthoromycosis
Erysipelas
Erysipeloid
Erythrasma
Exanthem
Folliculitis
Furuncle
Gas gangrene
Hidradenitis suppurativa
Immunocompromised hosts
Impetigo
Intertrigo
Leprosy
Lobomycosis
Methicillin-resistant
   Staphylococcus aureus
   (MRSA)
Molluscum contagiosum
Mycetoma
Nodular lymphangitis
Necrotizing fasciitis
Orf virus
Paronychia
Petechiae
Phaeohyphomycosis
Purpura fulminans
Pyoderma
Rhinosporidiosis
Scarlet fever
Shock
Tinea
Toxic shock syndrome
Vasculitis
Vesicle
Zoonoses

The skin is the body's first line of defense against microbial invasion. As a dynamic physical barrier, the skin continually undergoes epithelial cell turnover, removing substances as well as potentially pathogenic microorganisms on its surface. In addition, the skin is colonized with a variety of resident microbes that perform a protective function.

This chapter discusses the following:
- The role of the indigenous skin flora and other organisms in the pathogenesis of skin infection
- The clinical features and causes of various primary skin and soft tissue infections
- The dermatologic manifestations of systemic infections
- The diagnosis and management of skin and soft tissue infections

ANATOMY OF THE SKIN

The skin consists of three layers: the epidermis, dermis, and subcutaneous layers (Figure 33-1). The *epidermis* is the outermost layer and is composed of several layers of epithelial cells. The *stratum corneum,* the outermost layer of the epidermis, contains dead cells consisting of a protein called *keratin.* The second skin layer, the *dermis,* is a thick layer composed of connective tissue. Sweat gland ducts, hair follicles, and oil gland ducts are found in the dermis and penetrate into the subcutaneous layer. These structures also provide potential passageways through which microbes can enter the skin. Sebum and perspiration are able to provide moisture and nutrients necessary for the growth of certain microbes. However, the proliferation of other pathogenic microorganisms can be inhibited by salt and lysozymes contained in perspiration and in the fatty acids found in sebum.

Skin Biota

The usual flora of the skin consists of those microbes able to adapt to its high salt concentration and relative lack of moisture. Important skin microflora that are also common agents of skin infection are the gram-positive cocci including staphylococci and streptococci. Coagulase-negative staphylococci such as *Staphylococcus epidermidis* are permanent skin residents; coagulase-positive *Staphylococcus aureus* is typically a transient colonizer. Other normal biota are diphtheroids such as *Propionibacterium acnes* and *Corynebacterium xerosis* and the yeasts *Candida* and *Pityrosporum.* Although vigorous washing reduces the amount of surface skin flora, it does not eliminate resident flora colonization.

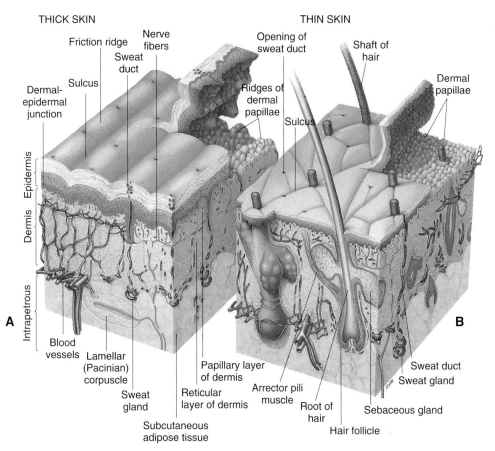

THICK SKIN

Friction ridge
Nerve
fibers
Sweat
duct
Sulcus
Dermal-
epidermal
junction

Epidermis
Dermis
Intrapetrous

A

Blood
vessels
Lamellar
(Pacinian)
corpuscle
Sweat
gland
Reticular
layer of dermis
Subcutaneous
adipose tissue
Papillary layer
of dermis

THIN SKIN

Opening of
sweat duct
Shaft of
hair
Dermal
papillae
Ridges of
dermal
papillae
Sulcus

B

Sweat duct
Sweat gland
Sebaceous gland
Hair follicle
Root of
hair
Arrector pili
muscle
Dermal
papillae

FIGURE 33-1   Anatomy of the skin. (From Patton KT, Thibodeau GA: *Anatomy and physiology,* ed 7, St Louis, 2010, Mosby.)

LOCALIZED BACTERIAL AND FUNGAL SKIN INFECTIONS

An extensive list of infections can involve the skin (Box 33-1).

Categorizing these infections is problematic because some may involve more than one soft tissue structure (e.g., skin, subcutaneous tissue, fascia, muscle) and different organisms can produce infections with the same clinical manifestations. Infections therefore may be classified in a variety of ways. One method classifies skin and soft tissue infections according to the morphology of the skin lesion, which is an important clue to the etiology of the infection and causative organisms, as noted in Box 33-1. Infections also may be classified, as they are in this chapter, according to the skin and soft tissue structure affected, the etiologic organisms (e.g., bacterial, viral, mycobacterial, fungal, parasitic), and whether the infection occurs as a primary process or a manifestation of systemic disease. It is also notable that a variety of the pathogens described may cause infection by gaining access to the skin as a result of another preexisting skin problem (Table 33-1).

The first section of the chapter examines the clinically important and prevalent infections of skin and soft tissues that typically occur in localized areas of the body. They are presented in order from the most superficial infections to the deeper, more serious infections, and they are predominantly the result of bacteria and fungi infection. Additional sections describe skin manifestations of systemic infections caused by

bacteria, fungi, viruses, and parasites, as well as immune- or toxin-mediated dermatologic diseases caused by infections.

Dermatitis

Dermatitis is a general term that describes an inflammation of the skin. It is characterized by areas of redness, swelling, and sometimes pruritus. There are many causes, only some of which are related to infection. The section below focuses on some of the common infectious etiologies of dermatitis.

Intertrigo and Superficial Candidiasis

Intertrigo is an inflammatory cutaneous condition that occurs in body areas subjected to heat, moisture, and friction, which work together to cause maceration and skin breakdown. Infectious agents enhance this process. Intertrigo occurs most frequently in the skin folds of infants and obese adults and often can be found in the axillae, perineum (e.g., diaper rash), beneath the breasts, and in abdominal folds. The most common organism present in these areas is *Candida*, although *S. aureus* and coliforms also may play a role.

Intertrigo is one form of superficial candidiasis, but *Candida* can affect the skin and mucous membranes in other forms. Thrush is a type of candidiasis involving the oral mucosa and is characterized by white, curd-like patches on the tongue, palate, or buccal mucosa. These patches adhere to the mucosa but can be removed by scraping, leaving a raw, erythematous base. A similar process can occur in the

BOX 33-1 Some Infectious Causes of Skin Lesions and Their Morphologic Manifestations

Macular, Papular, or Maculopapular Rashes
Rubeola (measles)
Rubella (German measles)
Roseola
Other viral exanthems
Scarlet fever
Toxic shock syndrome (TSS)
Secondary syphilis

Smooth Papules
Molluscum contagiosum
Condyloma latum (secondary syphilis)

Verrucous Papules or Plaques
Condyloma acuminata (venereal warts)
Viral warts
Cutaneous tuberculosis
Blastomycosis
Coccidioidomycosis
Chromomycosis
Wheals
Urticaria
Scabies
Cercarial dermatitis (swimmer's itch)
Pruritic papules
Scabies
Folliculitis
Erythematous patches or nodules
Erythema infectiosum (fifth disease)
Bacterial cellulitis
Necrotizing (gangrenous) cellulitis, fasciitis, myonecrosis
Disseminated mycoses

Serpiginous or Annular Plaques
Erythema multiforme
Erythema chronicum migrans (Lyme borreliosis)
Cutaneous larval migrans ("creeping eruption")

Vesicles or Bullae
Herpes simplex
Herpes zoster
Varicella (chickenpox)
Hand-foot-mouth disease

Herpangina
Staphylococcus scalded-skin syndrome

Pustules
Folliculitis
Impetigo
Acne
Disseminated gonococcal infection
Furuncles, carbuncles
Kerion
Herpetic whitlow
Ecthyma contagiosum (orf)
Milker's nodule
Hidradenitis suppurativa

Petechiae, Purpura, and Ecchymoses
Rocky Mountain spotted fever (RMSF)
Other rickettsial infections
Meningococcemia
Gonococcemia
Infective endocarditis
Plague
Dengue and other hemorrhagic fever viruses
Enteroviral infections
Leptospirosis

Ulcers or Necrosis
Primary syphilis
Herpes simplex
Chancroid
Lymphogranuloma venereum
Granuloma inguinale
Impetigo
Ecthyma gangrenosum
Sporotrichosis
Atypical mycobacteria
Nocardiosis
Histoplasmosis
Anthrax
Ecthyma contagiosum (orf)
Tularemia
Leishmaniasis

TABLE 33-1 Infections Secondary to Preexisting Skin Lesions

Infection	Major Pathogen
Surgical-wound infection	
Clean	*Staphylococcus aureus,* gram-negative bacilli
Contaminated, such as colon	Plus anaerobes, streptococci
Intravenous infusion sites	*S. aureus,* coagulase-negative staphylococci
Trauma	
Soil contamination	*Pseudomonas aeruginosa, clostridia*
Freshwater contamination	*Aeromonas, Plesiomonas*
Saltwater contamination	*Vibrio vulnificus*
Bites	
Human	Oral aerobes and anaerobes, *S. aureus*
Dog, cat	*Pasteurella multocida, S. aureus,* anaerobes
Rat	*Streptobacillus moniliformis, Spirillum minus (minor)*
Decubitus ulcer	Streptococci, *S. aureus,* coliforms, *Pseudomonas,* anaerobes including *Bacteroides fragilis*
Foot ulcer in diabetic patients	*S. aureus,* streptococci, coliforms, *P. aeruginosa,* anaerobes
Hidradenitis suppurativa	*S. aureus,* streptococci, coliforms, *Pseudomonas,* anaerobes
Burns	*S. aureus, Candida, P. aeruginosa*

vulvovaginal area, leading to *Candida* vaginitis. Balanitis, an inflammation of the glans penis that can spread to the thighs, scrotum, and buttocks is commonly caused by *Candida* as well. Thrush and *Candida* vaginitis can be the result of antibiotic use, because antibiotics alter the balance of the flora of the body and allow an overgrowth of yeast that is normally present and thus causes colonizing of the skin and mucous membranes. These syndromes can also occur more commonly in persons with impaired immune function. *Candida* can also cause paronychia, an inflammation of the folds of the skin bordering the nail beds (discussed further below), or onychomycosis, an infection of the nail itself.

Superficial forms of candidiasis are often treated successfully with topical antifungal agents such as nystatin or clotrimazole. Oral antifungal agents such as ketoconazole, itraconazole, or fluconazole may be necessary for treatment of more severe infections.

Erythrasma

Erythrasma is a superficial, chronic skin infection that manifests as pruritic, reddish-brown macules that are lightly scaled and wrinkled. The lesions are found most commonly in intertriginous areas, especially the groin, inner thighs, and toe webs. Axillae, intergluteal folds, and inframammary regions are less often affected. The infection occurs more often in men, obese individuals, and patients with diabetics and is generally localized and benign, but can become widespread in persons with impairment of the immune system. *Corynebacterium minutissimum,* a normal skin flora resident, is the causative organism and can be observed with a Gram stain of samples taken from the stratum corneum. The lesions also produce a coral-red fluorescence when examined under a Wood's lamp. Topical clindamycin and oral erythromycin are useful in the management of erythrasma.

Dermatophytes

Dermatophytes are moulds that colonize only keratinized surfaces of the body including hair, nails, and skin. These organisms can invade the stratum corneum of the skin, causing superficial infection in various regions of the body with the feet, groin, scalp, and nails most often affected. Three genera (*Trichophyton, Epidermophyton,* and *Microsporum*) and more than 30 species cause infection. The mode of transmission is generally through direct skin-to-skin contact or indirect contact via contaminated fomites or environmental surfaces. However, it seems that all persons are not equally susceptible to infection. For most dermatophytoses, humans are the primary reservoir; occasionally infections are acquired from infected domestic animals.

The classic lesion of a dermatophyte infection is a circular scaly patch of erythema with a raised border (Figure 33-2). Often the edges are more inflamed than the center. These infections are also known as *ringworm*, reflecting the tendency of some lesions to expand annularly. The term **tinea** is also used to denote a dermatophyte infection; the term is attached to a descriptor of the site of infection. For example, tinea cruris (jock itch) is a dermatophyte infection of the groin and perianal region, tinea pedis (athlete's foot) involves the feet, and tinea capitis is infection of the scalp (Figure 33-3). In

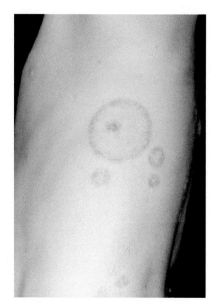

FIGURE 33-2 Tinea corporis.

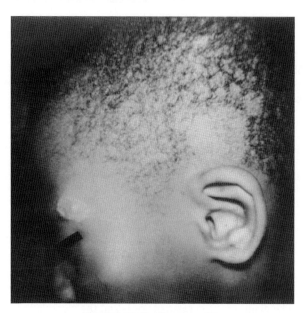

FIGURE 33-3 Tinea capitis.

addition to *Candida,* dermatophytes are another cause of onychomycosis; *tinea unguium* is the term used for this infection, which can result in significant thickening and discoloration of the nails. Tinea corporis is a dermatophyte infection of the body in general, and often involves the trunk and legs.

Tinea versicolor, or pityriasis versicolor, is an extremely common dermatophytosis that occurs worldwide (Figure 33-4). The disease is caused by *Malassezia furfur,* a lipophilic yeast and normal skin commensal. The characteristic skin manifestation of tinea versicolor is a diffuse distribution of hypopigmented or, less commonly, hyperpigmented macules principally located on the trunk and proximal portions of the extremities. The lesions are usually nonpruritic and often coalesce to form scaly plaques. Spontaneous remission may

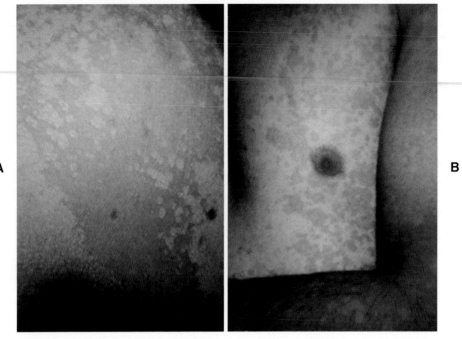

FIGURE 33-4 Hypopigmented **(A)** and hyperpigmented **(B)** rash of tinea versicolor.

TABLE 33-2 Common Primary Pyodermas

Infection	Organism	Comments
Impetigo	*Streptococcus pyogenes,* occasionally; *Staphylococcus aureus,* if bullous	Children affected most; communicable; no fever
Erysipelas	*S. pyogenes,* occasionally; other β-streptococci or *S. aureus*	Distinct raised borders; fever common
Cellulitis	*S. pyogenes, S. aureus; Haemophilus influenzae* in children	Erythema, tenderness, pain, edema, warmth; fever common
Folliculitis	*S. aureus;* gram-negative bacilli or *Candida* if predisposing conditions	Papules around hair follicles; areas exposed to whirlpool bath (*Pseudomonas aeruginosa*)
Furuncle	*S. aureus*	Fluctuant, painful nodules often in intertriginous areas
Carbuncle	*S. aureus*	Multiple abscesses
Paronychia	*S. aureus,* gram-negative bacilli, *Candida*	Periungual swelling

occur in some patients; for others, topical ketoconazole cream or selenium sulfide lotion is usually curative.

The diagnosis of **dermatophytosis** and the identification of its etiologic agents can generally be accomplished by microscopic examination of 10% potassium hydroxide preparations of involved skin, hair, and nails, or detritus beneath the nails. Skin or nails can be scraped with a scalpel blade, or nails can be clipped to obtain material for identification. Scrapings can be observed under a Wood's lamp, where certain dermatophytes (*Microsporum*) will fluoresce yellow-green. Precise mycologic etiology can be confirmed by culturing infected material on Sabouraud's agar. Dermatophytosis is treated with topical antifungal powders, ointments, and creams containing medications such as miconazole or clotrimazole. Nail infections often require oral systemic antifungal therapy for treatment (e.g., griseofulvin, terbinafine, itraconazole).

Pyoderma

The **pyodermas** are a group of inflammatory skin disorders caused by bacteria that produce pus. The terms *impetigo* and *pyoderma* have been used interchangeably by authors and in clinical practice, but there are other forms of pyoderma, as discussed below and as listed in Table 33-2.

Impetigo

Impetigo is a common pyoderma that is most often seen in children (Figure 33-5). Historically, the majority of cases were caused by group A streptococci (GAS; *Streptococcus pyogenes*) although *S. aureus* has become the predominant pathogen over the last 15 years. Group B *Streptococcus* occasionally causes impetigo in newborns secondary to acquisition of colonizing vaginal flora from the mother. Impetigo is common in hot and humid climates and is highly contagious, particularly in areas of crowding or poor hygiene. Initially, the lesions of impetigo begin as small **vesicles** that become pustules that rupture. The discharge is thick and yellow and dries to form the classic golden crusts. The lesions are superficial and painless and do not scar. They can be pruritic and easily spread by scratching. A bullous form of impetigo accounts for approximately 10% of cases. It is caused by strains of

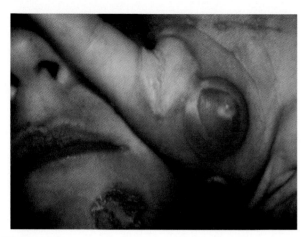

FIGURE 33-5 Bullous impetigo caused by *Staphylococcus aureus.*

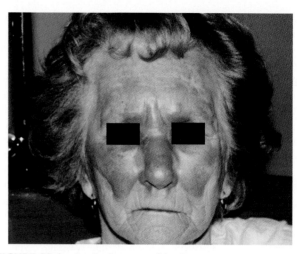

FIGURE 33-6 Erysipelas caused by *Streptococcus pyogenes.*

S. aureus that produce exfoliative toxins leading to the formation of **bullae** that quickly rupture and form a transparent light brown crust. The diagnosis of impetigo can be made from a Gram stain and culture of vesicle contents. Oral penicillin is efficacious for streptococcal impetigo, but because many cases involve *S. aureus,* penicillinase-resistant oral penicillins such as dicloxacillin or an antistaphylococcal cephalosporin such as cephalexin are better options for empiric treatment. If the patient is allergic to penicillin, erythromycin may be used. Because of the rising prevalence of community-acquired methicillin-resistant *S. aureus* infection (CA-MRSA; discussed further under Cellulitis), antibiotics with activity against these organisms, such as clindamycin or trimethoprim-sulfamethoxazole, may be preferable if a significant level of CA-MRSA is circulating in the community.

Erysipelas

Erysipelas is a type of superficial cellulitis (see Cellulitis below) that involves not only the epidermis but also the underlying dermis and lymphatic channels. Erysipelas is most often seen in children and older adults. In the past, the infection typically occurred on the face (Figure 33-6), but now it much more frequently is seen in the lower extremities. Predisposing factors in adults include diabetes mellitus, alcohol abuse, venous stasis, trauma, skin ulcers or chronic inflammatory skin conditions, and lymphatic obstruction. The lesions of erysipelas are characterized as painful, indurated areas of inflammation with raised borders that are sharply demarcated from adjacent normal skin. The involved skin is usually a bright red to crimson hue, and patients often have fever. Most uncomplicated cases remain confined to the dermis and lymphatics, but deeper extension with abscess formation or deep cellulitis can occur, and bacteremia is found in a minority of cases, making erysipelas a potentially life-threatening infection. Most infections are caused by GAS, although *S. aureus* has rarely been implicated. Usually the diagnosis is based on the clinical presentation because it is difficult to isolate GAS from the skin lesions. On occasion, aspiration of the advancing edge of a lesion with culture of the aspirate has been successful in identifying the organism. Penicillin or erythromycin are generally used for therapy.

Erysipeloid

Erysipeloid is a superficial soft tissue infection caused by *Erysipelothrix rhusiopathiae.* It is an occupational hazard of handlers of animals, meat, poultry, hides, and saltwater fish. Because it is typically introduced by trauma, the fingers and dorsum of the hand are the most frequent sites of infection. Mimicking erysipelas, the erysipeloid lesion is red and painful with raised borders. Septic arthritis and bacteremia may occur as complications. The organism is difficult to see on Gram stain but may be isolated in culture. Penicillin G is the preferred treatment.

Anthrax

Bacillus anthracis, the agent of anthrax, is a gram-positive rod that can cause ulcerative skin lesions. This form of anthrax is more common than pulmonary or systemic infection. The skin lesions most often occur in wool handlers or persons working with other animal products that are contaminated with *B. anthracis* spores. Lesions are most often seen on the face, neck, or arms at sites of minor abrasions. They begin as painless papules that vesiculate and are surrounded by significant erythema and a gelatinous type of edema. The vesicle evolves into a hemorrhagic and then necrotic lesion, and an eschar forms, although the skin lesions remain painless. Regional lymphadenopathy can be present, and bacteremia may occur with fever and hypotension. The diagnosis is often suspected clinically given the characteristic skin lesions, but biopsy and culture should be performed for confirmation. Penicillin has long been the drug of choice for the treatment of anthrax, but with the bioterrorism cases that occurred in the United States in 2001, concerns have arisen that strains can be deliberately altered so that they are resistant to commonly used antibiotics. Therefore treatment with ciprofloxacin or doxycycline has been recommended as initial therapy.

Cellulitis

Cellulitis is a diffuse inflammation and infection of both the superficial skin layers and subcutaneous tissues. It extends deeper than erysipelas and appears as an area of painful erythema, warmth, and edema of the skin with poorly demarcated margins. Depending on its extent and severity, cellulitis may or may not be accompanied by fever and other clinical or laboratory features of systemic infection (e.g., malaise, rigors, headache, elevated white blood cell count). Predisposing factors include surgery or other trauma and underlying skin disorders such as ulcers or dermatitis. Blood cultures are usually negative, and the diagnosis is often made clinically, based on the appearance of the affected area. The most common etiologic agents are GAS and *S. aureus,* so antistreptococcal and antistaphylococcal antibiotics are the treatment of choice, as discussed previously for impetigo. Patients with chronic open wounds, such as diabetic patients with foot ulcers, may develop surrounding cellulitis because of a mixture of gram-positive and gram-negative organisms and anaerobes (discussed further below).

Recurrent Cellulitis. Lymphedema, obesity, venous stasis, and untreated tinea pedis are associated with an increased risk of developing recurrent skin and soft tissue infection. Impaired lymphatic drainage leads to higher bacterial counts and difficulty with clearance of organisms. Sometimes patients are placed on long-term suppressive antibiotic regimens in an attempt to decrease the rate of infection.

MRSA Infections

Staphylococcus aureus is the most common etiology of skin and soft tissue infections in the United States, with **methicillin-resistant *Staphylococcus aureus* (MRSA)** isolates accounting for the majority of cases. MRSA is pervasive in the hospital, where 70% of *S. aureus* isolates from intensive care units are methicillin-resistant. MRSA is also increasing in community settings. Several different strains of community-acquired MRSA (CA-MRSA) are known, but strain USA 300 is the most prevalent and has been associated with severe disease including bacteremia, necrotizing pneumonia, and severe soft tissue infection. Of note, this strain is being found as a cause of disease even among patients with "hospital-acquired" infection. Studies are ongoing to determine whether strategies for eliminating MRSA colonization of the body are helpful in various settings to prevent initial or recurrent infection.

Paronychia. **Paronychia** is an infection of the cuticle surrounding the nail bed. Cases generally follow minor trauma, such as removing a hangnail. The involved part of the finger at the nail margin becomes painful, red, warm, and swollen, and pus may be expressed from around the nail bed. Staphylococci or *Candida* are usually the causative organisms. Paronychia usually responds to warm soaks, which often lead to spontaneous drainage of pus and resolution. Systemic antimicrobials and surgery typically are not required.

Folliculitis. **Folliculitis** is an inflammation and infection of hair follicles. *S. aureus* is the most common etiologic agent of folliculitis, although *Pseudomonas aeruginosa* has been implicated in cases acquired from contaminated swimming pools or whirlpools. A folliculitis caused by *Candida* spp. or gram-negative bacteria may occur in **immunocompromised hosts.** Lesions appear as small, erythematous papules and often evolve to form pustules with a whitish or yellowish central zone. Sycosis barbae is a form of folliculitis occurring in bearded men.

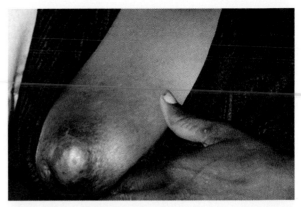

FIGURE 33-7 *Staphylococcus aureus* furuncle of the breast.

Furuncles and Carbuncles. Folliculitis can sometimes progress to form deeper inflammatory nodules called **furuncles** (Figure 33-7), especially in warm, moist areas of the body and areas subjected to friction. Certain individuals are predisposed to the development of furuncles, including those with diabetes mellitus, obesity, or defects in immune function. Furuncles are initially red and firm but soon become painful and fluctuant, and they generally drain spontaneously. *S. aureus* is the most common causative pathogen. Furuncles usually can be managed by the application of moist heat and systemic antimicrobial therapy.

A **carbuncle** is a more serious lesion that extends into the subcutaneous fat and consists of multiple coalescing abscesses that can drain at several adjacent sites along hair follicles. Carbuncles commonly occur at the nape of the neck and on the back of the thighs and are often associated with fever and systemic symptoms. Bacteremia can be a complicating event, and surgical drainage is needed for most carbuncles. Purulent drainage should be cultured to confirm the organism, which is typically *S. aureus.* Carbuncles can be treated with an oral penicillinase-resistant penicillin (e.g., dicloxacillin) or antistaphylococcal cephalosporin (e.g., cephalexin), with erythromycin or clindamycin as alternatives. CA-MRSA has become a prevalent cause of skin and soft tissue infections over the last several years (see above), although clindamycin, trimethoprim-sulfamethoxazole, and tetracyclines often retain good activity against it. MRSA should also be suspected if the patient has recently been exposed to a health care environment. Hospital-acquired MRSA infections typically are caused by multidrug-resistant *S. aureus,* and these infections therefore generally require vancomycin, linezolid, or daptomycin for treatment.

Hidradenitis Suppurativa. **Hidradenitis suppurativa** is a difficult-to-treat recurrent infection of the apocrine sweat glands. For unclear reasons, chronic obstruction of these glands, particularly ones in the axillae and groin, occurs in certain individuals, and this predisposes them to a secondary mixed bacterial infection of skin and skin structures. Organisms such as staphylococci, streptococci, gram-negative bacteria including *E. coli* and *Pseudomonas,* and anaerobic bacteria are commonly involved. The disease manifests as nodular, tender, erythematous swellings that become fluctuant and drain, often associated with fever and tender lymphadeni-

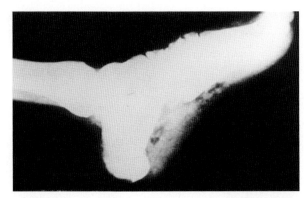

FIGURE 33-8 Diabetic foot infection with soft tissue gas formation.

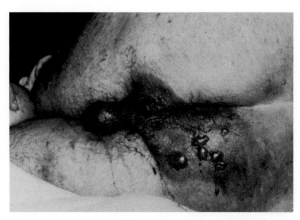

FIGURE 33-9 Clostridial myonecrosis (gas gangrene). (From Upjohn monogram: *Anaerobic infections*, Kalamazoo, Mich, 1986, The Upjohn Co.)

tis. Resolution of the lesions is typically accompanied by scarring of the involved areas. Individual episodes of infection are treated with local moist heat, broad-spectrum antibiotics, and frequently with surgical incision and drainage. Multiple recurrences of infection are often seen and this can lead to tissue fibrosis, sinus tract formation, and disfigurement.

Other Soft Tissue Infections

Diabetic Foot Infections

Foot infections are a very common occurrence in persons with diabetes mellitus, and they account for a significant amount of morbidity. Risk factors for foot infection include the presence of peripheral neuropathy, inadequate blood sugar control, compromise of the peripheral vascular circulation caused by diabetes, and improper foot care. Manifestations that can occur include cellulitis, typically caused by streptococci or staphylococci as described in the section on cellulitis above, acute or chronic soft tissue ulceration with or without underlying osteomyelitis, and gangrene (Figure 33-8). Ulcerative lesions and gangrene may, like cellulitis, be the result of staphylococci and streptococci but often are mixed infections and include gram-positives, Enterobacteriaceae, *Pseudomonas,* and anaerobic bacteria. The impairment of host defenses seen in diabetic persons can also allow low virulence organisms such as coagulase-negative staphylococci and diphtheroids to be pathogens in the skin. Cultures of open wounds are most helpful when they are obtained from deep tissues or from collections of pus beneath the skin surface. Superficial swabs yield little information because diabetic foot ulcers are often colonized with multiple bacteria that may not necessarily be the agents causing infection. Cellulitis can be treated with antibiotics active against staphylococci and streptococci whereas foot ulcers should be treated with agents that also have gram-negative and anaerobic activity. Most diabetic foot wounds require debridement, and they may even result in amputation if blood flow to the area is poor and/or a nonresponse to wound care and antibiotics is seen.

Infectious Gangrene

Infections that produce tissue necrosis and soft tissue gas represent an important subset of skin and soft tissue infection cases. Rapidly progressing and frequently life-threatening,

these soft tissue infections can be classified according to their level of soft tissue involvement (e.g., superficial, epidermal, or dermal structures, fascia, or muscle) and according to the causative microbiologic agent or agents. Subtypes of infectious gangrene include polymicrobial **necrotizing fasciitis,** typically caused by Enterobacteriaceae and anaerobes (type I; see Case in Point), streptococcal gangrene caused by *S. pyogenes* (type II), and **gas gangrene** (also known as clostridial myonecrosis) caused by *Clostridia* species, usually *C. perfringens* (Figure 33-9). Often these infections begin at a site of trauma, including surgery, but may also occur without any obvious portal of entry or as the result of a bacteremia with secondary involvement of the skin and soft tissues.

As described in the Case in Point, as infectious gangrene progresses from superficial to deep, the patient appears more acutely ill and toxic, has more soft tissue pain, and can exhibit a progressively worsening and fulminant course with fever, leukocytosis, and **shock.** Initially pain of the involved site is out of proportion to the physical findings. Hemorrhage and necrosis of the skin ensue, with bullae formation and palpable gas (crepitus) caused by tissue ischemia from thrombosed blood vessels. Loss of sensation of the involved area of skin and soft tissue may occur. Gangrenous soft tissue infections represent true medical and surgical emergencies; immediate surgical exploration is required to determine the degree and level of soft tissue spread, excise all devitalized tissue, and obtain deep tissue specimens for microbiologic processing. Prior to obtaining culture results, these infections must be treated with a combination of agents active against aerobic gram-positive cocci, Enterobacteriaceae, and anaerobes to ensure adequate coverage.

Mycetoma

Mycetoma (also called *Madura foot* or *maduromycosis*) is a chronic skin and subcutaneous infection caused by fungi such as *Madurella* spp., *Aspergillus* spp. or *Pseudoallescheria boydii* (eumycetoma or *true* fungal infection), or higher bacteria including actinomycetes such as *Nocardia* or *Actinomadura* spp. (actinomycetoma) (Table 33-3).

It is characterized by swelling and suppuration of subcutaneous tissues and formation of sinus tracts, with visible

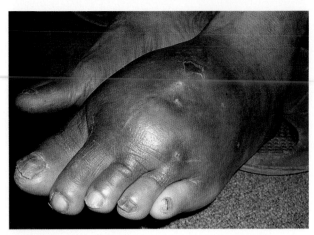

FIGURE 33-10   Madura foot. (Courtesy Dr. Gail Reid, University of Illinois at Chicago.)

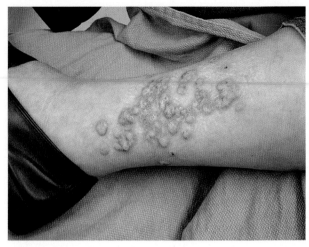

FIGURE 33-11   Chromoblastomycosis of the leg. (Courtesy Dr. Gail Reid, University of Illinois at Chicago.)

TABLE 33-3   Major Etiologic Agents of Subcutaneous Mycoses

Disease	Principal Organism(s)
Mycetoma	*Madurella mycetomatis, Madurella grisea, Scedosporium apiospermum, Leptosphaeria senegalensis, Exophiala jeanselmei, Pyrenochaeta romeroi, Fusarium* spp., *Acremonium* spp., *Pseudoallescheria boydii, Aspergillus nidulans, Neotestudina rosatii, Actinomadura madurae, Actinomadura pelletieri, Nocardia brasiliensis, Nocardia asteroides, Nocardia caviae, Streptomyces somaliensis*
Chromomycosis	*Phialophora verrucosa, Fonsecaea pedrosoi, Fonsecaea compacta, Cladophialophora carrionii, Rhinocladiella aquaspersa*
Phaeohyphomycosis	Dematiaceous fungi
Sporotrichosis	*Sporothrix schenckii*
Rhinosporidiosis	*Rhinosporidium seeberi*
Rhinoentomophthoromycosis	Conidiobolus, Basidiobolus
Lobo's disease	*Lacazia loboi (Loboa loboi)*

granules formed by aggregates of organisms in the pus draining from these fistulae (Figure 33-10). The disease process is slowly progressive and destructive, with extension to muscle and bone. Soil and decaying vegetation are reservoirs for the etiologic organisms. The disease is often seen in outdoor laborers and may be a result of lack of protective clothing including shoes; it develops as a consequence of skin trauma with an object contaminated with fungal elements (e.g., thorns, splinters) or introduction of organisms into preexisting abrasions. There is no person-to-person transmission. Lesions usually appear on the foot and lower leg but can involve other sites such as the hand, shoulder, and back, rarely the face. The involved areas are usually nontender, and no systemic signs of infection occur. Mycetoma is rare in the continental United States but common in tropical and subtropical parts of the world, especially where people go barefoot. Treatment with antibiotics alone may not be successful. Surgery is often times the only curative measure. Eumycetomas best respond to azole antifungal agents such as itraconazole or voriconazole. Actinomycetoma may be treated with combination antimicrobial treatment including streptomycin with trimethoprim-sulfamethoxazole or dapsone.

Mycetoma may be difficult to distinguish from chronic osteomyelitis and botryomycosis, the latter being a clinically and pathologically similar entity caused by a variety of bacteria, including staphylococci and gram-negative bacteria. Specific diagnosis depends on visualizing the granules in fresh preparations or histopathologic sections and isolating the causative actinomycete or fungus in culture. Different etiologic agents produce different color granules, helping to determine the causative organism in the laboratory.

Chromoblastomycosis

Chromoblastomycosis, or chromomycosis, is a chronic spreading mycosis of the skin and subcutaneous tissues (Figure 33-11). It produces localized scaly lesions, usually of a lower extremity or, less commonly, the hand or back. The disease has been found worldwide but, similar to mycetoma, it is most common in tropical and subtropical regions of the world. The mode of transmission is also similar to mycetoma, with skin inoculation of organisms via minor trauma. Progression is slow, over a period of years, with eventual large warty or cauliflower-like masses and obstruction of lymphatic drainage leading to marked swelling in some cases. Unlike mycetoma, chromoblastomycosis generally does not involve muscle or bone. Infectious agents include the dark-walled (dematiaceous) fungi found in soil and decaying vegetation. *Fonsecaea pedrosoi* is most frequently isolated, although infection caused by *F. compacta, Phialophora verrucosa, Cladophialophora carrionii,* and *Rhinocladiella aquaspersa* also occur. Microscopic examination of scrapings or biopsies from lesions reveals characteristic brown, thick-walled, rounded cells that divide by fusion in two planes. Confirmation of the diagnosis is made by biopsy and culture of the causative fungus. Therapy with antifungal agents such as itraconazole or terbinafine and local debridement or application of liquid nitrogen has been effective in treating this disease.

Other Uncommon Fungi

Phaeohyphomycosis is a term used to define infections caused by fungi that produce dark cell walls. These fungi are also termed *dematiaceous* because of their dark pigmentation. In addition to causing some cases of mycetoma and chromoblastomycosis, the agents of phaeohyphomycosis can cause subcutaneous nodules. *Bipolaris, Exophiala, Phialophora,* and *Wangiella* are some of the common genera isolated from skin lesions, although many others comprise this group. They are found in soil and decaying organic matter and on plants, and are usually introduced into the body in a manner similar to that described above for mycetoma and chromoblastomycosis. Subcutaneous phaeohyphomycosis starts as an isolated erythematous nodule, often on the extremities, and can expand to involve deep tissues including bone. The infection can spread locally with the formation of additional nodules and extension to bone. Immunocompromised persons are at highest risk for this infection, and in this setting, the infection can disseminate to other regions of the body, including the brain. Surgical debridement is generally necessary for cure; several antifungal agents produce activity against these organisms, including amphotericin B (usually reserved for life-threatening cases), itraconazole, voriconazole, and posaconazole.

Fungi of the order Entomophthorales (in the class Zygomycetes) are also present in organic debris and can cause a chronic subcutaneous form of infection, **entomophthoromycosis,** that often occurs as the result of traumatic implantation of the organisms in the skin. Entomophthoromycosis is caused by *Conidiobolus coronatus, Conidiobolus incongruous,* and *Basidiobolus ranarum* (previously known as *Basidiobolus haptosporus*). *B. ranarum* causes subcutaneous infection of the proximal limbs in children and is characterized by rubbery masses that can be large and ulcerate. They may be found on the shoulders, hips, and thighs. *Conidiobolus* infection is localized to the facial area, predominantly in adults. *Conidiobolus* infections occur after inhalation of fungal spores, which subsequently invade the sinuses and facial soft tissues and cause painless swelling of the lips and face that can be very deforming. Occasionally these infections may disseminate to other areas of the body, particularly in immunocompromised persons. Entomophthoromycosis is most often seen in tropical regions, especially in Africa, India, and Latin America. Diagnosis can be made clinically based on the typical skin and soft tissue findings but should be confirmed with biopsy and culture. Itraconazole is active against these organisms, although fluconazole, terbinafine, and amphotericin B have also been effective.

Rhinosporidiosis is a chronic, usually painless infection of humans and animals that occurs as mucosal polyps of the nasopharynx and conjunctiva. Formerly believed to be a fungus, the causative agent *Rhinosporidium seeberi* has never been cultured, but nucleic acid analysis has shown that it is a protist related to other aquatic protistan parasites. Protists are eukaryotic organisms that are usually unicellular and are neither plant, animal, nor fungi; protozoa and algae are members. Rhinosporidiosis occurs worldwide although most cases have been reported from India and Sri Lanka. The habitat of *R. seeberi* is unknown but is thought to be freshwater; for example, swimming in ponds, lakes, and rivers has been linked to disease. Patients can present with nasal obstruction or nosebleeds, and lesions increase in size over months to years. Rarely, polyps occur in the vagina, urethra, or penis. *R. seeberi* forms round, thick-walled cysts (sporangium) in the submucosa that are sometimes visible in the mucosa as white dots. The diagnosis is made by biopsy and finding the distinctive appearance of the organisms on microscopy. The treatment of choice is surgery, although recurrences are common.

Finally, **lobomycosis** is a chronic fungal infection of the skin caused by *Lacazia loboi* (previously known as *Loboa loboi*). This infection is mainly found in the tropics of South and Central America, and the organisms are thought to reside in soil or vegetation and infect humans via skin trauma. Farmers, hunters, and jungle workers are affected more than others. Dolphins can also be infected, so it is presumed that *L. loboi* exists in bodies of water. The disease occurs as slowly forming skin nodules of various sizes that occur on the face, arms, legs, and feet. The lesions can vary in appearance, and can be flat or nodular, warty or ulcerated. Infection can exist over a period of years with slow progression of the disease, which is relatively asymptomatic. Biopsy of a lesion is required to confirm the diagnosis because a characteristic appearance of the fungi is shown only with special stains. *L. loboi* has never been isolated in culture. The only effective treatment is surgical excision, although clofazimine may be partially effective.

Nodular Lymphangitis

Nodular lymphangitis, or lymphocutaneous syndrome, is an entity characterized by inflammatory nodules that occur along lymphatic vessels that drain an area of primary skin infection (Figure 33-12). Certain organisms are commonly associated with nodular lymphangitis including *Sporothrix*

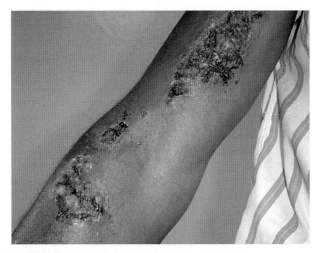

FIGURE 33-12 Nodular lymphangitis caused by sporotrichosis with ulceration of the overlying skin. (Courtesy Dr. Gail Reid, University of Illinois at Chicago.)

---

schenckii, Nocardia, and mycobacteria, although other more unusual infections can be associated as well (Box 33-2).

Sporotrichosis

Sporothrix schenckii is the most frequently recognized cause of nodular lymphangitis. This organism is known as a dimorphic fungus because it is capable of existing in both a yeast form (at higher temperatures, as in human tissue) and a hyphal form (in the environment, at temperatures below 37° C). Sporotrichosis is classically an occupational disease of gardeners, farmers, and horticulturalists. Introduction of the fungus through the skin occurs by pricks of thorns or barbs; the handling of sphagnum moss or slivers from wood, lumber, and other material contaminated with the organism have also been identified as risks for infection.

Sporotrichosis is usually localized to the skin and subcutaneous tissues, although dissemination to bone and other organs can occur in immunocompromised persons, and pulmonary disease can occur when *S. schenckii* conidia are inhaled. Cutaneous disease begins as an erythematous painless nodule at the inoculation site, which may ulcerate and remain confined (cutaneous form) or grow and spread proximally with surrounding satellite nodules along the lymphatic channels (lymphocutaneous form or nodular lymphangitis). Laboratory confirmation of sporotrichosis is made by culture of pus or exudate, preferably aspirated from an unopened lesion. The characteristic oval to cigar-shaped yeasts are rarely visualized by direct smear of pus because the organisms are often few in number, but Gomori methenamine silver and other fungal stains of biopsied tissue are useful in identifying the fungus. Oral potassium iodide is an effective treatment in many cases of soft tissue sporotrichosis; more extensive or refractory infections may be treated with itraconazole or amphotericin B. Heating tissues to 42° to 43° C has also been effective in decreasing the size of lesions because *S. schenckii* grows best in cooler temperatures.

Nocardia

Nocardia spp. are ubiquitous in the environment and may be found in soil, water, and vegetation. They can cause localized or disseminated infection with the latter occurring more often in immunocompromised hosts. In the skin and soft tissue form of nocardiosis, which results from direct cutaneous inoculation, manifestations range from lymphocutaneous syndrome to subcutaneous abscesses, cellulitis, and mycetoma. Although the *N. asteroides* complex causes the majority of noncutaneous invasive disease, *N. brasiliensis* is the most common species causing cutaneous nocardiosis. *N. transvalensis* and *N. otitidiscaviarium* can also cause cutaneous disease. Direct smears from nocardial skin lesions will show grampositive, beaded, branching filaments. The organisms are acid-fast negative but can be seen with a modified acid-fast stain that uses a weaker acid to decolorize the carbol fuchsin stain. This feature as well as its aerobic growth can distinguish *Nocardia* from organisms such as *Actinomyces,* which is acid-fast and modified acid-fast negative and grows anaerobically. *Nocardia* spp. may take as long as 2 weeks to grow on blood culture media. The treatment of choice is trimethoprim-sulfamethoxazole, although other antimicrobials such as imipenem and amikacin also have good activity and there are species differences in antimicrobial susceptibilities.

Mycobacteria

Many species of mycobacteria, including *Mycobacterium tuberculosis,* have been noted to cause cutaneous disease (discussed further below), including nodular lymphangitis. However, the marine organism *Mycobacterium marinum* is the mycobacterial species most often associated with nodular lymphangitis. This infection, also known as "swimming pool granuloma," develops in individuals with a history of cleaning fish tanks or exposure to saltwater or nonchlorinated swimming pools. The microorganism enters through an open wound or through traumatic inoculation of skin. The lesions are initially solitary and located on the hands or arms 2 to 3 weeks after exposure. They are papular or nodular and can become wart-like or ulcerated. The infection can then progress to a lymphocutaneous syndrome characterized by the development of more proximal lesions along the path of lymphatic drainage of the initial site of infection. The diagnosis is made by biopsy and culture of a skin lesion in association with obtaining a history suggestive of exposure. *M. marinum* grows best at 25° to 32° C. Treatment involves systemic antimycobacterial therapy (e.g., rifampin plus ethambutol or clarithromycin or doxycycline monotherapy) for several months until resolution of the lesions occurs. Applying local heat has also been used as an adjunctive therapy.

Nontuberculous Mycobacteria. Nearly all nontuberculous *Mycobacteria* (NTM) have been shown to cause cutaneous disease. Some nontuberculous mycobacterial skin diseases, like that caused by *M. marinum,* are the result of primary skin

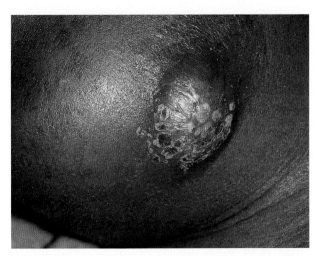

FIGURE 33-13 Actinomycosis of the jaw following dental infection. (Courtesy Dr. Gail Reid, University of Illinois at Chicago.)

infection via trauma and others are related to hematogenous spread (discussed further below). Puncture wounds, motor vehicle accidents, injections, and surgery can lead to infection. Aside from *M. marinum, M. abscessus, M. fortuitum, M. chelonae,* and *M. ulcerans* are the most common species causing localized skin infections. The lesions caused by these NTM can appear as nodules, papules, plaques, and ulcers. *M. chelonae* is seen most often in immunocompromised patients. *M. ulcerans* infection usually occurs as a single, pruritic ulcer with undermined edges, also known as a *Buruli ulcer. M. ulcerans* infection is associated with swamps and may be a chronic infection in tropical climates. Diagnosis of cutaneous NTM infections is made by culture of skin biopsy or drainage material. Antituberculous antimicrobials do not have significant activity against most of these NTM, but antibiotics such as fluoroquinolones, clarithromycin, aminoglycosides, and cephalosporins may be used, depending on the species.

Mycobacterium tuberculosis. Inoculation of the skin with *M. tuberculosis* can lead to tuberculosis verrucosa cutis (TVC). TVC lesions develop as purple papules that become wart-like, and they occur in areas of the body prone to trauma. Historically, this manifestation of *M. tuberculosis* was seen in physicians and anatomists. In the tropics, TVC is seen in children who walk barefoot in soil that is contaminated with tuberculous sputum. Tuberculous chancre, a skin ulcer, is another localized dermatologic manifestation of *M. tuberculosis* following traumatic inoculation of the skin with the organisms. Biopsy and culture will make the diagnosis.

Actinomycosis

Actinomycosis is a chronic disease characterized by the formation of abscesses, fibrosis of tissues, and draining sinuses that discharge sulfur granules (masses of organisms). It is caused by non–spore-forming anaerobic or microaerophilic bacterial species, especially *Actinomyces israelii*. Once thought to be fungi because of their branching, *Actinomyces* spp. and the closely related *Nocardia* spp. are classified as higher prokaryotic bacteria. *Actinomyces* spp. are gram-positive, pleomorphic, and diphtheroidal, or more commonly, delicately

filamentous. Although there are thoracic, abdominopelvic, and central nervous system (CNS) forms of the disease, involvement of the face and neck is the most common manifestation (Figure 33-13) and often follows dental sepsis or manipulation, trauma, tonsillitis, otitis, or mastoiditis. Cervicofacial actinomycosis may extend to the underlying mandible or facial bones, leading to osteomyelitis. Penicillin is the preferred treatment.

DERMATOLOGIC MANIFESTATIONS OF SYSTEMIC BACTERIAL AND FUNGAL INFECTIONS

Systemic infections can produce skin lesions that may provide important diagnostic clues. This phenomenon may be seen with a variety of bacterial, fungal, parasitic, and viral infections. In this section, some important dermatologic findings associated with systemic bacterial and fungal infections are discussed. Skin lesions associated with viral and parasitic infections are described in separate sections later in the chapter.

Bacteria

Pseudomonas

A characteristic skin lesion associated with *Pseudomonas* bacteremia is ecthyma gangrenosum. These lesions begin as painless, flat erythematous areas that progress to nodules and then bullae, which subsequently ulcerate and form a black eschar on the surface with surrounding erythema. Although **ecthyma gangrenosum** has classically been associated with *Pseudomonas sepsis*, these types of lesions have also been reported in the setting of sepsis caused by other gram-negative bacteria and *Candida*. Ecthyma gangrenosum is the result of bacterial invasion of dermal veins leading to hemorrhage and necrosis. Biopsy of the lesions will reveal bacteria on Gram stain.

Vibrio and Aeromonas

Vibrio vulnificus is part of the ocean flora and can cause very severe disease with a high fatality rate, particularly in persons with underlying liver disease. Infection occurs through ingestion of contaminated shellfish such as raw oysters or exposure of an existing wound to seawater containing the organisms. Patients with *V. vulnificus* sepsis can develop widespread skin lesions that are characterized by the formation of hemorrhagic bullae that evolve into ulcers with skin necrosis. *V. vulnificus* grows well on MacConkey agar (MAC) but can be overlooked among other gram-negatives because it is a lactose fermenter. In addition, *Vibrio* spp. can be isolated from stool specimens, but in many laboratories, this identification is not routinely performed and must be specifically requested.

Aeromonas spp., which are present in fresh or brackish water, can cause skin lesions similar to those of *V. vulnificus,* but they are often localized to an area of skin trauma and cellulitis. Skin infections are generally the result of contamination of a wound with water containing the organisms. Aeromonads cause a variety of infections in addition to cellulitis including gastroenteritis, peritonitis, and cholangitis. These infections may be complicated by bacteremia and sepsis, and patients with underlying liver disease are at higher

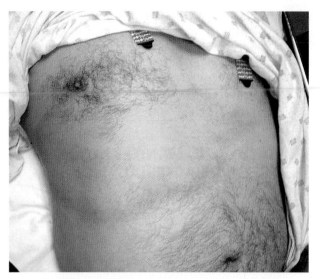

FIGURE 33-14 Erythema migrans rash of Lyme disease. (Courtesy Dr. Gail Reid, University of Illinois at Chicago.)

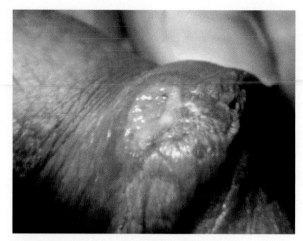

FIGURE 33-15 Penile syphilitic chancre caused by *Treponema pallidum* subsp. *pallidum.*

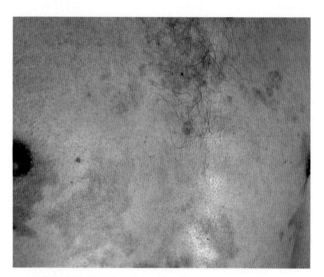

FIGURE 33-16 The rash of secondary syphilis.

risk for invasive *Aeromonas* infection. *Aeromonas* skin infection is typically rapidly progressing with hemorrhagic bullae formation and skin necrosis. Osteomyelitis and myonecrosis with gas formation in the tissues may ensue, and debridement is required in this setting. *Aeromonas* infection is also a well-recognized complication of medicinal leech therapy used in reimplantation or flap procedures, because aeromonads are symbionts within the leech gut. *Aeromonas* spp. can be cultured on MAC and are oxidase-positive, which distinguishes the organisms from Enterobacteriaceae.

Borrelia

The tick-borne spirochete of Lyme disease, *Borrelia burgdorferi,* characteristically produces a distinctive bulls-eye or target skin lesion called *erythema migrans (EM)* at the inoculation site, 1 to 2 weeks after infection (Figure 33-14). The lesions average 15 cm in size and may become hemorrhagic or necrotic in the center. EM is the most useful diagnostic marker of Lyme disease, and over a period of weeks, multiple secondary EM lesions can occur in various regions of the body as the spirochetes disseminate. Other manifestations of Lyme disease include arthritis, carditis, and neurologic disease. A number of antibiotics, including ceftriaxone, penicillin G, amoxicillin, erythromycin, and tetracycline are useful in the treatment of Lyme disease.

A nonspecific petechial, macular, or papular skin rash is commonly seen during the end of the primary febrile episode of relapsing fever caused by *Borrelia recurrentis*. The disease is transmitted by either human body lice or by ticks. Diagnosis of relapsing fever is made by demonstration of *Borrelia* organisms in the peripheral blood of febrile patients using dark-field microscopy or Giemsa- or Wright-stained thick and thin blood smears.

Treponema

Syphilis is an acute and chronic treponemal venereal disease. It is characterized clinically by a primary lesion, a secondary eruption involving skin and mucous membranes, long periods of latency, and late tertiary lesions of the skin, bone, central nervous, and cardiovascular systems, and other viscera. The primary lesion usually appears as a papule at the inoculation site about 3 weeks after the initial exposure. Erosion and ulceration then occur, forming the characteristic painless syphilitic chancre (Figure 33-15), which is indurated or rubbery, in contrast to the painful "soft chancre" of chancroid caused by *Haemophilus ducreyi*. Spontaneous resolution of the primary lesion occurs in 4 to 6 weeks and is followed by a secondary eruption involving skin, mucous membranes, and sometimes, internal viscera such as the liver. The rash of secondary syphilis is characterized as a diffuse, painless, maculopapular rash (Figure 33-16), and systemic complaints, including fever and malaise, commonly accompany secondary syphilis.

Both primary and secondary lesions are typically teeming with spirochetes and thus are infectious. Secondary manifestations also disappear spontaneously within weeks. Subsequently, the infection remains clinically latent for weeks to years and may evolve into tertiary disease affecting predominantly the central nervous system and heart. Diagnosis can be made based on physical findings, or by serologic tests. Sometimes spirochetes can be seen on silver-stained biopsy materials, but *Treponema pallidum* cannot be grown on media.

Mycoplasma

Mycoplasma organisms are prokaryotes that lack a cell wall. *Mycoplasma pneumoniae* is a cause of pneumonia but is also associated with a variety of extrapulmonary complications involving the central nervous system, heart, and skin. *Mycoplasma* can cause a variety of dermatologic findings including maculopapular and vesicular rashes, urticaria, and the hypersensitivity reactions erythema nodosum and erythema multiforme (EM), including EM major (Stevens-Johnsons syndrome). EM major is characterized by erythematous bullae and vesicles of the skin with involvement of mucocutaneous tissues such as the oral mucosa, conjunctivae, and gastrointestinal tract. *Mycoplasma*-associated EM lesions have been reported both with and without apparent respiratory disease. Diagnosis can be made by obtaining acute and convalescent antibody titers or by detection of *Mycoplasma* antigens or nucleic acids (the latter using polymerase chain reaction [PCR] assay) in respiratory specimens, because isolation of the organism is difficult. The presence of cold agglutinins in the serum can also be suggestive of *Mycoplasma* infection, although this finding is not sensitive. Because of the lack of cell walls, *Mycoplasma* organisms are resistant to penicillin and are treated with macrolides, tetracyclines, or fluoroquinolones.

Zoonoses

Zoonotic diseases are those transmitted to humans by wild or domestic animals. There are hundreds of zoonotic diseases; this section examines some of the more common systemic bacterial **zoonoses** that have significant dermatologic manifestations.

Rickettsiae. Rickettsiae are gram-negative intracellular pathogens that reside within endothelial cells and macrophages. Rickettsiae have various types of animal reservoirs and are transmitted to humans through a number of species-specific insect vectors (e.g., ticks, mites, lice, fleas). There are two general groups of rickettsiae: the spotted fever group, which is predominantly the tick-borne rickettsial diseases, and the typhus group, transmitted by insects.

Clinical symptoms common to rickettsial infections include high fever, chills, malaise, headache, myalgias, skin rash, and conjunctival injection. Systemic and cutaneous disease manifestations are the result of widespread inflammation of small blood vessels **(vasculitis).** Dermatologically, rickettsial infections are characterized by the type and distribution of the associated skin rash (e.g., petechial or vesicular, centripetal or centrifugal) and the presence or absence of a black eschar at the vector bite inoculation site.

Rocky Mountain spotted fever (RMSF), caused by *Rickettsia rickettsii*, is the most frequently seen rickettsial infection in the United States and is transmitted by several different types of ticks, depending on geographic location. A maculopapular rash appears on the extremities around the third day after exposure. It usually includes the palms and soles and spreads rapidly and centripetally to most of the body. **Petechiae** and purpura represent extravasation of blood out of blood vessels into the skin and evolve as a result of the cutaneous vasculitis. RMSF is fatal within 1 to 2 weeks if appropriate therapy is not administered. The clinical syndrome of RMSF may be confused with atypical measles, meningococcal bloodstream infection, other forms of bacterial sepsis, secondary syphilis, typhoid fever, enteroviral infection, and leptospirosis. Diagnosis is made based on clinical presentation and serology, because culture of these organisms is difficult. *R. rickettsii* is resistant to many common antibiotics, but the infection is generally successfully treated with either a tetracycline or chloramphenicol if therapy is given early in the course of the disease.

Boutonneuse fever, caused by *R. conorii*, is characterized by the *tache noir* (black spot) or eschar at the site of the tick vector bite. This illness is not endemic in the United States but can be seen in returning travelers from destinations such as India, Pakistan, Africa, and eastern and southern Europe. The skin lesion is the result of endothelial injury in soft tissues with necrosis and perivascular edema. Rickettsialpox, caused by *R. akari*, is also one of the spotted fever group of rickettsial diseases, but it is transmitted by the bite of mites, rather than ticks, and mice are the reservoir. The organism occurs worldwide but was initially found in New York City. Clinical findings include fever, rash, and eschar; the eschar develops from a papule that vesiculates. The rash spares the palms and soles, is papular and vesicular, and leaves black crusts. These illnesses are treated similarly to RMSF, with doxycycline or chloramphenicol.

Leptospirosis. Leptospirosis is a zoonotic disease caused by *Leptospira interrogans* and carried in the renal systems of rodents and other mammals including dogs and livestock. Humans become infected after contact with the urine or tissues of infected animals in vegetation, soil, or water. It is found throughout the world, and the highest incidence in the United States is in Hawaii. Leptospirosis can be a self-limited illness or may be fatal with renal and liver failure and pneumonia. The rash of leptospirosis is maculopapular and may become hemorrhagic. The diagnosis of leptospirosis is usually made serologically, and penicillin G and doxycycline are generally recommended for this disease.

Bartonella. The most common forms of bartonellosis are caused by *Bartonella henselae* and *B. quintana*. *B. henselae* is the cause of cat-scratch disease, and both species can cause bacteremia and endocarditis as well as the main dermatologic disease of bartonellosis, bacillary angiomatosis (BA), which is predominantly seen in human immunodeficiency virus (HIV)–infected persons. Cat fleas are a vector for *B. henselae*; *B. quintana* is transmitted by louse vectors. These organisms cause febrile systemic infections with hepatosplenomegaly, lymphadenopathy, anemia, and cutaneous manifestations. BA is caused by new blood vessel formation in the skin or other organs such as the liver (peliosis hepatis). The skin lesions occur in crops, are generally nodular, are red or purple in color, and can ulcerate. The size of the lesions ranges from several millimeters to centimeters, and they bleed easily with trauma. They are most prominent on the extensor surfaces of the limbs. The organism may be cultured from the skin and subcutaneous lesions or occasionally from the blood. Diagnosis can also be made by histopathologic demonstration of organisms in tissue specimens using Warthin-Starry staining.

Rat-Bite Fever. Two bacterial diseases, rare in the United States, are included under the general term *rat-bite fever*: streptobacillosis, caused by *Streptobacillus moniliformis,* and spirillosis, caused by *Spirillum minus* (minor). Rat-bite fever is usually transmitted by bites or scratches from rodents or carnivores that ingest rodents. The diseases share clinical and epidemiologic characteristics. An abrupt onset of fever and chills, headache, and muscle pain is followed shortly by a maculopapular or sometimes petechial or pustular rash that is most marked in the extremities, may become purpuric, and can lead to desquamation. Joint swelling and pain often occur in association with the rash. Laboratory confirmation is made by isolation of the causative organism after inoculating material from the primary lesion, lymph node, blood, joint fluid, or pus into culture media or laboratory animals. Pleomorphic bacilli may be seen with Giemsa or Gram stain. Serum antibodies may be detected by agglutination tests. Penicillin G is the treatment of choice.

Francisella. *Francisella tularensis,* a gram-negative coccobacillus, causes several forms of tularemia, including glandular, oculoglandular, pulmonic, and septicemic or typhoidal forms. The disease is transmitted to humans by direct inoculation of skin through handling of infected rabbits and other wild or, less commonly, domestic animals or by the bite of infected fleas, ticks, deerflies, and mosquitoes. The ulceroglandular type of tularemia is most common. It presents as an indolent ulcer, often on the hand, accompanied by painful swelling of the regional lymph nodes. Some patients can have nodular lymphangitis. The other forms of tularemia can also be associated with maculopapular or vesicular rash as well as erythema nodosum, urticaria, and erythema multiforme. Diagnosis of tularemia is most commonly made by a rise in specific antibodies in the patient's serum, although cross-reactivity with *Brucella, Proteus,* and heterophile antibodies can occur. Examination of ulcer exudates, lymph node aspirates, and other clinical specimens using a fluorescent antibody test may provide a rapid diagnosis, although the organism is not often seen on Gram stain. *Francisella* does not grow on routine media but can be identified by culture on buffered charcoal yeast extract agar or by inoculation of laboratory animals with material from lesions, blood, or sputum; great care must be exercised with this approach, however, because this highly infectious agent poses an occupational hazard for laboratory workers. Streptomycin with or without tetracycline is the usual treatment.

Mycobacteria

Nontuberculous Mycobacteria and Tuberculosis. As noted previously, NTM can cause localized cutaneous infection, generally as the result of skin inoculation via trauma with resulting contained disease of the skin and adjacent soft tissues, sometimes extending to bone and joints. These infections can also become disseminated (Figure 33-17). This typically occurs in the setting of impaired immune function, as in persons with HIV and cancer. Patients with central venous

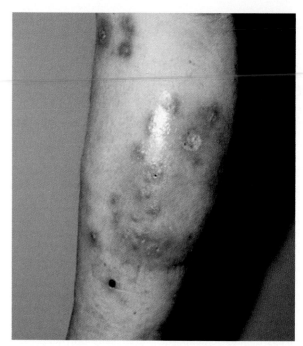

FIGURE 33-17 Subcutaneous nodules and cellulitis caused by disseminated *Mycobacterium chelonae.*

catheters may get NTM catheter-related infections, which can disseminate hematogenously to various organs including the skin. These infections are most often the result of *Mycobacterium fortuitum, M. chelonae,* and *M. abscessus.* The characteristics of the skin lesions and their treatments are similar to those noted above for localized cutaneous disease caused by NTM.

M. tuberculosis can spread to the skin through the lymphatic system, bloodstream, or by contiguous spread from adjacent tissues and can cause a variety of skin manifestations. Extension from the lymph nodes or bones to the skin is called *scrofuloderma.* This is most often seen in the region of the cervical lymph nodes with draining sinus tracts from the node or ulceration of the overlying skin. Hematogenous spread to cutaneous sites leads to nodular swellings of the skin known as *tuberculous gummas* or *lupus vulgaris,* which is the most common form of cutaneous tuberculosis (TB). Lupus vulgaris is characterized by circumscribed red-brown plaques of the head and neck. Other forms of cutaneous TB are the result of hypersensitivity reaction rather than significant skin infection with the organism. For example, erythema induratum of Bazin can develop in patients with extracutaneous TB and is characterized by multiple tender, indurated nodules, typically on the legs. Biopsy of these lesions shows inflammatory changes including vasculitis and panniculitis, but organisms may not be detected. However, the lesions do respond to antituberculous therapy.

Leprosy. Leprosy (also known as *Hansen's disease*) is found in South Asia, Africa, and South America. Cases reported from the United States are typically in immigrants from these endemic areas. The classic skin manifestation of *M. leprae,* the causative agent of leprosy, is a circumscribed, hypopigmented, or less commonly, hyperpigmented macule

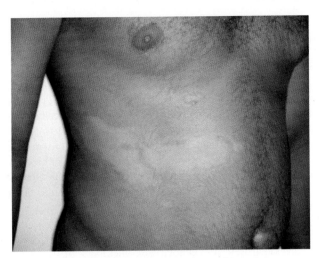

FIGURE 33-18 Hypopigmented macules of leprosy. (Courtesy Dr. Gail Reid, University of Illinois at Chicago.)

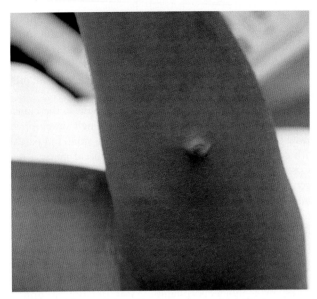

FIGURE 33-19 Nodular skin lesion caused by *Blastomyces dermatitidis*. (Courtesy Dr. Gail Reid, University of Illinois at Chicago.)

(Figure 33-18). Two main types of leprosy occur: tuberculoid or lepromatous, with gradations occurring between these two extremes. Tuberculoid leprosy is characterized by few skin lesions with a paucity of mycobacteria in the lesions because of a host TH1 immune response (interleukin [IL]-2 and interferon-gamma production). Patients with lepromatous leprosy have a large number of lesions with many mycobacteria and infiltration of peripheral nerves, and a TH2-type response in the host (IL-4, IL-5, and IL-10 production). Because the peripheral nerves are infiltrated with organisms, these lesions are painless. *M. leprae* has a predilection for the cooler parts of the body, such as the ears and nose, and the main mode of transmission is via respiratory or nasal secretions. Acid-fast bacilli and granulomas can be seen in tissue biopsy specimens, but *M. leprae* cannot be cultured in vitro. Effective treatment usually involves combination chemotherapy with agents such as rifampin, dapsone, and clofazimine.

Fungi

Candida

Skin lesions can be a clue to the diagnosis of invasive forms of *Candida* infection such as candidemia. An erythematous maculopapular, pustular, or nodular rash may be associated with systemic *Candida* infection. The lesions represent subcutaneous *Candida* abscesses. Skin biopsy will reveal fungal pseudohyphae with inflammatory cells and *Candida* can be grown from culture of the aspirate or biopsy.

Endemic Fungi and Moulds

Sporothrix schenckii (discussed previously), *Histoplasma capsulatum*, *Blastomyces dermatitidis*, and *Coccidioides immitis* are the major "endemic fungi." They are fungi that often cause disease in healthy hosts, as opposed to the opportunistic fungi such as *Aspergillus*, and they exhibit different forms at varying temperatures, existing as moulds in the environment at 25° to 30° C but as yeasts at body temperature. In addition, *Histoplasma*, *Blastomyces*, and *Coccidioides* are distributed in specific geographic areas of the Americas. These three genera

most often enter the body via the respiratory tract but can become systemic infections that may produce secondary skin lesions through hematogenous spread. *Blastomyces* commonly produces well-circumscribed nodules (Figure 33-19) or plaques that may be verrucous and can ulcerate. They may be mistaken for pyoderma gangrenosum, nontuberculous mycobacterial infections, or other fungal infections. *Histoplasma* is less often associated with skin lesions, but when they do occur they can be papular, nodular, or ulcerated. Histoplasmosis may also manifest as oral ulcerations. One of the most common areas of the body *Coccidioides* disseminates to is the skin. Lesions can be maculopapular, verrucous, ulcerated, or fluctuant abscesses, and there is a predilection for the nasolabial fold. Diagnosis of these endemic fungal infections can be made by biopsy and culture of the skin lesions in addition to serologic testing and sometimes blood cultures. Systemic antifungal therapy with amphotericin B or azoles is generally effective treatment.

Disseminated mould infections including those caused by *Aspergillus*, Zygomycetes (e.g., *Rhizopus*, *Mucor* or *Rhizomucor* spp.), and *Fusarium* often produce black, necrotic skin lesions and eschars. These infections generally occur in severely immunocompromised persons and have a poor prognosis.

VIRAL INFECTIONS

Viruses are a diverse group of microorganisms that require the presence of a cell to replicate. Viruses can produce localized or disseminated disease and in some cases cause chronic infection by evading the host immune system (e.g., HIV, hepatitis C virus). The viruses commonly associated with skin and soft tissue infection are discussed in this section.

Rubeola

Rubeola, also known as *measles*, is caused by a paramyxovirus (genus *Morbillivirus*, family Paramyxoviridae) and is spread by direct contact with respiratory secretions of infected persons. Measles is one of the most communicable of all infectious diseases but because of vaccination, less than 150 cases are reported per year in the United States. Most cases in the United States occur in unvaccinated persons from other countries.

After an incubation period of 10 to 14 days, the clinical features of coryza, conjunctivitis, and cough develop, followed by the appearance of Koplik's spots, small red patches with central bluish-gray specks, on the buccal mucosa near the second molars. Shortly thereafter a maculopapular rash occurs. The rash spreads from the face downward to the trunk and extremities and affects the palms and soles. Patients with measles are most infectious during the late prodromal phase of the illness, when cough and coryza are at their peak. However, the disease is probably contagious from several days before onset of the rash to several days after its onset. Measles can be complicated by secondary bacterial pneumonia, otitis media, or meningoencephalitis. Viral isolation is difficult because of slow growth of the virus and the limited number of cell types in which it can grow. The diagnosis is usually based on signs and symptoms or by serologic testing for antibody titers.

Rubella

Rubella, also known as *German measles,* is a viral infection of children and adults that resembles measles. It is characterized by fever, rash, and lymphadenopathy. The virus is in the Togaviridae family (genus *Rubivirus*). Rubella virus is spread in droplets shed from the respiratory secretions of infected persons. The period of contagion extends from about 10 days before the appearance of the rash to 15 days after its onset. Many rubella infections are subclinical, and most infections in the United States occur in unvaccinated immigrants or travelers, similar to measles. For symptomatic persons, a nonspecific maculopapular rash begins on the face and moves down the body and often is accompanied by cervical and occipital lymphadenopathy and, at times, splenomegaly. The disease is clinically milder than measles, although arthritis and encephalitis can be complications, and serious congenital defects can be a consequence when the infection occurs during pregnancy. Diagnosis may be made by isolating the virus from urine, throat, or nasopharyngeal specimens, or by serologic testing to detect the development of antibodies. Congenital rubella infection is often diagnosed by detecting viral nucleic acids in the infant via a PCR assay.

Parvovirus B19

Erythema infectiosum, or fifth disease, is one of the common viral **exanthems** of childhood. It is caused by the human parvovirus B19 (genus *Erythrovirus,* family Parvoviridae), which replicates in erythrocyte precursor cells. The primary mode of transmission is thought to be via the respiratory route. Fifth disease is characterized by a bright red rash of the face (the so-called "slapped cheek appearance") followed in 1 to 4 days by a fine, lace-like rash on the trunk or extremities. The rash may fade quickly, only to recur during the ensuing 2 to 3 weeks on exposure to sunlight or heat. Infection is generally not associated with fever, although mild constitutional symp-

toms may precede the rash. **Scarlet fever** and rubella are other childhood diseases to be distinguished from fifth disease. Complications are more common in adult infection where patients (particularly women) can get a symmetric arthralgia and arthritis. In persons with hemolytic disorders and in immunosuppressed persons such as those with HIV, parvovirus B19 can cause marked inhibition of red blood cell formation with extremely low blood counts. Parvovirus B19 infection in pregnancy can lead to hydrops fetalis and miscarriage. Diagnosis is often made by detection of the virus in blood or bone marrow with PCR. Serious manifestations of infection are treated with intravenous immunoglobulin and blood transfusion.

Enteroviruses

Coxsackieviruses and echoviruses, members of the genus *Enterovirus* (family Picornaviridae), cause a variety of exanthems. Enteroviral infections are more prevalent in summer and autumn months in temperate climates and occur year-round in tropical regions. Most infections occur in children, particularly infants, and mucocutaneous features are also found more commonly in infants and children than in adults. Enteroviruses are predominantly spread via the fecal-oral route but at times may be spread by respiratory secretions. Most enteroviral infections are asymptomatic or result in brief febrile illnesses, but coxsackie and echoviruses can cause more serious disease including aseptic meningitis or encephalitis, hemorrhagic conjunctivitis, pericarditis, myocarditis, and pleuritis. Enteroviruses are also the cause of many different exanthems, some of which have oral mucosal involvement. These are generally benign diseases and can resemble other viral causes of rash. They are grouped as rubelliform or morbilliform (resembling rubella or measles), roseoliform (resembling roseola), or herpetiform (resembling herpes) exanthems. Enteroviruses can also produce petechial or purpuric type rashes resembling meningococcal bloodstream infection. One common rash caused most often by coxsackievirus A16 is the herpetiform hand-foot-and-mouth (HFM) disease. HFM is primarily seen in young children and is characterized by fever, throat pain, and red macules on the palate, tonsils, and tongue that ulcerate. Vesicles that resemble herpes simplex or varicella-zoster lesions can also occur on the lateral aspects of the feet, dorsal fingers, and toes and sometimes the buttocks and genitalia. Herpangina is another herpetiform disease typically caused by coxsackie A viruses. Herpangina is characterized by fever, throat pain, and vesicular lesions on the soft palate and posterior oropharynx. Viral culture of stool, throat, or involved tissue can be performed to make a diagnosis. Serologic testing demonstrating a fourfold increase in antibody titer can also be employed.

Herpesviridae

There are more than 100 Herpesviridae viruses although only eight are common causes of human infection. All eight can lead to dermatologic disease, but some, such as varicella-zoster virus and herpes simplex virus, are associated with more prominent skin findings. These viruses are described further below.

Varicella-Zoster Virus

Varicella infection, or chickenpox, is a common childhood illness acquired by respiratory inhalation of the varicella-zoster virus (VZV). The skin lesions of primary VZV infection become apparent approximately 2 weeks after initial exposure. The lesions begin as vesicles or small blisters on an erythematous base. The lesions become pustular or rupture and form eschars over a period of several days. The rash starts on the trunk and face and then spreads to the extremities. A characteristic of chickenpox is the presence of lesions in various stages of evolution. When primary varicella infection occurs in adults, it tends to be more severe and systemic, involving the lungs, CNS, and liver.

Treatment with the antiviral agent acyclovir is recommended in immunosuppressed individuals and patients with visceral involvement. In recent years, routine administration of varicella vaccine to children in the United States has resulted in a reduction of greater than 90% in the annual incidence of varicella and a 66% reduction in mortality.

Varicella-zoster virus is a herpesvirus that exhibits, like other members of the family Herpesviridae, lifelong latency in the human host. After primary infection, the virus enters peripheral nerves and establishes persistence within the dorsal root ganglia. The virus may be reactivated under various conditions, most importantly by immunosuppression associated with age, certain diseases, or drug therapies (e.g., corticosteroids and cytotoxic chemotherapy). With reactivation, the virions move along peripheral sensory nerves of the skin and produce a vesicular eruption in a unilateral dermatomal distribution (Figure 33-20). The resulting condition is called *herpes zoster* or *shingles*. The vesicles are similar to those of chickenpox but remain localized along sensory nerves. The disease is generally benign but may lead to postherpetic neuralgia, a syndrome of lingering pain at the site of the healed rash. In addition, when the face is involved, the virus may spread along the ophthalmic branch of the trigeminal nerve to the eye (zoster ophthalmicus), resulting in sight-threatening disease. In immunosuppressed patients, the virus may disseminate widely to the skin and to internal viscera such as lungs, meninges, brain, and liver.

The diagnosis of chickenpox or herpes zoster is made by viral culture of a scraping from the base of a vesicular lesion. Direct fluorescent antibody testing is also available to make a rapid diagnosis from a tissue scraping. Acyclovir is the drug of choice for treatment of complicated zoster or to prevent dissemination of localized disease in immunosuppressed hosts.

Herpes Simplex Virus

Herpes simplex virus (HSV) types 1 and 2 cause some of the most common skin and mucous membrane infections affecting humans. HSV infections occur after contact of mucous membranes or abraded skin with infected secretions. Initial infection may lead to the characteristic vesicular skin lesions at the site of infection or may be asymptomatic. After penetrating the skin or mucosa, the virus enters nearby neurons and leads to a lifelong latent infection in neuronal ganglia that can reactivate under various conditions, particularly immunosuppression, and cause recurrent disease. Both HSV type 1 (HSV-1) and HSV type 2 (HSV-2) can cause oral or genital infection, but HSV-1 more commonly causes orofacial infection and HSV-2 tends to cause genital infection. Clinical findings cannot distinguish HSV-1 from HSV-2, and cutaneous HSV lesions are also indistinguishable from those caused by VZV, although HSV skin lesions generally do not follow a dermatomal pattern. In severely immunosuppressed hosts, such as persons with hematologic and lymphoreticular malignancies and organ transplant recipients, a disseminated and life-threatening form of herpes simplex can occur, with diffuse cutaneous lesions and lung, liver, or other visceral organ involvement.

Primary HSV-1 infection may present as severe ulcerative gingivostomatitis and pharyngitis and typically occurs in children younger than 5 years. This initial bout of infection is often accompanied by fever and systemic toxicity. Oral vesicles involving the soft palate, buccal mucosa, tongue, lips, and roof and floor of the mouth quickly ulcerate and may coalesce. Primary herpetic gingivostomatitis can resemble bacterial pharyngitis, herpangina caused by coxsackie A virus, aphthous stomatitis, erythema multiforme major (Stevens-Johnson syndrome), infectious mononucleosis, and chemotherapy-induced mucositis. Herpes labialis, a condition commonly known as *fever blisters* or *cold sores*, is the most common manifestation of HSV reactivation. Lesions begin as superficial clear vesicles on an erythematous base and occur on the lips or in the oropharynx. The lesions heal spontaneously and may recur in the same area. Recurrent herpes labialis is generally unaccompanied by systemic complaints, in contrast to primary infection.

Other notable cutaneous manifestations of HSV infection include eczema herpeticum, a vesicular eruption that involves areas of chronic eczema or burns and can be quite severe (Figure 33-21), and erythema multiforme (EM), an acute hypersensitivity reaction that manifests as "target"-type erythematous skin lesions that may involve mucous membranes. HSV DNA has been identified in biopsies of EM skin lesions, and it is thought that HSV precipitates the majority of cases

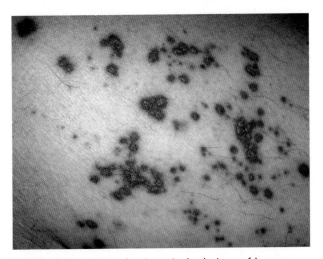

FIGURE 33-20 Hemorrhagic vesicular lesions of herpes zoster. (Courtesy Dr. Gail Reid, University of Illinois at Chicago.)

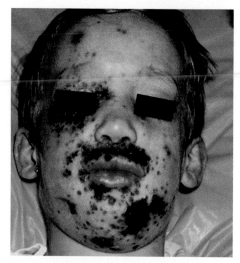

FIGURE 33-21 Eczema herpeticum caused by herpes simplex virus.

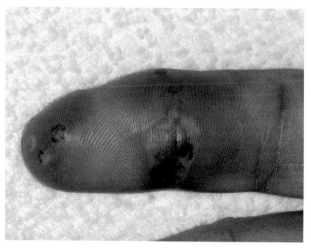

FIGURE 33-22 Herpes whitlow.

of recurrent EM. An additional presentation of cutaneous HSV is herpetic whitlow, or primary herpetic lesions of the finger (Figure 33-22). This can be caused by either HSV-1 or HSV-2. Usually a single digit is involved, with the appearance of one or more deep vesicles that may coalesce. Fever and intense local pain are often present. The condition may be misdiagnosed as bacterial paronychia, and unnecessary incision may be performed. Recurrent herpetic whitlow can be a difficult occupational problem among medical, paramedical, and dental personnel. Herpetic whitlow in newborns (following finger sucking) and serious disseminated infection are two important neonatal herpes syndromes. Infants are infected during passage through the infected maternal genital tract.

HSV-2 in adults is transmitted primarily by sexual contact, resulting in primary and recurrent herpes genitalis and peri-rectal infections. Initial infection may be accompanied by fever, myalgias, and inguinal lymphadenopathy. Vesicles and ulcerations occur in the genital and/or perirectal regions. Urethritis and aseptic meningitis are potential complications.

HSV-1 can also cause genital infection but typically causes fewer recurrences compared to HSV-2.

The diagnosis of HSV infection is made by viral culture of a vesicular or ulcerated skin lesion or biopsy and culture of tissue from an affected visceral organ. Direct fluorescent antibody techniques are also available to detect HSV antigens in tissues. Type-specific serologic testing can also be performed to ascertain whether a patient has been infected with HSV-1, HSV-2, or both. Acyclovir or the oral pro-drugs valacyclovir and famciclovir are the drugs of choice for herpes simplex infections requiring treatment. Intravenous acyclovir is given for severe manifestations of disease.

Other Herpesviruses

Mononucleosis syndromes caused by Epstein-Barr virus (EBV) and cytomegalovirus (CMV) can sometimes be associated with nonspecific rashes. These are most often maculopapular. EBV can also cause petechial or urticarial rashes and may be a trigger for erythema multiforme. The administration of penicillin therapy during mononucleosis very often precipitates an immunologic reaction that leads to a pruritic, erythematous maculopapular rash.

Human herpesvirus 6 (HHV-6) is the major cause of roseola infantum (also known as *exanthem subitum* or *sixth disease*), a febrile syndrome that occurs in infants and children. High fever is present over a period of several days and is followed by a maculopapular rash that begins on the trunk and spreads outward. The symptoms are usually benign although febrile seizures may be associated. The diagnosis is usually made clinically, but serologic testing can be performed to confirm the diagnosis. The related human herpesvirus 7 likely causes a minority of exanthem subitum cases. In immunocompetent persons, treatment for mononucleosis syndromes and HHV-6 and 7 infections is supportive.

Kaposi's sarcoma herpesvirus (KSHV), or human herpesvirus 8 is the most recently described herpesvirus. It was discovered in association with HIV-associated Kaposi's sarcoma (KS) and has since been found to have a role in the development of other malignancies. KSHV is spread mainly through sexual contact among men who have sex with men, although nonsexual transmission also occurs, possibly via saliva. KS is a vascular neoplasm, and its cutaneous form is characterized by the appearance of erythematous or purplish nodules and plaques that are indurated and may be disfiguring (Figure 33-23). KS may spread to the lungs, gastrointestinal tract, or other organs. AIDS-related KS may regress in response to reconstitution of the immune system with antiretroviral therapy for HIV infection, but local or systemic chemotherapy is sometimes required for treatment.

Molluscum Contagiosum

Molluscum contagiosum is a common skin disease caused by a poxvirus and is characterized by small firm, waxy papules, often with umbilicated centers; occasionally giant lesions may be seen (Figure 33-24). The virus replicates in the lower layers of the epidermis and extends upwards Molluscum contagiosum is transmitted directly from person to person, in many instances by sexual contact. It can also be spread from one area of the body to another by contact. The disease most

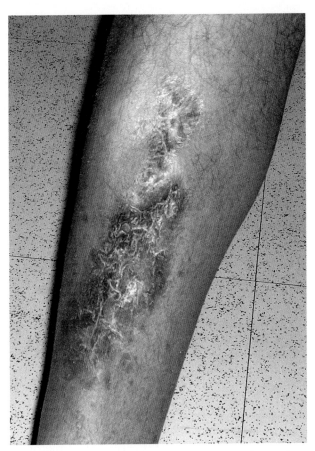

FIGURE 33-23 Large hyperpigmented plaque of Kaposi's sarcoma.

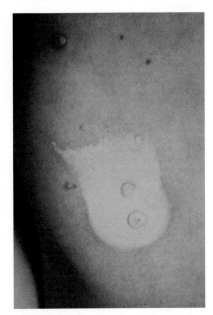

FIGURE 33-24 Giant molluscum contagiosum.

often appears on the genitalia, face, or perirectal area. It tends to be self-limited and benign, although lesions can be removed for cosmetic reasons by curettage or by using liquid nitrogen cryotherapy.

Orf and Milker's Nodule

Parapoxviruses (family Poxviridae) can cause a pustular dermatitis in humans. Two of the species that infect humans are parapoxvirus ovis **(orf virus)** and parapoxvirus bovis (milker's nodule virus; MNV), also known as *pseudocowpox*. These viruses normally cause disease in sheep, cattle, and goats and thus are zoonotic occupational diseases of farmers, veterinarians, slaughterhouse workers, and others exposed to infected animals. The skin lesion is usually a solitary papule, pustule, or nodule that may have central crusting and can be associated with local lymphadenitis. The lesions are often located on the hands, arms, or face and can be confused with human anthrax. Person-to-person spread is rare, and there is no specific treatment; the illness usually resolves in several weeks without scarring.

Human Papillomavirus

Papillomaviruses (family Papovaviridae) cause a variety of skin and mucous membrane lesions that range in severity from benign growths to malignancies. There are over 100 types of human papillomaviruses (HPV), with most human infections being asymptomatic or leading to warts, benign proliferations of skin, or mucosal cells. Common warts (circumscribed, hyperkeratotic, rough-textured, painless papules varying in size from several millimeters to large masses), plantar warts (flat, hyperkeratotic lesions of the plantar surface of the feet that may be painful), and flat warts (smooth, slightly elevated, usually multiple lesions varying in size from 1 millimeter to 1 centimeter) are typical cutaneous manifestations. They often resolve spontaneously over time. Certain HPV strains preferentially affect the oral cavity and have been linked to oral cancers. Genital lesions associated with HPV include venereal warts, or condyloma acuminata (cauliflower-like fleshy growths seen most often in the moist genital and perianal regions) and flat papillomas of the cervix. Transmission of HPV from mother to infant via infection of the birth canal can lead to laryngeal papillomas on the vocal cords and epiglottis of children. Some forms of cancer, namely skin, cervical, and anorectal cancers, may be associated with oncogenic types of papillomavirus (most commonly HPV 16 and 18). Treatment of warts is generally with topical chemical therapy or cryotherapy. A vaccine is now licensed that offers protection against HPV-6, HPV-11, HPV-16, and HPV-18; these HPV types cause 70% of cervical cancers and 90% of genital warts.

Hemorrhagic Fever Viruses

A number of viruses of the Togaviridae (e.g., chikungunya, O'nyong-nyong, and Ross River viruses), Flaviviridae (e.g., yellow fever, dengue virus), Arenaviridae (e.g., Junin, Lassa, and Machupo viruses), Bunyaviridae (e.g., Hantavirus, Crimean-Congo hemorrhagic fever [CCHF], Rift Valley fever viruses), and Filoviridae (e.g., Ebola, Marburg) families may cause a characteristic viral syndrome including fever, headache, myalgias, nausea and vomiting, abdominal pain, and prostration that can be accompanied by severe bleeding manifestations such as nasal or gastrointestinal bleeding and hematuria. Bleeding into the skin also occurs and results in

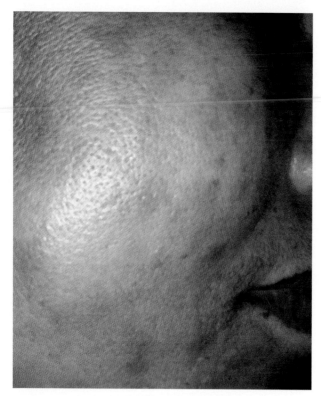

FIGURE 33-25   Facial rash of dengue fever. (Courtesy Dr. Gail Reid, University of Illinois at Chicago.)

petechiae, purpura, and ecchymoses. These viruses are found in the tropics and many are zoonotic, having a rodent reservoir or an arthropod vector, with humans as accidental hosts. Treatment is generally supportive, although the antiviral ribavirin has been useful in some cases, particularly with Lassa fever and CCHF. Preventive measures include rodent vector control and isolating persons infected with viruses for which person-to-person transmission occurs, such as Lassa fever, CCHF, and Marburg and Ebola viruses.

Dengue is one of the more common hemorrhagic fever viruses and is endemic to the Caribbean, areas of the Middle East, South America, sub-Saharan Africa, and Asia. It is an acute illness manifested by fevers, severe headache, and muscle aches, the latter giving rise to its nickname, "breakbone fever." As the fever disappears, a macular rash occurs, which spares the palms and soles and often involves the neck and face (Figure 33-25). Dengue hemorrhagic fever is a severe manifestation of disease that occurs in persons who have been previously infected with a different serotype of the virus; petechiae and purpura are common, as are thrombocytopenia, disseminated intravascular coagulation, and shock. PCR and viral culture of blood during viremia can be performed for diagnosis, or serologic testing can confirm the diagnosis in a recovering patient. Treatment for dengue is supportive.

PARASITIC INFECTIONS

Three main categories of human parasitic infections are helminthic, protozoal, and ectoparasitic. These infections are most often encountered in tropical and subtropical regions of the world and cause an enormous burden of disease in developing countries. Helminths (derived from the Greek term for "worms") are large, multicellular organisms that are extremely prevalent worldwide. Protozoa are unicellular organisms that can either be free-living or parasitic, and those that infect the blood of humans are transmitted by arthropod vectors. **Ectoparasites** are organisms that live on, rather than in, the human body and include fleas, lice, ticks, and mites. Many of these parasitic infections have major or minor dermatologic manifestations as part of the illnesses they cause. Some of the more common of these infections are discussed below.

Helminths

Schistosoma

Schistosomes are trematode flatworms (flukes). Dermatitis caused by schistosomes is most often seen when the infective larvae of bird and animal schistosomes infect humans. Free-living larvae, or cercariae, that have developed in snails penetrate the skin of humans bathing or swimming in infected waters. This results in an intensely pruritic, papular eruption known as cercarial dermatitis or "swimmer's itch." These nonhuman schistosomes do not mature in humans and they die in the skin. Such infections can be prevalent among bathers in lakes in many parts of the world, including the Great Lakes region of North America and certain coastal beaches. The diagnosis is usually made clinically and the dermatitis is self-limited. Acute schistosomiasis caused by human schistosomes (Katayama fever) is sometimes associated with a similar pruritic rash related to skin penetration by cercariae. This disease is encountered in Asia, Africa, the Middle East, and South America.

Strongyloides

The intestinal helminth *Strongyloides stercoralis* is a nematode (round worm) found in Southeast Asia, Latin America, Africa, and areas in the southeastern United States. Free-living larvae in soil penetrate the skin of humans and may cause a transient dermatitis as they migrate to the vasculature on their way to the lung and then gastrointestinal tract. In chronic infection, adult *Strongyloides* worms reside in the large intestine and produce larvae that may autoinfect the skin, causing a rash known as *larva currens*, characteristically a migratory, serpiginous, and very pruritic eruption. Urticaria may appear, and the buttocks, groin, and thighs are often involved as the larvae penetrate the skin in the perianal area. *Strongyloides* infection may persist for decades. The antiparasitic medication ivermectin is effective treatment.

Filaria

Filariasis is caused by nematodes that reside in the lymph nodes, lymphatic vessels, and subcutaneous tissues. Three main species cause most human infections: *Wuchereria bancrofti, Brugia malayi,* and *Onchocerca volvulus.* The former two are transmitted by the bite of mosquitoes and cause lymphatic filariasis. Onchocerca is transmitted by blackflies and causes subcutaneous nodules and river blindness.

W. bancrofti is found in tropical areas of the world, and *B. malayi* is seen in Asia. Lymphatic filariasis is often asymp-

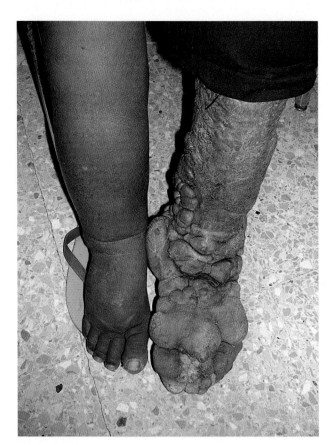

FIGURE 33-26 Disfiguring lower extremity swelling and marked thickening of the skin caused by lymphatic filariasis. (Courtesy Dr. Gail Reid, University of Illinois at Chicago.)

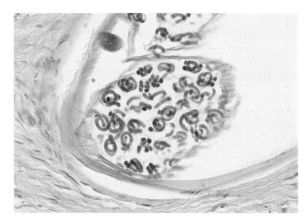

FIGURE 33-27 Tissue cross-section of a nodule containing *Onchocerca volvulus* microfilariae.

of microfilariae through skin leads to an intensely itchy rash and skin edema. Depigmentation or thickening of the skin can occur over time. Laboratory diagnosis of the cutaneous disease can be made by superficial skin biopsies ("skin snips"), with demonstration of microfilariae by microscopic examination although the sensitivity of this method may not be as good as serologic testing or urine testing for filarial antigens. If present, cutaneous nodules can also be excised to confirm the presence of adult worms. Ivermectin kills microfilariae but has limited effect on adult worms. Because it can therefore control the disease but may not cure it, ivermectin is often given as an initial single dose with periodic retreatment on a quarterly or yearly basis. This can reduce morbidity and interrupt transmission of the parasite.

Hookworm

The human hookworms include two nematode species, *Ancylostoma duodenale* and *Necator americanus,* which are found worldwide but predominantly in areas with warm, moist climates including Africa, Asia, the Middle East, and the Americas. Eggs are shed into the environment and infective larvae develop in soil. When they come in contact with human skin, the larvae quickly penetrate and can cause a dermatitis known as "ground-itch," particularly in persons previously exposed to hookworm. The larvae then pass through the bloodstream into the lungs and eventually to the intestine where they reside.

Larvae of the dog and cat hookworms, *Ancylostoma caninum* and *Ancylostoma braziliense,* respectively, can also penetrate the skin of humans but are unable to develop further. They produce a self-limited dermatitis known as *cutaneous larva migrants (CLM)* or "creeping eruption." The dermatitis is characterized by larval migration in the skin with associated serpiginous, elevated tunnels, and indurated, itchy papules. The skin lesions can become superinfected with bacteria such as staphylococci and streptococci. CLM is endemic in the developing world and in the United States can be found in southeastern states. The disease is often seen in children who play in sandboxes frequented by cats and dogs, and it is an occupational hazard of workers who crawl or work in areas with damp, sandy soil contaminated by dog or cat feces. Spontaneous cure is the rule, although CLM can persist for

tomatic for many years, but some patients experience obstruction of the lymphatic vessels in the lower extremities and genital region with resulting "elephantiasis" (Figure 33-26). Fever and inflammation of associated lymph nodes can occur and may be the result of secondary bacterial or fungal infection; these secondary infections are facilitated by the compromised lymphatic function. The parasites can be found in the bloodstream and identified by Giemsa or hematoxylin and eosin stains of blood smears. Filarial antigen detection assays and PCR are also available. Albendazole and diethylcarbamazine are effective in killing the adult-stage parasites and can improve elephantiasis.

Onchocerciasis is a chronic, nonfatal disease caused by *Onchocerca volvulus,* which is confined geographically to parts of West Africa, Mexico, Central and South America, and the Middle East. After being introduced into the body by blackflies, the larvae develop into adult worms in subcutaneous tissues, particularly over bony prominences in the head and shoulders, hips, and lower extremities. These subdermal nodules are known as "onchocercomata" (Figure 33-27). The worms shed thousands of microfilariae that migrate through the skin and have an affinity for the eye. The most important manifestation of onchocerciasis, river blindness (so named because transmission is most often in rural villages near rapidly flowing streams), is the result of this infiltration of the eye by the organisms. This leads to an inflammatory response that causes visual disturbances and blindness. The migration months or occasionally years. Albendazole, ivermectin, and thiabendazole are all effective treatments; thiabendazole may also be effective topically.

Leishmania

There are few protozoal diseases that cause significant skin infection, but *Leishmania* is one that can manifest predominantly as a cutaneous or mucosal disease. It can also cause visceral infection, known as *kala-azar*. *Leishmania* is endemic throughout Latin America, Asia, the Middle East, and southern Europe; is maintained in mammal reservoirs (dogs, rodents, humans); and is transmitted by the bite of sandflies. Most *Leishmania* infections are limited to the skin and adjacent lymph nodes. Cutaneous leishmaniasis develops days to months after the bite of an infected sandfly and is characterized by a painless papule that enlarges and may ulcerate (Figure 33-28). Some lesions remain smooth or become hyperkeratotic, and the appearance of the lesions can vary according to the infecting *Leishmania* species. Local dissemination of infection can occur with the development of additional skin lesions in a sporotrichoid or nodular lymphangitis pattern. Hematogenous dissemination may also occur with widespread

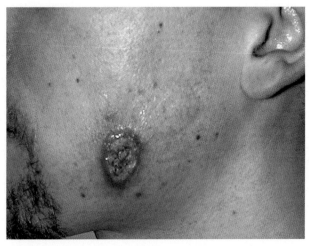

FIGURE 33-28 Facial ulceration caused by *Leishmania* infection.

cutaneous lesions that are often associated with mucosal involvement. Cutaneous leishmaniasis can be complicated by scarring that is disfiguring and secondary infection. The diagnosis is made by identifying amastigotes in a scraping or biopsy of a skin lesion; culture and/or PCR can also be performed on the tissue. Spontaneous cure of cutaneous lesions is typical over a period of months. Treatment can be given to speed healing and to prevent scarring, dissemination, and relapse. Pentavalent antimony is the most active drug but is relatively toxic and expensive. Depending on the species of *Leishmania,* fluconazole, amphotericin, miltefosine, and pentamidine may produce activity against these organisms.

Ectoparasites

A number of ectoparasites may cause human infection, including lice (pediculosis), mites (scabies), fleas, flies, ticks, chiggers, and bedbugs (Figure 33-29). Ectoparasites attach or burrow in the skin and can remain there for weeks to months. The dermatologic features of these infestations include severe itching and the formation of papules, vesicles, nodules, linear burrows, and excoriations of the skin and scalp. *Sarcoptes scabiei,* the mite that causes scabies, is too small to be seen by the naked eye and burrows in the stratum corneum, laying eggs that hatch and mature. The rash frequently occurs in the genital region and in the webs between fingers. Norwegian scabies is a particularly severe infestation that occurs in immunocompromised individuals and causes a psoriasis-type dermatitis (Figure 33-30). Scrapings of affected areas of skin with microscopy can confirm the diagnosis, and treatment consists of topical lindane or permethrin. Oral ivermectin is often given for Norwegian scabies.

Lice are blood-sucking insects. Different types of *Pediculus* lice cause infestation of different parts of the body (head, body, or pubic region). Lice are transmitted by close contact, and transmission is facilitated by poor hygiene. The disease is characterized by intense itching and local erythema, papules, and excoriations of the skin. The diagnosis is made by identifying live lice, which are 1 to 3 millimeters in size, and nits (eggs). Topical permethrin, malathion, and lindane are effective treatments, and oral antihelminths such as ivermectin or albendazole may be given for severe infestations.

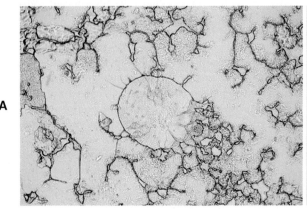
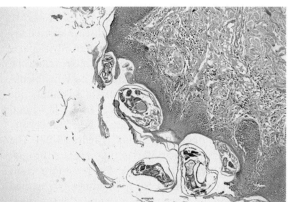

FIGURE 33-29 **A,** *Sarcoptes scabiei* adult showing short legs and conical spines. **B,** Tissue cross-section of scabies lesion showing larvae burrowed into the epidermal layer of the skin.

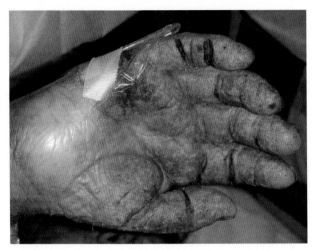

FIGURE 33-30 Thick scaly plaques of Norwegian scabies. (Courtesy Dr. Gail Reid, University of Illinois at Chicago.)

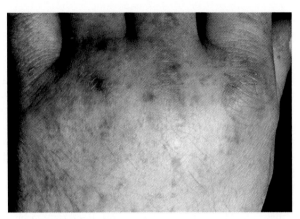

FIGURE 33-31 Petechial lesions in meningococcemia.

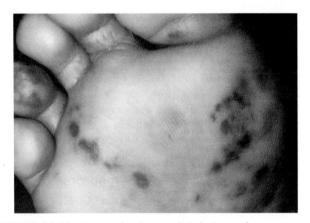

FIGURE 33-32 Hemorrhagic vasculitic lesions of *Staphylococcus aureus* endocarditis.

IMMUNE- OR TOXIN-MEDIATED DERMATOLOGIC MANIFESTATIONS OF INFECTIOUS AGENTS

As described in previous sections of this chapter, many different local and systemic infections caused by bacteria, fungi, viruses, and parasites produce diseases of the skin. Skin lesions resulting from direct cutaneous infection and those resulting from hematogenous spread to the skin have been described above. Additional dermatologic manifestations of infection can result from either the body's immune response to the infecting organism or from toxin production by the organism. Some of the more common of these syndromes are described below.

Immune-Mediated Cutaneous Disease

Disseminated Intravascular Coagulation

Dysregulation of the blood coagulation system frequently occurs during sepsis from any cause and, when severe, can manifest as disseminated intravascular coagulation (DIC). In the past it was thought that lipopolysaccharides on the surface of gram-negative bacteria directly activated the coagulation system, but it is now known that cytokines released in response to infection play an important intermediary role in this process. The cascade initiated by these events leads to low levels of antithrombin and activated protein C, alteration in endothelial cells, and widespread intravascular fibrin and microthrombi deposition in the liver, lungs, brain, and kidneys. Some of the coagulation factors can in turn activate additional inflammatory responses. This process manifests clinically as venous thromboses, petechiae of the skin (Figure 33-31), thrombocytopenia, bleeding, and multiorgan dysfunction. Bacterial sepsis such as that caused by *Neisseria meningitidis,* streptococci, or enteric gram-negatives is the most common setting in which to encounter infection-related DIC, but it can occur with other types of pathogens including, for example, the hemorrhagic fever viruses.

An additional skin manifestation of DIC is **purpura fulminans.** This syndrome has classically been associated with meningococcemia, but bloodstream infections with *S. aureus, Streptococcus pneumoniae,* and *Haemophilus influenzae* have also been associated. It is characterized by rapidly developing skin hemorrhage and necrosis and peripheral gangrene accompanied by shock syndrome. Death or amputation often result. It appears that purpura fulminans can be the result of autoimmune protein C or S deficiency.

Vasculitis

Many types of infections may trigger immune-mediated damage to small blood vessels in dermal tissues, resulting in a vasculitis that most often manifests as palpable purpura, typically over the lower extremities. Some of these cutaneous findings have been mentioned briefly in earlier sections in this chapter. It is estimated that approximately 20% of all cutaneous vasculitis is caused by infection due to bacteria, fungi, viruses, protozoa, and helminths. Viruses such as hepatitis B and C, adenoviruses, parvovirus and herpesviruses, and bacteria including streptococci, staphylococci (Figure 33-32), *Mycoplasma pneumoniae, Legionella, Rickettsiae,* and *Yersinia* are some of the organisms more commonly described as causing vasculitis. Hepatitis C can also be associated with a cutaneous vasculitis that results from the production of cryoglobulins, immunoglobulins that precipitate in cold temperatures.

Immune Complex Disease

Infection-related immune complex–induced cutaneous disease is commonly seen in endocarditis (as is vasculitis, described above). Painful, small skin nodules located on the pads of the fingers and toes and on the thenar eminence, known as Osler's nodes, are the result of the deposition of immune complexes in soft tissues. The other characteristic skin finding in endocarditis, the Janeway lesion, actually represents septic microemboli to the skin rather than deposition of immune complexes. These lesions are flat, painless hemorrhagic macules located on the palms and soles. Bacteria can be cultured from biopsies of Janeway lesions. Staphylococci and streptococci are typically associated with the aforementioned skin manifestations, although gram-negative bacteria and *Candida* may produce similar lesions.

Toxin-Mediated Cutaneous Disease

Certain bacteria, particularly staphylococci and streptococci, are capable of producing toxins that affect the skin, resulting in distinct clinical syndromes. These infections may start as primary skin and soft tissue infections or may initially affect another site with subsequent involvement of the skin caused by the effects of circulating toxin.

Staphylococcal Scalded-Skin Syndrome

In staphylococcal scalded-skin syndrome (SSSS), *S. aureus* produces exfoliative toxins that result in fever, skin tenderness, and a scarlatiniform rash, followed by extensive bullae formation and exfoliation similar to that seen in burn patients. This is a syndrome predominantly of children, although it can occasionally be seen in immunocompromised adults. The toxins act exclusively on the stratum granulosum of the epidermis and thus do not affect mucosal tissues. The Nikolsky sign is characteristic, which is separation of the epidermal layer upon gentle stroking. Large flaccid blisters form and rupture, causing skin to denude and peel off in sheets and leaving areas of bright red underlying skin exposed. Scarring generally does not occur. Nosocomial epidemics of SSSS have been reported in newborn nurseries. SSSS treatment involves administration of antistaphylococcal antibiotics, hydration, and local wound care.

Toxic Shock Syndrome

Cutaneous desquamation occurs in **toxic shock syndrome** (TSS) because of the production of staphylococcal exotoxins. These include a unique group of exotoxins that are referred to as "superantigens" because of their ability to cause widespread non–antigen-specific activation of T lymphocytes. Superantigens include toxic shock syndrome toxin-1 (TSST-1) and staphylococcal enterotoxins. The activation produced by these superantigens results in the rapid release of cytokines by lymphocytes and macrophages. Originally described among children by Todd in 1978, TSS subsequently gained notoriety in 1980 when a number of cases were reported among women who had used superabsorbent tampons. The tampons apparently provided an environment favorable for TSST-1 production. There are many different settings in

which nonmenstrual TSS occurs as well. It has, for example, been described postpartum, following influenza infection, and in association with surgical wound infections and contaminated nasal packing in patients with nosebleeds. Menstrual and nonmenstrual TSS have similar clinical presentations: a diffuse sunburn-like erythroderma appears early in the course and is accompanied by fever, hypotension, and evidence of multiorgan dysfunction. Desquamation of skin, especially on the palms and soles, occurs during the convalescent stage of the illness. Blood cultures may be positive for *S. aureus,* and staphylococci may be cultured from the initial site of infection. Treatment includes antistaphylococcal antibiotics and supportive care with hydration, vasopressors, and debridement of any infected tissue. Recurrences have been described in as many as 30% to 40% of cases.

A streptococcal TSS caused by group A streptococcus (GAS; *S. pyogenes*) began appearing in the late 1980s and has become more prevalent in recent years, with the resurgence of invasive and complicated streptococcal infections. Like its staphylococcal counterpart, streptococcal TSS may occur whenever exotoxin-producing strains of GAS infect or colonize the skin or mucous membranes, particularly strains producing streptococcal pyrogenic exotoxin (SPE)-A, although other exotoxins have been implicated. The majority of streptococcal TSS cases have been in young, otherwise healthy adults, and it is thought that lack of protective immunity is a risk factor. The portal of entry is typically the skin with cellulitis that progresses rapidly. The subsequent clinical signs and symptoms of GAS TSS are similar to those of staphylococcal TSS. Blood cultures are more often positive in streptococcal than staphylococcal TSS. Treatment is with antistreptococcal antibiotics, debridement of infected tissues, and supportive measures.

Scarlet Fever

Scarlet fever is a form of GAS disease that can occur when the infecting strain produces SPEs. It occurs mostly in children and concomitantly with pharyngeal infection, although it can also be seen with infections at other sites. Fever is typically present, and the rash starts on the chest and spreads outward. The red, sandpaper-textured rash is often better felt than seen and appears most often on the neck and chest and in skin folds. Typically, the rash does not involve the face, but there is a flushing of the skin with circumoral pallor, and the patient may have a strawberry tongue (a bright red tongue with dots of white papillae). During convalescence, desquamation of the skin occurs, especially on the hands and feet. The diagnosis is usually made clinically, and treatment is with antistreptococcal antibiotics such as penicillins, macrolides, or cephalosporins.

LABORATORY DIAGNOSIS

In the management of skin infections, the surface of broken or ulcerated skin is often swabbed by clinicians for purposes of Gram staining and culture. However, this technique provides little clinically useful information. Swabs of surface wounds or skin are likely to yield colonizing or contaminating bacteria, and there is a lack of correlation between surface colonization and below-the-surface infection. Swabs may also lead to false-negative Gram stains and cultures because they do not contain sufficient amounts of material for culture, organisms may adhere to the swabs, and bacteria do not survive as well on a swab as they do within fluid or a tissue sample. Therefore deep aspirates or biopsies of involved tissue are generally much more informative. For example, if pustules or vesicles are present, the roof or crust should be removed with a sterile blade, and any pus or exudate should be Gram stained and cultured. It is possible to obtain a specimen in a patient with cellulitis by injecting a small amount (about 3 mL) of preservative-free, physiologic saline into the advancing margin of the affected skin, aspirating back, and then culturing the fluid that is withdrawn. Alternatively, a punch biopsy of the skin can be performed and submitted for Gram stain and culture.

Laboratory diagnosis of bacterial skin infections should consist of a direct smear examination and culture of the affected site, which may reveal the causative agent(s). Exuded pus or wound dressings should always be examined for the presence of granules and branching filaments, suggestive of infections with actinomycetes or fungi. Smears prepared from exudative material and subsequently Gram stained may show the presence of inflammatory cells and the characteristic morphology that may lead to an initial diagnosis. Results of the direct smear examination are especially important to the clinician, although Gram staining is relatively insensitive for detecting bacteria and culture is still the best clinically available method of diagnosing cutaneous infections. It is also important to note that organisms may not appear the same on a Gram stain of tissue as they do in pure culture; staphylococci, for example, may not be found in clusters and streptococci may not form chains. In addition to Gram stain, it may be appropriate to perform a wet mount with the addition of potassium hydroxide to enhance the appearance of any fungi that may be present. Calcofluor white (CW) stain may also be used when fungal infections are suspected; CW allows yeasts and moulds to fluoresce and be identified. In addition, if mycobacterial disease is suspected, a Ziehl-Neelsen or Kinyoun acid-fast stain may be performed that will make mycobacteria appear as red bacilli under light microscopy. Fluorescent stains (rhodamine and auramine dyes) are also available that bind mycobacterial cell walls and are a more sensitive method of staining mycobacteria. To identify *Nocardia* species, a modified acid-fast stain can be performed, using a weaker decolorizing agent than the aforementioned acid-fast stains. As noted in the section on herpesviruses, certain viral pathogens such as HSV and VZV can be detected in rapid fashion by obtaining scrapings of new vesicular or ulcerated lesions and performing a direct fluorescent antibody test on the specimen to detect viral antigens.

Infectious agents are recovered in routine culture using both primary, nonselective media such as blood and chocolate agars and selective media. MAC is a selective medium that is designed to grow gram-negative bacilli and identify those that ferment lactose; phenylethyl alcohol (PEA) and colistin-nalidixic acid (CNA) are selective media that preferentially grow gram-positive organisms (see Chapter 6). For the growth of anaerobic organisms, samples must be collected from infected tissue and transported properly, using an anaerobic transport medium to maximize recovery. Because many anaerobic infections are polymicrobial, samples must be inoculated on culture media that are selective for gram-positive and gram-negative bacteria. There are ranges of pH, temperature, oxygen levels, and nutrients that are required for the growth of various types of organisms. Therefore communication between the clinician and microbiology laboratory is essential for optimizing the information obtained from a clinical specimen.

Once organisms are growing in culture, identification of isolates is performed using a variety of methods, some of which may be automated. A Gram stain provides the morphologic characteristics of bacterial organisms growing in culture and further information is gleaned from the appearance of the bacterial colonies and the presence of hemolysis on blood agar. Biochemical tests such as those for catalase, coagulase, oxidase, bile solubility, and a number of others can then pinpoint the identity of the organism. Antimicrobial susceptibility testing is subsequently performed on isolates when the susceptibility cannot reliably be predicted based on the organism identity. For example, group A streptococci have been uniformly susceptible to penicillin, so antibiotic testing for this organism is typically presumed unnecessary. Standards have been published and are updated regularly on the performance and interpretation of antimicrobial susceptibility testing based on the correlation of testing results with clinical outcomes. In some cases there are inadequate data on which to define the drug concentrations at which certain organisms are susceptible to various antimicrobials, particularly for unusual or fastidious organisms.

Other media and techniques are used to culture nonbacterial organisms. *Candida* spp. will grow on blood agar plates, but Sabouraud's agar is a selective fungal medium that has an acidic pH, which is preferred for optimizing fungal growth and antibiotics that suppress the growth of bacteria. Lowenstein-Jensen or Middlebrook media are the solid media that support the growth of mycobacteria. Certain mycobacteria such as *M. chelonae* and *M. abscessus* grow quickly in culture, but more slowly growing species such as *M. tuberculosis* may take as long as 8 weeks to grow. Studies have demonstrated that mycobacteria grow more quickly in liquid media, with certain liquid media speeding the growth of *M. tuberculosis* to 2 weeks. Nucleic acids probes are available for several of the mycobacterial species including *M. tuberculosis*, and these can make an identification to the species level once growth is present on solid media.

Because viruses are intracellular pathogens, they cannot be cultured using the above techniques and generally require a medium containing living cells (tissue culture). Specimens should be transported in special viral medium that contains antibiotics to suppress the growth of nonviral organisms. After inoculation of the specimen into a tissue culture, the presence of virus is revealed by the observation of a "cytopathic effect" (CPE), or a lysing of the cells and separation from the tissue culture dish. The identity of the virus can then be confirmed by the addition of specific fluorescent antibodies directed against various viruses or related immunoassay techniques. The "shell vial" technique is a more rapid and economical version of viral culture; the specimen to be cultured is centrifuged onto a monolayer of cells on a removable glass cover slip at the bottom of a small vial.

The glass cover slip can then be removed and observed for CPE.

BIBLIOGRAPHY

Bailey MS, Lockwood DN: Cutaneous leishmaniasis, *Clin Dermatol* 25:203, 2007.

Baird JK, Wear DJ: Cercarial dermatitis: the swimmer's itch, *Clin Dermatol* 5:88, 1987.

Bisno AL, Stevens DL: Streptococcal infections of skin and soft tissues, *New Engl J Med* 334240, 1996.

Botelho-Nevers E, Raoult D: Fever of unknown origin due to rickettsioses, *Infect Dis Clin North Am* 21:997, 2007.

Bratton RL et al: Diagnosis and treatment of Lyme disease, *Mayo Clin Proc* 83:566, 2008.

Bravo FG, Gotuzzo E: Cutaneous tuberculosis, *Clin Dermatol* 25:173, 2007.

Bray M: Highly pathogenic RNA viral infections: challenges for antiviral research, *Antiviral Res* 78:1, 2008.

Brook I: Secondary bacterial infections complicating skin lesions, *J Med Microbiol* 51:808, 2002.

Brown-Elliott BA, Wallace RJ: Infections caused by nontuberculous mycobacteria. In Mandell GL, Bennett JE, Dolin R, editors: *Principles and practice of infectious diseases*, ed 6, Philadelphia, 2005, Churchill Livingstone, pp 2909-2916.

Burd EM: Human papillomavirus and cervical cancer, *Clin Microbiol Rev* 16:1, 2003.

Buttner M, Rziha HJ: Parapoxviruses: from the lesion to the viral genome, *J Vet Med B Infect Dis Vet Public Health* 49:7, 2002.

Carlson JA, Chen KR: Cutaneous vasculitis update: small vessel neutrophilic vasculitis syndromes, *Am J Dermatopathol* 28:486, 2006.

Carneiro SC et al: Viral exanthems in the tropics, *Clin Dermatol* 25:212, 2007.

Cherry JD, Hurwitz ES, Welliver RC: Mycoplasma pneumoniae infections and exanthems, *J Pediatr* 87:369, 1975.

Davis MD, Dy KM, Nelson S: Presentation and outcome of purpura fulminans associated with peripheral gangrene in 12 patients at Mayo Clinic, *J Am Acad Dermatol* 57:944, 2007.

Dinubile MJ: Nodular lymphangitis: a distinctive clinical entity with finite etiologies, *Curr InfectDis Rep* 10:404, 2008.

Dodiuk-Gad R et al: Nontuberculous mycobacterial infections of the skin: A retrospective study of 25 cases, *J Am Acad Dermatol* 57:413, 2007.

Eliasson H et al: Tularemia: current epidemiology and disease management. *Infect Dis Clin N Am* 20:289-311, 2006.

Fakhry C, Gillison ML: Clinical implications of human papillomavirus in head and neck cancers, *J Clin Oncol* 24:2606, 2006.

Fatahzadeh M, Schwartz RA: Human herpes simplex virus infections: epidemiology, pathogenesis, symptomatology, diagnosis, and management, *J Am Acad Dermatol* 57:737, 2007.

Fridkin SK et al: Methicillin-resistant *Staphylococcus aureus* disease in three communities, *New Engl J Med* 352:1436, 2005.

Ganem D: KSHV infection and the pathogenesis of Kaposi's sarcoma, *Annu Rev Pathol* 1:273, 2006.

Gershon AA: Varicella-zoster virus infections, *Pediatr Rev* 29:5, 2008.

Goh BT: Syphilis in adults, *Sex Transm Infect* 81:448, 2005.

Gould EA, Solomon T: Pathogenic flaviviruses, *Lancet* 371:500, 2008.

Hay RJ: Dermatophytosis and other superficial mycoses In Mandell GL, Bennett JE, Dolin R, editors: *Principles and practice of infectious diseases*, ed 6, Philadelphia, 2005, Churchill Livingstone, pp 3051-3062.

Herold BC et al: Community-acquired methicillin-resistant *Staphylococcus aureus* in children with no identified predisposing risk, *JAMA* 279:593, 1998.

Heukelbach J, Feldmeier H: Epidemiological and clinical characteristics of hookworm-related cutaneous larva migrans, *Lancet Infect Dis* 8:302, 2008.

Hospenthal DR: Uncommon fungi. In Mandell GL, Bennett JE, Dolin R, editors: *Principles and Practice of infectious diseases*, ed 6, Philadelphia, 2005, Churchill Livingstone, pp 3068-3079.

Hospenthal DR: Agents of mycetoma. In Mandell GL, Bennett JE, Dolin R, editors: *Principles and practice of infectious diseases*, ed 6, Philadelphia, 2005, Churchill Livingstone, pp 2991-2995.

Hotez PJ et al: Hookworm infection, *New Engl J Med* 351:799, 2004.

Huang CM: Human papillomavirus and vaccination, *Mayo Clin Proc* 83:701, 2008.

Kaplan SL: Implications of methicillin-resistant *Staphylococcus aureus* as a community-acquired pathogen in pediatric patients, *Infect Dis Clin North Am* 19:747, 2005.

Kauffman CA: Endemic mycoses: blastomycosis, histoplasmosis, and sporotrichosis, *Infect Dis Clin North Am* 20:645, 2006.

Kauffman CA et al: Clinical practice guidelines for the management of sporotrichosis: 2007 update by the Infectious Diseases Society of America, *Clin Infect Dis* 45:1255, 2007.

Kingston ME, Mackey D: Skin clues in the diagnosis of life-threatening infections, *Rev Infect Dis* 8:1, 1986.

Klevens RM et al: Changes in the epidemiology of methicillin-resistant *Staphylococcus aureus* in intensive care units in US hospitals, 1992-2003, *Clin Infect Dis* 42:389, 2006.

Klevens RM et al: Invasive methicillin-resistant *Staphylococcus aureus* infections in the United States, *JAMA* 298:1763, 2007.

Kravitz GR et al: Purpura fulminans due to *Staphylococcus aureus*, *Clin Infect Dis* 40:941, 2005.

Lai-Cheong JE et al: Cutaneous manifestations of tuberculosis, *Clin Exp Dermatol* 32:461, 2007.

Levett PN: Leptospirosis, *Clin Microbiol Rev* 14:296, 2001.

Levi M et al: Infection and inflammation and the coagulation system, *Cardiovasc Res* 60:26, 2003.

Lipsky BA et al: Diagnosis and treatment of diabetic foot infections, *Clin Infect Dis* 39:885, 2004.

Lupi O, Tyring SK, McGinnis MR: Tropical dermatology: fungal tropical diseases, *J Am Acad Dermatol* 53:931, 2005.

Mahanty S, Bray M: Pathogenesis of filoviral haemorrhagic fevers, *Lancet Infect Dis* 4:487, 2004.

Manders SM: Toxin-mediated streptococcal and staphylococcal disease, *J Am Acad Dermatol* 39:383, 1998.

Miller LG et al: Necrotizing fasciitis caused by community-associated methicillin-resistant *Staphylococcus aureus* in Los Angeles, *New Engl J Med* 352:1445, 2005.

Moran GJ et al: Methicillin-resistant *S. aureus* infections among patients in the emergency department, *New Engl J Med* 355:666, 2006.

Murray HW et al: Advances in leishmaniasis, *Lancet* 366:1561, 2005.

Nguyen HQ, Jumaan AO, Seward JF: Decline in mortality due to varicella after implementation of varicella vaccination in the United States, *New Engl J Med* 352:450, 2005.

Orion E, Matz H, Wolf R: Ectoparasitic sexually transmitted diseases: scabies and pediculosis, *Clin Dermatol* 22:513, 2004.

Parola P, Paddock CD, Raoult D: Tick-borne rickettsioses around the world: emerging diseases challenging old concepts, *Clin Microbiol Rev* 18:719, 2005.

Pfaller MA, Diekema DJ: Unusual fungal and pseudofungal infections of humans, *J Clin Microbiol* 43:1495, 2005.

Plouffe JF: Importance of atypical pathogens of community-acquired pneumonia, *Clin Infect Dis* 31(Suppl 2):S35, 2000.

Sadick NS: Current aspects of bacterial infections of the skin, *Dermatol Clin* 15:341, 1997.

Saliba EK, Oumeish OY, Oumeish I: Epidemiology of common parasitic infections of the skin in infants and children, *Clin Dermatol* 20:36, 2002.

Schalock PC et al: Erythema multiforme due to *Mycoplasma pneumoniae* infection in two children, *Pediatr Dermatol* 23:546, 2006.

Scott LA, Stone MS: Viral exanthems, *Dermatol Online J* 9:4, 2003.

Seybold U et al: Emergence of community-associated methicillin-resistant *Staphylococcus aureus* USA300 genotype as a major cause of health care-associated blood stream infections, *Clin Infect Dis* 42:647, 2006.

Siddiqui AA, Berk S: Diagnosis of *Strongyloides stercoralis* infection, *Clin Infect Dis* 33:1040, 2001.

Sladden MJ, Johnston GA: Common skin infections in children, *BMJ* 329:95, 2004.

Smego RA Jr, Castiglia M, Asperilla MO: Lymphocutaneous syndrome: a review of non-sporothrix causes, *Medicine* 78:38, 1999.

Somer T, Finegold SM: Vasculitides associated with infections, immunization, and antimicrobial drugs, *Clin Infect Dis* 20:1010, 1995.

Stalkup JR, Chilukuri S: Enterovirus infections: a review of clinical presentation, diagnosis, and treatment, *Dermatol Clin* 20:217, 2002.

Stevens DL et al: Practice guidelines for the diagnosis and management of skin and soft-tissue infections, *Clin Infect Dis* 41:1373, 2005.

Stevens DL et al: Severe group A streptococcal infections associated with a toxic shock-like syndrome and scarlet fever toxin A, *New Engl J Med* 321:1, 1989.

Swartz MN: Clinical practice: cellulitis, *New Engl J Med* 350:904, 2004.

Swartz MN, Pasternack MS: Cellulitis and subcutaneous tissue infections. In Mandell GL, Bennett JE, Dolin R, editors: *Principles and practice of infectious diseases*, ed 6, Philadelphia, 2005, Churchill Livingstone, pp 1172-1194.

Turetz ML et al: Disseminated leishmaniasis: a new and emerging form of leishmaniasis observed in northeastern Brazil, *J Infect Dis* 186:1829, 2002.

Udall DN: Recent updates on onchocerciasis: diagnosis and treatment, *Clin Infect Dis* 44:53, 2007.

Ulbrecht JS, Cavanagh PR, Caputo GM: Foot problems in diabetes: an overview, *Clin Infect Dis* 39(Suppl 2):S73, 2004.

Update: measles—United States, January-July 2008, *MMWR* 57:893, 2008.

Wagner D, Young LS: Nontuberculous mycobacterial infections: a clinical review, *Infection* 32:257, 2004.

Weber DJ, Cohen MS, Rutala WA: The acutely ill patient with fever and rash. In Mandell GL, Bennett JE, Dolin R, editors: *Principles and practice of infectious diseases*, ed 6, Philadelphia, 2005, Churchill Livingstone, pp 729-746.

Wilson ML, Winn W: Laboratory diagnosis of bone, joint, soft-tissue, and skin infections, *Clin Infect Dis* 46:453, 2008.

Wolfson JS, Sober AJ, Rubin RH: Dermatologic manifestations of infections in immunocompromised patients, *Medicine* 64:115, 1985.

Points to Remember

- The skin, skin structures, and normal microbiologic flora play a significant role in protecting the host against microbial invasion and disease.
- The normal skin flora can be involved in the pathogenesis of skin and skin structure infections, particularly if the integrity of the skin is compromised.
- There is an extensive variety of skin and soft-tissue infections, which can be classified according to the type of skin lesion produced, the etiologic organism, or the pathogenesis of the infection (e.g., as a primary entity or secondary to a preexisting infection or systemic manifestation).
- Bacteria, viruses, fungi, and parasites are all important causes of skin and soft tissue infection.
- Virulence factors of disease-producing organisms (e.g., toxins) can enable the organisms to evade host defense mechanisms, and this can result in severe manifestations of infection.
- A compromised immune system can lead to more severe or unusual manifestations of infection and can allow normally innocuous organisms to be pathogenic.
- The occurrence of disease in a host is a function of both the underlying host immunity and the virulence of the pathogen.
- The method and site of collection, the quality of the clinical specimen, and the clinical context are all important factors to consider when distinguishing between colonization and infection.
- Proper specimen collection and laboratory processing of specimens are factors critical to the success of making a microbiologic diagnosis of infection.

Learning Assessment Questions

1. A healthy young man developed a leg abrasion while playing football. The area became warm, red, and swollen. Exudate from the wound revealed gram-positive cocci on Gram stain. What are the likely microbiologic causes of this scenario?
2. What is/are the microbiologic agents involved in intertrigo and what conditions lead to its development?
3. What is the characteristic appearance of tinea infections?
4. What are the typical organisms found in diabetic foot infections and gangrene?
5. What is a mycetoma and what organisms cause it?
6. What is nodular lymphangitis and what organisms cause it?
7. What is a zoonotic disease and what are some of the zoonoses that can cause skin and soft tissue infection?
8. Which bacteria produce cutaneous manifestations as a result of toxin production?
9. Which of the common childhood viral infections are life-long and can manifest in adults after a period of latency?
10. What are the causes of "swimmer's itch," "creeping eruption," and "ground itch"?
11. Which organisms are characterized by the formation of granules and branching filaments in wound exudates?

Gastrointestinal Infections and Food Poisoning

Maximo O. Brito, Jennifer E. Layden-Almer, Connie R. Mahon, George Manuselis

- ■ GENERAL CONCEPTS IN EVALUATING GASTROINTESTINAL INFECTIONS AND FOOD POISONING
- ■ ANATOMIC CONSIDERATIONS
- ■ A PRACTICAL APPROACH TO DIAGNOSIS OF THE PATIENT WITH DIARRHEA
  History
  Physical Examination
  Laboratory Studies
- ■ CLINICAL PRESENTATIONS AND PATHOGENIC MECHANISMS OF ACUTE DIARRHEA
  Enterotoxin-Mediated Diarrhea
  Diarrhea Mediated by Invasion of the Bowel Mucosal Surface
  Diarrhea Mediated by Invasion of Full Bowel Thickness with Lymphatic Spread

- ■ COMMON VIRAL, BACTERIAL, AND PARASITIC PATHOGENS
  Viral Pathogens
  Bacterial Pathogens
  Parasitic Pathogens
- ■ DIARRHEA IN SPECIAL CIRCUMSTANCES
  Toxic Agents of Food Poisoning
  The Returning Traveler
  The Immunocompromised Host
- ■ LABORATORY DIAGNOSIS OF GASTROINTESTINAL PATHOGENS
  Specimen Collection and Handling
  Direct Microscopic Examination
  Culture
- ■ TREATMENT AND PREVENTION OF DIARRHEA

OBJECTIVES

After reading and studying this chapter, you should be able to:

1. Explain the normal host defenses at each level of the gastrointestinal tract in preventing infection.

2. Explain the major mechanisms by which bacteria can cause diarrhea.

3. Describe the various methods by which *Escherichia coli* can cause diarrhea.

4. Explain several means by which infectious diarrhea differs between the immunocompromised and the immunocompetent patient.

5. Describe the common etiologies of traveler's diarrhea.

6. For each of the bacterial agents described, discuss the predicted results of direct microscopy of the stool specimen and the selective media for the maximal recovery of the pathogen.

Case in Point

A 32-year-old healthy man from the United States was visiting a small village in Mexico. The patient consumed some of the local fare and drank the water. Four days after arriving, he experienced sudden onset of diarrhea. The diarrhea occurred more than 10 times the first day and was accompanied by nausea with several episodes of loose, watery stool. The stool contained no gross blood, pus, or mucus. The patient was afebrile but complained of crampy abdominal pain with stooling and dizziness when standing. His heart rate was rapid (120 beats/minute).

Issues to Consider

After reading the patient's case history, consider:

- ■ The travel, food intake, and medical history of the patient
- ■ Clinical symptoms at the time of presentation, the duration, and the time of onset of symptoms
- ■ Possible sources of infection

Acute diarrheal illness is one of the most common problems evaluated by clinicians. It has been estimated that in the United States there are 211 million to 375 million episodes per year, which leads to more than 900,000 hospitalizations and 6000 deaths. Worldwide, diarrheal illnesses are an even larger problem.

Although most otherwise healthy people suffer a self-limited illness lasting only a few days, others can experience chronic symptoms, bacteremia and metastatic infections, dehydration, and serious sequelae. It is important to identify those individuals who require treatment early in their clinical course to limit morbidity and mortality. This chapter reviews both host and pathogen factors that lead to illness; presents a clinical and laboratory approach to making the diagnosis; discusses common bacterial, viral, and parasitic pathogens; and summarizes treatment and prevention strategies.

GENERAL CONCEPTS IN EVALUATING GASTROINTESTINAL INFECTIONS AND FOOD POISONING

The first step in evaluating an individual presenting with acute diarrheal illness is the history and physical examination. A careful history gives clues leading to the appropriate laboratory workup to give a diagnosis. Because most infections are acquired by ingesting the offending organism, a careful dietary history may point to a diagnosis. History should include other individuals in contact with the patient who have also become ill. Recent travel history is also important, in that travelers to underdeveloped areas are at risk for various types of infections. Other recreational activities, including hiking or backpacking and even swimming in public pools, have also been associated with outbreaks of infectious diarrhea. These are the major points to consider when evaluating a patient with gastrointestinal disease.

Other key questions:

- **Does the patient have a history of previous gastrointestinal symptoms?** A positive history may suggest other illnesses, such as inflammatory bowel disease or irritable bowel syndrome, rather than an infectious cause.
- **Does the patient have an underlying illness?** For example, patients with acquired immunedeficiency syndrome (AIDS) or who are immunosuppressed due to chemotherapy or organ transplantation are at risk for organisms not routinely considered as pathogens in otherwise healthy individuals.
- **Is the patient taking any medications?** Some medications (e.g., several common antidepressant medications, medications for human immunodeficiency virus) are known to cause gastrointestinal side effects. A recent history of antibiotic use may also suggest an infection with *Clostridium difficile*.

The differential diagnosis of acute diarrheal illness is among the broadest in medicine. A variety of viral, bacterial, and parasitic pathogens may be involved. Preformed toxins may be the cause of diarrhea; there are numerous noninfectious causes for both acute and chronic diarrhea as well. Evaluating all patients for all possible causes of diarrhea would be prohibitively expensive, so clinical clues must play a role in guiding the most efficient workup. It is the role of the physician to determine the most appropriate workup and therefore limit not only morbidity and mortality for the patient, but also secondary transmission of the infection. The role of the microbiologist is no easier: It can be extremely difficult to recover and isolate the pathogen from the usual colonizing bacteria.

ANATOMIC CONSIDERATIONS

Although there are exceptions, diarrheal pathogens are usually acquired by ingesting a contaminated food or beverage. Figure 34-1 is a diagram of the gastrointestinal tract; there are host defenses against infection at many levels. When the microorganisms enter the stomach, they are usually exposed to a very acidic environment resulting in a substantial reduction in the number of bacteria that reaches the more distal gastrointestinal tract. Some pathogens are resistant to the action of gastric acids, most notably the cyst phase of some parasites and some bacterial spores.

The small intestine has a different mechanism to prevent infection. It is constantly in motion (peristalsis). Organisms that rely on adhering to the intestinal wall in order to cause infection may be hampered by the peristaltic movements. The colon also has defense mechanisms. Antibody, primarily immunoglobulin A (IgA), is produced locally, which may have some effect against pathogenic organisms. There is also an enormous number of other bacteria already living in the colon (the host's normal gut flora)—an estimated 1012 organisms of normal biota per gram of fecal material. Most of these are anaerobic bacteria, which outnumber the facultative aerobic bacteria by a factor of 1000:1. Table 34-1 lists the microorganisms frequently found in the large intestine. These established organisms compete with possible pathogens for nutrients as well as places to attach to the colon wall. The normal host flora can also, in some cases, produce substances toxic to potential pathogens. Several factors determine the risk of being infected with a gastrointestinal pathogen. The first factor is the number of ingested organisms, which is typically estimated by the **median infectious dose (ID_{50}),** the number of organisms that must be ingested to cause a diarrheal illness in 50% of exposed individuals. Even with the best defenses, if an overwhelming number of organisms are ingested, disease can occur. The second factor relates to host defenses. Patients with inadequate stomach acidity (**achlorhydria**: absence of hydrochloric acid in gastric secretions [normal

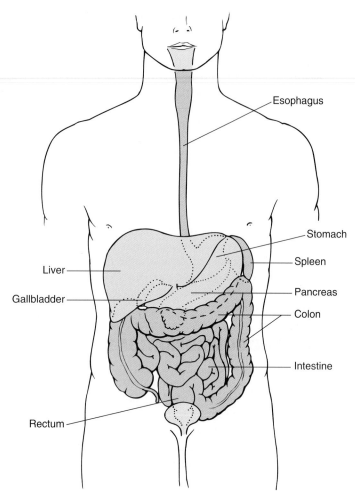

FIGURE 34-1 Anatomy of the gastrointestinal tract.

TABLE 34-1 Microbial Flora Found in the Large Intestine

Bacterial Species*	Incidence (%)
Strict anaerobes	
Gram-negative	
Bacteroides fragilis	100
Bacteroides spp.	100
Fusobacterium spp.	100
Gram-positive	
Lactobacilli	20-60
Clostridium perfringens	25-35
Clostridium spp.	1-35
Peptostreptococcus spp.	Common
Peptococcus spp.	Common
Facultative anaerobes	
Gram-positive cocci	
Staphylococcus aureus	30-50
Enterococcus spp.	100
β-Hemolytic streptococci, groups B, C, F, and G	0-16
Gram-negative bacilli (Enterobacteriaceae)	
Escherichia coli	100
Klebsiella spp.	40-80
Enterobacter spp.	5-55
Proteus spp.	3-11
Salmonella enteritidis (1400 serotypes)	3-7
Shigella, groups A–D	0-1
Pseudomonas aeruginosa	3-11
Candida albicans	15-30

Modified from Sommers HM: The indigenous microbiota of the human host. In Youmans GP, Paterson PY, Sommers HM, editors: *The biologic and clinical basis of infectious diseases*, ed 2, Philadelphia, 1980, Saunders.
*Strict anaerobes are present in ratio of 1000:1 with facultative aerobes.

pH is 1.6]), whether primary or as a result of medications (e.g., proton-pump inhibitors, which can dramatically alter gastric pH), are more likely than individuals with normal gastric acidity to become ill. Recent antibiotic exposure can also alter the normal biota of the colon, perhaps also predisposing to infection with an enteric pathogen.

A PRACTICAL APPROACH TO DIAGNOSIS OF THE PATIENT WITH DIARRHEA

A differential diagnosis for diarrhea can usually be determined on the basis of clinical history, physical examination findings, and examination of a stool specimen. Table 34-2 summarizes some of the common pathogens involved in diarrhea and the relative frequency of fever, nausea and vomiting, bloody diarrhea, and fecal evidence of inflammation.

History

Recent food ingestion, travel, recreational activities and exposure to other sick individuals are particularly important elements in the history of a patient with diarrhea. Travel to countries with less effective sewage facilities increases the risk of acquiring an enteric pathogen. **Traveler's diarrhea** is most commonly caused by enterotoxigenic *Escherichia coli*. This disease has a short incubation period (usually less than 24 hours) and normally lasts between 1 and 3 days. If a diarrheal illness lasts longer or develops in the days or weeks after a traveler returns home, then the patient more likely has a different pathogen. In this case, a parasitic infection, such as *Giardia lamblia* or *Entamoeba histolytica*, would be much more likely. Consider the patient in the Case in Point. An important aspect of the patient's case history is travel outside the United States and the timing of the diarrhea onset. Later, history of food consumed by the patient will help determine the cause of the illness.

Because most diarrheal pathogens are acquired by ingesting a contaminated food or beverage, a detailed food history extending at least 3 days before onset of symptoms is helpful. Water, unpasteurized milk, poultry, beef, and shellfish are often involved in infection. Table 34-3 lists foods that are commonly implicated in infectious diarrhea and the organisms that are often involved. The duration of the illness can also be helpful in narrowing the differential diagnosis. Patients with an invasive bacterial pathogen and bloody stools usually present much earlier than a patient with *Giardia* or other parasitic infections. Some patients with toxin-mediated illness may either present very early in the course of symp-

TABLE 34-2 Common Pathogens Involved in Diarrhea

Pathogen	Fever	Nausea/Vomiting	Bloody Stool	Fecal Inflammation
Campylobacter spp.	Common	Occurs	Occurs	Common
Salmonella spp.	Common	Occurs	Occurs	Common
Shigella spp.	Common	Common	Occurs	Common
Enterohemorrhagic *Escherichia coli*	Atypical	Occurs	Common	Often not found
Clostridium difficile	Occurs	Not characteristic	Occurs	Common
Yersinia enterocolitica	Common	Occurs	Occurs	Occurs
Entamoeba histolytica	Occurs	Variable	Variable	Variable
Cryptosporidium spp.	Variable	Occurs	Not characteristic	None to mild
Cyclospora	Variable	Occurs	Not characteristic	Not characteristic
Giardia lamblia	Not characteristic	Occurs	Not characteristic	Not characteristic
Viruses	Variable	Common	Not characteristic	Not characteristic

Modified from Thielman NM, Guerrant RL: Clinical practice. Acute infectious diarrhea, *N Engl J Med* 350:38, 2004.

TABLE 34-3 Common Food Vehicles for Specific Pathogens or Toxins

Vehicle	Pathogen or Toxin
Undercooked chicken	*Salmonella* spp., *Campylobacter* spp.
Eggs	*Salmonella* spp. (especially *S. enteritidis*)
Unpasteurized milk	*Salmonella*, *Campylobacter* spp., and *Yersinia* spp.
Water	*Giardia lamblia*, **Noroviruses,** *Campylobacter* spp., *Cryptosporidium* spp., *Cyclospora*
Fried rice	*Bacillus cereus*
Fish	
Shellfish	*Vibrio cholerae, V. para-haemolyticus, V. vulnificus,* other Vibrio spp., neurotoxic shellfish poisoning, paralytic shellfish poisoning, Norwalk virus
Tuna, mackerel, mahi-mahi	Scombroid poisoning
Grouper, amberjack, snapper	Ciguatera
Sushi	*Anisakis* spp.
Beef, gravy	*Salmonella* spp., *Campylobacter* spp., *Clostridium perfringens*

Modified from Goodman LJ: Diagnosis, management, and prevention of diarrheal diseases, *Curr Opin Infect Dis* 6:88, 1993.

toms or never present to a clinician at all because of the relatively brief course of these illnesses. Medications that the patient is currently taking are important in the history of diarrheal illness. One of the most common side effects from almost any prescription medication is gastrointestinal upset. If the patient is currently taking or has recently completed taking antibiotics, then *C. difficile* would be an important consideration.

The patient should also be asked about other medical conditions because diarrhea can be from noninfectious causes, such as inflammatory bowel disease or radiation therapy. If the patient is immunosuppressed from AIDS, chemotherapy, organ transplantation, or other medical reasons, pathogens that would not normally be considered may be a cause of diarrhea.

Physical Examination

The first step in the physical examination of a patient with a diarrheal illness is to determine the patient's state of hydration, because dehydration is the most common cause of death in patients with diarrhea. Several signs on physical examination point toward dehydration; for instance, the patient may

have a sunken appearance to the eyes, dry oral membranes, and a loss of skin resiliency known as *skin tenting.* This is best tested by gently pinching the skin on the back of the hand or over the sternum. In a dehydrated patient, the skin remains in a pinched or "tented" position. Patients may also have a decrease in blood pressure or an increase in heart rate upon moving from a supine to a seated or standing position **(orthostatic changes).** If the dehydration is severe enough, the patient may have changes in mental status or dysfunction of other organ systems (e.g., kidney failure). If the patient has a fever, it may be a clue that the patient is infected with an invasive pathogen.

Examination of the abdomen may also help lead to a diagnosis. Frequently, the abdomen is diffusely tender. Examination with a stethoscope reveals that bowel sounds are present, sometimes hyperactive in quality. If the pain is localized to only one part of the abdomen, if there is severe pain on palpation of the abdomen, or if bowel sounds are absent, the patient should be evaluated for complications of diarrheal infection (e.g., **toxic megacolon,** intestinal perforation) or a different disease process such as appendicitis, pancreatitis, or ovarian torsion.

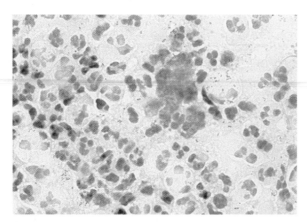

FIGURE 34-2 Gram stain of a direct fecal smear to show the presence of white blood cells, indicative of an invasive process and not an enterotoxin.

Laboratory Studies

Evaluation of the patient's peripheral blood count may reveal a leukocytosis in invasive infections. Anemia may be present in cases of severe gastrointestinal blood loss or a hemolytic infection. Thrombocytopenia (low platelet count) may be present in some infections. Evaluation of the patient's blood chemistries can show electrolyte abnormalities from the diarrhea and is a good indicator of the hydration status of the patient. Examination of the stool for red blood cells and evidence of inflammation (either white blood cells in the stool called **fecal leukocytes** [Figure 34-2] or fecal lactoferrin testing [a neutrophil marker that is associated with inflammation]) may help differentiate those patients who have invasive disease and those patients suffering from toxin-mediated illnesses, viral illnesses, or parasitic infections. For example, the patient in the Case in Point produced stool that contained no blood, pus, or mucus. In addition, the patient was afebrile. The absence of fever and cellular materials is indicative of a toxin-mediated illness.

CLINICAL PRESENTATIONS AND PATHOGENIC MECHANISMS OF ACUTE DIARRHEA

On the basis of history, physical examination, and preliminary laboratory findings, the clinician should be able to shorten the list of potential pathogens. The workup of the patient can then be completed in conjunction with the microbiologist to determine appropriate methods of diagnosis.

There are many ways to work up the etiology of acute diarrhea. Taking a careful history using the questions mentioned earlier can help formulate a differential of expected pathogens. This alone may shorten the likely differential to a small group of pathogens. Another classic approach is to categorize acute diarrhea by pathogenic mechanisms. Based on certain signs/symptoms and stool sampling, diarrhea can be characterized as enterotoxin-mediated or invasive. Although there may be significant overlap between these groups, a division such as this is useful as an initial diagnostic approach.

Enterotoxin-Mediated Diarrhea

Case Study

A 25-year-old woman recently attended a picnic gathering at a family reunion. A few hours after returning home, she experienced the sudden onset of vomiting and frequent diarrhea with abdominal cramping. She denied any fever. She felt lightheaded when standing and had a rapid heart rate (130 beats/minute). The stool was watery without any pus or gross blood. Her symptoms resolved the following day. It is determined that several other family members who attended the reunion developed similar symptoms.

The lack of fever and absence of blood or pus in the stool points toward an enterotoxin-mediated illness. The bacteria associated with enterotoxin production do not invade the gut wall, and the toxin does not elicit an inflammatory response, so microscopic examination of the stool does not reveal any red or white blood cells. Because there is no systemic inflammatory response, patients usually do not have a fever.

In the Case Study, the patient's symptomatic lightheadedness, coupled with rapid heart rate, suggests significant volume depletion. Initial treatment should be aimed at rehydrating the patient, either through drinking fluids if tolerated or with intravenous fluids.

The rapid onset of symptoms after food ingestion suggests that the illness in this case is enterotoxin-mediated. The preformed toxin is usually present in the contaminated food and is then ingested by the patient, leading to the symptoms. Because toxin may already be present and can act fairly proximally in the bowel (the small intestine), incubation period is relatively short, usually less than 12 hours. When patients present to a physician, they usually report an illness that started either the day of, or the day before, presentation. They typically have a large number (sometimes more than 20 per day) of nonbloody, watery stools and frequently have vomiting and abdominal cramping, particularly during defecation. Stool examination will be negative for red and white blood cells. There are several causative organisms for classic **enterotoxin-mediated diarrhea**. Enterotoxigenic *E. coli* accounts for the largest percentage of cases of diarrhea in travelers to underdeveloped areas. Other organisms responsible for enterotoxin-mediated disease are *Vibrio cholerae, Staphylococcus aureus, Clostridium perfringens,* and *Bacillus cereus.* When *S. aureus* is the culprit, the source of infection can often be traced to food handlers with small, localized abscesses in the nailbeds known as *paronychias.* There can be similar clinical syndromes from some other bacterial pathogens (e.g., *Plesiomonas, Aeromonas*), or viral gastroenteritis. Noninvasive parasitic infections such as giardiasis, cryptosporidiosis, or infection with *Isospora belli* can also produce an afebrile diarrhea with a negative microscopic stool examination. However, patients with these infections typically have fewer stools per day than those infected with enterotoxin-mediated disease, and they usually have more prolonged illnesses.

Diarrhea Mediated by Invasion of the Bowel Mucosal Surface

Case Study

A 56-year-old man was being treated with clindamycin for a skin infection. After 4 days of the antibiotics, he developed a fever and about 15 episodes of diarrhea per day. A peripheral blood count revealed a new leukocytosis. Stool examination revealed fecal white blood cells as well as the presence of *Clostridium difficile* toxin. The patient was treated with oral metronidazole with resolution of symptoms.

As opposed to the enterotoxin-mediated illnesses mentioned previously, organisms that invade the bowel mucosal surface cause an inflammatory response. This is manifested by the presence of fecal leukocytes and may cause fever and leukocytosis in peripheral blood. The most common organisms that fall into this category are *Salmonella* spp., *Campylobacter* spp., *Shigella* spp., some *E. coli,* and *Entamoeba histolytica.*

These organisms exert their effects in the colon, usually affecting the mucosal surface of the bowel wall. Although possible, deeper invasion of the bowel wall and extension to regional lymph nodes is unusual. Because the organisms (except *C. difficile*) must pass through the stomach and small intestine, begin multiplication in the colon, and then invade the mucosal surface, the incubation period (usually 1 to 3 days) for illness is usually longer than with enterotoxin-mediated illness. Microscopic examination of the stool of patients with diarrhea from invasion of the bowel mucosal surface frequently reveals both red and white blood cells. Because these infections usually involve only the superficial mucosal surface, patients usually do not present with bacteremia or metastatic infection. Patients with bowel mucosal invasion are also the most likely of those with diarrheal infections to present with true dysentery syndrome, characterized by gross blood and pus in the stool. Enterohemorrhagic *E. coli* infections can also cause gross blood in the stool, but systemic fever and fecal white blood cells are less common than with the other pathogens in this group. *E. histolytica* causes a clinical syndrome similar to the bacterial pathogens in this group, although the incubation period is usually much longer (ranging from 1 to 3 weeks).

Diarrhea Mediated by Invasion of Full Bowel Thickness with Lymphatic Spread

Case Study

A 30-year-old woman returning from South America presented with high temperature. Laboratory studies showed a mild anemia, low platelet count, and mild neutropenia. Blood cultures were sent to the laboratory. In the next week, the patient developed a watery diarrhea, and stool cultures were sent to the laboratory. Both stool and blood cultures were positive for *Salmonella typhi.* The patient was treated with ciprofloxacin with improvement in symptoms after several days.

The most common invasive enteric organisms are *Salmonella typhi* and *Yersinia enterocolitica.* Incubation period, similar to the organisms that invade only the mucosal surface, is about 1 to 3 days. These organisms can invade through the bowel wall, cause bacteremia, and cause a mesenteric lymphadenitis that may be confused with appendicitis. Diarrhea is often not the presenting symptom, and patients may actually have constipation at the onset of illness. Stool examination often reveals both red and white blood cells, and gross blood can sometimes be present (about 25% of patients with *Y. enterocolitica* infection). *S. typhi* infections may also cause a chronic carrier state in affected patients, leading to spread of the infection to others (e.g., "Typhoid Mary").

COMMON VIRAL, BACTERIAL, AND PARASITIC PATHOGENS

The number of possible agents involved in diarrheal illness can make diagnostic testing challenging. In addition to the known agents as causes of illness, other agents continue to be implicated as causes of diarrheal disease (e.g., *Cyclospora cayetanensis* and new species of *Helicobacter*). This section identifies some of the major known viral, bacterial, and parasitic causes of infectious diarrhea.

Viral Pathogens

Case Study

A 2-year-old boy who attends daycare developed vomiting and diarrhea. He had a low-grade fever of 100.0° F (37.8° C). When the parents questioned the daycare employees, they learned that several of the other daycare children also had similar symptoms, and several children had been absent from the daycare due to illness. Stool examination from the patient did not reveal any fecal leukocytes. The child was encouraged to drink copious fluids, and his symptoms resolved after a few days.

Viruses were suspected to be a cause of gastroenteritis since the 1940s, but no pathogen was identified in feces of ill individuals until 1972. Since then, the number of identified viral pathogens has steadily increased. Viruses pose a challenge to the microbiologist for diagnostic workup. The viruses are far too small to see with a conventional light microscope, so secondary tests are needed for evaluation. These include culture in various cell lines, monoclonal antibody testing, use of electron microscopy, antigen detection, and molecular biology techniques including polymerase chain reaction (PCR) amplification of the viral genome. However, many of these techniques are not readily available or are extremely cumbersome to use, so there is often no firm diagnosis as to the causative agent of viral gastroenteritis. The viruses characterized in the following sections are but a few of the total number of viruses associated with gastrointestinal illness.

Rotaviruses

Members of the Reoviridae family, **rotaviruses** are nonenveloped and have a 70-nm-diameter icosahedral structure. They are classified into groups, subgroups, and serotypes based on the antigens of the capsid proteins. These viruses infect cells of the villi of the small intestine, leading to epithelial atrophy and proliferation of cells with secretory capacity. This may decrease the absorptive capacity of the bowel, contributing to diarrhea. The enteric nervous system is also stimulated by infection, increasing diarrhea by increasing the amount of intestinal water and electrolytes. Rotaviruses are the major cause of diarrhea in children younger than 5 years of age, causing an estimated 130 million episodes of illness worldwide each year.

Enteric Adenoviruses

Adenoviruses, members of the Adenoviridae family, are non-enveloped, 70-nm viruses with icosahedric symmetry. Adenoviruses have been implicated in many illnesses ranging from the common cold and epidemic keratoconjunctivitis (pink eye) to infectious diarrhea. Two adenovirus serotypes, 40 and 41, are most frequently associated with infectious diarrhea. It is thought that diarrhea results from a similar mechanism as that of the rotavirus. These agents are thought to be the cause of 1% to 8% of cases of diarrhea in the developed world.

Calciviruses

Members of the Calciviridae family, the calciviruses are characterized by 32 cup-shaped depressions along the surface. There are two genus associated with gastrointestinal disease: the noroviruses (formerly Norwalk-like virus), and the sapovirus (formerly Sapporo-like viruses). The noroviruses are named after the original strain Norwalk virus, which was first isolated in patients from a town with that name in Ohio in 1968. These viruses cause an acute, self-limited diarrheal illness associated with vomiting and low-grade fever. This disease is highly contagious and is transmitted by the fecal-oral route, by fecally contaminated food or water, by environmental fomites, and person-to-person. There is also evidence to suggest that this agent could be transmitted by aerosolization of vomitus. Recent outbreaks have been reported aboard cruise ships.

Astroviruses

These viruses express different morphologies depending on the pH of the media to which they are exposed. The original characterization as a small, 28-nm virus that appears as a five- or six-pointed star is the morphology at alkaline pH; the virus has a 41-nm icosahedric appearance with defined spikes at other pH values. The cause of diarrhea from these agents is not yet certain, but animal studies suggest that an osmotic diarrhea may develop from inflammatory infiltrates in the lamina propria and intestinal villus atrophy. These agents usually cause infection in the elderly or the very young.

Bacterial Pathogens

Case Study

A 30-year-old man hosted a barbecue for a football weekend at which he served chicken. On the Tuesday following the event, the patient and several other people who attended the barbecue developed fever and diarrhea. Stool studies from the patient revealed red blood cells and fecal leukocytes as well as numerous curved, gram-negative rods. After several days, both the patient and other attendees recovered without complications.

Bacterial agents are a common cause of infectious diarrhea. Several agents are known to cause infectious diarrhea with mechanisms of illness that range from toxin production (either preformed in the food or produced in the intestine) to mucosal invasion. Antibiotics are often used for the treatment of some of these illnesses. The microbiologist has an important role in isolating these organisms to lead to a diagnosis.

Campylobacter jejuni

Various *Campylobacter* species have been isolated as a cause of diarrhea, and *Campylobacter jejuni* is the most common bacterial cause of gastroenteritis in the world. For most cases, antibiotics are not necessary. Possibly because of the widespread use of antibiotics, these organisms are developing significant resistance to the most commonly used class of antibiotics for diarrheal illnesses, the fluoroquinolones. There can be serious sequelae to *C. jejuni* infections; for example, rarely, Guillain-Barré syndrome may result (about 1 in 1000 cases) from infection. There can also be resultant reactive arthritis.

Infection with this organism usually results in a self-limited disease characterized by fever, abdominal cramping, and diarrhea. The incubation period is normally 2 to 5 days, but in some cases has extended up to 10 days. Diarrhea is often preceded by a period of febrile malaise with myalgias and abdominal pain. Stools may have gross blood and pus present. It is also frequently possible to identify the organism on direct Gram stain of stool. The diarrhea usually lasts 2 to 3 days, but abdominal discomfort can last for several days after resolution of the diarrhea. The pathogen can usually continue to be cultured from stools for several weeks after the illness has subsided. The environmental reservoir of *Campylobacter* includes both wild and domestic animals, and most frequently birds. This is usually a food-borne infection, often with poultry as the source. Other outbreaks have been traced to contaminated meat, contaminated water, and unpasteurized milk. Although there is prolonged fecal shedding of the organism, there is little person-to-person transmission of the infection. If antibiotics are to be used for infection (in the cases of the immunocompromised patient or severe or prolonged illness), a macrolide antibiotic is frequently used due to the emerging rates of fluoroquinolone resistance. Because domesticated poultry are almost universally colonized with these bacteria, efforts in prevention have been aimed at reducing antibiotic resistance and transmission of the disease to humans. Because the organism is heat-sensitive, thorough cooking of meat and poultry is effective at preventing human infection. There have also been efforts at decreasing the amount of antibiotics given to domesticated poultry in an effort to limit the rate of fluoroquinolone resistance. Although food irradiation may be effective in decreasing the amount of bacteria present in uncooked food, this process has been met with public apprehension in many areas.

Salmonella Species

Gastroenteritis and Food Poisoning. Nontyphoidal *Salmonella* spp. can lead to gastroenteritis through ingestion of contaminated meat, poultry, eggs, and dairy products, as well as aquaculture-farmed fish and shellfish. There is a wide variety of nontyphoidal *Salmonella* serotypes in animal hosts, most notably birds and reptiles.

Symptoms usually start between 6 and 48 hours after ingestion of contaminated foods and consist of nausea, vomiting, and diarrhea. Patients may also develop fever, headaches, and myalgias. The illness is usually self-limited and normally resolves within a few days. Antibiotics are not generally recommended in most cases, because they do not shorten the course of the illness and they can prolong the time period of pathogen shedding in the stool, placing other persons at risk of contracting disease.

Enteric Fever. *Salmonella typhi* causes the most severe form of **enteric fever**—typhoid fever. Unlike the other serotypes of *Salmonella* mentioned previously, humans are the only known host for this pathogen. The infection is normally spread through fecally contaminated food or water, and many fewer organisms are required to establish an infection.

In the initial stages of infection, the pathogens invade the small and large bowel walls, creating an inflammatory response, but there is no initial diarrhea (many patients may actually have constipation). The invading bacteria are ingested by host immune cells (monocytes), but are resistant to the cell's normal mechanisms of killing bacterial pathogens. The bacteria survive in the host immune cells, and are therefore called *intracellular pathogens*. The bacteria are transported to regional lymphatic tissue and the bloodstream, spreading throughout the body. Unlike the other enteric pathogens, the initial symptoms of infection are headache, fever, general malaise, and sometimes abdominal tenderness. Once the organism has spread throughout the body, it reaches the gallbladder and Peyer patches in the colon; infection of these areas can cause the diarrheal stage of the illness. The organism can frequently be recovered from both blood and stool cultures. Appropriate antibiotic use results in clinical improvement; however, stool cultures often remain positive, which can serve as a source of infection for other individuals. Some patients can also develop chronic colonization of their gallbladder and biliary tree, leading to persistent shedding of the organism and infections in many other people (the classic "Typhoid Mary" case).

Shigella Species

Very closely related to *Escherichia* spp., the *Shigella* species can be responsible for a diarrheal illness characterized by both gross blood and pus. There are four *Shigella* spp. recognized: *S. sonnei* (the most common in the United States), *S. flexneri*, *S. dysenteriae*, and *S. boydii*. Because the ID_{50} of this organism is very low (possibly less than 100 organisms), it is among the most easily communicable bacterial diarrhea pathogens. Invasion into the intestinal mucosa leads to ulceration and a marked inflammatory response; the organism usually does not invade past the mucosa or disseminate into the bloodstream. The bacteria produce several toxins, one of which is the shiga toxin, which can have cytotoxic, enterotoxic, and neurotoxic effects.

The incubation period for disease can range from 1 day to 1 week, but most patients have symptoms develop within 12 to 50 hours after exposure. Initial symptoms are fever, malaise, fatigue, and anorexia. A watery diarrhea with abdominal cramping and tenesmus then develops, which may progress to having gross blood and pus in the stool. Although the disease is often self-limited, antibiotics can hasten clinical improvement. Because there is increasing resistance to various antibiotic classes, however, fluoroquinolones are used as initial empirical therapy when antibiotics are required.

Escherichia coli

Although this species is a normal inhabitant of the human gastrointestinal tract, five different groups of *E. coli* have been associated with disease (Table 34-4).

Enterotoxigenic *Escherichia coli*. Enterotoxigenic *E. coli* (ETEC) produce both adhesins to bind to intestinal mucosa and enterotoxins, which are either heat-stable (ST) or heat-labile (LT) and are responsible for the diarrhea. LT toxin is similar to *V. cholerae* toxin (discussed next). ST toxin binds to guanylate cyclase, leading to increased intracellular cGMP levels and active efflux of water and electrolytes from the

TABLE 34-4 Diarrheagenic *Escherichia coli*

Group	Major Virulence Factors	Reported Food Sources
ETEC	Adhesins LT and ST toxins	Fresh fruits and vegetables, scallops, tuna paste, soft cheeses
EIEC	Invasion proteins	Cheese, guacamole
EHEC	Intimin (adherence to intestinal mucosa) Shiga toxins	Undercooked beef, sausage, chicken, lunch meats, deer jerky, lettuce, radishes, alfalfa sprouts, potatoes, milk, apple juice, cider, cheese curds
EPEC	Intimin (adherence to intestinal mucosa) Bundle-forming pili Surface-associated filaments Translocated intimin receptor	Fresh fruits and vegetables, likely infant formula
EAEC	Aggregative adherence fimbriae Dispersin Plasmid-encoded toxin	Likely food-borne, possibly fruits and vegetables, other food sources uncertain

ETEC, Enterotoxigenic *E. coli*; *LT*, heat-labile; *ST*, heat-stable; *EIEC*, enteroinvasive *E. coli*; *EHEC*, enterohemorrhagic *E. coli*; *EPEC*, enteropathogenic *E. coli*; *EAEC*, enteroaggregative *E. coli*.

intestinal cells. Clinically, patients have a watery diarrhea that lacks red blood cells and fecal leukocytes. This is a common cause of traveler's diarrhea.

Enteroinvasive *Escherichia coli*. Enteroinvasive *E. coli* (EIEC) produce an infection similar to *Shigella*. Patients usually first develop a watery stool similar to that produced by ETEC. Some patients then progress to an invasive-type diarrheal syndrome with fever, abdominal cramping, and bloody stools. Fecal leukocytes are abundant.

Enterohemorrhagic *Escherichia coli*. Enterohemorrhagic *E. coli* (EHEC) usually start as a watery diarrhea. However, over the next day or two, abdominal pain increases and stools become bloody. Stool may contain some fecal leukocytes, so there may be some confusion between this infection and EIEC or *Shigella*. Although the disease is usually self-limited, patients can develop *hemolytic-uremic syndrome* (HUS), characterized by hemolytic anemia, low platelet count, and kidney failure. The *E. coli* strain O157:H7, among others, falls into this category. It is uncertain whether antibiotic therapy will decrease the probability of developing HUS, and there is some concern that subtherapeutic antibiotic dosing may actually increase the risk of developing HUS by stimulating bacterial toxin production.

Enteropathogenic *Escherichia coli*. Enteropathogenic *E. coli* (EPEC) are also referred to as the enteroadherent *E. coli* in some classification schemes. Although the mechanism of diarrhea is not completely understood, it seems that the organisms express various factors allowing adherence to the intestinal cells. This causes disruption and destruction of the brush border of the cells and other intestinal cell derangements, reducing the absorptive capacity of the cells and leading to electrolyte abnormalities and diarrhea. These organisms can commonly affect children in nurseries and daycare centers; patients often have low-grade fever, vomiting, and diarrhea, which may contain a great deal of mucus.

Enteroaggregative *Escherichia coli*. Enteroaggregative *E. coli* (EAEC) also adhere to the intestinal surface, like the EPEC, but in a more clumped or aggregative fashion. An emerging pathogen, these organisms apparently first adhere to the intestinal wall via various adhesive molecules, cause an increase in the production of mucus, and then induce an inflammatory response by host cytokine release. These organisms are being increasingly recognized as a cause of traveler's diarrhea. Infections with these organisms can range from asymptomatic to a chronic, watery diarrhea.

Vibrio Species

Vibrio species are curved, gram-negative rods, similar in appearance to *Campylobacter*. These organisms are usually found in water environments and are therefore a risk for contaminating fish and shellfish.

Although there are many species of *Vibrio* implicated in human disease, one of the best known is *V. cholerae*, the causative agent of **cholera.** This organism creates a well-studied enterotoxin that consists of two subunits (a core "A" subunit surrounded by five "B" subunits). The B subunits permit attachment to the small bowel mucosa; the A subunit then enters the cell. Once in the cell, through various enzymatic effects, the toxin results in an increase in the amount of cyclic adenosine monophosphate (cAMP), which causes the cell to secrete large amounts of water and electrolytes. This increased secretion causes the "rice-water stools" characteristic of cholera. Many liters of stool per day can be produced, and patients without adequate medical care are at risk of death from dehydration. Although the quantity of diarrhea can be impressive, it is toxin-mediated and noninflammatory, so the stools are free of red and white blood cells. There are many serogroups (serovars) of *V. cholerae;* serogroups O1 and O139 have been implicated as causes of epidemic cholera. The other serogroups can also cause illness but have not been associated with the epidemic form of the disease. Two other *Vibrio* species that can cause illness are *V. parahaemolyticus* and *V. vulnificus*, although other species have been implicated as well. *V. parahaemolyticus* is the most common *Vibrio* species responsible for disease in the United States and is fairly common worldwide. Patients with this infection, unlike those with classic cholera, can have fever and evidence of fecal inflammation, suggesting that there is some potential for mucosal invasion. *V. vulnificus* is the most virulent of all noncholera vibrios, causing an often fulminant illness characterized by sepsis and bullous skin lesions in patients with a recent ingestion of shellfish (i.e., raw oysters). This *Vibrio* species is part of the marine flora, making it a common colonizer of a large percentage of oysters harvested in the warmer months. Compromised patients, particularly those with liver disease, are more susceptible to development of fulminant disease.

Yersinia enterocolitica

Related to the organism responsible for bubonic plague, *Yersinia enterocolitica*, a gram-negative bacillus, can produce gastroenteritis. Infections with this organism, which are more common in the winter months, have been linked to meat, unpasteurized milk, other dairy products, and chitterlings. Refrigeration does not prevent growth of this organism, because it can survive and grow at 4° C.

Patients can present with a self-limited enteritis consisting of fever, nausea, diarrhea, and abdominal pain or can develop a more invasive disease with spread of the organism to the mesenteric lymph nodes. This mesenteric lymphadenitis can be mistaken for appendicitis. Stool studies will show both red and white blood cells. Because the organism has the ability to invade and spread throughout the body, distant foci of infection and abscesses can also develop.

Clostridium difficile

First identified in 1935 as an anaerobic gram-positive spore- and toxin-producing organism, *C. difficile* was later observed to be a causative agent of antibiotic-associated diarrhea. *C. difficile*–associated disease (CDAD) was initially reported in patients receiving clindamycin; however, almost all classes of antibiotics have been linked to this infection.

The initial event in the pathogenesis of the disease is the antibiotic-induced disruption of the indigenous bacterial flora of the colon, which allows for the overgrowth of *C. difficile*. The organism produces two different exotoxins, toxin A and toxin B, that bind to surface epithelial cell receptors, leading to inflammation, mucosal injury, and diarrhea. The development of characteristic pseudomembranes, composed of neutrophils, fibrin, mucin, and cellular debris, in the colonic mucosa, is pathognomonic of CDAD. In mild cases, these pseudomembranes are usually absent.

Other important risk factors for asymptomatic colonization and infection with this bacterium include a recent hospitalization and residence in a long-term care facility. Cases of community-acquired disease unrelated to antimicrobial use have also been described. The organism is transmitted from person to person via the fecal-oral route and can easily be passed from a colonized patient to other patients in the hospital by health care personnel who do not observe proper hand hygiene. *C. difficile* has been cultured from inanimate hospital surfaces.

The clinical presentation of CDAD ranges from a mild watery diarrhea to a life-threatening toxic megacolon, which requires surgical intervention. Patients with severe disease often present with abdominal pain, leukocytosis, and fever, in addition to the diarrhea . A new epidemic and more virulent strain of *C. difficile* has been recently identified. This strain is typically resistant to fluoroquinolones and produces larger amounts of toxins, which causes a more aggressive form of the disease when compared to the non-epidemic strains.

Diagnosis of CDAD is often made on clinical grounds or by detecting the presence of *C. difficile* toxins in a stool sample. The finding of pseudomembranes during rectosigmoidoscopy is highly suggestive of the disease. Oral metronidazole or vancomycin remain the mainstay of therapy.

Listeria monocytogenes

A gram-positive, non–spore-forming facultative anaerobic bacillus, *L. monocytogenes* is best known for causing systemic disease, such as meningitis. However, several outbreaks of gastroenteritis have implicated this intracellular pathogen. Presence of this organism in an asymptomatic individual is not necessarily a cause for concern, because between 5% and 10% of healthy adults transiently carry *L. monocytogenes* in the bowel at any given time.

Helicobacter Species

Not thought to be a cause of diarrheal illness, *H. pylori* nonetheless is a significant cause of disease. Living in the stomach and duodenum, *H. pylori* (Figure 34-3) has been associated with ulcer disease. This infection is common, in that many patients have detectable antibody against this organism. When the organism is recovered from a gastric or duodenal ulcer, there is evidence that patients have faster, more durable ulcer recovery with antibiotic therapy. Active infection can be diagnosed by detecting the organism on an endoscopically derived biopsy specimen or through breath testing (Figure 34-4). This testing is based on the fact that the organism shows high urease activity; urea labeled with either ^{13}C or ^{14}C will, when ingested, rapidly produce labeled CO_2 in the patient's breath if the organism is present.

Other *Helicobacter* spp. (e.g., *H. cinaedi*, *H. fennelliae*) are thought to rarely play a role in diarrheal illnesses.

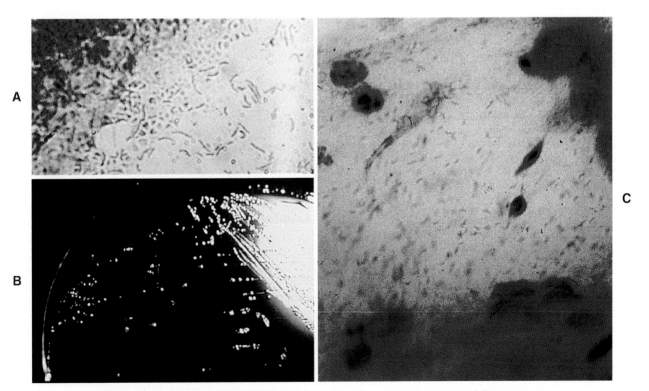

FIGURE 34-3 Microscopic morphology of *Helicobacter pylori* Gram-stained from a colony. **A,** Gram stain culture. **B,** Gray, translucent *H. pylori* colonies grown on agar culture medium. **C,** Gram stain on gastric mucus. (Courtesy American College of Gastroenterology and DiaSorin, Inc.)

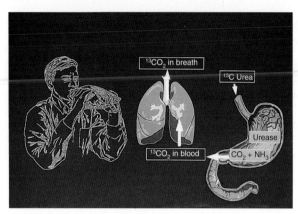

FIGURE 34-4 The urea breath test. (Courtesy American College of Gastroenterology and DiaSorin, Inc.)

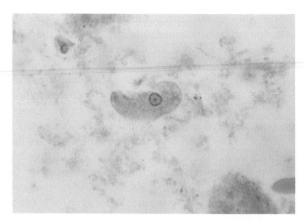

FIGURE 34-5 *Entamoeba histolytica* trophozoites.

Other Bacterial Pathogens

Aeromonas species and *Plesiomonas shigelloides*, related to *Vibrio*, have been associated with a watery diarrhea, although *Aeromonas* is much more likely to be involved in soft tissue infections. *Edwardsiella tarda*, associated with fish and shellfish, is a rare cause of gastroenteritis.

Organisms responsible for sexually transmitted diseases (STDs) can also cause gastrointestinal diseases. *Neisseria gonorrhoeae*, *Chlamydia trachomatis*, *Treponema pallidum* (the agent of syphilis), and herpes simplex virus (HSV) may all cause a proctitis with loose stools and pain on defecation, most frequently in patients infected through receptive anal intercourse. As these agents would not be routinely identified with standard culture techniques, the history obtained from the patient is key in screening for these pathogens.

Parasitic Pathogens

Case Study

A 21-year-old man recently spent 2 weeks backpacking through the Appalachian Mountains. One week after his return, he developed cramping abdominal pain, increased flatulence, and diarrhea. Otherwise, he felt well and had no other symptoms. Stool examination did not reveal any red blood cells or fecal leukocytes, but did show cysts consistent with *Giardia lamblia*, and antigen detection confirmed the diagnosis. He was successfully treated with metronidazole.

Parasitic infections account for a small percentage of diarrheal illnesses in the United States. They frequently have a longer incubation period than the bacterial and viral pathogens and have a longer clinical course, although the severity of the symptoms may be less. Examination of the stool for the pathogens is important in the diagnosis, although there are antigen detection methods for some of the parasites.

Giardia lamblia

The most commonly identified intestinal pathogen in the United States, *G. lamblia* is usually acquired by ingestion of contaminated water or person-to-person spread. As the organism lives well in mountain streams, campers and others

who engage in outdoor activities are at risk if they inadequately purify their water supply. After an incubation period of 1 to 2 weeks, patients can develop nausea, vomiting, flatulence, cramping, and diarrhea. As the organism is not invasive, the patients typically do not have fever or fecal leukocytes on examination. Examination of the stool can reveal a characteristic trophozoite or cyst; yield of duodenal aspirates (obtained either through endoscopy or string test) may be higher. Antigen detection tests are available.

Entamoeba histolytica

Amebiasis from *E. histolytica* (Figure 34-5) can cause both gastrointestinal and disseminated disease. Because of the potentially invasive nature of *E. histolytica*, when this organism causes gastrointestinal disease it may be characterized by fever and grossly bloody diarrhea. However, the range of illness is broad and may present only as a mild, watery diarrhea, complicating diagnosis. Both trophozoites and cysts may be identified in the stool, and antigen detection and serologic tests for diagnosis are also available. The organism is morphologically similar to the nonpathogenic *Entamoeba dispar*, also found in the intestinal tract, which has led to much confusion when calculating how frequently this organism is responsible for disease. The trophozoites of *E. histolytica* are able to leave the intestine and can cause metastatic illness, most frequently as a liver abscess.

Cryptosporidium parvum and hominis

In otherwise healthy individuals, cryptosporidial diarrheal illness, after a 1-week incubation period, can produce an illness characterized by abdominal cramping, watery diarrhea, vomiting, fever, and anorexia. Symptoms generally last about 10 days, and there may be recurrent symptoms after initial improvement. This organism is fairly resistant to chlorine, so public swimming pools can be a source of an outbreak. Other sources of exposure include fecally contaminated food or water, international produce, and person-to-person spread. Several outbreaks have been associated with potable water in developed countries. In developing countries, the most common manifestation is childhood diarrhea. Because this organism is acid-fast, stool specimens should be prepared with this staining technique for identification.

Cyclospora cayetanensis and *Isospora belli*

C. cayetanensis has been associated with outbreaks of diarrhea from contaminated water, food, and produce. Illness in the immunocompetent patient generally consists of an acute onset of watery diarrhea, which usually lasts for about 10 days. Patients also may have a prodromal syndrome of myalgias and arthralgias; other symptoms can include cramping, fever, profound fatigue, nausea, and vomiting. In healthy individuals, diarrheal disease from *I. belli* is similar to other parasitic infections. Most are self-limited and consist of watery diarrhea and abdominal cramps. In the United States most cases are seen in individuals who have traveled to highly endemic areas.

Microsporidia

Enterocytozoon bieneusi and *Encephalitozoon intestinalis* comprise the microsporidia. These pathogens can cause illness similar to *C. parvum* and *C. cayetanensis*. Disease can range from asymptomatic to a self-limited diarrhea disease in healthy individuals. This organism is an important cause of diarrhea in immunocompromised individuals, particularly in patients with AIDS. Special staining of stool specimens is needed to see these organisms under light microscopy. Occasionally, they will stain acid-fast positive.

Other Parasitic Infections

In addition to the protozoal parasitic infections mentioned earlier, there are many other organisms that can cause human disease, most of which are rare in the United States. Some of these organisms responsible for infection include *Ascaris lumbricoides* (common roundworm), *Strongyloides stercoralis*, *Ancylostoma* and *Necator* spp. (hookworms), *Trichuris trichiura* (whipworm), and *Enterobius vermicularis* (pinworm). Others include *Capillaria philippinensis*, which is most frequently found in Thailand, Iran, Egypt, and the Philippines, and *Trichinella spiralis*, which is obtained by eating poorly cooked pork. There have also been cases of *Anisakis* infection associated with eating contaminated sushi or sashimi. The parasitic organisms listed here are a sampling of the identified human parasites; a complete discussion of these organisms is beyond the scope of this chapter. For most organisms, examination of the stool for ova and parasites aids in the diagnosis.

DIARRHEA IN SPECIAL CIRCUMSTANCES

Toxic Agents of Food Poisoning

> **Case Study**
>
> A 32-year-old woman ate a fish dinner at a restaurant. Before she returned home from the restaurant, she began to feel warm. She developed a headache, abdominal cramping with some diarrhea, and was generally flushed. Symptoms continued for a few hours and then abated.

A food-borne outbreak is defined as the occurrence in multiple people of gastrointestinal or neurologic symptoms within 72 hours of a common meal. The most commonly identified bacterial agents involved in food-borne outbreaks are *Salmonella* spp., *C. jejuni*, *S. aureus*, *Clostridium botulinum*, and *C. perfringens*. *G. lamblia*, *Cryptosporidium*, and *Cyclospora* have also been associated with outbreaks, usually associated with a contaminated fruit, vegetable, or other food source. There have also been outbreaks of viral gastroenteritis, often associated with contaminated shellfish.

Chemical intoxications are often associated with fish exposure. The case mentioned is typical for **scombroid.** The syndrome, which consists of flushing, headache, and crampy abdominal pain with diarrhea, is due to ingesting contaminated fish (often tuna, mackerel, and yellow jack). The tissues of the fish contain histamine and enzyme inhibitors, which cause the symptoms. Symptom onset is rapid, usually within 1 hour of ingestion, and usually only lasts several hours. **Ciguatera** is due to ciguatoxin, produced by dinoflagellates. This toxin accumulates in fish as it passes up the food chain, and most cases of illness are associated with snapper, sea bass, grouper, or barracuda. The symptoms include diarrhea, abdominal pain, weakness, paresthesias, and headache. Symptoms often begin within 1 to 2 hours of eating the contaminated fish and may progress to respiratory failure and hypotension. Because no antitoxin exists, patients are treated supportively. Paralytic shellfish poisoning is associated with contaminated clams, mussels, and scallops. Usually occurring during the summer months, paralytic shellfish poisoning produces a syndrome similar to ciguatera. One of the deadliest toxins, tetrodotoxin, which can be found in the puffer fish, leads to mortality in more than half of patients exposed. The contaminated food appears normal in each of these cases of toxin-mediated food poisoning. Prevention is aimed at locating and removing sources of contaminated fish. Table 34-5 outlines several of the common food-borne organisms and characteristics of illness.

The Returning Traveler

Traveler's diarrhea is a common problem in patients visiting developing countries. Although most cases are often mild and self-limited, it can lead to significant morbidity and disrupt the traveler's itinerary. Traveler's diarrhea most often occurs within the first 2 weeks of travel onset. Symptoms vary by causative agent, but all are heralded by the presence of diarrhea. Other symptoms can include malaise, abdominal pain, fever, nausea and vomiting, and occasionally blood in the stool. The travel destination impacts one's risk of acquiring traveler's diarrhea. The Centers for Disease Control and Prevention (CDC) has classified the risk of developing the disease by geography, as can be seen in Figure 34-6. The destinations holding the highest risk for traveler's diarrhea include Asia, Africa (excluding South Africa), Central America, and Mexico. The infectious etiologies of traveler's diarrhea are broad, including many of the bacterial, viral and parasitic organisms already described. Most often the culprit is bacterial, with ETEC being the most common known cause. Other causes include EAEC, *Salmonella*, *C. jejuni*, and *Shigella* species. Rotaviruses are the most common viral pathogen. Parasitic infections are less commonly associated with typical traveler's diarrhea. However, travelers to certain areas are more at risk for such infections—for instance, travelers to

TABLE 34-5 Compendium of Common Food-Borne Diseases

Average Incubation Period	Organism	Average Duration	Implicated Foods	Typical Symptoms	Comments
2-16 hours	*Bacillus cereus*	1 day	Boiled and fried rice, meats, vegetables	Nausea, vomiting, (emetic) abdominal cramping, watery diarrhea	Produces two toxins; one emetic form that causes nausea and vomiting within hours, and one diarrheic form. Common year round. Isolation of large numbers from implicated foods and patient stool
6-72 hours	*Vibrio parahaemolyticus*	3 days	Shellfish	Pain, vomiting, fever, watery diarrhea	Blood sometimes in stool. Common spring, summer, fall in the coastal states. Stool culture using TCBS media is recommended
6-72 hours	*Vibrio cholerae*	3-7 days	Seafood, water	"Rice water" stools, severe diarrhea, no fever	No blood or mucus in stool, mechanism of action in vivo enterotoxin production. No tissue invasion. Stool culture using TCBS media is recommended
<8 hours	*Staphylococcus aureus*	<1 day	Egg salads, meat, poultry, pastries	Abrupt onset of nausea, pain and projectile vomiting, infrequent diarrhea	Mechanism of action is preformed enterotoxin in foods. Common in summer. ELISA or reverse passive latex agglutination enterotoxin test; gel electrophoresis in lieu of phage typing
8-22 hours	*Clostridium perfringens*	1 day	Beef, poultry, gravy, fish	Abdominal cramping, watery diarrhea; vomiting and fever uncommon	In vivo enterotoxin production; unlike *Staphylococcus aureus*, viable organisms must be ingested for disease to occur. Common in fall, winter, spring
12-48 hours	*Salmonella* spp.	3 days	Eggs, dairy products, fowl, beef	Fever, abdominal cramping, diarrhea, mild vomiting	WBCs in stool. Common in summer. Culture and serologic identification
16-48 hours	*Yersinia enterocolitica*	1 day to 4 weeks	Milk, pork	Fever, severe abdominal pain, diarrhea	WBCs and RBCs in stool. Common in winter
18-36 hours	*Clostridium botulinum*	Weeks-months	Vegetables, fruits (canned foods), fish, honey (infants)	Nausea, vomiting, diarrhea, paralysis	Mechanism of action is a preformed neurotoxin. Common in summer and fall
24-72 hours	*Shigella* spp.	3 days	Egg and tuna salads, lettuce, milk	Fever, abdominal cramping, diarrhea, occasional vomiting	WBCs, RBCs, and mucus in stools. Tissue invasion common mechanism of action. Common in summer. Culture and serologic identification
24-72 hours	Enterotoxigenic *Escherichia coli* (ETEC)	3 days	Fruits, meats, pastries, salads	Abdominal cramping, watery diarrhea, no vomiting or fever	In vivo enterotoxin, major cause of "traveler's diarrhea," year-round distribution, patient history includes travel to Mexico and other developing countries
24-72 hours	Enterohemorrhagic *E. coli* (EHEC)	3 days	Undercooked ground beef, cider	Watery diarrhea progressing to bloody diarrhea, abdominal cramping, no fever or vomiting	Implicated shiga-toxin producing *E. coli*, organisms disappear rapidly from stool. Culture of sorbitol-negative *E. coli* from stool using SMAC plate recommended

TCBS, Thiosulfate-citrate–bile salts–sucrose; *ELISA*, enzyme-linked immunosorbent assay; *WBCs*, white blood cells; *RBCs*, red blood cells; *SMAC*, Sorbitol-MacConkey.

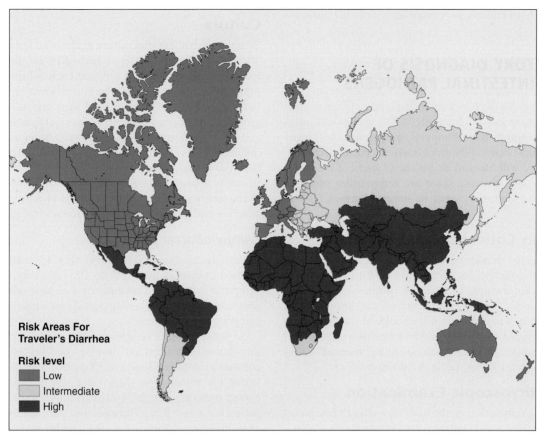

FIGURE 34-6   Geographic distribution of risk for traveler's diarrhea. (Courtesy Centers for Disease Control and Prevention, Atlanta, Ga.)

mountainous regions, especially if they are camping and drinking spring water, are at increased risk for *G. lamblia*. The two geographic areas with the highest rates of giardia infection are the country of Nepal and St. Petersburg in Russia.

The Immunocompromised Host

The immunocompromised host consists of individuals with AIDS; cancer patients, especially while on chemotherapy; those who have received either a solid organ or bone marrow transplant; and any individual with a chronic disease requiring the administration of immunosuppressive agents. Although all of the previously described pathogens can cause diarrhea in the immunocompromised host, these patients are also at risk for developing infections with "opportunistic" organisms. These **opportunistic pathogens** generally do not cause disease in an otherwise healthy individual, but can cause significant, occasional deadly disease in a susceptible host. Numerous opportunistic pathogens exist that can lead to diarrhea, which will be briefly described later.

Mycobacterial disease typically causes pulmonary disease. However, in immunocompromised patients, disseminated and extrapulmonary disease is possible and more likely to occur. The two most common mycobacterial human pathogens are *Mycobacterium tuberculosis* (TB), *and Mycobacterium avium* complex (MAC). In patients infected with human immunodeficiency virus (HIV), MAC is rarely seen unless the CD4 count drops below 100 cells/mL. When these bacteria invade the

gastrointestinal system, they can lead to abdominal pain and diarrhea, which sometimes may turn bloody. Other symptoms such as weight loss, fevers, and night sweats are often present.

Cytomegalovirus (CMV) is an opportunistic virus that can lead to diarrhea. CMV can infect many organ systems; commonly described problems include retinitis, pulmonary disease, and gastrointestinal disease. CMV can affect any part of the gastrointestinal system. It can create ulcers in the esophagus, leading to painful swallowing and esophagitis. It can also invade the colon, leading to colitis. Typical symptoms consist of watery diarrhea, pain, and blood in the stool. Fever is often present.

Numerous opportunistic parasitic infections exist that can lead to diarrhea. Many of the previously discussed parasitic pathogens that can lead to diarrheal disease in immunocompetent patients also cause disease in immunocompromised individuals. However, whereas in healthy patients the diarrhea is usually mild and self-limited, in immunocompromised patients the disease can be chronic, more severe, and cause significant dehydration and malabsorption.

The diagnostic workup of diarrhea in an immunocompromised host can be more difficult. Typical pathogens can be diagnosed using traditional techniques. For parasitic and protozoal infections including *Cryptosporidium, Cyclospora, Isospora,* and microsporidia, special stains, including a modified acid-fast, are needed. The laboratory must be notified when there is suspicion for these pathogens so that the appropriate stains can be completed. When mycobacterial or viral disease are suspected, an endoscopic procedure with tissue biopsy is often needed.

LABORATORY DIAGNOSIS OF GASTROINTESTINAL PATHOGENS

It is not enough for the physician to just send a stool specimen to the laboratory and ask for analysis. The proper tests must be requested before the laboratory can prepare the proper analysis. In most cases, if the stool is sent for bacterial culture, the laboratory will attempt to isolate *C. jejuni, Salmonella,* and *Shigella* spp. Because there are many other potential pathogens, the laboratory must be informed which tests to perform.

Specimen Collection and Handling

Stool specimens should be transported to the laboratory quickly after collection, avoiding refrigeration if possible. If there are to be attempts at bacterial cultures, preservatives must be avoided. On the other hand, if the stool is to be examined for ova and parasites, it should be transported in preservative media containing preservatives such as polyvinyl alcohol or formalin. If rectal swabs are to be processed, Cary-Blair or similar transport media should be used.

Direct Microscopic Examination

Microscopic examination of the stool may reveal white blood cells if the patient has an inflammatory diarrhea (e.g., *Salmonella, Shigella, Yersinia, Campylobacter,* EIEC, and various *Vibrio* species). Red blood cells may be present due to intestinal wall bleeding.

The bacterial pathogen may be visible on direct microscopic examination of the stool. If gram-negative, curved rods with a "seagull-wing" appearance (Figure 34-7) are present, the patient may have a *Campylobacter* or *Vibrio* infection. If wet mount or hanging-drop preparations are performed in a patient with *C. jejuni* infection, characteristic darting motility may be seen. *E. histolytica* may also be seen on direct examination in patients with bloody diarrhea.

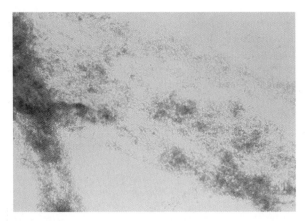

FIGURE 34-7 Gram stain of *Campylobacter* colony showing the typical microscopic morphology described as "seagull wings."

Culture

Selective and differential culture media are commonly used to attempt to identify bacterial pathogens in stool. Selective media limit the numbers of different bacterial species that will grow, often by containing different antibiotics or chemicals to limit the growth of normal fecal flora and to enhance the growth of pathogens. Without the normal fecal flora to mask growth, identification of the pathogens becomes easier. The differential aspect of the media often allows differentiation of bacterial species based on colony morphology; the differences in colony appearance are usually due to different biochemical characteristics of the organisms. Table 34-6 lists some of the selective media used to isolate gastrointestinal pathogens.

Campylobacter jejuni

Campylobacter jejuni grows best at 42° C in an atmosphere of reduced oxygen content (5% to 10%), making them microaerophilic organisms. Laboratories may have special gas supplies and culture chambers to provide an atmosphere for best culturing this organism.

C. jejuni colonies on growth media form a characteristic morphology described as "running" or "wet-looking" as the colonies seem to run together. Examination of the organisms under the microscope shows characteristic gram-negative curved rods (see Figure 34-7). This appearance helps differentiate *C. jejuni* from *Pseudomonas aeruginosa,* which can grow under similar environmental conditions.

Salmonella Species

In patients with typhoid fever, blood cultures are most likely to be positive in the first week of infection, whereas stool cultures are more likely to be positive in the third and fourth weeks of infection. In patients with nontyphoid *Salmonella* gastroenteritis, the organisms may be recovered from stool. Routine microbiologic media such as sheep blood agar (SBA) and MacConkey agar (MAC) can be used; highly selective media such as Hektoen enteric (HE) agar (Figure 34-8) and xylose-lysine-deoxycholate (XLD) agar may also be used.

Shigella Species

Relatively fragile organisms, these bacteria do not survive well outside the host for long periods of time. Culture recovery is therefore enhanced by rapid transport of the specimen to the microbiology laboratory and by prompt processing of the specimen. Media that can successfully recover *Salmonella* spp. are also useful for the recovery of *Shigella* spp. (Figure 34-9).

Escherichia coli

Escherichia coli is a normal inhabitant of the human gastrointestinal tract, and diarrheogenic *E. coli* appear no different on culture media than do their more benign counterparts. A few diagnostic tests help differentiate pathogenic from nonpathogenic *E. coli*. For example, many EHEC will not ferment the sugar sorbitol. These can therefore be differentiated from sorbitol-fermenting *E. coli* with the use of a differential medium such as sorbitol-MAC (Figure 34-10). EIEC have morphology and biochemical reactions similar to those of *Shigella* species.

TABLE 34-6 Selective Media Commonly Used to Recover Diarrheal Agents

Culture Medium	Purpose	Characteristic Morphology	
		Pathogens	**Colon Flora**
MacConkey agar	To recover Enterobacteriaceae and other nonfastidious gram-negative bacilli Inhibits gram-positive organisms and some fastidious gram-negative bacilli	*Salmonella, Shigella* (with few exceptions) organisms *Edwardsiella* organisms appear clear and colorless	Lactose fermenters, such as *Escherichia coli, Klebsiella* spp., *Enterobacter* spp., and certain *Citrobacter* spp., appear dark pink to red Late or slow lactose fermenters, such as *Citrobacter* spp., *Serratia* spp., and *Hafnia* spp., appear colorless in 24 hours and slightly pink after 24-48 hours Nonlactose fermenters, such as *Citrobacter* spp., *Proteus* spp., *Providencia* spp., and *Morganella* spp. appear clear and colorless
Hektoen enteric (HE) agar	A highly selective medium to recover primarily *Salmonella* and *Shigella* spp. Inhibits common colon flora Contains indicators to detect hydrogen sulfide (H$_2$S) production	*Salmonella* spp. appear green to blue-green with black centers because of H$_2$S production *Shigella* spp. appear green without black centers, because they do not produce H$_2$S	Lactose fermenters, such as *E. coli*, are slightly inhibited and appear orange to salmon pink *Proteus* spp. are slightly inhibited; small, clear colonies with black centers may appear
Xylose-lysine deoxycholate (XLD) agar	A differential and selective medium to isolate *Salmonella* spp. and *Shigella* spp. from stool Inhibits most colon flora and most gram-positive bacteria Certain *Shigella* spp. (*S. dysenteriae* and *S. flexneri*) may be slightly inhibited	*Salmonella* spp. appears red with black centers owing to the production of H$_2$S; *Salmonella* does not ferment lactose or sucrose but does ferment xylose, which is essential in decarboxylating lysine to revert the acid pH (yellow from sucrose fermentation) to an alkaline pH (red from lysine decarboxylation) *Shigella* spp. do not ferment any of these carbohydrates and appear red or clear	Enterobacteriaceae that may not be completely inhibited, such as *Proteus vulgaris*, appear yellow (from sucrose) with black centers *Citrobacter freundii*, which produces H$_2$S, appears yellow with black centers owing to the inability to decarboxylate lysine Other intestinal flora that may grow ferment one or all of the carbohydrates in this medium, resulting in yellow colonies
Campylobacter blood agar (CAMPY-BA)	An enrichment-selective medium primarily to isolate and cultivate *Campylobacter* spp. from stool	*Campylobacter jejuni* appears pinkish gray, moist, and runny when incubated at 42° C	
Cefsulodin-Irgasan-novobiocin (CIN)	A selective medium to primarily isolate and recover *Yersinia enterocolitica* *Aeromonas* spp. and *Plesiomonas shigelloides* may also be recovered Inhibits most gram-positive cocci, except for enterococci, and most gram-negative bacilli, particularly the Enterobacteriaceae	*Y. enterocolitica* produce colonies that look like "bull's-eyes": the center is red and the periphery appears colorless *Aeromonas* species also ferment mannitol present in the medium, like *Yersinia*; *P. shigelloides* does not	Except for *Pseudomonas aeruginosa, Citrobacter,* and *Serratia*, most colon flora are inhibited
Thiosulfate-citrate–bile salts–sucrose agar (TCBS)	A highly selective medium to recover *Vibrio* spp., including *Vibrio cholerae*, from stool and food Inhibits most colon flora because of the high pH (preferred by vibrios) and high bile salts content *Aeromonas* spp. may be recovered from this medium	TCBS contains sucrose, so sucrose-fermenting *Vibrio* spp. such as *V. cholerae* and *V. alginolyticus* produce yellow colonies Nonsucrose fermenters, such as *V. parahaemolyticus* and *V. vulnificus*, produce blue-green colonies	Inhibitory to most colon flora, except for occasional *Pseudomonas* isolates, which may also appear blue-green
Cycloserine-cefoxitin-fructose agar (CCFA), anaerobic incubation required	A selective medium to primarily isolate *Clostridium difficile* from stool of patients suspected of antibiotic-associated diarrhea or pseudomembranous colitis Inhibits most colon flora, both gram-positive and gram-negative bacteria	*C. difficile* appears yellow from fructose fermentation	Colon flora are inhibited
Sorbitol-MacConkey (SMAC)	A differential medium to detect sorbitol-negative *Escherichia coli*. Contains sorbitol instead of lactose	*E. coli* O157:H7 appears colorless; does not ferment sorbitol	Most appear pink

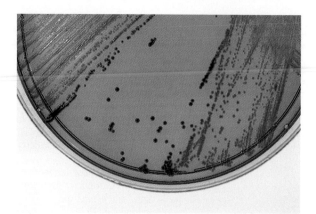

FIGURE 34-8 *Salmonella* colonies growing on Hektoen enteric agar showing black centers resulting from the production of hydrogen sulfide.

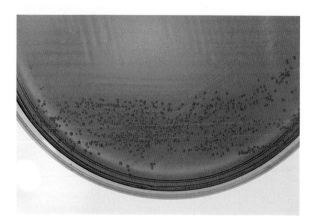

FIGURE 34-9 *Shigella* colonies growing on Hektoen enteric agar showing clear green colonies.

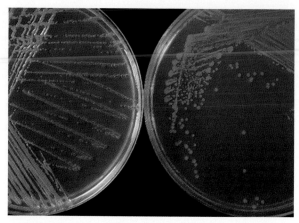

FIGURE 34-10 *Left, Escherichia coli* iO157:H7 growing on MacConkey agar (MAC). *Right, E. coli* O157:H7 on sorbitol MAC. *E. coli* O157:H7 does not ferment sorbitol, whereas most other *E. coli* serotypes do ferment sorbitol.

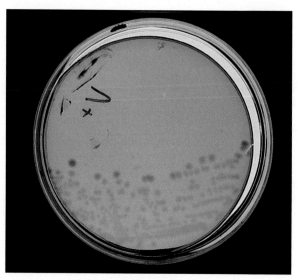

FIGURE 34-11 *Vibrio vulnificus* growing on TCBS (thiosulfate–citrate–bile salts–sucrose). *V. vulnificus* is a non–sucrose-fermenting Vibrio species.

Yersinia Species

Yersinia species grow well at cooler temperatures of 25° C. This may be used in the microbiology laboratory by plating and incubating specimens at this temperature to enhance recovery of this organism. The use of certain selective media, such as cefsulodin–irgasan–novobiocin (CIN), can allow ready isolation of these species. Recovery of the organism can be increased by placing fecal samples in isotonic saline and keeping them at 4° C before inoculation onto the selective medium.

Vibrio Species

Vibrio species require highly selective media for recovery. If these pathogens are suspected, the initial stool specimen should be transported to the laboratory in Cary-Blair or similar transport media. The sample can then be inoculated on thiosulfate–citrate–bile salts–sucrose (TCBS) agar for maximal yield. This medium not only inhibits the normal colonic flora but also differentiates sucrose-fermenting from non–sucrose-fermenting *Vibrio* spp. (Figure 34-11). The salt requirement for growth may also help differentiate *V. cholerae* from more halophilic *Vibrio* spp. In certain areas, especially in places where cholera is endemic, antisera are available to identify outbreak strains of *V. cholerae*.

Clostridium difficile

An anaerobe, *C. difficile* produces yellow, ground glass colonies on cycloserine-cefoxitin-fructose agar. However, culture is not frequently used to diagnose this pathogen, because patients may be colonized with non–toxin-producing strains. Instead, stool specimens are often examined for the presence of the *C. difficile* toxin.

TREATMENT AND PREVENTION OF DIARRHEA

The most important factor to consider in treating a patient with acute diarrhea is hydration status. Volume depletion and electrolyte derangements are the major sources of morbidity and mortality from diarrheal illnesses. As patients lose electrolytes in diarrheal stools, rehydration cannot occur with pure water alone. The best rehydration solution contains both glucose and sodium, in that transport of these are coupled in the intestinal wall. Although most patients can be treated effectively with oral rehydration, some will require intravenous infusion of isotonic solutions (e.g., 0.9% saline, 5% dextrose in 0.9% saline, Ringer's lactate).

Antibiotic therapy is ineffective against the viral causes of gastroenteritis. Patients with viral gastroenteritis should be given supportive care with adequate hydration. Measures should also be taken to prevent the spread of the pathogen to others. In severe cases, antibiotics may be used against some of the bacterial pathogens. However, in several cases, this may be associated with an increased time of shedding of the organism in the stool, placing other people at risk of contracting the disease. There is also concern that treating EHEC infections may increase the chance of developing HUS. Antibiotic therapy can be effective in shortening the duration of illness associated with some, but not all, of the parasitic pathogens. Antidiarrheal medications such as diphenoxylate with atropine (Lomotil) or loperamide may decrease the frequency of stool for some patients. However, there is some concern in using these agents for invasive diarrhea. Although several studies have conflicting data, there is the possibility that these agents may increase the severity of invasive disease, possibly due to increased contact time of the pathogen with the intestinal wall. These medications are most frequently used with enterotoxin-mediated diarrhea or viral gastroenteritis. Both antibiotics and other agents are frequently used in traveler's diarrhea. Bismuth subsalicylate (Pepto-Bismol) can be effective in shortening the course of traveler's diarrhea, especially that resulting from ETEC, possibly by binding the toxin. Many people traveling to areas known to be associated with traveler's diarrhea will often bring antibiotics (usually fluoroquinolones) and antimotility agents with them. Although this may be effective at reducing the duration of illness, most cases of traveler's diarrhea are self-limiting without this therapy. The increasing prevalence of antibiotic-resistant organisms is likely to further limit the utility of this relatively expensive practice. Travelers to high-risk areas should be advised to drink only bottled beverages as well as to avoid high-risk foods and ice. High-risk foods include any foods prepared by another person and served uncooked (e.g., salad, fruits, vegetables), dips and other foods left standing at room temperature, and raw or partially cooked fish or shellfish. For the nontraveler, pathogens are best avoided by thoroughly cooking all meats and poultry, ensuring that the cooked meats or poultry do not come in contact with surfaces contaminated by the raw food, and by thoroughly washing all fruits and vegetables. To prevent secondary infections, patients infected with acute gastroenteritis should practice careful handwashing and avoid preparing food for others. They also may wish to avoid confined public swimming places (e.g., community swimming pools) for several weeks following infection, depending on the pathogen.

BIBLIOGRAPHY

Adachi JA et al: Enteroaggregative *Escherichia coli* as a major etiologic agent in traveler's diarrhea in 3 regions of the world, *Clin Infect Dis* 32:1706, 2001.

Allos BM: *Campylobacter jejuni* infections: update on emerging issues and trends, *Clin Infect Dis* 32:1201, 2001.

Brown GH, Rotschafer JC: *Cyclospora*: review of an emerging parasite, *Pharmacotherapy* 19:70, 1999.

Butzler JP: *Campylobacter*, from obscurity to celebrity, *Clin Microbiol Infect* 10:868, 2004.

Centers for Disease Control and Prevention: Outbreak of *Escherichia coli* O157-H7 infection associated with eating fresh cheese curds—Wisconsin, June 1998, *MMWR* 40:911, 2000.

Centers for Disease Control and Prevention: Protracted outbreaks of cryptosporidiosis associated with swimming pool use—Ohio and Nebraska, 2000, *MMWR* 20:406, 2001.

Centers for Disease Control and Prevention: Shigellosis outbreak associated with an unchlorinated fill-and-drain wading pool—Iowa, 2001, *MMWR* 37:797, 2001.

Centers for Disease Control and Prevention: Neurologic illness associated with eating Florida pufferfish, *MMWR* 15:321, 2002.

Centers for Disease Control and Prevention: Outbreak of *Campylobacter jejuni* infections associated with drinking unpasteurized milk procured through a cow-leasing program—Wisconsin, 2001, *MMWR* 25:548, 2002.

Centers for Disease Control and Prevention: Multistate outbreak of *Salmonella* serotype typhimurium infections associated with drinking unpasteurized milk—Illinois, Indiana, Ohio, and Tennessee, 2002-2003, *MMWR* 26:613, 2003.

Centers for Disease Control and Prevention: Norovirus activity—United States, 2002, *MMWR* 3:41, 2003.

Centers for Disease Control and Prevention: Outbreaks of *Salmonella* serotype entiritidis infection associated with eating shell eggs—United States 1999-2001, *MMWR* 51:1149, 2003.

Centers for Disease Control and Prevention: *Yersinia enterocolitica* gastroenteritis among infants exposed to chitterlings—Chicago, Illinois, 2002, *MMWR* 40:956, 2003.

Centers for Disease Control and Prevention: Cholera epidemic associated with raw vegetables—Lusaka, Zambia, 2003-2004, *MMWR* 34:783, 2004.

Centers for Disease Control and Prevention: Outbreak of cyclosporiasis associated with snow peas—Pennsylvania, 2004, *MMWR* 37:876, 2004.

Centers for Disease Control and Prevention: An outbreak of Norovirus gastroenteritis at a swimming club—Vermont, 2004, *MMWR* 34:793, 2004.

Chen XM et al: Cryptosporidiosis, *N Engl J Med* 346:1723, 2002.

Clark DP: New insights into human cryptosporidiosis, *Clin Microbiol Rev* 12:554, 1999.

Didier ES, Weiss LM: Microsporidiosis: current status, *Curr Opin Infect Dis* 19:485, 2006.

Fox JG: The non-*H. pylori* helicobacters: their expanding role in gastrointestinal and systemic diseases, *Gut* 50:273, 2002.

Gilligan PH: *Escherichia coli*. EAEC, EHEC, EIEC, ETEC, *Clin Lab Med* 19:505, 1999.

Huang DB et al: Enteroaggregative *Escherichia coli:* an emerging enteric pathogen, *Am J Gastroenterol* 99:383, 2004.

Janda JM, Abbott SL: Unusual food-borne pathogens. *Listeria monocytogenes, Aeromonas, Plesiomonas,* and *Edwardsiella* species, *Clin Lab Med* 19:553, 1999.

Jong E: Intestinal parasites, *Prim Care* 29:857, 2002.

Kosek M et al: Cryptosporidiosis: an update, *Lancet Infect Dis* 1:262, 2001.

Kucik CJ, Martin GL, Sortor BV: Common intestinal parasites, *Am Fam Physician* 69:1161, 2004.

Leber AL: Intestinal amebae, *Clin Lab Med* 19:601, 1999.

Loo VG et al: A predominantly clonal multi-institutional outbreak of *Clostridium difficile*–associated diarrhea with high morbidity and mortality, *N Engl J Med* 353:2442, 2005.

McDonald LC et al: An epidemic toxin gene–variant strain of *Clostridium difficile*, *N Engl J Med* 353:2433, 2005.

Mentec H et al: Cytomegalovirus colitis in HIV-1-infected patients: A prospective research in 55 patients, *AIDS* 8:461, 1994.

Okhuysen PC: Travelers' diarrhea due to intestinal protozoa, *Clin Infect Dis* 33:110, 2001.

Poutanen SM, Simor AE: *Clostridium difficile*–associated diarrhea in adults, *CMAJ* 171:51, 2004.

Powell JL: *Vibrio* species, *Clin Lab Med* 19:537, 1999.

Sack DA et al: Cholera, *Lancet* 363:223, 2004.

Shlim DR: Update in traveler's diarrhea, *Infect Dis Clin North Am* 19:137, 2005.

Thielman NM, Guerrant RL: Clinical practice. Acute infectious diarrhea, *N Engl J Med* 350:38, 2004.

von Sonnenburg F et al: Risk and aetiology of diarrhoea at various tourist destinations, *Lancet* 356:133, 2000.

Widdowson MA et al: 2004 Outbreaks of acute gastroenteritis on cruise ships and on land: identification of a predominant circulating strain of norovirus—United States, 2002, *J Infect Dis* 190:27, 2004.

Widdowson M, Monroe SS, Glass RI: Are noroviruses emerging? *Emerg Infect Dis* 11:735, 2005.

Wilhelmi I et al: Viruses causing gastroenteritis, *Clin Microbiol Infect* 9:247, 2003.

Points to Remember

- Factors that predispose patients to diarrheal illnesses include previous history of gastrointestinal disease, immunosuppression or other immunocompromised state, and medication intake.
- Travel history and food intake provide significant information in determining the cause of the diarrheal disease. Certain foods such as meat, shellfish, and poultry serve as vehicles of food-borne disease.
- Food-borne diseases are transmitted and acquired by ingestion of contaminated food and beverage.
- Clinical presentations can be characterized as enterotoxin-mediated diarrhea, invasion of bowel mucosa, or invasion with lymphatic or metastatic spread of infection.
- Food poisoning may be caused by chemical intoxications from fish or shellfish consumption.
- Appropriate laboratory diagnosis may include the use of direct microscopy and selective culture media to recover and identify the suspected etiologic agent.

Learning Assessment Questions

1. What are the major host defense mechanisms located in the stomach? The small bowel? The colon?

2. What are the key elements to obtain in history when interviewing a patient with diarrheal illness?

3. What initial laboratory findings aid in the diagnosis of acute diarrhea?

4. Which viruses, usually not associated with diarrheal illness in immunocompetent patients, may result in diarrhea in AIDS patients?

5. Which parasite may cause a bloody diarrhea and disseminated infection?

6. What are some toxin-mediated forms of illness associated with fish and shellfish?

7. What are some life-threatening complications associated with bacterial diarrheal infections?

8. Which diarrheal infection is associated with prior antibiotic use?

9. Which serotypes of *Vibrio cholerae* are associated with epidemic diarrhea?

10. How can travelers best avoid traveler's diarrhea?

Infections of the Central Nervous System

Sumati Nambiar, Kalavati Suvarna*

- **GENERAL CONCEPTS RELATED TO INFECTIONS OF THE CENTRAL NERVOUS SYSTEM**
  Anatomic Organization
  Cerebrospinal Fluid Characteristics
  Host-Pathogen Relationships
- **INFECTIONS OF THE CENTRAL NERVOUS SYSTEM**
  Meningitis
  Meningoencephalitis and Encephalitis

Brain Abscesses
Bacterial Pathogens
Fungal Pathogens
- **LABORATORY DIAGNOSIS OF CENTRAL NERVOUS SYSTEM INFECTIONS**

OBJECTIVES

After reading and studying this chapter, you should be able to:

1. Describe the production and distribution of cerebrospinal fluid (CSF).

2. Describe the characteristics of normal CSF.

3. Describe the collection, transportation, and processing of CSF samples.

4. List the common bacterial pathogens in meningitis along with one host-related factor and one virulence-related factor for each pathogen.

5. List the common bacterial, fungal, and parasitic pathogens associated with brain abscess.

6. List fungi that typically produce meningitis, and compare virulence and host factors of two fungi that typically produce intracerebral lesions.

7. List two viruses associated with meningitis, encephalitis, and paralysis.

8. Compare and contrast the physical, chemical, and cellular features of bacterial, mycobacterial (tuberculous), fungal, syphilitic, viral, and parasitic central nervous system (CNS) infections.

Case in Point

A 3-year-old boy with a recent history of acute otitis media arrived at the emergency department; on examination, he was febrile to 103° F (39.4° C) and lethargic. No skin rash was present. Examination of a complete blood count showed leukocytosis with a total leukocyte count of 21,000/μL with a left shift. Lumbar puncture revealed cloudy CSF with a cell count of 210 leukocytes/mm³ with 85% neutrophils. The CSF glucose was decreased at 15 mg/dL, and the CSF protein was elevated at 450 mg/dL. The child received intravenous ceftriaxone, and the cerebrospinal fluid (CSF) sample was sent to the microbiology laboratory for Gram stain and culture. A cytocentrifuged CSF smear revealed moderate intracellular gram-positive cocci in pairs. Culture of the CSF grew a mucoid strain of *Streptococcus pneumoniae*. Susceptibility studies were performed, and the following minimal inhibitory concentrations (MICs) were obtained:

penicillin 2.0 μg/mL, ceftriaxone 0.012 μg/mL, and vancomycin less than 1.0 μg/mL.

Issues to Consider

After reading the patient's case history, consider the following:

- Host-related risk factors of the patient
- Bacterial, fungal, or parasitic agents that may be involved based on the clinical presentation, onset of infection, and possible source of infection
- Physical, chemical, and cellular features of CSF
- Specimen collection, transport, and processing for maximum recovery of causative agent
- Rapid diagnostic methods that can facilitate presumptive diagnosis and institution of therapy

---

*This chapter was prepared by the authors in their private capacities. No official support or endorsement by the FDA is intended or implied.

Infections of the **central nervous system (CNS)** are serious and potentially life threatening. These infections may be caused by bacteria, fungi, viruses, or parasites. Positive laboratory findings are "critical values" communicated directly to the clinician. The physician arrives at a presumptive diagnosis based on the patient's age, physical examination, local epidemiology of CNS infections, **cerebrospinal fluid (CSF)** analysis, and often radiologic studies. Specific etiologic diagnosis is arrived at by laboratory testing.

The epidemiology of bacterial meningitis has changed over the decades. Since the introduction of vaccination against *Haemophilus influenzae* type b in the 1980s, there has been a dramatic reduction in the incidence of meningitis due to this organism. With the inclusion of pneumococcal vaccination in the routine immunization schedule for children and the availability of newer meningococcal vaccines, there has been a further reduction in the incidence of meningitis. The mortality rate ranges from less than 5% for *H. influenzae* meningitis to around 10% for meningococcal meningitis and around 20% for those with pneumococcal meningitis. In the United States, approximately 3000 cases of meningococcal disease occur each year. The rates are severalfold higher in sub-Saharan Africa ("the meningitis belt"), extending from Senegal in the west to Ethiopia in the east. Although mortality rates have decreased as a result of improved medical management of CNS infections, some children may develop learning disabilities, behavioral problems, and developmental delay. Thus infections of the CNS are a cause of both immediate and long-term health concerns.

This chapter discusses the following:
- The interplay of host-related risk factors and virulence factors associated with the pathogens
- Characteristics of the CSF
- Microbial agents of infections of the CNS
- Laboratory diagnosis of CNS infections

GENERAL CONCEPTS RELATED TO INFECTIONS OF THE CENTRAL NERVOUS SYSTEM

Anatomic Organization

The CNS encompasses the brain, spinal cord, and cranial nerves, but not the peripheral nerves (Figure 35-1). The brain and spinal cord are protected by the skull, vertebral column, and three layers of meninges: the dura, arachnoid, and pia mater. The dura mater is a thick, fibrous, white membrane that is firmly adherent to the overlying skull. Deep to dura mater is the arachnoid mater, followed by the pia mater.

The subarachnoid space between the arachnoid and pia mater is occupied by surface blood vessels and CSF. The CSF is produced by both filtration and secretion from specialized capillary tufts of the choroid plexus within the four ventricles of the brain. CSF flows from the two lateral ventricles to the third ventricle and enters the fourth ventricle via the aqueduct of Sylvius. From here the CSF enters the basal cisterns and circulates over the cerebellum and convexities of the cerebral hemispheres. The CSF is absorbed primarily by the arachnoid villi through tight junctions of the endothelium.

Cerebrospinal Fluid Characteristics

Cerebrospinal fluid is a clear, colorless, and sterile fluid. In normal adults the CSF volume ranges from 90 to 150 mL, the protein level is 15 to 45 mg/dL, and the CSF glucose level is 40 to 80 mg/dL (CSF glucose : serum glucose ratio of 0.6). In adults normal CSF contains 0 to 7 leukocytes/microliter, with a differential count of 60% to 80% lymphocytes, 10% to 40% monocytes, and 0% to 15% neutrophils. Compared with adults, normal newborns have higher CSF concentrations of protein (15 to 150 mg/dL), glucose (30 to 120 mg/dL), and cells (0 to 30 leukocytes/mL), with a greater percentage of monocytes and neutrophils. The paucity of leukocytes and protein (including immunoglobulins) within the CSF provides little initial defense against invading organisms. Infections of the CNS are frequently, but not invariably, associated with an increase in CSF cell count **(pleocytosis)** and alteration in glucose and protein levels.

Host-Pathogen Relationships

Infection results from the complex interplay among the host, the organism, and the environment. Host risk factors that predispose to infection include extremes of age; nutritional and immunologic status; and comorbidities such as alcoholism, diabetes mellitus, sickle cell anemia, and malignancy. Structural components of the organism—such as surface encapsulation, pili, and fimbriae—that mediate adherence to respiratory tract epithelial cells play an important role in meningeal infection. Additionally, the bacterial capsule can resist neutrophil phagocytosis and complement-mediated bactericidal activity, thus enhancing survival in the bloodstream. Host factors that attempt to limit infection include the presence of mucosal immunity—mediated via immunoglobulin A (IgA) antibody, complement activation, and the presence of organism-specific antibodies.

INFECTIONS OF THE CENTRAL NERVOUS SYSTEM

Meningitis

Acute **meningitis** is commonly caused by bacteria (e.g., *Streptococcus pneumoniae*, *Neisseria meningitidis*, *H. influenzae*) or viruses (e.g., enteroviruses, herpes virus, mumps virus). Less commonly, it is caused by other organisms, such as spirochetes (e.g., *Treponema pallidum*, *Borrelia burgdorferi*), proto-

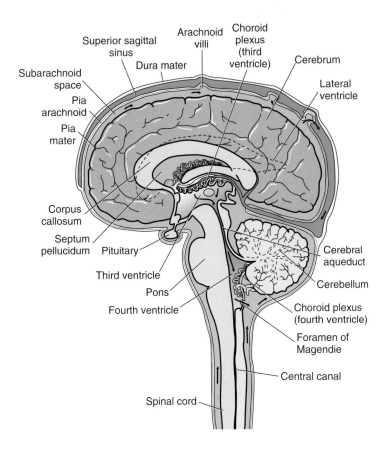

FIGURE 35-1 Components of the central nervous system (CNS) and flow pattern of cerebrospinal fluid (CSF).

zoa (e.g., *Naegleria fowleri*) or helminths (e.g., *Angiostrongylus cantonensis*). Patients with acute meningitis usually have fever, headache, vomiting, photophobia, and altered mental status. In infants and children, irritability, restlessness, and poor feeding may be the only signs of meningitis. Untreated meningitis can result in obtundation (use of a substance, such as a narcotic, to blunt pain), coma, and death.

Bacterial Meningitis

The likely etiologic agents of bacterial meningitis depend on the age of the patient (Box 35-1) and on host factors such as immune status, presence of a cerebrospinal leak, presence of a foreign body such as a ventriculoperitoneal shunt, or prolonged hospitalization.

Pathogenesis. The first step in the development of a meningeal infection involves nasopharyngeal colonization by one of the meningeal pathogens, followed by local invasion across the mucosal barrier and entry into the bloodstream. Despite the presence of host defense mechanisms, bacteria are able to gain access to the meninges. The exact mechanism by which bacteria gain access to the CNS or the exact site of entry in the CNS remains unclear. In the subarachnoid space, bacteria replicate, release bacterial components, and cause an inflammatory reaction.

H. influenzae type b, a gram-negative coccobacillus, is an important cause of bacterial meningitis. In addition to

---

BOX 35-1   Bacteria Involving the Central Nervous System

Bacterial Meningitis Related to Age

Neonates (<1 Month)
Gram-negative bacilli (*Escherichia coli, Klebsiella* spp., *Enterobacter* spp.)
Streptococcus agalactiae (group B)
Listeria monocytogenes

Infants (1-23 Months)
Streptococcus agalactiae (group B)
Escherichia coli
Haemophilus influenzae
Streptococcus pneumoniae
Neisseria meningitidis

Children (>2 Years) and Adults
Streptococcus pneumoniae
Neisseria meningitidis

Older Adults (>65 Years)
Streptococcus pneumoniae
Neisseria meningitidis
Listeria monocytogenes
Aerobic gram-negative bacilli

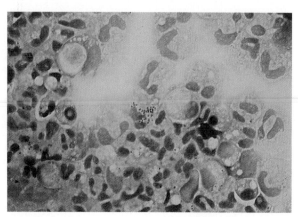

FIGURE 35-2 Direct smear of the cerebrospinal fluid (CSF) from a high-school student showing clusters of gram-negative diplococci consistent with *Neisseria meningitidis* within polymorphonuclear leukocytes. Note the increased cellularity of the smear in this cytocentrifuge preparation. Gram stain; high-power view.

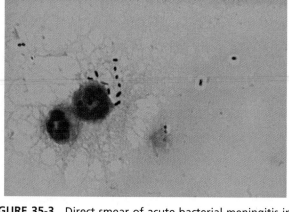

FIGURE 35-3 Direct smear of acute bacterial meningitis in an adult showing the lancet-shaped, gram-positive diplococci characteristic of *Streptococcus pneumoniae*. The polysaccharide capsule produces a prominent "halo" around organisms. Gram stain; noncytocentrifuge preparation; high-power view.

meningitis, it can cause otitis media, pneumonia, and epiglottitis. *H. influenzae* was previously the most common cause of bacterial meningitis, especially in young children. Most cases were due to the capsular type b strains. Since the adoption of routine use of conjugate vaccines against *H. influenzae* type b, there has been a marked reduction in the number of cases of *H. influenzae* meningitis. In developing countries with limited vaccine coverage, however, it continues to be an important cause of bacterial meningitis. *N. meningitidis*, a gram-negative diplococcus (Figure 35-2), is classified into 12 serogroups based on antigenically distinct, non–cross-reactive capsular polysaccharides. Serogroups A, B, C, Y, and W-135 account for most cases of meningococcal disease throughout the world. Serogroups B, C, and Y account for most cases in Europe and the United States. Disease attributable to serogroup A is seen in Asia and Africa but is rare in industrialized countries. Disease caused by serogroups A and C can occur in epidemics. Outbreaks have also been reported with the W135 serogroup. Individuals deficient in terminal components of complement (C5-9) or properdin are at a higher risk for meningococcal infections. A meningococcal polysaccharide vaccine containing polysaccharides A, C, Y, and W-135 is available for use in individuals older than 2 years. A quadrivalent meningococcal diphtheria-conjugate vaccine was recently approved for use in 2- to 55-year-olds. *S. pneumoniae*, a gram-positive diplococcus, is the most common cause of meningitis in adults and the second most common cause of meningitis in children (Figure 35-3). In patients with a CSF leak resulting from a basilar skull fracture, pneumococcus is the most likely etiologic agent. Of more than 90 serotypes, only a few serotypes—including 4, 6B, 9V, 14, 18C, 19 F, and 23F—account for most cases of invasive childhood pneumococcal infections in the United States. Patients with sickle cell anemia, splenectomy or asplenia, malignancy, malnutrition, and chronic renal or liver disease are more likely to develop serious pneumococcal disease. Two pneumococcal vaccines are available for use: the heptavalent pneumococcal conjugate

vaccine (PCV7), which is composed of purified polysaccharides of seven serotypes conjugated to a diphtheria protein, and the 23-valent vaccine (PS23), composed of 23 purified capsular polysaccharides. The PCV7 vaccine is part of the routine immunization schedule of children. *Listeria monocytogenes* is a gram-positive rod. Infection by this organism is more commonly seen in neonates, older adults, alcoholics, and immunosuppressed individuals. Outbreaks of *Listeria* infection have been associated with consumption of contaminated coleslaw, milk, ice cream, and cheese. *Streptococcus agalactiae* or group B streptococcus (GBS) is a gram-positive coccus that is often isolated from rectal or vaginal cultures of asymptomatic pregnant women. It is a common cause of meningitis in neonates and infants up to 3 months of age. Neonatal acquisition most commonly results from vertical transmission from mother to infant. Nosocomial transmission via the hands of health care workers has also been described. Most cases of neonatal meningitis are caused by serotype III. Risk factors for GBS infection in adults include age greater than 60 years, diabetes mellitus, and underlying malignancy. Aerobic gram-negative bacilli such as *Escherichia coli*, *Klebsiella* (Figure 35-4), *Serratia*, or *Salmonella* organisms, can cause meningitis. Besides neonates, older adults, patients with head trauma, or those who have undergone neurosurgical procedures are also at risk of meningitis with these organisms. Most strains of *E. coli* that cause meningitis possess the K1 antigen.

Other Bacteria. Meningitis from *Staphylococcus aureus*, coagulase-negative staphylococci, or *Abiotrophia* and *Granulicatella* species usually occurs in patients who have undergone recent neurosurgical procedures or in those with CSF shunts, whereas meningitis from enterococci or group A streptococci are not commonly seen. Meningitis from anaerobic streptococci, *Bacteroides* spp. (Figure 35-5), and *Fusobacterium* spp. are uncommon and usually associated with a concurrent **brain abscess** or a contiguous focus of infection.

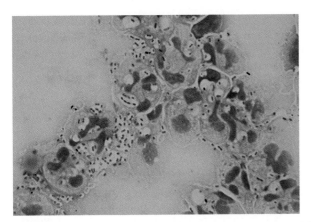

FIGURE 35-4 Direct smear of posttraumatic, acute bacterial meningitis showing numerous intracellular and extracellular gram-negative bacilli with the prominent capsules characteristic of *Klebsiella pneumoniae*. Gram stain; cytocentrifuge preparation; high-power view.

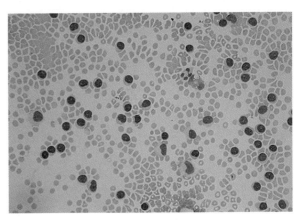

FIGURE 35-6 Cytocentrifuge preparation of cerebrospinal fluid (CSF) in a case of "aseptic" meningitis. Lymphocytes are present, and in this case the background is bloody. No organisms are seen; Wright stain.

Viral Infections

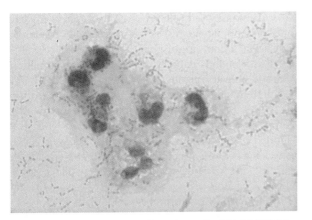

FIGURE 35-5 Direct smear of cerebrospinal fluid (CSF) from a newborn delivered to a woman with amnionitis secondary to premature rupture of the membranes. Numerous short, gram-negative bacilli in chains consistent with a *Bacteroides* sp. are seen. The organism could easily be confused with a *Streptococcus* sp. if the Gram stain was improperly decolorized. Gram stain; noncytocentrifuge preparation; high-power view.

CSF Shunt Infections. Generally CSF shunts are placed in patients with hydrocephalus or other lesions of the CNS that interfere with the flow of CSF. The proximal end of the shunt is in the CSF space and the distal end is in the peritoneal, pleural, or vascular space. Patients with shunts in place are at risk of developing infections. Staphylococci account for two thirds of CSF shunt infections, with coagulase-negative staphylococci being the most common, followed by *S. aureus.* Gram-negative organisms such as *E. coli, Klebsiella* spp., and *Proteus* spp. also can cause shunt infections. Recently an increasing incidence of shunt infections from *Propionibacterium acnes* has been reported. Immunosuppressed patients can develop shunt infections with *Candida* spp. Shunts terminating in the peritoneal cavity have a greater risk of infection with gram-negative organisms; mixed infections are seen when the catheter perforates a hollow viscus.

Case Study

A 36-year-old male with human immunodeficiency virus (HIV) infection presented to an emergency department with complaints of inability to urinate for 3 days. He also reported numbness and weakness in his right leg for 7 months, a 25-lb weight loss, and bowel incontinence. Physical examination revealed an afebrile, dehydrated, emaciated male with bilateral lower extremity weakness and decreased deep tendon reflexes. Lesions of Kaposi sarcoma, thrush, and perianal herpetic vesicles were observed. A magnetic resonance imaging (MRI) scan revealed no evidence of spinal cord compression, and a presumptive diagnosis of polyradiculopathy secondary to acquired immune deficiency syndrome (AIDS) was made. A lumbar puncture was performed. The CSF showed an increased protein level (326 mg/dL) and leukocyte count of 1720 cells/mL with 86% neutrophils.

Viruses are the most frequent cause of **aseptic meningitis,** a condition characterized by a lymphocytic pleocytosis in the CSF and a lack of an identifiable etiologic agent after routine stains and culture of the CSF (Figures 35-6 and 35-7). The most common viruses producing aseptic meningitis include the enteroviruses and herpesviruses. Less common causes of viral aseptic meningitis include mumps virus, lymphocytic choriomeningitis virus, and the human immunodeficiency virus (HIV) (Box 35-2). Viral pathogens colonize various mucosal surfaces in the body, such as the respiratory or gastrointestinal tract. Some viruses—for example, enteroviruses, adenoviruses, and parvovirus—can resist inactivation by gastric acid. After initial replication at the site of mucosal colonization, viremia develops, followed by invasion of the CNS. Early viral infections may show a predominance of neutrophils in the CSF, but the pleocytosis rapidly progresses to a lymphocytosis.

Enteroviruses. Enteroviruses (EVs) belong to the family Picornaviridae and include the polioviruses, coxsackieviruses A and B, echoviruses, and the newly numbered EVs. The EVs that are frequently associated with neurologic illness include coxsackievirus B and echoviruses. Although many different

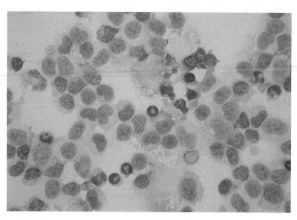

FIGURE 35-7 Cytocentrifuge preparation of cerebrospinal fluid (CSF) in meningitis resulting from tularemia. Reactive lymphocytes with "monocytoid" features are the only clue that this is not a viral infection. No organisms are seen. Cultures were positive; Wright stain.

BOX 35-2 Viral Agents Involving the Central Nervous System

Enteroviruses
Coxsackieviruses A and B
Echoviruses
Polioviruses
Arboviruses (arthropod-borne viruses)
Eastern equine encephalitis
Western equine encephalitis
Venezuelan equine encephalitis
St. Louis encephalitis virus
La Crosse virus
Colorado tick fever virus

Herpesviruses
Herpes simplex (HSV-1 and HSV-2)
Epstein-Barr virus
Cytomegalovirus
Varicella-zoster virus

Others
Lymphocytic choriomeningitis virus
Human immunodeficiency virus (HIV)
Mumps virus
Nipah virus
Rabies virus

---

serotypes can cause meningitis, coxsackie virus serotypes B2 and B5 and echovirus serotypes 4, 6, 9, 11, 16, and 30 are the most common.

In temperate climates, enteroviral infections are more common in the summer, but in subtropical areas no marked seasonality is observed. These infections are acquired by the fecal-oral route. Most cases of enteroviral meningitis are uncomplicated, with signs and symptoms resolving in 2 to 7 days. Human parechoviruses (HPeVs) are members of the Picornaviridae family. HPeV3 is associated with neonatal sepsis and meningitis. Most poliovirus infections are asymp-

tomatic or cause aseptic meningitis, but a small proportion of infections progress to destruction of motor neurons in the anterior spinal cord, resulting in paralysis. Although the incidence of paralytic poliomyelitis has decreased dramatically since effective vaccines became available, outbreaks continue to occur in some parts of the world.

Arboviruses. Arboviruses include a group of viruses transmitted by arthropod vectors such as mosquitoes, ticks, sandflies, and other biting arthropods. Several of these viruses cause **encephalitis,** but aseptic meningitis and **meningoencephalitis** can also occur. The common arboviruses causing aseptic meningitis include St. Louis encephalitis virus, La Crosse virus, Eastern and Western equine encephalitis virus, and West Nile virus. Japanese encephalitis virus, a mosquito-borne flavivirus, is endemic in parts of Asia. It can produce a severe encephalitis characterized by coma, seizures, paralysis, and abnormal movements. About a third of patients die, and serious sequelae are common in a significant proportion of survivors.

Mumps Virus. The mumps virus, a member of the Paramyxoviridae family, is an RNA virus that commonly causes parotitis. Aseptic meningitis is the most common neurologic complication. Symptoms of meningitis occur in up to 30% of patients with mumps parotitis (infection or inflammation of the parotid salivary glands) within 4 to 10 days of illness. Occasionally meningeal symptoms can precede parotitis by up to 7 days. Mumps meningitis is not associated with parotitis in almost half the cases. Infection of the CNS is usually self-limited and associated with complete recovery. Mumps virus vaccine is a live-attenuated vaccine that is usually given as part of the combined mumps-measles-rubella (MMR) vaccine.

Lymphocytic Choriomeningitis Virus. Lymphocytic choriomeningitis virus (LCMV) is a member of the Arenaviridae family. It is an RNA virus that is an uncommon cause of aseptic meningitis in humans. The virus is shed in the urine and other excretions of infected rodents and hamsters. Humans are infected by aerosol or by ingestion of dust or food contaminated with the urine, feces, blood, or nasopharyngeal secretions of infected rodents. Individuals living in rodent-infested dwellings, pet store owners, and laboratory workers who work with rodents are at risk for infection. There have been reports of transmission of LCMV through organ transplantation. As many as 50% of symptomatic patients will develop neurologic manifestations ranging from aseptic meningitis to severe encephalitis. LCMV infection during pregnancy can lead to fetal death or a congenital syndrome characterized by chorioretinitis, hydrocephalus, and microcephaly or macrocephaly.

Herpes Virus. Herpesviruses are DNA viruses and include herpes simplex virus (HSV-1 and HSV-2), Epstein-Barr virus (EBV), cytomegalovirus (CMV), varicella-zoster virus (VZV), and human herpesviruses 6, 7, and 8. Herpesviruses account for 0.5% to 3% of all cases of aseptic meningitis. Although aseptic meningitis can occur with any of these viruses, only meningitis associated with HSV appears to be of numeric significance. The clinical outcome in patients with aseptic meningitis resulting from herpes virus is indistinguishable from other causes, and the outcome is uniformly good. It is important, however, to differentiate between herpes simplex encephalitis, a potentially fatal disease, and the self-limited HSV aseptic meningitis.

Human Immunodeficiency Virus. Human immunodeficiency virus is a member of the Retroviridae family. Meningitis associated with HIV infection may occur as part of the primary infection, or it may occur in a patient who is already infected. Patients with acute infection usually have aseptic meningitis as part of the mononucleosis-like syndrome. Patients presenting with chronic meningitis often have other associated symptoms, such as cranial neuropathies. In addition, patients with HIV can present with CNS involvement attributable to opportunistic pathogens.

The determination of a specific etiologic virus associated with a CNS infection is not practical in most cases, particularly in mild or self-limited disease. Specific diagnosis is difficult because (1) a large number of different viruses involve the CNS, (2) viruses may come from endogenous reactivation or exogenous infection, (3) many viruses produce a spectrum of neurologic complaints, and (4) the magnitude of any neurologic illness resulting from viruses may depend on the age and immune status of the patient as well as other undefined factors. The determination of a specific viral etiology can often be made through a careful patient history; selected serologic tests (determination of virus-specific immunoglobulin M [IgM] or of a fourfold or greater rise in antibody titer between acute and convalescent sera); viral culture or polymerase chain reaction (PCR) for selected viruses; or tissue biopsy for routine light microscopy, immunofluorescence, or ultrastructural studies. Viruses isolated from body sites other than the CNS may be implicated in CNS syndromes. Appropriate specimens for culture include nasopharyngeal swabs, urine, stool, tissue, and occasionally blood. Cultures should generally be obtained within the first 5 days following onset of a viral syndrome (aseptic meningitis, meningoencephalitis, or paralytic symptoms).

Mycobacterial Infections

Mycobacteria are acid-fast bacilli with a thick cell wall containing lipids, peptidoglycans, and arabinomannans. The bacilli enter the body through respiratory droplets and multiply in the alveolar spaces or macrophages. Spread to extrapulmonary sites occurs via blood.

The most common mycobacterial infection of the CNS is **tuberculous meningitis** caused by *Mycobacterium tuberculosis.* Other mycobacteria associated with CNS infections include *Mycobacterium avium, Mycobacterium intracellulare, Mycobacterium kansasii, Mycobacterium fortuitum, Mycobacterium abscessus,* and *Mycobacterium africanus.* HIV infection is a risk factor for tuberculous meningitis. Tuberculous meningitis results when the brain tubercle ruptures into the subarachnoid space. Both the meninges and the brain itself are frequently involved, with a resulting thick exudate especially at the base of the brain. The clinical presentation of tuberculous meningitis is subacute and includes fever, headache, **meningismus,** and mental changes. Vomiting and other signs of increased intracranial pressure may occur.

Spirochetal Infections

The two spirochetes associated with CNS infection are *T. pallidum* and *B. burgdorferi. T. pallidum,* the causative agent of syphilis, enters the nervous system during early infection and can be isolated from CSF in patients with primary syphilis. Many cases of neurosyphilis are reported in patients with HIV infection. Manifestations of neurosyphilis can occur at any stage of infection, especially in patients with HIV infection. Syphilitic involvement of the CNS can take one of four forms: syphilitic meningitis, meningovascular syphilis, parenchymatous neurosyphilis, and gummatous neurosyphilis.

Involvement of the CNS can occur in patients with Lyme disease. It is usually seen in patients with early disseminated disease and is less likely during late disease. Not all cases of Lyme meningitis are preceded by the characteristic erythema migrans rash. Besides signs of meningeal irritation, some patients with Lyme meningitis can have other neurologic manifestations of Lyme disease such as cranial nerve neuropathy (commonly the seventh nerve) and radiculoneuritis.

Fungal Infections

Fungi are rare causes of CNS infection (Box 35-3). The most common organisms in CNS fungal infections are *Cryptococcus neoformans, Coccidioides immitis, Histoplasma capsulatum,* and *Blastomyces dermatitidis.* Rare cases of meningeal sporotrichosis caused by *Sporothrix schenckii* have been reported. The clinical presentation is usually of chronic meningitis. The risk factors for CNS fungal infections include acquired immunodeficiency syndrome (AIDS), organ transplantation, diabetes, or indwelling intravascular catheters. The

---

BOX 35-3 Fungal Organisms Involving the Central Nervous System

Common
Cryptococcus neoformans
Coccidioides immitis

Uncommon
Histoplasma capsulatum
Candida spp.
Aspergillus spp.
Blastomyces dermatitidis

Rare
Paracoccidiodes brasiliensis
Pseudallescheria boydii
Mucorales (*Mucor, Rhizopus, Absidia,* and *Cunninghamella* spp.)
Sporothrix schenckii
Trichosporon beigelii
Penicillium spp.
Fusarium spp.
Alternaria spp.
Curvularia spp.
Acremonium spp.
Fonsecaea spp.
Bipolaris spp.
Drechslera biseptata

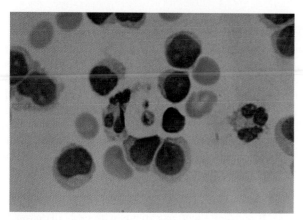

FIGURE 35-8 Cytocentrifuge preparation of cerebrospinal fluid (CSF) showing a single yeast with narrow-based budding and prominent surrounding capsule characteristic of *Cryptococcus neoformans*. Cryptococcal meningitis in partially immunocompetent hosts may show only rare organisms mixed with an inflammatory background of lymphocytes, monocytes, and eosinophils. Wright stain; high-power view.

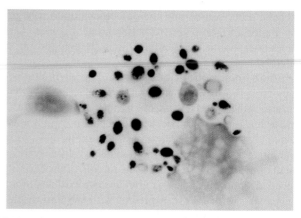

FIGURE 35-9 In contrast, cryptococcal meningitis in immunosuppressed hosts may show numerous organisms and scarce or absent inflammation. Notice the variation in size, variable Gram staining, and narrow-based budding. The organisms are evenly spaced because of their abundant polysaccharide capsules. Gram stain; cytocentrifuge preparation; medium-power view.

white blood cell count is usually moderately elevated with a predominance of lymphocytes. A predominance of eosinophils may occur in infections due to *Coccidioides* organisms.

Case Study

A 52-year-old white male arrived at an emergency department in a disoriented and poorly responsive state with labored breathing. The patient's history included poorly controlled diabetes and chronic obstructive pulmonary disease secondary to cigarette smoking. Current medications included steroids for his pulmonary disease. Physical examination showed that the patient was febrile, lethargic, and in respiratory failure. A lumbar puncture was performed. Direct smear using calcofluor reagent showed encapsulated budding yeasts. Despite aggressive therapy with amphotericin B and 5-flucytosine, the patient's condition failed to improve and he died on the third day of hospitalization.

Cryptococcus neoformans is an encapsulated basidiomycetous yeast. It can spread hematogenously to the CNS from pulmonary foci and cause chronic meningitis, particularly in patients with AIDS. There are two varieties of *C. neoformans*: var. neoformans and var. gattii. *C. neoformans* var. neoformans is the major isolate in patients with AIDS and consists of serotypes A and D. *C. neoformans* var. gattii is restricted to tropical and subtropical regions and consists of serotypes B and C. The number of organisms in the CSF may be small in immunocompetent patients (Figure 35-8) but large in immunosuppressed patients (Figure 35-9). *C. immitis* is a dimorphic fungus that causes chronic meningitis. Infections due to *C. immitis* are limited to endemic regions, mainly the southwestern United States, Mexico, and Central and South America. Human infection occurs via inhalation of arthroconidia.

Blastomyces dermatitidis is a dimorphic fungus. Inhalation of conidia results in pulmonary infection, which may disseminate to the CNS and cause an abscess or fulminant meningitis. It is endemic in the Mississippi and Ohio River basins. *H. capsulatum* is also a dimorphic fungus. In rare cases of disseminated histoplasmosis, involvement of CNS is observed. Like *B. dermatitidis*, it is endemic in the Mississippi and Ohio River basins. *Candida* spp. are causes of both fungal meningitis and cerebral abscesses. It is mainly seen in patients with invasive or disseminated candidiasis. Candidiasis may be acquired as a nosocomial infection in patients with indwelling catheters or those receiving antibacterial therapy. Central nervous system infection with *Candida* spp. can occur in patients with ventriculoperitoneal shunts. Patients with low peripheral blood neutrophil counts secondary to chemotherapy are at risk for candidal infections. *Candida albicans*, *Candida tropicalis*, and *Candida parapsilosis* are the most commonly identified species.

Parasitic Infections

Although uncommon, both protozoa and helminths can invade the CNS and cause meningitis. Some parasites cause CNS lesions without obvious meningeal inflammation. They are discussed briefly in this section.

Protozoa. The free-living amebae that can infect humans include *Naegleria fowleri*, *Acanthamoeba* spp., and *Balamuthia mandrillaris*. Trophozoites invade the nasal epithelium and migrate to the CNS via the olfactory nerve. *N. fowleri* can cause a rapidly progressive and almost always fatal **primary amebic meningoencephalitis**. *Acanthamoeba* spp. and *B. mandrillaris* usually cause granulomatous amebic encephalitis with a more insidious onset. *N. fowleri* is found in warm freshwater and moist soil. Most cases of infection have been associated with swimming in warm natural bodies of water. *Acanthamoeba* spp. are found in soil, fresh and brackish water, and sewage. No environmental sources have been identified for *B. mandrillaris*.

Helminths. Infection by the larval forms of the nematode *Angiostrongylus cantonensis* can cause eosinophilic meningitis. *A. cantonensis* infection is fairly common in certain parts of the world (e.g., Thailand, Malaysia, Vietnam). Humans become infected when they ingest larvae in snails or slugs or by eating green, leafy vegetables contaminated by these parasites. In the CNS, the larvae usually do not complete their life cycle and eventually die surrounded by an eosinophilic infiltrate. Both peripheral and CSF eosinophilia is usually seen in these patients.

Cerebral malaria is an acute illness that occurs due to sequestration of the parasite *Plasmodium falciparum* in CNS and is characterized by changes in mental status, seizures, motor defects, and coma. Human infection is initiated when the sporozoite stage of *P. falciparum* is injected into the bloodstream during mosquito feeding. The pathogenesis of cerebral malaria is not completely understood. Parasitized red blood cells develop knobs with cytoadherent properties on their surface, causing them to adhere to the endothelium of capillaries and venules in the brain. *Toxoplasma gondii* is a coccidian obligate intracellular protozoan. Humans acquire infection by eating raw or undercooked meat containing tissue cysts or by contact with feral or domestic cats. Organ transplant recipients may acquire toxoplasmosis from a donated organ. The seroprevalence of toxoplasmosis is higher in Europe and South America than in the United States. Sporozoites released from the ingested oocyst or tissue cysts invade the human small intestine, spread hematogenously, and invade cells of the viscera and possibly the brain. In immunocompromised patients, toxoplasmosis may result from primary infection or reactivation of a latent infection and commonly affects the CNS. The CSF findings (Figure 35-10) are nonspecific and include a mild lymphocytic pleocytosis and an increased CSF protein level. The diagnosis of toxoplasmosis is usually serologic, although immunocompromised patients may not demonstrate a humoral immune response to the infection. In such cases, especially if there is a focal brain lesion, diagnosis can be obtained by brain biopsy. In AIDS patients, the brain lesions have characteristic radiologic features, and the diagnosis is often confirmed by clinical response to specific therapy. Trypanosomes that infect humans include *Trypanosoma brucei* subsp. gambiense, *Trypanosoma brucei* subsp. rhodesiense, and *Trypanosoma cruzi*. The first two are found

predominantly in Africa. Humans are infected by the bite of tsetse flies. *T. brucei* gambiense results in a chronic meningoencephalitis more commonly known as sleeping sickness. CNS infection with *T. brucei* rhodesiense results in a more acute disease, often resulting in death. *T. cruzi*, the causative agent of Chagas' disease, is found in Central and South America. In immunosuppressed patients, encephalitis due to *T. cruzi* is observed.

Gnathostoma spinigerum, a gastrointestinal parasite of wild and domestic dogs and cats, may cause eosinophilic meningoencephalitis. *G. spinigerum* is common in Southeast Asia, China, and Japan. Humans acquire the infection following ingestion of undercooked infected fish and poultry. *Baylisascaris procyonis* is an ascarid parasite that is prevalent in the raccoon population in the United States and has emerged as a causative agent of human eosinophilic meningoencephalitis. Human infections occur following ingestion of food products contaminated with raccoon feces. Neurocysticercosis is a major cause of brain lesions in certain parts of the world. It is caused by the larvae of the pig tapeworm *Taenia solium*. Humans become infected by ingestion of food or water contaminated with eggs of *T. solium*. Larvae released from the eggs migrate through the intestinal wall to the CNS and form cysts in the subarachnoid space. The CSF may be normal, or it may show pleocytosis with predominance of neutrophils or eosinophils and a decreased CSF glucose level. The diagnosis is confirmed by radiographic studies and demonstration of cyst antigen in the CSF or serum using an enzyme-linked immunoelectron transfer blot test. *Paragonimus westermani*, the oriental lung fluke, is known to cause brain lesions. Human infection is confined to Japan, South Korea, Thailand, China, and the Philippines. Infection occurs by ingestion of raw or improperly cooked crustaceans. Neurologic symptoms such as epilepsy and paralysis are observed when the brain is infected. Serologic assays may be useful for the detection of *P. westermani*. *Echinococcus granulosus*, a tapeworm, causes formation of hydatid cysts in humans. Humans are infected during contact with the intermediate hosts for the parasite, such as sheep and dogs. Although the liver and lungs are the most commonly affected organs, the brain may be invaded by the parasite, resulting in seizures. Human visceral larva migrans results from ingestion of eggs of *Toxocara canis* or *Toxocara cati*. Although most of the larval stages are seen in the liver, some larvae reach the CNS and cause lesions in the brain.

Meningoencephalitis and Encephalitis

Patients with meningoencephalitis or encephalitis have involvement of the cerebral cortex. The diagnosis of encephalitis is usually inferred from the clinical presentation. Because of diffuse involvement of the cerebral cortex in patients with encephalitis, mental status changes and other focal or diffuse neurologic signs, such as seizures, are common. The most common causes of encephalitis are viruses, including herpes viruses, enteroviruses, and arboviruses. Acute meningoencephalitis due to paramyxoviruses such as Nipah virus have been reported in abattoir workers. Nonviral causes include *L. monocytogenes*, *Rickettsia*, *Bartonella*, *Mycoplasma*, *B. burgdorferi*, and *T. gondii*.

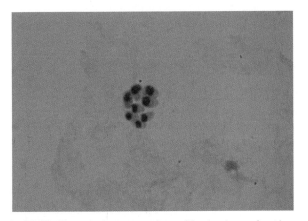

FIGURE 35-10 Touch preparation of brain tissue showing typical "floret" of *Toxoplasma gondii* trophozoites. The organisms are not typically seen in preparations of cerebrospinal fluid. Wright stain; high-power view.

Clues to the etiology of the encephalitis are sometimes available on physical examination, such as the rashes of Lyme disease, Rocky Mountain spotted fever (RMSF), or herpes zoster. History of tick bite may suggest a diagnosis of RMSF, Colorado tick fever, Lyme disease, or ehrlichiosis. Herpes simplex encephalitis in adults may follow primary herpesvirus infection or result from reactivation of a previous herpesvirus infection. Neonatal herpes simplex meningoencephalitis usually reflects disseminated herpetic disease. Beyond the neonatal period, HSV encephalitis is usually caused by HSV-1. Patients usually have fever, altered sensorium, and focal neurologic symptoms consistent with temporal lobe involvement. Encephalitis from other herpes viruses is less common.

Arboviruses (arthropod-borne viruses) are RNA viruses that demonstrate strong tropism for the CNS. These viruses are transmitted to humans by mosquitoes, ticks, or sandflies. Important arboviruses in the Western Hemisphere include members of the α-viruses (eastern equine encephalitis [EEE], western equine encephalitis [WEE], and Venezuelan equine encephalitis [VEE] viruses), *Flavivirus* (St. Louis encephalitis virus [SLE]), *Bunyavirus* (La Crosse [LAC] virus), and *Coltivirus* (Colorado tick fever virus). The incidence of these infections can vary with the geographic region. EEE, the most severe arthropod-borne encephalitis in the United States, is typically a fulminant disease leading to coma and death in one third of cases and serious neurologic sequelae in another third. It is endemic along the entire East Coast of the United States. Infections are most common in young children and the elderly. WEE occurs predominantly in the midwestern and western United States. The clinical severity of WEE is intermediate, with a case fatality of 5%. VEE is endemic in Central America and Florida. WEE and VEE are difficult to distinguish from EEE on clinical grounds, and infants and young children are at greatest risk for infection. Fortunately the risk of fatal encephalitis is much lower (about 10% in WEE and 0.6% in VEE). Despite its name, SLE has been reported throughout the United States. Children and older adults experience more severe illness. It can present with confusion, fever, slow disease progression, lack of focal neurologic findings, generalized weakness, and tremors. The risk of fatal encephalitis is estimated at about 10%. LAC is the most commonly isolated member of the California serogroup of bunyaviruses. Encephalitis resulting from LAC virus occurs most commonly in Ohio, Illinois, Wisconsin, and Minnesota. Children are most commonly afflicted. LAC virus and the other California serogroup viruses are relatively benign arboviral infections, with a mortality rate of less than 1%. West Nile virus (WNV) is a mosquito-borne flavivirus that commonly causes a self-limited febrile illness, often associated with a rash. In 1999 the virus was introduced in the United States and has since spread rapidly. Neurologic involvement includes aseptic meningitis, myelitis, and fatal encephalitis. The mortality rate is about 5%, and death occurs mainly in older patients. Colorado tick fever virus belongs to the *Coltivirus* genus of Reoviridae. In addition to meningoencephalitis, Colorado tick fever virus shows a peculiar tropism for the bone marrow, and infection is often accompanied by leukopenia and thrombocytopenia. Rabies is a zoonosis caused by a bullet-shaped RNA virus of the genus *Lyssavirus*. Infection occurs following bites from infected animals, such as skunks, raccoons, bats, and foxes, as well as unimmunized domesticated animals such as dogs. Initial symptoms include fatigue, gastrointestinal symptoms, and pain at the bite wound. Rabies can present as acute encephalitis indistinguishable from other viral encephalitides or with the classic syndrome of agitation, emotional lability, seizures, and hallucinations (furious rabies). Less commonly, rabies may manifest as paralysis followed by coma and death (dumb rabies). Diagnosis is confirmed by demonstration of rabies antigen (by immunofluorescence) in neck skin biopsies or by demonstration of rabies antigen or characteristic inclusions (Negri bodies) in neurons of the brains of patients or infected animals.

Brain Abscesses

In contrast to the superficial meningeal inflammation seen in meningitis, brain abscesses are circumscribed areas of tissue destruction containing organisms and inflammatory cells. A cerebral abscess begins as a focal area of acute inflammation, followed by the development of a necrotic center and the presence of macrophages and fibroblasts in the periphery. Eventually there is a diminution in the necrotic center and formation of a collagenous capsule.

Most cerebral abscesses occur as a result of spread from a contiguous focus of infection in the middle ear, mastoid cells, or paranasal sinuses. Brain abscesses secondary to ear infections are usually localized in the temporal lobe or cerebellum, and those attributable to spread from paranasal sinuses or from dental infections are seen in the frontal lobe. The second common mechanism for development of brain abscess is by hematogenous spread from a distant focus of infection such as lung abscess, bronchiectasis, empyema, infective endocarditis, and intra-abdominal infections. Brain abscess can also develop secondary to trauma with dural breach or following neurosurgery. In some patients none of these pathogenic mechanisms is evident. The microorganism isolated from brain abscess often depends on the predisposing condition. In patients with brain abscess secondary to ear or sinus infection, the common organisms include streptococci, *Bacteroides,* and *Prevotella,* whereas in patients with penetrating trauma or infective endocarditis, *S. aureus* is more likely to be identified. Neutropenic or transplant patients are more susceptible to developing infections by fungi such as *Aspergillus* or *Mucorales* spp., and patients with HIV are more likely to have infection from *T. gondii, Nocardia* spp., or *Mycobacterium* spp.

Bacterial Pathogens

The most common organism isolated from nontraumatic brain abscesses include aerobic, anaerobic, and microaerophilic streptococci (Figure 35-11). Streptococci such as *S. anginosus, S. intermedius,* and *S. constellatus* are isolated in 50% to 70% of cases. Mixed infections are seen in 30% to 40% of cases. Anaerobes commonly identified from brain abscess include *Bacteroides* spp. and *Prevotella* spp. Enteric gram-negative aerobes such as *E. coli, Proteus* spp., and *Enterobacter* organisms can sometimes cause brain abscess. *Citrobacter diversus* meningitis is often associated with brain abscess. In neonates, *E. sakazakii* has been reported to cause brain

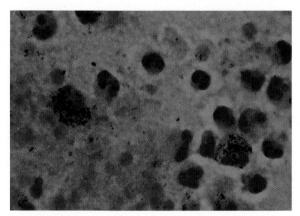

FIGURE 35-11   Direct smear of aspirated brain abscess contents. Clusters of intracellular gram-positive cocci in groups are consistent with microaerophilic streptococci. Gram stain; noncytocentrifuge preparation; high-power view.

abscesses. *Actinomyces* and *Nocardia* spp. may also be isolated from patients with brain abscess. Nocardial abscess is more common in patients with HIV, organ-transplant patients, or those on corticosteroid therapy.

Fungal Pathogens

The increasing use of immunosuppressive drugs and broad-spectrum antimicrobials has contributed to the increasing incidence of fungal brain abscess. Besides *Candida* spp., *Aspergillus* and zygomycetes (*Mucor, Rhizopus,* and *Absidia*) are the common fungi that can cause brain abscess. Invasive candidiasis is more common in patients with indwelling catheters, in those receiving hyperalimentation, or those on chronic steroid therapy. *Aspergillus* infection results from dissemination of the organism from a primary focus, usually the lung, or by direct extension, such as from the paranasal sinuses. Mucormycosis is more commonly seen in patients with diabetic ketoacidosis, transplant or hematologic malignancies. The organism enters the nervous system from the paranasal sinuses by eroding the frontal bone to reach the CNS (rhinocerebral mucormycosis) or by hematogenous dissemination. Other fungi occasionally isolated from cerebral abscesses include *B. dermatitidis, C. neoformans, Coccidioides* spp., and *Pseudallescheria boydii.*

LABORATORY DIAGNOSIS OF CENTRAL NERVOUS SYSTEM INFECTIONS

The diagnosis of CNS infections is based on examination of CSF samples obtained by lumbar puncture. Blood cultures are often helpful in identifying the causative microorganism. The CSF sample is obtained by inserting a sterile, hollow needle into the spinal subarachnoid space in the lower (lumbar) back (Figure 35-12). Lumbar puncture is often performed after obtaining computed tomography (CT) scan in cases with elevated intracranial pressure or focal neurologic lesions because of the risk of brain herniation. In patients with brain abscess, aspirates and tissue samples are helpful because CSF may be normal.

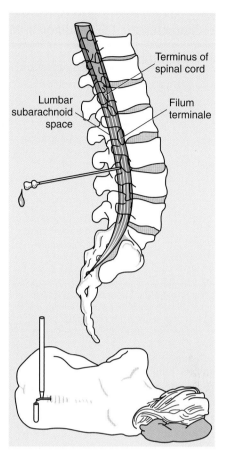

FIGURE 35-12   Lumbar puncture. The cerebrospinal fluid is obtained by inserting a long, sterile, hollow needle into the spinal subarachnoid space in the lumbar region.

Cerebrospinal Fluid Transport and Analysis

The CSF samples should be transported to the laboratory without delay and processed as soon as possible to prevent loss of viability of the causative agent. If delay cannot be avoided, CSF samples should be stored at room temperature until processed (within 24 hours). For viral testing, CSF samples may be stored at 2° to 8° C short term (less than 48 hours) and at −70° C long term. When large volumes (greater than 1 mL) of CSF sample are available, concentration by centrifugation improves yield of microorganism for microscopic examination and culture. It is standard to obtain three to four tubes of CSF, each containing 1 or 2 mL of fluid. Cultures are performed using samples that have the least likelihood of contamination (second or third tube). The CSF is analyzed for glucose and protein concentration, cell counts, and identification of etiologic agent by Gram stain, culture, antigen detection, and PCR. Meningitis is suspected from the presenting clinical symptoms and initial CSF studies, including visual inspection, chemical analysis, and cell counts. The characteristic CSF laboratory findings are compared for a variety of infectious disorders in Table 35-1.

Culture

Isolation of fastidious organisms would require special medium and incubation conditions. Anaerobic bacteria rarely

TABLE 35-1 Characteristic CSF Findings in Meningitis

	Bacterial	Fungal	Tuberculous	Syphilitic	Viral	Parasitic
Organisms seen in CSF	Usually	Less common	Rare	None	None	Rare
Cell count (leukocytes/microliter)	100-100,000 neutrophils predominate	Normal-500 lymphocytes predominate*	50-500 lymphocytes predominate[†]	100-750 lymphocytes predominate	Normal-200 lymphocytes predominate[‡]	Normal-200 lymphocytes and/or eosinophils predominate
Protein (mg/dL)	100-500	Normal-250	Normal-150	50-250	Frequently normal	Usually increased
Glucose	Usually markedly decreased	Normal to decreased	Usually decreased	Normal	Normal	Normal to decreased
Additional findings	Bacterial antigen test	Calcofluor concentrated specimen; latex agglutination (i.e., *Cryptococcus neoformans*)	Polymerase chain reaction, auramine-rhodamine on concentrated specimen	Positive VDRL	Serology, polymerase chain reaction, culture, biopsy	Serology, biopsy

CSF, Cerebrospinal fluid; *VDRL*, Venereal Disease Research Laboratory.
*May have normal CSF cell count with *C. neoformans*. Eosinophils may predominate in *C. immitis* infection.
[†]Neutrophils may predominate in early meningitis.
[‡]CSF cell count may be more than 1000 leukocytes/mL in lymphocytic choriomeningitis virus infection. Neutrophils may predominate in early meningitis.

cause meningitis but are commonly associated with brain abscess. Transport media such as the modified Stuart's medium or Amies medium are generally sufficient for isolation of most microorganisms including anaerobes. Sheep blood and chocolate agar incubated in 3% to 5% CO_2 is usually used for bacterial culture of CSF. When CSF samples are collected from shunts, broth media should also be inoculated.

Bacterial Infections

In acute bacterial meningitis, the CSF is turbid or cloudy as protein levels are significantly raised. Glucose levels are very low (i.e., less than 40% of the serum glucose concentration) in most patients with bacterial meningitis. The gold standard for diagnosis of bacterial meningitis is culture of CSF. Staining techniques are rapid but less sensitive than culture. The sensitivity of Gram stain ranges from 40% to 90%, depending on whether the patient received antimicrobial therapy prior to lumbar puncture. Latex agglutination tests for the detection of *H. influenzae* type b, *S. pneumoniae,* group B streptococci, and *N. meningitidis* are available; however, these kits do not detect group B meningococci and coagulase-negative staphylococci. False-positive results can occur because of cross-reactivity with other bacterial species. False-negative results have been observed in specimens from pregnant women and infants. Routine use of antigen detection methods for diagnosis of bacterial meningitis is of limited value because the performance of the antigen test is similar to Gram stain and finding of a positive antigen test usually does not alter the course of therapy. However, bacterial antigen testing may be beneficial in instances where cultures are negative and the clinical suspicion of bacterial meningitis is high or in cases of partially treated meningitis with sterile cultures. The Limulus amebocyte lysate (LAL) test has also been used on a limited basis to screen CSF for gram-negative agents of meningitis. The LAL uses hemolymph from the horseshoe crab, which

clots on exposure to small amounts of lipopolysaccharide (endotoxin) present in the cell wall of gram-negative bacteria; however, the assay does not distinguish between the different gram-negative bacteria. Multiplex PCR assay for the simultaneous detection of the different *N. meningitidis* serogroups (A, B, C, W-135, and Y) is being developed.

Viral Infections

In viral infections, the number of lymphocytes in the CSF is increased. The diagnosis of viral meningitis is based on detection of viral genome by PCR or antigen detection by fluorescent antibody or enzyme immunoassay. The sensitivity of viral culture is only 14% to 24% compared with 88% to 94% with PCR, making PCR the method of choice for detection of viral causes of meningitis. The sensitivity and specificity of PCR assays can vary in relation to the virus being tested. Cell culture is recommended for enteroviruses. Recently, the GeneXpert enterovirus assay, a real-time multiplex PCR assay for detection of enterovirus RNA in CSF, has become available. A positive result with the GeneXpert enterovirus assay does not rule out other causes of meningitis. The results from this assay should be interpreted in conjunction with available clinical and laboratory information. Real-time PCR assays are available for detection of HPeV. For HSV, diagnosis includes detection of HSV DNA in CSF by PCR, growth of HSV on culture, antigen detection in brain biopsy samples, and demonstration of antibody in CSF and serum. The antigen and antibody assays have low sensitivity and are positive in the later stage of the disease. Although the PCR assay is highly sensitive, a false-negative result may be obtained in CSF samples obtained within the first 48 hours of illness. Repeat testing is helpful in such cases. In the case of infections from WNV, detection of IgM antibodies confirmed by the WNV plaque reduction neutralization antibody test is used for diagnosis along with PCR and culture. The laboratory diagnosis of JE virus is based on virus isolation, detection of viral RNA by PCR, and virus-specific antibodies. The diagnosis of Japanese encephalitis by serum and CSF immunoglobulin M (IgM) antibody capture ELISA (MAC ELISA) is widely accepted.

Mycobacterial Infections

Tuberculous meningitis is characterized by excess of lymphocytes, elevated protein, and reduced glucose. The gold standard for diagnosis is identification of mycobacteria in the CSF by acid-fast staining and culture. Broth medium (e.g., Middlebrook 7H9, Dubos) and solid agar medium (e.g., Middlebrook 7H11, Löwenstein-Jensen) are used routinely to culture mycobacteria but require a long incubation period. Use of the mycobacterial growth indicator tube or other automated systems such as the MB/BacT (Organon Teknika, Durham, N.C.), ESP (Trek Diagnostic System, Westlake, Ohio), BACTEC9000 TB series or BACTEC460 can improve recovery and reduce the time to detection of mycobacteria in CSF. Staining is positive in 10% to 22% of cases, and cultures are positive in 38% to 88% of cases. The number of mycobacteria in the CSF is usually small; therefore concentration of the CSF sample is useful in improving recovery of the bacteria. Other techniques may be helpful, such as the detection of mycobacterial antigen, antimycobacterial antibodies, or the detection of mycobacterial DNA by PCR. Commercial PCR assays are available for detection of *M. tuberculosis* in sputum and bronchial aspirates. These PCR assays have also been used for detection of mycobacteria in CSF; however, false-positive results do occur, and a negative test does not exclude tuberculous meningitis. The PCR assays should be used in conjunction with culture.

Fungal Infections

Direct microscopic examination of Gram-stained or India ink–stained CSF samples, calcofluor-stained tissue samples, and culture are used for diagnosis of fungal causes of CNS infection. Concentration methods can improve the sensitivity of fungal staining and culture. Several media are available for fungal cultures of CSF or CNS tissue. All fungal cultures should be incubated for 4 to 6 weeks. Antigen detection by latex agglutination test is useful in the case of infections due to *C. neoformans* and *H. capsulatum*. The latex agglutination tests for *C. neoformans* show false-positive results with rheumatoid factor and in patients with infections due to *Trichosporon* spp., *Stomatococcus mucilaginosus,* or *Capnocytophaga canimorsus*. False-negative results may be observed because of infection with a poorly encapsulated strain or low fungal burden. The CSF and serum galactomannan levels are useful for the diagnosis of *Aspergillus* infections. Antibody detection using the complement fixation assay and immunodiffusion is useful for diagnosis of *C. immitis*. PCR tests for routine detection of fungal DNA are not standardized.

Parasitic Infections

The identification of parasitic causes of CNS infections is usually based on microscopic examination of Giemsa- or Calcofluor-stained aspirate or biopsy samples. Culture using agar with bacterial overlay is recommended for free living ameba such as *Naegleria* and *Acanthamoeba* but not for *B.*

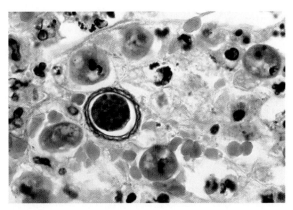

FIGURE 35-13   This photomicrograph shows a magnified view of brain tissue within which is a centrally located *Acanthamoeba* sp. cyst. (Courtesy George Healy, Ph.D., Centers for Disease Control and Prevention, Atlanta, Ga: http://phil.cdc.gov/phil/details.asp.)

mandrillaris (Figure 35-13). Serology and PCR testing are available for detection of *Toxoplasma*. Antibody detection by immunoblot is used as an adjunct serologic test for confirmation of radiologic diagnosis in patients with neurocysticercosis. Diagnosis of human trypanosomiasis is mainly by examination of unstained and Giemsa-stained blood smears, lymph node aspirates, marrow, or CSF for trypomastigotes. Other methods such as the card agglutination trypanosomiasis test (CATT), various concentration techniques, and PCR have been developed for detection of trypanosomes but are mainly used as research tools. Concentration techniques using the quantitative buffy coat analysis tubes improve the sensitivity of detection of the parasite. Hematocrit centrifugation and anion-exchange column chromatography also improve the sensitivity of parasite detection. Examination of CSF processed by a double-centrifugation technique often reveals trypanosomes in patients with late stage of the disease.

BIBLIOGRAPHY

American Academy of Pediatrics: Pneumococcal infections. In Pickering LK, editor: *Red book: 2003 report of the Committee on Infectious Diseases*, ed 26, Elk Grove Village, Ill, 2003, American Academy of Pediatrics.

Connolly KJ, Hammer SM: The acute aseptic meningitis syndrome, *Infect Dis Clin North Am* 45:99, 1990.

Food and Drug Administration: *Safety alert: risks of devices for direct detection of group B streptococcal antigen*, Washington, DC, 1997, Department of Health and Human Services.

Gamboa F et al: Direct detection of *Mycobacterium tuberculosis* complex in nonrespiratory specimens by Gen-Probe amplified mycobacterium tuberculosis direct test, *J Clin Microbiol* 35:307, 1997.

Gray LD, Fedorko DP: Laboratory diagnosis of bacterial meningitis, *Clin Microbiol Rev* 5:130, 1992.

Perkins MD, Mirrett S, Reller LB: Rapid bacterial antigen detection is not clinically useful, *J Clin Microbiol* 33:1486, 1995.

Pfyffer GE et al: Diagnostic performance of amplified *Mycobacterium tuberculosis* direct test with cerebrospinal fluid, other nonrespiratory, and respiratory specimens, *J Clin Microbiol* 34:834, 1995.

Rosenstein NE et al: Meningococcal disease, *N Engl J Med* 344:1378, 2001.

Saez-Llorens X, McCracken GH: Bacterial meningitis in neonates and children, *Infect Dis Clin North Am* 4:623, 1990.

Swartz MN: Bacterial meningitis—a view of the past 90 years, *N Engl J Med* 351:1826, 2004.

Thomson RB, Bertram H: Laboratory diagnosis of central nervous system infections, *Infect Dis Clin North Am* 15:1047, 2001.

Tunkel AR, Scheld WM: Acute meningitis. In Mandell GL, Bennett JE, Dolin R, editors: *Principles and practice of infectious diseases*, vol 1, ed 6, Philadelphia, 2005, Elsevier.

Wolthers KC et al: Human parechoviruses as an important viral cause of sepsis like illness and meningitis in young children, *Clin Infect Dis* 47:358, 2008.

Points to Remember

- Host-related risk factors and pathogen-specific virulence factors are important in the pathogenesis of central nervous system (CNS) infections.
- The characteristics of the cerebrospinal fluid (CSF) such as chemical and cellular features, may provide presumptive diagnostic clues to the etiology of CNS infection.
- The age and immune status of the host will help to determine likely causative pathogens.
- Virulence factors of disease-producing organisms enable them to evade host defense mechanisms and cause clinical infection.
- The prevalence of different viral pathogens varies according to seasonal changes.
- The occurrence of opportunistic disease in patients with HIV infection is a function of underlying host immunodeficiency as well as pathogen virulence.
- Immunocompromised patients, including those who have had bone marrow or organ transplants, are at increased risk for certain types of meningitis.

Learning Assessment Questions

1. How is cerebrospinal fluid (CSF) produced and distributed in the central nervous system (CNS)?

2. How would you characterize normal CSF?

3. What are the common bacterial pathogens causing meningitis? What are the host-related and virulence-related factors associated with each pathogen?

4. How would you compare the physical, chemical, and cellular findings of the CSF during bacterial, fungal, tuberculous, and viral meningitis?

5. Which fungal species are typically associated with intracerebral abscesses?

6. Which fungal species are associated with meningitis?

7. Why should you examine CSF specimens as soon as they are received?

8. How would you initially evaluate the CSF sample?

9. What types of culture media should be used to recover bacterial pathogens?

10. What rapid and other ancillary methods are useful in evaluating CNS infections?

Bacteremia and Sepsis

Maribeth L. Flaws

OBJECTIVES

After reading and studying this chapter, you should be able to:

1. Define bacteremia and differentiate this condition from septicemia.

2. Classify each type of bacteremia and describe when each condition occurs.

3. Discuss the epidemiology and pathogenesis of bacteremia.

4. Associate specific organisms with each type of bacteremia.

5. Explain the pathophysiology of sepsis and septic shock.

6. List the most common organisms isolated from blood cultures and evaluate the significance of these organisms when recovered from blood culture samples.

7. Describe the proper procedure for blood culture collection.

8. Discuss the methods for the detection of bacteremia, including the following:
   - Media
   - Blood culture additives
   - Methods of removing antimicrobials
   - Advantages and disadvantages of each procedure described

9. Name the methods that are used to isolate viruses, fungi, and fastidious and unusual bacteria from the blood.

10. Describe therapies for sepsis and septic shock.

Case in Point

A 4-year-old boy with acute lymphocytic leukemia was undergoing induction chemotherapy administered via an indwelling Hickman catheter and was hospitalized because of fever and granulocytopenia. His admission white blood cell and platelet counts were 600 µL and 55,000 µL, respectively, and his temperature was 103° F (39.4° C). Blood cultures were drawn before antibiotics were administered. He was immediately given ceftazidime and vancomycin. Blood cultures yielded gram-positive cocci in clusters after 24 hours of incubation. Removal and culture of the Hickman catheter and culture tip yielded gram-positive cocci in clusters with the same susceptibility pattern as those isolated from the blood.

Key Terms

Antibiotic removal device (ARD)

Bacteremia

Community-acquired bacteremia

Continuous bacteremia

Disseminated intravascular coagulation (DIC)

Fungemia

Intermittent bacteremia

Nosocomial bacteremia

Occult (unsuspected) bacteremia

Polymicrobial bacteremia

Primary bacteremia

Pseudobacteremia

Secondary bacteremia

Sepsis

Septicemia

Septic shock

Sodium polyanetholsulfonate (SPS)

Systemic inflammatory response syndrome (SIRS)

Transient bacteremia

Viremia

Bacteremia is the presence of viable bacteria in the blood. Although bacteremia may be a transient, self-limited phenomenon without clinical consequences, it frequently reflects the presence of serious infection. Life-threatening infections caused by bacteremia are a particular concern in patients who are immunocompromised, either through drug or chemotherapeutic intervention or as the result of preexisting disease and subsequent immunosuppression. Bacteremia is often associated with hospitalization, insertion of foreign bodies such as catheters into blood vessels, and other kinds of procedures.

This chapter begins with general concepts pertinent to bacteremic infections, including definitions of conditions relating to bacteremia and how each condition manifests. This chapter then does the following:

- Discusses the epidemiology, risk factors for, and pathogenesis of bacteremia
- Describes infections associated with bacteremia
- Presents diagnostic laboratory procedures
- Explains treatment modalities

GENERAL CONCEPTS RELATED TO BACTEREMIC INFECTIONS

Definitions

The presence of viable bacteria in the blood, as determined by its growth in a blood culture, is known as **bacteremia.** As such it is a laboratory finding that may or may not indicate

infection. Blood cultures may also be positive as a result of contamination of blood samples during phlebotomy, leading to false-positive results, a phenomenon termed **pseudobacteremia.** Such contamination is most often due to skin commensals, such as coagulase-negative staphylococci (CoNS). Pseudobacteremia is not an indication of infection and does not require therapy. Growth of CoNS or other skin flora from a blood culture does not always represent pseudobacteremia, however, and may indicate true bacteremia, depending on the clinical situation.

Even when growth of an organism from a blood culture reflects a true-positive result, bacteremia may not be associated with any physical signs or symptoms of severe infection, a condition known as **occult (unsuspected) bacteremia.** Occult bacteremia frequently occurs in children younger than 2 years of age and is most often due to *Streptococcus pneumoniae.* Because of the lack of clinical evidence for serious infection in such patients, the diagnosis of bacteremia may be overlooked, with potentially catastrophic consequences if treatment is delayed.

Usually, however, bacteremia that reflects true infection results in systemic physiologic responses that indicate the presence of a serious infection. In the past, the term **septicemia** was used to indicate bacteremia plus a clinical presentation of physical signs and symptoms of bacterial invasion and toxin production. *Septicemia* is still a term used clinically and in the collection of epidemiologic data on causes of death. Because of its imprecision in defining a disease state, however, it is not suitable for categorizing all patients who have bacteremia-related infections or for designing clinical trials. To facilitate the study of the pathogenesis and treatment of the consequences of severe infections, including those associated with bacteremia, an international consensus conference of the American College of Chest Physicians and the Society of Critical Care Medicine devised standardized definitions of the response to infection, shown in Table 36-1. The **systemic inflammatory response syndrome (SIRS)** comprises a spectrum of increasingly severe conditions ranging from **sepsis** (infection with a systemic inflammatory response) to severe sepsis (sepsis accompanied by organ dysfunction, hypotension, or tissue hypoperfusion) to **septic shock** (sepsis accompanied by refractory hypotension). As might be expected, the risk of death progressively increases as patients move along this continuum. Although bacteremia may result in sepsis, severe sepsis, or septic shock, these responses are not automatically associated with bacteremia; for example, blood cultures may be negative in more than 70% of septic patients, despite clear clinical signs of infection.

Classification of Bacteremia

Classification by Site of Origin

Bacteremia may be classified by its site of origin. **Primary bacteremia** occurs when the bacteria are present in an endovascular source such as an infected cardiac valve or an infected intravenous catheter, whereas **secondary bacteremia** occurs when the bacteria are coming from an infected extravascular source, such as the lung in patients with pneumonia. A case in which the source of bacteremia remains undefined is termed

TABLE 36-1 Definition of Terms Related to Severe Infection

Term	Definition
Systemic inflammatory response syndrome	Systemic response to a variety of clinical insults. Criteria include at least two of the following: Temperature > 38° C or <36° C Heart rate > 90 beats/minute Respiratory rate > 20 breaths/minute, or $PaCO_2$ < 32 mm Hg White blood cell count > 12,000/mm^3 or <4000/mm^3, or >10% band forms
Sepsis	Infection with systemic inflammatory response
Hypotension	Systolic blood pressure < 90 mm Hg, mean arterial pressure < 70 mm Hg, or reduction > 40 mm Hg from baseline
Severe sepsis	Sepsis associated with organ dysfunction, hypoperfusion, or hypotension
Septic shock	Sepsis with hypotension despite adequate fluid resuscitation and requiring pressor therapy, along with perfusion abnormalities

bacteremia of unknown origin. Classification in this manner has important clinical consequences because it determines the appropriate therapy and prognosis. For example, a secondary bacteremia from an infected focus, such as an abscess, may require surgical therapy to remove the abscess or source of infection in addition to antimicrobials to achieve cure of the infection. Bacteremias of unknown origin generally have a poorer prognosis than primary or secondary bacteremia.

Classification by Causative Agent

Bacteremia may also be categorized by the general class of microorganism or specific pathogen that has invaded the bloodstream. Gram-positive bacteremia is due to organisms such as *Streptococcus pneumoniae, Staphylococcus aureus,* or *Enterococcus faecium,* whereas gram-negative bacteremia is due to organisms such as *Escherichia coli* or *Pseudomonas aeruginosa.* Anaerobic bacteremia is due to organisms such as *Bacteroides fragilis,* whereas **polymicrobial bacteremia** is due to a mixture of organisms. General classification of bacteremias in this fashion can provide initial clues to the underlying source of a bacteremia and guide therapy even before organisms have been speciated. For example, CoNS bacteremia in a hospitalized patient is frequently due to infection of an indwelling vascular device, whereas polymicrobial bacteremia with a mixture of enterococci and gram-negative organisms is frequently due to invasion of the bloodstream by gastrointestinal flora from bowel perforation.

Classification by Place of Acquisition

Bacteremia can also be categorized by its place of acquisition. **Community-acquired bacteremia,** as the term suggests, occurs in individuals living in the general community, whereas **nosocomial bacteremia** occurs in patients who are hospitalized or living in a nursing home or other facility. In order to avoid misclassification of bacteremia that began just at the time of hospital admission as nosocomial when it is really community-acquired, nosocomial bacteremia is conventionally defined as any bacteremia occurring more than 72 hours after hospital admission. Certain bacteremias are more often community-acquired; for example, more than 90% of cases of *S. pneumoniae* bacteremia are acquired in the community. Others, such as those due to *P. aeruginosa* or *Enterococcus* species, are much more likely to be nosocomial. The place of acquisition may thus be extremely significant in guiding initial therapy; for example, nosocomial bacteremia is more likely to be due to resistant organisms that express β-lactamases or other resistance factors that inactivate first-line antimicrobial agents.

Classification by Duration

Bacteremia may also be classified by the duration of a bacteremic episode. Bacteremic episodes may be transient, intermittent, or continuous. The frequency, time, and number of blood cultures to be collected may depend on the type of bacteremic episode the patient is experiencing. **Transient bacteremia** usually occurs after a procedural manipulation of a particular body site that is colonized by indigenous flora causing the organisms to enter the blood. Such sites include the mouth and the gastrointestinal and urogenital tracts. Transient bacteremia may appear for a brief period following dental, colonoscopic, or cystoscopic procedures. The organisms are normally rapidly cleared by the host immune defense and so their presence is rarely symptomatic. **Intermittent bacteremia** can occur because of the presence of abscesses somewhere in the body or as a clinical manifestation of certain types of infections, such as meningococcemia and gonococcemia or pneumonia. In intermittent bacteremia, organisms are periodically released from the primary site of infection into the blood. **Continuous bacteremia** occurs when the organisms are coming from an intravascular source and are consistently present in the bloodstream. Infective endocarditis is the most common clinical manifestation associated with continuous bacteremia, although other endovascular sources such as infected intravascular catheters or septic thrombi can also result in continuous bacteremia.

EPIDEMIOLOGY

Incidence and Mortality

Brill reported the first case of bacteremia (due to *Bacillus pyocyaneus,* now *Pseudomonas aeruginosa*) in 1899. Ten years later fewer than 40 cases had been reported worldwide, with fewer than 30 additional cases in the following 15 years. Between 1950 and 2003, however, the mortality rate due to septicemia increased almost 40-fold. Septicemia (defined based on ICD-10) was the 10th leading cause of death overall in the United States in 2006 (1.4% of total deaths). There was a significant decrease in the rate of death due to septicemia, though, in 2006 as compared with 2005 (1.8%), but the overall death rate was 1.9% lower during that same time period or 2.8% lower when the rate is adjusted for changes in age distribution over time. Bacterial sepsis was the eighth leading cause of death among infants, causing 2.8% of infant deaths in 2006.

The incidence of septic shock in bacteremic patients varies from 10% to 30%, depending on the pathogen, the source of bacteremia, the presence of immunosuppression, and the presence or absence of comorbid conditions, but, once present, septic shock is associated with a mortality rate of 40% to 50%. Mortality rates in patients with bacteremia without shock range from 10% to 20%, depending on the underlying source of the bacteremia. Patients with severe sepsis and septic shock who have three or more failing organs have a mortality rate of 70%. Factors associated with an unfavorable outcome in bacteremia include age greater than 70 years; polymicrobial bacteremia; presence of malignancy, acquired immune deficiency syndrome (AIDS), or renal failure; origin of the bacteremia in the respiratory tract or bowel; unknown origin of bacteremia; and inappropriate antimicrobial therapy.

Risk Factors

The increased incidence of bacteremia during the past 25 years may be due to the following, some of which have also changed over the same time period:

- Decreased immune competency of selected patient populations
- Increased use of invasive procedures
- Age of the patient
- Antimicrobial resistance
- Diagnostic criteria and coding practices

Decreased Immune Competency of Selected Patient Populations

Bacteremias are more frequent among persons with neoplasia (abnormal growth of new cells that may be benign or malignant), especially those with hematologic malignancies, those receiving immunosuppressive chemotherapy, and those undergoing bone marrow transplantation. This is due in part to the decrease in circulating neutrophils in such patients as well as to disruption in the gastrointestinal mucosa attributable to chemotherapy, allowing invasion of normal flora into the bloodstream. Persons with other chronic underlying diseases (e.g., diabetes, cirrhosis) and those receiving immunosuppressive therapy (e.g., those receiving glucocorticoids for rheumatoid arthritis) are also at increased risk for bacteremia. Infection with human immunodeficiency virus (HIV) also predisposes patients to increased bacteremias because of the immunosuppression caused by the virus.

Increased Use of Invasive Procedures

Increased use of indwelling devices, respirators, and invasive diagnostic procedures may play a role in the occurrence of bacteremia. The widespread use of semipermanent vascular catheters to administer chemotherapy to cancer patients or to provide vascular access for hemodialysis in patients with end-stage renal disease increases the risk of bacteremia by breaking the normal integrity of the skin and permitting colonization of a foreign body in direct contact with the bloodstream. More than 80,000 bacteremias occur annually in the United States due to infected central venous catheters. Indwelling urethral catheters, suprapubic catheters, and intravenous (IV) pyelograms also predispose patients to catheter infections by penetrating otherwise sterile areas, encouraging colonization with bacteria from surrounding tissue. Surgery involving the urinary, gastrointestinal, and biliary tracts may also result in bacteremia because of the disruption of mucosal barriers that normally function to block the spread of resident flora.

Age of the Patient

Bacteremias are more prevalent in people at the extremes of age, with infants and adults older than 50 years being most susceptible. Both infants and older adults have decreased immune system function as compared with people from ages 1 to 50 because in very young patients a competent immune response has not yet fully developed. In older adult populations, there is a general decrease in immune competency with age. The presence of comorbid conditions such as diabetes, hypertension, chronic obstructive pulmonary disease, and congestive heart failure in older adults and neoplastic disorders, HIV infection, and low and very low birth weights in neonates and infants significantly increased the incidence of bacteremia in these groups.

Antimicrobial Resistance

The indiscriminate administration of broad-spectrum antimicrobials reduces susceptible normal microbiota and favors colonization and invasion by resistant bacteria. A recent survey of hospitals around the United States revealed that on average 36% of *S. aureus* isolates were resistant to methicillin (oxacillin), 10% of *Enterococcus* was resistant to vancomycin, 5% of *Klebsiella* species were resistant to ceftazidime, and 6% of *E. coli* isolates were resistant to ciprofloxacin. In addition, 66% of the hospitals responding to the survey reported that their rate of methicillin-resistant *S. aureus* had increased over the previous 3 years, whereas 4% of responding hospitals reported a decrease in the percentage of *S. aureus* isolates that were resistant to methicillin. An increasing population of antimicrobial resistant organisms results in bacteremias that are harder to treat and thereby increases mortality rates.

Diagnostic Criteria and Coding Practices

The factors just described have been shown to lead to a real increase in the incidence of bacteremia. There may be some artifactual increase in the incidence of bacteremia because of variations in the diagnostic criteria of bacteremia and how bacteremias are coded in the patient record. It is difficult to compare rates from one study to another because of these changes over time (e.g., pre-consensus conference to post-consensus conference) and changes from hospital to hospital and physician to physician. In addition, there are multiple *International Classification of Diseases* (ICD) codes that may apply to bacteremia; for example, bacteremia, septicemia, septicemic, disseminated fungal infection, disseminated candida infection, and disseminated fungal endocarditis are all assigned separate ICD-9 codes. Investigators in different studies may consider some or all of these when evaluating bacteremia rates. Finally, each revision of the ICD is slightly different. Since 1994 hospitals have been using the 10th revision of ICD.

ETIOLOGY

Over the past 25 years, the pattern of organisms responsible for bacteremia has shifted. In the 1960s and 1970s, gram-negative organisms such as *E. coli* and *P. aeruginosa* predominated in prospective studies of bacteremia. In the 1980s and 1990s, the pattern shifted so that most bacteremias were due to gram-positive organisms such as *S. aureus*, CoNS, and *Enterococcus* spp., although gram-negative organisms still represented a large proportion of cases. More recently, in addition to bacterial invasion of the bloodstream, cases attributable to fungal invasion of the bloodstream **(fungemia)** caused by organisms such as *Candida albicans* have become increasingly important. Table 36-2 shows the frequencies of bacteremia caused by different organisms in a recent hospital-based prospective survey. These changes in the microbiology are likely due to the risk factors discussed already, particularly the widespread use of indwelling vascular catheters (readily colonized by CoNS), along with immunosuppressive cancer chemotherapy, which renders patients receiving such treatments susceptible to infection by CoNS and other commensals that normally do not cause disease in immunocompetent individuals.

In addition to the shift in organisms responsible for bacteremia, the susceptibility patterns of pathogens causing bacteremia have also changed. Bacteremia caused by methicillin-resistant *Staphylococcus aureus* (MRSA), a rare entity in the 1970s, now accounts for more than 40% of all hospitalizations for *S. aureus* bacteremia, and the incidence of bacteremia caused by vancomycin-resistant enterococci (VRE) has also increased. In addition, gram-negative organisms expressing extended-spectrum β-lactamases (ESBLs) have become more prevalent, complicating the therapy of patients with bacteremia resulting from these organisms. These shifts are thought to be due to the increasing use (and misuse) of broad-spectrum antimicrobials, resulting in selection of multidrug-resistant pathogens.

The microbiology of bacteremia is also marked by an increasing incidence of polymicrobial bacteremia. In the 1930s, virtually every case of bacteremia involved a single organism. By the early 1990s, 10% of bacteremias involved more than one organism. Polymicrobial bacteremia is generally associated with a higher mortality than is monomicrobial bacteremia. The predisposing factors in polymicrobial bacteremia include IV drug use, burns, and gastrointestinal tract sources. Especially at risk are immunocompromised patients, particularly those with alcoholism, granulocytopenia, extensive burns, diabetes mellitus, and chronic renal failure, and patients with vascular insufficiency attributable to ischemia. *B. fragilis* often has been associated with polymicrobial infections. Given the resistance of *B. fragilis* to many antimicrobials, its involvement in bacteremia carries an increased risk for mortality.

Finally, some organisms have become less prevalent causes of bacteremia because of immunization practices that have decreased the risk of infection with such pathogens. For example, the incidence of infection with *Haemophilus influenzae* type b (Hib), formerly a major cause of bacteremia and sepsis in children, decreased by more than 95% after introduction of the conjugate Hib vaccine. Similarly, implementation of the *Streptococcus pneumoniae* vaccine resulted in an 84% reduction of bacteremia due to *S. pneumoniae*, as well as, interestingly, a 67% reduction in bacteremia in general in the 3- to 36-month-old children in the study.

PATHOGENESIS

The pathogenesis of bacteremia depends in part on the infecting pathogen, the portal of initial entry, and the immune status of the patient. In general, however, bacteremia occurs because of disruption of normal skin or mucosal barriers leading to bacterial invasion of the bloodstream. Such disruption may occur via trauma, burns, or ischemia giving rise to breaks in the skin that allow access to the microvasculature; via an antecedent viral infection that disrupts the epithelial lining (e.g., influenza virus infection involving the upper respiratory tract) and allows resident flora to invade the bloodstream via capillaries; or iatrogenic disruptions, such as surgery, instrumentation, or placement of an indwelling device. Alternatively a focal bacterial infection (e.g., bacterial pneumonia) may lead to bacteremia via local inflammation, edema, and tissue destruction that disrupts nearby vascular structures and allows bloodstream invasion.

Once bacteremia occurs, the patient's immune system attempts to control infection via antibodies, which opsonize organisms and activate complement-mediated killing, as well as by phagocytosis. In addition, filtering mechanisms in the lymphatics and large vascular beds in the liver and spleen may sequester organisms and facilitate their destruction by phagocytic cells. If, however, these defenses are unsuccessful, two major complications may ensue: metastatic infection and septic shock. Invasion of the bloodstream may result in spread of organisms throughout the body, causing seeding of multiple sites and leading to widely disseminated infection. For example, bacteremia that is due to *S. pneumoniae* may lead to infection of the meninges, resulting in pneumococcal meningitis, a catastrophic infection with a mortality rate as high as 25%, even with optimal treatment. Other infections associated with a period of bacteremia as part of the disease process include salmonellosis, infective endocarditis, and

TABLE 36-2 Most Common Organisms Associated with Nosocomial Bacteremias

Organism	Percentage of Bacteremias (N = 20,978)
Coagulase-negative staphylococci	31.3
Staphylococcus aureus	20.2
Enterococcus spp.	9.4
Candida albicans	9.0
Escherichia coli	5.6
Klebsiella spp.	4.8
Pseudomonas aeruginosa	4.3
Enterobacter spp.	3.9
Serratia spp.	1.7
Acinetobacter baumannii	1.3

acute hematogenous osteomyelitis. *S. aureus* is particularly likely to cause metastatic infection or abscess formation as a consequence of bacteremia; *S. aureus* bacteremia may lead to endocarditis, osteomyelitis, septic arthritis, hepatic abscess, or pyomyositis. Sepsis and septic shock are also potential consequences of bacteremia. Although gram-negative bacteremias were once thought to be more likely to cause septic shock than those caused by gram-positive organisms, the risk of sepsis, severe sepsis, septic shock, and death is now known to be similar between these two classes of bacteremia. In both cases, a bacterial membrane component (lipopolysaccharide [LPS], also known as *endotoxin,* in the case of gram-negative organisms; lipoteichoic acid and peptidoglycan in the case of gram-positive organisms) interacts with macrophages and causes release of tumor necrosis factor (TNF), interleukin-1 (IL-1), IL-6, and other proinflammatory cytokines, increasing endothelial activation, vascular permeability, blood flow, and recruitment of neutrophils. These responses are directed at controlling infection and are normally counterregulated by anti-inflammatory mediators to prevent a destructive systemic inflammatory reaction. In sepsis and septic shock, however, an imbalance in regulation leads to an unopposed proinflammatory state, leading to microvascular abnormalities and endothelial injury; in turn, these derangements lead to decreased tissue perfusion, complement activation, and **disseminated intravascular coagulation (DIC),** which cause multiorgan dysfunction, eventually leading to septic shock and death.

CLINICAL ASPECTS OF BACTEREMIA

Clinical Syndromes Associated with Bacteremia

Numerous sources can give rise to bacteremia. The most common sites associated with bacteremia and sepsis are infected intravascular catheters, the urinary tract, the lung, and the abdomen.

Catheter-Related Bloodstream Infections

Intravascular catheters have become indispensable for modern medical and surgical therapy. Most of these are temporary catheters placed in peripheral veins and are intended for short-term use in the administration of medications and fluids. Semipermanent catheters (referred to as Hickman, Broviac, Quinton, or Tenckoff catheters, after the names of their developers) are placed in central veins and remain in place for weeks or months to administer chemotherapy to patients with cancer or to perform hemodialysis in patients with end-stage renal disease. Still other catheters are placed in arteries or, via central veins, the pulmonary artery or right-sided chambers of the heart, where they may be left for days for hemodynamic monitoring.

As useful as these devices are, they are exquisitely vulnerable to colonization and infection by organisms such as CoNS, *S. aureus,* and *Enterococcus,* with subsequent spread to the bloodstream to cause bacteremia; frequently the strains causing catheter-related bloodstream infections (CRBSIs) are resistant to multiple antibiotics. More than 250,000 cases of

CRBSI occur in the United States every year, and more than 50% of these are due to CoNS. CRBSI accounts for about 19% of all symptomatic bacteremias. Production of a polysaccharide biofilm by CoNS is one mechanism that has been associated with CRBSI. The biofilm may serve as a ligand during initial surface adhesion and colonization, or it may be produced after the organism has established a focal presence by adhering to the surface. The biofilm also protects the organism from host defenses by inhibiting phagocytosis, chemotaxis, and oxidative metabolism and by suppressing the lymphoproliferative response. It may also significantly increase the concentrations of antimicrobials required to inhibit the growth of CoNS attached to the catheter. Although CoNS are of relatively low virulence, bacteremias due to these organisms in patients with compromised immune systems (e.g., cancer patients made neutropenic through chemotherapy) are associated with mortality rates of 13% to 18%. Bacteremias due to *S. aureus* are associated with even higher mortality rates, in part because the virulence of this organism as well as the ease with which it adheres to native cardiac valves and causes endocarditis. Occasionally fluids administered via these catheters become contaminated via a break in infusion lines, causing bacteremia; organisms associated with such infusion-associated bacteremias are typically gram-negative organisms such as *P. aeruginosa* and *Enterobacter cloacae.*

Urinary Tract Infections

Urinary tract infections account for roughly 17% of all bacteremias. Infection of the upper urinary tract (acute pyelonephritis) leads to bacteremia in as many as 40% of affected patients. *E. coli* is the most common cause of bacteremia in this setting. These infections are most common in elderly patients.

Pneumonias

Lower respiratory tract infections represent about 12% of bacteremic infections. The most common organisms in pneumonia that produce a concurrent bacteremia include *S. pneumoniae, H. influenzae, S. aureus, P. aeruginosa,* and *E. aerogenes.* Of patients with pneumococcal pneumonia, 25% will have positive blood cultures; the risk of mortality is higher in such patients.

Intra-Abdominal Infections

Intra-abdominal infections account for about 5% of bacteremias. Primary peritonitis, which frequently occurs in patients with cirrhosis, is associated with bacteremia in 75% of cases involving aerobic bacteria; common pathogens include *E. coli, K. pneumoniae, S. pneumoniae,* and enterococci. Secondary peritonitis arising from perforation of the gastrointestinal tract may give rise to intra-abdominal abscesses, resulting in intermittent bacteremia due to *E. coli,* anaerobes, and enterococci. In some instances, intra-abdominal abscesses may be due to seeding of the liver or spleen by a transient bacteremia arising from outside the abdomen, most often due to *S. aureus.*

Skin Infections

Cellulitis due to *S. aureus, Streptococcus pyogenes,* or *Streptococcus agalactiae* can lead to bacteremia in about 2% of patients. Skin breakdown in bedridden patients or peripheral vascular disease from diabetes are common causes of infected skin ulcers, which can provide a portal of entry for bacterial invasion of the bloodstream, often resulting in polymicrobial bacteremia. Some of the most commonly reported offending organisms are *Proteus mirabilis*, *E. coli*, *S. aureus*, *B. fragilis*, *Pseudomonas* spp., *Clostridium* species, and anaerobic *Peptostreptococcus*.

A number of infections resulting from transient bacteremias can subsequently become the source of bacteremia, including the following infections.

Infective Endocarditis

Transient bacteremia (from dental procedures or a superficial skin infection) can seed cardiac valves with bacteria. These organisms multiply within a dense vegetation composed of bacteria and fibrin, protected from killing by neutrophils, and give rise to a continuous bacteremia, which can then seed other organs. Continued growth can lead to valvular damage and congestive heart failure. Organisms commonly associated with endocarditis include viridans streptococci, *S. aureus*, and in the case of prosthetic heart valves, CoNS.

Musculoskeletal Infections

Acute osteomyelitis is often associated with transient bacteremia due to *S. aureus*; frequently the portal of entry is an otherwise unnoticed minor skin infection. The organisms seed end-loop capillaries in bone, where blood flow is slow, and begin to multiply, causing destruction of bone and giving rise to intermittent bacteremia in about 50% of cases. Prosthetic joints, particularly those implanted in the hip, can be hematogenously seeded by organisms such as *S. aureus* and CoNS and then give rise to bacteremia. Occasionally prosthetic joint infections are caused by intraoperative contamination, although this risk has decreased considerably because of the use of perioperative prophylaxis and ultraclean operating rooms. Prosthetic joint infection with virulent organisms such as *S. aureus* or group A β-hemolytic streptococci can lead to florid sepsis and death. Bacteremia caused by *S. aureus* or *Neisseria gonorrhoeae* can result in seeding of joints and cause acute septic arthritis, an infectious disease emergency that requires prompt drainage of pus from the joint and aggressive antimicrobial therapy.

Central Nervous System Infections

Acute bacterial meningitis is generally caused by transient bacteremia due to *S. pneumoniae* or *Neisseria meningitidis*; these organisms may colonize the nasopharynx in normal individuals and occasionally invade the bloodstream to cause disease. Occasionally meningitis is caused by bacteremia resulting from sinusitis or otitis due to *S. pneumoniae*.

Clinical Signs and Symptoms

The classic signs and symptoms of bacteremia include abrupt onset of shaking chills, fever, or hypothermia. About 14% of patients with bacteremia will have hypotension, and about 40% of patients experience prostration and diaphoresis (profuse sweating). Tachypnea (abnormal rapid breathing) is an early sign of bacteremia, and adult respiratory distress

syndrome occurs in 18% of patients with culture-positive septic shock. Other symptoms may include delirium, stupor, or agitation (evidence of decreased central nervous system perfusion), along with nausea and vomiting. As many as 38% of patients with bacteremia and sepsis will have acute renal failure, with oliguria or anuria. Ecthyma gangrenosum, a central necrotic area surrounded by an erythematous base, is classically associated with *Pseudomonas* bacteremia. The failure of the body to mount an elevated temperature is also associated with increased mortality among newborns and older adults. Altered clinical laboratory values that may be indicative of bacteremia include the following:

- Thrombocytopenia
- Leukocytosis or leukopenia
- Lactic acidosis
- Hypoglycemia or hyperglycemia
- Abnormal liver function tests (especially hyperbilirubinemia)
- Coagulopathy
- DIC
- Elevations in C-reactive protein, haptoglobin, and fibrinogen

LABORATORY DIAGNOSIS

Specimen Collection

It is important to remember that even though antiseptic technique is used in the collection of blood, somewhere between 1% and 3% of blood cultures become contaminated with organisms such as coagulase-negative staphylococci, *Corynebacterium* spp., *Bacillus* spp. (not *B. anthracis*), α-hemolytic streptococci, and *Propionibacterium acnes*, which are skin colonizers, resulting in pseudobacteremia. However, in some patients, such as those receiving cancer chemotherapy, such organisms can represent true pathogens, making it essential to distinguish between blood culture results that reflect true bacteremia and those that represent pseudobacteremia.

Therefore it is most important to prepare the skin properly before venipuncture for blood culture. There are several acceptable protocols. Palpation for the vein can be checked with a gloved finger. Cleansing the skin with 80% to 95% ethanol or isopropyl alcohol, followed by an iodine-based compound (povidone-iodine or tincture of iodine) scrubbed in a concentric fashion around the venipuncture site, is a common practice. Other substances such as chlorhexidine may be substituted for iodine in cases of known skin hypersensitivity. For decontamination to be effective, the iodine should be left on the skin for at least 1 minute. After the venipuncture, the disinfecting agent should be removed with an alcohol pad.

When blood is collected for culture it is critical that the blood not be allowed to clot. The formation of a clot will trap the bacteria and reduce the ability to detect them. Thus the blood should be inoculated directly into blood culture bottles or inoculated into a tube containing anticoagulants. Tubes containing heparin, ethylenediaminetetraacetic acid (EDTA), and sodium citrate have been shown to inhibit the growth of many different organisms and should not be used.

Tubes containing 0.025% to 0.050% of **sodium polyanetholsulfonate (SPS)** are the best tubes to use for collecting blood for culture.

Blood for blood culture should be obtained by venipuncture and not from indwelling IV or intra-arterial lines. There is more risk of isolating skin flora from indwelling lines than from venipuncture. If blood is collected from an indwelling line, a second sample collected via venipuncture should be cultured for comparison. For patients who have IV lines through which they are getting fluids and/or medications, blood must be drawn below the line because blood drawn above the line will be diluted with the fluid being transfused. Best practice, though, is to not draw blood from the extremity that has an IV line, but to perform venipuncture on an extremity that does not have an indwelling line.

General Principles in Determining the Volume, Frequency, and Number of Blood Cultures

Density of Bacteremia in Adults versus Neonates.
Bacteremia may involve a large number of microorganisms in the blood; however, more commonly, only a relatively small number of bacteria per unit volume of blood (as low as 1 bacterium per milliliter) are seen in patients with bacteremia that is clinically significant. The detection methods common in most laboratories produce positive results in adult patients with bacteremias if organisms are present in the range of 10 to 15 bacteria per milliliter of blood; however, there are many circumstances in which patients have fewer than this number, and this must be taken into consideration when choosing how much blood to collect per blood culture bottle and how many blood cultures to perform.

Studies that have examined the relationship between volume of blood collected and rate of positivity have demonstrated that as the volume of blood cultured is increased from 2 to 20 mL of blood per culture, the yield of positive culture results increases from 30% to 50%. One study in particular clearly demonstrated the advantage of culturing 10 mL of blood per blood culture bottle as compared with 5 mL of blood/bottle, finding that 7.2% more cases of bacteremias were detected in the bottle inoculated with 10 mL of blood and that the organisms were detected sooner than in the bottles inoculated with only 5 mL of blood. If inoculating more blood into the blood culture bottle increases the sensitivity and rate of detection, why not inoculate even more blood into each bottle? Taking excessive amounts of blood from a patient can be difficult depending on the health of the patient and the underlying illness and can induce anemia in the patient, and, according to at least one study, inoculating more than 10 mL per bottle did not increase the rate of positivity and in fact decreased it.

The reason more blood inoculated into the blood culture bottle resulted in fewer bacteremic episodes detected, as previously mentioned, is probably because of the increase in the amount of inhibitors in the bottle. Blood naturally contains many inhibitors of bacterial growth from complement and lysozyme to white blood cells. In addition, although blood should be collected before antibiotics are given, it is likely that many patients from whom blood is drawn are already receiving antimicrobial treatment that also inhibits the growth of bacteria in blood culture bottles. Thus the blood and the inhibitors present in the blood need to be diluted by the blood culture medium. The optimal ratio of blood to culture medium is about 1:5 to 1:10. The dilution aids in negating the bactericidal effect of normal serum. In cases in which a 1:5 dilution cannot be achieved, 0.025% to 0.050% of SPS can be added to the bottle, which serves to inhibit complement, coagulation, and phagocytosis within the bottle.

Newborns tend to be more septic as a result of the incomplete development of their immune defense mechanisms and generally have higher numbers of microorganisms per milliliter of blood. On the other hand, it is not uncommon to see low levels of bacteremia in children as are seen in adults. Because newborns and children have a smaller volume of total blood, it is not safe to take as much blood from a newborn or child as can be taken from an adult. As a general rule, about 4% of a patient's total blood volume can be taken safely for culture, and this has been shown to be an optimal amount for the detection of most bloodstream infections in newborns and children. The following age-volume protocol therefore has been recommended:

Age	Amount
Younger than 10 years	1 mL of blood for each year of life
10 years or older	20 mL
10 years or older (poor veins)	Less than 20 mL

Another scheme uses the weight of the newborn or child to determine how much blood can be safely drawn for culture where 2 mL of blood can be safely collected from a newborn weighing less than 1 kg (less than 2.2 lb); 4 mL total from a newborn weighing up to 2 kg (up to 4.4 lb); 6mL total from a child up to 12.7 kg (27 lb); and 10 mL total from a child up to 36.3 kg (up to 80 lb). A child who weighs more than 36.3 kg (more than 80 lb) can have as much blood drawn as an adult (20 to 30 mL). Because less blood is typically drawn from newborns and children as compared with adults, most commercial blood culture systems have pediatric bottles that contain less blood culture medium into which less blood is inoculated. The ratio of blood to broth is kept at 1:5 to 1:10, and some pediatric bottles may be supplemented with X and V factors to enhance the recovery of *H. influenzae*, which is more likely (or was more likely before implementation of the Hib vaccine) to be isolated from children than adults.

Frequency of Bacteremic Episodes versus Time and Frequency of Collection.
The frequency of bacteremic episodes is another factor to consider in determining the time, frequency, and volume of blood collection for culture. Because bacteremias can be transient, intermittent, or continuous with respect to the presence of microorganisms in the peripheral circulation, collection of samples may depend on the type of bacteremia suspected.

In patients with transient bacteremia, organisms are immediately cleared from the peripheral system by the reticuloendothelial system (RES). In such patients, clinical symptoms, especially fever, may not occur until after bacteria are cleared from the bloodstream. Because these symptoms serve as the signal to obtain blood cultures, bacteremia may go undetected because of delays in obtaining blood cultures relative to the time of peak concentrations of circulating bacteria. Therefore, in suspected cases of intermittent bacteremia, it is recommended that blood culture specimens be collected before an anticipated temperature rise to ensure maximum recovery. In patients with continuous bacteremia, on the other hand, the organisms are constantly released into the bloodstream and therefore are likely to be isolated whenever the blood culture specimen is taken. Although a single set of blood culture bottles may yield the etiologic agent, two and maybe three or even four sets of blood cultures are highly recommended (a set may consist of one bottle for aerobic incubation and another for anaerobic incubation) for a few reasons as explained next.

Rationale for Multiple Blood Collections. There are a few reasons for drawing multiple blood cultures. One study revealed that about 80% of bacteremias are discovered in the first set of blood culture specimens taken, 90% are detected if two sets of specimens are taken, and as many as 99% are diagnosed if a third set is taken. Other studies have duplicated these results and further found that it is not so much the number of blood cultures that are collected that improves the detection of bacteremias; it is the total volume of blood that is cultured. In the past, guidelines for the collection of blood for culture stated that multiple blood cultures should be submitted where blood is collected from multiple different venipuncture sites with 30 to 60 minutes in between draws. Although it is best to collect blood when the patient spikes a temperature, or before, because this is when more organisms are present in the blood, not all patients have fever when microorganisms are in the blood, and it is almost impossible to predict when fever will occur. Because organisms can be present in the blood transiently or intermittently and there is no way to know when the organisms are present, yielding a positive blood culture, or not present, giving a negative culture, collecting blood can be a hit-or-miss procedure.

Yet bacteremia is a very serious clinical condition that requires rapid treatment, so methods for almost guaranteeing its detection need to be determined. Therefore studies have been performed to determine the best practice for when and how much blood to collect that will yield the highest percentage of positive cultures. These studies have come to the conclusion that the volume of blood collected is more important than the number of sets, and that multiple sets can be inoculated with blood drawn at the same time instead of from multiple different collections. At least 30 mL of blood should be collected in a 24-hour period, and if 10 mL of blood is inoculated into one bottle, two sets of two bottles each will satisfy the volume requirement and will most likely result in the detection of bacteremia if it is present.

Another reason for inoculating multiple bottles is to aid in the determination of whether an isolated organism is a true pathogen or a contaminant. The collection of one single sample should be strongly discouraged because the volume of blood cultured is not sufficient for detecting some infections, as discussed previously. In addition, the significance of the isolation of CoNS or other skin flora, for example, from one culture is hard to interpret. Its presence could represent true infection, or it could be a result of contamination. It is not until there are repeat isolations of the same organism from multiple cultures that the significance can be determined.

Most blood culture systems as described later have separate bottles for the isolation of aerobic and anaerobic bacteria. Typically a blood culture consists of a set of two bottles, one aerobic and one anaerobic. This practice has been questioned in light of the fact that the incidence of bacteremia due to obligate anaerobes was found to be decreasing in some studies. Therefore some investigators have recommended that two aerobic bottles be inoculated instead to maintain the necessary volume of blood that should be collected and to increase the ability to detect the aerobic and facultative anaerobes that are more commonly isolated. Additional studies into the incidence of anaerobic bacteremia, however, have shown that anaerobes are not infrequent isolates, that their presence is difficult to predict based on analysis of clinical predictors, and that antimicrobial resistance is increasing among anaerobes, making these infections important to detect. Thus the inoculation of separate aerobic and anaerobic bottles remains the standard procedure for blood cultures, although this can vary from institution to institution depending on their isolation rates of anaerobes.

Multiple blood cultures are necessary to detect bacteremia, but there is a limit to the number that should be collected. Repeat blood cultures or daily collections of blood for culture are not necessary. If at least 30 mL of blood has been cultured and antimicrobial therapy has begun, it is best to wait for the results of the initial sets of cultures before collecting more blood. Most organisms will grow within 3 days in the continuous monitoring systems that are used in most laboratories, so it is best to wait at least 3 days before collecting additional blood for culture. If no organisms grow in the blood cultures, it is more reasonable to consider other causes of symptoms rather than culturing more blood.

Blood Culture Methods

Culture Media Used in Conventional Broth Systems

A blood culture set typically includes a bottle or tube designated for aerobic recovery and another for anaerobic recovery of microorganisms. The typical aerobic culture bottle contains media that is multipurpose and nutritionally enriched and can be a soybean casein digest broth, peptone broth, tryptic or trypticase soy broth, brain-heart infusion, *Brucella* agar, or Columbia broth base. Although typical anaerobic broth media may contain the same types of basic media as the aerobic culture systems, 0.5% cysteine may have been added to permit the growth of certain thiol-requiring organisms, and the media may be prereduced to decrease the oxidation-reduction potential in the media to help support the growth of anaerobes. Unvented blood culture bottles generally can be used to support anaerobic organisms.

Neutralization of Inhibitors. In specimens from patients receiving clinical amounts of β-lactam antimicrobial agents, penicillinase may be added to the medium to inactivate these agents, although it is not added as often anymore. Some commercially available automated blood culture systems have blood culture bottles containing an **antibiotic removal device**

(ARD), a resin that nonspecifically absorbs any antimicrobial agent present in the patient's blood, whereas other systems incorporate activated charcoal for this purpose. The yield of both bacteria and yeast increases with the incorporation of these inhibitors into the culture medium.

Anticoagulants and Other Additives. SPS, one of the commonly used additives, performs the following functions:
- Anticoagulation (effective at a 0.03% concentration)
- Neutralization of the bactericidal activity (i.e., complement and lysozyme) of human serum
- Prevention of phagocytosis
- Inactivation of certain antimicrobial agents (streptomycin, kanamycin, gentamicin, polymyxin B)

Despite its usefulness in blood culture media, SPS inhibits the growth of certain organisms, notably *Peptostreptococcus anaerobius*, *N. gonorrhoeae*, *N. meningitidis*, and *Gardnerella vaginalis*. If these organisms are suspected, 1.2% gelatin added to the blood culture bottle may help to neutralize the inhibitory effect of SPS.

Other anticoagulants and supplements are available for use in blood culture systems, but are not better than SPS. Sodium amylosulfate (SAS) is a structural relative of SPS that is less effective in neutralizing serum bactericidal activity and is inhibitory to *Klebsiella pneumoniae*. Sodium citrate (0.5% to 1.0%), an anticoagulant, is inhibitory to some gram-positive cocci. Sucrose (10% to 30%) is sometimes used as an osmotic stabilizer. Sucrose is especially helpful in dealing with bacteria that have undergone cell wall damage to some extent, and the resultant hypertonicity counteracts the normal bactericidal effect of blood. Other supplements, such as the anticoagulants ammonium-potassium or sodium oxalate and ethylenediaminetetraacetic acid (EDTA), are not recommended.

Incubation Conditions. Continuous-monitoring blood culture instruments, as described later, contain an incubator as a part of the system; an incubator used to incubate agar media plates can be used to incubate blood culture media of the manual systems. Blood culture bottles are incubated at $35 \pm 2°$ C for 5 days typically for the automated systems and may be held for 7 days for the manual systems. During incubation of the bottles in a continuous-monitoring blood culture system, the aerobic bottles and, on some systems, the anaerobic bottles as well are agitated during incubation. The agitation can take the form of a rocking motion (BacT/ALERT and BACTEC) or a rotary motion with the formation of a vortex (VersaTREK). The agitation of the bottles increases oxygenation of the broth, enhancing the detection of microorganisms in the bottles and decreasing the time to detect growth in the bottles. The head space of the bottles contains ambient air, sometimes with increased CO_2 in the aerobic bottles. The anaerobic bottles will have increased N_2 and CO_2 replacing all of the O_2 in the bottle to facilitate isolation of obligate anaerobes.

Blood Culture Systems

Manual Systems

A broth-slide system (Septi-Chek [Becton Dickinson, Sparks, Md.) was designed from the original biphasic (solid agar and broth combination) blood culture medium called the *Casta-* *ñeda culture bottle.* Septi-Chek consists of a slide paddle containing chocolate (CHOC), MacConkey (MAC), and malt extract agars (selective for yeast and fungi) attached to the top of a standard broth bottle. Once these bottles have been inoculated, they should be tipped daily or at least twice weekly to bathe the slide paddle with the broth culture medium, thereby allowing frequent blind subcultures without the use of needles and syringes. Bacterial growth appears either as small, discrete colonies or as a confluent growth on the slide paddle. Most organisms will grow within 48 hours of inoculation, but the bottles are incubated for 7 days before they are discarded and reported as negative. This system has the advantage of providing more rapid recovery of facultative bacteria and isolated colonies for identification and susceptibility testing. However, there are certain disadvantages, including a slightly higher cost of materials and contamination rate. An additional unvented bottle is still required for adequate isolation of anaerobes.

The Oxoid Ltd. (Thermo Fisher Scientific, Waltham, Mass.) Signal system is another manual blood culture system in which blood is inoculated into a bottle containing a liquid medium that will support the growth of aerobes, anaerobes, and microaerophiles. A clear plastic signal device is then attached to the top of the bottle. The signal device has a long needle that extends down into the bottle below the level of the liquid. When microorganisms grow in the bottle, they generate CO_2 that accumulates in the head space of the bottle. The increase of gas in the atmosphere of the bottle increases pressure on the liquid, forcing it up through the needle and into the clear plastic signal device. The presence of fluid in the signal device can be seen by the microbiologist during daily inspection of the bottles and indicates the growth of bacteria. The fluid from the signal device can then be removed for gram staining and plating. The inoculated Oxoid bottles are incubated at $35 \pm 2°$ C, agitated on a shaker, for the first 24 hours. Bottles are held for a total of 7 days with a terminal blind subculture performed and examined before the culture is reported as negative.

The lysis-centrifugation method (DuPont Isolator; Isostat; Wampole, Inverness Medical Professional Diagnostics, Princeton, N.J.) has been shown to provide optimal recovery of unusual fastidious bacteria such as *Bartonella,* yeasts, and dimorphic fungi and mycobacteria that are causing systemic infections. This method produces a concentrated sample of blood for direct inoculation onto appropriate solid agar media, as opposed to the two previously described systems where the blood is inoculated and incubated in a broth medium. The Isolator tube contains a mixture of saponin, propylene glycol, SPS, and EDTA. This mixture causes lysis of white and red blood cells, releasing intracellular organisms; prevents clotting; and neutralizes complement. Microorganisms are concentrated through high-speed centrifugation (3000 *g* for 30 minutes). The sediment containing the organisms is directly inoculated on a solid culture medium including fungal and mycobacterial media.

Examination of Blood Culture Bottles in a Manual System

Blood culture bottles are examined macroscopically with transmitted and reflected light for evidence of turbidity, hemolysis, gas production, or bacterial colonies in or on the blood layer. If visible growth is observed, 0.25 mL of blood should be aspirated with a sterile needle and syringe. A smear is prepared for Gram stain and then plated to a solid medium. In addition to examining the blood culture fluid for evidence of microbial growth, the Septi-Chek paddle is examined daily for the presence of colonies; the Oxoid bottle signal device is examined each day for the presence of fluid indicating microbial growth in the medium.

Any finding of microbial growth should be reported immediately by telephone to a physician.

Continuous-Monitoring Blood Culture Systems

The BACTEC System (BACTEC 460; Becton Dickinson Microbiology Systems, Sparks, Md.), was the first automated growth detection system for blood cultures that detected the growth of microorganisms using radiolabeled carbon (^{14}C) in the broth medium. When the organism in the blood culture bottle used the ^{14}C-labeled substrate, $^{14}CO_2$ was released. The instrument monitored $^{14}CO_2$ production by aspirating gas into an ionization chamber using sterile needles injected into the bottle. In the ionization chamber, the amount of $^{14}CO_2$ produced was measured as a growth index and compared with an established threshold level. If the patient's blood culture showed a growth index that exceeded the threshold level, the instrument sent a signal indicating that the bottle was positive. The automated radiometric blood culture system had the advantage of early detection of bacterial growth, especially of slow-growing bacterial species (e.g., *Mycobacterium tuberculosis*). The disadvantages included the high initial cost of the instrument, high contamination rate (the result of inadequate needle sterilization between bottles), and the hazards and expense associated with radioisotope disposal. Development of subsequent automated blood culture instruments kept the detection of CO_2 as an indication of microbial growth.

BACTEC 9000 Series. In order to eliminate radioactive isotopes as a growth detection mechanism, Becton Dickinson introduced the BACTEC 9000 series. Three models are currently available: the 9240 (holds 240 bottles/module), the 9120 (holds 120 bottles/module), and the 9050 (holds 50 bottles/module). These are noninvasive, continuous-monitoring blood culture instruments that use fluorescence to detect CO_2. When microorganisms grow in the bottle, they produce CO_2. Carbon dioxide is detected using a gas-permeable sensor on the bottom of each vial as described below. When a bottle is placed into the instrument, a baseline reading of the sensor is taken, and this reading is used as a reference for subsequent readings.

Carbon dioxide produced by an organism diffuses into the sensor, generating hydrogen ions. The increase in hydrogen ion concentration increases the fluorescence output of the sensor. Using photodetectors, the instrument measures the amount of fluorescence every 10 minutes, which corresponds to the amount of CO_2 produced by the microorganism. A computer program then interprets these data using several algorithms to determine when to flag a bottle as positive. If a bottle contains a microorganism, the indicator continuously changes. The sensor detects the increase in fluorescence as well as the increase in the rate of fluorescence until they reach

a point at which the bottle is flagged as positive. The instrument alerts the microbiologist to the presence of a positive vial by displaying a message on the computer monitor and with an audible alarm. Figure 36-1 illustrates the BACTEC 9000 schematic.

VersaTREK (TREK Diagnostic Systems, Cleveland, Ohio). The former Difco ESP system has been replaced by the VersaTREK automated detection system. VersaTREK differs from the other continuous-monitoring systems in that it detects the consumption or production of multiple gases (CO_2, H_2, and O_2) by organisms growing in the culture medium. These gases are detected by monitoring changes in head-space pressure. The advantages to this system include the detection of multiple different gases that may be produced or consumed by an organism present in the bottle and not just production of CO_2, and earlier detection of growth by detecting the consumption of gas as organisms enter the log phase of growth and before they start to produce CO_2. An internal computer algorithm monitors the changes in pressure, plots the pressure against time to derive a growth curve, and determines when to flag the bottle as positive.

BacT/ALERT 3D System (bioMérieux Industry, Hazelwood, Mo.). A fully automated, nonradiometric blood culture system, the BacT/ALERT 3D System consists of aerobic and anaerobic bottles with pH-sensitive membranes placed in the bottom of the bottles. Microbial growth causes a release of CO_2, which changes the pH in the sensor as indicated by a change in color from gray to yellow. The color change is measured by reflected light. The instrument measures CO_2 production colorimetrically without going into the bottles. An advantage to this system is that the changes in the color of the sensor can be detected and verified if necessary. Another advantage to this system is that in 2003, bioMérieux released gas-impermeable *plastic* blood culture bottles that are safer and lighter than traditional glass bottles and do not interfere with microorganism growth or metabolism.

Recovery of Other Types of Organisms from Blood

The most common organisms that were isolated in one study of nosocomial bacteremia were listed in Table 36-2. All of the organisms listed in this table are easily recovered from traditional routine blood culture methods as described earlier. There are other organisms, however, that can be found in blood that require special conditions in order to be detected. Communication with the physician will be critical in deciding when and what extraordinary procedures are performed.

- *Francisella tularensis,* the causative agent of tularemia, is best recovered from a liquid blood culture medium to which L-cysteine and dextrose have been added.
- *Leptospira* spp. are recovered during the first week of disease, with one to three drops of freshly drawn blood placed in 5 mL of Fletcher medium. The blood culture is incubated at 30° C for 28 days in the dark and examined weekly by dark-field microscopy.
- *Brucella* spp. requires extended incubation times, and when *Brucella* is suspected, blood culture media should be held for up to 30 days at 35 ± 2° C and subcultured periodically.

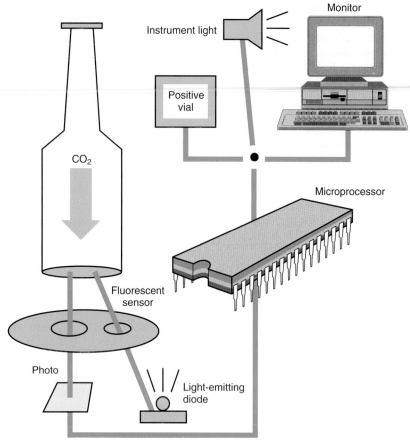

FIGURE 36-1 BACTEC 9000 schematic.

- Nutritionally deficient streptococci (*Abiotrophia* and *Granulicatella*) are adequately recovered using standard broth culture bottles because of the vitamin B_6 present in human blood. However, pyridoxal-containing blood agar medium, or a "staph streak," is necessary for subculture to recover this group of streptococci. The "staph streak" test is performed with a confluent growth of the organism on a blood agar plate. A single line of *S. aureus* is streaked across the middle of the plate. Following 24 hours of incubation, the plate is observed for tiny colonies growing near the *S. aureus*.

- *Campylobacter* spp. can be isolated from blood. Although the *Campylobacter* may grow in the blood culture bottles, subcultures of the broth will have no growth unless the broth is subcultured onto selective media and incubated in a microaerophilic environment required by the *Campylobacter* to grow. A clue that the bottle contains a *Campylobacter* will be the presence of curved gram-negative rods in the blood culture broth.

- *Coxiella burnetii* is the most common fastidious bacterium reported in the literature as causing endocarditis. *Coxiella* can be isolated in cell culture, but this should not be attempted unless the laboratory is equipped to handle dangerous pathogens. Instead, *Coxiella* is better diagnosed by serology.

- *Bartonella* spp. are best isolated using lysis centrifugation and plating the concentrated blood onto freshly prepared media containing 5% horse or rabbit blood. Plates have to be incubated for at least 3 weeks in a humid atmosphere. Because the isolation of *Bartonella* spp. is difficult, serology and molecular methods of detection are preferred.

- Members of the HACEK group of gram-negative bacilli are known causes of endocarditis and will grow well in blood culture bottles, but may require extended incubation times to be detected.

- The isolation of mycobacteria from the blood requires the use of lysis centrifugation to lyse the cells and concentrate the blood. The concentrated blood then needs to be inoculated onto media selective for the isolation of mycobacteria. These plates must be held and examined for 6 to 8 weeks before the presence of mycobacteria can be ruled out.

- *Fungemia* is the presence of fungi in the blood. The incidence of fungemia is increasing, with *C. albicans* being isolated as frequently as gram-negative bacilli. Although the yeast may grow in the continuous-monitoring blood culture systems, the best way to recover yeast and fungi in the blood is to use the lysis centrifugation system and culture the blood onto fungal media. Yeasts and dimorphic fungi are the most common fungi isolated from the blood.

- **Viremia** is the presence of viruses in the blood. Most of the time, the presence of viruses is determined using serology or molecular-based detection systems. Blood can be cultured to determine the presence of viruses. Blood for viral culture should be collected in a green-top (heparin) tube. Viruses that can be isolated from the blood include cytomegalovirus and enterovirus.

Contamination in Blood Cultures

A contamination rate of 2% to 3% can be expected, with *Staphylococcus epidermidis, Micrococcus,* diphtheroids, and *P. acnes* as common contaminants. However, any organism cultured from two or more blood culture bottles should not be overlooked as a contaminant. Any of the organisms previously mentioned can also be responsible for bacterial endocarditis. Contamination rates should be monitored, and if they increase above 3%, an examination of phlebotomy practices should be performed along with re-education of phlebotomists and nurses with regard to appropriate methods for collecting blood for culture.

Other sources of contamination causing pseudobacteremia include IV catheters as well as various skin disinfectant solutions. Benzalkonium chloride has been demonstrated to be occasionally contaminated with *Burkholderia cepacia* and *Enterobacter* spp. Alcohol or iodine as a skin disinfectant has been preferred. However, contamination of certain iodine solutions, such as povidone-iodine, with *B. cepacia* has also been reported. Contamination with *S. marcescens* and *Moraxella* species has been reported in certain evacuated blood collection tubes.

In the past, contamination was more clear-cut. The media and volume of blood used now are more sensitive and grow more contaminants. It is difficult to determine when a pathogen is isolated and when contamination occurs. As the volume of blood increases, the number of positive blood culture results increases. Microbiologists cannot make this determination (true pathogen or contaminant) in the laboratory; physician input and patient history are needed. Criteria that can be used to determine whether an isolate from a blood culture is a pathogen or contaminant include the following:

- Identify of the microorganism. *S. aureus, E. coli* and other members of the Enterobacteriaceae, *S. pneumoniae, P. aeruginosa,* and *Candida albicans* when isolated almost always indicate true infection, whereas CoNS, diphtheroids, and other skin flora when isolated should be questioned.
- More than one blood culture bottle growing the same organism usually indicates that the isolate is significant, whereas growth of an organism, especially one associated with skin flora, in a single bottle when multiple bottles are inoculated usually indicates that the isolate is a contaminant.
- Isolation of the same organism in the blood and from a normally sterile site usually indicates that the organism isolated from the blood is a pathogen.

Rapid Identification of Microorganisms Growing in Blood Cultures

Automated continuous-monitoring blood culture systems have taken the labor out of reading blood culture bottles for the presence of microbial growth, but these systems can only determine that something is growing in the bottle. The micro-

biologist must remove a flagged bottle from the instrument and process the fluid to determine whether a viable microorganism is present and identify what it is. A small amount of fluid is removed from the bottle and used to make a smear to be gram-stained and plated onto appropriate media, usually blood, CHOC, and MAC agars and, if the anaerobic bottle is positive, an anaerobic blood agar plate. The Gram-stained smear can be examined quickly, and the physician can be notified of the positive blood culture along with the type of organism growing; for example, gram-positive cocci or gram-negative rods. Definitive identification and susceptibility results will not be available until there are colonies growing on the subcultured plates to test and therefore will take 24 to 48 hours. During this time, the patient will be put on empiric antimicrobial therapy that may or may not be optimally effective for the isolate. It is clear that the sooner the patient is treated with an effective antimicrobial agent, the better the outcome for the patient. In order to decrease the time it takes to identify a microorganism growing in a blood culture, a few rapid methods are available:

- Direct tube coagulase can be used to determine whether gram-positive cocci in clusters that are growing in a blood culture are *S. aureus* (coagulase positive) or CoNS. A small portion of the blood culture fluid is inoculated into a tube containing rabbit plasma, incubated at 35° C for 4 hours, and then examined for the presence of a clot (positive). The result can be communicated to the physician, who will determine the best course of therapy.
- Fluorescence in situ hybridization (FISH) targets rRNA in an organism using either an oligonucleotide or peptide nucleic acid (PNA) probe with a fluorescent label. Although this is a molecular method, there is no amplification of nucleic acid involved. The procedure takes about 4 hours to perform, and the sensitivity of species-specific probes in one study was reported to be 97% with 95% specificity. Many different probes are available that target the most common organisms that are isolated from blood cultures.
- Nucleic acid amplification (NAA) methods, such as polymerase chain reaction (PCR), that can identify microorganisms growing in a blood culture are increasing in availability. A common target is methicillin-resistant *Staphylococcus aureus* (MRSA). Not only can the organism be identified as *S. aureus* by NAA , but the susceptibility of the isolate to β-lactamase-resistant-β-lactams such as oxacillin can also be determined in one assay within a few hours.

TREATMENT

With such a complex disorder, it would be expected that there would be many therapeutic attempts to alleviate this devastating clinical event. In fact, there are several treatment modalities that have been tried, but some have not shown positive results, as follows.

Antimicrobial Therapy

Antibiotics remain the mainstay of treatment of bacteremia. Because of the potentially devastating consequences of untreated bacteremia, therapy is frequently instituted empirically on the basis of clinical signs and symptoms, before bacteremia has been confirmed by a positive blood culture or before the causative agent has been definitively identified. The choice of initial therapy is based on the likely identity of the infecting microorganism (based on the patient's clinical syndrome), the presence of comorbid conditions that might affect the risk of infection with particular bacterial species (e.g., cancer), the patient's immune status, recent environmental exposures (e.g., hospitalization that might have resulted in colonization by resistant organisms), and prior antimicrobial therapy that might have selected for resistant pathogens. Broad-spectrum agents are frequently used for initial empiric therapy, and a combination of agents may be used to ensure coverage of possible pathogens.

After identification of organisms cultured from blood and determination of their antimicrobial susceptibility, the initial therapy may be more narrowly targeted, thus allowing use of the agent most effective against the responsible pathogen while minimizing the potential for adverse reactions and emergence of antimicrobial resistance. For bacteremia due to some pathogens (e.g., *E. faecium, P. aeruginosa*), a cell-wall active agent such as a β-lactam is combined with an aminoglycoside, resulting in a synergistic antimicrobial effect and an improved clinical outcome. Along with antimicrobial therapy, adjunctive measures, such as drainage of infected fluid collections or removal of an infected intravascular catheter, may be essential to achieving cure of the infection. Treatment of comorbid conditions such as diabetes is helpful in gaining control of infection. Finally, measures aimed at restoring immune competence—such as administration of cytokines that increase the number of circulating neutrophils in patients who are immunosuppressed due to cancer chemotherapy—are critical in complementing antimicrobial therapy.

Antisepsis Therapy

Because of the high mortality of septic shock, whether accompanied by bacteremia or not, a number of therapies aimed at blocking the cascade of events that result in sepsis, shock, and death have been studied. These therapies are invariably used in combination with antimicrobial agents.

Physiologic Support

Resuscitation with IV fluids to maintain tissue perfusion is a fundamental method for management of the septic patient. In patients with septic shock who do not respond to fluid support, pressor agents may be used to ensure an adequate blood pressure. Along with fluids, respiratory therapy with oxygen is used to support septic patients.

Anticoagulation Agents

Because the consequences of bacteremia and sepsis may include activation of the coagulation cascade, with resultant DIC and decreased tissue perfusion, use of anticoagulants have been studied in the treatment of sepsis. One agent, drotrecogin alfa, also known as activated protein C, has been shown in clinical trials to decrease mortality in patients with septic shock. Drotrecogin alfa inhibits factors Va and VIIIa of the coagulation cascade, thereby inhibiting coagulation.

Drotrecogin alfa may also decrease chemotaxis of white blood cells by interfering with the interaction between the leukocytes and the endothelium of blood vessels. Because of the potential bleeding complications from this therapy, however, its use is restricted to patients who are at the highest risk of death; it is not effective in less severely ill patients. Other anticoagulant therapies, such as antithrombin III, have not been shown to be effective in the treatment of sepsis.

Glucocorticoids

Because of their potent anti-inflammatory action, glucocorticoids have long been of interest in the treatment of sepsis. Although early studies of high-dose glucocorticoids appeared to show benefit in septic patients, a randomized controlled trial in the late 1980s showed no advantages to use of glucocorticoids over placebo in severely ill patients with sepsis, and their use was largely abandoned. More recently, however, the use of glucocorticoids has made a cautious comeback, based on controlled trials of low doses of these agents used to treat adrenal insufficiency associated with sepsis rather than to block inflammation.

Anticytokine Therapies

A large number of investigational agents aimed at blocking the action of TNF and other cytokine mediators of sepsis have been studied in the treatment of sepsis. Despite an apparently sound theoretical rationale and promising results in animal models, these therapies have not proved effective in clinical trials.

PREVENTION

Prevention of community-acquired bacteremias is largely based on immunizations; pneumococcal vaccination has been effective in preventing invasive infection due to *S. pneumoniae*, and influenza and varicella vaccinations have helped lower the incidence of invasive secondary infections due to pathogens such as *S. aureus* and *S. pyogenes*. In the hospital setting, prevention of nosocomial bacteremias revolves around minimizing iatrogenic infections from indwelling intravascular or urinary catheters by following recommended infection control practices. Use of antibiotic-coated central venous catheters has been shown to decrease rates of CRBSI.

BIBLIOGRAPHY

ACCP. American College of Chest Physicians/Society of Critical Care Medicine Consensus Conference: Definitions for sepsis and organ failure and guidelines for the use of innovative therapies in sepsis, *Crit Care Med* 20:864, 1992.

Allary J, Annane D: Glucocorticoids and sepsis, *Minerva Anestesiol* 71:759, 2005.

Angus DC, Wax RS: Epidemiology of sepsis: an update, *Crit Care Med* 29:S109, 2001.

Annane D et al: Effect of treatment with low doses of hydrocortisone and fludrocortisone on mortality in patients with septic shock, *JAMA* 288:862, 2002.

Aronson MD, Bor DF: Blood cultures, *Ann Intern Med* 106:246, 1987.

Bernard GR et al: Efficacy and safety of recombinant human activated protein C for severe sepsis, *N Engl J Med* 344:699, 2001.

Baron JE et al: *1C blood cultures IV, cumitech*, Washington, DC, 2005, ASM Press.

BD Diagnostics: product pamphlet, Sparks, Md, 2005, Becton-Dickinson.

Brill NE, Libman E: *Pyocyaneus* bacillemia, *Am J Med* 118:153, 1899.

Brouqui P, Raoult D: Endocarditis due to rare and fastidious bacteria, *Clin Microbiol Rev* 14:177, 2001.

Centers for Disease Control and Prevention: Impact of vaccines universally recommended for children—United States, 1990-1998, *MMWR* 48:243, 1999.

Cooper GS et al: Polymicrobial bacteremia in the late 1980s: predictors of outcome and review of the literature, *Medicine (Baltimore)* 69:114, 1990.

Diekema DJ et al: Antimicrobial resistance trends and outbreak frequency in United States hospitals, *Clin Inf Dis* 38:78, 2004.

Fenner L et al: Is the incidence of anaerobic bacteremia decreasing? Analysis of 114,000 blood cultures over a ten-year period, *J Clin Microbiol* 46:2432, 2008.

Heron M et al: Deaths: Final Data for 2006, National Center for Health Statistics, *National Vital Statistics Reports* 57:14, 2009.

Herz AM et al: Changing epidemiology of outpatient bacteremia in 3- to 36-month-old children after the introduction of the heptavalent-conjugated pneumococcal vaccine, *Pediatr Infect Dis J* 25:293, 2006.

Hotchkiss RS, Karl IE: The pathophysiology and treatment of sepsis, *N Engl J Med* 348:138, 2003.

Hoyett DL et al: Deaths—Preliminary data for 2003. National Center for Health Statistics, *National Vital Statistics Report* 53:4, 2005.

Isenberg HD, editor: *Clinical microbiology procedures handbook*, ed 2, Washington, DC, 2004, ASM Press.

Karchmer AW: Nosocomial bloodstream infections: organisms, risk factors, and implications, *Clin Infect Dis* 31:S139, 2000.

Kellogg JA et al: Frequency of low-level bacteremia in children from birth to fifteen years of age, *J Clin Microbiol* 38:2181, 2000.

Kiyoyama T et al: Isopropyl alcohol compared with isopropyl alcohol plus povidone-iodine as skin preparation for prevention of blood culture contamination, *J Clin Microbiol* 47:54, 2009.

Kuehnert MJ et al: Methicillin-resistant-*Staphylococcus aureus* hospitalizations, United States, *Emerg Infect Dis* 11:868, 2005.

Lamy B et al: What is the relevance of obtaining multiple blood samples for culture? A comprehensive model to optimize the strategy for diagnosing bacteremia, *Clin Infect Dis* 35:842, 2002.

Lassmann B et al: Reemergence of anaerobic bacteremia, *Clin Infect Dis* 44:895, 2007.

Levy MM, et al: 2001 SCCM/ESICM/ACCP/ATS/SIS International Sepsis Definitions Conference, *Crit Care Med* 31:1250, 2003.

Li J, et al: Effects of volume and periodicity on blood cultures, *J Clin Microbiol* 32:2829, 1994.

Lombardi DP, Engleberg NC: Anaerobic bacteremia: incidence, patient characteristics, and clinical significance, *Am J Med* 92:53, 1992.

Malani A et al: Review of clinical trials of skin antiseptic agents used to reduce blood culture contamination, *Infect Control Hosp Epidemiol* 28:892, 2007.

Martin GS et al: The epidemiology of sepsis in the United States from 1979 through 2000, *N Engl J Med* 348:1546, 2003.

McBean M, Rajamani S: Increasing rates of hospitalization due to septicemia in the US elderly population, 1986-1997, *J Infect Dis* 183:596, 2001.

Mirrett S et al: Controlled clinical comparison of VersaTREK and BacT/ALERT blood culture systems, *J Clin Microbiol* 45:299, 2007.

Morris AJ et al: Rationale for selective use of anaerobic blood cultures, *J Clin Microbiol* 31:2110, 1993.

Nguyen HB et al: Severe sepsis and septic shock: Review of the literature and emergency department management guidelines, *Ann Emerg Med* 48:28, 2006.

O'Grady NP et al: Guidelines for the prevention of intravascular catheter-related infections, *Infect Control Hosp Epidemiol* 23:759, 2002.

Panlilie AL et al: Infections and pseudoinfections due to povidone-iodine solution contaminated with Pseudomonas cepacia, *Clin Infect Dis* 14:1078, 1992.

Peters RPH et al: Faster identification of pathogens in positive blood cultures by fluorescence in situ hybridization in routine practice, *J Clin Microbiol* 44:119, 2006.

Richter SS et al: Minimizing the workup of blood culture contaminants: implementation and evaluation of a laboratory-based algorithm, *J Clin Microbiol* 40:2437, 2002.

Sands KE et al: Epidemiology of sepsis syndrome in 8 academic medical centers, *JAMA* 278:234, 1997.

Stoll ML, Rubin LG: Incidence of occult bacteremia among highly febrile young children in the era of the pneumococcal conjugate vaccine, *Arch Pediatr Adolesc Med* 158:671, 2004.

Washington JA: Collection, transport, and processing of blood cultures, *Clin Lab Med* 14:59, 1994.

Watson RS et al: The epidemiology of severe sepsis in children in the United States, *Am J Resp Crit Care Med* 167:695, 2003.

Weinstein MP et al: The clinical significance of positive blood cultures: a comprehensive analysis of 500 episodes of bacteremia and fungemia in adults. I. Laboratory and epidemiologic observations, *Rev Infect Dis* 5:35, 1983.

Weinstein MP et al: Controlled evaluation of 5 versus 10 milliliters of blood cultured in aerobic BacT/Alert blood culture bottles, *J Clin Micro* 32:2103, 1994.

Weinstein MP: Current blood culture methods and systems: clinical concepts, technology, and interpretations of results, *Clin Infect Dis* 23:40, 1996.

Weinstein MP et al: The clinical significance of positive blood cultures in the 1990s: a prospective comprehensive evaluation of the microbiology, epidemiology, and outcome of bacteremia and fungemia in adults, *Clin Infect Dis* 24:584, 1997.

Wilson ML, editor: *Clinics in laboratory medicine*, Philadelphia, 1994, Saunders.

Wisplinghoff H et al: Nosocomial bloodstream infections in US hospitals: analysis of 24,179 cases from a prospective nationwide surveillance study, *Clin Infect Dis* 39:309, 2004.

Points to Remember

- Patients who are immunocompromised are at greatest risk for bacteremia and the systemic complications that may follow.
- Most bacteremias are due to gram-positive organisms, although gram-negative organisms still represent a large proportion of cases.
- Fungal agents are becoming significant causes of bacteremia (fungemia).
- Instrumentation for laboratory diagnosis of bacteremia has become more sensitive in the detection of organisms present in blood culture samples.
- Antibiotics remain the mainstay of treatment of bacteremia.

Learning Assessment Questions

1. What form of bacteremia is demonstrated by the Case in Point?

2. What condition has placed the patient at an increased risk for bacteremia?

3. What other risk factors favor bacteremic episodes in certain patient populations?

4. What are the most common sources of bacteremia?

5. Which bacterial pneumonias produce concurrent bacteremia?

6. What are the major consequences of bacteremia?

7. What are the major means of treatment of bacteremia?

8. Who is at risk for polymicrobial bacteremia?

9. Why is it important to keep the blood to culture medium ratio to 1:10?

10. How many sets of blood cultures should be used, and how often are they collected for maximum recovery of infecting agents?

Urinary Tract Infections

Gail Reid, Vanessa Sarda

OBJECTIVES

After reading and studying this chapter, you should be able to:

1. Discuss the variety of infections that occur in the urinary system.

2. Describe the clinical signs, symptoms, and parameters that define each of the disease manifestations.

3. Identify the epidemiology and risk factors associated with the development of a urinary tract infection (UTI).

4. Identify the organisms associated with UTIs.

5. Discuss the interpretation of urinalysis results based on bacterial colony count, pyuria, and symptoms and signs presented by the patient.

6. Understand the laboratory diagnosis of UTIs, including specimen collection, screening methods, and interpretation of colony counts.

Case in Point

A 77-year-old surgical patient, who had been discharged to a long-term care facility 6 months earlier, developed delirium and elevated temperature (39.9° C), low blood pressure (90/60 mm Hg), and mildly elevated peripheral white blood cell (WBC) count (12,000 WBC/μL). Peripheral blood culture and clean-catch urine specimens were collected. The urine specimen was sent on ice to a reference laboratory. A screening urinalysis yielded a positive result on the leukocyte esterase test. At 100× oil immersion, a Gram stain performed on spun urine revealed several gram-negative rods of similar morphotype and a few white cells. Cultures performed at 24 hours showed 100,000 colony-forming units (CFU)/mL of *Escherichia coli*. Blood cultures were reported as growing gram-negative rods.

Issues to Consider

After reading the patient's case history, consider:
■ The difference between single-episode UTI and recurrent UTI
■ The different ways patients present with a UTI
■ The value of the urinalysis and the Gram-stain procedure
■ The common etiologic agents of UTIs
■ The wide variety of methods for urine collection

Key Terms

Acute urethral syndrome
Bacteriuria
Cervicitis
Cystitis
Dysuria
Prostatitis
Pyelonephritis
Pyuria
Urethritis
Urinary tract infection (UTI)

Urinary tract infections (UTIs) are considered to be one of the most common bacterial infections. UTIs accounted for more than 1.8 million emergency department visits between 1995 and 2005. Accurately assessing the incidence of UTIs is difficult, because they are not reportable diseases. Diagnosis depends on the symptoms, urinalysis, and urine culture. In the outpatient setting, however, diagnosis is usually made without the latter. UTIs occur more frequently in women than in men. Half of all women will have a UTI during their lifetime. Others at risk for UTI include the elderly, pregnant women, patients who have had renal transplantation, patients with spinal cord injuries, patients with catheters, and patients with genitourinary (GU) tract abnormalities.

The pathogenesis and course of UTIs are greatly influenced by the anatomy of the organs involved (Figure 37-1), which includes the urethra, bladder, ureters, prostate, and kidneys. It is therefore practical to separate UTIs into upper and lower UTIs. Upper UTIs involve the renal parenchyma (pyelonephritis) or the ureters (ureteritis). Lower UTIs involve the bladder (cystitis), the urethra (urethritis) and, in males, the prostate (prostatitis).

The heterogeneity of disease presentation, management, and prognosis is reflected in the terminology of UTIs. Box 37-1 lists terms and definitions frequently used in connection with UTIs. Each has specific criteria and must be used appropriately.

There are two clinical schemas for classifying UTIs: single episode versus recurrent, and complicated versus uncomplicated. A single-episode UTI occurs once and does not recur. Patients with chronic or recurrent UTIs have repeated episodes of bacteriuria with or without clinical manifestations. These episodes are arbitrarily divided into relapse and reinfection. The former involves the same organism and implies a focus of infection in the renal or prostatic parenchyma; the latter implies a different organism and usually is limited to the bladder.

Uncomplicated UTIs occur primarily in sexually active young women with normal GU tracts and no prior instrumentation and are usually caused by antibiotic-susceptible bacteria. Complicated UTIs occur in individuals who have one or more structural or functional GU abnormalities or have indwelling catheters and whose conditions cannot be controlled with therapy.

Bacteriuria, which can be symptomatic or asymptomatic, is the presence of bacteria in the urine. Asymptomatic bacteriuria (ASB) is the isolation of bacteria from the urine in

---

BOX 37-1   Definitions of Terms and Abbreviations Commonly Used for Urinary Tract Diseases

Urinary tract infection (UTI)
A spectrum of diseases caused by microbial invasion of the genitourinary (GU) tract that extends from the renal cortex of the kidney to the urethral meatus (see Figure 37-1).

Upper urinary tract infection (U-UTI)
A GU tract infection that is limited to the renal parenchyma (pyelonephritis) or the ureters (ureteritis). It is often accompanied by lower urinary tract (L-UTI) symptoms in addition to costovertebral (CV) flank pain or tenderness and fever. At times, L-UTI precedes the appearance of fever and U-UTI by 24 to 48 hours.

Lower urinary tract infection (L-UTI)
A GU tract infection that is limited to the urethra (urethritis), bladder (cystitis), and, in males, the prostate (prostatitis). These infections generally appear in adults with dysuria (pain on urination), increased frequency, urgency, and occasionally suprapubic tenderness.

Acute urethral syndrome
Includes dysuria and pyuria. Defined as more than 8 leukocytes per cubic millimeter (mm^3) of uncentrifuged urine or approximately 2 to 5 leukocytes/high-power field (hpf) in centrifuged urine sediment.

Prostatitis
A GU infection in males that involves the prostate; fever often is present.

Cervicitis
Inflammation of the cervix; it may occur as an acute or a chronic presentation. Causative agents include sexually transmitted organisms, such as *Neisseria gonorrhoeae* and *Chlamydia trachomatis*. Symptoms include dysuria, urgency, vaginal discharge, and low back pain.

Bacteriuria
The presence of detectable bacteria in the urine. Patients may be symptomatic or asymptomatic (e.g., geriatric or pregnant patients).

Urethritis
Inflammation of the urethra, presenting as dysuria and discharge. Causative agents include *Neisseria gonorrhoeae*, *Chlamydia trachomatis*, and *Ureaplasma urealyticum*. Other causes include trauma, allergic, or chemical.

Cystitis
Inflammation of the bladder, presenting as dysuria, urinary frequency, and urgency. It is often due to gram-negative bacilli, such as *E. coli*, *Proteus*, and *Klebsiella*. It occurs more frequently in women than men. It can also be caused by medication and certain viruses, such as adenovirus.

Pyelonephritis
Infection in the kidney. This is often due to infection in the lower tract ascending to the kidney. Symptoms include fever, chills, nausea, vomiting, and lower back tenderness, as well as dysuria. It can be accompanied by bacteremia.

ANATOMY	TERM	DISEASE
	U-UTI	Pyelonephritis
Diaphragm	L-UTI	Cystitis
Adrenal gland / Adrenal gland		Cervicitis
Right kidney / Left kidney		Urethritis
Ureters		Prostatitis
Bladder		Vaginitis
Orifices of ureters / Trigone		
Urethra		
MALE Prostate / FEMALE Cervix		

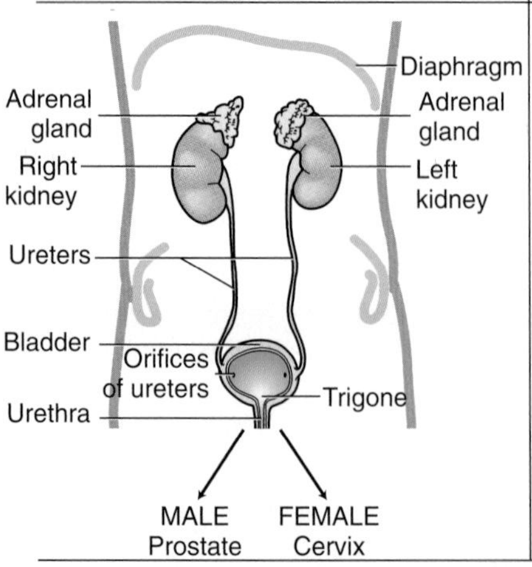

FIGURE 37-1   Anatomy of the urinary tract with corresponding terms and diseases.

significant quantities, but without GU signs or symptoms of infection. ASB requires treatment only in some populations, such as pregnant women and patients about to undergo instrumentation of the GU tract. Disease occurs when the multiplication of organisms in the urinary tract interferes with the normal function of the involved organ. It is important to remember that infection is defined by clinical parameters and urinalysis and not solely by quantitation or identification of microbes.

THE URINARY SYSTEM

Except for the urethral mucosa and the renal medulla, which appear to be relatively susceptible to infection, the normal urinary tract is resistant to colonization and subsequent infection by bacteria. The urinary tract efficiently and rapidly eliminates both virulent and avirulent microorganisms.

Although urine is frequently considered a good culture medium, the extremely high urine osmolarity (concentration) and low pH levels inhibit the growth of many uropathogens and almost all normal biota of the urethra. In addition, very dilute urine fails to support the growth of most bacterial species. In terms of antibacterial activity, urine from men is more inhibitory than urine from women because of the pres-

ence of prostatic fluids in the urine of men, as well as the difference in pH and osmolarity.

However, conditions such as high ammonia concentration, hyperosmolarity, lowered pH, and sluggish blood flow in the renal medulla can contribute to reduced leukocyte chemotaxis and bactericidal activity of white blood cells (WBCs), resulting in lowered infection resistance. Urine itself has also been shown to inhibit the migrating, adhering, agitating, and killing function of polymorphonuclear cells. But the presence of acid-labile mucopolysaccharides, which inhibit bacterial adherence, and the flushing action of the bladder provide additional defensive mechanisms along the lower urinary tract that overcome these immunosuppressive effects. Table 37-1 lists the comparative physiologic parameters of normal urine for different populations.

EPIDEMIOLOGY AND RISK FACTORS

Age

Pediatrics

Urinary tract infection in children is associated with great morbidity and long-term medical problems, including

TABLE 37-1 Comparative Parameters for Urine in Control Subjects and Patients with Urinary Tract Infections

Parameter	Normal	Ranges Abnormal Cystitis	Ranges Abnormal Pyelonephritis
Chemistries			
Specific gravity	1.001-1.035		
Volume (average/24 hr)			
Child (1-14 yr)	500-1400		
Adult (younger than 60 yr)	600-1800		
Adult (older than 60 yr)	250-2400		
pH range	4.7-8.0 (6.0 average)		
Protein	Negative to trace		Increased
WBC esterase	Negative		
Nitrite	Negative	Positive	Positive
Microscopic			
WBCs			
Male	0-3/hpf	Variable	Elevated to greatly increased
Female/child	0-5/hpf	Variable	Elevated to greatly increased
RBCs	0-2/hpf	Variable	Variable to greatly increased
Epithelial cells			
Squamous			Variable/hpf
Renal	0-1/hpf		
Transitional	0-2/hpf		
Crystals	Variable	Negative	Negative
Mucus	Variable	Negative	Negative
Casts			
Hyaline	0-2/lpf		
Granular	0-1/lpf		
WBC	Negative	Negative	Positive
Microorganisms			
Bacteria	Less than 1/hpf	Variable	Positive
Yeast	Negative	Variable	Variable
Trichomonas spp.	Negative	Variable	Negative

WBCs, White blood cells; *RBCs,* red blood cells; *hpf,* high-power field; *lpf,* low-power field.

impaired renal function, hypertension, end-stage renal disease, and complications of pregnancy as an adult. This necessitates extensive evaluation to identify underlying functional or anatomic abnormalities.

During the neonatal period, about 1% of all babies have bacteria in bladder urine; the incidence is higher in boys, and bacteremia often is present. In addition, autopsies have shown a predominance of infection in infant boys with pyelonephritis. Strong evidence exists that shows there is a protective effect of circumcision against UTIs in male infants. Noncircumcised males younger than 6 months of age have a 12-fold increased risk of UTI compared with circumcised cohorts. Among preschool-aged children, girls develop UTIs more often than boys, and infection frequently is associated with severe congenital abnormalities. These infections are often asymptomatic. It is believed that most of the renal damage caused by a UTI occurs in this age group. Among school-aged girls in whom UTIs go into long-term remission, either spontaneously or through antibacterial therapy, many develop symptomatic infection after they marry or become pregnant, and these infections occur at a far higher rate than that of the general population. Thus the presence of bacteria in the urine in childhood defines a population at higher risk for the development of UTIs in adulthood.

Adults to Age 65

From adulthood to age 65, the incidence of UTIs in men is extremely low. When infections do occur, they often are associated with anatomic abnormalities or prostatic disease and the consequent instrumentation, such as catheterization. Among women in this age group, however, as many as one fifth experience a symptomatic UTI.

Geriatrics

The diagnosis and management of UTI in the geriatric population can be challenging. Older adults frequently have an atypical clinical presentation including delirium, fevers alone, or failure to thrive. Geriatric patients also have more comorbidities (two or more unrelated diseases or coexisting medical problems), and an increased risk of drug interactions.

In patients older than 65 years of age, the incidence of UTIs increases dramatically for both genders, and the female-to-male ratio progressively declines. The increased incidence of UTIs in men arises from obstructive uropathologic conditions caused by the prostrate and from the loss of the bactericidal activity of prostate secretions. In women, bladder prolapse contributes to the occurrence of infection, as does soiling of the perineum from fecal incontinence in women afflicted with dementia. In both genders, neuromuscular disease and increased instrumentation and bladder catheterization are contributing factors. The time course of UTIs is shown in Figure 37-2. The epidemiology of UTIs is influenced by the pathophysiology of the infections and by other factors, such as the virulence of the infecting organisms and their inherent mechanisms of pathogenicity, the person's immune status, and other selective external pressures. Box 37-2 lists well-defined microbial virulence factors, and Table 37-2 presents both nonspecific and GU-specific factors that affect host defense and the immune system's ability, both humoral and

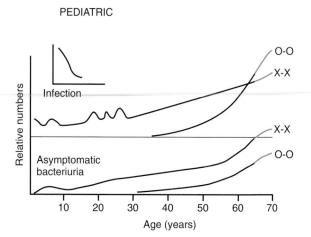

FIGURE 37-2   Frequency of urinary tract infection over time. *X-X,* Females; *O-O,* males.

BOX 37-2   Microbial Virulence Factors

Adherence (bacterial adhesions)
Calculi formation (kidney stones)
Toxin production
Lipopolysaccharides
Capsular polysaccharide
Hemolysins
Biofilms

---

cellular, to resist infection. A dynamic interaction that exists among these factors is continually changing. The severity of infection cannot be defined by the type of invading organism or by colony counts alone; the total clinical situation must be assessed. Predisposing factors that may affect a person's immune status include pregnancy; the presence of an indwelling catheter or intermittent catheterization; urinary tract instrumentation, manipulation, or obstruction; and underlying disorders such as diabetes mellitus. Other underlying risk factors include sexual activity in younger women and incontinence in the geriatric age group. Nonspecific factors that can significantly enhance the virulence of bacteria, either directly or indirectly, include smoking and the use of birth control pills, alcohol, or antibiotics.

Institutionalized Care

Hospitalized patients and those residing in long-term care facilities develop UTIs more often than outpatients. The generally ill condition of the institutionalized population, higher probability of urinary tract instrumentation, and higher incidence of GU tract anatomic or functional abnormalities, are major contributors to this difference.

ASB is a common and usually benign condition in this population. Neurogenic bladder and incontinence increase the frequency of ASB. It can be difficult to distinguish ASB from a symptomatic infection. In one study of nursing home patients with fever, only 10% had UTI as the cause. However, a majority of the patients had a positive urine culture caused by underlying ASB. A serious cause of fever, such as pneumonia, bacteremia, or abdominal infection, can be missed if

TABLE 37-2 Host Defenses and External, Selective Pressures That Influence the Outcome of Interaction Between Bacteria and the Urinary Tract

	Nonspecific	Genitourinary Specific
Host defense (resistance)	Intact skin	Diabetes mellitus
	WBC function	Pregnancy
	Age	Sickle cell (black women)
	Neoplasia	Neuromuscular diseases
	Immune competence	Structural abnormality
	Hormonal changes	Gout (?)
	Pregnancy	Hypertension (?)
	Malnutrition	Potassium deficiency (?)
	Malaria, diabetes	
	Psychologic state	
	Attitude	
	Immunodeficiency syndrome	
Selective pressures	Birth control pill	Sexual activity
	Smoking	Incontinence
	Alcoholism	Bladder catheterization, indwelling or intermittent
	Anesthesia	
	Drug addiction	
	Immunosuppressive drugs	Instrumentation
	Irradiation, therapeutic	Urinary stone
	Antibiotics	

WBC, White blood cell.

the clinical assessment stops with a urinalysis and a positive urine culture.

Pregnancy

Pregnant women are at higher risk for UTI for several reasons. Hormonal changes lead to changes in the ureter and urethra, making them more susceptible to bacterial adherence and infection. In addition, the enlarging uterus can put pressure on the bladder and impair urinary flow. Asymptomatic bacteriuria in pregnant women should be treated because infection can lead to premature labor. Susceptibility testing is particularly important in this patient population because not all antibiotics can be given to pregnant women. This is particularly true for drugs such as fluoroquinolones, which have been a standard of treatment for urinary tract infections.

Renal Transplant

The number of kidney transplants in the United States has increased during the past 12 years to a current peak of 16,224 in 2007, for which the most recent data is available. Although kidney transplant can be life saving and improve quality of life, significant complications accompany it, including infection of the urinary tract system. Several factors contribute to this increased risk of UTI, including significant immunosup-

pression; foreign bodies, such as stents and urinary catheters; stricture, obstruction, or other abnormalities of the ureter and urethra; graft trauma; and diabetes mellitus. In addition, because these patients are on trimethoprim-sulfamethoxazole prophylaxis for *Pneumocystis* pneumonia, as well as for UTIs, they can have infection with organisms that are resistant to this antibiotic.

Urinary tract infections in kidney transplant recipients most often present as cystitis, however, pyelonephritis may occur in almost 25% of them and can lead to allograft injury. In addition, UTIs may be responsible for more than 50% of bacteremias in this population.

The pathogens identified as the cause of UTI in kidney transplant recipients include gram-negative bacilli, namely *E. coli,* in as many as 90% of culture positive infections. Some transplant centers are now reporting a rise in enterococcal UTIs, particularly in the first month post-transplantation.

Bladder Catheterization

Urinary tract infections are the most common hospital-acquired infections, affecting an estimated 560,000 patients per year. Most of these infections, up to 95%, are related to bladder catheterization. The risk for a catheterized patient of acquiring a UTI depends on the duration of catheterization, appropriate catheter care, and host susceptibility. Bacteriuria will inevitably occur given enough time because mechanisms of infection and colonization involve intra- and extra-luminal migration of bacteria. The most common pathogens include enteric gram-negative bacteria, enterococci and yeast. Candiduria is a common finding in long-term catheterized patients, and its clinical relevance is difficult to determine and controversial, particularly in asymptomatic patients. The CDC has published guidelines to aid in the prevention of catheter-associated UTIs including recommendations for proper collection of urine specimens.

CLINICAL SIGNS AND SYMPTOMS

Neonates and children younger than 2 years with UTIs usually have nonspecific symptoms, including failure to thrive, vomiting, lethargy, and fever. Children older than 2 years are more likely to display localized symptoms, such as dysuria, frequency, and abdominal or flank pain.

Adults with uncomplicated lower UTIs limited to the urethra or bladder present primarily with dysuria, often in combination with frequency, urgency, suprapubic pain, and hematuria. Each episode of uncomplicated UTI in women is usually associated with 1 week of symptoms. Acute complicated UTI presents with the same symptoms seen in uncomplicated UTIs. However, the symptoms and signs of complicated UTI in the elderly and in patients with spinal cord injury are often subtle. Patients with upper UTIs, such as pyelonephritis, present with flank pain, nausea, vomiting, fevers, chills, night sweats, and costovertebral angle tenderness. These symptoms may occur in the presence or absence of symptoms of cystitis. At times, the lower urinary tract symptoms precede the appearance of fever and upper urinary tract symptoms by 1 or 2 days. Bacteremia, when present,

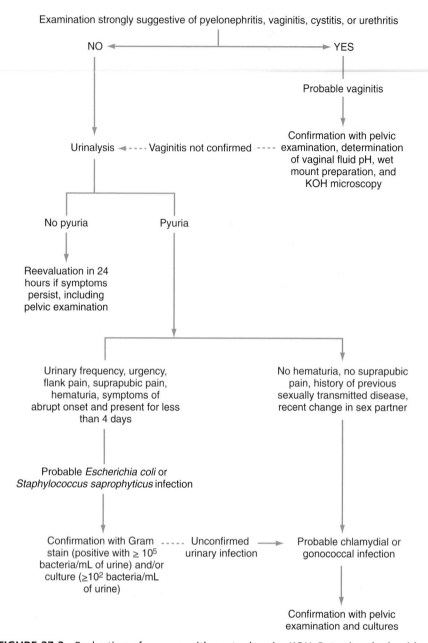

FIGURE 37-3 Evaluation of women with acute dysuria. *KOH,* Potassium hydroxide.

may help confirm a diagnosis of pyelonephritis. It is critically important to remember that these presentations can vary widely. Cases of pyelonephritis may be asymptomatic, may manifest symptoms similar to those in lower UTIs, or may present as life-threatening sepsis. Most elderly patients have atypical presentations such as delirium, failure to thrive, or weakness.

Although dysuria is the most common reason for obtaining a urine culture, this clinical presentation is neither sensitive nor specific. Dysuria may be present in infections with herpes simplex virus, *Chlamydia trachomatis,* or *Neisseria gonorrhoeae.* These organisms are not detected by the routine bacteriologic culture of urine. Many noninfectious conditions, including urethral inflammation from physical or chemical agents or from trauma, may have similar symp-

toms. Flank pain and fever without lower urinary tract symptoms, and bacteremia without any urinary tract symptoms, can be seen in patients with indwelling urinary catheters. Figure 37-3 shows an evaluation schema for women with acute dysuria.

ETIOLOGY OF URINARY TRACT INFECTIONS

Pathogenesis of Urinary Tract Infections

Bacteria gain access to the urinary tract by three routes: the ascending route, the hematogenous (descending) route, and the lymphatic pathways. Women acquire UTIs most frequently via the ascending route. Because of the shorter ureter in women, bacteria are easily introduced into the bladder by sexual intercourse. Once established in the bladder, bacteria ascend the ureters, probably aided in many cases by vesicoureteral reflux or by peristaltic dilated ureters caused by intraluminal infection, an inflammation of the GU tract musculature.

Infection of the renal parenchyma by many species of gram-positive bacteria (particularly in patients with staphylococcal bacteremia or endocarditis), mycobacterial infection, *Candida* infection, and other fungal infections clearly occurs by the hematogenous route. Gram-negative infections rarely occur by the hematogenous route. Increased pressure on the bladder can cause lymphatic flow to be directed to the kidney. However, evidence for a significant role for renal lymphatics in the pathogenesis of pyelonephritis is unimpressive. Of the three possible routes of infection, the ascending route is of paramount importance, and the hematogenous route is a less frequent, but significant pathway.

Etiologic Agents of Urinary Tract Infections

The normal bacterial flora of the paraurethral area consists mostly of *Staphylococcus epidermidis*. Table 37-3 presents the organisms that do not grow well in urine and are not common causes of UTIs, arranged in descending order by age or patient status. Those listed first are most commonly found, and those at the end are less frequently isolated.

Box 37-3 lists the more readily recognized agents of UTIs, as well as emerging uropathogens that need to be recognized, given the dynamics of urinary tract pathogens, the population at risk, and selected pressures, as outlined earlier. These organisms present unique challenges to clinical microbiologists.

Gram-Negative Bacilli

Of the Enterobacteriaceae, antibiotic-susceptible strains of *E. coli* that emanate from the patient's own fecal flora cause most uncomplicated UTIs. Multiple antibiotic-resistant members of the Enterobacteriaceae derived from the hands of hospital personnel and contaminated solutions colonize and subsequently infect hospitalized patients with indwelling bladder instruments. As the duration of hospitalization and catheterization increases, *E. coli* is less likely to be encountered than organisms such as *Pseudomonas, Proteus, Klebsiella, Acinetobacter,* and *Enterobacter* spp. Complicated infections often are polymicrobic, involve renal stones, and can yield urine cultures that are positive for multidrug-resistant organisms.

Gram-Positive Cocci

Among the gram-positive cocci, enterococci and *Staphylococcus saprophyticus* are the most commonly encountered causative agents. Enterococcal UTIs occur primarily in older men, particularly in association with urinary tract manipulation or instrumentation or prostatic hypertrophy. *S. saprophyticus,* on the other hand, is found predominantly in symptomatic sexually active women younger than 40 years of age. Staphylococci that are neither *Staphylococcus aureus* nor *S.*

TABLE 37-3 Flora of Normal Voided Urine* Defined by Patient's Age and Status

Patient Age/Status	Usual Flora
Newborn	Sterile
1-3 days old	Staphylococci
	Enterococci
	Diphtheroids
	Mycobacterium smegmatis
Prepubertal	Micrococci
	Streptococci (α-hemolytic and nonhemolytic)
	Coliforms
	Diphtheroids
Adult	*L. acidophilus*
	Staphylococcus epidermidis
	Streptococci (α-hemolytic and nonhemolytic)
	Escherichia coli
	Diphtheroids
	Yeasts
	Anaerobic streptococci
	Listeria spp.
	Clostridium spp.
Pregnancy	Increase in *L. acidophilus*
	Yeasts
	S. epidermidis
Postmenopausal	Similar to prepubertal flora

*Usually sterile or fewer than 1000 colonies/mL.

BOX 37-3 Recognized Microbial Agents of Urinary Tract Infections

Common
Enterococci (including vancomycin-resistant enterococci)
Streptococcus agalactiae (group B streptococci)
Enterobacteriaceae
Pseudomonas spp.
Streptococcus pyogenes (group A streptococci)
Staphylococcus aureus
Staphylococcus saprophyticus
Candida spp.

Less Common
Gardnerella vaginalis
Ureaplasma urealyticum
Mycoplasma hominis
Mobiluncus spp.
Leptospira spp.
Mycobacterium spp.
Chlamydia trachomatis (males)

Often Associated with Multisystem Diseases
Salmonella spp. (with gastroenteritis)
Schistosoma haematobium
Cryptococcus neoformans
Trichosporon beigelii
Trichomonas vaginalis
Aspergillus spp.
Penicillium spp.
Adenovirus
Herpes simplex virus

TABLE 37-4 UTIs Caused by Coagulase-Negative Staphylococci

Characteristics of Infections	Organism	
	S. epidermidis	*S. saprophyticus*
Sex and age of affected patients	Men and women equally	Women 95%, 16-35 years of age
Population at risk	Hospitalized patients with urinary tract complications	Healthy outpatients
Incidence	Common; 20% or more of all UTIs for hospitalized patients older than 50 years	Uncommon: 3.5% or fewer of all UTIs in hospitalized patients
Presentation	90% asymptomatic	90% symptomatic; indistinguishable from *Escherichia coli* UTIs
Therapy	Often resistant to multiple drugs	Responds readily to traditional urinary tract antimicrobials except nalidixic acid
Outcome	Bacteriuria often persists after therapy	Relapse rare; occasional reinfection

UTI, Urinary tract infection.

saprophyticus frequently are identified as *S. epidermidis,* which commonly is found in hospitalized patients older than 50 years of age. These individuals most often have had recent urinary tract surgery, have indwelling urinary catheters, or have chronic urinary tract disease. *S. epidermidis* is associated with UTI in only about 20% of cases. Table 37-4 highlights important features of coagulase-negative staphylococcal UTIs.

Gram-Positive Bacilli

Isolation of *Bacillus* spp. can almost always be considered contamination. UTIs truly caused by the organism are exceedingly rare. The significance of *Clostridium* spp. is as difficult to assess in urine as it is in blood. The evidence in the literature concerning clostridial UTIs or the recovery of clostridia in urine with a soft tissue abscess is insufficient to support a definitive statement of significance. Mycobacteria infrequently may be seen in Gram-stained specimens of urine and appear as gram-positive bacilli. Mycobacteria have been associated with UTIs and may have added significance in patients infected with the human immunodeficiency virus (HIV) or those who are otherwise immunosuppressed. In rare cases, *Listeria monocytogenes* may be isolated from the urine of infants who acquired a perinatal infection with this organism, and in 1% of patients with a systemic infection or renal transplant. Diphtheroids, mycobacteria, and *L. monocytogenes* all cause diseases, predominantly in highly selected patient populations and almost always in association with bacteremia. If any of these organisms are recovered from urine or seen on smears, consultation with the physician permits some assessment of the significance. Within selected populations, blood cultures or cultures from other sites may help determine the significance of the isolate.

Fungi

Candiduria is rare in healthy adults, however, it is commonly seen in hospitalized patients. As many as 10% of patients in tertiary care facilities have *Candida* in their urine. Over the past 20 years, nosocomial candidal UTIs have increased. This is a result of several factors, including critically ill patients, increasing incidence of urinary instrumentation, and increasing use of broad-spectrum antibiotics. A majority of candidal UTIs are acquired by the ascending route.

On agar medium, young colonies of *Candida albicans* can resemble colonies of coagulase-negative staphylococci and may be misidentified if Gram-stained smears are not examined. A wet mount preparation examined under 10× magnification also can provide a rapid identification. Because *Candida* spp. often are recovered from hospitalized patients with indwelling catheters, incorrect identification results in a susceptibility report indicating broad antimicrobial resistance. *Candida* and *Cryptococcus* spp. usually are evident in culture within 2 to 5 days. Unless dimorphic fungi are suspected, fungal urine cultures can be discarded as having a negative result after 2 weeks. Cultures of dimorphic fungi may require 4 to 6 weeks for colonies to appear. Predisposing factors include diabetes mellitus, antibiotic and corticosteroid therapy, female gender, and disturbance of urine flow. The isolation of any other classic pathogenic fungi, such as *Cryptococcus neoformans, Blastomyces dermatitidis, Coccidioides immitis,* and *Histoplasma capsulatum* in the urine is a highly significant finding indicative of disseminated infection. Optimal management of candiduria is still debated. There is a paucity of data regarding efficacy of fungal agents. A recent study involving hospitalized patients with candiduria (asymptomatic or minimally symptomatic) showed that fluconazole, an antifungal agent, was effective for short-term eradication, but long-term eradication rates were disappointing. Experience has shown that removal of catheters is effective in eliminating candiduria in catheterized patients.

Although findings of candiduria may not require antifungal therapy, particularly in catheterized patients, properly collected urine specimens yielding *Candida* spp. should be considered abnormal. Candiduria may be an indication of bladder or renal parenchymal infection, a urinary tract fungus ball, or disseminated candidiasis. Predisposing factors include diabetes mellitus, antibiotic and corticosteroid therapy, female sex, instrumentation, and disturbance of urine flow.

Other Agents of Urinary Tract Infections

Other significant organisms may be encountered in urine cultures. Anaerobes, which are common flora in the urethra, are not usually responsible for UTIs but may be considered significant when isolated from suprapubic aspirates. *C. trachomatis* and *N. gonorrhoeae* can cause the symptoms of **urethritis, cystitis,** and **prostatitis.** This is particularly an issue with women, because in women it is clinically difficult to distinguish between urethritis and **cervicitis.** Recently, *Mycoplasma* and *Ureaplasma* organisms have been associated with UTIs, particularly in neonates from lower socioeconomic groups.

The isolation of *Gardnerella vaginalis* in urine commonly represents vaginal contamination, but this organism is also an emerging urinary tract pathogen. Although the role of *G. vaginalis* in UTIs has not been clearly established, repeated cultures in which this microbe is the primary isolate should not be ignored. Certain organisms, particularly *Salmonella* spp., are involved with multiple organ systems; these may be part of a primary disease or may arise secondarily. Viral agents, especially adenovirus and herpes simplex virus, also have been associated with cystitis and must be identified when the clinical situation warrants. Table 37-5 presents organisms associated with UTIs, listing the uropathogens most often associated with a particular clinical presentation or disease syndrome.

TABLE 37-5 Most Common UTI Etiologic Agents Associated with Frequent Clinical Presentation (Disease Syndromes)

Clinical Presentation	Common Etiologic Agents
Upper urinary tract infections	
Acute pyelonephritis	Enterobacteriaceae
	Staphylococcus aureus
Subclinical pyelonephritis	Coagulase-negative staphylococci
	Candida spp.
	Mycobacterium spp.
	Mycoplasma hominis
Lower urinary tract infections	
Acute bacterial cystitis	*Escherichia coli*
	Klebsiella spp.
	Other Enterobacteriaceae
	Enterococci
	Coagulase-negative staphylococci
Urethritis	
Acute urethral syndrome	*Chlamydia trachomatis*
	Neisseria gonorrhoeae
	Ureaplasma urealyticum
Other infections	
Gonococcal urethritis	*N. gonorrhoeae*
Chlamydial urethritis	*C. trachomatis*
Vaginitis	
Prostatitis	
Symptomatic bacteriuria	
Catheter-associated (hospital-associated) UTI	*E. coli*
	Klebsiella spp.
	Proteus mirabilis
	Pseudomonas spp.
	Candida spp.
Chronic or recurrent (inpatient/outpatient) UTI	Adherent *E. coli*

UTI, Urinary tract infection.

LABORATORY DIAGNOSIS

Significance of Colony Counts: A Historical Background

The urinary tract, above the urethra in normal, healthy individuals is sterile, as is urine, unlike the urethra, which is colonized with many normal microbiota (see Fig. 37-1). In women, it is important to note that the microbiota that colonize the vagina may contaminate the urine. Many of these organisms that colonize the vagina are also implicated in UTIs. Therefore it would be difficult to know whether growth in urine cultures was indicative of infection or contamination.

Since 1956, the interpretation of quantitative urine cultures has been considered one of the more straightforward and simpler laboratory tests to diagnose UTIs. It was "dogma" that a finding of 100,000 (10^5) colony-forming units per milliliter (CFU/mL) or more was a "positive" test result symbolizing infection. In his 1956 classic study, Edward Kass showed a clear separation between the number of bacteria in the urine of asymptomatic or symptomatic women with pyelonephritis and those who were uninfected. Significantly, 95% had colony counts higher than 10^5 CFU/mL when infected.

In retrospect, this study had some very definitive parameters, namely that all specimens were collected by *catheterization,* not voided, that most asymptomatic women had counts below 10^3 CFU/mL, and that the prevalence of infection was only 6%. With this low prevalence rate, the number of false positives would be higher, hence the 10^5 CFU/mL so-called "cut off" positive infection point. The sensitivity was only 51% for women with clinical pyelonephritis who had colony counts above 10^5 CFU/mL (see Chapter 5 for review of definitions). In the 1960s and 1970s, additional studies began to challenge Kass's original work. A number of investigators showed that for women with symptomatic, acute lower UTIs (urethra, bladder, or both), 29% to 45% had colony counts lower than 10^5 CFU/mL by *suprapubic aspiration.* These women had **dysuria** and **pyuria,** yet unexpectedly "negative cultures" by the traditional "Kass-based" criterion (e.g., more than 10^5 CFU/mL signifying infection). In 1980, the **acute urethral syndrome,** or urethritis, was more clearly defined as one of the three causes of acute dysuria with pyuria. The other causes were vaginitis and cystitis. The causative organisms included classic coliforms and *S. saprophyticus* at colony counts above 10^3 but below 10^5 CFU/mL. Simultaneously implicated in sexually active women were the emerging nongonococcal urethritis pathogens, *Chlamydia trachomatis* and *Ureaplasma urealyticum.* Thus in women with UTIs, as many as half had urethral syndrome—not cystitis—and were "culture-negative" by traditional "laboratory" methods.

In 1982, Stamm and co-workers restudied the diagnostic criteria for women with acute symptomatic lower UTIs. In contrast with Kass's classic work, Stamm's study included coliforms at counts above 10^2 CFU/mL. The criteria of 10^2 CFU/mL provided a sensitivity of 0.95 and a specificity of 0.85. The presence of pyuria in uncentrifuged urine specimens was a sensitive adjunct. The prevalence of coliform infections was 36% in women evaluated by Stamm et al. (1982), compared with Kass's 6%. Because of this higher prevalence of infection, the positive predictive value (PPV) of infection also increases, and the number of false positives decrease. Stamm was able to use a low "cutoff" of 10^2 CFU/mL to differentiate infection from contamination. Finally, in the late 1980s, because of the emerging significance of pyuria, investigators reevaluated the accuracy of the classic urinary sediment microscopic examination (urinalysis). All agreed that urinalysis screening for detection of UTI was inherently inaccurate, was not reproducible, and did not correlate with clinically proven UTIs. It was thought that microscopic examination of urine specimens should be reserved for the detection of casts and crystals. Furthermore, investigators could not correlate urinalysis determinations of WBCs with the actual leukocyte excretion rate of WBCs per cubic millimeter measured by hemocytometer chamber count. When clinical studies using the latter method of determining pyuria were reviewed, the following conclusions emerged:

- A leukocyte count of $10/mm^3$ or higher occurs in fewer than 1% of asymptomatic, nonbacteriuric patients but in more than 96% of symptomatic men and women with significant bacteriuria.
- Most symptomatic women with pyuria but without significant bacteriuria either have UTIs with bacterial uropathogens present in colony counts lower than 10^5 CFU/mL (more than 10^2 to less than 10^5 CFU/mL) or have infections with *C. trachomatis/U. urealyticum*.
- Women with ASB probably should be divided into those with true asymptomatic infection associated with pyuria and those with transient self-limited bladder colonization and no pyuria.
- Most patients with catheter-associated bacteriuria also have pyuria, hence, infection.
- Simultaneously, an impregnated paper strip that measured urine leukocyte esterase was introduced and found to correlate well with hemocytometer chamber counts. The leukocyte esterase test (LET) was inexpensive and quick (1 minute) and required no technical skills or equipment, just the classic "dipstick."

What did all this mean, and how did it fit into the laboratory faced with myriad problems in interpreting uropathogen colony counts? Until recently, the colony count was regarded as the gold standard for determining whether a patient had a real and treatable UTI; the fact is, however, that the urine bacterial colony count cannot stand alone as a single criterion when evaluating for the presence or absence of UTI. Urine cultures are requested not only in connection with the symptoms of acute UTI but also in the absence of specific symptoms, as a test of cure, to evaluate the effectiveness of antimicrobial therapy, to detect ASB in pregnant women, and to evaluate for bacteremia or fever or both, to name a few. Furthermore, the criteria that determine whether a UTI is present must include the presence or absence of symptoms, predisposing factors, the patient population, and the type of organism or organisms isolated. The outcome of a urine culture therefore must be evaluated together with other laboratory and clinical data; attempts to attach significance to the colony count should be restricted to the original patient population in which that significance was established: asymptomatic individuals with pyelonephritis.

Specimen Collection

Preventing contamination by normal vaginal, perianal, and interior urethral flora is the most important consideration in collecting a clinically relevant urine specimen. Nonetheless, it is still an important fact that physicians rely on colony counts. Therefore all necessary precautions should be taken to ensure that the colony count represents the numbers of organisms present at the time the specimen was collected. It is incumbent on the laboratory directors to define specific criteria for collection and transport and, within their realm of responsibility, to ensure that these protocols are followed. A wide variety of methods can be used for collecting urine samples.

Voided Midstream Specimen Collection

The voided midstream collection, in which the patient collects the urine specimen, is the most commonly used method in clinical practice. The urine is contaminated with bacteria from the urethra unless the first portion of the voided specimen is discarded. Voided urine collection kits should contain instructions to the patient on proper specimen procurement, and these instructions should be read slowly to the patient rather than merely supplied. Patient education should be part of the specimen processing, because proper collection has a considerable influence on the result of subsequent laboratory procedures. It has also been reported that stick figure diagrams showing the manner in which a specimen should be collected are much more easily understood by the patient than written instructions.

Catheterized Specimen Collection

Catheterized specimen collection, which is an invasive technique, reduces the risk of contamination of urine with the urethral flora; however, because the catheter is passed through the urethra, some contamination may occur. Before collecting urine with a single, straight catheter, the urethral opening or vaginal vault is cleansed with a soap solution and rinsed with sterile water. The initial urine flow is discarded because it may contain organisms acquired as the catheter passed through the urethra. When specimens are collected from an existing, indwelling urinary catheter, the catheter collection port should be cleaned with an alcohol pad and punctured directly with a needle and syringe. The specimen should never be collected from the drainage bag. Samples obtained from an ileoconduit are collected from the stomal opening after the area has been swabbed with an alcohol wipe. The urine on the external appliance is never used for culture, because it is similar to the urine in a drainage bag in patients with indwelling catheters. The bacteriologic results of separate urine specimens collected by cystoscopy (bilateral urethral catheterization) or by bladder washout are used to localize the infection to the upper or lower urinary tract and, in the former case, to the left or right kidney. Specimens obtained by straight catheterization, by bilateral urethral catheterization, by bladder washout, or from an ileoconduit may be submitted in a tube or broth unless an assessment of pyuria is necessary. When such a specimen arrives at the laboratory, it must be labeled as to location or timing, and this information must accompany the results for proper interpretation.

Suprapubic Aspiration

Suprapubic aspiration is the definitive method for collecting uncontaminated specimens. Although most consider any organism isolated on these specimens to be clinically significant, this may not be correct because transient colonization of the bladder can occur. Suprapubic aspirations are collected primarily from infants and patients in whom the interpretation of the results of voided specimens is difficult. Suprapubic aspiration urine specimens are the only ones suitable for anaerobic culture. With the bladder full, the urine is collected with a needle and syringe following skin antisepsis.

Other Considerations. In addition to the manner in which the specimen is collected, other parameters may have an impact on the suitability of the specimen including the following:

- *Urine volume.* The volume of urine received is rarely a problem for routine bacteriologic culture. Detection of significant pyuria by sediment examination requires at least 10 mL of specimen. Alternative methods of pyuria detection may be needed when smaller volumes are received. As much as 20 mL of urine may be required to recover mycobacteria or fungi. If these agents are strongly suspected and previous specimens of lesser volume tested negative, a request for a single collection of at least 20 mL should be forwarded to the physician. It must be remembered that 24-hour collections for urine specimens in microbiology are totally unsatisfactory.
- *The number of specimens and timing of collection.* The number of specimens and the timing of urine collection depend on the patient's clinical state and the method used. A single clean voided specimen or a single specimen obtained by catheterization in a patient with specific symptoms is sufficient if significant pyuria is demonstrable and culture yields a recognized uropathogen. In symptomatic patients, antimicrobial therapy often is instituted immediately after urine collection and is not withheld to allow the procurement of subsequent specimens. For purposes of optimal quantitation, it has been recommended that only first morning specimens be processed or, if such specimens are not available, that the urine be allowed to incubate in the bladder for as long as possible (with a minimum of 4 hours) before collection to increase the bacterial density. This procedure appears to be rather imprecise and probably unnecessary because of the insignificance of colony counts in symptomatic patients and the need for antimicrobial therapy.

In the absence of symptoms, a single first morning voided urine specimen from a pregnant woman is sufficient to detect ASB. In this case, one or two more first morning specimens may be collected on separate days to demonstrate the significance of the isolates. Because quantitation is necessary for the diagnosis of ASB and because an asymptomatic condition does not require immediate therapeutic intervention, these specimens should be limited to first morning collections. Urine specimens from other asymptomatic patient populations, except those demonstrating significant pyuria, cannot be reliably interpreted.

Additives

Additives to urine are designed primarily to preserve the bacterial density present at collection. These additives maintain the original colony count during ambient temperature transport until quantitative cultures can be accomplished, obviating a need for refrigerated transportation. An example is sodium borate, which maintains the sample integrity for as long as 48 hours at room temperature. Sodium borate also helps prevent overgrowth without causing toxicity to existing pathogens. Liquid preservatives have been associated with dilution errors and decreased recovery of organisms at 24 and 48 hours. Lyophilized preservation is less inhibitory and requires a urine volume of at least 3 mL to avoid dilution effect. The effects of preservatives on the detection of pyuria have not been adequately determined. Regardless of the preservative used, the maximum time from collection to processing should not exceed 24 hours. In addition, the effect of preservatives on selected manual and automated methods, which are discussed later in the chapter, has not been extensively evaluated.

The importance of the determination of pyuria in many cases and the lack of evidence that urine preservatives allow an accurate leukocyte count after 2 hours argue against the use of preservatives for specimens from symptomatic patients. The dip-slide urine collection container offers a more reliable method of preserving bacterial density in specimens from asymptomatic pregnant women or from patients for whom quantitative cultures are required; it also allows quicker detection of the etiologic agent. This method may be particularly suited to physicians' offices. In the current cost-conscious environment, it is recommended that all urine specimens in physicians' offices be cultured with the dip-slide method and held for 48 hours. If the patient does not respond to empirical therapy, these original specimens can be forwarded to the laboratory for identification and susceptibility testing. If the appropriate antibiotic is selected, the specimens can be discarded.

Specimen Transport

Urine is an excellent supportive medium for the growth of most uropathogens and therefore must be immediately refrigerated or preserved. Generally, urine should be refrigerated, received, and processed in the laboratory within 2 hours. Longer delays render examination for significant pyuria unreliable, and the extremes of pH and urea concentration and the presence of antimicrobial agents may adversely affect the recovery of uropathogens.

A specimen submitted on a dip-slide transported at room temperature may be received up to 18 hours after collection. Liquid urine submitted for diagnosis of ASB for which an examination for pyuria is not requested may be refrigerated for a maximum of 18 hours before processing. Except for specimens submitted for the sole purpose of isolating mycobacteria or fungi, or the diagnosis of ASB, refrigeration is not an optimal, or to some, an acceptable method of preserving urine specimens. Refrigeration cannot preserve the number of leukocytes beyond 2 hours, and there is no need to stabilize the bacterial density in urine for symptomatic patients for the purpose of quantitative culture.

MICROBIAL DETECTION

Specimen Screening: Rapid, Nonculture Methodologies

The ideal urine screening system should identify all urine specimens from infected patients at a high negative predictive value and be rapid and cost effective. Toward this goal, a number of manual and automated methods have been developed. To maximize the benefits of the screening method, preliminary reports should be produced as soon as possible. Preliminary reports should consist of the degree of pyuria and, depending on the method used, the presence or absence of bacteria or fungi. These results should reach the physician within 2 hours after collection of a urine specimen.

The report also should indicate whether additional identification methods are being used and their turnaround time. Ideally, the report should also include guides to appropriate antimicrobial therapy based on in-house laboratory antibiograms tabulated over the past 6 months. However, the need for screening and the extent of identification and susceptibility testing of isolates depend on the method of collection and the purpose for which the urine was submitted. Hence a uniform and consistent means of communicating that purpose to the laboratory must be developed so that information useful to the physician can be produced in the timeframe required. Additionally, a number of key points need to be remembered when using screening methods:

- Screening methods capable of detecting bacterial densities of 10^5 CFU/mL or higher are appropriate for the detection of ASB in pregnant women.
- False-positive results occur more often with methods that test for more than one parameter (e.g., bacteria and WBC counts).
- Methods of detecting significant pyuria and bacteriuria with sensitivities of 50 to 100 leukocytes/mm^3 and 10^2 CFU/mL may be appropriate for screening voided

urine specimens or specimens from indwelling urinary catheters in symptomatic patients.
- Screening methods are not appropriate for urine collected by straight catheterization, cystoscopy, suprapubic aspiration, or bladder washout or for testing of cure specimens and specimens collected from ileoconduits.

Manual Urine Screening Methods

Table 37-6 lists various manual screening methods that are useful in detecting bacteria and leukocytes in urine.

Microscopy.

Detection of Bacteria When Pyelonephritis Is Suspected. Gram staining of urine samples should be performed, because it may reveal the etiologic agent. Uncentrifuged urine samples may be used for a stained smear. Cytospin technology has been found to be remarkably applicable to rapid urine microscopy. The presence of one or more bacterial cells per oil immersion field in at least five fields in a smear of uncentrifuged urine correlates with more than 10^5 CFU/mL. If the uncentrifuged preparation tests negative, the sedimented preparation for leukocyte examination should be stained. Bacterial cells seen in this preparation indicate a density of fewer than 10^5 organisms/mL and, in the presence of clinical findings of acute pyelonephritis, may suggest urinary obstruction or perinephric abscess. The presence of gram-positive or gram-negative bacteria or fungi assists in the selection of an appropriate antibiotic therapy. Acridine orange stain decreases the detectable threshold from 10^5 CFU/mL to 10^4 CFU/mL.

Detection of Pyuria. Detection of leukocytes may be performed by microscopic examination of a wet mount of a urinary sediment resulting from centrifugation of 10 mL of a specimen at 200 rpm on a tabletop centrifuge for 5 minutes. At least five fields should be examined, and each leukocyte seen per high-power field (hpf) (40×) represents approximately 5 to 10 cells per cubic millimeter of urine. In this way, 5 to 10 leukocytes/hpf in the sediment is the upper limit of normal, representing 50 to 100 cells/mm^3. If a more precise method is

---

TABLE 37-6 Various Manual Screening Methods, Principles of Assay, and Threshold of Detection for UTI

Screens	Principle	Reported Threshold of Detection (CFU/mL)
Manual		
Microscopy	Recognition of organism morphotypes and Gram stain	≥1 organism/OIF = ≥10^5
Direct, uncentrifuged or centrifuged (cytospin)		
Chemical		
Enzymatic dipstick		
Nitrate reductase (Griess test)	Gram-negative bacteria reduce nitrates to nitrites	
WBC/leukocyte esterase	Measures presence of WBC enzyme	Equivalent to 5 WBC/hpf
Chemstrip LN	Combination testing of both nitrate and esterase assays	>10^4 to 10^5
Enzyme tube		
Uriscreen	Measures catalase present in both bacteria and somatic cells	<10^4 to 10^5
Colorimetric particle filtration		
FiltraCheck—UTI	Combination testing of both bacteria and WBCs by membrane filtration and detection using safranin O dye	>10^4

UTI, Urinary tract infection; *CFU*, colony-forming unit; *OIF*, oil immersion field; *WBC*, white blood cell; *hpf*, high-power field.

required, the technique described by Brumfitt may be used. This involves the examination of a fresh, uncentrifuged specimen in a hemocytometer chamber. More than 8 to 10 leukocytes/mm^3 indicates significant pyuria.

Detection of Fungi and Mycobacteria. The cells of yeasts can usually be readily identified by Gram stain, but the cells of other fungi, because of their varying size and unique forms, may be difficult to discern. If fungi are suspected clinically or from the Gram stain, a smear can be stained using fluorescent microscopy and calcofluor white. This stain preferably binds chitin present in the cell walls of fungi and makes visualization and identification easier. Cotton swabs may not be used to apply the specimen to the microscope slide, however, because the stains bind to the cotton fibers and fluoresce.

Examination of urine for acid-fast bacilli is productive only if restricted to a particular patient population. Because of the presence of nonpathogenic mycobacteria in the smegma, smears that test positive must be confirmed with culture.

Chemical Methods. Chemical screening techniques include a variety of procedures, such as the nitrate reductase (Griess) test, WBC leukocyte esterase test, and Chemstrip (Roche Diagnostics, Basel, Switzerland). As with manual microscopy, these methods may be labor intensive and insensitive for low-grade significant bacteriuria.

Recently, tube enzyme (catalase) and colorimetric particle filtration (safranin O dye) have been reintroduced into the clinical setting with modified, updated protocols. Both measure a combination of bacteria and extracellular products of WBCs.

Automated Urine Screening Methods

Table 37-7 summarizes various automated screening methods for bacterial detection in urine samples. Bioluminescence systems detect bacterial adenosine triphosphate. Such systems may be expensive, frequently require batching of specimens (therefore time delays), and have not been adequately evaluated for their efficacy in detecting low-grade bacteriuria and funguria. The popularity of automation has grown, however, as more laboratories search for quick, same-day results and the means to eliminate negative urine culture results.

A number of photometry methods, including the Vitek system (bioMérieux Vitek, Hazelwood, Mo.) have been developed to measure growth. If a significant number of organisms are present in the urine specimens, rapid growth is detected in the nutrient medium. The clinical evaluations of all these systems are less than optimal because sensitivity for a low-grade bacteriuria has not been assessed. These systems are relatively expensive. Particle filtration systems, such as Bac-T-Screen 2000 (bioMérieux Vitek, Hazelwood, Mo.) are used to trap organisms and WBCs on filters and then selectively stain the cells. These systems are very sensitive even for low-grade infections, are somewhat nonspecific, yield many false-positive results, and are relatively expensive.

Rejection Criteria

It is imperative that the laboratory establish, in concert with the various medical services, criteria for obtaining optimal specimens. Specimens may be rejected because of an inadequate or inappropriate method of collection or transport. These criteria demand strict adherence to guidelines for collection and transport of specimens. If the specimen does not meet these tailored guidelines for each institution, it is incumbent on the laboratory (as soon as possible) to inform the service or physician (or both) of the inadequacy of the specimen and the fact that the specimen will not be processed. Antibiotic therapy may not have been initiated, and a better specimen still may be collected. Samples to be rejected include 24-hour urine specimens and Foley catheter tips; these should not be processed.

Culture for Etiologic Agents of Urinary Tract Infections

Generally, routine urine culture should include plating onto one selective (e.g., MAC) and one nonselective medium. Calibrated loops of 0.01 mL should be used, not 0.001 mL (1 μL) loops, because quantitation is difficult to obtain with a low inoculum. The urine specimen should be mixed thoroughly and the calibrated loop should be inserted vertically; inserting the loop in a more horizontal position may increase the volume beyond calibration; it should also be observed visually for bubbles that would decrease the volume. Routine specimens incubated longer than a full 24 hours yield "noise"

TABLE 37-7 Various Automated Screening Methods, Principle of Assay, and Threshold of Detection for UTI

Automated	Principle	Threshold of Detection (CFU/mL)
Bioluminescence		
UTI screen	Detected bacterial ATP using enzymatic bioluminescent reaction of ATP with luciferin and luciferase	>10^4 to 10^5
Photometry	If a significant number of organisms are present in the urine specimen, they will grow in the medium to a detectable concentration using photometry	>10^4 to 10^5
Colorimetric particle filtration		
Bac-T-Screen	Automated combination testing for both bacteria and WBCs by membrane filtration and detection using safranin O dye	>10^4 to 10^5

UTI, Urinary tract infection; *CFU,* colony-forming unit; *ATP,* adenosine triphosphate; *WBC,* white blood cell.

or background urethral flora that increase cost and may impair the clinical usefulness of the urine culture.

Two important factors govern the selection of culture methods for urine specimens. First, some circumstances may account for the presence of a low number of bacteria in specimens; such circumstances include pyelonephritis with obstruction, perinephric abscess, the period before the start of antimicrobial therapy, and bacterial persistence while the patient is undergoing antimicrobial therapy. In these cases, methods with appropriate sensitivity are necessary to detect the low densities. Second, organisms in deep-seated infections, such as upper UTIs, often are in a hydrophilic state and do not emerge on direct plating of the specimen on agar. A suspicion that certain etiologic agents may be present may also dictate the method of processing for culture. For example, media should include detection of *N. gonorrhoeae* and *U. urealyticum* if these organisms are suspected. If fungal cells or hyphae are seen on wet mount or Gram stain or if fungal infection is suspected, media such as Sabouraud dextrose agar (Emmons modification) may be inoculated. If mycobacteria are suspected, the specimen should be decontaminated and inoculated to one Bactec bottle (Becton Dickinson, Cockeysville, Md.) and one Löwenstein-Jensen slant. The specimens are then processed according to the standard protocol for acid-fast bacilli culture.

Use of agar dipsticks and biplates should be reserved for clinics and physicians' offices, circumstances in which retrieval of specimens after therapy may be less than optimal, and only cultures from patients who are not responding to therapy would need a complete identification. The method also needs to be adjusted to the specimen source and the underlying disease process.

Asymptomatic Bacteriuria

If the patient is asymptomatic, immediate microbial therapy is not necessary, unless the patient is pregnant or undergoing GU surgery. Identification and susceptibility testing of isolates can be achieved by any conventional or automated method. The colony count should accompany any positive culture result to indicate the diagnosis of ASB. Because the organisms most frequently identified include *E. coli* and other rapidly growing members of Enterobacteriaceae, 24 hours of incubation at 35° C is sufficient.

Pyelonephritis

Urine specimens submitted from patients suspected of having pyelonephritis generally contain high numbers of bacteria. Microscopic examination of urine for leukocytes and bacteria quickly provides therapeutically useful information. Because the antibiotic susceptibilities of the responsible organisms are variable and unpredictable, culture should be designed for optimal recovery. Plates should be incubated for 48 hours at 35° C, and the method may include a drop of specimen inoculated into trypticase soy broth for optimal recovery.

Lower Urinary Tract Infections

Specimens from patients with symptoms of lower UTI should be processed in the same manner as for suspected cases of pyelonephritis. If significant pyuria is found in a symptomatic

patient and no recognized urinary pathogen is detected, the laboratory should consider the presence of *C. trachomatis*, *Mycoplasma* spp., *U. urealyticum*, and *N. gonorrhoeae*.

Suprapubic Aspirates

Aspirates may contain bacteria that are likely to be present in low numbers and may include anaerobic species. Such specimens should be routinely inoculated on a blood agar plate, a MacConkey agar plate, and a trypticase soy broth for up to 48 hours. For recovery of *G. vaginalis*, chocolate agar is acceptable. Anaerobic bacteria are recovered in approximately 1% of cases and therefore need only be sought after consultation.

Catheterized Specimens

Urine specimens obtained by straight catheterization, by bilateral ureteral catheterization, by bladder washout, or from ileoconduits require inoculation of both agar plates and liquid medium for maximum recovery.

Prostatic Secretions

The etiologic agent of acute prostatitis is usually recovered from catheterized specimens, which should be cultured in the same manner as for specimens from symptomatic men. In cases of chronic prostatitis, prostatic secretions are submitted, as well as urethral urine and midstream-voided urine specimens obtained before and after prostatic massage. Quantitative cultures are necessary for proper interpretation.

Historically, yeasts have been detected within 24 hours, but certain forms may need a total of 48 hours of incubation. When isolated, the numbers of yeast should be reported. Low colony counts may be just as significant as higher colony counts. When mycobacteria are suspected, the specimen should be decontaminated and inoculated to one Bactec bottle (Becton Dickinson) and one Löwenstein-Jensen slant and processed according to the standard acid-fast bacilli protocol. Use of agar dipsticks and biplates should be avoided, if possible, because isolated colonies may not be available, thus delaying final identification and antimicrobial susceptibility testing. These methods should be reserved for clinics or physicians' offices where retrieval of specimens following therapy may be less than optimal and only cultures from patients not responding would need detailed identification.

INTERPRETATION OF RESULTS

Routine workup of isolates and susceptibility testing must be tailored according to the patient at risk and the specimen type submitted. Figure 37-4 shows a flow diagram that takes into account three features considered in all UTIs:

- Colony count of a pure or predominant organism
- Measurement of pyuria
- Presence or absence of symptoms (dysuria and frequency)

It is important to recognize, however, that no one scheme can fit all situations. This figure is organized into a cascade scheme using a dichotomous key. This allows the final laboratory selection from 12 clinical categories, depending on knowledge of symptoms and recognizing the need for physi-

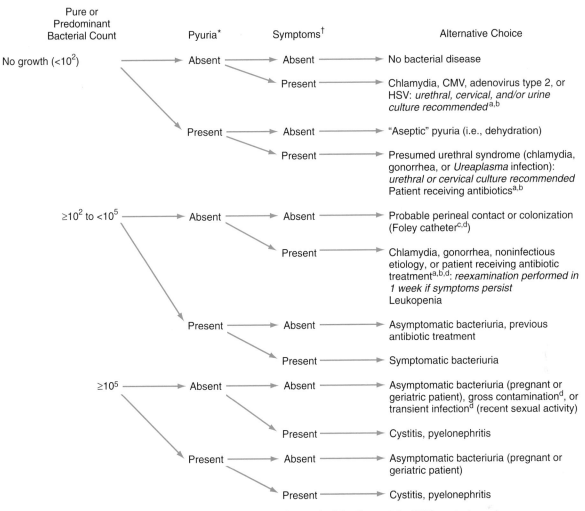

a. If patient is receiving antibiotic treatment, the result of the Gram stain, WBC analysis, and culture may not agree.
b. Quantitation of organisms and white cells by urinalysis of a centrifuged specimen is of no comparative value for the measurement of leukocyte esterase and bacteria done by microbiologic study, which is performed routinely on a noncentrifuged specimen.
c. Interpretation for indwelling catheter has not been established.
d. Plates held 72 hours for consultation.

*Leukocyte esterase (+); equivalent to 5 WBC/hpf.
†Clinical dysuria and frequency.

FIGURE 37-4 Interpretation of urine culture results using algorithm based on bacterial colony count, pyuria, and symptoms. *CMV,* Cytomegalovirus; *hpf,* high-power field; *HSV,* herpes simplex virus; *WBC,* white blood cell.

cian input. Historically most guidelines suggested that laboratory evaluation and culture setup should depend on previous knowledge of symptoms. Because this is often unrealistic, given the general lack of communication between physicians and the laboratory, the schema presented allows the final differentiation to be made by the physician, based on his or her knowledge of the patient's symptoms. Figure 37-4 also takes into account ASB. Furthermore, if the patient is receiving antibiotic therapy, the Gram stain, WBC analysis, and culture results may not agree. Last, quantitation of organisms and white cells by urinalysis of a centrifuged specimen has no comparative value for the measurement of leukocyte esterase

and bacteria done by microbiologic study, which is performed routinely on a noncentrifuged urine specimen.

This figure particularly addresses the "acute urethral syndrome" and the recognition that cystitis and urethritis are clinically difficult to differentiate, particularly in the female patient. It is imperative that clinicians recognize that routine urine cultures do not include isolation and identification of *C. trachomatis, N. gonorrhoeae,* or *U. urealyticum.* It is also important to recognize that given the high propensity of negative cultures sent to the laboratory (i.e., approximately 50%), reevaluation of the patient with a negative culture may require consideration of a sexually transmitted disease (STD). Table

TABLE 37-8 Guidelines for Interpretation of Urine Culture Results and Subsequent Workup

Colony Count (CFU/mL)*	Symptoms, Clinical Disease, or Patient Population[†]	Urine Source[‡]	Number of Organism Types Isolated	Laboratory Workup Suggested[§] (Inpatient)
<10[†]		CV/CA	None	None[¶]
≥10[†]	Pediatric	Suprapubic	≤2 organisms by anaerobic culture	ID & AST
≥[†]	Symptomatic female, urethritis	CV	Pure culture	ID & AST
≥[‡]	Symptomatic male, prostatitis	CA	≤2 organisms	ID & AST
		CA	Pure culture	ID & AST
≥10[‡]		Bladder washout		ID & AST
≥10[¶]	Cystitis/pyelonephritis	CV	Pure culture	ID & AST
			2-3 organisms	Q & SID
			>3 organisms	Q & M or Q & GS

*Inoculation of 0.01 mL of urine is required to detect 10^2 CFU/mL.
[†]See Table 37-1 for description of clinical diseases, symptoms, and patient population.
[‡]*CV,* Clean; *CA,* straight catheterized.
[§]Workup required. Any yeast may be quantitated and reported (regardless of number); >100,000 needed to identify to species.
[¶]See figures and text for suggested comments and educational information helpful to physicians.
CFU, Colony-forming unit; *ID & AST,* perform identification and antimicrobial susceptibility testing; *Q & SID,* quantitate and perform sight identification, identification and sensitivity not indicated, hold plates 72 hours; *Q & M,* quantitate total amount of bacteria and report as "mixed urethral flora"; *Q & GS,* quantitate and report Gram stain morphotypes.

37-8 lists guidelines for the interpretation of urine cultures and suggests subsequent workup. In summary, these guidelines suggest the following, remembering that cost-effective strategies may define different algorithms for inpatient and outpatient cases:

- Specimens with multiple uropathogens (i.e., three or more) indicate probable contamination.
- One or two significant uropathogens present (i.e., 10^5 CFU/mL or more) should routinely be identified. Susceptibility tests should be performed for inpatients. Outpatient cases may use a different algorithm that does not routinely call for susceptibility tests; rather, it emphasizes empirical selection based on antibiograms.
- One or two uropathogens present in small numbers (i.e., 10^2 CFU/mL or more) should be routinely identified (10^2 or more to less than 105 CFU/mL) if the clinical situation warrants, such as in acute urethral syndrome or cases of previous antibiotic therapy.

SUSCEPTIBILITY REPORTING

With the growing number of emerging uropathogens and the simultaneous increase in newer antibiotics, it is mandatory that laboratories use standardized methods and report only appropriate antibiotics for UTIs. Antimicrobial agents approved by the Food and Drug Administration (FDA) for routine testing and reporting by clinical microbiology laboratories for urinary tract isolates are listed as Group U supplemental for urine only in the 2006 CLSI *Performance Standards for Antimicrobial Disk Susceptibility Tests,* 9th edition, Approved Standard CLSI Document M2-A9.

A number of laboratories have tailored susceptibility testing according to the needs of the clinical setting: outpatient versus inpatient; pediatric versus adult; intensive care versus nonintensive care. Nevertheless, it is imperative to remember that attainable antibiotic blood levels and urine levels are often different; this will have an impact on the interpretation of some semiquantitative susceptibility results or the quantitative minimal inhibitory concentration of inhibitory antimicrobials. Recently, given the cost-conscious environment, an additional strategy has been developed and implemented in certain laboratories; that is, they use antibiograms to select outpatient empirical therapy and do not routinely perform culture and susceptibility studies. This implies that laboratories monitor carefully over selected time intervals for emerging resistance and maintain a national electronic surveillance.

Urinary Tract Infection Antibiograms

Historically, one of the primary functions of the clinical microbiology laboratory has been to measure antibiotic resistance trends. This was most often accomplished by using an annual antibiogram that established cumulative percentage susceptibilities for selected UTI bacterial-antibiotic combinations. Today this is even more important and requires "focused" antibiograms that tailor these historical resistance fingerprints to selected patient locations, inpatient versus outpatient status, disease type, and age. Most importantly, these should be evaluated more frequently than yearly, perhaps quarterly, and should be formulated to help clinicians choose empirical therapy. Often outpatient urine isolates have a stable and predictable pattern.

BIBLIOGRAPHY

Abbott KC et al: Hospitalizations for bacterial septicemia after renal transplantation in the United States, *Am J Nephrol* 21:120, 2001.

Alangaden GJ et al: Infectious complications after kidney transplantation: current epidemiology and associated risk factors, *Clin Transplant* 20:401, 2006.

Bowden RA, Ljungman P, Paya CV, editors: *Transplant infections*, ed 2, Philadelphia, 2003, Lippincott Williams & Wilkins.

Brumfitt W: Urinary cell counts and their value, *J Clin Pathol* 118:550, 1965.

Doshi M et al: *Symptomatic urinary tract infections in renal transplant recipients: risk factors and current epidemiology* (abstract 1493), 7th Annual Joint Meeting of the Society of Transplant Surgeons and the American Society of Transplantation, San Francisco, Calif, May 5-7, 2007, American Transplant Congress 2007.

Ergin F et al: Urinary tract infections in renal transplant recipients, *Transplant Proc* 35:2685, 2003.

Clinical and Laboratory Standards Institute: *Performance standards for antimicrobial disk susceptibility tests: approval standard*, ed 9, M2-A9, vol 26, Wayne, Pa, 2006, CLSI.

Clarridge JP, Pezzlo M, Vosti KL: Cumitech 2A. In Wessfield AL, editor: *Laboratory diagnosis of urinary tract infections*, Washington DC, 1987, American Society for Microbiology.

Foxman B: Epidemiology of urinary tract infections: incidence, morbidity, and economic costs, *Am J Med* 113:5S, 2002.

Gupta K, Scholes D, Stamm WE: Increased prevalence of antimicrobial resistance among uropathogens causing acute uncomplicated cystitis in women, *JAMA* 281:736, 1999.

Hooten TM et al: Randomized comparative trial and cost analysis of 3-day antimicrobial regimens for treatment of acute cystitis in women, *JAMA* 273:41, 1995.

Jinnah F et al: Drug sensitivity pattern of *E. coli* causing urinary tract infection in diabetic and nondiabetic patients, *J Int Med Res* 24:296, 1996.

Johnson JR, Stamm WE: Urinary tract infections in women: diagnosis and treatment, *Ann Intern Med* 111:906, 1989.

Kass EH: Asymptomatic infections of the urinary tract, *Trans Assoc Am Physicians* 69:56, 1956.

Kierkegaard H et al: Falsely negative urinary leucocyte counts due to delayed examination, *Scand J Clin Lab Invest* 40:259, 1980.

Klevens RM et al: Estimating health care-associated infections and deaths in U.S. hospitals, 2002. *Public Health Rep* 122:160, 2007.

Kunin CM: *Detection, prevention, and management of urinary tract infections*, Philadelphia, 1997, Williams and Wilkins.

Maartens G, Oliver SP: Antibiotic resistance in community-acquired urinary tract infections, *S Afr Med J* 84:600, 1994.

Mandell GL, Bennett JE, Dolin R: *Principles & practice of infectious diseases*, ed 6, New York, 2005, Churchill Livingstone.

Beers MH, Porter RS, Jones TV: *Merck Manual*, ed 18, Rahway, NJ, 2006, Merck.

Murray PR et al, editors: *Manual of clinical microbiology*, ed 9, Washington, DC, 2007, ASM Press.

Nawar EW, Niska RW, Xu J: National Hospital Ambulatory Medical Care Survey: 2005 emergency department summary, *Adv Data* (386):1, 2007.

Nicolle LE: Urinary infection in the elderly: symptomatic or asymptomatic? *Int J Antimicrob Agents* 11:265, 1999.

Norden CW, Kass EH: Bacteriuria of pregnancy: a critical appraisal, *Annu Rev Med* 19:431, 1968.

Pezzlo M: Detection of urinary tract infections by rapid methods, *Clin Microbiol Rev* 1:268, 1988.

Pezzlo M: Urine and culture procedure. In Isenberg HD, editor: *Clinical microbiology procedures handbook*, ed 2, Washington, DC, 2007, ASM Press.

Richards MJ et al: Nosocomial infections in medical intensive care units in the United States. National Nosocomial Infections Surveillance System, *Crit Care Med* 27:887, 1999.

Schaeffer AJ: Urinary tract infections in urology: a urologist's view of chronic bacteriuria, *Infect Dis Clin North Am* 1:875, 1987.

Senger SS et al: Urinary tract infections in renal transplant recipients. *Transplant Proc* 39:1016, 2007.

Shortliffe LM, McCue JD: Urinary tract infection at the age extremes: pediatrics and geriatrics, *Am J Med* 113:55S, 2002.

Sobel JD et al: Candiduria: a randomized, double-blind study of treatment with fluconazole and placebo, *Clin Infect Dis* 30:19, 2000.

Stamery TA: *Pathogenesis and treatment of urinary tract infections*, Baltimore, 1981, Williams & Wilkins.

Stamm WE et al: Causes of the acute urethral syndrome in women, *N Engl J Med* 303:409, 1980.

Stamm W et al: Diagnosis of coliform infections in acutely dysuric women, *N Engl J Med* 307:463, 1982.

Stamm WE, Hooten TM: Management of urinary tract infections in adults, *N Engl J Med* 329:1328, 1993.

Thomson KS, Sanders WE, Sanders CC: USA resistance patterns among UTI pathogens, *J Antimicrob Chemother* 33:9, 1994.

Trautner BW, Darouiche RO: Catheter-associated infections: pathogenesis affects prevention. *Arch Intern Med* 164:842, 2004.

US Preventative Services Task Force: Recommendations on screening for symptomatic bacteriuria by dipstick urinalysis, *JAMA* 262:1220, 1989.

Valera B et al: Epidemiology of urinary infections in renal transplant recipients, *Transplant Proc* 38:2414. 2006.

Winn WC Jr: Diagnosis of urinary tract infection: a modern procrustean bed, *Am J Clin Pathol* 99:117, 1993.

Winstanley TG et al: A 10-year survey of the antimicrobial susceptibility of urinary tract isolates in the UK: the Microbe Base Project, *J Antimicrob Chemother* 40:591, 1997.

Wong ES: Guideline for prevention of catheter-associated urinary tract infections, *Am J Infect Control* 11:28, 1983.

Points to Remember

- Urinary tract infections (UTIs) occur frequently, especially in women. Half of all women will have a UTI in their lifetime.
- The pathogenesis and course of UTIs depend upon the organs involved and the patient's state of health.
- Lower UTI involves the bladder (cystitis), the urethra (urethritis), or the prostate (prostatitis). Symptoms of lower UTIs may include dysuria, hematuria, or changes in urinary frequency.
- Upper UTI involves the kidneys (pyelonephritis) or the ureters (ureteritis). Symptoms may include fevers, chills, night sweats, nausea, vomiting, flank pain, and costovertebral angle tenderness.
- Common etiologic agents of UTIs include coagulase-negative staphylococci, *E. coli*, *Klebsiella* spp., Enterobacteriaceae, and Enterococci. *Pseudomonas* spp., *Proteus mirabilis*, and *Candida* spp. are also seen, especially in hospital- or catheter-associated UTIs.
- Urinalysis and culture is an important component in the evaluation of UTI. The presence of bacteriuria and pyuria indicates infection.

Learning Assessment Questions

1. How would the urine culture described in the Case in Point be worked up and reported?

2. Where do these organisms originate?

3. What is the significance of the patient's clinical symptoms and the positive blood culture results?

4. What is the difference between single-episode urinary tract infection (UTI) and recurrent UTI?

5. What is the value of the screening urinalysis and the Gram-stain procedure?

6. What is the optimum incubation period for routine urine culture?

7. What may occur if routine urine cultures are incubated longer than 24 hours?

8. What is the definition of a contaminated urine culture?

9. Why is it important for clinicians to reevaluate negative urine culture results on specimens from symptomatic patients?

10. Should a susceptibility test be performed for all organisms isolated from urine?

11. A patient with a kidney transplantation 6 weeks ago develops fever, chills, nausea and vomiting, and dysuria. What laboratory tests should be performed to aid in the diagnosis of this patient's condition?

12. In the above patient, indicate four possible reasons that he developed this infection.

Genital Infections and Sexually Transmitted Diseases

Edward F. Keen, Wade K. Aldous

OBJECTIVES

After reading and studying this chapter, you should be able to:

1. Describe the clinical manifestations produced by the following agents:
   - *Neisseria gonorrhoeae*
   - *Chlamydia trachomatis*
   - *Candida albicans*
   - *Gardnerella vaginalis*
   - *Trichomonas vaginalis*
   - *Treponema pallidum* subsp. pallidum
   - *Haemophilus ducreyi*
   - Herpes simplex virus (HSV)
   - *Klebsiella granulomatis*
   - Human immunodeficiency virus (HIV)
   - Human papillomavirus (HPV)

2. Discuss the epidemiology and pathogenesis of each of the infections caused by the aforementioned agents.

3. Describe the proper specimen collection and laboratory methods used to diagnose the diseases caused by each of the previously listed organisms.

4. Discuss how the advent of molecular testing has affected the identification of sexually transmitted disease.

5. Differentiate the clinical characteristics between gonococcal and nongonococcal urethritis.

6. Interpret both specific and nonspecific serologic test results used to diagnose syphilis.

7. Recognize the common clinical manifestations, complications, and treatment for pelvic inflammatory disease.

Case in Point

A 19-year-old college freshman presents to the student health center complaining of a burning sensation when he urinates. He has had these symptoms for the past few days following several chance encounters of unprotected sex at a social party. There is no identifiable penile discharge or exudate noted. His doctor uses a swab to sample the inside of his urethra and submits it to the laboratory for molecular testing. Additionally, the patient is provided with oral antibiotics and encouraged to notify all of his sexual partners.

Issues to Consider

After reading the patient's case history, consider the following:

- What different organisms could be causing this infection
- Urethritis can be caused by dual infections of *Neisseria gonorrhoeae* and *Chlamydia trachomatis*
- How the infection is diagnosed and what considerations need to be made on diagnosis
- What type of sample is collected for laboratory testing
- Complications of infection without adequate treatment

Key Terms

Acquired immune deficiency syndrome (AIDS)

Bacterial vaginosis (BV)

Chancroid

Chlamydia

Donovan bodies

Genital herpes

Gonorrhea

Granuloma inguinale

Human immunodeficiency virus (HIV)

Nontreponemal (nonspecific) antibody tests

Nongonococcal urethritis (NGU)

Pelvic inflammatory disease (PID)

Syphilis

Treponemal antibody tests

Trichomoniasis

Vulvovaginal candidiasis

Genital and sexually transmitted infections (STIs) are caused by organisms normally present in the reproductive tract, or introduced from the outside during medical procedures or during sexual contact. STIs are spread primarily through intimate person-to-person sexual contact, including vaginal intercourse, oral sex, and anal sex. Several STIs, in particular human immunodeficiency virus (HIV), chlamydia, and gonorrhea can also be transmitted from mother to child during pregnancy and childbirth and through blood products and tissue transfer. There are more than 30 different sexually transmissible bacteria, viruses, epizoa, fungi, and parasites. Sexually transmitted diseases (STDs) are a diverse group of infectious diseases with a wide variety of pathogens and wide-ranging clinical manifestations (Table 38-1). The term *STI* is more commonly used because it has a broader range of meaning; a person may be infected, and may potentially infect others, without showing signs of disease.

STIs continue to be a major health threat in both the United States and worldwide. According to the World Health Organization (WHO), more than 340 million new cases of sexually transmitted bacterial and protozoal infections occur throughout the world every year. In the United States alone, about 19 million cases of STDs are diagnosed annually; almost half are youth from 15 to 24 years of age. Many people still engage in risky sexual behavior even after being diagnosed with an STI, which can be correlated with increased drug use. Recently, it has been demonstrated that African-American teens are at the greatest risk of infection in the United States. The rate of infections still rises annually for syphilis and chlamydia. Screening and prevention programs have been shown to be cost effective and beneficial to the public, but clearly more has to be done to stem the tide.

In 2006, 3 of the top 10 reportable diseases in the United States were STDs (chlamydia, gonorrhea, and syphilis [Table 38-2]). The Centers for Disease Control and Prevention

TABLE 38-1 Sexually Transmitted Diseases and Causative Agents

Disease	Agent(s)
AIDS	HIV-1
Bacterial vaginosis	*Gardnerella vaginalis, Mobiluncus* spp., etc.
Chlamydia	*Chlamydia trachomatis*
Chancroid	*Haemophilus ducreyi*
Cytomegalovirus disease	Cytomegalovirus
Genital warts	Human papillomavirus
Gonorrhea	*Neisseria gonorrhea*
Donovanosis	*Klebsiella granulomatis*
Leukemia, lymphoma	HTLV I, II or myelopathy
Lymphogranuloma venereum	*Chlamydia trachomatis*
Molluscum contagiosum	Molluscum contagiosum virus
Nongonococcal urethritis	*Mycoplasma genitalium, Ureaplasma urealyticum*
Pubic lice	*Phthirus pubis*
Scabies	*Sarcoptes scabei*
Syphilis	*Treponema pallidum* subsp. pallidum
Trichomoniasis	*Trichomonas vaginalis*

AIDS, Acquired immune deficiency disease; *HIV,* human immunodeficiency virus; *HTLV,* human T-cell leukemia virus.

TABLE 38-2 Top 10 Reportable Diseases in 2006

Disease/Organism	Reported per 100,000
Chlamydia	347.80
Gonorrhea	120.90
Varicella	28.65
Salmonellosis	15.45
Syphilis total, all stages	12.46
Streptococcus pneumoniae	11.93
Giardiasis	7.28
Coccidioidomycosis	6.79
Lyme disease	6.75
Shiigellosis	5.23

Modified from Centers for Disease Control and Prevention: *Sexually transmitted disease surveillance, 2006,* Atlanta, Ga, November 2007, U.S. Department of Health and Human Services.

(CDC) has developed new technology and methodologies to upgrade its national surveillance data management system for **human immune deficiency virus (HIV)** and **acquired immunedeficiency syndrome (AIDS).** Though the incidence of HIV/AIDS was not included in the 2006 CDC assessment, in past years it too was ranked among the top 10 reportable diseases. CDC's first estimates using the new system indicate that the HIV epidemic is worse than previously believed. Approximately 56,300 new HIV infections occurred in the United States in 2006, roughly 40% higher than the CDC's former estimate of 40,000 infections per year. In 2006, the estimated rate of HIV/AIDS cases in the 33 states with confidential name-based HIV infection reporting was 18.5 per 100,000 persons. In addition to the potentially devastating health impact of these infections, STDs create an immense economic burden, with direct medical costs as high as $14.7 billion per year. Although the STIs are diverse, this chapter focuses on the common exudative (gonorrhea, chlamydia, vulvovaginitis), ulcerative (syphilis, chancroid, genital herpes), and other (HIV, human papillomavirus [HPV]) STIs.

URETHRITIS

Etiology

Urethritis is the most common STD syndrome recognized in men and is often seen in women with coinciding cervicitis. Urethritis is an inflammation of the urethra, which can be caused by mechanical injury (catheterization), chemical irritation (antiseptics), or infectious disease. Infectious urethritis is more commonly associated with organisms that cause sexually transmitted disease, such as *Neisseria gonorrhoeae* and *Chlamydia trachomatis.* Cases can be divided into two types based on its causation, gonococcal urethritis (GU) and **nongonococcal urethritis (NGU).** GU is diagnosed based on the presence of gram-negative intracellular diplococci suggestive of the bacterium *N. gonorrhoeae.* NGU is diagnosed when inflammation is detected without the presence of *N. gonor-*

rhoeae and has both infectious and noninfectious etiologies. The etiology of a majority of NGU cases is unknown. *C. trachomatis* is the most common cause of NGU (15%-55% of cases) followed by *Ureaplasma urealyticum* and *Mycoplasma genitalium.* Other potential etiologic agents of NGU include *Trichomonas vaginalis,* herpes simplex virus (HSV), and adenovirus. The two types of urethritis are not mutually exclusive because coinfection with both *N. gonorrhoeae* and *C. trachomatis* is as high as 20% in men and 42% in women.

Epidemiology

Gonorrhea is the second most commonly reported infectious disease in the United States, and the CDC estimates that more than 700,000 people contract new gonorrheal infections each year. Only half of these new infections are reported. Following the implementation of the national gonorrhea control program in 1975, the incidence of gonorrhea in the United States declined 74.3% through 1997. After a small increase in 1998, the rate remained at a relatively steady level of around 350,000 reported cases per year (Figure 38-1). Recent data indicate that rates of gonorrhea in the United States have increased for the second consecutive year. In 2006, the CDC determined that 358,366 cases of gonorrhea were reported in the United States. The rate of reported gonorrheal infections was 120.9 per 100,000 persons, an increase of 5.5% from the rate in 2005 (114.6 per 100,000 persons). The incidence of gonorrhea continues to remain high for sexually active adolescents and young adults with the overall gonorrhea rate highest for the 20- to 24-year-old age group (527.7 per 100,000 persons). Gonorrhea rates among African Americans increased by 6.3% from 2005 to 2006 and were 18 times higher than for whites. Worldwide, gonorrhea rates also have continued to rise during the last 20 years, with an estimated 62 million new cases annually. Many of these infected people are asymptomatic (80% of women, 10% of men), which does cause concern for both treatment and control. In addition, people with gonorrhea can more easily contract HIV, the virus that causes AIDS. Patients with both

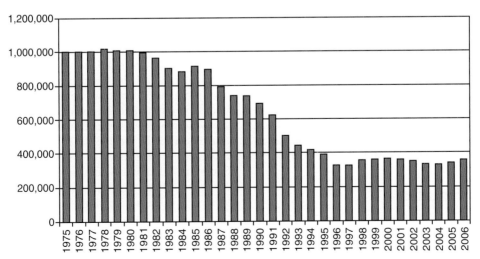

FIGURE 38-1 Reported cases of gonorrhea since 1975. (Modified from Centers for Disease Control and Prevention: *Sexually transmitted disease surveillance, 2006,* Atlanta, Ga, November 2007, U.S. Department of Health and Human Services.)

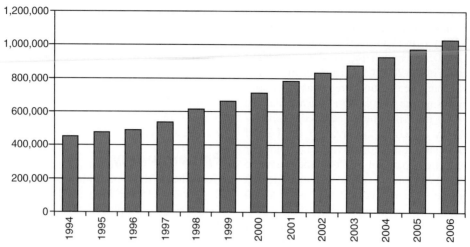

FIGURE 38-2 Reported cases of chlamydia since 1994. (Modified from Centers for Disease Control and Prevention: *Sexually transmitted disease surveillance, 2006,* Atlanta, Ga, November 2007, U.S. Department of Health and Human Services.)

HIV and gonorrhea are more likely to transmit HIV to someone else.

Chlamydia is the most commonly reported infectious disease in the United States. In 2006, the CDC estimates that over one million cases of genital *C. trachomatis* infection were reported. The national rate of reported chlamydia was 347.8 cases per 100,000 persons, representing a 5.6% increase from 2005. Rates of reported chlamydial infections among women have been steadily increasing since the late 1980s when public programs for screening and treatment of women were first established to avert **pelvic inflammatory disease (PID)** and related complications. The continued increase in reported chlamydia infections during the past decade reflects an expansion of screening activities, use of more sensitive diagnostic testing, increased case reporting, and improvements in national reporting systems (Figure 38-2). The continued increase in chlamydia case reports in 2006 may also reflect a true increase in morbidity. Chlamydia rates for females in 2006 were three times higher than for males (515.8 versus 173.0). The incidence of chlamydia remains high for sexually active adolescents and young adults, with the overall chlamydia rate highest for the 15- to 19-year-old age group (2862.7 per 100,000 persons). African-American females (1,760.9) are disproportionately affected with infection rates (1,760.9) seven times higher than for white females (237.0) and more than twice that of Hispanic females (761.3). Worldwide, chlamydia rates have continued to rise during the last 20 years, with about 97 million new cases annually. Chlamydial infection rates continue to increase globally with as many as 92 million new cases in 1999.

Clinical Manifestations

Gonococcal urethritis causes an acute infection with dysuria and urethral discharge. *N. gonorrhoeae* binds specifically to columnar epithelial cells of the genitourinary tract, including the urethra, cervix, endocervix, and Bartholin glands. The organism also attaches to columnar epithelial cells of the anal canal, pharynx, and conjunctiva. From time of exposure to

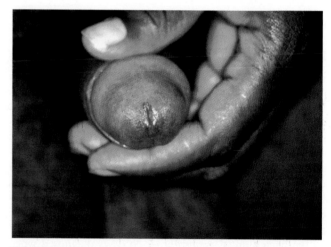

FIGURE 38-3 A case of nonspecific urethritis with accompanying mild meatitis and mucoid urethral discharge. (Courtesy Jim Pledger, Centers for Disease Control and Prevention, Atlanta, Ga.)

the onset of symptoms, the incubation period averages 2 to 7 days. After this period 95% or more of males experience a purulent urethral discharge, with the remaining 5% being asymptomatic. Infected women often have no symptoms for weeks or months, and the disease may be discovered only after she is examined as a sexual contact of a male partner who has tested positive for the disease. The incubation period of NGU is between 7 and 21 days, with symptoms arising less abruptly. Symptoms of urethritis in women include dysuria or pyuria and, less often, urethral discharge. Because urethritis in women is often accompanied by cervicitis (70% to 90%), a woman may also experience abnormal cervicovaginal discharge, intermenstrual bleeding, and pain during or after vaginal sex. Patients with NGU are much more likely to be asymptomatic than patients with GU. In symptomatic patients, NGU often results in a urethral discharge that is less profuse and more mucoid compared with GU (Figure 38-3).

Dysuria may be present without urethral discharge in these patients.

If left untreated, most cases of urethritis in males will resolve on their own; however, complications of ascending infection include acute prostatitis, epididymitis (a painful inflammation of the coiled tube [epididymis] at the back of the testicle), and urethral stricture. Ascending infection occurs in 10% to 20% of women with undiagnosed infections. These women are in danger of developing pelvic inflammatory disease (PID) presenting as salpingitis (infection of the fallopian tubes), endometritis, and internal abscesses and chronic pelvic pain. Women with PID do not always have symptoms, but when symptoms are present, they can be very severe and can include lower abdominal pain, abnormal cervical discharge and bleeding, and fever. According to the CDC, about 1 million women each year in the United States develop PID and about 100,000 of them become infertile. In 0.5% to 3% of untreated cases of gonococcal urethritis, *N. gonorrhoeae* will invade the bloodstream and result in disseminated gonococcal infection. Perinatal exposure to *N. gonorrhoeae* and *C. trachomatis* can result in severe disease in newborns including sepsis, pneumonia, inclusion conjunctivitis, and ophthalmia neonatorum, which can result in perforation of the globe of the eye and blindness.

Laboratory Diagnosis

Urethritis can be diagnosed based on the presence of mucopurulent or purulent urethral discharge, demonstrating 5 or more leukocytes per high-power field in a smear of urethral exudate, and a positive leukocyte esterase test on first-void urine or microscopic examination of more than 10 white blood cells (WBC) per high-power field of first-void urine sediment. The CDC recommends that all patients who have confirmed or suspected urethritis be tested for both gonorrhea and chlamydia. A Gram stain of male urethral exudate that demonstrates WBC with gram-negative intracellular diplococci is considered diagnostic (99% specific and 95% sensitive) for *N. gonorrhoeae* in symptomatic men (Figure 38-4). The sample is usually obtained by passing a small swab a few

centimeters into the urethra. Because of the lower sensitivity, a negative Gram stain result should not rule out gonococcal infection in asymptomatic males. If none of these criteria are present, the patient should be tested for *N. gonorrhoeae* and *C. trachomatis* and followed closely if test results are negative. Testing methods available for the most common organisms associated with urethritis include enzyme immunoassay, direct fluorescence assay, nucleic acid hybridization, and nucleic acid amplification test (NAAT). Both *N. gonorrhoeae* and *C. trachomatis* can be isolated in culture. *N. gonorrhoeae* is a fastidious organism that requires a selective growth medium (Thayer-Martin, Martin-Lewis, New York City media) in a CO_2-rich environment for culture. Cell culture using McCoy cells is considered the gold standard for chlamydia diagnosis; however, molecular testing is proving to be more sensitive and specific. There are several Food and Drug Administration (FDA)-approved NAAT assays available with very high rates of sensitivity and specificity (more than 95%) and allow combination testing for *N. gonorrhoeae* and *C. trachomatis* (Table 38-3). Acceptable specimens for gonorrhea and chlamydia testing include a swab of urethral exudate; alternatively, a first-void urine sample may be tested for these organisms using a NAAT. The ability to submit a urine specimen instead of a urethral swab should greatly increase the amount of testing performed and will hopefully provide an earlier diagnosis and treatment of individuals.

Treatment

Treatment of patients presenting with urethritis should be initiated right away. Fluoroquinolones (i.e., ciprofloxacin, ofloxacin, levofloxacin) have been recommended for the treatment of gonococcal urethritis since 1993 because of their efficacy, availability, and use as a single-dose, oral therapy. Prevalence of quinolone-resistant *Neisseria gonorrhoeae* (QRNG) remained less than 1% from 1990 to 2001; however, fluoroquinolone resistance in *N. gonorrhoeae* has been increasing and is becoming widespread in the United States, necessitating changes in treatment regimens. Based on preliminary data from the 2006 Gonococcal Isolate Surveillance Project (GISP), the CDC no longer recommends the use of fluoroquinolones to treat gonorrhea. Cephalosporins are the only class of antibiotics recommended for treatment of gonococcal infections. The CDC currently recommends a single intramuscular dose of ceftriaxone or a single oral dose of cefixime. A majority of patients with gonorrhea are also infected with *C. trachomatis*. For this reason, the CDC recommends that patients with *N. gonorrhoeae* infections be treated with a regimen that is effective against both pathogens. Azithromycin and doxycycline are effective treatment options for chlamydial urethritis, and most isolates of *N. gonorrhoeae* in the United States are also susceptible. Analysis of clinical trials comparing the use of azithromycin versus doxycycline for treatment of chlamydia demonstrated that both are equally effective; however, *Mycoplasma genitalium* infections may respond better to azithromycin. Patients should return for a follow-up evaluation if symptoms continue despite therapy or recur after its completion. Sex partners of these patients should be notified and treated. To avoid re-infection, partners are encouraged to abstain from sexual intercourse until therapy is completed.

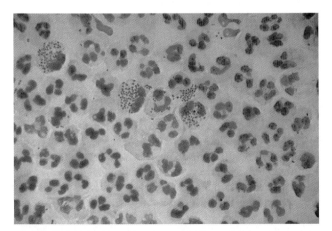

FIGURE 38-4 Gram-stain of an acute case of gonococcal urethritis demonstrating gram-negative intracellular diplococci within leukocytes. (Courtesy Joe Millar, Centers for Disease Control and Prevention, Atlanta, Ga.)

TABLE 38-3 FDA-Approved Molecular Tests for Gonorrhea and Chlamydia

Test	Manufacturer	Test Name	Method
Chlamydia trachomatis	Qiagen, Germantown, Md.	HC2® CT ID	Hybrid capture
	Gen-Probe, Inc., San Diego, Calif.	APTIMA CT® Assay	TC, TMA, DKA
		PACE® 2 CT	HPA
		Probe Competition Assay	
	Roche Molecular Diagnostics, Pleasanton, Calif.	AMPLICOR®CT/NG Test for *Chlamydia trachomatis*	PCR
		COBAS AMPLICOR® CT/NG Test for *C. trachomatis*	PCR
Neisseria gonorrhoeae	Qiagen, Germantown, Md.	HC2® GC ID	Hybrid capture
	Gen-Probe, Inc., San Diego, Calif.	APTIMA® GC Assay	TC, TMA, DKA
		PACE® 2 GC	HPA
		Probe Competition Assay	
	Roche Molecular Diagnostics, Pleasanton, Calif.	AMPLICOR®CT/NG Test for *Neisseria gonorrhoeae*	PCR
		COBAS AMPLICOR® CT/NG Test for *Neisseria gonorrhoeae*	PCR
Chlamydia trachomatis/ Neisseria gonorrhoeae	Becton, Dickinson & Company, Sparks, Md.	BD ProbeTec™ ET *C. trachomatis* and *N. gonorrhoeae* amplified DNA Assay	SDA
	Qiagen, Germantown, Md.	HC2® CT/GC Combo Test	Hybrid capture
	Gen-Probe, Inc., San Diego, Calif.	APTIMA Combo 2® Assay	TC, TMA, DKA
		PACE® 2C CT/GC	HPA
	Roche Molecular Diagnostics, Pleasanton, Calif.	AMPLICOR® CT/NG Test	PCR
		COBAS AMPLICOR™ CT/NG Test	PCR

FDA, Food and Drug Administration; *TC,* target capture; *TMA,* transcription mediated amplification; *DKA,* dual kinetic assay; *HPA,* hybridization protection assay; *PCR,* polymerase chain reaction; *SDA,* Strand displacement amplification.
Modified from FDA-Cleared/Approved Molecular Diagnostics Tests table current through Aug 20, 2008; Association for Molecular Pathology (www.amp.org).

CERVICITIS

Etiology

Cervicitis is an inflammation of the columnar and subepithelial cells of the endocervix, which can be caused by both infectious and noninfectious means. The infectious cases are much more common and are almost always caused by infection with organisms causing STDs such as *C. trachomatis* and *N. gonorrhoeae*. Other less common microorganisms such as *Mycoplasma* and *Ureaplasma* have also been identified. The noninfectious route of inflammation comes from injury to the cervix, usually from a foreign object inserted into the vagina, such as a birth control device, a douche, or a tampon. Chemical irritation can also occur from using these products.

Epidemiology

Cervicitis is a very common condition with more than half of all women developing this condition sometime in their adult lives. It is the most common STD in adolescent females. Common risk factors for development of disease include beginning sexual activity at an early age, engaging in high-risk sexual behaviors, having a history of sexually transmitted diseases, and having multiple sex partners. It is considered to be the silent partner of male urethritis because symptoms are not always obvious. The lack of well-recognized symptoms and signs of cervicitis make its diagnosis very difficult. In cases where symptoms are not noted or recognized, no treatment is provided and serious complications such as pelvic inflammatory disease, infertility, ectopic pregnancy, chronic pelvic pain, spontaneous abortion, and even cervical cancer may occur.

Clinical Manifestations

Symptoms of cervicitis, when present, may start out fairly mild and then progress over time. The most common symptom is a vaginal discharge that may be grayish or yellow, possibly with an odor. Other signs include bleeding, itching, irritation of the external genitals, pain during intercourse, bleeding or spotting after intercourse, dysuria, and sometimes lower back or abdominal pain. Severe cases will demonstrate a profuse, almost pus-like discharge accompanied with vaginal itchiness or abdominal pain.

Laboratory Diagnosis

Diagnosis of cervicitis is mainly clinically performed; however, microscopic analysis showing more than 10 WBC per high-power field of exudate has been associated with chlamydial and gonococcal infection of the cervix. Whereas gram-negative intracellular diplococci from urethral exudates are diagnostic in men, Gram stains of cervical exudates are at most 50% accurate and are not commonly used. Most women presenting with symptoms of cervicitis are assessed for signs of pelvic inflammatory disease and tested for *C. trachomatis* and *N. gonorrhoeae*. However, because the female genital tract is contiguous, there is some overlap between vulvovaginitis and cervicitis. Thus, if warranted, individuals should also be evaluated for bacterial vaginosis and trichomoniasis. Culture for any of these organisms lacks sensitivity compared with nucleic acid based assays. The most common are the amplified tests with very high rates of sensitivity and specificity (more than 95%). There are several FDA-approved assays available in automated and nonautomated formats (see Table 38-3). Fluorescent antibody tests can be used for detection of the elementary bodies of *C. trachomatis*. Rapid antigen tests are also available for point-of-care testing or physician office laboratories for *Chlamydia, Neisseria,* and bacterial vaginosis, but not for the Mycoplasmataceae. Although useful, in the physician office setting, the lack of sensitivity may require additional testing for confirmation of infection.

Treatment

Treatment options vary according to the organisms suspected or detected. Empiric therapy should be provided for high-risk patients (age 25 years or younger, new or multiple sex partners, and unprotected sex), especially if there is a possibility that they will be lost to follow-up. In the past, patients with gonorrhea were treated with penicillin, but with the advent of penicillinase-producing *N. gonorrhoeae* (PPNG), that regimen was switched to a fluoroquinolone. Now, there are quinolone-resistant strains of *N. gonorrhoeae* (QRNG). As discussed previously, patients with *N. gonorrhoeae* and/or *C. trachomatis* are usually treated with multiple agents including a cephalosporin, doxycycline, and an aminoglycoside such as azithromycin or erythromycin, thus providing coverage for both organisms and lessening the chances of garnering resistance. Studies indicate that roughly half of all infections with either of these two organisms are actually a coinfection of both organisms. Cases of trichomoniasis or bacterial vaginosis will usually be treated with metronidazole. Women with persistent cervicitis should be evaluated for a possible re-exposure to an STD or perhaps switched to a different antibiotic regimen. Follow-up is recommended to ensure eradication of the organism(s). Sex partners should also be notified and treated. To avoid re-infection, partners are encouraged to abstain from sexual intercourse until therapy is completed.

VULVOVAGINITIS

Etiology

Vaginal infections account for more than 10 million visits to a health care provider annually. Vaginitis occurs when the mucosal lining of the vagina becomes inflamed and irritated. Bacteria, yeast, or viruses are the main infectious causes, but chemical or mechanical irritants such as feminine hygiene products, soaps, contraceptives, and clothing can also cause vaginitis. Typical signs include vaginal discharge, vulvar itching and irritation, and often odor. Three commonly associated diseases with these symptoms include bacterial vaginosis, trichomoniasis, and candidiasis. The distinction between these syndromes can be made by observations of the vaginal discharge.

Bacterial Vaginosis

Epidemiology

Bacterial vaginosis (BV) is the most prevalent cause of vaginal discharge or malodor; however, more than 50% of women with BV are asymptomatic. The prevalence of BV was determined to be 29.2% of women surveyed in the United States from 2001 to 2004; corresponding to 21.4 million women. Prevalence varies significantly by sociodemographic characteristics, earlier age of first sexual contact, higher numbers of sex partners, and a previous female sex partner. Other risk factors for developing BV include having multiple sex partners or new sex partners, frequent douching, or even a lack of protective lactobacilli. Sexually naïve women are rarely affected. It is unclear whether BV results from acquisition of a sexually transmitted pathogen; however, women who have never been sexually active are rarely affected.

Clinical Manifestations

BV occurs when the delicate balance of the bacterial flora is disrupted, allowing overgrowth of specific organisms. The healthy vagina maintains a pH between 3.8 and 4.5 and has a normal microbiota consisting mainly of *Lactobacillus* spp. These organisms produce the enzyme catalase to help preserve acidity and prevent the overgrowth of other vaginal flora (hormonal changes such as menstrual periods and pregnancy will also reduce vaginal acidity). When vaginal pH increases, various species of *Prevotella, Porphyromonas, Peptostreptococcus, Mobiluncus, Gardnerella vaginalis, Mycoplasma hominis,* and *Ureaplasma* spp. will overwhelm the lactobacilli. This mix of organisms leads to the vaginal discharge and distinct odor. Discharge is often more apparent and odorous after intercourse, after exposure to male ejaculate. Patients with BV demonstrate a discharge that is usually a milky homogeneous thin liquid adhering to the walls of the vagina.

Laboratory Diagnosis

Bacterial vaginosis can be diagnosed by observing and performing tests on the vaginal discharge. The discharge can be observed microscopically to look for the presence of "clue cells," which are vaginal squamous epithelial cells coated with *G. vaginalis*. These clue cells are identified by microscopic examination of a vaginal wet mount preparation. Normal vaginal squamous epithelial cells have distinct cell margins and lack granularity, whereas clue cells show coccobacillary organisms attached in clusters on the cell surface, making the border indistinct or stippled (Figure 38-5). Polymorphonuclear leukocytes (PMNs) can also be demonstrated on the normal vaginal wet mount preparation, whereas they are rare in cases of BV in the midst of clue cells. Additional criteria for the diagnosis of BV include an increased pH greater than 4.5, the lack of visible lactobacilli, and a positive "whiff" test. The whiff test demonstrates a typical fishy odor on addition of one or two drops of 10% KOH to vaginal discharge because of the presence of volatile amines. The demonstration of at least three of these conditions is diagnostic for bacterial vaginosis.

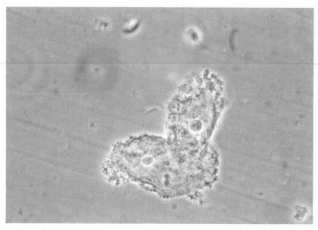

Figure 38-5 Microscopic saline preparation of vaginal squamous epithelial cells with numerous attached bacteria (*Gardnerella vaginalis*). Combined, these are identified as "clue cells" and are key indicators of bacterial vaginosis. (Courtesy M. Rein, Centers for Disease Control and Prevention, Atlanta, Ga.)

There are other conventional methods for detecting BV. Culture of *G. vaginalis* is possible, but identification is usually presumptive and requires the use of specialized media; thus it is discouraged because of lack of specificity. The DNA hybridization test, Affirm VPIII (Becton Dickinson) detects the most common causes of vaginosis, *G. vaginalis, Candida* spp., and *Trichomonas vaginalis*. This test is easy to perform and can be completed in less than 1 hour, but it requires technical expertise and additional equipment. Although more expensive than other tests of this category, it definitively identifies the causative organism, thus providing focused therapy for the patient. Rapid antigen tests are also available for the detection of *G. vaginalis* proline aminopeptidase activity in vaginal fluid specimens. This type of assay can easily be used in a physician office laboratory.

Treatment

Bacterial vaginosis is usually treated with an oral or a topical antibiotic such as metronidazole or now tinidazole. Metronidazole therapy is a twice-daily, 7-day course, whereas tinidazole therapy is a shorter course, thus improving patient compliance. The bacterial infection usually resolves within a few days, but if recurrences occur, a longer therapeutic period may become necessary. Treatment is provided to relieve the symptoms and reduce the risk of infectious complications with other organisms. Bacterial vaginosis in pregnancy can lead to the adverse outcome of preterm delivery; thus women who are at high risk (previous preterm birth) should be managed carefully.

Case Study

A 24-year-old female notes vaginal itching and irritation with a slight discharge. Previously, she developed a yeast infection that was treated with over-the-counter medications and resolved. Thinking that this was a recurrence, she again self-treated. This time, however, the symptoms did not resolve, and now there is a pungent odor along with a frothy discharge. She presents to her HMO for diagnosis, and the nurse practitioner takes a swab of the secretions in order to perform a rapid point-of-care test and microscopy. A wet mount of the swab demonstrates "swimming" organisms.

Trichomoniasis

Epidemiology

Trichomonas vaginalis, a parasitic protozoan, is the causative agent of trichomoniasis, another common manifestation of vaginitis. Humans are the only natural host of *T. vaginalis*. **Trichomoniasis,** considered an STD, is an extremely common infection in the United States, with an estimated annual incidence of 7.4 million new cases. Because this infection is easily cured and is not a reportable disease, it receives little emphasis from public health STD control programs and has a much lower priority compared with chlamydia and gonorrhea infections. *T. vaginalis* infections are commonly associated with other STDs, in particular, cases of bacterial vaginosis or gonorrhea. The number of cases of trichomoniasis is evenly distributed throughout all age groups and may be considered a useful marker for risky sexual behavior.

Clinical Manifestations

Trichomonas infections demonstrate generalized symptoms of vaginal discharge, pruritus, and irritation. Classical signs of infection include a greenish to yellow frothy vaginal discharge, odor, and erythema (Figure 38-6). The vaginal discharge also demonstrates an elevated pH. Patients may also present with a "strawberry cervix," but this is best detected by colposcopy and rarely during routine examination. Other complaints may include dysuria and lower abdominal pain. The urethra is also infected in the majority of women. Nearly half of all infections are asymptomatic, making screening very important in reducing overall infection. Severity of symptoms depends on a multitude of factors that influence the host inflammatory response such as hormonal levels, the coexisting vaginal flora, and the strain and relative concentration of the organisms present in the vagina. Additionally, this organism possesses many virulence factors. Male sexual partners can also be infected with *Trichomonas* but will present with symptoms of nongonococcal urethritis. A number of complications are associated with infection with *T. vaginalis*. Cellulitis has been shown in some patients following hysterectomies. A significant correlation has been found between infection and low birth weight, premature rupture of membranes, and preterm delivery. African studies also confirm increased potential for HIV acquisition with a *Trichomonas* infection.

Laboratory Diagnosis

Trichomoniasis can be easily determined through visualization of motile trichomonads in a saline preparation of the vaginal fluid (Figure 38-7). Many physicians may perform this test within the clinic because organisms lose viability quickly after collection of the sample. This is allowable under Clinical Laboratory Improvement Act (CLIA) rules as provider performed microscopy (PPM). Despite the ease of the test, it has

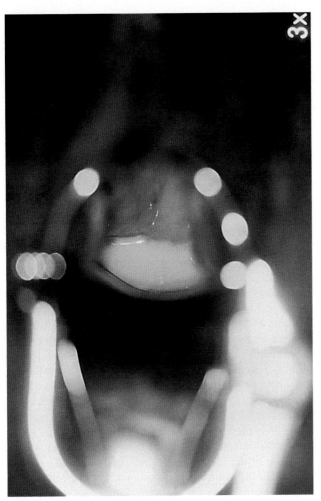

FIGURE 38-6 Yellowish green frothy purulent discharge emanating from the cervical os, demonstrative of *trichomonas vaginitis*. (Courtesy Centers for Disease Control and Prevention, Atlanta, Ga.)

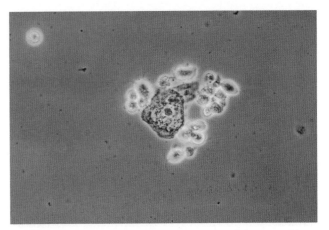

FIGURE 38-7 Phase contrast wet mount micrograph of a vaginal discharge revealing the presence of *Trichomonas vaginalis* protozoa surrounding a squamous epithelial cell. (Courtesy Centers for Disease Control and Prevention, Atlanta, Ga.)

limited sensitivity, ranging from 60% to 70%. Culture is still considered the "gold standard," which requires Diamond's medium, although this is not widely available. A commercially available pouch system (BioMed Diagnostics) has been shown to be as good as culture, and has been used successfully with both clinician-obtained and self-obtained specimens. A delayed-inoculation technique is possible, allowing for initial reading of the wet preparation and then inoculation of the culture pouch if the wet preparation is negative. Swab specimens may sit at room temperature for up to 30 minutes prior to pouch inoculation. Newer commercially available methods for diagnosis include an office-based oligonucleotide probe test, Affirm VPIII (Becton Dickinson), which has been described above, and point-of-care rapid antigen detection tests, OSOM® Trichomonas Rapid Test licensed (Genzyme Corp). The approximate sensitivity of this assay is roughly 80% compared with culture. This test may be of value in settings where microscopy is not possible. polymerase chain reaction (PCR)-based tests for *T. vaginalis* currently exist only as home-brew laboratory assays and are performed by select

laboratories. Development of FDA-approved assays is still in progress.

Treatment

Metronidazole is the drug of choice for treating trichomoniasis cases. Approximately 2.5% to 5% of all cases display some level of resistance to treatment with metronidazole, although this can usually be overcome with higher oral doses. Occasionally patients are allergic to metronidazole; thus a newer agent, tinidazole, is also available with a longer half-life for a shorter therapeutic duration. All sexual partners should be treated along with patients with asymptomatic infection. Otherwise, if left untreated, they may later become symptomatic, and transmission of infection will continue.

Candidiasis

Epidemiology

Vulvovaginal candidiasis is symptomatic vaginitis usually caused by infection with the yeast *Candida*. Almost all cases of infection are caused by *C. albicans*, with only a small percentage caused by nonalbicans species (*C. glabrata, C. parapsilosis, C tropicalis, C. krusei*). Yeast infections are also termed *vaginal thrush* or *moniliasis*. Infection is very common, with nearly 75% of all adult women having had at least one genital "yeast infection" in their lifetime. *Candida* is always present in the body in small amounts, so when an imbalance occurs, such as changes in the normal acidity of the vagina, symptoms occur. Vaginal candidiasis is not considered a true STD, but because it causes very similar symptoms in the female genital tract as the other organisms described above, it is included in this discussion. Rare candidal infections can be passed sexually to male partners, but these infections are not very serious and respond well to treatment.

Yeast infections are the most common genital infections affecting women. Infections occur as a result of many different changes in vaginal flora. In many cases, infection may follow a course of broad-spectrum antibiotics that were pre-

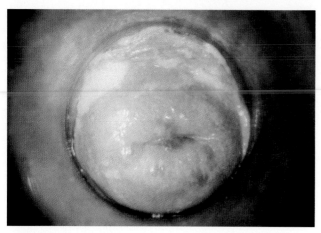

FIGURE 38-8 Candidal cervicitis, caused by the fungus *Candida* sp. The cervical discharge is white, thick, and curd-like. (Courtesy Centers for Disease Control and Prevention, Atlanta, Ga.)

scribed for another purpose that inadvertently eliminated the normal biota. Hormonal causes of yeast infections include pregnancy, ovulation, menopause, oral contraceptives, or women prescribed with estrogen replacement therapy. Immunosuppressive conditions such as diabetes mellitus, iron deficiency, or HIV infection will also lead to an increased infection rate. Finally, various skin conditions (psoriasis, lichen planus, or lichen sclerosus) can also lead to infection. The highest prevalence of infections occur typically in women of child-bearing age who are producing ample amounts of estrogen, which causes the lining of the vagina to mature and to contain glycogen, a preferred growth substrate for *C. albicans*.

Clinical Manifestations

Women with vulvovaginal candidiasis usually experience genital itching or burning, with an abnormal vaginal discharge ranging from a slightly watery, white discharge to a thick, white, curd-like discharge (Figure 38-8). Additional signs and symptoms include vulvar inflammation and redness sometimes spreading widely in the groin to include pubic areas, inguinal areas and thighs, pain with intercourse, and painful urination. Males who develop genital candidiasis demonstrate an itchy rash on the penis.

Laboratory Diagnosis

Diagnosis of yeast infections are typically done personally or clinically. Discharge can be submitted for microscopy and culture to rule out other causative agents of vaginosis. Microscopic evaluation of a yeast infection would demonstrate budding yeast forms in both the Gram stain and a KOH prep. The pH of the vaginal fluid stays approximately normal as opposed to elevated for BV and trichomoniasis.

Treatment

Yeast infections are typically treated with over-the-counter (OTC) medications or prescription antifungal agents. In most cases, symptoms usually disappear completely with adequate treatment; however, recurrences do happen, which may signal

some other underlying health issues such as immunosuppression. Numerous antifungal drugs, both prescription and OTC medications, are available to treat yeast infections, but all are azole antifungal agents, either in suppositories, topical creams or lotions, and oral pills. The agent used may depend on whether or not the infection is self-diagnosed versus provider diagnosed. Duration of therapy is agent specific and can be as little as a single dose or treatments lasting up to 7 days. Women with first-time infections should seek advice from their provider, as should those who seem to have a chronic or recurrent form of disease (four or more proven episodes). Women with a weakened immune system may require a longer therapeutic regimen and should consult their providers before self-treating as well.

Despite therapy, chronic or recurrent infections may still occur. This may be from inadequate initial treatment or perhaps a secondary infection may develop as a result of prolonged scratching, causing the skin of the vulva to become cracked and raw. In many cases, women will opt to self-treat as opposed to visiting their health care provider in order to save time and money. But, unless women are fully aware of the signs and symptoms of candidiasis, their diagnosis may be incorrect. A high percentage of all OTC drugs sold to treat candidiasis were probably used by women without the disease, thus increasing the resistance rate. It is now thought that women who experience recurrent yeast infections suffer from persistent infection and not re-infection.

Methods of prevention suggested to reduce the incidence rate of yeast infections include wearing cotton undergarments and loose-fitting clothing to avoid persistent and excessive moisture in the genital area. Additionally, women should not wear wet bathing suits or exercise clothing for long periods of time. Women who may be prone to recurrent infections are recommended to soak in a salt bath, using a non-soap cleanser or aqueous cream for washing or to apply hydrocortisone cream to reduce itching. They may also self-treat with an antifungal cream before each menstrual period and before antibiotic therapy to prevent relapse. Prescription oral medications may also be taken regularly based on the recommendations of their provider. Interestingly, there are also a number of "don'ts," such as treating the sexual partner; switching to a low-sugar, low-yeast, or high-yogurt diet; putting yogurt in the vagina; and trying natural remedies.

GENITAL ULCER DISEASE

Etiology

Genital ulcer disease is characterized by a disruption of the skin and/or mucosal layer of the genital region. In the United States, the majority of patients who present with genital ulcers have herpes, syphilis, or chancroid. Less common causes of genital ulcers include lymphogranuloma venereum and donovanosis. The frequency of each infection can differ by geographic area and patient population; however, genital herpes is the most prevalent of these diseases. More than one of these diseases can be present in a patient who has genital ulcers. Agent-specific diagnosis based solely on clinical evaluation of the ulcers is often confounded by the overlapping patterns of clinical presentation and the occurrence of multiple and mixed infections. Successful treatment of genital ulcer disease is becoming increasingly important, because multiple studies have demonstrated that its presence increases the risk of HIV susceptibility and transmission. The following sections will describe the common etiologic agents of genital ulcer disease.

Case Study

A 14-day-old female is brought to her pediatrician with a 2-week history of eye discharge. Following delivery, the infant continued to squint, only opening her eyes in the dark. She was referred to an ophthalmologist who noted large bilateral corneal ulcers. These ulcers were scraped and submitted for culture. The infant was delivered vaginally and at full term. The patient's mother noted a scabby labial rash and dyspareunia ("abnormal pain during sexual intercourse caused by a spasm") during the pregnancy, which resolved after about 1 week.

Genital Herpes

Epidemiology

Genital herpes is a chronic viral infection caused by the herpes simplex virus (HSV) and is the most common ulcerative STI in the United States. HSV contains a double-stranded, linear DNA genome encased within an icosahedral capsid. There are two serotypes of HSV, HSV-1 and HSV-2, and both can cause genital herpes. Infections with HSV-2 typically affect the genital area, and transmission is usually through sexual contact. In contrast, HSV-1 commonly causes oropharyngeal infection, and transmission is primarily through nongenital personal contact. Both serotypes are capable of causing either genital or oropharyngeal infection and can produce mucosal ulcers that are clinically indistinguishable from one another. Reports from a variety of clinical settings reveal that genital herpes is the most common patient request for treatment of symptomatic genital ulcers in the United States. According to National Health and Nutrition Examination Surveys (NHANES), the prevalence of HSV-2 infection increased dramatically from 1976 to 1988. Recent studies suggest that the upward trend of HSV-2 seroprevalence has been reversed; however, genital herpes caused by HSV-1 may be increasing in the United States and other developed countries.

The CDC estimates that more than 50 million people in the United States 12 years of age and older, or 20% of the total adolescent and adult population, are infected with genital herpes. Case reporting data for HSV infection are not available and trend data are limited to estimates of the initial office visits in physicians' office practices from the National Disease and Therapeutic Index (NDTI) (Figure 38-9). These data indicate that despite reported declines in seroprevalence in HSV, genital herpes trends suggest recent increases. The incidence of HSV-2 antibodies has gradually increased, with about 22% of the general population being seropositive. According to the CDC, genital HSV-2 infection is more common in women than in men (25% versus 12.5%). This disparity is most likely due to male to female transmission being more prevalent than female to male transmission. It is estimated that 1.6 million new HSV-2 cases are transmitted each year, with approximately 640,000 infections in the 15- to 24-year age category. As many as 70% to 90% of individuals may be unaware of their infections because they are asymptomatic or have only vague symptoms. Many patients with subclinical disease have episodes of viral shedding from anogenital sites and represent a significant reservoir of transmission. The estimated cost of genital herpes infections in the United States in 2000 was $1.8 billion, but if the incidence of infection continues to increase, the estimated cost could be as high as $2.7 billion by 2025.

Clinical Manifestations

HSV infection of oral or genital tissue is initiated from an active (either primary or recurrent) infection of another

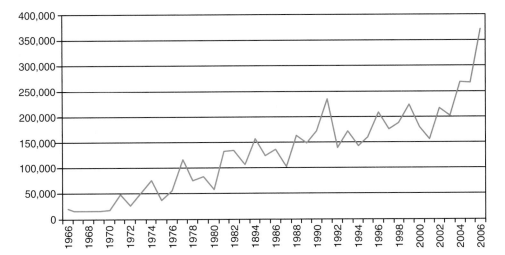

FIGURE 38-9 Genital herpes—initial visits to physicians' offices: United States, 1966–2006. (Modified from Centers for Disease Control and Prevention: *Sexually transmitted disease surveillance, 2006*, Atlanta, Ga, November 2007, U.S. Department of Health and Human Services.)

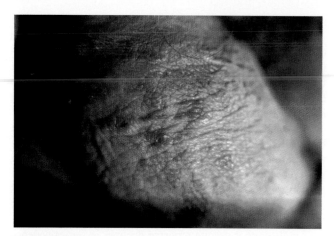

FIGURE 38-10 Vesicles of herpetic lesions on the penile shaft due to herpes simplex virus 2. (Courtesy Centers for Disease Control and Prevention, Atlanta, Ga.)

individual. The virus enters the body through the direct sexual contact of skin or mucous membranes with the secretions or mucosal surfaces of an infected person. Incubation periods range from 1 to 26 days after the initial exposure. Most individuals infected with genital herpes are asymptomatic or show minimal signs or symptoms and have not been diagnosed with genital herpes. Despite a lack of symptoms, these patients continue to shed HSV into the genital tract intermittently. Therefore the disease is often transmitted by those who are unaware that they are infected or who are asymptomatic when transmission occurs.

In symptomatic patients, primary infection with HSV-2 manifests with extensive, painful vesicles, fever, myalgia, malaise, dysuria, and inguinal lymphadenopathy. These systemic effects are usually limited to the primary episode. Primary lesions last 2 to 6 weeks and vesicles, appearing approximately 6 days after exposure, contain large quantities of infectious HSV particles (Figure 38-10). In primary infections viral shedding can last 15 to 16 days with new lesions continuing to form up to 10 days post-exposure. Asymptomatic viral shedding can continue for up to 1 year following resolution of the primary clinical presentation, increasing the risk of transmission to sexual partners. Lesions of primary genital herpes typically ulcerate and heal inward from the periphery without scarring within 3 weeks. Ulcers that form on dry surfaces (buttocks or thighs) heal more rapidly than those on mucocutaneous surfaces (vagina, cervix, glans of the penis). Women tend to suffer from more severe disease caused by genital herpes infection, including constitutional symptoms and complications, than do men. This disparity between the sexes may be due to the larger affected surface area of the female genital tract and the ability of HSV to spread more easily over the abundant moist surfaces.

Following recovery from primary infection, HSV ascends along the sensory nerve roots to the dorsal root ganglion and establishes latency. Reactivation of the virus occurs upon exposure to stressors including extensive exposure to sunlight, menstruation, malnutrition, fatigue, anxiety, and subsequent viral infections. With reactivation, the virus travels from the dorsal root ganglion back down the nerve root to create a

recurrent outbreak of symptoms. Although clinical presentation is indistinguishable, recurrent disease caused by HSV-1 generally recurs less regularly than genital infections with HSV-2. Recurrent disease typically results in milder symptoms compared with primary infection, and the lesions heal more quickly. Approximately 90% of patients with genital herpes have at least one recurrence during the first year following primary infection. The median recurrence rate for genital HSV-2 is four episodes per year with an average of 50 days to first recurrence. Over time the frequency of recurrence lessens.

The most serious complication of genital herpes is neonatal transmission. Neonatal infection with HSV most often occurs during delivery (85%) but can also occur congenitally (5%) or postnatal (10%). Symptoms of neonatal HSV disease acquired during delivery usually appear in the first 9 to 11 days of life. Exposure to vaginal secretions containing HSV can result in a variety of clinical manifestations, including localized disease of the skin, eyes, and mucosa; central nervous system (CNS) involvement; or disseminated disease. The mortality rate for neonates with CNS or disseminated disease can be as high as 80%. Risk of infection transmission from mother to child during delivery is high (30% to 50%) among women who acquire the disease during the third trimester and is low (less than 1%) among women with histories of recurrent herpes at term or who acquire genital HSV infection during the first half of pregnancy. It is thought that maternal antibodies from the recurrent infection protect the neonate from serious disease. Other serious complications of genital HSV infection include corneal infection and fatal sporadic encephalitis in immunocompromised hosts.

Laboratory Diagnosis

Viral isolation is the most common method for the diagnosis of HSV infections. The best specimens for culture are vesicle fluids collected with a syringe or swab. Cervical swabs and mucosal surface swabs are also acceptable. The sensitivity of viral culture is relatively low, especially for recurrent lesions. Specimens for culture must be taken as early as possible in the disease process from mucocutaneous lesions. The likelihood that a herpetic lesion will produce a positive culture diminishes with each day after the appearance of the lesion. Specimens should be placed in viral transport medium, shipped cold, and should not be frozen. If crusting lesions are the only possible specimen for culture, then vigorously collected specimens containing epithelial cells from the lesion help improve sensitivity of culture. Viral samples can be stored at 4° C; however, specimens being kept for longer periods of time should be stored at −70° C. HSV grows rapidly on numerous cell culture lines, and the cytopathic effect (CPE) in culture can be seen within the first 24 hours in most cases, but some isolates can take as long as 14 days to develop CPE. The most common cell lines used for viral culture include mink lung cells, rhabdomyosarcoma cells, MRC-5, HEp-2, and A549 cells. Infected cells develop intracellular granulation, enlarge, and then display intracellular inclusions (Figure 38-11). Viral culture is a reliable method to detect HSV because it is highly specific and relatively inexpensive. However, the sensitivity ranges from 30% to 95%, depending

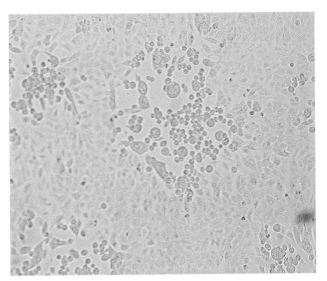

FIGURE 38-11 Culture results of a genital specimen inoculated into A549 cells. Cytopathic effects demonstrate rounded, swollen, refractile cells. BAMC (Courtesy Bonnie Hill, Brooke Army Medical Center, San Antonio, Tx.)

on the stage of the lesion and whether it is a primary infection or recurrence.

Because of the potential for low sensitivity of viral culture and because other viruses can mimic the CPE of HSV, confirmation using monoclonal antibodies against type-specific epitopes is recommended. Many direct fluorescent antibody (DFA), indirect fluorescent antibody (IFA), or cytospin DFA assay commercial kits are available for this purpose. In many clinical laboratories, this type of test is routinely set up in conjunction with culture to save time and provide a more clinically relevant result. The CDC recommends serotyping viral culture isolates to determine whether infection is due to HSV-1 or HSV-2. Serologic assays are based on HSV-specific glycoprotein G2 (HSV-2) and glycoprotein G1 (HSV-1). FDA-approved serotyping assays include HerpeSelect™ HSV-1 or HSV-2 enzyme-linked immunosorbent assay (ELISA) IgG, HerpeSelect™ 1 and 2 Immunoblot IgG (Focus Technology, Inc., Herndon, Va.), and HSV-2 ELISA (Trinity Biotech USA, Berkeley Heights, N.J.). Other confirmatory tests that are available include genetically engineered cell lines, enzyme immunoassays (EIAs), and molecular methods such as in situ hybridization and PCR. PCR assays specific for HSV DNA are more sensitive; however, PCR tests are not FDA-approved for routine clinical testing of genital specimens.

Treatment

Genital herpes is a chronic, life-long viral infection for which there is no cure. Antiviral chemotherapy is widely used to treat mucocutaneous and genital herpes, offering some clinical benefits to the majority of symptomatic patients. Clinical trials have demonstrated that acyclovir, valacyclovir, and famciclovir are effective antivirals for the treatment of genital herpes. These drugs can reduce the signs and symptoms of genital herpes when used to treat primary infection and recurrent episodes. No treatment currently exists that will eradicate

latent virus or reduce the risk, frequency, or severity of recurrences after therapy is discontinued. Suppressive therapy can reduce the frequency of recurrences by 70% to 80% in patients who have more than six recurrences per year. Safety and efficacy of suppressive therapy has been demonstrated among patients receiving daily therapy with acyclovir up to 6 years and with valacyclovir or famciclovir for 1 year. Not only does daily therapy decrease the frequency and duration of recurrences, but it also limits viral shedding, reducing disease transmission rates. Clinicians also use suppressive therapy to prevent the transmission of HSV from mother to child during delivery. Neonates exposed to HSV infection during delivery should be closely monitored for symptoms of disease. Treatment with intravenous antiviral chemotherapy can reduce the overall morbidity and mortality of neonatal herpes. The CDC recommends intravenous acyclovir for treatment of neonatal herpes (20 mg/kg body weight IV) every 8 hours for 21 days for disseminated and CNS disease or for 14 days for disease limited to the skin and mucous membranes.

> ### Case Study
>
> A 23-year-old homeless female crack cocaine addict is arrested during a drug bust and brought to prison. During her in-processing physical, she admits to routinely exchanging sex for drugs to continue her habit. A full physical notes a rash on both her palms and her soles. The lesions are sampled and identified through dark-field microscopy. A serum sample is also taken and submitted to the laboratory for screening and conformational tests for syphilis.

Syphilis

Epidemiology

Syphilis is a genital ulcer disease caused by the spirochete *Treponema pallidum* subsp. pallidum *(T. pallidum)*. *T. pallidum* is an obligate parasite of humans and does not have any other known animal hosts or environmental reservoirs. Despite the existence of effective prevention measures, such as barrier prophylaxis, and treatment options, syphilis remains a global problem with an estimated 12 million people infected each year. The incidence of syphilis in the United States immediately following World War II was close to 500,000 cases per year. The number of reported infections declined during the 1990s, and in 2000 the rate was the lowest since reporting began (Figure 38-12). Primary and secondary (P&S) syphilis rates increased from 2001 to 2006, and the CDC reported 9756 infections in 2006, up from 8724 reported in 2005. Overall increases were observed primarily among men (from 3.0 cases per 100,000 persons to 5.7 cases per 100,000 persons); however, the rate of P&S syphilis among women did increase slightly from 0.8 cases per 100,000 persons in 2004 to 1.0 case per 100,000 persons in 2006. The average yearly rate of congenital syphilis declined 14.1% from 1996 to 2005, representing a total decline of 74.2% decrease overall during that time period. Unfortunately, the rate of congenital syphilis increased 3.7% between 2005 and 2006 (from 8.2 to 8.5 cases per 100,000 live births). The increase in the number of cases (339 to 349) may represent the slight increase in the

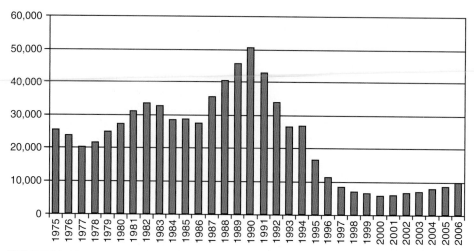

FIGURE 38-12 Reported cases of primary and secondary syphilis since 1975. (Modified from Centers for Disease Control and Prevention: *Sexually transmitted disease surveillance, 2006,* Atlanta, Ga, November 2007, U.S. Department of Health and Human Services.)

number of women with P&S syphilis. Most reportable cases of syphilis occur in the southern United States and urban areas in other areas of the country. Beginning in 2005 the CDC required all state health departments to report the sex of partners of persons with syphilis. These data indicate that the highest number of syphilis cases in 2006 occurred in men who have sex with men (MSM). The CDC estimated that the proportion of P&S syphilis cases attributable to MSM increased 58% from 2000 to 2004.

Clinical Manifestations

Syphilis is a multistage disease with diverse and wide-ranging clinical manifestations. *T. pallidum* subsp. pallidum is an invasive organism that can enter the host through any site and initiate infection. The three stages in the pathogenesis of syphilis are primary, secondary, and tertiary (or late) syphilis. The incubation period from initial exposure to development of the primary chancre ranges between 10 to 90 days. Infection occurs when *T. pallidum* penetrates dermal microabrasions or intact mucous membranes, typically producing a single lesion, also called *chancre,* at the site of inoculation (Figure 38-13). Appearance of the initial chancre, usually in the anogenital region, signals primary syphilis. Moderate regional lymphadenopathy is associated with the primary stage. The chancre usually becomes indurated and will progress to ulceration but typically is not purulent. In some cases syphilis occurs without a visible ulcer. The chancre has an indurated, raised edge. Usually there is only one chancre per infection. The painless, nonsuppurative lesion is extremely infectious. The lesion will spontaneously heal in 3 to 6 weeks (but can be as long as 12 weeks) if the patient does not receive antimicrobial therapy. The disappearance of the chancre does not signal an end to the infection.

Treponemes gain access to the bloodstream in untreated patients, and this spirochetemia is responsible for the signs and symptoms of secondary syphilis, which begins about 6 weeks to 6 months after infection. Clinical manifestations of secondary syphilis include, but are not limited to, skin rash,

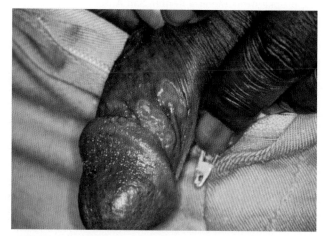

FIGURE 38-13 Chancres on the penile shaft due to a primary syphilitic infection caused by *Treponema pallidum* bacteria. Painless lesions are indurated with raised edges. (Courtesy M. Rein, MD, Centers for Disease Control and Prevention, Atlanta, Ga.)

mucocutaneous lesions, and lymphadenopathy (Figure 38-14). This is the period when the organisms are at their highest numbers. The hematogenous spread of the treponemes causes fever, lymphadenopathy, myalgia, and anorexia. Almost any organ can be involved in secondary syphilis. Signs of organ system involvement include hepatitis, osteitis, and keratitis. CNS involvement can occur during the secondary phase. Most patients develop macular or papular skin lesions involving the trunk, soles of the feet, and palms. Fluid from these "nickel and dime" lesions is extremely infectious. Another result of secondary syphilis is the appearance of condylomata lata, which are mucoid, fleshy wart-like growths. These lesions often occur in the perianal region but can occur in other moist regions of the body. Even without treatment, the symptoms of secondary syphilis disappear within a few weeks of onset, and the patient enters the latent phase. Patients are no longer

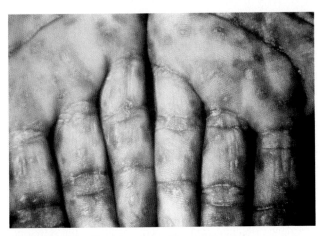

FIGURE 38-14 Close-up view of keratotic lesions on the palms of a patient's hands due to a secondary syphilitic infection. Each lesion is full of treponemes. (Courtesy Centers for Disease Control and Prevention, Atlanta, Ga.)

infectious after secondary syphilis lesions heal; however, relapses occur in about 25% of untreated patients during the first year following infection.

Latent syphilis is divided into two stages, early latent and late latent syphilis. Patients within the first year following infection are considered to have early latent syphilis, whereas late latent syphilis is defined as asymptomatic infection of longer than 1 year or unknown duration. Serologic testing during the late latent stage is positive and the patient is asymptomatic. Sexual transmission of disease is unlikely during the latent period, but organisms may enter the bloodstream intermittently and can infect the developing fetus during pregnancy. Latent syphilis is characterized by cerebrospinal fluid (CSF) abnormalities in the absence of symptoms. Indicators include elevated protein levels, depressed glucose levels, or pleocytosis (the presence of white blood cells in the CSF). Many untreated patients relapse during the first year of the latent period and will suffer a recurrence of the symptoms associated with secondary syphilis. Other patients may never relapse, and a third group of patients will experience late or tertiary syphilis. Tertiary syphilis is associated with immune sequelae of the primary and secondary syphilis, rather than the direct presence of treponemes. These patients may develop neurologic symptoms, cardiovascular effects, or experience late benign syphilis. In the latter condition, the patient develops nonspecific granulomatous lesions, called *gummas*. Gummas can occur in skin, bone, or viscera and cause a localized form of tissue and bone destruction. The lesions rarely resolve without appropriate antibiotic therapy. The late stages of syphilis develop in about 15% of untreated patients and can occur decades after they initially acquired the disease.

T. pallidum can cross the placenta and cause congenital infection in neonates. Congenital syphilis occurs when a live or stillborn infant is born to a mother with untreated or improperly treated syphilis. Infection across the placenta is most likely to occur during the primary or secondary stages of syphilis, but the fetus can be infected at anytime during pregnancy. Congenital syphilis is divided into two stages,

early and late disease. At birth, neonates with early congenital syphilis usually develop symptoms 2 to 10 weeks after delivery and show signs of secondary syphilis, including hepatosplenomegaly, jaundice, rash, condylomata lata, meningitis, and periostitis. Untreated children can go on to develop late congenital syphilis. These patients are asymptomatic at birth but can develop blindness, deafness, and deformed long bones or Hutchinson's teeth as young children. To prevent congenital syphilis, routine serologic screening of pregnant women during the first prenatal visit is recommended.

Laboratory Diagnosis

Treponema pallidum does not survive outside of a mammalian host and all attempts to continuously propagate the organism in vitro have been unsuccessful. Dark-field microscopy and DFA for *T. pallidum* (DFA-TP) examination tests of patient specimens are considered the definitive methods for diagnosing early syphilis from lesion exudates. Antibodies produced in response to infection with *T. pallidum* are detectable during primary syphilis and continue to concentrate as the disease progresses to the secondary stage. Serologic tests for the diagnosis of syphilis are divided into two general types: the **nontreponemal (nonspecific) antibody tests** and the treponemal (specific) antibody test. The nontreponemal antibody tests, such as the rapid plasma reagin (RPR), regain screen test (RST), unheated serum regain (USR), toluidine red unheated serum test (TRUST), and Venereal Disease Research Laboratory (VDRL) are used as screening tests and detect the presence of antibodies to cardiolipin and other lipoidal indicators of tissue damage. These tests are not highly specific but usually correlate with disease activity. Febrile infections, pregnancy, and autoimmune disorders may produce biologically false-positive reactions with nontreponemal tests. A fourfold change in titer is considered necessary to demonstrate a clinically significant difference between two nontreponemal test results that were obtained by the same methods. Clinicians can use quantitative nonspecific tests to follow the efficacy of treatment because these antibody levels decrease and ultimately disappear with the successful treatment of syphilis.

Patients with reactive nontreponemal test results are then tested with tests that use specific treponemal antigens to confirm the diagnosis. These confirmatory tests are specific **treponemal antibody tests** and include the EIAs, fluorescent treponemal antibody absorption (FTA-ABS*)*, and *T. pallidum* particle agglutination (TP-PA) tests. The most common tests performed in the United States are the TP-PA test and EIA. These tests help distinguish true- and false-positive nontreponemal test results and the diagnosis of late latent or tertiary syphilis. Treponemal antibody tests cannot be used to follow therapy because these antibodies do not disappear following the successful treatment of the disease. Most patients remain seropositive throughout their lives regardless of the treatment or its success; however, 15% to 25% of patients who received treatment early in the disease revert to being serologically nonreactive within 2 to 3 years. Additional assays are in development or becoming available for detection of specific treponemal antigens. These tests include EIA and molecular methods such as Western blotting and PCR. Most of these methods are considered experimental and are not performed in routine clinical laboratories. Rapid antigen tests are available internationally but not in the United States.

The diagnosis of congenital syphilis is complicated by the ability of maternal nontreponemal and treponemal immunoglobulin G (IgG) antibodies to cross the placenta. This passive transfer of antibodies makes serologic test interpretation in neonates difficult. To differentiate maternal antibody from the infant antibody to syphilis, an IgM-specific FTA-ABS test may be useful. Current testing recommendations suggest that infants born to mothers who have reactive serologic test results should be evaluated with a quantitative nontreponemal serologic test (RPR or VDRL) performed on infant serum. Confirmation of congenital syphilis includes clinician suspicion based on symptoms and history, along with the demonstration of treponemes in body tissues or fluids.

Treatment

Antibiotic susceptibility testing of *T. pallidum* is impractical given the inherent difficulty of culturing the organism in vitro. The CDC recommends a single intramuscular dose of penicillin G for the treatment of primary and secondary syphilis. Penicillin therapy has been the mainstay of treatment for over 50 years because *T. pallidum* isolates appear to be uniformly susceptible to β-lactam drugs. Current guidelines suggest multiple doses of aqueous or procaine penicillin G for suspected cases of neurosyphilis. A single dose of penicillin G is not as effective as multiple doses because low levels of the drug are maintained in CSF. Ceftriaxone, amoxicillin, and ampicillin are also effective for treatment of early syphilis. For patients allergic to penicillin, the CDC recommends doxycycline (100 mg orally twice daily for 14 days) or tetracycline (500 mg four times daily for 14 days) as an alternative regimen. Tetracycline and doxycycline are not recommended during pregnancy because of concerns of cosmetic staining of fetal primary dentition. Pregnant patients who are allergic to penicillin should be desensitized and treated with penicillin. The use of macrolides, such as azithromycin and erythromycin, for treatment of syphilis is not recommended due to reported resistance.

Chancroid

Epidemiology

Chancroid, or soft chancre, is an STI caused by the fastidious gram-negative bacterium *Haemophilus ducreyi*. Chancroid is a major cause of genital ulcerative disease in Africa, Southeast Asia, the Caribbean, and Latin America and is of increasing concern in the United States. The WHO estimates that there are more than 7 million cases of chancroid worldwide. Studies from regions where chancroid is endemic revealed that most cases of the disease occurred in patients with direct exposure to a commercial sex worker. The disease was endemic throughout many parts of the world well into the 20th century. Prevalence of chancroid declined steadily in the developed world before the discovery of antibiotics, largely because of a reduction in mass migrations and tighter regulation of the commercial sex industry. According to the CDC, reported cases of chancroid declined steadily from 1987 to 2006 when 33 cases were reported in the United States (Figure 38-15). This trend most likely reflects a decline in the incidence of this disease; however, rates of infection may be underreported because *H. ducreyi* is very difficult to culture. Like other etiologic agents of genital ulcer disease, chancroid is associated with increased transmission of HIV. Many patients with chancroid are also coinfected with *T. pallidum* or HSV.

Clinical Manifestations

Chancroid is characterized by painful genital ulceration inflammatory inguinal adenopathy, and bubo formation. The pathogen enters through microabrasions in the skin following sexual intercourse. Human inoculation experiments demonstrated that a dose of one colony-forming unit will result in infection at 50% of inoculation sites. A tender erythematous papule develops at the site of infection 4 to 7 days after exposure before progressing to the pustular stage. Once the papule develops into a pustule, it will usually rupture 2 to 3 days later to form painful, shallow ulcers with granulomatous bases and purulent exudates. The chancroid usually develops on the

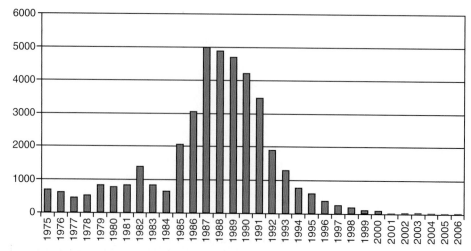

FIGURE 38-15 Reported cases of chancroid since 1975. (Modified from Centers for Disease Control and Prevention: *Sexually transmitted disease surveillance, 2006,* Atlanta, Ga, November 2007, U.S. Department of Health and Human Services.)

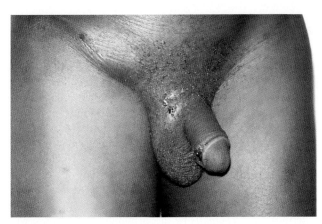

FIGURE 38-16 Chancroid lesion of the groin and penis affecting the ipsilateral inguinal lymph nodes. Chancroid lesions are painful and have ragged or uneven edges. (Courtesy Jim Pledger, Centers for Disease Control and Prevention, Atlanta, Ga.)

external genitalia of both men and women. The sites of infection in men include the prepuce, coronal sulcus, glans, and shaft; in women, the labia, clitoris, vaginal wall, and cervix can be involved. Chancroid ulcers must be differentiated from chancres and herpetic lesions. The chancroid is usually a more painful lesion than the chancre, and the chancroid typically has ragged or uneven edges. This ulcer may persist for weeks or months with slow resolution in the absence of antibiotic therapy. Painful, tender inguinal lymphadenitis occurs in nearly half of all chancroid cases. Lymphadenopathy in these patients is usually unilateral and is more frequently observed in men. If left untreated, swollen lymph nodes can develop into fluctuant buboes (Figure 38-16), which can rupture spontaneously if not drained. Extragenital manifestations of chancroid are rare, but lesions have been observed on the inner thighs, breasts, and fingers.

Laboratory Diagnosis

Clinical diagnosis and laboratory culture of *H. ducreyi* are considered the "gold standards" for the diagnosis of chancroid. Ulcer lesion material and/or bubo aspirate may be submitted for direct smear examination and culture. Microscopically, *H. ducreyi* are pleomorphic, gram-negative coccobacilli that occasionally occur in chains or "school-of-fish" formations. Gram stains are not a sensitive or specific tool for the diagnosis of chancroid, because the specimen often includes numerous bacterial contaminants. *H. ducreyi* is extremely fastidious and requires relatively expensive media for growth. Some clinical isolates grow well on chocolate agar, but enriched media can increase the sensitivity of culture. Two commercially available varieties of enhanced media contain gas chromatography (GC) agar base, hemoglobin, IsoVitalex, and fetal calf serum, and another has Mueller-Hinton agar with chocolate horse blood and IsoVitalex. Most *H. ducreyi* strains grow well at 33° C to 35° C in a 5% CO_2 atmosphere. It is critical that specimens be sent as quickly as possible to the laboratory for successful culture. Even with the optimal combination of media and timely deliver to the laboratory, culture is only about 80% sensitive.

Alternative testing methodologies to culture, such as PCR and immunoassays, are being developed to improve the sensitivity of chancroid diagnosis. Currently, no FDA-approved PCR assays are commercially available in the United States. Multiplex PCR assays specific for multiple agents of genital ulcer disease have been developed and are performed in a few laboratories that have completed validation studies. Preliminary studies indicate that these assays can be more rapid and sensitive than culture. Serologic detection of chancroid has been demonstrated by enzyme immunoassays that contain antibodies against *H. ducreyi* lipooligosaccharide and antigen detection using direct immunofluorescence. These assays are not widely available and suffer from cross-reactivity problems. Given the limitations of alternative testing methods, culture remains the primary diagnostic test performed by most microbiology laboratories for suspected cases of chancroid.

Treatment

Antibiotic therapy for treatment of patients with chancroid resolves the clinical symptoms, prevents transmission to others, and cures the disease. Current treatment guidelines include a single oral dose of azithromycin, oral ciprofloxacin (twice a day for 3 days), oral erythromycin base (four times a day for 7 days), or a single intramuscular dose of ceftriaxone. Patients with underlying immunosuppression or HIV infection and uncircumcised men should be carefully managed. Genital ulcers heal more slowly in these patients, and persistence of *H. ducreyi* in the lesions has been documented. In uncircumcised men, lesions under the foreskin also take longer to heal. Given the difficulty of culturing *H. ducreyi* and the limitation of sensitive testing methodologies, presumptive treatment for chancroid should be considered if HSV and syphilis are ruled out. Chancroid should also be considered if the patient lives in or has traveled to an endemic area or an outbreak is underway.

Lymphogranuloma Venereum

Epidemiology

Lymphogranuloma venereum (LGV) is a sexually transmitted disease caused by serovars L1, L2, L2a, L2b, and L3 of the intracellular bacterium *C. trachomatis*. Serovars A-K are restricted to mucosal columnar epithelial cells of the genital tract and are the predominant strains involved in human genital and ocular infection. Compared with serovars A-K, LGV strains are more virulent in experimental animal models of infection and more invasive in humans. LGV rarely occurs in the United States and other industrialized countries, but higher rates of disease can be found in Africa, Southeast Asia, Central and South America, and Caribbean countries. Prevalence of the disease is unclear because of the difficulty in clearly distinguishing it from other causes of genital ulceration and bubo formation such as chancroid. During the past few years, health care providers in Europe have reported outbreaks of LGV in MSM. Signs and symptoms associated with rectal infection can be misdiagnosed as ulcerative colitis. Because the signs and symptoms of LGV are not always obvious, the actual number of cases in the United States is unknown.

Clinical Manifestations

Whereas serovars A-K are largely confined to mucosal columnar epithelial surfaces of the genital tract and eye, LGV serovars predominantly infect monocytes and macrophages, pass through the epithelial surface to regional lymph nodes, and may cause disseminated infection. Clinical LGV infection has three stages: primary, secondary, and tertiary. The primary lesion produced by LGV usually presents as a small genital or rectal lesion, which can ulcerate at the site of transmission. It is possible for a primary lesion to not occur, or it may simply go unnoticed within the urethra, vagina, or rectum. Symptoms typically occur after a 3- to 30-day incubation period following exposure. Proctitis can occur as a primary manifestation of infection following direct inoculation of the rectal mucosa, and symptoms may arise within days of exposure.

The secondary stage of LGV involves the spread of *C. trachomatis* from the initial site of inoculation via the lymphatics to regional lymph nodes. This stage begins 2 to 6 weeks after the initial lesion develops and primarily affects the inguinal lymph nodes. Characteristic of the inguinal form of LGV is the presence of unilateral inguinal and/or femoral lymphadenopathy. Pressure from the inguinal ligament separating the groin lymph nodes gives rise to the "groove sign," once believed to be diagnostic for LGV, but only occurring in 20% of cases. Affected nodes can coalesce to form buboes, which may then ulcerate and discharge pus from multiple points. The inguinal form of LGV is more common in men because lymphatic drainage from the penis is to the inguinal lymph nodes. In women, lymphatic drainage of the vagina and cervix is to the retroperitoneal lymph nodes. As a result of enlargement and suppuration of the perirectal and pelvic lymphatics, LGV will commonly present as backache in women, with initial lesions on the cervix/upper vagina or in the rectal area in men who engage in receptive anal intercourse with men. Rectal involvement presents as an acute ulcerative proctitis with bloody purulent rectal discharges, pain, tenesmus, and constipation. Systemic symptoms such as fever, malaise, and headache can occur during the secondary stage of LGV. Infection with LGV serovars is not restricted to the genital region. Submaxillary and cervical gland lymphadenitis can result from exposure to *C. trachomatis* organisms during oral sex. Ocular inoculation causes conjunctivitis along with preauricular lymphadenopathy.

In tertiary stage disease, untreated infections can lead to chronic inflammation and destruction of affected tissues. Patients with untreated LGV proctitis may develop rectal damage, strictures, and in women, the formation of rectovaginal fistulae. If LGV continues untreated, lesions caused by *C. trachomatis* often lead to fibrosis and granulomas. Fibrosis can lead to lymphatic obstruction, causing elephantiasis of the genitalia in either sex, esthiomene in women, which results in a destructive, hypertrophic, granulomatous enlargement of the vulva and subsequent ulceration. Tertiary stage sequelae do not typically disappear once antibiotic therapy is initiated, and surgical intervention is required to correct many late complications, such as rectal stricture.

Laboratory Diagnosis

Diagnosis of LGV is based on clinical presentation, epidemiologic information, and the exclusion of other etiologies of genital or rectal ulcers, inguinal lymphadenopathy, and/or proctitis. *C. trachomatis* can be identified in bubo aspirates or in ulcer material by tissue culture, direct fluorescent microscopy, EIAs, or nucleic acid amplification tests (NAATs). Isolation of viable *C. trachomatis* from specimens requires tissue culture using HeLa-229 or McCoy cell lines. Tissue culture used to be considered the "gold standard," but the technique is no longer widely used because of its difficulty to perform and sensitivity issues. Genital and lymph node smears may be tested for *C. trachomatis* by direct immunofluorescence with a fluorescently labeled monoclonal antibody. Serologic assays for *C. trachomatis* infection, with complement fixation titers greater than 1:64 indicating a positive result, support LGV diagnosis in an appropriate clinical context. LGV serologic test interpretation is not standardized, tests have not been validated for anorectal specimens, and *C. trachomatis* serovar–specific serologic tests are not widely available. The diagnostic utility of serologic methods other than complement fixation and some microimmunofluorescence procedures has not been established.

NAATs have rapidly become the preferred diagnostic method for detecting genital *C. trachomatis* infections because of their sensitivity and specificity. Another advantage of NAATs is the ability to test self- or clinician-collected vaginal swabs or urine, eliminating more invasive procedures. PCR and nucleic acid hybridization assays are available for the diagnosis of genital infections but have not been well evaluated for the diagnosis of LGV. Although a number of real time–PCR assays have been validated to detect LGV in rectal specimens, currently no FDA-approved NAATs are commercially available. Detection of *C. trachomatis* in bubo or lymph node material by any of these diagnostic methods is highly suggestive of LGV; however, detection of the organism in ulcer material can only support the diagnosis if the strain is identified by sequencing or typing assays. Most identification algorithms reflex positive *C. trachomatis* PCR results for genotyping PCR-based restriction fragment length polymorphism (RFLP) analysis and/or sequencing of the conserved region of DNA.

Treatment

Current CDC treatment guidelines recommend the use of doxycycline, twice a day for 21 days, to treat cases of LGV. A longer course of therapy, at least 3 weeks, is recommended because of the deep tissue penetration by the organism. Doxycycline is not recommended for use in pregnant or lactating women. An alternative treatment recommended for these patients is erythromycin four times a day for 21 days. Azythromycin may prove useful for treatment of LGV in pregnancy, but minimal clinical data are available on the effectiveness of azithromycin in the treatment of LGV. Anorectal lymphogranuloma venereum has an excellent prognosis if the disease is diagnosed and treated early. Delays in treatment can lead to serious complications such as abscesses, fistulae, and rectal strictures. The CDC recommends treating patients that present with symptoms consistent with LGV, including proctitis, genital ulcer disease, or inguinal lymphadenopathy, in settings without access to specific diagnostic LGV testing.

Patients coinfected with both LGV and HIV should receive the same treatment regimen as those who are HIV-negative. Prolonged antibiotic therapy may be required for HIV-positive patients, and symptoms may resolve more slowly. Sexual contacts of patients diagnosed with LGV should be notified within 60 days of symptom onset to be evaluated and treated. Prompt treatment can prevent symptom development and lessens the risk of the original patient becoming reinfected. Sexual intercourse should be avoided until the course of treatment is completed and symptoms have completely disappeared.

Donovanosis

Epidemiology

Donovanosis, or **granuloma inguinale** as it is sometimes referred to, is a genital ulcerative disease caused by the intracellular gram-negative bacterium *Klebsiella granulomatis* (formerly *Calymmatobacterium granulomatis*). The disease is rare in the United States, but it is endemic in some tropical and developing areas, including India, Papua, New Guinea, central Australia, Brazil, and southern Africa. Ulcers are more common in uncircumcised men with poor standards of genital hygiene. Disseminated donovanosis may spread to bone and liver and is often associated with pregnancy and cervical infection. Cases that occur in the United States typically involve someone who is from or recently traveled to an endemic region.

Clinical Manifestations

Donovanosis is thought to be spread by direct contact with lesions during sexual activity; however, nonsexual transmission has been documented. Donovanosis often produces a firm papule or subcutaneous nodule that ulcerates at the primary site of inoculation. Ulcerative lesions usually develop in the genital region but may occur at oral, anal, or other extragenital sites. Lesions frequently appear in warm, moist surfaces such as the folds between the thighs, perianal region, scrotom, or labia. Local lymphadenopathy can occur, which may lead to ulcerative lesions developing in the skin overlying the infected lymph nodes. Four different types of donovanosis have been described in the literature: (1) ulcerogranulomatous—nonfriable, beefy red, nontender ulcers that bleed readily when touched and may become quite extensive if left untreated (Figure 38-17); (2) hypertrophic or verrucous ulcer—growth of the ulcer is usually with an irregular edge, sometimes completely dry; (3) necrotic, foul-smelling, deep ulcer that progresses to tissue destruction; (4) dry, sclerotic, or cicatricial lesion with fibrous tissue and scar tissue.

In men, donovanosis frequently affects the penis, the scrotum, the glans, and/or the anus. In women, the disease primarily affects the labia minora, fourchette, and less often, the cervix and upper genital tract. Pregnant women have a higher risk for developing disseminated donovanosis with spread to bone and liver predominating. Extragenital exposure may result in ulceration of the lips, cheeks, and gums. If

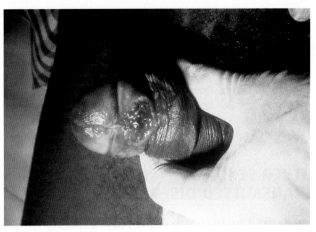

FIGURE 38-17 Progressively ulcerative, highly vascular "beefy red" lesions caused by *Klebsiella granulomatis* (donovanosis). (Courtesy Centers for Disease Control and Prevention, Atlanta, Ga. Slide provided by Dr. Tabua, Chief Medical Officer from, Port Moresby, Papua, New Guinea.)

left untreated, the disease process may result in extensive destruction of the genitalia and spread to distant sites by autoinoculation. It is considered to be only mildly contagious, and repeated exposure may be necessary for clinical infection to occur.

Laboratory Diagnosis

Diagnosis of donovanosis is usually determined clinically based on a detailed history and physical exam findings of ulcerative lesions on a patient with sexual contact in an endemic region. The diagnosis can be confirmed by identifying characteristic intracellular **Donovan bodies** within Giemsa or Wright's stains of macrophages. Smears obtained directly from tissue or biopsy samples can be examined. Donovan bodies measure 0.5 to 0.7 × 1 to 1.5 mm in diameter and may or may not be capsulated. *K. granulomatis* is an extremely fastidious organism, and culture is beyond the capability of most clinical laboratories. PCR assays have been developed to detect *K. granulomatis,* but no FDA-approved test is commercially available. An indirect immunofluorescent assay was developed using antigen derived from donovanosis lesions. These assays have low sensitivity for detecting early infection and are not widely available.

Treatment

Very few studies on donovanosis treatment have been reported in the literature. Effective treatment halts the progression of destructive ulcers, but therapy should continue until granulation and re-epithelialization of the lesions occurs. The CDC recommends doxycycline taken orally twice a day for 3 weeks or until symptoms resolve. Alternative antibiotics include azithromycin, ciprofloxacin, erythromycin, and trimethoprim-sulfamethoxazole. Doxycycline and ciprofloxacin are contraindicated in pregnant women. Pregnant and lactating women should be treated with erythromycin and a parenteral aminoglycoside, such as gentamicin. Individuals diagnosed with both donovanosis and HIV should receive the same treatment regimen as those who are HIV-negative. Addition of an aminoglycoside should be considered to increase the chances of successful resolution. Patients should be followed clinically until symptoms of the disease have resolved. Recurrence of symptoms can occur 6 to 18 months after symptom resolution, even after apparently effective therapy was completed. Sexual contacts within the 60 days preceding the onset of symptoms should be identified and examined for disease. Once the lesions have healed, extensive deformity and functional disability may require surgical intervention to repair.

OTHER SEXUALLY TRANSMITTED DISEASES

Human Immunodeficiency Virus

Epidemiology

When human immunodeficiency virus (HIV) was first described, it was mainly considered to be a sexually transmitted disease amongst the male homosexual population. Male homosexuals still garner most of the infections and the rate increases annually. However, in today's society, nearly one third of the new HIV infections are found in heterosexuals engaging in risky behaviors. African-American men and women account for approximately 50% of all new infections, basically a sevenfold greater incidence rate than the Caucasian population. Currently, there are more than 1 million individuals in the United States infected with HIV, of whom approximately 25% do not realize that they are infected. HIV infection leads to development of acquired immune deficiency syndrome (AIDS), for which no cure has yet to be found.

Clinical Manifestations

AIDS weakens the immune system such that an individual has a difficult time fighting off infections. When someone develops various infections and demonstrates a low T-cell count, they are said to have AIDS. The initial symptoms of HIV infection are fairly nonspecific, resembling a mononucleosis-like illness that may resolve normally. Unless individuals recognize the approximate risks (intravenous drug use, exchanging sex for drugs, unprotected sex, sex with multiple or anonymous partners, previous STD infections) that they are subjected to, they may not realize an infection has occurred until they develop advanced symptoms of AIDS. Such symptoms include rapid weight loss, dry cough, fever or night sweats, lymphadenopathy, diarrhea, pneumonia, or neurologic disorders.

Laboratory Diagnosis

Multiple methods are available for diagnosising HIV infection. Antibodies directed against HIV are common targets for screening assays. Tested specimens can be blood, serum, plasma, urine, or even oral fluid. Some tests are rapid point-of-care (POC) type that can be performed within the clinic, some can be self-collected specimens and mailed in for testing, and other tests are collected and sent off to a laboratory for screening. Typically, the rapid tests have the lowest sensitivity of detection. Testing is always done in two parts using an initial screening assay followed by a secondary assay to confirm infection. This method is used to improve overall

diagnosis; as singly performed, these assays can be still be faulty. The Western blot assay is the conventional confirmatory assay that detects a number of conserved protein regions produced by the virus. In the United States, a combination of glycoproteins representative of the group antigen (gag—gp55, gp 40, gp 24, gp18), reverse transcriptase (pol—gp68, gp 53, gp 32), and envelope (env—gp160, gp 120, gp 41) gene products confirms infection by HIV. Unfortunately, these tests are time consuming, subjective, and expensive. Recently a new testing algorithm has been introduced that uses currently licensed tests and compares favorably with the conventional algorithm in detecting and confirming established HIV infection. HIV testing should be followed up with counseling to help the patient understand the results, either positive or negative, and receive education on preventive measures.

Treatment

Once an individual has a confirmed infection, he needs to see a licensed health care provider, even if he does not feel sick, so that he can begin immediate therapy. This helps achieve maximum benefit from the antiretroviral agents. Because the person will be prone to several potentially devastating infections, it is important to be tested for tuberculosis and other STDs. Patients should begin to practice safe sex to avoid spreading and acquisition of other infectious agents. Patients should also try to live a healthier lifestyle, such as quitting smoking, reducing alcohol intake, and eliminating usage of illegal drugs. The health care provider will also want to get an idea of the patient's viral load throughout therapy to determine antiretroviral efficacy and whether or not to change treatment regimens.

Advances in antiretroviral therapy have improved the outlook for infected patients. Initially, the stigma of infection meant an eventual downward spiral culminating in full-blown AIDS and death. The mortality rate in developed countries with good access to health care has even dropped. Although a cure has yet to be found, infected individuals are leading more active lifestyles with sometimes many years passing by before development of AIDS. Many people have become more casual in their approach to HIV infection, thinking that a cure will be found before they develop AIDS. The internet has even helped increase these risky behaviors by individuals setting up anonymous meetings online. The annual rate of new HIV infections continues to increase every year. Additionally, there is a marked increase in antiretroviral resistance, because of noncompliance, which is becoming a significant health issue. Monitoring of patients may soon be required. Clearly, there is a need for greater prevention programs in an effort to reduce the overall spread of disease.

Case Study

A 16-year-old female presents to her pediatric clinic for a routine sports physical. During the checkup, her doctor discusses common teenage sexual infections and diseases noted within her community. Although she is not sexually active, her doctor discusses the effects of human papilloma virus (HPV) infections and offers to provide a vaccination for protection against four of the most common types of HPV causing cervical cancer and genital warts.

Human Papillomavirus

Epidemiology

Human papillomavirus (HPV) is the most common sexually transmitted viral disease in the United States. An estimated 6.2 million individuals become infected annually. There are several different genotypes of HPV, which are usually distinguished into two separate groupings. Certain genotypes cause various forms of cancer within the genital area, in particular within the cervix. However, the second group causes genital warts, which are the expression of a sexually transmitted disease. Two specific genotypes within this second group, HPV types 6 and 11, are attributed to approximately 90% of all genital warts. A recent study showed that 5.6% of the 18- to 59-year-old population had been diagnosed with genital warts; women have a higher infection rate than males. Factors associated with increased risk of infection include gender, age, ethnicity, number of lifetime partners, and use of illicit drugs. Indeed, HPV infections are the most common STD in individuals aged 24 or less.

Clinical Manifestations

Humans are the only known reservoir for HPV. The virus affects skin and mucous membranes and causes development of warts in the moist and dry areas of the genitals that can be variable in size and shape. They are typically small bumps that can be raised or flat, single or in groups, small or large, and sometimes cauliflower shaped (Figure 38-18). The manifestation of the cauliflower-shaped genital warts in moist regions is called *condylomata accuminata*. Genital locations include the vulva, vagina, anus, cervix, penis, scrotum, and groin or thigh. Infection is spread through intimate contact, most often during vaginal and anal sex. In homosexual males, anal warts occur more often than genital warts.

Diagnosis

Diagnosis of genital warts is clinically made upon physical exam. Flat warts, which are not as visible, can be diagnosed by using a weak acetic acid solution to suspected areas of genital tissue; the solution causes infected areas to whiten, making them more visible. Tissue biopsies may also be performed to confirm HPV infection.

Treatment

There is no permanent cure for HPV, and recurrences may be found in skin nearby to the initial site. Depending on the genotype detected, these infections could potentially lead to cancer. Several methods of treatment are available including cryotherapy with liquid nitrogen, electrocautery using trichloracetic acid, laser surgery, and various topical medications that are immune response modifiers. In some cases, no therapy is used to see whether the warts will disappear on their own. α-Interferon can also be injected directly into the warts that have returned after removal using other traditional methods. Over-the-counter cures for warts should not be used near the genitals because severe irritation can occur. Sexual contact should be avoided until the warts are treated.

A few recommendations are given in order to prevent infection from occurring. Abstinence is the safest way to

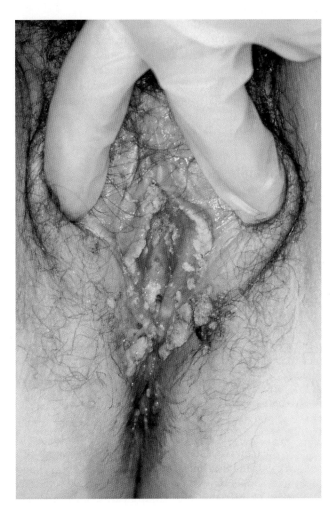

FIGURE 38-18 Genital warts on the labia. (Courtesy Joe Millar, Centers for Disease Control and Prevention, Atlanta Ga.)

prevent an infection. When that is not possible, individuals should utilize safe sex practices using barriers to prevent transmission and limiting sexual contact. Additionally, women who have regular pap smears can potentially detect infection earlier and then get proper treatment. The newest preventive measure is a newly created HPV vaccine. This vaccine is quadrivalent and is directed against the most common genotypes to cause cervical cancer (16, 18) as well as the common genotypes for genital warts (6, 11). Studies to date demonstrate the reduction of disease and may substantially decrease public STD clinic workloads. The vaccine is recommended for young women ages 9 to 26. Although not currently available for vaccination of males, it is becoming recommended within the medical community.

Pelvic Inflammatory Disease

Epidemiology

Pelvic inflammatory disease (PID) is a grouping of syndromes affecting the female reproductive organs. It is a common complication of cervicitis in women who have mainly been infected with the bacterial sexually transmitted diseases chlamydia and gonorrhea. More than 1 million women annually are estimated to develop PID, of whom 100,000 may become infertile. PID develops as bacteria ascend up the female genital tract into the reproductive organs. Sexually active women of childbearing age and women under 25 are generally at the greatest risk of developing PID. Several risk factors in developing PID include having multiple partners, frequent douching, and intrauterine use. Previous episodes of disease also increase the risk of developing PID and further complications.

Clinical Manifestations

PID is vaguely defined and can be a conglomeration of several diseases of the female upper genital tract such as endometriosis, salpingitis, tuboovarian abscess, and pelvic peritonitis. Symptoms are variable, ranging from nonexistent to severe. The full complement of commonly recognized symptoms of lower abdominal pain, fever, vaginal discharge, painful intercourse, pain on urination, and irregular menstrual bleeding should alert the provider to check for evidence of infection with gonorrhea or chlamydia. Because symptoms may be vague and nonspecific, it's estimated that PID goes unrecognized about two thirds of the time, leading to multiple complications caused by permanent damage to the reproductive organs.

Diagnosis

PID is very difficult to diagnose because of a lack of specific symptoms. There are no specific tests for PID, so the health care provider must usually make the diagnosis based on a physical exam and the clinical findings described above. Laboratory tests should be ordered to confirm infection with causative agents. A pelvic ultrasound or laparoscopy can also be used to view the pelvic area to determine whether any inflammatory processes are occurring within any of the reproductive organs. PID causes scarring within these organs, leading to serious complications including chronic pelvic pain, infertility, ectopic pregnancy, and in rare cases, spreading of the disease to in the peritoneum and formation of scar tissue on the liver (Fitz-Hugh-Curtis syndrome).

Treatment

PID is treated with antibiotics that are specific against the causative organisms. Broad-spectrum antibiotics are used in an effort to promote action against multiple infectious agents. Typically, ceftriaxone and doxycycline are recommended for chlamydia and gonorrhea. Patients should be tracked following treatment to ensure antibiotic effectiveness. In severe cases, a patient may need to be hospitalized for therapy. PID can be prevented by practicing various risk reduction methods. Abstinence or changes in social behavior and barrier methods all help to decrease the probability of infection. When women are able to identify any abnormal changes or recognize a potential infection, they should see their physician immediately. The CDC recommends yearly screening for all sexually active women 25 years and younger, all women in high-risk groups (e.g., multiple partners), and all pregnant women. The military recommends screening women for chlamydia at the basic entry level and until age 25 to reduce the level of PID in its female service members. Any positive confirmed results can then be treated immediately, as can any partners, to reduce the chance of spread of disease.

Molluscum Contagiosum

Molluscum contagiosum is a common skin disease caused by the molluscum contagiosum virus. This is a poxvirus that can easily be spread through direct skin to skin contact or through contact with contaminated objects. It is considered to be an STD when found in the genital area. This disease is common in HIV patients and may signal immunosuppression. Common symptoms are a small umbilicated papule that can become red and inflamed. These papules can be easily removed when scratched or rubbed, thus spreading disease to other areas of the body. Diagnosis is clinical and can be confirmed by microscopic analysis. Treatment is removal of the papules by scraping, freezing, or laser therapy. Avoidance of sexual contact is recommended until the infection is completely resolved.

Epididymitis

Epididymitis is inflammation of the epididymis affecting males most commonly between the ages of 19 and 35. This is generally a complication of infection with chlamydia or gonorrhea. Common signs and symptoms include scrotal inflammation, testicle pain and tenderness, pain on urination or intercourse, chills and fever, lymphadenopathy, penile discharge, or blood in the semen. Men who engage in high-risk sexual behaviors and have had STD infections previously are at great risk of developing this condition. Diagnosis is clinically based but should include STD screening tests to confirm the causative agent(s). Antibiotics are provided for the confirmed infectious agent.

Case Study

A 21-year-old gay male presents to the local STD clinic with complaints of tenesmus, rectal discomfort, bloody stools, and a purulent discharge. Social history indicates that he has had multiple partners since a breakup with his boyfriend more than 6 months ago. He routinely chats with potential partners online to arrange anonymous encounters. He reports commonly participating in receptive anal intercourse and anilingus. His provider takes a rectal swab and submits it to the laboratory for identification. Additionally, the patient is referred to a local gastroenterologist for a flexible sigmoidoscopy.

Proctitis

Proctitis is recognized as inflammation of the rectal lining and is most common in people who engage in anal or oral-anal intercourse. It is mainly caused by the STDs chlamydia, gonorrhea, syphilis, herpes simplex, and HPV. Symptoms include rectal bleeding, mucus passage, anal and rectal pain, diarrhea, and pain with bowel movements. When presenting to the physician for these complaints, additional STD screening should be performed. Antibiotics or antivirals can then be provided based on the confirmed infectious agent.

BIBLIOGRAPHY

Alfa M: The laboratory diagnosis of *Haemophilus ducreyi*, *Can J Infect Dis Med Microbiol* 16:31, 2005.

Allsworth JE, Peipert JF: Prevalence of bacterial vaginosis: 2001-2004 National Health and Nutrition Examination Survey Data, *Obstet Gynecol Oncol* 109:114, 2007.

Al-Tawfiq JA et al: Cumulative experience with *Haemophilus ducreyi* in the human model of experimental infection, *Sex Transm Dis* 27:111, 2000.

Amsel R et al: Nonspecific vaginitis, diagnostic criteria and microbial and epidemiologic associations, *Am J Med* 74:14, 1983.

Al-Tayyib AA et al: Health care access and follow-up of chlamydial and gonococcal infections identified in an emergency department, *Sex Transm Dis* 35:583, 2008.

Bangsberg DR: Preventing HIV antiretroviral resistance through better monitoring of treatment adherence, *J Infect Dis* 197:S272, 2008.

Beauman JG: Genital herpes: a review, *Am Fam Physician* 72:1527, 2005.

Benedetti J, Corey L, Ashley R: Recurrence rates in genital herpes after symptomatic first-episode infection, *Ann Intern Med* 121:847, 1994.

Bertagnolio S et al: World Health Organization/HIVResNet Drug Resistance Laboratory Strategy, *Antivir Ther* 13:49, 2008.

Bertozzi SM et al: Making HIV prevention programmes work, *Lancet* 372(9641):831, 2008.

Bhalla P et al: Simultaneous detection of *Neisseria gonorrhoeae* and *Chlamydia trachomatis* by PCR in genitourinary specimens from men and women attending an STD clinic, *J Commun Dis* 39:1, 2007.

Bhaskaran K et al: Changes in the risk of death after HIV seroconversion compared with mortality in the general population, *JAMA* 300:51, 2008.

Bloom MS et al: Incidence rates of pelvic inflammatory disease diagnoses among Army and Navy recruits potential impacts of Chlamydia screening policies, *Am J Prev Med* 34:471, 2008.

Bowden FJ et al: Pilot study of azithromycin in the treatment of genital donovanosis, *Genitourin Med* 72:17, 1994.

Bowden FJ: National Donovanosis Eradication Advisory Committee: Donovanosis in Australia: going, going, *Sex Transm Infect* 81:365, 2005.

Bradshaw CS et al: Etiologies of nongonococcal urethritis: bacteria, viruses, and the association with orogenital exposure, *J Infect Dis* 193:336, 2006.

Burd EM: Human papillomavirus and cervical cancer, *Clin Microbiol Rev* 16:1, 2003.

Chen CY et al: The molecular diagnosis of lymphogranuloma venereum: evaluation of a real-time multiplex polymerase chain reaction test using rectal and urethral specimens, *Sex Transm Dis* 34:451, 2007.

Centers for Disease Control and Prevention: Lymphogranuloma venereum among men who have sex with men—Netherlands, 2003-2004, *MMWR Morb Mortal Wkly Rep* 53:985, 2004.

Centers for Disease Control and Prevention (CDC): Sexually transmitted diseases treatment guidelines, 2006, *MMWR Morb Mortal Wkly Rep* 55:1, 2006.

Centers for Disease Control and Prevention (CDC): Update to CDC's sexually transmitted diseases treatment guidelines, 2006: fluoroquinolones no longer recommended for treatment of gonococcal infections, *MMWR Morb Mortal Wkly Rep* 56:332, 2007.

Centers for Disease Control and Prevention (CDC): Availability of cefixime 400 mg tablets—United States, *MMWR Morb Mortal Wkly Rep* 57:435, 2008.

Centers for Disease Control and Prevention (CDC): Summary of notifiable diseases—United States, 2006, *MMWR Morb Mortal Wkly Rep* 55:1, 2008.

Centers for Disease Control and Prevention (CDC): False-positive oral fluid rapid HIV tests—New York City, 2005-2008, *MMWR Morb Mortal Wkly Rep* 57:660, 2008.

Centers for Disease Control and Prevention (CDC): HIV/AIDS surveillance report, 2006, Atlanta, Ga, U.S. Department of Health and Human Services, *Centers for Disease Control and Prevention* 18:1, 2008. www.cdc.gov/hiv/topics/surveillance/resources/reports/

Centers for Disease Control and Prevention (CDC): Persons tested for HIV—United States, 2006, *MMWR Morb Mortal Wkly Rep* 57:845, 2008.

Centers for Disease Control and Prevention (CDC): *Sexually transmitted disease surveillance, 2006*, Atlanta, Ga, 2006, U.S. Department of Health and Human Services, Centers for Disease Control and Prevention.

Centers for Disease Control and Prevention (CDC): Trends in HIV- and STD-related risk behaviors among high school students—United States, 1991-2007, *MMWR Morb Mortal Wkly Rep* 57:817, 2008.

Chesson HW et al: The estimated direct medical cost of sexually transmitted diseases among American youth, 2000, *Perspect Sex Reprod Health* 36:11, 2004.

Collins L, White JA, Bradbeer C: Lymphogranuloma venereum, *BMJ* 332:66, 2006.

Cook JA et al: Crack cocaine, disease progression, and mortality in a multicenter cohort of HIV-1 positive women, *AIDS* 22:1355, 2008.

Corey L: First-episode, recurrent, and asymptomatic herpes simplex infections, *J Am Acad Dermatol* 18:169, 1988.

Corey L et al: Genital herpes simplex virus infections: clinical manifestations, course, and complications, *Ann Intern Med* 98:958, 1983.

Cotch MF et al: *Trichomonas vaginalis* associated with low birth weight and preterm delivery, The Vaginal Infections and Prematurity Study Group, *Sex Transm Dis* 24:353, 1997.

Cunningham KA, Beagley KW: Male genital tract chlamydial infection: implications for pathology and infertility, *Biol Reprod* 79:180, 2008; Epub May 14, 2008.

D'Costa LJ et al: Prostitutes are a major reservoir of sexually transmitted diseases in Nairobi, Kenya, *Sexually Transmitted Diseases* 12:64, 1985.

Decker MR et al: Sex purchasing and associations with HIV/STI among a clinic-based sample of US men, *J Acquir Immune Defic Syndr* 48:355, 2008.

Dempsey AF et al: Using risk factors to predict human papillomavirus infection: implications for targeted vaccination strategies in young adult women, *Vaccine* 26:1111, 2008; Epub Dec 26, 2007.

Dinh TH et al: Genital warts among 18- to 59-year-olds in the United States, national health and nutrition examination survey, 1999-2004, *Sex Transm Dis* 35:357, 2008.

Draper D et al: Detection of *Trichomonas vaginalis* in pregnant women with the InPouch TV culture system, *J Clin Microbiol* 31:1016, 1993.

Dunne EF et al: Prevalence of HPV infection among men: a systematic review of the literature, *J Infect Dis* 194:1044, 2006; Epub 2006 Sep 12.

Espy MJ et al: Comparison of shell vials and conventional tubes seeded with rhabdomyosarcoma and MRC-5 cells for the rapid detection of herpes simplex virus, *J Clin Microbiol* 29:2701, 1991.

Evans DT et al: A retrospective audit of the management and complications of pelvic inflammatory disease, *Int J STD AIDS* 19:123, 2008.

Farage MA, Miller KW, Ledger WJ: Determining the cause of vulvovaginal symptoms, *Obstet Gynecol Surv* 63:445, 2008.

Fine D et al: Region X Infertility Prevention Project: Increasing chlamydia positivity in women screened in family planning clinics:

do we know why? *Sex Transm Dis* 35:47, 2008. Comment in: *Sex Transm Dis* 35:53, 2008.

Fisman DN et al: Projection of the future dimensions and costs of the genital herpes simplex type 2 epidemic in the United States, *Sex Transm Dis* 29:608, 2002.

Fleming DT et al: Herpes simplex virus type 2 in the United States, 1976 to 1994, *N Engl J Med* 337:1105, 1997.

Freinkel AL et al: A serological test for granuloma inguinale, *Genitourin Med* 68:269, 1992.

Frenkl TL, Potts J: Sexually transmitted infections, *Urol Clin North Am* 35:33, 2008.

Garland SM et al: Quadrivalent vaccine against human papillomavirus to prevent anogenital diseases, *N Engl J Med* 356:1928, 2007.

Gardner HL, Dukes CD: *Haemophilus vaginalis* vaginitis: a newly defined specific infection previously classified non-specific vaginitis, *Am J Obstet Gynecol* 69:962, 1955.

Giuliano AR: Human papillomavirus vaccination in males, *Gynecol Oncol* 107:S24, 2007.

Gjestland T: The Oslo study of untreated syphilis; an epidemiologic investigation of the natural course of the syphilitic infection based upon a re-study of the Boeck-Bruusgaard material, *Acta Derm Venereol Suppl* 35(Suppl 34):3, 1955; Annex I-LVI.

Goldberg J: Studies on granuloma inguinale. V. Isolation of a bacterium resembling Donovania granulomatis from the faeces of a patient with granuloma inguinale, *Br J Vener Dis* 38:99, 1962.

Grulich AE, Kaldor JM: Trends in HIV incidence in homosexual men in developed countries, *Sex Health* 5:113, 2008.

Guan M: Frequency, causes, and new challenges of indeterminate results in Western blot confirmatory testing for antibodies to human immunodeficiency virus, *Clin Vaccine Immunol* 14:649, 2007; Epub Apr 4, 2007.

Gur I: The epidemiology of molluscum contagiosum in HIV-seropositive patients: a unique entity or insignificant finding? *Int J STD AIDS* 19:503, 2008.

Hall HI et al: Estimation of HIV incidence in the United States, *JAMA* 300:520, 2008.

Hammerschlag MR et al: Single dose of azithromycin for the treatment of genital chlamydial infections in adolescents, *J Pediatr Adolesc Gynecol* 122:961, 1993.

Havlir DV et al: Opportunities and challenges for HIV care in overlapping HIV and TB epidemics, *JAMA* 300:423, 2008.

Herring A, Richens J: Lymphogranuloma venereum, *Sex Transm Infect* 82:iv23, 2006.

Hill LV, Embil JA: Vaginitis: current microbiologic and clinical concepts, *CMAJ* 134:321, 1986.

Hobbs MM et al: *Trichomonas vaginalis* as a cause of urethritis in Malawian men, *Sex Transm Dis* 26:381, 1999.

Holguín A et al: Performance of three commercial viral load assays: Versant HIV-1 RNA bDNA v3.0, COBAS AmpliPrep/COBAS AmpliPrep/COBAS TaqMan HIV-1 Test, and Nuclisens HIV-1 EasyQ v1.2 Testing HIV-1 non-B subtypes and recombinant variants, *J Clin Microbiol* 46(9):2918, 2008.

Holland-Hall C: Sexually transmitted infections: screening, syndromes, and symptoms, *Prim Care* 33:433, 2006.

Horner P et al: Role of *Mycoplasma genitalium* and *Ureaplasma urealyticum* in acute and chronic nongonococcal urethritis, *Clin Infect Dis* 32:995, 2001.

Jin F et al: Risk factors for genital and anal warts in a prospective cohort of HIV-negative homosexual men: the HIM study, *Sex Transm Dis* 34:488, 2007.

Kahn RH et al: *Chlamydia trachomatis* and *Neisseria gonorrhoeae* prevalence and coinfection in adolescents entering selected US juvenile detention centers, 1997-2002, *Sex Transm Dis* 32:255, 2005.

Kerani RP et al: Rising rates of syphilis in the era of syphilis elimination, *Sex Transm Dis* 34:154, 2007. Comment in: *Sex Transm Dis* 34:162, 2007.

Kimberlin D: Herpes simplex virus, meningitis and encephalitis in neonates, *Herpes* 11:65A, 2004.

Klausner JD, Kohn R, Kent C: Etiology of clinical proctitis among men who have sex with men, *Clin Infect Dis* 38:300, 2004; Epub Dec 19, 2003.

Krieger JN et al: Diagnosis of trichomoniasis: comparison of conventional wet-mount examination with cytologic studies, cultures, and monoclonal antibody staining of direct specimens, *JAMA* 259:1223, 1988.

James AB, Simpson TY, Chamberlain WA: Chlamydia prevalence among college students: reproductive and public health implications, *Sex Transm Dis* 35:529, 2008.

Lafond RE, Lukehart SA: Biological basis for syphilis, *Clin Microbiol Rev* 19:29, 2006.

Laga M et al: Non-ulcerative sexually transmitted diseases as risk factors for HIV-1 transmission in women: results from a cohort study, *AIDS* 7:95, 1993.

Lau CY, Qureshi AK: Azithromycin versus doxycycline for genital chlamydial infections: a meta-analysis of randomized clinical trials, *Sex Transmit Dis* 29:497, 2002.

Lewis DA: Chancroid: clinical manifestations, diagnosis, and management, *Sex Transm Infect* 79:68, 2003.

Lima VD et al: Expanded access to highly active antiretroviral therapy: a potentially powerful strategy to curb the growth of the HIV epidemic, *J Infect Dis* 198:59, 2008.

Lister NA et al: Validation of Roche COBAS Amplicor assay for detection of *Chlamydia trachomatis* in rectal and pharyngeal specimens by an omp1 PCR assay, *J Clin Microbiol* 42:239, 2004.

Liu AY et al: Detection of pathogens causing genital ulcer disease by multiplex polymerase chain reaction, *Chin Med Sci J* 20:273, 2005.

Lossick JG: Epidemiology of urogenital trichomoniasis. In Honigberg BM, editor: *Trichomonads parasitic in humans*, New York, 1990, Springer-Verlag.

Lukehart SA et al: Macrolide resistance in *Treponema pallidum* in the United States and Ireland, *N Engl J Med* 351:154, 2004.

Lyerla R, Gouws E, Garcia-Calleja JM: The quality of sero-surveillance in low- and middle-income countries: status and trends through 2007, *Sex Transm Infect* 84:i85, 2008.

Lynch CM et al: Lymphogranuloma venereum presenting as a rectovaginal fistula, *Infect Dis Obstet Gynecol* 7:199, 1999.

Lyss SB et al: *Chlamydia trachomatis* among patients infected with and treated for *Neisseria gonorrhoeae* in sexually transmitted disease clinics in the United States, *Ann Intern Med* 139:178, 2003.

Mabey D, Peeling RW: Lymphogranuloma venereum, *Sex Transm Infect* 78:90, 2002.

Mackay IM et al: Detection and discrimination of herpes simplex viruses, *Haemophilus ducreyi, Treponema pallidum,* and *Calymmatobacterium (Klebsiella) granulomatis* from genital ulcers, *Clin Infect Dis* 42:1431, 2006.

Marrazzo JM, Handsfield HH, Whittington WL: Predicting chlamydial and gonococcal cervical infection: implications for management of cervicitis, *Obstet Gynecol* 100:579, 2002.

Marrazzo JM et al: Risk factors for cervicitis among women with bacterial vaginosis, *J Infect Dis* 193:617, 2006.

Martin DH et al: A controlled trial of a single dose of azithromycin for the treatment of chlamydial urethritis and cervicitis, The Azithromycin for Chlamydial Infections Study Group, *N Engl J Med* 327:921, 1992.

Masaro CL et al: Perceptions of sexual partner safety, *Sex Transm Dis* 35:566, 2008.

Mayeaux EJ Jr, Dunton C: Modern management of external genital warts, *J Low Genit Tract Dis* 12:185, 2008.

McLean CA, Stoner BP, Workowski KA: Treatment of lymphogranuloma venereum, *Clin Infect Dis* 44:S147, 2007.

Mehrany K et al: Disseminated gonococcemia, *Int J Dermatol* 42:208, 2003.

Merson MH et al: The history and challenge of HIV prevention, *Lancet* 372:475, 2008; Epub Aug 5, 2008.

Minkoff H et al: The relationship between cocaine use and human papillomavirus infections in HIV-seropositive and HIV-seronegative women, *Infect Dis Obstet Gynecol* 2008:587082, 2008.

Nilsen A et al: A double blind study of single dose azithromycin and doxycycline in the treatment of chlamydial urethritis in males, *Genitourin Med* 68:325, 1992.

O'Farrell N: Donovanosis, *Sex Transm Infect* 78:452, 2002.

Owen SM et al: Alternative algorithms for human immunodeficiency virus infection diagnosis using tests that are licensed in the United States, *J Clin Microbiol* 46:1588, 2008; Epub Mar 5, 2008.

Peipert JF et al: Bacterial vaginosis, race, and sexually transmitted infections: does race modify the association? *Sex Transm Dis* 35:363, 2008.

Powell K et al: Survival for patients with human immunodeficiency virus admitted to the intensive care unit continues to improve in the current era of highly active antiretroviral therapy, *Chest* 135(1):11-7, 2009.

Richards J et al: Healthcare seeking and sexual behavior among patients with symptomatic newly acquired genital herpes, *Sex Transm Dis* 35(12):1015, 2008.

Richens J: Donovanosis (granuloma inguinale), *Sex Transm Infect* 82:iv21, 2006.

Risser WL et al: Incidence of Fitz-Hugh-Curtis syndrome in adolescents who have pelvic inflammatory disease, *J Pediatr Adolesc Gynecol* 20:179, 2007.

Romanowski B et al: Serologic response to treatment of infectious syphilis, *Ann Intern Med* 114:1005, 1991.

Rosser BR et al: HIV risk and the Internet: results of the Men's INTernet Sex (MINTS) Study, *AIDS Behav* 13(4):746, 2009.

Satterwhite CL et al: Estimates of *Chlamydia trachomatis* infections among men: United States, *Sex Transm Dis* 35(11 Suppl):53, 2008.

Schlicht MJ et al: High prevalence of genital mycoplasmas among sexually active young adults with urethritis or cervicitis symptoms in La Crosse, Wisconsin, *J Clin Microbiol* 42:4636, 2004.

Schmid GP et al: Enhanced recovery of *Haemophilus ducreyi* from clinical specimens by incubation at 33° versus 35° C, *J Clin Microbiol* 33:3257, 1995.

Schmid G et al: Prevalence of metronidazole-resistant *Trichomonas vaginalis* in a gynecology clinic, *J Reprod Med* 46:545, 2001.

Schumacher CM, Ellen J, Rompalo AM: Changes in demographics and risk behaviors of persons with early syphilis depending on epidemic phase, *Sex Transm Dis* 35:190, 2008.

Schwebke JR, Burgess D: Trichomoniasis, *Clin Microbiol Rev* 17:794, 2004.

Schwebke JR, Morgan SC, Pinson GB: Validity of self-obtained vaginal specimens for diagnosis of trichomoniasis, *J Clin Microbiol* 35:1618, 1997.

Schwebke JR, Venglarik MF, Morgan SC: Delayed versus immediate bedside inoculation of culture media for diagnosis of vaginal trichomonosis, *J Clin Microbiol* 37:2369, 1999.

Shamos SJ et al: Evaluation of a testing-only "express" visit option to enhance efficiency in a busy STI clinic, *Sex Transm Dis* 35:336, 2008.

Shew ML et al: Association of condom use, sexual behaviors, and sexually transmitted infections with the duration of genital human papillomavirus infection among adolescent women, *Arch Pediatr Adolesc Med* 160:151, 2006.

Smith MA et al: The predicted impact of vaccination on human papillomavirus infections in Australia, *Int J Cancer* 123:1854, 2008.

Soper DE, Bump RC, Hurt WG: Bacterial vaginosis and trichomoniasis vaginitis are risk factors for cuff cellulitis after abdominal hysterectomy, *Am J Obstet Gynecol* 163:1016; discussion 1021, 1990.

Steen R: Eradicating chancroid, *Bull World Health Organ* 79:818, 2001.

Sturm AW et al: Clinical and microbiological evaluation of 46 episodes of genital ulceration, *Genitourin Med* 63:98, 1987.

Tang JW et al: Failure to confirm HIV infection in two end-stage HIV/AIDS patients using a popular commercial line immunoassay, *J Med Virol* 80:1515, 2008.

Tapsall J: Antibiotic resistance in *Neisseria gonorrhoeae* is diminishing available treatment options for gonorrhea: some possible remedies, *Expert Rev Anti Infect Ther* 4:619, 2006.

Tarr ME, Gilliam ML: Sexually transmitted infections in adolescent women, *Clin Obstet Gynecol* 51:306, 2008.

Torian LV et al: Risk factors for delayed initiation of medical care after diagnosis of human immunodeficiency virus, *Arch Intern Med* 168:1181, 2008.

Totten PA et al: Etiology of genital ulcer disease in Dakar, Senegal, and comparison of PCR and serologic assays for detection of *Haemophilus ducreyi*, *J Clin Microbiol* 38:268, 2000.

Wagner EK, Bloom DC: Experimental investigation of herpes simplex virus latency, *Clin Microbiol Rev* 10:419, 1997.

Wald A et al: Polymerase chain reaction for detection of herpes simplex virus (HSV) DNA on mucosal surfaces: comparison with HSV isolation in cell culture, *J Infect Dis* 188:1345, 2003.

Wasserheit JN: Epidemiological synergy: interrelationships between human immunodeficiency virus infection and other sexually transmitted diseases, *Sex Transm Dis* 19:61, 1992.

Weinstock H, Berman S, Cates W Jr: Sexually transmitted diseases among American youth: incidence and prevalence estimates, 2000, *Perspect Sex Reprod Health* 36:6, 2004.

White J, Ison C: Lymphogranuloma venereum: what does the clinician need to know? *Clin Med* 8:327, 2008.

Whitley RJ: Herpes simplex virus infections of women and their offspring: implications for a developed society, *Proc Natl Acad Sci U S A* 91:2441, 1994.

Winer RL et al: Condom use and the risk of genital human papillomavirus infection in young women, *N Engl J Med* 354:2645, 2006.

Wilson C: Recurrent vulvovaginitis candidiasis; an overview of traditional and alternative therapies, *Adv Nurse Pract* 13:24; quiz: 30. 2005.

Workowski KA, Berman SM: Centers for Disease Control and Prevention sexually transmitted diseases treatment guidelines, *Clin Infect Dis* 44:S73, 2007.

Wølner-Hanssen P et al: Clinical manifestations of vaginal trichomoniasis, *JAMA* 261:571, 1989.

World Health Organization: *Global prevalence and incidence of selected curable sexually transmitted diseases: overview and estimates, WHO/HIV_AIDS/2001.02*, New York, 2001, WHO.

World Health Organization: *Global strategy for the prevention and control of sexually transmitted infections: 2006-2015: breaking the chain of transmission*, New York, 2007, WHO.

Xu F et al: Trends in herpes simplex virus type 1 and type 2 seroprevalence in the United States, *JAMA* 296:964, 2006.

Zhang Y et al: Negative results of a rapid antibody test for HIV in a 16-month-old infant with AIDS, *Ann Clin Lab Sci* 38:293, 2008.

Zule WA et al: Methamphetamine use and risky sexual behaviors during heterosexual encounters, *Sex Transm Dis* 34:689, 2007.

Points to Remember

- Sexually transmitted diseases (STDs) are caused by a wide variety and diverse group of organisms, including bacteria, viruses, protozoan, epizoa, and fungi.
- Clinical manifestations and presentations of the diseases are varied; some may be described as exudative, but others produce nonexudative lesions.
- The epidemiology and pathogenesis of each of the infections may serve as useful tools in providing guidance with regard to specimen collection, transport, and handling as well as methods for identification.
- The method and site of collection, the quality of the clinical specimen, and the clinical presentation are all important factors to consider when diagnosing the etiologic agent of STDs.
- Molecular testing methods demonstrate increasing sensitivity of detection. Using noninvasive sampling such as voided urine, more patients and contacts will present for screening assays.

Learning Assessment Questions

1. Describe the signs and symptoms and the long-term effects of pelvic inflammatory disease (PID).
2. What are the different causes of vulvovaginitis and how are they distinguished clinically?
3. Why is it important to perform trace contacting of sexual partners of an affected individual?
4. Why is it important to screen for additional STDs besides that for which the patient is presenting?
5. Why is it necessary to perform confirmatory testing for several STDs?
6. What methods of prevention can be undertaken to reduce the overall spread of STDs?
7. What are the differences in clinical presentations and etiology of chancroids and chancres?
8. How has the advent of molecular testing advanced the detection of various STDs?
9. What are the distinguishing characteristics between gonococcal and nongonococcal urethritis?
10. What genotypes are utilized in the HPV vaccine and for what purpose?

Infections in Special Populations

Maribeth L. Flaws

- ■ MALIGNANCY
  Infections in Neutropenic Patients
  Infections in Cancer Patients
  Infections in Patients with Hodgkin Disease
- ■ ACQUIRED IMMUNE DEFICIENCY SYNDROME
- ■ COMPLEMENT DEFICIENCY
- ■ BURNS
- ■ ORGAN TRANSPLANTATION

- ■ POSTSPLENECTOMY
- ■ CYSTIC FIBROSIS
- ■ VENTILATOR-ASSOCIATED PNEUMONIA
- ■ DIABETES
- ■ AGING
- ■ PREGNANCY, THE FETUS, AND THE NEONATE

OBJECTIVES

After reading and studying this chapter, you should be able to:

1. Describe the various conditions that compromise the host's immune status.

2. Discuss the various infections that occur in each population.

3. Determine the risk factors associated with each condition.

4. Associate the various infectious agents that affect special populations with the conditions that predispose these patients to a particular infection.

Case in Point

A 32-year-old woman was vacationing out of town when she was involved in a serious car accident. She had extensive bruising on her abdominal region. She was sent by medevac helicopter to a trauma hospital, where an emergency splenectomy was performed. Surgery and postsurgery recovery were uneventful, and the patient was discharged and returned home. Two weeks later, the patient had flulike symptoms of fever, malaise, epigastric discomfort, shortness of breath, and nonproductive cough. She was rushed to the hospital nearest her home. The attending physician noted a large scar above the patient's abdomen and immediately ordered laboratory tests. She was admitted to the hospital, and laboratory tests suggested that the patient was significantly septic. Cultures of her blood and sputum grew *Streptococcus pneumoniae*.

Issues to Consider

After reading the patient's case history, consider the following:

- ■ Characteristics of the organism causing the infections
- ■ Risk factors for the acquisition of the organism

Key Terms

Acquired immune deficiency syndrome (AIDS)

Adaptive immune response

Bacterial interference

Cellular immune response

Complement

Congenital

Endogenous

Epstein-Barr virus (EBV)

Exogenous

Granulocytopenia

Hodgkin disease (HD)

Human immunodeficiency virus (HIV)

Humoral immune response

Immunocompetent

Immunocompromised

Immunosenescence

Immunosuppression

Innate immune response

Neutropenia

Opportunistic

Perinatal

Postsplenectomy

Septicemia

The presence of certain types of underlying disease can make people more susceptible to infection. On the other hand, people can be more susceptible to infection just because of their age (very young or very old) or because of pregnancy. All of these situations, whether normal (age) or abnormal (underlying disease), have in common some

TABLE 39-1 Opportunistic Pathogens Most Often Identified in the Compromised Host

Bacteria	*Staphylococcus aureus*
	Streptococcus pneumoniae
	Pseudomonas aeruginosa
	Escherichia coli
	Klebsiella pneumoniae
	Salmonella spp.
	Serratia spp.
	Burkholderia spp.
	Haemophilus influenzae
	Legionella pneumophila
	Aeromonas hydrophila
	Nocardia spp.
	Listeria monocytogenes
	Mycobacterium tuberculosis
	Mycobacterium avium
	Murine vibrios (halophilic)
Parasites	*Toxoplasma gondii*
	Strongyloides stercoralis
	Cryptosporidium
	Microsporidia
Fungi	*Candida* spp.
	Aspergillus spp.
	Zygomycetes
	Pneumocystis jiroveci (carinii)
	Cryptococcus neoformans
	Histoplasma capsulatum
	Fusarium
Viruses	Herpes simplex virus
	Varicella-zoster virus
	Cytomegalovirus
	Epstein-Barr virus
	Hepatitis B virus
	Adenovirus
	Papovaviruses
	Enteroviruses
	Influenza virus

form of **immunosuppression** that makes the host more susceptible to infections. The organisms found in these situations are, for the most part, **opportunistic** organisms. Opportunistic organisms are ones that typically do not cause disease in an **immunocompetent** host. Bacteria, fungi, parasites, and viruses can all cause opportunistic infections. Table 39-1 lists the major organisms that are isolated from immunocompromised hosts.

Many of the organisms listed in Table 39-1 are very common in the environment or are members of the host normal microbiota. Thus opportunistic infections can have an **endogenous** or **exogenous** source. An endogenous infection occurs when an indigenous member of the host microbiota invades, a body site where it is not normally found and causes disease; for example, viridans streptococci in the mouth. This organism can gain access to the bloodstream and cause endocarditis when the patient has poor dental hygiene or when a dental procedure is performed on the mouth that disrupts the normal mucous-membrane barrier. In an exogenous infection, an organism present in the environment enters the body through inhalation, ingestion or traumatic inoculation and causes disease; for example, fungal conidia present in the soil are inhaled and may cause a respiratory tract infection.

The normal host immune response, whether it is the nonspecific barriers to infection, such as intact skin and mucus membranes, the **innate immune response** of which macrophages and neutrophils are a major part, or the **adaptive immune response** in which B and T lymphocytes are active, are usually able to eliminate most of the organisms. When one or more parts of the immune response are deficient, however, organisms that are normally cleared start to proliferate and cause disease (see immune response, Chapter 2).

The term **immunocompromised** is used to describe patients who have serious disease that affects the immune system, making them highly predisposed to infections by a variety of opportunistic bacterial, fungal, parasitic, and viral pathogens. The number of immunocompromised patients has increased steadily during the past 30 years, reflecting increased use of immunosuppressive therapy, instrumentation, and organ transplantation. Unfortunately, the potential gain in years of useful life for many patients through successful management and treatment of diseases is offset by serious adverse effects on the immune system. As a result, infection, rather than the primary illness, becomes the leading cause of death in immunocompromised patients.

The primary predisposing factor in these patient populations is the presence of underlying disease that affects host defense mechanisms. Examples of compromised defense mechanisms include the following:
- Leukocyte number or functions, as in aplastic anemia and leukemia
- Humoral and cell-mediated immune functions, as in B-cell and T-cell abnormalities
- Reticuloendothelial system function, as in splenectomized patients

Other underlying disease states are burns, diabetes mellitus, renal failure, and autoimmune diseases. Table 39-2 summarizes the various conditions that compromise the host's immune status and the pathogens usually encountered in infections associated with them.

Immunosuppression may also predispose patients to severe infections. Infection with the **human immunodeficiency virus (HIV)** and immunosuppressive therapy such as chemotherapy and radiation, particularly in organ transplant patients, frequently leads to an immunocompromised condition.

Secondary factors that facilitate infection include the use of invasive devices, such as indwelling intravenous catheters, which breach the usual skin and mucosal protective barriers and introduce organisms into the bloodstream. One or a combination of any of these underlying conditions leaves a person less able to cope with infections.

MALIGNANCY

A variety of deficiencies in the **humoral** (involving B cells and antibodies) and **cellular** (involving T cells) **immune responses** occur in patients with malignancy. Deficiencies can be caused directly by the tumor cells, either because of the cell type that has become malignant (e.g., leukemias and lymphomas, which are tumors of the immune system that are more associated

TABLE 39-2 Organisms Associated with Immunocompromised Patients

Immune Status	Examples of Conditions	Commonly Encountered Pathogen(s)
↓Leukocyte number or function	Myelocytic leukemia Chronic granulomatous disease Granulocytopenia Acidosis Burns	*Staphylococcus* spp. *Serratia* spp. *Pseudomonas* spp. *Candida* spp. *Aspergillus* spp. *Nocardia* spp. *Legionella* spp. *Mycobacterium* spp.
↓Humoral immune response and complement deficits	Lymphocytic leukemia Multiple myeloma Nephrosis Antimetabolite therapy Hypogammaglobulinemia	*Streptococcus pneumoniae* *Haemophilus influenzae* *Streptococcus pyogenes* *Pseudomonas* spp. *Pneumocystis jiroveci* Enteroviruses *Staphylococcus aureus*
↓Cellular immune response	Hodgkin disease Steroid therapy Uremia Antimetabolite therapy Acquired immune deficiency syndrome (AIDS) Malnutrition	*Mycobacterium* spp. *Candida* spp. *Coccidioides immitis* *Histoplasma capsulatum* *Blastomyces dermatitidis* *P. jiroveci* *Cryptococcus neoformans* *Cryptosporidium* Herpes viruses Adenoviruses Cytomegalovirus *Toxoplasma gondii* *Legionella* spp. *Listeria monocytogenes*
↓Reticuloendothelial system function	Splenectomy Chronic hemolysis	*Streptococcus pneumoniae* *Salmonella* spp. *L. monocytogenes*

Modified from Drew WL: Infections in the immunocompromised patient. In Ryan KJ, Ray CG, editors: *Sherris medical microbiology: an introduction to infectious diseases*, ed 4, New York, 2004, McGraw-Hill.

with defects in the host immune response than tumors of other cell types), or because of immunosuppressive molecules (cytokines) secreted by the tumor cells. In addition, cytotoxic drugs administered to cancer patients to kill the tumor cells contribute substantially to the breakdown of mucosal barriers and decrease cell-mediated immune (CMI) reactivity in these patients, further suppressing their immune response.

Granulocytopenia, or a reduction in granulocytes to 500 cells/mm³, is commonly demonstrated in patients with hematologic malignancies and in those receiving chemotherapy. Once the granulocyte count drops below 500 to 1000 cells/mm³, the risk of infection increases steadily with the degree and duration of immunosuppression. In patients with a neutrophil count below 500 cells/mm³, the mortality rate may be as high as 60%. The fatality rate among patients whose neutrophil count is lower than 100 cells/mm³ during the first week of infection may be as high as 80%.

In addition to the decrease in the number of neutrophils, inadequate neutrophil function, including the inability to migrate to sites of inflammation, impaired phagocytosis, and reduced killing of ingested organisms, predisposes patients suffering from chronic leukemia and **Hodgkin disease (HD)** to infections. Most of these infections are caused by bacteria of endogenous origin, that is, gastrointestinal (GI) tract, mucosal, or cutaneous flora. Fungi are also likely to invade the granulocytopenic host.

Infections in Neutropenic Patients

Septicemia is most likely to occur in patients with **neutropenia** because neutrophils play an important role in containing infections to the local site. *Escherichia coli, Klebsiella pneumoniae,* and *Pseudomonas aeruginosa* account for most of the gram-negative bacilli infections. *Staphylococcus aureus,* coagulase-negative *Staphylococcus,* and *Enterococcus* are the gram-positive organisms most commonly involved in sepsis. Emerging pathogens that cause disease in the neutropenic patient include the gram-negatives *Stenotrophomonas, Legionella, Burkholderia cepacia, Capnocytophaga,* and *Methylobacterium* and the gram-positive viridans streptococci.

Pneumonia, especially when caused by gram-negative bacilli, is a major problem for the neutropenic patient. Because such a patient cannot mount an adequate immune response, pulmonary infection may spread rapidly and extensively. Infections with these organisms are particularly serious because they cause extensive necrosis and have a high fatality rate. Because of the lack of an inflammatory response to infection, neutropenic patients fail to develop the characteristic symptoms of pneumonia and may remain undiagnosed until after the infection has disseminated.

Infections in Cancer Patients

Factors responsible for the high incidence of infections among cancer patients vary with the underlying malignancy. For example, tumors that outgrow their blood supply may become necrotic and infected. A GI tumor may ulcerate, providing a focus for invasion by enteric pathogens. Tumors may also obstruct the drainage of the tracheobronchial tree or the urinary tract, permitting infection distal to the obstruction to become established.

Septicemia accounts for nearly 50% of the fatal infections in patients with genitourinary and GI tumors and for less than 10% in patients with lung cancer. Pneumonia accounts for 75% of fatal infections in patients with cancer of the head, neck, and lungs and for less than 40% in patients with genitourinary and other tumors. Aspiration of oral secretions probably accounts for the pneumonia in patients in this last group, whereas pneumonia in those with solid tumors is usually a consequence of primary or metastatic tumor invasion of the lung.

Skin infections are also common in cancer patients for several reasons. Cancer patients often develop decubitus ulcers because they are constantly bedridden. These patients also develop catheter-associated infections, cellulitis, and local necrosis involving the extremities, sometimes due to venipunctures, intravenous lines, and other procedures.

Patients with hematologic malignancies and those who have undergone surgery for tumors involving the head and spine may suffer from central nervous system (CNS) infections. In these patients, meningitis accounts for 75% of infections, 30% of which are caused by *Cryptococcus neoformans*. Gram-negative bacilli are responsible for another 40%. Fungal agents such as *Aspergillus* spp. and *Mucor* spp. are commonly associated with brain abscesses that occur in patients with leukemia. Oropharyngeal candidiasis occurs in about 5% of cancer patients. Superficial GI candidiasis is also found in patients with acute leukemia and lymphoma. Although candidiasis can involve any portion of the GI tract, it is found most often in the esophagus and stomach. Other areas sometimes affected are the kidneys, liver, spleen, and lungs.

Other types of infections that occur in cancer patients include those caused by viral and parasitic agents. The most serious viral infections occurring in cancer patients are caused by members of the herpesvirus group. Characteristically these viruses infect young patients, resulting in lifelong immunity; such immunity contributes toward maintaining latent infections that occur in immunocompetent people. The lack of cellular immunity, in particular, in immunosuppressed cancer patients results in the reactivation of latent virus and the potential for serious disseminated disease.

Herpes zoster or shingles occurs upon reactivation of latent varicella-zoster virus (VZV). It is seen in 3% to 15% of patients with lymphoma, myeloma, and chronic lymphocytic leukemia. Chemotherapy has been shown to cause a twofold increase in the frequency of zoster infection. VZV disseminates in 20% to 40% of cancer patients. Dissemination of VZV to the lungs, liver, pancreas, adrenals, and CNS occurs in nearly 30% of children undergoing chemotherapy. The mortality rate from VZV is about 5%, and death is usually associated with pneumonitis.

Herpes simplex infections of the lip may result in extensive cellulitis as a result of superinfection with mixed bacterial and fungal organisms (especially *Candida* spp. and gram-negative bacilli) in cancer patients.

Children with cancer are more susceptible to cytomegalovirus (CMV) infection than are adults. The most common manifestation is pneumonia, which may be unilateral or bilateral and is usually accompanied by a more severe bacterial or fungal infection. Dissemination of CMV affects the lungs, kidneys, lymph nodes, heart, adrenals, spleen, pancreas, and bone marrow. Death sometimes occurs from myocarditis, renal failure, or adrenal insufficiency.

Pneumocystis jiroveci (carinii) and *Toxoplasma gondii* are other agents that affect patients with malignancy. Infections with either organism may represent reactivation or primary exposure. *P. jiroveci* accounts for as many as 45% of cases of interstitial pneumonia in cancer patients. Similarly, *T. gondii,* an obligate intracellular parasite, causes pneumonia, chorioretinitis, and a mononucleosis-like infection. It is seen most commonly in HD, but also occurs in patients with lymphoma and leukemia.

Strongyloides stercoralis infections have been reported in patients with chronic lymphocytic leukemia and lymphoma. Serious manifestations caused by *Strongyloides* infection may occur in patients receiving adrenal corticosteroids or antitumor therapy. Ulceration may result when the rhabditiform larvae penetrate the GI tract. Larval migration to the lungs may cause a pulmonary infiltrate. Interestingly, in many cases, the *Strongyloides* infection is not symptomatic, nor is it diagnosed, until the patient becomes immunosuppressed.

Infections in Patients with Hodgkin Disease

Historically HD has been associated with impairment of CMI. Patients with HD are especially susceptible to infections caused by facultative intracellular parasites, such as *Mycobacterium tuberculosis, Listeria monocytogenes,* and *C. neoformans.* These intracellular organisms are resistant to bactericidal agents within the phagocytic cell and are able to multiply within the cells.

As the number of circulating lymphocytes decreases, patients with HD who are receiving chemotherapy become more susceptible to infections. Chemotherapy inhibits inflammation, reduces capillary permeability, and decreases cellular exudation. It also interferes with the diapedesis of leukocytes, inhibits antibody production, and impairs reticuloendothelial function.

ACQUIRED IMMUNE DEFICIENCY SYNDROME

Acquired immune deficiency syndrome (AIDS) is caused by HIV, a virus that infects and destroys CD4$^+$ helper T cells. The helper T cells are critical for stimulating B cells to produce antibody, cytotoxic T cells to lyse target cells, and macrophages to phagocytize and destroy ingested organisms. Because of the integral role for this cell type in almost every arm of the immune response, the lack of this cell causes a profound immunosuppression that seriously undermines the body's ability to defend itself from infection and disease. HIV, if not treated, can cause an infected person to be vulnerable to many different opportunistic infections. As a result of its importance, HIV/AIDS is discussed extensively in Chapter 29.

COMPLEMENT DEFICIENCY

The **complement** system is a series of proteins that, when activated, increase the activation and function of many different cells involved in the immune response. Complement is particularly important in the opsonization or coating of microorganisms that enhances the phagocytosis of the organism by the phagocytic cell such as a neutrophil or macrophage. Complement is also directly lytic for microorganisms, helping to kill them directly.

A complement deficiency can be inherited or acquired and typically involves a lack of one particular protein of the system. Disorders involving deficiencies of a complement system protein include increased susceptibility to infections such as pneumonia or meningitis caused by *Streptococcus pneumoniae* or *Neisseria meningitidis* or development of autoimmune disease, such as systemic lupus erythematosus.

Patients with C3 deficiency are particularly susceptible to sepsis with pyogenic (pus-forming) bacteria such as *S. aureus* or *Streptococcus pyogenes*. Deficiency in the terminal components of the complement cascade C56789 results in an inability to lyse gram-negative bacteria, and patients are especially susceptible to developing recurrent bacteremia caused by *N. meningitidis* or *N. gonorrhoeae*. Deficiency of the alternative complement pathway leads to serious *S. pneumoniae* infections, including meningitis.

BURNS

Each year about 500,000 Americans seek medical attention for burns; about 40,000 require hospitalization, and 4000 die annually. About one third of burn patients are children younger than 1 year of age. Most deaths occur at the scene of the fire or shortly thereafter. Infection is a major cause of morbidity and mortality in those who survive and seek medical care. The risk of infection in a burn patient is directly proportional to the extent of the burn and reflects the combined effect of the impairment of all aspects of the host defense system. As a result of systemic immunologic impairment, infection in sites other than the burn wound itself remains the most common cause of death of burn patients. Pneumonia is the most common infection seen in burn patients; burn wound infections have decreased as a result of vigilant wound care. The balance between host defense capacity and invasiveness of the microorganism in burn patients provides the optimal example of the susceptibility to infection in an immunocompromised patient.

In normal patients, **bacterial interference** (potential pathogens being inhibited by the nonpathogenic resident microbiota) plays a significant role in controlling cutaneous colonization of the skin. In burn patients, anatomic barriers have been breached. The normal skin flora are destroyed or removed by desquamation. The denatured protein of the burn eschar and the avascularity of the tissue provide an excellent environment for microbial growth.

The immune defense mechanisms in burn patients, both humoral and cell-mediated defenses, are suppressed. Immunoglobulins, especially IgG, are depressed. Fibronectin levels are also reduced. Fibronectin, a dimeric α-glycoprotein found in plasma and the extracellular matrix of most tissues, is necessary for normal reticuloendothelial cell function and opsonizes *S. aureus*. A decrease in fibronectin levels precedes sepsis. The risk of fungal infections is increased with wound maceration, acidosis, lack of competitive bacterial pressure, and antibiotic therapy. Methicillin-resistant *S. aureus, Enterococcus, P. aeruginosa, Klebsiella, Acinetobacter, Serratia, Candida, Aspergillus,* and *Mucor* spp., as well as herpes simplex virus, are major causes of infections in burn patients.

ORGAN TRANSPLANTATION

The transplantation of solid organs as well as hematopoietic stem cells from bone marrow, peripheral blood, or umbilical cord blood has increased greatly over the past few years, with solid organ transplants in particular increasing 20% when the period 1998 to 2002 is compared to 1993 to 1997. In order to maintain the viability of the graft, immunosuppressive agents are given to organ transplant recipients to prevent immune-mediated destruction or rejection of the graft. Unfortunately, the immunosuppression is not limited to inhibiting the immune cells that recognize the engrafted organ. All cells of the immune system will be adversely affected by these drugs, rendering the patient unable to respond to infection.

Organ transplant patients may develop specific types of infections at certain intervals after transplantation occurs. During the first month after transplantation, postoperative bacterial infections are most common. Approximately 1 to 6 months after transplantation, opportunistic infections caused by CMV, *M. tuberculosis, L. monocytogenes, Nocardia* and *Aspergillus* spp., *P. jiroveci (carinii),* **Epstein-Barr virus (EBV),** varicella-zoster virus, parvovirus B19, and polyomaviruses BK and JC are most likely to be reported.

Immunosuppressive therapy reactivates latent CMV infection, which is probably the most significant cause of mortality and morbidity among transplant patients; 60% to 90% of renal transplant patients develop CMV 1 to 4 months after transplantation.

Infection caused by EBV in transplant patients has also increased during recent years. EBV has been recognized as a causative agent of B-cell lymphoma, the pathogenesis of which is related to immunosuppressive therapy. Furthermore, in patients who acquire primary EBV infection after transplantation, EBV-associated lymphoproliferative disease is likely to occur. This has become a major concern because primary EBV infection develops most commonly in children; hence children who are transplant recipients are at greatest risk for EBV-associated lymphoproliferative disease. Central nervous system infections caused by *L. monocytogenes, C. neoformans, T. gondii,* and *Aspergillus* spp. also occur in these patients.

Bone marrow transplant patients are susceptible to similar infections, especially by fungal agents. *Aspergillus* spp. and respiratory viruses are possibly inhaled from the environment, whereas *Pseudomonas* and *Legionella* spp. can be acquired from water sources.

Infections that occur more than 6 months after transplantation are usually associated with community-acquired organisms, such as viral influenza, secondary bacterial pneumonia, food-borne illnesses (acquired during travel to locations with poor sanitary conditions), and mycotic infections from specific geographic areas that may result in dissemination. Precautions about travel to underdeveloped areas and unfamiliar places are given to transplant patients to help them avoid unnecessary exposure to community-acquired infections.

POSTSPLENECTOMY

The major risk following splenectomy is overwhelming bacterial infection or **postsplenectomy** sepsis, resulting from the body's decreased ability to clear bacteria from the bloodstream and decreased levels of IgM in blood plasma. The loss of splenic function puts patients at risk of infection with encapsulated organisms such as *S. pneumoniae, Haemophilus influenzae,* and *N. meningitidis,* and also with the protozoans *Plasmodium* and *Babesia.* The greatest risk of infection is in children, in patients with malignant disease, and during the 2 years after splenectomy. Patients must be aware that they are at increased risk of infection and should therefore seek medical advice at the onset of any fever.

CYSTIC FIBROSIS

Cystic fibrosis (CF) is an autosomal recessive disorder caused by a mutation in the cystic fibrosis transmembrane conductance regulator (CFTR), which codes for a transmembrane protein that controls the movement of chloride anions across the cell membrane of cells, especially in the exocrine glands. Normally cyclic adenosine monophosphate (cAMP) regulates the transport of chloride across this protein. The lack of CFTR function results in a decrease in the amount of chloride secretion and the increased reabsorption of sodium and water by the epithelial cells. The lack of water in the mucus causes the mucus to be very thick and sticky. The thickness of the secretions adversely affects the function of the respiratory and gastrointestinal tracts, sweat glands, and other exocrine glands.

The thick secretions in the lung in particular make the patient highly susceptible to chronic infections. The organism isolated most frequently from CF patients and the most prob-

lematic is *P. aeruginosa.* In CF patients, *P. aeruginosa* is more likely to be resistant to antimicrobial agents and forms a biofilm in a polysaccharide matrix that makes it harder for antimicrobial agents to gain access to the organism. Newer research shows that the production of the polysaccharide and the resistance to antimicrobial agents are linked genetically.

Other organisms that are isolated frequently from the lungs of CF patients include *S. aureus, H. influenzae,* and *B. cepacia. B. cepacia* is particularly problematic because infection with *B. cepacia* is associated with higher mortalities. Patients may lose their eligibility for a lung transplant because of adverse outcomes after transplantation when the patient is infected with *B. cepacia* prior to transplantation.

VENTILATOR-ASSOCIATED PNEUMONIA

Ventilator-associated pneumonia (VAP) is a nosocomial pneumonia that occurs in patients who have been on a mechanical respirator for more than 48 hours. In 2002, the Centers for Disease Control and Prevention's National Nosocomial Infection Surveillance System reported that the rate of VAP was 2.2 per thousand ventilator days in a pediatric intensive care unit (ICU) and 14.7 per thousand ventilator days in a trauma ICU. Being on a mechanical ventilator increases the risk of developing nosocomial pneumonia by as much as 21 times as compared with the development of pneumonia while not on a ventilator.

Signs of VAP include fever, leukocytosis greater than 12×10^9/mL, and appearance of new or progressive pulmonary infiltrates or purulent tracheobronchial secretions. The diagnosis of VAP can be made using a quantitative culture of bronchoalveolar lavage (BAL) fluid or fluid collected using a protected specimen brush. Detection of 10^3 colony-forming units (CFU)/mL or greater may be considered diagnostic. Blood cultures (two sets) may also be helpful in determining the cause of the VAP. There are multiple strategies in place for diagnosing VAP from the collection of different types of respiratory tract samples (invasive versus noninvasive), to using non- or semiquantitative cultures, to using a clinical score system. Studies comparing various methods have not yet revealed the optimal diagnostic strategy.

Organisms associated with VAP include *S. pneumoniae, H. influenzae, S. aureus, P. aeruginosa, Klebsiella, Enterobacter, Serratia, Acinetobacter, Stenotrophomonas,* and *B. cepacia.*

DIABETES

In diabetes, patients either have insufficient insulin produced by the pancreas (type I) or insulin resistance of cells (type II), causing glucose not to enter cells to be utilized for energy. Because cells do not use up the glucose, body fluids contain increased levels of glucose. High levels of glucose lead to ketoacidosis, where ketones and organic acids accumulate in the blood, lowering the pH (called *acidemia*). The high levels of glucose are immunosuppressive, decreasing neutrophil function as well as cell-mediated immunity. The immune system suppression can be reversed by decreasing the blood glucose levels and increasing the pH.

Infections that are more common in diabetic patients include:

- Pneumonia
- Pyelonephritis
- Soft tissue infections (especially of the extremities, most often caused by *S. pyogenes* and *S. aureus*)
- Mucocutaneous *Candida* infections

Infections that are almost exclusively seen in diabetic patients include:

- Invasive otitis externa caused primarily by *P. aeruginosa*
- Rhinocerebral mucormycosis caused by *Rhizopus, Mucor,* and *Absidia* spp.
- Emphysematous pyelonephritis (formation of gas in the kidney)

AGING

Diverse changes in immune function occur with normal aging. Age-induced alterations of the immune system are often more qualitative (i.e., involving lymphocytic function) than quantitative (i.e., involving cell number or immunoglobulin levels). **Immunosenescence,** in which naïve T cells are no longer available to be stimulated by antigen, leads to the decline of the immune response over time. In addition, older adults may be immunosuppressed because they have undiagnosed underlying disease, are on immunosuppressive medications for diagnosed disease, or are malnourished. Further, good personal hygiene deteriorates and many older adults may be in group housing conditions, both of which increase the exposure of the patient to infectious microorganisms.

Infections, autoimmune disease, and malignancy increase among elderly patients as a result of immunologic decline. Organ function declines with age, and the presence of underlying disease, especially malignancy and diabetes, which are found more commonly in older adults, increases the susceptibility of the older adult to infection. Infections in older adults are most frequently in the respiratory (pneumonia and aspiration pneumonia) or urinary tracts (especially catheter- and enlarged prostate–related infections), soft tissues (infection of pressure ulcers), abdominal cavity, or endocardium. Bacteremia of unknown source may also occur.

The organisms most often isolated as pathogens in older adults are *S. pneumoniae* and enteric gram-negative bacilli, *E. coli* in particular. Tuberculosis also increases in incidence with age. Not only are older adults more likely to have serious infections than younger adults, but the older adults are more likely to die from those infections. The mortality of pneumonia is 3 times higher in older adults than in younger patients. Older adults have a 5 to 10 times higher mortality rate due to pyelonephritis and a 10 times higher rate of mortality due to tuberculosis than younger patients.

PREGNANCY, THE FETUS, AND THE NEONATE

Infections in pregnant women are of concern not just to the patient, but to her fetus. Infections can cause preterm birth, spontaneous abortion, birth defects, and developmental disabilities in the fetus as well as lead to increased morbidity and mortality for the woman. Pregnant women are naturally immunosuppressed so that the antigenically different fetus is not rejected, leaving the woman more susceptible to infection and to more serious disease. The immune system in the fetus and neonate is immature, rendering them immunosuppressed as well.

The most common infection in pregnant women is urinary tract infections, most often caused by *E. coli* and other gram-negative bacilli. Vaginal yeast infections caused by *Candida* spp. are more common in pregnancy. Pregnant women with bacterial vaginosis are more likely to have premature rupture of the membranes or premature delivery, and the baby may then have a low birth weight because of the premature delivery.

Organisms associated with causing **congenital** (acquired in utero when the organism infecting the woman crosses the placenta to infect the fetus) infections are listed here. Congenital infections with these organisms can lead to developmental problems and even death:

- *Toxoplasma gondii*
- Rubella virus
- Cytomegalovirus
- Herpes simplex virus
- Varicella-zoster virus
- HIV
- Parvovirus B19
- Hepatitis B virus
- *Treponema pallidum*
- *Streptococcus agalactiae*
- *Listeria monocytogenes*

Other organisms can be transmitted during labor and delivery (the **perinatal** period) and are also associated with adverse outcomes for the baby. Most of the organisms listed here are sexually transmitted diseases that are acquired as the baby moves through the infected birth canal:

- *Neisseria gonorrhoeae*
- *Chlamydia trachomatis*
- *Streptococcus agalactiae*
- *Escherichia coli*
- Human papillomavirus
- Cytomegalovirus
- Herpes simplex virus

BIBLIOGRAPHY

Chaparro C et al: Infection with *Burkholderia cepacia* in cystic fibrosis, *Am J Respir Crit Care Med* 163:43, 2001.

Chastre J et al: Evaluation of bronchoscopic techniques for the diagnosis of nosocomial pneumonia, *Am J Respir Crit Care Med* 152:231, 1995.

Chastre J et al: Prospective evaluation of the protected specimen brush for the diagnosis of pulmonary infections in ventilated patients, *Am Rev Respir Dis* 130:924, 1984.

Church D et al: Burn wound infections, *Clin Microbiol Rev* 19:403, 2006.

Donowitz GR et al: Infections in the neutropenic patient—new views of an old problem, *Hematology* 1:113, 2001.

Drew WL: Infections in the immunocompromised patient. In Sherris J, editor: *Medical microbiology*, ed 4, Ohio, 2004, McGraw-Hill.

Edwards-Jones V, Greenwood JE: What's new in burn microbiology? James Laing Memorial Prize Essay 2000, *Burns* 29:15, 2003.

Erice A et al: Ganciclovir treatment of cytomegalovirus disease in transplant recipients and other immunocompromised hosts, *JAMA* 257:3082, 1987.

Fishman JA: Infection in solid-organ transplant recipients, *N Engl J Med* 357:2601, 2007.

Froland S: Bacterial infections in the compromised host, *Scand J Infect Dis Suppl* 43:7, 1984.

Hibberd P, Rubin RH: Infections in transplant patients and the role of the microbiology laboratory, *Clin Microbiol Newsl* 13:161, 1991.

Jacobs P: The immunocompromised host, *South Am Med J* 71:371, 1987.

Karasek M editor: *Aging and age-related diseases: The basics*, 2006, Nova Science.

Klastersky J, Aoun M: Opportunistic infections in patients with cancer, *Ann Oncol* 15:329, 2004.

Koenig SM, Truwit JD: Ventilator-associated pneumonia: diagnosis, treatment and prevention, *Clin Micro Rev* 19:637, 2006.

Kotton CN: Donor-derived infections in transplant patients, *Clin Micro Newsletter* 31:63, 2009.

Lipschitz DA et al: Influence of aging and protein deficiency on neutrophil function, *J Gerontol* 41:690, 1986.

Martins PNA et al: Age and immune response in organ transplantation, *Transplantation* 79:127, 2005.

Mayhall CG: Ventilator-associated pneumonia or not? Contemporary diagnosis, *Emerg Inf Dis* 7:200, 2001.

Mehta S, Fantry L: Gastrointestinal infections in the immunocompromised host, *Curr Opin Gastroenterol* 21:39, 2005.

Meunier F: Prevention of mycoses in immunocompromised patients, *Rev Infect Dis* 9:408, 1987.

Munster AM: Immunologic response of trauma and burns: an overview, *Am J Med* 77:142, 1984.

Murray C, Hospenthal DR: Burn wound infections, Medscape Emedicine. Available at: www.emedicine.medscape.com/article/213595-overview. Accessed May 19, 2009.

Okabayashi T, Hanazaki K: Overwhelming postsplenectomy infection syndrome in adults—a clinically preventable disease, *World J Gastroenterol* 14:176, 2008.

O'Toole GA: Microbiology: a resistance switch, *Nature* 416:695, 2002.

Powers DC et al: Immune function in the elderly, *Postgrad Med* 81:335, 1987.

Pruitt BA, McManus AT: The changing epidemiology of infection in burn patients, *World J Surg* 16:57, 2005.

Rasmussen SA, Hayes EB: Public health approach to emerging infections among pregnant women, *Am J Public Health* 95:1942, 2005.

Rogers TR: Investigation of infection in immunocompromised patients [editorial], *Br J Haematol* 61:195, 1985.

Rouse BT, Horohov DW: Immunosuppression in viral infections, *Rev Infect Dis* 8:850, 1986.

Schaberg DS, Norwood JM: Case study: infections in diabetes mellitus, *Diabetes Spectrum*, 15:37-40, 2002.

Sharma GD: Cystic fibrosis, Medscape Emedicine. Available at: www.emedicine.medscape.com/article/1001602-overview. Accessed May 20, 2009.

Sheagren JM: Treatment of skin and skin structure infections in the patient at risk, *Am J Med* 76:180, 1984.

Singh N, Paterson DL: Aspergillus infections in transplant recipients, *Clin Micro Rev* 18:44-69, 2005.

Skinhoj P: Herpesvirus infection in the immunocompromised patient, *Scand J Infect Dis Suppl* 47:121, 1985.

Sutton RNP et al: Virus infections in immunocompromised patients: their importance and their management, *J R Soc Med* 78:100, 1985.

Vesosky B, Turner J: The influence of age on immunity to infection with *Mycobacterium tuberculosis*, *Immunol Rev* 205:229, 2005.

Viscoli C, Varnier O, Machetti M: Infections in patients with febrile neutropenia: epidemiology, microbiology, and risk stratification, *Clin Infect Dis* 40(suppl 4):240, 2005.

Weiner LP, Fleming JO: Viral infections of the nervous system, *J Neurosurg* 61:207, 1984.

Wolfson JS et al: Dermatologic manifestations of infections in immunocompromised patients, *Medicine (Baltimore)* 64:115, 1985.

Points to Remember

- Immunocompromised patients are susceptible to bacterial, fungal, and viral infections that healthy immune systems usually conquer.
- Defects in the immune system can be either inherited or acquired.
- Successful treatment of infections in the compromised patient depends on recognition of the deficit, early diagnosis, and prompt intervention.

Learning Assessment Questions

1. What is the most likely sequence of events that led to the febrile condition of the patient in the opening case study?

2. What is the likely connection between infections and malignancy?

3. What other hematologic conditions may predispose patients to various infections?

4. What organisms are of concern in pregnant women?

5. Why are infections and malignancy common among the elderly?

6. Which organisms are more likely to cause infections in patients with cystic fibrosis and VAP?

Zoonotic Diseases

Carl Brinkley

OBJECTIVES

After reading and studying this chapter, you should be able to:

1. Associate the animal hosts or vectors associated with the following infections:
  ■ Anthrax
  ■ Plague
  ■ Erysipeloid
  ■ Leptospirosis
  ■ Tularemia
  ■ Lyme borreliosis

2. Correlate the pathogen (genus and species) that causes the diseases listed below. Discuss the epidemiology and describe the clinical manifestations associated with each disease condition.
  ■ Anthrax
  ■ Plague
  ■ Erysipeloid
  ■ Leptospirosis
  ■ Tularemia
  ■ Lyme borreliosis

3. For the following human rickettsial diseases, link the causative agent and compare the mode of transmission to humans:
  ■ Rocky Mountain spotted fever
  ■ Rickettsialpox
  ■ Murine typhus
  ■ Louse-borne typhus

4. Compare and contrast infections caused by *Ehrlichia* versus *Anaplasma*.

5. Discuss the three factors that define zoonotic infections as a growing medical problem.

6. Discuss the impact of emerging zoonotic pathogens in the public health community.

Case in Point

A 16-year-old female resident of western Colorado experienced pain in the left axilla and arm with numbness in the arm. One or two days later she developed chills and fever, and she had multiple episodes of vomiting. She went to the emergency department of a local hospital. Examination there found that she had a normal temperature, elevated pulse (100 beats/minute), normal blood pressure, and a normal chest radiograph. She reported falling from a trampoline 4 days earlier and was diagnosed as having a possible brachial plexus injury related to this incident. She was treated with analgesics and given an appointment with a neurologist. Two days after she was seen in the emergency department, she was found semiconscious at home and was taken to the hospital. Upon examination, she had a temperature of 32.9° C (102.5° F), a pulse of 170 beats/minute, blood pressure of 130/70 mm Hg, and mental status of confusion, along with pain in the neck and generalized soreness. Less than 1 hour after her arrival at the hospital, she experienced respiratory arrest and was intubated. Numerous gram-positive diplococci were found in a blood smear, and a chest radiograph showed bilateral pulmonary edema. She was treated with 2 g ceftriaxone intravenously and transferred to a referral hospital. There she was diagnosed with septicemia, disseminated intravascular coagulation, acute respiratory distress syndrome, and possible meningitis. Sputum, blood, and cerebrospinal fluid (CSF) were taken for microbiologic studies. A Gram stain of CSF showed white blood cells but no bacteria. She was treated for gram-positive sepsis.

Her condition deteriorated rapidly and she died later that day. Additional cultures of CSF grew unidentified gram-negative rods and *Streptococcus pneumoniae*. In addition, cultures of blood and respiratory aspirates produced *Yersinia pseudotuberculosis*, identified by a rapid microidentification method. The blood culture isolate was identified as *Yersinia pestis* by the reference state laboratory. It was later revealed that adjacent to the patient's residence an extensive prairie dog die-off had recently occurred. Four of five family dogs and one of three family cats had high titers to *Y. pestis* F1 antigen. Investigators concluded that the patient had been infected by direct contact with abscess material from the pet cat while providing the cat's care.

Issues to Consider

After reading the patient's case history, consider:
- Zoonotic infections are common; as many as 61% of organisms pathogenic to humans are zoonotic in origin.
- A key piece of information in a patient examination is exposure to animals.
- Although some zoonoses are asymptomatic or are characterized by mild symptoms, others are associated with high mortality.
- A surge in some atypical infections could reflect a larger change that has occurred in local animal populations.
- Detection of certain infections in humans, such as West Nile, anthrax, monkeypox, and avian influenza might indicate an emerging public health threat.

Key Terms

Anthrax
Brill-Zinsser disease
Buboes
Bubonic plague
Emerging zoonoses
Erythema migrans (EM)
Eschar
Human granulocytic anaplasmosis (HGA)
Human monocytic ehrlichiosis (HME)

Leptospirosis
Morulae
Pneumonic plague
Rocky Mountain spotted fever (RMSF)
Taches noires
Tularemia
Undulant fever
Weil syndrome
Woolsorter's disease
Zoonoses

Zoonotic infections are those that can naturally jump from animals to humans. The term *zoonotic* was used first by a German physician in 1855. Infections can be transmitted from animals to humans through a variety of routes, including vectors, skin to skin contact, animal bites, inhalation of respiratory droplets, and ingestion of contaminated animal products. Many bacterial zoonotic infections are foodborne or waterborne. A new spin and appreciation for the zoonoses came to light after a publication by Cleaveland in 2001. In this paper, the author describes 1415 microbial species that cause infections in humans. Her data included 217 prions and viruses, 538 bacteria and rickettsiae, 307 fungi, 66 protozoa, and 287 helminths. Amazingly, 868 of these pathogenic agents (61%) are zoonotic. To further emphasize the importance of **zoonoses** to human health, of the 175 emerging infections defined, a full 75% are zoonotic. Clearly, the majority of the pathogenic agents described in this textbook are likely to be classified as zoonotic agents.

The increasing importance of zoonotic infections is occurring for many reasons. More humans are on the planet than ever before, and as these people move into previously unpopulated areas, there is increased exposure of people to animals and their infections. Wild animals are often transported by humans to areas that are new for the animals, increasing the microbial exchanges between humans and animals. As wild animals are moved, they sometimes have more interaction with livestock and domestic animals. And, of course, technology allows for the detection of novel agents of disease previously impossible to grow and characterize. Some zoonotic infections occur normally in animal populations and rarely jump to humans. Occasionally, once these rare infections are introduced into a human population, the zoonotic pathogen can be transmitted from human to human, resulting in a sustained persistence of the agent in the human population. Some zoonotic agents that have done this include human immunodeficiency virus (HIV), influenza virus, Ebola virus, and severe acute respiratory syndrome associated coronavirus. Other zoonotic agents are transmitted from animals to humans, but the resulting disease is generally not contagious from one person to another, so humans essentially represent dead-end hosts. Some zoonotic infections of this type include West Nile virus, rabies, ehrlichiosis, bubonic plague,

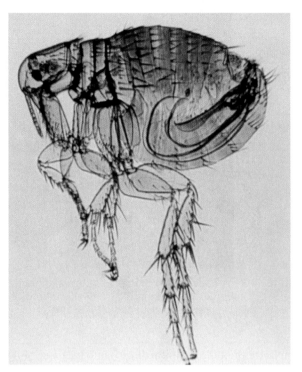

FIGURE 40-1 Rodent fleas carry zoonotic infections such as plague and murine typhus. (Courtesy Centers for Disease Control and Prevention, Atlanta, Ga.)

tularemia, brucellosis, leptospirosis, and Lyme borreliosis. Because zoonotic agents and infections are so common, this chapter summarizes major sources of zoonoses, giving examples of each.

ZOONOTIC INFECTIONS TRANSMITTED BY SCRATCHES, BITES, AND OTHER CONTACT WITH DOMESTIC OR WILD ANIMALS

Plague

Etiology

Plague is caused by the gram-negative bacillus *Yersinia pestis*. This genus is named for Alexander Yersin, a French microbiologist who isolated the plague bacillus during an epidemic in Hong Kong in 1894. Historically three pardemics occurred; "Black Death," the notorious second pandemic, caused 25 million deaths (approximately 30% of the European population.) Rats are the natural host for the vectors (e.g., ticks, insects, other arthropods) that transmit the disease from one organism to another by means of a bite, and humans are accidental hosts. The vectors are fleas, *Xenopsylla cheopis*, (Figure 40-1) that normally infest the brown *(Rattus norvegicus)* and black *(Rattus rattus)* rats. In the United States, most cases are in the Southwest. The organism persists in this region through the sylvatic cycle, being passed among fleas and their rodent hosts. *Y. pestis* can survive for months in animal burrows, and uninfected rodents can get the infection

from this reservoir. The disease is spread to humans by rodents, when contaminated rural areas come in contact with areas of human habitation. Humans can also become infected from domestic cats that hunt rodents.

Life Cycle of *Yersinia pestis*

Fleas develop yersiniosis when they take a blood meal from an infected animal host. The yersiniae multiply in the gut of the flea, eventually reaching such a high concentration that they block the flea's gut. This blockage impairs the flea's ability to feed, and it responds by infesting a wider range of hosts and biting more often. Humans living near rats can be infected by the fleas. Infection is begun when the fleas regurgitate the plague bacilli into the bite wound during feeding.

Clinical Manifestations

Plague has two major manifestations: the bubonic and the pneumonic forms. **Bubonic plague** is an acute, febrile disease with an incubation time of 1 to 7 days. The disease is usually characterized by a lesion in a regional lymph node that drains the infected area. The resulting painful **buboes** usually occur in the groin, axilla, or subauricular area. In the case in point, the patient complained of painful axilla and numbness in her arm. This may have been the beginning of bubo formation. Within 3 to 6 days after the onset of infection, the patient develops signs of septic shock. If the disease goes untreated, the organism can be disseminated hematogenously, leading to septicemia. However, septicemic plague may occur without the bubonic form. The mortality rate of septicemic plague is nearly 100%, with death occurring within 1 to 3 days.

Septicemic plague may lead to a secondary pneumonia, referred to as pneumonic plague. **Pneumonic plague** is almost always the result of hematogenously spread bubonic or septicemic plague. Two forms of pneumonic plague exist: primary and secondary. Primary pneumonic plague occurs when the patient acquires the organism by infectious droplets, whereas secondary pneumonic plague results from the plague bacillus entering the lungs of the same patient who has either bubonic or septicemic plague.

Lyme Borreliosis

Case Study

A 28-year-old woman with shaking chills and perspiration was seen at an emergency department. She explained that before the fever, she had swollen and painful ankles, knees, wrists, and elbows. Her temperature was 38°C, and synovitis was noted in the wrists, elbows, knees, and ankles. She had no rash or lymphadenopathy. She admitted to a family history of osteoarthritis and rheumatoid arthritis. She lived in a rural area and had evidence of multiple insect bites, although she could not remember any recent tick bites. The patient was treated with naproxen and doxycycline for polyarthritis, systemic lupus erythematosus, and late-stage Lyme disease.

Etiology

Lyme borreliosis, caused by *Borrelia burgdorferi*, is an arthropod-borne disease in which humans are accidental hosts (see Chapter 24). The disease is most commonly trans-

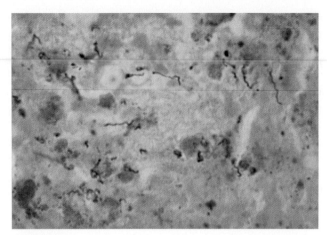

FIGURE 40-2   The spirochete form of *Borrelia burgdorferi* in a Dieterle silver stain preparation. (Courtesy Centers for Disease Control and Prevention, Atlanta, Ga.)

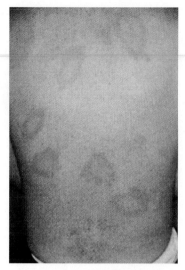

FIGURE 40-3   A patient with multiple erythema migrans lesions. (From Berger BW: Dermatologic manifestations of Lyme disease, *Rev Infect Dis* 2[suppl 6]:S1476, 1989.)

mitted by ticks, including *Ixodes dammini, Ixodes pacificus* (the black-legged tick), *Ixodes ricinus* (the European sheep tick), and *Amblyomma americanum* (the common wood tick, also known as the Lone Star tick), although other insects can also harbor the spirochete. *B. burgdorferi* organisms are gram-negative spirochetes about 0.18 to 0.25 μm × 4 to 30 μm in size (Figure 40-2).

Epidemiology

Lyme borreliosis is the most common vector-borne disease in the United States, with approximately 20,000 cases reported annually. There are about 60,000 cases each year in Europe. The disease that would eventually be named Lyme borreliosis was probably first noted in Sweden in 1908. At that time, erythema chronicum migrans (ECM; recently simplified to **erythema migrans, EM**) was described as a rash that could expand its margins. Red circles ringed a white, hard center of the rash, resulting in a "bull's eye" appearance (Figure 40-3). The next several decades saw more appearances of EM in Europe. Some cases were even associated with tick bites, but no in-depth research was done on the infection. The first report of a similar phenomenon in the United States was in 1970. In 1975, an outbreak of juvenile rheumatoid arthritis occurred in Lyme and Old Lyme, Connecticut. The clustered outbreak of juvenile rheumatoid arthritis appeared suspicious, and thanks to some family members who thought that some infectious agent might be involved, an investigation was begun by health officials. It was the accidental discovery by Willy Burgdorfer of spirochetes in the blood of ticks recovered from the Old Lyme area that ultimately led to the description of Lyme disease. In 1984, the name *B. burgdorferi* was proposed for these organisms.

Life Cycle

Ixodid ticks have a 2-year life cycle, requiring blood meals to pass from the larval stage to the nymph stage, and from the nymph stage to the adult stage. Nymphs and larvae feed primarily on the white-footed mouse, whereas adult ticks usually infest the white-tailed deer. This horizontal transmission ensures maintenance of the pathogen in the wild. Infected nymphs transmit the organism directly into the tissue of hosts (including humans) by regurgitating during feeding. Nymphs transmit the disease primarily in spring and summer. Their very small size poses the greatest threat because they are very hard to see.

Clinical Manifestations

Lyme borreliosis usually has an early stage and a late stage, although patient staging can be difficult. Some patients may not exhibit symptoms during the early phase, whereas other patients may never progress to the late phase. In other patients, the two phases may overlap. In about two thirds of infected patients, the early stage is characterized by a red papule at the site of the bite within the first 30 days of infection. The papules, referred to as *erythema migrans,* can expand to form erythematous concentric rings with central clearing. Spirochetemia can cause flulike symptoms, lymphadenopathy, oligoarthritis, carditis, and neurologic manifestations. Secondary lesions may appear weeks after the initial lesion. Because the concentration of bacteria in the host remains low, it is possible that many of the effects seen in Lyme borreliosis result from the host immune response, including attraction of macrophages to synovial fluid and production of interleukin-1 by host monocytes.

The Lyme spirochetes are rarely isolated from the blood or other body fluids of infected patients. Apparently the organism prefers solid tissue rather than fluid. The spirochete has a nonspecific adhesion that allows it to attach to the endothelial cells of blood vessels. This ability may enhance the migration of the organism from the bloodstream into the basement membrane, resulting in vascular damage that can lead to carditis, arthritis, and central nervous system disease. Late-stage Lyme borreliosis is characterized by relapsing arthritis, and chronic synovitis can occur months to years after the initial symptoms. The joints most commonly affected are the knees, shoulders, and elbows. Untreated patients may have decreasingly severe attacks with the passage of time, until the symptoms eventually disappear. It is difficult to isolate the Lyme spirochete during the late stage. The arthritis may be mediated by the host immune system, rather than by the organism.

Pasteurellosis

Case Study

Parents took their lethargic and irritable 6-month-old daughter to an emergency department. The child had a low-grade fever and a non-erythematous nodule on the right upper arm, but no sign of rash or lymphadenopathy was present. Two shallow abrasions, possibly scratches from the family's pet cat, were near the nodule. The results of the patient examination and laboratory tests were as follows:

Temperature: 38.9°C
Pulse: 200 beats/minute
Respiration: 60 breaths/minute
WBC: 2.2×10^9/L
57% polymorphonuclear neutrophils; 20% band neutrophils
12% lymphocytes; 6% monocytes
Hematocrit: 28%
Cerebrospinal fluid: 3 RBCs/μL; 327 WBCs/μL
75% polymorphonuclear neutrophils
12% lymphocytes
Glucose: 48 mg/dL
Protein: 79 mg/dL

Etiology

Pasteurella multocida is a pleomorphic ovoid to filamentous gram-negative bacillus, about 0.5 to 1.0 μm in size. It can be a primary pathogen or secondary invader. It is pathogenic for a wide range of hosts and occurs in the oral cavities of most dogs and cats (see Chapter 18).

Clinical Manifestations

Pasteurellosis occurs worldwide and encompasses a wide range of endemic diseases of fowl and nonhuman mammals. The most common manifestation of human pasteurellosis is cellulitis, primarily from the bites or scratches of dogs and cats. Cats are usually more often involved than dogs. Although most *P. multocida* infections are transmitted directly from the animal bite to the human, animals can infect pre-existing abrasions by licking them. The infected site becomes inflamed within 48 hours, but the presence of pus is rare. Typically, the patient with pasteurellosis is afebrile and does not have inflamed lymph nodes.

Other clinical manifestations include upper and lower respiratory tract infections, endophthalmitis, and genitourinary tract infections. Rare complications of human infection with *P. multocida* can occur in the absence of animal bites or scratches. These include sepsis, meningitis, septic arthritis, peritonitis, and osteomyelitis. The pathogenesis of *P. multocida* infection in humans is not fully understood, but the antiphagocytic capsule and an outer membrane antiphagocytic protein apparently help the dissemination of the pathogen in avians. These factors are probably responsible for the microbe's virulence in humans as well. Some serogroups of *P. multocida*, including some human isolates, produce an exotoxin.

Erysipeloid

Case Study

A 67-year-old man who fell from a ladder experienced fever and lower back and bilateral leg pain. He went to an emergency department 10 days later and was admitted to the hospital. He was afebrile on admission, but examination revealed a pruritic erythema of the trunk and extremities. The patient explained that the rash had started as a papule that had spread, showing central clearing. The patient also worked in the vicinity of hog pens. Blood cultures were collected, and routine laboratory tests were done. Radiographs showed no bone damage, and the urinalysis was normal.

On hospital day 2, the laboratory reported gram-positive cocci isolated from the blood of the patient. The isolated organism was preliminarily identified as an α-hemolytic *Streptococcus*. The patient received penicillin.

Data from Gorby GL, Peacock JE Jr: *Erysipelothrix rhusiopathiae* endocarditis: microbiologic, epidemiologic, and clinical features of an occupational disease, *Rev Infect Dis* 10:317, 1988.

Etiology

Erysipelothrix rhusiopathiae is the causative agent of the zoonosis erysipelas, seen primarily in pigs (rose disease) and is characterized by fever, skin lesions, arthritis, and sudden death. In humans, *E. rhusiopahtiae* causes syndromes referred to as Rosenbach erysipeloid; erysipelotrichosis; rose disease; and fish-handler's disease. *E. rhusiopathiae* is a thin, facultatively anaerobic gram-positive bacillus, 0.2 to 0.4 μm × 0.8 to 2.5 μm, which can grow singly, in short chains, or in long filaments (see Chapter 16).

Epidemiology

Often isolated from contaminated water and soil, *E. rhusiopathiae* is important in veterinary medicine, causing infections in swine, poultry, small mammals, fish, and crustaceans. The organism occurs worldwide. Swine erysipelas is an important economic disease in North America, South America, and Europe.

Clinical Manifestations

The most common clinical manifestation of infection with *E. rhusiopathiae*, erysipeloid, occurs as a result of handling infected animals or animal products. Three clinical manifestations may occur in humans. The first is a localized cutaneous form (also known as Rosenbach erysipeloid) where the site of infection is usually an abrasion or wound of the hands or fingers (Figure 40-4). The infection is mild, localized, and self-limiting. An edematous lesion forms 1 to 7 days after infection. Erythema and itching might also be present. The lesion usually heals without treatment within 1 month. The second type is a more diffuse cutaneous form, and the third is a generalized systemic infection with bacteremia. Patients with structural valvular disease, alcoholism, or other predisposing conditions may develop sepsis and endocarditis.

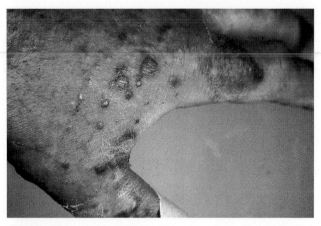

FIGURE 40-4 Erysipeloid. An infection of the hands caused by *Erysipelothrix rhusiopathiae* characterized by blue-red patches of the skin. (From Conlon CP, Snydman DR: *Mosby's color atlas and text of infectious disease*, London, 2000, Mosby.)

Capnocytophaga canimorsus Infection

Case Study

A 47-year-old woman entered an emergency department with weakness, diarrhea, and a facial rash. The patient had a pulse of 80 beats/minute, temperature of 36.5° C, and blood pressure of 80 mm Hg. She had an eschar on the left hand with no evidence of cellulitis. The facial rash covered the nose and cheeks. There were ecchymoses on her extremities. Her arms and legs were cold to the touch. Lung, cardiac, and central nervous system function were normal. The patient was admitted to the intensive care unit.

A dog had bitten her on the left hand 5 days before admission. She had seen a local physician shortly after the bite, and he treated her for an allergic reaction with corticosteroids. The patient received empirical amoxicillin-clavulanic acid and amikacin and then later received ceftazidime and amikacin. One aerobic blood culture bottle (using Bactec NR-660) was positive, with a thin, gram-negative bacillus. The blood was subcultured onto brain-heart infusion agar supplemented with 10% horse blood, and a small colony appeared after 48 hours of incubation in carbon dioxide. The laboratory identified the isolate as CDC group DF-2.

Data from Hantson P et al: Fatal *Capnocytophaga canimorsus* septicemia in previously healthy women, *Ann Emerg Med* 20:126, 1991.

Etiology

Capnocytophaga canimorsus, previously known as dysgonic fermenter-2 (CDC group DF-2), is a thin, nonsporing, non-motile, oxidase- and catalase-positive gram-negative bacillus, 1 to 3 µm long. The organism grows poorly on laboratory media. This pathogen causes a wide range of clinical manifestations, ranging from a mild, self-limiting localized infection to fulminant septicemia with involvement of several organs.

Infection occurs as the result of handling dogs. The carrier rates for this organism in dogs seem to be low, but inadequate recovery techniques may have influenced this finding.

Clinical Manifestations

Capnocytophaga canimorsus is a normal inhabitant of canine and feline oral biota, and infections occur as the result of bites. Dissemination and septicemia occur more often than the self-limiting lesions. About 90% of infections are found in patients who are splenectomized, have cancer, or abuse drugs. The most severe infections are seen in splenectomized patients, who develop an endotoxin-mediated Shwartzman-like phenomenon with purpura, septic shock, and disseminated intravascular coagulation (DIC). Infection of previously healthy individuals is rare, probably because of the susceptibility of the organism to normal serum killing.

Cat Scratch Disease

Etiology

There are currently 18 species within the genus *Bartonella*. Approximately half of those species are capable of causing disease in humans, usually as a result of a bite by an arthropod vector. Some species that infect humans (with vectors and/or animal hosts listed in parentheses) are *B. henseleae* (flea, cat), *B. clarridgeiae* (flea, cat), *B. vinsonii* subsp. vinsonii (vole ear mites), *B. vinsonii* subsp. berkhoffii (ticks, dogs, coyotes), and *B. vinsonii* subsp. arupensis (ticks). The genus *Afipia* contains several species, including *A. felis*.

Clinical Manifestations

Cat scratch disease (CSD) was first described in 1889 and was first associated with cats in 1939, when the term *cat scratch disease* was first used. However, no causative agent was found for the disease until 1983. Researchers at the Armed Forces Institute of Pathology in Washington, DC, described coccobacilli on patient tissue sections that had been processed using the Warthin-Starry silver stain. After almost a decade of study, the new pathogen was named *Afipia felis*. Serologic data and gene amplification tests were used to determine that most CSD infections were not due to *A. felis*, but rather to *Rochalimaea henselae* (later reclassified as *Bartonella henselae*) with some cases probably also due to *B. clarridgeiae*. Approximately 25,000 cases of CSD are diagnosed in the United States each year, although the disease may be underdiagnosed. Almost all patients with CSD report exposure to felines, and the majority of those patients recall a scratch or bite by the feline. Infection is likely transmitted among cats and kittens via fleas.

The disease in humans is usually mild and self-limiting, lasting anywhere from 6 to 12 weeks in untreated patients. Patients usually develop a lesion within a few days after the bite or scratch. Lymphadenopathy occurs at the lymph nodes involved in the draining of the infected area 1 to 2 weeks after appearance of the lesion. Patients may also experience flulike symptoms, including fever, malaise, and anorexia.

ZOONOTIC INFECTIONS TRANSMITTED BY DIRECT CONTACT OR INHALATION

Anthrax

Case Study

A 57-year-old male patient, employed as an electrician, had felt ill and feverish before reporting to the hospital and had collapsed at home when he tried to stand. He had been bitten by an insect on the upper left chest the previous day while at work. He was taking no medications and had no travel history. Examination of the patient detected hypotension, a fever (temperature of 38.2° C), and a necrotic lesion at the site of the insect bite on the chest with edema and erythema. Streptococcal cellulitis and septicemia were diagnosed, and he was admitted to the hospital. He was treated with intravenous benzyl penicillin and flucloxacillin. Subsequent laboratory values were as follows:

Hemoglobin: 17.9 g/dL
WBC: 10.9×10^9/L
Platelets: 262×10^9/L
Serum creatinine: 117 μmol/L
Serum creatinine phosphokinase elevated to 883 IU/L (reference < 235)
Anti-streptolysin O: 240 units/mL (reference < 200 units/mL)
Urea concentration: 4.9 mmol/L

Data from Mallon E, McKee PH: Extraordinary case report: cutaneous anthrax, *Am J Dermatopathol* 19:79, 1997.

Etiology

Anthrax, also known as **woolsorter's disease** and *malignant pustule*, is caused by *Bacillus anthracis*, a large (2.5 × 10 μm), gram-positive, spore-forming bacillus. This organism occurs naturally in the soil and is a pathogen of herbivores, such as cattle, sheep, and goats. Human infections occur as the result of direct or indirect contact with animals or animal products.

Epidemiology

Bacillus anthracis survives well in soil that is neutral or mildly alkaline. Areas with alternating dry and wet seasons enhance anthrax. Floods tend to concentrate spores, which remain in the grasses after flood waters drain. These spores have been known to last in fields for as long as 20 years. Animals are then infected by grazing in a contaminated area.

Anthrax occurs worldwide, commonly in agricultural regions such as Central and South America, Africa, and the Middle East. Anthrax is rare in the United States. Recurrences of anthrax are prevented by containing the spores and eliminating their spread through the environment. Because the anthrax bacteria in tissues do not sporulate until they are exposed to oxygen, infected animal carcasses are usually incinerated whole or are buried in deep pits and covered with lime.

Vaccines are available for humans and for cattle. A cell-free vaccine, prepared from the protective antigen of *B. anthracis,* is used for people in high-risk occupations. Another vaccine, made with an avirulent, nonencapsulated strain of *B. anthracis,* is available for animals.

Clinical Manifestations

Human anthrax manifests as cutaneous, intestinal, or pulmonary. The route of transmission determines the incubation period and symptoms.

Cutaneous Anthrax. The most common form of anthrax is the cutaneous form (95% of cases), which mimics many other cutaneous infections. It is most common in nonindustrialized countries. The spores enter the host through abraded skin and then germinate. After 48 to 72 hours, a papule is formed; it darkens and ruptures, leaving a painless crater-like ulcer, which progresses to a necrotic **eschar.** The infection usually remains localized and self-limiting, and the eschar heals without scarring. In about 20% of patients with cutaneous anthrax, the immune system is unable to contain the infection, and *B. anthracis* enters the bloodstream and disseminates. With treatment, death is rare.

Gastrointestinal Anthrax. The gastrointestinal form, the second most common form of anthrax, is also found more frequently in nonindustrialized nations. It is caused by the ingestion of meat or meat products contaminated with spores. Once the spores are ingested, they germinate, and the organisms gain entry through preexisting intestinal mucosa lesions. Dissemination of the bacteria then occurs via the lymphatics. Clinically, the patient will be febrile and have bloody stools and can lose as much as 12 L of fluid per 24-hour period. Septicemia and death may result.

Pulmonary (Inhalation) Anthrax. The pulmonary form occurs as a result of inhaling spores, usually from contaminated animal products. This form of anthrax is more common in industrialized countries. Macrophages ingest the spores and then concentrate them in lymph nodes. Eventually, the spores germinate and sepsis occurs. The result of this form of infection is usually death of the patient within 24 hours, regardless of the treatment.

B. anthracis produces three virulence factors: glutamic acid, which inhibits phagocytosis; lethal factor (LF); and edema factor (EF). In order for LF and EF to become biologically active toxins, they must first combine with the *B. anthracis* protective antigen (PA), which binds to the host cell. PA is also a transport protein, which carries both EF and LF into the host cell. EF is an adenylate cyclase that causes characteristic edema. Necrosis occurs as the result of increased capillary permeability and destruction of the phagocytic cells. Edema can be remarkable and may cause the patient to suffocate by literally swelling the neck shut. Excessive edema of the neck, thorax, and mediastinum signals the beginning of a rapidly fatal course.

Tularemia

Case Study

A 63-year-old man noticed swelling and localized pain in the dorsum of his left thumb 5 days after a cat bite. He was treated with oral penicillin and cloxacillin for 3 days. He continued to experience pain, general malaise, fever, and vomiting, and he was admitted to the hospital. The patient was lethargic, his temperature was 38.7° C,

Continued

chest was clear, and he was hemodynamically stable, with a 3- × 5-cm indurated, erythematous region on the dorsal aspect of the base of his left thumb and hand. Because this was considered to be a possible abscess, the physician performed an incision and drainage, but no abscess was found. Swabs from the infected region grew coagulase-negative staphylococci.

The patient was treated with intravenous penicillin and cloxacillin. Five days after admission the patient developed shortness of breath and had patchy pneumonic infiltrates of the right middle and lower lobes of the lung. Seven days after admission, lymphangitic streaking on the upper left extremity and tender axillary lymphadenopathy were detected. The patient's therapy was changed to clindamycin and gentamicin. The patient defervesced, and his respiratory status improved.

A swab from the wound was plated onto sheep blood and chocolate agar plates and incubated in CO_2. After 3 days, small, smooth, gray colonies were visible. Gram-negative coccobacilli were identified as *Francisella tularensis* by fatty acid analysis and slide agglutination by specific antisera. Acute and convalescent sera samples were 1 : 800 and 1 : 3200, respectively. The patient's cats were adopted strays that lived outdoors and probably fed on wild rodents.

Etiology

Tularemia is caused by *Francisella tularensis*, a strictly aerobic gram-negative bacillus about 0.2 μm × 0.2 to 0.7 μm. The first isolation of the bacterium was in 1911 during an epizootic outbreak of plaguelike ground squirrel disease. The organism was named *Bacterium tularense* after Tulare County, California, the site of the outbreak. In 1944, researchers defined the role of cottontail and jackrabbits in the transmission of the disease to humans. Since 1945 the proportion of vector-borne (*Dermacentor andersoni*, *Dermacentor variabilis*, and *A. americanum*) transmission has increased, while transmission from vertebrate reservoirs has decreased. In 1959, the genus name of the organism was changed to *Francisella* in honor of Edward Francis, who first isolated the organism.

Epidemiology

The two biovars *F. tularensis* biovar tularensis (type A) and *F. tularensis* biovar palaearctica (type B) occur in different parts of the world. In North America, the predominant biovar is type A, the more virulent strain in humans. Humans are usually infected with this strain by rabbits or ticks, although more than 100 species of vertebrate and invertebrate natural reservoirs can transmit the infection. Type B also occurs in North America, but it is more often recovered in Europe and Asia. It is less virulent than type A and is more often transmitted by rodents and mosquitoes. Types A and B differ from each other biochemically and genetically but not serologically.

Clinical Manifestations

Tularemia is an acute, febrile, granulomatous disease characterized by rapid onset and flulike symptoms. The most common presentations are ulceroglandular (ulcers and lymphadenopathy), oropharyngeal (pharyngeal ulcer and lymphadenopathy), oculoglandular (conjunctival ulcer and lymphadenopathy), glandular (lymphadenopathy without ulcer), pleuropulmonary (no ulcer, possible lymphadenopa-

thy), and typhoidal (no ulcers or lymphadenopathy). The ulceroglandular, oculoglandular, and glandular types usually occur as the result of direct contact with infected vertebrate or invertebrate reservoirs. Typhoidal and oropharyngeal cases of tularemia usually occur after eating contaminated food.

Pneumonic tularemia may result from exposure to aerosols. The symptoms associated with tularemia include fever, chills, headache, and myalgia. Typhoidal tularemia, especially when complicated with pneumonia, has a high fatality rate. In the United States, most cases of tularemia are ulceroglandular. These infections are usually caused by direct contact with contaminated game or by insect bites. The incubation period of tularemia is 3 to 10 days. A papule, which forms at the site of infection, eventually ulcerates. Patients usually have only one lesion, although multiple lesions can occur. The actual site of the lesion is indicative of the transmission; lesions of the hands or arms often indicate infection by direct contact with infected mammals, whereas lesions on the head or the back indicate transmission by an insect vector.

Brucellosis

Case Study

A 25-year-old man complaining of headache, malaise, arthralgia, and a 6-kg weight loss was admitted to the hospital. His symptoms first started during the last 3 months after his return from a trip to Syria. He reported having eaten fresh goat's cheese. On admission he was in moderate distress and had the following laboratory results:
WBC: 5.3×10^9/L
C-reactive protein: 10.7 mg/dL (normal < 1.0 mg/dL)
Malaria smear: Negative
Serology for *Salmonella* spp.: Negative
Blood culture: Positive for *Brucella abortus*
Serology for *B. abortus*: Positive, titer 1 : 10,000

The patient was treated with doxycycline, 400 mg daily, and rifampin, 600 mg daily. The patient improved, he became afebrile, and his C-reactive protein level returned to normal after a few days. The patient's girlfriend developed the same symptoms 2 months later and was admitted to the hospital. Blood cultures were positive for *B. abortus*. She was successfully treated and recovered without complications.

The authors believe this to be the first case of possible sexual transmission of *B. abortus* in humans. The female had no travel history or other risk factors. The couple had unprotected sexual intercourse, and sexual transmission was considered to be the most likely route of infection.

Data from Thalhammer F et al: Unusual route of transmission for *Brucella abortus*, *Clin Infect Dis* 26:763, 1998.

Etiology

Brucellosis has many synonyms, including Mediterranean fever, Malta fever, Gibraltar fever, Bang disease, Neapolitan fever, Cyprus fever, and **undulant fever.** The genus name comes from Sir David Bruce, who in 1887 was the first to describe these agents as the cause of undulant fever.

Epidemiology

Four species, which originate from animal reservoirs, are pathogenic to humans:

Brucella melitensis (goats)
Brucella abortus (cattle)
Brucella canis (canines)
Brucella suis (swine)

The most pathogenic species for humans, in descending order, are *B. melitensis*, *B. suis*, *B. abortus*, and *B. canis*. Other species not known to cause human disease are *B. neotomae* (desert wood rat) and *B. ovis* (sheep). In the animal hosts, the brucellae can induce spontaneous abortion secondary to bacteremia in pregnant females. The urine and milk of infected animals contain the infective organisms. *B. melitensis*, the most common agent of human brucellosis, occurs in many areas of the world, including Mexico, Central and South America, southeastern Europe, countries bordering the Mediterranean, Africa, southern Russia, India, Iran, and central Saudi Arabia.

Clinical Manifestations

In the United States, the brucellae infect humans primarily through contact with infected animals and animal products. Veterinarians, meat packers, sheepherders, and abattoir workers are at risk for infection.

The organism can enter the body through abraded skin, mucous membranes, or the conjunctivae. In experiments, *B. abortus* has penetrated intact skin. After an incubation period of 1 to 3 weeks, the brucellae are disseminated hematogenously, where circulating monocytes ingest them. The brucellae are facultative intracellular parasites. Monocytes transport the brucellae to lymph nodes. From there, the bacteria are disseminated to the spleen and the liver. *B. abortus* usually causes granuloma formation, whereas *B. melitensis* usually causes formation of microabscesses. *B. melitensis* is also able to inhibit phagosome-lysosome fusion in phagocytic cells, allowing intracellular bacterial replication. Normal human serum is bactericidal to *B. abortus*, but not to *B. melitensis*, accounting for the relative differences in their pathogenicity. The symptoms of acute brucellosis are chills, fever, sweating, weakness, and fatigue.

Leptospirosis

Case Study

A 48-year-old man, employed as a river dredger, presented with headache, fever, dark urine, arthralgia, diarrhea, breathlessness, and confusion, which had become worse over the past 4 days. The patient was hypoxic, and chest x-ray study showed a rapid deterioration with shadowing in all regions of the lungs. He was treated with doxycycline and erythromycin. His condition continued to deteriorate and he was given mechanical respiratory support. Methylprednisolone was prescribed in addition to the antimicrobials. Chest x-ray studies showed continued deterioration for a period of 7 days before showing gradual clearance. Renal function also returned to normal. He was discharged after 21 days. He was determined to have culture-positive leptospirosis with severe pulmonary hemorrhage. The date of the positive culture was not reported.

Record reviews of the Tropical Public Health Unit showed 149 cases of leptospirosis reported; 24 of those patients were hospitalized and 5 had life-threatening pulmonary hemorrhage. Although not frequently reported, this complication is worth noting because of its

serious consequences. In a 1995 outbreak in Nicaragua, 40 of 2000 patients died because of pulmonary hemorrhage.

In the experience of these authors with the five cases, all patients gave nonspecific histories of malaise, myalgia, and fever. Renal impairment and jaundice, considered to be hallmarks of leptospirosis, were absent in two of the five patients.

Data from Simpson FG et al: Leptospirosis associated with severe pulmonary haemorrhage in Far North Queensland, *Med J Aust* 169:151, 1998.

Etiology

Leptospires are helical cells, about 6 to 20 μm × 0.1 μm (Figure 40-5). They are motile and have two subterminal flagella. The cells have characteristic hooks on the ends. The genus *Leptospira* contains a large group of serologically diverse organisms. There are 12 species within the genus. As many as 250 serovars are organized into 23 serogroups.

Epidemiology

Until recently, **leptospirosis** was not considered a widely common infection. Current thought suggests this infection is one of the most common zoonoses, primarily as a result of exposure during recreational activity. It is most often reported in the United States from southeastern, Gulf, and Pacific coastal states and Hawaii. Recreational activities that involve contact with water or moist soil are most often associated with transmission. In Hawaii, some homes use rainwater catchment systems and these have also been reported as a risk factor. As many as 5% to 10% of leptospirosis infections are fatal.

Rodents and domestic animals are the primary reservoirs for the organism. Other animals, including cows, horses, mongoose, and frogs, can harbor the leptospires. Humans may be directly infected from animal urine or indirectly by contact with soil or water that is contaminated with urine from infected animals. The patient in the case in point worked as a

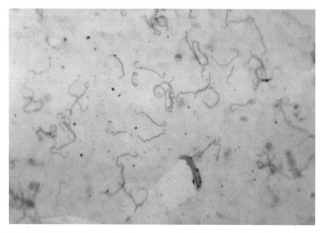

FIGURE 40-5   A photomicrograph of *Leptospira* taken from a liver preparation from a patient with fatal leptospirosis. (Photograph by Dr. Martin Hicklin; courtesy Centers for Disease Control and Prevention, Atlanta, Ga.)

river dredger and doubtless had frequent repeated contacts with untreated water. Infected humans can shed leptospires in urine for up to 11 months, cows for $3\frac{1}{2}$ months, dogs for 4 years, and infected rodents possibly for their full lifetime. Veterinarians, abattoir workers, fish and poultry processors, and dairy workers are at risk for leptospirosis. Agricultural workers and soldiers are also at risk because of contact with soil and mud.

Leptospirosis is endemic in most areas of the world, although the incidence of disease can be underreported because of undiagnosed infections. The infection is more prevalent in areas with warm climates, especially in late autumn and early winter. The treatment of choice is doxycycline or penicillin.

Clinical Manifestations

The number of diagnosed leptospiral infections has increased in recent years. Leptospiral infections can range from subclinical to lethal. The organisms enter the host through mucous membranes or abraded skin. The incubation period ranges from 5 to 14 days.

Anicteric leptospirosis is usually a biphasic disease. In the first phase, the patient has sudden temperature spikes, severe headaches, nausea, vomiting, and muscle aches. Patients often experience confusion, secondary to dehydration. The majority of patients develop vivid pink eyes. During this period, the leptospires are recoverable from the patient's blood and cerebrospinal fluid (CSF). This phase of leptospirosis lasts for about 3 weeks.

In the second phase of anicteric leptospirosis, the leptospires disappear from the circulatory system and CSF of the patient. This change occurs after the appearance of specific IgM antibodies. Symptoms may subside for a few days, but a limited febrile episode may follow. Patients can also develop aseptic meningitis and severe headaches. During this stage of infection, the urine contains leptospires, but the blood of the patient does not. The length of this stage depends on the serotype of the infecting leptospire.

Leptospira interrogans serovar icterohaemorrhagiae can cause *icteric leptospirosis,* also known as **Weil syndrome**. This form of leptospirosis is more life-threatening than the anicteric form. Weil syndrome starts in the same way as does anicteric leptospirosis. On about the third day of the illness, however, the patient develops hemolysis, jaundice, and renal failure. These symptoms occur as the leptospires multiply in the liver and the kidney. In Weil syndrome, mortality ranges from 15% to 40%. In fatal cases, renal failure is the usual cause of death. In nonfatal cases, the leptospires clear from the patient's kidneys, brain, and eyes as antibodies appear.

THE RICKETTSIAE

The term *rickettsiae* can specifically refer to the genus *Rickettsia* or it can refer to a group of organisms included in the order Rickettsiales. Significant reorganization in the order Rickettsiales has occurred in recent years. The order includes the families Rickettsiaceae and Anaplasmataceae. The family Rickettsiaceae includes the genera *Rickettsia* and *Orientia*. All members of the family Rickettsiaceae are obligate intracellular bacteria and can grow only in the cytoplasm of host cells. They spend at least part of their life cycle in an arthropod. The family Anaplasmataceae includes the genera *Ehrlichia, Anaplasma, Cowdria, Wolbachia,* and *Neorickettsia*. As a result of this reorganization, *Coxiella* has been removed from the family Rickettsiaceae.

With few exceptions, rickettsiae are not agents of zoonoses in the same sense as the organisms presented earlier in this chapter. Most of the members of the rickettsial group are arthropod-borne, obligately intracellular pathogens. The arthropod hosts generally serve as both reservoirs (transovarial transmission) and vectors (transmission between mammalian hosts) for members of the genus *Rickettsia*.

Genus *Rickettsiaceae*

Rickettsia are short, nonmotile, gram-negative bacilli about 0.8 to 2.0 μm × 0.3 to 0.5 μm in size. The members of the genus *Rickettsia* have been grown in monolayer cell lines and embryonated eggs. However, due to their infectious nature, it is not recommended to try to cultivate them in clinical laboratories without proper equipment and training. The rickettsiae are divided into groups according to the types of clinical infections they produce. The typhus group consists of *R. prowazekii* and *R. typhi*. The spotted fever group includes the *R. rickettsii* group, *R. japonica, R. montana,* the *R. massiliae* group, *R. helvetica, R. felis,* and the *R. akari* group. Both *R. bellii* and *R. canada* are excluded from either group.

Rocky Mountain Spotted Fever

Rocky Mountain spotted fever (RMSF), caused by *R. rickettsii,* is the most severe of the rickettsial infections and the most common in the United States. Humans acquire the infection by tick bites. A number of species of ticks can transmit the disease, with the most common being *D. variabilis* in the southeastern United States and *D. andersoni* in the western part of the country. Rodents and ticks serve as reservoirs. The bacteria preferentially infect the endothelial cells, where they replicate primarily in the cytoplasm of the host cell. The rickettsiae spread hematogenously throughout the host and induce vasculitis in internal organs, including the brain, heart, lungs, and kidneys.

After an incubation period of approximately 7 days, the patient presents with flulike symptoms that include fever, headache, myalgia, nausea, vomiting, and rash. The rash begins as erythematous patches on the ankles and wrists during the first week of symptoms then extends to the palms of the hands and soles of the feet. However, it normally does not affect the face. The maculopapular patches eventually consolidate into larger areas of ecchymoses. Other symptoms include hypotension and DIC. With rapid diagnosis and appropriate therapy, the mortality rate is 3% to 6%. The mortality rate without treatment can be 20% or higher.

Rickettsialpox

Rickettsialpox, caused by *R. akari,* occurs in Korea and the Ukraine as well as in the eastern United States. The disease was first reported in the United States in an apartment in the borough of Queens, New York City in 1946. Outbreaks have occurred in several large cities including New York City, Cleveland, and Philadelphia. The reservoir is the common house mouse, and the vector is the mouse mite. The infections occur in crowded urban areas where rodents and their mites exist. Rickettsialpox is similar to RMSF but milder. After an incubation period of about 10 days, a papule forms at the site of inoculation. The papule progresses to a pustule, then to an indurated eschar. Additional symptoms include headache, nausea, and chills. Unlike RMSF, the rash of rickettsialpox appears on the face, trunk, and extremities and does not involve the palms of the hands or soles of the feet. Rickettsialpox symptoms resolve without medical attention.

Murine Typhus

Rickettsia typhi causes murine (endemic typhus) typhus. The arthropod vector is the oriental rat flea, and the rat is the reservoir. The cat flea can also serve as a reservoir. Because this flea infests a large number of domestic animals, it may be an important factor in the persistence of infection in urban areas. The rickettsiae also survive in nature, to a lesser extent, by transovarial transmission.

In the 1940s, approximately 5000 cases of endemic typhus were reported annually in the United States. Although it is no longer a reportable disease in the United States, fewer than 100 cases are reported annually. The disease essentially occurs only in southern Texas and southern California. Worldwide, it continues to be a problem in areas where rats and their fleas are present in urban settings. As with RMSF, the clinical course of murine typhus includes fever, headache, and rash. Unlike RMSF, however, murine typhus does not always produce a rash; slightly more than one half of the cases are characterized by a rash. When the rash is present, it usually occurs on the trunk and extremities. Patients often have an eschar at the site of inoculation. Complications are rare, and recovery usually occurs without incident.

Louse-Borne Typhus

Rickettsia prowazekii causes louse-borne (endemic typhus) typhus. Vectors include the human louse, the squirrel flea, and the squirrel louse. The reservoirs are primarily humans and flying squirrels located in the eastern United States. Unlike vectors of other rickettsiae, the louse often dies of its rickettsial infection.

Louse-borne typhus is still found commonly in areas of Africa and Central and South America where overcrowding and poor sanitation promote the presence of body lice. As demonstrated during World War II, epidemic typhus can occur even in developed countries when sanitation is disrupted. More than 20,000 cases of louse-borne typhus were documented during the 1980s, with the vast majority originating in Africa.

Lice are infected with *R. prowazekii* when feeding on infected humans. The organisms invade the cells lining the gut of the louse and spill into the lumen of the gut when infected cells are lysed. When the louse feeds on another human, it defecates, and the infected feces are scratched into the skin. The disease progression resembles RMSF, including a rash involving the palms of the hands and soles of the feet. Unlike RMSF, the face may also be affected by the rash. Mortality rates in treated patients are very low; however, the mortality rates for untreated patients can approach 40%. **Brill-Zinsser disease,** or recrudescent typhus, is a reactivation of louse-borne typhus. The bacteria can lie dormant in the lymph tissue of the human host for several years after the primary infection. Recrudescent typhus is milder than louse-borne typhus, and death is rare. Patients with latent infections constitute an important reservoir for the organism.

Anaplasmataceae

Case Study

A 65-year-old white man experienced fever, headache, myalgia, and anorexia for 5 days. When he went to his personal physician, his temperature was 38.3° C, his blood pressure was 128/60 mm Hg, and he was dehydrated. There was no sign of rash or lymphadenopathy.

Serial blood cultures were negative, as were routine serology tests. The patient received intravenous doxycycline for 3 days. He then received oral doxycycline. His fever resolved after 6 hours of therapy. Following are the laboratory test results:

WBC: 2.5×10^9/L
Platelet: 57,000/µL
Hematocrit: 41.1%
Hemoglobin: 11.6 g/dL
AST (aspartate aminotransferase): 167 U/L
Creatine phosphokinase: 403 U/L
Alkaline phosphatase: 173 IU/L
Total bilirubin: 1.7 mg/dL

Data from Taylor JP et al: Serological evidence of possible human infection with *Ehrlichia* in Texas, *J Infect Dis* 158:217, 1988.

Members of the genera *Ehrlichia* and *Anaplasma* are the most important pathogens within the family Anaplasmatacieae. *Ehrlichiosis* was first noted to cause lethal infection in dogs in the 1930s. Postmortem examination revealed rickettsial-like inclusions in the monocytes. The bacteria were named *Rickettsia canis*. They differ from the other members of the rickettsiae in that they multiply in the phagosomes of host leukocytes and not in the cytoplasm of endothelial cells. In addition, they do not appear to be transmitted transovarially in ticks. Because of these differences, they were reclassified into the new genus, *Ehrlichia*, in 1945. They were eventually named *E. chaffeensis*.

The ehrlichiae, like the chlamydiae, possess an infective form known as the elementary body, which replicates in the phagosome. As the bacteria divide, they develop **morulae** (mulberry-like bodies; see Figure 24-7). As the host cell ruptures, the morulae break into many individual elementary bodies that continue the infective cycle. *Ehrlichia chaffeensis* causes **human monocytic ehrlichiosis (HME).** The infection occurs worldwide. In the United States most cases are found in the southeastern and south central states, as well as in the mid-Atlantic States. Fewer than 2000 cases have been definitely or presumptively identified since the disease description in 1986; however, cases may be underreported. Natural hosts of the organism include dogs and deer, as well as humans, with the Lone Star tick *(A. americanum)* being the primary vector.

Anaplasma phagocytophilum, formerly known as *Ehrlichia phagocytophilum,* causes a disease now referred to as **human granulocytic anaplasmosis (HGA).** In 1994, molecular amplification and DNA sequencing showed that the causative agent of HGA was distinct from *E. chaffeensis.* There were 16 cases per 100,000 population reported in northern Wisconsin from 1990 to 1995. In 2007, nationally 834 cases (0.31/100,000 population) were reported; that is equivalent to HME. Both diseases are probably underreported. Deer, rodents, horses, cattle, and humans are natural hosts. Tick vectors include *Ixodes scapularus* and *I. pacificus.*

HME and HGA cases are similar clinically and many patients may experience asymptomatic infection. The organisms have an incubation period of 5 to 10 days. Disease is clinically variable, but most patients with HGA have a moderately severe febrile illness. The most frequent manifestations are malaise (94%), fever (92%), myalgia (77%), and headache (75%). A minority of patients have arthralgia or involvement of the gastrointestinal tract (nausea, vomiting, diarrhea), respiratory tract (cough, pulmonary infiltrates, acute respiratory distress syndrome), liver, or central nervous system. Rash is observed in about 6% of the patients.

As many as 60% of the pediatric patients infected with *E. chaffeensis* may have a rash, although adults with the same infection rarely experience rash. Patients may also have evidence of leukopenia, thrombocytopenia, and elevated liver enzymes. Patients can experience severe complications, including illness similar to toxic shock–like syndrome, central nervous system involvement, and adult respiratory distress syndrome. Mortality rates are approximately 2% to 3%.

EMERGING ZOONOSES

The impact of infectious diseases on human populations has to be respected. Approximately 5 million deaths occur on the planet each year just from tuberculosis, malaria, and acquired immunodeficiency syndrome; knowing that those are diseases for which there are therapeutics forces one to understand the power of "Mother Nature." Currently, the United States and other nations are preparing for the possibility of pandemic influenza (avian flu), the possibility of which is greater now than in the past several decades. Preparations are being made with a limited availability of neuraminidase inhibitors for therapy and with only enough vaccine to inoculate a few million humans. One factor that will help determine whether the influenza virus spreads further than Asia and Eastern Europe is the behavior of migrating birds that are able to expose new populations in new countries to this high-pathogenicity avian influenza strain. The risk for mutation and adaptation to humans increases as the countries with infected birds and poultry increases. The planning for an influenza pandemic is similar to the planning that was done when the spread of severe acute respiratory syndrome (SARS) was considered an important health risk.

The similarity is that both avian influenza and SARS are examples of **emerging zoonoses.** The term implies the discovery of a new agent, discovery of a known agent that has moved to a new geographic location, discovery of a known pathogen that has become drug resistant, or some other modification. These emerging zoonoses can expose human susceptibility to novel agents that jump from animal populations into the human population. The majority of these emerging zoonotic diseases are caused by pathogens transmitted directly or indirectly through arthropod vectors.

By definition, some of the zoonotic agents already discussed fall into the category of emerging pathogens, including *B. burgdorferi, E. chaffeensis, A. phagocytophilum, A. felis,* and *B. henselae.* Other chapters in this textbook discuss the following zoonotic agents: Lake Victoria Marburgvirus, Zaire, Reston, Sudan, and Tai Forest Ebola viruses; Rift Valley fever virus; Henipaviruses; monkeypox virus; SARS-associated coronavirus; West Nile virus; and high-pathogenicity avian influenza. Additional chapters discuss the suspected origin of zoonotic diseases. For example, hepatitis E (HEV) is transmitted by the fecal-oral route. Cattle, rats, sheep, monkeys, goats, and especially pigs are vulnerable to HEV infection. In Nepal, most outbreaks have occurred after monsoon rains and flooding, fecal contamination of well water, and untreated raw sewage entering city water supplies.

BIBLIOGRAPHY

Aguero-Rosenfield ME et al: Diagnosis of Lyme Borreliosis, *CMR* 18(3):484, July 2005.

Beninati T et al: First detection of spotted fever group rickettsiae in *Ixodes ricinus* from Italy, *Emerg Infect Dis* 8:983, 2002.

Bengis RG et al: The role of wildlife in emerging and re-emerging zoonoses, *Rev Sci Tech* 23:497, 2004.

Brown C: Emerging zoonoses and pathogens of public health significance—an overview, *Rev Sci Tech* 23:435, 2004.

Childs JE, Gordon ER: Surveillance and control of zoonotic agents prior to disease detection in humans, *Mt Sinai J Med* Oct; 76:421, 2009.

Cleaveland S et al: Diseases of humans and their domestic mammals: pathogen characteristics, host range and risk of emergence, *Phil Trans R Soc Lond* 356:991, 2001.

Dumler JS et al: Reorganization of the genera in the families Rickettsiaceae and Anaplasmataceae in the order Rickettsiales: unification of some species of *Ehrlichia* with *Anaplasma, Cowdria* with *Ehrlichia* and *Ehrlichia* with *Neorickettsia,* description of six new species combinations and designation of *Ehrlichia canis* and "HGE agent" as subjective synonyms of *Ehrlichia phagocytophila, Int J Syst Bacteriol* 51:2145, 2001.

Flicek BF: Rickettsial and other tick-borne infections, *Crit Care Nurs ClinNorth Am* Mar; 19:27, 2007.

Higgins R: Emerging or re-merging bacterial zoonotic diseases: bartonellosis, leptospirosis, Lyme borreliosis, plague, *Rev Sci Tech* 23:569, 2004.

Kahn RE, Clouser DF et al: Emerging infections: a tribute to the one medicine, one health concept. *Zoonoses Public Health,* May 20, 2009 (Epub ahead of print). www.ncbi.nlm.nih.gov/pubmed. Accessed 11/20/2009.

Krusell A et al: Rickettsial pox in North Carolina: a case report, *Emerg Infect Dis* 8:727, 2002.

Olano JP, Aguero-Rosenfeld ME: *Ehrlichia, Anaplasma,* and related intracellular bacteria. In Murray PR et al, editors: *Manual of clinical microbiology,* ed 9, Washington, DC, 2007, ASM Press.

Slingenbergh J et al: Ecological sources of zoonotic diseases, *Rev Sci Tech* 23:467, 2004.

Trevejo RT, Barr MC et al: Important emerging bacterial zoonotic infections affecting the immunocompromised, *Vet. Res* 36:493, EDP Sciences, 2005.

Torres-Velex F, Brown C: Emerging infections in animals—potential new zoonoses? *Clin Lab Med* 24:825, 2004.

Walker DH, Bouyer DH: *Rickettsia* and *Orientia.* In Murray PR et al, editors: *Manual of clinical microbiology,* ed 9, Washington, DC, 2007, ASM Press.

World Health Organization Zoonotic Infections. www.who.int/vaccine_research/diseases/zoonotic/en/print. Accessed August 31, 2009.

Points to Remember

- Zoonotic infections represent a significant percentage of workload in a clinical microbiology laboratory.
- Animal exposure and insect bites are important clues as to possible causes of a patient's infection.
- Zoonotic agents can be bacterial or viral, as well as parasitic or mycotic.

- Not all zoonotic infections are contagious. In several zoonotic infections, the pathogens transmit efficiently to humans but do not spread easily from person to person.
- For the past 30 years, emerging infections have been recorded, including the discovery of previously unknown pathogens. Of these, 75% have zoonotic origin.

Learning Assessment Questions

1. Erythema migrans is a rash associated with which zoonotic infection?

2. Late-stage Lyme borreliosis is usually characterized by what type of clinical manifestation?

3. Which two animals are most often associated with human cases of pasteurellosis?

4. List two preexisting medical conditions that might increase the risk of *Capnocytophaga canimorsus* infections in humans.

5. Name the most likely organism associated with cat scratch disease (CSD). What is another organism that also can cause CSD?

6. What is the most common form of anthrax? Which type of anthrax has the highest associated mortality rate?

7. Which toxins are responsible for life-threatening edema in pulmonary anthrax?

8. Name the four species of brucellae that are pathogenic to humans and the normal hosts for these organisms.

9. Explain the differences between icteric and anicteric leptospirosis.

10. The order Rickettsiales includes which two families? What is the major route of transmission of these organisms to humans?

11. Which species are included in the typhus group of the genus *Rickettsia?*

12. What is the most severe rickettsial disease? Symptoms of Rocky Mountain spotted fever are primarily associated with damage to which tissue?

Ocular Infections

Darlene Miller

OBJECTIVES

After reading and studying this chapter, you should be able to:

1. Identify common ocular structures and their functions.

2. Discuss the role of normal biota in protecting ocular structures.

3. List the most frequent ocular infections and their causative agents.

4. Describe laboratory procedures for recovery and identification of ocular pathogens.

5. Compose a list of commercial topical antimicrobials.

A healthy 20-year-old woman with no history of ocular disease had been wearing disposable contact lenses for 3 months. She replaced them every 7 to 10 days. The patient developed blurred vision, pain, photophobia, and redness in her right eye during the twelfth week. An examination revealed edema and four small ulcers with a green, mucopurulent discharge. Gram and Giemsa stains were prepared from the mucopurulent discharge. Cultures were performed from corneal scrapings and from the contact lens and solution.

Issues to Consider

After reading the patient's case history, consider:

- The role insertion and removal of the contact lens may have in establishing ocular infections
- The need for rapid diagnosis in this case
- Common pathogens involved in this type of infections

Key Terms

Blepharitis	Keratitis
Canaliculitis	Orbital cellulitis
Conjunctivitis	Preseptal cellulitis
Dacryoadenitis	Retinitis
Dacryocystitis	Scleritis
Endophthalmitis	Uveitis
Keratoconjunctivitis	

Any organism capable of gaining entrance to ocular structures can cause disease. Ocular infections range from the relatively mild, self-limiting episodes of conjunctivitis and blepharitis to the more severe and sight-threatening conditions of keratitis and endophthalmitis. Surrounding soft tissues, sclera, lacrimal system, and bony orbit are also subject to microbial invasion. Bacteria, fungi, viruses, and protozoa all play prominent roles in the pathogenesis of ocular disease. The selection of specific microbiologic procedures is dependent upon the severity of symptoms, the site of infection, and the likely pathogen.

GENERAL CONCEPTS RELATED TO OCULAR INFECTIONS

Ocular Structures

Figure 41-1 outlines the most important ocular structures. The visual system is composed of the eyeball, muscles, fat, nerves, orbital bones, and neural pathways that carry and translate electrical impulses into vision. This system does not actually "see" but rather acts as a receptor for sensory light stimuli that are translated to neural impulses by the retina and then processed by the occipital lobe of the brain. In a sense, the eye is a frontal extension of the brain.

Conjunctiva

The conjunctiva is a mucous membrane, similar to those in the mouth and nose. It lines the upper and lower lids and constitutes the front line of defense against invading organisms. The tears that keep the conjunctiva moist contain many enzymes and other factors (IgG, IgM, β-lysin, lysozyme, lactoferrin) that protect the conjunctiva from microbial invasion.

Lids

The eyelids are thin elastic layers, or folds, of tissue that help protect the structures of the orbit. They are the thinnest skin covering in the body. The blinking action of the lids and conjunctivae helps keep the cornea and sclera lubricated and sweeps away debris and potential pathogens. The cilia, or lashes, act as a filtering and monitoring system that alert the brain to potentially harmful agents.

Cornea

The cornea is considered the "window" of the eye. Its size and function are similar to those of a crystal on a wristwatch. The internal ocular structures can be viewed through the cornea. The function of the curved corneal surface is to refract, collect, and focus light onto the retina. A layer of tears (the tear film) blankets the cornea to provide optical clarity, lubrication, and nutrition. Many free nerve endings are located in the corneal epithelium. When there is a break in or an injury to the epithelium, the patient usually complains of considerable pain. Infections and injury to the cornea are considered true ocular emergencies.

Sclera

Known as the "white of the eye," the sclera protects and provides structural support to the internal ocular structures. It consists of tough, interlacing collagen fibers, which gives it an opaque appearance.

Orbit

The "closed-box" structure of the bony orbit protects the soft tissues of the eye. The pyramid-shaped bones are connected on several sides with the maxillary, ethmoid, sphenoid, and frontal sinuses. The ocular structures actually occupy only about one fifth of the orbital cavity, with fat and muscle filling the rest of the space. This unit protects the internal structures from blunt trauma.

Lacrimal Apparatus

The lacrimal gland, tear sac, accessory glands, canaliculi, puncta (lacrimal points), and nasolacrimal duct constitute the lacrimal apparatus. The function of this system is to provide tears to lubricate the epithelial lining of the conjunctivae, cornea, and sclera. The tears play a protective role in warding off potential pathogens. When one area of this system is

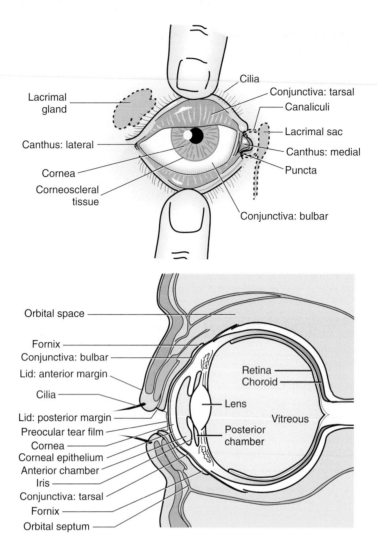

FIGURE 41-1 Common ocular structures. (Modified from Jones DB et al: Laboratory diagnosis of ocular infections. In Washington JA, editor: *Cumitech 13*, Washington, DC, 1981, American Society for Microbiology.)

clogged, the resulting malfunction may result in too many or too few tears, exposed epithelium, or gross swelling of the lids. All these conditions can lead to infection.

Anterior Chamber

The anterior chamber is the fluid-filled (aqueous humor) chamber at the front of the eye, divided by the iris into anterior and posterior cavities. Its function is to maintain the intraocular pressure. When the production of aqueous humor alters, glaucoma may result. The matrix of the aqueous humor is similar to that of the serum.

Vitreous Chamber

The vitreous chamber is filled with a gelatinous material (comprising 99% water, collagen fibers, and hyaluronic acid) and makes up about two thirds of the volume of the eye. Its major function is to maintain the elliptical shape of the eyeball. If lost (trauma, surgery), the vitreous humor must be replaced with injection of saline, gas, or other artificial substances to prevent collapse of the intraocular chambers. Vitre-

ous fluid serves as a magnificent culture medium for the growth of invading microorganisms.

Uveal Tract

The uveal tract is the middle layer of the ocular system and consists of the iris, ciliary body, and choroids. The ciliary body produces the aqueous humor that fills the chamber at the front of the eye. The iris is an extension of the ciliary body and divides this chamber into the anterior and posterior cavities. It is attached to the lens and controls the amount of light that enters the eye. The choroid is predominantly composed of blood vessels and functions to nourish the retina.

Retina

The retina is the light-sensitive, neural tissue of the eye. It is multilayered and functions as a receptor of the light stimuli, transcribing these into electrical impulses and then sending these impulses along the optic nerve to the brain.

Cones and rods are located in the retinal pigmented epithelium. Cones play a role in sharpening vision and color

TABLE 41-1 Ocular Resident Flora from Noninflamed Eyes

Organisms*	Incidence (%)
Coagulase-negative staphylococci[†]	34-94
Propionibacterium acnes[†]	40-86
Corynebacterium spp.[†]	3-83
Staphylococcus aureus	0-30
Haemophilus influenzae	0-25
Micrococcus spp.	2-22
Streptococcus pneumoniae	0-5
Viridans streptococcal group	0-12
Gram-negative rods (*Proteus* spp., *Escherichia coli, Klebsiella pneumoniae, Enterobacter* spp.)	0-5
Moraxella spp. (including *Moraxella catarrhalis*)	0-3
Bacillus spp. (*Bacillus cereus, Bacillus subtilis*)	0-4
Neisseria spp. (*Neisseria sicca, Neisseria flavescens*)	0-7
Fungi (any saprophyte, depends on locale)	0-24
Anaerobic flora other than *Propionibacterium acnes* (*Peptostreptococcus* spp., *Bacteroides* spp., *Clostridium* spp.)	1-5
β-Hemolytic streptococci, including *Streptococcus pyogenes*	0-3
Sterile	9-47

*Source is usually the conjunctivae and lids; organism isolated depends on age of patient, geographic locale, season, previous and current therapy, and underlying condition (e.g., diabetes, epithelial disease). Most common isolates usually reflect that of the surrounding tissue.
[†]Can also cause mild to severe disease in immunocompromised patients.

discrimination. Rods are important in night and peripheral vision.

Role of Indigenous Ocular Microbial Flora

Coagulase-negative staphylococci and *Corynebacterium* spp. make up 80% to 90% of indigenous flora recovered from uninflamed eyes. However, depending on the age of the patient, season, location, and underlying conditions, *Staphylococcus aureus, Streptococcus pneumoniae, Haemophilus influenzae,* and other potential pathogens may be recovered from uninfected eyes (Table 41-1). The presence of a resident flora on the conjunctivae and lids acts as a protective mechanism, inhibiting invasion and colonization by more harmful organisms.

Discriminating Between Indigenous Microbiota and Pathogens

The distinction between indigenous microbiota and ocular pathogens is blurred. Coagulase-negative staphylococci, *Propionibacterium acnes,* and *S. aureus* are responsible for a majority of intraocular and corneal infections. The presence of biomaterials, use of steroids, and antimicrobials can predispose ocular tissues to infection with indigenous flora.

Differentiating Between Colonization and Infection

Organisms may be recovered from the conjunctival sac and eyelids that do not cause disease. Quantitative ocular cultures have been used to establish a threshold to differentiate between

infection and colonization. A threshold is set for each organism. Infection is established when organisms reach or exceed the threshold numbers. Treatment efficacy of new antibacterials has also been documented using this method.

Long-term use of antimicrobials, diets, and other therapeutics can impact the usual ocular microbiota. The normal resident conjunctival and lid microbiota also changes with age. It is important to remember that once the epithelium of the conjunctiva or cornea is compromised, any organism gaining entrance can result in disease.

Host Immune Status

Because of their location, external ocular structures and surfaces, such as the conjunctivae and cornea, are frequently challenged by a variety of microorganisms. Whether an infection or damage ensues depends on the structure, immune status of the host, integrity of the underlying tissues, character of the invading organism, and immune response of the host.

Protection of ocular structures is partly supported by a defense system that includes local and systemic, specific and nonspecific, and humoral and cellular mechanisms that join together to prevent microbial colonization or invasion. Protection of these structures is further supported by an anatomic arrangement that leaves the inner ocular structures well sequestered. The intact epithelia of the lid, conjunctiva, and cornea provide a protective barrier against invasion by most microbial invasion. Tears and the tear film contain high concentrations of IgA, lysozyme, and lactoferrin. All three have antimicrobial properties. IgA coats bacteria and aids in complement fixation and phagocytosis. Lysozyme attacks bacterial cell walls by splitting bonds in the peptidoglycan layer. Lactoferrin inhibits the growth of bacteria by competing for and binding to iron. The blinking action and the flow of tears also protect the eye from infection by removing bacteria and debris from the ocular surface. Cooler ocular surface temperatures also inhibit survival of many microorganisms.

Risk factors associated with ocular infections include age, sex, race, socioeconomic status, behavior, geographic location, occupation, and underlying disease. Acute bacterial and viral conjunctivitis occurs more frequently in childhood, whereas chronic conjunctivitis and varicella-zoster virus (VZV) conjunctivitis occurs most frequently in the elderly. *S. aureus* and *Candida albicans* are most often recovered from keratitis in cooler climates; *Pseudomonas aeruginosa* and filamentous fungi are the main pathogens recovered from patients in warmer climates. Farmers and agricultural workers are diagnosed with fungal or traumatic keratitis. *Streptococcus pneumoniae* and *Moraxella* spp. are recovered from alcoholics and homeless people. Women are more likely than men to be associated with trachoma, whereas chlamydial inclusion conjunctivitis has most often been identified in men.

Virulence Factors of Ocular Pathogenic Organisms

Several microbes can penetrate the intact epithelium of the conjunctiva or cornea, including *Neisseria gonorrhoeae, Neisseria meningitidis, S. pneumoniae, Listeria monocytogenes,* and *Corynebacterium diphtheriae.*

For other microbes to enter and establish disease, a break must occur in the protective epithelial barrier. Once the intact epithelium is breached (e.g., by trauma, by insertion or removal of a contact lens), an intrusion by pathogenic and saprophytic organisms can occur. Many ocular pathogens process adhesions and enzymes that aid in adherence, multiplication, and dissemination in ocular tissues. *S. aureus, P. aeruginosa,* and coagulase-negative staphylococci may persist in ocular tissue or biomaterials in a biofilm, which protects them from host defenses, high levels of antibiotics, and eradication.

When an infection has started in one layer of the eye, spread to adjacent layers and tissues can occur rapidly. Dissemination of the infection within ocular structures can result in devastating and permanent damage to the functional integrity of the eye. Box 41-1 lists organisms recovered from ocular infections. Any organism that can gain entrance to the internal structures of the eye is capable of causing infection. The list is long and varied. Organisms considered "contaminants" or "colonizers" are the most frequent pathogens. The eye does not exist in a vacuum, and many systemic illnesses, such as tuberculosis, diabetes, hypertension, and acquired immune

---

BOX 41-1 Microorganisms Associated with Ocular Infectious Disease

Bacteria
Gram-negative (aerobic)
Alcaligenes spp.
Acinetobacter spp.
Actinobacillus actinomycetemcomitans
Achromobacter xylosoxidans
Aeromonas hydrophila
Bartonella henselae
Borrelia burgdorferi (Lyme disease)
Borrelia tularensis
Brucella spp.
Chlamydia trachomatis
Chlamydophila pneumoniae
Chlamydophila psittaci
Coxiella burnetii
Eikenella corrodens
Enterobacteriaceae
Flavobacterium spp.
Francisella tularensis
Haemophilus aegyptius
Haemophilus influenzae
Haemophilus parainfluenzae
Kingella spp.
Neisseria gonorrhoeae
Neisseria meningitidis
Moraxella catarrhalis
Moraxella lacunata
Moraxella spp.
Pseudomonas aeruginosa
Other pseudomonads
Rickettsia akari
Rickettsia prowazekii
Rickettsia rickettsii
Rickettsia tsutsugamushi
Treponema pallidum

Gram-negative (anaerobic)
Bacteroides spp.
Capnocytophaga spp. (capnophilic)
Fusobacterium spp.
Prevotella spp.

Gram-positive (aerobic)
Bacillus cereus
Bacillus spp.
β-Hemolytic streptococci (A, B, C, F, G)
Coagulase-negative staphylococci spp.
Corynebacterium spp.
Enterococcus faecalis
Enterococcus spp.

Listeria monocytogenes
Micrococcus spp.
Staphylococcus aureus
Staphylococcus epidermidis
Streptococcus pneumoniae
Streptococcus viridans group

Gram-positive (anaerobic)
Actinomyces israelii
Actinomyces spp.
Clostridium spp.
Peptostreptococcus spp.
Propionibacterium acnes
Propionibacterium propionicus

Mycobacterium spp.
Mycobacterium abscessus
Mycobacterium avium-intracellulare
Mycobacterium chelonae
Mycobacterium fortuitum
Mycobacterium gordonae
Mycobacterium leprae
Mycobacterium mucogenicum
Mycobacterium nonchromogenicum
Mycobacterium triviale
Mycobacterium tuberculosis

Parasites
Acanthamoeba spp.
Ascaris lumbricoides
Leishmania spp.
Loa loa
Microsporidia spp.
Oestrus ovis
Onchocerca volvulus
Phthirus pubis
Plasmodium spp.
Schistosoma haematobium
Taenia solium
Toxocara canis and *cati*
Toxoplasma gondii
Trichinella spiralis
Trypanosoma spp.
Vahlkampfia spp.
Wuchereria bancrofti

Viruses
Adenovirus
Coxsackievirus
Cytomegalovirus
Enterovirus

Epstein-Barr virus
Herpes simplex virus types 1 and 2
Human herpesviruses 6, 7, and 8
Human immunodeficiency virus
Human papillomavirus
Influenza virus
Measles virus
Molluscum contagiosum virus
Mumps virus
Newcastle disease virus
Vaccinia virus
Varicella-zoster virus

Fungi (moulds)
Acremonium spp.
Alternaria spp.
Aspergillus spp.
Bipolaris spp.
Blastomyces dermatitidis
Cladosporium spp.
Coccidioides immitis
Colletotrichum spp.
Curvularia spp.
Cylindrocarpon spp.
Drechslera spp.
Exophiala jeanselmei
Fusarium oxysporum
Fusarium solani
Fusarium spp.
Helminthosporium spp.
Histoplasma capsulatum
Lasiodiplodia spp.
Neurospora spp.
Paecilomyces spp.
Penicillium spp.
Phialophora spp.
Scedosporium apiospermum
Sporothrix schenckii
Volutella spp.
Zygomycetes

Fungi (yeasts)
Candida albicans
Candida spp., other *C. albicans*
Cryptococcus neoformans
Rhodococcus spp.
Torulopsis glabrata

Aerobic actinomycetes
Nocardia spp.
Streptomyces spp.

deficiency syndrome (AIDS), also have ocular symptoms and presentations. The organism most likely to be encountered depends on the season, climate, age of the patient, and underlying disease.

INFECTIONS OF THE CONJUNCTIVAE (CONJUNCTIVITIS)

Conjunctivitis is the most common ocular complaint, includes all age groups, and occurs worldwide. Symptoms may include itching, tearing, foreign body sensation, discharge (purulent, watery), and hyperemia or "red eye." Red eye constitutes more than 50% of the office visits to ophthalmologists and is the most common ocular source for microbiologic evaluation. Conjunctivitis may be acute, hyperacute, subacute, or chronic. The etiologic agents are usually bacterial or viral, although some patients have fungal or parasitic infections (Box 41-2).

Acute bacterial conjunctivitis is generally self-limiting and resolves within 10 to 14 days. If treated, the condition may resolve in 1 to 3 days. Corneal involvement may follow conjunctivitis and compromise vision. The conjunctiva may also be the entry site for *N. meningitidis* and lead to meningitis and septicemia. Chronic infections are more difficult to manage and result in long-term ocular morbidity and compromised vision.

Bacteria

Acute Bacterial Conjunctivitis

In warm climates, *S. aureus* is the most frequently isolated pathogen, whereas *S. pneumoniae* may be the most common isolate in areas with cooler temperatures. *H. influenzae, S. aureus, S. pneumoniae,* and other *Streptococcus* spp. and members of the Enterobacteriaceae are the most frequently isolated organisms from infants and children with acute conjunctivitis. *N. gonorrhoeae* (Figure 41-2) and *N. meningitidis* cause a hyperacute conjunctivitis that produces huge amounts of exudate that runs down the face of the patient. Infants acquire *N. gonorrhoeae* as they travel down an infected birth canal. Symptoms may appear within 5 to 7 days after exposure to the pathogen. It is believed that adults acquire gonococcal conjunctivitis through self-inoculation. Meningococcal conjunctivitis may result from contiguous spread from the respiratory tract.

Chronic Bacterial Conjunctivitis

The etiologic agents in chronic conjunctivitis are less clear. The microorganisms that have been isolated include coagulase-negative staphylococcal species, *S. aureus,* and *Propionibacterium acnes.* Chronic conjunctivitis may result from an

---

BOX 41-2 Microorganisms Associated with Conjunctivitis

Bacteria
Gram-negative
Acinetobacter spp.
Bartonella henselae
Borrelia burgdorferi
Enterobacteriaceae (e.g., *Escherichia coli, Proteus mirabilis,*
   Shigella spp.)
Francisella tularensis
Haemophilus influenzae
Haemophilus ducreyi
Moraxella catarrhalis
Moraxella lacunata (other *Moraxella* spp.)
Neisseria gonorrhoeae
Neisseria meningitidis
Pseudomonas aeruginosa
Rickettsia spp. (*R. rickettsii, R. typhi*)
Treponema pallidum
Yersinia enterocolitica

Gram-positive
β-Hemolytic streptococci (A, B, C, G)
Corynebacterium diphtheriae
Corynebacterium spp.
Listeria monocytogenes
Mycobacterium tuberculosis
Staphylococcus aureus
Staphylococcus epidermidis
Streptococcus pneumoniae
Viridans streptococci

Viruses
Adenovirus
Human coronavirus

Herpesviruses (1 to 8)
Influenza virus
Paramyxoviruses (measles, mumps, Newcastle disease)
Picornaviruses (echovirus, enterovirus, coxsackievirus, polio)
Poxviruses (molluscum contagiosum, vaccinia, variola)

***Chlamydia* and related spp.**
Chlamydophila pneumoniae
Chlamydia psittaci
Chlamydia trachomatis

Fungi (rare)
Candida spp.
Coccidioides immitis
Rhinosporidium seeberi
Sporothrix schenckii

Parasites (rare)
Ascaris lumbricoides
Fly larvae (*Oestrus ovis,* myiasis)
Loa loa
Microsporidia
Onchocerca volvulus
Pthirus pubis
Schistosoma haematobium
Taenia solium
Thelazia californiensis
Trichinella spiralis
Toxocara canis
Wuchereria bancrofti

interplay between the organism and the aggressive ocular immune response.

Bacterial conjunctivitis can also be caused by instillation of contaminated cosmetics or medications. The organisms encountered in such infections are *S. aureus, Staphylococcus epidermidis, Corynebacterium* spp., *P. aeruginosa,* and *Proteus mirabilis.* Allergic and chemical conjunctivitis can sometimes be confused with microbial infections.

Laboratory Diagnosis. Laboratory tests can be of assistance in differentiating acute, allergic, and chronic conjunctivitis. Conjunctival scrapings are collected using a Kimura spatula, blade, or sterile swab and plated directly onto slides and culture media. Routine stains (Gram, Giemsa) and culture should reveal the etiologic agent in most acute cases. Smears and cultures should be collected in all cases of purulent, membranous, or pseudomembranous conjunctivitis. Laboratory workup is mandatory for all neonatal and infant conjunctivitis. Culture and smears may be of less value in establishing the etiologic agent in chronic conjunctivitis.

Treatment. The majority of bacterial conjunctivitis cases are self-limiting and resolve without antibiotics. Antibiotics may reduce symptoms and prevent secondary infections. Empirical topical therapy is often started before antibiotic

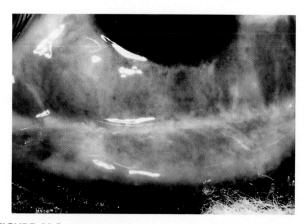

FIGURE 41-2 Gonococcal conjunctivitis. Note the copious discharge in response to invasion by *Neisseria gonorrhoeae.*

sensitivity testing. Targeted therapy is then adjusted based on the isolated organism.

Chlamydial Ocular Infections

Chlamydia trachomatis causes a myriad of ocular infections, including neonatal conjunctivitis, inclusion conjunctivitis (Figure 41-3, *A*), lymphogranuloma venereum (LGV), and trachoma. Currently, 15 serotypes (A, B, Ba, C through K, L1 through L3), or serovars, of *C. trachomatis* exist. Certain serovars are associated with certain clinical entities. Trachoma, which is "as old as recorded history," is usually caused by serotypes A, B, or C, whereas immunotypes D to K are usually associated with oculogenital (inclusion conjunctivitis) chlamydiae. Neonatal conjunctivitis occurs when the infant is infected while traveling down a contaminated birth canal. Infection becomes apparent within 8 to 10 days. LGV (serotypes LGV 1, 2, 3) is strictly a sexually transmitted disease (STD) and conjunctival inoculation is accidental.

Case Study

A sexually active 17-year-old girl presented with a 2-week history of pain, redness, and purulent discharge affecting both eyes. The patient had vaginitis, inguinal and cervical lymphadenopathy, a history of *N. gonorrhoeae* infection, and Sjögren's syndrome. The conjunctivae were puffy and displayed a mixed papillary and follicular reaction. Oculoglandular syndrome was diagnosed. Conjunctival smears and cultures collected from both eyes were submitted to rule out bacteria, chlamydia, and fungi. Serum was collected to rule out *Rickettsia* and tularemia, and to determine HIV status. *Chlamydia trachomatis* serovar L2 was isolated from the patient. The diagnosis was lymphogranuloma venereum (LGV) with ocular involvement. IgG chlamydia titers were 1 : 1024. A microimmunofluorescent assay was used to determine the serovar.

C. trachomatis inclusion conjunctivitis can lead to pharyngitis, otitis media, and interstitial pneumonitis in the newborn. Chronic conjunctivitis with cornea involvement is a consequence of untreated or inadequately treated inclusion conjunctivitis. Trachoma is an ancient disease and is a leading cause of world blindness. Regional variation in prevalence

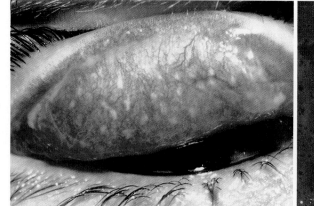
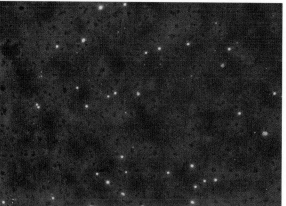

FIGURE 41-3 **A,** White spots on the conjunctiva represent pockets of *Chlamydia* organisms in tissue. **B,** Immunofluorescence stain of scrapings from neonatal conjunctivitis, confirming the presence of chlamydial elementary bodies.

and severity occurs. Worldwide, 400 million people in Africa, Asia, Latin America, Australia, and the Pacific Islands suffer from the disease. In the United States, it affects mainly the poor or those with poor personal hygiene. The initial conjunctivitis is follicular conjunctivitis, followed by repeat infections, which lead to scarring and blindness. Nasolacrimal duct obstruction and dacryocystitis (infection of the lacrimal sac caused by obstruction; usually seen in children) are complications that follow trachoma.

A chronic conjunctivitis leading to scarring and chronic keratitis may follow trachoma and inclusion conjunctivitis.

Laboratory Diagnosis. Direct detection of the chlamydial inclusions or elementary bodies in scrapings or on impression cytology membranes are among the most sensitive methods for confirming ocular *Chlamydia* (see Figure 41-3, *B*). Cultures using McCoy or Hep-2 cells may be used to confirm the diagnosis, especially in cases of suspected trachoma. Other nonculture detection methods—polymerase chain reaction (PCR), ligase chain reaction (LCR), and enzyme immunoassay (EIA)—may also be used to detect ocular *Chlamydia*. A combination of smear and culture with PCR, LCR, or EIA may offer the best system in populations with high and low rates of STD and in areas where trachoma remains endemic.

The prevalence rates for ocular chlamydial infection parallel those of genital disease. In areas with high rates of STD, ocular disease rates are also high. Populations with the highest incidence of disease include neonates and sexually active adolescents and adults. The incidence can range from 20% to 90%, depending on the age group. In areas with low rates of STD, ocular chlamydial infection rates also are low.

Treatment. Topical treatment alone is inadequate. Current Centers for Disease Control and Prevention (CDC) treatment recommendations for ocular chlamydia are as follows:
- *Adults*—doxycycline: 100 mg twice a day for 7 days; or, azithromycin: 1 g by mouth as a single dose
- *Neonates*—erythromycin syrup: 50 mg/kg/day by mouth in four doses for 14 days

Chlamydia psittaci ocular infections are due to incidental transmission from infected birds. *Chlamydophila pneumoniae* was originally isolated from the conjunctiva of a child. Most adults will have antibodies against this organism. Acute ocular infections with this organism are rare. It has been isolated most often in lower respiratory tract infections.

Both of these organisms can be isolated in tissue culture, but molecular detection and serology are most often used for confirmation. Erythromycin, doxycycline, and tetracycline are first-line drugs for ocular management of these infections.

Viruses

Viral conjunctivitis is the most commonly recognized ocular infectious disease. It may also present as an acute or chronic illness, ranging from a mild, self-limiting condition to a severe, destructive disease resulting in impaired vision. Corneal involvement often follows viral infection of the conjunctiva.

Nosocomial transmission of adenoviruses may occur during ocular examinations, and the virus persists in solutions or on tonometer tips. Use of unit dose packages or sterile drops augmented with frequent handwashings can reduce the risk of transmission to patients and health care providers. The tonometer tips should be cleaned with alcohol, rinsed with sterile water, and allowed to dry. Patients exposed to contaminated body fluids, fomites, or vesicular fluids are at increased risks for infection with herpes simplex virus (HSV), VZV, or epidemic **keratoconjunctivitis** (EKC).

Acute Viral Conjunctivitis

Acute viral infections are attributed mainly to adenoviruses, herpesviruses, or enteroviruses. The adenoviruses are responsible for two distinct ocular viral syndromes.

The first, EKC, is quite contagious and associated with adenovirus types 8 and 19, but recovery of serovars 7, 9, 10, 11, 14, and 16 has also been documented. The second syndrome, pharyngoconjunctival fever (PCF), is caused regularly by adenovirus type 3 and occasionally by serovars 1, 2, 4, 5, 6, 8, and 14. Both syndromes are self-limiting and have no specific treatment; PCF lasts about 10 days, and EKC lasts 3 to 4 weeks at most. A highly contagious disease, EKC may be spread by direct contact or fomites and is not uncommonly spread by physicians. It is usually responsible for outbreaks in ophthalmic offices and clinics, school locker rooms, or college dormitories. Acute hemorrhagic conjunctivitis (Figure 41-4), or epidemic hemorrhagic conjunctivitis (EHC), is an acute short-lived infection that is caused by enterovirus 70, coxsackievirus A24, and on rare occasions, adenovirus type 11. It is often called the Apollo XI conjunctivitis because it was first recognized in Ghana during the time of the Apollo XI moon mission. The onset of symptoms usually occurs within 8 to 48 hours of exposure, with patients complaining of pain, sensitivity to light, copious tears, and subconjunctival hemorrhages. It is self-limiting and has no outlined treatment program. Recovery occurs within 5 to 7 days. Because EHC is highly contagious and easily spread from person to person, patients should be isolated or sent home until the condition has resolved. Herpes simplex blepharoconjunctivitis is responsible for the majority of severe ocular viral infections. This disease usually occurs in young children. It is important to make the distinction between HSV and adenovirus etiologies,

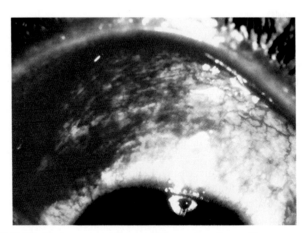

FIGURE 41-4 Acute hemorrhagic conjunctivitis. The etiologic agent is usually enterovirus 70 or coxsackievirus A24. Other members of the enterovirus group may also be recovered. Note the heavy conjunctival hemorrhaging.

because HSV can be treated with specific ocular antiviral medications, whereas an adenovirus infection must run its course. More than 90% of cases of this herpes simplex blepharoconjunctivitis are caused by HSV-1, but HSV-2 has been isolated from infants and adults. VZV may also cause conjunctivitis. This condition is usually a manifestation of the systemic disease chickenpox or a complication of herpes zoster ophthalmicus. Cytomegalovirus can usually cause conjunctivitis when it becomes disseminated or is transmitted through tears from another patient. Epstein-Barr virus (EBV) conjunctivitis may result as a complication of infectious mononucleosis.

Chronic Viral Conjunctivitis

Chronic viral conjunctivitis may result from molluscum contagiosum or vaccinia, a complication of smallpox vaccination.

Laboratory Diagnosis. Conjunctival scrapings may be stained with monoclonal antibodies to confirm infections with the ocular viral pathogens. The most common pathogens may be grown in tissue culture and serotyped with monoclonal antibodies or neutralization tests.

Treatment. Currently there is no treatment for adenoviral and/or enteroviral ocular infections. Cold compresses may help alleviate some of the symptoms. Oral acyclovir can be used to treat severe cases of HSV and VZV infections.

Rickettsia

All pathogenic human rickettsiae are capable of causing conjunctivitis. The conjunctiva is often the portal of entry for Rocky Mountain spotted fever, scrub typhus, Q fever, endemic murine typhus, and Marseilles fever. This type of conjunctivitis is usually mild but can be a severe complication of the systemic disease. Isolation of rickettsiae is difficult, and confirmation is usually by serologic methods. The most sensitive and specific tests for confirmation of rickettsial infection are microimmunofluorescence, microagglutination, complement fixation, and PCR. Treatment with chloramphenicol or tetracycline can inhibit rickettsial organisms long enough for the body to clear them from the system.

Fungi

Although various fungi can be isolated from the uninflamed eye, fungal conjunctivitis is relatively rare. The organisms that have been recovered from fungal conjunctivitis are *Candida* spp. and *Sporothrix schenckii*. Systemic fungal infections caused by *Coccidioides immitis, Histoplasma capsulatum,* and *Cryptococcus neoformans* may extend to the conjunctival tissue and cause disease. A high index of suspicion is needed by the physician to diagnose fungal conjunctivitis, and the laboratory must be alerted to ensure the proper setup for recovery of these organisms. Laboratory diagnosis includes recovery on routine media and detection on Gram and Giemsa stains. Natamycin and amphotericin B ocular preparations are used to treat common infections.

Parasites

Parasitic infestation of the conjunctiva is rare. The conjunctiva is among the least affected ocular sites and is usually a secondary complication. Ophthalmomyiasis ("fly larvae conjunctivitis") or ocular myiasis is caused by the deposit of fly larvae (maggots) into the conjunctival sac. This infestation occurs frequently in the tropics but can occur wherever people and flies coexist. The maggots may be removed by paralyzing them with 10% cocaine and lifting them out with tweezers.

Loa loa, the "eye worm," is one of the leading causes of blindness in West Africa (river blindness). Clinical symptoms are caused by the continuous migration of the adult worms into the subcutaneous tissues and blood vessels. Onchocerciasis, which is transmitted by the bite of the blackfly, is also a leading cause of blindness in Africa and is now endemic in South and Central America. Ocular complications result from the discharge of large numbers of microfilariae by the adult female and their subsequent local invasion and tissue damage. Recovery and diagnosis of ocular involvement depends on observing and removing the actual protozoans and confirming their presence through histologic stains, isolating the organisms from blood or tissues, or confirming their presence by serologic means. Diethylcarbamazine is the drug of choice.

INFECTIONS OF THE LIDS (BLEPHARITIS)

Blepharitis (inflammation of the lid margins) and inflammation of the conjunctivae are not mutually exclusive. Conjunctivitis usually presents as a blepharoconjunctivitis. Therefore any organism that causes conjunctivitis can affect the lids. However, each site has unique organisms and conditions. The skin covering of the lids is among the thinnest on the body. Any organisms capable of initiating skin infections can also cause blepharitis.

Bacteria

Staphylococcus aureus and members of the coagulase-negative staphylococcal family are the most frequently isolated bacteria from the lid margins. Blepharitis involving these organisms is a low-grade inflammation associated with functional disease of the seborrheic glands (seborrheic blepharitis). In this mixed infection, dry (staphylococcal) and greasy (seborrheic) scales are attached to the lashes, with various areas of ulcerations that cause the lashes to fall out. Antibiotics are given to cure the staphylococcal disease. Because the scalp, eyebrows, and lids are all involved in seborrhiasis, all must be kept clean with a medicated shampoo.

Four types of glands are located in the lids: the meibomian gland, the glands of Moll and Zeis, and the accessory lacrimal glands. Acute infection of the glands of Zeis or Moll with staphylococci results in an external hordeolum (stye). A stye is an abscess with pus formation in the lumen of the affected gland. Hot soaks assist in the continuous drainage of the abscess. Topical erythromycin or tetracycline may be applied as supplementary therapy. An internal hordeolum caused by staphylococci is a little larger and affects the meibomian gland. Additional lid glandular disorders include formation of a chalazion, a sterile granulomatous inflammation of the meibomian gland that usually subsides spontaneously. Meibomianitis is inflammation of multiple glands; its etiology is unknown. Only rarely does the laboratory receive a request for lid culture. If such a request is received, it is to confirm the presence of staphylococci and determine whether therapy is adequate. Other microbial agents recovered from patients with blepharitis are listed in Box 41-3. *Bacillus anthracis* causes carbuncle-like lesions on the lid margins, which are eradicated with penicillin. *Actinomyces* spp. may spread from the facial skin to the lids. *Mycobacterium* spp. that cause ocular infections are listed in Box 41-1.

Viruses

Viral blepharitis may be caused by HSV-1 or -2, VZV, poxvirus, papovavirus, or vaccinia. HSV infection usually occurs during early childhood. Vesicles appear on the lid margins and the skin around the eye. The vesicles break open and form crusted secondary lesions, which then may become superinfected by skin organisms. Direct detection with immunofluorescence or immunoperoxidase can be done by scraping the base of a freshly opened vesicle. Vesicular fluids are collected for culture. Ninety-five percent or more of cultures grow HSV within 72 hours or less.

When the face is involved during episodes of chickenpox (varicella), vesicles may appear on the upper or lower lid margins. Molluscum contagiosum is a wartlike lesion of the lid margins that is produced by poxvirus. The lesion is waxy and pearly white with an umbilicated center. Expression (squeezing) of the white center to allow blood into the lesion is usually adequate management. Vaccinia infection of the lids results from direct inoculation from a smallpox vaccination. Other viruses that produce ocular warts are members of the papillomavirus family.

Fungi

Fungal blepharitis is rare and is usually a complication of systemic disease, especially involving *Candida* spp. and *Blastomyces dermatitidis.*

Parasites

Parasitic lid complications may be observed in patients with cutaneous leishmaniasis, African or American trypanosomiasis, *Loa loa* infections, and dirofilariasis. The crab, or pubic louse *(Phthirus pubis),* infests the cilia and lid margins of the eyelids. The patient's main complaint is pruritus, or itching. All members of the patient's family must be treated. Treatment consists of application of a 1% γ-benzene hexachloride (lindane) ointment or shampoo to the affected areas. Laboratory studies and treatment are as for conjunctivitis.

INFECTIONS OF THE CORNEA (KERATITIS)

Microbial **keratitis** is considered a true ocular emergency. Few organisms can invade the intact cornea. If the cornea epithelium is breached by trauma, by contact lens insertion and removal, or by surgery, organisms can enter and cause infections. Infection begins in the most superficial layer (the epithelium); if not checked, infection advances through the Bowman zone, the stroma (excellent culture media), and the Descemet's membrane to the endothelium (the innermost layer). Perforation of the Descemet's membrane compromises vision and must be treated aggressively with antimicrobials and/or surgical intervention.

In the United States, contact lens wear is the greatest risk factor for development microbial keratitis. Incidence of contact lens related keratitis ranges from 1.0 to 4.2 per 10,000 population for daily contact lens wearers to 2.7 to 36.8 per 10,000 population for extended wearers. Additional risk factors for microbial keratitis include trauma and refractive surgery.

Bacteria

Geographic variations in the etiology of bacterial and fungal ulcers are evident for certain regions of the United States. Historically, *P. aeruginosa,* the most frequent isolate recovered from contact lens–associated keratitis, constitutes as much as 50% of the cases of keratitis reported in Florida; however, *S. aureus* is the most frequent pathogen in other regions of the country (Figure 41-5). Cases include patients wearing soft, daily, extended-wear, and disposable contact lenses (Figure 41-6, *A*). Figure 41-6, *B*, shows the recent trends in the types of bacteria recovered from contact lenses and solutions.

Mycobacterium chelonae, Mycobacterium abscessus, and other rapid growers are being isolated with increasing fre-

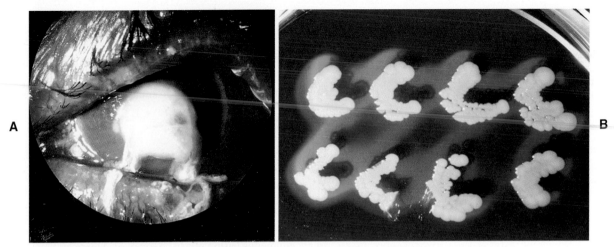

FIGURE 41-5 **A,** Corneal melt caused by bacterial invasion. **B,** C streaks of *Staphylococcus aureus* from infected cornea. The enzymes produced by some strains of *S. aureus* and *Pseudomonas aeruginosa* can liquefy the cornea within 48 hours.

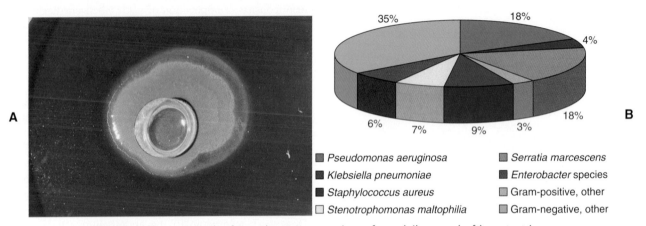

- Pseudomonas aeruginosa
- Klebsiella pneumoniae
- Staphylococcus aureus
- Stenotrophomonas maltophilia
- Serratia marcescens
- Enterobacter species
- Gram-positive, other
- Gram-negative, other

FIGURE 41-6 **A,** Growth of *Pseudomonas aeruginosa* from daily-wear (soft) contact lens. Patient had an ulcerative keratitis. The corneal culture also grew *P. aeruginosa.* **B,** Recent trends in bacteria recovered from contact lenses and solutions.

quency from patients with keratitis (Figure 41-7). Risk factors include refractive surgery (LASIK), trauma, and contact lens use. Reservoirs include contaminated instruments and/or exposure to contaminated soil and water. Less frequently encountered corneal isolates are listed in Box 41-4.

Laboratory Diagnosis

Laboratory assistance with diagnosis is mandatory in all cases of suppurative keratitis or keratitis not responding to therapy. Scrapings for smears and cultures are collected by an ophthalmologist and inoculated directly onto slides and culture plates and sent immediately to the laboratory for evaluation. Scrapings for stains can afford the physician an early indication of the offending organism and assist in the selection of appropriate therapy. The cornea may also be invaded via metastatic spread from the conjunctiva or systemic lesions.

Treatment

Therapy is often selected on the basis of the smear results and or chosen empirically for the most likely pathogen. Manage-

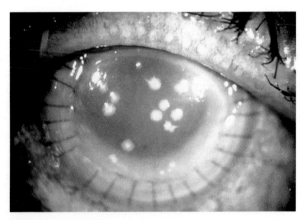

FIGURE 41-7 Colonies of *Mycobacterium fortuitum* growing on infected corneal graft tissue.

BOX **41-4** MOTT Keratitis Isolates

Mycobacterium abscessus
Mycobacterium asiaticum
Mycobacterium avium-intracellulare
Mycobacterium chelonae
Mycobacterium fortuitum
Mycobacterium gordonae
Mycobacterium mucogenicum
Mycobacterium nonchromogenicum
Mycobacterium szulgai
Mycobacterium triviale

Note: *Mycobacterium tuberculosis* and *Mycobacterium leprae* are ocular pathogens and are usually an extension of systemic disease. Isolates are frequently recovered from patients who wear contact lenses, have a history of eye trauma from soil or water, or have undergone refractive surgery.
MOTT, Mycobacteria other than tubercle bacilli.

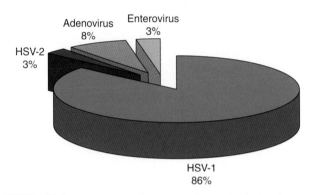

FIGURE 41-8 Frequency of common keratitis viral isolates in southern Florida. *HSV-1,* Herpes simplex virus type 1; *HSV-2,* herpes simplex virus type 2.

ment includes topical antibiotic drops or ointments supplemented with oral or systemic antimicrobials.

Viruses

Herpes simplex viruses are the leading cause of infectious blindness and ocular morbidity in the United States and other industrialized countries. Approximately 500,000 new cases occur each year. Keratitis caused by HSV may result from direct inoculation or reactivation of latent virus in the trigeminal ganglion. The majority of the ocular lesions are caused by HSV-1, but HSV-2 has been recovered from cases involving both infants and adults. Figure 41-8 shows the frequency of common keratitis viral isolates in southern Florida. Scarring and blindness result from repeat outbreaks and surgical interventions. The lesions caused by these two are indistinguishable.

Laboratory diagnosis includes direct detection using monoclonal antibodies, DNA probes, commercial kits, PCR, and/or growth in tissue culture. Treatment includes debridement when possible, topical antivirals, and corneal transplants. Other viral agents that cause keratitis are listed in Box 41-5.

BOX **41-5** Microorganisms Associated with Keratitis

Bacteria
Gram-negative isolates
Haemophilus influenzae
Moraxella spp.
Proteus mirabilis
Pseudomonas aeruginosa
Serratia marcescens

Gram-positive isolates
Corynebacterium spp.
Staphylococcus aureus
Staphylococcus epidermidis and other coagulase-negative staphylococci
Streptococcus pneumoniae
Streptococcus viridans group

Uncommon Keratitis Isolates
Nocardia spp.
Capnocytophaga spp.
Propionibacterium acnes
Mycobacteria other than tubercle bacilli
Acanthamoeba, other free-living amebae

Viruses
Adenovirus
Cytomegalovirus
Enterovirus
Epstein-Barr virus
Herpes simplex virus types 1 and 2
Human immunodeficiency virus (tears and stroma)
Measles
Mumps
Newcastle disease virus
Vaccinia
Varicella-zoster virus

Fungi
Acremonium spp.
Alternaria spp.
Aspergillus spp.
Bipolaris
Candida spp. (*Candida parapsilosis* and *Candida tropicalis*—most common)
Colletotrichum spp.
Curvularia spp.
Cylindrocarpon spp.
Fusarium spp. (*Fusarium solani* and *Fusarium oxysporum*—most common)
Lasiodiplodia theobromae
Paecilomyces spp.
Phialophora spp.
Pseudallescheria boydii
Trichosporon beigelii

Fungi

Fungal infections of the cornea are associated most often with opportunistic or saprophytic organisms. More than 70 genera have been documented as etiologic agents in fungal keratitis. Filamentous species, mainly *Fusarium* and *Aspergillus* spp., are common pathogens in warm climates, whereas *Candida* spp. are most often recovered in cooler climates. Patients commonly have a history of trauma involving soil or plant material. Long-term antibiotic treatment may also predispose patients to fungal colonization and invasion. All cases of fungal keratitis must be confirmed by the laboratory. Fungal keratitis agents are listed in Box 41-5.

Laboratory Diagnosis

Samples for culture must be collected from multiple scrapings of the involved, actively advancing edges of the ulcer. Sometimes a biopsy is necessary to isolate the fungi. Giemsa and calcofluor white preparations from scrapings can confirm hyphal elements or budding yeast. Antifungal therapy can be instituted once a fungal etiology has been established.

Treatment

Topical antifungals include amphotericin B, natamycin, nystatin, and imidazole compounds. Topical preparations from systemic antifungals may be used to manage fungal keratitis. Selection depends on the organism. Often corneal transplant is necessary to restore sight.

Parasites

Infection of the cornea by free-living amebae (e.g., *Acanthamoeba* spp., *Naegleria* spp., and *Vahlkampfia* spp.) is a painful and sight-threatening consequence of injury or exposure to contaminated water, contact lenses, or soil. *Acanthamoeba* spp. are the most frequent isolates. Homemade saline solution associated with contact lens wear was the original identified risk factor. This factor seems to play a lesser role in the diagnosis of amebic keratitis today. Currently, trauma and swimming in contaminated pools, lakes, or rivers are the most frequently identified risk factors. Amebic keratitis is often mistaken for viral or fungal keratitis, and a diagnosis of amebic keratitis is made only when all other cultures (bacterial, fungal, and viral) are negative.

Laboratory Diagnosis

Scrapings are collected and placed in the center of two nonnutrient agar plates. A few drops containing heat-killed or "live" *Escherichia coli* are placed over the tissue. The plates are sealed with tape, and one is placed at room temperature and the second in the incubator (35°C). If only one plate is collected, it should be incubated at 35°C. Scrapings also may be inoculated into tissue culture, and maintenance media may be added. The amebae cause a generalized destruction of the tissue culture cells. A third method of cultivation is to grow free-living amebae in broth (axenic) culture. *Acanthamoeba* spp. may also be confirmed using molecular techniques.

Depending on the quality of the scrapings and the infectious dose of the organism, *Acanthamoeba* trophozoites may be seen on agar within 48 hours. The polygonal, double-walled cysts may be detected on a direct smear with either Giemsa or calcofluor white stain. Trophozoites are much less discernible on smear and are best seen in "tracts" on the agar (Figure 41-9).

Treatment

Treatment includes debridement in early disease and topical propamidine isethionate (1%) solution supplemented with

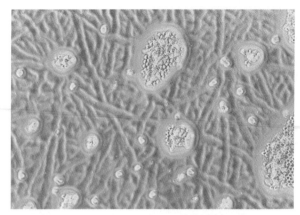

FIGURE 41-9 "Tracts" of *Acanthamoeba* trophozoites. The meandering trophozoites are at the end of the tracts. The large clusters of organisms contain trophozoites and cysts.

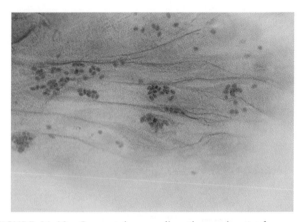

FIGURE 41-10 Gram stain revealing the oval cyst of *Microsporidia* spp. Organisms can also be detected with Giemsa, acid-fast, and calcofluor white stains.

neomycin drops or polyhexamethylene biguanide (0.01% to 0.02% solution). Corneal transplants are often necessary.

Microsporidian keratitis, seen in immunocompromised patients, is a disease that has appeared fairly recently. Microsporidiosis is usually a disease associated with bees or other insects. The microsporidians are intracellular, spore-forming protozoans. In humans, both ocular and nonocular diseases have been reported. Currently, this is an emerging disease in patients with AIDS. The protozoan is an obligate intracellular parasite that infects ocular conjunctivae and corneal tissue. Its size may range from 1 to 20 μm, and it has a round or spherical shape (Figure 41-10). The organism develops in two stages, the schizogenic and the sporulation, or sporogenic, phase. Infection is by the fecal-oral route. Spores may be detected on Gram, Giemsa, acid-fast, or calcofluor white stains. Electron microscopy is usually required for classification and confirmation. No uniform treatment is used.

Detection of ocular parasites is based on (1) observing and removing the actual protozoan, (2) confirming the presence of the organism with histologic or other stains, and (3) isolating the organisms from blood, tissues, or body fluids. Treatment depends on the organism and the availability of an effective anti-infective.

BOX 41-6 Microorganisms Associated with Scleritis

Bacteria
Borrelia burgdorferi
Moraxella spp.
Mycobacterium chelonae
Mycobacterium fortuitum
Mycobacterium leprae
Mycobacterium tuberculosis
Nocardia spp.
Other Enterobacteriaceae
Pseudomonas aeruginosa
Staphylococcus aureus
Staphylococcus epidermidis
Serratia marcescens
Streptococcus pneumoniae, other streptococci
Treponema pallidum

Fungi
Aspergillus spp.
Curvularia spp.
Fusarium spp.
Paecilomyces spp.

Viruses
Herpes simplex virus 1 and 2
Mumps
Varicella-zoster virus

Parasites
Acanthamoeba spp.
Toxoplasma gondii
Toxocara spp.

INFECTIONS OF THE SCLERA AND EPISCLERA (SCLERITIS AND EPISCLERITIS)

The sclera is composed of tough collagen fibers, and few organisms can penetrate this strong protective coat. Infections are protracted, painful, and quite destructive. **Scleritis** is usually a local manifestation of systemic connective tissue disease (e.g., rheumatoid arthritis, lupus) or the result of contiguous spread from adjacent ocular tissues. The presentation may be acute (pyogenic) or chronic (granulomatous). The episclera is a thin layer of elastic vascular tissue that overlies the sclera. Inflammation of this tissue is termed *episcleritis*. Episcleritis is more common than scleritis and has an undetermined etiology in 70% of cases. Etiologic agents of scleritis are listed in Box 41-6.

Laboratory diagnosis includes collection of tissue or discharge from the site and plating on routine and special media to rule common and infrequent isolates. Treatment is dependent on organisms. Surgical intervention may be necessary to retard progression.

INFECTIONS OF THE ORBIT (PRESEPTAL AND ORBITAL CELLULITIS)

Preseptal cellulitis is infection of the eyelids and soft tissues surrounding the orbit. It is a medical emergency in children.

Infection can lead to blindness or death if not treated immediately and aggressively in all age groups. Predisposing factors include trauma, lower respiratory infections, impetigo, and herpetic diseases. *S. aureus, H. influenzae, S. pneumoniae,* and *S. pyogenes* are recovered in the majority of preseptal cellulitis. Laboratory workup includes Gram stains, aerobic cultures, and anaerobic cultures. Antibiotic choice depends on the organisms. Broad-spectrum coverage is for *S. aureus, H. influenzae, S. pneumoniae,* and *S. pyogenes,* which constitute 95% of the microorganisms recovered from cases of preseptal cellulitis.

Infections of the orbit and associated structures may have a devastating effect on vision and ocular structural integrity. The close proximity of the orbit and related tissues to the parasinuses, the absence of an effective drainage system from this "closed-box" construction, and the unique structure of the lids all predispose this area to invasion by various microorganisms. Microorganisms can gain entry into the orbital tissue through trauma or injury to the eyelids or orbit resulting from surgery, infections of the eyelids and adjacent skin, upper respiratory tract infections, and dental caries. Parasites may also invade the orbital tissue and cause considerable destruction. Orbital infections are also considered extensions of bacterial or fungal sinus infections. Because of the close proximity of the orbital cavity to the parasinuses, any organisms that initiate sinusitis will also cause **orbital cellulitis.** Various anaerobic organisms are isolated from samples from patients with orbital cellulitis associated with long-standing chronic sinusitis. The majority of these infections are caused by bacteria, but saprophytic fungi may also be involved (Box 41-7). Usually both aerobic and anaerobic bacteria are isolated from these infections. Chronic orbital cellulitis may be caused by *Mycobacterium* spp., *Nocardia* spp., and *Actinomyces* spp. Bacterial infections associated with orbital implants or prostheses present increasing threats to useful vision. The organisms recovered include *M. chelonae, Nocardia* spp., *S. epidermidis, Capnocytophaga* spp., *Candida parapsilosis,* and *P. acnes.* Trichinosis, caused by the nematode *Trichinella spiralis,* can invade the extraocular muscles and result in periorbital edema and pain on movement. It is the ophthalmologist who usually makes the diagnosis of trichinosis, because invasion of the ocular muscles is usually the first sign of this disease.

Other parasitic infections are rare. The larvae of *Echinococcus granulosus* may invade orbital tissue, inducing a hydatid cyst that must be surgically exposed and whose contents must be aspirated. Maggots (fly larvae) may occasionally be deposited in the orbit and associated tissues.

Laboratory Diagnosis

Aspirations for smears and cultures are collected onto slides by an ophthalmologist and sent immediately to the laboratory for evaluation. Stains from tissues and/or aspirations can afford the physician an early indication of the offending organism and assist in the selection of appropriate therapy.

Treatment

Systemic therapy should be instituted as soon as appropriate culture samples (conjunctiva, nasal, and blood) are collected.

BOX 41-7 Microorganisms Associated with Orbital Cellulitis

Bacteria
Actinomyces spp.
Capnocytophaga spp.
Fusobacterium spp.
Eikenella corrodens, Pasteurella multocida (associated with dog bites)
Haemophilus influenzae
Moraxella catarrhalis
Mycobacterium tuberculosis
MOTT (*Mycobacterium chelonae, Mycobacterium fortuitum*—most frequent)
Nocardia spp.
Propionibacterium acnes
Staphylococcus aureus
Staphylococcus epidermidis
Streptococcus pneumoniae
Streptococcus pyogenes, other β-streptococci

Fungi
Aspergillus spp.
Bipolaris spp.
Candida parapsilosis
Curvularia spp.
Mucor, Rhizopus, and *Absidia* spp.
Penicillin spp.
Sporotrichum spp.

Parasites
Echinococcus granulosus
Fly larvae (maggots)
Trichinella spiralis

BOX 41-8 Microorganisms Associated with Lacrimal Apparatus Infections

Bacteria
Staphylococcus aureus
Streptococcus pneumoniae
Streptococcus pyogenes
Haemophilus influenzae
Pseudomonas aeruginosa
Proteus mirabilis
Chlamydia trachomatis
Treponema pallidum
Actinomyces israelii
Propionibacterium acnes, Propionibacterium propionicus
Capnocytophaga spp.
Fusobacterium spp.
Mycobacterium tuberculosis
Mycobacterium leprae

Viruses
Coxsackie A virus
Cytomegalovirus
Echovirus
Epstein-Barr virus
Herpes simplex virus types 1 and 2
Influenza
Measles
Varicella-zoster virus

Fungi
Aspergillus spp.
Candida albicans
Rhizopus, Mucor, Rhizopus spp.

Parasites
Cysticercus cellulosae
Onchocerca volvulus
Schistosoma haematobium

Therapy should provide coverage for both aerobic and anaerobic pathogens.

INFECTIONS OF THE LACRIMAL APPARATUS

The lacrimal glands, accessory glands, puncta, canaliculi, tear sac, and nasolacrimal duct together are known as the *lacrimal apparatus,* which has two functions. First, the lacrimal and accessory glands produce the aqueous component of the tear film. Second, the puncta, canaliculi, lacrimal sac, and nasolacrimal duct drain the tears from the conjunctiva cul-de-sac to the nasal cavity. Disorders and infections of the lacrimal apparatus are caused by blockage or underproduction or overproduction of tears.

Dacryoadenitis, inflammation of the main lacrimal gland, may be infectious or noninfectious. Organisms are seeded into the gland via the bloodstream. Blunt trauma also predisposes the gland to infection. Bacterial isolates include *N. gonorrhoeae, S. aureus,* and *Streptococcus* spp. Chronic bacterial infections of the gland involve tuberculosis, syphilis, or leprosy. Mucormycosis and aspergillosis may result from contiguous spread from infections of the orbit. Mumps and infectious mononucleosis are the common viral infections associated with the lacrimal gland. Subclinical or inapparent infections have occurred in patients with HSV, VZV, cytomegalovirus, coxsackievirus A, and echovirus. Other viruses implicated in lacrimal gland infections are measles and influenza viruses. Parasitic invasions with *Schistosoma haematobium, Onchocerca volvulus,* and *Cysticercus cellulosae* have been reported. **Canaliculitis,** a disease exclusively found in adults, is a low-grade inflammation that affects the lower canaliculus more than the upper. Purulent, cheesy material may be expressed from the lumen. Etiologic agents are diverse and include bacteria, fungi, and viruses. Bacterial infections consist of mixed aerobic and anaerobic flora; *S. aureus* and streptococci are among the aerobes recovered (Box 41-8). Aerobic isolates also include gram-negative rods and *C. trachomatis.* The predominant microbiota recovered include the gram-positive anaerobes such as *Actinomyces israelii, Propionibacterium propionicus,* and *P. acnes. Nocardia, Fusobacterium,* and *Capnocytophaga* spp. may also be recovered. Fungal isolates include *C. albicans* and *Aspergillus* spp. Both herpes simplex and zoster may inflame the canaliculi.

Inflammation of the lacrimal or tear sac—**dacryocystitis**—is the most common infection of the lacrimal apparatus. Infections are usually seen in infants, and are associated with obstruction of the nasolacrimal sac. Infections are characterized by tearing and discharge from the eye, an inflamed sac, and pain (Figure 41-11). Thus any organisms that colonize

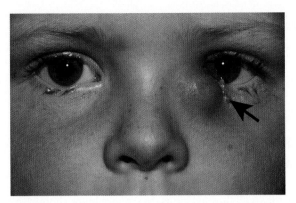

FIGURE 41-11 Dacryocystitis (infection of the lacrimal sac) of the left eye *(arrow)* in a young child. (From Zitelli BJ, Davis HW: *Atlas of pediatric physical diagnosis*, ed 5, Philadelphia, 2008, Mosby.)

the nasolacrimal sac could be responsible for lacrimal sac infections (see Box 41-8). *C. trachomatis* may cause a recurrent, chronic inflammation of the tear sac. *Aspergillus* spp., *Candida* spp., and *Actinomyces* spp. may also be recovered.

Laboratory Diagnosis

Submitted materials for microbiologic evaluation include drainage material, pus, and cheesy exudate. Direct smears for bacteria and fungi should be prepared from this material. Often the etiologic agents (e.g., *Actinomyces* spp.) and fungal hyphae are seen in large numbers. Infections with mixed organisms are also evident. Media should be inoculated so that aerobic and anaerobic organisms as well as fungi will be recovered.

Treatment

Systemic antibiotics are used to treat infections of the lacrimal system. Topical drops or ointments are used to control chronic disease. Removal of artificial tear duct biomaterials may be necessary to resolve the infection.

INFECTIONS OF THE INTRAOCULAR CHAMBERS (ENDOPHTHALMITIS)

Infectious **endophthalmitis,** inflammation of intraocular tissues or cavities, is a catastrophic development resulting from complications of surgery, contiguous spread of infection from infected tissues, use of contaminated medications, or penetrating ocular trauma. It is the most serious and sight-threatening of all ocular infections. Any organism that gains entry into the inner chambers of the eye can result in disease. The etiologic agents include bacteria, viruses, fungi, and parasites. Endophthalmitis may also be caused by instillation of contaminated eyedrops and implantation of contaminated biomaterials.

Bacteria

Etiologic agents of endophthalmitis, which include bacteria, viruses, and fungi, are listed in Box 41-9. *S. epidermidis* and other coagulase-negative staphylococci are the most frequent

---

BOX 41-9 Microorganisms Associated with Endophthalmitis

Bacteria
Achromobacter xylosoxidans
Actinomyces spp.
Bacillus spp.
Capnocytophaga spp.
Coagulase-negative staphylococci
Enterobacteriaceae
Enterococcus faecalis
Haemophilus influenzae
Moraxella spp.
Mycobacterium chelonae
Propionibacterium acnes
Proteus mirabilis
Pseudomonas aeruginosa
Serratia marcescens
Staphylococcus aureus
Staphylococcus epidermidis
Streptococcus viridans group

Viruses
Cytomegalovirus
Enterovirus
Herpes simplex virus types 1 and 2
Varicella-zoster virus

Fungi
Aspergillus spp.
Candida spp. (*Candida albicans*—most common)
Cryptococcus neoformans
Curvularia spp.
Fusarium spp.
Paecilomyces spp.

Parasites
Onchocerca volvulus
Toxoplasma gondii
Toxocara spp.

---

pathogens. Contamination of intraocular chambers and/or intraocular lens with conjunctival flora is the common reservoir for these infections. Bacterial endophthalmitis is often associated with infected biomaterials (intraocular lens, scleral buckles) following cataract and or retinal surgery. *Bacillus cereus* and other *Bacillus* spp. are the most frequently isolated organisms from endophthalmitis resulting from traumatic injuries. The onset of symptoms is sudden, and the course is fulminant. Release of necrotizing enzymes can result in loss of the eye within 48 hours. A high index of suspicion and aggressive therapy are required to retain useful vision.

Fungi

Mycotic endophthalmitis is mostly an extension of keratitis. However, it may also result from hematogenous spread from a remote focus and from implantation of contaminated intraocular lenses. The most frequent isolates are *C. albicans* and other *Candida* spp. Saprophytes that infect the cornea may extend into the intraocular cavities. The filamentous species recovered include *Aspergillus* spp., *Fusarium solani, Paecilomyces* spp., *Curvularia* spp., and *S. schenckii*. Other reported species recovered in cases of endophthalmitis include *Monosporium apiospermum, Cephalosporium* spp., *Volutella* spp., *C. immitis, H. capsulatum, C. neoformans,* and *B. dermatitidis. Pneumocystis jiroveci (carinii)* may be isolated from patients with AIDS and human immunodeficiency virus (HIV).

Parasitic Endophthalmitis

Intraocular parasites usually affect the retina or choroid or are transient invaders from adjacent ocular structures. *Onchocerca* spp., *Toxocara* spp., and *Toxoplasma gondii* are the most frequent intraocular pathogens.

Laboratory Diagnosis

Rapid recovery and identification of the invading organism, complemented by an early, specific, and aggressive therapy, are mandatory to prevent loss of useful vision and preserve internal ocular structures. Specimens include aspirated anterior chamber or vitreous fluids (usually less than 5 mL) and washings from the flushing out of vitreous chambers (usually more than 10 mL). Intraocular fluids are plated directly onto selected media. Drops are placed on slides for Gram, Giemsa, or calcofluor white stains. Vitreous washings are filtered through a 0.45-μm Teflon filter, sectioned, and placed on selected media (Figure 41-12).

Treatment

Therapy includes injection of intravitreal antibiotics for both gram-positive and gram-negative pathogen coverage. Ceftazidime and vancomycin are the drugs of choice, but other combinations are available. Antivirals are also placed inside the eye to manage viral infections.

INFECTIONS OF THE UVEAL TRACT (UVEITIS)

Uveitis is a general term for inflammatory disorders of one portion or all three portions (iris, ciliary body, choroid) of the uveal tract. Inflammation of the uveal tract results from ocular trauma or dissemination of systemic disease. Connective tissue diseases, such as juvenile rheumatoid arthritis, Reiter's syndrome, and systemic lupus erythematosus, are associated with uveitis. Iritis and iridocyclitis are referred to as *anterior uveitis,* whereas choroiditis or chorioretinitis is termed *posterior uveitis.* The etiology of anterior uveitis is considered nongranulomatous and is nonmicrobial. Posterior uveitis is classified as a granulomatous disease, and its etiology may be bacterial, fungal, viral, or parasitic.

Mycobacterium tuberculosis, Treponema pallidum, and *Mycobacterium leprae* all are involved in chronic disease of

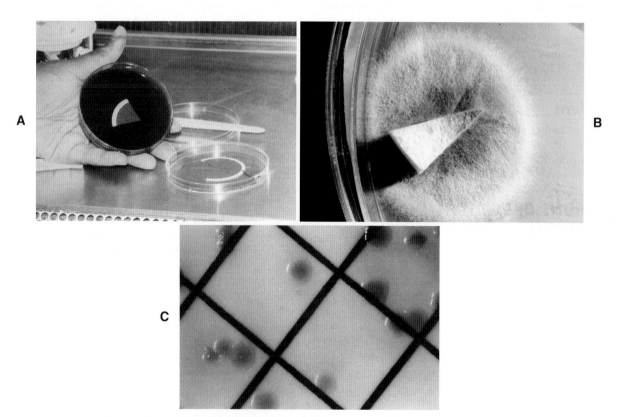

FIGURE 41-12 **A,** Section from filter used to concentrate vitreous fluids. Once filtered, the 0.45-μm filter is then sectioned and placed on selected media. **B,** *Curvularia* spp. from intraocular fluids on 0.45-μm filter section. **C,** *Burkholderia cepacia* on a filter from a vitrectomy specimen.

the uveal tract. Members of the herpes group (HSV, cytomegalovirus, and VZV) may be involved in necrotizing disease. Such disease is usually associated with **retinitis.** Chorioretinitis may be a better description of the syndrome. *H. capsulatum, Aspergillus* spp., *Nocardia asteroides,* and *Candida* spp. all cause granulomatous disease of the uveal tract. Infections involving the uveal tract usually manifest as chorioretinitis. Recovery in culture is difficult. Serologic assessment via enzyme-linked immunosorbent assay (ELISA), immunofluorescence, or complement fixation may be of greater value in identifying the causative agent. Genomic amplification (PCR) or DNA probes may also assist in some cases. Viral isolation is attempted by cocultivation of the fluids or tissues with fibroblasts. Treatment includes control of the inflammation with corticosteroids and antimicrobials as appropriate.

INFECTIONS OF THE RETINA (RETINITIS)

The retina is a multilayered, neural tissue that transforms images and relays impulses to the brain so that the individual can see. Insults to the retina, whether infectious or noninfectious, result in irreversible damage. Microbial infections are rare but can be devastating. Microbial infections may occur via hematogenous or contiguous spread. The bacterial and fungal infections are usually the same as those found in uveitis. *P. jiroveci* invades the retina, resulting in classic "cotton wool spots" during systemic disease. Viral and parasitic organisms are responsible for syndromes that are unique to the retina. Microbial agents recovered in retinitis are shown in Box 41-10.

BOX **41-10** Microbes Associated with Retinitis

Bacteria
Mycobacterium leprae
Mycobacterium tuberculosis
Nocardia asteroides
Treponema pallidum

Viruses
Cytomegalovirus
Herpes simplex viruses types 1 and 2
Human immunodeficiency virus
Rubella
Rubeola
Subacute sclerosing panencephalitis (SSPE)
Varicella-zoster virus

Fungi
Aspergillus spp.
Candida spp.
Histoplasma capsulatum

Parasites
Cysticercus cellulosae
Pneumocystis jiroveci (carinii)
Toxoplasma gondii
Toxocara spp.

Viruses

Viral syndromes are rare but devastating, resulting in unilateral or bilateral decreased vision. The immunocompromised patient is often at risk for viral retinitis. Increased disease (e.g., cytomegalovirus retinitis) is seen in individuals with AIDS. HSV, VZV, and cytomegalovirus all cause viral retinal disease. In the United States, HSV is the leading cause of blindness. Both HSV-1 and -2 cause posterior uveitis. Acute necrotizing retinitis is usually seen in the newborn as a result of acquiring the virus during passage through an infected birth canal. Adults may acquire the disease from recurrent episodes of viral keratitis. Varicella-zoster retinitis may be a manifestation of reactivation of the virus in herpes zoster ophthalmicus.

Cytomegalovirus infections may affect the newborn or the immunocompromised patient and especially patients who have had transplants or have AIDS. Cytomegalovirus retinitis with loss of vision (Figure 41-13) is often indicative of AIDS. Acyclovir, ganciclovir, and foscarnet are antivirals used to treat and modulate these episodes. Both rubeola and rubella cause retinopathy. About 30% of patients with subacute sclerosing panencephalitis (SSPE), which may appear years after an attack of clinical measles, also have chorioretinitis on examination. The ocular complications of congenital rubella include cataracts and glaucoma.

Ocular Manifestations in Patients with Human Immunodeficiency Virus

Ocular involvement occurs in 50% to 75% of patients infected with HIV during the course of their illness. Symptoms appear with advancing disease. HIV has been isolated or amplified from tears, conjunctiva, and corneal and retinal tissues. The virus may also be recovered from contact lenses of infected patients. The route by which HIV reaches the ocular surface tissues and tears remains uncertain. Cytomegalovirus retinitis is the second most common condition in patients with full-blown AIDS and can affect both eyes even in the absence of systemic disease. This retinitis is listed as an indicator infec-

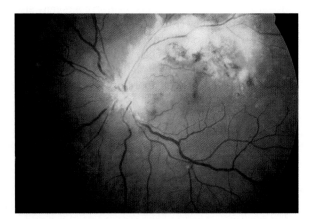

FIGURE 41-13 Acute cytomegalovirus retinitis with optic nerve involvement in a 40-year-old patient who is HIV positive. Active viral particles are seen in satellite lesions temporal to the main infection *(yellow).*

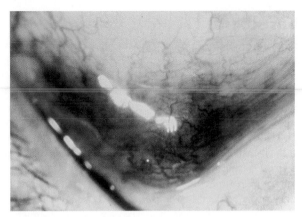

FIGURE 41-14 Kaposi sarcoma (raised dark spots) on the conjunctiva of a patient who has AIDS.

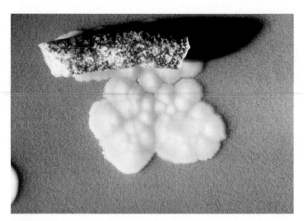

FIGURE 41-16 Extruded scleral buckle on blood agar plate with growth of *Candida albicans*.

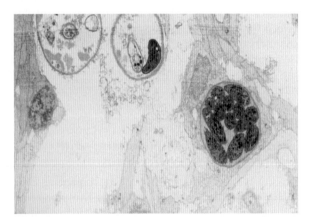

FIGURE 41-15 *Toxoplasma gondii* trophozoites and cysts in retinal tissue. This protozoan has a predilection for ocular tissue. This disease is now more common in HIV patients than in the general U.S. population.

tion in the differential diagnosis of AIDS. Patients may have a history of sudden loss or impairment of vision. Cotton wool spots—fluffy, white lesions—are the ocular lesions most often seen in patients with AIDS. Retinal hemorrhages may also be present. Kaposi sarcoma (Figure 41-14) appears on the ocular tissues of 10% of infected patients. *P. jiroveci (carinii)* and *T. gondii* retinitis are also ocular sequelae associated with patients who have AIDS.

Laboratory Diagnosis. Laboratory diagnosis of retinal pathogens is usually confirmed by serology and/or PCR. Routine microbiology cultures may be compromised by the small volume available for smears and culture.

Treatment. Treatment is similar to that for endophthalmitis.

Parasites

Toxoplasma gondii is a protozoan with a predilection for ocular tissues (Figure 41-15). Ocular infection is a late manifestation of congenital toxoplasmosis. This infection is now more prevalent in patients with AIDS than in the general population. *Cysticercus cellulosae* and *Toxocara* spp. are found in 10% to 13% of intraocular infections. Other proto-

zoal infections that may cause transient retinitis include malaria (retinal hemorrhage); babesiosis—a rare disease similar to malaria but having distinct differences—which is seen mainly in the northern United States in the New England area; and infection with *Loa loa,* the eye worm, which can enter the intraocular cavities and cause inflammation in its migration through the ocular tissues. The laboratory support for these infections is the same as that for uveitis.

SCLERAL BUCKLE INFECTIONS

Scleral buckles, sponges, and bands are biomaterials employed to realign detached retinas. All of these serve as good substrates for biofilm formation. They may also become expressed and partially extruded from the surgical site. Once exposed, they are subject to bacterial colonization, which can lead to infections of the conjunctivae, sclera, or intraocular cavities. The most frequently isolated bacteria are coagulase-negative staphylococcal species. *S. aureus, P. mirabilis,* and *P. aeruginosa* have also been recovered. MOTT (mycobacteria other than tubercle bacilli), in particular *M. chelonae* and *Mycobacterium fortuitum,* have been recovered from these materials at an alarming rate during the last few years. Additional isolates include *Candida* spp., *Corynebacterium* spp., and *Citrobacter koseri* (Figure 41-16). Management includes removing the infected materials along with any remaining necrotic tissue when possible.

BIOFILM-CENTERED OCULAR INFECTIONS

Microorganisms in biofilms are causative agents in a variety of ocular infections (Table 41-2). These include contact lens–associated and crystalline keratitis, late-onset postoperative endophthalmitis, scleral buckle and orbital implant infections, and uveitis. Biomaterial-centered infections have also been documented for ocular keratoprosthesis, glaucoma shunts, and ocular sutures.

Biofilms may form on a variety of ocular biomaterials and or on damaged ocular tissues. The most frequent ocular biomaterials predisposed to biofilm formation include contact

TABLE 41-2 Biofilm-Associated Ocular Disease

Clinical Disease	Biomaterial and/or Biofilm Origin	Recovered or Common Organisms
Contact lens–associated keratitis	Hydrogel and silicone (soft) contact lens PMMA (hard) contact lens	*Pseudomonas aeruginosa* *Staphylococcus aureus* Coagulase-negative staphylococci
Crystalline keratitis	Damaged tissue	*Streptococcus* viridans group *Candida* spp.
Diffuse lamellar keratitis Radial keratotomy Intracorneal rings	Damaged tissues Damaged ocular tissue Damaged-tissue implant	Endotoxins/microbial products released from biofilms *Streptococcus* viridans group *Serratia marcescens* *Pseudomonas aeruginosa*
Endophthalmitis	Intraocular lenses	Coagulase-negative staphylococci (*S. epidermidis*—most frequent) *Propionibacterium acnes* *Candida albicans*
Scleral buckle/explant infections	Damaged tissue Buckle material	*Staphylococcus epidermidis* *Mycobacterium chelonae* *Mycobacterium fortuitum* *S. aureus*
Orbital implant infections	Implant Orbital tissues	*S. aureus*
Glaucoma drainage	Implant Damaged tissue	*S. aureus* *Mycobacterium* spp.
Punctual plugs	Implant Damaged tissue	*Staphylococcus epidermidis*
Lacrimal plugs	Implant Damaged tissue	*Mycobacterium chelonae* *S. aureus*

PMMA, Polymethylmethacrylate.

lenses, intraocular lenses, scleral buckles, glaucoma, and corneal and orbital implants. Common pathogens include coagulase-negative staphylococci, *S. aureus, P. acnes, Candida albicans,* and *P. aeruginosa* (Figure 41-17). Biofilm-centered ocular infections are recalcitrant to antimicrobial therapy, and the sequestered biofilm-encased organisms are protected against the host's humoral and cellular immunity. Complications include chronic infections, decreased vision, and blindness. Removal of the biomaterial is often necessary to resolve the infection or inflammation.

LABORATORY DIAGNOSIS OF OCULAR INFECTIONS

Specimen Collection

The keys to proper collection of ocular specimens are similar to those for any other microbiologic specimen. Materials or scrapings for cultures should be collected as soon as possible after the onset of infection (24 to 48 hours for bacteria and 3 to 7 days for viruses) and before the instillation of antimicrobials or steroids. The sample must be collected from the actual site of the infection; for example, conjunctival and lid cultures are inadequate to assess corneal involvement. All ocular fluids, tissues, sponges, and other surgical material must be submitted in sterile, leakproof containers that are properly labeled.

The ophthalmologist must communicate with the hospital or reference laboratory personnel performing the microbiologic evaluation of the specimen to ensure isolation of ocular

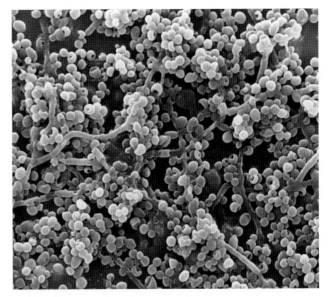

FIGURE 41-17 Fungal (yeast) biofilm on contact lens. Culture grew *Candida albicans.*

pathogens. Media and the accompanying requisitions must be properly labeled with complete patient information and should indicate any antibiotics, antivirals, steroids, or antifungals the patient is currently receiving. It should also be noted whether the patient is a contact lens wearer. For best results, ocular materials must be inoculated directly onto the appropriate media. Scant recovery is the norm when Culturettes

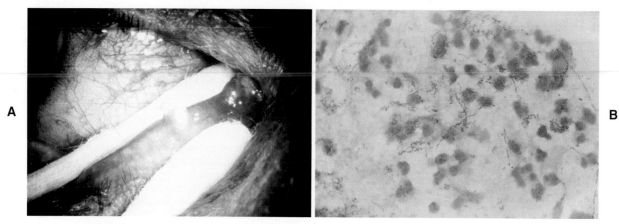

FIGURE 41-18   A, Concretions being expressed from canaliculi. **B,** "Smashed" and stained concretions, revealing gram-positive, slender, branching rods *(Actinomyces israelii).*

(Becton Dickinson, Sparks, Md.) or swabs are submitted for recovery of ocular pathogens. The type of swab used can further reduce organism recovery. Cotton-tipped swabs inhibit the growth of some bacteria and HSV because of the fatty acids released during sterilization. Dacron or calcium alginate swabs may be used to collect ocular samples. Furthermore, the calcium alginate swab may be lethal to some viral ocular pathogens. Expressed materials from areas such as canaliculi are preferred to rule out infection (Figure 41-18). Materials are inoculated directly onto the media. Smears are also prepared from the material. Collection by direct aspiration or scraping is performed by the ophthalmologist. Media to recover aerobic and anaerobic organisms must be included. Vitreous washings (with a volume greater than 10 mL) may be injected into blood culture bottles or viral transport media or may be sent to the laboratory for concentration through a 0.22- or 0.45-μm filter (see Figure 41-12). Biopsy tissue must be minced or ground. Media to recover aerobic and anaerobic bacteria, fungi, and mycobacteria should be inoculated. If free-living amebae are suspected, two nonnutrient (agar) plates should be included.

Direct Microscopic Examination

Conjunctiva and cornea scrapings, intraocular fluids, and aspirations are collected by an ophthalmologist using a Kimura spatula, blade, or sterile swab.

Scrapings and fluid aspirations from the involved ocular site, complemented with the appropriate stains, can afford the physician circumstantial as well as definite information concerning the identity of the invading organisms. Table 41-3 provides a summary of stains that are routinely used in ocular microbiology and appropriate applications of each procedure. Gram and Giemsa stains (Figure 41-19) should be collected for all cases of bacterial conjunctivitis, keratitis, and endophthalmitis. The calcofluor white stain should be added to rule out fungal or parasitic disease. A fluorescent or conventional acid-fast stain is used to detect the presence of acid-fast organisms. Direct antigen detection in cases of viral or chlamydial disease may be the only confirmation test available. In addition, impression cytology using 0.45-μm Teflon-coated

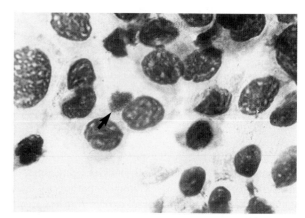

FIGURE 41-19   Giemsa stain of conjunctival epithelial cells with chlamydial inclusions *(arrow).* The Giemsa stain also provides information on the types and numbers of inflammatory cells and the condition of the epithelial cells.

TABLE 41-3 Smear Guide

	Gram	Giemsa	IF	IC	CFW
Bacteria	+	+			
Fungi	+	+			+
Viruses		+	+	+	
Chlamydia		+	+	+	
Parasites	+	+		+	+

IF, Immunofluorescent stains—monoclonals for chlamydia, herpes simplex virus, adenovirus, enterovirus, varicella-zoster virus, and cytomegalovirus; *IC,* impression cytology—collected cells remain intact, and test can track disease progress; *CFW,* calcofluor white stain—used to detect fungi or parasites in ocular tissue.

membrane filters to collect conjunctival and corneal tissue may increase bacterial, fungal, viral, and protozoan detection by as much as 50%. The advantage with this technique is that cells remain intact with characteristic morphology and microbial infestation and invasion (Figure 41-20).

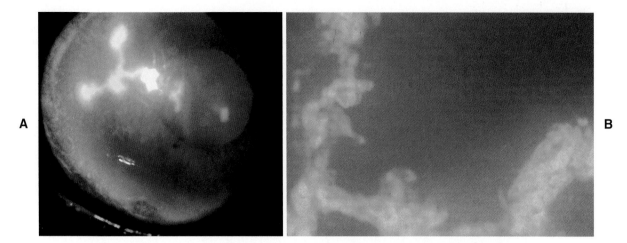

FIGURE 41-20 A, Cornea stained with rose bengal to outline dendrite infected with herpes simplex virus (HSV). HSV is the virus most often isolated from corneal dendritic infections. **B,** Dendrite on membrane filter collected by impression cytology. The filter was stained with a monoclonal antibody against HSV-1. Almost all the HSV-infected cells of the dendrite "lit up" when stained. The uninfected cells do not stain and appear red.

Culture and Identification

Most of the bacterial and fungal ocular isolates may be recovered on chocolate and blood agar when they are incubated under the proper conditions of temperature (35° to 37°C) and atmosphere (5% to 10% CO_2, aerobic) or in an anaerobic jar or bag. Table 41-3 shows a general plating guide that may be followed to recover all possible agents of ocular infections. Table 41-4 shows a minimal plating guide for bacteria and fungi. The addition of thioglycollate broth, Thayer-Martin agar, Sabouraud agar with gentamicin (Figure 41-21), viral and chlamydial transport media, Löwenstein-Jensen slants, and nonnutrient agar plates allows for the recovery of most pathogens involved in ocular disease. All thioglycollate tubes are held for 10 days or for 21 days if *Actinomyces* spp. or *P. acnes* is suspected.

Interpretation of growth from ocular samples is based on the same sound microbiologic criteria used in general hospital microbiology laboratories. Quantitation of growth is particularly important. Samples from patients receiving anti-infective agents, steroids, or other medications may have reduced flora, which should be taken into consideration when evaluating the culture. Special considerations are involved in corneal and intraocular fluid cultures. Traditionally, corneal scrapings are inoculated in a C streak fashion. Each row of C streaks represents a separate scraping of a corneal ulcer. The dilution effect is from left to right. Generally more colonies of bacteria or fungi appear on the first C streaks of each row. Each successive C streak progresses from the superficial to the deep layers of the cornea. The greater the number of corneal streaks with growth, the more involved and serious the infection (Figure 41-22). Any growth from intraocular fluids appearing on the inoculation sites or filter should be assessed and reported. The physician correlates the organism's pathobiology with the patient's clinical picture and diagnosis. The coagulase-negative staphylococci, the most common isolates

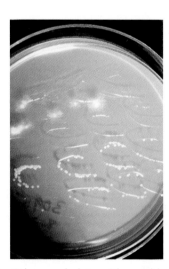

FIGURE 41-21 Sabouraud plate with mould and yeast. Patient had a mixed fungal keratitis. *Top,* The superficial layer of the cornea was infected with a mould *(Fusarium oxysporum). Bottom,* The deeper layers were infected with a yeast *(Candida albicans).*

and normally considered "contaminants," are the ones most frequently involved in microbial intraocular infections (Figure 41-23). Stains, impression cytology, and tissue cultures are routinely used to confirm ocular chlamydia and viral pathogens.

Molecular Techniques

DNA probes and PCR help in confirming clinical diagnosis for difficult or unusual ocular pathogens. This method may be ideal for detecting microbes in ocular samples because of the small volume. Molecular techniques have been used to detect *Chlamydia,* herpesviruses, toxoplasma, and Whipple's disease.

TABLE 41-4 General Ocular Plating Guide*

Clinical Presentation	Minimum Media to Inoculate									Stains					Common Isolates
	Chocolate Agar	5% Sheep Blood Agar	Sabouraud Agar	Thioglycollate	Agar/Agar	Anaerobic Blood Agar	Löwenstein-Jensen Slant	Blood Culture Bottles	Viral and or *Chlamydia* Transport Media	Gram Stain	Giemsa	Calcofluor White Stain	Immunofluorescent stain		
Conjunctivitis															
Bacterial	X	X								X					*Staphylococcus aureus, Haemophilus influenzae, Streptococcus pneumoniae*
Chlamydial	X								X	X	X		X		*Chlamydia trachomatis*
Viral	X								X				X		Adenovirus, HSV-1, -2, Enterovirus
Blepharitis															
Same as for conjunctivitis															Same as above
Keratitis															
Bacterial	X	X		X						X					*Pseudomonas aeruginosa, S. aureus, Serratia marcescens*
Fungal	X	X	X	X						X	X	X			*Fusarium* spp., *Candida* spp., *Aspergillus* spp.
Viral	X								X				X		HSV-1, -2, VZV, adenovirus
Free-living ameba	X	X			X					X		X			*Acanthamoeba* spp., *Vahlkampfia* spp.
Contact lenses	X		X		X							X			*P. aeruginosa, S. aureus,* ameba
Atypical	X	X	X	X	X	X	X			X	X				MOTT, *Nocardia* spp.
Endophthalmitis															
Bacterial	X	X		X		X		X		X					CNS, *S. aureus, Propionibacterium acnes*
Fungal	X	X	X	X						X					*Candida* spp., *Aspergillus* spp.
Viral	X								X				X		HSV, VZV, CMV (PCR preferred)
Orbital cellulitis															
Bacterial	X	X		X		X				X					*S. aureus,* anaerobes, *H. influenzae*
Fungal	X		X	X						X					*Aspergillus* spp., *Mucor* spp., *Rhizopus* spp.
Preseptal cellulitis															
Same as for orbital cellulitis															
Dacryocystitis															
Bacterial	X	X		X		X				X					*S. aureus, Actinomyces* spp., anaerobes

HSV, Herpes simplex virus; *MOTT*, mycobacteria other than tubercle bacilli; *CNS*, central nervous system; *VZV*, varicella-zoster virus; *CMV*, cytomegalovirus; *PCR*, polymerase chain reaction.
*Additional procedures include AFB stains, DNA probes, *Limulus* lysate, and filtration.

Special Procedures for Recovering Ocular Pathogens

Limulus Lysate

The *Limulus* lysate test can be used as a rapid means of detecting the presence of endotoxins in corneal tissues or intraocular fluid. The *Limulus* lysate is a mixture of the amebocytes of the horseshoe crab. When these cells are mixed with fluids or substances containing endotoxins (e.g., cell walls of gram-negative organisms), they form a gel clot, much like that of the coagulase test. Both tests are enzymatic tests. The assay is set up, incubated, and read in 1 hour.

Agar-Agar Medium

Agar-agar is a nonnutrient agar that is first inoculated with ocular materials and then overlaid with an aliquot of heat-killed or live *E. coli,* which serve as food for the excysting *Acanthamoeba* organisms. The amebic trophozoites are identified by locating them at the end of the "tracts" they generate as they eat through the *E. coli.* Cysts are identified by their refractile, double-walled, polygonal shape and are best seen using calcofluor white stains and the fluorescent microscope. Recovery of any parasite from corneal scrapings is significant and should be reported. Usually cultures of free-living amebae contain both cysts and trophozoites (see Figure 41-9).

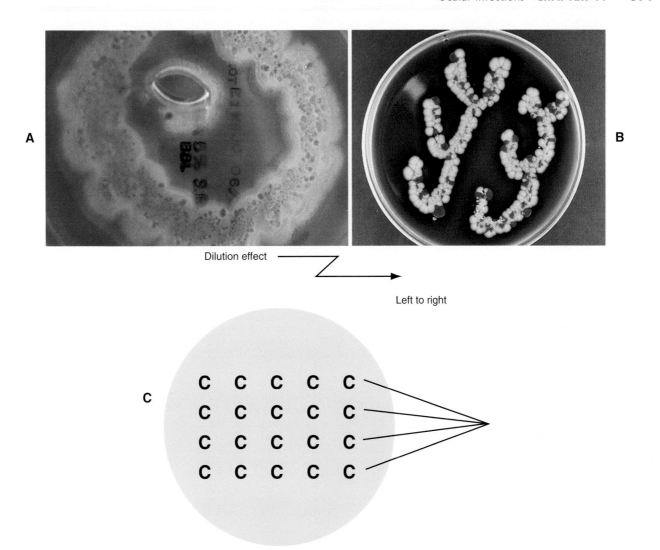

Dilution effect

Left to right

FIGURE 41-22 **A,** Contact lens and lens solution on 5% sheep blood agar surrounded by growth of *Pseudomonas aeruginosa*. **B,** C streaks growing pigmented and nonpigmented *Serratia marcescens*. **C,** Corneal scrapings. (Note: Each row of C streaks represents a separate corneal scraping.)

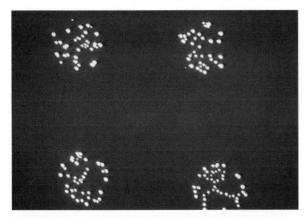

FIGURE 41-23 *Staphylococcus epidermidis* recovered from vitreous fluids (drops) on a blood agar plate. Samples may be inoculated onto a chocolate or blood agar plate and allowed to dry or may be streaked out as for a routine microbiology specimen.

Blood Culture Bottles for Intraocular Fluids

Blood culture bottles are used when blood cultures are requested and to culture intraocular fluids. Vitreous washings may be placed in the traditional (i.e., 50- to 70-mL) bottles; fluids from direct vitreous or anterior chamber taps should be inoculated into the pediatric (10- to 20-mL) bottles. Bottles are then incubated for 5 to 7 days.

Sabouraud Agar with Gentamicin

The very fungi that traditional mycology media aim to inhibit (saprophytes) are the agents most often recovered in mycotic ocular disease (e.g., *Fusarium* spp., *Paecilomyces* spp., *Aspergillus* spp., and *Penicillium* spp.).

Special Culture Techniques

Contaminated Ocular Medications

Ophthalmic drops (e.g., antibiotics, analgesics) are easily contaminated when improperly handled by patients or ophthal-

---

BOX 41-11 Microbes Recovered from Contaminated Ocular Medications

Acanthamoeba spp.
Alcaligenes spp.
Aspergillus spp.
Candida spp.
Citrobacter freundii
Coagulase-negative staphylococci
Enterobacter cloacae
Klebsiella spp.
Micrococcus spp.
Morganella morganii
Mycobacterium chelonae
Non–glucose-fermenting gram-negative rods
Ochrobactrum anthropi
Proteus mirabilis
Pseudomonas aeruginosa
Pseudomonas spp.
Serratia spp.
Staphylococcus aureus
Stenotrophomonas maltophilia
Zygomycetes

BOX 41-12 Microorganisms Recovered from Contact Lenses, Solutions, and Cases

Acanthamoeba spp.
Achromobacter spp.
Acinetobacter baumannii complex
Aeromonas spp.
Agrobacterium tumefaciens
Alcaligenes spp.
Bacillus spp.
Brevundimonas vesicularis
Burkholderia cepacia
Candida spp.
Chryseobacterium spp.
Citrobacter spp.
Comamonas spp.
Enterobacter spp.
Escherichia coli, Escherichia hermanii
Flavimonas spp.
Flavobacterium spp.
Fusarium spp.
Gemella spp.
Haemophilus spp.
Klebsiella spp.
Mycobacterium spp.
Neisseria spp.
Ochrobactrum anthropi
Paecilomyces spp.
Propionibacterium spp.
Proteus spp.
Pseudomonas aeruginosa
Pseudomonas spp.
Serratia spp.
Staphylococcus aureus
Staphylococcus epidermidis, other CNS
Stenotrophomonas maltophilia
Streptococcus pneumoniae
Streptococcus viridans group
Trichoderma spp.
Vahlkampfia, other free-living amebae

CNS, Coagulase-negative staphylococci.

---

mic personnel. Inappropriate handling can contribute to ongoing ocular disorders and to initiation of new infections. Even though most ocular medications are prepared with preservatives to inhibit the growth of microorganisms, once the preservative's threshold has been breached, microbes survive, multiply, and are dispensed with the next drop of medication. Medications should be collected from patients with conjunctivitis, keratitis, or endophthalmitis and sent to the laboratory for culture.

The medications most often contaminated and associated with concurrent patient infection, in descending order, include steroids, β-blockers, antiglaucoma drugs, antibiotics, and artificial tears. Box 41-11 shows the microbes recovered from contaminated ocular medications.

Contact Lenses and Solutions

Contact lenses are major risk factors for microbial keratitis. Keratitis associated with contact lenses (soft, daily wear, extended wear, or disposable) is being documented with increasing frequency. Gram-negative rods (especially and predominantly *P. aeruginosa* and *S. marcescens*) are common isolates in southern Florida and other warm climates, whereas *S. aureus* is the most frequent in other part of the country and cooler regions.

Acanthamoeba spp., MOTT, and gram-positive cocci have also been recovered. Sources include contact lenses as well as contact lens solutions (Box 41-12) and cases. Contamination of the soft contact lenses is usually caused by failure to follow manufacturer's recommended procedures or poor hygiene. Organisms attach to and form biofilm. Placement of the lenses on the cornea delivers a high microbial load and facilitates attachment and entrance into the cornea. The cornea stroma serves as an excellent media for microbial proliferation and spread. Wearers of hard contact lenses are less susceptible to infection from microbial contamination. This might be related to the type of biomaterials used to make this type of lens.

Cornea Storage Media and Tissue Culture

Replacement of diseased or opacified corneas is a common operation performed by ophthalmic surgeons. The new corneal tissue is obtained from donors within 24 hours of death and is preserved in McCarey and Kaufman (MK) or Dexsol medium. After surgery, the container with the medium and remaining corneal rim is sent to the laboratory for culture. Bacteriologic evaluation of the donor tissue is paramount in reducing the transmission of host-carried disease to the recipient. Viral studies of corneal transplantation tissue have been limited.

Gram-positive organisms (i.e., coagulase-negative staphylococci and *P. acnes*) are the most frequently isolated organisms, but gram-negative organisms, yeasts, or moulds may also be recovered from these media. The actual correlation between isolates and resultant disease is less than 1%. All positive cultures should be reported directly to the surgeon and a final report sent to the eye bank and the physician.

ANTIBIOGRAM Jan.-Dec. 2004	Total Isolates	Common Antibiotics % Susceptible						
		Cefazolin	Ceftazidime	Ciprofloxacin	Levofloxacin	Gentamicin	Tobramycin	Polymyxin B/Trimethoprim
Acinetobacter sp.	**12**	0	50	67	64	69	69	100
Alcaligenes sp.	**14**	0	93	40	78	20	13	71
Haemophilus influenzae	**36**	78	93	100	NT	NT	NT	100
Haemophiles parainfluenzae	**14**	79	100	100	NT	NT	NT	100
Klebsiella pneumoniae	**10**	100	100	100	100	100	100	100
Proteus mirabilis	**14**	86	100	100	100	100	100	93
Pseudomonas aeruginosa	**136**	0	99	99	100	99	100	98
Serratia marcescens	**21**	0	95	100	100	100	95	100
Gram-Negative Isolates (all ocular)	**341**	**46**	**85**	**83**	**87**	**91**	**91**	**91**
Staphylococcus aureus-MSSA	**99**	100	100	96	96	94	NT	100
Staphylococcus aureus-MRSA	**40**	0	0	20	20	85	NT	92
Staphylococcus epidermidis	**23**	57	57	54	54	83	NT	83
Streptococcus pneumoniae	**29**	NT	NT	NT	100	NT	NT	72
Streptococcus viridans group	**24**	NT	NT	NT	92	NT	NT	90
Gram-Positive Isolates (all ocular)	**236**	**66**	**66**	**71**	**79**	**94**	**NT**	**94**
Conjunctiva Isolates	**154**	59	59	81	82	93	89	80
Cornea Isolates	**198**	21	21	85	87	97	97	43
Vitreous Isolates	**28**	68	68	65	70	86	NT	76
Total Ocular Isolates	**577**	**57**	**57**	**77**	**85**	**92**	**91**	**92**

FIGURE 41-24 Antibiogram for common ocular isolates. *NT*, Not tested.

OCULAR THERAPY

The therapeutic agents used in ophthalmology are applied to the diagnosis of ocular disorders, the treatment of ophthalmic disease, and the prevention of postoperative infections. They differ from drugs used in other areas of medicine in delivery routes, antibiotic and antiviral combinations, dosing intervals, and toxicity. The traditional routes of administration of drugs may be implemented to supplement ocular management.

For ophthalmic drugs to be effective, they must reach ocular tissues in relatively high concentrations. Therefore

---

BOX 41-13 Ocular Anti-Infectives

Antibacterials

Amikacin	Neomycin*	Foscarnet	Antimony sodium gluconate
Ampicillin	Ofloxacin	Ganciclovir	Diethylcarbamazine
Bacitracin*	Penicillin G	Zidovudine (azidothymidine	Iodoquinol
Carbenicillin	Polymyxin B*	[AZT])	Ivermectin
Cefazolin	Polytrim*		Mebendazole
Cephalothin	Sulfacetamide*	**Antifungals**	Metronidazole
Chloramphenicol*	Sulfisoxazole*	Amphotericin B	Minocycline
Ciprofloxacin*	Tetracycline*	Clotrimazole	Niridazole
Clindamycin*	Tobramycin*	Fluconazole	Paromomycin
Colistin*	Trimethoprim	Flucytosine	Pentamidine isethionate
Erythromycin*	Trimethoprim-sulfamethoxazole	Griseofulvin	Propamidine isethionate
Gatifloxacin*	Vancomycin	Hydroxystilbamidine	Physostigmine
Gentamicin*	Antivirals	Ketoconazole	Pyrimethamine
Levofloxacin*	Idoxuridine (IDU)*	Miconazole	Spiramycin
Moxifloxacin*	Trifluridine*	Natamycin*	Surinam quassia
Methicillin	Vidarabine (ara-A)*	Potassium iodine	Thiabendazole
	Acyclovir*	Antiparasitics	

*Commercially available ocular preparations (drops or ointment).

Ocular preparations may be single antibiotics or combinations of one or two antibiotics and/or anti-inflammatories. Only natamycin has been approved by the U.S. Food and Drug Administration for topical treatment of ocular fungal pathogens.

---

ocular formulations include drugs in concentrations 10 to 100 times (i.e., fortified) that of drugs prepared for intramuscular or intravenous delivery. The routes of administration of ophthalmic drugs include topical (which is the most common and may include drops or ointments), periocular, intracameral, and intravitreal.

Drugs are dispensed as either drops or ointments, with topical administration being the most common route. Alternative or traditional routes are required for the treatment of disease involving the retina, optic nerve, and intraocular cavities. Ocular medications usually contain preservatives to inhibit the growth of contaminating microorganisms. Once the etiologic agent has been identified, susceptibility studies should be generated as quickly as possible. Traditional microbiologic methods are used to determine susceptibility patterns. Box 41-13 outlines the most common types of anti-infective agents commercially available to ophthalmologists. Pharmacists with training in ocular therapy can prepare ocular doses for most intravenous or intramuscular drugs. An antibiogram for common ocular isolates is shown in Figure 41-24.

BIBLIOGRAPHY

Alfonso EC et al: Fungal keratitis. In Krachmer, et al, editors: *Cornea—fundamentals, diagnosis and management*, ed 2, Philadelphia, 2005, Elsevier.

Biswell R: Cornea. In Riordan EP, Whitcher JP, editors: *Vaughn D. & Asbury's general ophthalmology*, ed 16, New York, 2004, Lange Medical Books/McGraw-Hill.

Buss DR et al: Lymphogranuloma venereum conjunctivitis with a marginal corneal perforation, *Ophthalmology* 95:799, 1988.

Cunningham ET, Shetlar DJ: Uveal tract & sclera. In Riordan EP, Whitcher JP, editors: *Vaughn D & Asbury's general ophthalmology*, ed 16, New York, 2004, Lange Medical Books/McGraw Hill.

Dursun et al: Advanced *Fusarium* keratitis progressing to endophthalmitis, *Cornea* 22:300, 2003.

Elder MJ et al: Biofilm-related infections in ophthalmology, *Eye* 9(Pt 1):102, 1995.

Frietas D et al: An outbreak of *Mycobacterium chelonae* infection after LASIK, *Ophthalmology* 110:276, 2003.

Garcia-Ferrer FJ et al: Conjunctivitis. In Riordan EP, Whitcher JP, editors: *Vaughn D & Asbury's general ophthalmology*, ed 16, New York, 2004, Lange Medical Books/McGraw-Hill.

John T, Velotta E: Nontuberculous (atypical) mycobacterial keratitis after LASIK: current status and clinical implications, *Cornea* 24:245, 2005.

Jones DB et al: Laboratory diagnosis of ocular infections. In Washington JA, editor: *Cumitech 13*, Washington, DC, 1981, American Society for Microbiology.

Kean BH et al, editors: *Color atlas of ophthalmic parasitology*, New York, 1991, IgakuShoin.

Kodjikian L et al: Intraocular lenses, bacterial adhesion and endophthalmitis prevention: a review, *Biomed Mater Eng* 14:395, 2004.

Lloyd AW et al: Ocular biomaterials and implants, *Biomaterials* 22:769, 2005.

Mah-Sadorra JH et al: Trends in contact lens-related corneal ulcers, *Cornea* 24:51, 2005.

Miller D: *Comparison of laboratory tests and risk factors for ocular chlamydia*, MPH thesis, May 1997, University of Miami.

Miller D, Alfonso EC: Comparative in vitro activity of levofloxacin, ofloxacin, and ciprofloxacin against ocular streptococcal isolates, *Cornea* 23:289, 2004.

Miller D et al: Utility of tissue culture for detection of *Toxoplasma gondii* in vitreous humor of patients diagnosed with toxoplasmic retinochoroiditis, *J Clin Microbiol* 38:3840, 2000.

Miller JJ et al: Acute-onset endophthalmitis after cataract surgery (2000-2004): incidence, clinical settings, and visual acuity outcomes after treatment, *Am J Ophthalmol* 139:983, 2005.

O'Brien T: Conjunctivitis. In *Mandell, Douglass, and Bennett's principles and practice of infectious disease*, ed 5, vol 1, Philadelphia, 2000, Churchill Livingstone.

O'Brien T: Endophthalmitis. In *Mandell, Douglass, and Bennett's principles and practice of infectious disease*, ed 5, vol 1, Philadelphia, 2000, Churchill Livingstone.

O'Brien T: Keratitis. In *Mandell, Douglass, and Bennett's principles and practice of infectious disease*, ed 5, vol 1, Philadelphia, 2000, Churchill Livingstone.

O'Brien T: Periocular infections. In *Mandell, Douglass, and Bennett's principles and practice of infectious disease*, ed 5, vol 1, Philadelphia, 2000, Churchill Livingstone.

Palma LA et al: The microbial flora in patients with keratoprosthesis, *Anales del Instituto Barraquer* 28(Suppl):67, 1999.

Pepose JS et al: *Ocular infection & immunity*, St Louis, 1996, Mosby.

Seal D: Treatment of *Acanthamoeba* keratitis, *Expert Rev Anti Infect Ther* 2:205, 2003.

Seal DV et al: *Ocular infection: investigation and treatment in practice*, St Louis, 1998, Mosby.

Tabbara KF, Hyndiuk RA: *Infections of the eye*, ed 2, Boston, 1996, Little, Brown and Company.

Wilhelmus KR et al: *Laboratory diagnosis of ocular infections, Cumitech 13A*, Washington, DC, 1994, ASM Press.

Zegans ME et al: The role of bacterial biofilms in ocular infections, *DNA Cell Biol* 21:415, 2002.

Points to Remember

- The external ocular surface is constantly challenged by microbes.
- Ocular infections may be mild or sight threatening.
- Surface defenses and intact cornea and globe prevent invasion by most microorganisms.
- Any organism gaining entry to the eye can establish infection.
- Inflammatory response can damage ocular structures.
- Infections of the cornea and intraocular structures are medical emergencies.

Learning Assessment Questions

1. _____is the most common gram-positive ocular pathogen.
   a. *P. acnes*
   b. Coagulase-negative staphylococci
   c. *S. aureus*
   d. *S. pneumoniae*
   e. *Micrococcus*

2. _____elicits enzymes that can "melt down" the cornea within 48 hours.
   a. *S. marcescens*
   b. *P. aeruginosa*
   c. *P. mirabilis*
   d. *H. influenzae*
   e. *E. coli*

3. _____and_____ are unusual pathogens that may invade compromised cornea tissue.
   a. *Microsporidia* and *Aspergillus* spp.
   b. *A. xylosoxidans* and *Penicillin* spp.
   c. *Fusarium* spp. and *G. lamblia*
   d. *Acanthamoeba* and *Microsporidia* spp.

4. The _____are the most frequent group of viruses to be involved in ocular disease.
   a. Herpesviruses
   b. Adenoviruses
   c. Enteroviruses
   d. Poxviruses

5. Name two microbiologic techniques that are unique to ocular microbiology.

6. Culture requests are received most often from which ocular site or sites? Which organisms are most likely to be recovered? Which media and/or stains should be included in the initial setup?

7. List the types of smears used to identify ocular pathogens.

8. Which is the most common route of administration for antibiotic treatment of common ocular infections?

9. Name two sexually transmitted diseases that also affect the eye.

10. List two biofilm-related ocular infections.

A

Selected Bacteriologic Culture Media

Maribeth L. Flaws

A wide variety of basal, enrichment, selective, and differential media are available to the clinical microbiology laboratory. Each of these media is intended to aid the technologist in the isolation, cultivation, and identification of clinically significant organisms from patient specimens. Efficient performance of these functions depends not on maintaining a vast array of media for routine use, but rather on the ability to make wise choices when selecting a routine media menu—choices that should be dictated by the factors discussed in Chapter 6. This appendix provides the reader with information about a select number of bacteriologic media cited in the bacteriology section of this text. Most media detailed in this appendix are commercially available in either dehydrated or finished form. Sterility and performance tests (quality controls) should be performed as discussed in Chapter 5.

ACETATE AGAR

Acetate agar is a differential medium used to distinguish *Escherichia coli* from *Shigella* spp. by determining the ability of an isolate to use acetate as the only available carbon source. Organisms capable of using acetate also use the medium's ammonium salt as a nitrogen source. The breakdown of the ammonium salt results in a shift of the pH into the alkaline range. At alkaline pH, the incorporated pH indicator, bromthymol blue, shifts from green (negative) to blue (positive). *Escherichia* spp. and many other members of the Enterobacteriaceae are positive, whereas *Shigella, Proteus,* and *Providencia* spp. are negative. The slant should be inoculated and incubated at 35° C for up to 4 days, monitoring daily for the expected color change.

ALKALINE PEPTONE WATER

Alkaline peptone water is an enrichment medium useful in the recovery of *Vibrio* and *Aeromonas* spp. from stool specimens. The alkaline pH of this medium allows uninhibited replication of these species while temporarily suppressing the replication rate of many commensal intestinal bacteria.

Some formulations recommend adjusting to pH 9.0 and adding sodium chloride to a concentration of 0.5% to 1.0% to recover the vibrios specifically. Alkaline peptone water cultures should be incubated at 35° C and subcultured to thiosulfate citrate, bile salts, sucrose (TCBS) agar within 12 to 18 hours.

BACTEROIDES BILE-ESCULIN AGAR

Bacteroides bile-esculin (BBE) agar is a selective, differential agar used for the isolation and identification of members of

the *Bacteroides fragilis* group. The incorporation of oxgall (bile salts) separates bile-resistant species (growth) from bile-sensitive ones (no growth), whereas the 1% esculin, in conjunction with ferric ammonium citrate, differentiates between the isolates that do grow based on the isolate's ability (positive) or inability (negative) to hydrolyze esculin. Products of esculin hydrolysis (esculetin) react with the ferric ammonium citrate to form an insoluble iron salt that is deposited within the medium surrounding the positive colonies, causing it to turn dark brown or black. Plated medium should be inoculated, streaked for isolation, and incubated anaerobically at 35° C.

BILE ESCULIN AGAR

Bile esculin agar is a selective, differential agar used to isolate and identify group D streptococci and the enterococci. Oxgall (bile salts) is the selective ingredient that inhibits the growth of most gram-positive organisms, whereas esculin is the differential component. All group D streptococci and enterococci can grow in the presence of bile and also hydrolyze esculin. Products of esculin hydrolysis (esculetin) react with ferric citrate in the medium to produce insoluble iron salts. Deposition of the iron salts results in a blackening of the medium. Test results must be interpreted in conjunction with Gram stain morphology because *Listeria monocytogenes* and a small number of other organisms also produce positive reactions.

The addition of vancomycin to the traditional bile esculin medium can be used to detect vancomycin-resistant streptococci and enterococci that will grow in the presence of vancomycin and hydrolyze the esculin. Azide is added to other formulations to inhibit gram-negative organisms. When azide is added, the concentration of bile is decreased to make the medium less inhibitory to non–group D streptococci. Bile esculin medium should be inoculated, incubated aerobically at 35° C, and observed for growth. Darkening of the medium indicates esculin hydrolysis.

BISMUTH SULFITE AGAR

Bismuth sulfite agar is a selective medium for the isolation of *Salmonella* spp. The selective ingredients are bismuth sulfite and brilliant green, which inhibit the growth of gram-positive bacteria, most lactose-fermenting intestinal normal flora, and *Shigella*. Although this is not a differential medium in the strictest sense, the ferrous sulfate in this medium is reactive with hydrogen sulfide to produce ferric sulfide, which is deposited within the bacterial colony as a black, insoluble precipitate. Typically *Salmonella* serotype typhi colonies are black and surrounded by a metallic sheen, whereas *Salmonella* serotype gallinarum, *Salmonella* serotype choleraesuis, and *Salmonella* serotype paratyphi colonies are light green on this medium. When bismuth sulfite agar is used to isolate *Salmonella* from feces and other clinical specimens, the parallel use of a less inhibitory medium is recommended, as bismuth sulfite agar may inhibit or partially inhibit the growth of some *Salmonella* strains.

This medium cannot be autoclaved and must be used on the day it is prepared. Plated medium should be inoculated with fecal or enrichment broth materials, streaked for isolation, and incubated at 35° C for 48 hours.

BLOOD AGAR, ANAEROBIC, CDC*

CDC anaerobic blood agar is an enrichment medium useful for the isolation of fastidious anaerobes. It is better for the isolation of anaerobic gram-positive cocci than for other anaerobes. It has a tryptic soy agar base and contains yeast extract, L-cysteine, hemin, sheep blood, and vitamin K_1.

This medium can be stored for up to 6 weeks if it is sealed in a cellophane bag and stored at 4° C. Plates should be inoculated, streaked for isolation, and incubated anaerobically at 35° C for 48 hours.

BLOOD AGAR, ANAEROBIC, BRUCELLA BASE, WADSWORTH

Wadsworth *Brucella* base anaerobic blood agar is a useful enrichment medium for the isolation of moderately fastidious, obligate anaerobes. Sheep blood provides the enrichment. Vitamin K_1 and hemin are also added to this medium.

Plated medium should be sealed in bags and stored at 4° C for up to 2 weeks. Usable plates are inoculated, streaked for isolation, and incubated anaerobically at 35° C for 48 hours.

BLOOD AGAR, ANAEROBIC, WITH KANAMYCIN AND VANCOMYCIN

Kanamycin and vancomycin (KV) blood agar is a variation of CDC anaerobic blood agar made semiselective by the addition of the antimicrobials kanamycin and vancomycin. It is useful in the primary isolation of obligate gram-negative anaerobes, particularly *Bacteroides* spp., from specimens with a mixed bacterial population.

KV blood agar plates sealed in bags can be stored at 4° C for up to 4 weeks. Usable plates should be inoculated, streaked for isolation, and incubated anaerobically at 35° C for 48 hours. Inoculated plates that lack growth at 48 hours may be reincubated, depending on the particular situation.

BLOOD AGAR, ANAEROBIC, LAKED, WITH KANAMYCIN, VANCOMYCIN, AND VITAMIN K

Anaerobic, laked blood agar with kanamycin, vancomycin, and vitamin K (KVKL) is a selective enrichment medium

recommended for the isolation of species of *Bacteroides* and *Prevotella* from clinical specimens. Although appropriate for the isolation of any *Bacteroides* spp., this medium is particularly helpful in the isolation of *Prevotella melaninogenica* as pigment production is enhanced. Laked erythrocytes and vitamin K constitute the enrichment ingredients, whereas the antibiotics inhibit all cocci and facultative gram-negative bacilli except the pseudomonads.

Plated medium should be inoculated, streaked for isolation, and incubated anaerobically at 35° C for a minimum of 48 hours.

BLOOD AGAR, RABBIT

Rabbit blood agar is an enrichment medium particularly useful in the recovery and the demonstration of β-hemolysis by *Haemophilus* spp. and *Gardnerella vaginalis*.

BLOOD AGAR, SHEEP

Sheep blood agar (SBA) is a routine medium used to cultivate a wide variety of moderately fastidious bacterial organisms. An infusion agar or tryptic soy agar base can be enriched by the addition of 5% to 10% defibrinated sheep, rabbit, or human blood. Sheep blood, however, has proved to be the most versatile enrichment additive. Incorporation of the blood not only provides enrichment for the growth of the bacterial organisms, but also allows the detection and characterization of hemolytic activity. Usable plates should be inoculated, streaked, and incubated as dictated by the specific application.

BLOOD PHENYLETHYL ALCOHOL AGAR, ANAEROBIC, CDC

Blood phenylethyl alcohol agar (PEA) is a selective enrichment medium that is useful in the isolation of *Bacteroides, Prevotella,* and other obligate anaerobes from specimens containing a mixture of obligate and facultative anaerobes. Enrichment is provided by yeast extract, hemin, vitamin K, and defibrinated sheep blood. Selectivity is provided by the incorporation of phenylethyl alcohol, which inhibits facultative gram-negative anaerobes by suppressing DNA synthesis and cell division.

Plated medium should be sealed in plastic bags for storage. Bagged plates can be stored for up to 4 weeks at 4° C. Usable plates should be inoculated, streaked for isolation, and incubated anaerobically at 35° C for at least 48 hours.

BLOOD PHENYLETHYL ALCOHOL AGAR, WADSWORTH

Wadsworth blood phenylethyl alcohol agar is an alternative to the CDC formulation of blood phenylethyl alcohol agar. Like the CDC formulation, it is a selective medium for the isolation of *Bacteroides* and *Prevotella* spp. The inoculation, incubation, and interpretation of growth on this medium are the same as those for the CDC blood phenylethyl alcohol agar discussed previously.

---

*Center for Disease Control, Atlanta, Ga.

BORDET-GENGOU BLOOD AGAR

Bordet-Gengou (B-G) blood agar is a selective enrichment medium for the isolation of *Bordetella pertussis* and *Bordetella parapertussis* from clinical specimens. Peptone is used in the base medium and is enriched by the addition of glycerol, potato infusion, and sterile, defibrinated sheep blood. Increased selectivity of the medium has been achieved by adding penicillin, methicillin, or cephalexin to the medium.

The antibiotic should be added aseptically just before the addition of the blood enrichment. Blood enrichment between 15% and 30% (3 to 6 mL/20-mL tube) is appropriate. The source of the sterile, defibrinated blood obtained is not critical, but properly prepared plates should be cherry red, moist, and bubble-free. Complete plated medium should be used immediately if possible. If for some reason this is not possible, plates can be maintained for about 1 week at 4° C if they are tightly sealed. Usable, complete medium can be inoculated by rolling the nasopharyngeal swab specimen over one third of the plate surface and then streaking for isolation with a platinum loop. The specimen should be inoculated in this fashion onto B-G plates without antibiotic and B-G plates with antibiotic. Inoculated plates should be incubated at 35° to 37° C with 5% to 10% CO_2 and increased humidity and then examined at 48 hours. Plates that have no growth at 48 hours should be reincubated. Plates must be held for 5 days, but not more than 7 days, before they can be regarded as negative for the organism.

BRAIN-HEART INFUSION BROTH

Brain-heart infusion (BHI) broth is an enriched medium suitable for the cultivation of a number of nonfastidious and moderately fastidious microorganisms. This broth medium is recommended for cultivation of pneumococci for the bile solubility test. Brains and beef heart provide nutrients, and peptones, glucose, sodium chloride, and buffers are also added. This formulation is often used as a blood culture medium. NaCl (6.5%) can be added to differentiate the salt-tolerant enterococci from the streptococci that are inhibited by the high salt concentration. This broth can also be used to prepare inocula for antimicrobial susceptibility testing.

BUFFERED CHARCOAL-YEAST EXTRACT AGAR

Buffered charcoal-yeast extract agar (BCYE) is an enrichment medium that is useful in the isolation of *Legionella* spp. from clinical specimens. Ferric pyrophosphate provides iron that is required by the organism. Yeast extract, α-ketoglutarate, and L-cysteine enhance the growth of *Legionella* organisms. Activated charcoal is incorporated to absorb toxic compounds that either accumulate as the result of the organism's metabolism or are present following preparation of this medium. This medium can also be used to isolate *Francisella* and *Nocardia* spp.

Usable plated medium can be stored in plastic bags, away from light, at 4° C for up to 4 weeks. Plated medium should be inoculated, streaked for isolation, and incubated at 35° C in a carbon dioxide incubator. Cultures should be checked daily for up to 2 weeks, and incubator humidity should be monitored to prevent excessive drying of plates. *Legionella* colonies may not be grossly visible until 3 to 5 days after inoculation.

Several modifications of BCYE exist. In one formulation, L-cysteine is omitted. Because *Legionella* spp. require L-cysteine, they will not grow on this medium. Comparison of growth on this L-cysteine–deficient medium with that on regular BCYE can help to determine whether an isolate is *Legionella* spp. or another type of gram-negative rod. The addition of antibiotics to BCYE will make the medium more selective. Commonly used antibiotics include cefamandole to inhibit gram-positive organisms; polymyxin B to inhibit gram-negative bacilli, especially pseudomonads; and anisomycin for fungal inhibition. The Wadowsky-Yee modification uses glycine and polymyxin B to inhibit gram-negative organisms, vancomycin to inhibit gram-positive cocci, and anisomycin to inhibit fungi. This medium is useful in recovering *Legionella* organisms from body sites that contain mixed flora. The Wadowsky-Lee modified BCYE also has bromcresol purple and bromthymol blue serving to differentiate between colonies. *L. pneumophila* colonies are light blue with a pale green tint.

BURKHOLDERIA CEPACIA SELECTIVE AGAR

Burkholderia cepacia selective agar (BCSA) is used to select for the isolation of *B. cepacia* in respiratory specimens taken from patients with cystic fibrosis. The base consists of trypticase peptone, yeast extract, sucrose, lactose, and sodium chloride. Polymyxin B, gentamicin, vancomycin, and crystal violet are the selective agents. *B. cepacia* has variable colony morphology on this medium, from smooth to rough, dry or moist, or purple owing to absorption of crystal violet. In addition, colonies may have a surrounding yellow zone because of carbohydrate fermentation or a pink zone because of peptone breakdown. BCSA is better for selectively isolating *B. cepacia* than *P. cepacia* selective agar (PCSA) or oxidative-fermentative polymyxin B–bacitracin-lactose (OFPBL) media. Inoculated BCSA plates should be incubated aerobically at 35° C and checked every 24 hours for growth. Plates should be incubated for at least 72 hours before they are discarded if there is no growth.

CAMPYLOBACTER BLOOD AGAR (CAMPY-BA)

Campylobacter blood agar (Campy-BA) is a selective enrichment medium that is useful in the isolation and cultivation of *Campylobacter* spp. from stool specimens. *Brucella* agar serves as the base medium for Campy-BA because it contains sodium bisulfite, which lowers the redox potential, thereby enhancing the recovery of microaerophilic organisms such as *Campylobacter* spp. Ten percent sheep blood enriches the basal medium, and an antibiotic mixture makes the medium selective. Although minor variations exist in the composition of the antibiotic mixture, most formulations have incorporated vancomycin to inhibit gram-positive cocci, trimethoprim to inhibit swarming strains of *Proteus,* polymyxin B to inhibit gram-negative bacilli, and amphotericin B to inhibit filamentous fungi and yeasts. Currently cefoperazone is being promoted to replace cephalothin. Cefoperazone has antipseudomonal activity (lacking in cephalothin) and is more effective against members of Enterobacteriaceae. This medium once inoculated with stool should be incubated in a microaerophilic environment. *Campylobacter* species generally grow as flat, gray, nonhemolytic colonies, or they may be raised and mucoid. Some isolates may be tan or slightly pink. The colonies may appear swarming or spreading across the surface of the plate.

CAMPYLOBACTER CHARCOAL DIFFERENTIAL AGAR

Campylobacter charcoal differential agar is less inhibitory for *Campylobacter* spp. than other selective media used to isolate *Campylobacter* and also more inhibitory for organisms found as normal fecal flora. Preston agar is the base that is supplemented with beef extract and peptones. Cefoperazone is added as a selection agent instead of cephazolin. Blood is not added to this formulation. Once inoculated with stool, this plate should be incubated in a microaerophilic environment.

CAMPYLOBACTER CHARCOAL SELECTIVE MEDIUM

This medium is used to select and enrich for the isolation of *Campylobacter* spp. from stool specimens. A Columbia agar base is supplemented with activated charcoal and hematin to substitute for the blood components. Vancomycin, cefoperazone, and cycloheximide are added to inhibit the growth of other organisms.

CAMPYLOBACTER THIOGLYCOLATE BROTH

Campylobacter thioglycolate broth (Campy-Thio) is a selective liquid medium used to enhance the isolation of *Campylobacter* spp. The base medium is thioglycolate broth with 0.16% agar, and the selective component is the antibiotic formulation used in Campy-BA.

CARBOHYDRATE FERMENTATION MEDIA, ANAEROBIC

Carbohydrate broths are differential media that are useful in determining the ability of an isolate to ferment specific carbohydrates. This formulation, based on a carbohydrate medium base (Difco, Detroit, Mich.), is useful in determining carbohydrate fermentations carried out by anaerobic isolates. Tubes containing various carbohydrates should be inoculated using a capillary pipette delivering the inoculum near the bottom of the tube without introducing air. One pipette can be used to inoculate multiple tubes.

All cultures should be incubated anaerobically, with the caps loosened, at 35° C for up to 7 days. Tubes should be examined on days 1, 2, and 7 for fermentation with produc-

tion of acid. Three different color reactions may occur. If fermentation occurs, the pH decreases to 6.0 or lower and the bromthymol blue indicator turns yellow, indicating a positive fermentation reaction. If fermentation does not occur, the bromthymol blue indicator remains blue to blue-green (negative reaction). If the cultured organism can reduce the bromthymol indicator, the medium becomes colorless. If this occurs, a sterile pipette can be used to transfer two to three drops of material from the involved tube(s) to a spot plate. Two to three drops of dilute indicator should then be added to the transferred material and observed for color change. NOTE: Rapid test systems are available that include carbohydrate fermentations with a bromcresol purple indicator. Correlation between fermentation and color change is similar, as is the problem of indicator reduction and the method for detecting acid in the presence of reduced indicator.

CARBOHYDRATE FERMENTATION MEDIA FOR GRAM-POSITIVE COCCI

Carbohydrate broths are differential media that are useful in determining the ability of a variety of aerobic bacteria to ferment specific carbohydrates. The base is heart infusion broth, which provides sufficient nutrients to support the growth of gram-positive cocci, including streptococci.

The sterile carbohydrate is added to the sterile basal medium (cooled to 50° C) to give a final concentration of 1%. Tubed carbohydrate fermentation medium should be inoculated and incubated aerobically at 35° C. A positive reaction (acid production) is indicated by a color change from purple to yellow.

CARBOHYDRATE FERMENTATION MEDIA FOR AEROBIC GRAM-NEGATIVE BACILLI

Carbohydrate fermentation medium of this formulation does not contain sufficient quantities of complex nutrients to support the growth of fastidious aerobic bacteria. It is, however, sufficient to support the less fastidious Enterobacteriaceae; thus it is the formulation of choice to determine the fermentative patterns of suspected Enterobacteriaceae isolates. Andrade pH indicator detects acid production. A positive result (acid production) is indicated by a color change from yellow or colorless (alkaline) to pink or red. Alternatively, phenol red is used as a pH indicator in carbohydrate fermentation media. With phenol red as an indicator, when acid is produced on fermentation of the test carbohydrate, the decrease in pH is seen as yellow, whereas with the lack of fermentation, the phenol red remains a reddish color.

CASEIN MEDIUM

Casein medium is a differential medium used to demonstrate proteolytic activity by *Actinomycetes* spp. Proteolysis is seen as a clearing of the medium around the inoculum growth. Sterile plated medium should be inoculated by the cut streak or point inoculation method. Each run should include the setup of the unknown and three known controls (*Streptomy-*

ces spp., *Nocardia asteroides, Nocardia brasiliensis*) using one half of the plate for each organism. Inoculated plates should be incubated at room temperature and observed for proteolysis over a 14-day period. *Streptomyces* spp. typically hydrolyze the incorporated casein within 2 to 5 days. *N. brasiliensis* typically hydrolyzes casein within 7 to 10 days; *N. asteroides* does not hydrolyze casein.

CEFSULODIN-IRGASAN-NOVOBIOCIN

Cefsulodin-Irgasan-novobiocin (CIN), also known as *Yersinia*-selective agar, is used to select for the isolation of *Yersinia enterocolitica* in stool samples. Peptones, beef, and yeast extracts are added as sources of nutrition. Sodium desoxycholate, cefsulodin, novobiocin, Irgasan, and crystal violet are added to inhibit the growth of other organisms found in stool. Mannitol is the differentiating agent, and neutral red is added as a pH indicator. *Yersinia* grows on this medium and ferments mannitol, forming clear colonies with a red center described as a "bull's-eye." *Aeromonas* spp. will also grow and ferment mannitol, but the *Aeromonas* colonies have a pink center and an uneven clear periphery. Most other organisms will not grow on this medium.

CETRIMIDE AGAR

Cetrimide agar, also known as pseudosel agar or *Pseudomonas*-selective medium, is used to select for *Pseudomonas aeruginosa* in specimens with mixed flora. Also, because it inhibits other *Pseudomonas* spp. (except *P. fluorescens*) and closely related organisms, this test can be useful in the differentiation of non-glucose-fermenting gram-negative rods.

This medium contains cetrimide, also called *cetyl trimethyl ammonium bromide* or *hexadecyltrimethyl ammonium bromide*. Produced from bromine, cetrimide is highly inhibitory and has been used as an antiseptic. If the organism can tolerate cetrimide, it will grow on the medium. Magnesium chloride and potassium sulfate stimulate the production of pyocyanin, the green pigment characteristically produced by *P. aeruginosa*. Under ultraviolet light, colonies of *P. aeruginosa* will fluoresce a yellow-green because of pyoverdin production stimulated by the low iron content of the medium.

CHOCOLATE AGAR

Chocolate agar (CHOC) is an enrichment agar that is especially useful in promoting the growth of *Haemophilus* and other fastidious bacterial species. This medium, a variation of sheep blood agar, may be made by adding sheep blood while the basal medium is warm enough to release the red cell hemoglobin and nicotinamide-adenine dinucleotide (NAD). Alternatively, sheep blood may be replaced by 2% hemoglobin and a chemical supplement solution, such as Iso-Vitalex (BBL, Cockeysville, Md.). The enrichment used must result in the complete medium containing cell-free hemoglobin and NAD. The temperature at which either enrichment is added results in a chocolate-brown medium. Plated medium can be stored at 4° C. Usable plates should be inoculated, streaked for isolation, and incubated at 35° C in CO_2.

CHROMAGARS

CHROMagars are selective/differential chromogenic media that have been developed for the isolation and identification of yeast, *Staphylococcus aureus, E. coli* O157:H7, and other organisms. Peptone and glucose are present in the basal nutrient agar, to which are added proprietary chromogenic mixtures, antibiotics, and other additives. As a result, particular colonies will have a typical and predictable colored colony that can be distinguishable from other colonies. These media can be used as primary isolation plates, such as the CHROMagar Orientation that is suggested for urine cultures in place of a blood agar plate, MacConkey agar, or both.

CITRATE AGAR, SIMMONS

Simmons citrate agar is useful in differentiating gram-negative enteric bacilli. Similar in principle to acetate agar, citrate replaces acetate in this medium, and differentiation is based on the isolate's ability or inability to use citrate as its sole source of carbon. Organisms capable of using the citrate also use the medium's ammonium salt as a nitrogen source. The breakdown of the ammonium salt results in a shift of the pH into the alkaline range. At alkaline pH, the incorporated pH indicator bromthymol blue shifts from green to blue.

This medium should be inoculated by streaking the organisms onto the slant with a sterile loop or needle. A light inoculum should be used because dead organisms from a heavy inoculum can be a carbon source, producing a false positive reaction. Inoculated slants should be incubated at 35° C for up to 4 days and monitored daily for the expected color change. Organisms that can utilize citrate (positive) will grow on the slant and produce a blue color in the slant. Organisms that cannot utilize citrate (negative) will not grow on the slant.

COLUMBIA AGAR WITH AND WITHOUT 5% SHEEP BLOOD

Columbia agar is a basal nutrient agar that contains peptones derived from casein and meat as well as beef and yeast extracts. The basal medium is suitable for cultivation of a number of aerobic and anaerobic bacterial organisms found in clinical materials. Additionally it provides an efficient base for preparation of a variety of enrichment agars that support the growth of more fastidious aerobes and anaerobes. For example, 5% sheep blood can be added to support the growth of more fastidious organisms. The addition of sheep blood allows for the detection of hemolytic reactions, although sometimes the β-hemolytic streptococci may look α-hemolytic because of the high carbohydrate content of this medium. Further, the sheep blood will provide X factor for organisms that require it, but NADase present in the blood will destroy the V factor, so organisms requiring V factor will not grow on this medium.

COLUMBIA AGAR WITH ANTIBIOTICS

Columbia agar with antibiotics (Columbia CNA agar) is a selective enrichment medium suitable for the isolation of gram-positive cocci from specimens that might also be expected to contain gram-negative bacilli, especially *Proteus* spp. Sheep blood is the usual enrichment ingredient, whereas colistin and nalidixic acid are incorporated to inhibit gram-negative overgrowth of desired gram-positive isolates.

COOKED MEAT (OR CHOPPED-MEAT GLUCOSE) MEDIUM

Cooked meat medium is useful in the cultivation of anaerobes, especially pathogenic species of *Clostridium*. This medium contains solid meat particles and is excellent for initiating growth from a very small inoculum as well as sustaining culture viability over long periods. It is useful for cultivation of mixed cultures because all organisms are supported while overgrowth by the more rapid growers is retarded. Dehydrated medium containing peptones, beef heart, and dextrose is suspended in tubes according to the manufacturer's directions and allowed to stand until thoroughly moistened (approximately 15 minutes) before sterilizing by autoclaving (121° C for 15 minutes). Tubed medium should be stored at room temperature, but stored tubes should be placed in flowing steam or a boiling water bath for 10 minutes, so as to drive off dissolved gases, and then cooled rapidly before inoculating. Cooled tubed media should be inoculated and incubated in a manner appropriate for the species being isolated or subcultured. The digestion of the meat particles indicates the proteolytic activity of cultured organisms. Saccharolytic clostridial species typically produce acid with gas.

CYSTINE TRYPTIC AGAR WITH SUGAR

Cystine tryptic (tryptophan/trypticase) agar (CTA-sugar) is a semisolid base medium that contains no meat or plant extracts and is free from fermentable carbohydrates. It may be made differential by the addition of a carbohydrate (CTA-sugar). CTA-sugars are recommended for the determination of fermentation reactions by fastidious organisms.

Alternatively, carbohydrates are available in the form of differentiation disks that can be aseptically added to the base tubed medium as needed. Sterile, tubed CTA-sugars should be inoculated with a heavy inoculum, stabbing to a depth of approximately 2 mm below the medium surface. The caps should be tightly closed and the tubes incubated at 35° C for 24 hours. With phenol red as the pH indicator, fermentation is indicated by a color change in the medium from red to yellow.

CYCLOSERINE CEFOXITIN FRUCTOSE AGAR

Cycloserine cefoxitin fructose agar (CCFA) is a selective, differential medium that is useful in the isolation and identification of *Clostridium difficile* from stool specimens of patients suspected of having antibiotic-associated diarrhea with pseudomembranous colitis. The selective antibiotic ingredients, cycloserine and cefoxitin, inhibit the growth of intestinal normal flora by interfering with cell wall synthesis in both gram-positive and gram-negative bacteria. Indigenous bacteria are inhibited, but *C. difficile* is not. Although cycloserine and cefoxitin are incorporated for their selective properties,

fructose and a pH indicator, neutral red, are included to confirm that the isolates can ferment this sugar.

NOTE: A variation of this medium is made with mannitol rather than fructose and uses bromthymol blue indicator. A second variation adds egg yolk suspension so that lecithinase and lipase activities can be detected. *C. difficile* grows as a yellow colony and turns the surrounding medium yellow. If the colonies are viewed under an ultraviolet light, *C. difficile* will fluoresce a gold-yellow color.

DECARBOXYLASE TEST MEDIUM (MOELLER)

Decarboxylase test medium with an incorporated amino acid is a differential medium that is useful in the identification of fermentative and nonfermentative gram-negative bacteria. The differential ingredient is one of three amino acids: lysine, arginine, or ornithine. Decarboxylation of the amino acids yields alkaline end products, which are detected by a change in the color of an incorporated pH-sensitive dye, bromcresol purple. The tubed basal medium (no amino acid) serves as a control for reading the reactions.

Decarboxylase tubes and a control tube should be inoculated from a 24-hour slant culture using a loop. Inoculated tubes should be overlaid with 4 to 5 mm of sterile mineral oil to avoid oxidative deamination of available protein, which would be falsely interpreted as a positive reaction. Inoculated, overlaid tubes should be incubated at 35° C for up to 4 days. Incubating tubes should be checked daily. Early in the incubation, fermentative organisms will ferment glucose, turning the control and all decarboxylase tubes yellow. For these organisms, as the pH drops, the hydrogen ion concentration becomes optimal for decarboxylase activity in the decarboxylase tubes; the subsequent conversion of the amino acid to amines raises the pH, reversing the yellow to purple, whereas the control tube remains yellow. Nonfermenters do not produce the initial yellow color change, and use of the amino acid is indicated when the amino acid–containing tube becomes a deeper purple than the control.

DEOXYRIBONUCLEASE (DNASE) TEST AGAR WITH OR WITHOUT INDICATOR DYE

DNase test agar is a differential medium that is used to detect the production of an active DNase exoenzyme by aerobic bacterial species. The differential ingredient is incorporated DNA. Methods available for the detection of DNA degradation include hydrochloric acid precipitation of undegraded DNA and color change of an incorporated metachromatic dye, such as toluidine blue or methyl green.

Sterile plated medium should be inoculated using a 1- to 2-cm streak or a spot inoculum approximately 5 mm in diameter. Inoculated plates should be incubated aerobically at 35° C for 18 to 24 hours. Following incubation, DNase activity is detected in one of the following ways:

1. If a basal medium without a metachromatic dye was inoculated, flood the plate with 1 N HCl and look for a zone of clearing around the bacterial growth. If the incorporated DNA is undegraded, it is precipitated by the 1 N HCl and the medium becomes opaque. If the incorporated DNA is degraded, the nucleotide fragments dissolve in the 1 N HCl and the medium remains clear.

2. If the medium includes toluidine blue, the blue, DNA-bound dye is released from nucleotide fragments, producing a color change to rose. The medium remains clear blue in negative reactions.

3. If the medium includes methyl green, the green, DNA-bound dye is released from nucleotide fragments, resulting in a loss of color. The medium remains green in negative reactions.

DESOXYCHOLATE CITRATE AGAR

Desoxycholate citrate agar is a selective, differential medium that is useful in the isolation of enteric pathogens directly from feces and urine specimens or indirectly from enrichment broths, such as selenite-F. The selective ingredients are sodium citrate and sodium desoxycholate at concentrations that can inhibit most nonpathogenic enteric bacilli as well as gram-positive organisms. The differential ingredients are lactose to detect fermentation and ferric ammonium citrate to detect the production of H_2S. Nonfermenting enteric pathogens appear as colorless colonies. Those lactose fermenters that do overcome the inhibitors appear as pink to red colonies as the result of the pH change that accompanies lactose fermentation. Colonies that produce H_2S will have a black center.

This medium is not autoclaved. Plates may be stored under refrigeration for several days. Plated medium should be inoculated, streaked for isolation, and incubated at 35° C in ambient air (not in CO_2) for up to 48 hours. A heavy inoculum is recommended if the specimen is feces, urine, or other direct bodily materials, whereas a light inoculum is recommended if the subculture is from an initial enrichment broth.

DILUTE GELATIN MEDIUM (0.4%)

Dilute gelatin medium is a differential medium useful in the differentiation of *Nocardia* spp. from one another and from *Streptomyces* spp. on the basis of growth and colonial morphology. In this medium, *N. asteroides* does not grow or grows poorly with a thin, flaky appearance. Conversely, *N. brasiliensis* grows well, forming compact, rounded colonies, whereas *Streptomyces* spp. produce poor to good growth with a stringy or flaky morphology.

The medium should be inoculated with a very small fragment of growth from a Sabouraud-dextrose agar slant and incubated at room temperature (or 37° C if the suspected strain grows better at 37° C). Inoculated tubes should be examined daily for growth for up to 21 to 25 days.

EGG YOLK AGAR, CDC FORMULATION

Egg yolk agar (EYA), also known as modified McClung-Toabe agar, is a differential medium that is useful in the detection of lecithinase, lipase, and protease activity. Incorporated egg emulsion provides the lecithin, lipids, and proteins to be degraded by these enzymes. On EYA, exoenzyme activity is detected as follows: Lecithinase activity produces a zone of opacity immediately around the growth streak; lipase activity results in an iridescent sheen on or around the surface of colonies; and protease activity is seen as a clearing of the medium around and just beyond the streaked growth area. A given organism may produce one or all of these exoenzymes.

Plated medium is inoculated as a single streak across the plate and incubated anaerobically at 35° C for 24 to 72 hours. If the Nagler test is to be performed, half of the plate surface should be smeared with a few drops of *Clostridium perfringens* type A antitoxin before inoculation. The inoculation streak should then extend across both halves (no antitoxin/antitoxin) of the plate. Inoculated plates should be incubated anaerobically at 35° C for 24 to 48 hours. A positive test result is the inhibition of lecithinase activity on the half of the plate with antitoxin. Plated medium not used immediately can be stored at 4° C if it is sealed in plastic bags.

EOSIN–METHYLENE BLUE AGAR

Eosin–methylene blue (EMB) agar is a selective, differential medium that is useful in the isolation and identification of gram-negative enteric bacteria. Eosin Y and methylene blue dyes, the selective ingredients, are incorporated to inhibit the growth of gram-positive bacteria while allowing the growth of gram-negative ones. The carbohydrates lactose and sucrose are incorporated to allow differentiation of isolates based on lactose or sucrose fermentation. Fermentation is detected by color changes and precipitation of the incorporated dyes as the pH drops. Sucrose serves as an alternative carbohydrate source for slow lactose fermenters, allowing their timely elimination from consideration as possible pathogens. *E. coli,* a coliform lactose fermenter, typically forms blue-black colonies with a metallic greenish sheen. Other coliform fermenters, such as *Enterobacter,* form pink colonies. Nonfermenter colonies are translucent, being either amber-colored or colorless.

ESCULIN AGAR

Esculin agar is a differential medium used to determine the ability of an organism to hydrolyze esculin. The hydrolytic products from esculin react with the ferric salt present in this medium to precipitate iron compounds and produce a gray to black discoloration of the medium.

Slanted medium should be inoculated, incubated aerobically at 35° C, and observed for growth, with darkening of the medium indicative of esculin hydrolysis.

FLETCHER SEMISOLID MEDIUM FOR *LEPTOSPIRA*

Fletcher semisolid medium is an enrichment medium recommended for detection of leptospiral species in blood, spinal fluid, and urine specimens as well as possibly contaminated water and other materials. The enrichment component of this medium is rabbit serum containing some hemoglobin.

The lyophilized rabbit serum with natural hemoglobin is commercially available as Leptospira Enrichment, or sterile, pooled, fresh natural rabbit serum may be added. The medium should be aseptically dispensed into sterile screw-capped tubes (5 mL/tube) and stored at room temperature overnight. The medium must be inactivated by placing tubes in a 56° C water bath for 1 hour on the day following preparation. Cooled inactivated medium should be inoculated with one or two drops of the fluid specimen, using a sterile, plugged Pasteur pipette. Small inocula introduced into multiple tubes are recommended to optimize pathogen recovery and minimize any interference by developing antibody titers in the body fluid specimens. Inoculated tubes should be incubated with caps loosened at 25° to 30° C for 4 to 5 weeks and examined weekly for growth in the form of turbidity at the top of the medium. A loopful of fluid from any tube showing turbidity should be placed on a clean slide, a coverslip added, and the specimen examined by dark-field microscopy.

GELATIN MEDIUM (NUTRIENT)

Gelatin medium is a differential medium used to determine a bacterial isolate's ability to produce gelatinase and thereby hydrolyze gelatin. A variety of gelatin-containing media can be used for this purpose, including starch-gelatin agar, Kohn modified gelatin for the Kohn gelatin method, and nutrient gelatin.

Sterile tubed medium can be stored at 4° C. The medium is inoculated and incubated, along with an uninoculated control tube, at 35° C for 18 to 24 hours. Following incubation, both the inoculated tube and the control tube are refrigerated for 30 minutes before reading. The control tube should gel, whereas the consistency of the inoculated tube will depend on the isolate's ability or inability to hydrolyze gelatin. If the inoculated tube gels, the isolate is gelatinase negative. If the gelatin in the inoculated tube remains liquid, the isolate is gelatinase positive.

GRAM-NEGATIVE BROTH

Gram-negative (GN) broth is a selective enrichment medium used to enhance the chance of recovering enteric pathogens, such as *Salmonella* and *Shigella* spp., from fecal specimens. The selective ingredients are desoxycholate and citrate salts, which inhibit the growth of gram-positive bacteria while allowing the growth of aerobic gram-negative bacteria. Enrichment is provided by increasing the concentration of mannitol, which temporarily favors the growth of mannitol-fermenting, gram-negative rods (*Salmonella* and *Shigella*) over that of the non–mannitol fermenters (e.g., *Proteus*).

Sterile, tubed media should be inoculated with fecal material and incubated, with caps loosened, at 35° C. Incubated GN broth cultures should be subcultured onto selective, differential plated media after 6 to 8 hours and again after 18 to 24 hours.

HAEMOPHILUS TEST MEDIUM

Susceptibility testing of *Haemophilus* isolates is performed on the enriched *Haemophilus* test medium. This medium has a clear agar base and includes beef, yeast, and casein extracts, as well as hematin and NAD. This formulation can also be made as a liquid and used for broth minimal inhibitory concentration (MIC) determinations of *Haemophilus* organisms.

HEKTOEN ENTERIC AGAR

Hektoen enteric (HE) agar is a selective, differential medium used for direct isolation of enteric pathogens from feces and for indirect isolation from selective enrichment broth. The selective ingredients are bile salts at concentrations that not only inhibit the growth of gram-positive bacteria but also inhibit the growth of many gram-negative organisms that are part of the normal intestinal flora. The differential ingredients include lactose, salicin, and sucrose to determine fermentation patterns, detected by the pH indicator bromthymol blue, and ferric salts (sodium thiosulfate and ferric ammonium citrate) to detect the production of hydrogen sulfide gas.

This medium should not be autoclaved, and overheating should be avoided. Plated medium should be inoculated, streaked for isolation, and incubated aerobically (not in CO_2) at 35° C for 18 to 24 hours. Most nonpathogens ferment one or both of the sugars, and colonies appear bright orange to salmon-pink owing to the low-pH interaction with incorporated dyes. Nonfermenters, such as *Salmonella* and *Shigella* spp., typically produce green to blue-green colonies. Hydrogen sulfide gas production is seen as a black precipitate that accumulates within colonies.

HIPPURATE BROTH

Hippurate broth is a differential broth that is useful in the identification of group B streptococci. The differential ingredient is 1% sodium hippurate, which the group B streptococci hydrolyze to glycine and benzoic acid. In this method, hydrolysis is detected by the addition of ferric chloride, which reacts with the benzoic acid to produce ferric benzoate, which precipitates.

The broth should be inoculated with the isolate and incubated at 35° C for more than 20 hours. Following incubation, 0.8 mL of supernatant is removed and placed into another tube, to which 0.2 mL of ferric chloride reagent is added. A positive reaction yields grossly visible precipitate that persists for 10 minutes or longer after the addition of ferric chloride. A negative reaction produces no precipitate or only a faint precipitate that disappears in less than 10 minutes after the addition of ferric chloride. A rapid method available uses a 1% aqueous solution of sodium hippurate dispensed in 0.4-mL quantities. Colonies of the isolate are emulsified in the solution until it is very cloudy and are then incubated in a 37° C water bath for 2 hours. Hydrolysis is detected by adding five drops of ninhydrin reagent (triketohydrindene hydrate) without shaking the tube and continuing to incubate for a minimum of 10 minutes, but not longer than 30 minutes. Positive reactions are deep purple, and negative reactions show no color change.

HYDROGEN SULFIDE, LEAD ACETATE

Lead acetate is one differential method used to detect the production of hydrogen sulfide (H_2S) from sulfur-containing amino acids. The organism is cultured in a nutrient broth or on an agar medium with sufficient protein to ensure the presence of sulfur-containing amino acids. As the organism metabolizes these amino acids, H_2S gas is released. Lead acetate–impregnated paper strips suspended over the culture during incubation detect the liberated gas. The H_2S reacts with the lead acetate to produce lead sulfide, a black insoluble salt, causing the strip to blacken.

KLIGLER'S IRON AGAR

Kligler's iron agar (KIA) can be used to determine whether a gram-negative rod is a glucose or lactose fermenter or both. The medium also tests for gas production during carbohydrate fermentation and hydrogen sulfide production, both of which are useful in the differentiation of gram-negative rods belonging to the family Enterobacteriaceae.

KIA contains glucose and lactose (fermentable carbohydrates), where lactose is present at 10 times the glucose concentration; phenol red (pH indicator); peptone (carbon/nitrogen source); and sodium thiosulfate plus ferric ammonium sulfate (sulfur source and hydrogen sulfide indicator, respectively). KIA resembles triple sugar iron agar (TSI) except it lacks sucrose. When reading the reactions, by convention the following shorthand is used: the reaction of the slant is put over the reaction in the butt; "K" is used for alkaline and "A" for acid. The following three carbohydrate fermentation patterns are possible:

1. Alkaline (red) slant and acid (yellow) butt (K/A) indicate the organism ferments glucose but not lactose. This organism ferments glucose by the Embden-Meyerhof-Parnas (EMP) pathway to produce organic acids, changing the pH indicator from red to yellow. Once the glucose has been consumed, the organism then breaks down peptones, producing ammonia. The breakdown of peptones happens only aerobically and results in an increase in pH, and thus the slant reverts to red.
2. Acid (yellow) slant and acid (yellow) butt (A/A) indicate that the organism ferments both glucose and lactose. The organism ferments glucose, producing acid products. Once the glucose is consumed, it ferments lactose, breaking it down into glucose and galactose, causing the pH in the slant portion to remain acidic.
3. Alkaline (red) slant and alkaline (red) butt (K/K) indicate that the organism cannot ferment glucose or lactose and therefore produces no acidic products. The slant may become redder owing to peptone catabolism. Often, with the lack of glucose fermentation, the butt is the same color as the butt of an uninoculated tube. Therefore some sources prefer the designation "no change" (NC) as opposed to alkaline.

If there are gas bubbles in the butt, splitting of the medium, or displacement of the medium from the bottom of the tube, the organism is aerogenic; that is, it is able to produce carbon dioxide and hydrogen gases during fermentation. This designation is noted in the shorthand designation as "g" (e.g., A/Ag). Any blackening in the butt indicates that the organism produces hydrogen sulfide gas from thiosulfate. The hydrogen sulfide combines with iron salt to produce ferrous sulfide, a black precipitate. H_2S is added after the slant/butt shorthand

to signify that the organism produces H_2S (e.g., K/A H_2S). With an inoculating needle that has a sample of a pure culture of the isolate, inoculate the medium by stabbing the butt and streaking the slant. The cap should be slightly loose. If the cap is screwed on too tightly, there will not be sufficient air for peptone catabolism and, as a result, gram-negative rods able to ferment only glucose may appear as lactose fermenters. Reactions should be interpreted at 18 to 24 hours. If the medium is read earlier, organisms able to ferment only glucose may appear to be lactose fermenters. If the medium is read later, lactose fermenters may consume the lactose and begin to catabolize peptones, with the slant reverting to red. A yellow slant and red butt may indicate failure to stab the butt or inoculation of the medium with gram-positive organisms. Examination of the medium for stab line or performance of Gram stain should clarify this situation. The hydrogen sulfide indicator system in KIA is not as sensitive as the lead acetate method or as sensitive as that found in other media, such as sulfide indole motility agar. A black butt should be read as acid even though yellow color may be obscured. If hydrogen sulfide is reduced, this indicates that an acid condition does exist and can be assumed. Critical to understanding how this medium works is the fact that glucose is present in one tenth the amount of lactose. Organisms use the simplest carbohydrate, glucose, first; once this is consumed, the organisms attack the more complex carbohydrate, lactose. If the organisms lack the appropriate enzymes, they move on to protein catabolism. There is sufficient lactose in the medium to prevent breakdown of peptone, provided it is read at the appropriate time.

LIM BROTH

Lim broth is used for the isolation of *Streptococcus agalactiae*, most often from vaginal or rectal swabs obtained from pregnant women who are being screened for carriage of group B streptococci prior to delivery. Lim broth is a modified Todd-Hewitt broth. The Lim broth contains peptones, yeast extract, and dextrose to support the growth of the streptococci. Colistin and nalidixic acid are added to inhibit the growth of gram-negative organisms.

Lim broth is inoculated with the vaginal/rectal swab and incubated at room temperature for 18 to 24 hours. At this time, the broth is subcultured to a blood agar plate, then incubated at 35° to 37° C in 5% CO_2 for 24 hours. The plate is then examined for the presence of β-hemolytic colonies. If no such colonies are present after the first incubation, the plate should be reincubated and reexamined after another 24-hour incubation period.

LOEFFLER COAGULATED SERUM SLANT

Loeffler coagulated serum slant is used primarily for recovery and identification of *Clostridium diphtheriae*. This medium can be used for primary recovery of *C. diphtheriae* from nose and throat specimens and for subculture purposes. Because Loeffler medium is so enriched, *C. diphtheriae* grows well within 12 to 16 hours and produces nondistinctive translucent to gray-white colonies. The medium promotes the development of characteristic metachromatic granules that can be detected microscopically with methylene-blue stains. High serum content, as well as the incorporation of eggs, enables the detection of proteolytic activity. Positive organisms produce colonies surrounded by small holes containing liquefied medium. The entire slant may eventually turn to liquid and produce a foul odor.

Loeffler serum slant should be inoculated as soon as possible after specimen collection, and more selective media containing tellurite should always be used as well. Smears for *C. diphtheriae* should be prepared and examined after 8 to 24 hours of incubation. Although granule formation is typical of *Corynebacterium* spp., other organisms can produce a similar microscopic appearance. Therefore additional testing must be performed for confirmation of this organism.

LÖWENSTEIN-JENSEN MEDIUM

Löwenstein-Jensen (LJ) medium is used to cultivate *Mycobacterium* spp. Most media contain ingredients that can inhibit the growth of mycobacteria. The potato flour, egg, and glycerol included in LJ medium help to detoxify this medium and also to supply nutrients required for growth of these organisms. Asparagine is included for maximum production of niacin by certain *Mycobacterium* spp. The malachite green inhibits the growth of other bacteria that may be present in specimens.

LJ medium is good for 1 month if tightly capped to prevent moisture loss and stored at 4° to 6° C. LJ medium must be kept out of direct light because malachite green is light-sensitive. Decontaminated, digested, or untreated specimens are inoculated onto the medium and incubated in a carbon dioxide incubator (5% to 10% CO_2) for 6 to 10 weeks. It is important to leave caps loosened for proper gas exchange. LJ medium can be prepared as deeps to be used in semiquantitative catalase testing for ascertaining the particular species of *Mycobacterium*. LJ medium with 5% NaCl may be prepared to aid in identifying rapid growers. This medium is the same as LJ except 5 g of NaCl is added per each 100 mL of medium. The additional salt allows for testing the ability of certain mycobacteria to tolerate and grow in presence of high salt concentration. The Gruft modification makes this medium more selective through the addition of penicillin (50 U/mL) and nalidixic acid (35 µg/mL) before dispensing into tubes. This formulation also includes 0.05 µg/mL of ribonucleic acid, which increases the rate of mycobacterium isolation over the standard LJ formulation. In the Petran and Vera modification, cyclohexamide, lincomycin, and nalidixic acid are added to make LJ more selective. Both modifications can permit gentler decontamination or digestion procedures.

LYSINE-IRON AGAR

Lysine-iron agar (LIA) measures three parameters that are useful in identifying species of Enterobacteriaceae: lysine decarboxylation, lysine deamination, and hydrogen sulfide production.

LIA contains lysine (amino acid), glucose (carbohydrate source), a small amount of protein, bromcresol purple (pH indicator), and sodium thiosulfate/ferric ammonium citrate (sulfur source and hydrogen sulfide indicator). The shorthand similar to that used for KIA is used to record LIA reactions. The difference is that a purple color denotes an alkaline environment and thus gets the "K". Also, an "R" is used for the Bordeaux red color.

Three lysine use patterns are possible:
1. Alkaline (purple) slant and alkaline (purple) butt (K/K) indicate that the organism decarboxylates lysine but cannot deaminate it. Initially the organism ferments glucose, causing production of acid and changing the indicator in the butt to yellow. The organism then decarboxylates lysine to produce cadaverine, an alkaline product, which causes the pH indicator to change from yellow back to purple.
2. Alkaline (purple) slant and acid (yellow) butt (K/A) indicate that the organism fermented the glucose but was unable to deaminate or decarboxylate the lysine.
3. Bordeaux red slant and acid (yellow) butt (R/A) indicate that the organism deaminated lysine but could not decarboxylate it. The yellow butt is caused by glucose fermentation. The red slant results from the product of lysine deamination combining with ferric ammonium citrate and flavin mononucleotide to form a burgundy color on the slant.

Any blackening in the butt indicates production of hydrogen sulfide from sodium thiosulfate. This gas reacts with ferric salt to produce the black precipitate, ferrous sulfide. This medium appears purple before use. LIA is inoculated by stabbing the butt twice and streaking the slant with an inoculating needle. The cap should be left slightly loose because oxygen is required for detection of deamination. Reactions should be read after 18 to 24 hours of incubation at 35° C. The medium may be incubated for up to 48 hours if needed. LIA is not as sensitive as other media for hydrogen sulfide detection. Typically hydrogen sulfide–producing *Proteus* spp. may appear negative. Also, *Morganella morganii* produces a variable lysine deamination reaction after 24 hours of incubation. This medium can be used only with organisms that can ferment glucose. LIA is not a true replacement for the Moeller decarboxylase tests.

MACCONKEY AGAR

MacConkey agar (MAC) is a selective, differential primary plating medium. It selects for Enterobacteriaceae and other gram-negative rods in the presence of mixed flora and differentiates them into lactose fermenters and non–lactose fermenters.

Bile salts and crystal violet inhibit most gram-positive organisms but permit growth of gram-negative rods. Lactose serves as the sole carbohydrate source. Gram-negative rods that ferment lactose produce pink or red colonies, which may be surrounded by precipitated bile. Acid production from lactose fermentation causes the neutral red dye absorbed into the colonies to change to red and can also cause the bile salts to become insoluble. Non–lactose-fermenting gram-negative rods produce colorless or transparent colonies. Plates are streaked for isolation and incubated in ambient air, not in a carbon dioxide incubator, for 18 to 24 hours at 35° C. Weak or slow lactose fermenters may produce colorless colonies at 24 hours or appear slightly pink in 24 to 48 hours. Plates should not be incubated longer than 48 hours because this can lead to confusing results. Some gram-negative rods may fail to grow on the medium, whereas with prolonged incubation, gram-positives such as *Enterococcus* spp. may produce tiny colonies. Room-temperature incubation may enhance recovery of *Yersinia enterocolitica*. The agar concentration may be increased to prevent swarming of *Proteus* spp. A formulation of MAC without crystal violet has been used to aid in identifying mycobacteria.

MACCONKEY SORBITOL AGAR

MacConkey sorbitol agar contains the same components as MAC except D-sorbitol is substituted for lactose. This medium has been used to isolate *E. coli* O157:H7, which does not ferment sorbitol very rapidly. Plates should be incubated at 37° C for 24 hours. Sorbitol-negative colonies will appear colorless on this medium, may indicate possible *E. coli* O157:H7, and should be tested further. Most other clinical isolates of *E. coli* produce a pink to red color on this medium.

MALONATE BROTH

Malonate broth is used in the identification of species of Enterobacteriaceae, particularly *Salmonella*. The broth contains sodium malonate (the primary carbon source), small quantities of glucose and yeast extract (nutrients), bromthymol blue (pH indicator), various salts, and a buffering system. Organisms producing a Prussian blue color are able to use malonate as a carbon source. If they can use malonate as a carbon source, they also employ ammonium sulfate as a nitrogen source, thereby producing alkaline products that cause a rise in pH and a change in the color of the medium to blue. Organisms unable to use malonate as a carbon source usually fail to grow, and the medium stays green. Because malonate resembles succinate, it competitively binds to succinic dehydrogenase, which catalyzes the succinate to fumarate reaction in the Krebs cycle. The inhibition of this enzyme, coupled with the inability to use malonate as a carbon source, prevents growth of the malonate-negative organism.

Malonate broth should be inoculated from triple sugar iron agar, KIA, or broth culture of the organism. The inoculum should be light. Cultures should be incubated at 35° C, checked at 18 to 24 hours, and checked again at 48 hours for production of a blue color. Some organisms produce only small amounts of alkalinity. Any trace of blue should be considered positive. Comparison with an uninoculated tube may be useful. Production of a yellow color is a negative reaction and is probably due to fermentation of the small amount of glucose in the medium.

MANNITOL SALT AGAR

Mannitol salt agar is a selective and differential primary culture medium that is useful in recovery and identification of staphylococci from specimens containing mixed flora.

High salt concentration (7.5%) inhibits most gram-negative and gram-positive bacteria except *Staphylococcus* spp. *S. aureus* is able to ferment mannitol, the sole carbohydrate in the medium, to produce acid products. This lowers the pH and changes the color of the pH indicator, phenol red, to yellow. Colonies of *S. aureus* typically appear yellow, surrounded by a yellow zone. Other *Staphylococcus* and *Micrococcus* spp. usually do not ferment mannitol and therefore produce reddish colonies that may exhibit a red to purple surrounding zone as a result of peptone breakdown. Plates are streaked for isolation and incubated at 35° C for 24 to 48 hours in ambient air. *Enterococcus* may be able to grow on mannitol salt agar and weakly ferment mannitol. Differentiation is readily accomplished through Gram stain and catalase test. With prolonged incubation, organisms other than staphylococci may begin to grow and ferment mannitol. Some strains of *S. aureus* may be slow in fermenting mannitol, so plates should not be discarded until after 48 hours of incubation. All colonies suggestive of *S. aureus* should be further tested for coagulase or with an alternative acceptable procedure. Subculture to less selective agar is preferable before performing this testing. Some formulations recommend inclusion of 20 mL of sterile egg yolk. Coagulase-positive staphylococci also produce a lipase that causes formation of an opaque precipitate around the colonies. Non–coagulase-producing staphylococci do not produce this egg yolk lipase and therefore lack these zones.

MES (*UREAPLASMA* AGAR)

MES [2-(*N*-morpholino)ethanesulfonic acid] agar is used for the isolation of *U. urealyticum*. This medium contains horse serum, which supplies the cholesterol necessary for stabilizing these organisms because they lack cell walls. Yeast dialysate serves as a growth factor and supplies preformed nucleic acid precursors. Urea is a required nutrient for *Ureaplasma*. Phenol red serves as a pH indicator, and MES or 2-(*N*-morpholino) ethanesulfonic acid acts as a buffer. The antibiotics penicillin and lincomycin inhibit normal flora but permit the growth of *Ureaplasma*. After the components are mixed together, the medium is poured into Petri dishes (5 mL per plate). The plates are stored in plastic for up to 2 weeks under refrigeration. Inoculated plates should be incubated in a carbon dioxide incubator or under anaerobic conditions. At 48 hours colonies of *Ureaplasma* show a "fried-egg" appearance. If a solution of 1% urea and 0.8% manganese chloride is poured over these colonies, they will turn dark brown owing to the production of urease.

METHYL RED–VOGES-PROSKAUER MEDIUM

Methyl red–Voges-Proskauer medium (MRVP) broth is used for performing the methyl red and Voges-Proskauer tests. These procedures are useful in distinguishing among members of the Enterobacteriaceae. For example, *E. coli* is methyl red positive and Voges-Proskauer negative; *Enterobacter aerogenes, Enterobacter cloacae,* and *Klebsiella pneumoniae* show the reverse reactions.

Members of Enterobacteriaceae can be divided into two groups based on the way they metabolize glucose. One group produces large amounts of mixed acids (lactic, formic, succinic, and acetic). When methyl red reagent is added to one of these cultures, a red color is produced owing to the acidic pH. The other group produces predominantly neutral end products, acetoin or acetylmethylcarbinol, by the butylene glycol pathway. When α-naphthol and 40% potassium hydroxide are added to the broth culture containing a member of this latter group, acetoin (if present) is oxidized to diacetyl in the presence of air and base. α-Naphthol catalyzes a reaction between the diacetyl and guanidine components of peptone to produce a pink-red color.

For the methyl-red test, the broth culture is inoculated with a light inoculum and must be incubated for 48 hours. The Voges-Proskauer test was originally designed to be performed after 5 days of incubation at 30° C. By using 0.5 to 1 mL of broth per tube, the test can be done after 18 to 24 hours of incubation at 35° C. Shaking aerates the broth culture and enhances the reaction.

MIDDLEBROOK 7H10 AND 7H11 AGARS

Middlebrook 7H10 and 7H11 agars are used to cultivate *Mycobacterium* spp. Isoniazid-resistant strains grow better on these media, especially Middlebrook 7H11, than on egg-based media such as LJ. The Middlebrook agars are also more chemically defined than the LJ formulations.

Middlebrook 7H10 and 7H11 are similar, except 7H11 contains casein hydrolysate, which stimulates growth of drug-resistant *Mycobacterium tuberculosis*. Both media contain growth factors, such as amino acids, glycerol, and inorganic salts, that encourage recovery of mycobacteria. In addition, both formulations include OADC (oleic acid–dextrose-catalase) enrichment, which chemically simulates egg components. The oleic acid is a fatty acid that is used by the mycobacteria. Albumin is added to inhibit toxic agents that might be present and to provide a source of protein. The added dextrose is for the mycobacteria to use to generate energy. Finally, the exogenous catalase neutralizes toxic peroxides. Malachite green is also added, although at a lower concentration than in LJ, and it gives some selectivity to the medium. Thin pour Middlebrook 7H11 plates are commercially available that have a reduced volume of medium in the plate. These thin pour plates are used to detect mycobacterial colonies faster than on standard pour plates. The thin pour plate is inoculated with a specimen and examined microscopically every 2 days for the appearance of microcolonies.

MITCHISON 7H11 SELECTIVE AGAR

Mitchison 7H11 selective agar is prepared by adding antibiotics to the Middlebrook 7H11 formulation, thereby making the medium more selective for mycobacteria. Amphotericin B, carbenicillin, polymyxin B, and trimethoprim are typically incorporated to make Mitchison 7H11 selective agar more inhibitory to gram-negative rods in particular, as well as yeast.

MODIFIED THAYER-MARTIN

Modified Thayer-Martin (MTM) agar is a selective enrichment medium used for recovering *Neisseria gonorrhoeae* and *N. meningitidis* from specimens that have mixed flora. MTM agar is highly enriched to support the growth of the more fastidious *Neisseria* spp. A chocolate agar base and added growth factors such as hemoglobin, vitamins, diphosphopyridine nucleotide, L-cysteine, NAD, and glutamine constitute the main constituents of MTM. Cornstarch is also included to absorb any inhibitory substances that might be present. The modified formulation has less agar and dextrose than the original Thayer-Martin medium. These changes seem to result in improved recovery of *Neisseria* spp. MTM and Thayer-Martin media both contain antibiotics that allow for the growth of pathogenic *Neisseria* spp. and prevent the growth of most other organisms. Both media contain vancomycin to inhibit the growth of gram-positive cocci, colistin to inhibit gram-negative rods, and nystatin to prevent the growth of fungi. MTM differs from the original Thayer-Martin formulation by the addition of trimethoprim, which prevents *Proteus* spp. from swarming.

Martin-Lewis agar was developed as a modification of the MTM formulation. In Martin-Lewis agar, anisomycin (20 μg/mL) is substituted for nystatin as the antifungal agent. In addition, the vancomycin concentration (4 μg/mL) is higher than in the MTM formulation. When using MTM plates, the microbiologist should incubate them in a carbon dioxide incubator or candle jar for several days. Because some strains of *N. gonorrhoeae* can be inhibited by vancomycin and trimethoprim, a chocolate plate should be used in conjunction with an MTM plate.

MOTILITY TEST MEDIUM

The purpose of the motility test medium is to determine whether an organism is motile or nonmotile. This test is particularly useful in the identification of members of the Enterobacteriaceae, in which two genera, *Shigella* and *Klebsiella*, are always nonmotile, and certain *Yersinia* spp. show motility at room temperature but not at 35° C. *L. monocytogenes* gives a classic umbrella-shaped motility pattern, and the non–glucose-fermenting gram-negative rods can be differentiated based in part on their motility.

Nonmotile organisms, which lack flagella, grow only along the stab line, and the surrounding medium remains clear. Motile organisms, which usually possess flagella, move out from the stab line, and the medium appears cloudy. Low agar concentration makes the medium semisolid and permits better detection of motility. The medium is inoculated using an inoculating needle to stab the middle of the medium straight up and down once without going all the way to the bottom of the medium. It is important to be careful and remove the inoculating needle along the initial stab line. Motility media should be incubated at 35° C. Because flagellar protein is not formed as well at higher temperatures, some microbiologists prefer incubation at 18° to 20° C. For *Yersinia,* noting the motility reaction at room temperature is particularly useful. Triphenyl-tetrazolium chloride (TTC) may be added to the basic motility medium to enhance detection of motility. A 1% solution of TTC is prepared and filter sterilized, and 5 mL of this solution is added to 1 L of motility medium. If TTC is used, bacteria incorporate colorless TTC and reduce it to a red formazan pigment. The medium shows reddening where there is growth. Other media such as SIM (sulfide indole motility) and MIO (motility indole ornithine) can be used to detect motility in addition to other reactions.

MUELLER-HINTON AGAR

Mueller-Hinton agar is a transparent medium that is useful in testing the susceptibility of organisms to antibiotics. The medium also has been used for testing starch hydrolysis. Because Mueller-Hinton agar contains animal infusion, casein extract, and starch, it supports the growth of most organisms. In addition, sheep blood may be added to the basic formulation to perform susceptibility testing on streptococci, in particular *Streptococcus pneumoniae*. The addition of heated or chocolatized sheep blood to Mueller-Hinton agar makes an enriched medium that can be used for susceptibility testing of fastidious organisms, such as *Haemophilus* and *Neisseria*. Starch is included in the medium for two reasons: it may protect the organisms against toxic substances, and it also serves as an energy source. Ca^{++} and Mg^{++} concentrations are critical in the testing of *Pseudomonas* isolates with aminoglycoside antibiotics. Usually Mueller-Hinton agar contains sufficient amounts of bivalent cations, but it may be necessary to add these substances to Mueller-Hinton broth.

MUELLER-HINTON AGAR WITH 2% NaCl

The addition of 2% NaCl to the basic Mueller-Hinton medium results in a medium that is selective for staphylococci. This formulation is thus used to test the susceptibility of *Staphylococcus* spp. to nafcillin and oxacillin using the Kirby-Bauer method or Etest. Once inoculated, the medium should be incubated at 35° C for a full 24 hours to detect more accurately the heteroresistant methicillin-resistant isolates.

MUELLER-HINTON AGAR WITH 4% NaCl AND 6 µg OXACILLIN

For this variation, 4% NaCl and 6 µg oxacillin are added to the basic Mueller-Hinton medium to selectively screen *S. aureus* isolates for resistance to oxacillin or nafcillin. The inoculated plate should be incubated for 24 hours at 35° C in ambient air and examined using transmitted light for the presence of colonies.

NEW YORK CITY MEDIUM

The purpose of New York City (NYC) medium is to isolate *N. gonorrhoeae* and *N. meningitidis* from specimens containing mixed normal flora. This medium will also support the growth of some mycoplasmas as well as *Ureaplasma urealyticum*.

NYC medium is enriched with hemoglobin from lysed horse erythrocytes, yeast dialysate, and horse plasma to support the growth of *N. gonorrhoeae* and *N. meningitidis*. Selectivity for these two organisms is accomplished by incorporating four antibiotics that inhibit normal flora. Vancomycin prevents the growth of gram-positive bacteria, colistin inhibits gram-negative rods, and amphotericin B prevents growth of yeast and

molds. Trimethoprim is included to prevent swarming of *Proteus* spp. Inoculated NYC plates should be incubated in increased carbon dioxide for several days. Also, a nonselective agar, such as CHOC, should also be inoculated because 5% of gonococci are inhibited by the antibiotics, particularly vancomycin and trimethoprim, found in this medium.

NITRATE REDUCTION BROTH

The purpose of nitrate reduction broth is to determine whether an organism can reduce nitrate to nitrite or to gaseous end products, such as nitrogen. The test is useful in the recognition of members of Enterobacteriaceae, and differentiation of non–glucose-fermenting gram-negative rods, *Neisseria* spp., and *Moraxella catarrhalis*.

The nitrate broth is inoculated with the test organism and incubated for 18 to 24 hours at 35° C. The determination of nitrate reduction is performed in two parts. Sulfanilic acid and N,N-dimethyl-α-naphthylamine reagents are added first. If nitrate has been reduced to nitrite, nitrite will react with these reagents to form a red diazonium dye, *p*-sulfobenzene-azonaphthylamine, and the test is read as positive. If there is no color change, then either nitrate was not reduced or the nitrate was reduced to nitrogen gas. In this situation zinc dust is added. Zinc reduces the remaining nitrate to nitrite, forming a red color. If nitrates are still present and a red color appears after the addition of zinc, then the organism is nitrate reduction negative. However, if nitrate was reduced to nitrogen gas, no color change occurs and the test is interpreted as positive. The presence of gas can be detected by putting a Durham tube into the broth before incubation. Gas produced during nitrate reduction will be captured in the tube and seen as a bubble. This test needs to be performed correctly to avoid incorrect interpretations. The results should be immediately determined after the addition of the reagents because the color fades quickly. If it is necessary to add zinc, avoid using large amounts. Too much zinc can result in the formation of hydrogen gas, which can cause reduction and decrease the color reaction. The medium may need to be supplemented with serum and incubated for up to 5 days in testing for *Neisseria* organisms.

NUTRIENT AGAR

Nutrient agar has been used to distinguish between the non-fastidious, less pathogenic *Neisseria* spp. and pathogenic *Neisseria* spp, such as *N. gonorrhoeae* and *N. meningitidis*.

Nutrient agar contains minimal nutrients and an especially low concentration of protein. Growth of an isolate on this medium means that it is not very fastidious and does not require special supplements. The less fastidious neisseriae grow on nutrient agar, whereas the more pathogenic species do not. Nutrient agar also has been used for the maintenance of stock cultures.

OXIDATIVE-FERMENTATIVE MEDIUM (HUGH AND LEIFSON FORMULATION)

Oxidative-fermentative (OF) medium is used to determine whether a gram-negative non–glucose-fermenting rod is oxidative, fermentative, or biochemically inert. Three modifications over traditional media make this medium useful in testing nonfermenting gram-negative rods. A low concentration of peptone prevents formation of alkaline products that might neutralize the small quantities of acid produced through oxidation. The high concentration of carbohydrate increases the potential amount of acid that can be formed, and the lower concentration of agar makes the medium semisolid, permitting acids formed on the surface to diffuse throughout the medium. Bromthymol blue serves as the pH indicator for acid detection.

The classic method for using this medium involves the stabbing of two tubes with the organism. The medium in one tube is covered with vaspar (a mixture of petrolatum and paraffin) or melted paraffin. Sterile mineral oil has been used for this purpose, but it is not recommended because it does not block oxygen as well. Results are interpreted after incubation at 35° C. Several days of incubation may be required because of the slower growth of some nonfermenting gram-negative rods. A color change to yellow in both tubes means the organism is fermentative (i.e., it can produce acid in the absence of oxygen). Color change to yellow in the uncovered tube only means that the organism is oxidative (requires oxygen to use the carbohydrate). If neither tube changes in color or the covered tube shows no change while the uncovered tube turns blue, the organism cannot use the carbohydrate oxidatively or fermentatively and is considered inert. A one-tube modification of this test has been described. One tube is stabbed, and it is not covered. Color change to yellow near the top of the medium only indicates the oxidative use of glucose. If the entire tube changes to yellow, fermentation is suggested. Because the medium is semisolid, motility may be observed in this medium. NOTE: Sometimes OF medium is used for differentiating staphylococci (fermentative) from micrococci (oxidative). This testing requires a different formulation.

OXIDATIVE-FERMENTATIVE POLYMYXIN B–BACITRACIN-LACTOSE AGAR

Oxidative-fermentative polymyxin B–bacitracin-lactose agar (OFPBL) is a selective and differential medium used for the isolation of *Burkholderia cepacia* from the respiratory samples of patients with cystic fibrosis. Polymyxin B and bacitracin are added to inhibit the growth of most gram-negative and gram-positive organisms. The medium differentiates between colonies that grow based on the ability or inability of the isolate to ferment lactose. *B. cepacia* can ferment lactose and appears as a yellow colony. Non–lactose-fermenting colonies that grow appear green. OFPBL plates should be inoculated with the specimen and incubated aerobically at 30° C.

PEPTONE–YEAST EXTRACT–GLUCOSE BROTH

Peptone–yeast extract–glucose (PYG) broth is useful for culturing anaerobes. PYG broth culture of an anaerobic isolate may be used in gas-liquid chromatography procedures that detect metabolic end products.

PYG broth contains several nutrients and supplements that encourage the growth of anaerobes. These enrichments include vitamin K (required for pigment-producing *Prevotella* and *Porphyromonas*), yeast extract, hemin, and glucose. Cysteine helps keep the medium more reduced and anaerobic. Resazurin serves as an anaerobic indicator. Pink color means that oxygen is present.

PHENYLALANINE DEAMINASE AGAR

Phenylalanine deaminase (PAD) agar is used to detect an organism's ability to deaminate phenylalanine. A positive reaction is most useful for distinguishing *Proteus, Providencia,* and *Morganella* spp. from other members of the family Enterobacteriaceae. This test also can be used to distinguish *Moraxella* organisms that are phenylpyruvate-positive from other *Moraxella* organisms.

PAD agar includes the following: phenylalanine; yeast extract, a nitrogen and carbon source; various salts; and agar (a solidifying agent). Protein hydrolysates and meat extracts are not included because these substances contain a variable amount of phenylalanine. The PAD slant is inoculated with the test organism, and the slant is incubated at 35° C for 18 to 24 hours. At the end of the incubation period, a few drops of 12% $FeCl_3$ are added to the tube so that they run down the slant. If an organism produces phenylalanine deaminase, it converts phenylalanine to the α-keto acid, called *phenylpyruvic acid*. This acid reacts with the added ferric chloride reagent to form a dark-green complex. The immediate appearance of a dark-green slant on addition of ferric chloride reagent is a positive reaction; no color change upon addition of reagent is a negative reaction.

PHENYLETHYL ALCOHOL AGAR

The purpose of phenylethyl alcohol (PEA) agar is to isolate gram-positive cocci, such as staphylococci and streptococci, from specimens having mixed flora. Most gram-positive rods will also grow on this medium, except *Bacillus anthracis,* which is unique among the *Bacillus* spp. in its lack of growth on this medium.

PEA agar is similar to sheep blood agar except PEA contains phenylethyl alcohol. This component inhibits facultative gram-negative rods, especially swarming *Proteus* spp., but permits the growth of gram-positive cocci. Phenylethyl alcohol is volatile, and plates should be tightly sealed in plastic bags and stored in the refrigerator. Hemolytic reactions are not dependable on this medium because of the action of phenylethyl alcohol on cell membranes. Gram-negative rods may grow on PEA agar, but colonies are smaller than usual and can be readily differentiated from those of gram-positive rods. *P. aeruginosa* is not inhibited by this medium. Some gram-positive cocci may require more than 24 hours of incubation to grow well on PEA agar. An anaerobic formulation can be achieved by adding phenylethyl alcohol to CDC anaerobic agar before autoclaving or by supplementing the formulation with vitamin K and sheep blood after sterilization of basal medium. The anaerobic formulation of this medium selects for gram-negative and gram-positive nonsporulating anaerobes while inhibiting the facultatively anaerobic gram-negative rods and other anaerobes.

PPLO AGAR

PPLO agar is used to isolate *Mycoplasma* spp. PPLO is derived from the original name for *mycoplasmas, pleuropneumonia-like organism*. Nutrients in this medium are provided by yeast-enriched peptones, serum, and heart infusion. Sodium chloride is added to maintain the osmotic balance. Agar is added to solidify the medium, but at a lower concentration than in other solid agar plates. With less agar, the medium is softer so that the mycoplasmas can grow into the medium and grow only slightly on top of the plate. Antibiotics can be added to inhibit the growth of contaminating bacteria. The medium should be inoculated with the specimen and incubated at 35° C in 5% to 10% CO_2. Plates should be examined under a microscope for the growth of small (0.01- to 0.5-mm diameter) colonies that have a dense center surrounded by a less dense periphery ("fried-egg"-like). Plates should be saved for at least 7 days before they are discarded as negative.

PSEUDOMONAS CEPACIA AGAR

Pseudomonas cepacia (PC) agar was developed to isolate selectively *B. cepacia* from respiratory specimens collected from patients with cystic fibrosis. *B. cepacia* grows more slowly than do other bacterial organisms and has variable colony morphologies on routine media. As a result other organisms would often overgrow the *B. cepacia,* and, because the colonies were often different, isolation and detection of *B. cepacia* were problematic. Crystal violet, bile salts, polymyxin B, and ticarcillin are incorporated to inhibit most gram-positive and gram-negative organisms. These selective agents are added to a medium containing inorganic salts, peptones, pyruvate, and phenol red. *B. cepacia* can grow on this medium and utilize the pyruvate. The breakdown of pyruvate results in the production of alkaline by-products. The increased pH changes the phenol red indicator from dull yellow to hot pink.

REGAN-LOWE MEDIUM

Regan-Lowe medium is enriched and selective for the isolation of *B. pertussis*. The nutritional base comprises beef extracts, horse blood, niacin, and pancreatic digests. Cephalexin is the selective agent. Charcoal and starch are added to neutralize the inhibitors, especially fatty acids and peroxides that might be present in the medium.

Inoculated plates should be incubated aerobically at 35° to 37° C in a moist environment for 5 to 7 days. *B. pertussis* colonies are domed, shiny, transparent, and tiny. The colonies are described as resembling mercury droplets. Regan-Lowe transport medium is also available. The transport medium differs from the isolation medium in that the transport medium uses lysed horse blood, whereas whole horse blood is used in the isolation medium. In addition, the transport medium contains half as much charcoal as the isolation medium.

SALMONELLA-SHIGELLA AGAR

Salmonella-Shigella (SS) agar is used to select for *Salmonella* and some strains of *Shigella* from stool specimens. SS agar is also differential in that these organisms produce characteristic colonies on the medium.

SS agar contains bile salts, sodium citrate, and brilliant green, which inhibit the growth of gram-positive and many lactose-fermenting gram-negative rods normally found in stool. Lactose is the sole carbohydrate source in the medium, and neutral red is the pH indicator. If an organism grows on the medium and ferments lactose, it will produce acid and change the indicator to pink-red. Sodium thiosulfate is added as a source of sulfur for the production of hydrogen sulfide. If hydrogen sulfide is produced, it reacts with the ferric ammonium citrate present in the medium, forming a black precipitate in the center of the colony. A heavy inoculum of stool can be planted on SS agar because the formulation is so inhibitory; however, strains of *Shigella* may not grow on SS agar, and this medium should not be used as the sole primary plating medium when *Shigella* is the potential isolate. *Shigella* colonies appear colorless on SS agar because these organisms do not ferment lactose or produce hydrogen sulfide. *Salmonella* colonies are colorless with a black center because these organisms usually make hydrogen sulfide but do not ferment lactose. Pink to red colonies indicate that the organism ferments lactose; if there is a black center, it also produces hydrogen sulfide. If *Proteus* grows on this medium, swarming is inhibited.

SCHAEDLER'S AGAR

Schaedler's agar is an enriched medium used for the isolation of anaerobic bacteria. Vegetable and meat peptones, yeast extract, and dextrose provide nutrients for the anaerobes. The growth of more fastidious anaerobes is aided by the addition of vitamin K, sheep blood, and hemin. Facultative anaerobes will also grow on this medium, so aerotolerance testing should be performed on all isolated colonies to determine their oxygen dependency.

SELENITE BROTH

Selenite broth is an enrichment broth used for the recovery of low numbers of *Salmonella* and some strains of *Shigella* from stool and other specimens containing large amounts of mixed bacteria. The sodium selenite present in this medium inhibits the growth of many gram-negative rods and enterococci but permits recovery of *Salmonella* and some *Shigella* species. Selenite is most effective at a neutral pH. Reduction of selenite during bacterial growth produces alkaline products that may inhibit the growth of the salmonella and also reduce the toxicity of the selenite for other organisms, so lactose and phosphate buffers have been included in this medium to maintain a neutral pH. Lactose fermenters produce acid, which neutralizes these alkaline products and returns the medium to a neutral pH, at which selenite works most effectively.

Approximately 1 to 2 g of stool should be inoculated into the broth, which is then incubated at 35° to 37° C. The broth should be subcultured to enteric media after it has incubated 12 to 18 hours (some references suggest 6 to 12 hours). Beyond this time frame, overgrowth with normal flora is likely because the inhibitory effect of the selenite decreases after 12 hours. A variation of the selenite broth formulation includes the addition of cystine to increase the recovery of *Salmonella*.

SODIUM CHLORIDE BROTH, 6.5%

Sodium chloride (NaCl) broth is useful in the differentiation of streptococci, particularly those producing β-hemolytic and nonhemolytic colonies. Primarily it distinguishes *Enterococcus* spp. (positive) from group D streptococci (negative), both of which produce a positive bile-esculin reaction. In addition, viridans streptococci can be distinguished from *Enterococcus* (which may sometimes appear α-hemolytic) because the viridans streptococci, like group D streptococci, cannot grow in this medium.

Sodium chloride broth is prepared from heart infusion broth, a general-purpose medium that already contains 0.5% NaCl. When 6% NaCl is added to this medium, the salt concentration becomes 6.5%. Sodium chloride broth also contains glucose as a carbohydrate source, and some formulations add bromcresol purple, a pH indicator. If the organism can tolerate this high concentration of salt, it will grow in the medium and produce cloudiness. Fermentation of glucose produces acid and may cause the medium to turn from purple to yellow if the pH indicator is present. To use this medium, several colonies are inoculated into the broth and incubated overnight at 35° C. Any growth in the broth is considered positive even if the indicator does not change color. To avoid a false-negative result, the broth should be gently mixed before interpretation. Inoculating the broth too heavily may give a false-positive result. Organisms other than enterococci, such as group B streptococci and aerococci, can produce positive results.

SP-4 BROTH/AGAR

SP-4 broth and SP-4 agar serve as primary isolation media for *Mycoplasma* spp. SP-4 media contain yeast products that serve as growth factors for *Mycoplasma* and supply preformed nucleic acid. Fetal bovine serum supplies the cholesterol necessary for stabilizing these organisms because they lack cell walls. Various antibiotics inhibit normal flora that may be present in the specimen. Penicillin is included to prevent the growth of gram-positive bacteria; amphotericin B inhibits fungi; and polymyxin B inhibits gram-negative rods. Biphasic media provide both microaerophilic and moist conditions, which some *Mycoplasma* spp. prefer.

SP-4: ARGININE, GLUCOSE, AND UREA BROTHS

SP-4 broths are useful in the identification of *Mycoplasma* and *Ureaplasma* spp. Yeast products included in SP-4 broth supply nutrients required for the growth of *Mycoplasma* and *Ureaplasma* organisms. Fetal bovine serum contains cholesterol, which helps to stabilize these organisms because they lack cell walls. Penicillin prevents the growth of gram-positive cocci but does not affect the mycoplasmas because they do not possess cell walls. Phenol red serves as a pH indicator. In SP-4 arginine broth, utilization of arginine results in the production of alkaline products and a color change to red. This reaction is characteristic of *Mycoplasma hominis*. In SP-4 urea broth, removal of an amino group from urea, characteristic of *Ureaplasma* spp., causes formation of ammonia and a similar color change to red. SP-4 glucose broth detects glucose fermentation. Acid is produced, which lowers the medium's pH and changes its color to yellow. This reaction is typical of *Mycoplasma pneumoniae*, as well as a few other *Mycoplasma* spp.

STREPTOCOCCUS-SELECTIVE AGAR

Streptococcus-selective agar is a selective medium used to isolate streptococci, primarily to detect β-hemolytic streptococci in throat swabs. Columbia agar is the base to which ribonucleic acid and maltose are added to enhance the production of streptolysin S. Polymyxin B and neomycin are added to inhibit the growth of gram-positive and gram-negative organisms that are found as normal oral flora. An alternate formulation incorporates colistin and oxolinic acid to suppress the normal flora. Nonselective media (e.g., a blood agar plate) should also be inoculated with the specimen, and the growth on both plates should be compared.

TELLURITE BLOOD AGAR WITH OR WITHOUT CYSTINE

Tellurite blood agar is a selective-differential enrichment agar that is useful in isolating *C. diphtheriae*. All formulations include animal blood as a source of enrichment. Some formulations also incorporate cystine to further enhance the growth of fastidious organisms, including *C. diphtheriae*. Potassium tellurite is the selective and differential ingredient responsible for inhibiting the growth of gram-negative organisms, staphylococci, and streptococci while allowing the growth of *C. diphtheriae* and diphtheroids. *C. diphtheriae* reduces the tellurite, resulting in a black colony. This isolate also breaks down the cystine, which is seen as a brown halo in the medium surrounding the colony.

Tubes of base medium can be stored and melted to make the complete medium as culture plates are needed. Freshly plated medium should be inoculated, streaked for isolation, and incubated at 35° C. On this medium, colonies of *C. diphtheriae* are dull gray-black, whereas diphtheroids are light gray-green with dark centers. Some *Staphylococcus* spp., gram-negative bacilli, and yeasts may overcome inhibition and grow on this medium. The *Staphylococcus* colonies are large, glistening, and jet black, whereas those of the gram-negative bacilli and yeast are dull gray-black but larger than the *C. diphtheriae* colonies.

TETRATHIONATE BROTH

Tetrathionate broth is an enrichment medium used for recovery of low numbers of *Salmonella* spp. from stool specimens.

Tetrathionate is produced when an iodine–potassium iodide solution is added to the basal broth. Bile salts in conjunction with thiosulfate and the added iodine-iodide solution inhibit the growth of most gram-negative rods and gram-positive organisms except *Salmonella*. Some formulations also include brilliant green or crystal violet, which increases the inhibitory nature of the medium. The medium must be used within 24 hours of preparation. Because the basal medium may be stored in the refrigerator indefinitely, some microbiologists prefer to dispense 10 mL of basal medium per tube. Just before use, 0.2 mL of iodine solution can be added to each tube. A heavy inoculum of stool can be added to the broth. After 12 to 24 hours of incubation at 35° C, the broth should be subcultured to enteric media to prevent overgrowth with normal flora. This medium inhibits most *Shigella* spp. and should not be used for recovering *Salmonella typhi*.

THIOGLYCOLATE BROTH, BASAL AND ENRICHED

Thioglycolate broth is an all-purpose medium that can be used to isolate a wide range of bacteria. It is often used as a backup broth and inoculated along with culture plates. In this case, it helps detect either organisms that are present in low numbers or anaerobes that are present in the original specimen. When glucose is omitted, thioglycolate broth can be used in fermentation studies of anaerobes.

Nutrients are provided by the incorporation of casein and soy proteins. Thioglycolate, cystine, and sodium sulfite act as reducing agents in this medium, and the low concentration of agar prevents downward diffusion of oxygen, allowing for the growth of anaerobic organisms toward the bottom of the tube. Various supplements can be added to support the growth of more fastidious organisms. These include hemin (5 μg/mL), vitamin K (0.1 μg/mL), and sodium bicarbonate (1 mg/mL), which can be autoclaved in the medium. Supplements that must be added after autoclaving include rabbit or horse serum (10% vol/vol) and Fildes enrichment (5% vol/vol), which are given as final concentrations in the medium. Thioglycolate broth should be stored at room temperature, then boiled and cooled before use. When used as a backup broth, the medium is incubated at 35° C for 3 to 7 days and examined for turbidity. Gram stains of broth are compared with growth obtained on primary culture plates. If something different appears to be growing in the broth, subcultures should be performed.

THIOSULFATE CITRATE BILE SALTS SUCROSE AGAR

Thiosulfate citrate bile salts (TCBS) sucrose agar is a selective medium used to isolate *Vibrio* spp. from stool specimens having mixed flora. TCBS agar is also differential in that *Vibrio* spp. produce characteristic colonies. *Vibrio* spp. grow poorly on media designed for isolation of *Salmonella* and *Shigella* but produce colorless colonies on MAC. TCBS agar includes sodium citrate, sodium thiosulfate, and oxgall (10% solution equivalent to full-strength bile), which together inhibit many gram-positive cocci and gram-negative rods nor-

mally present in stool specimens. In addition, the high pH of TCBS agar encourages the growth of *Vibrio* spp. while inhibiting other organisms. The ability or inability of an organism to ferment sucrose is the basis for differentiating between various species of *Vibrio*. Bromthymol blue and, in some formulations, thymol blue are incorporated to indicate the pH. For example, *Vibrio cholerae* and *Vibrio alginolyticus* produce yellow colonies because they can ferment sucrose, whereas *Vibrio parahaemolyticus* and *Vibrio vulnificus* usually produce blue-green colonies because they do not ferment sucrose. Organisms that can produce hydrogen sulfide from sodium thiosulfate have black centers because of the reaction of this gas with ferric citrate. *Vibrio* spp. do not produce hydrogen sulfide. Oxgall and sodium cholate or bile salts (8 g/L) can be used in place of oxgall alone.

When using TCBS agar, a heavy inoculum should be applied because *Vibrio* spp. die off quickly, and this medium is very inhibitory. A fresh specimen is best because these organisms are sensitive to drying out, sunlight, and acid pH. If there is a delay in planting, Cary-Blair semisolid transport medium should be inoculated with the stool specimen rather than buffered glycerol transport medium. Plates should be incubated at 35° C for 18 to 24 hours and up to 48 hours. Oxidase testing cannot be performed on colonies isolated on TCBS agar. Occasionally strains of *V. cholerae* produce blue-green colonies on this medium because of delayed sucrose fermentation. Some *Vibrio* spp. do not grow well on this medium. Also, other organisms, such as *Pseudomonas, Plesiomonas*, and *Aeromonas*, can grow on TCBS agar and usually produce blue colonies; therefore these must be distinguished from *Vibrio* spp.

TINSDALE AGAR

Tinsdale agar is a selective, differential medium useful in isolating and identifying *C. diphtheriae* from specimens containing mixed flora. Tinsdale agar contains a high concentration of potassium tellurite, which inhibits the growth of most normal flora but permits *Corynebacterium* spp., especially *C. diphtheriae*, to grow. All *Corynebacterium* spp. growing on the medium produce gray to black colonies owing to the reduction of tellurite to tellurium. In addition, *C. diphtheriae* colonies are surrounded by a brown halo. The brown halo is produced from the interaction of tellurite with the hydrogen sulfide produced by the organism from cystine and thiosulfate. The basal medium can be stored indefinitely; tellurite and serum can be added just before use. Once prepared, the medium has a shelf life of 4 days.

When using Tinsdale agar, the plates are streaked for isolation and the medium is stabbed in several areas. Sometimes browning occurs in these stabbed areas before it can be seen around colonies. Plates should be incubated at 35° C for 24 to 48 hours in ambient air. Increased carbon dioxide can slow down the production of the brown halo. It may require 48 hours for some *C. diphtheriae* strains to produce the characteristic halo. In addition, *Corynebacterium ulcerans* and *C. pseudodiphtheriticum* may also produce a dark halo on this medium and must be differentiated from *C. diphtheriae*. Other organisms occasionally grow on Tinsdale agar. *Proteus* produces mucoid colonies and tends to blacken the medium. Rare streptococci and staphylococci can produce dark colonies with a surrounding halo but could be distinguished from the corynebacteria by performing a Gram stain.

TODD-HEWITT BROTH WITH GENTAMICIN AND NALIDIXIC ACID

Todd-Hewitt broth is typically used to isolate group B streptococci from vaginal and rectal swabs. It can be used, however, to isolate any β-hemolytic streptococcus from a clinical specimen that has mixed flora. Nutrients are provided by peptones and BHI, dextrose is added as an energy source, and gentamicin and nalidixic acid are added to inhibit the growth of gram-negative rods. This broth is inoculated with the vaginal or rectal swab and incubated at room temperature for 18 to 24 hours. The broth is then subcultured to a blood agar plate, incubated for 24 hours at 35° to 37° C in 5% CO_2, and examined for the presence of β-hemolytic colonies.

TRIPLE-SUGAR IRON AGAR

Triple-sugar iron (TSI) agar can be used to determine whether a gram-negative rod is a glucose-fermenter or non–glucose-fermenter, a fundamental characteristic in the initial classification of gram-negative rods. The medium also tests for sucrose and/or lactose fermentation, gas production during glucose fermentation, and hydrogen sulfide production, all of which are useful in the differentiation of gram-negative rods belonging to the family Enterobacteriaceae.

TSI agar contains glucose, sucrose, and lactose (fermentable carbohydrates) where sucrose and lactose are each present at 10 times the glucose concentration; phenol red (pH indicator); peptone (carbon/nitrogen source); and sodium thiosulfate plus ferric ammonium sulfate (sulfur source and hydrogen sulfide indicator, respectively). TSI agar resembles KIA except TSI contains sucrose. Carbohydrate fermentation patterns are similar to those with KIA; however, an acid (yellow) slant and acid (yellow) butt (A/A) in the TSI indicate that an organism ferments glucose and sucrose or lactose or both. Gas bubbles and blackening mean the same thing in TSI agar as in KIA. Precautions concerning the inoculation and incubation outlined in the KIA description also apply to TSI.

TRYPTICASE SOY AGAR

Trypticase soy agar (TSA) is an all-purpose medium that supports the growth of many organisms. It is frequently used as the basal medium for sheep blood agar plates. TSA contains peptones from soybeans and casein as a nutrient source and sodium chloride as an osmotic stabilizer. Agar serves as solidifying agent.

If TSA with sheep blood is to be prepared, the TSA should be cooled to 50° C before 5% defibrinated sheep blood is added. In most cases, agar can be added to a broth formulation to produce solid agar plates; however, the commercial TSA product does not contain glucose, which makes it suitable for a blood agar base. Adding agar to trypticase soy broth does not accomplish the same thing. Trypticase soy broth contains glucose, a fermentable carbohydrate, which can interfere with the expression of β-hemolysis on sheep blood agar plates.

TRYPTICASE SOY BROTH

Trypticase soy broth (TSB) is an all-purpose medium that supports the rapid growth of most organisms, including streptococci, without added supplements. Trypticase soy broth contains soybean and casein digests as protein sources, sodium chloride for osmotic stability, glucose as a fermentable carbohydrate, and dipotassium phosphate as a buffer.

Trypticase soy broth contains glucose, which when fermented can lower pH. This can cause acid-sensitive organisms such as *S. pneumoniae* to die off at 24 hours of incubation. This broth is used as a medium in blood culture bottles, to make an inoculum to be used for Kirby-Bauer susceptibility testing, and as a medium for sterility testing.

TRYPTOPHAN BROTH (1%)

Tryptophan broth is used for performing the indole test, a procedure that is particularly useful in identifying species of Enterobacteriaceae and in identifying non–glucose-fermenting, gram-negative rods. This broth contains trypticase, a peptone rich in tryptophan, and sodium chloride, which serves as an osmotic stabilizer. Some bacteria possess an enzyme system called *tryptophanase*, which hydrolyzes and deaminates tryptophan, producing indole, pyruvic acid, and ammonia. When Ehrlich's or Kovac's reagent is added to a tryptophan broth culture, any indole produced by the organism reacts with the aldehyde portion of dimethylaminobenzaldehyde, the primary chemical in these reagents, to form a red color.

Tryptophan broth should be inoculated with a few colonies from a pure culture and incubated for 24 hours at 35° C. Five drops of Kovac's reagent are added to the medium; a red color in the reagent layer or at the interface of the reagent and broth signifies the presence of indole (positive). If Ehrlich's reagent is used, 1 mL of xylene or ether is added to the broth culture at the end of the incubation period. The tube is shaken and five drops of the reagent are added. Kovac's reagent is generally used in testing members of the Enterobacteriaceae and Ehrlich's when testing non–glucose-fermenting gram-negative rods and anaerobes. Other media have been developed to detect the production of indole from tryptophan. These include sulfide indole motility (SIM) agar, indole nitrate broth, and motility indole ornithine (MIO) medium. A spot test using filter paper saturated with paradimethylaminocinnamaldehyde reagent also has been used for indole determination. In this case, the organism is rubbed onto the surface of filter paper saturated with the spot indole reagent; the appearance of a blue color indicates a positive test.

UREA AGAR AND BROTH

Urea media detect an organism's ability to hydrolyze urea. This characteristic is particularly useful in identifying species of Enterobacteriaceae. In these media, urea is hydrolyzed to form carbon dioxide, water, and ammonia. The ammonia then reacts with components in the medium to form ammonium carbonate. This compound causes a rise in pH, which changes the pH indicator, phenol red, to pink. Neither the agar nor broth formulations contain much protein, which prevents the formation of alkaline products from the breakdown of peptones and could result in false-positive results. The broth formulation contains monopotassium phosphate and disodium phosphate, which make the medium highly buffered. In addition, the broth formulation lacks glucose and peptone. Only organisms (e.g., *Proteus* spp.) that are strong urease producers and not very fastidious will appear positive in this type of medium. The agar formulation is less buffered, so smaller amounts of urease activity can be detected. Also, glucose and peptone, which help support growth, are included in these media.

To inoculate a urea slant, the slant is streaked with a sterile inoculating loop or needle that has a small amount of the organism and incubated at 35° C for 18 to 24 hours. If urease is produced, the medium will turn pink. Rapid urease producers such as *Proteus* spp. turn the entire tube pink and may be detectable in a few hours. Slow urease producers, such as *Klebsiella,* only turn the slant pink. If the organism does not produce urease, there will be no color change. Stuart urea broth is incubated at 35° C for 18 to 24 hours. A positive reaction is red color throughout the broth.

VAGINALIS AGAR

Vaginalis (V) agar is a selective or nonselective (depending on the addition of antimicrobial agents or not) enrichment medium that is useful in the isolation of *G. vaginalis.* V agar is essentially a Columbia agar base with added peptone to provide nutrients, cornstarch as an energy source, and human blood, rather than sheep blood, to detect hemolysis. *G. vaginalis* produces diffuse β-hemolysis only on media containing human blood. V agar can be made selective by the addition of colistin, nalidixic acid, and nystatin, which will inhibit many of the organisms that are found as normal vaginal flora.

Inoculated V agar plates are incubated in 5% CO_2 at 35° C. Plates might be observed at 24 hours, but often 48 to 72 hours is required for *Gardnerella* to grow. The organism produces tiny dome-shaped colonies surrounded with zones of diffuse β-hemolysis.

XYLOSE-LYSINE-DESOXYCHOLATE AGAR

Xylose-lysine-desoxycholate agar (XLD) is a selective, differential primary plating medium that is used to isolate *Salmonella* and *Shigella* spp. from stool and other specimens containing mixed flora. *Salmonella* and *Shigella* spp. produce characteristic colonies on XLD, which aids in their recognition. XLD agar contains sodium desoxycholate, which inhibits gram-positive cocci and some gram-negative rods that are

found in stool as normal flora. Because XLD agar has a lower concentration of bile salts than other formulations of enteric media, such as SS and HE agars, it is less selective but permits better recovery of *Shigella.* XLD agar contains three fermentable carbohydrates: sucrose and lactose, which are present in excess concentration, and xylose, which is present in lower amounts. Phenol red serves as a pH indicator. The amino acid lysine is included to detect lysine decarboxylation. Sodium thiosulfate acts as a sulfur source from which organisms can make hydrogen sulfide. The hydrogen sulfide combines with ferric ammonium citrate to produce ferrous sulfide, a black precipitate.

Four types of colonies are produced on XLD agar. Yellow colonies are produced by organisms such as *E. coli* that ferment the excess carbohydrates to produce a great deal of acid and change the pH indicator to yellow. Because there is excess carbohydrate, these organisms do not decarboxylate the lysine, even though they may possess lysine decarboxylase. Bacteria that ferment only xylose and do not decarboxylate lysine also produce yellow colonies. Yellow colonies with black centers are organisms that ferment the excess carbohydrate and also produce hydrogen sulfide. Examples of organisms that produce this colony type are *Citrobacter* and some *Proteus. Shigella* and *Providencia,* which neither ferment xylose, lactose, or sucrose nor produce hydrogen sulfide, produce colorless or red colonies. *Salmonella* and *Edwardsiella* produce red colonies with black centers. *Salmonella* and *Edwardsiella* ferment xylose to make acid, producing a yellow colony; but because xylose is present in limiting concentrations and gets used up, these organisms will then decarboxylate the lysine to produce cadaverine, which is an alkaline product that causes the colony to revert back to red. Blackening is caused by hydrogen sulfide production. XLD agar should be incubated at 35° C for 24 hours in ambient air. Some investigators have recommended incubating plates for up to 48 hours to enhance blackening in *Salmonella* colonies. With any prolonged incubation, the delicate balance of this medium may be altered, and distinguishing normal flora from potential pathogens becomes more difficult. *Shigella dysenteriae* and *Shigella flexneri* may occasionally be inhibited on XLD agar. Some strains of *Salmonella* may fail to produce hydrogen sulfide and therefore resemble *Shigella* colonies. On this medium, blackening is more likely to occur when alkaline conditions exist.

BIBLIOGRAPHY

Murray PR et al, editors: *Manual of clinical microbiology,* ed 9, Washington, DC, 2007, American Society for Microbiology.

Forbes BA et al: *Bailey & Scott's diagnostic microbiology,* ed 12, St Louis, 2007, Mosby.

Difco Laboratories: *Difco manual,* ed 11, Sparks, Md, 1998, Difco Laboratories.

Shepard M, Lunceford C: Differential agar medium (A7) for identification of *Ureaplasma urealyticum* (human T mycoplasmas) in primary cultures of clinical material, *J Clin Microbiol* 3:613, 1976.

Selected Mycology Media, Fluids, and Stains

Maribeth L. Flaws

FUNGAL MEDIA

A variety of enrichment and selective media is available to the clinical laboratory for the isolation and identification of pathogenic fungi. This appendix is included to provide the reader with information about a select number of mycology media cited in the mycology section of this text. Most media detailed in this appendix are commercially available in either dehydrated or finished form. Recommendations as to general use of the media, either enrichment or selective, or combinations of each type, are outlined in the mycology section of this text.

Antifungal Susceptibility Testing Media

The M27-A3 Clinical and Laboratory Standards Institute (CLSI) document describes the procedure for determining the susceptibility of yeast to antifungal agents by a broth dilution method. The medium that is recommended is an RPMI 1640 medium that does not have sodium bicarbonate but does have L-glutamine. Morpholinepropanesulfonic acid (MOPS) is added as a buffer to maintain the pH of the medium at 7.0. The yeast nitrogen base broth with 2% glucose can also be used for broth dilution procedures.

Assimilation Base for Carbohydrates (Modified Yeast Nitrogen Base)

Modified yeast nitrogen base is a synthetic basal medium that provides sufficient sources of nitrogen to support the growth of fungi. Fungal isolates are plated for confluent growth, and carbohydrate disks are dispensed onto the surface to provide the specific carbohydrates for assimilation testing. The plates are incubated at 30° C for 48 to 72 hours and examined for growth around each disk. Good growth around a disk indicates assimilation of that carbohydrate, whereas scant or no growth around a disk indicates no assimilation. A dextrose disk serves as the growth control.

Alternatively, the basal media can be prepared as a broth to which individual carbohydrates are added in separate tubes. The yeast is inoculated into the series of tubes, the tubes are incubated, and if the yeast can assimilate the carbohydrate, there will be turbidity in the tube. The pattern of carbohydrate assimilation is used to identify the yeast.

Birdseed Agar (Modified Staib Agar or Niger Seed Agar)

Birdseed agar is a differential enrichment medium designed for the isolation and preliminary identification of *Cryptococcus neoformans*. The ground seeds of *Guizotia abyssinica* provide enrichment, whereas biphenyl provides a substrate for the detection of phenol oxidase activity. On this medium, *C. neoformans* colonies typically darken to a rich brown as phenol oxidase activity results in the deposition of melanin in yeast cell walls. The colonies of other *Cryptococcus* spp. and other yeasts remain cream-colored. Chloramphenicol is added to inhibit the growth of bacteria.

Brain-Heart Infusion Agar/Blood Agar With or Without Antibiotics

Brain-heart infusion (BHI) agar with 10% sheep blood is an enrichment agar that is useful in the isolation of pathogenic yeast and the dimorphic fungi (in yeast form) from clinical specimens. The addition of antibiotics (either chloramphenicol and gentamicin or penicillin and streptomycin) makes the medium selective by inhibiting the growth of bacteria.

Candida Bromcresol Green Agar

Candida bromcresol green agar (BCG) is used to isolate and differentiate between species of *Candida*. Nutrition is provided by the inclusion of glucose, yeast extract, and peptones. Neomycin is added as a selection agent to inhibit the growth of bacteria. Bromcresol green is a pH indicator that turns from blue-green to yellow in the presence of acid produced when the yeast utilizes the glucose. Each species of *Candida* has a particular pattern of surface and base colony colors that can be used presumptively to identify the species. For example, *C. albicans* has base and surface colony colors that are yellow to bluish green, whereas *C. tropicalis* has an intense blue-green color of the submerged growth, a lighter base color, with a pale yellowish-green surface color.

CHROMagar *Candida*

CHROMagar *Candida* is used for the isolation of fungi from clinical material. The medium is selective like Sabouraud's dextrose for fungi and differentiates between species of *Candida* based on the breakdown of chromogenic substrates. *C. albicans* colonies are a light to medium green; *C. tropicalis* appears dark blue to metallic-blue; and *C. krusei* is a light mauve to mauve-colored colony.

Cornmeal Agar

Cornmeal agar is typically made as any one of three variations on a basal formulation. Each formulation is useful in the cultivation of fungi. Each variation is recommended for the cultivation or enhancement of particular fungal characteristics. Cornmeal agar without added dextrose is recommended for the cultivation of chlamydospore-bearing *C. albicans,* with chlamydospore production further enhanced by the addition of 1% Tween-80. On the other hand, cornmeal agar with 0.2% added dextrose is not recommended for production of chlamydospores. Rather, it favors more luxuriant growth and improves pigment production that is used to differentiate *Trichophyton rubrum,* which produces a red pigment, from *Trichophyton mentagrophytes,* which does not.

Each plate should be inoculated with a known *C. albicans* control and the unknown isolate(s) as single streaks cut deep into the agar or as surface streaks with the streak lines and then covered with a flame-warmed coverslip. The plate should be incubated at room temperature and examined with a low-power lens of a microscope daily for up to 1 week. Isolates may become positive for chlamydospores (macroconidia) within 48 hours but cannot be considered negative before the fifth day of culture.

Dermatophyte Test Medium

Dermatophyte test medium is used to isolate dermatophytes from cutaneous specimens. Cycloheximide, chloramphenicol, and gentamicin are incorporated to inhibit the growth of bacteria. This medium turns from yellow to red when dermatophytes grow. The microscopic characteristics of the dermatophyte can be seen from the colonies growing on this medium.

Inhibitory Mold Agar

Inhibitory mold agar is used to selectively isolate fungi that are susceptible to cycloheximide and thus will not grow on Mycosel/mycobiotic agar. Chloramphenicol and gentamicin are added to inhibit bacterial growth.

Littman Oxgall Agar

Littman oxgall agar is a general-purpose medium used to isolate fungi, especially dermatophytes. It is similar to inhibitory mold agar in that it does not contain cycloheximide. Glucose is added as a carbon source, oxgall prevents the spreading of fungal colonies so that yeasts and molds form distinct colonies and can be isolated in pure culture, and crystal violet and streptomycin are added to inhibit growth of bacteria.

Modified Potassium Nitrate Assimilation Medium (MKA)

Potassium nitrate assimilation medium provides a differential medium useful in assessing the ability of a yeast isolate to assimilate potassium nitrate (KNO_3). The modified medium is a solid, slanted medium containing KNO_3, yeast carbon base, Nobel agar, and bromthymol blue. A single colony of the cultured isolate is picked using a sterile applicator stick,

inoculated over the entire MKA slant surface, and incubated at 25° to 30° C. The ability to assimilate potassium nitrate is indicated by a color change of the medium from greenish yellow to blue or blue-green.

Mycosel/Mycobiotic Agar (Cycloheximide-Chloramphenicol Agar)

Mycosel/mycobiotic agar is a selective medium used to isolate pathogenic fungi, both dermatophytes and systemic pathogens. The cycloheximide suppresses the growth of saprophytic fungi, whereas the chloramphenicol inhibits bacterial contaminants.

Potato Dextrose Agar

Potato dextrose agar is the recommended plating medium for the cultivation, enumeration, and identification of yeasts and molds from dairy and other food products as well as from clinical specimens. The potato infusion encourages growth of and sporulation by fungi. Dermatophyte pigment production is enhanced on this medium. This medium is commonly used in the slide culture technique to visualize the microscopic morphology of fungi.

Potato Flakes Agar

Potato flakes agar is used to induce sporulation in fungi. It is easier to prepare and is more stable than potato dextrose agar. Cycloheximide and chloramphenicol are incorporated to make the medium more selective for fungi, especially dermatophytes.

Rice Extract Agar

Rice extract agar without additional dextrose is useful in the cultivation of *C. albicans,* with enhancement of chlamydospore production. Rice extract agar with 2% dextrose has been shown to enhance pigment production by *T. rubrum,* facilitating its differentiation from *T. mentagrophytes.*

The medium should be inoculated by cutting through the agar surface similar to that described for the inoculation of cornmeal agar. The cut streaks should be covered with a flame-warmed coverslip to stimulate chlamydospore production. All cultures should be incubated at room temperature for 18 to 72 hours.

Rice Grains Medium

Rice grains medium is useful in the differentiation of *Microsporum audouinii* from other dermatophytes, especially *Microsporum canis.* On this medium, *M. audouinii* grows poorly and discolors the medium. Other dermatophytes and most other fungi grow well and sporulate on this medium with no discoloration of the medium. Sterile rice grains should be spot-inoculated to prevent confusion in differentiating between discoloration and actual growth.

Sabouraud–Brain-Heart Infusion Agar

Sabouraud–brain-heart infusion agar (SABHIA) is a general-purpose medium used to isolate fungi. It is made from a combination of Sabouraud's dextrose and BHI ingredients. This medium is particularly useful for the isolation of dimorphic fungi from clinical specimens. The addition of blood further increases the isolation of dimorphic fungi and promotes the conversion to the yeast stage. Antibiotics such as chloramphenicol, cycloheximide, streptomycin, and penicillin can be added to increase the selectivity of the medium for fungi.

Sabouraud Dextrose Agar or Broth (Emmons Modification)

Sabouraud dextrose agar and Sabouraud dextrose broth are nutrient media suitable for the cultivation of fungi, especially those associated with cutaneous and mucocutaneous infections. The formulations are identical with the exception of the agar. To make a solid plated medium, 1.5% to 2% agar is added to the broth formulation.

The Emmons-modified Sabouraud dextrose agar is the formulation commonly used today. It has 2% dextrose and a neutral pH as opposed to 4% dextrose and an acidic pH that were in the original formulation. Antibiotics can be added to this medium to make it more selective for fungi.

FUNGAL MOUNTING FLUIDS

KOH-Glycerin

Potassium hydroxide (or sodium hydroxide) and glycerin solution are used as a mounting fluid in the preparation of wet mounts to visualize fungi in clinical material. The KOH (or NaOH) aids in clearing the specimen of nonfungal materials, and the glycerol retards the dissolution of the fungal elements. A modification of this basic principle involves combining the KOH with dimethyl sulfoxide (DMSO) rather than glycerol. The DMSO facilitates the penetration of KOH into the specimen materials and speeds the clearing process.

FUNGAL STAINS

Calcofluor White Stain

The use of calcofluor white stain with 10% KOH enhances visualization of fungi in clinical specimens of skin, hair, and nails. Fungal elements take up the fluorescent dye because it binds to cellulose and chitin, which are found in fungal cell walls only and, depending on the combination of filters used, appear brilliant green-yellow or blue-white, whereas the background fluoresces a dim red.

For examination of clinical samples, one drop of calcofluor white solution and one drop of 10% KOH are added to the specimen on a microscope slide. A coverslip is placed on top of the mixture, and the preparation is examined using a fluorescence microscope. The microscope must have either a K532 excitation filter–BG 12 barrier filter or a G-35 excitation filter–LP420 barrier filter combination.

India Ink

The India ink method is useful in demonstrating the presence of a capsule. It is especially recommended for the demonstration of *C. neoformans* in clinical specimens, particularly cerebrospinal fluid. In this method the capsule displaces the colloidal carbon particles in the ink; thus the capsule appears as a clear halo around the body of the microorganism.

Lactophenol Aniline Blue

Lactophenol aniline blue (formerly lactophenol cotton blue) is a mounting medium that is useful in examining the microscopic morphology of an isolated fungus. It aids in staining hyphal elements (aniline blue) and preserving fungal materials (lactic acid), and it enhances visualization by staining all chitin-containing structures a light blue. To use the medium, a small drop of the stain is placed onto a slide; the fungal material is either added directly and teased apart or placed on the surface of cellophane tape, topped with a coverslip, and examined. Some manufacturers now add 10% polyvinyl alcohol as a fixative so that permanent smears can be prepared.

BIBLIOGRAPHY

Murray PR et al, editors: *Manual of clinical microbiology*, ed 9, Washington, DC, 2007, American Society for Microbiology.

Difco Laboratories: *Difco manual*, ed 11, Sparks, Md, 1998, Difco Laboratories.

Fisher F Cook N: *Fundamentals of diagnostic mycology*, Philadelphia, 1998, WB Saunders.

Forbes BA et al: *Bailey & Scott's diagnostic microbiology*, ed 12, St Louis, 2007, Mosby.

Howard B et al: *Clinical and pathogenic microbiology*, ed 2, St Louis, 1994, Mosby.

Pincus D et al: Modification of potassium nitrate assimilation test for identification of clinically important yeasts, *J Clin Microbiol* 26:366, 1988.

Rohde P et al: *BBL Manual of products and laboratory procedures*, ed 5, Cockeysville, Md, 1968, Becton Dickinson.

Answers to Learning Assessment Questions

CHAPTER 1

1. The Gram stain needed to be repeated because the *E. coli* quality control slide gave a false gram-positive reaction. Because of this quality control result, the smear made from the clinical sample could not be accurately interpreted.

2. The most likely cause of the false gram-positive result for *E. coli* was insufficient decolorization time. Crystal violet, the primary stain, was not removed from the bacterial cells.

3. Pili, made up of pilin protein, aid in bacterial attachment to solid surfaces such as mucous membranes. Flagella, consisting of flagellin protein, are responsible for motility.

4. Capsules help microorganisms resist phagocytosis. Phagocytic cells are less able to bind to the capsular polysaccharide than they are to surface proteins. In addition, capsules hide antigens on the surface of bacteria, preventing them from interacting with antibodies produced by an animal in response to an infection.

5. If Gram's iodine is inadvertently omitted from the staining procedure, gram-positive bacteria will decolorize more readily, producing a false gram-negative reaction. The iodine forms a complex with crystal violet, aiding the retention of the dye during the decolorization step.

6. LPS is also known as endotoxin. This molecule is toxic to animals, inducing nonspecific effects such as fever, inflammation, hypotension, and shock.

7. The thick peptidoglycan layer of gram-positive bacteria is responsible for retention of the crystal violet–iodine complex during decolorization.

8. Older bacterial cells are decolorized more easily than younger cells, because as cells age their cell walls become "leaky" and allow molecules to pass more readily out of the cell. In the Gram stain, the crystal violet–iodine complex is more readily lost during the decolorization step.

9. c

10. Bacterial spores have a thick protein coat that makes them highly resistant to chemical agents, temperature change, starvation, dehydration, ultraviolet and gamma radiation, and desiccation.

11. The three ways in which genetic material may be transferred from one bacterium to another are transformation, transduction, and conjugation.

Transformation is the uptake and incorporation of naked or free DNA into a bacterial cell. Transduction is the transfer of bacterial genes by a bacteriophage from one cell to another. Conjugation is the transfer of genetic material from a donor bacterial strain to a recipient strain. Conjugation requires close contact between the two cells.

12. 3′ TTACGGACAAC 5′
    5′ AATGCCTGTTG 3′

13. Uracil

CHAPTER 2

Section A

1. The antimicrobial therapy eliminated her indigenous flora, which gave the opportunistic member of the flora (yeast) the opportunity to proliferate and initiate an infectious process.

2. Resident flora are organisms that occupy a specific body site indefinitely for a long time (months to years). Transient flora are those that inhabit a site for a short time, or temporarily.

3. A carrier is a host that may be colonized by a potentially pathogenic organism without causing clinical symptoms in the host.

4. The carrier becomes a source of infection and can transmit the infecting organism to a susceptible individual.

5. The nutritional status of the site, pH, oxidation-reduction potential, and presence and interference of already established organisms all determine the composition.

6. A symbiotic relationship.

7. The usual microbial flora help to (1) prime the host immune system, (2) produce substances toxic to more pathogenic species, and (3) decrease the numbers of pathogenic organisms by competing for nutrients.

Section B

1. Immune response is compromised because of HIV infection.

2. *Cryptococcus neoformans* is an encapsulated fungus that stimulates or requires cellular immune responses. The patient had a reduced ability to respond because of his HIV infection, and he was not able to defend himself from this infecting organism.

3. True pathogens are organisms that cause disease in susceptible hosts. An opportunistic pathogen in an

organism is usually a member of the indigenous flora of the host; when the host immune system is compromised or changed, the organism takes the opportunity to cause disease.

4. Inflammation occurs when the body detects a foreign body or when an injury takes place. During inflammation, a large number of phagocytic cells and leukocytes accumulate at the site of injury. Phagocytes digest and engulf the foreign material, and the leukocytes release mediators to facilitate phagocytosis and in turn the killing of an invading organism.

5. Exotoxins are extracellular substances produced by an organism that has acquired a toxin gene encoded by phage, plasmids, or transposons. Endotoxins comprise the lipopolysaccharide component of the cell wall of gram-negative bacteria. The toxicity is cause by the lipid A portion of the lipopolysaccharide.

6. See the following table for the cells and soluble mediators that are involved in the innate immune response versus the adaptive immune response and humoral versus cellular.

	Cells	Soluble Mediators
Innate immune response	Macrophages Natural killer cells Neutrophils Eosinophils	Complement Cytokines
Adaptive immune response	Lymphocytes	Antibodies Cytokines
Humoral immune response	T helper cells B lymphocytes	Antibodies
Cellular immune response	Cytotoxic T cells Helper T cells Macrophages Natural killer cells	Cytokines

7. Microorganisms can evade the immune response by producing a capsule to inhibit phagocytosis, by going intracellular to evade antibodies, and by changing their antigens to stay ahead of the immune response.

8. Organisms are transmitted by ingestion, inhalation, and injection.

9. The major immune response against extracellular bacteria is antibodies binding and inducing complement-mediated lysis and phagocytosis. The major immune response against intracellular bacteria is delayed-type hypersensitivity where TH1 cells activate macrophages to phagocytose and destroy infected cells. The major immune response against viruses is cytotoxic T cells and natural killer cells. Antibodies are only effective in preventing viruses from attaching to and entering host cells.

10. These are the steps involved in phagocytosis and how microorganisms can evade each step:
    - Contact between the phagocytic cell and microorganism. Organisms can evade this step by preventing opsonization with antibody and complement and masking its antigens.
    - Formation of the phagosome. The phagocytic cell extends pseudopodia around the microorganism.
    - Fusion of phagosome with lysosomes to form a phagolysosome. Organisms can evade this step by leaving the phagosome and residing in the cytoplasm.
    - Digestion of organism. Some organisms secrete enzymes such as catalase and superoxide dismutase that break down the oxygen-reactive intermediates that are present to digest the organism. The production of these enzymes makes the organism resistant to digestion.

11. IgG is only monomer, and it activates complement and phagocytosis. IgG is the predominant immunoglobulin in the serum and is a marker of immunity or past infection with an organism. IgM can be a monomer or a pentamer. As a pentamer, IgM is the best at agglutinating particles to help get rid of them. Pentameric IgM can activate complement. IgM is the first immunoglobulin isotype produced in an immune response and is a marker of an acute infection with an organism.

12. Zoonoses are diseases that are acquired from animals. The following organisms are some of those that are considered zoonotic: *Brucella* spp., *Francisella* spp., *Bacillus anthracis*, *Salmonella* spp., *Yersinia* spp., *Campylobacter*, and *Escherichia coli* O157:H7.

CHAPTER 3

1. a
2. b
3. b
4. c
5. d
6. c
7. d
8. b
9. d
10. d

CHAPTER 4

Section A

1. Sterilization is a chemical or physical process resulting in the destruction of living organisms. Disinfection is the physical but usually chemical method that reduces the number of viable cells.

2. An antiseptic is used to reduce the number of microorganisms on living tissue before an invasive procedure, such as venipuncture or surgery.

3. False. Boiling water will not kill spores. Water boils at a temperature that is too low to inactivate spores.

4. High-level disinfectants and autoclaving kill bacterial endospores.

5. Phenolics are commonly found in germicidal soaps.

6. A disinfectant is used to reduce the number of microorganisms on an inanimate object, whereas an

antiseptic is milder and is used to reduce the number of bacteria on living tissue.

7. c

8. Alcohols inactivate microorganisms by denaturing proteins. Aldehydes denature proteins and inactivate nucleic acids. Iodine and chloride compounds are active based on oxidative effects. Heavy metals (e.g., silver, mercury, zinc, copper) are less commonly used today because of their toxicity; they work by combining with proteins, thereby inactivating them. The antimicrobial action of cationic detergents (e.g., benzalkonium chloride, cetylpyridinium chloride) is mediated through disruption of the cellular membrane, resulting in leakage of cell contents. Phenolics, molecules derived from phenol, work by denaturing proteins and disrupting plasma membranes. The killing mechanism of ethylene oxide is the alkylation, and subsequent inactivation, of nucleic acids.

9. b

10. The Antimicrobial Division of the EPA regulates the registration on the use, sale, and distribution of antimicrobial pesticide products for certain inanimate, hard, nonporous surfaces, or pesticide products incorporated into substances under the pesticide law, the Federal Insecticide, Fungicide and Rodenticide Act (FIFRA). An EPA registration number is granted only when the requirement of laboratory test data, toxicity data, product formula, and label copy are approved. The disinfectant label should indicate several highlighted points important in selecting the appropriate agents for the designated use. The FDA approves antiseptics through two processes: the new drug application (NDA) process or the over-the-counter (OTC) drug review known as the *monograph system.* NDAs are defined by law as being recognized as safe and effective (RASE). The approved NDA is manufacturer-specific and allows only that particular sponsor to market the product.

11. The main goal of handwashing is to eliminate transient flora. Health care workers can acquire microbes, including methicillin-resistant *Staphylococcus aureus* (MRSA), during direct contact with patients or contaminated surfaces. The purpose of the surgical hand scrub and waterless surgical handrubs is to eliminate the transient flora and most of the resident flora. Resident flora can be persistently isolated from the hands of most people. These organisms include coagulase-negative staphylococci, *Corynebacterium* (diphtheroids or coryneforms), *Propionibacterium,* and *Acinetobacter* spp. The goal of preoperative skin preparation formulations is to degerm an intended surgical site rapidly as well as provide a high level of bacterial inactivation and persistent antimicrobial activity, up to 6 hours after skin preparation. Preoperative skin preparation product is defined as fast-acting, broad-spectrum, and persistent antiseptic containing preparation that significantly reduces the number of microorganisms on intact skin.

12. d

Section B

1. True
2. c
3. b
4. b
5. d
6. c
7. a
8. The NFPA hazard-rating diamond states risk for flammability, reactivity, and health. Each criterion is rated on a scale of 0 to 4, from stable or safe to highly dangerous.
9. b
10. Although hazardous chemicals that are present in microbiology laboratories vary, the following are frequently found: acetone, ethanol, hydrogen peroxide, hydrochloric acid, sulfuric acid, acetic acid, and sodium hydroxide.

CHAPTER 5

Section A

1. b
2. b
3. a
4. a
5. c
6. c
7. d
8. a
9. d
10. d

Section B

1. b
2. a
3. 89.3%
4. 95%
5. Efficiency of tests

CHAPTER 6

1. The specimen in the Case in Point is unacceptable because it has been collected onto a culture plate in which the medium is expired and obviously dried out. JEMBEC plates are used to culture *Neisseria gonorrhoeae*, and this fastidious organism will not be able to grow on inappropriate culture medium. If this specimen were accepted, the culture would not be able to yield growth of this potential pathogen. The microbiology technologist must notify the office where the specimen was collected and inform them that the medium is not acceptable. If necessary, the specimen must be recollected.

2. Subcutaneous infections are below the external surface of the skin and into the connective tissues. A swab specimen will collect material only from the external cutaneous surface and will not be representative of the infectious process. The sample should be collected via needle aspiration.

3. c

4. b
5. d
6. a
7. d
8. c
9. b
10. a

CHAPTER 7

1. True
2. a
3. e
4. c
5. b
6. b
7. True
8. b

CHAPTER 8

1. The organism is a lactose fermenter.
2. BAP is a nonselective medium that supports the growth of both gram-positive and gram-negative bacteria. MAC is a selective medium that inhibits the growth of gram-positive bacteria and allows gram-negative bacilli to grow.
3. *Streptococcus*
4. They generally produce clear, colorless colonies on MAC.
5. β-Hemolysis is complete hemolysis of the red blood cells in the agar showing a clear zone around the colony. α-Hemolysis is incomplete hemolysis of the red blood cells and shows a green discoloration around the colony.
6. "Puffballs" in the broth medium usually suggests the presence of certain streptococcal species.
7. *Proteus* spp.
8. d
9. c
10. b

CHAPTER 9

1. a
2. d
3. b
4. c
5. d
6. a
7. b
8. The red slant indicates alkaline pH cause by peptone utilization; therefore the bacteria are unable to ferment lactose or sucrose. The black butt indicates H_2S production. Because H_2S production requires an acid environment, it can be assumed that the bacteria produced acid from glucose.
9. Two important enzymes necessary for the rapid metabolism of lactose are lactose (β-galactoside) permease and β-galactosidase. The permease enzyme facilitates the uptake of lactose. Delayed lactose fermenters lack permease but contain β-galactosidase.

It takes delayed lactose fermenters longer to transport lactose across the cell wall and plasma membrane. Acid formation can be delayed until 48 to 72 hours.
10. No color change after the addition of the reagents indicates that nitrite (NO_2) is not present. Two explanations are that the bacterium was unable to reduce nitrate (NO_3) or the bacterium reduced nitrate to nitrite, then to nitrogen gas (N_2). Zinc dust reduces nitrate to nitrite. If after the addition of zinc dust the broth still does not change color, then the nitrate had been totally reduced by the bacterium to nitrogen gas. If color forms after the addition of zinc dust, then the nitrate had not been reduced by the bacterium, and this is a true negative result.

CHAPTER 10

1. High titers of IgM indicate a recent infection. In this case, IgM to CMV in a neonate indicates a congenital infection. Congenital CMV infections typically have serious consequences.
2. Monoclonal antibodies arise from a single clone of lymphocytes and recognize a single epitope. Monoclonal antibodies are therefore very specific. Polyclonal antibodies contain a mixture of antibodies recognizing similar but different epitopes. Polyclonal antibodies are less specific but generally more sensitive.
3. False-negative test results can be the result of (1) immunocompromised patients not being able to produce detectable antibody levels, (2) the sample being collected too early in the course of the infection (in some diseases it may take a long time to form antibodies), or (3) the diagnostic kit having too high a concentration of antigen (postzone phenomenon).
4. Double immunodiffusion is a precipitation reaction performed in an agarose matrix. The antigen and specific antibody are placed in separate nearby wells, and they both diffuse through the agarose. At the zone of equivalence, a visible precipitate is formed. With single radial immunodiffusion, antibody is evenly distributed in an agarose matrix. Corresponding antigen is added to wells in the agar. The antigen diffuses through the agar, and a concentration gradient is formed. At the zone of equivalence, a visible precipitate is formed. The diameter of the precipitation ring is proportional to the concentration of the antigen.
5. During passive agglutination, an antigen is bound to a carrier particle, such as latex beads or red blood cells. When the carrier particles are mixed with a clinical sample, agglutination will occur if the corresponding antibody is present. With reverse passive agglutination, antibody is fixed to the surface of a carrier particle. When the carrier particles are mixed with a clinical sample containing the corresponding antigen, agglutination occurs.
6. In the antistreptolysin-O (ASO) neutralization assay, the last dilution with no hemolysis is the endpoint. In

this example that would be 1:16. The ASO titer is reported in Todd units; therefore the result is 16 Todd units. Remember that Todd units are used only for the ASO test.

7. In an indirect immunofluorescent assay for detecting antibody, the conjugate is an antihuman IgG and/or IgM antibody with a fluorescent label.

8. Western blots use a number of different proteins from an infectious agent separated by electrophoresis. The banding pattern produced in the assay allows laboratory scientists to determine which antibodies to the different antigens are present.

9. The RPR test uses nontreponemal antigens. Although this test is very sensitive, it is not highly specific. A confirmatory test, such as the fluorescent *Treponema pallidum* antibody absorbance (FTA-ABS) assay or the *Treponema pallidum*–particulate agglutination (TP-PA) test, must be performed next.

10. Antibodies from humans that agglutinate sheep and horse red blood cells is highly suggestive of infectious mononucleosis, a disease caused by Epstein-Barr virus. Antibodies produced against viral antigens also bind to antigens found on certain red blood cells. These are examples of heterophile antibodies.

CHAPTER 11

1. b
2. c
3. a
4. c
5. d
6. a
7. c
8. b
9. d
10. a

CHAPTER 12

1. d
2. c
3. e
4. d
5. a
6. e
7. c
8. b
9. d
10. True

CHAPTER 13

Section A

1. Viridans streptococci are normal flora in the throat. Reporting antimicrobial susceptibility test results often suggests to the physician that the isolated organism is clinically significant and antimicrobial therapy should be considered. Reporting antimicrobial susceptibility results on viridans streptococci from the throat may lead to inappropriate use of antimicrobial agents and

may also prevent the physician from seeking the true answer to the patient's problem.

2. 1.5×10^8
3. Oxacillin
4. b
5. c
6. b
7. b
8. a
9. d
10. c
11. a, True; b, false; c, false; d, true; e, false
12. b

Section B

1. Endocarditis is a serious infection and is located at a body site where immune defense mechanisms are not abundant. Therefore it is essential for the antimicrobial agent to kill the bacteria in order to effect a cure.

2. 99.9%
3. Logarithmic
4. False
5. a
6. Schlichter
7. a
8. c
9. b
10. d

CHAPTER 14

1. Although this organism has had a lengthy association with hospitalized and nursing home patients, recovery in community populations, including pediatric populations, has increased. *S. aureus* has been associated with toxin-mediated diseases and infections of the skin, soft tissues, and deep sites.

2. *S. aureus* is noted for causing skin infections such as impetigo, bullous impetigo, furuncles (boils), carbuncles, mastitis, cellulitis, and wound infections associated with trauma, surgery, and burns, as well as pneumonia, organ abscesses, bacteremia, endocarditis, osteomyelitis, and septic arthritis.

3. Protein A is able to bind the Fc portion of an immunoglobulin, thereby interfering with phagocytosis.

4. Toxic shock syndrome (TSS) is associated mainly with TSST-1. However, some cases of TSS have been linked to enterotoxin B or C.

5. Exfoliative toxin or epidermolytic toxin causes staphylococcal scalded skin syndrome.

6. Enterotoxins A to E and G to J, and most commonly A and D, are associated with staphylococcal food poisonings.

7. Although not all CoNS are considered clinically significant, those CoNS associated with indwelling devices and immunocompromised patients are considered potential pathogens. Urinary tract infections caused by *S. saprophyticus* are also clinically significant.

8. The clinically significant CoNS are *S. epidermidis* and *S. saprophyticus*. More recently, infections

(e.g., endocarditis, septicemia, peritonitis) due to *S. haemolyticus* and *S. lugdunensis* have become more common.

9. Cell-bound coagulase or clumping factor can be detected by a slide coagulase and latex slide agglutination assays. Free or extracellular coagulase is detected with a tube coagulase test.

10. A positive coagulase test would differentiate *S. aureus* from most other staphylococci.

11. A disk diffusion test using a 5-μg novobiocin disk can be used. *S. saprophyticus* will be resistant, whereas most other CoNS will be susceptible.

12. An oxacillin-resistant *S. aureus* isolate is considered resistant to all penicillinase-stable penicillins and is commonly referred to as a methicillin-resistant *S. aureus* (MRSA).

13. Oxacillin had been commonly used to predict methicillin resistance. Cefoxitin is now recommended for determining oxacillin resistance in staphylococcal species. For the most accurate detection of methicillin resistance, molecular tests for *mec*A or tests that detect the *mec*A product, PBP2, may be used. For detection of clindamycin resistance, an induction test (D test), as described in the CLSI/NCCLS M100-S15 document, using disk diffusion testing of clindamycin and erythromycin should be used. Not all susceptibility methods are able to detect VISA or VRSA. Recently the CLSI and CDC have recommended the addition of a vancomycin agar plate, which can be used as a supplemental plate when testing MRSA isolates. Most VISA and VRSA, thus far, have been detected in these more resistant *S. aureus* strains.

14. Some strains of *S. lugdunensis, S. schleiferi,* and *S. sciuri* will produce positive results in a slide coagulase test for clumping factor or a latex agglutination test for clumping factor and/or protein A. These species, however, are coagulase negative. Although nearly all strains of *S. aureus* are positive for clumping factor, occasional strains are also fibrinolytic. This means that they could lyse a clot, formed as the result of coagulase activity, producing a false-negative reaction.

CHAPTER 15

1. The child in the Case in Point was found to have a group A *Streptococcus (S. pyogenes)* infection. Three tests that would be useful in the identification of this organism are bacitracin susceptibility (sensitive), SXT susceptibility (resistant), and an immunoassay for detection of the group A antigen.

2. b
3. c
4. d
5. a
6. Penicillin is the drug of choice for the treatment of *S. pyogenes* pharyngitis. Patients allergic to penicillin are often treated with erythromycin.

7. *S. pyogenes* has been linked to necrotizing fasciitis. Streptococcal toxic shock syndrome is a systemic disease mediated by a soluble toxin. The infection is not necessarily invasive. Rheumatic fever and acute glomerulonephritis are immunological sequelae and not invasive infections.

8. *S. pneumoniae* is the most common cause of community-acquired pneumonia and is the most common cause of bacterial pneumonia overall.

9. Group B streptococci *(S. agalactiae)* are rarely associated with disease in healthy adults; however, they are a significant cause of morbidity and mortality in neonates. Neonates can acquire infection in utero following premature rupture of the membrane or during delivery. Pregnant women are often screened for group B streptococci as part of the prenatal workup.

10. Members of the genera *Granulicatella* and *Abiotrophia,* formerly referred to as the nutritionally variant streptococci, have a requirement for pyridoxal. Isolates are generally able to grow in blood cultures, but to sustain growth on solid media, agar needs to be supplemented with pyridoxal. Alternatively, the bacteria can grow as small pinpoint colonies around colonies of *Staphylococcus aureus,* which secretes small amounts of pyridoxal during growth.

CHAPTER 16

1. b
2. c
3. In the spore stain, vegetative cells are red, but the spores stain green.
4. a
5. d
6. b
7. *Streptococcus agalactiae* (group B *Streptococcus*) and *Enterococcus* spp. can produce clinical laboratory findings similar to those for *L. monocytogenes*. Initial differentiation between *L. monocytogenes* and similar microorganisms can be made by the Gram stain, catalase test, and esculin hydrolysis.
8. b
9. a
10. b

CHAPTER 17

1. b
2. d
3. d
4. c
5. b
6. a
7. d
8. c
9. The presence of gram-negative diplococci of commensal *Neisseria* and *Moraxella* species makes diagnosis difficult. Culture using selective media is imperative.
10. PID is an acute or recurring acute infection of the oviducts and ovaries with surrounding tissue involvement. It includes inflammation of the cervix (cervicitis), uterus (endometritis), fallopian tubes (salpingitis), and ovaries, and it can spread to adjacent

connective tissue. Sterility, ectopic pregnancy, and Fitz-Hugh-Curtis syndrome are additional complications. *Neisseria gonorrhoeae* and *Chlamydia trachomatis* are the etiological agents.

CHAPTER 18

Section A

1. *H. influenzae* will grow only where both X and V factors are present; therefore the bacteria will grow between the two strips where the two factors have diffused.
2. a
3. d
4. *H. ducreyi* is fastidious and requires enriched media for growth. GC agar supplemented with 1% hemoglobin, 5% fetal calf serum, 1% IsoVitaleX, and 3 mg/L of vancomycin is recommended. The plates need to be incubated in an atmosphere of increased humidity and CO_2 (5% to 10%) and at a temperature of about 32° C.
5. Both *H. aegyptius* and *H. influenzae* biogroup aegyptius are noted for causing conjunctivitis. *H. influenzae* biogroup aegyptius, however, is associated with a more invasive disease known as Brazilian purpuric fever (BPF) that is characterized by conjunctivitis, high fever, vomiting, petechiae, purpura, septicemia, and shock.
6. b
7. d
8. The most likely identification is *Pasteurella multocida*. This microorganism is noted for causing skin infections following cat and dog bites. *P. multocida*, the most common *Pasteurella* spp. isolated is an oxidase negative bacterium that grows on SBA but not MacConkey agar.
9. *Brucella melitensis* will grow on SBA and does not require X or V factor, whereas *H. influenzae* will not grow on SBA and does require X and V factors.
10. *Francisella tularensis* is the most likely causative agent. The primary reservoirs for *F. tularensis* are rabbits. Although some infections are acquired by ingestion, it is more common to find ulceroglandular infections following direct contact with rabbits.

Section B

1. *Mycoplasma pneumoniae, Chlamydophila (Chlamydia) pneumoniae,* and *Legionella pneumophila* are the three most common causes of community-acquired atypical pneumonia.
2. Age (elderly), smoking, alcohol consumption, and immunocompromised state are risk factors that contribute to severe infections caused by *Legionella* spp.
3. Crowded conditions and a high-humidity environment contribute to infections by *Legionella.*
4. Advantages of DFA testing include rapid, moderately sensitive, and specific results. Disadvantages are requirement for trained personnel for rapid tests offered on all shifts, high monetary cost, the possibility of false positives due to cross-reactivity, and requirement for culture confirmation when a test is negative.
5. Buffered charcoal yeast extract (BCYE) agar with L-cysteine is the preferred medium for the recovery of *Legionella* spp.
6. Urine for the urine antigen test is the best nonrespiratory specimen for the detection of *Legionella* spp.
7. Chlorine tolerance below 2 to 3 mg/L, ability to grow at 20° to 43° C and survival for varying periods at 40° to 60° C, capacity to adhere to components of piped water systems, ability to survive in the presence of environmental bacteria and algae, and ability to multiply within free-living protozoa are factors contributing to human infections caused by *Legionella* spp.
8. Presumptive identification methods include Gram staining a suspicious colony growing only on BCYE medium and finding thin, gram-negative rods that may show size variation from 2 to 20 μm in length. Also, testing for L-cysteine requirement by subculturing to BCYE and to SBA should be performed. Smears prepared from colonies that require L-cysteine for growth are tested with DFA conjugates.
9. *Legionella* spp. are pleomorphic, weakly staining gram-negative rods that are approximately 1 to 2 by 0.5 μm in size but can elongate. On BCYE medium, colonies appear grayish-white or blue-green, convex, and glistening measuring approximately 2 to 4 mm in diameter (see Figure 18-30). Young colonies have a "ground-glass" appearance and are light gray and granular, whereas the periphery appears pink and/or light blue or with bottle-green bands. Illumination with a long-wave ultraviolet light (366 nm) can show differences in colony autofluorescence (see Box 18-1).
10. c

Section C

1. The pertussis vaccination series consists of five doses from age 6 weeks to 6 years, although evidence suggests an additional booster should be administered in adolescence. A child might miss one or more doses because of disruption in public health during political upheaval.
2. No, adults are not immune; however, infections in adults are normally mild or asymptomatic. Adults serve as reservoirs for disease in children and adolescents. Immunity wanes within a few years after vaccination.
3. Nasopharyngeal aspirates and calcium alginate swabs are the clinical samples of choice for the diagnosis of *B. pertussis* infection.
4. Amies, 1% casein hydrolysate, and Regan-Lowe with cephalexin transport media are the most appropriate for the maximum recovery of *B. pertussis*.
5. Direct fluorescent antibody testing is the preferred method for the detection of *Bordetella* in nasopharyngeal smears.
6. The PCR assay was recently accepted for rapid detection of *B. pertussis*.

7. On charcoal–horse blood, young colonies of *B. pertussis* are smooth, glistening, and silver, resembling mercury droplets. Colonies turn whitish-gray as they age.

8. Six doses of vaccination are required for protection against pertussis: four in the initial infant series and two boosters (before the age of 6 years and in adolescence). However, immunity is not lifelong.

9. Both species cause pertussis in children; however, pertussis caused by *B. parapertussis* tends to be milder.

10. No, serology is not widely available, but it can be used as a retrospective epidemiological tool.

CHAPTER 19

1. Most members of the family Enterobacteriaceae are able to ferment glucose, are oxidase negative (except for *Plesiomonas shigelloides*), and are able to reduce nitrate to nitrite (except for *Photorhabdus* spp. and *Xenorhabdus* spp.).

2. a, D; b, C; c, A; d, B

3. c

4. a

5. b

6. a

7. d

8. b

9. c

10. d

CHAPTER 20

1. b

2. c

3. a

4. d

5. c

6. a

7. b

8. c

9. Appropriate specimens for the isolation of enteric campylobacters are stool samples and rectal swabs; stool samples are preferred. Two categories of media are available for isolation: blood-based media and charcoal-based media. A commonly used blood-based medium is CAMPY-BAP. This is a *Brucella* agar–based medium with 10% sheep red blood cells and a combination of antimicrobials. Charcoal cefoperazone deoxycholate agar is an alternative. The addition of antimicrobial agents and incubation of the plates at 42° C inhibits normal fecal flora. Because the campylobacters require oxygen at a concentration less than room air, they must be incubated in a microaerophilic atmosphere.

10. The most commonly used nonculture method for the diagnosis of *H. pylori* is the noninvasive ^{13}C- or ^{14}C-labeled urea breath test. The patient is given an oral dose of labeled urea. Urease activity by *H. pylori* results in the formation of radioactive-labeled CO_2, which is absorbed into the bloodstream, then exhaled. Other nonculture methods include microscopic examination of stained gastric tissue, direct fecal antigen detection, polymerase chain reaction, and urease activity of gastric biopsy material.

CHAPTER 21

1. Fermentative gram-negative bacilli are able to metabolize carbohydrates to derive energy under anaerobic conditions. Phenotypically, these bacteria can produce an acid "butt" in specific media (i.e., triple sugar iron [TSI] agar or Kligler's iron agar [KIA]). Nonfermenters are gram-negative bacilli that cannot ferment sugars and are not able to acidify the butt of TSI or KIA.

2. Most nonfermenters exist in the environment, often a moist or aquatic environment. They are not usually part of the normal human flora. Nonfermenters may also be found in soil and on plants, as well as in hospital environments on countertops, on equipment, and occasionally in contaminating biological liquids used for dispensing medications.

3. Nonfermenters rarely cause infections outside of the hospital environment, except when traumatically implanted (e.g., into the skin from soil, vegetation, or water sources). In the hospital, nonfermenters may be the cause of nosocomial urinary tract infections, postsurgical wound infections, pneumonia, or bacteremia. The incidence of infection is greater in the immunocompromised patient.

4. Risk factors for infection by nonfermenters include immunocompromised states from cancer or cancer chemotherapy, transplantation, and steroid use. In the immunocompetent individual, infections are associated with burns, catheters, prior use of broad-spectrum antimicrobial agents, metabolic disorders (e.g., diabetes mellitus), and foreign body implantation either traumatically or via transplanted organs.

5. *Pseudomonas aeruginosa* is the most common nonfermenter associated with clinical infections, especially nosocomial (hospital-acquired) infections. *Acinetobacter baumannii* complex and *Stenotrophomonas maltophilia* are often isolated from hospitalized patients, especially from respiratory specimens, but they are more often "colonizers" and not always clinically significant. The isolation of a nonfermenter from a single blood culture, or as part of a polymicrobial infection, often indicates that the organism is acting as a colonizer or a laboratory contaminant rather than a relevant pathogen. However, if one of the nonfermenters is seen on a Gram stain from a sterile site, is the only organism isolated, and is present in high numbers, clinical significance needs to be considered.

6. Many of the nonfermenters, especially *P. aeruginosa, A. baumannii* complex, and *S. maltophilia,* can be resistant to agents used to treat infections caused by fermentative gram-negative bacilli. They are resistant to penicillin, ampicillin, most third-generation cephalosporins (except ceftazidime), and macrolides,

lincosamides, and agents active against gram-positive bacteria. There is variability of their in vitro and in vivo response to aminoglycosides; quinolones; aminopenicillins, such as piperacillin and ticarcillin; and SXT. Specific susceptibility tests need to be performed if the nonfermenter is considered clinically relevant.

7. Most nonfermenters will grow on media selective for gram-negative bacilli, such as MacConkey agar, but will remain lactose-negative. In addition, many of the nonfermenters will be oxidase-positive. The Gram stain of many nonfermenters is that of thin bacilli, often a little longer than the rods of the fermenters, such as *E. coli* and other Enterobacteriaceae. When a nonfermenter is placed on media to determine carbohydrate utilization, such as TSI or KIA, there will be no acidification of the butt. This result will enhance the suggestion of a nonfermenter.

8. The ability to grow at 42° C and the presence of a blue-green pigment diffusing through the media are characteristics of *P. aeruginosa* that can be used to differentiate this organism from other members of the fluorescent pseudomonad group. In addition, the distinct grape-like odor of *P. aeruginosa* may be a clue.

9. *Acinetobacter* spp. are gram-negative coccobacillary organisms rather than true bacilli. They are oxidase-negative, which is uncharacteristic of most other nonfermenters. In addition, they have a bluish-purple appearance on MacConkey agar and are often susceptible to the antimicrobial combination of ampicillin and sulbactam, which is unusual for many other nonfermenters.

10. Both *B. pseudomallei* and *P. stutzeri* may produce very "wrinkled" colonies. *B. pseudomallei* may require a longer time to grow and will oxidize lactose, whereas *P. stutzeri* will not.

CHAPTER 22

1. B, C, D, A, E
2. D
3. C
4. B
5. D
6. A
7. B
8. F
9. F
10. T
11. T
12. T

CHAPTER 23

1. The spirochetes are slender, flexuous, helically shaped, unicellular bacteria ranging from 0.1 to 0.5 μm wide and from 5 to 20 μm long, with one or more complete turns in the helix. They differ from other bacteria in that they have a flexible cell wall around which several fibrils are wound.

2. Geographic location, season, outdoor exposure, and a history of tick bites are risk factors for endemic relapsing fever.

3. *B. burgdorferi* is the *Borrelia* sp. associated with Lyme disease (Lyme borreliosis) characterized by a skin rash, fever, "flu-like" symptoms, joint and bone pain, and symptoms resembling viral meningitis.

4. Pathogen transmission is more probable the longer the vector is attached.

5. Peripheral blood smear stained with Giemsa stain is the test of choice for the laboratory diagnosis of relapsing fever borreliosis.

6. Most cases are contracted in Hawaii. Because the incubation period is typically 10 to 12 days, it is likely that visitors to Hawaii can become infected but not show symptoms until they return home.

7. Primary, secondary, and tertiary are the three stages of syphilis. In the United States, the tertiary stage of the disease is not seen often because most patients are adequately treated with antimicrobial agents before the tertiary stage is reached.

8. *T. pallidum* subsp. *pallidum* (syphilis), *T. pallidum* subsp. *pertenue* (yaws), *T. carateum* (pinta), and *T. pallidum* subsp. *endemicum* (endemic syphilis [bejel])

9. The classic "target" or "bulls-eye" skin lesion of Lyme disease normally found at the site of the tick bite is called *erythema chronicum migrans*. It begins as a red macule and expands to form a large annular erythema with partial central clearing.

10. The treponemal tests for syphilis detect antibodies specific for treponemal antigens. The nontreponemal tests are nonspecific and detect reaginic antibodies that develop against lipids released from damaged cells. The two categories of tests have approximately equal sensitivities; however, the treponemal antigen tests are more specific and are used as confirmatory tests.

CHAPTER 24

1. The two most common causes of neonatal conjunctivitis are *Neisseria gonorrhoeae* and *Chlamydia trachomatis*. The prophylactic use of erythromycin eye drops has helped to control this serious disease.

2. Although the Giemsa stain is easy to perform on eye scrapings, it is not very sensitive and requires expertise. A direct fluorescent antibody stain is more reliable. Alternatively, an antigen detection assay or nucleic acid amplification test could be performed.

3. The infant in the Case in Point was infected with *C. trachomatis*. This organism can cause a variety of infections in neonates including pneumonia and vaginal, pharyngeal, and enteric infections.

4. Lymphogranuloma venereum (LGV)

5. LGV differs from other diseases caused by *C. trachomatis* because the serovars causing this disease are more invasive. These serovars are able to survive inside mononuclear cells and are carried into the lymphoid tissue, where they produce a strong inflammatory response.

6. *Chlamydophila pneumoniae* is thought to be a common cause of pharyngitis and pneumonia. Recently the organism has been linked to atherosclerosis and coronary heart disease.

7. Psittacosis is an infection caused by *Chlamydophila psittaci*; it typically manifests as pneumonia. Because of the highly contagious nature of *C. psittaci*, cultures are not recommended. Diagnosis is best made by detecting antibodies to the bacterial antigens.

8. Serologic assays are the most commonly used testing method for the diagnosis of rickettsial diseases. Unfortunately, antibodies are generally detected in convalescent specimens too late to affect treatment. The Weil-Felix test is a nonspecific agglutination assay infrequently used in the United States. This test uses antigens from various strains of *Proteus*. The immunofluorescent antibody test is the methodology most commonly used.

9. *Ehrlichia* spp. generally infect monocytes and macrophages. They prevent phagolysosome formation and survive within phagosomes. The *Anaplasma* are unusual in that they preferentially infect granulocytes. They too prevent phagosome-lysosome fusion and survive within phagosomes.

10. *Coxiella burnetii* is an obligate intracellular parasite that develops within the phagolysosome of infected cells. The *Rickettsia* spp. prevent phagolysosome formation and develop within a phagosome. *C. burnetii* forms spores while *Rickettsia* spp. do not. In addition, although *C. burnetii* is known to infect more than 12 genera of ticks and other arthropods, it is generally not transmitted by arthropods.

CHAPTER 25

1. The infant in the Case in Point most likely most likely acquired the infection passing through the birth canal; however, studies have demonstrated neonatal infections following cesarean deliveries.

2. Because of the fastidious nature of the mycoplasma, routine prenatal cultures would not have detected most organisms. *M. hominis* will grow on routine media, but it forms pinpoint colonies after 48 hours of incubation that could be missed easily.

3. The mollicutes lack a cell wall; therefore they do not Gram stain.

4. Primary atypical pneumonia is milder than pneumococcal pneumonia and more often seen in young adults compared with the elderly. In addition, unlike pneumococcal pneumonia, primary atypical pneumonia does not have a seasonality incidence. Numbers of infection do not increase in the winter.

5. The four species of mollicutes associated with the urogenital tract of humans are *Mycoplasma hominis, M. genitalium, Ureaplasma urealyticum,* and *U. parvum.*

6. The Dienes or methylene blue stains are used to stain suspected mycoplasmal colonies.

7. A7 and A8 are selective and differential media for the isolation of *M. hominis* and *U. urealyticum*. In addition,

Shepard's 10B arginine broth can also be used. *M. hominis* and *M. pneumoniae* can be grown on SP4 broth, if arginine is added for the latter. *M. hominis* is the least fastidious of the mollicutes and will grow on sheep blood and chocolate agars.

8. The cold agglutinin test detects antibodies that agglutinate red blood cells incubated at 4° C. Historically, the test had been used to aid in the diagnosis of primary atypical pneumonia caused by *M. pneumoniae*. However, it is not very sensitive (only about 50% of the patients infected are positive) or specific.

9. Complement fixation assays had been the primary serologic method to detect anti–*M. pneumoniae* antibodies. Because of technical problems, enzyme immunoassays and immunofluorescent-antibody methods are now more commonly used.

10. The mycoplasmas lack a cell wall and are therefore inherently resistant to the β-lactams: penicillins and cephalosporins.

CHAPTER 26

1. A number of mycobacterial species, both saprophytes and potential pathogens, may be isolated from humans. Historically, mycobacteria have been identified by growth characteristics and biochemical testing. More recently, molecular biology assays have been developed. These assays include mycolic acid analysis of bacterial cell walls and DNA probe technology and DNA sequencing. Genetic probe technology offers tremendous promise in microbial identification at a variety of levels—family, genus, species, and subspecies. The most common probe technology is the commercially available single-stranded, acridinium ester–labeled DNA probe for the detection of rRNA (Gen-Probe, Inc.). Probes specific for the *M. tuberculosis* complex (*M. tuberculosis, M. bovis, M bovis* BCG, *M. africanum, M. canettii,* and *M. microti*), *M. kansasii, M. gordonae,* and separate probes for *M. avium* and *M. intracellulare* are available. Laboratories should perform identification according to the level of service for which they are qualified. All isolates should be identified to the species level.

2. Slowly growing *M. tuberculosis* has the extraordinary ability to persist and replicate in the harsh environment of the alveolar macrophage. The organism has evolved effective mechanisms to survive most macrophage defense activities, and infection, once established, may lead to the formation of lung granulomas. The pathogenic mycobacteria are slow growers, which also lends to drug resistance. Antimicrobial agents are more active against rapidly growing bacteria. The American Thoracic Society, the Centers for Disease Control and Prevention, and the International Union Against Tuberculosis and Lung Disease recommend a 6-month regimen of isoniazid and rifampin, supplemented by pyrazinamide for the first 2 months, for the treatment of tuberculosis. Multidrug-resistant tuberculosis, defined as an isolate resistant to at least isoniazid and

rifampin, may be treated with a combination of antimicrobial agents. The treatment regimen may include the administration of antimicrobial agents such as isoniazid, rifampin, pyrazinamide, and ethambutol. Long-term treatment is necessary to ensure a cure, and the use of multiple drugs maintains antibacterial activity in case the bacteria become resistant to one of the drugs.

3. Mycobacteriologic services have spread to many laboratories. Clinical laboratory functions that contribute to the diagnosis and management of tuberculosis have been divided into the following three major categories of service offered.
   - Level 1: collection and transport of specimens, preparation and examination of smears for acid-fast bacilli
   - Level 2: procedures of Level 1, plus isolation and identification of *M. tuberculosis*
   - Level 3: all procedures of Level 2, plus identification of mycobacteria other than *M. tuberculosis*

   The determination of drug susceptibility may be performed at Level 2 and should be performed at Level 3. A laboratory may choose to develop or maintain the skills defined under one of the levels just described, depending on the frequency with which specimens are received for isolation of mycobacteria, the nature of the clinical community being served, and the availability of specialized referral service. All laboratories that perform clinical mycobacteriology should participate in recognized proficiency testing programs, and levels of service should be established and limited by the quality of performance demonstrated in these examinations.

4. Most clinical specimens contain an abundance of nonmycobacterial contaminants. Unless an attempt is made to inhibit these usually fast-growing contaminants, they can quickly overgrow the more slowly growing mycobacteria. The organic debris (tissue, serum, and other proteinaceous material) surrounding the organism in the specimen also must be liquefied so that decontaminating agents will kill undesirable microbes and surviving mycobacteria can gain access to the growth media.

   Mycobacteria are more refractory to harsh chemicals; therefore chemical digestion and decontamination procedures have been used with success to enhance the recovery of acid-fast bacteria from clinical specimens. NaOH digests and decontaminates specimens, whereas *N*-acetyl-L-cysteine effectively digests the specimen but does not decontaminate.

5. Because low levels of mycobacteria organism may be found in clinical samples, meticulous care must be practiced during the processing of specimens for the demonstration and isolation of mycobacterial organisms. False-negative results may occur if processing protocols are not followed appropriately. Prolonged decontamination may have a negative effect by killing the mycobacteria. Improper centrifugation

force may also lead to false-negative results. If insufficient force is applied, the mycobacteria may remain in the interface of the processed specimen and may be inadvertently discarded during processing. Care must be applied during culturing of the specimen.

False-positive results may occur through carryover from the mouths of containers used to transfer processing agents; introduction of the organism from environmental sources, such as water; or the introduction of organisms from aerosols produced when specimen containers are opened. When making slides, care must be taken to prevent carryover from one side to another. Slides should never come in contact with one another.

Cross-contamination between specimens may occur if instruments are not properly maintained.

6. The mycobacteria are easily spread by the airborne route; therefore it is important to avoid aerosol-generating procedures. In addition, mycobacterial laboratories should be under negative air pressure, so that when doors to the laboratory are opened, air flows inward. Specimen processing should be conducted in a biological safety cabinet; laboratory scientists must wear laboratory coats, eye protection, and a respirator (not a surgical mask). When disposable inoculating loops and needles are not used, electric incinerators should be used instead of open flames for sterilizing metal loops and needles. When specimens are centrifuged, they must be in a screw-capped tube in a secondary screw-capped container.

7. a
8. c
9. d
10. b

CHAPTER 27

1. *Blastomyces dermatitidis:* Microscopic examination of cultures grown at 37° C reveals large, broad-based budding yeast. At 22° C, the microscopic examination of the mold reveals conidia that are borne on short lateral branches that are ovoid to dumbbell-shaped and vary in diameter from 2 to 10 μm. *Coccidioides immitis:* Microscopic examination of secretions may reveal the spherules containing the endospores. At 22° C, the microscopic examination of the mold reveals alternating (separated by a disjunctor cell), hyaline arthroconidia. *Histoplasma capsulatum* var. capsulatum: Microscopic examination of cultures grown at 37° C reveals small yeast cells. The yeast cells measure 2 to 3 μm by 4 to 5 μm. At 22° C, the microscopic examination of the mold reveals both nondescript spherical microconidia and characteristic tuberculate macroconidia. *Sporothrix schenckii:* Microscopic examination of cultures grown at 37° C reveals small, cigar-shaped yeast. Microscopic examination of the mold phase reveals conidia developing in a "rosette" pattern at the ends of delicate conidiophores in addition to dark-walled conidia being produced along the sides of the hyphae.

2. *Microsporum gypseum:* Microscopic examination reveals fusiform, moderately thick-walled conidia measuring 8 to 15 µm by 25 to 60 µm with as many as six cells. In some isolates, the distal end of the macroconidium may bear a thin, filamentous tail. *Microsporum cani:* Microscopic examination reveals spindle-shaped macroconidia with echinulate, thick walls measuring 12 to 25 µm by 35 to 110 µm with 3 to 15 cells. The tapering, sometimes elongated, spiny distal ends of macroconidia are key features that distinguish this species. *Trichophyton rubrum:* Microscopic examination reveals clavate or peg-shaped microconidia formed along undifferentiated hyphae. Rare macroconidia may be formed. Both the urease and hair perforation tests are negative. *Trichophyton mentagrophytes:* Globose microconidia are found primarily in clusters described as grape-like or engrape. Macroconidia are thin-walled, smooth, and cigar-shaped with four to five cells separated by parallel cross-walls. Both urease and hair perforation tests are positive.

3. *Trichophyton rubrum* is urease positive, whereas *T. mentagrophytes* is typically negative. Wedge-shaped perforations in the hair shaft (positive) are characteristic of *T. mentagrophytes* as well as *T. canis* and *M. gypseum.* Species negative for hair perforation include *T. rubrum, T. audouinii,* and *M. praecox.*

4. Saprobes are usually environmental contaminants and are not considered human pathogens. However, saprobes may cause disease in individuals with impaired immune systems. When a saprobe is recovered from an immunocompromised patient, the laboratory should work closely with the physician to help determine if the isolate is indeed an environmental contaminant, or if it is possibly causing disease.

5. *Penicillium* spp. and *A. fumigatus* may both form blue-green colonies, but they may be differentiated microscopically in that conidia in the aspergilli are formed from phialides attached to a vesicle or metula, whereas conidia in the penicillia are formed from branched conidiophores bearing phialides at their tips. *Fusarium* spp. are typically white to pink to purple colonies that produce large, hyaline, thin canoe- to green bean–shaped macroconidia. *Curvularia* spp. have black colonies that produce wide, dematiaceous crescent to moon-shaped conidia.

6. Lesions of chromoblastomycosis most often appear as verrucous nodules that may become ulcerated and crusted. Long-standing lesions have a cauliflower-like surface. Brown, round sclerotic bodies, which are nonbudding structures occurring singly or in clusters, are seen in tissues. These sclerotic bodies reproduce by dividing in various planes, resulting in multicellular forms. Lesions of mycetoma are characterized by tumefaction, draining sinuses, and granules. Mycetomas are localized infections that involve both the cutaneous and subcutaneous tissue, and possibly bone. Granules are released through the draining sinus tracks.

7. Fungi are eukaryotic and possess a true nucleus with nuclear membrane and mitochondria. Bacteria are prokaryotic and lack these structures. Unlike plants, fungi do not possess chlorophyll and must absorb nutrients from the environment. In addition, fungal cell walls are made of chitin, whereas those of plants contain cellulose.

8. Fungal colonies, although occurring in many colors, may be generally divided as hyaline or dematiaceous. Hyaline molds are lightly colored, whereas dematiaceous fungi are darkly pigmented. This pigmentation is a result of melanin in the cell wall of the organism. The Fontana-Masson stain will detect dematiaceous hyphae in the tissues because it stains melanin.

9. The teleomorph is the sexual stage of a fungus, whereas the anamorph is the stage that reproduces asexually. In certain species, more than one asexual stage is associated with the same teleomorph. When more than one anamorph exists, they are called *synanamorphs.*

10. The germ tube test would be positive within 2.5 to 3 hours, and the cornmeal agar would result in both true and pseudohyphae with rare chlamydoconidia.

CHAPTER 28

1. The most likely identification is *G. lamblia;* these parasites are pathogenic for humans.

2. Both thick and thin smears are routinely performed on blood specimens to detect parasites. Because the thick smear is made with a larger volume of blood, it is more sensitive than a thin smear. However, species identification is made from the thin smear because the red blood cells are intact and parasites have a more characteristic morphology.

3. The eggs of *Taenia* spp. are round, approximately 35 µm in diameter, have a striated border, and contain a hexacanth oncosphere. The eggs of *T. solium* and *T. saginata* cannot be differentiated. *A. lumbricoides* eggs are either fertilized or unfertilized. The fertilized eggs are slightly oval with a thick mammillated coat, and they measure about 75 µm long by 50 µm wide. The unfertilized eggs are more oval and are as long as 90 µm with a thick mammillated coat or an extremely minimal mammillated layer. Eggs of *T. trichiura* are oval with plugs on both poles; they are about 52 µm long and 22 µm wide. Hookworm eggs are oval with broad ends, have a clear space between the thin shell and the embryo, and measure 55 to 75 µm long by 35 to 40 µm wide. The eggs of the two human hookworm species, *A. duodenale* and *N. americanus,* cannot be differentiated.

4. The gravid females of *E. vermicularis* (pinworm) migrate out of the anus to deposit eggs; therefore stool samples are not the specimen of choice. The best method for detection of pinworm eggs is to use the scotch tape or sticky paddle technique.

5. *C. cayetanensis* oocysts are round and average 8 to 10 µm in diameter. On a wet mount, they appear nonrefractile with a cluster of granules. The organisms

are not readily distinguishable on trichrome-stained smears and may appear as round, wrinkled, clear objects. With modified acid-fast stain, the organisms stain variably from a dark pink to almost colorless and may have a wrinkled or distorted shape. Oocysts of *Cyclospora* autofluoresce under ultraviolet light, blue at a wavelength of 365 nm and green at 450 nm. *C. parvum* oocysts are round and approximately 4 to 6 μm in diameter. Because of their small size, they are not distinguishable either on wet mounts or in permanent stained smears. With a modified acid-fast stain they are dark pink and round. Direct fluorescent antibody techniques that detect the oocyst in the feces are available.

6. The most likely identification is *E. histolytica* trophozoite. If no ingested erythrocytes had been seen, the organism would have been reported as *E. histolytica/E. dispar* because the organisms are morphologically identical. The presence of ingested erythrocytes indicates it is *E. histolytica*. This parasite is considered pathogenic for humans. Patients with *E. histolytica* infection can suffer from amebic dysentery, which can manifest as fever and intense colicky abdominal pain.

7. *C. parvum* produces two types of oocysts: thin-walled and thick-walled. The thick-walled oocysts are passed out in the feces and are infective for others. The thin-walled oocysts are involved in autoinfection. These structures rupture in the intestine and release sporozoites that reinfect intestinal cells. With *S. stercoralis* infection, the eggs rupture in the intestine and release rhabditiform larva that mature to filariform larva in the intestine. The filariform larvae burrow into the intestinal wall and gain access to the circulation and then complete the life cycle.

8. The organism belongs to the genus *Trypanosoma*. The morphologic form is the trypomastigote. Members of the genus *Trypanosoma* cause African sleeping sickness, transmitted by tsetse flies, and Chagas disease, transmitted by kissing or reduviid bugs.

9. PAM is caused by *Naegleria fowleri*. Young, healthy individuals are most commonly infected and present with a history of swimming in warm, stagnant water. The trophozoite gains direct access to the brain via the nasal olfactory nerve when water is forced into the nose. The infection has a rapid onset (within 2 to 7 days) after exposure, and symptoms resemble those of bacterial meningitis: photophobia, headache, vomiting, and stiff neck. Death usually occurs within a week of onset of symptoms. Diagnosis can be made by observing the ameboid trophozoite in a wet mount of the CSF sediment. Trophozoites may be found in biopsy tissue of the brain. GAE is a chronic infection caused by *Acanthamoeba* spp. and is usually found in individuals with underlying conditions such as lymphoma or diabetes. The organism may enter through the skin or be inhaled and spreads hematogenously to the brain. It may take years for symptoms to develop. Symptoms include headache,

dizziness, mental confusion, and seizures. Often the infection is detected at autopsy. Both trophozoite and cyst forms can be identified on biopsy specimens.

10. Toxoplasmosis in the immunocompetent host is usually asymptomatic or presents as a transient flulike illness. The immunocompromised patient often develops encephalitis or pneumonia. *Cryptosporidium* infection in the immunocompetent host causes diarrhea that is self-limiting. In the immunocompromised host, the diarrhea is prolonged and severe (partially due to the autoinfective part of the life cycle). The patient may lose as much as 10 L of fluid per day and develop electrolyte problems. Long-term infection may lead to malabsorption syndrome. *Strongyloides* infection in the immunocompetent host may also be asymptomatic or present with vague abdominal symptoms that can mimic those of an ulcer. In the immunocompromised host, hyperinfection (dissemination) may result with filariform larvae migrating to multiple body organs.

CHAPTER 29

1. Some opportunistic infections and conditions associated with AIDS include candidiasis, cryptococcal meningitis, cryptosporidiosis, histoplasmosis, persistent HSV infections, mycobacterial infections, recurrent pneumonia, and Kaposi sarcoma.

2. Testing for HIV-specific antigens and antibodies is important in the diagnosis of HIV infection, including antibodies to viral antigens p24, p31, gp41, and gp120/160.

3. EBV causes infectious mononucleosis. EBV has been associated with Burkitt lymphoma, nasopharyngeal carcinoma, and development of a B-cell lymphoproliferative disorder or lymphoma. Other EBV complications include splenic hemorrhage, hepatitis, thrombocytopenia purpura with hemolytic anemia, Reye syndrome, and encephalitis.

4. Signs and symptoms of acute HBV infection include fever, anorexia, and hepatic tenderness, with jaundice occurring in 30% to 50% of infected older children and adults. The immune response slowly clears HBV from the body, and the majority of patients become noninfectious. Some patients become HBV carriers for more than 6 months, and these patients are very likely to carry the virus for much longer. Patients with chronic hepatitis have a higher risk of cirrhosis or hepatic carcinoma. Acute hepatitis patients resolve as HBsAg clears, and anti-HBsAg can be detected. As the infection resolves, HBeAg fades, and anti-HBeAg appears. In chronic hepatitis patients, HBsAg persists, and the corresponding antibody cannot be detected. Likewise, HBeAg can persist.

5. Dengue fever (DF) is a fairly mild, self-limiting disease, with patients experiencing fever, headache, myalgia, and bone pain. Dengue hemorrhagic fever is a serious infection. These patients develop the symptoms of classic DF, along with thrombocytopenia, hemorrhage, and shock. Death can result from the infection.

6. One of the classic methods for the diagnosis of rabies is to detect Negri bodies, eosinophilic cytoplasmic inclusions, in neurons; however, fluorescent antibody and ELISA methods are also available for the rapid detection of rabies in brain tissue.

7. Erythema infectiosum is also referred to as *fifth disease* because it is the fifth childhood viral rash, after rubeola, rubella, varicella, and exanthem subitum. The causative agent for fifth disease is parvovirus B19.

8. The enteroviruses, found in the genus *Enterovirus,* include the polioviruses, coxsackieviruses A, coxsackieviruses B, echoviruses, and enteroviruses.

9. Arenaviruses (family Arenaviridae) are ssRNA viruses that have a sandy appearance (*arena* is Latin for "sand"). Several species, including Lassa virus, in the family cause hemorrhagic fever.

10. Many human papillomaviruses (HPVs) cause plantar, common, and genital warts. Some strains are associated with a rare autosomal disease called *epidermodysplasia verruciformis,* and some HPVs, especially HPVs 16 and 18, are associated with cervical cancer.

11. The viruses most noted for latency are the herpesviruses.

12. Influenza viruses mutate often as a result of replication errors. These mutations cause antigenic drift, ensuring antigenic variability of strains each year. Health agencies predict the most likely strains to predominate the next season. Trivalent influenza vaccines are proposed and made available prior to the start of the influenza season. Although this process is extremely successful, occasionally an unexpected strain will predominate, and the vaccine may not provide exact coverage for that strain.

CHAPTER 30

1. Sepsis and respiratory distress with radiographic evidence of mediastinitis is the most typical clinical presentation for a patient who was a target of a criminal release of anthrax spores.

2. Serum, blood, tissue, and body fluids are the specimens most appropriate to detect *C. burnetii* from potentially exposed patients.

3. Pneumonia with sepsis is the most typical clinical presentation for a patient who was a target of a criminal release of *Y. pestis.*

4. Botulinum toxin is the most toxic known biological compound.

5. *B. anthracis, Y. pestis, F. tularensis,* botulinum toxin, variola virus, and the hemorrhagic fever viruses (Ebola virus, Lassa fever virus, Junin virus, Machupo virus, Rift Valley fever virus, and Omsk hemorrhagic fever virus) are examples of biothreat Level A agents.

6. Nonmotile, nonhemolytic gram-positive bacilli isolated from blood cultures are characteristics leading to a presumptive identification of *B. anthracis.*

7. Sentinel laboratories use CDC protocols to rule out isolates as biothreat agents. If they are unable to rule out an isolate as a potential agent of bioterror, then the laboratory must notify the state laboratory and refer the isolate to a reference laboratory. Reference laboratories use rapid tests and conventional culture to confirm or rule out the identity of potential biothreat agents. National laboratories perform forensic work and definitive characterization on biothreat agents. There are three such laboratories, two of which have BSL-4 facilities.

8. Mediastinitis is the widening of the mediastinum, the area essentially located in the middle of the chest. It is usually associated with inhalation anthrax.

9. Modified smallpox is a case of smallpox seen in a person with partial immunity. The disease is usually minor and resembles chickenpox.

10. Descending flaccid paralysis is the major clinical manifestation of a patient with botulinum toxin exposure.

CHAPTER 31

1. The planktonic phenotype is adapted for a free-swimming or free-floating lifestyle. The organisms tend to be motile and express attachment (adhesion) molecules and pili. The sessile microorganisms have adapted to existence on a solid surface in a community of cells. Sessile organisms are generally nonmotile, and many species have the ability to produce an exopolysaccharide. Sessile microorganisms form cell aggregates.

2. The first stage in biofilm formation is attachment to a solid surface. This stage is irreversible and is mediated by attachment molecules and pili. The next stage is characterized by the formation of small cell aggregates and loss of motility. Once the biofilm contains multilayers of cells and has reached a thickness of about 10 mm, it is considered to be in stage III. Once the biofilm reaches its maximum thickness, generally about 100 mm, it is in stage IV. The fifth and final stage begins when cells are dispersed from the biofilm. These cells can presumably establish a biofilm downstream.

3. Biofilms aid microbial attachment because of the production of exopolysaccharide (EPS) by some members of the community and the cell-to-cell interactions resulting in the formation of cell aggregates.

4. A mature multispecies biofilm will consist of many microcolonies containing different species of microorganisms in several layers. The microcolonies are described as being mushroom-shaped and anchored to the substratum. The microcolonies are surrounded by a matrix consisting of EPS, DNA, and other molecules. Flowing around the microcolonies are water channels that can carry nutrients, DNA, and bacteria.

5. Biofilms can increase antimicrobial resistance by acting as barriers to penetration. Nutrients, antimicrobial agents, and other molecules may be trapped by the matrix and diffuse slowly; they may not even reach the cells in the lower layers. In addition, because the bacteria near the substratum have fewer nutrients and may be in an anaerobic environment, they are growing slowly, and slow-growing microorganisms are more

resistant to antimicrobial agents. Lastly, the environment within a biofilm facilitates the exchange of genetic material, and drug-resistant genes can be readily transferred from one organism to another.

6. Virulence mechanisms of biofilms include aiding microbial attachment, increasing the efficiency of community metabolism, enhancing antimicrobial drug resistance, protecting against host defenses, facilitating gene transfer, and allowing the spread of microorganisms to other body sites.

7. The acquired pellicle is a coating of host proteins and glycoproteins on the enamel surface of teeth. Pellicle formation is the first step in biofilm formation in the oral cavity. Once the pellicle is in place, normal oral flora can adhere to the tooth surface by binding to the pellicle via adhesion molecules and pili.

8. The primary cause of inflammation during gingivitis is the formation of a biofilm in the sulcus, a space between a tooth and the gingiva at the base of the tooth. Pathogenic bacteria in the biofilm can release exotoxins, lipopolysaccharide, and other inflammatory mediators. Some of the microorganisms can produce adhesion molecules allowing them to adhere to and invade cells of the gingiva. Polymorphonuclear cells arrive at the site and degranulate, causing more inflammation. Cell-mediated and humoral-mediated immune responses are generated.

9. Indwelling medical devices increase the risk of infection by providing a substratum for microbial attachment. Many microorganisms can readily adhere to plastics and polymers, inducing the formation of a biofilm. Once a biofilm is established, cells can "break off" and establish an infection downstream.

10. Areas of concern for clinical microbiologists when dealing with biofilms include false-negative cultures, viable but nonculturable organisms, underestimated colony counts, inappropriate specimen collection, and increased antimicrobial resistance.

11. One method for studying potential biofilm formation in vitro is based upon the staining of microorganisms attached to a solid surface, such as wells of a microtiter plate or the inside of test tubes. The color intensity of the stained cells can be read by a spectrophotometer. Alternatively, bacteria can be allowed to grow in the presence of silicone disks. Growth on the disk is measured by a colorimetric method.

12. When a biofilm in an individual is disrupted by treatment, bacteria can be released. These bacteria can establish an infection elsewhere in the host. It is important for physicians to monitor patients after treatment for such an occurrence.

CHAPTER 32

1. The normal flora of the respiratory tract plays an important role in protecting the host from infection. Isolation of normal flora from a microbiologic specimen will have less clinical significance than the isolation of pathogenic microorganisms capable of causing disease.

2. Immunocompromised hosts are at risk to develop infection with opportunistic pathogens. These organisms are of low virulence and generally are not pathogenic in hosts with intact immune system. Opportunistic pathogens are so named because they generally do not cause disease in normal hosts but require the "opportunity" of an impairment of host defense mechanisms to cause disease.

3. Certain pathogens exhibit seasonal variation and are more common during certain times of year. Awareness of seasonal trends helps to narrow the possible etiologies of infection, thereby facilitating a more accurate and timely diagnosis. This trend is seen in the winter when there is an upswing in viral infections, such as influenza and parainfluenza, and thus influenza vaccination is for susceptible patient populations.

4. Examples of what are termed "emerging viral infections" are the SARS coronavirus that caused the SARS outbreak and other viruses, such as metapneumovirus and bocavirus, that are increasingly recognized as important respiratory tract pathogens.

5. The common bacterial pathogens that cause community acquired pneumonia are *Streptococcus pneumoniae, Haemophilus influenzae, Moraxella catarrhalis,* and increasingly *Staphylococcus aureus.* Patients who come from the community but have had recent contact with health care, nursing home, or other medical facilities must also be considered to be a risk for disease caused by gram-negative bacterial pathogens, which are more common causes of hospital-acquired pneumonia. Atypical pneumonia is a commonly used (but questionable) term for pneumonia caused by *Mycoplasma pneumoniae, Chlamydia pneumoniae,* and *Legionella pneumoniae.* One must also consider pneumonias caused by respiratory viruses (e.g., influenza, respiratory syncytial virus, parainfluenza virus) in this spectrum of pathogens. So-called atypical pneumonia usually presents as a less dramatic, milder form of illness compared with disease caused by the common bacterial pathogens, which is generally more rapid in onset and severe in intensity. However, there are overlaps in these presentations that can make it difficult to distinguish these etiologies on clinical grounds, especially in immunocompromised patients or those with a variety of chronic, underlying conditions.

6. Influenza viruses are constantly changing genetically. The changes can be slowly evolving in the population, as a result of mutations caused by the error-prone viral RNA polymerase. This process is termed *antigenic drift* and is associated with influenza of the same HN phenotype (e.g., H3N2) that has subtle changes in these viral antigens that can render existing host immunity less effective. Antigenic drift is the basis for the need to produce a new multiple-strain vaccine (containing influenza A H3N2, influenza A H1N1, and influenza B) for each year's influenza epidemic. In contrast, *antigenic shift* is a term used for a relatively sudden appearance

in the global population of an influenza strain that has resulted from genetic recombination (so-called gene segment reassortment) among multiple viruses. Whereas genetic drift occurs almost annually, genetic shift is an uncommon epidemiological event, having occurred only a half-dozen times since the 1800s. Antigen shifts are unpredictable and have the major problem of a much higher transmission rate because of the lack of immune recognition of these "new" viruses by most people in the global community. Influenza A can undergo both types of genetic changes, whereas influenza B changes mostly by genetic drift.

7. There is a difference between the groups of pathogens that cause community-acquired and nosocomial (hospital-acquired) pneumonias that make diagnosis and management different for pneumonias in these two settings. For example, community-acquired pneumonia is more likely to be caused by streptococci, whereas nosocomial pneumonia is more likely to be caused by gram-negative bacilli, such as *Pseudomonas* and *Enterobacter*. The pathogens that cause nosocomial pneumonias are more likely to be resistant to antibiotics and thus more difficult to treat.

8. The absolute CD4 cell count is a surrogate marker for assessing the level of immunosuppression and the risk of HIV-associated complications. With CD4 cell counts greater than $500/mm^3$, there is an increased risk of infections with virulent, such as *S. pneumoniae* or *M. tuberculosis*. When the CD4 cell count falls to less than $200/mm^3$, the risk of opportunistic pathogens, such as *Pneumocystis jiroveci*, significantly increases.

9. In patients such as the one described in the question, tuberculosis should be suspected. Because TB can be a presenting illness in HIV-infected patients, all patients new diagnosed with active TB should also be tested for HIV infection.

10. *Bacillus anthracis, Yersinia pestis, Coxiella burnetii,* and *Francisella tularensis* have been identified as bacterial pathogens that might be used as agents of bioterrorism. The diagnostic microbiology laboratory needs to be alerted if these agents are suspected in the diagnosis of pneumonia, because culture isolation of these microorganisms poses a risk to laboratory personnel and must be done under conditions of biocontainment, usually through a facility in the Laboratory Response Network that is prepared for such studies.

CHAPTER 33

1. The patient appears to have cellulitis, a diffuse inflammation and infection of skin and subcutaneous tissues that is often preceded by trauma to the affected area. The most common causative agents of cellulitis are group A *Streptococcus* and *Staphylococcus aureus,* and the Gram stain result is consistent with either of these possibilities.

2. Intertrigo is an inflammatory skin condition that occurs in areas of heat, moisture, and friction, such as in skin folds of infants and obese adults. The result is maceration and skin breakdown, and the process is accelerated by infectious agents. The most common organism present is *Candida,* although *S. aureus* and coliforms also may play a role.

3. The classic tinea infection, caused by dermatophytes, is a circular scaly patch of erythema with a raised border, often with more inflammation of the edges than the center. These infections are also known as *ringworm,* reflecting the tendency of some lesions to expand outward in a ring. Examples are tinea cruris (jock itch) of the groin and tinea pedis (athlete's foot) involving the feet.

4. Diabetic foot infections can range from cellulitis, typically due to streptococci or staphylococci, to acute or chronic soft tissue ulceration with or without associated osteomyelitis, or gangrene. Ulcerative lesions and gangrene may also be due to staphylococci and streptococci but often are mixed infections and include gram-positives, Enterobacteriaceae, *Pseudomonas,* and anaerobic bacteria. Even low-virulence organisms such as coagulase-negative staphylococci and diphtheroids can be pathogens in these infections.

5. Mycetoma, also known as *Madura foot* or *maduromycosis,* is a chronic skin and subcutaneous infection caused by fungi including *Madurella* spp., *Aspergillus* spp., or *Pseudallescheria boydii* (eumycetoma or "true fungal" infection). A similar process known as *actinomycetoma* is caused by actinomycetes such as *Nocardia* or *Actinomadura* spp. These infections are characterized by swelling of subcutaneous tissues and formation of sinus tracts that drain pus and visible granules formed by aggregates of organisms. The disease process can extend to muscle and bone.

6. Nodular lymphangitis is also known as *lymphocutaneous syndrome.* It is characterized by inflammatory nodules that occur along lymphatic vessels that drain an area of primary skin infection. Certain organisms such as *Sporothrix schenckii, Nocardia,* and mycobacteria are classically associated with nodular lymphangitis, but other, more unusual infections can be associated as well; for example, *Francisella tularensis* and *Leishmania* spp.

7. Zoonotic diseases are those transmitted to humans by wild or domestic animals. There are hundreds of zoonotic diseases, but some of the more common ones that cause skin and soft tissue infection include Rocky Mountain spotted fever (caused by *Rickettsia rickettsii*), leptospirosis, bartonellosis, and tularemia.

8. *Staphylococcus aureus* may produce toxins that cause the exfoliating skin condition known as *staphylococcal scalded skin syndrome,* and toxin production by *S. aureus* or *Streptococcus pyogenes* may produce a diffuse erythroderma associated with toxic shock syndrome. Toxin production by *S. pyogenes* may also result in scarlet fever, which is characterized by a red, sandpaper-textured rash.

9. Members of the Herpesviridae family of viruses are characterized by the establishment of lifelong

infection. The initial infection is often accompanied by symptoms, but this is usually followed by a prolonged asymptomatic period during which the virus latently infects the host. The herpesviruses that are most likely to reactivate in adulthood after a period of latency include varicella-zoster and herpes simplex viruses.

10. "Swimmer's itch" is an intensely pruritic, papular rash caused by bird or animal schistosomes. They penetrate the skin of humans who are bathing or swimming in infected waters. These nonhuman schistosomes do not mature in humans, and they die in the skin. "Creeping eruption" or "ground itch" are common terms for the dermatitis known as *cutaneous larva migrans* (CLM). The CLM syndrome is due to subcutaneous migration of larvae of animal nematodes such as the dog and cat hookworms, *Ancylostoma caninum,* and *Ancylostoma braziliense,* respectively. The larvae of these and other worms can penetrate the skin of humans and produce a self-limited itchy, indurated dermatitis.

11. Infections due to *Actinomyces* and *Nocardia* can be characterized by the formation of "sulfur granules," yellow particles consisting of masses of tangled filamentous bacteria. Analysis of the granules microscopically by staining and by culture can identify the infecting organism.

CHAPTER 34

1. Major host defenses of the stomach include gastric acids and digestive enzymes. The small bowel is protected by peristalsis, a layer of mucus lining the cells of the small intestines, secretory antibody (primarily IgA), and normal bacterial flora. The colon is protected by the same mechanisms as the small intestines; however, there is a larger amount of normal bacterial flora present.

2. A patient's history should include determining whether other individuals in contact with the patient have also become ill. Additional important items include recent travel history; recreational activities, including hiking or backpacking and even swimming in public pools; and duration of illness. Other questions to ask include: does the patient have a history of gastrointestinal symptoms, does the patient have an underlying illness, and is the patient taking any medications?

3. Evaluation of the patient's peripheral blood count may reveal a leukocytosis in invasive infections. Anemia may be present in cases of severe gastrointestinal blood loss or a hemolytic infection. Thrombocytopenia may be present in some infections. Evaluation of the patient's blood chemistries can show electrolyte abnormalities from the diarrhea and is also a good indicator of the hydration status of the patient. Examination of the stool for red blood cells and evidence of inflammation (either fecal leukocytes or fecal lactoferrin testing) can be helpful.

4. Immunocompromised patients are at risk from viral agents that normally would not cause gastrointestinal disease in immunocompetent individuals. These viruses include cytomegalovirus (CMV), Epstein-Barr virus (EBV), picobirnavirus, and torovirus.

5. *Entamoeba histolytica* is an intestinal parasite that can cause bloody diarrhea and extraintestinal infections.

6. Chemical intoxications are sometimes associated with fish exposure, including scombroid. The syndrome is caused by ingesting contaminated fish (e.g., tuna, mackerel, yellow jack). The tissues of the fish contain histamine and enzyme inhibitors, which cause the symptoms. Ciguatera is caused by ciguatoxin produced by dinoflagellates. This toxin accumulates in fish as it passes up the food chain.

7. A number of complications are associated with diarrheal diseases. Volume depletion and electrolyte imbalance from diarrhea have been associated with kidney failure, liver failure, myocardial infarction, and death. When the colon is severely inflamed, toxic megacolon can develop. Reiter syndrome (characterized by a triad of urethritis, conjunctivitis, and arthritis) can develop following some diarrheal or sexually transmitted diseases. Hemolytic uremic syndrome (HUS) from enterohemorrhagic *E. coli, Shigella,* or some viral infections can lead to permanent renal failure or death. *Campylobacter* has been associated with Guillain-Barré syndrome, an ascending neuromuscular paralysis, that can result in death or permanent disability.

8. Pseudomembranous colitis, caused by *Clostridium difficile,* is associated with prior antimicrobial therapy.

9. *V. cholerae* serogroups O1 and O139 have been implicated as causes of epidemic cholera.

10. Travelers to high-risk areas should be advised to drink only bottled beverages and to avoid high-risk foods and ice. High-risk foods include any foods prepared by another person and served uncooked (e.g., salad, fruit, vegetables), dips and other foods left standing at room temperature, and raw or partially cooked fish or shellfish.

CHAPTER 35

1. The cerebrospinal fluid (CSF) is produced by both filtration and secretion from specialized capillary tufts of the choroid plexus within the four ventricles of the brain. The CSF flows from the two lateral ventricles to the third ventricle and enters the fourth ventricle via the aqueduct of Sylvius. From there, the CSF enters the basal cisterns and circulates over the cerebellum and convexities of the cerebral hemispheres. The CSF is absorbed primarily by the arachnoid villi through tight junctions of their endothelium.

2. CSF is a clear, colorless, and sterile fluid. In normal adults the protein level is 15 to 45 mg/dL, and the glucose level is 40 to 80 mg/dL (CSF glucose:serum glucose ratio of 0.6). Normally, few white blood cells are present.

3. The common bacteria causing acute meningitis include *Streptococcus pneumoniae, Neisseria meningitidis,*

Streptococcus agalactiae, (group B *Streptococcus*), *Haemophilus influenzae,* and *Listeria monocytogenes.* Patients with sickle-cell anemia, splenectomy or asplenia, malignancy, malnutrition, and chronic renal or liver disease are more likely to develop serious *S. pneumoniae* infection. Individuals who are deficient in terminal components of complement (C5–C9) or properdin are at a higher risk for *N. meningitidis* infection. *S. agalactiae* is a common cause of meningitis in neonates and infants up to 3 months of age. Neonatal acquisition most commonly results from vertical transmission from mother to infant. Before the widespread use of a conjugated vaccine, *H. influenzae* was a common cause of invasive illness in young children. The incidence of invasive disease by this organism has been substantially reduced. Infection due to *L. monocytogenes* is more commonly seen in neonates, elderly patients, alcoholics, and immunosuppressed individuals.

4. In acute bacterial meningitis, the CSF is turbid or cloudy as protein levels and white blood cell counts are significantly raised. Primarily the neutrophils are increased. Glucose levels are very low (less than 40% of the serum glucose concentration) in most patients with bacterial meningitis. In viral infections, the number of lymphocytes is increased in the CSF, and protein concentrations are slightly elevated while glucose concentration is near the reference range. Fungal and tuberculous meningitis is characterized by increased lymphocytes, elevated protein, and decreased glucose.

5. *Candida* spp., *Aspergillus* spp., and *Zygomycetes* spp. are the common fungi that can cause brain abscesses. *Blastomyces* dermatitidis is also associated with abscesses.

6. *Cryptococcus neoformans, Coccidioides immitis, Histoplasma capsulatum, Blastomyces dermatitidis,* and *Candida* spp. are associated with meningitis.

7. CSF specimens should be examined as soon as they are received because some of the infectious agents are fastidious and can become nonviable if specimens are not processed quickly. In addition, some infectious agents found in CSF can be diagnosed by rapid assays, facilitating proper treatment of life-threatening disease.

8. Initial examination of a CSF specimen includes a macroscopic description (i.e., turbidity) and microscopic examination by a Gram stain. Many laboratories will also perform an antigen detection assay for *Cryptococcus neoformans*. In the case of a neonate, an antigen detection assay for *Streptococcus agalactiae* should also be done.

9. Sheep blood and chocolate agar media incubated in 3% to 5% CO_2 at 35° C are usually used for bacterial culture of CSF.

10. Tests performed on CSF for the diagnosis of infectious agents include blood chemistry (protein and glucose), cell counts and white blood cell differential, direct antigen detection, polymerase chain reaction assays, and cultures for bacteria, fungi, and viruses. In addition, it is sometimes relevant to test for antibodies to common pathogens found in the central nervous system.

CHAPTER 36

1. Because no other associated site of infection is identified, this case is an example of a primary bacteremia.

2. The patient has granulocytopenia that placed him at risk for all types of bacterial infections—in particular, bacteremia. Neutropenic patients are usually at risk for gram-negative bacteremia.

3. The following conditions also place patients at an increased risk for bacteremia: reduced immune competency, increased use of invasive procedures and instrumentation, aging, and administration of immunosuppressive therapy and other drugs.

4. Sources of bacteremic spread include peritoneal dialysis, pericarditis, bacterial pneumonia, bedsores, prosthetic devices and instrumentation, and skeletal, skin, and soft tissue infections.

5. Bacterial pneumonias that usually produce a concurrent bacteremia include *Staphylococcus aureus, Streptococcus pneumoniae, Pseudomonas aeruginosa, Haemophilus influenzae,* and *Enterobacter aerogenes.*

6. Sepsis, septic shock, renal failure, and eventually death

7. Antimicrobials, antisepsis therapy physiologic support, and anticoagulation agents have been used.

8. Those at risk for polymicrobial bacteremia include immunocompromised patients, especially those with alcoholism, granulocytopenia, extensive burns, diabetes mellitus, and renal failure. Patients with vascular insufficiency resulting from ischemia are also at risk.

9. It has been suggested that 10 mL of blood should be drawn from adult patients and placed in 90 mL of diluting fluid (1:10 dilution). This ratio helps reduce the bactericidal effect of serum. Sodium polyanetholsulfonate (SPS) in the culture medium serves as anticomplement and anticoagulant.

10. The number of samples and time of collection could be highly dependent on the type of bacteremia suspected. In general, collecting three sets within a 24-hour period at 1-hour intervals is appropriate, especially in suspected cases of subacute endocarditis.

CHAPTER 37

1. The patient's urine analysis revealed pyuria, and the culture was positive for a single organism. These results should be worked up further and susceptibilities performed so that the patient can be treated appropriately.

2. The organism *(E. coli)* likely originated from the patient's own fecal flora.

3. The patient's deteriorating symptoms (delirium, hypotension, fever), in addition to the laboratory findings of leukocytosis and positive urine and blood cultures, signify urosepsis. The patient should be treated aggressively with empiric antimicrobials, until susceptibility results of the blood and urine cultures return.

4. A single-episode UTI occurs only once and resolves after antimicrobial therapy, whereas recurrent UTI occurs repeatedly. Recurrent UTI may involve the same organism (relapse) or a different organism (reinfection).

5. Gram-stained smears of uncentrifuged urine may reveal the etiologic agent of UTI. The presence of white blood cells also would be detected, indicating infection. Other screening methods are used to detect the presence of pyuria and bacteruria, which provides the clinician information on how to proceed with patient care.

6. Urine specimens for routine culture should be incubated for a full 24 hours at 37° C.

7. Background urethral flora may appear after 24 hours. This appearance may result in costly identification and confusion of the clinical purpose of the urine culture.

8. Specimens with multiple uropathogens (three or more) likely represent contamination.

9. Routine urine cultures do not include the recovery of *Neisseria gonorrhoeae, Chlamydia trachomatis,* or *Ureaplasma urealyticum,* all of which are sexually transmitted agents. Symptoms produced by these organisms are difficult to differentiate from that of a true urinary tract infection.

10. One or two uropathogens present in greater than 10^5 CFU/mL should be identified and susceptibility tests should be performed.

11. Urinalysis, urine culture, and blood culture should be performed.

12. Reasons the patient developed this infection include immunosuppression, diabetes mellitus, foreign body (stent, urinary catheter), stricture, graft trauma, and obstruction.

CHAPTER 38

1. Pelvic inflammatory disease usually presents with vague symptoms that vary by the individual. Many women are asymptomatic, whereas common signs include fever, unusual vaginal discharge, foul odor, painful intercourse, painful urination, irregular bleeding, and abdominal pain. Untreated PID can cause permanent damage to the female reproductive organs to cause infertility, ectopic pregnancy, or chronic pelvic pain.

2. Vulvovaginitis can be divided into three distinct entities. Bacterial vaginosis is usually caused by *G. vaginalis* and *Mobiluncus* spp. that have overgrown the normal vaginal flora to increase the overall vaginal pH. Women usually present with an abnormal vaginal discharge that is positive by the whiff test, negative viewing on KOH prep, and typically clue cells seen on wet prep. Trichomoniasis is caused by the organism *T. vaginalis* to produce a yellowish-green frothy discharge, which may also be positive by whiff test. Motile trichomonads seen on wet prep are diagnostic. Candidiasis presents with a cheese curd–like clumpy discharge and is typically caused by *C. albicans,* although other candidal species may also be involved. The vaginal pH remains normal, and pseudohyphae and budding yeast cells are recognized on KOH prep.

3. Trace contacting of partners is important to get them tested and treated before they can spread infection to additional partners. Such contacting will slow the spread of disease to other persons.

4. Many patients presenting to a clinic with such complaints also have a secondary infection with another organism that may not be presenting symptoms. Because prescribed therapy may be targeted only for a single organism, it allows the provider to prescribe broad agents to cover all infections. Additionally, infection with a single agent often predisposes an individual to infection by another agent; for example, HSV2 and *T. vaginalis.*

5. Laboratory testing for several of these infectious agents is very expensive. In an effort to reduce costs, many screening tests are performed, which have the advantage of lower costs with the drawback of decreased sensitivity. A more expensive confirmatory test can then be performed on those positive screening results. Additionally, because the diagnosis of an STD may sometimes have economic and social consequences, having two independent positive test results should help minimize any implications.

6. Education has been one of the mainstays of preventing STDs, especially within high-risk groups. If individuals are provided with an understanding of the potential consequences of infection, it is hoped that they will practice the recommended precautionary measures such as abstinence, condom usage, and other safe sexual practices. In some areas, outreach programs are going into the community to perform organized screening allowing for earlier detection and elimination of spread. Additionally, the HPV vaccine is currently available for females ranging in age from 9 to 26.

7. Both the chancre and chancroid are ulcerative genital lesions, but the biggest difference is whether or not pain is involved. Chancroid is caused by infection with *Haemophilus ducreyi,* and patients present with painful ulcers and a fluctuant adenopathy, prompting the adage, "You do cry with ducreyi." Chancres are painless nontender ulcers with nonfluctuant adenopathy.

8. The molecular tests typically demonstrate greater sensitivity than culture-based methods. Due to the increased sensitivity, many invasive sampling methods are no longer required (swab versus urine) allowing for greater compliance in getting patients and contacts tested. More people are volunteering for testing so that preventive measures can be instituted when positive results occur.

9. In males, gonococcal urethritis is diagnostic with a mucopurulent urethral discharge and a demonstration of gram-negative intracellular diplococci within leukocytes. Males presenting with symptoms of urethritis but no discharge may represent a nongonococcal infection. In females, due to the lack of many visible signs and symptoms, a clinical diagnosis is much more difficult, requiring further laboratory testing to confirm infection.

10. The HPV vaccine is quadrivalent representing genotypes 6, 11, 16, and 18. Genotypes 6 and 11 cause approximately 90% of all genital warts, whereas genotypes 16 and 18 are known to cause approximately 70% of all cervical cancers. Although this vaccine is not comprehensive, it provides a measure of protection against the most common causes of HPV disease.

CHAPTER 39

1. The treatment for the gastrointestinal malignancy that the patient received placed the patient at an increased risk for infections. The patient became neutropenic, making him susceptible to endogenous microflora. Septicemia is not uncommon among neutropenic patients.

2. *Pseudomonas aeruginosa* is a member of the normal colonic flora. If a malignancy occurred at this particular site, cytotoxic drugs taken by the patient may have contributed to the breakdown of mucosal barriers, providing access for the organism to gain entrance into the bloodstream.

3. Although a decrease in the number of neutrophils is the most commonly demonstrated hematologic disturbance, inadequacy of neutrophil functions, such as the inability to migrate to sites of inflammation, is another cause of increased infections among such patients. The inability of the neutrophils to phagocytize or kill the ingested organisms also predisposes patients with this type of malignancy and places them at risk of infections from endogenous organisms.

4. There are many organisms of concern in pregnant women. *E. coli* and other gram-negative bacilli can cause urinary tract infections, while *Candida* spp can cause vaginal yeast infections. A number of organisms can cause congenital infections, including *Toxoplasma gondii*, rubella virus, cytomegalovirus, herpes simplex virus, varicella zoster virus, HIV, parvovirus B19, hepatitis B virus, *Treponema pallidum*, *Streptococcus agalactiae*, and *Listeria monocytogenes*. Finally, several organisms can be transmitted during labor and delivery and may adversely affect the baby, including *Neisseria gonorrhoeae*, *Chlamydia trachomatis*, *Streptococcus agalactiae*, *Escherichia coli*, human papilloma virus, cytomegalovirus, and herpes simplex virus.

5. Several changes in the immune function occur as the human body ages, increasing its susceptibility to infections and malignancy. The qualitative decline of cellular immune defenses (function) predisposes elderly individuals to various types of infections, including respiratory, gastrointestinal, urinary tract, and soft tissue infections. Because of decreased tumor surveillance by immune and nonimmune mechanisms,

the occurrence of malignancy in this population is also increased.

6. Organisms associated with causing infection in patients with cystic fibrosis include *P. aeruginosa*, *S. aureus*, *H. influenzae*, and *Burkholderia cepacia*. Organisms associated with causing infection in patients with VAP include *S. pneumoniae*, *H. influenzae*, *S. aureus*, *P. aeruginosa*, *Klebsiella*, *Enterobacter*, *Serratia*, *Acinetobacter*, *Stenotrophomonas*, and *B. cepacia*.

CHAPTER 40

1. Lyme borreliosis
2. Relapsing arthritis and chronic synovitis
3. Cats and dogs
4. Splenectomy, cancer, substance abuse
5. *Bartonella henselae*; *Afipia felis* or *B. clarridgeiae*
6. Cutaneous; inhalation
7. The virulence factors present in *B. anthracis* include the lethal factor (LF) and the edema factor (EF). In order for LF and EF to become biologically active toxins, they must first combine with the *B. anthracis* protective antigen (PA), which is also a transport protein that allows entry of the toxins into the host cell.
8. *B. melitensis*, *B. abortus*, *B. suis*, *B. canis*; goats, cattle, pigs, dogs
9. In icteric leptospirosis, the patients show the same initial symptoms, but they also develop jaundice, hemolysis, and renal failure. Icteric leptospirosis has a mortality rate of 15% to 40%. In anicteric leptospirosis, patients develop fever, myalgia, headaches, and nausea for about 3 weeks. These symptoms subside, after which the patient may develop CNS symptoms.
10. Rickettsiaceae and Anaplasmataceae; arthropod vectors
11. *R. typhi* and *R. prowazekii*
12. Rocky Mountain spotted fever (RMSF); blood vessels

CHAPTER 41

1. c
2. b
3. d
4. a
5. *Limulus* lysate, acanthamoeba culture, contact lens culture
6. Conjunctiva; *S. aureus*, *H. influenzae*, *S. pneumoniae*; chocolate agar, blood agar, Gram stains
7. Gram, Giemsa, immunofluorescent (IF), calcofluor white stain (CFW), acid-fast bacillus (AFB)
8. Topical
9. *Chlamydia*, HIV, syphilis, HSV
10. Keratitis, endophthalmitis, uveitis, scleral buckle infections

Selected Procedures

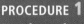

PROCEDURE 1
Bacitracin Susceptibility

PURPOSE
To differentiate *Streptococcus pyogenes* from other β-hemolytic streptococci

PRINCIPLE
Group A streptococci are susceptible to low levels (0.04 units) of bacitracin, whereas other groups of β-hemolytic streptococci are resistant. Rare strains of group A streptococci are resistant (approximately 1%), whereas some strains of groups B, C, and G streptococci are sensitive (5% to 10%). Sensitivity to bacitracin presumptively identifies an isolate as *S. pyogenes*. This procedure was designed for use only with pure cultures.

SPECIMEN
Isolated colonies of test organism on sheep blood agar

MEDIA
5% sheep blood agar plate

REAGENT
Bacitracin disk (0.04 units)

PROCEDURE
1. Streak surface of agar plate to obtain isolated colonies.
2. Aseptically place bacitracin disk onto inoculated surface. Press down gently on the disk to ensure complete contact with the agar surface.
3. Invert and incubate plates at 35° C for 18 to 24 hours in a CO_2 incubator.

INTERPRETATION
Susceptible = Any zone of inhibition around the bacitracin disk

Resistant = Uniform lawn of growth up to the edge of the disk (see Figure 15-17)

CONTROLS
Positive: *S. agalactiae*
Negative: *S. pyogenes*

PROCEDURE 2
CAMP Test

PURPOSE
To differentiate *Streptococcus agalactiae* from other β-hemolytic streptococci

PRINCIPLE
Streptococcus agalactiae produces CAMP factor that enhances the lysis of sheep red blood cells by staphylococcal β-lysin. A positive reaction can be observed in 5 to 6 hours with incubation in CO_2 (18 hours with incubation in ambient air).

SPECIMEN
1. Isolated colonies of test organism on sheep blood agar
2. β-Lysin–producing *S. aureus* on sheep blood agar

MEDIUM
Sheep blood agar plate

PROCEDURE
1. Inoculate *S. aureus* along a line down the center of the agar plate.
2. Inoculate the streptococcal isolates along a thin line 2 cm long and perpendicular to, but not touching, the *S. aureus* streak.
3. Incubate plate at 35° C for 18 hours.

INTERPRETATION
Positive result = Arrowhead-shaped area of enhanced hemolysis where the two streaks (staphylococcal and streptococcal) approach each other (see Figure 15-18)

Negative result = No enhanced hemolysis

CAMP inhibition reaction (reverse CAMP positive) = Inhibition of hemolysis by *S. aureus* where the two streaks approach each other. This reaction is characteristic of *Arcanobacterium haemolyticum*.

CONTROLS
Positive: *S. agalactiae*
Negative: *S. pyogenes*

PROCEDURE 3
Hippurate Hydrolysis Test

PURPOSE
To differentiate *Streptococcus agalactiae* from other β-hemolytic streptococci

PRINCIPLE
The enzyme hippuricase hydrolyzes hippuric acid to form sodium benzoate and glycine. Subsequent addition of ninhydrin results in the release of ammonia from the oxidative deamination of the α amino group in glycine as well as the reduced form of ninhydrin, hydrindantin. The ammonia reacts with residual ninhydrin and hydrindantin to produce a purple-colored complex. Some isolates of group D streptococci also hydrolyze hippurate; however, these isolates are less likely to be β-hemolytic, and their colony morphology is different from that of group B streptococci. An isolate that is hippurate positive and bile esculin negative has a very high probability of being *S. agalactiae*.

SPECIMEN
Isolated colonies of test organism on sheep blood agar

REAGENTS

Sodium hippurate (1%)

Sodium hippurate	1 g
Distilled water	100 mL

Dispense 0.5-mL aliquots in small capped vials. Store at −20° C. Storage life is 6 months.

Ninhydrin reagent

Ninhydrin	3.5 g
Acetone-butanol mixture (1 : 1)	100 mL

Store at room temperature. Storage life is 12 months.

PROCEDURE
1. Inoculate the solution of sodium hippurate heavily with colonies 18 to 24 hours old until a milky suspension is obtained.
2. Incubate tube for 2 hours at 35° C.
3. Add 0.2 mL of ninhydrin reagent.
4. Mix and incubate for 10 to 15 minutes at 35° C.

INTERPRETATION
Positive result = Deep purple color, indicates hippurate hydrolysis
Negative result = No color change or very slight purple color

CONTROLS
Positive: *S. agalactiae*
Negative: *S. pyogenes*

PROCEDURE 4
PYR Hydrolysis Test

PURPOSE
To differentiate those gram-positive cocci that will hydrolyze the substrate L-pyrrolidonyl α-naphthylamide (PYR) from those that are PYR negative

PRINCIPLE
PYR-impregnated disks serve as the substrate to produce α-naphthylamine, which is detected in the presence of D-dimethylaminocinnamaldehyde (DMCA) by the production of a red color.

SPECIMEN
Isolated colonies of test organism on sheep blood agar

PROCEDURE
1. Lightly moisten a PYR-impregnated disk with sterile water.
2. Using a sterile loop, rub one or more isolated colonies onto the surface of the disk.
3. NOTE: Incubation time and temperature varies slightly by manufacturer. Incubate disk as indicated in the manufacturer's instructions, generally 2 to 15 minutes.
4. Add a drop of color developer and observer for a red color on the disk within 5 minutes.

INTERPRETATION
Positive result = Red color
Negative result = Colorless

CONTROLS
Positive: *Enterococcus faecalis*
Negative: *Streptococcus agalactiae*

PROCEDURE 5
Bile Esculin Hydrolysis

PURPOSE
To differentiate group D streptococci and enterococci from other gram-positive cocci

PRINCIPLE
Group D streptococci and enterococci grow in the presence of bile and also hydrolyze esculin to esculetin and glucose. Esculetin diffuses into the agar and combines with ferric citrate in the medium to produce a black complex.

SPECIMEN
Isolated colonies of test organism on sheep blood agar

MEDIA
Bile esculin agar

PROCEDURE
1. Pick one or two isolated colonies from the sheep blood agar plate and inoculate to bile esculin agar medium.
2. Incubate plate or slant at 35° C for 18 to 24 hours. NOTE: A positive result is often seen within 4 hours. A negative result should be incubated for an additional 24-hour period.

INTERPRETATION
Positive result = Blackening of the agar
Negative result = No blackening of the agar. NOTE: Growth alone does not constitute a positive result.

CONTROLS
Positive: Group D *Streptococcus*
Negative: Viridans *Streptococcus*

PROCEDURE 6
Salt-Tolerance Test

PURPOSE
To differentiate gram-positive cocci that will grow in 6.5% NaCl from those that are inhibited by this salt concentration

PRINCIPLE
Enterococcus, Aerococcus, and some species of *Pediococcus* and *Leuconostoc* can withstand a higher salt concentration than other gram-positive cocci.

SPECIMEN
Isolated colonies of test organism on sheep blood agar

MEDIUM
6.5% NaCl broth (nutrient broth base)

PROCEDURE
1. Pick one or two isolated colonies from the sheep blood agar plate and lightly inoculate 5 mL of NaCl broth.
2. Incubate broth at 35° C for 3 days. Check daily for growth.

INTERPRETATION
Positive result = Turbidity
Negative result = No turbidity

CONTROLS
Positive: *Enterococcus faecalis*
Negative: Viridans *Streptococcus*

PROCEDURE 7
X- and V-Factor Requirement

PURPOSE
To differentiate *Haemophilus* spp. based on their requirement for X and/or V factors

PRINCIPLE
A suspension of bacteria to be tested is lawned onto the surface of a minimal medium. Disks or strips impregnated with X, V, and X and V factors are placed on the surface of the medium. After incubation, the pattern of bacterial growth determines which factor(s) the bacteria require.

SPECIMEN
Isolated colonies on chocolate agar

MEDIUM
Trypticase soy broth
Mueller-Hinton or trypticase soy agar plate
X, V, and X and V factors

PROCEDURE
1. Make a suspension of the isolate in trypticase soy broth. The suspension is then incubated at 35° C for about 2 hours to exhaust any X and V factors carried over from the plating medium.
2. A swab is used to inoculate the broth onto plated medium devoid of X and V factors; Mueller-Hinton or trypticase soy agars are acceptable.
3. After the plates dry, sterile forceps are used to gently place a strip or disk containing X factor on the plate. A V factor strip or disk is placed parallel to the X factor strip or disk approximately 15 mm away. A greater distance away, a strip or disk containing both X and V factor is placed onto the medium.
4. The plate is incubated at 35° C in 5% to 10% CO_2 for 18 to 24 hours. The plates are then examined for growth around and/or between the strips.

INTERPRETATION
V factor only required = Growth entirely around the V factor disk or strip and the disk or strip containing both X and V factors

X factor only required = Growth entirely around the X factor disk or strip and the disk or strip containing both X and V factors

X and V factors both required = Growth between the X and V disks or strips and the disk or strip containing both X and V factors

CONTROLS
V factor only required: *Haemophilus parainfluenzae*
X and V factors both required: *Haemophilus influenzae*

PROCEDURE 8
NALC-Sodium Hydroxide Digestion-Decontamination

PURPOSE
To enhance the recovery of mycobacteria from clinical specimens by reducing the number of contaminating or commensal bacteria

PRINCIPLE
Sodium hydroxide (NaOH) acts as both a decontaminating agent and a digestant. Because of the toxicity of NaOH to mycobacteria, the agent should be used at the lowest concentration that inhibits growth of contaminating bacteria. N-acetyl-L-cysteine (NALC) is a mucolytic agent, which allows for a lower concentration of NaOH to be used and thereby optimizes the recovery of mycobacteria from the specimen.

REAGENTS
NALC-NaOH digestant: Combine equal volumes of 2.94% sodium citrate dihydrate (0.1 M) and 4% NaOH. Just before use, add 0.5 g of powdered NALC per 100 mL of mixture. Refrigerate when not in use; discard after 24 hours.

Phosphate buffer (0.067 M, pH 6.8) or sterile, distilled water, 30 to 40 mL per specimen

Bovine albumin fraction V, 0.2% in sterile saline

PROCEDURE
1. Working within a biological safety cabinet, transfer 10 mL (or total specimen if volume is less than 10 mL) to 50-mL screw-cap centrifuge tube. If specimen volume is greater than 10 mL, select most purulent-appearing material. Add an equal volume of NALC-NaOH digestant to each sample.
2. Tighten caps and mix on a vortexer until liquefied (5 to 20 seconds), inverting each tube to ensure that NALC-NaOH solution contacts any untreated particles on the upper part of the tube.
3. Let tubes stand at room temperature for 15 minutes. If more decontamination is desired, increase the concentration of NaOH rather than the time the specimen is exposed to the digestion-decontamination mixture.
4. Dilute the digested-decontaminated specimens to the 50-mL mark with sterile distilled water or sterile phosphate buffer to minimize the continuing action of the NaOH and lower the specific gravity of the specimen. Tighten caps and invert or swirl to mix.
5. Centrifuge at 3000 × g for 15 minutes (or the appropriate combination of relative centrifugal force and time to give 95% sedimentation) using aerosol-free safety cups or in an aerosol-controlled vented centrifuge.
6. Holding the tube so that the sediment is on the upper side of the tube, pour off supernatant into a splashproof discard container of disinfectant.
7. Holding the tube in a horizontal position to keep the sediment as dry as possible, use a sterile applicator stick to remove a small part of the sediment and place it on a marked microscope slide. The smear should be about 1 × 2 cm.
8. Resuspend sediment in 1 to 2 mL of sterile 0.2% bovine albumin solution. If media will be inoculated immediately, the sediment may be resuspended in sterile water or sterile saline.
9. An optional step is to prepare a 1:10 dilution using 0.5 mL of the resuspended sediment in 4.5 mL of sterile water. Dilution decreases the concentration of toxic substances that may inhibit growth of mycobacteria. Inoculate diluted and undiluted specimens to solid media.

PROCEDURE 9
Slide Culture for the Identification of Fungi

PURPOSE

To aid in the identification of moulds by microscopic appearance

PRINCIPLE

Isolated fungi are inoculated onto a block of agar. The agar block is covered with a coverslip and incubated until mature growth of the fungi is noted. The coverslip is removed and the material attached to the coverslip is stained and examined microscopically. Microscopic morphology is an important characteristic in the identification of fungi, particularly moulds.

SPECIMEN

Isolated cultures of test fungi

MEDIUM

Sabouraud dextrose agar or other fungal medium

PROCEDURE

Prepare slide cultures within a properly operating biological safety cabinet. Fungi suspected of being pathogens are not recommended for observation in slide cultures.

1. Place a piece of filter paper into the bottom of a 100-mm sterile Petri dish.

2. Place a bent glass rod, two pieces of plastic tubing, or the bent end of a flexible straw on the filter paper.
3. Lay a clean, flamed glass microscope slide on top of the bent glass rod, two pieces of plastic tubing, or the bent end of a flexible straw.
4. Cut a 1 × 1-cm square block of fungal medium, such as Sabouraud dextrose agar, from a Petri dish, and aseptically transfer the block to the microscope slide.
5. Inoculate the four sides of the agar block with the desired fungus by using a heavy-gauge teasing needle or sterile wooden applicator stick.
6. Cover the block with a flamed sterile coverglass.
7. Moisten the filter paper with sterile water and place the lid on the Petri dish.
8. Incubate the slide culture at room temperature (22° C). Examine the culture periodically for growth, and add more water as necessary. The Petri dish can be placed on a microscope stage and the culture examined with the 10× objective.
9. When conidia or spores are evident, carefully lift the coverglass off the agar with a forceps, and place the coverglass into a drop of lactophenol cotton blue on another microscope slide for examination.

PROCEDURE 10
Germ Tube Production for the Identification of Yeast

PURPOSE

To differentiate among the pathogenic yeast based on the ability to produce a germ tube

PRINCIPLE

When grown in serum or plasma at 35° C, some yeasts have the ability to form hyphae. This is an important characteristic in the identification of *Candida albicans*.

SPECIMEN

Isolated cultures of test yeasts

MEDIUM

Rabbit plasma or serum or fecal calf serum

PROCEDURE

1. Make a light suspension by adding one yeast colony to 0.5 mL of sterile serum. Germ Tube Solution (Remel,

Lenexa, Kan.), composed of fetal bovine serum and trypticase soy broth, may be used as an alternative. This alternative substrate eliminates the risk of human immunodeficiency virus and hepatitis viruses that can be present in human serum.

2. Incubate the suspension at 35° C for 2.5 to 3 hours.
3. Place one drop of the suspension on a microscopic glass slide and add a coverslip.
4. Observe microscopically for the presence of germ tubes.

CONTROLS

A known germ tube positive isolate of *C. albicans* can serve as the positive control; as a negative control, *Cryptococcus* spp. can be used.

PROCEDURE 11
Cornmeal Agar for the Identification of Yeast

PURPOSE
To aid in the identification of pathogenic yeasts by microscopic morphology

PRINCIPLE
Isolated yeasts are inoculated onto the surface of an agar plate. The inoculum is covered with a coverslip and incubated 3 days. The yeasts on the plate are examined microscopically. Microscopic morphology is an important characteristic in the identification of yeasts.

SPECIMEN
Isolated cultures of test yeasts

MEDIUM
Cornmeal-Tween 80 plate; one third or one fourth of a plate can be used for each yeast.

PROCEDURE
1. Pick up a small amount of a yeast colony with an inoculating loop.
2. Make one streak of the yeast in the center of the agar surface. Do not cut the agar.
3. Make three or four streaks across the original streak to dilute the inoculum, being careful not to cut into the agar.
4. Cover the inoculum with a sterile coverslip and incubate at room temperature in the dark for 3 days.
5. Remove the lid from the Petri dish and examine the yeast with the low- (10×) and high- (40×) power objectives for the presence of hyphae, pseudohyphae, arthroconidia, chlamydoconidia, and blastoconidia.

CONTROLS
Candida albicans is used to demonstrate hyphae and chlamydospores.
Cryptococcus sp. is used to demonstrate blastoconidia.

PROCEDURE 12
Calibration of the Ocular Micrometer

PURPOSE
To calibrate an ocular micrometer to determine the size of parasites and formed elements examined microscopically

PRINCIPLE
Size is an important criterion in the identification of parasites, especially those found in clinical specimens from the digestive tract. Calibrating an ocular micrometer allows laboratory scientists to determine the size of objects seen during a microscopic examination of clinical material.

PROCEDURE
1. Insert the ocular micrometer in the eyepiece of the microscope so that the zero of the scale is on the left side.
2. Place the calibrated stage micrometer on the stage and focus on the scale using the low power (10× objective). The stage micrometer is divided into major lines separated by 0.1 mm (100 μm) and minor lines separated by 0.01 mm (10 μm).
3. While using low power, align the left-hand zero of the stage micrometer with the left-hand zero of the ocular micrometer. Do not move the stage micrometer after this point.
4. Scan the two scales for a point where a division line on the ocular micrometer directly aligns with a division line (minor line) on the stage micrometer.
5. Count the number of stage units and ocular units at this point. Divide the number of stage units by the number of ocular units and multiply the result by 10. This gives the value (in micrometers) for one ocular unit on low power.

$$\text{Micrometers/ocular unit} = \frac{\text{\# stage units}}{\text{\# ocular units}} \times \frac{10 \text{ micrometers}}{\text{stage unit}}$$

6. Repeat the procedure at high power (40× objective) and with the 100× objective to get the value of one ocular unit at each of those magnifications. To calculate the size of an organism, count the number of ocular units, multiply by the value for an ocular unit at that magnification, and report the value in micrometers.

Glossary

5′ nuclease assay A real-time polymerase chain reaction detection technique, also called the *Taqman assay*. This assay uses a probe labeled on the 5′ end with a fluorophore and on the 3′ end with a quencher. The probe binds to target DNA and is dissociated by the action of DNA polymerase when primer extension occurs. The dissociation of the probe results in fluorescence as the fluorophore and quencher are removed from close proximity.

A

accuracy The degree of conformity of a measurement to a standard or a true value.

achlorhydria Absence of hydrochloric acid from the gastric juice.

acid-fast See **acid-fastness.**

acid-fast bacteria Microorganisms or their parts that are resistant to the washing out of carbolfuchsin stain with acidified alcohol are designated as acid-fast bacteria. Mycobacteria and related species with waxes and phospholipids in their cell walls share this characteristic.

acid-fastness Ability of bacteria, such as the *Mycobacterium* spp., to retain dye when treated with mineral acid or an acid-alcohol solution.

acquired immune system See **adaptive immunity.**

acquired immunedeficiency syndrome (AIDS) AIDS is the most severe clinical manifestation of the disease spectrum caused by infection with human immunodeficiency virus (HIV).

acquired resistance See **adaptive immunity.**

actinomycosis A chronic, granulomatous infectious disease characterized by the development of sinus tracts and fistulae, which erupt to the surface and drain pus containing sulfur granules. It is caused by *Actinomyces israelii* and related anaerobic organisms.

actinomycotic mycetoma Mycetoma caused by aerobic actinomycetes.

acute glomerulonephritis A post-streptococcal disease that occurs after a cutaneous or pharyngeal infection that results from antigen-antibody complexes deposited in the glomeruli.

acute phase The early stage of a disease preceding the adaptive phase of the immune response.

acute sinusitis Disease that results from infection of one or more of the paranasal sinuses.

acute urethral syndrome A condition wherein patients experience dysuria and frequency with bacterial urine colony counts fewer than 105 organisms per milliliter of urine.

adaptive immune response See **adaptive immunity.**

adaptive immunity An immune response elicited by a specific stimulus from a foreign molecule that causes antigen recognition by B, TH, or TC cells and results in proliferation and differentiation of the stimulated cells into effector cells and memory cells. An immunity resulting from a previous encounter of the host and an antigenic stimuli.

adenylate cyclase toxin Virulence factor of *Bordetella* spp. that inhibits host epithelial and immune effector cells by inducing supraphysiologic concentrations of cyclic adenosine monophosphate.

adhesin Thin, filamentous protein structures, including proteinaceous capsular antigens (fimbrial antigens), that mediate the adhesion of bacteria to surfaces and play a role in pathogenesis. They have a high affinity for various epithelial cells.

aerobe A microorganism that lives and grows in the presence of oxygen.

aerotolerance test A test used to determine whether an isolate is a strict anaerobe or a facultative anaerobe.

aerotolerant anaerobe A microorganism that grows best in the absence of oxygen but can tolerate low concentrations of oxygen.

agar dilution minimal inhibitory concentration (agar dilution MIC) A minimal inhibitory test wherein a specific concentration of antimicrobial agent is incorporated into an agar medium contained in a Petri plate. As many as 36 bacterial isolates from individual patients and quality control strains are tested on a series of agar dilution plates, each containing a different concentration of antimicrobial agent.

agarose gel electrophoresis Method used to separate nucleic acid molecules. Agarose is made from seaweed and acts as a molecular sieve. Nucleic acids migrate through the agarose gel when an electrical current is applied. Nucleic acids are naturally negatively charged and will migrate to a positive pole. This migration separates the molecules.

amastigote A life-cycle stage found in humans that is characteristic of blood and tissue flagellates. It is a small oval intracellular body with a prominent nucleus and small kinetoplast.

aminoglycoside An antibiotic that has a six-membered ring with amino group substituents, aminocyclitol. The term *aminoglycoside* results from the glycosidic bonds between the aminocyclitol and two or more amino-containing or non–amino-containing sugars.

δ-aminolevulinic acid A substrate used in biochemical testing of *Haemophilus* spp. to determine X factor (hemin) requirement.

amorphous debris Debris without form or shape that is made up of necrotic tissue or cells, protein fluids, or mucus.

amplicon The amplified DNA that results from several cycles of the polymerase chain reaction (PCR). Also known as *PCR product.*

anaerobe An organism that does not require oxygen for life and reproduction.

anaerobic chamber An incubation system that provides an oxygen-free environment for inoculating media and incubating cultures.

anaerobic transport system Systems designed to maintain the viability of anaerobic bacteria from the time of collection to processing of the specimen. The vials are gassed out with oxygen-free carbon dioxide or nitrogen and contain an oxygen tension indicator.

analytical activity The process of analyzing the sample.

analytical sensitivity The ability of a test to detect a particular analyte or a small change in its concentration.

analytical specificity The ability of a test to detect substances other than the analyte of interest.

anamnestic immune response The stronger, quicker response on subsequent exposure to an immunogen.

anamnestic response A subsequent exposure to the same antigen results in a more rapid production of antibodies, in greater amounts, and for a longer period of time.

anamorph A fungus that reproduces asexually but has been linked to a fungus that reproduces sexually.

anneal Pairing, utilizing hydrogen bonding, of complementary of RNA and DNA sequences to form a double-stranded molecule. Describes the binding of a short probe or primer.

antagonism Occurs when the antimicrobial activity of a combination of antimicrobial agents is less than the activity of the individual agents alone.

anthrax Disease of livestock in which humans are accidentally infected. In humans it can take three clinical forms: cutaneous, gastrointestinal, and inhalational (pulmonary anthrax). An infection associated with *Bacillus anthracis*.

antibiogram The compilation of selected microorganisms and the percent susceptibility to selected antimicrobial agents.

antibiotic Substance used to prevent or treat an infection caused by bacteria and other pathogenic microorganisms.

antibiotic removal device (ARD) A resin that nonspecifically absorbs any antimicrobial agent present in the patient's blood.

antibody A protein, which in the monomer form has two heavy and two light chains, consisting of a hypervariable region capable of recognizing a particular binding site on another molecule; an immunoglobulin molecule characterized by specific amino acid sequence produced by the host as a result of a specific antigenic stimulation.

antibody titer The reciprocal of the highest dilution of a clinical sample that can be detected in a reaction with the corresponding antigen.

anticodon The triplet of bases on the tRNA that bind the triplet of bases on the mRNA. It identifies which amino acid will be in a specific location in the protein.

antigen Any substance that produces sensitivity and initiates an immune response from the host when it comes in contact with or is introduced to the host cell. A molecule that exhibits reactivity with an immunologic effector such as an antibody or T-cell receptor.

antigenic drift The phenomenon of slight antigenic change seen in influenza viruses over time as a result of minor mutations in the ssRNA.

antigenic shift The phenomenon by which an often unexpected change occurs in influenza virus strains. This antigenic change is often so drastic that it triggers pandemics.

antigenic variation Systematic change in surface antigens while organisms such as *Borrelia recurrentis* are in the host during the course of a single infection.

antimicrobial agent See **antibiotic.**

antimicrobial assay A method to measure the amount of antimicrobial agent in serum or body fluid.

antisepsis Destruction of microorganisms to prevent infection.

antiseptic Substance that inhibits, destroys, or reduces the bacterial load of living tissues or microorganisms. No sporicidal activity is implied. Used specifically for substances applied to living tissue.

antiseptic drug Considered to be a representative germicide, except in the case of a drug purporting to be, or represented as, an antiseptic for inhibitory use as a wet dressing, ointment, dusting powder, or other use that involves prolonged contact with the body.

arbovirus Virus transmitted between vertebrate hosts by arthropods.

archaea See **archaeobacteria.**

archaeobacteria Group of living microorganisms that exist in the absence of oxygen; produce methane; and live only in bodies of highly concentrated saltwater, hot, acidic waters of sulfur springs, and temperatures near 80° C and pH levels as low as 2.

arthroconidium Asexual spore formed by the breaking of a hypha at the point of septation. Arthroconidia can be adjacent or separated by a dysjunctor cell.

asaccharolytic A microorganism that is unable to metabolize carbohydrates in the presence or absence of oxygen and that must rely on other carbon sources for energy.

ascospore Sexual spore produced by fusion of a male nucleus into a female cell in an ascus.

ascus A saclike structure usually containing two to eight ascospores.

aseptic meningitis A syndrome characterized by signs and symptoms of meningeal inflammation with the presence of inflammatory cells in the cerebrospinal fluid without bacteria or fungi recovered from cultures. Occasionally associated with meningitis caused by viruses.

asexual reproduction Reproduction by methods such as fission, in which the nucleus and cytoplasm are split to form two new, separate organisms.

aspiration pneumonia Pulmonary inflammation resulting from the abnormal entry of fluid, particulate substances, or endogenous secretions into the lower airways.

atypical pneumonia See **primary atypical pneumonia.**

auramine/auramine-rhodamine fluorochrome stains Fluorochrome stains (either auramine or auramine-rhodamine) are acid-fast stains that are more sensitive than carbolfuchsin stains.

autotrophs Organisms that produce organic compounds from carbon dioxide as a carbon source, using either light or reactions of inorganic chemical compounds as a source of energy.

avidity The strength of binding between an antibody molecule and an antigen with multiple epitopes.

B

Babès-Ernst granules Metachromatic granules of *Corynebacterium diphtheriae* that stain more intensely than other parts of the bacterial cell.

bacteremia The presence of viable bacteria in the blood evidenced by their recovery in blood cultures.

bacteria Also referred to as *eubacteria;* single-celled microorganisms that lack a true cell nucleus and multiply by binary fission.

bacterial interference Potential pathogens being inhibited by the nonpathogenic resident microbiota.

bacterial vaginosis (BV) A syndrome characterized by vaginal symptoms that include inflammation, perivaginal irritation, vaginal odor described as "fishy," and mild to moderate discharge. The organism *Gardnerella vaginalis* has been recovered from most patients with bacterial vaginosis.

bactericidal An antimicrobial that kills a microorganism.

bactericidal effect Killing effect or amount of antimicrobial agent required to kill.

bacteriocin Proteins produced by some bacteria that inhibit the growth of other strains of the same organism or related species. Genes for bacteriocins may reside on plasmids.

bacteriophage A virus that infects bacteria.

bacteriostatic An antimicrobial that inhibits bacterial growth but does not kill the bacteria.

bacteriuria The presence of bacteria in the urine.

bamboo rods Term that describes the microscopic appearance of *Bacillus anthracis* in a Gram stain, referring to the cells' arrangement and the unstained central spore.

baseline data Surveillance data that represent the normal endemic level of infections in a health care setting; used to gauge when an outbreak occurs.

Bayes' theorem The formulas for calculating positive and negative predictive values are commonly referred to as *Bayes' theorem,* which was published posthumously in 1763.

benchmarking A reference point obtained by using an industry's or a profession's best practices to imitate and improve processes.

bias The mean difference of test results from an accepted reference method by systemic errors.

bile solubility A test that determines the ability of bacterial cells to lyse in the presence of bile salts; it is used to differentiate *Streptococcus pneumoniae* (bile soluble) from other α-hemolytic streptococci (bile insoluble).

biofilm Communities of microorganisms attached to a solid surface.

biofouling The undesirable accumulation of microorganisms, plants, algae, and/or animals on wetted structures. For example, biofilms can form in pipes carrying drinking water, making the water unsafe to drink.

biosafety cabinet A portable safety station for the handling of aerosols and particulates; provides laboratory personnel protection.

biosafety level The maintenance of safe conditions in biological research to prevent harm to workers, nonlaboratory organisms, or the environment. The CDC established guidelines for four biosafety levels.

bioterrorism The intentional use of biological agents (bacteria, viruses, or toxins) to cause illness or death as a tact of terrorism.

bipolar staining The distinctive "safety-pin" appearance that results from the staining with a polychromatic stain such as Wayson or Wright-Giemsa.

black death Another name for the plague, a disease caused by *Yersinia pestis*. Victims have a dark color caused by cyanosis and petechiae.

blackwater fever Syndrome associated with *Plasmodium falciparum* infection characterized by reddish to black urine resulting from hemoglobinuria.

blastoconidium Conidium formed by budding yeast and along hypha or pseudohypha.

blepharitis Inflammation of the eyelids.

blood-borne pathogens Pathogenic microorganisms that are present in human blood and can cause disease in humans. These pathogens include, but are not limited to, hepatitis B virus (HBV) and human immunodeficiency virus (HIV).

borderline oxacillin-resistant isolates A subtle type of oxacillin resistance in *Staphylococcus aureus* that lack the *mecA* gene and have oxacillin minimal inhibitory concentrations right above (or zones of inhibition right below) the breakpoint for susceptibility.

borderline oxacillin-resistant *Staphylococcus aureus* (BORSA) See **borderline oxacillin-resistant isolates.**

Bordet-Gengou potato infusion agar A medium supplemented with glycerol, peptones, and horse or sheep blood for isolation of *Bordetella* spp.

botulism A serious form of food poisoning caused by the ingestion of preformed botulinum toxin produced by *Clostridium botulinum*.

bradyzoite *Toxoplasma gondii* life-cycle stage that forms within a cyst-like structure. The organisms multiply slowly but may be transformed into tachyzoites when the host's immune system activity is impaired.

brain abscess An abscess within the brain tissue caused by inflammation and collection of infected material coming from local (ear infection, infection of paranasal sinuses, infection of the mastoid air cells of the temporal bone, epidural abscess) or remote (lung, heart, kidney etc.) infectious sources.

branched DNA (bDNA) detection A technique that amplifies signal after probes have annealed to target nucleic acid. A capture probe attached to a solid support anneals to target nucleic acid. Then target probes also anneal to the nucleic acid and to preamplifier probes. Amplifier probes then bind to the preamplifier probes, resulting in the formation of branched DNA (bDNA) structures. Label probes then bind to the bDNA structures, resulting in massive signal amplification.

breakpoint (cutoff) Minimal inhibitory concentration or zone diameter value used to indicate susceptible, intermediate, or resistant for an antimicrobial agent as defined by the interpretive criteria used in Clinical and Laboratory Standards Institute standards.

breakpoint panel A variation of the standard broth microdilution MIC panel is the breakpoint panel, in which only one or a few concentrations of each antimicrobial agent are tested on a single panel.

Brill-Zinsser disease Also called *recrudescent typhus*, this is a reactivation of *Rickettsia prowazekii* in patients who have had epidemic typhus. The reactivation disease is normally milder than epidemic typhus.

brittle Adjective used in defining colony consistency; splinters.

bronchiolitis An infectious disease of infants usually caused by respiratory viruses, characterized by inflammation of the bronchioles, and clinically expressed as a febrile upper respiratory tract infection with concurrent signs of lower respiratory tract airway obstruction.

bronchitis An illness characterized by inflammation of the bronchi and clinically expressed as cough, usually with sputum production, and evidence of concurrent upper airway infection.

bronchoalveolar lavage A procedure in which saline or some other physiologic fluid is instilled into the alveoli and recovered for the purpose of culture or cytology examination.

broth macrodilution minimal inhibitory concentration A minimum inhibitory concentration (MIC) test performed in test tubes, usually with 1.0- to 2.0-mL volumes of antimicrobial solutions.

broth media Liquid medium used as a supplement to agar plates to detect small numbers of most aerobes, anaerobes, and microaerophiles.

broth-macrodilution MIC Broth dilution MIC tests performed in test tubes are referred to as *broth-macrodilution MIC* or *tube-dilution MIC* tests. Generally a twofold serial dilution series, each containing 1 to 2 mL of antimicrobial agent, is prepared.

broth microdilution MIC A minimum inhibitory concentration (MIC) test performed in multiwell polystyrene microdilution trays, usually with 0.1-mL volumes of antimicrobial solutions.

bubo (buboe) Inflammation of a lymph node, characterized by swelling and ulceration, resulting from infection, especially in the area of the armpit or groin, that is characteristic of certain infections such as bubonic plague. Inflamed, tender swelling of a lymph nodes.

bubonic plague The most common form of plague, which usually results from the bite of a flea infested with *Yersinia pestis*. A common result is the formation of a bubo.

buffered charcoal yeast extract (BCYE) Recommended medium for isolation of *Legionella* spp.

bulla (plural *bullae*) A blister more than 5 mm (about 3/16 inch) in diameter with thin walls that is full of fluid.

bullous impetigo A form of impetigo in which the skin lesions are bullae instead of vesicles. The crusts are thin and greenish yellow. Infection is treated with oral anti-staphylococcal antibiotics. Exfoliative toxin has also been implicated in bullous impetigo. See also **impetigo**.

Buruli ulcer An infectious disease caused by *Mycobacterium ulcerans* characterized by painless swelling that later develops into a lesion.

butyrous Adjective used in defining colony consistency; creamy.

C

CAMP test A test used for the presumptive identification of group B streptococci (*S. agalactiae*). A positive result is determined by enhanced, arrowhead, β-hemolysis from the interaction of CAMP factor from group B streptococcus and the β-lysin from certain strains of *Staphylococcus aureus*.

canaliculitis Inflammation of the canaliculus.

capnophile Microorganism that grows best in the presence of carbon dioxide.

capnophilic Term used to describe microorganisms that require an increased concentration of CO_2, usually between 5% and 10%.

capsid The protein covering a virus.

capsule An organelle in some prokaryotic cells, such as a bacterial cell located outside the cell wall of bacteria. It is usually made up of polysaccharides but could be composed of other materials. Used by microorganisms as a protective structure against phagocytosis and physical and chemical effects of the environment.

carbuncles A cluster of furuncles caused by a subcutaneous spread of a staphylococcal infection.

carrier An individual or animal that harbors a potentially pathogenic organism of infectious agent without the host showing signs of the disease but that serves as source of infection to susceptible individuals.

carrier state A condition in which an individual or animal harbors a potentially pathogenic organism of infectious agent without the host showing signs of the disease but serves as source of infection to susceptible individuals.

Cary-Blair transport media Semisolid medium used for maintenance of various pathogens, including enteric bacteria such as *Salmonella, Shigella,* and *Campylobacter* spp. in stool specimens.

case definition Description establishing parameters that define a case in an outbreak investigation.

catalase An enzyme present in staphylococci; useful for distinguishing staphylococci from streptococci.

catarrhal phase Initial phase of pertussis. Symptoms are nonspecific and include sneezing, mild cough, runny nose, and sometimes conjunctivitis.

category A agents Bacteria, viruses, and toxins that, if used as bioterror agents, would cause significant public health disruption.

catheter-related bloodstream infection (CR-BSI) Bloodstream infections related to the presence of an intravascular device in a major vessel, generally ending at or near the heart.

cell culture Cells removed from an organism and grown in complex medium for several purposes, including growth of viruses.

cell wall deficient Refers to gram-positive or gram-negative bacteria lacking a cell wall, also called *L-forms.* Exposure to antimicrobial agents that inhibit cell-wall synthesis (e.g., penicillin) can lead to this condition. The mycoplasma inherently lack the ability to produce a cell wall; so, when they were first discovered, they were referred to as *cell-wall deficient.*

cellular immune response An immune response that involves the activation of macrophages and natural killer cells, the production and release of antigen-specific cytotoxic T-lymphocytes, and the release of various cytokines in response to an antigenic stimulus. It does not require antibodies.

cellulitis A serious, even life-threatening, skin infection that involves deep tissues and can be accompanied by bacteremia or sepsis.

Centers for Disease Control and Prevention (CDC) The CDC is a federal agency established for the protection of the health and safety of people, both at home and abroad, providing credible information to enhance health decisions and promoting health.

central line–associated bloodstream infections (CLA-BSIs) One of multiple acute-care hospital acquired infections; occur because of instrumentation, increased use of antimicrobial agents, breaks in aseptic techniques, and lack of hand hygiene.

central nervous system (CNS) The largest part of the nervous system that is made up of the brain and the spinal cord.

cercaria The "tailed" stage in the life cycle of flukes that is produced from rediae that develop in snail tissue. This stage is released into the water.

cerebrospinal fluid (CSF) The clear fluid formed by the choroid plexus or the ventricles that fills the subarachnoid space in the brain and serves as a "cushion" for the cortex.

cervicitis Inflammation of the tissues surrounding the cervix; can be caused by an infection of a variety of agents, such as *Chlamydia* and *Neisseria gonorrhoeae.*

cervicofacial actinomycosis An infectious disease caused by the anaerobic *Actinomyces,* which can occur in the mouth, lungs, and digestive tract. Abscesses may penetrate the surrounding bone and muscle to the skin, where they break open and leak large amounts of pus. When it occurs in the mouth, it is called *cervicofacial.*

chancre The lesion characteristic of primary syphilis. It is typically a single, firm, painless erythematous ulcer with a clean surface and raised border.

chancroid A sexually transmitted disease caused by *Haemophilus ducreyi.*

chemiluminescent immunoassay A type of labeled assay when a chemical reaction emits light.

chemotactic agent A protein that is able to direct the migration of a specific cell.

chemotaxis Movement of cells in response to chemical stimulant.

chlamydiosis An infection caused by *Chlamydia* spp.

cholera An acute infectious diarrheal illness caused by *Vibrio cholerae* that may occur in an epidemic proportion.

choleragen A powerful enterotoxin produced by organism *Vibrio cholerae;* also called *cholera toxin.*

cholera toxin A powerful enterotoxin produced by *Vibrio cholerae.* Also referred to as a *choleragen.*

chromatoidal bars RNA that has been condensed into a barlike structure within the cyst of some protozoan organisms.

chromogenic substrate A molecule that is initially colorless; when cleaved by a specific enzyme, it becomes a colored compound.

chromomycosis A chronic fungal infection of the skin and subcutaneous tissues, also called *chromoblastomycosis.* The most commonly associated fungi are *Fonsecaea pedrosoi, Phialophora verrucosa, Cladophialophora carrionii,* and *Fonsecaea compacta.*

chromosomally mediated resistant *Neisseria gonorrhoeae* (CMRNG) Type of penicillin resistance in *N. gonorrhoeae* attributable to genes located on the chromosome that code for an alteration in penicillin-binding proteins.

-cidal A suffix used to indicate that a substance destroys microorganisms (e.g., *bactericidal, virucidal*).

ciguatera A form of food poisoning from ciguatera toxin produced by dinoflagellates; passed up the food chain; ingested in snapper, sea bass, or grouper.

citrate test A bacteriologic test to determine an organism's ability to use citrate as a sole carbon source.

Clark and Lub's medium A classic bacteriologic medium used for the methyl red, Voges-Proskauer test.

clean-catch midstream urine specimen Technique to collect urine specimen while reducing contaminant skin flora; patient cleanses external genitalia and begins voiding urine, collecting the midstream sample.

Clinical and Laboratory Standards Institute (CLSI; formerly NCCLS) An international, interdisciplinary, nonprofit, standards-developing, and educational organization that promotes the development and use of voluntary consensus standards and guidelines within the health care community.

Clinical Laboratory Improvement Act of 1988 (CLIA) Law establishing quality standards for all laboratory testing to ensure accuracy, reliability, and timeliness of patients' test results.

clinical (diagnostic) sensitivity The proportion of positive test results obtained when a test is applied to patients known to have a disease.

clinical (diagnostic) specificity The proportion of negative results obtained when a test is applied to patients known to be free of a disease.

clumping factor A cell-bound coagulase that is able to clot plasma and may be used to screen for *Staphylococcus aureus*.

coagglutination A particulate agglutination assay using *Staphylococcus aureus* to bind the Fc portion of antibodies.

coagulase A clotting enzyme (staphylocoagulase) that is useful in differentiating coagulase-positive staphylococci, such as *Staphylococcus aureus,* from coagulase-negative staphylococci.

coagulase-negative staphylococci (CoNS) Staphylococci that lack the enzyme coagulase.

codon The gene sequence inscribed in DNA and in RNA composed of trinucleotide units.

cold enrichment Incubating broth cultures at 4° C for several days to select for bacteria, such as *Listeria* and *Yersinia* organisms, that grow well at this temperature.

cold-agglutinating antibody Antibody that agglutinates antigens at 4° C; if present, suggestive of infection caused by *Mycoplasma pneumoniae.*

College of American Pathologists (CAP) The CAP is the principal organization of board-certified pathologists that serves and represents the interest of patients, pathologists, and the public by fostering excellence in the practice of pathology and laboratory medicine.

colonial morphology Colony characteristics and form.

colonization The formation of a population of microorganisms within the host that does not cause disease.

colony-forming units (CFU) The number of microbes that grow from a measured inoculation. Bacteria are easily seen in direct smears at concentrations of 10×5 CFU/mL following cytocentrifugation.

commensal An organism that lives in a relationship in which one organism derives food or other benefits from another organism without hurting or helping it.

commensalism A relationship between different species (host and organism) wherein one (organism) benefits from the other (host) without causing harm. The host species does not benefit from the relationship or organism.

communal living Community living programs; might include prisons and behavioral health facilities. In these facilities, infections might be found that are spread by contact (illicit tattooing) or by intimate contact with blood and body fluids.

community-acquired bacteremia Bacteremia that occurs in individuals living in the general community.

community-acquired infections Infections that start in the community and are not acquired within a health care setting.

community-associated methicillin-resistant *Staphylococcus aureus* (CA-MRSA) See also **methicillin-resistant *Staphylococcus aureus* (MRSA).** Since the 1990s CA-MRSA infections have risen and can be found in patients who lack traditional health care–associated risk factors such as recent hospitalization, long-term care, dialysis, or indwelling devices. CA-MRSA infections and outbreaks have been reported among athletes, correctional facility inmates, military recruits in close contact environments, pediatric patients, and tattoo recipients.

competency The quality of being well qualified both physically and intellectually to perform all assigned duties.

competent As in an immunocompetent patient, the state of well-being in which the immune system is functioning properly and is able to protect the individual from infectious diseases.

complement Plasma proteins that function either as enzymes or as binding proteins; plays an essential role in host defense against infectious agents and in the inflammatory process.

complement deficiency The lack of any one or more of the proteins that make up the biochemical cascade of the immune system.

complement fixation Activation of complement proteins.

congenital Acquired in utero when the organism infecting the woman crosses the placenta to infect the fetus.

conidium Asexual fungal reproductive structure usually formed at the side of hyphae. It is not contained in a sac-like structure; small and usually single-celled conidia are called *microconidia,* and larger multiceled conidia are called *macroconidia.*

conjugate A substance formed by combining two different molecules, specifically in immunologic assays, adding an enzyme or fluorochrome to an antibody or antigen.

conjugation The transfer of genetic material between bacteria through cell-to-cell contact.

conjunctivitis Inflammation of the conjunctiva.

consistency A degree of density, firmness, viscosity, and so on.

continuing education Educational resources that presents professional continuing education seminars and training.

continuous bacteremia Occurs when the organisms are coming from an intravascular source and are consistently present in the bloodstream.

continuous cell culture A culture capable of a virtually unlimited number of passages, sometimes referred to as an *immortal cell culture.*

convalescent phase In pertussis, the third and final phase, generally beginning within 4 weeks of onset of infection. There is a decrease in the frequency and severity of the coughing spells; complete recovery occurs in weeks to months.

creamy See **butyrous.**

creeping eruption The rash caused by the movement of hookworm larvae beneath the surface of the skin.

cross-functional teams Teams composed of members from different departments.

Curschmann's spirals Condensed bronchial secretions that take on the shape and size of bronchial passageways, particularly if there is constriction or obstruction.

cumulative antibiogram The report generated by analysis of individual susceptibility results on isolates from a particular institution in a defined period that represents the percentage of isolates of a given species susceptible to the antimicrobial agents commonly tested against the species.

customer concepts The view or perception each laboratory customer holds in regard to quality and their own expectations.

cycling probe technology A technique that amplifies signal after a DNA:RNA:DNA chimeric probe is incubated with target nucleic acid. The probe has a 5′ fluorophore and a 3′ quenching molecule; the result is no fluorescence until the probe anneals to target nucleic acid. RNase H digests the RNA in the probe after annealing has occurred, resulting in fluorophore release from the quencher. This then results in an increase in fluorescent signal. A new probe molecule will then anneal to the same target nucleic acid, and the process repeats for more fluorescence.

cyst The infective form of a protozoan; characterized by the formation of a thick protective wall that is resistant to environmental factors.

cysticercus The larval stage of *Taenia* spp. It is a fluid-filled sac that contains the scolex of the tapeworm.

cystine tellurite blood agar (CTBA) A selective and differential medium for the recovery of *Corynebacterium diphtheriae* and related organisms.

cystitis Inflammation of the urinary bladder.

cytocentrifugation A mechanical process in which centrifugal force is used in a machine to deposit cells on a glass slide for staining and viewing.

cytolytic toxins Exotoxins that can affect erythrocytes, leukocytes, macrophages, and platelets.

cytopathic effect Visible changes in cell cultures resulting from toxins or infection by a virus.

D

D-zone test Test used to detect inducible clindamycin resistance in staphylococci and β streptococci. An erythromycin disk is placed next to a clindamycin disk on a standard disk diffusion plate; flattening of the clindamycin zone between the two disks indicates inducible clindamycin resistance.

dacryoadenitis Infection of the lacrimal gland.

dacryocystitis Infection of the lacrimal sac.

darting motility A distinct type of rapid motility, characteristic of *Campylobacter* spp., observed under a wet preparation owing to their long polar flagellum.

data mining Computer-based search of data to indicate areas of potential concern for an Infection Control Practitioner (ICP); implies in-depth correlation of computer data.

deaminase Enzyme that removes amine groups (NH_2) from amino acids.

decarboxylase An enzyme capable of removing a carboxy group (CO_2) from an amino acid.

definitive host The individual in which a parasite has either its adult and or sexual reproductive stage.

denaturation Dissociation of double-stranded nucleic acid molecules into single strands. Denaturation is usually accomplished in molecular biology techniques with high heat (–95° C) so that primers or probes may then anneal to target nucleic acid sequences.

dendrogram A branching tree-like diagram frequently used to show the interrelationships between a group of organisms.

density The degree of opacity of a substance, medium, or similar that transmits light.

deoxynucleotide triphosphates (dNTPs) Individual nucleic acid bases used by enzymes such as DNA polymerase to synthesize new nucleic acid strands. Adenine (dATP), cytosine (dCTP), guanine (dGTP), and thymidine (dTTP) are used by DNA polymerase to synthesize new DNA strands.

dermatophyte Fungus able to use keratin and infect the skin, hair, and nails of humans; they belong to the genera *Epidermophyton*, *Microsporum*, and *Trichophyton*.

dermatophytosis An infection caused by a dermatophyte.

destruction See **sterilization.**

detection limit Analytical sensitivity is usually defined at the 0.95 confidence level (±2 standard deviations [SD]) and may be referred to as the *detection limit*. In microbiology the detection limit may be correlated to the number of colonies in the culture or to the lowest quantity of antigen or antibody a test can detect.

diapedesis The passage of inflammatory cells and other formed elements in the blood through the endothelial walls of the blood vessel.

differential media Media that allows grouping of microbes based on different characteristics demonstrated on the medium.

differential stains Stains such as the Gram stain that stain components of the smear differently so that each component can be recognized (i.e., gram positive, gram negative).

diffusely adherent *Escherichia coli* (DAEC) Enteropathogenic and uropathogenic *E. coli* strains defined by their attachment to HEp-2 cells.

dimorphic fungi Existing as either a yeast/spherule or mold, depending on growth conditions.

diphtheria Disease caused by *Corynebacterium diphtheriae*.

diphtheria toxin Potent toxin produced by *Corynebacterium diphtheriae* that causes tissue necrosis, exudate formation, and systemic effects involving the heart, kidneys, and nervous system.

diploid Finite cell lines containing two copies of each chromosome. Diploid is the normal genetic makeup for eukaryotic cells.

diploid cell culture Cells used for the growth of viruses that contain the normal number of chromosomes.

direct agglutination test An agglutination assay in which the antigen naturally occurs on a cell.

direct fluorescent antibody test An assay using a fluorochrome-labeled primary antibody to detect an antigen in a clinical specimen or culture isolate.

direct microscopic examination Examination of the specimen under the microscope, with or without staining.

direct sandwich immunoassay An assay in which an antigen is captured by an antibody affixed to a solid phase. A second labeled antibody is added that is able to bind to the antigen.

disinfectant A substance designed to be used on inanimate objects to kill or destroy disease-producing microorganisms, including spores in some cases.

disinfection Removal from an environment of microbes that may cause disease.

disseminated intravascular coagulation (DIC) A pathological activation of blood clotting mechanisms that occurs in response to a variety of diseases, which leads to the formation of small blood clots inside the blood vessels throughout the body.

dissemination Spread to other sites.

DNA microarray A technique used to assay the entire expression of genes in cells; it can also be used to identify organisms from samples, identify mutations, iden-

tify new genes, and for other purposes. Microscopic spots of DNA are placed on a solid support in an array, and unknown samples are fluorescently labeled and hybridized to the DNA on the array. A scanner is used to identify hybrids and to indicate positive samples or high levels of gene expression.

DNA polymerase An enzyme that synthesizes new strands of DNA. DNA polymerase uses dNTPs and primers to synthesize the new strands. The most common DNA polymerase in use in molecular diagnostics methods is *Taq* DNA polymerase, a thermostable enzyme that can withstand the denaturation temperatures used in the polymerase chain reaction and other methods.

DNA replication The copying of a double-stranded DNA strand in a cell, prior to cell division.

DNA transcription The process through which a DNA sequence is enzymatically copied by an RNA polymerase to produce a complementary RNA.

DNase An enzyme capable of hydrolyzing double-stranded DNA.

Donovan bodies The diagnosis of donovanosis can be confirmed by identifying characteristic intracellular "Donovan bodies" within Giemsa or Wright's stains of macrophages. Donovan bodies measure 0.5 to 0.7 by 1 to 1.5 mm in diameter and may or may not be capsulated. See also **granuloma inguinale.**

double indirect fluorescent antibody An assay in which antibody in a patient's serum binds to a known antigen. A second unlabeled anti-human antibody is added, and multiple molecules can bind to the patient's antibody. A third fluorochrome-labeled antibody directed against the second antibody is added.

dual-probe FRET A real-time polymerase chain reaction (PCR) detection method. Dual-probe FRET uses two probes, one with a donor fluorophore on the 3′ end and the other with an acceptor fluorophore on the 5′ end. The two probes anneal head-to-tail to accumulated PCR products. Light from the real-time PCR instrument excites the donor fluorescent dye, and this energy is transferred to the acceptor dye by FRET. The acceptor dye then gives off this energy, and it is read by the instrument. As PCR amplicon accumulates, fluorescence increases.

dysgonic fermenter (DF) Gram-negative fermentative bacillus that has difficulty growing on routine media. At one time, these were referred to by the Centers for Disease Control and Prevention as DF-1, DF-2, and DF-3; all have now been placed in the genus *Capnocytophaga*.

dysuria Difficulty in urination.

E

ecthyma gangrenosum A cutaneous infection most commonly associated with a *Pseudomonas aeruginosa* bacteremia.

ectoparasite Organisms that live on, rather than in, the human body and include fleas, lice, ticks, and mites.

edema factor (EF) One of three proteins that make up the anthrax toxin. Edema results from the combination of protective antigen with this factor.

efflux pumps Proteins located in the bacterial cell membrane that transport molecules out of the cell.

electroendosmosis The movement of buffer ions toward the cathode causing antibody molecules, which have a weak net negative charge, to be carried toward the cathode.

Elek test An immunodiffusion test originally described by Elek for detecting the toxin produced by *Corynebacterium diphtheriae*.

elementary body Metabolically inactive infectious form of *Chlamydia*.

elevation An elevated place, thing, or part; an eminence. The elevation should be determined by tilting the culture plate and looking at the side of the colony. Elevation may be raised, convex, flat, umbilicate (depressed center, concave, an "inny"), or umbonate (raised or bulging center, convex, an "outy").

El Tor A strain of *Vibrio cholerae* belonging to the serotype O1.

Embden-Meyerhof pathway An energy-yielding pathway converting one molecule of glucose to two molecules of pyruvate. Also called *Embden-Meyerhof-Parnas pathway*.

emergency response plan A plan established by each health care setting to deal with the potential of some emergency, such as a bioterror event.

emerging pathogens Pathogens that are newly recognized.

emerging zoonoses Infectious agents that fulfill the definition of zoonotic agents that are newly discovered agents, modified agents, or previously known agents that move to a new geographic location.

empirical antimicrobial therapy Institution of treatment based on practical experience in the absence of culture data.

employee right-to-know OSHA laboratory chemical hygiene plan and a hazard communication standard (29 CFR 1910.1200, Hazard Communication Standard [HCS]) that states that all clinical laboratory personnel have both a need and a right to know the hazards and identities of the chemicals they are exposed to when working. They also need to know what protective measures are available to prevent adverse effects from occurring.

empyema A collection of purulent fluid in the pleural space between the lung and the chest wall.

encapsulated Strains of bacteria and yeast that produce a capsule.

encephalitis Inflammation of the brain.

endemic relapsing fever Tick-borne relapsing fever caused by *Borrelia* spp.

endemic syphilis A nonvenereal spirochetal disease of the Middle East or Africa caused by *Treponema pallidum* subsp. *endemicum*. Clinical disease closely resembles yaws and is also known as *bejel*.

endogenous Originating from within an organism.

endogenous anaerobe An anaerobe that exists inside the bodies of animals (a member of the indigenous microflora).

endophthalmitis Inflammation of the intraocular fluids and tissues.

endotoxin Lipopolysaccharide (LPS) component of gram-negative cell walls is composed of lipid A + core polysaccharide + O antigen (O polysaccharide side chain) and is released upon lysis of the cell during infection. Lipid A component is responsible for endotoxin activity effects on the host; O side chain is the antigenic portion of the LPS molecule.

endotracheal Within the trachea.

engineering controls Controls that isolate or remove the hazard from the workplace.

enriched media Media that contain nutritional enhancement to allow growth of fastidious microbes.

enrichment broth Liquid medium designed to encourage the growth of small numbers of a particular organism while suppressing other flora present.

enteric fever A systemic bacterial infection characterized by diarrhea and prolonged fever and associated with *Salmonella* organisms.

enterics Members of the family Enterobacteriaceae consisting of organisms that all ferment glucose, nearly all fail to produce the cytochrome oxidase, and nearly all reduce nitrates to nitrites. Most are resident flora of the gastrointestinal tract.

enteritis necroticans *Clostridium perfringens* type C food poisoning.

enteroaggregative *Escherichia coli* (EAEC) Pathogenic *E. coli* strains defined by their attachment to HEp-2 cells; they cause persistent pediatric diarrhea.

enterohemorrhagic *Escherichia coli* (EHEC) Diarrheagenic *E. coli* strains producing Shiga toxins, also called *verotoxins*.

enteroinvasive *Escherichia coli* (EIEC) Diarrheagenic *E. coli* strains that invade the intestinal mucosa and cause dysentery similar to that caused by *Shigella* spp.

enteropathogenic *Escherichia coli* (EPEC) Diarrheagenic *E. coli* strains that cause severe infantile diarrhea.

enterotoxigenic *Escherichia coli* (ETEC) Diarrheagenic *E. coli* strains producing toxins similar to those produced by *Vibrio cholerae*.

enterotoxin The protein exotoxins secreted by either living or lysed bacteria that alter cell function or damage membranes of the gastrointestinal tract.

enterotoxin-mediated diarrhea Diarrheal illness that manifests primarily owing to the toxin produced by the infecting organism.

entomophthoromycosis Fungi of the order Entomophthorales (in the class Zygomycetes) present in organic debris can cause this chronic subcutaneous form of infection. It often occurs as the result of traumatic implantation of the organisms in the skin. Entomophthoromycosis is caused by *Conidiobolus coronatus, Conidiobolus incongruous,* and *Basidiobolus ranarum* (previously known as *Basidiobolus haptosporus*).

envelope See **enveloped virus**.

enveloped virus Virus surrounded by a phospholipid membrane.

environmental cultures Cultures taken of the environment, such as air, water, or surfaces.

Environmental Protection Agency (EPA) The EPA is the agency of the U.S. government that is responsible for regulating environmental pollution and environmental quality.

epidemic relapsing fever Louse-borne relapsing fever caused by *Borrelia* spp.

epidemiologic curve A graph plotted in an outbreak investigation so that the number of events (cases) can be compared with the time of their development.

epiglottitis A rapidly progressive infection of the epiglottis and adjacent structures usually caused by bacteria.

epitope A specific region of an antigen that binds to an antibody or T-cell receptor, also called an *antigenic determinant*.

Epstein-Barr virus (EBV) Also called *Human herpesvirus 4* (HHV-4), it can cause infectious mononucleosis. Epstein-Barr virus primarily infects B cells, where it forms a latent infection that persists for life.

erysipelas An acute spreading skin lesion that involves the subcutaneous tissues. The lesion is intensely erythematous with a plainly demarcated but irregular edge.

erysipeloid An infection in humans caused by *Erysipelothrix rhusiopathiae*.

erythema chronicum migrans Classic target-shaped or bull's-eye skin lesion normally found at the site of the tick bite during infections by *Borrelia burgdorferi*.

erythrasma A skin disease that can result in pink patches, which can turn into brown scales.

erythrocytic phase Part of the life cycle of malaria occurring within red blood cells.

eschar The dark area where necrosis occurs in the center of the necrotic lesion characteristically seen in patients with cutaneous anthrax.

***Escherichia/Citrobacter*-like organisms** Produce a dry, pink colony with a surrounding "halo" of pink, precipitated bile salts.

Etest A commercial minimal inhibitory concentration (MIC) test that uses plastic strips impregnated with a gradient of antimicrobial concentrations. The strips are placed on an agar plate that has been inoculated with the test bacteria and, following overnight incubation, the MIC is noted where the ellipse intersects the scale imprinted on the top of the strip.

etiologic agent The microorganism causing a disease.

eugonic fermenter (EF) Gram-negative bacillus or coccobacillus that ferments glucose or other carbohydrates and grows on routine media, as compared with the dysgonic fermenters, which do not grow on routine media. The designation *EF* means that it has yet to be placed into a specific genus.

eugonic oxidizer Gram-negative bacillus or coccobacillus that does not ferment glucose but can oxidize it; it grows on routine media but are not yet placed into a specific genus.

eukarya See **eukaryote.**

eukaryote An organism with complex cell (cells) structures in which the genetic material is organized into a membrane-bound nucleus (nuclei).

eumycotic mycetoma Mycetoma caused by fungal organisms, usually comprising wide septate hyphae.

exanthema A skin eruption or rash that may have specific diagnostics features of an infectious disease. Chickenpox, measles, roseola infantum, and rubella are usually characterized by a particular type of exanthem.

exfoliative toxin A toxin that affects the epidermal layers of the skin.

exoerythrocytic phase Part of the life cycle of malaria that begins when the sporozoites are injected into humans from the mosquito. The sporozoites first invade liver cells.

exogenous Originating outside of an organism, as opposed to an endogenous factor.

exogenous anaerobe An anaerobe that exists outside of the body.

exopolysaccharide A carbohydrate substance secreted by a number of microorganisms; it is used for attachment and is a major component of biofilms.

exotoxin A toxic protein produced by a bacterium and released into its environment. It may exert adverse effects quite remote from the site of infection.

expectorated sputum Material from the lower respiratory tract produced by a deep cough.

exposure control plan The OSHA Blood-borne Pathogen Standard safety requirement that the employer must have in place to protect the employee from blood-borne pathogens; must be annually reviewed and updated and available to all employees.

extended-spectrum β-lactamase (ESBLs) β-Lactamase produced by *Escherichia coli, Klebsiella* spp., *Proteus mirabilis,* and other Enterobacteriaceae that hydrolyze and render inactive penicillins, cephalosporins, and aztreonam.

F

facilitator A person with no vested interest in a problem whose role is to use problem-solving skills and experience to help team members resolve a problem.

facultative anaerobe A microorganism that does not require oxygen for growth but will use oxygen and grow better if it is present.

false-negative A negative test result in an individual with the disease in question.

false-positive A positive result in an individual without the disease in question.

family In biological classification, a rank or a taxon in the rank between an order and genus. Next to species and genus, it is the most important rank in taxonomy.

fast-acting A term used to describe an antimicrobial property that exhibits the most rapid action of antiseptics; usually the rapid action of antiseptic is expressed in seconds to minutes.

fastidious Hard to grow, requires additional growth factors.

fecal leukocytes White blood cells found in stool.

fermentation Process in which a molecule is oxidized to produce energy without an exogenous electron acceptor. Organic molecules usually serve as both electron donors and acceptors.

fermentative Bacteria that are able to utilize glucose or other carbohydrates in the absence of oxygen by using an organic molecule as a final electron acceptor.

filamentous Composed of or containing filaments.

filamentous hemagglutinin Virulence factor of certain *Bordetella* spp. believed to facilitate attachment of bacteria to ciliated epithelial cells.

filariform larva The larval stage infective for the definitive host.

filtration Filtration of liquids is accomplished through the use of thin membrane filters composed of plastic polymers or cellulose esters containing pores of a certain size. The liquid is pulled (vacuum) or pushed (pressure) through the filter matrix. Organisms larger than the size of the pores are retained.

fimbriae Nonflagellar, sticky, proteinaceous, hairlike appendages that adhere some bacterial cells to one another and to environmental surfaces; plural of *fimbria.*

Fitz-Hugh-Curtis syndrome Perihepatitis occurring as a complication of *Neisseria gonorrhoeae* infection, characterized by fever, upper quadrant pain, and tenderness and spasm of the abdomen.

flagella Exterior protein filaments that rotate and are used by microorganisms for motility.

fluorescein isothiocyanate Fluorescent molecule commonly bound to antibody and used in diagnostic tests.

fluorescence resonance energy transfer (FRET) Fluorescence resonance energy transfer (FRET) occurs between two dye molecules held in very close proximity to each other. One dye is a donor, the other an acceptor. Two dyes may be used in conjunction to generate fluorescence, as in dual-probe FRET, or a fluorescent dye and a quenching molecule may be used in conjunction to keep fluorescence low until the two molecules are separated from each other, as in the 5' nuclease assay.

fluorochrome A chemical used in fluorescent immunoassays that absorbs light of one wavelength and emits light of a different wavelength.

fluorogenic substrate A nonfluorescent molecule that becomes fluorescent when cleaved by a specific enzyme.

fluorophore A fluorescent dye molecule attached to probes used in molecular assays.

focused monitors A process created to monitor a suspected problem.

folliculitis An inflammation involving the hair follicles as a result of infection or irritation.

Food and Drug Administration (FDA) The FDA is a federal agency in the Department of Health and Human Services established to regulate the release of new foods, drugs, and health-related products.

form External appearance of a clearly defined area, as distinguished from color or material; configuration; shape; mold.

fungemia Fungal invasion of the bloodstream.

furuncles Also called *boils,* they are the result of staphylococcal infections that involve a hair follicle.

fusiform Spindle-shaped or tapered at each end.

G

β-galactosidase An enzyme capable of hydrolyzing lactose to glucose and galactose.

β-galactoside permease A bacterial membrane protein facilitating the uptake of β-galactosides.

gamete One of two cells, a male and a female, whose union is necessary in sexual reproduction.

gametocyte The sexual cell of Apicomplexa; the female (macrogametocyte) and male (microgametocyte) that develop into gametes.

gas gangrene A bacterial infection that produces gas within tissues and may lead to myonecrosis and sepsis. A medical emergency.

gelatinase A proteolytic enzyme that breaks down gelatin to amino acids.

genital herpes A viral infection in the genitals caused by herpes simplex virus.

genital ulcer disease (GUD) Group of sexually transmitted diseases causing ulcers on the genital area. Diseases include syphilis and genital herpes, among others.

genotype The genetic makeup of an organism.

genus A taxonomic grouping in classifying microorganisms. A genus may consist of one or more species.

germ theory The theory that all infectious diseases are caused by the activity of microorganisms.

germ tube Tube-like projection from a blastoconidium or spore without a constriction at its base.

glanders The disease caused by *Burkholderia mallei.*

glycolysis The sequence of reactions that converts glucose into pyruvate with the concomitant production of a relatively small amount of adenosine triphosphate. Glycolysis can be carried out anaerobically (in the absence of oxygen) and is thus an especially important pathway for organisms that can ferment sugars.

glycopeptide A class of antibiotic drugs that consists of glycosylated cyclic or polycyclic peptide. Examples include vancomycin and teicoplanin. This class of antibiotics inhibits the synthesis of cell walls in susceptible microbes by inhibiting peptidoglycan synthesis.

glycylcycline A class of antibiotic drugs derived from the tetracyclines. Similar to tetracyclines, this class of antibiotics binds to the 30S ribosomal subunit to prevent the aminoacyl tRNA from binding to the A site of the ribosome.

gonorrhea A sexually transmitted disease caused by the bacterium *Neisseria gonorrhoeae.*

gonorrheal ophthalmia neonatorum When caused by *Neisseria gonorrhoeae,* a form of conjunctivitis acquired by a newborn during birth when the baby's eyes are contaminated during passage through the birth canal when the mother is infected with *N. gonorrhoeae. Chlamydia trachomatis* can produce a similar infection.

gram-negative bacteria Bacteria that do not retain the crystal violet complex and are stained red by the safranin counterstain.

gram-negative intracellular diplococci (GNID) Gram-negative cocci in pairs found inside a phagocyte or polymorphonuclear cell.

gram-positive bacteria Bacteria that retain the crystal violet–iodine complex and appear blue-black on gram-stained smears.

Gram stain The method of staining microorganism using a violet stain, followed by an iodine solution; decolorizing with an alcohol or acetone solution; and counterstaining with safranin. The retention of either the violet color or the stain or the pink color of the counterstain serves as a primary means of identifying and classifying bacteria.

granulocytopenia An abnormally low concentration of granulocytes in the blood.

granuloma inguinale A genital ulcerative disease caused by the intracellular gram-negative bacterium *Klebsiella granulomatis* (formerly *Calymmatobacterium granulomatis*); also called *donovanosis.*

ground-glass appearance Colonial morphology resembling ground glass, characteristic of *Legionella* spp.

GRASE A term used to describe nonprescription drug products that are "generally recognized as safe and effective."

gummas Granulomatous lesions in skin, bones, and liver. Symptom of tertiary syphilis.

H

H antigen The flagellar antigen.

HACEK Specific species of the genera *Haemophilus, Aggregatibacter (Actinobacillus), Cardiobacterium, Eikenella,* and *Kingella* have been grouped together to form the acronym HACEK (first letter of each genus).

halophilic "Salt loving"; an organism that grows best in media with an increased concentration of NaCl.

hand hygiene Techniques used to ensure that hands are clean and microbe free. Hand hygiene involves washing with soap and water if the hands are soiled or using alcohol handrubs if the hands are not soiled.

health care antiseptic drug product An antiseptic-containing drug product applied topically to the skin to help prevent infection or help prevent cross contamination.

health care–associated infections Infections that are acquired within a health care setting.

health care personnel handwash An antiseptic-containing preparation designed for frequent use; it reduces the number of transient microorganisms on intact skin to an initial baseline level after adequate washing, rinsing, and drying; it is broad-spectrum, fast acting, and, if possible, persistent.

hemagglutinin A glycoprotein antigen on influenza viruses that facilitates attachment of the virus to susceptible host cells. The antigen gets its name from also being able to clump erythrocytes.

α-hemolysin A cytolytic toxin produced by *Staphylococcus aureus* that can damage erythrocytes, platelets, and macrophages.

β-hemolysin A cytolytic toxin, also known as *sphingomyelinase C,* that acts on the sphingomyelin membrane component of erythrocytes.

hemolysis "Lysis," dissolution or breaking apart; "hemo" pertains to red blood cells. A reaction, especially caused by enzymatic or toxin activity of bacteria, observed in the medium immediately surrounding or underneath the colony.

α-hemolysis A partial lysing of erythrocytes in a blood agar plate around and under the colony that results in a green discoloration of the medium.

β-hemolysis Complete clearing of erythrocytes in a blood agar plate around or under the colonies because of the complete lysis of red blood cells.

hemolytic-uremic syndrome A clinical syndrome characterized by the destruction of red blood cells; damage to the lining of blood vessel walls; and, in severe cases, kidney failure.

heterophile antibody An antibody produced in an individual in response to one antigen that can also bind to a different but similar antigen.

heteroploid Cells used for the growth of viruses that contain an abnormal and variable number of chromosomes that is not a multiple of the normal haploid number.

heteroresistant A population of cells in which some cells appear susceptible and others appear resistant.

heterotroph An organism that requires organic substrates as a source of carbon for growth and development.

hexacanth embryo (oncosphere) The first larval stage of most tapeworms; it is found within the egg and is characterized by the presence of six hooklets.

hidradenitis suppurativa A skin disease that affects areas that maintain apocrine sweat glands and hair follicles, such as the axillae, groin, and buttocks and under the breasts of women.

high-level aminoglycoside resistance In enterococci, indicates resistance to high concentrations of aminoglycosides (gentamicin or streptomycin) that usually result from production of aminoglycoside-modifying enzymes. Enterococci with high-level gentamicin resistance do not show synergism with ampicillin, penicillin, or vancomycin; streptomycin performs similarly.

hippurate hydrolysis A test used for the presumptive identification of group B streptococci *(Streptococcus agalactiae)*. The hippuricase enzyme found in group B streptococci hydrolyzes sodium hippurate to sodium benzoate and glycine.

Hodgkin disease A type of lymphoma characterized by swollen lymph nodes and the presence of large malignant cells called *Reed-Sternberg cells*, which are either multinucleated or bilobed nucleus (thus resembling an "owl's eye" appearance) with prominent eosinophilic inclusion-like nucleoli.

homogenization Preparation of tissue for microbiology culture by grinding to release microbes from cells and produce an even suspension.

hospital-associated MRSA (HA-MRSA) See **methicillin-resistant *Staphylococcus aureus* (MRSA).**

housekeeping gene Genes that code for basic functional proteins for cells. They are always turned on, so they are always expressed. They are good targets for internal controls from clinical specimens.

human blood bilayer Tween (HBT) agar The medium of choice for *Gardnerella vaginalis.*

human granulocytic anaplasmosis (HGA) An infectious disease caused by *Anaplasma phagocytophilum* (formerly known as *Ehrlichia phagocytophilum*). The symptoms closely resemble HME; fewer than 11% of infected individuals have a rash.

human granulocytic ehrlichiosis (HGE) An infection caused by *Anaplasma phagocytophilum.*

human immunodeficiency virus (HIV) A retrovirus that infects components of the human immune system, primarily CD4+T cells, macrophages, and dendritic cells.

human monocytic ehrlichiosis (HME) A disease caused by *Ehrlichia chaffeensis.*

humoral immune response A type of immune response that involves circulating antibodies.

hyaluronidase An enzyme, also referred to as *spreading factor,* that solubilizes the ground substance of mammalian connective tissues (hyaluronic acid).

hybrid capture A signal amplification method. An RNA probe is annealed to target DNA; then a capture antibody binds the DNA:RNA hybrid to a solid surface. A probe labeled with alkaline phosphatase (AP) then anneals to the hybrid, and the AP substrate is added to the system; cleavage of the substrate results in light emission detected by a luminometer.

hybridoma A cell formed from the fusion of a normal B cell to a myeloma cell, a cancerous plasma cell, such that the resulting cell is able to secrete antibodies and is immortal.

hydroxyl radical OH⁻. This is a short-lived molecule but is the most potent biological oxidant known.

hypha A long strand of fungal cells with or without cross walls; filaments that interweave to form mats called *mycelia* (plural: *hyphae*).

I

iatrogenic Pertains to an event caused by a medical intervention.

iatrogenic infection Conditions actually caused by medical interventions.

immune complex Antigen-antibody complexes.

immune response The resultant action of the immune system such as antibody production to an antigen; response of the immune system to an antigen.

immune system The organ system that protects an organism from outside biological influences.

immunocompetent Term used to describe the ability of an immune system to mobilize and deploy its antibodies and other responses to stimulation by an antigen.

immunocompromised Term used to describe an individual with deficient function of the immune system.

immunocompromised hosts See **immunocompromised.**

immunodiffusion Movement of antigens or antibodies through a matrix such as agarose.

immunogen Molecules capable of stimulating an immune response.

immunoglobulin A complex group of serum proteins that are produced by B cells in response to foreign antigens. In humans there are five isotypes: IgG, IgM, IgA, IgD, and IgE.

immunoglobulin A (IgA) The antibody defined by the α heavy chain. This is the immunoglobulin found in secretions and is associated with innate immunity.

immunoglobulin E (IgE) The antibody defined by the γ heavy chain. IgE is primarily attached to mast cells and serves as the antigen recognition for type I hypersensitivity reactions to allergens and immunity to parasites.

immunoglobulin G (IgG) The antibody defined by the γ heavy chain. This is the primary immunoglobulin found in human serum.

immunoglobulin M (IgM) The antibody defined by the μ heavy chain. Found in human serum as a pentamer, but monomers are embedded into mature B-cell membranes.

immunosenescence Naïve T cells are no longer available to be stimulated by antigens, which leads to the decline of the immune response over time.

immunosuppression The term used to describe the state of an immune system that is suppressed.

impetigo A localized skin disease that begins as small vesicles and progresses to weeping lesions.

incidence The number of new cases of a disease over a period of time (e.g., weeks, months, years).

index case The first case in an outbreak investigation.

indifference Occurs when the antimicrobial activity of a combination of antimicrobial agents is equal to the activity of the individual agents.

indigenous microflora Microorganisms of low virulence that are normally found in or on body sites. Synonymous with *normal flora.*

indirect agglutination An agglutination assay in which an antigen is artificially attached to a carrier particle, such as latex beads.

indirect fluorescent antibody test An immunoassay using a known antigen affixed to a microscope slide that binds antibody in patient's serum. A second fluorochrome-labeled anti-human antibody is then added.

indirect sandwich immunoassay An immunoassay using a known antigen affixed to a microscope slide that binds antibody in patient's serum. A second labeled anti-human antibody is then added.

indole test A bacteriologic test determining an organism's ability to form indole from tryptophan with the enzyme tryptophanase.

induced sputum Material from the lower respiratory tract collected following aerosol induction.

infection control practitioner (ICP) An individual within a health care setting whose responsibility it is to institute outbreak investigations, develop procedures to prevent the acquisition of infections, and implement infection control practices.

infection control risk assessment (ICRA) Review of a situation, such as new construction, to determine any infection control risks that may be present.

infection rate Calculations indicating the occurrence of infections within a given at-risk population, expressed as a percentage or as a rate per 1000 device days.

inflammation Physiologic reaction of vascularized tissue to injury involving physical symptoms of pain, redness, swelling, and tenderness due to accumulation of plasma and white blood cells.

inhalation anthrax The form of anthrax that results from inhaling anthrax spores. This is the most likely form of anthrax that would result from a release of anthrax spores into the air.

initial body in _Chlamydia_ species The chlamydial intracellular form that is larger, with a thinner cell wall, that divides by fission.

innate immune response See **innate immunity.**

innate immune system See **innate immunity.**

innate immunity Natural form of host protection; nonspecific and not stimulated by specific antigenic stimuli.

insertion sequence Mobile genetic elements known to encode only functions involved in insertion events.

in situ amplification (ISA) A technique that couples polymerase chain reaction amplification with in situ hybridization. The method is used to amplify DNA directly from tissue specimens, intact cells, or chromosomal material. It is used to increase the sensitivity and specificity of in situ hybridization reactions.

in situ hybridization A hybridization method wherein target DNA or RNA is detected directly in intact cells, tissue, or chromosomal material with a labeled probe.

integron A mobile DNA element that can capture and carry genes, especially those that carry antibiotic resistance.

interferon A class of mediators that increase the resistance of cells to viral infection by inhibiting viral replication and the growth of some euplastic cells.

interleukin (IL) A type of cytokine originally thought both to be produced by and to act upon leukocytes; however, it has since been discovered that other types of cells can elaborate some interleukins and that interleukins also have effects on cells other than leukocytes.

intermediate Interpretation of susceptibility test results that implies that the agent might be effective for infections located at body sites where the drugs are physiologically concentrated or when a high dosage of drug can be used. The intermediate category also includes a buffer zone, which should prevent small, uncontrolled technical factors from causing major discrepancies in interpretations.

intermediate host The individual in which a parasite has either its larval and or asexual reproductive stage.

intermittent bacteremia Occurs as the result of abscesses present at a particular site or as a clinical manifestation of certain types of infections.

intertrigo A yeast infection of skin folds caused by _Candida albicans_.

intervention The implementation of procedures to stop the spread of an infection or an outbreak.

intravascular device A device such as a catheter that is inserted into a blood vessel.

intrinsic resistance A type of antimicrobial resistance that is an inherent genotypic characteristic disseminated horizontally to progeny. Mechanisms that mediate intrinsic resistance to antibiotics include cell-wall impermeability, efflux, biofilm formation, and the expression of genes mediating inactivating enzymes.

isolation streak Technique to spread specimen inoculum over the surface of agar plates so that individual colonies can be obtained and a semiquantitative analysis can be performed.

J

Jarisch-Herxheimer reaction A systemic reaction of fever, chills, headache, myalgias, and exacerbation of cutaneous lesions believed to be caused by the rapid release of endotoxin from organisms shortly after initiation of antimicrobial therapy.

JEMBEC system (James E. Martin Biological Environmental Chamber) Commercial system for collection of specimens for _Neisseria gonorrhoeae;_ contains selective agar and a CO_2 generating tablet.

The Joint Commission (TJC) (formerly The Joint Commission on Accreditation of Healthcare Organizations [JCAHO]) A health care accrediting organization whose mission is to improve the safety and quality of care provided to the public.

K

K antigen Capsular surface antigen possessed by some strains of Enterobacteriaceae, particularly _Salmonella enterica_ serotype Typhi, where it is called the Vi antigen.

Kanagawa phenomenon A heat-stable hemolysin, produced by most strains of _Vibrio parahaemolyticus,_ able to lyse human red blood cells in a special high-salt mannitol medium (Wagatsuma agar). Production of β-hemolysis on this agar is called the _Kanagawa phenomenon._

karyosome The spherical chromatin mass within the nucleus of protozoa.

keratitis Inflammation of the surface or connective tissues of the cornea.

keratoconjunctivitis Inflammation of the ocular external surfaces (conjunctiva and cornea epithelia).

kinetoplast A structure found in some blood and tissue protozoans that is composed of the granule from which either

the flagellum or undulating membrane arises and a mitochondrion.

Kinyoun stain Procedure often used for acid-fast staining. Like the Ziehl-Neelson stain, Kinyoun stain is a carbolfuchsin method; however, it does not involve heat application.

Kirby-Bauer test A type of antimicrobial susceptibility test in which filter-paper disks impregnated with antimicrobial agents are placed on the surface of an agar plate that has been inoculated with the test bacteria. Following overnight incubation, zones of inhibition of growth are measured and results for each agent tested are interpreted as susceptible, intermediate, or resistant based on predefined Clinical and Laboratory Standards Institute criteria.

Klebsiella/Enterobacter-like organisms Produce large, mucoid, pink colonies that occasionally have cream-colored centers.

Kliger's iron agar A bacteriologic medium that aids in determining carbohydrate fermentation (glucose and lactose) and H_2S formation.

Koplik's spots White spots that appear on the mucous membranes of measles patients approximately 1 day before the appearance of the typical measles rash.

L

Laboratory Response Network (LRN) National program for detection and identification of biothreat agents.

β-lactam antibiotic An antibiotic that contains the β-lactam ring, the structure essential for the antibacterial activity of the antibiotic in this class.

β-lactamases Enzymes produced by bacteria that destroy the activity of β-lactam agents by hydrolyzing the β-lactam ring portion of the β-lactam molecule. There are many types of β-lactamases that affect specific β-lactam agents.

lactoferrin A multifunctional protein with antimicrobial activity that is part of the innate defense proteins mainly at mucoses. Found in mucosal secretions such as tears. This protein is present in secondary granules of polymorphonuclear neutrophils. Belongs to the transferrin family of proteins showing a high affinity by iron (ferric state).

lactose fermenters Easily detected by the color change they produce on media; as the pH changes when lactose is fermented, the organisms produce pink, dark pink, to red colonies. Colonies of nonfermenters remain clear and colorless.

Lancefield classification A classification of streptococci based on a surface antigen, the C carbohydrate.

latent phase In syphilis, the period in secondary syphilis when it passes into a silent period, which may last for many years. This phase permits the infection to evolve without any obvious external symptoms.

Legionnaires' disease Febrile disease with pneumonia caused by *Legionella* organisms.

leprosy An infection of the skin, mucous membranes, and peripheral nerves caused by *Mycobacterium leprae*.

leptospirosis A zoonotic disease in humans caused by *Leptospira interrogans*.

lethal factor One of three proteins that make up the anthrax toxin. The combination of lethal factor with protective antigen results in cell death.

leucine aminopeptidase A test used in the presumptive identification of the streptococci. Leucine aminopeptidase is a peptidase that hydrolyzes peptide bonds adjacent to a free amino group. It is called *LAP* because it reacts most quickly with leucine.

leukocidin Toxins secreted by certain bacterial species that are toxic to leukocytes. An example is Panton-Valentine leukocidin produced by *Staphylococcus aureus*.

L-forms Bacteria that have temporarily lost their cell wall as a result of environmental conditions.

Lister Joseph Lister (1827–1912) introduced the concept of aseptic surgery.

lobomycosis A chronic fungal infection of the skin caused by *Lacazia loboi* (previously known as *Loboa loboi*); mainly found in the tropics of South and Central America. The organisms are thought to reside in soil or vegetation and infect humans via skin trauma.

Loeffler medium (Loeffler agar) A nonselective medium containing serum; most often used for growing *Corynebacterium* spp.

Löwenstein-Jensen medium Egg-based, opaque, solid medium commonly used in clinical laboratories for growth of tubercle bacilli.

Lyme borreliosis Systemic, multistage illness, also known as *Lyme disease*, caused by *Borrelia burgdorferi* infection following a tick bite.

lymphocyte A type of white blood cell that develops not only in the bone marrow but also in other areas such as the thymus, spleen, and lymph nodes.

lymphogranuloma venereum A severe invasive sexually transmitted disease associated with specific serovars (L1, L2, L2a, and L3) of *Chlamydia trachomatis*.

lymphokines Chemical messengers produced by lymphocytes that carry messages between the cells of the immune system. Examples include interferon, which initiates defensive reactions to viruses, and the interleukins, which activate specific immune cells.

lysine iron agar A bacteriologic medium determining lysine metabolism and the ability to produce H_2S.

lysogeny Incorporation of the genetic material of a bacteriophage with that of the host bacterium.

lysozyme An enzyme that destroys bacterial cell walls by hydrolyzing the polysaccharide component of the cell wall. Lysozyme can be found in the mucosal membranes that line the human nasal cavity and tear ducts.

M

M protein An antigen found in the cell wall of *Streptococcus pyogenes*, not found in the other Lancefield group streptococci, that is important for virulence.

macroconidium The larger of two types of conidia produced by fungi, typically multicelled.

macrolide A class of antibiotic drugs, such as erythromycin, clarithromycin, and azithromycin, that target the 50S subunit specifically by binding to the peptidyl-transferase cavity in the proximity of the A and P loops, near adenine 2058 of 23S rRNA.

macroscopic observation Gross appearance or physical characteristics of the specimen.

major outer membrane protein A predominate protein present in the outer membrane of bacteria. These proteins often exhibit antigenic variation, allowing serogrouping of bacteria, such as with *Chlamydia trachomatis*.

malonate test A bacteriologic test determining an organism's ability to utilize malonate as a sole carbon source.

margin A border or edge.

material safety data sheets (MSDSs) Provided by the manufacturer or distributor for hazardous chemicals.

McFarland turbidity standards Suspensions of latex particles or barium sulfate prepared at various densities to represent specific numbers of bacteria. For example, the turbidity of a McFarland 0.5 standard is comparable to the turbidity of a bacterial suspension containing 1.5×10^8 colony-forming units per milliliter.

mecA The gene that codes for penicillin-binding protein 2a, which confers oxacillin resistance in staphylococci.

median infectious dose (ID50) The average amount or number of organisms that will cause an infection in 50% of those who acquire the organism.

mediastinitis The widening of the mediastinum. Although not specific for anthrax, it is a common radiologic finding in patients with inhalation anthrax.

medusa head Phrase used to describe the colonial appearance of *Bacillus anthracis*.

melioidosis The disease caused by *Burkholderia pseudomallei*.

melting curve analysis A real-time polymerase chain reaction (PCR) method used to determine whether nonspecific PCR products or primer-dimers have formed. The method is also used to determine the identity of a target. Fluorescence is observed in real-time PCR when a fluorophore is annealed to a PCR product. When the temperature of an assay is increased for melting curve analysis, the fluorophore will be released from the PCR product by denaturation. This causes a sudden decrease in fluorescence, which can be read as a peak—the temperature that a fluorophore is released from the target sequence.

melting temperature (T_m) The temperature at which a double-stranded nucleic acid molecule is 50% hybridized and 50% dissociated. A temperature below the T_m is often used for hybridization reactions, including the polymerase chain reaction.

meningismus The term used when nuchal rigidity, headache, and photophobia are present without the presence of inflammation or infection but are seen in concordance with other acute illness in children.

meningitis (leptomeningitis) An infectious disease characterized by the inflammation of the meninges.

meningococcemia The presence of meningococci (*Neisseria meningitidis*) in the bloodstream.

meningoencephalitis The presence of inflammation in the meninges and the brain.

merozoite Parasitic form produced during schizogony. In malaria, these structures are released from a ruptured erythrocyte and invade other erythrocytes at the end of an asexual reproductive cycle. Some merozoites differentiate into gametocytes.

mesophile An organism that grows best in moderate temperature, neither hot nor cold (25° to 40° C.)

metacercaria For most flukes this is the life-cycle stage infective for humans. It develops after the cercaria invades the tissue of the second intermediate host or contacts water vegetation, loses its tail, and develops a protective wall.

metagenomics The study (genomic analysis) of the genetic material of all microorganisms recovered directly from environmental samples using molecular techniques.

methicillin-resistant *Staphylococcus aureus* (MRSA) The term used to describe *S. aureus* spp. that contain *mecA* and PBP2a and are resistant to methicillin or any of the other β-lactamase–resistant penicillins such as oxacillin or nafcillin.

methicillin-resistant *Staphylococcus epidermidis* (MRSE) *S. epidermidis* isolates that are resistant to methicillin or β-lactamase resistant penicillins.

methyl red–Voges-Proskauer tests Bacteriologic test determining the end products of glucose fermentation: methyl red, mixed acids; Voges-Proskauer, stable neutral products.

microaerophile Microorganism that grows with reduced oxygen and increased carbon dioxide.

microaerophilic Microorganisms that require environments containing concentrations of oxygen lower than that present in the atmosphere (about 20%).

microbial load Total number of organisms present (bioburden).

microbial morphotypes Organisms have size, shape, and internal structure. Categories of microorganisms can be recognized by their form. Gram-positive cocci in pairs, tetrads, and grape-like clusters are a staphylococcal morphotype.

microbiota Microscopic organisms of a region (e.g., respiratory, urinary, GI) harbored by normal, healthy individuals.

microconidium The smaller of two types of conidia produced by fungi; they are usually single-celled and rarely two-celled.

Middlebrook 7H10 and 7H11 agars Serum albumin–based clear agar media used to support the growth of mycobacteria.

minimal bactericidal concentration (MBC) Lowest concentration of antimicrobial agent that kills 99.9% of the test bacteria.

minimal inhibitory concentration (MIC) Lowest concentration of antimicrobial agent that inhibits the growth of a bacterium.

minimal medium A laboratory growth medium whose contents are simple and completely defined; not usually used in the diagnostic microbiology laboratory.

Moeller decarboxylase base medium A classic bacteriologic medium used to detect decarboxylase activity.

moist heat Heat under steam pressure; the agent used in autoclaves.

molecular beacons A real-time polymerase chain reaction (PCR) detection technique. A molecular beacon probe is a hairpin loop structure with a fluorophore on the 5′ end and a quencher on the 3′ end. During the denaturation step of PCR, the molecular beacon probe dissociates, as does formed PCR product. The probe anneals to the PCR product, and when this occurs the fluorophore and the quencher are no longer in close proximity. Fluorescence thus increases as PCR product accumulates.

molluscum contagiosum A common skin disease caused by a poxvirus; characterized by small, firm, waxy papules, often with umbilicated centers; occasionally giant lesions may be seen.

monoclonal antibody An antibody solution with specificity to a single epitope.

monograph Developed for therapeutic classes of ingredients that are generally recognized as safe and effective. A manufacturer wanting to market a product containing an ingredient covered under the over-the-counter monograph need not seek the Food and Drug Administration's prior approval.

monomicrobial One microbe morphotype is present, and if it is the likely pathogen in an infection, the infection is monomicrobial.

morula An intracellular inclusion suggestive of infection with *Ehrlichia* spp.

motility-indole-ornithine medium A bacteriologic medium determining motility, the ability to form indole from tryptophan, and ornithine metabolism.

mold A fungus characterized by hyphae, also known as *filamentous fungi*.

mRNA translation Messenger RNA that encodes and carries information from DNA during transcription to sites of protein synthesis to undergo translation to yield a gene product. Translation is a step in the process of protein biosynthesis.

multilocus enzyme electrophoresis (MLEE) A nonamplified strain typing method. Proteins are isolated from the strain of interest and separated in a gel. A probe is then used to detect a specific protein. Differences in protein migration patterns are mutations, and different strains can be identified in this manner.

multilocus sequence typing (MLST) A strain typing method that uses polymerase chain reaction to amplify several different genetic loci. The resulting fragments are separated by electrophoresis and analyzed. The same strain will have the same pattern.

multilocus variable number of tandem repeat analysis (MLVA) A typing method that takes advantage of repetitive DNA sequences in genomes. MLVA amplifies regions of DNA that contain repeats. When there are different numbers of repeats at a given locus, it is referred to as *variable number of tandem repeats (VNTR)*. MLVA maps VNTRs among bacterial strains by using polymerase chain reaction.

multiplex PCR A polymerase chain reaction (PCR) method that utilizes two primer sets in the same tube. Each primer set is specific for a different target.

mycelia Intertwined hyphae that form a mat on the surface of a fungal colony.

mycetoma Localized subcutaneous abscesses caused by *Nocardia* spp. and other aerobic actinomycetes.

***Mycobacterium tuberculosis* complex** Organisms that cause the disease known as *tuberculosis*. Five closely related organisms are grouped together to form the *Mycobacterium tuberculosis* complex: *M. tuberculosis, M. bovis, M. africanum, M. canettii,* and *M. microti.*

mycolic acids Complex branched-chain fatty acids with large numbers of carbon atoms that are components of the *Mycobacterium tuberculosis* cell wall.

mycosis A disease caused by fungi.

myonecrosis Necrosis of the muscle. Synonymous with *gas gangrene.*

N

nanobiotechnology (nanotechnology) The use of nanotechnology (sometimes called *nanobiotechnology* when used for biological purposes) in molecular diagnostics is also called *nanomolecular diagnostics*. Although there are different definitions of *nanotechnology*, it is useful to consider it as a technology that uses atomic and/or molecular properties to build structures starting at the molecular level, at the nanometer scale (a nanometer is a billionth of a meter).

narrow spectrum In antimicrobial activity, a limited range of activity of an antibiotic.

National Fire Protection Association (NFPA) hazard-rating diamond The National Fire Protection Association (NFPA 704) system uses a diamond-shaped diagram of symbols and numbers to indicate the degree of hazard associated with a particular chemical or material. These diamond- shaped symbols are placed on containers of chemicals or materials to identify the degree of hazard associated with the chemical or material.

National Nosocomial Infection Surveillance System A federal agency whose goal is to monitor the incidence of health care–associated (nosocomial) infections and their associated risk factors and pathogens at the national level, correlating data from multiple health care settings across the United States.

necrotizing fasciitis A rapidly progressing and frequently life-threatening soft tissue infection that is a subtype of infectious gangrene typically due to Enterobacteriaceae and anaerobes.

negative predictive value (NPV) See **predictive value.**

nested polymerase chain reaction (nested PCR) A sensitive PCR technique that uses two PCR assays. The first assay produces PCR amplicon that is then used as template in the second PCR assay.

neutropenia An abnormally reduced concentration or number of neutrophils in the bloodstream.

new drug application (NDA) An NDA requires that the drugs be proven safe and effective for human use before being marketed.

nitrate reduction test A bacteriologic test determining an organism's ability to form nitrite or nitrogen gas by reducing nitrate.

***o*-nitrophenyl-β-D-galactopyranoside (ONPG)** A chromogenic substrate that is initially colorless but is cleaved by β-galactosidase, producing the yellow compound *o*-nitrophenyl.

nodular lymphangitis An entity characterized by inflammatory nodules that occur along lymphatic vessels that drain an area of primary skin infection (also called *lymphocutaneous syndrome*).

nonchromogenic *Mycobacterium* spp., such as *M. tuberculosis,* that do not produce pigmentation.

nonencapsulated Strains of bacteria and yeast that do not produce a capsule.

nonfermentative Bacteria that are unable to utilize glucose or other carbohydrates in the absence of oxygen. Oxidative bacteria in this group require molecular oxygen as final electron acceptor as a result of oxidative carbohydrate metabolism.

nongonococcal urethritis (NGU) An infectious condition of the urethra in males that is not caused by gonorrheal infection.

nonlactose fermenter See **lactose fermenters.**

nonoxidizers Bacteria that neither oxidize nor ferment glucose or other carbohydrates. They derive their energy from carbon compounds other than carbohydrates.

nonphotochromogenic The characteristic appearance of some *Mycobacterium* spp. in which exposure to light does not stimulate pigment production.

nonporous surface A smooth, unpainted solid surface that limits penetration of liquid.

nonselective media Media that support the growth of most nonfastidious aerobes.

nonsusceptible This reporting category is used when there are no "Intermediate" or "Resistant" interpretive criteria, only a "Susceptible" interpretive criterion, and the MIC or disk diffusion zone size for classifying the organism as susceptible is not achieved.

nontreponemal (nonspecific) antibody tests A series of tests for syphilis that detect antibodies to nontreponemal antigens. Generally these tests are used to screen for disease and confirmed using treponemal antibody tests.

nontuberculosis mycobacteria (NTM) Mycobacteria not associated with tuberculosis; some are nonpathogenic, whereas others have been commonly implicated as opportunistic pathogens; they are ubiquitous in the environment.

normal biota Microbes normally present in an organ or region of the body; may act to help fight infection.

normal microbial flora Organisms that exist in a symbiotic relationship with the host. These organisms are isolated from the host in the absence of disease.

Northern blot A procedure that detects RNA with a specific, labeled probe. The RNA is separated by electrophoresis and then transferred to a solid membrane. The probe is labeled and detected by a variety of methods.

nosocomial Of or being a secondary disorder associated with being treated in a hospital but unrelated to the patient's primary condition.

nosocomial bacteremia Occurs in patients who are hospitalized or living in a nursing home or other facility.

nosocomial infection An infection acquired within 72 hours of a stay in a health care facility.

novobiocin susceptibility Test useful in differentiating novobiocin-resistant *Staphylococcus saprophyticus* from other coagulase-negative staphylococci.

nucleic acid hybridization The ability of two nucleic acid species to anneal, or bind, to each other and form a hybrid, or duplex. Nucleic acid molecules hybridize when they are complementary to each other.

nucleic acid sequence–based amplification (NASBA) An amplification assay that occurs at one temperature that produces transcript from target nucleic acid. This method uses a pair of primers and reverse transcriptase, RNase H, and T7 RNA polymerase to synthesize many transcript copies from each target nucleic acid sequence.

nucleocapsid The genome of a virus enclosed in a protein coat (the capsid).

numeric codes A number generated by a series of biochemical tests in a commercial identification kit that can be compared with numbers in a database to determine the identification of an organism.

nutrient media Culture media that are complex and made of extracts of meat or soybeans.

O

O antigen Heat-stable somatic cell antigens of the Enterobacteriaceae, notably identified in *Escherichia coli* and *Salmonella* spp.

obligate aerobe A microorganism that requires oxygen for growth.

obligate anaerobe A microorganism that can live and reproduce only in a strict anaerobic environment (0% oxygen).

obligate intracellular parasite Microorganism or virus unable to live independently outside a living cell.

occult (unsuspected) bacteremia Bacteremia not associated with any physical signs or symptoms of severe infection.

O/F basal medium A bacteriologic medium used in determining the ability of bacteria to use carbohydrates oxidatively or fermentatively.

Ohara disease Another name for *tularemia,* which is caused by *Francisella tularensis.*

oligonucleotide A small nucleic acid molecule that is used either as a primer or a probe in molecular diagnostic techniques. Oligonucleotides are synthetic, single-stranded nucleic acids that are complementary to target sequences.

onychomycosis Infections caused by fungi involving the nails.

opaque Not transparent or translucent; impenetrable to light; not allowing light to pass through.

ophthalmia neonatorum Severe eye infection in infants caused by *Neisseria gonorrhoeae,* acquired during natural delivery.

opportunist Microorganisms that usually do not produce disease but are capable of causing disease in an individual whose immune system is compromised.

opportunistic infection Disease caused by a microorganism with low virulence that becomes pathogenic in a host with low immunologic resistance.

opportunistic pathogen See **opportunist.**

opsonin Complement fragment that enhances phagocytosis.

opsonization The process by which microorganisms are changed so that they are more easily and readily engulfed by phagocytes and macrophages.

optochin test A test that determines an organism's susceptibility to optochin (ethylhydrocupreine); it is used to differentiate *Streptococcus pneumoniae* (sensitive) from other α-hemolytic streptococci (resistant).

orbital cellulitis Infections of the orbital tissues.

orf A contagious viral skin disease acquired from infected sheep and goats, characterized by painless vesicles that may progress to red, weeping nodules and finally to crusting and healing; caused by parapox virus (parapoxvirus ovis).

organ culture The maintenance or growth of organ fragments.

orthostatic changes Changes that occur while in an erect posture or position.

ORYX A Joint Commission initiative requiring health care organizations to submit performance measurements to be analyzed and compared with similar institutions.

osteomyelitis A chronic or acute infection of the bone or the bone structures as a result of an infective process.

over-the-counter (OTC) drugs Nonprescription drugs that are considered to be safe and effective for consumers to use without professional supervision, provided the required label directions and warnings are followed.

otitis media Disease that results from infection of the middle ear and characterized by the presence of middle ear inflammation and fluid.

outbreak The occurrence of events, such as infections, that exceeds the normal and expected numbers.

outbreak investigation The epidemiologic investigation of an outbreak.

outcome monitors Measurements of the result of a process.

oxacillin screen plate Agar plate containing 6 µg/mL of oxacillin and 4% NaCl that is used for detecting oxacillin-resistant *Staphylococcus aureus.*

oxazolidinone A class of azoles with the carbon between the nitrogen and oxygen oxidized to a ketone.

oxidase test A bacteriologic test determining the presence of the intracellular enzyme oxidase, which is part of the electron transport system.

oxidation A chemical process whereby electrons are donated. In bacteria, oxygen is frequently used as the terminal electron acceptor during glucose oxidation; however, other inorganic molecules can also be used.

oxidizers Bacteria that require molecular oxygen as final electron acceptor; glucose or carbohydrates are metabolized only in the presence of oxygen.

P

Panton-Valentine leukocidin (PVL) A staphylococcal cytolytic toxin that can act on polymorphonuclear leukocytes.

paradoxic (eagle) effect As related to minimal bactericidal concentration testing, decreased bactericidal activity of an antimicrobial agent at higher concentrations of antimicrobial agent as demonstrated by more colonies growing on subcultures at higher concentrations than at lower concentrations.

paraffin bait technique Technique used to recover *Nocardia* spp. and aerobic actinomycetes from contaminated samples. It is based on the principle that these organisms can utilize simple carbon sources for nutrition.

parasite An organism that lives in or on and takes its nourishment from another organism. A parasite cannot live independently. Parasitic diseases include infections by protozoa, helminths, and arthropods.

parasitism The relationship between species (host and organism) wherein one of the species (parasite) benefits at the expense of the other (host).

paronychia An inflammation of the folds of the skin bordering the nail beds.

paroxysmal phase The second phase of pertussis characterized by the sudden attack of severe, repetitive coughing followed by a "whoop" as the individual gasps for air, sometimes followed by vomiting.

pasteurization Method of disinfection used mostly in the food industry; eliminates food-borne pathogens as well as organisms responsible for food spoilage. It is carried out at 63° C for 30 minutes. The main advantage of pasteurization is that treatment at this temperature reduces spoilage of food without affecting its taste.

pathogen A microorganism that causes disease.

pathogenic bacteria See **pathogenic microorganisms.**

pathogenic microorganisms Organisms capable of causing disease.

pathogenicity The ability of a microorganism to cause disease.

patient preoperative skin preparation A fast-acting, broad-spectrum, and persistent antiseptic-containing preparation that significantly reduces the number of microorganisms on intact skin.

pelvic inflammatory disease (PID) An acute or recurring acute infection of the oviducts and ovaries with surrounding tissue involvement. It includes inflammation of the cervix (cervicitis), uterus (endometritis), fallopian tubes (salpingitis), and ovaries, which can spread to adjacent connective tissue. The most common causes are *Chlamydia trachomatis* and *Neisseria gonorrhoeae.*

penicillin-binding proteins (PBP) Transpeptidase enzymes important in bacterial cell-wall formation. These proteins have various affinities to the β-lactam antimicrobials and play an important role in resistance to these agents when altered.

penicillinase-producing *Neisseria gonorrhoeae* (PPNG) Type of penicillin resistance in *N. gonorrhoeae* that is due to genes located on the plasmids that code for penicillinase (a type of β-lactamase) production.

penicillinase-resistant penicillins Group of agents resistant to hydrolysis by staphylococcal β-lactamase, including oxacillin, methicillin, nafcillin, cloxacillin, and dicloxacillin.

performance improvement Continuous analysis of processes or procedures and continual implementation of improvements.

perinatal Organisms that transmitted during labor and delivery of a baby.

peripheral chromatin DNA present on the nuclear membrane of some protozoa.

periplasmic flagella Fibrils around which the spirochete flexible cell wall is wound; also known as the *axial fibrils, axial filaments, endoflagella,* and *periplasmic fibrils.* Responsible for motility.

persistent Prolonged or extended antimicrobial activity that prevents or inhibits the proliferation or survival of microorganisms after product application.

persisters As related to minimal bactericidal concentration testing, the growth of small numbers (but greater than 0.1% of the test inoculum) of colonies from several concentrations of antimicrobial agent above the minimal inhibitory concentration.

persistor cell A microbial cell that is alive but weakly metabolic; it has the potential to return to an actively growing state.

personal protective equipment Specialized clothing or equipment that is worn by an employee for protection.

pertussis An acute infectious inflammation of the airways characterized by recurrent bouts of spasmodic coughing, followed by a noisy inspiratory stridor or "whoop." The infection is caused by *Bordetella pertussis* or *Bordetella parapertussis.*

pertussis toxin A protein exotoxin of *Bordetella pertussis* that produces a wide variety of responses in vivo. The main activity of pertussis toxin is modification of host proteins by ADP-ribosyltransferase, which interferes with signal transduction.

petechiae Red spots or discoloration on the skin caused by minor bleeding underneath the skin. See also **purpura.**

phaeohyphomycosis A term used to define infections caused by fungi that produce dark cell walls.

phagocyte A mobile or fixed cell in a multicellular organism that is able to ingest debris. Phagocytes are present as "housekeepers" in all multicellular organisms. Neutrophils, macrophages, and histiocytes are the major human phagocytes.

phagocytosis The process of engulfing or ingesting and digesting foreign particles.

pharyngitis An upper respiratory tract infection affecting the pharynx that may be caused by a virus or bacterium; acute bacterial pharyngitis is often caused by *Streptococcus pyogenes* and is characterized by sore throat, malaise, fever, and headache.

phenotype Observable or measurable characteristics of an organism.

pheromone Extracellular molecules passed between bacteria, allowing communication. When pheromones bind to specific receptors on bacteria, gene expression is altered.

photochromogenic The characteristic appearance of *Mycobacterium* spp. in which exposure to light stimulates pigment production.

photochromogens *Mycobacterium* spp. that produce carotene pigment upon exposure to light.

phyla (phylum) In biological classification, a subset or category.

pigment A coloring matter or substance.

pili Nonmotile, long, hollow, protein tubes that connect two bacterial cells and mediate DNA exchange; also known as *conjugation pili*.

pinta A nonvenereal skin disease caused by *Treponema carateum* found in the tropical regions of Central America and South America.

planktonic Free-floating microorganisms.

plasmid Extrachromosomal, circular pieces of DNA found in many strains of bacteria. Plasmids often carry virulence genes and antibiotic resistance genes.

plasmid profile analysis A nonamplified typing method that analyzes the plasmid DNA profile from bacterial isolates.

pleocytosis The presence of white blood cells in cerebrospinal fluid.

pleomorphic Demonstrating a variety of shapes and forms; for a Gram stain, neither distinctly coccoid nor rod shaped. Also used to describe the Gram-stain morphology of bacteria that exhibit a combination of cocci, bacilli, coccobacilli, and filamentous forms in a single stained smear.

pleuropneumonia-like organism (PPLO) The first mycoplasmata were isolated from cows with pleuropneumonia. Subsequently, when the first human mycoplasma was isolated, it was referred to as *pleuropneumonia-like organism.*

pneumonia A disease characterized by inflammation of the lungs, typically associated with fever, respiratory symptoms, and the presence of parenchymal involvement detected either by physical examination or by the presence of infiltrates on chest radiography.

pneumonic plague *Yersinia pestis* infection involving either primary or secondary infection of the lungs.

pneumonic tularemia Pneumonia resulting from inhaling *Francisella tularensis*. This is the form that would most likely occur as a result of a bioterror release of this agent, although inhalation tularemia can occur naturally.

polyclonal A mixture of antibodies recognizing different antigens and epitopes with different binding affinities.

polyclonal antibody A mixture of antibodies able to bind the same antigen but recognize different epitopes.

polymerase chain reaction (PCR) A popular molecular method that produces an exponential amount of product from a target nucleic acid sequence. PCR consists of denaturation, primer annealing, and primer extension, and it uses several components, including DNA polymerase, primers, target nucleic acid, a buffer, deoxynucleotides, and a thermal cycler.

polymicrobial Two or more microbial morphotypes are present and, if they are likely pathogens in an infection, the infection is polymicrobic.

polymicrobial bacteremia Bacteremia that involves more than one microbial organism.

polymorphic fungi A fungus that has both yeast and mold states present when cultured under the same growth conditions.

polyvinyl alcohol (PVA) A plastic resin often used in stool fixatives to adhere fecal material to a slide before staining.

Pontiac fever Mild febrile disease without pulmonary symptoms caused by *Legionella* organisms.

population analysis profiles (PAP) Detection method done by plating increasing numbers of organisms on plates containing various concentrations of vancomycin and then dividing the number by the area under the curve.

porin Transmembrane structures made up of proteins large enough to facilitate passive diffusion.

porphyrin An intermediate formed during the biosynthesis of hemin.

positive predictive value (PPV) See **predictive value.**

postanalytical activity Processes that occur after the sample has been analyzed, such as result review, transcription, or the reporting of results.

postsplenectomy After removal of the spleen.

postzone A phenomenon resulting from an antibody solution that is too dilute to demonstrate agglutination or precipitation; also referred to as *antigen excess.*

Pott disease Name given to tuberculosis of the spine.

preanalytical activity Processes that occur before the sample being analyzed, such as patient identification and sample ordering.

precipitation An immunologic reaction between soluble antigens and antibodies forming a visible macromolecular complex that falls out of solution.

precision The measure of exactness of a test.

predictive value The probability that a positive result (positive predictive value [PPV]) accurately indicates the presence of an analyte or a specific disease or that a negative result (negative predictive value [NPV]) accurately indicates the absence of an analyte or a specific disease. Predictive values vary significantly with the prevalence of the disease or analyte unless the test is 100% sensitive (for NPV) or specific (for PPV).

preseptal cellulitis Inflammation of the periorbital tissues.

prevalence of disease The frequency of a disease at a designated single point in time in the population being studied.

preventive maintenance Procedures performed on equipment designed to keep the equipment operating at optimal performance and to extend its lifetime.

primary amebic meningoencephalitis An infection caused by a free-living ameba called *Naegleria fowleri*.

primary atypical pneumonia A pneumonia that differs from the typical pneumonia caused by *Streptococcus pneumoniae*. Primary atypical pneumonia is most often caused by *Mycoplasma pneumoniae*.

primary bacteremia Bacteremia that arises from an endovascular source such as an infected cardiac valve or an infected intravenous catheter.

primary cell culture A culture started from cells, tissues, or organs taken directly from organisms.

primary syphilis The first stage of syphilis that is marked by the development of a chancre and spread of the causative spirochete in the tissues of the body.

primer annealing The second step of polymerase chain reaction, in which primers anneal to denatured target nucleic acid strands. This hybridization reaction usually occurs at a temperature of 5° C lower than the melting temperature (T_m) of the primers.

primer extension The third step of polymerase chain reaction. Once primers have annealed to template nucleic acid, DNA polymerase uses free deoxynucleotides and synthesizes new strands of DNA from the primers.

primer-dimers Primers that anneal to each other and form hybrids during polymerase chain reaction or other amplification procedures.

primers Small, single-stranded oligonucleotides used in polymerase chain reaction and other molecular diagnostics methods. Primers anneal to target sequences, and DNA polymerase starts synthesis of new DNA strands from the primers.

prion A protein particle similar to a virus but lacking the nucleic acid. These agents are known to cause degenerative diseases of the nervous system, such as Creutzfeldt-Jakob disease in humans.

probe An oligonucleotide with an attached label for detection. The label can be either a radionucleotide or a chemical. Probes anneal to target sequences in many molecular diagnostic reactions.

probe-mediated stains Antibody- or nucleotide-mediated identity reactions made visible by relatively simple chemical stains.

process monitors Ongoing data collection that can be used to establish trends or to spot problems when trends are disrupted.

proficiency testing The testing of carefully designed "unknown" samples used to evaluate analytical processes.

proglottid One segment of a tapeworm. Each proglottid contains both male and female reproductive organs.

prokaryote Microorganisms that lack a true nucleus and nuclear membrane.

prostatitis Inflammation in the prostate.

protective antigen One of three proteins that make up the anthrax toxin. Protective antigen is necessary for edema factor and lethal factor to bind to and penetrate host cells.

protein A A cellular component of *Staphylococcus aureus* that can bind immunoglobulin and prevent phagocytosis.

protein expression Also called *gene expression*. The process by which a gene's DNA sequence is converted into the structures and functions of a cell.

proteomics A large-scale analysis of protein expression, often at the cellular level. The method is often used to analyze proteins expressed in various disease states.

prozone A phenomenon resulting from a high concentration of antibody preventing agglutination or precipitation; also referred to as *antibody excess*.

pseudobacteremia When bacteria are recovered from blood cultures that might be caused by contamination of blood samples during phlebotomy, leading to false-positive results.

pseudogerm tube Tube-like projection from a blastoconidium or spore with a constriction at its base.

pseudohypha Chain of elongated fungal cells with constrictions at points of attachment resembling true hyphae.

pseudomembranous colitis A disease characterized by damage to the lining of the colon; most often caused by *Clostridium difficile*.

pseudomonad A gram-negative, nonfermentative, oxidase-positive bacillus, possessing polar flagella, found in most aquatic environments and not usually part of the human normal flora.

psychrophiles Bacteria that grow best at cold temperatures (optimal growth at 10° to 20° C).

public health A health care setting that provides services to the public.

pulsed field gel electrophoresis (PFGE) A commonly used strain typing method. A restriction enzyme is used to digest chromosomal DNA, and the resulting fragments are separated in an agarose gel in a pulsed electrical field. Strains show unique banding patterns.

purified protein derivative (PPD) A diagnostic skin test for tuberculosis.

purpura A purplish discoloration that appears under the skin and is caused by bleeding underneath the skin. Small spots are called *petechiae,* and large areas are referred to as *ecchymoses.*

purpura fulminans A skin manifestation of disseminated intravascular coagulation (DIC) classically associated with meningococcemia, but bloodstream infections with *Staphylococcus aureus, Streptococcus pneumoniae,* and *Haemophilus influenzae* have also been associated. It is characterized by rapidly developing skin hemorrhage and necrosis and peripheral gangrene accompanied by shock syndrome.

purulence Sample component consisting of neutrophils, protein, and necrotic debris. Purulence is seen grossly as "pus."

pyelonephritis Infection that involves the kidneys.

pyocyanin A water-soluble blue pigment, characteristic of *Pseudomonas aeruginosa.* When combined with the fluorescein pigment of *P. aeruginosa,* it forms blue-green colonies on a variety of solid media.

pyoderma A skin infection characterized by the appearance of necrosis in tissues.

pyogenic streptococci See ***Streptococcus pyogenes.***

pyoverdin Fluorescein pigment of members of the *Pseudomonas* fluorescent group. Fluorescein can be seen with ultraviolet light. When combined with the pyocyanin (blue) pigment of *P. aeruginosa,* a blue-green colony results.

pyrosequencing A sequencing-by-synthesis technique that does not require labeled nucleotides or primers and also does not require a postreaction electrophoresis step. It is a rapid sequencing technique that generates approximately 20 to 50 base sequences per primer; thus this technique is best used for short sequences. Pyrosequencing utilizes the enzymes DNA polymerase, ATP sulfurylase, luciferase, and apyrase, and the substrates adenosine 5′-phosphosulfate (APS) and luciferin.

pyrrolidonyl-α-naphthylamide (PYR) hydrolysis A test used for the presumptive identification of group A streptococci and enterococci. The substrate is hydrolyzed to β-naphthylamine.

pyuria The presence of white blood cells (leukocytes) in the urine. More than 8 to 10 leukocytes/mm³ indicates significant pyuria.

Q

Q fever See **query fever.**

Q-probes An external peer comparison program sponsored by the College of American Pathologists that addresses process, outcome, and structure-oriented quality assurance issues.

QRNG Fluoroquine-resistant *Neisseria gonorrhoeae.*

quality control (QC) A system for detecting and correcting analytical errors by establishing performance limits and ensuring the maintenance of proper standards, especially by periodic random inspection of the product.

quantitative isolation Technique in which a measured amount of specimen is inoculated to an agar plate to determine the quantity of microbes in the specimen.

query fever The original name of Q fever, which is caused by *Coxiella burnetii.*

quinolone A class of broad-spectrum antibiotics that act by inhibiting the bacterial enzyme DNA gyrase or topoisomerase IV enzyme, thereby inhibiting DNA replication and killing the organism.

quorum sensing A process whereby bacteria communicate by means of extracellular molecules called *pheromones.*

R

radioimmunoassay (RIA) An immunoassay that uses radioactive isotopes to detect antigen-antibody complexes in vitro.

random amplified polymorphic DNA (RAPD) An amplified strain-typing procedure that uses primers with random sequences that anneal to random chromosomal DNA sequences of the strain of interest. Polymerase chain reaction is used to amplify DNA, and strains have unique patterns of fragments.

rapid plasma reagin (RPR) test A nontreponemal serologic test for syphilis.

RASE A term used to describe prescription drug products that are recognized as safe and effective.

reagin antibody Antibody produced during *Treponema pallidum* infection against nontreponemal antigens. Immunoglobulin E antibodies cause a type 1 hypersensitivity reaction; also referred to as *reagin.*

real-time PCR A commonly used detection method for polymerase chain reaction (PCR) amplicons. A probe or fluorescent dye is used for detection. The real-time PCR platform analyzes the accumulation of fluorescence after every PCR cycle so that the results can be observed on a computer screen in "real time." Thus PCR and detection are coupled from the same tube.

reemerging pathogens Microbial pathogens, once thought to be eliminated or greatly reduced in numbers, that are once again seen or potentially seen.

Regan-Lowe transport medium Recommended transport medium for suspected *Bordetella pertussis* when overnight or several-day transport is required; contains charcoal (half-strength from charcoal horse blood agar isolation media), 10% horse blood, and 40 mg/L cephalexin.

Reiter's syndrome Causes urethritis, conjunctivitis, polyarthritis, and mucocutaneous lesions; in adults it is believed to be caused by *Chlamydia trachomatis*.

repetitive palindromic extragenic elements polymerase chain reaction (Rep-PCR) A form of strain typing using primers that are complementary for repetitive palindromic sequences that occur throughout chromosomes. PCR is used to amplify DNA between the palindromic sequences. Strains have unique fragment patterns.

resident microbial flora Microorganisms usually found at a particular body site of healthy individuals and that remain at the site for long periods or indefinitely.

resistant In therapeutic terms, resistant strains are not inhibited by the usually systemic concentrations of the antimicrobial agent with normal dosage schedules or fall in the range where specific microbial resistance mechanisms are likely and clinical efficacy has not been reliable in treatment studies.

respiration The efficient energy-generating process in which molecular oxygen is the final electron acceptor; also called *oxidation*.

respiratory burst The release of reactive oxygen species (superoxide radical and hydrogen peroxide) from different types of cells. Usually it denotes the release of these chemicals from immune cells (e.g., neutrophils, macrophages) as they come into contact with different bacteria or fungi.

restriction enzyme An enzyme that cuts DNA at specific sequences. Many unique restriction enzymes are commercially available. They are used in various molecular techniques, such as Southern blotting. Restriction enzymes are also called *restriction endonucleases*.

reticulate body Metabolically active non-infectious form of *Chlamydia*.

retinitis Inflammation of the retina.

reverse passive agglutination test An agglutination immunoassay where antibodies are attached via the Fc portion of the antibody to a carrier particle such as latex.

reverse transcription–polymerase chain reaction (RT-PCR) A type of PCR that uses reverse transcriptase to produce cDNA copies of transcript. The cDNA is then used in a standard PCR assay using specific primers. RT-PCR is used to assay for RNA viruses and to analyze transcript.

rhabditiform larva The feeding but noninfective larval stage. This stage hatches from the egg.

rheumatic fever A complication of *Streptococcus pyogenes* pharyngitis characterized by fever and inflammation of the heart, joints, blood vessels, and subcutaneous tissues.

rheumatoid factor Autoantibody, usually immunoglobulin M, directed against immunoglobulin G antibodies.

rhinosporidiosis A chronic, usually painless infection of humans and animals that occurs as mucosal polyps of the nasopharynx and conjunctiva. The causative agent is *Rhinosporidium seeberi*.

rhizoid Rootlike hypha.

ribonuclease H (RNase H) A ribonuclease that degrades RNA in DNA-RNA hybrids.

ribotyping A method that detects rRNA restriction fragment length polymorphism patterns by Southern blotting.

ribotyping When rRNA RFLP patterns are detected by Southern blotting, the technique is called *ribotyping*. The genes that code for rRNA are conserved in different species of organisms and appear in conserved positions of a species chromosome. For this reason, ribotyping displays excellent reproducibility and discriminatory power.

risk group Categorization for infectious agents based on hazardous characteristics and relative risk.

Ritter disease Also known as *staphylococcal scalded skin syndrome*.

river blindness Also called *onchocerciasis*, it is a disease caused by *Onchocerca volvulus*.

rotavirus A member of the Reoviridae family that infects cells of the villi of the small intestine, leading to epithelial atrophy and proliferation of cells with secretory capacity. This may decrease the absorptive capacity of the bowel, contributing to diarrhea. Rotaviruses are the major cause of diarrhea in children younger than 5 years of age, causing an estimated 130 million episodes of illness worldwide each year.

S

saprobe An environmental fungus that derives nutrients from dead organic material; generally nonpathogenic for humans.

satellitism Small colonies of bacteria growing around another colony; the small colonies derive an essential nutrient secreted by the other colony. A phenomenon exhibited by some *Haemophilus* spp. on sheep blood agar.

scalded skin syndrome (SSS) A toxin-mediated exfoliative dermatitis associated with *Staphylococcus aureus*, superficially resembling a burn injury.

scarlet fever A disease characterized by a diffuse red rash that appears on the upper chest and spreads to the trunk and extremities; this disease is caused by strains of *Streptococcus pyogenes* that produce an erythrogenic toxin.

schizogony The asexual life cycle of the Apicomplexa. In malaria, it is characterized by splitting of the nucleus into multiple segments and the formation of merozoites.

schizont Parasitic form producing merozoites during schizogony. In malaria, it is part of the erythrocytic asexual life cycle.

Schüffner's stippling Malarial pigment characterized as tiny red staining dots in infected red blood cells infected with either *Plasmodium vivax* or *P. ovale*.

scleritis Inflammation of the sclera.

scolex The anterior end of the tapeworm that contains structures such as suckers or hooklets used for attachment to the host.

scombroid A form of food poisoning from ingestion of heat-stable toxins produced by bacteria in contaminated fish, often tuna, mackerel, or yellow jack.

Scorpion primers A detection method for real-time polymerase chain reaction (PCR). A Scorpion primer is a hairpin loop structure with a fluorophore on the 5′ end and a quencher on the 3′ end. Also attached to the 3′ end is a small primer sequence specific for the target of interest. The primer anneals to target nucleic acid and primer extension occurs. Denaturation dissociates the PCR product and the Scorpion primer. A portion of the primer is complementary to the PCR product and anneals to it, physically separating the fluorophore from the quencher, and an increase in fluorescence is observed.

scotochromogenic *Mycobacterium* spp. produces pigment in either light or dark growth environments.

secondary bacteremia Bacteremia that arises from an infected extravascular source such as the lung in patients with pneumonia.

secondary syphilis The second stage of syphilis that appears 2 to 6 months after primary infection and that is marked by lesions, especially in the skin, but also in organs and tissues; lasts from 3 to 12 weeks.

select biological agent Microbial agents classified by the Centers for Disease Control as potential agents of bioterrorism because of their dissemination potential and ability to cause disease and/or death in humans, animals, and plants.

selective media Media that support the growth of one type or one group of microbes but not of another.

selective reporting Following testing of a clinical isolate, reporting of results for certain antimicrobial agents based on defined criteria such as organism identification, body site, and overall susceptibility profile. Secondary (broader spectrum, most costly, more toxic) agents are only reported if primary agents are resistant or if they offer significant clinical advantages for the particular isolate and patient.

Semmelweis Ignaz Semmelweis (1816–1865) is considered to be an important pioneer for the promotion of asepsis. More than 100 years ago, Semmelweis demonstrated in a Vienna maternity hospital that routine handwashing can prevent the spread of disease.

sentinel laboratories Part of the Laboratory Response Network; comprise most of the hospital-based microbiology laboratories and are divided into two levels.

sepsis Systemic response to bacterial infection.

septic shock Sepsis accompanied by refractory hypotension.

septicemia See **sepsis.**

sequencing In genetics and biochemistry, *sequencing* means to determine the primary structure of an unbranched biopolymer. Sequencing results in a symbolic linear depiction, known as a *sequence,* which succinctly summarizes much of the atomic-level structure of the sequenced molecule. DNA sequencing is the process of determining the nucleotide order of a given DNA fragment.

seroconversion Demonstration of detectable antibodies to an immunogen, such as an infectious agent or vaccine.

serology The study of serum or, more specifically, the use of immunologic assays to detect antibodies for the purpose of diagnosing an infectious disease.

serotype The antigenic constituency of an organism.

serotyping An example of phenotypic testing used with biochemical testing for identifying different strains of bacteria within a species. Serotyping uses antibodies to detect specific antigens on the surface of bacteria; also called *serogrouping.*

serum bactericidal test (SBT) A method for determining the highest dilution or titer of a patient's serum that is inhibitory to and the highest dilution or titer that is bactericidal to the patient's own infecting bacterial isolate.

sessile Microorganisms attached to solid surface, usually found in a community of cells called a *biofilm.*

sexual reproduction Union of a male and a female cell to produce a zygote.

Shiga toxin (Stx) One of two toxins produced by *Shigella* and enterohemorrhagic *Escherichia coli* strains, toxic to African green monkey kidney cells.

shock A serious, life-threatening medical condition where insufficient blood flow reaches the body tissues.

simple stains Chemical stains that are water or alcohol based that can be used directly on a fixed or air-dried sample without additional preparation or complex steps. Gram, Wright's, and acridine orange are simple stains.

skipped wells As related to broth-dilution minimal inhibitory concentration testing, growth at higher concentrations and no growth at one or more of the lower concentrations of antimicrobial agent in the series of concentrations tested.

small colony variants Rare, fastidious strains of staphylococci requiring CO_2, hemin, or menadione for growth; grow on media containing blood, forming colonies about $\frac{1}{10}$ the size of wild-type strains after at least 48 hours' incubation.

sodium polyanetholsulfonate (SPS) Anticoagulant used in collection of microbiology specimens. In addition to preventing clot formation, it is anticomplementary and antiphagocytic.

Southern blot A hybridization procedure in which chromosomal DNA is digested with a restriction enzyme and the fragments are separated by agarose gel electrophoresis. A specific, labeled probe is then used to detect target DNA.

species In microbiology (biology), the basic unit of biodiversity. In classifying organisms, it is assigned a two-part name in Latin. The genus is listed first, followed by a specific species epithet.

specificity The probability that an individual without a condition or disease will test negative. The ability of an antibody to discriminate between closely related epitopes.

spirochetes Slender, flexuous, helically shaped, unicellular bacteria ranging from 0.1 to 0.5 μm wide and from 5 to 20 μm long, with one or more complete turns in the helix.

sporangiophore Asexual stalk that bears a sporangium; it may be branched or unbranched.

sporangiospore Asexual spore produced by cleavage inside a sporangium.

sporicidal An antimicrobial that kills spores.

sporoblast Structure within an immature oocyst that ultimately develops into the sporocyst.

sporocyst The structure within the oocyst that contains the sporozoites.

sporogony The sexual life cycle of malaria that takes place in the gut of the mosquito and results in production of sporozoites; the infective stage for humans.

sporozoite An elongated cell that develops within an oocyst. In malaria it is the stage transmitted to humans when the mosquito takes a blood meal. In other members of the Apicomplexa, it is contained within the oocyst that is passed in the feces.

standard precautions Infection-control precautions that assume that all patients are potentially infected and that implement practices to prevent contact with blood and body fluids.

staphylococcal scalded skin syndrome A toxin-mediated exfoliative dermatitis associated with *Staphylococcus aureus,* superficially resembling a burn injury.

static A term that indicates that a substance inhibits the growth of an organism but that on removal the organism might grow again.

sterile pyuria The presence of 10 white blood cells per high-power field seen in centrifuged urine samples without any uropathogens recovered from urine cultures.

strain A variant of a plant, virus, or bacterium.

streamers Growth of an organism in liquid media represented by vines and puffballs.

Streptococcus pyogenes A species of streptococcus with many strains that are pathogenic to humans. It causes suppurative (pus-forming) diseases, such as scarlet fever and strep throat.

streptogramin A mixture of two structurally distinct compounds, type A and type B, that are separately bacteriostatic but bactericidal in appropriate ratios. These antibiotics act at the level of inhibition of translation through binding to the bacterial ribosome. Quinupristin and dalfopristin are both streptogramins.

streptolysin O An oxygen-labile hemolysin produced by *Streptococcus pyogenes* that is responsible for hemolysis on sheep blood agar plates incubated anaerobically.

streptolysin S A streptococcal hemolytic exotoxin that is oxygen stable, lyses leukocytes, and is nonimmunogenic. The hemolysis seen around colonies that have been incubated aerobically is due to streptolysin S.

string of pearls Phrase that describes the microscopic appearance of *Bacillus anthracis* after short-term exposure to penicillin. The presence of large spherical organisms in chains is useful for a presumptive identification.

suboptimal specimen Specimen that is not properly selected, collected, or transported such that a microbiology workup will lead to misleading results.

sulfide-indole-motility medium (SIM) A bacteriologic medium used to determine whether an organism is motile and has the ability to produce H_2S and to form indole from tryptophan.

sulfur granules The yellow-orange coloration of masses of filamentous organisms seen in certain mycetomas.

superoxide anion An oxygen free radical, O_2^-, toxic to cells.

superoxide dismutase An enzyme composed of metal-containing proteins that converts superoxide radicals into less toxic agents.

suppurative Forming or discharging pus.

surgical hand scrub An antiseptic-containing preparation that significantly reduces the number of microorganisms on intact skin; it is broad spectrum, fast acting, and persistent.

surgical site infection An infection that occurs at a surgical site.

surveillance Ongoing, systematic collection of data and the analysis and interpretation of details surrounding a disease or event.

susceptible In therapeutic terms, implies that an infection caused by the bacterial strain tested may be appropriately treated with the dosage of antimicrobial agent recommended for that type of infection and infecting species.

swarming A hazy blanket of growth on the surface that extends well beyond the streak lines.

swimmer's itch A dermatitis caused by the larvae of certain schistosomes of birds and mammals that may penetrate the human skin.

SYBR Green A dye that binds to nucleic acids and that fluoresces green after exposure to ultraviolet light. SYBR Green I is used to stain DNA, and SYBR Green II is used to stain RNA.

symbionts Organisms that share a relationship in which at least one member of the pair benefits from the relationship.

symbiosis The relationship between species (host and organism) in which each benefits from each other and from the relationship.

synanamorph Two different fungi that reproduce asexually but have been linked to the same sexual fungus.

syncytia Giant multinucleated cells formed from cell fusion as a result of virus infection.

synergism Occurs when the antimicrobial activity of a combination of antimicrobial agents is greater than the activity of the individual agents alone.

syphilis Multistage sexually transmitted disease caused by *Treponema pallidum* subsp. *pallidum*.

syphilitic chancre The initial lesion of syphilis that is painless and nonsuppurative but infectious; its appearance signals primary syphilis. The chancre appears at the site of inoculation, usually the genitalia.

systemic inflammatory response syndrome (SIRS) An inflammatory state affecting the whole body related to sepsis, SIRS comprises a spectrum of increasingly severe conditions ranging from sepsis to severe sepsis to septic shock.

T

T-helper cells Cells that express CD4 and a T-cell receptor on their surfaces and respond to antigen presentation by antigen-presenting cells (APCs).

tache noires Literally "black spots," the characteristic lesions that can form when either *Rickettsia conorii* or *Orientia tsutsugamushi* organisms infect humans.

tachyzoite Motile, replicating intracellular stage of *Toxoplasma gondii*.

target The nucleic acid species studied in molecular diagnostics assays. The target is single-stranded and complementary to primers and/or probes.

targeted surveillance Surveillance of specific, preidentified events of concern or importance.

taxa Term that denotes categories of microorganisms.

taxonomy The orderly classification and grouping of organisms into taxa or categories.

teleomorph A fungus that reproduces sexually.

temperate The phage DNA that becomes incorporated into the bacterial genome, where it is replicated along with the bacterial chromosomal DNA.

template The target nucleic acid for molecular diagnostics assays.

tertiary syphilis The third stage of syphilis that develops after the disappearance of the secondary symptoms and that is marked by ulcers in and gummas under the skin and commonly by involvement of the skeletal, cardiovascular, and nervous systems.

test validation The ongoing process providing information that a test is performing correctly.

tetanospasmin The neurotoxin that causes the characteristic signs and symptoms of tetanus produced by *Clostridium tetani*.

tetanus A disease that acts on the central nervous system and is characterized by muscular contractions.

tetracycline A broad-spectrum antibiotic produced by the *Streptomyces* species, indicated for treatment of various bacterial infections. It inhibits cell growth by inhibiting translation by binding to the 30S ribosomal subunit and preventing the aminoacyl tRNA from binding to the A site of the ribosome.

thermal cycler A programmable instrument that cycles temperatures for polymerase chain reaction assays.

thermophile Bacteria that grow best at high temperatures (optimal growth at 50° to 60° C).

thiosulfate citrate bile salts sucrose agar (TCBS) A selective medium used for isolation of *Vibrio* spp. Sucrose-fermenting species are yellow, and nonsucrose-fermenting organisms are green.

time-kill assays A method for measuring the rate of killing of a bacterial isolate by an antimicrobial agent by examining the number of viable bacteria remaining at various intervals after exposure to the agent.

tinea The term used to denote superficial fungal diseases of various parts of the body. Also called *ringworm*.

tissue culture The maintenance or growth of complex tissue.

T$_M$ See **melting temperature.**

tolerance As related to minimal bactericidal concentration (MBC) testing, the lack of bactericidal activity at several concentrations above the minimal inhibitory concentration (MIC), often defined as an MBC:MIC ratio of 32 or greater.

total surveillance Surveillance of all events within a health care setting.

toxic epidermal necrolysis (TEN) A clinical manifestation with multiple etiologies and often caused by a drug or chemical reaction but that may resemble scalded skin syndrome.

toxic megacolon A life-threatening complication of other intestinal conditions characterized by a very inflated colon, abdominal distention, fever, pain, and shock.

toxic shock syndrome (TSS) A potentially fatal multisystem disease caused by toxins, primarily TSST-1, produced by *Staphylococcus aureus*.

toxic shock syndrome toxin-1 (TSST-1) An exotoxin acting as a superantigen, most commonly associated with toxic shock syndrome.

tracheal cytotoxin Virulence factor of certain *Bordetella* spp. that contributes to pathogenesis by causing ciliostasis, inhibiting DNA synthesis, and promoting cell death.

trachoma A chronic severe eye infection associated with specific serovars (A, B, Ba, and C) of *Chlamydia trachomatis*.

trailing As related to broth dilution minimal inhibitory concentration testing, growth at lower concentrations followed by one or more wells or tubes that show greatly reduced growth in the form of a small button or a light haze.

transcript Messenger RNA (mRNA), the expressed product of a gene.

transcription-mediated amplification (TMA) An amplification assay that is very similar to nucleic acid sequence–based amplification.

transduction The transfer of bacterial genes by a bacteriophage (a bacterial virus) from one cell to another.

transformation Uptake and incorporation of naked DNA into a bacterial cell.

transient bacteremia Occurs after a procedural manipulation of a particular body site that is colonized by indigenous flora.

transient flora Organisms picked up from contact with the environment or from other persons and not part of the established normal flora.

transient microbial flora Microorganisms that reside at body sites for short periods, sometimes for days or weeks.

transillumination Passing of bright light through the bottom of the plate to determine whether the organism is hemolytic. This technique can be also used on clear media (e.g., MacConkey), to see slight differences in the color of non–lactose-fermenting bacilli.

translucent Permitting light to pass through but diffusing it so that objects on the opposite side are not clearly visible.

transparent Having the property of transmitting rays of light through its substance so that bodies situated beyond or behind can be distinctly seen.

transport media Liquid or semisolid medium meant to preserve and maintain the integrity of the specimen for the period between specimen collection and laboratory processing of the sample.

transposon A segment of DNA that can become integrated at many different sites along a chromosome, especially a segment of bacterial DNA that can be translocated as a whole.

traveler's diarrhea An acute diarrheal illness generally acquired when travelers ingest contaminated food or water; often caused by enterotoxigenic *Escherichia coli*; also known as *turista*.

treponemal antibody tests A series of tests for syphilis that detect specific antibodies to treponemal antigens used to confirm a nontreponemal antibody screening test.

trichomoniasis An extremely common STD and common manifestation of vaginitis; *Trichomonas vaginalis* is the causative agent of trichomoniasis.

triple sugar iron (TSI) agar A bacteriologic medium that aids in the determination of carbohydrate fermentation (glucose, lactose, and sucrose) and H_2S formation.

trophozoite The feeding, motile, noninfective form of a protozoan. This form replicates in the host and is responsible for causing damage.

true pathogen A microorganism capable of producing disease in both immunocompetent and immunocompromised individuals.

trypomastigote A life-cycle stage found in humans that is characteristic of blood and tissue flagellates. It is a long, spindle-shaped organism with a flagellum, undulating membrane, prominent nucleus, and kinetoplast.

T-strain mycoplasma The original name given to the *Ureaplasma* spp. because they produce tiny colonies compared with the *Mycoplasma* spp.

tube-dilution MIC See **broth macrodilution minimal inhibitory concentration.**

tuberculous meningitis Meningitis or inflammation of the meninges due to an infection caused by *Mycobacterium tuberculosis*.

tularemia The disease caused by the bacterium *Francisella tularensis*.

tumbling motility Characteristic "end-over-end" motility of *Listeria* spp.

turbidity Cloudiness of liquid media caused by growth of microorganisms.

turista See **traveler's diarrhea.**

type B gastritis Type of chronic gastritis usually associated with *Helicobacter pylori* infections.

U

ulceroglandular tularemia The most common form of tularemia.

umbilicate Depressed center, concave, an "inny."

umbonate Raised or bulging center, convex, an "outy."

undulant fever A synonym for brucellosis.

uracil-*N*-glycosylase (UNG) An enzyme that prevents replication of DNA strands synthesized with uracil instead of thymine. UNG is sometimes used as a contamination prevention measure.

urea breath test A rapid diagnostic procedure used to identify infections by *Helicobacter pylori*, a bacterium implicated in gastritis, gastric ulcer, and peptic ulcer disease.

urease test A bacteriologic test to determine an organism's ability to break down urea with the enzyme urease.

urethritis Inflammation of the urethra.

urinary tract infection (UTI) An infection occurring in or associated with the urinary tract.

usual or indigenous microbial flora Microorganisms usually found at body sites without causing disease; certain species may produce disease, given the opportunity, or when the host's immune system is weakened.

uveitis Inflammation of the iris, ciliary body, and choroidal tissues.

V

V factor (NAD) A growth factor that some *Haemophilus* spp. require in media for growth, also known as *nicotinamide adenosine dinucleotide (NAD)*.

vaccinia virus Virus strain used to vaccinate humans against smallpox.

vasculitis Widespread inflammation of small blood vessels.

vancomycin agar screen plate Brain-heart infusion agar plate containing 6 μg/mL of vancomycin that is used for detection of vancomycin-resistant enterococci, vancomycin-intermediate *Staphylococcus aureus*, and vancomycin-resistant *S. aureus*.

vancomycin-intermediate *Staphylococcus aureus* (VISA) Those *S. aureus* isolates that show reduced susceptibility levels to vancomycin and fall in the intermediate range of 8 to 16 μg/mL.

vancomycin-resistant enterococci (VRE) Common term used to describe enterococci that have vancomycin minimal inhibitory concentration in the resistant range of ≥32 μg/mL.

vancomycin-resistant *Staphylococcus aureus* (VRSA) Common term used to describe *S. aureus* organisms that have vancomycin minimal inhibitory concentration in the resistant range of ≥32 μg/mL.

variola major Severe form of smallpox with approximately 30% mortality.

variola minor A milder form of smallpox with approximately 1% mortality.

Venereal Disease Research Laboratory (VDRL) test A nontreponemal antigen test commonly used for the diagnosis of syphilis, named after the Venereal Disease Research Laboratory where the test was developed.

vector The organism responsible for transmitting a parasite from an infected host to a noninfected host.

ventilator-associated pneumonia (VAP) A pneumonia whose cause has been associated with a ventilator device, such as an endotracheal tube or a tracheotomy.

verotoxin See **Shiga toxin.**

vesicles Liquid-filled sacs.

Vi antigen See **K antigen.**

viremia The presence of viruses in the blood.

virion A complete virus particle.

virucidal An antimicrobial that kills viruses.

virulence The degree of pathology caused by the organism. The extent of the virulence is usually correlated with the ability of the pathogen to multiply within the host and may be affected by other factors. The disease-evoking power of a microorganism.

Voges-Proskauer (VP) Test A test that detects acetoin production from glucose.

vulvovaginal candidiasis Symptomatic vaginitis usually caused by infection with the yeast *Candida*.

W

Waterhouse-Friderichsen syndrome A complication of *Neisseria meningitidis* infection involving hemorrhage of the adrenal glands and characterized by a sudden onset of fever, cyanosis, petechial hemorrhages of the skin and mucous membranes, and coma.

Weil disease Severe systemic form of leptospirosis that includes renal failure, hepatic failure, and intravascular disease and may result in death.

Weil syndrome Synonym for *icteric leptospirosis*.

Whipple disease A rare, intestinal disease caused by *Tropheryma whipplei*;

characterized by severe intestinal malabsorption.

whooping cough See **pertussis.**

woolsorter disease Name given to inhalation (pulmonary) anthrax describing anthrax disease associated with occupational exposure to *Bacillus anthracis* spores as a result of handling contaminated animal products.

work practice controls Altering the manner in which a task is performed in order to reduce the likelihood of exposure to infectious agents.

X

X factor A growth factor that some *Haemophilus* spp. require in media for growth, also known as *hemin*.

Y

yaws A nonvenereal spirochetal disease of the tropics resembling syphilis caused by *Treponema pallidum* subsp. *pertenue*.

yeast A fungus that reproduces by budding.

Z

Ziehl-Neelson stain Procedure often used for acid-fast staining. It is a carbolfuchsin method that involves the application of heat.

Ziemann's dots Malarial pigment characterized as tiny, red staining dots, smaller than Schüffner's stippling, in red blood cells infected with *Plasmodium malariae*.

zone of equivalence Portion of a precipitin or agglutination curve when antibody and antigen concentrations are optimal for lattice formation.

zone of inhibition As related to disk diffusion testing, this zone is a clear area surrounding an antimicrobial disk following overnight incubation that results from diffusion of the antimicrobial molecules into the agar and inhibition of growth of the test bacterium.

zoonosis A disease that humans acquire from exposure to infected animals or products made from infected animals.

zoonotic Pertains to diseases that can be transmitted from animals to humans.

Index